OXFORD MEDICAL PUBLICATIONS

Textbook of Adverse Drug Reactions

Textbook of
Adverse Drug Reactions

Fourth Edition

Edited by

D.M. DAVIES, FRCP, FRCP Ed

Consultant Physician, Editor of the *Adverse Drug Reaction Bulletin*

OXFORD   NEW YORK   TOKYO
OXFORD UNIVERSITY PRESS
1991

Oxford University Press, Walton Street, Oxford OX2 6DP

Oxford   New York   Toronto
Delhi   Bombay   Calcutta   Madras   Karachi
Petaling Jaya   Singapore   Hong Kong   Tokyo
Nairobi   Dar es Salaam   Cape Town
and associated companies in
Berlin   Ibadan

Oxford is a trade mark of Oxford University Press

Published in the United States
by Oxford University Press, New York

© Oxford University Press, 1977, 1981, 1985, 1991

First edition 1977
Second edition 1981
Third edition 1985
Fourth edition 1991

A catalogue record for this book is
available from the British Library

Library of Congress
(Cataloging data is available)
ISBN 0–19–262045–2

Typeset by Meditext, Weybridge, Surrey
Printed in Great Britain by
Butler & Tanner Ltd, Frome, Somerset

Dedicated to the memory of
FRANCIS T. ROBERTS of the United States of America,
LEOPOLD MEYLER of the Netherlands, and
SIR DERRICK DUNLOP of the United Kingdom,
who did so much to remind doctors that drug
therapy could at times be harmful as well as
beneficial.

Foreword to the first edition

by the late SIR DERRICK DUNLOP, MD, FRCP
First Chairman of the Committee on Safety of Drugs and, later, of the Medicines Commission.

This considerable volume — a tribute principally to the Newcastle Medical School which supplies 22 of its 32 contributors — is the most comprehensive account published of adverse reactions to drugs, and also supplies a very complete bibliography on the subject. Its unsentimental but unavoidably somewhat horrific contents might well give the average reader an aversion to drugs in general, but this would be unjustified. Although modern drugs are formidable agents, if prescribed and used with skill, wisdom, and propriety their benefits far exceed their occasional adverse effects. It is appropriate, therefore, that a foreword to a book on the dangers of drugs should be prefaced by a reminder of the great blessings they have conferred upon society.

Since the beginning of this century the average expectation of life at birth in this and most other European countries has increased by about 25 years. In the early part of the century this improving expectation of longevity was largely the result of better hygiene, housing, and nutrition but during the last 30 or 40 years it has been mostly due to modern medicines (a term taken to include bacteriological products and hormones). Quite apart from their favourable effect on mortality statistics, the relief from suffering resulting from their purely symptomatic used, and the saving to national economies in diminished morbidity — less time lost from work, fewer and shorter admissions to hospital — is vast but more difficult to compute. It is becoming hard for older physicians to remember and it must be difficult for young ones to imagine what it was like to practise medicine when there was no insulin, vitamin B_{12}, sulphonamides, antibiotics, specifics for tropical diseases, hypotensives, anticoagulants and potent hormones, diuretics and anticonvulsants. Further, few of us would be callous enough to practise medicine without anesthetics, narcotics, hypomania, and analgesics.

No revolution, however, no matter how salutary, ever occurs without being harmful to some and the revolution in medicinal therapeutics of the last 50 years is no exception to this rule. Just as the old horse and buggy, though very slow, caused few fatal accidents whereas the modern automobile, though very fast, is a lethal instrument, so the old-fashioned bottle of medicine, elaborately compounded, meticulously bottled, elegantly flavoured, and exquisitely labelled, though relatively ineffective, was also comparatively innocuous whereas modern drugs, like atomic energy, are powerful for good but also for evil. The ill health that may result from their use — 'iatrogenic illness' as it is called or, more optimistically, if a little ironically, 'illness due to medical progress' — has become a new dimension in the aetiology of disease: perhaps up to 10 per cent of patients suffer to a greater or lesser extent from efforts to treat them. Our powers over Nature in this as in other respects have advanced so far that Nature seems to have become retaliatory and to be exacting a massive retribution. A drug that can modify or repress biological processed in invaluable in treatment but if it has this capacity it is bound also to cause adverse effects from time to time. Those who say that nothing but the complete safety of drugs will suffice demand the impossible: a drug without any side-effects is probably an ineffective one. The public who require progress must be prepared for some risk: it has always accepted the not inconsiderable risks of surgery to which some modern drugs are equivalent in efficacy. While shuddering at a death rate of, say, one in 40 000 patients dying as the result of taking a usually valuable remedy (and which surgeon, incidentally, would not be enchanted with such statistics for the most minor operation?) we are much more complacent about the far greater dangers of cigarette smoking, alcoholism, or road accidents. Yet were all drugs invariably prescribed and used properly, and sensible governmental controls were enforced, the dangers would be small, for the majority of their adverse reactions — though by no means all — are due to their well-recognised and predictable side-effects.

The medical profession has not been entirely guiltless in their use of drugs. We must confess that there has been a good deal of excessive, and occasionally ignorant and irresponsible prescribing for which there are many reasons.

Firstly, there are too few doctors in most countries for their increasing populations, so that most are busy and some overworked. Although it takes a long time to elucidate an accurate clinical history, to carry out a careful, physical examination, and to give wise advice, it only takes a moment to write a prescription which often satisfies both patient and doctor that some positive action has been taken. Most excessive prescribing is 'placebo' prescribing for which there is a limited justification — the patient expects some treatment or the doctor wants to give his patient hope. When genuine placebos are prescribed they should be cheap, innocuous, and pharmacologically largely inactive. The old 'tonics' we used to prescribe fulfilled these criteria, but the modern psychotropic drugs do not. The latter have of course changed the whole atmosphere and length of stay in our mental hospitals, have done much to prevent anguish of mind and suicide, and have brought the merciful dispensation of sleep to many in need of it. Nevertheless, they are overprescribed: all the anxieties, frustrations, and disappointments in life do not necessarily demand drug treatment. A good doctor should be a placebo in himself.

Secondly, ignorant prescribing may often be due to inadequate instruction about drugs. In most medical schools pharmacology has traditionally been taught as a pre-clinical subject — a valuable scientific academic discipline, using drugs to illustrate physiological problems — an 'acetylcholine' type of pharmacology, so to speak; but it is impossible at this stage in an undergraduate's career to teach the therapeutic use of drugs: the student is not familiar with pathology, bacteriology, or patients. Fortunately, the relatively new discipline of clinical pharmacology has now been introduced into most medical schools and plays an important part in the undergraduate curriculum and in the continuing education of the postgraduate, instructing them in the therapeutic use of the powerful tools of their trade.

Thirdly, excessive prescribing may be encouraged by the insistent and skillful promotion of drugs by the pharmaceutical industry, some of which, in the past at any rate, has been subject to justifiable criticism. The pharmaceutical industry seems to possess most of the conventional commercial virtues: a high rate of investment; satisfactory labour relations; good quality control; an admirable record of supplying customers during epidemics or individual emergency; generous benefactions to charities and to medical, dental, veterinary, and agricultural research; and a brilliant record of commercial success which in 1975 contributed over £300 million to our export drive. It is therefore a little surprising that few other industries have been subjected to so much adverse

criticism, jealous political antagonism, or stringent bureaucratic controls. It must be confessed that in the creation of this atmosphere the industry itself has not been entirely blameless: in its period of most rapid development from the 1940s till the early 1960s it sometimes got carried away by its success and salesmanship occasionally took precedence over what was best for medicine. It would be idle to deny that commercialism sometimes dictated the marketing of a product before it had been completely investigated or that research workers in industry were occasionally subjected to commercial pressures. Of course, equally, academic research workers are sometimes carried away by their enthusiasms and the medical profession — or any other for that matter — have not always had their actions dictated by motives of pure altruism. In some future Utopia non-profit-making motivations may achieve the same brilliant results without side-effects. Till then we must take the world as we find it and remember that since the October Revolution the state-owned industries in the USSR and its satellites have hardly produced a single new product of real therapeutic importance.

In the old days medicines did not greatly influence the natural history of disease and it was not sufficiently stressed that an account of what drugs a patient had recently been taking should be an invariable and important part of any clinical history. Neglect of drug history taking often persists even in this chemotherapeutic era. Many adverse reactions to drugs exquisitely simulate the signs and symptoms of naturally occurring disorders. Thus complicated, often disagreeable, and expensive investigations are frequently undertaken when a few simple questions about the patient's recent consumption of drugs would have rendered these attempts to elucidate obscure symptoms unnecessary. Further, it is undesirable to anaesthetize or operate on a patient taking certain drugs — corticosteroids for example — without taking precautions; and the danger of giving unsuitable drugs to patients already being given, particularly, monoamine oxidase inhibitors, anticoagulants, or oral hypoglycaemic agents is considerable. When the taking of a drug history has become a routine part of a clinical history a significant advance will have been made in the prevention of adverse reactions to drugs.

Though science does not always lend itself to legislative or regulatory manipulation, modern drugs are such potent weapons that there is a general consensus that the sole responsibility for their production and use can no longer be left entirely to the manufacturer or prescriber. Yet it is difficult to know how far Government should attempt to control their production and prescription without undue interference with the advance of scientific therapeutics, the well-being of the pharmaceutical industry, and the cherished freedom of the doctor, dentist, or veterinary surgeon to prescribe as he thinks best. Inadequate regulation may prejudice public safety but excessive regulation can also be prejudicial in stultifying innovation and delaying the introduction of valuable remedies. The thoughtful legislator must direct his efforts between these two extremes and protect the public from inadequately tested and dangerous drugs, but at the same time permit an orderly progress of research, development, and marketing by the pharmaceutical industry. The operation of controls must be efficient, economical, and expeditious for otherwise the public are denied new and useful drugs. Finally, labelling, while excluding exaggerated and dangerous claims must be sufficiently elastic to permit the physician to exercise his judgement in the use of drugs. Very restrictive or directive types of labelling might result in a so-called learned profession being reduced to signing forms entitling their patients to receive such drugs for such purposes as the regulatory agencies permit.

One of the most urgent tasks confronting us today is to place adverse drug reactions on a sound epidemiological basis. No matter how meticulous the preparatory work of the pharmacologist and clinician may have been before a drug is marketed or how careful a licensing authority may have been in reviewing its protocols, nothing can replace experience of its use in practice over many years. Thus, the computerized collection, tabulation, and analysis of suspected adverse reactions on a national and ultimately on an international scale is of paramount importance and in recent years many countries, including Britain as a pioneer, have established monitoring systems of this nature. Their success depends on the co-operation of the medical profession in reporting suspected adverse reactions., especially to new drugs. It took many decades before the deleterious effects of aspirin on the alimentary canal became apparent and almost as long before it was recognised that the protracted abuse of phenacetin could produce renal papillary necrosis; 35 years elapsed before it became clear that amidopyrine could cause agranulocytosis; and several years before the association of phocomelia with thalidomide became obvious. Had a register of adverse reactions then existed these effects would have become apparent much earlier than was the case. The frequency of even major adverse reactions to drugs is not as yet really well known nor is their cause invariably well understood. A proper understanding of the dangers involved is the first step to their intelligent prevention. This book admirably supplies such an understanding.

Preface

In the preface to the first edition I wrote: 'In recent years a vast amount has been written about adverse reactions to drugs in a multitude of medical books and journals; yet, paradoxically, this surfeit of information has made it more difficult for the clinician to obtain prompt and unambiguous answers to his questions. He now requires help to find his way through the jungle of toxicological fact and theory, and it seemed to us that there was a need for a 'map' arranged in the style of orthodox textbook of medicine and written by doctors able to view the problems posed by adverse reactions in perspective against the background of their own experience.

'Our desire to be comprehensive has been tempered by our wish to produce a book of reasonable size, and we hope that our compromise will satisfy our readers. In a book with so many contributors it is not easy to ensure that each topic is given as much attention as it warrants, but no more than it deserves. We have tried very hard to achieve such a balance, and where a section seems disproportionately long it will usually be found that it deals with matters of fundamental importance or with subjects that have been particularly well studied.'

All this remains true of this fourth edition, though some changes have again become necessary. To accommodate the amount of new information that has become available since the last edition, without increasing the size of the book unduly, it has been necessary to prune severely, and the material chosen for omission is that now readily available elsewhere in books devoted solely to the subjects concerned. Thus, the chapters on assessment of quality and safety of drugs, detection and investigation of adverse drug reactions, and medico-legal aspects and implications, and the appendix on adverse reactions attributed to drug excipients have been removed. But the second appendix in the third edition, listing adverse reactions discussed elsewhere in the text, has now been upgraded to a chapter, to allow more detailed dissection of interactions that are of undoubted clinical importance from those that are mainly of theoretical interest.

In addition to these changes, all surviving chapters have been carefully revised and many have been completely rewritten, some by new authors. Eighteen of the 39 contributors to the third edition have decided to hand over their burdens to others; I am sad to lose them and anxious to thank them for helping to make this book the success it has been. I am satisfied that their successors have maintained the high standards they set.

I still believe that our approach — by clinical feature rather than by drug — matches the way the problem usually presents itself to the clinician. This approach has met with the approval of most reviewers, and I must respectfully reject the criticism of those few who have complained that it is necessary to spend hours wading through the book to discover the full spectrum of adverse reactions to a particular drug or drug group, for our very detailed index enables the reader to obtain this information within seconds.

The contributors again express their gratitude to the medical secretaries and librarians who helped them with their chapters; and I, as Editor, am very much indebted to Miss Jean Hill, Assistant Editor of the *Adverse Drug Reaction Bulletin*, for her assistance at all stages of dealing with manuscripts and proofs and for sharing the enormous task of compiling the index; and to Dr Hugh de Glanville for his meticulous copy-editing and typesetting, his skilled literary guidance, and his invariably good-humoured tolerance of the Editor's inadequacies and idiosyncrasies.

May 1991   *DMD*

Contents

List of contributors

G. Ansell, MD, FRCP, FRCR, DMRD, formerly Senior Consultant Radiologist, Whiston Hospital; Lecturer in Radiodiagnosis, University of Liverpool.

E-S.K. Assem, MB, ChB, Dip Med (Cairo), FRCP Ed, FRCP Glas, MRCP, FRCPath, DCH (Cairo), Honorary Consultant Physician (Allergy and Clinical Pharmacology), University College Hospital; Senior Research Fellow, Department of Pharmacology, University College, University of London.

M.W. Baig, MB, BS, MRCP, Senior Registrar in Cardiology, The General Infirmary at Leeds; Lecturer in Cardiology, University of Leeds.

D.N. Bateman, BSc, MD, FRCP, Consultant Physician, Freeman Hospital; Reader in Therapeutics, University of Newcastle upon Tyne.

L. Beeley, MA, BM, BCh, FRCP, Director, Drug and Therapeutics Unit, and Consultant Clinical Pharmacologist, The Queen Elizabeth Hospital, Birmingham.

P.G. Blain, B Med Sci, MB, BS, PhD, MRCP, CBiol, FIBiol, MFOM, Honorary Consultant Physician, Newcastle Health Authority; Professor of Environmental Medicine, University of Newcastle upon Tyne.

N.P. Bown, BA, Senior Scientific Officer, Department of Human Genetics, University of Newcastle upon Tyne.

P.J. Carey, MB, BS, MRCP, MRCPath, Consultant Haematologist, The Royal Infirmary, Sunderland.

M.J.D. Cassidy, MB, BS, MRCP, Consultant Nephrologist, Royal Postgraduate Medical School, Hammersmith Hospital, London.

J.C.N. Chan, MB, ChB, MRCP, Lecturer in Clinical Pharmacology, Chinese University of Hong Kong.

C.S. Cockram, BSc, FRCP, FRCP Ed, Honorary Consultant Endocrinologist, Prince of Wales Hospital; Reader in Medicine, Chinese University of Hong Kong.

J.C. Cowan, MA, BM, BCh, DPhil, MRCP, Honorary Consultant Cardiologist, The General Infirmary at Leeds; Senior Lecturer in Cardiology, University of Leeds.

S.I. Davidson, MB ChB, FRCS, FC Ophth, DO, formerly Consultant Ophthalmologist, St Paul's Eye Hospital; Director of Studies in Ophthalmology, University of Liverpool.

D.M. Davies, FRCP, FRCP Ed, Honorary Consultant Physician, Shotley Bridge General Hospital and Emeritus Consultant Physician, Newcastle Health Authority; formerly Director, Northern Regional Clinical Pharmacology Unit, Newcastle upon Tyne; Professor of Clinical Pharmacology, Chinese University of Hong Kong; Member of the Subcommittee on Safety, Efficacy, and Adverse Reactions, Committee on Safety of Medicines.

M. Davis, MD, FRCP, Consultant Physician and Gastroenterologist, Royal United Hospital, Bath.

K. Davison, FRCP, FRCP Ed, FRCPsych, Emeritus Consultant Psychiatrist, Newcastle Health Authority; Honorary Lecturer in Psychiatry, University of Newcastle upon Tyne.

C. Diamond, MB, ChB, FRCS Glas, Consultant Ear, Nose, and Throat Surgeon, Freeman Hospital; Clinical Lecturer in Ear, Nose, and Throat Studies, University of Newcastle upon Tyne.

J.F. Dunne, B.Sc., MB, BS, PhD, Programme Manager, Pharmaceuticals, World Health Organization, Geneva.

R.H. Felix, MA, MB, BChir, FRCP, Consultant Dermatologist, Frimley Park Hospital, Camberley.

R.E. Ferner, MSc, MD, MRCP, Consultant Physician and Clinical Toxicologist, West Midlands Poisons Unit, Dudley Road Hospital; Honorary Senior Lecturer in Clinical Pharmacology, University of Birmingham.

F. HASSANYEH, MB, BS, FRCPsych, Consultant Psychiatrist, St Nicholas Hospital; Clinical Lecturer in Psychiatry, University of Newcastle upon Tyne.

M. HICKEY-DWYER, MB, BCh, FRCS Glas, DO, Senior Registrar in Ophthalmology, St Paul's Eye Hospital, Liverpool.

G.H. JACKSON, MA, MB, BS, MRCP, Registrar in Medicine, Royal Victoria Infirmary, Newcastle upon Tyne.

N.P. KEANEY, BSc, MB, BCh, PhD, Consultant Physician, The Royal Infirmary, Sunderland.

D.N.S. KERR, MSc, MB, ChB, FRCP, FRCP Ed, Honorary Consultant Physician, Hammersmith and Queen Charlotte's Special Health Authority; Dean, Royal Postgraduate Medical School, London; Professor of Renal Medicine, University of London.

R.J.M. LANE, BSc, MD, MRCP, Consultant Neurologist, Regional Neurosciences Centre, Charing Cross Hospital, London.

D.H. LAWSON, MD, FRCP, FFPM, Consultant Physician, Glasgow Royal Infirmary; Visiting Professor of Clinical Pharmacology, University of Strathclyde; Chairman, Committee on Review of Medicines.

J.S. MALPAS, DPhil, FRCP, FRCR, FFPM, Honorary Consultant Physician, St Bartholomew's Hospital; Professor of Medical Oncology, University of London.

M.L'E. ORME, MA, MD, FRCP, Honorary Consultant Physician, The Royal Liverpool Hospital; Professor of Pharmacology and Therapeutics, University of Liverpool.

S.J. PROCTOR, MB, BS, FRCP, FRCPath, Consultant Haematologist, Royal Victoria Infirmary; Senior Lecturer in Medicine and Haematology, University of Newcastle upon Tyne.

M.D. RAWLINS, BSc, MD, FRCP, FRCP Ed, FFPM, Honorary Consultant Clinical Pharmacologist, Royal Victoria Infirmary and Freeman Hospital; Professor of Clinical Pharmacology, University of Newcastle upon Tyne; Chairman, Subcommittee on Safety, Efficacy, and Adverse Reactions, Committee on Safety of Medicines.

D.F. ROBERTS, ScD, Professor of Human Genetics, University of Newcastle upon Tyne.

P.A. ROUTLEDGE, MD, FRCP, Honorary Consultant Physician, Llandough Hospital, Penarth; Professor of Clinical Pharmacology, University of Wales College of Medicine, Cardiff.

R.A. SEYMOUR, BDS, PhD, FDS, RCS Ed, Honorary Consultant in Restorative Dentistry, Newcastle Health Authority; Reader in Dental Pharmacology, University of Newcastle upon Tyne.

H.G.M. SHETTY, BSc, MB, BS, MRCP, Honorary Senior Registrar in Medicine, Llandough Hospital, Penarth; Lecurer in Pharmacology, University of Wales College of Medicine, Cardiff.

A.G. SMITH, MD, MRCP, Consultant Dermatologist, City General Hospital, Stoke-on-Trent.

J.M. SMITH, BPharm, PhD, MRPharmS, MCPP, MI Inf Sci, Regional Pharmaceutical Adviser, Northern Regional Health Authority; Pharmaceutical Director, Northern Drug and Therapeutics Centre; Honorary Lecturer in Clinical Pharmacy, University of Newcastle upon Tyne.

R. SWAMINATHAN, MSc, MB, BS, PhD, MRCPath, FRCPA, Honorary Consultant Chemical Pathologist, Prince of Wales Hospital; Professor of Chemical Pathology, Chinese University of Hong Kong.

L-B. TAN, BSc (Hons), MB, BChir, DPhil, MRCP, Honorary Consultant Cardiologist, Killingbeck Hospital; Senior Lecturer in Cardiology, University of Leeds.

J.W. THOMPSON, MB, BS, PhD, FRCP, Director of Studies and Honorary Physician, St Oswald's Hospice; Emeritus Consultant Clinical Pharmacologist, Newcastle Health Authority; Emeritus Professor of Pharmacology, University of Newcastle upon Tyne.

J.G. WALTON, BDS, Emeritus Consultant in Restorative Dentistry, Newcastle Health Authority; formerly Senior Lecturer in Restorative Dentistry and Lecturer in Dental Pharmacology, University of Newcastle upon Tyne.

R. WILLIAMS, MD, FRCP, FRCP Ed, FRCS, Consultant Physician and Director, Institute of Liver Studies, King's College Hospital School of Medicine and Dentistry, London.

K.W. WOODHOUSE, Honorary Consultant Physician, Cardiff Royal Infirmary and University Hospital of Wales; Professor of Geriatric Medicine, University of Wales School of Medicine, Cardiff.

V.T.F. YEUNG, MB, BS, MRCP, Lecturer in Medicine, Chinese University of Hong Kong.

1. History

D. M. DAVIES

Adverse reactions to drugs are as old as Medicine. Some of the earliest writings bear witness to the potential dangers of contemporary medical treatment, and the punishments prescribed for incompetent practitioners. The Babylonian *Code of Hammurabi*, of 2200 BC, ordained that a physician who caused a patient's death should lose his hands, and the *Hermetic Books of Thoth* outlined therapeutic paths from which the physician strayed only at his peril.

In the course of medical history many laymen and doctors were to advise caution in therapeutics and to criticize the materia medica and those who used it. Among the first was Homer (*c.* 950 BC), who said of drugs that there were 'many excellent when mingled, and many fatal' (*Odyssey*, IV). Hippocrates (460–370 BC) pleaded 'Do not harm'; Galen (131–201) warned against the dangers of badly written and obscure prescriptions; and Rhazes (860–932) advised 'if simple remedies are effective do not prescribe compound remedies'.

Most of the drugs then in use were of plant or animal origin, but mercury, arsenic, and antimony were also used. The toxic effects of arsenic were well recognized from its deliberate use as a poison, and the dangers of mercurial inunction were also familiar, but toxic properties of antimony attracted less attention.

As time passed, the questionable purity of remedies began to exercise the minds of both civil and professional authorities. In the ninth century, Arabian authorities appointed an official, the *mutasib*, a guardian of public morals whose duties were later to embrace the supervision of the makers of drugs and syrups to ensure the purity of their wares: 'it is necessary that the *mutasib* make them fearful, try them, and warn them against imprisonment. He must caution them with punishment. Their syrups and drugs may be inspected at any time without warning after their shops are closed for the night' (Leve 1963). In the tenth century the school of Salerno, in Italy, was empowered to inspect drugs for adulteration, with dire penalties for transgressors:

'whosoever shall have or sell any poison or noxious drug not useful or necessary to his art, let him be hanged' (Withington 1894).

In 1224 the Hohenstaufen Emperor, Frederick II, ordered the regular inspection of the drugs and mixtures prepared by apothecaries, and pronounced that the life of a purveyor of a poison, a magic elixir, or a love potion would be forfeit if a consumer died; and in the same century the Oath for apothecaries in Basle, Switzerland, included an undertaking to provide for physicians drugs 'of such good quality and of such usefulness that he knows, upon his oath, that it will be good and useful for the confection which the physician is making' (Mez-Mangold 1971). For many years after the foundation of the Royal College of Physicians, in 1518, its Fellows concerned themselves with the quality control of drugs; and the authors of the first *London Pharmacopoeia* (1618) spoke harshly in their preface of 'the very noxious fraud and deceit of those people who are allowed to sell the most filthy concoctions . . . under the name and title of medicaments. . . . Ironically, they themselves were content to include worms, dried vipers, and fox lung in their catalogue of acceptable remedies. In 1599 a charter granted by James VI of Scotland to what was to become the Royal College of Physicians and Surgeons of Glasgow made provisions for the supervision of the sales of drugs and poisons (Mann 1989).

In the seventeenth century, for the first time, a named drug was proscribed because of its toxicity: members of the Paris Faculty of Physicians were forbidden to use antimony. But the ban could not be maintained after the drug was credited with the cure of an attack of typhoid suffered by Louis XIV in 1657.

Not until 1745, when Sir William Heberden published his *Antitheriaca, Essay on Mithridatium and Theriaca*, was the value of compound remedies and animal extracts seriously questioned. Even so, physicians were very slow in improving their standards of treatment and they long continued to deserve Voltaire's stricture that they 'poured drugs of which they knew little into bodies of which they knew less'.

Perhaps the most elegant and definitive of descriptions of an adverse drug reaction was William Withering's account of digitalis toxicity in 1785: 'The Foxglove, when given in very large and quickly repeated doses, occasions sickness, vomiting, purging, giddiness, confused vision, objects appearing green or yellow, increased secretion of urine with frequent motions to part with it, and sometimes inability to retain it; slow pulse, even as low as 35 in a minute, cold sweats, convulsions, syncope and death'.

At about this time, epidemics of yellow fever in some American states brought to mercury both fame and notoriety. Believing that in this disease 'the gastrointestinal tract was filled with putrid and fermenting biliary substances' and that their expulsion was the key to cure, some physicians advocated large doses of calomel (mercurous chloride) often mixed with other purgatives (Risse 1973). Many patients were apparently unharmed by this heroic therapy, possibly because the vomiting caused by the infection drastically reduced the systemic absorption of the mercury. Others were less fortunate and developed clinical mercurialism with intense salivation; loosening of the teeth; and ulceration, even gangrene, of the mouth and cheeks, and osteomyelitis of the mandible (Risse 1973). Nevertheless, by the next century calomel had become a 'cure-all' in febrile illness, the 'Sampson of the Materia Medica'. But if most doctors had come to view the drug through rose-coloured spectacles, some laymen regarded it (and its prescribers) in a different light:

> Since calomel's become their boast,
> How many patients have they lost,
> How many thousands they make ill,
> Of poison with their calomel.

Some physicians now added their protests. One wrote of 'Calomel considered as a poison' (Mitchell 1844–5), and another, with calomel in mind, commented: 'if the whole materia medica, as it is now used, could be sunk to the bottom of the sea, it would be all the better for mankind — and all the worse for the fishes' (Holmes 1861). Despite such broadsides, calomel remained in favour among physicians for years to come and is believed to have paved the way for such unorthodox (but, at the time, gentler) systems of healing such as homoeopathy, osteopathy, chiropractic, Thompsonianism, and Grahamism.

The nineteenth century saw the appearance in several countries of important new pharmacopœias that for the first time laid down standards of drug purity. In 1848, the first statute was passed to control the quality of drugs in America after quinine imported for the Army was found to have been adulterated.

In the closing years of the nineteenth century and the early years of the twentieth came other innovations. There were formal enquiries into suspected adverse reactions to drugs; the first concerned with sudden deaths during chloroform anæsthesia (McKendrick et al. 1880), and the second with jaundice following arsenical treatment of syphilis (Medical Research Council 1922). Then the American Medical Association established the Council on Pharmacy and Chemistry and its publication *New and Nonofficial Remedies*, 'a mighty service for American medicine' (Leake 1929). Next, the American Food, Drug and Insecticide Administration (later the Food and Drug Administration) was established. But much remained to be done. In 1929 Leake drew attention to the inadequacy of existing testing procedures for new drugs: 'many drug firms make the mistake of believing that their chemists can furnish trustworthy pharmacologic opinion. Indeed some eminent chemists impatient with careful pharmacologic technic have ventured to estimate for themselves the clinical possibilities of their own synthetics . . . There is no short cut from the chemical laboratory to the clinic except one that passes too close to the morgue.' His words were prophetic: 107 people died in 1937 as a result of poisoning by an elixir of sulphanilamide containing as a solvent diethylene glycol (Geiling and Cannon 1938). The manufacturers had not troubled to enquire whether the solvent was safe for its purpose; yet the toxic effects of diethylene glycol and closely related compounds were already documented (von Oettingen and Jirouch 1931; Barber 1934). In the wake of the disaster came a Federal Act that forbade the marketing of new drugs until they had been cleared for safety by the Food and Drug Administration.

In France, a disaster of similar magnitude occurred in 1954 when 100 people died from poisoning by Stalinon, an organic compound of tin used in the treatment of boils (Wade 1970).

Major catastrophes of this kind focused attention on the problem of drug toxicity, but awareness and concern were only transient. The profession's threshold of stimulation remained too high and its latent period before reaction too long. It had taken some 47 years to discover that amidopyrine was a potent marrow poison (Wade 1970). Fifteen years had passed before it was appreciated that cinchophen caused jaundice (Worster-Drought 1923) and 11 years more before this fact gained recognition (Wade 1970). Aspirin had been in use for 39 years before it was incriminated as a cause of gastric haemorrhage (Douthwaite 1938) and for another 20 before the news spread adequately (Alvarez and Summerskill

1958). The dangers of chloramphenicol were first appreciated in the early 1950s, yet some two decades later the Chairman of a US Senate Subcommittee had good cause to complain that warnings of these dangers had gone unheeded (*Journal of the American Medical Association* 1968). Until the 1950s textbooks of medicine devoted comparatively little space to adverse drug reactions, and that only to the ill-effects of one or two drugs. Few medical teachers had much to say on the subject. Epidemiological studies of adverse drug reactions were almost unknown.

Then the climate began to change. In 1952 appeared the first book to concern itself entirely with adverse drug reactions (Meyler 1952). In the same year the council on Pharmacy and Chemistry of the American Medical Association set up an organization to monitor drug-induced blood dyscrasias. A little while later, the first report of epidemiological studies of adverse drug reactions was published; and in 1960 the Food and Drug Administration began to collect reports of adverse reactions and sponsored new hospital drug-monitoring programmes.

In the winter of 1961 came news of the thalidomide disaster — a sudden upsurge in the number of babies born with the deformities of phocomelia or micromelia. Thalidomide had been prescribed as a 'safe' hypnotic. It had not been tested in animals for teratogenicity, but thousands of babies born to mothers who had taken the drug during pregnancy provided the missing data.

As a result of this horrifying epidemic, many countries established agencies concerned with drug safety such as our own Committee on Safety of Drugs; and later the World Health Organization set up an international bureau to collect and collate information from national drug-monitoring organizations. Such agencies have done much to identify and prevent illness caused by drugs; but they provide no absolute guarantee against outbreaks of novel and quite unpredictable reactions such as those produced by practolol.

Periodicals dealing solely with adverse reactions to drugs, such as *Clin-Alert* in 1962, the *Adverse Drug Reaction Bulletin* in 1966, now began to appear.

In the mid-1960s a somewhat different aspect of drug therapy came under repeated scrutiny. In Britain this had been prompted by the report of the Aitken Committee (1958), set up to examine systems of prescribing, administration, and storage of drugs in hospitals. The Committee concluded that all was not well, and made recommendations for improving matters; and later many physicians, pharmacists, and nurses in several countries made detailed studies of the diverse and complex problems of hospital prescribing and devised new procedures

intended to solve them. These various studies and recommendations have been reviewed in detail by Haslam (1988). But making recommendations and rules is one thing, getting them accepted and obeyed is another; and years later drug prescribing and administration in hospitals remains far from perfect (Haslam 1987; Davies 1988; Bonati *et al.* 1990).

In Great Britain the Medicines Act of 1968 provided new and comprehensive safeguards covering most aspects of drug development, production, and use. The beneficial effects of these measures on drug safety have been supplemented by the wealth of information on rational therapeutics and drug toxicity provided by general and specialized medical journals and books, by the formation of drug and therapeutics committees in many hospitals in this country (George and Hands 1983) and elsewhere, and by teachers of clinical pharmacology and toxicology.

More recently the relatively new (at least in the United Kingdom) schemes for 'medical audit' hold promise of improvements in medical care, both in hospitals (Royal College of Physicians 1989, McKee *et al.* 1989) and general practice (Royal College of General Practitioners 1985; Wilmot 1990); and it is to be hoped that audit protocols will strongly emphasize the importance of the detailed and accurate writing of prescriptions and of records of drug administration.

It is apparent from what has been said here that governments, medical colleges and faculties, editors, research workers, and teachers have done a great deal to improve drug safety. It remains for prescribing doctors, patients, and the pharmaceutical industry to match their efforts. Experienced clinicians with open eyes and an interest in therapeutics know that many powerful and potentially dangerous drugs are used with insufficient thought and caution and continue to be given when they might be withdrawn without detriment and, indeed, with benefit to the patient's condition. They would point out that many illnesses are short-lasting and do not require the drug that is often given; that simple and innocuous remedies can provide greater and quicker relief than the more complex remedies usually employed; that the safest drug is not always used when there is a choice; that where one drug would have sufficed, more have often been given; and that a doctor has sometimes prescribed a drug without knowing what other drugs the patient is taking, or used a mixture not knowing precisely what it contained and the pharmacological actions of its ingredients.

There can be little doubt that much modern medicinal treatment is unnecessary, and the blame for this state of affairs must be shared between doctors, patients, and the pharmaceutical industry. Doctors are probably 'unduly concerned with satisfying the public's "wants" rather than what we think are its "needs" ' (Dunlop 1970), and are oversusceptible to the blandishments and misplaced 'generosity' of drug salesmen (Editorial 1989a). Patients have come to believe that the mildest of symptoms, even the ordinary trials and tribulations of everyday life, must be matched by a drug. The pharmaceutical industry still has grave shortcomings as far as its promotional activities are concerned. These are most blatant in third-world countries with less well-developed or poorly enforced legislation controlling promotion, supply, and use of drugs (Medawar 1989; Editorial 1989b, 1990; Lee 1990), but devious promotional methods are still encountered in countries with stringent drug regulation, such as Britain (*Drug and Therapeutics Bulletin*, 1990).

We have made considerable progress towards the goal of making drug therapy as safe as is possible (it is unlikely that *complete* safety will ever be attained), but we shall only reach that goal when the providers, prescribers, and recipients of therapeutic drugs begin at last to take drug treatment *seriously*.

References

Aitken, J.K. (1958). *Report of the joint subcommittee on the control of dangerous drugs and poisons in hospitals*. HMSO, London.

Alvarez, A.S. and Summerskill, W.H.J. (1958). Gastrointestinal haemorrhage and salicylates. *Lancet* ii, 920.

Barber, H. (1934). Haemorrhagic nephritis and necrosis of the liver from dioxane poisoning. *Guy's Hosp. Rep.* 84, 267.

Bonati, M., Marchetti, F., Zullini, M.T., Pistotti, V., and Tognoni, G. (1990). Adverse drug reactions in neonatal intensive care units. *Adverse Drug React. Acute Poisoning Rev.* 9, 107.

Davies, D.M. (1988). Data provided for the review of Haslam, R. (1988). Drug safety and medication systems in hospitals. *Adverse Drug React. Acute Poisoning Rev.* 3, 133.

Douthwaite, A.H. (1938). Some recent advances in medical diagnosis and treatment. *Br. Med. J.* i, 1143.

Drug and Therapeutics Bulletin (1990). Product licences and devious promotion. *Drug Ther. Bull.* 28, 20.

Dunlop, Sir D. (1970). The use and abuse of psychotropic drugs. *Proc. R. Soc. Med.* 63, 1279.

Editorial (1989a). On physicians' samples and gifts. *Drug, Disease, Doctor* 2, 73.

Editorial (1989b). Quackery — the ubiquitous game. *Drug, Disease, Doctor* 2, 25.

Editorial (1990). Right to information — of doctors? *Drug, Disease, Doctor* 3, 1.

Geiling, E.M.K. and Cannon, P.R. (1938). Pathogenic effects of elixir of sulfanilamide (diethylene glycol) poisoning. *JAMA* iii, 919.

George, C.F. and Hands, D.E. (1983). Drug and therapeutics committees and information pharmacy services: the United Kingdom. *World Development* ii, 229.

Haslam, R. (1987). Thesis for the degree of Master of Science, University of Newcastle upon Tyne.

Haslam, R. (1988). Drug safety and medication systems in hospitals. *Adverse Drug React. Acute Poisoning Rev.* 3, 133.

Holmes, O.W. (1861). *Currents and countercurrents in medical science, with other addresses and essays,* p. 167. Boston.

Journal of the American Medical Association (1968). Medical News — a report of a U.S. Senate investigation. *JAMA* 203, 54.

Leake, C.D. (1929). The pharmacologic evaluation of new drugs. *JAMA* 93, 1632.

Lee, D. (1990). Continued marketing of a useless drug ('Varidase') in Panama. *Lancet* 335, 667.

Levey, M. (1963). Fourteenth century medicine and the Hisba. *Medical History* 7, 176.

McKee, C.M., Lauglo, M., and Lessof, L. (1989). Medical audit: a review. *J. R. Soc. Med.* 82, 474.

McKendrick, J.G., Coats, J., and Newman, D. (1880). Report of the action of anaesthetics. *Br. Med. J.* ii 957.

Mann, R.D. (1989). The historical development of medicines regulations. In *International medicines regulations* (ed. S.R. Walker and J.P. Griffin), p. 5. Kluwer, London.

Medawar, C. (1989). On our side of the fence. In *Side effects of drugs, Annual 13,* p xix. Elsevier, Amsterdam.

Medical Research Council (1922). Toxic effects following the employment of arsenobenzol preparations. *Special Report Series*, No. 66.

Meyler, L. (1952). *Side effects of drugs*. Elsevier, Amsterdam.

Mez-Mangold, L. (1971). *A history of drugs,* p. 83. F. Hoffmann-La Roche and Co., Basle.

Mitchell, T.D. (1844–5). Calomel considered as a poison. *N. Orleans Med. Surg J.* i, 28.

Risse, G.B. (1973). Calomel and the American Medical Sects during the nineteenth century. *Mayo Clinic Proc.* 48, 57.

Royal College of General Practitioners (1985). *What sort of doctor? Report from general practice 23*. Royal College of General Practitioners, London.

Royal College of Physicians (1989). *Medical audit — a first report: what, why, and how?* Royal College of Physicians of London.

von Oettingen, W.F. and Jirouch E.A. (1931). Pharmacology of ethylene glycol and some of its derivatives. *J. Pharmacol Exp. Ther.* 42, 355.

Wade, O.L. (1970). *Adverse reactions to drugs*. Heinemann. London.

Wilmot, J. (1990). Review of medical audit. *J. R. Soc. Med.* 83, 58.

Withering, W. (1785). *An account of the foxglove and some of its medicinal uses; with practical remarks on dropsy and other diseases*. London.

Withington, E.T. (1894). *Medical history from earliest times*, (reprint 1964). The Holland Press, London. *via* Penn, R.G. The state control of medicines: the first 3000 years. *Br. J. Pharmacol.* 8, 293.

Worster-Drought, C. (1923). Atophan poisoning. *Br. Med. J.* i. 148.

2. Epidemiology

D. H. LAWSON

Definition

Epidemiology is the study of the distribution and determinants of health-related events in populations and the application of this study to the control of health problems (Last 1983).

Epidemiological studies tend to be grouped into three major categories: (1) the descriptive type, which investigates the occurrence of a specific disease entity within subgroups of the population, paying particular regard to basic characteristics such as age, sex, race, occupation, geographic location, and social class; (2) the analytical type, which usually involves a hypothesis-testing approach to investigating possible associations between disease and a variety of possible causative factors; such studies are usually observational and may involve the techniques of cohort follow-up or case–control analysis; (3) there is the experimental type of epidemiological study which is usually hypothesis-testing and uses techniques such as randomized controlled clinical trials.

Possible adverse drug reactions have been studied using all three epidemiological strategies. These studies are, however, not easy to conduct, since the definition of an 'adverse drug reaction' is complicated by the fact that the external manifestations of such reactions are not unique. Both humans and animals have a limited number of ways in which they can react to noxious stimuli. Even as clear-cut an event as phocomelia occurring in the offspring of mothers exposed to thalidomide in the early stages of pregnancy is not invariably drug-induced. Indeed, there is a magnificent painting by Goya on display in the Prado museum in Madrid that portrays a child suffering from phocomelia — an occurrence which had clearly taken place long before the development of thalidomide.

All major adverse reactions for which drugs have been withdrawn in the recent past — for example, aplastic anaemia (chloramphenicol), Guillain–Barré syndrome (zimeldine), endometrial cancer (unopposed oestrogen replacement therapy), lactic acidosis (phenformin), and acute haemolytic anaemia (nomifensine) — occur naturally in the absence of exposure to drugs. It follows that unless there is a dramatic increase in the observed incidence of such events, as was the case with thalidomide and phocomelia, formal studies are required in order to clarify the drug–disease relationship. While this is true of major events such as have been described, it is also true of minor events such as fatigue, inability to concentrate, nasal congestion, pains in muscles, headaches, skin rash, bizarre dreams, dry mouth, pain in joints, etc, all of whichoccur naturally in the population. They have been reported, for example, to a varying extent among a sample of 670 healthy university students and hospital staff taking no medications at the time. The observers concluded that the experience with this group indicated the clear need for proper controls in all studies of potential adverse drug reactions (Reidenberg and Lowenthal 1968).

For the practising physician, these observations lead to the conclusion that,while it is easy to decide that a patient has experienced an adverse event, it is not easy to determine the causative noxious stimulant. Similar problems were encountered in the context of the developing understanding of the bacterial aetiology of disease. They were solved by the application of Koch's postulates which should be met before a causative relationship can be accepted between a particular bacterial parasite or disease agent and a disease in question. These are:

1. the agent must be shown to be present in every case of the disease, by isolation in pure culture;
2. the agent must not be found in cases of other diseases;
3. once isolated, the agent must be capable of reproducing the disease in experimental animals;
4. the agent must be recoverable from the experimental disease produced.

Later, Evans (1976) expanded the Koch postulates and applied them more generally to the aetiology of disease. The so-called Evans's postulates are:

1. the prevalence of disease should be significantly higher in those exposed to the hypothesized cause than in controls not so exposed;
2. exposure to the suspected cause should be more frequent amongst those with the disease than in controls without the disease, when all other risk factors are held constant;
3. the incidence of the disease should be significantly higher in those exposed to the purported cause than in those not so exposed, as shown by prospective studies;
3. the disease should follow exposure to the hypothesized causative agent with a distribution of incubation periods in a bell-shaped curve;
5. the spectrum of host responses should follow exposure to the hypothesized agent along a logical biological gradient from mild to severe;
6. a measurable host response following exposure to the hypothesized cause should have a high probability of appearing in those lacking it before exposure, or should increase in magnitude if present before exposure. This response pattern should be infrequent in unexposed persons;
7. experimental reproduction of the disease should occur more frequently in animals or man appropriately exposed to the hypothesized cause than in those not so exposed. This exposure may be deliberate in volunteers, experimentally induced in the laboratory, or may represent a regulation of natural exposure;
8. elimination of modification of the hypothesized cause should decrease the incidence of the disease;
9. prevention or modification of the host response on exposure to the hypothesized cause should decrease or eliminate the disease;
10. all the relationships and findings should make biological and epidemiologic sense.

Clearly, neither Koch's postulates nor the updated Evans's postulates are fulfilled for most hypotheses about drug-related disease. Indeed, in many reports of suspected adverse reactions we know little about pre-exposure status and the stability of this status with time. We often have scant information, poorly described, about the timing and dose of the hypothesized causative agent. The event that was thought to be drug-related is often incompletely described. Finally, it is very rare for there to be a rechallenge or re-exposure study.

Appreciation of the limitations of these postulates in the everyday world of suspected adverse drug reactions has led to a move to develop structures for obtaining reproducible operational identification of adverse drug reactions (Karch and Lasagna 1977; Kramer et al. 1979; Hutchinson et al. 1979) together with studies to determine the reproducibility of judgements of trained observers (Blanc et al. 1979). Although such approaches are theoretically beneficial, they have proven cumbersome in use and have not been widely adopted. Thus the literature on adverse drug reactions is a relatively murky area of substantial subjectivity, where the truth is often difficult to elucidate and supporting data are at best approximations. Because of the evanescent nature of much drug therapy, this difficulty is to be expected, but it must be kept in mind when reviewing individual studies.

Classification of reactions

The Rawlins and Thompson classification of adverse drug reactions into predictable pharmacological reactions (Type A) and unpredictable idiosyncratic reactions (Type B) is now generally accepted to be a helpful way of looking at this problem (Rawlins and Thompson 1977 and see Chapter 3), and is used in this book. Unfortunately, most collected information on adverse reactions ignores this classification or does not provide the necessary detail to allow its derivation. An assumption frequently made by academic pharmacologists is that the pharmacological type of reaction is primarily attributable to inappropriate prescribing and hence intrinsically less 'interesting' or relevant than the idiosyncratic type of reaction, which presents a much greater intellectual challenge. None the less, it is clear from several major studies that pharmacological reactions, whether or not due to inappropriate prescribing, constitute the bulk of adverse drug reactions experienced by the population.

Studies based in medical wards all indicate that unwanted pharmacological actions of drugs are the most common cause of suspected adverse reactions, accounting for approximately 80 per cent of notified drug-related events (Ogilvie and Ruedy 1967; Hurwitz and Wade 1969; Miller 1974; Caranasos et al. 1974). The remaining events are most likely to be idiosyncratic or allergic in nature. Hurwitz and Wade (1969) separated pharmacological reactions into those in which an unwanted secondary pharmacological action was the cause of the undesired effect (60 per cent) and those where an excessive effect of the principal pharmacological action was the cause (25 per cent), while the remaining 15 per cent of results were non-pharmacological in nature.

Descriptive studies

Drug use

In a WHO European Monograph on studies of drug utilization, published in 1979, Graham Dukes (1979) began by stating that 'one of the most puzzling features of the world of medicines at the present day is the astonishing and, in some respects, disastrous lack of information about the way in which drugs are used and misused. In most major countries of the world it is still impossible to find out how many medicines are on sale, much less what the turnover of these products might be. Where this basic information is to be found, one is left wondering which physicians are using these products for which patients and why.' Eleven years on, similar sentiments could still be expressed. Even crude information on sales is not generally available to the medical profession or to the public. Individual studies have reported wide disparities in drug use between countries and within individual countries, for example, studies on the use of oral antidiabetic agents saw 10-fold to 20-fold differences between individual European countries (Bergman 1979; Dukes 1979). Similar studies on variations of psychotropic drug use in Nordic countries have appeared from time to time. Lawson and Jick (1976), in an interesting 'fall-out' from the Boston Collaborative Drug Surveillance Program (BCDSP) medical inpatient studies, reported that the use of drugs in hospitalized patients in the United States was twice that in a matched comparison group in Scotland. The reasons for such differences are not clear, but relate more to physician behaviour than patient need. Perhaps a more striking example of this is the major disparity in the use of intravenous fluids between two hospitals with otherwise virtually identical drug use reported from Glasgow (Lawson 1977). The hospital with the greater prevalence of intravenous fluid use showed a substantially lower volume of infusion per patient indicating that the difference in prescribing habits was not readily explicable on the basis of patient need.

With increasing economic constraints on drug prescribing, health care providers are likely to require much more information on drug-use patterns than heretofore — a development that is to be given every encouragement, being greatly overdue.

Reactions during hospital admission

Reported incidence of adverse drug reactions varies from 1 per cent or less to 28 per cent (MacDonald and Mackay 1964; Reidenberg and Lowenthal 1968; Miller 1974). In most studies, the figure, however, lies somewhere between 10–20 per cent (Seidl et al. 1965; Smith et al. 1966; Ogilvie and Ruedy 1967; Hurwitz and Wade 1969; Gardner and Watson 1970). These wide differences reflect variations in the particular definition of adverse reactions used and in the methods used to detect and report suspected reactions; when investigators have

relied on others to notify them of suspected reactions the yields have been low, but when they have undertaken a detailed search using independent research workers the yields have been much higher. Although, theoretically, these differing figures could be reconciled if the spontaneous reports related to more severe adverse reactions and those from more detailed surveys included milder reactions, such interpretation is difficult to substantiate, relatively mild reactions being reported in both types of survey. Clearly, controlled observations of symptoms and signs before the administration of drugs would not be practical in this type of approach. Although, theoretically, information about non-exposed individuals could assist in providing comparison, such information is rarely available and is itself subject to substantial bias. Thus the available data provide at best only a rough estimate of the overall incidence of adverse drug reactions in hospital.

Most studies so far have concentrated on medical inpatients. There have been a number of small studies looking at surgical inpatients (Armstrong et al. 1976; Danielson et al. 1982), paediatric wards (BCDSP 1972a; Mitchell et al. 1979, 1982) and psychiatric wards (Swett 1974). These reviews tend to record a lower incidence of reactions than are seen in medical inpatients, probably reflecting the lesser severity of the underlying illness rather than a lower intrinsic toxicity of drugs in these populations.

In an attempt to analyse the situation more rigorously, several workers have reported on the frequency of severe reactions by restricting their analysis to include only reactions of life-threatening severity or those that resulted in death (Shapiro et al. 1971; Armstrong et al. 1976; Caranasos et al. 1976; Porter and Jick 1977). Overall, these workers report a death rate attributable to drug treatment of some 2 per 10 000 surgical patients and 9 per 10 000 medical patients, the drugs most frequently implicated being cardiac glycosides, anticoagulants, and intravenous fluids.

Reactions in outpatients

Few workers have formally studied the overall incidence of adverse effects in outpatients. Mulroy (1973) reported that one in 40 consultations was due to drug-induced disease. Kellaway and his colleagues in Auckland (1973) reported an overall incidence of 32 per cent in 200 patients discharged from hospital who were followed for the ensuing 6 months. Martys (1979) reported that 41 per cent of patients receiving drug treatment developed some type of reaction.

Even fewer investigators have conducted substantive drug-specific studies in outpatients. Halsey and Cardoe (1982) reviewed the events occurring in some 300 patients in their practice who had received benoxaprofen, then a new non-steroidal anti-inflammatory agent. They confirmed the toxic potential of this drug for the skin and gastrointestinal tract.

Time of onset of adverse drug reactions

Various investigators have attempted to pinpoint the most likely time of onset of adverse drug reactions. Their estimates vary from the first day of hospitalization (Seidl *et al.* 1966) to the second day (Miller 1974), the first two days (Hurwitz and Wade 1969), and a fairly constant rate throughout the first nine days (Ogilvie and Ruedy 1967). Clearly, figures such as these are of limited value. What is important is the known clinical pharmacology of the drug and the date of initial exposure. In an interesting review of 2656 patients receiving heparin sodium therapy, within the BCDSP data, the average cumulative risk of bleeding during 7 days of treatment was 9 per cent (Walker and Jick, 1980). The exposed individual was at greatest risk on the third day of heparin administration, but the daily incidence figures remained relatively consistent at 1–2 per cent throughout some 18 days of follow-up. Regrettably, longitudinal data of this nature are available for few commonly used drugs.

Spontaneous reports to regulatory authorities

Most investigators looking at large series of prospective patients in medical wards report that the commonest adverse reactions recorded were attributable to aspirin and the non-steroidal anti-inflammatory agents, antibiotics, cardiac glycosides, anticoagulants, diuretics, and steroids. Similar conclusions arise from analyses of spontaneous reports to drug regulatory authorities (McQueen 1974; ADRAC 1980; Bem *et al.* 1988). The UK spontaneous report scheme for suspected adverse drug reactions has been an effective, inexpensive, and useful tool to aid regulatory authorities to come to judgements about drug toxicity (Rawlins 1986). There is, however, substantial under-reporting of adverse reactions. Such under-reporting has been studied in general practice (Walker and Lumley 1986; Lumley *et al.* 1986), but not in any detail in hospitals, towards which one might expect the majority of patients with serious adverse reactions to gravitate. In an analysis of drug-related deaths reported to the UK Committee on Safety of Medicines, Girdwood (1974) found that the leading causes of suspected drug-related death at that time were oral contraceptives, phenylbutazone, chlorpromazine, and corticosteroids. By the late 1980s, this picture had changed substantially, partly as a result of the reduction in oestrogen content of the oral contraceptive preparations now available, partly to withdrawal of phenylbutazone, and partly to the emergent widespread use of a variety of non-steroidal anti-inflammatory agents.

Detailed analysis of cumulative spontaneous reports of adverse reactions is fraught with difficulty (Griffin and Weber 1985, 1986, 1989; Rawlins 1986, 1988*a,b*). The non-steroidal anti-inflammatory agents illustrate this most efficiently. The information available to the UK Committee on Safety of Medicines was analysed in 1986 (CSM 1986). The numbers of suspected serious gastrointestinal reactions to non-steroidal anti-inflammatory agents during 1964–85 were reviewed. The results were considered not only in terms of absolute numbers of reports, but also as the number of reports per million recorded prescriptions. The available data allowed grouping of the non-steroidal agents into three major groups of serious suspected reactions per million prescriptions:

1. ibuprofen, which appeared to have the lowest rate of serious reactions per million prescriptions (13.2). This drug has subsequently become available in pharmacies without prescription;
2. benoxaprofen, fenclofenac, indoprofen, feprazone and the Osmosin formulation of indomethacin, which showed high total reaction 'rates' of between 132 and 555 per million prescriptions. These drugs have been withdrawn from the marketplace;
3. the remaining drugs with rates between 35 and 87 per million prescriptions. These are difficult to separate one from the other and have remained available by prescription.

Of considerable interest are the differences between these reporting rates and the substantially lower rates for the same drugs reported in the United States (Sachs and Bortnichak 1986; Rossi *et al.* 1987). In an analysis of 15 spontaneous reporting schemes for adverse drug reaction monitoring throughout the world, Griffin (1986) clearly showed the wide variability in reporting rates in different countries. Thus, great care should be taken before attempts are made to collate such disparate data resources and to draw any conclusion. Edwards and his colleagues emphasize this in a review of the World Health Organisation's International Collaborative Programme on Drug Monitoring (Edwards *et al.* 1990).

They claim that such a system has strengths as a signal generator or hypotheses-generating system, but has no value as a hypotheses-testing resource.

Augmented spontaneous reports of suspected adverse reactions

Several groups have endeavoured to surmount both the under-reporting and the numerous distortions inherent in spontaneous reporting schemes. Notable among these are the augmented spontaneous reporting schemes developed in New Zealand (Coulter and McQueen 1982; Edwards 1987), prescription event monitoring designed by Professor Inman and his group in Southampton (1988), and a number of *ad hoc* studies undertaken by individual drug firms, examples of which would include those of ketotifen (Maclay *et al.* 1984) and captopril (Chalmers *et al.* 1987). In these approaches, detailed studies encouraging reports either of suspected adverse reactions or of events experienced by drug recipients together with feedback, either documentary or via computer terminals, allow a better understanding and quantitation of suspected reactions than has been possible hitherto with spontaneous schemes reporting directly to regulatory authorities.

Analytical studies

Case registries

Case registries first came into vogue as a method of quantitating suspected adverse reactions with the discovery that chloramphenicol could be associated with the development of aplastic anaemia (Yunis 1973). Similar techniques were adopted in the search for a possible aetiological agent in the outbreak of vaginal adenocarcinoma in premenarchal girls noted in the eastern seaboard of the United States (Herbst *et al.* 1971). This technique is of great value where a drug commonly causes an otherwise very rare disease which is clearly defined and not subject to diagnostic confusion. The drug must be in reasonably widespread use and the suspect condition must be virtually non-existent in the absence of the drug.

It is perhaps surprising that this technique has not been adopted more extensively since these demonstrations of its potential. There is a strong argument for mounting a series of case registries for otherwise rare events that are frequently drug-related: examples of these would include acute renal failure, acute hepatic necrosis, Guillain-Barré syndrome, aplastic anaemia, and agranulocytosis (Lawson 1990).

Cohort studies

Recently the United Kingdom Committee on Safety of Medicines has reviewed its experience of drug-related problems and has concluded that, for new drugs used in relatively benign conditions in domiciliary practice, some form of surveillance ought to be in continuous operation for the early years following marketing. In essence, the technique that can most readily address this problem is the cohort study. Several such cohort studies have been undertaken and published, a classic example being that in which some 9928 consecutive cimetidine recipients were reviewed over a period of one year during which time all the diagnoses recorded during episodes of hospital contact, whether inpatient or outpatient, were analysed together with all deaths and the cause of those deaths. Thereafter, the names of patients were noted for future reference by the Central Registry of Deaths and they have now been followed up over a period of 10 years. Such a massive exercise has produced useful data on the patterns of adverse reaction experience with everyday use of H_2-blockers and has been of value in attempting to review the association between H_2-blocker use and upper gastrointestinal tract tumours (Colin-Jones *et al.* 1983, 1985*a,b*). These studies are expensive to operate, however, and the facility to undertake them is not widely available. Moreover, it is difficult to collect information on an appropriate comparator group. Indeed, doubts about the value of such comparison data have been raised in relation to the cost of undertaking the study. Such caveats may be less important in the future when record-linkage studies become more widely available (Beardon *et al.* 1988, 1989).

Case–control studies

Case–control studies are of considerable use in testing hypotheses about drug-related disease. The technique is not without its problems and its critics (Horowitz and Feinstein 1979); it is, however, a powerful tool for coming rapidly to a conclusion about suspected adverse drug reactions under certain strict conditions (Sartwell 1974; Jick and Vessey 1979). Used appropriately, this approach can be of great value in studying possible drug-related events in defined populations. Indeed, some investigators have gone so far as to undertake what is called case–control surveillance whereby they investigate a series of well-defined cases in a prospective manner as part of a hospital-based national surveillance programme (Slone *et al.* 1979). Examples of the type of information available from case–control studies include the associations between cholelithiasis and oral contraceptives (BCDSP 1973), venous thromboembolism and postmenopausal estrogen therapy (BCDSP 1974), and acute pancreatitis and thiazide diuretics (Bourke *et al.* 1978).

Record-linkage studies

Previously, cohort studies and case–control studies have tended to be done as and when required. The availability, however, of powerful computers, particularly in the United States, has led to record-linkage schemes whereby information regarding outcome of hospitalization and drug exposure within hospitals and, latterly, within general practice, is collated and analysed to give us a powerful tool for conducting aetiological research following drug exposure. Finney (1965) foresaw the use of such large databases to generate hypotheses about possible adverse drug effects while avoiding the likelihood of bias contained in physicians' judgements. At the time, however, the necessary computer power was not available. In an early attempt at analysing output from a large data resource, Skegg and Doll (1977) in Oxford reported their ability to identify an increased prevalence of eye and skin problems in practolol recipients when compared with propranolol recipients. These analyses were conducted following the discovery of the practolol syndrome; they confirmed, however, the potential of such large data sources for generating significant information on adverse drug effects. As computer facilities have become more widespread and are able to handle much more information, the possibilities foreseen by Finney in 1965 have become a reality. Foremost amongst such record-linkage studies are those conducted by the Boston Collaborative Drug Surveillance Program within the Group Health Co-operative Health Maintenance Organisation in Puget Sound (Jick *et al.* 1984; Porter *et al.* 1982). Other studies have been conducted using different data sources within the USA (Strom *et al.* 1985) and Canada (Guess *et al.* 1988). Wayne Ray and his colleagues in Tennessee (1987, 1989) have used Medicaid data to conduct inpatient studies into risk factors for hip fracture, indicating a positive association with long-term psychotropic drug use and a negative association with long-term thiazide diuretic use.

Within the United Kingdom, similar studies are beginning to be developed by the Medicines Evaluation and Monitoring Unit in Dundee (Beardon *et al.* 1989).

Experimental studies

Most small-scale, randomized, controlled clinical trials do not produce data of major interest to the pharmaco-epidemiologist. Only when one enters the area of large-scale multicentre studies do we see studies of sufficient size to be of potential value. A classic example of this was the use of clofibrate in the secondary prevention of myocardial infarction (Oliver *et al.* 1984).

Predisposing factors

Race and genetic polymorphism

Recently, considerable interest has been directed towards the role of genetic polymorphism in explaining interindividual variation in susceptibility to adverse drug reactions. Several important genetic polymorphisms have been discovered in the oxidation and acetylation pathways of drug metabolism. Examples include extensive and poor metabolisers of debrisoquine (Mahgoub *et al.* 1977). Poor metabolisers of debrisoquine tend to have reduced first-pass metabolism, increased plasma levels, and exaggerated pharmacological response to this drug, resulting in postural hypotension. By contrast, rapid metabolisers may require considerably higher doses for a standard effect. More recently, it has been shown that nortriptyline and desipramine are metabolised by mechanisms similar to those of debrisoquine (Mellstrom *et al.* 1981), as a result of which the steady-state plasma levels of these drugs are phenotype-dependent (Bertilsson and Aberg-Wistedt 1983). This problem may become most clinically relevant in subjects taking overdoses of these tricyclic antidepressants. Under such circumstances, the serious potential for cardiotoxicity is enhanced in poor metabolisers (Spiker *et al.* 1976).

Acetylator polymorphism is another clinically relevant example of genetic polymorphism. In this case, the drugs particularly affected are procainamide, isoniazid, hydralazine, and phenelzine. There are wide variations in the distributions of rapid acetylators in different races. Rapid acetylators predominate amongst Eskimos and Japanese and slow acetylators amongst Mediterranean Jews. Slow acetylators are more likely to develop peripheral neuropathy due to isoniazid, and lupus erythematosus associated with procainamide, isoniazid, or hydralazine (Lunde *et al.* 1983). Conversely, fast acetylators may be more susceptible to the toxicity associated with isoniazid (Mitchell *et al.* 1975).

Glucose 6-phosphate dehydrogenase deficiency, which predisposes to some drug-induced haemolytic anaemias, is commoner amongst Africans, Kurdish and Iraqi Jews, some Mediterranean people, and Filipinos, and is relatively infrequent amongst other races.

There is wide interracial variability in the distribution of human lymphocyte antigens (HLA), resulting in racial predisposition to those adverse reactions believed to be associated with HLA phenotype. Several examples of the association of HLA phenotype and adverse drug reaction have been reported, although the mechanisms by which such reactions are mediated have yet to be fully explained. Up till now, particular interest has concentrated in the higher prevalence of toxicity of drugs used in the treatment of rheumatoid arthritis. Whether this observation is a result of more frequent testing of HLA phenotypes in patients with rheumatoid disease is unclear. Veys and others (1978) reported an association with levamisole toxicity and HLA-B27. Bardin and colleagues (1982) reported cases of nephrotoxicity from penicillamine associated with the HLA-DR3 haplotype and Woolley and co-workers (1980) reported associations with toxicity from sodium aurothiomalate and penicillamine in patients with HLA-DR3,DR1.

Racial differences in the incidence of haemolytic anaemia induced by methyldopa have been reported. A positive direct antiglobulin test was found in 15 per cent of Caucasian patients under treatment; but no positive tests were found in 73 Indians and Africans who had been taking methyldopa for at least 3 months (Seedat and Vawda 1968) or in 58 Chinese patients who had received the drugs for at least 9 months (Burns-Cox 1970; Chen and Ooi 1971).

Women in Scandinavia and Chile appear to be particularly susceptible to the cholestatic jaundice induced by oral contraceptives, for reasons that are not clear (Reyes 1982).

Some types of porphyria are aggravated by drugs. These tend to vary in incidence between different races; for instance, acute intermittent porphyria is more frequent in people of Scandinavian, Anglo-Saxon, or German origin than amongst other ethnic groups, while the disease itself is very rare in negroes.

Jick and others (1969) reported that blood group has a significant influence on susceptibility to thromboembolic disease amongst oral contraceptive users, and to digoxin toxicity (BCDSP 1972b).

Sex

Several studies have shown that women are more likely to report adverse drug reactions than men (Seidl et al. 1966; Hurwitz 1969; Caranasos et al. 1974; Miller 1974). Although this could be explained largely by the greater susceptibility of the female skin and gut to noxious stimuli, women also appear to be more susceptible to the toxic effects of digoxin (Hurwitz and Wade 1969), hep-arin (Miller 1974), and captopril (Chalmers et al. 1987). Agranulocytosis caused by phenylbutazone or chloramphenicol is about three times commoner (D'Arcy and Griffin 1972), and aplastic anaemia due to chloramphenicol twice as common (Yunis and Bloomberg 1964) in women as in men. Drug-associated lupus erythematosus affects more women than men, as does the spontaneous disease (Lee and Siegal 1968; Batchelor et al. 1980).

Age

The elderly

Castleden and Pickles (1988) reviewed the reports of suspected adverse reactions accumulated by the UK Committee on Safety of Medicines during 1965–83. A greater than expected proportion of reports came from elderly subjects. There were 3350 reports concerning individual patients aged 75 years or over, the commonest serious problems affecting the gastrointestinal and haemopoietic systems. As with younger subjects, non-steroidal anti-inflammatory agents accounted for a large proportion of the notified reactions in this age group.

Several cross-sectional studies of the elderly in hospital have indicated they suffer from more adverse reactions than younger patients (Hurwitz 1969; Miller 1974; Caranasos et al. 1974; Levy et al. 1980). None the less, interpretation of such studies is limited by failure to control important age-related variables, including measurements of renal function, hepatic function, plasma protein levels, etc., and the number of medications that a patient was receiving. More recent studies suggest that of the four traditional elements of pharmacokinetics — absorption, distribution, metabolism, and excretion — only absorption appears to be substantially independent of age (Johnson et al. 1985). Drug distribution may vary substantially between the young and the old. An age-related increase in body fat may well account for the greater volume of distribution of lipid-soluble medications such as long-acting benzodiazepines, and drug elimination by the kidney may be considerably impaired in elderly subjects owing to age-related decline in renal function, although there is a large interindividual variability in such deterioration (Rowe et al. 1976). Coupled with these changes in pharmacokinetic variables, certain pharmacodynamic variables also appear to be affected by age processes. Thus there appears to be an increase in the sensitivity of receptors for many medications in the elderly.

Reidenberg and others (1978) showed an increasing effect in the elderly of a given dose of diazepam despite these subjects having significantly lower plasma levels of the drug at the time. Similar studies have been reported involving other benzodiazepines and opiates (Belville *et al.* 1971; Kaiko 1980). In a classic study using data from the BCDSP, Greenblatt and his colleagues reviewed information from 2542 consecutive flurazepam recipients and showed a strong age and dose effect in relation to the occurrence of undesired drowsiness with this drug (Greenblatt *et al.* 1977). In a large study based on Medicaid prescribing records, Avorn *et al.* (1986) showed that, among a sample of 143 253 recipients, depression (defined as receipt of a tricyclic antidepressant drug) appeared less common in older subjects as compared with younger subjects. This study also showed a higher prevalence of depression among female recipients of β-adrenoceptor blockers when compared with males.

It has been shown that a single dose of digoxin produces a higher plasma concentration and the plasma half-life of the drug is longer than with the same dose in younger people (Ewy *et al.* 1969). This may partly explain the high incidence of digoxin toxicity found in older patients (MacDonald and MacKay 1964; Ogilvie and Ruedy 1967; Hurwitz and Wade 1969), though potassium depletion induced by powerful modern diuretics in patients taking a poor diet may play a part, as may renal tubular excretory and secretory factors (Hall 1972).

Elderly patients are more likely to bleed during heparin treatment than are younger patients (Walker and Jick 1980). The anticoagulant effect of a single dose of warfarin appears to be greater in the old than in the young (Hewick *et al.* 1975), a finding in keeping with clinical experience. In a review of 321 patients attending a University Hospital, however, Gurwitz and others (1988) failed to show an association between age and bleeding reactions. Similar findings were recorded by Petty and colleagues (1986) in a large retrospective study of patients attending an anticoagulant clinic. Levine and co-workers (1989) surveyed some 171 studies of anticoagulant therapy but were unable to establish any association between age and bleeding, as insufficient information was recorded in many articles reviewed.

It has long been accepted that elderly patients are more sensitive to the effects of powerful analgesics than younger patients; and that they are apt to become confused and disturbed by barbiturates. Possible explanations for these clinical impressions are provided by experiments which show that after a standard single intravenous dose of pethidine the plasma concentration is higher and the half-life of the drug longer in old than in younger subjects (Chan *et al.* 1975); and that the rate of hydroxylation of amylobarbitone is reduced in the elderly (Irvine *et al.* 1974). Elderly patients are particularly prone to cerebral dysfunction when they take nitrazepam in the usual adult dose (Evans and Jarvis 1972).

Experimental studies also suggest that the old may be at greater risk of suffering adverse reactions to phenylbutazone (O'Malley *et al.* 1971) and propranolol (Castleden *et al.* 1975). They are more liable than the young to develop potassium depletion from diuretic therapy, postural hypotension caused by antihypertensive drugs and phenothiazines, urinary retention from anticholinergics and antiparkinsonian drugs, and spontaneous hypothermia associated with treatment with sedatives and tranquillizers (Hall 1972).

The young

In the neonate, especially when premature, several of the enzymes involved in drug metabolism and elimination are poorly developed, and consequently the risk of adverse reactions to some drugs is increased. The most hazardous drugs in this respect are chloramphenicol, sulphonamides, novobiocin, barbiturates, morphine and its derivatives, and vitamin K and its analogues. In the very young child, chloramphenicol may induce the grey syndrome, characterized by abdominal distension, vomiting, peripheral cyanosis, profound shock, respiratory failure, and death. Sulphonamides, novobiocin, and vitamin K analogues may induce or aggravate kernicterus; and barbiturates, morphine, and other narcotics may cause severe respiratory depression.

Some ototoxic antibiotics (e.g. streptomycin) are eliminated by the kidney more slowly in the young child than in the adult, and toxic effects may occur unless the dose is reduced. The increased sensitivity to digoxin in the first 2 weeks of life may be explained by a similar mechanism (Morselli *et al.* 1983).

The increased sensitivity of the newborn to morphine and its derivatives has been attributed to a poorly developed glucuronidation mechanism, upsets in cholinergic and adrenergic regulation, and the inefficiency of the immature blood–brain barrier. Poorly developed oxidation reactions or inadequate renal function, or both of these, may also account for the poor tolerance of the newborn to some barbiturates (Done and Jung 1970; Gadeke 1972).

Using the data from the UK spontaneous reporting scheme, Bateman and colleagues (1985) showed that extrapyramidal reactions with metoclopramide were reported significantly more often in young adults than expected, the highest rate being seen in young females (190 reports per million prescriptions), and the lowest rate in elderly males (3.5 reports per million prescriptions). This difference is of major clinical importance and appears not to be due to pharmacokinetic abnormalities but rather to different end-organ responses.

End-organ failure

Patients with impaired renal or liver function are at substantially greater than normal risk of developing adverse reactions to drugs eliminated by these organs. Epidemiological techniques have rarely been used in studies in this area, largely because of the complexity of most of the clinical cases surveyed.

Drug formulation

Changes in formulation resulting either in increased bioavailability or in patients being exposed to new excipients may be a cause of epidemics of drug toxicity. Classic examples of this are the development of phenytoin toxicity and of digoxin toxicity following reformulation of old products (Greenblatt *et al*. 1983; Neuvonen 1983). Further details of these incidents are given in a later chapter and the whole question of toxicity arising from excipients in medicines has been well reviewed by Golightly and colleagues (1988*a,b*).

Conclusions

Considering the relatively 'soft' nature of much of the information cited above and the intrinsic difficulty of assessing whether an event is drug-related or not, it is hardly surprising that different commentators have come to widely differing conclusions about the overall effect on public health of the hazards of drug therapy. Melmon (1971) from the western USA expressed the view that many lives were lost and much unnecessary hospitalization arose from adverse drug effects. By contrast, Jick (1974), based in Massachussets but using worldwide data, concluded that drugs were remarkably non-toxic, given their powerful nature and widespread use. Citing information from the BCDSP, he concluded that most adverse reactions were self-limiting and of little consequence to the clinical course of the patient's illness. Serious reactions were uncommon and tended to occur in patients who were ill and suffering from potentially fatal diseases. In his opinion, the main culprits in producing avoidable adverse reactions of major degree were the often uncritical use of intravenous fluids and of electrolyte replacement.

More recently, Inman (1984) has made an eloquent plea for investigators in this difficult area to pay some regard to the benefits of drug therapy and its hazards in relation to the expected life-span of the individual recipient. Such an approach is undoubtedly valid and merits more widespread adoption.

It is clear from the information presented that the use of powerful drugs has increased substantially in the last few decades. With this increase goes a potential for serious adverse reactions. To minimize these risks, prescribers have daily to consider the objectives of their treatment, how long it should continue, which drug they should choose, and how they can estimate the appropriate dose for their patient. Such concerns are important in all subjects, but become particularly clamant where the objective of therapy is not to alleviate symptoms of existing disease, but to prevent the development of complications in patients suffering from asymptomatic abnormalities such as hypertension or hyperlipidaemia. Such individuals are increasingly exposed to powerful medications in order to achieve long-term benefit in the form of reduction in disease progression and consequent prolongation of useful life. Great care must be taken to ensure that the treatment advocated should be as free as possible from risk to health, lest the treatment prove worse than the disease. In order to establish the true risks and benefits of such therapeutic interventions, long-term studies of an epidemiological nature will be required. The technology for such studies is now available. So far, however, we seem to lack the will to implement it widely, possibly because of perceived cost implications. The solution to these problems, however, must be increasing use of record-linkage facilities in the USA, and their development in Europe and Japan. It is to be hoped that efforts in this direction will be greatly increased in the coming decade.

Further reading

Hartzema, A.G., Porta, M.S., and Tilson, H.H. (1988). *Pharmacoepidemiology: an introduction*. Harvey Whitney, Cincinnati.

Inman, W.H.W. (1986). *Monitoring for drug safety* (2nd edn). Medical and Technical Press, Lancaster.

Strom, B.L. (1989). *Pharmacoepidemiology*. Churchill Livingstone, Edinburgh.

References

ADRAC (Adverse Drug Reactions Advisory Committee) (1980). ADRAC report for 1980. *Med. J. Aust.* 5, 416.

Armstrong, B., Dinan, B., and Jick, H. (1976). Fatal drug reactions in patients admitted to surgical services. *Am. J. Surg.* 132, 643.

Avorn, J., Everitt, D.E., and Weiss, S. (1986). Increased antidepressant use in patients prescribed beta-blockers. *JAMA* 255, 357.

Bardin, T., Dryll, A., Debeyre, N., Byckewaert, A., Legrand, L., Marcelli A., *et al.* (1982). HLA system and side effects of gold salts and D-penicillamine treatment of rheumatoid arthritis. *Ann. Rheum. Dis.* 41, 599.

Batchelor, J.R., Welsh, K.I., Mansilla-Tinoco, R., Dollery, C.T., Hughes, G.R.V., Bernstein, R. *et al.* (1980). Hydralazine-induced systemic lupus erythematosus: influence of HLA-DR and sex on susceptibility. *Lancet* i, 1107.

Bateman, D.N., Darling, W.M., and Rawlins, M.D. (1985). Extrapyramidal reactions to metoclopramide and prochlorperazine. *Q. J. Med.* 71, 307.

BCDSP (Boston Collaborative Drug Surveillance Program) (1972a). Drug surveillance: problems and challenges. *Pediatr. Clin. North Am.* 19, 117.

BCDSP (Boston Collaborative Drug Surveillance Program) (1972b). Relation between digoxin arrhythmias and ABO blood groups. *Circulation,* 45, 352.

BCDSP (Boston Collaborative Drug Surveillance Program) (1973). Oral contraceptives and venous thromboembolic disease, surgically confirmed gallbladder disease and breast tumours. *Lancet* i, 1399.

BCDSP (Boston Collaborative Drug Surveillance Program) (1974). Surgically confirmed gallbladder disease, venous thromboembolism, and breast tumors in relation to postmenopausal estrogen therapy. *N. Engl. J. Med.* 290, 15.

Beardon, P.H.G., Brown, S.V., and McDevitt, D.G. (1988). 4-year mortality among cimetidine takers in Tayside: results of a controlled study using record linkage. *Pharm. Med.* 3, 333.

Beardon, P.H.G., Brown, S.V., and McDevitt, D.G. (1989). Gastrointestinal events in patients prescribed non-steroidal anti-inflammatory drugs: a controlled study using record linkage. *Q. J. Med.* 71, 497.

Belville, J.W., Forrest, W.H., Miller, E., and Brown, B.W. (1971). Influence of age on pain relief from analgesics. *JAMA* 217, 1835.

Bem, J.L., Breckenridge, A.M., Mann, R.D., and Rawlins, M.D. (1988). Review of yellow cards (1986): report to the Committee on the Safety of Medicines. *Br. J. Clin. Pharmacol.* 26, 679.

Bergman, U. (1979). International comparisons of drug utilisation: use of antidiabetic drugs in 7 European countries. In *Studies in drug utilisation* (ed. U. Bergman, A. Grimsson, A.H.W. Wahba, and B. Westerholm). WHO Regional Publications No. 8. WHO, Copenhagen.

Bertilsson L. and Aberg-Wistedt, A. (1983). The debrisoquine hydroxylation test predicts steady-state plasma levels of desipramine. *Br. J. Clin. Pharmacol.* 15, 388.

Blanc, S., Leuenberger, P., Berger, J.P., Brooks, E.N., and Schelling, J.L. (1979). Judgement of trained observers on adverse drug reactions. *Clin. Pharmacol. Ther.* 25, 493.

Bourke, J.B., McIllmurray, M.B., Mead, G.M., and Langman, M.J.S. (1978). Drug-associated primary acute pancreatitis. *Lancet* i, 706.

Burns-Cox, C.J. (1970). Negative Coombs test in Chinese on methyldopa. *Lancet* ii, 673.

Caranasos, G.J., Stewart, R.B., and Cluff, L.E. (1974). Drug-induced illness leading to hospitalization. *JAMA* 228, 713.

Caranasos, G.J., May, F.E., Stewart, R.B., and Cluff, L.E. (1976). Drug-associated deaths of medical in-patients. *Arch. Intern. Med.* 136, 872.

Castleden, C.M. and Pickles, H. (1988). Suspected adverse drug reactions in elderly patients reported to the Committee on Safety of Medicines. *Br. J. Clin. Pharmacol.* 26, 347.

Castleden, C.M., Kaye, C.M., and Parsons, R.L. (1975). The effect of age on plasma levels of propranolol and practolol in man. *Br. J. Clin. Pharmacol.* 2, 303.

Chalmers, D., Dombey, S.L., and Lawson, D.H. (1987). Postmarketing surveillance of captopril (for hypertension): a preliminary report. *Br. J. Pharmacol.* 24, 343.

Chan, K., Kendall, M.J., Mitchard, M., Wells, W.D. E., and Vickers, M.D. (1975). The effect of ageing on plasma pethidine concentration. *Br. J. Clin. Pharmacol.* 2, 297.

Chen, B.T.M. and Ooi, B.S. (1971). Negative Coombs test in Chinese on methyldopa. *Lancet* i, 87.

Colin-Jones, D.G., Langman, M.J.S., Lawson, D.H., and Vessey, M.P. (1983). Postmarketing surveillance of the safety of cimetidine: 12 month mortality report. *Br. Med. J.* 286, 1713.

Colin-Jones, D.G., Langman, M.J.S., Lawson, D.H., and Vessey, M.P. (1985a). Postmarketing surveillance of the safety of cimetidine: 12 month morbidity report. *Q. J. Med.* 54, 253.

Colin-Jones, D.G., Langman, M.J.S., Lawson, D.H., and Vessey, M.P. (1985b). Postmarketing surveillance of the safety of cimetidine: mortality during second, third and fourth years of follow-up. *Br. Med. J.* 291, 1084.

Committee on Safety of Medicines (CSM) Update (1986). Non-steroidal anti-inflammatory drugs and serious gastrointestinal adverse reactions — 1. *Br. Med. J.* 292, 614.

Coulter, D.M. and McQueen, E.G. (1982). Postmarketing surveillance. Achievements and problems in the intensified adverse drug reaction reporting scheme. *N.Z. Family Physician* 1, 13.

Danielson, D.A., Porter, J.B., Dinan, B.J., O'Connor, P.C., Lawson, D.H., and Kellaway, G.S.M. (1982). Drug monitoring of surgical patients. *JAMA* 248, 1482.

D'Arcy, P.F. and Griffin, J.P. (ed.) (1972). *Iatrogenic diseases*, p. 3. Oxford University Press.

Done, A.K. and Jung, A.L. (1970). Neonatal pharmacology. In *Current pediatric therapy*, Vol. 4 (ed. S.S. Gellis and B.M. Kagan), p. 995. Saunders, Philadelphia.

Dukes, M.N.G. (1979). Drug utilisation studies in perspective. In *Studies in drug utilisation* (ed. U. Bergman, A. Grimsson, A.H.W. Wahba, and B. Westerholm). WHO Regional Publications No. 8. WHO, Copenhagen.

Edwards, R.I. (1987). Adverse drug reaction monitoring. The practicalities. *Med. Toxicol.* 2, 405.

Edwards, R.I., Lindquist, M., Wiholm, B-E., and Napke, E. (1990). Quality criteria for early signals of possible adverse drug reactions. *Lancet* 336, 156.

Evans, A.S. (1976). Causation and disease: the Henle–Koch postulates revisited. *Yale J. Biol. Med.* 49, 175.

Evans, J.G. and Jarvis, E.H. (1972). Nitrazepam and the elderly. *Br. Med. J.* iv, 487.

Ewy, G.A., Kapadia, G.C., Toa, L., Lullin, M., and Marcus, F.I. (1969). Digoxin metabolism in the elderly. *Circulation* 39, 449.

Finney, D.J. (1965). The design and logic of a monitor of drug use. *J. Chronic Dis.* 18, 77.

Gadeke, R. (1972). Unwanted effects of drugs in the neonate, premature and young child. In *Drug-induced diseases*, Vol. 4 (ed. L. Meyler and H. M. Peck), p. 585. Associated Scientific Publishers, Amsterdam.

Gardner, P. and Watson, L.J. (1970). Adverse drug reactions: a pharmacist-based monitoring system. *Clin. Pharmacol. Ther.* 2, 802.

Girdwood, R.H. (1974). Deaths after taking medicaments. *Br. Med. J.* i, 501.

Golightly, L.K., Smolinske, S.S., Bennett, M.C., Sutherland, E.W., and Rumack, B.H. (1988a). Pharmaceutical excipients: adverse effects associated with inactive ingredients in drug products — I. *Med. Toxicol.* 3, 128.

Golightly, L.K., Smolinske, S.S., Bennett, M.C., Sutherland, E.W., and Rumack, B.H. (1988b). Pharmaceutical excipients: adverse effects associated with inactive ingredients in drug products — II. *Med. Toxicol.* 3, 209.

Greenblatt, D.J., Allen, M.D., and Shader, R.I. (1977). Toxicity of high-dose flurazepam in the elderly. *Clin. Pharmacol. Ther.* 21, 355.

Greenblatt, D.J., Smith, T.W., and Koch-Weser, J. (1983). Bioavailability of drugs: the digoxin dilemma. In *Handbook of clinical pharmacokinetics* (ed. M. Gibaldi and L.F. Prescott), p. 1. ADIS Health Science Press, Australia.

Griffin, J.P. (1986). Survey of the spontaneous adverse drug reaction reporting schemes in 15 countries. *Br. J. Clin. Pharmacol.* 22, 83.

Griffin, J.P. and Weber, J.C.P. (1985). Voluntary systems of adverse reaction reporting. Part I. *Adverse Drug React. Acute Poisoning Rev.* 4, 213.

Griffin, J.P. and Weber. J.C.P. (1986). Voluntary systems of adverse reaction reporting. Part II. *Adverse Drug React. Acute Poisoning Rev.* 1, 23.

Griffin, J.P. and Weber, J.C.P. (1989). Voluntary systems of adverse reaction reporting. Part III. *Adverse Drug React. Acute Poisoning Rev.* 8, 203.

Guess, H.A., West, R., Strand, L.M., Helston, D., Lydick, E.G., Bergman, U., *et al.* (1988). Fatal upper gastrointestinal hemorrhage or perforation among users and nonusers of nonsteroidal anti-inflammatory drugs in Saskatchewan, Canada 1983. *J. Clin. Epidemiol.* 41, 35.

Gurwitz, J.H., Goldberg, R.J., Holden, A., Knapki, N., and Ansall, J. (1988). Age-related risks of long-term oral anticoagulant therapy. *Arch. Intern. Med.* 148, 1733.

Hall, M.R.P. (1972). Drugs and the elderly. *Br. Med. J.* iii, 582.

Halsey, P. and Cardoe, N. (1982). Benoxaprofen: side-effect profile in 300 patients. *Br. Med. J.* 284, 1365.

Herbst, A.L., Ulfelder, H., Poskanzer, D.C. (1971). Association of maternal stilboestrol therapy with tumor appearance in young women. *N. Engl. J. Med.* 284, 878.

Hewick, D.S., Moreland, T.A., Shepherd, A.M.M., and Stevenson, I.M. (1975). The effect of age on sensitivity to warfarin sodium. *Br. J. Clin. Pharmacol.* 2, 189P.

Horowitz, R.I. and Feinstein, A.R. (1979). Methodologic standards and contradictory results in case–control research. *Am. J. Med.* 66, 556.

Hurwitz N. (1969). Predisposing factors in adverse reactions to drugs. *Br. Med. J.* i, 356.

Hurwitz, N. and Wade, O.L. (1969). Intensive monitoring of adverse reactions to drugs. *Br. Med. J.* i, 531.

Hutchison, T.A., Leventhal, J.M., Kramer, M.S., Karch, F.E., Lipman, A.G., and Feinstein, A.R. (1979). An algorithm for the operational assessment of adverse drug reactions. II. Demonstration of reproducibility and validity. *JAMA* 242, 633.

Inman, W.H.W. (1984). Risks in medical intervention — balancing therapeutic risks and benefits. *P.E.M. News, 2,* 16.

Inman, W.H.W., Rawson, N.S., Wilton, L.V., Pearce, G. L., and Speirs, C.J. (1988). Postmarketing surveillance of enalapril. I: results of prescription-event monitoring. *Br. Med. J.* 297, 826.

Irvine, R.E., Grove, J., Toseland, P.A., and Trounce, J.R. (1974). The effect of age on the hydroxylation and amylobarbitone sodium in man. *Br. J. Clin. Pharmacol.* i, 41.

Jick, H. (1974). Drugs — remarkably nontoxic. *N. Engl. J. Med.* 291, 824.

Jick, H. and Vessey, M.P. (1979). Case-control studies in the evaluation of drug-induced illness. *Am. J. Epidemiol.* 107, 1.

Jick H., Slone, D., Westerholm, B., Inman, W.H.W., Vessey, M.P., Shapiro, S., *et al.* (1969). Venous thromboembolic disease and ABO blood type: a cooperative study. *Lancet* i, 539.

Jick, H., Madsen, S., Nudelman, P.M., Perera, D.R., and Stergachis, A. (1984). Postmarketing follow-up at Group Health Cooperative of Puget Sound. *Pharmacotherapy* 4, 99.

Johnson, S.L., Mayersohn, M., and Conrad, K.A. (1985). Gastrointestinal absorption as a function of age: xylose absorption in healthy adults. *Clin. Pharmacol. Ther.* 38, 331.

Kaiko, R.F. (1980). Age and morphine analgesia in cancer patients with postoperative pain. *Clin. Pharmacol. Ther.* 28, 823.

Karch, F.E. and Lasagna, L. (1977). Towards the operational identification of adverse drug reactions. *Clin. Pharmacol. Ther.* 21, 247.

Kellaway, G.S.M. (1973). Intensive monitoring for adverse drug effects in patients discharged from acute medical wards. *N.Z. Med. J.* 78, 525.

Kramer, M.S., Leventhal, J.M., Hutchison, T.A., and Feinstein, A.R. (1979). An algorithm for the operational assessment of adverse drug reactions. I. Background description and instructions for use. *JAMA* 242, 623.

Last, J.M. (1983). *Dictionary of epidemiology.* Oxford University Press.

Lawson, D.H. (1977). Intravenous fluids in medical inpatients. *Br. J. Clin. Pharmacol.* 4, 299.

Lawson, D.H. (1990). Postmarketing surveillance of drugs. *Proc. R. Coll. Physicians Edinb.* 20, 129.

Lawson, D.H. and Jick, H. (1976). Drug prescribing in hospitals: an international comparison. *Am. J. Public Health* 66, 644.

Lee, S.L. and Siegel, M. (1968). Drug-induced systemic lupus erythematosus. In *Drug-induced diseases*, Vol. 3 (ed. L. Meyler and H. M. Peck), p. 244. Associated Scientific Publishers, Amsterdam.

Levine, M.M., Raskob, R., and Hirsh, J. (1989). Hemorrhagic complications of long-term anticoagulant therapy. *Chest* 95 (suppl.) 265.

Levy, M., Kewitz, H. Altwein, W., Hillebrand, J., and Eliakim, M. (1980). Hospital admissions due to adverse drug reactions: a comparative study from Jerusalem and Berlin. *Eur. J. Clin. Pharmacol.* 17, 25.

Lumley, C.E., Walker, S.R., Hall, G.C., Staunton, N., and Grob, P.R. (1986). The under-reporting of adverse drug reactions seen in general practice. *Pharm. Med.* 1, 205.

Lunde, P.K., Frislid, K., and Hansteen, V. (1983). Disease in acetylator polymorphism. In *Handbook of Clinical Pharmacokinetics* (ed. M. Gibaldi and L.F. Prescott), p. 150. ADIS Health Science Press, Australia.

MacDonald, M.G. and MacKay, B.R. (1964). Adverse drug reactions. *JAMA* 190, 1071.

Maclay, W.P., Crowder, D., Spiro, S., and Turner, P. (1984). Postmarketing surveillance: practical experience with ketotifen. *Br. Med. J.* 288, 911.

Mahgoub, A., Idle, J.R., Dring, L.G., Lancaster, R., and Smith, R.L. (1977). Polymorphic oxidation of debrisoquine in man. *Lancet* ii, 584.

Martys, C.R. (1979). Adverse reactions to drugs in general practice. *Br. Med. J.* ii, 1194.

McQueen, E.G. (1974). New Zealand Committee on adverse drug reactions. *N.Z. J. Med.* 10, 305.

Mellstrom, B., Bertillson, L., Sawe, J., Schulz H-U., and Sjøqvist, F. (1981). E- and Z-10-hydroxylation of nortriptyline: relationship to polymorphic debrisoquine hydroxylation. *Clin. Pharmacol. Ther.* 30, 189.

Melmon, K.L. (1971). Preventable drug reactions — causes and cures. *N. Engl. J. Med.* 284, 1361.

Miller, R.R. (1974). Hospital admissions due to adverse drug reactions. *Arch. Intern. Med.* 43, 219.

Mitchell, A.A., Goldman, P., Shapiro S., and Slone, D. (1979). Drug utilisation and reported adverse reactions in hospitalized children. *Am. J. Epidemiol.* 110, 196.

Mitchell, A.A., Hartz, S.C., Shapiro, S., and Slone, D. (1982). Patterns of preadmission medication use among hospitalized children. *Pediatr. Pharmacol* 2, 209.

Mitchell, J.R., Thorgeirsson, U.P., Black, M., Timbrell, J.A., Snodgrass, W.R., Potter, W.Z., *et al.* (1975). Increased incidence of isoniazid hepatitis in rapid acetylators: possible relation to hydralazine metabolites. *Clin. Pharmacol. Exp. Ther.* 18, 70.

Morselli, P.L., Franco-Morselli, R., and Bossi, L. (1983). Clinical pharmacokinetics in newborns and infants: age-related differences and therapeutic implications. In *Handbook of clinical pharmacokinetics* (ed. M. Gibaldi and L. F. Prescott), p. 98. ADIS Health Science Press, Australia.

Mulroy, R. (1973). Iatrogenic disease in general practice: its incidence and effects. *Br. Med. J.* ii, 407.

Neuvonen, P.J. (1983). Bioavailability of phenytoin: clinical pharmacokinetic and therapeutic implications. In *Handbook of clinical pharmacokinetics* (ed. M. Gibaldi and L. F. Prescott), p. 24. ADIS Health Science Press, Australia.

Ogilvie, R.I. and Ruedy, J. (1967). Adverse drug reactions during hospitalisation. *Can. Med. Assoc. J.* 97, 1450.

Oliver, M.F., Heady, J.A., Morris, J.N., and Cooper, J. (1984). WHO cooperative trial on primary prevention of ischaemic heart disease with clofibrate to lower serum cholesterol: final mortality follow-up. Report of the Committee of Principal Investigators. *Lancet* ii, 600.

O'Malley, K., Crooks, J., Duke, E., and Stevenson, J.H. (1971). Effect of age and sex on human drug metabolism. *Br. Med. J.* iii, 607.

Petty, D.B., Strom, B.L., Melmon, K.L. (1986). Duration of warfarin anticoagulant therapy and probabilities of recurrent thromboembolism and hemorrhage. *Am. J. Med.*, 81, 255.

Porter, J. and Jick, H. (1977). Drug-related deaths among medical inpatients. *JAMA* 237, 879.

Porter, J.B., Hunter, J.R., Danielson, D.A., Jick, H., and Stergachis, A. (1982). Oral contraceptives and nonfatal vascular disease: recent experience. *Obstet. Gynecol.* 59, 299.

Rawlins, M.D. (1986). Spontaneous reporting of adverse drug reactions. *Q. J. Med.* 59, 531.

Rawlins, M.D. (1988a). Spontaneous reporting of adverse drug reactions. I: The data. *Br. J. Clin. Pharmacol.* 26, 1.

Rawlins, M.D. (1988b). Spontaneous reporting of adverse drug reactions. II: Uses. *Br. J. Clin. Pharmacol.* 26, 7.

Rawlins, M.D. and Thompson, J.W. (1977). Pathogenesis of adverse drug reactions. In *Textbook of adverse drug reactions* (ed. D.M. Davies), p. 10. Oxford University Press.

Ray, W.A., Griffin, M.R. Schaffner, W., Baugh, D.K., and Melton, L.J. (1987). Psychotropic drug use and the risk of hip fracture. *N. Engl. J. Med.* 316, 363.

Ray, W.A., Griffin, M.R., Downey, W., and Melton, L.J. (1989). Long-term use of thiazide diuretics and risk of hip fracture. *Lancet* i, 687.

Reidenberg, M.M. and Lowenthal, DT. (1968). Adverse non-drug reactions. *N. Engl. J. Med.* 279, 678.

Reidenberg, M.M., Levy, M., Warner, H., Coutinho, C.B., Schwartz, M.A., Yu, G., *et al.* (1978). Relationship between diazepam dose, plasma level, age and central nervous system depression in adults. *Clin. Pharmacol. Ther.* 23, 371.

Reyes, H. (1982). The enigma of intrahepatic cholestasis of pregnancy: lessons from Chile. *Gastroenterology* 2, 87.

Rossi, A.C., Hsu, J.P., and Faich, G.A. (1987). Ulcerogenicity of piroxicam: an analysis of spontaneously reported data. *Br. Med. J.* 294, 147.

Rowe, J.W., Andres, R., Tobin, J.D., Norris, A., and Shock, N. (1976). The effect of age on creatinine clearance in man: a cross-sectional and longitudinal study. *J. Gerontol.* 31, 155.

Sachs, R.M. and Bortnichak, E.A. (1986). An evaluation of spontaneous adverse drug reactions monitoring systems. *Am. J. Med.* 81 (5B), 49.

Sartwell, P.E. (1974). Retrospective studies: a review for the clinician. *Ann. Intern. Med.* 81, 381.

Seedat, Y.K. and Vawda, E.I. (1968). The Coombs test and methyldopa. *Lancet* i, 427.

Seidl, L.G., Thornton, G.F., and Cluff, L.E. (1965). Epidemiological studies of adverse drug reactions. *Am. J. Public Health* 65, 1170.

Seidl, L. G., Thornton, G.F., Smith, J.W., and Cluff, L.E. (1966). Studies on the epidemiology of adverse drug reactions. III — Reactions in patients on a general medical service. *Bull. Johns Hopkins Hosp.* 119, 299.

Shapiro, S., Slone, D., Lewis, G.P., and Jick, H. (1971). Fatal drug reactions among medical inpatients. *JAMA* 216, 467.

Skegg, D.C.G. and Doll, W.R.S. (1977). The frequency of eye complaints and rashes among patients receiving practolol and propranolol. *Lancet* ii, 475.

Slone, D., Shapiro, S. Miettinen, O.S., Finkle, W.D., and Stolley, P.D. (1979). Drug evaluation after marketing. *Ann. Intern. Med.* 90, 257.

Smith, J.W., Seidl, L.G., and Cluff, L.E. (1966). Studies on the epidemiology of adverse drug reactions. V — Clinical factors influencing susceptibility. *Ann. Intern. Med.* 65, 629.

Spiker, D. G., Weiss, A.N., Chang, S.S., Ruwich, J.F., and Biggs, J.T. (1976). Tricyclic antidepressant overdose: clini cal presentation and plasma levels. *Clin. Pharmacol. Ther.* 18, 539.

Strom, B.L., Carson, J.L., Morse, M.L., and Leroy, A. A. (1985). The computerised on-line Medicaid pharmaceutical analysis and surveillance system: a new resource for postmarketing drug surveillance. *Clin. Pharmacol. Ther.* 38, 359.

Swett, C. (1974). Drowsiness due to chlorpromazine in relation to cigarette smoking. *Arch. Gen. Psychiatry* 31, 211.

Veys, E.M., Miclants, H., and Verbruggen, G. (1978). Levamisole induced adverse reactions in HLA-B27 positive rheumatoid arthritis. *Lancet* i, 148.

Walker A. M. and Jick, H. (1980). Predictors of bleeding during heparin therapy. *JAMA* 244, 1209.

Walker, S.R. and Lumley, C.E. (1986). The attitudes of general practitioners to monitoring and reporting adverse drug reactions. *Pharm. Med.* 1, 195.

Woolley, P.H., Griffin, J. Panayi, G.S., Batchelor, J.R., Welsh, K.I., and Gibson, T.J. (1980). HLA-DR antigens and toxic reaction to sodium aurothiomalate and D-penicillamine in patients with rheumatoid arthritis. *N. Engl. J. Med.* 303, 300.

Yunis, A.A. (1973). Chloramphenicol-induced bone marrow suppression. *Semin. Hemat.* 10, 225.

Yunis, A.A. and Bloomberg, G.R. (1964). Chloramphenicol toxicity: clinical features and pathogenesis. *Prog. Hematol.* 4, 138.

3. Mechanisms of adverse drug reactions

M. D. RAWLINS and J. W. THOMPSON

Introduction

Previous editions introduced a classification of adverse drug reactions and interactions (Rawlins and Thompson 1977) that has been widely adopted in both experimental (Plaa 1978; Zbinden 1980) and clinical (Folbe 1980; Venning 1983; Gillies *et al.* 1986; Laurence and Bennett 1987; Breckenridge and Orme 1987) pharmacology and toxicology. By separating adverse reactions into those that are normal but *augmented* (or *attenuated*) actions of a particular drug (Type A reaction) and those that are totally abnormal, *bizarre* effects (Type B reactions) it is possible to construct a logical framework for considering the toxicity of drugs that has both theoretical and practical utility.

Type A (augmented) adverse drug reactions

These reactions are the result of an exaggerated, but otherwise normal, pharmacological action of a drug given in the usual therapeutic doses. Examples include bradycardia with β-adrenoceptor antagonists, haemorrhage with anticoagulants, or drowsiness with benzodiazepine anxiolytics. Type A reactions are largely predictable on the basis of a drug's known pharmacology. They are usually dose-dependent and although their incidence and morbidity in the community is often high their mortality is generally low.

Type B (bizarre) adverse drug reactions

These reactions are totally aberrant effects that are not to be expected from the known pharmacological actions of a drug when given in the usual therapeutic doses to a patient whose body handles the drug in the normal way. Malignant hyperthermia of anaesthesia, acute porphyria, and many immunological reactions fall into this category. They are usually unpredictable and are not observed during conventional pharmacological and toxicological screening programmes. Although their incidence and morbidity are usually low, their mortality may be high.

In individual patients the distinction between Type A and B reactions can usually be made on pharmacological and clinical grounds alone, but in a few instances two separate mechanisms may produce the same effect. Agranulocytosis after chloramphenicol administration, and halothane hepatotoxicity, are probable examples.

Mechanisms of Type A adverse drug reactions

When a group of individuals receive a drug, a spectrum of response is observed. This variability manifests itself either as differing doses required to produce the same effect, or as differing responses to the administration of a defined dose (Smith and Rawlins 1973) and forms the basis of Type A reactions.

In some instances, Type A reactions may be an excessive therapeutic effect (such as hypoglycaemia with antidiabetic drugs, or hypotension with antihypertensive agents). In others, the reaction may occur as a result of a drug's primary pharmacological action at some other site (such as peptic ulceration and haemorrhage with non-steroidal anti-inflammatory drugs, or osteoporosis with glucocorticoids). Many Type A reactions, however, are not due to the pharmacological action of a drug that mediates its therapeutic effect but to some other property that it possesses. Thus, some phenothiazines, many histamine H_1-antagonists, and most tricyclic antidepressants have anticholinergic properties which result in 'atropine-like' adverse reactions, including dryness of the mouth, difficulty with accommodation, and, occasionally, retention of urine. Other examples include the antiandrogenic actions of progestogens and cimetidine, the γ-aminobutyric acid (GABA) antagonist properties of some quinolones, the motilin agonist actions of erythromycin, and the effects on the thyroid of amiodarone.

Variability in response to the administration of a defined drug dose is typically seen with non-steroidal anti-inflammatory drugs (NSAID). Some degree of gastrointestinal bleeding can be observed in nearly everyone following single doses. In the majority this is relatively small (less than 5 ml per day), and can be readily accommodated by increased red cell production. A few individuals, however, lose appreciable amounts of blood, and when they receive NSAID regularly they may well develop frank iron-deficiency anaemia — particularly if their iron stores are minimal before they start treatment.

In contrast, the doses of an anticoagulant, such as warfarin, that are required to achieve therapeutic anticoagulation may vary 20-fold between individuals. The reasons for this particular form of interindividual variability are multifactorial. They are not solely due to differences in the manner by which the drug is distributed and metabolised: interpersonal differences in the sensitivity at the site of action (the hepatocyte) are also involved. There is thus considerable variation, between individuals, in the plasma warfarin concentrations required to produce similar degrees of anticoagulation (Routledge *et al.* 1979).

Type A reactions develop in individuals lying at the extremes of dose–response curves for pharmacological and toxicological effects. The reasons why they should occupy this disadvantageous position are three-fold: first, the pharmaceutical formulation may predispose some individuals to toxicity; secondly, the way in which some individuals handle drugs is quantitatively abnormal (i.e. a pharmacokinetic change); thirdly, genetic factors or disease may alter the sensitivity of 'target' organs to drugs (i.e. a pharmacodynamic change). In some individuals combinations of these causes may be responsible.

Pharmaceutical causes

The pharmaceutical characteristics of a dosage form may predispose to Type A reactions, either because of alterations in the quantity of drug present, or because of its release characteristics.

Drug quantity

In most developed countries, marketed pharmaceutical products must fulfil certain requirements laid down by drug regulatory authorities. These stipulate the limits (usually ±5 per cent or less) within which the content of active drug must fall in relation to the stated dose. In less developed countries, however, such regulations either

may not exist, or be poorly complied with (Adjepon-Yamoah 1980).

Drug release

The release of active drug from a pharmaceutical preparation may vary with particle size, the nature and quantity of excipients used, and the coating materials. The outbreaks of digoxin and phenytoin toxicity in the late 1960s and early 1970s are important reminders of such possibilities.

Release rates and formulation characteristics may determine local gastrointestinal toxicity (Bros 1987). Potassium salts are highly irritant to the gut mucosa, and the administration of potassium chloride tablets is accompanied by an unacceptably high incidence of haemorrhage, perforation, and cicatrization (Boley *et al.* 1965). When potassium chloride is given dispersed in a wax matrix, however, so that very high local concentrations are avoided, these problems are largely obviated, unless there is stasis of the gastrointestinal contents. The unexpectedly large number of reports to the UK Committee on Safety of Medicines (1983) of gastrointestinal bleeding and haemorrhage in patients receiving Osmosin (a rate-controlled preparation of indomethacin) was also probably due to the irritant effects of a very high concentration of the active ingredient on a localized area of intestinal mucosa (Rawlins and Bateman 1984). Adherence of tablets to the intestinal mucosa, particularly the oesophagus, may result in local damage when the drug itself is irritant: this seems the likely explanation for the reports of oesophageal ulceration and stenosis following the administration of certain preparations of emepronium bromide.

Sustained release formulations of drugs such as theophylline are designed to prolong the absorption phase so as to increase the interval between successive doses. Such products therefore usually contain larger quantities of the active drug substance than would normally be given as a single dose. The delayed release for some products is achieved by enclosing it in a pH-dependent membrane which is only disrupted in a neutral or alkaline medium. When swallowed on an empty stomach, the low intragastric pH thus results in the maintenance of the integrity of the product's coating membrane. If, however, the product is ingested on a full stomach, the membrane may rupture and the entire contents be released. Rapid, rather than sustained, absorption then occurs and may give rise to transient postprandial toxicity. This phenomenon, so-called 'dose-dumping', has been described in association with sustained release theophylline products (Hendeles *et al.* 1985). The phenomenon has also been reported with products that show pH-independent dissolution characteristics although the explanation is unclear (Steffensen and Pedersen 1986).

Pharmacokinetic causes

Pharmacokinetics is the study of the time-course of drug quantities and actions in biological tissues (Dost 1953). It is therefore particularly concerned with the absorption, distribution, and elimination of drugs. Quantitative alterations in these processes may give rise to abnormally high concentrations of the drug at its site of action and a correspondingly enhanced biological effect. Such alterations are therefore liable to produce exaggerated but otherwise predictable pharmacological responses, which are Type A adverse drug reactions. Alternatively, abnormally low drug concentrations may develop and result in therapeutic failure.

Drug absorption

Most drugs are administered orally, and absorption is possible anywhere from the mouth to the anal canal. Absorption occurs with greatest facility in the small intestine, where the huge mucosal surface and blood supply encourage diffusion of drug molecules across the lipoprotein cell membranes of the enterocytes. Lipid-soluble drugs, which can most readily cross cell membranes, are most easily absorbed. If these drugs are weak electrolytes (existing in ionized and non-ionized states), only the non-ionized moieties will dissolve in lipid and therefore be capable of being absorbed. The absorption of lipid-insoluble drugs is frequently incomplete and varies widely between individuals; the reasons for this are not always obvious. Complicating factors such as mucus, paracellular absorption, membrane permeability, and motility effects may also be important (Leahy *et al.* 1989).

Differences in both the *extent* and *rate* of drug absorption may have profound therapeutic implications. Type A adverse effects can follow changes in either of these.

Extent of absorption

The total amount of drug reaching the general circulation (bioavailability) is obviously dependent on the administered dose. In the case of drugs given by mouth, however, other factors are also important. They include not only the pharmaceutical formulation of the drug, but also the tendency to complex with other ingested agents, the motility of the gastrointestinal tract, the absorptive capacity of the gastrointestinal mucosa, and the ability of the gut wall and the liver to destroy drugs before they reach the systemic circulation.

The dose   Once a doctor has decided upon a specific drug dose, the actual quantity consumed by his patient is dependent on the accuracy with which he complies with the prescribed instructions. The compliance of patients with their prescribing instructions is notoriously variable. Factors associated with poor compliance include complexity of dosage regimens (once-daily dosing is much easier to remember than thrice-daily dosing), multiple drug therapy, social isolation, the development of adverse drug effects, and failure on the part of the patient to understand the nature of his disease or the reasons for treatment (Mucklow 1979). The most frequent problem, however, is partial compliance rather than non-compliance (Pullar *et al.* 1988; Cranmer *et al.* 1989) resulting in a reduced drug intake and hence therapeutic failure.

Influence of other drugs (drug interactions)   Other ingested substances may complex with orally administered drugs to yield non-absorbable derivatives (Welling 1984). This generally results in therapeutic failure. Charcoal and kaolin both absorb other drug molecules on to their surfaces. For this reason the use of charcoal has been advocated in the management of poisoning with salicylates (Levy and Tsuchiya 1971), as well as with paracetamol or nortriptyline. Cholestyramine, an ion-exchange resin used to bind bile salts in the gut, also binds oral anticoagulants and decreases both plasma drug levels and anticoagulant effect (Robinson *et al.* 1971). Salts of aluminium, magnesium, and iron all chelate with tetracyclines and impair their absorption (Kunin and Finland 1961). Oral iron, and antacid mixtures containing aluminium and magnesium oxides, also substantially impair the absorption of penicillamine (Osman *et al.* 1983).

All these interactions, however, occur only if the interacting agents are administered simultaneously or within 30–60 minutes of each other; they can be avoided by careful timing of drug doses. This, however, does not apply to an interesting interaction described between oral iron salts and doxycycline (Neuvonen and Pentilla 1974). This combination leads to enhanced doxycycline elimination, apparently because this tetracycline, unlike others, is highly lipid-soluble and is distributed very widely in various tissues and organs. This distribution includes the gastrointestinal contents where, in the lower regions of the small bowel, the drug may complex irreversibly with unabsorbed iron.

Gastrointestinal motility   Drug absorption from the stomach is slow compared with that in the small intestine. Changes in gastric emptying rate usually influence the rate rather than the extent of drug absorption (Prescott 1974). Some drugs, such as methyldigoxin, penicillins, and levodopa are metabolised or inactivated in the stomach, and if emptying is delayed they may be relatively ineffective (Bianchine *et al.* 1971).

Changes in the motility of the small intestine may have important consequences for the extent of drug absorption by altering the time available for equilibration to occur across the gastrointestinal mucosa (Davis 1989). Reduced motility following the administration of propantheline enhances digoxin absorption by allowing the drug to remain longer at sites of maximum absorption (Manninen *et al.* 1973).

Gastrointestinal mucosa   The effects of small bowel disease on drug absorption have not yet been adequately studied. In theory, malabsorptive states would be expected to impair, primarily, the absorption of lipid-insoluble compounds because the passage of the latter across the gut wall is already precarious. Certainly, the absorption of digoxin (Heizer *et al.* 1971) and practolol (Parson and Kaye 1974) is decreased in patients with coeliac disease. It appears, however, that the extent of absorption of many lipid-soluble drugs such as propranolol (Sandle *et al.* 1983) is unimpaired in coeliac patients even though the absorption rate is reduced.

'First-pass' elimination of drugs   With many drugs an appreciable fraction of an oral dose never reaches the general circulation, despite virtually complete absorption from the gastrointestinal tract. The reason for the reduced bioavailability of drugs such as chlorpromazine, isoprenaline, nortriptyline, lignocaine, and propranolol is that all undergo metabolism during their first 'passage' across the gut wall or through the liver (Gibaldi *et al.* 1971). Isoprenaline and chlorpromazine undergo metabolism in the gut wall, and with the former less than 1 per cent of an oral dose is systemically available. Drugs as diverse as lignocaine, propranolol, morphine, dextropropoxyphene, nortriptyline, paracetamol, and metoclopramide undergo significant metabolism by the liver before they reach the general circulation. Drugs undergoing significant first-pass metabolism are those that have high extraction ratios across the liver, and high systemic clearances. The extent of 'first-pass' hepatic metabolism of many drugs varies widely between individuals, and for drugs such as propranolol (Shand and Rangno 1972) and paracetamol (Rawlins *et al.* 1977) it is dose-dependent. Moreover, first-pass metabolism may be induced or inhibited by other drugs given at the same time (see below). The relevance of this to the present discussion lies in the fact that the process of first-pass elimination is one that varies considerably between individuals with the result that bioavailability differs from person to person.

Rate of drug absorption

The speed with which drugs are absorbed after ingestion or injection will determine the plasma concentration–time profile after single drug doses. Delayed absorption will result in a slower rise of plasma drug levels, a reduced peak plasma concentration, and a tendency for a more prolonged elimination phase. This may be advantageous if the intention is to produce prolonged pharmacological effects (as with slow-release oral preparations, or depot injections of insulin or corticotrophin). The slower appearance of drug in the circulation, however, may delay the onset and reduce the intensity of drug action. For example, intramuscularly administered phenytoin crystallizes out at its injection site. This results in such a slow rate of absorption that peak plasma levels after 1000 mg are rarely more than 2 mg per litre (Karlsson *et al.* 1974); since the therapeutic actions (either anticonvulsant or antiarrhythmic) occur only at levels of 10 mg per litre this route of administration is totally useless. When drugs are administered regularly, delayed absorption results in 'flattening' of plasma drug levels at steady-state during a dosage interval and has no effect on the average level during this period. This does not present any particular disadvantage except for those drugs (some antibiotics and cytotoxic agents) for which high peak plasma concentrations are required.

The rate of absorption of orally administered drugs is largely determined by the rate of gastric emptying (Prescott 1974), which is influenced by emotion and pain, by the nature of the gastric contents (volume, composition, and pH), by disease, and by drugs. Thus, ethanol or compounds with anticholinergic activity (atropine, tricyclic antidepressants, and propantheline) slow gastric emptying (Nimmo *et al.* 1973) and delay absorption, while metoclopramide has the opposite effect.

Drug distribution

Drug molecules that have reached the general circulation are distributed to various tissues and organs. The degree and extent of this will depend (Smith and Rawlins 1973) on regional blood flow, and the facility with which drugs can diffuse across cell membranes (dependent on lipid-solubility). In addition, drugs may be sequestered in body fat if they are highly lipid-soluble; they may bind to tissue macromolecules; or they may be actively transported across cell membranes or tissue planes.

The extent to which a drug is distributed may be estimated by its distribution volume. This volume relates the amount of drug in the body to its plasma concentration.

$$\text{distribution volume} = \frac{\text{amount of drug in body}}{\text{plasma concentration}}$$

and the greater the extent of distribution, the larger is the volume of distribution. It is important to realize, however, that the volume measured is an *apparent* one, and that it does not measure any particular anatomical space except in a few isolated instances.

Regional blood flow

Regional distribution of cardiac output and tissue perfusion rates are obviously important determinants of drug distribution. Our knowledge of the relevance of these processes — particularly in the presence of cardiovascular disease — to the distribution kinetics of particular drugs is scanty. There is increasing evidence, however, that for drugs whose hepatic metabolism is limited largely by liver blood flow (e.g. lignocaine), changes in hepatic perfusion may be extremely important. Thus, in cardiac failure (Thomson *et al.* 1973), after haemorrhage, during infusions of noradrenaline (Benowitz *et al.* 1974), or after β-blockade with propranolol (Ochs *et al.* 1980) or metoprolol (Conrad *et al.* 1983) liver blood flow is decreased and lignocaine clearance is reduced. In heart failure the central volume of distribution is, however, reduced and high drug concentrations may be observed after the administration of loading doses (Shammas and Dickstein 1988).

Disturbances in drug distribution can also be demonstrated in end-stage renal disease-possibly due to circulatory changes accompanying chronic anaemia. McLeod and others (1976) have shown that in these patients not only is pancuronium elimination reduced (as might be expected) but its distribution volume is increased. These findings may thus explain the clinical observations that patients with renal failure not only develop prolonged neuromuscular blockade following pancuronium but also require larger intravenous doses to produce adequate muscle relaxation.

Plasma protein binding

Many drugs bind loosely (reversibly) to plasma proteins. Acidic drugs bind predominantly to albumin, whilst basic drugs not only bind to albumin but more especially to the acute phase protein, α_1-acid glycoprotein. The bound drug is biologically inactive but in equilibrium with drug molecules free in plasma water. Only free (unbound) drug is available for distribution extravascularly, for producing biological effects and, in most in-

stances, for elimination either by the kidneys or the liver. For those drugs the extraction ratios of which across these organs are high, however, both free *and* bound molecules may be removed.

Binding of drugs to plasma proteins can alter in a number of circumstances. Decreased binding will occur in patients with hypoalbuminaemia (for acid drugs) irrespective of the cause (e.g. nephrotic syndrome, starvation, liver disease, ageing). Decreased binding is also seen if there is competition for binding sites with endogenous (e.g. bilirubin, free fatty acids) or exogenous (e.g. other drugs) ligands. Increased binding of basic drugs occurs when α_1-acid glycoprotein concentrations rise in association with inflammatory responses (e.g. infections, acute myocardial infarction). Binding to α_1-acid glycoprotein is reduced in individuals with a genetically determined variant form of the protein (Eap *et al.* 1990).

The consequences of altered plasma protein binding is the cause of much confusion (Smith and Rawlins 1973; Rawlins 1974*a*). When highly bound drugs are administered rapidly, and especially after intravenous injection, a decrease in binding will tend to result in elevated free drug concentrations in plasma, and an enhanced pharmacological effect. Such a phenomenon is observed after intravenous diazoxide, a highly protein-bound drug, which produces a greater fall in blood pressure in patients with reduced binding to plasma proteins (Pearson and Breckenridge 1976). When drugs are given more slowly, or on a regular basis, changes in protein binding will have less effect, because the potential for an increase in the free drug concentration will be offset by distribution to other organs, and by increased elimination. At worst, changes in the intensity of drug action will be transient, and in most instances will be without significant effect. Descriptions in the literature of an association between Type A adverse effects and hypoalbuminaemia (Lewis *et al.* 1971; BCDSP 1973; Greenblatt and Koch-Weser 1974) are probably due to alterations in hepatic metabolism. Similarly, the accounts of displacement interactions between warfarin and drugs such as phenylbutazone (Aggeler *et al.* 1967) were due to inhibition of the metabolism of the latter by the former.

The degree of drug protein binding is of greatest importance in the interpretation of plasma drug levels. Since most analytical techniques measure both bound and free drug in plasma, the validity of monitoring drug levels in clinical practice is dependent on the assumption that interpatient variation in binding is small. For highly bound drugs, and in circumstances where binding is likely to be reduced, appropriate corrections must be made to the interpretation of drug-level measurements.

Tissue binding

The relatively large apparent volume of distribution of drugs such as nortriptyline (20–50 litres per kg) can only be accounted for by extensive tissue binding. This process is now recognized as an important mechanism for producing some adverse drug reactions.

Tetracyclines chelate with newly formed bone producing a tetracycline–calcium orthophosphate complex. The half-life of tetracycline in bone is of the order of several months (Buyske *et al.* 1960) as compared with a few hours in plasma. Although in adults this is of little clinical consequence, in neonates it may result in a 40 per cent depression of bone growth (Cohlan *et al.* 1963), as well as discolouration and deformation of teeth.

A number of drugs, including chloroquine and phenothiazines, have a high affinity for melanin (Bernstein *et al.* 1964). *In vivo*, high concentrations accumulate in the melanin-containing tissues of the eye suggesting a causal relationship to the retinopathies produced by both these groups of drugs. The carcinogenicity of alkylating agents such as cyclophosphamide, azathioprine, and chlorambucil is due to binding to DNA.

Active transport of drugs

Although most drugs are distributed by passive transport, a few which resemble physiological compounds are actively transported across cellular membranes.

The adrenergic-neurone-blocking agents (guanethidine, bethanidine, debrisoquine) owe their antihypertensive properties to the fact that they reach high concentrations within sympathetic noradrenergic nerve terminals (Iversen 1967). This gradient is achieved by transport of the drugs across the membrane of the presynaptic neurones by an active process that normally transports noradrenaline. Drugs that inhibit this noradrenaline re-uptake (tricylic antidepressants, phenothiazines) also inhibit the transport of adrenergic-neurone-blocking agents and thereby antagonize their hypotensive properties (Mitchell *et al.* 1970). This interaction does not occur between tricyclic antidepressants and either methyldopa, thiazide diuretics, or β-adreno-ceptor-blocking agents (β-blockers). For as yet unexplained reasons, however, it does occur with clonidine (Briant *et al.* 1973).

Certain organic acids are actively transported from the cerebrospinal fluid to plasma across the choroid plexus (Davidson 1968). This 'pump' removes 5-hydroxy-indole acetic acid, salicylate, and penicillin; it can be blocked by perchlorate and probenecid. In animals, morphine is actively transported in a similar manner by a pump that is selective for organic bases (Wang and Takemori 1972). The clinical significance of these mech-

anisms is, as yet, unclear but they emphasize the complex nature of drug distribution, which may predispose to adverse drug reactions.

Drug elimination

Apart from volatile anaesthetics, drugs are excreted in the urine of bile, or metabolised by the liver to yield metabolites which are then eliminated by the kidneys. Changes in drug elimination rates are probably the most important cause of Type A adverse reactions. Reduced elimination leads to drug accumulation, with toxicity developing as a result of the elevated plasma and tissue levels. Conversely, enhanced elimination rates lead to reduced plasma and tissue drug levels, resulting in therapeutic failure.

Renal excretion

Drugs enter the proximal renal tubule by glomerular filtration. In addition, some organic acids are actively transported across the proximal tubular epithelium.

Glomerular filtration produces glomerular fluid drug concentrations identical with those in plasma water. Only unbound drug therefore appears in the filtrate and diminished protein binding may enhance renal excretion. Tubular secretory mechanisms also transport only unbound drug from the peritubular capillaries, but in contrast to glomerular filtration they reduce the concentration of drug in plasma water. Bound drug molecules therefore dissociate from plasma protein binding sites and so become available for transport. Active tubular secretion is therefore totally independent of protein binding and may result in complete extraction of drugs across the renal vascular bed (e.g. *p*-aminohippuric acid). Furthermore, interference with tubular secretion may seriously impair drug elimination.

Solute and water reabsorption along the course of the renal tubules will inevitably lead to a concentration gradient across the tubular epithelium. As a result, drugs will tend to diffuse from the nephron into peritubular capillaries, but their ability to cross cell membranes will be dependent upon their lipid solubility. Polar drugs, which are soluble in water (and therefore insoluble in lipid), will be unable to cross this membrane, and their clearances will approach glomerular filtration rate (or renal plasma flow if they undergo active secretion). Drugs that are lipid-soluble, however, will readily cross the tubular epithelium and reach equilibrium with free drug in plasma. Under these circumstances urinary drug levels and renal drug clearances will tend to be very low.

Glomerular filtration Impaired glomerular filtration inevitably leads to reduced elimination of drugs that are undergoing renal excretion. Reduced glomerular filtration occurs in infancy (West *et al.* 1948) and old age, as well as in hypovolaemic shock and intrinsic renal disease. As a result, all these groups of individuals are liable to develop Type A reactions to drugs that are mainly eliminated by the kidneys if given in 'usual' therapeutic doses. Of these, digoxin, aminoglycoside and glycopeptide antibiotics, angiotensin-converting-enzyme inhibitors, some Class 1 antiarrhythmic agents (flecainide, disopyramide), and many cytotoxic agents are the most important because they are the most toxic.

Renal drug clearances and glomerular filtration rates are linearly related (Dettli *et al.* 1971). It is therefore possible to calculate dosage requirements for individual patients on the basis of their renal function as assessed from serum creatinine concentrations or creatinine clearance. Such information is generally available in manufacturers' product literature and in national or regional formularies (e.g. *British National Formulary*). Drug toxicity due to accumulation in patients with renal impairment is thus an avoidable occurrence.

Active tubular secretion Some drugs are actively secreted by proximal tubular cells, against a concentration gradient, into the tubular fluid. Separate transport systems exist for acidic (penicillins, frusemide) and basic (amiloride, amphetamine) compounds. Competition between substances sharing the same transport system may reduce their renal clearance.

Competition between two drugs undergoing active tubular secretion is used to advantage when combining probenecid with penicillin. Less desirable, however, are the interactions between digoxin and both spironolactone and quinidine which impair the tubular secretion of this glycoside (Waldorff *et al.* 1978; Bussey 1982).

Competition may also occur between the tubular transport of drugs and endogenous materials such as urate. Hyperuricaemia and gout may be precipitated in patients receiving, for example, frusemide or thiazide diuretics, or low doses of aspirin or probenecid.

Tubular reabsorption Passive tubular reabsorption of drugs may be influenced by urine flow and by the pH of the tubular fluid.

Increases in urine flow rate will decrease the time available for drug in the tubular fluid to equilibrate with free drug in the plasma and interstitial fluid. Moreover, alterations in the solute content of the tubular fluid, which occur following the administration of most diuretics, may effectively reduce the concentration gradient across the tubular epithelium. Consequently, increased urine flow may result in significant increases in the renal clearance of some drugs, and limited use can be made of

this in the management of certain types of poisoning. Increased urinary flow rate, as a result of glomerulomegaly and increased kidney size, probably accounts for the enhanced renal elimination of some drugs in patients with cystic fibrosis (Prandota 1988).

The lipid-solubility (and therefore the ease with which drugs cross cell membranes) of drugs that are weak electrolytes is dependent upon the pH of the solution in which they are dissolved (Milne *et al.* 1958). The ionized fraction of a weak electrolyte is, for practical purposes, lipid-insoluble and so will not undergo passive tubular reabsorption. The non-ionized moiety, however, is lipid-soluble and therefore capable of passing across the tubular epithelium. Weak acids (e.g. salicylate) become ionized as pH *increases*, and tubular reabsorption tends to diminish as the tubular fluid becomes more alkaline. Salicylate clearances, which at urinary pH 5 are of the order of 10–20 ml per minute, increase to 150 ml per min at urinary pH 8. Similarly, the renal clearance of chlorpropamide increases from less than 0.1 ml per min (half-life 68.5±10.5 hours) at a urinary pH of 5, to 15 ml per minute (half-life 49.7±7.4 hours) at a urinary pH of 7 (Neuvonen and Karkkainen 1983). For weak bases (e.g. amphetamine) renal drug clearance increases with *decreasing* urinary pH. The effects of changes in urinary pH on the renal clearance of drugs are not only useful in treating some forms of acute toxicity but they may also account for substantial intraindividual and interindividual variations. Secretion of an alkaline urine may occur as a result of diet (e.g. in vegetarians), or because of other drugs (e.g. antacids, acetazolamide, thiazide diuretics), and an acidic urine is produced by a high-protein diet. In contrast, although drugs such as nortriptyline and propranolol (both weak bases) also undergo pH-dependent excretion, renal elimination plays such a small role in their overall disposal (less than 5 per cent) that changes in urinary pH can be confidently predicted to be of no clinical significance.

Biliary excretion

In experimental animals, biliary excretion of drugs and drug metabolites is a significant route of elimination for many foreign compounds (Smith 1973). The role of biliary drug excretion in man is less clear, but the existence of an enterohepatic circulation, which can be interrupted by repeated ingestion of activated charcoal, is strongly suggested for drugs such as phenobarbitone, carbamazepine, dapsone, and digitoxin (Neuvonen *et al.* 1980*a,b*; Pond *et al.* 1981). There may also be an important enterohepatic circulation for some drug conjugates, particularly glucuronides, with deconjugation (and subsequent reabsorption of the drug product) occurring as a result of the activity of flora in the large bowel. The implications of these processes remain largely unexplained but may be important in accounting for therapeutic failures in women receiving combined oral contraceptive agents who are treated with broad-spectrum antibiotics such as ampicillin, amoxycillin, or tetracyclines (Black *et al.* 1988). By an action on the gut flora, impaired deconjugation of ethinyloestradiol could result in a reduced enterohepatic circulation.

Drug metabolism

Renal excretion is an inefficient means of eliminating lipid-soluble drugs because these are extensively reabsorbed in the tubules. During the process of evolution, therefore, pathways have been developed to convert lipid-soluble compounds into lipid-insoluble agents which then undergo excretion by the kidneys. The metabolism of foreign compounds occurs predominantly in the liver, although other organs, including kidney, lung, skin, and gut, have some metabolising capacity. Drug metabolism has traditionally been regarded as a 'detoxification' pathway whereby many drug metabolites are rendered biologically inert. It is apparent, however, that many have pharmacological, therapeutic, or toxicological activity.

In man, drug metabolism can be conveniently divided into two phases (Williams 1967). Phase I (oxidation, reduction, or hydrolysis) exposes functionally reactive groups or adds them to the molecule. Phase II (glucuronidation, sulphation, methylation, acetylation) involves conjugation of the drug at the site of a reactive group produced during Phase I. A typical example of these phases is provided by the metabolism of phenacetin.

Drugs that already have reactive groups (e.g. morphine, paracetamol) undergo Phase II reactions only. Others are sufficiently water-soluble after Phase I to be eliminated by renal excretion. Each phase, however, tends to produce metabolites with increasing water solubility and decreasing lipid solubility.

Interindividual differences or alterations in the rate at which drugs are metabolised result in appropriate variations in elimination rates. As with renal excretion, reduced rates of metabolism will give rise to drug accumulation and increase the probability of Type A adverse reactions. Enhanced rates of metabolism may result in therapeutic failure. Some routes of metabolism are subject to wide interindividual differences, even among normal individuals, because of genetic and environmental influences. This particularly applies to oxidation, hydrolysis, and acetylation. Competition for glucuronidation may occur when two drugs metabolised by this pathway are given concurrently.

Microsomal oxidation   Drug oxidation occurs predominantly in the smooth endoplasmic reticulum of the hepatocytes via an electron transport chain whose terminal enzyme is a haem-containing protein, cytochrome P-450. Evidence now indicates the presence of multiple forms of cytochrome P-450 in the livers of various mammalian species, including man, that differ in the specificity of the reactions they catalyse (Nebert *et al.* 1989). Many common drugs are substrates for microsomal oxidation, including tricyclic antidepressants, oral anticoagulants, anticonvulsants, phenothiazines, benzodiazepines, antiarrhythmics, and some β_1-adrenoceptor antagonists. Drug oxidation rates are subject to enormously wide variation between normal individuals (Rawlins 1974*b*). As a result, individuals receiving 300 mg of phenytoin daily develop plasma phenytoin concentrations ranging from 4 mg per litre to 40 mg per litre (Loeser 1961). Type A adverse effects of phenytoin (ataxia, nystagmus) occur at plasma levels in excess of 20 mg per litre so that when patients are treated with conventional doses some will inevitably suffer adverse effects. Nortriptyline oxidation rates vary so widely that plasma levels vary from 10 μg per litre to 300μg per litre in patients receiving 75 mg daily (Sjöqvist *et al.* 1968), and Type A adverse effects occur at levels in excess of 140–160 μg per litre (Asberg *et al.* 1970).

Individual variations in rates of microsomal oxidation are due to genetic, biological, and environmental factors.

Some drugs show a genetic polymorphism for microsomal oxidation, of which the most notable is the

O.C$_2$H$_5$ → Phase I (oxidation) → OH → Phase II (glucuronidation) → O.C$_6$H$_9$O$_6$

NH.CO.CH$_3$ NH.CO.CH$_3$ NH.CO.CH$_3$

4-hydroxylation of debrisoquine (Mahgoub *et al.* 1977). Poor metabolisers are homozygous recessives for defective oxidation, and develop severe postural hypertension after small single doses. They constitute about 8–9 per cent of British (Evans *et al.* 1980), Canadian (Inaba *et al.* 1983), Ghanaian (Woolhouse *et al.* 1979), and Nigerian (Islam *et al.* 1980; Bertilsson *et al.* 1981) populations, but only 3 per cent of Swedes (Bertilsson *et al.* 1981), and 1 per cent of Saudi Arabians (Islam *et al.* 1980). Poor metabolisers of debrisoquine are poor metabolisers of other drugs including phenacetin, phenformin, metoprolol, timolol, nortriptyline, flecainide, and encainide. In general they appear to be particularly susceptible to Type A adverse reactions (Ayesh and Smith 1989). The abnormality is due to the defective expression of the so-called cytochrome P-450 IID6 isozyme (Nebert *et al.* 1989). Separate polymorphisms, unrelated to that of debrisoquine hydroxylation, have been described for other drugs including tolbutamide (Scott and Poffenbarger 1979) and methoin (mephenytoin) (Kupfer *et al.* 1979; Wilkinson *et al.* 1989). Defective stereospecific methoin hydroxylation is inherited as a recessive trait (Kupfer *et al.* 1984) and is due to the failure of expression of the cytochrome P-450 IIC9 isozyme (Nebert *et al.* 1989). The polymorphic control of tolbutamide hydroxylation requires confirmation.

While a genetic polymorphism may account for much of the individual variability in rates of microsomal oxidation of some drugs, for many others elimination rates are continuously distributed in the population. This could result either from involvement of several cytochrome P-450 isozymes, with overlapping specificities, in particular oxidation reactions; or it may be the combined effect of genetic and environment influences on rates of microsomal oxidation. In general, while twin studies have suggested high degrees of heritability, careful family studies have shown substantial, if not overwhelming, environmental control (Whittaker and Evans 1970; Blain *et al.* 1982).

Rates of microsomal oxidation may be altered in the young and old. In general, half-lives of oxidized drugs are longer in the newborn than in adults (Rane 1980), while older children have similar rates of oxidation. Indeed, maximum rates of phenytoin metabolism appear to be *greater* in children than in adults, when expressed in relation to body-weight, and this seems to be due to the relatively greater contribution of liver to total body-weight in this age group (Blain *et al.* 1981).

In the elderly, rates of microsomal oxidation of many drugs appear to decline with important consequences for increasing susceptibility to Type A adverse reactions (Woodhouse and Wynne 1988) with advancing years.

Careful studies have failed to demonstrate an age-related decline in the activities, or affinities, of drug metabolising enzymes in man (Woodhouse *et al.* 1984, 1988). There is, however, a marked reduction in liver mass and liver blood flow with increasing age, which appears to account for the reduced hepatic metabolism of drugs in the fit elderly (Woodhouse and Wynne 1988). Changes in enzyme activities may be of greater importance in the presence of disease or frailty.

Environmental factors known to influence rates of microsomal oxidation of at least some drugs include dietary constituents, environmental pollutants, and ethanol and other drugs. The relative contributions of dietary protein and carbohydrates (Kappas *et al.* 1976), anciferous vegetables (Pantuck *et al.* 1979), as well as the method of cooking (Kappas *et al.* 1978), influence the rates of oxidation of drugs such as theophylline, antipyrine, and phenacetin. These findings may explain some of the observed ethnic differences in rates of antipyrine metabolism (Fraser *et al.* 1979; Mucklow *et al.* 1982).

TABLE 3.1

Drugs and other substances known to induce hepatic microsomal drug oxidation in man

Group	Substance
Analgesics	Antipyrine
	Phenylbutazone
	Sulphinpyrazone
Antibiotics	Doxycycline
	Griseofulvin
	Rifampicin
Anticonvulsants	Carbamazepine
	Phenobarbitone
	Phenytoin
Diuretics	Spironolactone
Hypnotics	Barbiturates
	Dichloralphenazone
	Glutethimide
Insecticides	Dicophane
	Eldrin
	γ-Benzene hexachloride

A variety of drugs, environmental pollutants (Table 3.1), as well as cigarette smoking, can induce microsomal oxidation, giving rise to accelerated rates of elimination. The mechanism by which this occurs is not entirely clear, but it is associated with proliferation of the hepatic endoplasmic reticulum, and increased amounts of drug-oxidizing enzymes in the liver. When inducing agents are given to patients receiving oxidized drugs, decreased plasma levels and loss of therapeutic control may develop. This is typified by warfarin, the anticoagulant effect of which may be lost if a patient is given a hypnotic (Breckenridge *et al.* 1971). Stopping therapy with an enzyme-inducing agent may result in enhanced drug effects. This is frequently seen when patients, well controlled on warfarin in hospital, are discharged home and stop their ubiquitous nightly barbiturate sedation (Smith and Rawlins 1973). The inducing effects of the hypnotic wear off, so the elimination of warfarin becomes slower and plasma levels rise.

TABLE 3.2
Some drugs for which oxidation may be inhibited in man

Drug	Inhibited by
Cyclosporin	Ketoconazole
Diazepam	Cimetidine
Nortriptyline	Phenothiazines
Phenobarbitone	Valproate
Phenytoin	Cimetidine
	Dicoumarol
	Disulfiram
	Isoniazid
	Sulthiame
Propranolol	Cimetidine
Theophylline	Ciprofloxacin
	Erythromycin
Tolbutamide	Chloramphenicol
	Phenylbutazone
	Sulphaphenazole
Warfarin	Cimetidine
	Co-trimoxazole
	D-propoxyphene

Drug-induced *inhibition* of microsomal oxidation is theoretically a more dangerous interaction than induction and cimetidine is particularly potent (Somogyi and Muirhead 1987). Some of those known to do this are shown in Table 3.2. Their administration will clearly lead to accumulation of oxidized drugs and thus increase the likelihood of the patient developing Type A effects. The acute ingestion of alcohol, at doses consumed during 'social drinking', may also inhibit the oxidation of drugs such as warfarin, acetanilide (McKay *et al.* 1982), and amitriptyline (Dorian *et al.* 1983). Substrate competition for the active site of cytochrome P-450 is the likely mechanism for many inhibition reactions, but there are also other possible mechanisms (Murray and Reidy

1989). Moreover, while it is reasonable to predict that if a drug induces the metabolism of one oxidized drug it will induce the metabolism of others, such extrapolations are unwarranted in the case of enzyme inhibition (Rawlins and Smith 1973).

Mitochondrial oxidation   Alcohol and a variety of monoamines (noradrenaline, tyramine, phenylethylamine) undergo mitochondrial oxidation. Inhibition of monoamine oxidase (MAO) by inhibitors such as phenelzine, iproniazid, and tranylcypromine gives rise to serious Type A effects of agents that normally undergo first-pass metabolism by MAO in the liver (e.g. tyramine). Patients taking MAO inhibitors are therefore liable to develop hypertensive reactions if they take vasoactive amines such as tyramine or phenylpropanolamine. It is well known, however, that some patients can continue to eat tyramine (as cheese) with no adverse consequences. The reason for this is probably twofold: first, the tyramine content of a cheese declines towards its centre (Price and Smith 1971); secondly, some individuals may have an alternative pathway for tyramine metabolism (involving sulphate conjugation) which allows them to ingest tyramine with impunity in the presence of virtually complete MAO inhibition (Sandler 1973).

Patients taking MAO inhibitors are liable to develop severe adverse reactions to pethidine. These effects consist principally of hypotension and hyperpyrexia, and are reactions that are totally unlike the normal pharmacological effects of pethidine even in overdosage. They are therefore Type B reactions mediated via the central nervous system (Rogers and Thornton 1969).

Hydrolysis   The neuromuscular-blocking effects of suxamethonium are terminated by hydrolysis of the drug in plasma. Abnormalities of plasma pseudocholinesterase may result in impaired drug elimination and prolonged neuromuscular blockade. Plasma pseudocholinesterase is determined by genes of large effect (Smith and Rawlins 1973). Aberrant genes are occasionally encountered, and individuals homozygous for the atypical gene (E_1, E_1) are encountered in 1 in 2500 of the population (Harris 1964). Such individuals may develop prolonged neuromuscular blockade. Heterozygotes (E_0, E_1) who possess both the usual and atypical gene comprise 4 per cent of the population; they have normal sensitivities to suxamethonium *in vivo* but can be detected by *in vitro* tests. Phenotypic studies of patients with prolonged neuromuscular blockade after suxamethonium do not always reveal recognizable genetic abnormalities. In some instances these Type A reactions are secondary to liver or renal disease, both of which are associated with impaired plasma pseudocholinesterase activity. Further cases still remain, however, after all these causes have been eliminated (Simpson and Kalow 1966) and may account for 40 per cent of patients with suxamethonium apnoea.

Acetylation   Acetylation is the metabolic pathway by which a number of drugs, including many sulphonamides, dapsone, isoniazid, hydralazine, phenelzine, procainamide, and suphasalazine, are inactivated. Acetylation is under genetic control and shows a polymorphism: rapid acetylation is autosomally dominant. In the UK about half the population are rapid acetylators, but there are considerable racial differences. The incidence of rapid acetylation is highest amongst the Japanese and Eskimos (80–90 per cent) and lowest in an African tribe (!Kung) where only one rapid acetylator was found in 30 members examined.

Slow acetylators eliminate acetylated drugs much less rapidly than other people. Consequently, they are at greater risk from developing Type A adverse reactions. Thus, hydralazine-related systemic lupus erythematosus (Perry *et al.* 1967), isoniazid peripheral neuropathy (Devadatta *et al.* 1960), haematological adverse effects of dapsone (Ellard *et al.* 1974), and adverse effects of sulphasalazine (Schroder and Evans 1972) and procainamide (Woosley *et al.* 1978) occur more frequently in slow acetylators.

Glucuronidation   A number of drugs commonly used in clinical practice (e.g. morphine, paracetamol, salicylate, and salicylamide) are eliminated at least partially as glucuronide conjugates. Not only are these conjugates lipid-insoluble, but they are also weak acids and undergo active transport into the renal tubules. The glucuronidation of both salicylate and paracetamol (Levy 1971) can be inhibited by the concurrent administration of salicylamide at conventional dose levels, and this is perhaps the real rationale for adding salicylamide to paracetamol and salicylate preparations.

Effects of disease

Because of the central role of the liver in the drug metabolism, liver disease might be expected to impair drug detoxication and lead to Type A adverse effects. Indeed, there is an increased incidence of adverse reactions to conventional therapeutic doses of many drugs undergoing hepatic metabolism (Naranjo *et al.* 1978), which is at least partly due to altered rates of elimination. Acute liver damage produces impairment in a variety of pathways of drug metabolism, which broadly parallels the change in prothrombin time. Thus, after acute liver damage from paracetamol poisoning there is a decreased rate of paracetamol metabolism (which provides a prog-

nostic guide to the severity of the poisoning), but also slow metabolism of barbiturates, phenytoin, and antipyrine (Prescott *et al.* 1971; Prescott 1972). In chronic liver disease there is not only reduced *in vitro* activity of many of the enzymes concerned with drug metabolism (Brodie *et al.* 1981; Woodhouse *et al.* 1983) but also shunting of blood, which further reduces hepatic drug clearance. As a consequence, both first-pass hepatic metabolism, and systemic drug clearance (Blaschke 1977) are reduced to an extent which is correlated with the degree of hypoalbuminaemia. The changes do not, however, affect all metabolic pathways in parallel. Moreover, such is the regenerative power of the liver that induction by barbiturates may restore phenylbutazone metabolism to normal in the face of quite severe hepatic disease (Levi *et al.* 1968). This may explain the normal half-lives of phenylbutazone, salicylate, dicoumarol, and pentobarbitone that some workers (Sessions *et al.* 1954; Brodie *et al.* 1959) have observed in chronic liver disease.

Renal disease is associated with alterations in the hepatic clearance of some drugs, although the mechanisms involved are poorly understood and the extent of the problem is ill-defined. Thus, phenytoin oxidation is diminished in renal failure, and the conjugation of both metoclopramide (Bateman *et al.* 1981) and benoxaprofen (Aronoff *et al.* 1982) is reduced in patients with impaired renal function. The impairment of metoclopramide elimination in renal disease is probably causally related to the apparent increased risk of adverse reactions to the drug in this group of patients. Similar considerations may apply to benoxaprofen.

In patients with malnutrition, impairment of a variety of pathways of drug metabolism has been described, particularly in children (Buchanan *et al.* 1980; Eriksson *et al.* 1983).

Toxicity of drug metabolites   Although many products of drug metabolism are biologically inert, it is becoming increasingly apparent that many drug metabolites possess important pharmacological and toxicological properties (Garrittini 1985). Thus, the desmethyl metabolites of amitriptyline and imipramine contribute to the actions of their parent compounds. Similarly, carbamazepine epoxide and acetylprocainamide have pharmacological properties that contribute significantly to the overall effects of carbamazepine and procainamide respectively. Some drug metabolites, however, have purely toxic, and no therapeutic, actions. Thus, the urothelial toxicity of cyclophosphamide is mediated by its non-cytotoxic metabolite acrolein, while the anticoagulant action of certain cephalosporins (Lipsky 1983) may be mediated by a bacteriologically inactive metabolite (N-methyl-thio-tetrazole).

The accumulation, in patients with renal disease, of biologically active drug metabolites normally excreted by the kidney may predispose to severe Type A adverse reactions (Verbeeck *et al.* 1981). Examples include acebutolol (due to its acetyl metabolite), allopurinol (oxypurinol), pethidine (norpethidine), nitroprusside (thiocyanate), and propoxyphene (norpropoxyphene).

A further form of metabolite toxicity, and one which is probably of greatest importance, is mediated by production of highly reactive intermediates. During the course of certain forms of drug metabolism, particularly microsomal oxidation, highly reactive metabolites (peroxides, epoxides, and free radicals) are formed. Various cellular mechanisms for their inactivation are also present including epoxide hydrolase, superoxide dismutase, and glutathione transferases. Where the rate of formation of reactive metabolites, however, is enhanced (e.g. by increasing the dose, or when the activity of 'activating' enzymes is increased), or the rate of their removal is diminished (e.g. by cellular depletion of glutathione), then severe cellular damage may ensue.

Covalent binding of reactive intermediates to DNA may result in carcinogenicity (Jollow *et al.* 1977; Gelboin 1977). Thus, the oncogenic effects of aflatoxin and benz(α)pyrene are mediated by the formation of epoxides (by microsomal mono-oxygenases) that bind to DNA. The formation of reactive metabolites of organic solvents such as bromobenzenes and carbon tetrachloride is the mechanism by which this class of agent produces its hepatotoxic effect. The hepatotoxicity of such agents correlates with their capacity to bind covalently (Zampaglione *et al.* 1973) to cellular macromolecules (mainly protein): whether the binding to 'critical' macromolecules *per se* is responsible for cytotoxicity, or whether binding merely reflects other intracellular toxic events, is unclear.

The hepatotoxicity of paracetamol, after overdosage, is also mediated by the formation of a reactive intermediate (Hinson 1980). After therapeutic doses, paracetamol is metabolised primarily by conjugation with glucuronide and sulphate: only a small fraction of the dose is metabolised to a reactive product, and this is inactivated by conjugation with glutathione and excreted in urine as the mercapturate. Following overdosage, however, the sulphate and glucuronide pathways are saturated, and more of the drug (Mitchell *et al.* 1973*a,b*) is metabolised to the reactive, toxic intermediate. In the absence of sufficient glutathione to conjugate this intermediate, the latter produces cell damage and death — possibly by covalent binding to 'critical' macromolecules. The use of precursors of intrahepatic glutathione (cysteamine, methionine, and N-acetylcysteine) to replete intracellular stores (Prescott *et al.* 1974, 1977) is undoubtedly effective in preventing severe liver damage, provided it is given sufficiently early after poisoning.

The hepatotoxicity of other drugs is also probably mediated by the formation of reactive intermediates. Such drugs include halothane, phenytoin, isoniazid, methyldopa, and frusemide. In the case of phenytoin, the persistence of reactive toxic intermediates may be due to a genetically determined impaired ability to inactivate them further (Spielberg *et al.* 1981). The local formation of toxic intermediates may also account for pulmonary toxicity, such as that of nitrofurantoin (Boyd 1980) and the pancreatic toxicity of frusemide.

Pharmacodynamic causes

Many, if not most, Type A adverse drug reactions have a pharmacokinetic basis. Some, however, are undoubtedly due to enhanced sensitivity of target organs or tissues. Moreover, in some individuals, adverse drug reactions derive from a combination of these two.

The reasons why tissues from different individuals should respond differently to drugs are still largely unknown; but evidence is accumulating to show that target organ sensitivity is influenced by the drug receptors themselves, by physiological homoeostatic mechanisms, and by disease.

Drug receptors

Many drugs exert their pharmacological effects by combining with specific receptors (Paton 1970). These receptors may be on cell membranes, or within the cytoplasm or nucleus. Their normal function is to provide the means whereby endogenous extracellular substances may influence intracellular events. There are therefore specific receptors for neurotransmitters (e.g. noradrenaline, dopamine, and acetylcholine), hormones (e.g. glucocorticoids, corticotrophin [ACTH], and sex hormones), vitamins (e.g. vitamins D and K), and lipids (e.g. low-density lipoproteins). Specific receptors appear to be protein molecules and some, though not all, are enzymes. There are two ways in which the target organs of different individuals might respond differently to drugs acting through specific receptors. First, receptors might differ between individuals, some being less 'potent' than others. Secondly, different individuals might have different numbers of receptors in their tissues.

There is little direct evidence to support the first hypothesis. Hereditary warfarin resistance (O'Reilly *et al.* 1964, 1970), however, may be an example. This disorder, which has now been observed in two families, is manifested by extreme warfarin resistance so that huge doses and very high plasma levels are required to achieve therapeutic anticoagulation. Conversely, these individuals are extremely sensitive to the warfarin-antagonizing actions of vitamin K. Although these observations are compatible with the hypothesis that affected individuals possess abnormal warfarin–vitamin K receptors, there are other explanations (such as differences in clotting factor synthesis) that have yet to be excluded.

Indirect estimates have been made of the affinity constants (or pA_2 values) of the β-adrenoceptor antagonists propranolol (McDevitt *et al.* 1976) and labetalol (Sanders *et al.* 1979) in man. Both studies suggested that there may be differences between individuals, and in hypertension, but further work is required to confirm the heterogenicity in man. Reduced sensitivity of cardiac β-receptors to both agonists (isoprenaline) and antagonists (propranolol) has been observed in the elderly.

There is now both experimental and clinical evidence to indicate that the number of specific receptors in tissues may vary. Glucocorticoids exert their inhibitory effects on cell growth by combining with specific cytoplasmic protein receptors (Hackney *et al.* 1970). The steroid–receptor complex is then transported into the nucleus where the glucocorticoid combines with a second receptor. Nuclear steroid–receptor complexes modify the control of RNA and protein synthesis, leading to inhibition of cell growth. Cells with diminished amounts of cytoplasmic glucocorticoid receptors are resistant *in vitro* and *in vivo* to the inhibitory effects of steroids. In man, the presence of oestrogen and progestogen receptors in breast tumours appears to determine the *in vivo* response to endocrine therapy (McGuire *et al.* 1977).

Where the receptors for a particular drug are enzymes, qualitative differences may be important mechanisms of altering drug sensitivity. In bacteria, resistance to sulphonamides may be due to the presence of an enzyme with altered affinity for the drug, as shown by Pato and Brown (1963). These workers also showed, however, that certain resistant strains had normal enzymes, and suggested that resistance was due to failure of the drug to enter the cell.

Receptor sensitivity may also be affected by other drugs. The action of specific antagonists and agonists is well known. There is a suggestion, however, that some interactions involve a more subtle mechanism. Although norethandrolone, clofibrate, and thyroxine have no anticoagulant actions by themselves, they all potentiate the anticoagulant effects of warfarin by a mechanism that does not appear to be pharmacokinetic (Schrogie and

Solomon 1967). It has been suggested that these drugs all increase the affinity of anticoagulant for its hepatic receptor site (Solomon and Schrogie 1967).

Homoeostatic mechanisms

The actions of most drugs occur within the milieu of complex physiological control systems. The magnitude of a drug's effects may be dependent on such physiological factors. For example, intravenous atropine (an acetylcholine antagonist) produces a variable increase in heart rate and some individuals develop tachycardia of 160 beats per minute at a dose which is almost ineffective in others. The magnitude of the observed effect is dependent on the balance between parasympathetic and sympathetic cardiac tone which appears to be under genetic control (Bertler and Smith 1971).

Disease

Intercurrent disease may unmask pharmacological effects that are not apparent in normal individuals. Haemorrhage or perforation of peptic ulcers due to the anti-inflammatory actions of corticosteroids are a typical example. The bronchoconstriction which patients with obstructive airways disease develop when given unselective β-blockers (e.g. propranolol) is another. More subtle is the neuromuscular blockade that may be precipitated by streptomycin, neomycin, or kanamycin. These drugs have curare-like actions and reduce the sensitivity of motor end-plates to the depolarizing effects of acetylcholine. Their effects, however, are relatively feeble, and clinically inapparent in normal individuals.In patients already receiving muscle relaxants, or with myasthenia gravis, their pharmacological properties are unmasked and may produce paralysis (Toivakka and Hokkanen 1965).

Mechanisms of Type B adverse drug reactions

The distinguishing feature of Type B reactions is that they are aberrant, that is, inexplicable in terms of the normal pharmacology of the drug, and that they form a heterogeneous group. Pathogenetically they are characterized by the existence of some qualitative difference either in the drug, or in the patient, or possibly in both. The cause may be pharmacokinetic or pharmaceutical, or may lie in target organ response.

Pharmaceutical causes

There are three potential sources of Type B adverse reactions due to abnormalities of the drug: firstly, decomposition of the active constituents; secondly, effects of the additives, solubilizers, stabilizers, colourizers, and excipients, commonly incorporated in pharmaceutical preparations; and thirdly, effects from byproducts of the active constituents of chemical synthesis. Some drugs are chemically stable (e.g. lignocaine), while others are very unstable (e.g. adrenaline). Administration of a decomposed drug is most likely to result in therapeutic failure, particularly if the products are devoid of pharmacological properties. In certain rare instances, however, the decomposition products may be toxic and potentially lethal. Thus, paraldehyde decomposes to acetaldehyde, which is subsequently oxidized to acetic acid. A number of deaths due to this cause have been reported since paraldehyde was first introduced in 1889, and Sir Robert Hutchison (1930) gave a still unheeded warning of the dangers of decomposed paraldehyde. Paraldehyde that has been in stock for over 6 months should therefore be discarded, and all paraldehyde should be tested before use with litmus paper. Earlier formulations of tetracycline, when stored under warm conditions, change to a brown sticky mass. Degraded formulations of this kind produce a Fanconi-like syndrome (Ehrlich and Stein 1963; Gross 1963; Frimpter 1963) with aminoaciduria, glycosuria, acetonuria, albuminuria, pyuria, elevated plasma α-amino nitrogen, and photosensitivity (Sulkowski and Haserick 1964). Analysis of decomposed capsules showed them to contain 3.5% anhydrotetracycline and 0.5% epiandrotetracycline (Sulkowski and Haserick 1964). Moreover, citric acid, which has been used as a buffering agent for tetracycline preparations, has been shown to increase the degradation process and has therefore been removed; but even in the absence of citric acid, degradation of tetracycline occurs when it is stored at 37°C and 66 per cent relative humidity for 2 months (Walton et al. 1970).

Additives present in some pharmaceutical preparations are not entirely inert (Smith and Dodd 1982). Propylene glycol, which is used as a solvent for a variety of injected drugs, may be partially responsible for the hypotension observed following intravenous phenytoin (Solomon, personal communication). Many additives (including polypropylene glycol and carboxymethylcellulose) and agents combined with topical formulations may cause hypersensitivity reactions in man (Schneider et al. 1971; Wilkinson 1972). Certain drugs of low solubility are prepared for intravenous use by formulation with powerful non-ionic surfactants. These agents, for example Cremophor EL, are produced by the reaction of castor oil with ethylene oxide (epoxylation). The intravenous anaesthetic drugs Althesin (alphax-

alone and alphadolone) and propanidid (Epontol) have both been reported to cause anaphylactic reactions (Watkins et al. 1978; Watkins 1979; Dye and Watkins 1980). Similar reactions may be provoked by diazepam dissolved in Cremophor EL and given intravenously (Padfield and Watkins 1977). Furthermore, experiments in animals (miniature pig) have shown that Cremophor EL alone can cause anaphylactic reactions (Glen et al. 1979). The reactions to Althesin seem to be mediated predominantly by complement C3 activation but some appear to be mediated by an immune mechanism involving IgD or IgE (Watkins et al. 1978). An additional important point is that if Cremophor EL is given to patients over several days it can produce hyperlipidaemia and abnormal electrophoretic patterns of lipoprotein (Bagnarello et al. 1977) and also haematological changes (Niell 1977; Sung and Grendahl 1977; Sheth et al. 1977).

The eosinophilia–myalgia syndrome and L-tryptophan

During 1989, the possible relationship between a new clinical syndrome of eosinophilia with myalgia and the consumption of preparations containing L-tryptophan led the Food and Drug Administration to advise that sale of these preparations be stopped. The condition is characterized by intensive eosinophilia (>2000–$30\,000$ cells per mm^3) and myalgia (Flannery et al. 1990; Travis et al. 1990; Diggle 1990) with which may be associated arthralgia, swelling of the extremities, rash, fever, cough, interstitial lung disease, arrhythmias, ascending polyneuropathy, and sclerodermiform thickening of the skin (Diggle 1990; Kilbourne et al. 1990; Van Garsse and Boeykens 1990). Since all the initial reports came from the USA, it seemed likely that the syndrome was due to contaminants in the American preparations (Acheson 1989), but subsequently two Belgian patients receiving tryptophan from a source outside USA have developed the syndrome (Van Garsse and Boeykens 1990). The latter happening does not exclude the possibility that the syndrome is due to a similar, or the same, contaminant that may have caused problems in the American patients. Certainly it seems unlikely that L-tryptophan, a naturally occurring essential aminoacid, has suddenly become endowed with toxic properties. This latter conclusion is supported by the results of a recent investigation which showed that the syndrome may be related to the use of preparations containing a contaminant identified as a close chemical relative to L-tryptophan (Belongia et al. 1990). To date, over 1400 cases, including 19 deaths, have been reported to the Centres for Disease Control since it was first reported in New Mexico in 1989; and 60 cases have been seen in West Germany and an unknown number in France and Switzerland (*The Lancet* 1990). Five cases related to the use of health supplements have been reported in the UK (Diggle 1990). It is clearly a matter of urgency to find the cause of this potentially lethal condition. In the meantime, the diagnostic value of the eosinophil count is paramount.

Nebulizer solutions and paradoxical bronchoconstriction

A curious and as yet unexplained adverse reaction is paradoxical bronchoconstriction associated with the use of nebulized bronchodilator solutions. Between 1986 and 1987 the Committee on Safety of Medicines received 17 reports of paradoxical bronchoconstriction (CSM 1988) including two deaths (of a 2½-year-old boy and a 42-year-old woman). Bronchoconstriction usually occurred within 18 minutes of administration of the nebulizer. It seems likely that these reactions are due to the formulation of the nebulizer solutions, particularly since hypotonicity or hypertonicity, the presence of preservatives (e.g. benzalkonium, edetic acid, sulphites, and metabisulphite) can all cause bronchoconstriction. The possible role of any of these factors in the 17 reports remains unknown.

Pharmacokinetic causes

Theoretically, abnormalities of absorption, distribution, or elimination might give rise to Type B adverse effects. Both absorption and distribution, however, are predominantly passive processes (see above), and although changes in their kinetics may lead to Type A effects there are no documented Type B reactions that can be attributed to them.

As discussed in the preceding section, abnormalities of elimination generally reflect quantitative differences from the norm, and thus predispose to the development of Type A effects. Abnormalities of elimination giving rise to Type B effects might be expected to be due to the metabolism of a drug yielding an unusual or novel metabolite. One possible example concerns a family described by Shahidi (1967, 1968), some members of which developed severe methaemoglobinaemia following small doses of phenacetin; affected individuals were shown to have defective de-ethylation of the drug.

Pharmacodynamic causes

Qualitative abnormalities in the target organ occur for a number of reasons. Such factors as body-weight, age, sex, and route and time of administration all influence the final response of a patient to the dose of a particular drug. In general, changes in one or more of these are likely to produce quantitative and not qualitative differences in the response to drugs. In contrast, the presence of mental or physical illness (or both) may result in qualitative differences as well as a quantitative difference. For example, whereas an antidepressant drug will relieve depression in a patient suffering from this illness, the same drug will have no comparable effect in a mentally normal subject.

Qualitative differences in the response to drugs may be considered as genetic, immunological, or neoplastic and teratogenic.

Genetic causes for abnormal response

In the context of adverse drug reactions the term 'idiosyncrasy' has been used extensively as a label for those bizarre responses that were assumed to be due to some qualitative abnormality in the patient. Until recently, drug 'idiosyncrasies' have tended to form a dustbin for those adverse drug reactions that could not be classified under any other heading. This situation is now changing slowly as their mechanisms become clear, and it has become apparent that the majority have a genetic basis.

Erythrocyte glucose 6-phosphate dehydrogenase (G6PD) deficiency

Various enzyme deficiencies may affect tissue responses to drugs, and the best known of these is G6PD deficiency, which is a sex-linked, inherited defect of intermediate dominance, particularly common in American Negroes (10 per cent) but also occurring among coloured people of Africa, some Mediterranean races, Kurdish and Iraqi Jews, and some Filipinos. It is estimated that approximately 100 million individuals in the world are affected by this disorder (Weatherall and Hatton 1987). G6PD is normally responsible for maintaining cellular glutathione in the reduced form, and reduced glutathione prevents cellular damage by oxidizing agents. A deficiency of G6PD results in a corresponding deficiency of reduced glutathione, and under these vulnerable conditions oxidizing agents may denature intracellular proteins, including the globin part of the haemoglobin molecule (Frischer and Ahmad 1987; Fletcher *et al.* 1988). This ultimately leads to haemolysis, accompanied by a rapid fall in haemoglobin concentration, fever, prostration, and the formation of dark urine. Reticulocytosis occurs and Heinz bodies appear in erythrocytes. A large number of commonly used drugs with oxidant properties will cause haemolysis if there is a deficiency of G6PD, and these include 8-aminoquinolines (e.g. primaquine haemolysis), sulphonamides and sulphones, nitrofurans, analgesics (including aspirin and phenacetin), chloramphenicol, sodium aminosalicylate (PAS), probenecid, quinine, and quinidine (see Marks and Banks 1965; WHO 1967, 1973; Chan *et al.* 1976; Beutler 1984). Interestingly, slow acetylators of sulphamethazine are particularly susceptible to haemolysis while taking this sulphonamide (Woolhouse and Atu-Taylor 1982).

The prevention and treatment of haemolysis due to G6PD deficiency depends upon a knowledge of the genetic basis of this abnormality. There are two types of G6PD, known as A (abnormal) and B (normal). Since the gene for G6PD is located on the long arm of the X chromosome, G6PD deficiency is an X-linked trait, so that males and homozygous females with the deficiency have a single enzyme-deficient erythrocyte population. Heterozygous females possess two erythrocyte populations, one normal and one G6PD-deficient, with the ratio of the two populations varying from 1 to 99 per cent. Since only the G6PD-deficient cells are drug-sensitive (and in the typical heterozygous female only about half of the cells are affected), only about one-third of all heterozygous females possess a sufficiently high proportion of G6PD-deficient cells to predispose them to clinically significant haemolysis (WHO 1973).

Apart from sexual differences in the enzyme, there are striking racial differences, so that whereas the African type (A⁻) is characterized by a mild enzyme deficiency with a mean activity 8.8–20 per cent of normal, the Mediterranean type is characterized by severe deficiency leading to 0–4 per cent enzyme activity. Consequently, a potentially haemolytic drug is likely to be much less troublesome in patients with the African than with the Mediterranean type. Much work needs to be done to characterize other racial forms of G6PD deficiency but, as has been pointed out by the WHO Scientific Group on Pharmacogenetics (WHO 1973), the decision to use or to stop treatment with a potentially haemolytic drug must depend upon (a) the type of G6PD deficiency, (b) the sex of the patient, (c) the severity of the disease, (d) the need for the drug, and (e) the availability of alternative agents. Moreover, the degree of haemolysis induced by a particular drug can be accentuated by the presence of additional infection or disease. The detection of G6PD deficiency can be achieved by several different screening methods. The simplest method is to incubate red cells with glucose 6-phosphate, magnesium, and NADP, and then determine NADPH production spectroscopically.

A study in Chinese subjects has shown that, in the absence of oxidant drugs, those with the common G6PD variants (Canton, B(–) Chinese, Hong Kong-Pokfulam) have a compensated haemolytic state, so that in this population chronic haemolytic anaemia due to G6PD deficiency is exceedingly rare (Chan *et al.* 1976). In spite of this, haemolytic episodes can be provoked by drugs or illness in those with G6PD deficiency. Studies with co-trimoxazole have shown that those Chinese with the same variant of G6PD may nevertheless react differently because of variation in the metabolism of the drug, possibly as the result of coexisting disease that alters hepatic or renal function or some other undefined biochemical or metabolic characteristic (Chan *et al.* 1976). The list of agents that can provoke this Type B adverse drug reaction due to G6PD deficiency has grown, but reports based only on clinical observation must be accepted with reserve until specific tests such as the ^{51}Cr half-life G6PD erythrocytes (Chan *et al.* 1976) have been employed to define accurately the haemolytic effects of any drugs that come under suspicion.

Hereditary methaemoglobinaemia

This condition may occur in the presence of mutations affecting the haemoglobin molecule or the enzyme methaemoglobin reductase. Individuals with severe deficiency of methaemoglobin reductase deficiency (homozygotes) are more likely than normal persons to develop methaemoglobinaemia and cyanosis when they are given drugs that are oxidizing agents, which therefore cause an increase in methaemoglobinaemia. Thus, nitrites (or any of the drugs listed above as causing haemolysis in the presence of G6PD deficiency) may cause this effect (Cowan and Evans, 1964; Cohen *et al.* 1968). Heterozygotes possess about 50 per cent of the normal enzyme activity and are rarely susceptible to these adverse effects. They have a frequency in the population of 1 per cent. The importance of methaemoglobin reductase is well shown during infancy by the inverse relationship between age-dependent erythrocyte activity of the enzyme and prilocaine-induced methaemoglobinaemia (Nilsson *et al.* 1990).

Drug-sensitive haemoglobins

Certain mutations may affect the stability of the haemoglobin molecule. Thus, patients with Hb Zurich and Hb Torino may develop haemolysis in the presence of certain oxidising drugs. In those patients who are affected, the red cells can be shown to contain denatured haemoglobin present in the form of small inclusion bodies (Heinz bodies). Two small pedigrees have been described with haemoglobin Zurich in which arginine was found to be substituted for histidine at 63rd position of the β-chain of haemoglobin and approximately 150 cases of haemoglobin M in which the haemoglobin is composed of 4 β-chains (Vessell 1972).

Porphyria

Conditions due to inborn errors that occur at different

enzymic sites in the haem biosynthetic pathway cause rare metabolic disorders classified into acute and cutaneous porphyrias (Goldberg and Moore 1980). All the conditions are transmitted as autosomal dominants, with the exception of the rare congenital porphyria, which is recessive (Moore and Brodie 1985). The florid clinical condition of acute porphyria can be precipitated by drugs — ethanol and endogenous and exogenous steroid hormones. In contrast, cutaneous hepatic porphyria is most commonly precipitated by ethanol, although oestrogenic steroids have also been implicated. An acquired type may be caused by such organic chemicals such as hexachlorobenzene (Cain and Nigogosyan 1963; Kimbrough 1987). In the acute porphyrias, all patients show similar abdominal and neuropsychiatric disturbances. During an acute attack they excrete in their urine large amounts of the porphyria precursors 5-aminolaevulinic acid (ALA) and porphobilinogen (PBG). Earlier experiments failed to demonstrate pharmacological, electroencephalographic, cardiovascular, or behavioural effects of porphyrins (Goldberg et al. 1954, 1987) although more recent work has revealed that certain porphyrins can damage membrane proteins and enzymes (Dubbleman et al. 1980; Avner et al. 1983), which might explain some of the clinical effects. A number of commonly used drugs induce ALA synthase production in the liver, and these agents are usually potent enzyme inducers. Thus, barbiturates; sulphonamides; griseofulvin; oestrogens (including those in oral contraceptives); some anticonvulsants and tranquillizers; possibly, general anaesthetics; ethanol; chloroquine; chlorpropamide; and tolbutamide may all precipitate porphyria in susceptible patients (Matteis 1967; Moore and Brodie 1985). Nevertheless, it has become apparent that the sensitivities of patients who are liable to develop acute intermittent porphyria in response to drugs vary widely, with the result that whereas a single dose of a particular drug may trigger off an acute attack in one patient, another may require a number of relatively large doses of the same drug to produce any clinically significant effect.

It requires special studies to determine which drugs are potentially harmful in the different forms of hepatic porphyria and to obtain an estimate of the relative frequencies of the different reactions. In South Africa, Eales (1971) made a study from which he concluded that patients suffering from porphyria variegata should avoid the following drugs: barbiturates, non-barbiturate hypnotics (e.g. glutethimide, meprobamate), pyrazolone compounds (e.g. phenazone), anticonvulsants (e.g. phenytoin), sulphonamides, griseofulvin, synthetic oestrogens and progestogens, and ergot preparations. Other lists of dangerous and 'safe' drugs are also available (*Drug and Therapeutics Bulletin* 1976; Moore and Brodie 1985; and see Chapter 15).

Bleeding disorders

Patients with haemophilia or von Willebrand's disease are particularly sensitive to drugs that influence (albeit weakly) clotting and coagulation mechanisms. In particular, salicylates will prolong the bleeding time of haemophiliacs for several days after a single dose, and this outlasts the presence of detectable levels of aspirin (Weiss et al. 1968).

Malignant hyperthermia

Malignant hyperthermia (also known less appropriately as malignant hyperpyrexia) was first described in 1964 (Saidman et al. 1964); it can be summarized as a condition in which there is a rapid rise in the body temperature (at least 2°C an hour) occurring without obvious cause during anaesthesia, often in the presence of suxamethonium. Although the early cases were reported from North America, it has since appeared in all parts of the world and, in addition to the rapid rise of temperature, is characterized by stiffness of the skeletal musculature, hyperventilation, acidosis, hyperkalaemia, and signs of increased activity of the sympathetic nervous system, including tachycardia, vasoconstriction, hypertension, and raised blood glucose concentration. The condition is important because it carries a mortality of the order of 60–70 per cent. There is strong evidence that it is a primary disease of skeletal muscle that is inherited as an autosomal dominant trait. Many of those susceptible to the condition show evidence of myotonia or related muscle disorders (Harriman et al. 1973). Recent serological, biochemical, and pedigree studies (McPherson and Taylor 1982; Bender et al. 1990; MacLennan et al. 1990; McCarthy et al. 1990) provide strong evidence of a genetic basis for malignant hyperthermia, showing it to be linked to the q12–13.2 region of chromosome 19.

In the majority of affected families an elevated serum creatine phosphokinase level can be demonstrated (*The Lancet* 1973; Kelstrup et al. 1974). A more accurate prediction can be made, however, by testing specimens from a muscle biopsy *in vitro*, when it is found that those from individuals susceptible to malignant hyperthermia show heightened sensitivity to halothane, caffeine, suxamethonium, potassium chloride, and temperature change (Moulds and Denborough 1974a,b; Melton et al. 1989; Allen et al. 1990; Hackl et al. 1990). It is thus possible to distinguish those members of a family (with a history of malignant hyperthermia) who are not at risk.

When it occurs, it follows the administration of an inhalational general anaesthetic, most commonly halothane, and frequently in combination with suxamethonium; but it has been suggested by Ellis and others (1974) that nitrous oxide may act as a causative factor; and Britt and her co-workers (1974) have incriminated tubocurarine as a possible causative agent. Malignant hyperthermia may also present as heatstroke in subjects with the predisposing myopathy who are exposed to very severe physical stress (Denborough 1982). Several hypotheses have been suggested to explain the mechanism of the condition, but there is overwhelming evidence that the primary *trigger* is an abnormal calcium-induced release of intracellular ionized calcium (Moulds and Denborough 1974*a*; Ohnishi *et al.* 1986). Once released, it initiates a whole series of secondary changes that lead to the observed clinical changes and that also interact with each other and are thereby self-sustaining (Ording 1989).

It seems likely that fundamental to the condition is some inherited defect of cellular membranes, which would account for many of the other changes observed in malignant hyperthermia both clinically and experimentally. It is possible that there is a link between this disorder and the sudden infant death syndrome (SIDS) because Denborough (1981) found that 5 of 15 parents whose children died from SIDS had muscles that showed . changes indicating susceptibility to malignant hyperthermia. Prevention of malignant hyperthermia is obviously of major importance, and depends on awareness and vigilance by all doctors, especially anaesthetists. Treatment has been greatly facilitated by dantrolene, which inhibits the release of calcium from the sarcoplasmic reticulum and thereby halts the otherwise self-sustaining calcium release mechanisms that result in progressive and potentially fatal damage to susceptible subjects.

Glucocorticoid glaucoma

Since Francois (1954) first described a glaucoma-like rise in intraocular pressure following prolonged use of cortisone, the effect of glucocorticosteroid eye drops on intraocular pressure has been studied widely. In a randomly selected population the pressure change shows a trimodal distribution with relative frequencies of 66 per cent, 29 per cent, and 5 per cent for groups that exhibit low-, intermediate-, and high-pressure changes respectively in response to daily administration of glucocorticoid eye drops. Family studies established (Armaly 1965, 1966; Schwartz *et al.* 1972) that a two-allele model may explain the phenomenon, with genotypes $p^l p^l$, $p^l p^h$, and p^h, p^h. The allele p^l is responsible for low pressure and the allele p^h for high pressure, and the individuals with the genotype $p^l p^h$ appear to respond with a continuous rise in intraocular pressure following repeated administration of glucocorticoid eye drops, an effect that is completely reversible on withdrawal of the drug. On the other hand, a study of the effect of glucocorticoid eye drops on the intraocular pressure of 63 twins by Schwartz and others (1972) suggested that non-genetic factors may also play a major role in determining variation in the ocular responses to glucocorticoids. When administering glucocorticoid eye drops to patients it is obviously important to be aware of the fact that some individuals may respond with an increase in intraocular pressure which will require withdrawal of the drug. In case of doubt, there is obvious merit in checking intraocular pressure by means of tonometry. It should be noted that glaucoma induced by depot injection of triamcinolone may persist for as long as 10 months after the injection but may resolve promptly after the whitish plaque of residual steroid is removed (Mills *et al.* 1986).

Osteogenesis imperfecta

The production of general anaesthesia with halothane and suxamethonium may lead to a substantial increase of body temperature in patients suffering from osteogenesis imperfecta (Solomons and Myers 1972; Smith 1984). Fortunately, this elevation of body temperature is benign and can be controlled more satisfactorily and readily than in malignant hyperthermia (see above).

Periodic paralysis

This may be associated with several autosomal dominant conditions which are the result of an abnormality of the membrane of skeletal muscle. It is characterized by attacks of flaccid weakness during which either hyperkalaemia (lasting hours) or hypokalaemia (lasting days) may occur. Hyperkalaemic paralysis can be precipitated by the administration of potassium chloride and also by anaesthesia (Egan and Klein 1959; Gross *et al.* 1966; Layzer *et al.* 1967; Pearson and Kalyanaraman 1972). Hypokalaemic paralysis may be precipitated by a number of agents, including insulin, mineralocorticoids (not aldosterone), adrenaline, and ethanol. It has also been noted to follow the administration of ammonium glycyrrhizinate (licorice), and is presumably related to the mineralocorticoid properties of this compound (WHO 1973).

Familial dysautonomia (Riley–Day syndrome)

This condition affects Jewish families who originate from certain areas of Eastern Europe (Brunt and McKusick 1970) and is inherited as an autosomal recessive characteristic that gives rise to a wide variety of neurological disturbances. These patients produce exaggerated responses to drugs acting on the autonomic nervous system. Thus, the response to the parasympathomimetic drug methacholine is abnormal (Dancis 1968) and disturbances of blood-pressure regulation may develop during general anaesthesia. Patients also exhibit intolerance to halothane and methyoxyflurane (Meridy and Creighton 1971). If affected individuals require general anaesthesia, it is important to reduce the responses of the abnormal autonomic nervous system by prior administration of cholinergic-blocking and adrenergic-blocking agents, such as atropine and propranolol.

Chloramphenicol-induced aplastic anaemia

Chloramphenicol may induce thrombocytopenia, granulocytopenia, or aplastic anaemia, any of which may be dose-related and due to the effect of the drug on protein synthesis. In addition, there is a form of aplastic anaemia, induced by chloramphenicol, that appears to be idiosyncratic and which may be due to a genetically determined abnormality of DNA synthesis. Thus, while the other forms of blood dyscrasia, including the non-idiosyncratic form of aplastic anaemia, probably represent a normal and dose-related response of the bone marrow to chloramphenicol, the idiosyncratic form is an entirely separate entity, but like the other forms it calls for immediate withdrawal of the drug.

Cholestatic jaundice induced by oral contraceptives

It is well known that oral contraceptives (especially those with an alkyl substitution at the C_{17} position) may produce cholestatic jaundice. Evidence to date suggests that the familial and racial incidence of cholestatic jaundice following the administration of oral contraceptives may well have a genetic basis (Beeley 1975). It seems likely that oestrogen-induced changes in the composition of membrane lipids may play a major role in the production of cholestasis (Schreiber and Simon 1983). Further work requires to be carried out in order to clarify the underlying mechanisms.

Chlorpropamide–alcohol flushing (CPAF)

The first reports of facial flushing after ethanol in patients taking chlorpropamide (CPAF) occurred in the 1950s (Whitelock 1959), when it was estimated that it affected 15–30 per cent. A systematic study of 100 Type 2 diabetic patients taking chlorpropamide gave a frequency of 33 per cent (FitzGerald *et al.* 1962). Some authors have, however, suggested that CPAF is less common than previously suggested (Kobberling *et al.* 1980; DeSilva *et al.* 1981). The whole topic has been methodically reviewed by Johnston and others (1984*a,b*), and while there seems little doubt that CPAF exists, there is still uncertainty as to how best to test for it, its mechanism, whether it is inherited, and whether it is

associated with certain types of diabetes and with a relative freedom from diabetic vascular complications.

Johnston and others (1984*a*) describe CPAF thus: it consists of a flush of the face, sometimes spreading to the neck, which may be accompanied by injection of the conjunctivae. The flush is visible to observers as well as being felt by the subject. It may be so intense that it gives a burning sensation and, very rarely, a headache. CPAF is not accompanied by sweating or prostration (although in a few patients it is associated with wheezing), but it is often embarrassing. The reaction starts within 10 or 20 minutes of taking alcohol, reaches a peak at 30–40 minutes, and persists for 1–2 hours or more. CPAF is different from the flush due to alcohol alone; patients who have experienced both are in no doubt of their difference.

The original simple challenge test (chlorpropamide 250 mg, then two 40 ml glasses of sherry 12 and 36 hours, respectively, later [Leslie and Pyke 1978; Pyke and Leslie 1978]) is now known to be inadequate, because it has been found that the dose of chlorpropamide influences the frequency of a positive response. A satisfactory test probably requires (1) pretreatment with chlorpropamide 250 mg for 14 days; (2) flush assessment by patient and an observer (85 per cent agreement), (3) measurement of rise of facial skin temperature (significantly greater in 'flushers' in whom it is not simply due to differences in basal temperatures), and (4) the use of thermography, which is a better index of facial skin blood flow than thermometry (Johnston *et al.* 1984*a,b*).

Studies in 12 pairs of identical twins indicated that CPAF is an autosomal dominant inherited trait and is associated with non-insulin-dependent diabetes (especially where there is a strong family history), but not with insulin-dependent diabetes (Leslie and Pyke 1978; Pyke and Leslie 1978). Most of these studies, however, were made with the single-tablet challenge test of patients who were strongly positive flushers, and it is therefore possible that less responsive flushers might show a different pattern of response if they received a prolonged course of chlorpropamide (Johnston *et al.* 1984*a,b*).

The mechanism of CPAF is still not clear, but since flushers seem to be more sensitive than non-flushers to the effect of disulfiram (Antabuse), which inhibits the enzyme acetaldehyde dehydrogenase (ALDH), it seems possible that flushers may metabolise acetaldehyde more slowly than non-flushers. Furthermore, there is evidence that in chlorpropamide–alcohol-flushers the increase of plasma acetaldehyde is twice that in non-flushers (Johnston *et al.* 1984*a,b*) and this may be because ALDH is more sensitive to the inhibitory effect of chlorpropamide in flushers (Ohlin *et al.* 1982). The results of more recent work suggest the following:

(1) chlorpropamide is a major determinant of CPAF, which is associated with elevated blood acetaldehyde levels due to the inhibitions of ALDH by chlorpropamide (Groop *et al.* 1984*a,b*);

(2) ALDH activity is increased in Type 2 diabetics and determines CPAF. Furthermore, aldehyde concentration after chlorpropamide with ethanol is higher in patients with CPAF than in those without CPAF (Jerntop *et al.* 1986);

(3) in healthy non-diabetic adults CPAF appears to be a normal phenomenon (Hoskins *et al.* 1987);

(4) CPAF has a different enzymic basis from the ethanol flush reaction of oriental subjects. It seems likely that, in CPAF-positive subjects, ALDH may be particularly susceptible to inhibition by chlorpropamide (Johnston *et al.* 1986);

(5) while CPAF is associated with increased levels of plasma opioid peptides, especially metenkephalin (Leslie *et al.* 1979*a*; Medbak *et al.* 1981; Johnston *et al.* 1984*a*), it seems unlikely that CPAF is *caused* by this effect (Johnston *et al.* 1984*b*);

(6) there appears to be an association between fast acetylator phenotype and CPAF in Type 2, but not Type 1, diabetics; fast acetylators were more frequently CPAF-positive, while slow acetylators were more frequently negative. Furthermore, a linear relationship was found between acetylation rate and the speed of ascent of facial skin temperature after chlorpropamide and ethanol in Type 2 diabetics but not in Type 1 (Bonisolli *et al.* 1985).

Clearly, further studies are required to elucidate these mechanisms and relationships. It is possible that, in the Type B adverse drug reaction, CPAF is associated with a relative freedom from diabetic vascular complications (Leslie *et al.* 1979*b*; Barnett and Pyke 1980; Barnett *et al.* 1981), although not all workers agree with this suggestion (Micossi *et al.* 1982). There are many obvious reasons why every aspect of CPAF should be studied, not only because of the important light it may shed on the pathogenesis of Type 2 diabetes mellitus but also because it should explain the mechanism of this Type B drug reaction and so indicate how it can be avoided.

Immunological reasons for abnormal response

A most important group of qualitatively abnormal responses to drugs are those in which the cause is primarily immunological. In instances where the drug is immunogenic in its own right (e.g. antisera of animal origin) the reaction is obviously a Type A effect. Serum sickness is an example. Most allergic drug reactions, however, are not so obviously Type A responses, and in the absence of known mechanisms they can (perhaps temporarily) be categorized as Type B effects. The mechanisms involved in drug allergy are considered elsewhere in this book (Chapter 25). It seems possible that *human lymphocyte antigens* (HLA) may influence susceptibility to adverse drug reactions and thus could be an important factor in the determination of some Type B reactions. There is evidence that such a mechanism may be involved when patients with rheumatoid arthritis react adversely to levamisole (Schmidt and Mueller-Eckhardt 1977), gold therapy (Latts *et al.* 1980), and penicillamine (Wooley *et al.* 1980); and also in hypertensives who react adversely to hydralazine (Batchelor *et al.* 1980) (see also Chapter 2).

Neoplastic and teratological reasons for abnormal response

The possibility that a drug may be a significant factor in causing teratological or neoplastic changes is well known and these subjects are dealt with in detail in other chapters of this book (see Chapters 5 and 24). It is also important, however, to consider the possibility that a qualitatively abnormal response to a drug may occur as a result of the presence of some potentially neoplastic or teratological tissue in the organism. A preneoplastic condition may well be transformed into a frankly neoplastic state by the administration of a drug, such as an oestrogen or an androgen, which is given to treat some entirely unrelated condition.

TABLE 3.3
*Comparison between Type A and Type B
adverse drug reactions*

	A (Augmented/attenuated response)	B (Bizarre response)
Pharmacologically predictable	+	−
Dose-dependent	+	−
Incidence and morbidity	high	low
Mortality	low	high
Treatment	adjust dose	stop

Conclusion

In this chapter, we have used a classification of adverse drug reactions that divides them into those that are *quantitatively* abnormal (Type A) and those that are *qualitatively* abnormal (Type B). The main differences between these two classes of adverse reactions are summarized in Table 3.3.

In clinical practice, patients with Type A reactions, which are usually dose-related and predictable, can often be managed by either adjusting the dose, substituting a similar but more selective drug, or giving additional drugs to antagonize the unwanted effects of the primary agent. In contrast, in patients with Type B reactions it is usually necessary to withdraw therapy.

References

Acheson, D. (1989). L-tryptophan and eosinophilia–myalgia syndrome in the USA. Department of Health (PL/CMO (89)11), London.

Adjepon-Yamoah, K.K. (1980). Drugs for developing countries — the views of a practising doctor in the tropics. In *Proceedings of the first world conference on clinical pharmacology and therapeutics* (ed. P. Turner), p. 536. Macmillan, London.

Aggeler, P.M., O'Reilly, R.A., Leong, L., and Kowitz, P.E. (1967). Potentiation of anticoagulant effect of warfarin by phenylbutazone. *N. Engl. J. Med.* 276, 496.

Allen, G.C., Rosenberg, H., and Fletcher, J.E. (1990). Safety of general anesthesia in patients previously tested negative for malignant hyperthermia susceptibility. *Anesthesiology* 72, 619.

Armaly, M.F. (1965). Statistical attributes of the steroid hypertensive response in the clinically normal eye. 1. The demonstration of three levels of response. *Invest. Ophthalmol.* 4, 187.

Armaly, M.F. (1966). The heritable nature of dexmethasone-induced ocular hypertension. *Arch. Ophthalmol.* 75, 32.

Aronoff, G.P., Ozawa, T., Desante, K.A., Nash, J.F., and Ridolfo, A.S. (1982). Benoxaprofen kinetics in renal impairment. *Clin. Pharmacol. Ther.* 32, 190.

Asberg, M., Cronholm, B., Sjöqvist, F., and Tuck, D. (1970). Correlation of subjective side-effects with plasma concentrations of nortriptyline. *Br. Med. J.* iv, 18.

Avner, D.L., Larsen, R., and Berenson, M.M. (1983). Inhibition of liver surface membrane Na+, K-adenosine triphosphatase, Mg^2+-adenosine triphosphatase and 5-nucleotidase activities by protoporphyrin. *Gastroenterology* 85, 700.

Ayesh, R. and Smith, R.L. (1989). Genetic polymorphism in human toxicology. In *Recent advances in clinical pharmacology* (ed. P. Turner and G. Volans), p. 137. Churchill Livingstone, Edinburgh.

Bagnarello, A.G., Lewis, L.A., McHenry, M.C., Weinstein, A.J., Naito, H.K., McCollough, A.J., *et al.* (1977). Unusual serum lipoprotein abnormality induced by the vehicle of miconazole. *N. Engl. J. Med.* 296, 497.

Barnett, A.H. and Pyke, D.A. (1980). Chlorpropamide alcohol flushing and large vessel disease in non-insulin dependent diabetics. *Br. Med. J.* ii, 261

Barnett, A.H., Leslie, R.D.G., and Pyke D.A. (1981). Chlorpropamide alcohol flushing and proteinuria in non-insulin-dependent diabetics. *Br. Med. J.* 282, 522.

Batchelor, J.R., Welsh, K.I., Mansilla-Tinoco, R., Dollery, C.T., Hughes, G.R.V., Bernstein, R., *et al.* (1980). Hydralazine-induced systemic lupus erythematosus: influence of HLA-DR and sex on susceptibility. *Lancet* i, 1107.

Bateman, D.N., Gokal, R., Dodd, T.R.P., and Blain, P.G. (1981). The pharmacokinetics of single doses of metoclopramide in renal failure. *Eur. J. Clin. Pharmacol.* 19, 437.

BCDSP (Boston Collaborative Drug Surveillance Program) (1973). Diphenylhydantoin side effects and serum albumin levels. *Clin. Pharmacol. Ther.* 14, 529.

Beeley, L. (1975). Adverse reactions to drugs. *Medicine* 5, 207.

Belongia, E.A., Hedberg, C.W., Gleich, G.J., White, K.E., Nayeno, A.N., Loegering D.A., *et al.* (1990). An investigation of the cause of the eosinophilia–myalgia syndrome associated with tryptophan use. *N. Engl. J. Med.* 323, 357.

Bender, K., Seuff, H., Wienker, T.F., Spiess-Kiefer, C., and Lehmann-Horn, F. (1990). A linkage study of malignant hyperthermia (MH). *Clin. Genet.* 37, 221.

Benowitz, N., Forsyth, R.P., Melmon, K.L., and Rowland, M. (1974). Lidocaine disposition kinetics in monkey and man. II. Effects of haemorrhage and sympathomimetic drug administration. *Clin. Pharmacol. Ther.* 16, 99.

Bernstein, H., Zraifler, N., Rubin, M., and Manson, A.M. (1964). The ocular deposition of chloroquin. *Invest. Ophthalmol.* 2, 384.

Bertilsson, L., Mellström, B., Säwe, J., and Sjöqvist, F. (1981). Pharmacogenetic aspects of the metabolism of tricyclic antidepressants. In *New vistas in depression* (ed. S.Z. Langer). Pergamon Press, London.

Bertler, A.A. and Smith, S.E. (1971). Genetic influences in drug responses of the eye and heart. *Clin. Sci.* 40, 403.

Beutler, E. (1984). Sensitivity to drug-induced haemolytic anaemia in glucose-6-phosphate dehydrogenase deficiency. In *Banbury Report 16. Genetic variability in responses to chemical exposure* (ed. G.S. Omenn and H.V. Gelboin), p. 205. Cold Spring Harbor, New York.

Bianchine, J.F., Calimlin, L.R., Morgan, J.P., Dujurne, C.A., and Lasagna, L. (1971). Metabolism and absorption of L-3,4-dihydroxyphenylanine in patients with Parkinson's Disease. *Ann. N.Y. Acad. Sci.* 179, 126.

Black, D.J., Grimmer, S.F.M., Orme M.L'E., Proudlove, C., Mann, R.D., and Breckenridge, A.M. (1988). Evaluation of Committee on Safety of Medicines yellow card reports on oral contraceptive-drug interactions with anticonvulsants and antibiotics. *Br. J. Clin. Pharmacol.* 25, 527.

Blain, P.G., Mucklow, J.C., Bacon, C.J., and Rawlins, M.D. (1981). Pharmacokinetics of phenytoin in children. *Br. J. Clin. Pharmacol.* 12, 659.

Blain, P.G., Mucklow, J.C., Wood, P., Roberts, D.F., and Rawlins, M.D. (1982). Family study of antipyrine clearance. *Br. Med. J.* 284, 150.

Blaschke, T.F. (1977). Protein binding and kinetics of drugs in liver disease. *Clin. Pharmacokinet.* 2, 32.

Boley, S.J., Allen, A.C., Schultz, L., and Schwartz, S. (1965). Potassium-induced lesions of the small bowel. I. Clinical aspects. *JAMA* 193, 997.

Bonisolli, L., Pontiroli, A.E., De-Pasqua, A., Calderara, A., Maffi, P., Gallus, G., *et al.* (1985). Association between chlorpropamide-alcohol flushing and fast acetylator phenotype in type I and type II diabetes. *Acta Diabetol. Lat.* 22, 305.

Boyd, M.R. (1980). Biochemical mechanisms of pulmonary toxicity of furan derivatives. In *Reviews in biochemical toxicology*, Vol. 2 (ed. E. Hodgson, J.R. Bond, and R.M. Philpot), p. 71. Elsevier/North Holland, Amsterdam.

Breckenridge, A.M. and Orme, M.L'E. (1987). Principles of pharmacology and therapeutics. In *Oxford textbook of medicine* (2nd edn) (ed. D.J. Weatherall, J.G.G. Ledingham, and D.A. Warrell), p. 7.1 Oxford University Press.

Breckenridge, A., Orme, M. L'E., Thorgeirsson, S., Davies, D.S., and Brooks. R.V. (1971). Drug interactions with warfarin: studies with dichloralphenazone, chloral hydrate and phenazone (antipyrine). *Clin. Sci.* 40, 351.

Briant, R.H., Reid, J.L., and Dollery, C.T. (1973). Interactions between clonidine and desipramine in man. *Br. Med. J.* i, 522.

Britt, B.A., Webb, G.E., and LeDuc, C. (1974). Malignant hyperthermia induced by curare. *Can. Anaesth. Soc. J.* 21, 371.

Brodie, B.B., Burns, J.J., and Weiner, M. (1959). Metabolism of drugs in subjects with Laennec's cirrhosis. *Medna Exp.* 1, 290.

Brodie, M.J., Boobis, A.R., Bulpitt, C.J., and Davies, D.S. (1981). Influence of liver disease and environmental factors on hepatic mono-oxygenase activity *in vitro*. *Eur. J. Clin. Pharmacol.* 20, 39.

Bros, O. (1987). Gastrointestinal mucosal lesions: a drug formulation problem. Med. Toxicol. 2, 105.

Brunt, P.W. and McKusick, V.A. (1970). Familial dysautonomia. A report of genetic and clinical studies, with a review of the literature. *Medicine* 49, 343.

Buchanan, N., Davis, M., Danhof, M., and Breimer, D.D. (1980). Antipyrine metabolite formation in children in the acute phase of malnutrition and after recovery. *Br. J. Clin. Pharmacol.* 10, 363.

Bussey, H.I. (1982). The influence of quinidine and other agents on digitalis glycosides. *Am. Heart J.* 104, 289.

Buyske, D.A., Eisner, H.J., and Kelly, R.G. (1960). Concentration and persistence of tetracycline and chlortetracycline in bone. *J. Pharmacol. Exp. Ther.* 130, 150.

Cain, S. and Nigogosyan, G. (1963). Acquired toxic porphyria cutanea tarda due to hexachlorobenzene: Report of 348 cases caused by this fungicide. *JAMA* 183, 88.

Chan, T.K., Todd, D., and Tso, S.C. (1976). Drug-induced haemolysis in glucose 6-phosphate dehydrogenase deficiency. *Br. Med. J.* ii, 1227.

Cohen, R.J., Sachs, J.R., Wicker, Donna J., and Conrad, M.E. (1968). Methemoglobinemia provoked by malarial chemoprophylaxis in Vietnam. *N. Engl. J. Med.* 279, 1127.

Cohlan, S.Q., Berclander, G., and Tiansic, T. (1963). Growth of inhibition of prematures receiving tetracyclines: a clinical and laboratory investigation. *Am. J. Dis. Child.* 105, 453.

Conrad, K.A., Byers, J.M., Finley, P.R., and Burnham, L. (1983). Lidocaine elimination effects of metoprolol and propranolol. *Clin. Pharmacol. Ther.* 33, 133.

Cowan, W.K. and Evans, D.A.P. (1964). Primaquine and methemoglobin. *Clin. Pharmacol. Ther.* 5, 307.

Cranmer J.A., Mattson, R.H., Prevey, M.L., Scheyer, R.D., and Onellette, V.L. (1989). How often is medication taken as prescribed? *JAMA* 261, 3273.

CSM (Committee on Safety of Medicines) (1983). Osmosin (controlled release indomethacin). *Current Problems* No. 11. HMSO, London.

CSM (Committee on Safety of Medicines) (1988). Nebuliser solutions and paradoxical bronchoconstriction. *Current Problems* 22. HMSO, London.

Cunningham, J.L., Leyland, M.J., Delamore, I.W., and Evans, D.A.P. (1974). Acetanilide oxidation in phenylbutazone-associated hypoplastic anaemia. *Br. Med. J.* iii, 313.

Dancis, J. (1968). Altered drug response in familial dysautonomia. *Ann. N.Y. Acad. Sci.* 151, 876.

Davidson, H. (1968). *Physiology of the cerebrospinal fluid.* Churchill Livingstone, Edinburgh.

Davis S.S. (1989). Gastrointestinal transit and drug absorption. In *Novel drug delivery* (ed. L.F. Prescott and W.S. Nimmo), p. 89. Wiley, Chichester.

de Matteis, F. (1967). Disturbances of liver porphyrin metabolism caused by drugs. *Pharmacol. Rev.* 19, 523.

Denborough, M.A. (1981). Sudden infant death syndrome and malignant hyperpyrexia. *Med. J. Aust.* i, 649.

Denborough, M.A. (1982). Heat stroke and malignant hyperpyrexia. *Med. J. Aust.* i, 204.

DeSilva, N.E., Tunbridge, W.M.G., and Alberti, K.G.M.M. (1981). Low incidence of chlorpropramide-alcohol flushing in diet-treated non-insulin-dependent diabetics. *Lancet* i, 128.

Dettli, L., Spring, P., and Ryter, S. (1971). Multiple dose kinetics of drug dosage in patients with kidney disease. *Acta Pharmacol. Toxicol.* 29 (suppl. 3), 211.

Devadatta, S., Gangadharam, P.R.J., Andrews, R.H., Fox, W., Ramakrishnan, C.V., Selkon, J.B., *et al.* (1960). Peripheral neuritis due to isoniazid. *Bull. Wld Hlth Org.* 23, 587.

Diggle, G. (1990). The eosinophilia myalgia syndrome and L-tryoptophan. *Health Trends* 22, 2.

Dorian, P., Sellers, E.M., Reed, K.L., Warsh, J.J., Hamilton, C., Kaplan, H.C., *et al.* (1983). Amitriptyline and ethanol: pharmacokinetic and pharmacodynamic interaction. *Eur. J. Clin. Pharmacol.* 25, 325.

Dost, F.H. (1953). *Der Blutspiegelkinetik der Konzentrationsablaufe in der Kreislauffussigkeit.* Leipzig.

Drug and Therapeutics Bulletin (1976). Drugs and diet in the hereditary porphyrias. *Drug. Ther. Bull.* 14, 55.

Dubbleman, T.M., De Goeij, A.F., and van Steveninck, J. (1980). Protoporphyria-induced photodynamic effects on transport processes across the membrane of human erythrocytes. *Biophys. Acta* 595, 133.

Eales, L. (1971). Acute porphyria: the precipitating and aggravating factors. Proceedings of the national conference on porphyrin metabolism and porphyria. Cape Town, December 1970. *S. Afr. Lab. Clin. Med.* (special issue) 17, 120.

Eap C.B., Cuendet C., and Baumann, P. (1990).Binding of α-methadone, L-methadone, and DL-methadone to proteins in plasma of healthy volunteers: role of the variants of α₁-acid glycoprotein. *Clin. Pharmacol. Ther.* 47, 338.

Egan, T.J. and Klein, R. (1959). Hyperkalemic familial periodic paralysis. *Pediatrics* 24, 761.

Ehrlich, L.J. and Stein, H.S. (1963). Abnormal urinary findings following administration of achromycin V. *Pediatrics* 31, 697.

Ellard, G.A., Gammon, P.T., Savin, L.A., and Tan, R.S.H. (1974). Dapsone acetylation in dermatitis herpetiformis. *Br. J. Dermatol.* 13, 441.

Ellis, F.R., Clarke, I.M.C., Appleyard, T.N., and Dinsdale, R.C.W. (1974). Malignant hyperpyrexia induced by nitrous oxide and treated with dexamethasone. *Br. Med. J.* iv, 270.

Eriksson, M., Paalzow, L., Bolme, P., and Marian, T.W. (1983). Chloramphenicol pharmacokinetics in Ethiopian children of differing nutritional states. *Eur. J. Clin. Pharmacol.* 24, 819.

Evans, D.A.P., Mahgoub, A., Sloan, T.P., Idle, J.R., and Smith, R.L. (1980). A family and population study of the genetic polymorphism of debrisoquine oxidation in a white British population. *J. Med. Genet.* 17, 102.

FitzGerald, M.G., Gaddie, R., Malins, J.M., and O'Sullivan, D.J. (1962). Alcohol sensitivity in diabetics receiving chlorpropamide. *Diabetes* 11, 40.

Flannery, M.T., Wallach, P.M., Espinoza, L.R., Dohrenwend, M.P., and Moscinski, L.C. (1990). A case of the eosinophilia–myalgia syndrome associated with the use of an L-tryptophan product. *Ann. Intern. Med.* 112, 300.

Fletcher K.A., Barton, P.F., and Kelly, J.A. (1988). Studies on the mechanisms of oxidation in the erythrocyte by metabolites of primaquine. *Biochem. Pharmacol.* 37, 2683.

Folbe, P.I. (1980). *The safety of medicines.* Springer-Verlag, Berlin.

Francois, J. (1954). Cortisone et tension oculaire. *Ann. Oculist.* 187, 805.

Fraser, H.S., Mucklow, J.C., Bulpitt, C.J., Kahn, G.C., Mould, G., and Dollery, C.T. (1979). Environmental factors affecting antipyrine metabolism in London factory and office workers. *Br. J. Clin. Pharmacol* 7, 237.

Frimpter, G.W. (1963). Reversible 'Fanconi syndrome' caused by degraded tetracycline. *JAMA* 184, 111.

Frischer, H. and Ahmad, T. (1987). Consequence of erythrocyte glutathione reductase deficiency. *J. Lab. Clin. Med.* 109, 583.

Garrattini, S. (1985). Active drug metabolites: an overview. *Clin. Pharmacokinet.* 10, 216.

Gelboin, H.V. (1977). Cancer susceptibility and carcinogen metabolism. *N. Engl. J. Med.* 297, 384.

Gibaldi, M., Boyes, R.N., and Feldman, S. (1971). Influence of first-pass effect on the availability of drugs on oral administration. *J. Pharm. Sci.* 60, 1338.

Gillies, H.C., Roger, H.J., Spector, R.G., and Trounce, J.R. (1986). *A textbook of clinical pharmacology* (2nd edn). Hodder and Stoughton, London.

Glen, J.B., Davies, G.E., Thomson, D.S., Scarth, S.C., and Thompson, A.V. (1979). An animal model for the investigation of adverse responses to I.V. anaesthetic agents and their solvents. *Br. J. Anaesth.* 51, 819.

Goldberg, A. and Moore, M.R. (ed.). (1980). The porphyrias. In *Clinics in haematology* Vol. 9, p. 225. W.B. Saunders, London.

Goldberg. A., Paton, W.D.M., and Thompson, J.W. (1954). Pharmacology of the porphyrins and porphobilinogen. *Br. J. Pharmacol.* 9, 91.

Goldberg, A., Moore, M.R., McKoll, K.E.L., and Brodie, J.B. (1987). Porphyria metabolism and the porphyrias. In *Oxford textbook of medicine* (ed. D.J. Weatherall, J.G.G. Ledingham, and D.A. Warrell), p. 9.136. Oxford University Press.

Greenblatt, D.J. and Koch-Weser, J. (1974). Clinical toxicity of chlordiazepoxide and diazepam in relation to serum albumin concentration: a report from the Boston Collaborative Drug Surveillance Program. *Eur. J. Clin. Pharmacol.* 4, 259.

Groop, L., Eriksson, C.J., Huupponen, R., Ylikahri, R., and Pelkonen, R. (1984a). Roles of chlorpropamide, alcohol and acetaldehyde in determining the chlorpropamide–alcohol flush. *Diabetologia* 26, 34

Groop, L., Koskimies, S., and Tolppanen, E.M. (1984b). Characterisation of patients with chlorpropamide–alcohol flush. *Acta Med. Scand.* 215, 141

Gross, E.G., Dexter, J.D., and Roth, R.G. (1966). Hypokalemic myopathy with myoglobinuria associated with licorice ingestion. *N. Engl. J. Med.* 274, 602.

Gross, J.M. (1963). Fanconi syndrome (adult type) developing secondary to ingestion of outdated tetracycline. *Ann. Intern. Med.* 58, 523.

Hackl, W., Mauritz, W., Schemper, M., Winkler, M., Sporn, P., and Steinbereithner, K. (1990). Prediction of malignant hyperthermia susceptibility: statistical evaluation of clinical signs. *Br. J. Anaesth.* 64, 411.

Hackney, J.F., Gross, S.R., Aronow, L., and Pratt, W.B. (1970). Specific glucocorticoid-binding macromolecules from mouse fibroblasts growing *in vitro*. A possible steroid receptor for growth inhibition. *Mol. Pharmacol.* 6, 500.

Harriman, D.G., Summer, D.W., and Ellis, F.R. (1973). Malignant hyperpyrexia myopathy. *Q. J. Med.* 42, 639.

Harris, H. (1964). Enzymes and drug sensitivity. The genetics of serum cholinesterase deficiency in relation to suxamethonium apnoea. *Proc. R. Soc. Med.* 57, 503.

Heizer, W.D., Smith, T.W., and Goldfinger, S.E. (1971). Absorption of digoxin in patients with malabsorption syndromes. *N. Engl. J. Med.* 285, 257.

Hendeles, L., Weinberger, M., Milavetz, G., Hill, M., and Baughan, L. (1985). Food induced 'dose-dumping' from a once-a-day theophylline product as a cause of theophylline toxicity. *Chest* 87, 758.

Hinson, J.A. (1980). Biochemical toxicology of acetaminophen. In *Reviews in biochemical toxicology*, Vol. 2 (ed. E. Hodgson, J.R. Bland, and R.M. Philpot), p. 103. Elsevier/North Holland, New York.

Hoskins, P.J., Wiles, P.G., Volkmann, H.P., and Pyke D.A. (1987). Chlorpropamide alcohol flushing: a normal response? *Clin. Sci.* 73, 77.

Hutchison, R. (1930). A danger from paraldehyde. *Br. Med. J.* i. 718.

Inaba, T., Vinks, A., Ottou, S.V., and Kalow, W. (1983). Comparative pharmacogenetics of sparteine and debrisoquine. *Clin. Pharmacol. Ther.* 33, 394.

Islam, S.I., Idle, J.R., and Smith, R.L. (1980). The polymorphic 4-hydroxylation of debrisoquine in a Saudi Arabian population. *Xenobiotica*, 11, 819.

Iversen, L.L. (1967). *The uptake and storage of nor-adrenaline by sympathetic nerves.* Cambridge University Press.

Jerntop, P., Ohlin, H., Sundkvist, G., and Almer, L-O. (1986). Effects of chlorpropamide and alcohol on aldehyde dehydrogenase activity and blood acetaldehyde concentration. *Diabetes Res.* 3, 369.

Johnston, C., Wiles, P.G., and Pyke, D.A. (1984*a*). Chlorpropamide–alcohol flush: the case in favour. *Diabetologia* 26, 1.

Johnston, C., Wiles, P.G., Medbak, S., Bowcock, S., Cooke, E.D., Pyke, D.A., *et al.* (1984*b*). The role of endogenous opioids in the chlorpropamide–alcohol flush. *Clin. Endocrinol.* 21, 489.

Johnston, C., Saunders, J.B., Barnett, A.H., Ricciardi, B.R., Hopkinson, D.A., and Pyke, D.A. (1986). Chlorpropamide–alcohol flush reaction and isoenzyme profiles of alcohol dehydrogenase and aldehyde dehydrogenase. *Clin. Sci.* 71, 513.

Jollow, D.J. and Smith, C. (1977). Biological aspects of toxic metabolites. In *Biological reactive intermediates: formation, toxicity and inactivation* (ed. D.J. Jollow, J.J. Kocsis, R. Snyder, and H.Vainio), p. 44. Plenum, New York.

Jollow, D.J., Kocsis, J.J., Snyder, R., and Vainio, H. (1977). *Biological reactive intermediates: formation, toxicity and inactivation.* Plenum, New York.

Kappas, A., Anderson, K.E., Conney, A.H., and Alvares, A.P. (1976). Influence of dietary protein and carbohydrate on antipyrine and theophylline metabolism in man. *Clin. Pharmacol. Ther.* 20, 643.

Kappas, A., Alvares, A.P., Anderson, K.E., Pantuck, E.J., Pantuck, C.B., Chang, R., *et al.* (1978). Effect of charcoal-broiled beef on antipyrine and theophylline metabolism. *Clin. Pharmacol. Ther.* 23, 445.

Karlsson, E., Collste, P., and Rawlins, M.D. (1974). Plasma levels of lidocaine during combined treatment with phenytoin and procainamide. *Eur. J. Clin. Pharmacol.* 7, 455.

Kelstrup, J., Reske-Nielsen, E., Haase, J., and Jorni, J. (1974). Malignant hyperthermia in a family: a clinical and serological investigation of 139 members. *Acta Anaesth. Scand.* 18, 58.

Kilbourne, E.M., Swygert, L.A., and Philen, R.M. (1990). Interim guidance on the eosinophilia–myalgia syndrome. *Ann. Intern. Med.* 112, 85.

Kimbrough, R.D. (1987). Porphyrins and hepatotoxicity. In *Mechanisms of chemical-induced porphyrinopathies* (ed. E.K. Silbergeld and B.A. Fowler), p. 289. The New York Academy of Sciences.

Kobberling, J., Bengsch, N., Bruggersboer, B., Schwarck, H., Tillil, H., and Weber, M. (1980). The chlorpropamide–alcohol flush — lack of specificity for non-insulin-dependent diabetes. *Diabetologia* 19, 359.

Kunin, C.M. and Finland, M. (1961). Clinical pharmacology of the tetracycline antibiotics. *Clin. Pharmacol. Ther.* 2, 51.

Kupfer, A., Desmond, P., Schenka, S., and Branch, R. (1979). Family study of a genetically determined deficiency of mephenytoin hydroxylation in man. *Pharmacologist* 21, 173.

Kupfer, A., Desmond, P., Patwardham, R., Schenka, S., and Branch, R.A. (1984). Mephenytoin hydroxylation deficiency: kinetics after repeated doses. *Clin. Pharmacol. Ther.* 35, 33.

The Lancet (1973). Prevention of malignant hyperpyrexia. *Lancet* i, 1225.

The Lancet (1990). Contaminated L-tryptophan. *Lancet* 335, 1152.

Latts, J.R., Antel, J.P., Levinson, D.J., Arnason, B.G.W., and Medof, M.E. (1980). Histocompatibility antigens and gold toxicity. *J. Clin. Pharmacol.* 20, 206.

Laurence D.R. and Bennett, P.N. (1987). *Clinical Pharmacology* (6th edn). Churchill Livingstone, Edinburgh.

Layzer, R.B., Lovelace, R.E., and Rowland, L.P. (1967). Hyperkalemic periodic paralysis. *Arch. Neurol.* 16, 455.

Leahy, D.E., Lynch, J., and Taylor, D.C. (1989). Mechanisms of absorption of small molecules. In *Novel drug delivery* (ed. L.F. Prescott and W.S. Nimmo), p. 33. Wiley, Chichester.

Leslie, R.D.G. and Pyke, D.A. (1978). Chlorpropamide–alcohol flushing: a dominantly inherited trait associated with diabetes. *Br. Med. J.* ii, 1519.

Leslie, R.D.G., Pyke, D.A., and Stubbs, W.A. (1979*a*). Sensitivity to enkephalin as a cause of non-insulin-dependent diabetes. *Lancet* i, 341.

Leslie, R.D.G., Barnett, A.H., and Pyke, D.A. (1979*b*). Chlorpropamide–alcohol flushing and diabetic retinopathy. *Lancet* i, 997.

Levi, A.J., Sherlock, S., and Walker, D. (1968). Phenylbutazone and isoniazid metabolism in patients with liver disease in relationship to previous drug therapy. *Lancet* i, 1275.

Levy, G. (1971). Drug biotransformation interactions in man: non-narcotic analgesics. *Ann. N.Y. Acad. Sci.* 179, 32.

Levy, G. and Tsuchiya, T. (1971). Effect of activated charcoal on aspirin absorption in man. *Clin. Pharmacol. Ther.* 13, 317.

Lewis, G.P., Jusko, W.J., Burke, C.W., and Graves, L. (1971). Prednisone side effects and serum protein levels. *Lancet* ii, 778.

Lipsky, J.J. (1983). N-methyl-thio-tetrazole inhibition of the gamma carboxylation of glutamic acid: possible mechanism for antibiotic-associated hypoprothrombinaemia. *Lancet*, ii, 192.

Loeser, E.W. (1961). Studies on the metabolism of diphenylhydantoin (Dilantin). *Neurology*, 11, 424.

McCarthy, T.V., Healy, J.M., Haffron, J.J., Lehane, M., Deufel, T., Lehmann-Horn, F., *et al.* (1990). Localization of the malignant hyperthermia susceptibility locus to human chromosome 19q12–13.2. *Nature* 343, 562.

McDevitt, D.G., Frisk-Holmberg, M., Hollifield, J.W., and Shand, D.G. (1976). Plasma binding and the affinity of propranolol for a beta receptor in man. *Clin. Pharmacol. Ther.* 20, 152.

McGuire, W.L., Horwitz, K.D., Pearson, O.H., and Segaloff, A. (1977). Current status of estrogen and progesterone receptors in breast cancer. *Cancer* 39, 2934.

McKay, J., Rawlins, M.D., Cobden, I., and James, O.F.W. (1982). The acute effects of ethanol on acetanilide disposition in normal subjects, and in patients with liver disease. *Br. J. Clin. Pharmacol.* 14, 501.

MacLennan, D.H., Duff, C., Zorzato, F., Fujii, J., Phillips, M., Korneluk, R.G., et al. (1990). Ryanodine receptor gene is a candidate for predisposition to malignant hyperthermia. *Nature* 343, 559.

McLeod, K., Watson, M.K., and Rawlins, M.D. (1976). Pharmacokinetics of pancuronium in normal individuals and in patients with renal failure. *Br. J. Anaesth.* 48, 341.

McPherson, E. and Taylor, C.A. (1982). The genetics of malignant hyperthermia: evidence for heterogeneity. *Am. J. Med. Genet.* 11, 273.

Mahgoub, A., Dring, L.G., Idle, J.R., Lancaster, R., and Smith, R.L. (1977). Polymorphic hydroxylation of debrisoquine in man. *Lancet*, ii, 584.

Manninen, V., Apajalahti, A., Melin, J., and Karesoja, M. (1973). Altered absorption of digoxin in patients given propantheline and metoclopramide. *Lancet* i, 398.

Marks, P.A. and Banks, J. (1965). Drug-induced hemolytic anemias associated with glucose-6-phosphate dehydrogenase deficiency: a generally heterogeneous trait. *Ann. N.Y. Acad. Sci.* 123, 198.

Medbak, S., Wass, J.A.H., Clement-Jones, V., Cook, E., Bowcock, S., Cudworth, A.G., et al. (1981). Chlorpropamide alcohol flush and circulating metenkephalin: a positive link. *Br. Med. J.* 283, 937.

Melton, A.T., Martucci, R.W., Kien, N.D., and Gronert, G.A. (1989). Malignant hyperthermia in human-standardization of contracture testing protocol. *Anesth. Analg.* 69, 437.

Meridy, H.W. and Creighton, R.E. (1971). General anaesthesia in eight patients with familial dysautonomia. *Can. Anaesth. Soc. J.* 18, 563.

Micossi, R., Mannucci, P.M., Bozzini, S., and Malacco, E. (1982). Chlorpropamide-alcohol flushing in non-insulin dependent diabetes: prevalence of small and large vessel disease and risk factors for angiopathy. *Acta Diabetol. Lat.* 19, 141.

Mills, D.W., Siebert, L.F., and Climenhaga, M.D. (1986). Depot triamcinolone-induced glaucoma. *Can. J. Ophthalmol.* 21, 150.

Milne, M.D., Scribner, B.H., and Crawford, M.A. (1958). Non-ionic diffusion and the excretion of weak acids and bases. *Am. J. Med.* 24, 709.

Mitchell, J.R., Cavanaugh, J.H., Arias, L., and Oates, J.A. (1970). Guanethidine and related agents. III. Antagonism by drugs which inhibit the norepinephrine pump in man. *J. Clin. Invest.* 49, 1596.

Mitchell, J.R., Jollow, D.J., Potter, W.Z., Davis, D.C., Gillette, J.R., and Brodie, B.B. (1973a). Acetaminophen-induced hepatic necrosis. 1. Role of drug metabolism. *J. Pharmacol. Exp. Ther.* 187, 185.

Mitchell, J.R., Jollow, D.J., Potter, W.Z., Gillette, J.R., and Brodie, B.B. (1973b). Acetaminophen-induced hepatic necrosis. IV. Protective role of glutathione. *J. Pharmacol. Exp. Ther.* 187, 211.

Mitchell, J.R., Thorgeirsson, U.P., Black, M., Timbrell, J.A., Snodgrass, W.R., Potter, W.Z., et al. (1975). Increased incidence of isoniazid hepatitis in rapid acetylators: possible relation to hydrazine metabolites. *Clin. Pharmacol. Ther.* 18, 70.

Moore, M.R. and Brodie, M.J. (1985). The porphyrias. *Med. Int.* 2, 604.

Moulds, R.F.W. and Denborough, M.A. (1974a). Biochemical basis of malignant hyperpyrexia. *Br. Med. J.* ii, 241.

Moulds, R.F.W. and Denborough, M.A. (1974b). Identification of susceptibility to malignant hyperpyrexia. *Br. Med. J.* ii, 245.

Mucklow, J.C. (1979). Compliance. In *Topics in therapeutics*, Vol. 5 (ed. D.M. Davies and M.D. Rawlins), p. 47. Pitman Medical, Tunbridge Wells.

Mucklow, J.C., Caraher, M.T., Henderson, D.B., Chapman, P.H., Roberts, D.F., and Rawlins, M.D. (1982). The relationship between individual dietary constituents and antipyrine metabolism in Indo-Pakistan immigrants to Britain. *Br. J. Clin. Pharmacol.* 13, 481

Murray, M. and Reidy, G.F. (1989). Selectivity in the inhibition of mammalian cytochrome P-450 in chemical agents. *Pharmacol. Rev.* 42, 85.

Naranjo, C.A., Bristo, U., and Mardonics, R. (1978). Adverse drug reactions in liver cirrhosis. *Eur. J. Clin. Pharmacol.* 13, 429

Nebert, D.W., Nelson, D.R., Adesnik, M., Coon, M.J., Estabrook, R.W., Gonzales, F.J., et al. (1989). The P-450 superfamily: updated listing of all gases and recommended nomenclatures for the chromosomal loci. *DNA* 8, 1.

Neuvonen, P.J. and Elonen, E. (1980a). Effect of activated charcoal on absorption and elimination of phenobarbitone, carbamazepine and phenylbutazone. *Eur. J. Clin. Pharmacol.* 17, 51.

Neuvonen, P.J. and Karkkainen, S. (1983). Effects of charcoal, sodium bicarbonate, and ammonium chloride on chlorpropamide kinetics. *Clin. Pharmacol. Ther.* 33, 386.

Neuvonen, P.J. and Pentilla, O. (1974). Effect of oral ferrous sulphate on the half-life of doxycycline in man. *Eur. J. Clin. Pharmacol.* 7, 361.

Neuvonen, P.J., Elonen, E., and Mattila, M.J. (1980b). Oral activated charcoal and dapsone elimination. *Clin. Pharmacol. Ther.* 27, 823.

Niell, H.B. (1977). Miconazole carrier solution hyperlipidemia and hematologic problems. *N. Engl. J. Med.* 296, 1479.

Nilsson, A., Engberg, G., Henneberg, S., Danielson, K., and De-Verdier, C.H. (1990). Inverse relationship between age-dependent erythrocyte activity of methemoglobin reductase and prilocaine-induced methaemoglobinaemia during infancy. *Br. J. Anaesth.* 64, 72.

Nimmo, J., Heading, R.C., Tothill, P., and Prescott, L.F. (1973). Pharmacological modification of gastric emptying:

effects of propantheline and metoclopramide on paracetamol absorption. *Br. Med. J.* i, 587.

Ochs, H.R., Carstens, G., and Greenblatt, D.J. (1980). Reduction in lidocaine clearance during continuous infusions by coadministration of propanolol. *N. Engl. J. Med.* 303, 373.

Ohlin, H., Jerntorp, P., Bergstrom, B., and Almer, L. (1982). Chlorpropamide-alcohol flushing aldehyde dehydrogenase activity and diabetic complications. *Br. Med. J.* 285, 838.

Ohnishi, S.T., Waring, A.J., Fang, S-RG, Horiuchi, K., Flick, J.L., Sadanaga, K.K., *et al.* (1986). Abnormal membrane properties of the sarcoplasmic reticulum of pigs susceptible to malignant hyperthermia: Modes of action of halothane, caffeine, dantrolene, and two other drugs. *Arch. Biochem. Biophys.* 247, 294.

O'Reilly, R.A. (1970). The second reported kindred with hereditary resistance to oral anticoagulant drugs. *N. Engl. J. Med.* 282, 1448.

O'Reilly, R.A., Aggeler, P.M., Hoag, M.S., Leong, L.S., and Kropatkin, M.L. (1964). Hereditary transmission of exception resistance to coumarin anticoagulant drugs. The first reported kindred. *N. Engl. J. Med.* 271, 809.

Ording, H. (1989). Pathophysiology of malignant hyperthermia. *Ann. Fr. Anesth. Reanim.* 8, 411.

Osman, M.A., Patel, R.B., Schuna, A., Sundstrom, W.R., and Welling, P.G. (1983). Reduction in oral penicillamine absorption by food, antacid and ferrous sulphate. *Clin. Pharmacol. Ther.* 33, 465.

Padfield, A. and Watkins, J. (1977). Allergy to diazepam. *Br. Med. J.* i, 575.

Pantuck, E.J., Pantuck, C.B., Garland, W.A., Muir, B.H., Wattenburg, L.W., Anderson, K-E., *et al.* (1979). Stimulatory effects of Brussel sprouts and cabbage on human drug metabolism. *Clin. Pharmacol. Ther.* 25, 88.

Parson, R.L. and Kaye, C.M. (1974). Plasma propranolol and practolol in adult coeliac disease. *Br. J. Clin. Pharmacol.* 1, 348P.

Pato, M.L. and Brown, G.M. (1963). Mechanisms of resistance of *Escherichia coli* to sulphonamides. *Arch. Biochem. Biophys.* 103, 443.

Paton, W.D.M. (1970). Receptors as defined by their pharmacological properties. In *Molecular properties of drug receptors* (ed. R. Porter and M. O'Connor). Churchill Livingstone, Edinburgh.

Pearson, C.M. and Kalyanaraman, K. (1972). The periodic paralyses. In *The metabolic basis of inherited disease* (ed. J.B. Stanburg, J.B. Wyngaarden, and D.S. Fredrickson), p. 1181. McGraw-Hill, New York.

Pearson, R.M. and Breckenridge, A. (1976). Renal function, protein binding and pharmacological response to diazoxide. *Br. J. Clin. Pharmacol.* 3, 169.

Perry, H.M., Sakanoto, A., and Tan, E.M. (1967). Relationship of acetylating enzyme to hydrallazine toxicity. *J. Lab. Clin. Med.* 70, 1020.

Plaa, G.L. (1978). The problems of low-incidence response. In *Proceedings of the first international congress of toxicology* (ed. G.L. Plaa and W.A.M. Duncan), p. 207. Academic Press, New York.

Pond, S., Jacobs, M., Marks, J., Gamcu, J., Goldschlagu, N., and Hansen, D. (1981). Treatment of digitoxin overdose with oral activated charcoal. *Lancet* ii, 1177.

Prandota, J. (1988). Clinical pharmacology of antibiotics and other drugs in cystic fibrosis. *Drugs* 35, 542.

Prescott, L.F. (1972). The modifying effects of physiological variables and diseases upon pharmacokinetics and/or drug response. In *Liver disease* (Proceedings of the fifth international congress on pharmacology), p. 73. Iuphar, Basle.

Prescott, L.F. (1974). Gastric emptying and drug absorption. *Br. J. Clin. Pharmacol.* 1, 189.

Prescott, L.F., Wright, N., Roscoe, P., and Brown, S.S. (1971). Paracetamol half-life and hepatic necrosis in patients with paracetamol overdosage. *Lancet* i, 519.

Prescott, L.F., Newton, R.W., Swainson, C.P., Wright, N., Forrest, A.R.W., and Matthew, H. (1974). Successful treatment of severe paracetamol overdosage with cysteamine. *Lancet* i, 588.

Prescott, L.F., Park, J., Ballantyne, A., Adriaenssens, P., and Proudfoot, A.T. (1977). Treatment of paracetamol (acetaminophen) poisoning with *N*-acetylcysteine. *Lancet* ii, 432.

Price, K. and Smith S.E. (1971). Cheese reactions and tyramine. *Lancet* i, 130

Pullar, T., Peaker, S., Martin, H., Bird, H., and Feely, M. (1988). The use of a pharmacological indicator to investigate compliance in patients with a poor response to antirheumatic therapy. *Br. J. Rheumatol.* 27, 381.

Pyke, D.A. and Leslie R.D.G. (1978). Chlorpropamide–alcohol flushing: a definition of its relation to non-insulin-dependent diabetes. *Br. Med. J.* ii, 1521.

Rane, A. (1980). Drug metabolism in the young. In *Proceedings of the first world conference of clinical pharmacology and therapeutics* (ed. P. Turner), p. 98. Macmillan, London.

Rawlins, M.D. (1974*a*). Kinetic basis for drug interactions. *Adverse Drug React. Bull.* 46, 152.

Rawlins, M.D. (1974*b*). Variability in response to drugs. *Br. Med. J.* iv, 91.

Rawlins, M.D. and Bateman, D.N. (1984). Contribution of absorption to variation in response to drug. In *Drug absorption* (ed. L.F. Prescott). Adis Press, Auckland.

Rawlins, M.D. and Smith, S.E. (1973). Influence of allopurinol on drug metabolism in man. *Br. J. Pharmacol.* 48, 693.

Prescott, L.F., Wright, N., Roscoe, P., and Brown, S.S. (1971). Paracetamol half-life and hepatic necrosis in patients with paracetamol overdosage. *Lancet* i, 519.

Rawlins, M.D. and Thompson, J.W. (1977). Pathogenesis of adverse drug reactions. In *Textbook of adverse drug reactions* (ed. D.M.Davies), p. 44. Oxford University Press.

Rawlins, M.D., Henderson, D.B., and Hijab, A.R. (1977). Pharmacokinetics of paracetamol (acetaminophen) after intravenous and oral administration. *Eur. J. Clin. Pharmacol.* 11, 283.

Robinson, D.S., Benjamin, D.M., and McCormack, J.J. (1971). Interaction of warfarin and nonsystemic gastrointestinal drugs. *Clin. Pharmacol. Ther.* 12, 491.

Rogers, K.J. and Thornton, J.A. (1969). The interaction between monoamine oxidase inhibitors and narcotic analgesics in mice. *Br. J. Pharmacol.* 36, 470.

Routledge, P.A., Chapman, P.H., Davies, D.M., and Rawlins, M.D. (1979). Factors affecting warfarin requirements. *Eur. J. Clin., Pharmacol.* 15, 319.

Saidman, L.J., Havard, E.S., and Eger, E.I. (1964). Hyperthermia during anesthesia. *JAMA* 190, 1029.

Sanders, G.L., Routledge, P.A., Ward, A., Davies, D.M., and Rawlins, M.D. (1979). Mean steady-state plasma concentrations of labetalol in patients undergoing antihypertensive therapy. *Br. J. Clin. Pharmacol.* 8, 153.

Sandle, G.I., Ward, A., Rawlins, M.D., and Record, C.O. (1983). Propranolol absorption in untreated coeliac disease. *Clin. Sci.* 63, 81.

Sandler, M. (1973). New look at monoamine oxidase inhibitors: the new biochemical background. *Proc. R. Soc. Med.* 66, 946.

Schmidt, K.L. and Mueller-Eckhardt, C. (1977). Agranulocytosis, levamisole, and HLA-B27. *Lancet* ii, 85.

Schneider, C.H., de Weck, A.L., and Stanble, E. (1971). Carboxymethylcellulose additives in penicillins and the elicitation of anaphylactic reactions. *Experientia* 27, 167.

Schreiber. A.J. and Simon, F.R. (1983). Estrogen-induced cholestasis: pathogenesis and treatment. *Hepatology* 3, 607.

Schroder,H. and Evans, D.A.P. (1972). Acetylator phenotype and adverse effects of sulphasalazine in healthy subjects. *Gut* 13, 278.

Schrogie, J.J. and Solomon, H.M. (1967). The anticoagulant response to bishydroxy-coumarin. II. The effect of D-thyroxine, clofibrate and norethandrolone. *Clin. Pharmacol. Ther.* 8, 70.

Schwartz, J.T., Reuling, F.H., Feinleib, M., Garrison, R.J., and Collie, D.J. (1972). Twin heritability study of the effect of corticosteroids on intraocular pressure. *J. Med. Genet.* 9, 137.

Scott, J. and Poffenbarger, P.L. (1979). Pharmacogenetics of tolbutamide metabolism in humans. *Diabetes* 28, 41.

Sellers, E.M. and Koch-Weser, J. (1971). Kinetics and clinical importance of displacement of warfarin from albumin by acidic drugs. *Ann. N.Y. Acad. Sci.* 179, 213.

Sessions, J.T., Minkel, H.P., Bullard, J.C., and Ingelfinger, F.J. (1954). The effect of barbiturates in patients with liver disease. *J. Clin. Invest.* 33, 1116.

Shahidi, N.T. (1967). Acetophenetidin sensitivity. *Am. J. Dis. Child.* 113, 81.

Shahidi, N.T. (1968). Hematotoxic effects of acetophenetidin. *Hosp. Pract.* 3, 73.

Shammas F.V. and Dickstein, K. (1988). Clinical pharmacokinetics in heart failure: an update. *Clin. Pharmacokinet.* 15, 94.

Shand, D.G. and Rangno, R.E. (1972). The disposition of propranolol. 1. Elimination during oral absorption in man. *Pharmacology* 7, 159.

Sheth, N.K., Rose, N.O., and Krueger, J.A. (1977). Side effects of miconazole for systemic mycoses. *N. Engl. J. Med.* 297, 787.

Simpson, N.E. and Kalow, W. (1966). Pharmacology and biological variation. *Ann. N.Y. Acad. Sci* 134, 864.

Sjöqvist, F., Hammer, W., Indestrom, C-M., LInd, M., Tuck, D., and Asberg, M. (1968). Plasma levels of monomethyl-ated tricyclic antidepressants and side-effects in man. *Excerpta Med. (Amst.) International Congress Series* 145, 246.

Smith, J.M. and Dodd, T.R.P., (1982). Adverse reactions to pharmaceutical excipients. *Adverse Drug React. Acute Poisoning Rev.* 1, 93.

Smith, R. (1984). Osteogenesis imperfecta. *Br. Med. J.* 289, 394.

Smith, R.L. (1973). *The excretory function of bile.* Chapman and Hall, London.

Smith, S.E. and Rawlins, M.D. (1973). *Variability in human drug response.* Butterworths, London.

Solomon, H.M. and Schrogie, J.J. (1967). Change in receptor site affinity: a proposed explanation for the potentiating effect of D-thyroxine on the anticoagulant response to warfarin. *Clin. Pharmacol. Ther.* 8, 797.

Solomons, C.C. and Myers, D.N. (1972). Hyperthermia of osteogenesis imperfecta and its relationship to malignant hyperthermia. In *International symposium on malignant hyperthermia* (ed. R.A. Gordan, B.A. Britt, and W. Kalow), p. 319. Thomas, Springfield, Illinois.

Somogyi, A. and Muirhead, M. (1987). Pharmacokinetic interactions of cimetidine. *Clin. Pharmacokinet.* 12, 321.

Spielberg, S.P., Gordan G.B., Blake, D.A., Goldstein, D.A., and Herlong, E.F. (1981). Predisposition to phenytoin hepatoxicity. *N. Engl. J. Med.* 305, 722.

Steffensen, G. and Pedersen S. (1986). Food induced changes in theophylline absorption from a once-a-day theophylline product. *Br. J. Clin. Pharmacol.* 22, 571.

Sulkowski, S.R. and Haserick, J.R. (1964). Simulated systemic lupus erythematosus from degraded tetracycline. *JAMA* 189, 152.

Sung, J.P. and Grendahl, J.G. (1977). Side effects of miconazole for systemic mycoses. *N. Engl. J. Med.* 297, 786.

Thomson, P.D., Melmon, K.L., Richardson, J.A., Cohn, K., Steinbrunn, W., Cudihee, R., *et al.* (1973). Lidocaine pharmacokinetics in advanced heart failure, liver disease, and renal failure in humans. *Ann. Intern. Med.* 78, 499.

Toivakka, E. and Hokkanen, E. (1965). The aggravating effect of streptomycin on the neuromuscular blockade in myasthenia gravis. *Acta Neurol. Scand.* 41 (suppl. 13), 275.

Travis, W.D., Kalafer, M.E., Robin, H.S., and Luifel, F.J. (1990). Hypersensitivity vasculitis with eosinophilia in a patient taking an L-tryptophan preparation. *Ann. Intern. Med.* 112, 301.

van Garsse, L.G.M.M. and Boeykens, P.P.H. (1990). Two patients with eosinophilia myalgia syndrome associated with tryptophan. *Br. Med. J.* 301, 21.

Venning, G.R. (1983). Identification of adverse reactions to new drugs. *Br. Med. J.* 286, 458.

Verbeeck, R.K., Branch, R.A., and Wilkinson, G.R. (1981). Drug metabolites in renal failure: pharmacokinetic and clinical implications. *Clin. Pharmacokinet.* 6, 329.

Vesell, E.S. (1972). Drug therapy: pharmacogenetics. *N. Engl. J. Med.* 287, 904.

Waldorff, S., Damgaard-Anderson, J., Heeboll-Nielsen, N., Nielsen, O.G., Moltke, E., Sorrenson, U., *et al.* (1978). Spironolactone-induced changes in digoxin kinetics. *Clin. Pharmacol. Ther.* 24, 162.

Walton, V.C., Howlett, M.R., and Seltzer, G.B. (1970). An-hydrotetracycline and 4-epiandrotetracycline in market tetracyclines and aged tetracycline products. *J. Pharmacol. Sci.* 59, 1160.

Wang, J.H. and Takemori, A.E. (1972). Studies on the transport of morphine into the cerebrospinal fluid of rabbits. *J. Pharmacol. Exp. Ther.* 183, 41.

Watkins, J. (1979). Anaphylactoid reactions to i.v. substances. *Br. J. Anaesth.* 51, 51.

Watkins, J., Allen, R., and Ward, A.M. (1978). Adverse response to alphadolone/alphaxolone: possible role of IgD. *Lancet* ii, 736.

Weatherall, D.J. and Hatton, C.S.R. (1987). Congenital haemolytic anaemias. *Med. Int.* 2, 1712.

Weiss, H.J., Aledort, L.M., and Kochwa, S. (1968). The effect of salicylates on the hemostatic properties of platelets in man. *J. Clin. Invest.* 47, 2169.

Welling, P.G. (1984). Interactions affecting drug absorption. *Clin. Pharmacokinet.* 9, 404.

West, J.R., Smith, H.W., and Chassis, H. (1948). Glomerular filtration rate, effective renal blood flow, and maximal tubular excretory capacity in infancy. *J. Pediatr.* 32, 10.

Whitelock, O. (ed.) (1959). Chlorpropamide and diabetes mellitus (Symposium). *Ann. N.Y. Acad. Sci.* 74, 411.

Whittaker, J.A. and Evans, D.A.P. (1970). Genetic control of phenylbutazone metabolism in man. *Br. Med. J.* iv, 323.

Wilkinson, D.S. (1972). Sensitivity to pharmaceutical additives. In *Mechanisms in drug allergy* (ed. C.H. Dash and H.E.H. Jones), p. 75. Longman, London.

Wilkinson, G.R., Guengerich, F.P., and Branch, R.A. (1989). Genetic polymorphism of S-mephenytoin hydroxylation. *Pharmacol. Ther.* 43, 53.

Williams, R.T. (1967). Comparative patterns of drug metabolism. *Fed. Proc. Fedn Am. Soc. Exp. Biol.* 26, 1029.

Woodhouse, K.W. and Wynne, H.A. (1988). Age-related changes in liver size and hepatic blood flow: the influence in drug metabolism in the elderly. *Clin. Pharmacokinet.* 15, 287.

Woodhouse, K.W., Williams, F.M., Mutch, E., Wright, P., James, O.F.W., and Rawlins, M.D. (1983). The effect of alcoholic cirrhosis on the activities of microsomal aldrin epoxidase, 7-ethoxycoumarin o-de-ethylase and epoxide hydrolase, and on the concentrations of reduced glutathione in human liver. *Br. J. Clin. Pharmacol.* 15, 667.

Woodhouse, K.W., Mutch, E., Williams, F.M., and James, O.F.W. (1984). The effect of age on pathways of drug metabolism in human liver. *Age Ageing* 13, 328.

Woodhouse, K.W., Williams, F., Mutch, E., Wynne, H., Rawlins, M.D., and James, O.F.W. (1988). Phase I drug metabolism in ageing. In *Falk Symposium No 47, Ageing and the gastrointestinal tract*, p. 255. MTP Press, Lancaster.

Wooley, P.H., Griffin, J., Payani, G.S., Batchelor, J.R., Welsh, K.I., and Gibson, T.J. (1980). HLA-DR antigens and toxic reaction to sodium aurothiomalate and D-penicillamine in patients with rheumatoid arthritis. *N. Engl. J. Med.* 303, 300.

Woolhouse, N.M. and Atu-Taylor, L.C. (1982). Influence of double genetic polymorphism on response to sulfamethazine. *Clin. Pharmacol. Ther.* 31, 377.

Woolhouse, N.M., Andoh, B., Mahgoub, A., Sloan, T.P., Idle, J.R., and Smith, R.L. (1979). Debrisoquine hydroxylation polymorphism amongst Ghanaians and Caucasians. *Clin. Pharmacol. Ther.* 26, 584.

Woosley, R.L., Drayer, D.E., Reidenberg, M.M., Nies, A.S., Carr, K., and Oates, J.A. (1978). Effect of acetylator phenotype on the rate at which procainamide induces antinuclear antibodies and the lupus syndrome. *N. Engl. J. Med.* 298, 1157.

WHO (World Health Organization) (1967). Standardisation of procedures for the study of glucose-6-phosphate dehydrogenase. *WHO Tech. Rep. Ser.* 366.

WHO (World Health Organization) (1973). Pharmacogenetics. *WHO Tech. Rep. Ser.* 524.

Zampaglione, N., Jollow, D.J., Mitchell, J.R., Stripp, B., Harwick, M., and Gillette, J.R. (1973). Role of detoxifying enzymes in bromobenzene-induced liver necrosis. *J. Pharmacol. Exp. Ther.* 187, 218.

Zbinden, G. (1980). Predictive value of pre-clinical drug evaluation. In *Proceedings of the first world conference on clinical pharmacology and therapeutics* (ed. P. Turner), p. 9. Macmillan, London.

4. Chromosome damage

N. P. BOWN and D. F. ROBERTS

Clinical cytogenetics — the study of chromosome abnormalities in relation to human pathology — developed following technical advances made between the late 1950s and the early 1970s. That DNA damage inflicted by radiation or chemicals may have cytogenetic effects, and may be detectable in chromosome analysis, has been known for many years, but it is only during the last decade that the importance of cytogenetic studies in mutagenicity testing has gained full recognition. This has in part followed from deficiencies in the alternative bacterial gene mutation tests but also reflects the growing appreciation of the role of chromosome aberration in reproductive loss, congenital malformation, and carcinogenesis (Basler 1987).

The nature of chromosome damage

Damage to chromosomes is detected during cell division. In interphase, between mitotic divisions, the chromosomes are long and threadlike, and cannot be individually distinguished under the microscope, though the cell nucleus is very active metabolically. Interphase is divided into three periods, G_1, S, and G_2: in the S (synthesis) period the amount of chromosomal material in the nucleus is doubled, while G_1 and G_2 are periods of metabolic activity and growth. In prophase of mitosis, the chromosomes contract and become more readily visible, and each can be seen to consist of two chromatids. Shortening of the chromosomes continues into metaphase, with sister chromatids still held together at the centromeres; it is in this stage that detailed observation of chromosome morphology and structure can be made. At metaphase, the chromosomes are arranged on the equator of the cell with the spindle structure connecting the centromere of each chromosome to the poles of the cell. All the centromeres then divide, separating the sister chromatids, which migrate to opposite poles of the cell under the control of the spindle apparatus. As the two sets of daughter chromosomes separate, the cytoplasm divides. Subsequently, nuclear and cell membranes are formed, and the daughter nuclei pass into the next interphase. Opportunities for exogenous agents to interfere with the chromosomes arise first in interphase during the manufacture of the DNA required for the daughter chromosomes, secondly during prophase, when chromatids condense, and thirdly during anaphase when the sister chromatids separate.

Similarly, in meiosis (the production of gametes) there are opportunities for damage between cell divisions, during replication, and in the separation of chromosomes in each of the two consecutive divisions that are involved in the process.

Substances that cause chromosome damage are termed clastogens (after Shaw 1970).

Chromosome damage may be apparent in several forms:
1. gaps: small discontinuities in individual chromatids or in both chromatids of a single chromosome;
2. breaks: involving either a single chromatid, or both chromatids at the same point, and resulting in a deletion and an acentric fragment;
3. chromosome exchanges: translocations, rings, inversions, dicentrics, and other structural alterations;
4. pulverization: extensive destruction of the chromosomes resulting from large numbers of breaks.

In some studies the types of damage are classified as stable — that is, those that are retained over a series of cell divisions (Cs cells), and those that are unstable and disappear relatively rapidly (Cu). Diagrams of the effects of breaks are shown in Figure 4.1, and examples of damage in Figure 4.2.

Chromosome mutagenicity testing

The techniques of experimental examination fall into two categories. The first involves *in vitro* cultures, usually of peripheral blood lymphocytes stimulated to divide by phytohaemagglutinin (PHA). The amounts of damage inflicted on the chromosomes by the addition to such cultures of varying drug concentrations are then compared with control values. Secondly, *in vivo* damage may be examined, using metaphase cells — again, most conveniently blood lymphocytes — from patients undergoing drug therapy, and comparing their levels of chromosome damage with cells from matched controls not exposed to the drug. *In vivo* procedures have frequently been applied to animal studies, but cytogenetic data from such experiments cannot be directly extrapolated to humans because species differ in their drug metabolism both in terms of metabolic rates and by variations in biochemical pathways.

Scoring of gaps, breaks, and other forms of chromatid and chromosome lesions has been well established since the early days of human cytogenetics. The development of reliable chromosome banding techniques in the early 1970s allowed symmetrical chromosome rearrange-

ments, (i.e. exchanges that do not alter the shapes of the chromosomes), which were previously undetectable by solid staining, to be recorded. Subsequently, the development of more sophisticated techniques, most notably the sister chromatid exchange (SCE) method, has allowed new approaches to the study of chromosome damage. The SCE method involves incubation of cell cultures for two cycles of DNA replication in the presence of 5-bromodeoxyuridine (BudR) and differential staining to give the 'harlequin' pattern shown in Figure 4.2. SCE represents rearrangements of material within a given chromosome and provides a very sensitive indicator of genotoxicity, since they may often be induced at mutagen levels too low to produce classical chromosome aberrations. Only 70 per cent of studies show a close correlation between SCE frequencies and the incidence of classical chromosome abnormalities (Gebhart 1981). This suggests that different mechanisms of lesion for-

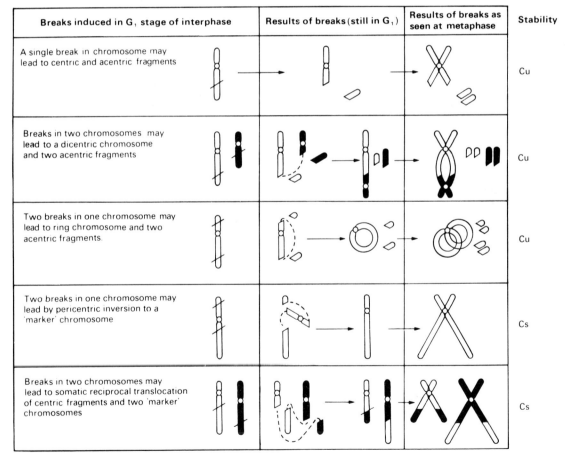

Breaks induced in G₁ stage of interphase	Results of breaks (still in G₁)	Results of breaks as seen at metaphase	Stability
A single break in chromosome may lead to centric and acentric fragments			Cu
Breaks in two chromosomes may lead to a dicentric chromosome and two acentric fragments			Cu
Two breaks in one chromosome may lead to ring chromosome and two acentric fragments.			Cu
Two breaks in one chromosome may lead by pericentric inversion to a 'marker' chromosome			Cs
Breaks in two chromosomes may lead to somatic reciprocal translocation of centric fragments and two 'marker' chromosomes			Cs

FIG. 4.1
Mechanisms of chromosome breakage and rearrangement. (After Stevenson *et al.* 1971.)

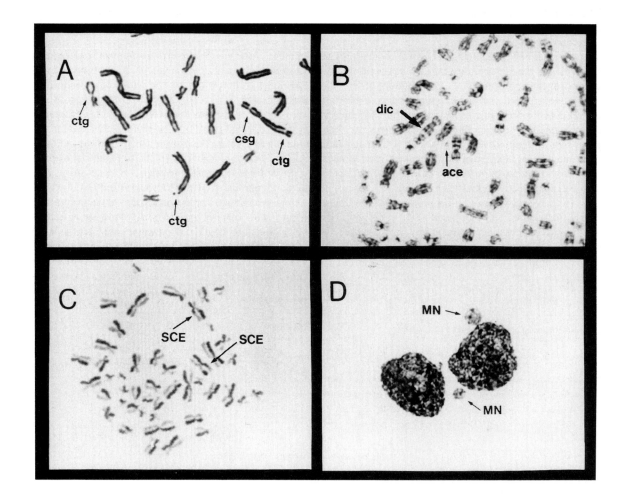

Fig. 4.2
Chromosome damage in human lymphocytes: (a) part of a metaphase cell showing chromosome and chromatid gaps;
(b) G-banded prearation showing a dicentric chromosome and an acentric fragment; (c) metaphase cell stained to demonstrate
sister chromatid exchanges; (d) micronuclei in a preparation treated with cytochalasin B.

mation may be involved in the two phenomena, with the implication that SCE techniques should be regarded as a useful addition to and not a replacement for traditional methods of measuring chromosome damage.

In recent mutagenicity testing the use of 'micronuclei' for *in vivo* damage scoring has been investigated. These result from the exclusion from daughter nuclei of acentric chromosome fragments (and also of whole chromosomes if the spindle apparatus has been damaged); in interphase, these fragments then appear as small micronuclei separate from the main nucleus (Heddle *et al.* 1983). By the use of cytochalasin B, which allows nuclear division but blocks cytoplasmic separation, cells with

micronuclei can be scored rapidly and reliably.

Very large numbers of cells could potentially be scored by the application of chromosome-specific DNA probes to interphase nuclei. This approach — using a Y chromosome-specific probe labelled either radioactively or by immunofluorescence — has recently been used by De Sario and others (1990) in an investigation of the *in vitro* effects of diethylstilboestrol, but only aneuploidy is detected and structural aberrations cannot be scored.

Classical chromosome damage, SCE, and micronuclei all occur spontaneously in normal cells; clastogenicity studies involve screening for excess damage superimposed on this background rate.

The significance of induced chromosome damage

The significance of induced chromosome damage lies in the role of chromosome aberration in both carcinogenesis and in reproduction.

The non-random involvement of chromosome changes in leukaemias and solid tumours, and the elucidation of chromosome rearrangement as a mechanism of oncogene activation, underlie concern about the carcinogenic potential of clastogenic agents. Susceptibility to genetic damage — or inability to repair such damage — is well known as the basis of the 'chromosome fragility syndromes' such as ataxia telangiectasia, Bloom's syndrome, and Fanconi's pancytopenia (Sandberg 1983). Furthermore, a number of studies demonstrate chromosome instability in cells from cancer patients; for example, Brown and colleagues (1985) investigated patients who had two or more primary tumours (and could therefore be regarded as having an inherent susceptibility to cancer) and found elevated levels of chromosome aberrations and SCE in lymphocytes from 6 of 11 cases. An association between increased rates of *in vivo* lymphocyte chromosome breakage and skin cancer has also been reported (Nordenson *et al.* 1984), while reduced ability to repair bleomycin-generated chromosome damage has been correlated with cancer risk in both a large family affected by high incidences of diverse cancers (Liang *et al.* 1989), and in lymphocytes of 19 patients with testicular cancer who showed elevated levels of chromosome damage compared with controls (Vorechovsky and Zaloudik 1989). Chromosome instability has also been documented in patients with testicular cancer who had not been exposed to chemotherapeutic drugs (van den Berg-de Ruiter *et al.* 1990). Thus, there appear to be strong grounds for concern that agents promoting somatic chromosome mutation could be involved in the initiation of human cancers.

The other main area in which induced chromosome damage may have a significant deleterious effect is in reproduction and embryogenesis. The induction of chromosome mutations in gametes or their precursors may result in either reduced fertility or in chromosomally abnormal offspring. Genetically unbalanced embryos may be either aneuploid as a result of damage to the meiotic spindle, or partially aneuploid as a result of recombination of a structural chromosome abnormality. Such embryos are likely to abort spontaneously and usually show congenital abnormalities if they survive to full-term and birth. Consequently, while the selection inherent in the processes of gametogenesis and in early embryo development probably eliminates the majority of germ cell mutations, the potential hereditary effects of induced chromosome damage are serious.

Genesca and others (1990) compared the incidence of structural chromosome aberration in both lymphocytes and spermatozoa from four treated cancer patients (two after chemotherapy, two after radiotherapy). In all four individuals there were elevated frequencies of cells showing chromosome damage in both tissues when compared with control series. The frequencies of damaged cells were very significantly higher in the spermatozoa than in the lymphocytes; this suggests that extrapolations from studies of somatic cell clastogenicity to potential effects on germ cells may not be straightforward.

The experience of aristolochic acid well illustrates the potential importance of clastogenicity testing of medicinal agents. This drug was in common use for a number of purposes until its abrupt withdrawal from the market in 1981 following evidence of potent carcinogenic effects in experimental rats. About 100 manufacturers of approximately 250 products were affected by the withdrawal of this drug. Abel and Schimmer (1983) subsequently investigated the *in vitro* chromosome-damaging properties of this substance to establish whether cytogenetic studies could have provided advance warning of genotoxic potential. Significant dose-dependent increases in both chromosome damage and SCE were apparent in lymphocyte cultures exposed to aristolochic acid.

Clastogenic compounds have been found in most of the major classes of drugs, including the cytostatic and antineoplastic agents, antibiotics, psychotropic drugs, anticonvulsants, immunosuppressants, and oral contraceptives, and also among drugs in social and illicit use.

The effect of drugs

Antibiotic and antineoplastic drugs

Of the therapeutic drugs, those on which the most investigation has been carried out are the antibiotic and antineoplastic agents, possibly because the action of many of these is directed through the DNA and RNA, and thus is likely to cause chromosome damage.

The clastogenic properties of cyclophosphamide have been recognized for many years, induced chromosome damage having been reported both *in vitro* (Urba 1971) and *in vivo* (Schmid and Bauchinger 1973; Dobos *et al.* 1974). The need to take physiological factors into account in considering genotoxic drug effects is illustrated by the work of Sargent and others (1987). These authors reported statistically significant increases in chromosome breakage in lymphocyte cultures exposed to

0.001–0.00001 μg per ml cyclophosphamide. Whole blood cultures, on the other hand, did not show chromosome instability even at 0.2 μg per ml since binding of the drug to red blood cells prevents activation.

An *in vitro* study by Raposa in 1978 of a range of cytostatic drugs demonstrated increased SCE frequencies after exposure to vincristine, cytosine arabinoside, and lycurium at doses too low to produce significant levels of classical chromosome damage. The number of gaps and breaks induced *in vitro* in lymphocyte cultures by treatment with busulphan and triaziquone, however, showed a distinct dependence on dose and on the stage of the cell cycle at the time of treatment (Gebhart 1971).

Lomustine (CCNU), used in melanoma cases, seems to cause prolonged and cumulative increases in SCE levels. In a study by Lambert and colleagues (1979), one patient demonstrated higher lymphocyte SCE frequencies 8 weeks after a second dose of lomustine than were found 6 weeks after the first dose.

Melphalan has been the subject of several investigations. Lambert and others (1984) examined lymphocyte chromosomes from 50 patients with ovarian cancer, and found that 5.4 per cent of the cells showed chromosome aberrations, compared with 2.3 per cent in the control group. Since chromosome aberrations were detected in circulating lymphocytes 7–8 years after treatment, this suggests that genetic damage had been inflicted on haematological progenitor cells — an interesting observation in view of the fact that the commonest secondary cancer in melphalan-treated patients is leukaemia. These findings have been strongly supported in a recent study of peripheral blood cells from 14 cancer patients; Mamuris and co-workers (1989) recorded an even more striking elevation in chromosome rearrangements, these being present in 21.5 per cent of patients' cells compared with 1.2 per cent of cells from healthy controls. Chromosomes 5 and 7 were the most frequently involved — these are also the chromosomes most frequently rearranged in secondary leukaemias.

Methotrexate is widely used as a prophylactic measure against CNS involvement in leukaemias. The clastogenic effects of this agent have long been recognized both *in vitro* (e.g. Mondello *et al.* 1984) and *in vivo* (Krogh Jensen and Nyfors 1979).

Dose-dependent clastogenic effects have been reported for cisplatinum both in human cells *in vitro* (Srb *et al.* 1986) and from an *in vivo* mouse study (Tandon and Sodhi 1985).

Neocarzinostatin has been shown to be a powerful inducer of chromosome and chromatid aberrations *in vitro*, but relatively poor at inducing SCE (Psaraki and Demopoulos 1988). A dose effect was noted for SCE induction, but only to a maximum of twice the control values.

Interferon is currently the subject of a clinical trial as a therapeutic agent in chronic myeloid leukaemia. There was no evidence for any clastogenic effect — either as chromosome aberrations or SCE — of interferon in a study of *in vitro* lymphocytes carried out by Vijayalaxmi in 1982.

Unusual forms of chromosome damage, such as 'uncompleted-packing mitotic figures' and 'free chromatin structures', were reported to be induced *in vitro* by the antitumour/antibiotic complex pingyanymycin (Heng *et al.* 1988).

Of the antibiotics used as antineoplastic agents, doxorubicin (adriamycin) — an inhibitor of nucleic acid synthesis — was shown by Neustad (1978) to cause a significant rise in lymphocyte SCE levels *in vitro* (9.6 SCE per cell, after exposure to 1 ng of doxorubicin compared with 4.8 SCE per cell for controls). The chromosome-damaging effect of bleomycin therapy was investigated by Bornstein and others (1971). Chromosomes from bone marrow preparations were screened for aberrations both before, on the last day of, and one month after bleomycin therapy in four carcinoma patients. All post-therapy samples were shown to contain a higher proportion of mitoses with chromosome abnormalities. The effect is specific to early interphase in the cell cycle (Dresp *et al.* 1978), since the main types of aberration after exposure early in the cycle were dicentrics and deletions, but in the G_2 phase were chromatid breaks: the amount of damage was linearly related to dose. The work of Vorechovsky and Zaloudik (1989) demonstrating enhanced susceptibility to bleomycin-induced chromosome damage in cancer patients has been mentioned above. Another intriguing result observed by Vijayalaxmi and Burkart (1989) was the acquisition of resistance to chromosome damage by cultured lymphocytes. Cells conditioned to a low concentration of bleomycin showed much less damage when subsequently challenged with a high dose of the drug or with X-rays, compared with cells not exposed to the conditioning regimen; the findings suggest that if therapeutic use involved appropriate concentrations and durations, the efficacy of the drug could be reduced, since its action depends on damaging the DNA of tumour cells.

RNA-inhibiting antibiotics, for example daunorubicin (Sinkus 1972), are clastogenic *in vitro*, while the work of Whang-Peng and others (1969) showed an increase of chromosome aberrations and exchanges in bone marrow metaphases of three out of seven patients receiving daunorubicin treatment.

The aminoglycoside antibiotic doxorubicin, a chemotherapeutic agent in the treatment of solid tumours and leukaemia, increases sister chromatid exchanges and chromosome aberrations *in vitro* and *in vivo*, though these disappear rapidly *in vivo* (Neustad 1978).

On the question of possible genotoxic hazards faced by medical staff in handling cytostatic and cytotoxic drugs, results have been mixed and contradictory; for example, Nikula and co-workers (1984) reported significantly raised numbers of chromosomally aberrant lymphocytes, compared with controls, in 11 nurses handling cytostatic agents, but Benhamou and others (1988), found no increase in SCE rates or chromosomal damage in 29 nurses handling these compounds.

A wide range of antibiotics has been assessed for clastogenic potential. Stevenson and Patel (1973*a*) reported an increase of gaps and breaks in lymphocyte cultures of patients treated with chlorambucil. There were similar findings (Palmer *et al*. 1984, 1985) in a group of 10 patients taking the drug for up to 68 months at doses of 2–6 mg per day. A highly significant elevation in SCE levels was noted, the excess correlating with both dose and length of treatment. Follow-up studies suggested that the damage was permanent, or at least very long-lasting.

Ampicillin and carbenicillin were investigated by Jaju and colleagues (1984) in human lymphocyte cultures. Chromosome damage was not observed at therapeutic plasma concentrations, but did appear at higher doses. SCE were not induced by either drug at any concentration tested.

Several antibiotics that inhibit DNA synthesis, such as mitomycin C (Cohen and Shaw 1964), produce chromosome breaks *in vitro*, even at low concentrations. Indeed, the reliable chromosome-damaging action of mitomycin C forms the basis of the cytogenetic diagnosis of Fanconi's pancytopenia — lymphocytes from patients with this chromosome fragility syndrome are less able to repair mitomycin-induced damage *in vitro* than lymphocytes from normal controls.

It is generally considered that the protein inhibitors puromycin, streptomycin, and the tetracyclines have no chromosome-breaking effect (Shaw 1970). The evidence for the genotoxicity of chloramphenicol was reviewed by Rosenkranz (1988). While clastogenic action has been reported in human cells in a number of studies involving both *in vivo* and *in vitro* exposure to chloramphenicol, negative results have been obtained in a number of other test systems for mutagenic potential, and Rosenkranz proposed that the chromosome-damaging properties of this antibiotic do not indicate genuine genotoxicity.

In 1982 the broad-spectrum antibiotic cephaloridine was shown to cause chromosome damage *in vitro* (Jaju *et al*. 1982). A dose effect was reported, and cephaloridine may be considered clastogenic at the upper levels of permissible therapeutic doses. Phleomycin has been reported to show similar properties (Jacobs *et al*. 1969).

Immunosuppressants

In 1979, Schuler and others investigated chromosome damage and SCE in patients with chronic renal disease receiving immunosuppressive drugs. Chromosome stability was tested by scoring breaks after exposure of lymphocytes to the alkylating agent lycurium. All treatments were found to produce significantly raised aberration frequencies, and dose effects were noted for all drug regimens except mercaptopurine monotherapy. The greatest clastogenic effects were recorded in patients receiving high doses of cyclophosphamide or chlorambucil, or a combination of vinblastine sulphate, cyclophosphamide, mercaptopurine, and prednisolone.

For azathioprine, there are contradictory results from various studies of chromosome stability. Apelt and others (1981) demonstrated no significant clastogenic properties *in vitro*, with SCE levels unchanged from control values at all concentrations tested. The *in vivo* study, on the other hand, did reveal a higher incidence of gross chromosome damage compared with controls.

An intriguing case report by Ostrer and colleagues (1984) described the simultaneous *de novo* occurrence of a deletion [del(7q)] and a reciprocal translocation [t(6;14)] in the constitutional karyotype of an infant with congenital abnormalities. The mother, who had lupus erythematosus, was receiving azathioprine and prednisone therapy at the time of conception and throughout pregnancy, but her lymphocytes showed no significant increase in chromosome damage or SCE. The authors proposed that, in view of the rarity of multiple *de novo* structural rearrangements, this karyotype might have been drug-induced.

Anticonvulsants

Initial cytogenetic studies of the anticonvulsant drugs phenytoin and ethotoin (e.g. Brogger 1970) suggested that these agents were non-clastogenic *in vivo*, although Muniz and others (1969) were able to induce structural chromosome aberrations in lymphocytes *in vitro* using phenytoin at clinically toxic doses.

Two subsequent studies of women treated with various anticonvulsant drugs and of their children exposed *in utero* (Neuhauser *et al*. 1970; Grosse *et al*. 1972) described increased numbers of metaphases with structural aberrations, but without apparent teratogenic effect. It seems that the fetal abnormalities known to occur after maternal treatment with these and related drugs do not derive directly from gross chromosome damage. A study in 1977 on bone marrow preparations from 22 epileptics suggested that phenytoin is non-clastogenic at therapeutic levels, the mean frequencies of classical chromosome aberrations being 0.5 per cent in patients and 0.4 per cent in the 20 healthy controls (Knuutila *et al.* 1977). These findings appear to differ from those of an *in vitro* study (Garcia Sagredo 1988) of phenytoin, ethosuximide, and phenobarbitone. Lymphocyte cultures were exposed to three drug concentrations ranging from 50 per cent to 300 per cent of therapeutic tissue levels, and significant dose-related increases in chromosome aberrations compared with control values were documented for all cultures.

SCE studies of antiepileptic drugs have produced similarly contradictory results. A trial carried out in 1982 in nine children receiving phenytoin therapy revealed a highly significant increase in mean SCE levels, with controls showing an average of 6.49 SCE per cell and patients 10.3 SCE per cell (Habedank *et al.* 1982). Riedel and Obe (1984), on the other hand, were unable to demonstrate induced SCE or chromosome aberrations after exposing cultured Chinese hamster ovary cells to phenytoin, primidone, and phenobarbitone.

Schaumann and colleagues (1985) investigated patients receiving carbamazepine (CBZ) therapy. No significant differences were found in *in vivo* SCE or chromosome damage in lymphocytes between nine patients and their controls. The *in vitro* study, scoring chromosome breaks in blood cultures from six healthy male donors, revealed a strong dose-related response starting at 10 μg per ml (therapeutic range in serum 4–12 μg per ml), but no induction of SCE at 5, 10, or 15 μg per ml. The authors suggested that the negative *in vivo* results are clinically more relevant than the positive *in vitro* result, since the latter arises from the failure of cultured lymphocytes metabolically to clear CBZ.

Psychotropic drugs

Nielsen and others (1968) reported increased damage to chromosomes in 17 patients treated with various psychotropic drugs, in particular, chlorpromazine, perphenazine, and LSD.

The effect of chlorpromazine was confirmed *in vitro* by Kamada and co-workers (1971). Cohen and colleagues (1972), however, investigating perphenazine and chlorpromazine, found no significant differences in chromosome damage between controls and patients before,

during, or after 6 weeks of treatment with the two drugs. In accounting for the discrepancies between their findings and those of previous trials, these authors pointed to the lack of established pretreatment damage levels in earlier studies, and to the use of orphenadrine in some patients — the clastogenic effect of which had not been investigated.

The tranquillizer trifluoperazine was shown by Jenkins (1970) to cause an increase in cells showing chromosome breaks in patients as compared with controls, the percentages being 27.7 and 10.2 respectively. Despite reports in 1969 that lithium might be a chromosome-breaking agent, Garson (1981) found no significant increase in SCE frequencies in 23 psychiatric patients when compared with 19 age-matched controls. Diazepam was found not to have any damaging effect at any concentration or exposure (Staiger 1969). Imipramine is a widely used antidepressant; there are isolated reports of an association with fetal skeletal defects, but *in vitro* study of cultures from seven donors showed no increase in chromosome breaks at any concentration (Fu and Jarvik 1977).

A significant clastogenic effect was reported for thioridazine (Saxena and Ahuja 1982); chromosome aberration frequencies were significantly elevated in psychiatric patients taking this drug when compared with both psychiatric and normal controls.

Contraceptive agents

Cytogenetic investigations of users of the contraceptive pill have produced controversial results.

Carr (1970) studied spontaneous abortions occurring within 6 months of discontinuing oral contraception and recorded a striking elevation in the incidence of polyploidy, with triploidy occurring four to five times more frequently in fetuses of the post-contraceptive group than in the controls, and a sixfold increase in tetraploidy.

McQuarrie and others (1970) found an increase in chromosome gaps and in the incidence of triploidy in babies born to mothers using oral contraception compared with those born to control mothers. There was no difference, however, in other aneuploidies or frequencies of chromosome breaks between the two groups of babies.

In 1975, a US investigation demonstrated significantly higher levels of chromosome breaks in the lymphocytes of nulligravid women taking the pill (7.8 per cent of metaphases showing breaks) compared with nulligravidae who had never used oral contraceptives (5.5 per cent) (Littlefield *et al.* 1975). These increased breakage frequencies could not, however, be correlated with the duration of contraceptive use. In contrast, Bishun (1976) concluded that the overall findings suggest no increase in chromosomal damage in women who had taken oral contraceptives at normal prescribed dosage for moderately long periods of time before conceiving.

An SCE investigation in 1979 of 15 normal women, 15 women in the third trimester of pregnancy, and 15 pill-users (taking a combined D-norgestrel/ethinyloestradiol prepaaration for between 6 and 24 months) showed a significantly (75 per cent) increased mean SCE per cell in the women using the oral contraceptives (Murthy and Prema 1979).

No significant induction of either chromosome abnormalities or of SCE in lymphocytes *in vitro* was observed in a 1985 study of diethylstilboestrol (DES) and oestradiol carried out by Banduhn and Obe. Micronuclei were noted, but were ascribed by the authors to mitotic spindle disruption rather than chromosome damage. Henderson and Regan (1985) exposed pregnant mice to high doses of diethylstilboestrol dipropionate and then examined maternal bone marrow and fetal liver for clastogenic effects. No increases were apparent in SCE, chromosome breakage, or micronuclei, although the levels of aneuploid and polyploid cells were elevated in both systems. The ability of DES to induce aneuploidy in cultured human cells has been confirmed by De Sario and others (1990). Using the *in situ* hybridization technique, these workers demonstrated a significant dose-related increase in hyperdiploidy in lymphocytes exposed to three concentrations of DES.

A more recent study compared peripheral lymphocyte chromosome aberrations in 44 women taking hormonal contraception for 7–98 months (mean 38 months) with those in 44 controls who had never used the pill (Pinto 1986). The women using hormonal contraception showed highly significant increases in both the proportions of abnormal cells and in numbers of chromosome aberrations per cell (p<0.0001 in both cases).

The antispermatogenic properties of gossypol, and its potential as a male contraceptive agent, have prompted several studies of its effects on human chromosomes. Tsui and colleagues (1983), for example, scored *in vitro* chromosome aberrations, SCE, and micronuclei in blood cultures exposed to gossypol — all with negative results (SCE frequencies did increase with increasing gossypol concentrations, but even at their highest levels were not significantly greater than in controls). These workers conceded that their results did not rule out effects on spermatogonial chromosomes. *In vitro* culture of seminiferous tubule segments allowed De-yu and others (1988) to study the mutagenic properties — as measured by micronucleus formation — of gossypol in

primary spermatocytes at the pachytene-diakinesis stage of meiosis. A small but significant increase in micronucleus formation was observed at subcytotoxic concentrations.

Fertility-enhancing drugs

Increasingly large numbers of couples affected by infertility are undergoing *in vitro* fertilization procedures. Most such techniques rely on the pharmacological induction of ovulation, and the potential adverse effects of the agents used are clearly a matter for concern.

Boue and Boue (1973) produced evidence that the ovulation-inducing drugs human menopausal gonadotrophin and human chorionic gonadotrophin could cause increased chromosome abnormalities in first-trimester abortions if conception occurred during the first two months after treatment. This was corroborated by a prospective study. From patients studied before and after clomiphene therapy, Charles and co-workers (1973) reported increased heteroploidy and chromatid lesions in endometrial tissue.

Bromocriptine, a dopamine agonist used against hyperprolactinaemic infertility, was the subject of cytogenetic investigations by Czeizel and others (1989). They compared peripheral blood lymphocytes from 31 children conceived after bromocriptine administration with those in 31 control children whose mothers had had no fertility problems. No evidence was found of chromosome mutagenic effects, although the study involved merely the recording of loss or gain of whole chromosomes.

Clastogenicity studies of other therapeutic drugs

The clastogenic properties of methotrexate *in vitro* are well established. Melnyk and others (1971) examined lymphocytes, fibroblasts, bone marrow, and testicular tissue from 27 male patients with psoriasis being treated with methotrexate: a significant increase in chromosome damage was found only in the bone marrow cells.

Stevenson and others (1971, 1973*a,b*) investigated a number of drugs thought likely to be clastogens. Positive *in vivo* results were obtained for phenylbutazone in lymphocytes from patients with osteoarthrosis, but no damage was recorded in patients taking trimethoprim or sulphamethoxazole.

Isoniazid, an antituberculous agent, has been extensively studied for evidence of chromosome-damaging ability. Early studies (e.g. Obe *et al.* 1973; Bauchinger *et al.* 1978) produced largely negative results. Isoniazid, however, is often used in combination with other drugs, and for at least two of these combinations evidence has emerged for a synergistic chromosome-damaging effect *in vivo*. In one study, chromosome damage in lymphocytes from 10 tuberculous patients receiving a combination of isoniazid and *p*-aminosalicylic acid was compared with that found in control groups of 10 healthy individuals and 10 patients not receiving therapy (Jaju *et al.* 1981); 11.3 per cent more damage — mostly single chromatid gaps and breaks — was recorded in the patients on combination therapy. A significant increase in the frequency of chromatid gaps and breaks was also reported for the isoniazid/thiacetazone combination (Ahuja *et al.* 1981), although the clastogenicity of thiacetazone itself was not determined.

The clastogenic effects of frusemide, a potent diuretic, were demonstrated by Jameela and others in 1979. Lymphocytes were exposed *in vitro* to three different frusemide concentrations for either 24 or 72 hours. A clear dose response was observed.

Initial studies of the analgesic drug aspirin either failed to demonstrate a chromosome-damaging action (Mauer *et al.* 1970), or showed a weak effect unlikely to be of *in vivo* significance (Loughman 1970). In a study based on long-term fibroblast cultures, however, Meisner and Inhorn (1972) recorded induction of chromosome rearrangements following exposure to 100 and 250 μg per ml. Thus, high concentrations of aspirin at the cellular level appear to be capable of exerting a mutagenic effect.

A strikingly positive clastogenic result was obtained by Gorla and others (1989) in an investigation of nifurtimox, a common treatment for Chagas' disease (trypanosomiasis). Six patients using this drug showed an average 13-fold increase in chromosome aberrations per cell compared with eight untreated patients (23.5 aberrations per 100 cells compared with 1.7 per 100 cells). The authors recommend limiting the use of this agent whenever possible in view of this genotoxic action.

MacKay and colleagues (1988) also reported strongly positive results with clear dosage correlations for the *in vitro* induction of both SCE and micronuclei by sulphasalazine in peripheral blood lymphocytes. It had previously been unclear whether the elevated chromosome damage and SCE reported in patients with inflammatory bowel disease being treated with this agent represented the effects of the disease itself or a by-product of treatment. The results of this *in vitro* study strongly implicated the treatment.

Watson and colleagues (1976) reported elevated frequencies of gaps, dicentrics and translocations in cultured lymphocytes of diabetic patients undergoing treatment with sulphonylurea. The subsequent demonstration of normal levels of structural chromosome aberrations and of SCE in untreated diabetics (Vormittag 1985) suggest that sulphonylurea drugs may have clastogenic potential.

Unambiguously negative results have been recorded for the antihypertensive serotonin derivative indorenate (Madrigal-Bujaidar and Rosas-Planaguma 1989), with no increases in SCE frequencies or levels of chromosome aberrations in either mouse bone marrow after *in vivo* exposure, or in human lymphocytes after *in vitro* exposure. Similarly, no evidence was obtained for any clastogenic effect of clodronate (dichloromethylene biphosphonate) in 10 patients with Paget's disease: frequencies of chromosome breaks and SCE did not alter significantly between cells examined before the start of therapy and after 2 months of therapy (Borgstrom *et al.* 1987). Finally, the use of feverfew by migraine sufferers appears not to be associated with any risk of chromosome damage, no meaningful differences being noted between SCE levels and chromosome aberrations in 30 patients taking feverfew preparations daily over a period of 11 months and in 30 matched controls (Anderson *et al.* 1988).

Penicillamine, used against rheumatoid arthritis, when tested for *in vitro* clastogenicity in bone marrow metaphases by Jensen and others (1979) produced no increase in either structural chromosome abnormalities or in erythroblast micronuclei. More recent work (e.g. Speit and Haupter 1987) has, however, demonstrated induction by this agent of both SCE and chromosome aberrations in cultured mammalian cells.

Drugs in social and illicit use

A very large amount of work on drug clastogenicity has been carried out on the hallucinogenic drugs, particularly LSD. The initial *in vitro* study was carried out by Cohen and others (1967*a,b*). A statistically significant increase in chromosome breaks was found at almost all concentrations and time periods tested. There followed a number of conflicting reports as several groups of workers repeated these experiments with mixed results. More recent work suggests that LSD causes chromosome damage only at concentrations far in excess of realistic tissue levels. Muneer, for example, in 1978, found no significant increase over control values in chromosome aberrations in lymphocytes exposed to LSD.

In parallel with the controversy over results of *in vitro* clastogenicity studies, investigations of *in vivo* chromosome damage in both illicit drug users and patients administered pure LSD for therapeutic purposes also proved contentious. Several groups examined lymphocyte metaphases from illicit LSD users; some found highly significant increases in chromosome abnormalities after relatively little drug exposure, while others could demonstrate no clastogenic effect even in users taking large doses of the drug. It was recognized that these investigations of illicit LSD users were hampered by a number of problems: for example, the accuracy of the information about doses and frequencies of use, the actual amounts of LSD in the compounds consumed, the pattern of multidrug abuse and the poor health and susceptibility to viral infection of the drug users.

In view of these problems, patients on therapeutic LSD were the subject of a number of chromosome studies. An extensive and well-controlled experiment was carried out in 1969 by Tjio and others. The chromosomes of 32 patients were studied before and after they had taken pure LSD; no increase in chromosome breakage was observed. Bender and Siva Sankar (1968) similarly found no increase over controls in chromosome damage in seven children treated with LSD. On the other hand, Hungerford and colleagues (1968) compared the amounts of chromosome breakage before and after three doses of LSD and also followed up four patients 1–6 months after treatment. The levels before treatment were the same as in controls. In the treated patients there was a transient increase in chromosome breakage which returned to the pretreatment level within 6 months after the final dose.

The chromosomes of children born to LSD users have also been analysed for breaks. Several reports have described individual cases showing elevated chromosome damage, but a study of 41 children born to drug users showed no overall significant increase in chromosomal breakage or rearrangement (Dumars 1971).

The consensus of opinion based on these studies is that high concentrations of LSD do produce chromosome damage *in vitro*, but that at the non-toxic concentrations found in the body there is no significant damage, and while LSD may have a transient and short-term effect on chromosomes *in vivo*, there is no proof that it inflicts long-term damage.

A similar problem of public interest concerns marijuana smoking. There is agreement that the addition of cannabis resin to human lymphocyte cultures does not increase the frequency of chromosomal abnormalities (e.g. Martin *et al.* 1973), but *in vivo* studies have produced both positive and negative findings. A prospective double-blind trial of the cumulative effects of medically supervised marijuana smoking failed to show any measurable effect (Matsuyama *et al.* 1977). Since then, however, evidence has been presented of a strongly positive effect in heroin/marijuana addicts; Chiesara and others (1983) described an incidence of chromosome

anomalies in cells of users of both drugs that was approximately eight times that found in users of marijuana alone, and approximately 21 times that in controls.

No clastogenic hazard was apparent in an *in vivo* study of peyote (mescaline) users carried out by Dorrance and co-workers in 1975, but another habit, the chewing of betel leaf, which is widespread in the tropics, may be deleterious; *in vitro* lymphocyte cultures from healthy donors showed an increase in chromosome damage related to the concentration of leaf extract applied to the culture (Sadasivan *et al.* 1978).

In 1978, Lambert and others reported a significant rise in SCE levels in cigarette smokers. This result was not unexpected since benzo(a)pyrene, the suspected precarcinogen in cigarette smoke, had previously been shown to double SCE levels in human lymphocytes *in vitro*. A dose effect was obvious when the smokers were subdivided according to consumption. The observation has been corroborated by other studies; for example, Kao-Shan and others (1987) found significantly elevated SCE levels in both bone marrow and peripheral blood metaphases, and also reported elevated expression of fragile sites at the cancer-associated breakpoints 3p14.2, 11q13.3, 22q12.2 and 11p13–p14.2. Tawn and Cartmell (1989) observed a fourfold increase in dicentric chromosomes in blood preparations from 12 moderate smokers compared to 12 age-matched controls. There was also a statistically significant increase in stable symmetrical aberrations (principally translocations). Since this type of damage is detectable only in banded preparations, the authors emphasize the importance of these techniques in studies of chronic clastogen exposure. The work of Sinues and colleagues (1990) on a series of 53 smokers compared with 41 non-smokers reinforces previous findings of dose-dependent damage.

Interestingly, cytogenetic damage has not been demonstrated in 'passive smokers'. A study of restaurant waiters showed no significant differences between smoking and non-smoking staff in terms of either chromosome aberrations or SCE (Sorsa *et al.* 1989). As part of the same study, these workers also measured SCE levels in cord-blood lymphocytes of newborn babies from 17 smoking and 25 non-smoking mothers. While a clear dose effect was apparent for SCE in the smokers themselves compared with the non-smokers, and while biochemical markers revealed tobacco smoke constituents at very nearly the same levels in maternal and fetal bloods at the time of birth, the SCE frequencies in the cord bloods were significantly lower for both groups. Thus the chromosome damage that has been well documented among active smokers cannot be demonstrated in those passively exposed in these two circumstances.

Ethanol, at realistic tissue concentrations, is probably a low-level mutagen. Alvarez and others (1980) exposed lymphocytes to 0.5 per cent ethanol (approximately half the blood level used to define intoxication in the United States) and recorded a 30 per cent rise in SCE frequency.

Finally, a drug that is in almost universal use in some measure — caffeine. Human lymphocytes in culture from volunteers after a regimen of 800 mg of caffeine daily for one month showed no significant increase in chromosome damage (Weinstein *et al.* 1972), the highest level of caffeine in the plasma was 30 μg per ml. *In vitro*, however, caffeine induced a high frequency of chromatid gaps and breaks. The damage was dose responsive: multiple exposure of lymphocytes to 30 μg per ml was without effect, but exposure to 250–750 μg per ml produced damage.

Caffeine also acts as a co-clastogen; that is, it enhances or even potentiates the chromosome-damaging properties of other clastogens. Increased frequencies of SCE and gross aberrations (including pulverized metaphases) are found in lymphocytes exposed to mitomycin C and other mutagens when caffeine is also present in the culture medium (Shiraishi *et al.* 1979; Faed and Mourelatos 1978).

Technical problems of measuring chromosome damage

It will be seen from the above that discrepancies between different reports of the damage done to chromosomes by a particular drug are very common. A number of factors contribute to this problem. Of primary concern is the question of controls. The normal controls used in different studies show wide variations in the frequency of chromosome damage, ranging from less than 1 per cent of cells being affected to perhaps 10 per cent. A survey of a large population has recently been published by Bender and others (1988). Chromosome damage and SCE were scored in lymphocytes from 493 subjects and correlations sought with age, race, smoking, and other variables. The only positive associations detected in this study were a strong effect of smoking on SCE levels, and a slight increase with age in the incidence of dicentrics (mean SCE levels in females were also found to be approximately 5 per cent higher than in males, but this simply corresponds to the extra chromosome material involved in the XX constitution compared with the XY). An overall average of eight SCE per cell was apparent in this sample. Schmickel (1967) found a chromosome breakage level of 1.21 per cent in 1569 normal individuals; this seems to correspond to the levels found by the majority of workers.

Variations may be attributable to several factors. First, there may be differences in the criteria on which measurements of damage are based, some workers including chromosome and chromatid gaps, while others exclude this type of aberration from the score of damage, and record only breaks and gross rearrangements.

Secondly, technical aspects of the tissue culture regimen — in particular the composition of the culture medium — can strongly influence the levels of chromosome damage. For example, Morita and colleagues (1989) established that pH changes in the tissue culture medium were capable by themselves of inducing chromosome damage in Chinese hamster ovary cells. This suggests that *in vitro* tests under non-physiological conditions may lead to false-positive results. Differences in the durations of cell culture can also cause discrepancies between different *in vitro* studies of a given drug — the action of the DNA and chromosome repair mechanisms do not allow direct comparisons between, for example, lymphocyte cultures harvested after 48 hours and similar cultures harvested after 72 hours. Differences between individuals in terms of the efficiency of DNA repair may also influence the levels of damage apparent after *in vivo* mutagen exposure — as a result of a number of studies (e.g. Vorechovsky and Zaloudik 1989), a spectrum of chromosomal stability is now envisaged among normal individuals quite apart from the clinically distinct chromosome breakage syndromes.

The findings of Schwartz and others (1990) have some serious implications for the design of SCE studies; while spontaneous SCE levels in their 24 subjects were relatively constant over time, significant variation between different sample days was apparent in the levels induced by bleomycin. This throws into question the validity of single observations of chemically induced SCE.

Another problem in the interpretation of chromosome mutagenicity data is that *in vitro* experiments do not necessarily reflect the condition *in vivo*. The body has complex mechanisms — which may not be available to cells in culture — for disposing of unwanted substances; for example, it was calculated by Loughman and colleagues (1967) that LSD is cleared from the body in about 4 hours. The drug is concentrated in the liver, where the highest level (five times that of the blood) will occur after 20 minutes, levelling off at a constant level of 3.5 times that of blood after 2 hours. For a 70 kg adult, a dose of 100 μg LSD would give a maximum concentration of 0.4 ng per g in blood and 1.2 ng per g in the liver. This is equivalent to the lowest of the *in vitro* levels, which produces no damage. In the same study, however, no increase was found in chromosome damage in a patient who had ingested 4000 μg the day before.

Schneider and Lewis (1982) compared the induction of SCE by four different mutagens in P388 tumour cells grown *in vitro* and *in vivo* in mice. The results showed that certain agents were more effective *in vitro*, while others were more potent *in vivo*, so that caution is necessary in comparing *in vitro* and *in vivo* mutagen screening data.

The most convincing demonstrations of the clastogenic actions of drugs are probably those *in vivo* studies in which the pretreatment levels of chromosome damage and SCE are established and compared with the levels following treatment. The scoring of large numbers of cells (from both the tissue exposed to the drug, and from carefully matched controls) allows greater confidence to be placed in the result, as does the examination of a range of different tissues — lymphocytes, bone marrow, fibroblasts, etc. After *in vivo* exposure, both lymphocytes and fibroblasts require some *in vitro* tissue culture before observation of metaphase cells is feasible. Bone marrow cell populations, on the other hand, are actively proliferating *in vivo* and only a minimal amount of *in vitro* culturing is necessary. For this reason, studies using a bone marrow system probably approximate most closely to the true *in vivo* action of the drug in question.

The detection of chromosome damage thus has implications for both carcinogenesis and teratogenesis, and clastogenicity testing using both SCE techniques and the scoring of large chromosome abnormalities is now established as an important part of drug safety evaluation. It is to be hoped that conflicting and equivocal results will become less common as the methods of cytogenetic analysis continue to improve, and as a degree of standardization emerges in terms of techniques and tissues used and types of damage recorded.

Mechanisms of drug action

The clastogenic drugs investigated exert their breaking effects by several different mechanisms. Those antibiotics which involve DNA inhibition (e.g. mitomycin C, a bifunctional alkylating agent) act by cross-linking the two backbones of the DNA by the formation of a covalent bond with a base. This is also the mechanism of the RNA-inhibiting drugs. The breaking of chromosomes that is observed can also be brought about by the direct scission of the DNA chain, as with some antineoplastic agents (e.g. bleomycin).

Many drugs do not act directly on the DNA molecule but exert an indirect effect. Methotrexate inhibits folic acid, which in turn inhibits inosine production, which inhibits purine synthesis, thus affecting the nucleic acid.

It is thought that the anticonvulsant drugs act either in this way or by inhibiting the synthesis of the proteins which are the constituents of the protein matrix. In the majority of drugs, however, the mechanism whereby chromosome damage is brought about remains unclear.

References

Abel, G. and Schimmer, O. (1983). Induction of structural chromosome aberrations and sister chromatid exchanges in human lymphocytes *in vitro* by aristolochic acid. *Hum. Genet.* 64, 131.

Ahuja, Y.R., Jaju, M., and Jaju, M. (1981). Chromosome damaging action of isoniazid and thiacetazone on human lymphocyte cultures *in vivo*. *Hum. Genet.* 57, 321.

Alvarez, M.R., Cimino, L.E., Cory, M.J., and Gordon, R.E. (1980). Ethanol induction of sister chromatid exchanges in human cells *in vitro*. *Cytogenet. Cell Genet.* 27, 66.

Anderson, D., Jenkinson, P.C., Dewdney, R.S., Blowers, S.D., and Johnson, E.S. (1988). Chromosomal aberrations and sister chromatid exchanges in lymphocytes and urine mutagenicity of migraine patients: a comparison of chronic feverfew users and matched non-users. *Hum. Toxicol.* 7, 145.

Apelt, F., Kolin-Gerresheim, J., and Bauchinger, M. (1981). Azathioprine, a clastogen in human somatic cells? Analysis of chromosome damage and SCE in lymphocytes after exposure *in vivo* and *in vitro*. *Mutat. Res.* 88, 61.

Banduhn, N. and Obe, G. (1985). Mutagenicity of methyl-2-benzimidazolecarbamate, diethyl-stilbestrol and estradiol: structural chromosome aberrations, sister-chromatid exchanges, C-mitoses, polyploidies and micronuclei. *Mutat. Res.* 156, 199.

Basler, A. (1987). Scientific justification of testing chromosome mutations and regulatory requirements for the assessment of mutagenicity. In *Cytogenetics* (ed. G. Obe and A. Basler). Springer-Verlag, Berlin.

Bauchinger, M., Gebhart, E., Fonatsch, Ch., Schmid, E., Muller, W., Obe, G., Beek, B., *et al.* (1978). Chromosome analysis in man in the course of chemoprophylaxis against tuberculosis and of antituberculosis chemotherapy with isoniazid. *Hum. Genet.* 42, 31.

Bender, L. and Siva Sankar, D.V. (1968). Chromosome damage not found in leucocytes of children treated with LSD 25. *Science* 159, 749.

Bender, M.A., Preston, R.J., Leonard, R.C., Pyatt, B.E., and Gooch, P.C. (1988). Chromosomal aberration and sister chromatid exchange frequencies in peripheral blood lymphocytes of a large human population sample. II. Extension of age range. *Mutat. Res.* 212, 149.

Benhamou, S., Pot-Deprun, J., Sancho-Garnier, H., and Chouroulinkov, I. (1988). Sister chromatid exchanges and chromosomal aberrations in lymphocytes of nurses handling cytostatic agents. *Int. J. Cancer* 41, 350.

Bishun, N.P. (1976). Chromosomes and oral contraceptives. *Proc. R. Soc. Med.* 69, 353.

Borgstrom, G.H., Elomaa, I., Blomqvist, C., and Porkaa, L. (1987). Cytogenetic investigations of patients on clodronate therapy for Paget's disease of bone. *Bone* 8 (suppl. 1), 585.

Bornstein, R.S., Hungerford, D.A., Haller, G., Engstrom, P.F., and Yarbro, J.W. (1971). Cytogenetic effects of bleomycin therapy in man. *Cancer Res.* 31, 2004.

Boue, J.G. and Boue, A. (1973). Increased frequency of chromosomal anomalies in abortions after induced ovulation. *Lancet* ii, 679.

Brogger, A. (1970). Anticonvulsant drugs and chromosomes. *Lancet* i, 979.

Brown, T., Dawson, A.A., McDonald, I.A., Bullock, I., and Watt, J.L. (1985). Chromosome damage and sister chromatid exchanges in lymphocyte cultures from patients with two primary cancers. *Cancer Genet. Cytogenet.* 17, 35.

Carr, D.H. (1970). Chromosome studies in selected spontaneous abortions — 1: conception after oral contraceptives. *Can. Med. Assoc. J.* 103, 343.

Charles, D., Turner, J.H., and Redmond, C.J. (1973). The endometrial karyotypic profiles of women after clomiphene citrate therapy. *J. Obstet. Gynaecol. Br. Commonw.* 80, 264.

Chiesara, E., Cutrufello, R., and Rizzi, R. (1983). Chromosome damage in heroin-marijuana and marijuana addicts. *Arch. Toxicol.* 53 (suppl. 6), 128.

Cohen, M.M. and Shaw, M.W. (1964). Effects of mitomycin C on human chromosomes. *J. Cell Biol.* 23, 386.

Cohen, M.M., Hirschhorn, K., and Frosch, W.A. (1967a). *In vivo* and *in vitro* chromosomal damage induced by LSD 25. *N. Engl. J. Med.* 277, 1043.

Cohen, M.M., Marinello, M.J., and Back, N. (1967b). Chromosomal damage in human leukocytes induced by lysergic acid diethylamide. *Science* 155, 1417.

Cohen, M.M., Lieber, E., and Schwartz, H.N. (1972). *In vivo* cytogenetic effects of perphenazine and chlorpromazine. *Br. Med. J.* iii, 21.

Czeizel, A., Kiss, R., Racz, K., Mohori, K., and Glaz, E. (1989). Case-control cytogenetic study in offspring of mothers treated with bromocriptine during early pregnancy. *Mutat. Res.* 210, 23.

De Sario, A., Vagnarelli, P., and De Carli, L. (1990). Aneuploidy assay on diethylstilbestrol by means of *in situ* hybridization of radioactive and biotinylated DNA probes on interphase nuclei. *Mutat. Res.* 243, 127.

De-yu, L., Lahdetie, J., and Parvinen, M. (1988). Mutagenicity of gossypol analysed by induction of meiotic micro-nuclei *in vitro. Mutat. Res.* 208, 69.

Dobos, M., Schuler, D., and Fekete, G. (1974). Cyclophosphamide-induced chromosome aberrations in non-tumorous patients. *Humangenetik* 22, 221.

Dorrance, D., Janiger, O., and Teplitz, L. (1975). Effect of peyote on human chromosomes. *JAMA* 234, 313.

Dresp, J., Schmid, E., and Bauchinger, M. (1978). The cytogenetic effect of bleomycin on human peripheral lymphocytes *in vitro* and *in vivo. Mutat. Res.* 56, 341.

Dumars, K.W. (1971). Parental drug usage effect upon chromosomes of progeny. *Pediatrics* 47, 1037.

Faed, M.J.W. and Mourelatos, D. (1978). Enhancement by caffeine of SCE frequency in lymphocytes from normal subjects after treatment by mutagens. *Mutat. Res.* 49, 437.

Fu, T.K. and Jarvik, L.F. (1977). The *in vitro* effects of imipramine on human chromosomes. *Mutat. Res.* 48, 89.

Garcia Sagredo, J.M. (1988). Effect of anticonvulsants on human chromosomes. 2. *In vitro* studies. *Mutat. Res.* 204, 623.

Garson, O. (1981). Chromosome studies of patients on long-term lithium therapy for psychiatric disorders. *Med. J. Aust.* ii, 37.

Gebhart, E. (1971). Experimental contributions to the problems of achromatic lesions (gaps). *Humangenetik* 13, 98.

Gebhart, E. (1981). Sister chromatid exchange (SCE) and structural chromosome aberration in mutagenicity testing. *Hum. Genet.* 58, 235.

Genesca, A., Barrios, L., Miro, R., Caballin, M.R., Benet, J., Fuster, C., *et al.* (1990). Lymphocyte and sperm chromosome studies in cancer-treated men. *Hum. Genet.* 84, 353.

Gorla, N.B., Ledesma, O.S., Barbieri, G.P., and Larripa, I.B. (1989). Thirteenfold increase of chromosome aberrations non-randomly distributed in chagasic children treated with nifurtimox. *Mutat. Res.* 224, 263.

Grosse, K.P., Schwanitz, G., Rott, H.D., and Wissmuller, HF. (1972). Chromosomenuntersuchungen bei Behandlung mit Anticonvulsiva. *Humangenetik* 16, 209.

Habedank, M., Esser, K.J., Brull, D., Kotlarek, F., and Stumpf, C. (1982). Increased sister chromatid exchanges in epileptic children during long-term therapy with phenytoin. *Hum. Genet.* 61, 71.

Heddle, J.A., Hite, M., Kirkhart, B., Mavournin, K., MacGregor, J.T., Newell, G.W., *et al.* (1983). The induction of micronuclei as a measure of genotoxicity. *Mutat. Res.* 123, 61.

Henderson, L. and Regan, T. (1985). Effects of diethyl stilboestrol dipropionate on SCEs, micronuclei, cytotoxicity, aneuploidy, and cell proliferation in maternal and fetal mouse cells treated *in vivo. Mutat. Res.* 144, 27.

Heng, H.Q., Chen, W.Y., and Wang, Y.C. (1988). Effects of pingyanymycin on chromosomes: a possible structural basis for chromosome aberration. *Mutat. Res.* 199, 199.

Hungerford, D.A., Taylor, K.M., Shagass, C., La Badie, G.U., Balaban, G.B., and Paton, G.R. (1968). Cytogenetic effects of LSD-25 therapy in man. *JAMA* 206, 2287.

Jacobs, N., Neu, R., and Gardner, L. (1969). Phleomycin-induced mitotic inhibition and chromosome abnormalities in cultured human leucocytes. *Mutat. Res.* 7, 251.

Jaju, M., Jaju, M., and Ahuja, Y.R. (1981). Combined action of isoniazid and para-aminosalicylic acid *in vitro* on human chromosomes in lymphocyte cultures. *Hum. Genet.* 56, 375.

Jaju, M., Jaju, M., and Ahuja Y.R. (1982). Effect of cephaloridine on human chromosomes *in vitro* in lymphocyte cultures. *Mutat. Res.* 101, 57

Jaju, M., Jaju, M., and Ahuja, Y.R. (1984). Evaluation of genotoxicity of ampicillin and carbenicillin on human lymphocytes *in vitro*: chromosome aberrations, mitotic index, satellite associations of acrocentric chromosomes and sister chromatid exchanges. *Hum. Toxicol.* 3, 173.

Jameela (Miss), Subramanyam, S., and Sadasivan, G. (1979). Clastogenic effects of frusemide on human leukocytes in culture. *Mutat. Res.* 66, 69.

Jenkins, E.C. (1970). Phenothiazines and chromosome damage. *Cytologia* 35, 552.

Jensen, M.K., Rasmussen, G., and Ingeberg S. (1979). Cytogenetic studies in patients treated with penicillamine. *Mutat. Res.* 67, 357.

Kamada, N., Brecher, G., and Tjio, J.H. (1971). *In vitro* effects of chlorpromazine and meprobamate on blast transformation and chromosomes. *Proc. Soc. Exp. Biol. Med.* 136, 210.

Kao-Shan, C.S., Fine, R.L., Whang-Peng, J., Lee, E.C., and Chabner, B.A. (1987). Increased fragile sites and sister chromatid exchanges in bone marrow and peripheral blood of young cigarette smokers. *Cancer Res.* 47, 6278.

Knuutila, S., Siimes, M., Simell, O., Tammisto, P., and Weber T. (1977). Long-term use of phenytoin: effects on bone marrow chromosomes in man. *Mutat. Res.* 43, 309.

Krogh Jensen, M. and Nyfors, A. (1979). Cytogenetic effect of methotrexate on human cells *in vivo*. Comparison between results obtained by chromosome studies on bone marrow cells and blood lymphocytes and by the micronucleus test. *Mutat. Res.* 64, 339.

Lambert, B., Lindblad, A., Nordenskjold, M., and Wereliu, B. (1978). Increased frequency of sister chromatid exchanges in cigarette smokers. *Hereditas* 88, 147.

Lambert, B., Ringborg, U., and Lindblad, A. (1979). Prolonged increase of sister chromatid exchanges in lymphocytes of melanoma patients after CCNU treatment. *Mutat. Res.* 59, 295.

Lambert, B., Holmberg, K., and Einhorn N. (1984). Persistence of chromosome rearrangements in peripheral lymphocytes from patients treated with melphalan for ovarian carcinoma. *Hum. Genet.* 67, 94.

Liang, J.C., Pinkel, D.P., Bailey, N.M., and Trujillo, J.M. (1989). Mutagen sensitivity and cancer susceptibility. *Cancer* 64, 1474.

Littlefield, L.G.J., Lewer, W., Miller, F., and Goh, K. (1975). Chromosome breakage studies in lymphocytes from normal women, pregnant women and women taking oral contraceptives. *Am. J. Obstet. Gynecol.* 121, 976.

Loughman WD. (1970). Acetyl salicylic acid and chromosome damage. *Science* 171, 829.

Loughman, W.D., Sargent, T.W., and Israelstam, D.M. (1967). Leukocytes of humans exposed to lysergic acid diethylamide: lack of chromosomal damage. *Science* 158, 508.

MacKay, J.M., Fox, D.P., Brunt, P.W., Hawksworth, G.M., and Brown, J.E. (1988). *In vitro* induction of chromosome damage by sulphasalazine in human lymphocytes. *Mutat. Res.* 222, 27.

McQuarrie, H.G., Scott, C.D., Ellsworth, H.S., Harris, J.W., and Stone, R.A. (1970). Cytogenetic studies on women using oral contraceptives and their progeny. *Am. J. Obstet. Gynecol.* 108, 659.

Madrigal-Bujaidar, E. and Rosas-Planaguma, E. (1989). *In vivo* and *in vitro* genotoxic evaluation of indorenate. *Mutat. Res.* 222, 317.

Mamuris, Z., Gerbault-Sereau, M., Prieur, M., Pouillart, P., Dutrillaux, B., and Aurias, A. (1989). Chromosomal aberrations in lymphocytes of patients treated with melphalan. *Int. J. Cancer* 43, 80.

Martin, P.A., Thorburn, M.J., and Bryant, JA. (1973). *In vivo* and *in vitro* studies of cytogenetic effects of *Cannabis sativa* in rats and man. *Teratology* 9, 81.

Matsuyama, S.S., Yen, F.S., Jarvik, L.S., Sparkes, R.G., Fu, T.K., and Fisher, H. (1977). Marijuana exposure *in vivo* and human lymphocyte chromosomes. *Mutat. Res.* 48, 255.

Mauer, I., Weinstein, D., and Solomon, H.M. (1970). Acetylsalicylic acid: no chromosome damage in human leukocytes. *Science* 169, 198.

Meisner, L.F. and Inhorn, S.L. (1972). Chemically induced chromosome changes in human cells *in vitro*. *Acta Cytol.* 16, 41.

Melnyk, J., Duffy, O.M., and Sparkes, R.S. (1971). Human mitotic and meiotic chromosome damage following *in vivo* exposure to methotrexate. *Clin. Genet.* 2, 28.

Mondello, C., Giorgi, R., and Nuzzo, F. (1984). Chromosomal effects of methotrexate on cultured human lymphocytes. *Mutat. Res.* 139, 67.

Morita, T., Watanabe, Y., Takeda, K., and Okumura, K. (1989). Effects of pH in the *in vitro* chromosomal aberration test. *Mutat. Res.* 225, 55.

Muneer, R. (1978). Effects of LSD on human chromosomes. *Mutat. Res.* 51, 403.

Muniz, F.E., Houston, R., Schneider, R., and Nusyowitz, M. (1969). Chromosomal effects of diphenylhydantoin. *Clin. Res.* 17, 28.

Murthy, P.B. and Prema, K. (1979). Sister-chromatid exchanges in oral contraceptive users. *Mutat. Res.* 68, 49.

Neilsen, J., Friedrich, U., and Tsuboi, T. (1968). Chromosome abnormalities and psychotropic drugs. *Nature* 218, 488.

Neuhauser, G., Schwanitz, G., and Rott, HD. (1970). Zur Frage mutagener und teratogener Wirkung von Antikonvulsiva. *Fortschr. Med.* 88, 819.

Neustad, NP. (1978). Sister chromatid exchanges and chromosomal aberrations induced in human lymphocytes by the cytostatic drug adriamycin. *Mutat. Res.* 57, 253.

Nikula, E., Kiviniitty, K., Leisti, J., and Taskinen, P.J. (1984). Chromosome aberrations in lymphocytes of nurses handling cytostatic agents. *Scand. J. Work Environ. Health* 10, 71.

Nordenson, I., Beckman, L., Liden, S., and Stjernberg, N. (1984). Chromosomal aberrations and cancer risk. *Hum. Hered.* 34, 76.

Obe, G., Beek, B., and Radenbach, K.L. (1973). Action of antituberculosis drugs on human leucocyte chromosomes *in vitro*. *Experientia* 29, 1433.

Ostrer, H., Stamberg, J., and Perinchief, P. (1984). Two chromosome aberrations in the child of a woman with systemic lupus erythematosus treated with azathioprine and prednisone. *Am. J. Med. Genet.* 17, 627.

Palmer, R.G., Dore, C.J., and Denman, A.M. (1984). Chlorambucil-induced chromosome damage to human lymphocytes is dose-dependent and cumulative. *Lancet* i, 246.

Palmer, R.G., Dore, C.J., and Denman, A.M. (1985). Chlorambucil-induced chromosome damage to human lymphocytes. *Lancet* ii, 1438.

Pinto, M.R. (1986). Possible effects of hormonal contraceptives on human mitotic chromosomes. *Mutat. Res.* 169, 149.

Psaraki, K. and Demopoulos, N.A. (1988). Induction of chromosome damage and sister chromatid exchanges in human lymphocyte cultures by the antitumour antibiotic Neocarzinostatin. *Mutat. Res.* 204, 669.

Raposa, T. (1978). Sister chromatid exchange studies for monitoring DNA damage and repair capacity after cytostatics *in vitro* and in lymphocytes of leukaemic patients under cytostatic therapy. *Mutat. Res.* 57, 241.

Riedel, L. and Obe, G. (1984). Mutagenicity of antiepileptic drugs. II. Phenytoin, primidone, and phenobarbital. *Mutat. Res.* 138, 71.

Rosenkranz, H.S. (1988). Chloramphenicol: magic bullet or double-edge sword? *Mutat. Res.* 196, 1.

Sadasivan, G., Rani, G., and Kumasi, C.K. (1978). Chromosome damaging effect of betel leaf. *Mutat. Res.* 57, 183.

Sandberg, A.A. (1983). *The chromosomes in human cancer and leukaemia*. Elsevier, New York.

Sargent, L.M., Roloff, B., and Meisner, L.F. (1987). Mechanisms in cyclophosphamide induction of cytogenetic damage in human lymphocyte cultures. *Cancer Genet. Cytogenet.* 29, 239.

Saxena, R. and Ahuja, Y.R. (1982). Clastogenic effect of the psychotropic drug thioridazine on human chromosomes *in vivo*. *Hum. Genet.* 62, 198.

Schaumann, B., Satish, J., Barden Johnson, S., Moore, K., and Cervenka, J. (1985). Effects of carbamazepine on human chromosomes. *Epilepsia* 26, 346.

Schmickel, R. (1967). Chromosome aberrations in leukocytes exposed *in vitro* to diagnostic levels of X-rays. *Am. J. Hum. Genet.* 19, 1.

Schmid, E. and Bauchinger, M. (1973). Comparison of chromosome damage induced by radiation and cytoxan therapy. *Mutat. Res.* 21, 271.

Schneider, E.L. and Lewis, J. (1982). Comparison of *in vivo* and *in vitro* SCE induction. *Mutat. Res.* 106, 85.

Schuler, D., Dobos, M., Fekete, G., Mitenyi, M., and Kalmar, L. (1979). Chromosome mutations and chromosome stability in children treated with different regimes of immunosuppressive drugs. *Hum. Hered.* 29, 100.

Schwartz, S., Astemborski, J.A., Budacz, A.P., Boughman, J.A., Wasserman, S.S., and Cohen, M.M. (1990). Repeated measurement of spontaneous and clastogen-induced sister-chromatid exchange. *Mutat. Res.* 234, 51.

Shaw, M.W. (1970). Human chromosome damage by chemical agents. *Annu. Rev. Med.* 21, 409.

Shiraishi, Y., Yamamoto, K., and Sandberg, A. (1979). Effects of caffeine on chromosome aberrations and sister chromatid exchanges induced by mitomycin C in BrdU-labelled human chromosomes. *Mutat. Res.* 62, 1 39.

Sinkus, A.G. (1972). Cytogenetic effect of rubomycin C in a culture of human lymphocytes. Chromosomal aberrations at the G_2 stage of the mitotic cycle. *Genetica* (Leningrad) 8, 138.

Sinues, B., Izquierdo, M., and Viguera, J.P. (1990). Chromosome aberrations and urinary thioethers in smokers. *Mutat. Res.* 240, 289.

Sorsa, M., Husgafvel-Pursiainen, K., Jarventus, H., Koskimies, K., Salo, H., and Vainio, H. (1989). Cytogenetic effects of tobacco smoke exposure among involuntary smokers. *Mutat. Res.* 222, 111.

Speit, G. and Haupter, S. (1987). Cytogenetic effects of penicillamine. *Mutat. Res.* 190, 197.

Srb, V., Kubzova, E., and Kubikova, K. (1986). Chromosome aberration and mitotic activity in human peripheral blood lymphocytes following *in vitro* action of platinum cytostatics *cis*-DDP and EM-Pt. *Neoplasma* 33, 465.

Staiger, G.R. (1969). Studies on the chromosomes of human lymphocytes treated with diazepam *in vitro*. *Mutat. Res.* 10, 635.

Stevenson, A.C., Patel, C.R., Bedford, J., Hill, A.G.S., and Hill, H.F.H. (1971). Chromosomal studies in patients taking phenylbutazone. *Ann. Rheum. Dis.* 30, 487.

Stevenson, A.C. and Patel, C.R. (1973a). Effects of chlorambucil on human chromosomes. *Mutat. Res.* 18, 333.

Stevenson, A.C., Clarke, G., Patel, C.R., and Hughes, D.T.D. (1973b). Chromosomal studies *in vivo* and *in vitro* of trimethoprim and sulphamethoxazole. *Mutat. Res.* 17, 255.

Tandon, P. and Sodhi, A. (1985). *cis*-Dichlorodiammine platinum (II) induced aberrations in mouse bone marrow chromosomes. *Mutat. Res.* 156, 187.

Tawn, E.J. and Cartmell, C.L. (1989). The effect of smoking on the frequencies of asymmetrical and symmetrical chromosome exchanges in human lymphocytes. *Mutat. Res.* 224, 151.

Tjio, J.H., Pahnke, W.N., and Kurland, A.A. (1969). LSD and chromosomes. A controlled experiment. *JAMA* 210, 849.

Tsui, Y.C., Creasy, M.R., and Hulten, M.A. (1983). The effect of the male contraceptive agent gossypol on human lymphocytes *in vitro*: traditional chromosome breakage, micronuclei, sister chromatid exchange, and cell kinetics. *J. Med. Genet.* 20, 81.

Urba, M. (1971). Changes in human chromosomes caused by drugs. *Cslka Oftal.* 27, 134.

van den Berg-de Ruiter, E., de Jong, B., Mulder, N.H., te Meerman, G.J., Schraffordt Koops, H., and Sleijfer, D.T. (1990). Chromosome damage in peripheral blood lymphocytes of patients treated for testicular cancer. *Hum. Genet.* 84, 191.

Vijayalaxmi (1982). Human leukocyte interferon does not induce sister chromatid exchanges in human blood lymphocytes. *Mutat. Res.* 105, 287.

Vijayalaxmi and Burkart, W. (1989). Resistance and cross-resistance to chromosome damage in human blood lymphocytes adapted to bleomycin. *Mutat. Res.* 211, 1.

Vorechovsky, I. and Zaloudik, J. (1989). Increased breakage of chromosome 1 in lymphocytes of patients with testicular cancer after bleomycin treatment *in vitro*. *Br. J. Cancer* 59, 499.

Vormittag W. (1985). Structural chromosome aberration rates and sister chromatid exchange frequencies in females with type 2 (non-insulin-dependent) diabetes. *Mutat. Res.* 1 43, 117.

Watson, W.A.F., Petrie, J.C., Galloway, D.B., Bullock, I., and Gilbert, J.C. (1976). *In vivo* cytogenetic activity of sulphonylurea drugs in man. *Mutat. Res.* 38, 71.

Weinstein, D., Mauer, I., and Solomon, H.M. (1972). The effect of caffeine on chromosomes of human lymphocytes. *In vivo* and *in vitro* studies. *Mutat. Res.* 16, 391.

Whang-Peng, J., Levanthal, B.G., Adamson, J.W., and Perry, S. (1969). The effect of daunomycin on human cells *in vivo* and *in vitro*. *Cancer* 23, 113.

5. Disorders of the fetus and infant

R. E. FERNER and J. M. SMITH

Introduction

Drugs given to the mother can in principle affect the developing child from the time the egg is fertilized until the baby is weaned from the breast. Effects on the chromosomes have already been considered in Chapter 4.

Cell division, tubular transport, and uterine implantation of the fertilized ovum may be affected. For example, high-dose oestrogens given shortly after conception result in loss of the conceptus, perhaps by affecting tubular motility, and also by altering the endometrium either directly or by inhibiting luteal function (*The Lancet* 1983*a*).

The loss rate during the implantation stage (days 0–6 from conception) is probably of the order of 50 per cent in pregnancies in the general population (Beckman and Brent 1986), so that it is very hard to know what effect drug therapy may have on the incidence. The cells are totipotent at this very early stage of development, and the outcome of damage is thought to be either loss of the conceptus or normal continuation of pregnancy (Beck and Lloyd 1965).

The embryo from the time of implantation until closure of the secondary palate, which marks the end of organogenesis, is vulnerable to outside agents that can disturb the programme of development. Cell division, programmed cell death, and interactions between cells, as well as cellular nutrition and metabolism, are potentially susceptible to malign external influences. Teratology (from τέραϭ, a monster or prodigy) is 'the name given by Geoffroy de St Hilare to the study or consideration of monsters or anomalies of organization' (Oxford English Dictionary). The possibility that chemical poisons could cause malformations has been recognized for some years, but only a few scattered observations were recorded up to 1960 (Willis 1962). After thalidomide was shown by Lenz and Knapp (1962) to be responsible for congenital defects there was heightened awareness of drugs as potential teratogens, that is, substances whose presence during embryonic or fetal life can induce abnormal postnatal structure or function.

Fetal health requires normal uterine and placental function and a normal amnion. Drugs that reduce placental blood flow or cause oligohydramnios can cause fetal harm. Fetal growth, from the closure of the secondary palate until delivery, can be retarded by the effects of drugs on cellular nutrition, metabolism, or division. Drugs that increase or decrease uterine contractility can cause premature or delayed labour. Neonatal well-being, which depends on physiological adaptation to the extra-uterine world, can also be compromised by drugs given to the mother before birth or transmitted in the breast milk after birth.

The susceptibility of the developing embryo and fetus to harm from drugs

The developing embryo is especially vulnerable to harm because:

1. the embryo contains relatively few differentiated cells, and therefore damage to small numbers of cells may have large consequences;
2. cells are dividing rapidly, and so the embryo is intolerant of interference with cell division;
3. groups of cells during organogenesis undergo processes, including migration, aggregation, cavitation, delamination, folding, closure, and fusion, which depend on precise localization in time and space and whose disruption leads to abnormal organ formation. Normal embryonic development depends on the programmed death of some cells. Excessive cell death in regions of programmed cell death may be important (Sulik *et al.* 1988);
4. the metabolizing enzymes of cells in the embryo may differ from those in mature animals. They may not be able to detoxify xenobiotic compounds as effectively, or may more readily transform non-toxic drugs into

teratogenic metabolites by bioactivation (Juchau 1989);
5. the immune system does not function during intra-uterine development.

The conceptus is also vulnerable, because of the specialized nature of its nutrition, through the metabolically active, vascular placenta. Interruption of nutrition or interference with metabolism can retard intrauterine growth.

Around the time of birth, the major adaptations of heart and lungs to extrauterine life are sensitive to agents (such as opioid analgesics) given to the mother and persisting in the neonatal circulation.

(See also Tyl 1988.)

How great a risk do drugs pose to the developing child?

The detection of harm, the association with a particular agent and the demonstration that this association is causal are all beset with difficulties.

The first suspicion that a drug may cause harm can come from experimental studies in animals, as, for example, with vitamin A (retinoic acid) derivatives (Teelmann 1988). It can come from cohort studies in which the maternal drug exposure and the incidence of malformations in a group of women are analysed, the best example being the Boston Collaborative Perinatal Project (Heinonen *et al.* 1977*b*) in which over 50 000 'mother–infant pairs' were studied and outcomes correlated with some 900 drugs to which they were exposed. Commonly, the earliest warning comes from case reports in which at most a few infants are observed with recognizable abnormalities after the mother has been exposed to a drug in pregnancy. The classical example is the observation (McBride 1961; Lenz and Knapp 1962) of phocomelic infants born to mothers who took thalidomide during the first trimester.

Case–control studies, in which the exposure to a putative causal agent is assessed in affected cases and in a control population matched as closely as possible for relevant factors other than exposure, can also provide helpful information, with the advantage that uncommon conditions can be studied much more effectively than in cohort studies.

Very substantial problems are associated with each method. Animal studies are notoriously difficult to extrapolate to man, as exemplified by the low teratogenicity of thalidomide in mice and rats. In contrast, cleft palate is easily induced in some strains of mice by administering corticosteroids to the mother, but there is no evidence that corticosteroids cause this defect in man.

Cohort studies contain a very low density of information: both exposure to unusual drugs and infants with unusual abnormalities are represented only infrequently, and so the method is insensitive. Since many comparisons are made in a search for possible associations in a study such as the Boston Collaborative Perinatal Project (Heinonen *et al.* 1977*b*), spurious associations will also occur. On average, 1 in 20 comparisons will show a significant association at $p<0.05$ purely by chance. Cohort studies are not therefore guaranteed to be either specific or sensitive.

The case–control study is retrospective. An association with *prior* exposure is sought *after* the affected case has occurred. This makes it extremely difficult to conduct such a study without bias, in the selection of cases or controls, or in the determination of prior exposure in the two groups. Sackett (1979) has enumerated potential causes of bias in comparative studies. A paticular selection bias is introduced by counting only live-born cases and controls (Hook 1982; Khoury *et al.* 1989). The teratogen and the condition with which it is putatively associated may affect prenatal mortality differently, and so the true degree of association can be overestimated or underestimated (Khoury *et al.* 1989).

Case reports can claim historical successes (Goldberg and Golbus 1986). The teratogenic effects of thalidomide (Lenz and Knapp 1962), warfarin (Kerber *et al.* 1968), and ethanol (Lemoine *et al.* 1968) were first described in case reports. The more unusual a case, the more likely is it to be described, so very bizarre or rare events are most likely to be detected. This poses a substantial problem, because intuitively the conjunction of two rare events suggests causality. For example, exposure to griseofulvin in the first 3 weeks of pregnancy has been recorded in two cases of conjoined twins (Rosa *et al.* 1987*a*). The chance of this specific event occurring on two occasions is obviously very low indeed. The chance, however, of exposure *in utero* to any one of several thousand chemicals being associated with any one of several thousand anomalies on two occasions, is several million times higher.

The conclusion is that no method can unequivocally demonstrate an association *ab initio*, it can only lead to the hypothesis that an association exists, a hypothesis which can be strengthened by further evidence, for example, from a case–control study designed specifically to examine that hypothesis. Much smaller numbers need to be studied to confirm that there is a high probability (say 95 per cent) that a hypothesis is true ($P_\alpha<0.05$) than are needed to refute the same hypothesis with the same degree of certainty ($P_\beta<0.05$). This means that once a hypothesis has been put forward it is more likely to be proved true than false; and so both 'true' and 'unproven' hypotheses remain. Very few drugs have been exonerated after the finger of suspicion has been pointed at them. Dicyclomine and the oral contraceptive pill may be rare examples (see below).

Measures of association between exposure to an agent and an adverse effect (for example, congenital anomaly in the offspring) are relative risk (risk ratio) and odds ratio. The relative risk is the ratio of *(the proportion affected in those exposed) : (the proportion affected in those unexposed)*. It therefore requires the complete enumeration of a (large) population, as may be obtained in a cohort study. The odds ratio can be derived from cohort or case–control studies, and is the ratio of *(exposed/unexposed in those affected) : (exposed/unexposed in those unaffected)*. When the proportion affected is small, the odds ratio gives an approximate value for the relative risk (Armitage and Berry 1987). The 95 per cent confidence intervals can be calculated for both ratios. These are often so wide as to include unity (no increased risk), and so are important in assessing a particular association.

An association does not prove a causal link. The human experience does not constitute a controlled experiment and so the population exposed to the drug often differs systematically from the unexposed population. This would be as true for antituberculous chemotherapy as for antineoplastic therapy. The disease process, rather than the drug, may be the cause of abnormalities in the offspring. This has been postulated for epilepsy and anticonvulsant drugs (Dodson 1989). Clearly, the demonstration that a hypothesized mechanism of action for the suspected teratogen pertains in one or more models strengthens the possibility that it is indeed deleterious, and the observation that an anomaly only occurs in the presence of a given drug and not in a patient with the disease state treated differently implicates it as a noxious agent, at least in the presence of that disease state (as with insomnia and thalidomide). It is salutary to note that none of the many possible mechanisms by which thalidomide is teratogenic has been confirmed (Stephens 1988), and that many drugs are suspected of causing malformations that also occur spontaneously.

Teratogens

Wilson (1977) formulated six general principles of teratogenesis, on which rather stringent criteria for the identification of teratogens can be based. They are summarized as:

1. the susceptibility of a conceptus to teratogenesis depends on its genotype — only certain genotypes are susceptible;

2. the susceptibility to teratogens varies with developmental stage at the time of exposure — organs are particularly sensitive during the critical period of their formation;
3. teratogens act by specific mechanisms — for example, by reducing the availability of a required substrate;
4. abnormal development can lead to death, malformation, growth retardation, or functional disorder;
5. the access of adverse environmental agents to developing tissues depends on the nature of the agents — but, for practical purposes, most drugs of molecular weight <800 can cross the placenta;
6. the observed effects of a teratogen depend on dose.

The understanding of human teratogens remains poor, but an animal model exemplifies the principles. Glucocorticoids can produce cleft palate in mice. Closure of the secondary palate in the mouse and other mammals requires contact of the apposing palatal shelves, adhesion of the epithelium, then epithelial breakdown along the line of adhesion, and fusion of the palatal mesenchyme. Cortisone is bound to tissue receptors and, in strains of mice susceptible to steroid-induced cleft palate, this binding is more extensive than in strains that are not susceptible. It is believed that the cortisone–receptor complex alters RNA transcription and suppresses the production of lysosomal enzymes. The reduced lysosomal enzyme production prevents the epithelial breakdown necessary for palatal fusion, and the palatal cleft persists (Goldman *et al.* 1983).

This specific example shows genetic and temporal susceptibility to a teratogen, which by specific processes causes a specific defect. Since cortisone is an endogenous hormone, it is clear, too, that effect depends on dose. Corticosteroids do not appear to be teratogenic in man.

Risk, uncertainty, and clinical practice

It is hard to estimate the risk that a given agent is teratogenic in man from survey data, for the reasons described above. This uncertainty colours clinical practice. A drug that could prevent serious harm to the mother (for example, a drug that is an effective prophylactic against malaria) will also potentially prevent harm to the fetus. A drug which is purely for symptomatic relief will not. Where more than one drug exists to treat a particular condition (for example, epilepsy) then their relative safety is of importance. This can be especially hard to determine, as lack of evidence does not prove lack of the potential to cause harm.

The general principle is that since risks of damage to the baby are uncertain and can be high, only drugs that confer clear benefits should ever be prescribed in pregnancy. This principle is only helpful in reducing the risks after pregnancy is diagnosed. Most currently used drugs, with the exception of vitamin A derivatives and cytotoxic drugs, seem unlikely to have a great propensity for causing abnormal babies.

Some reassurance can be derived from the small number of drugs that have clearly been shown to be teratogenic. Even with the most teratogenic drugs, the perceived risk may be greater than the true risk. After first-trimester exposure *in utero* to therapeutic doses of antimetabolite antineoplastic agents, for example, four out of five infants will be normal at birth. A number of reviews (Briggs *et al.* 1986; Hawkins 1987; Rubin 1987) provide useful guidance on drug therapy for pregnant women. Schardein's monograph (1985) includes comprehensive reviews of animal studies of teratogens.

The adverse reactions to drug exposure in the conceptus and neonate are now considered by time of exposure.

The first trimester

Gastrointestinal drugs

Antacids

The information on antacids is limited. The large prospective study of Heinonen and others (1977*b*) did not consider antacids at all. The retrospective survey by Nelson and Forfar (1971) recorded antacid consumption in 157/1369 women, and found that a greater proportion of women who had abnormal babies had taken antacids (12.4 per cent) than of women who had normal babies (11 per cent). Corresponding figures for the first trimester only were 5.9 per cent vs 2.6 per cent (p<0.01). When self-administered antacids where included, there was still a significant excess of antacid use in the women who were delivered of abnormal babies. No link with any particular antacid was found, and the possibility exists that antacids were taken for gastrointestinal symptoms associated with abnormal pregnancies. There was no significant excess of antacid use, taken over the whole of pregnancy, in women with abnormal babies. A subsequent study (RCGP 1976) failed to show an increased risk. The common symptom of heartburn ('acid reflux') during pregnancy usually occurs during the second and third trimesters, when there is no evidence for increased risk of antacids, though they are best avoided during the first trimester in favour of small meals and loose corsets (Feeney 1982).

Histamine H$_2$-antagonists

There are reports of four mothers who took ranitidine during the first trimester and subsequently had normal babies (Cipriani *et al.* 1983; Andrews and Souma 1989).

Cimetidine has been more extensively studied. In a postmarketing surveillance scheme (Jones *et al.* 1985), 20 cimetidine takers and 22 controls became pregnant. Two takers aged 23 had abnormal children: one baby had trisomy 21, and one had no congenital anomalies but had convulsions and died in the neonatal period, probably owing to intrauterine hypoxia. It was doubtful whether either abnormal pregnancy could be imputed to cimetidine. Three cases of women who took cimetidine during the first trimester and had normal babies are recorded (Corazza *et al.* 1982; Meggs *et al.* 1984).

These sparse data do not suggest that H$_2$-antagonists are major teratogens.

Sulphasalazine and mesalazine (5-aminosalicylic acid)

Inflammatory bowel disease affects young people, and the question often arises whether treatment should continue during pregnancy, particularly if the treatment is prophylactic. Miller (1986) reviewed 10 retrospective series of patients and found no evidence for an increase in congenital abnormalities due to the disease or due to sulphasalazine. However, there has been no controlled trial. There are reports of one case of cleft lip, cleft palate, and hydrocephalus in a baby born to a woman with ulcerative colitis in remission who had taken sulphasalazine throughout pregnancy (Craxi and Pagliarello 1980), of two cases of babies with coarctation and ventricular septal defect (Newman and Correy 1983; Hoo *et al.* 1988), and of a pair of stillborn twins with renal anomalies (Newman and Correy 1983). Three women treated with mesalazine throughout pregnancy had normal children (Habal and Greenberg 1987).

Sulphasalazine is a conjugate of sulphapyridine and mesalazine (5-aminosalicylic acid). It is well absorbed, and since its anti-inflammatory activity is due to the 5-aminosalicylic acid moiety, there is some logic in preferring mesalazine for prophylaxis in pregnant women with ulcerative colitis. The information on both agents is generally reassuring.

Antihistamine antiemetics

Neither prospective (Heinonen *et al.* 1977*b*) nor retrospective (Nelson and Forfar 1971) studies have demonstrated overall increased malformation rates in women taking chlorpheniramine or promethazine during the first trimester. Meclozine has been suggested to be a human teratogen (Watson 1962), but there were no overall increases in incidence of abnormalities in prospective studies of 1014 (Heinonen *et al.* 1977*b*) and 613 (Milkovich and van den Berg 1976) mothers taking meclozine during the first trimester, nor in a retrospective survey (Nelson and Forfar 1971).

A 'new thalidomide-style drug fear' (de St Jorre 1980*a*) was raised and allegations were made that preparations containing the antihistamine doxylamine (including Debendox in the UK and Bendectin in the US) caused deformities, when the manufacturers were sued by the parents of a boy who was born with Poland's anomaly (unilaterally absent pectoralis major and ipsilateral hand deformity) after his mother had taken Bendectin. The Court awarded damages against the manufacturer (de St Jorre 1980*b*), but the scientific evidence for any major teratogenic effect is lacking. Several large trials, all studying cohorts of more than 1000 patients (Bunde and Bowles 1963; Heinonen *et al.* 1977*b*; Newman and Dudgeon 1977; Shapiro *et al.* 1977; Jick *et al.* 1981; Gibson *et al.* 1981; Morelock *et al.* 1982; Smithells and Sheppard 1983; Shiono and Klebonoff 1989) have failed to find an increase in the overall rate of malformations. The 95 per cent confidence limits for relative risk of 0.76 and 1.04 admit of the possibility, however, that doxylamine is a low-grade teratogen, with a risk of a few per cent above background (Orme 1985). Several studies have suggested from subgroup analyses that significant associations might exist between the use of doxylamine and specific teratogenic effects. These have, however, involved different systems: genital tract anomalies (Gibson *et al.* 1981); oesophageal atresia or encephalocoele (Cordero *et al.* 1981); diaphragmatic hernia (Bracken and Berg 1983); pyloric stenosis (Eskanazi and Bracken 1982); congenital heart disease (Rothman *et al.* 1979); microcephaly, cataract, and pulmonary hypoplasia (Shiono and Klebonoff 1989). Since most of the papers report 20–60 subgroup analyses, statistical associations are expected by chance. Case–control studies have specifically failed to find evidence of a significantly increased risk of congenital heart disease (Mitchell *et al.* 1981; Zierler and Rothman 1985), congenital limb defects (Aselton and Jick 1983; McCredie *et al.* 1984), or oral clefts (Mitchell *et al.* 1981). The lack of any consistent evidence of an association with a unique group of malformations is reassuring (Check 1979; Brent 1983; Holmes 1983) and the lack of any observed change in malformation rates after the withdrawal of doxylamine preparations makes it most unlikely that Debendox/Bendectin does cause birth defects. The case of doxylamine shows the difficulty of proving that a small risk does not exist.

Anaesthetic gases

There is an increased rate of spontaneous abortion in women anaesthetists and theatre nurses (Ad Hoc Committee 1974; Pharoah *et al.* 1977; Vessey and Nunn 1980). Women undergoing general anaesthesia during the first or second trimester also have higher rates of spontaneous abortion than controls (Duncan *et al.* 1986). Nitrous oxide has been particularly implicated, because it inhibits methionine synthetase, and inactivates vitamin B_{12}. Clearly, unnecessary exposure to anaesthetic agents should be avoided in women who wish to become pregnant or are in the first or second trimester of pregnancy. Reassuring data from 550 pregnancies during which short anaesthetics with N_2O were administered during the first or second trimester (Aldridge and Tunstall 1986; Crawford and Lewis 1986) indicate that the risk is likely to be small. There is no evidence that nitrous oxide is teratogenic in man.

Anti-infective agents

Anthelmintic agents

Mebendazole

This drug may be teratogenic in man (Leach 1990). The manufacturers are aware of the outcome of 306 cases when mebendazole was taken during pregnancy, with 26 spontaneous abortions and 17 abnormal babies. Abnormalities included haemangiomata (4 cases), hypospadias (2 cases), and oesophageal atresia and imperforate anus (1 case) (T. Simonite, personal communication). There has been no relevant case–control study.

Piperazine

Administration of this drug from day 27 to day 33 after conception and again from day 41 to day 47 was associated with lobster-claw deformities of the hands and feet in the child delivered subsequently (Meyer and Brenner 1988). It is known that differentiation of the limbs occurs in the period 24–36 days after conception. New mutations and sporadic cases of lobster-claw deformity do, however, occur. In the absence of other evidence, it seems unlikely that piperazine is a common cause of lobster-claw deformity. Two other cases, one of anophthalmia and facial cleft and the other of an abnormal foot, have also been reported.

The anthelmintics should, if possible, not be used during the first trimester (Leach 1990).

Antibacterials

Aminoglycosides

Streptomycin and kanamycin, in common with other aminoglycosides, can cause damage to the eighth cranial nerve in treated subjects, and so it is not surprising that ototoxicity has been observed after exposure *in utero* to these antibacterials (Jones 1973; Donald and Sellars

1981). Similar considerations presumably apply to gentamicin and the newer aminoglycosides, although no cases have been reported. The incidence of other abnormalities is not apparently increased (Heinonen *et al.* 1977*b*).

Tetracyclines

Cases of discolouration of the cornea (Krejčf and Brettschneider 1983), congenital cataract (Harley *et al.* 1964), limb abnormalities (Carter and Wilson 1962, 1963), and multiple abnormalities (Corcoran and Castles 1977) have been reported after usage of tetracyclines in the first trimester, but prospective trials have shown no significant increase in fetal abnormalities (Elder *et al.* 1971; Heinonen *et al.* 1977*b*). These reports imply that the risks from inadvertently continuing low-dose tetracycline treatment for acne around the time of conception are likely to be small. Tetracyclines do have harmful effects, however, on fetal teeth and bones in later pregnancy.

Metronidazole

There is a theoretical risk that metronidazole, by inhibiting aldehyde dehydrogenase, might increase the chances of the fetal alcohol syndrome occurring in the offspring of women who drink during pregnancy (Dunn *et al.* 1979).

Antifungals

Griseofulvin

Exposure to this drug during early pregnancy had occurred in two cases of conjoined twins reported to a US Food and Drug Administration scheme (Rosa *et al.* 1987*a*). A possible association with spontaneous abortion was also noted. As fission of twins is normally complete by 20 days, only women bearing identical twins and given the drug before 20 days would be susceptible. No cases of griseofulvin exposure were recorded among mothers who gave birth to 39 conjoined twins in Hungary (Métneki and Czeizel 1987) or in 47 cases reported to an international monitoring scheme (Knudsen 1987), but the anomaly is so rare that the US cases should perhaps not be dismissed.

Antimalarials

Quinine

When quinine is taken by women as an abortifacient during the first trimester, and no abortion occurs, then the infant may be delivered with congenital defects of the central nervous system, limbs, face, heart, or other organs (Nishimura and Tanimura 1976). Auditory (Roberts 1870; Taylor 1934) and optic nerve (McKinna 1966) damage can also occur, as might be expected from the toxic effects in adults.

It is much less clear whether therapeutic use in falciparum malaria carries fetal risk, and the disease is so serious that it would not be logical to withhold treatment (*The Lancet* 1983*b,c*).

Chloroquine

There is a suggestion that high doses of chloroquine are ototoxic and retinotoxic (Hart and Naunton 1964), but a comparison of 169 infants exposed to maternal prophylaxis (300 mg per week) and 454 controls failed to find any evidence for a teratogenic effect (Wolfe and Cordero 1985).

Pyrimethamine

This is a folate antagonist and, as with other drugs of this class, it is reported to have caused birth defects — but only in one case of ectopic viscera (Morley *et al.* 1964). It has been suggested that folinic acid should be given concurrently to mothers taking malarial prophylaxis, at least throughout the first trimester (*The Lancet* 1983*c*).

Antituberculous drugs

A review of 1939 births from 10 series failed to find evidence for a major teratogenic effect of antituberculous therapy (Snider *et al.* 1980). *p*-Aminosalicylic acid treatment during the first trimester in 43 mothers was associated with congenital defects in five infants (Heinonen *et al.* 1977*b*), a result which may be due to chance.

Rifampicin

This is an enzyme-inducing agent, and therefore increases the rate of metabolism of oral contraceptive hormones, increasing the risk of unwanted pregnancy. In 226 women receiving rifampicin, pregnancy ended in spontaneous abortion or intrauterine death in 10, in neonatal death in 4, and in congenital abnormalities in 9, of whom 4 had limb abnormalities and 3 hydrocephalus or anencephaly (Steen and Stainton-Ellis 1977).

Isoniazid

Isoniazid may be linked to a number of central nervous system problems, including retardation and convulsions (Lowe 1964; Weinstein and Dalton 1968), but in 85 patients who received isoniazid during the first trimester there were 10 malformations, a non-significant increase (Heinonen *et al.* 1977*b*). Retrospective analysis of a placebo-controlled trial of isoniazid also failed to find a significant difference in fetal outcome (Ludford *et al.* 1973).

Anti-inflammatory agents

Salicylates

A case–control study (Zeirler and Rothman 1985) suggested that first-trimester aspirin use might be associated with cardiac defects, though a subsequent case–control study, in which adjustment was made for maternal age, family history, and certain other risk factors (Werler *et al.* 1989), failed to confirm an association.

Two cases of cyclopia in the offspring of women who had taken 3–4 g of salicylate daily during the first trimester (Benawra *et al.* 1980; Agapitos *et al.* 1986) are suggestive of a rare association, which is of theoretical interest. Early in embryogenesis, the forebrain cleaves in the midline and the paired structures of the face are formed. Cleavage defects, often associated with premaxillary agenesis, may be of any degree from cyclopia (no cleavage, single eyeglobe, arhinia) to failure of cleavage of the central incisor teeth. The cerebral anomaly results in a single 'holosphere', and the group of defects is called holoprosencephaly (Yakovlev 1959; Cohen 1982). An autosomal recessive form exists (McKusick 1988). As only the most severe form of cleavage defect has been reported and, as it is extremely rare, salicylates could only be responsible if they blocked the initiating process for midline cleavage in a very unusual, susceptible subgroup. Since congenital cytomegalovirus infection has been linked to cyclopia, it is possible that the salicylates were taken for that infection, which was itself the teratogen. This makes it less likely that salicylate is responsible for cyclopia, but there is a precedent: the plant *Veratrum californium* causes exactly this defect in sheep (Binns *et al.* 1965). It has been suggested (Webster *et al.* 1988) that cyclopia is the extreme form of the facial dysmorphogenesis seen with maternal ethanol abuse or anticonvulsant therapy.

Slone and colleagues (1976) failed to find any evidence of teratogenesis from heavy first trimester exposure to salicylates in 5128 pregnancies compared with 35 418 with no exposure and 9736 with intermediate exposure.

Penicillamine

Cutis laxa, that is, abnormally lax skin lacking normal elastic tissue, has been found in several cases where the mother had received penicillamine in pregnancy. (Laver and Fairley 1971; Mjølnerød *et al.* 1971; Solomon *et al.* 1977). In two cases (Linares *et al.* 1979; Harpey *et al.* 1983), the defect apparently resolved. This characteristic defect does not occur in the offspring of all women treated with penicillamine, and Lyle (1978) recounts 27 pregnancies: 26 with normal outcome after penicil-

lamine in the first trimester, and one with a 'small ventricular septal defect'.

Cardiovascular drugs

Antihypertensive agents

Minoxidil

Hypertrichosis, which is known to occur in patients taking minoxidil, was observed in the infants of two mothers who took the drug throughout pregnancy, together with other drugs (Kaler *et al.* 1987; Rosa *et al.* 1987*b*). One baby also had other abnormalities, including an omphalocele. In the only other case of intrauterine minoxidil exposure notified to the Food and Drug Administration, the baby died of cyanotic congenital heart disease.

Angiotensin-converting-enzyme (ACE) inhibitors

ACE inhibitors (captopril and enalapril) have been linked with a very rare skull ossification defect in three cases (Duminy and Burger 1981; Mehta and Modi 1989; Cunniff *et al.* 1990) and renal dysgenesis in two cases (Knott *et al.* 1989; Cunniff *et al.* 1990). Stillbirth, intrauterine growth retardation and perinatal death are more common, whether because of the ACE inhibitors or the pre-eclampsia that they are used to treat (Kreft-Jaïs *et al.* 1988).

Anticoagulants

Warfarin

Warfarin causes a specific pattern of developmental abnormalities, with nasal hypoplasia and calcific stripping of the epiphyses (chondrodysplasia punctata), in infants exposed during the first trimester. A similar disorder can occur as an autosomal recessive trait. There may also be optic atrophy and brain abnormalities (Warkany 1976). Two cases of diaphragmatic hernia have been reported in the infants exposed to warfarin *in utero* (Normann and Stray-Pedersen 1989). There is no critical period during organogenesis when exposure to warfarin results in defects: they can be manifest after exposure in the second or third trimester alone. Ginsberg and Hirsh (1988) were able to identify reports of 578 women given oral anticoagulants during pregnancy, of whom 31 had infants with warfarin embryopathy, and 21 suffered 'fetal wastage'. In a prospective study of 72 pregnancies in which warfarin was given during the first 6 weeks of pregnancy, 10 babies had warfarin embryopathy; all occurred in the 35 pregnancies in which warfarin therapy continued into weeks 8–12 (Iturbe-Alessio *et al.* 1986).

In a prospective study of 50 pregnancies in women with artificial heart valves treated with warfarin during the first and second trimesters, there were 18 deaths *in utero* or perinatally, and 2 cases of warfarin embryopathy (Sareli *et al.* 1989).

Warfarin inhibits the formation of carboxyglutamyl residues from glutamyl residues, and so reduces the binding of calcium to protein; this might explain the abnormal ossification of cartilage which it causes (Hall *et al.* 1980). This hypothesis is supported by the case of a boy with the typical somatotype of warfarin embryopathy who had not been exposed to warfarin *in utero* but who had decreased activities of vitamin-K-dependent coagulation factors (Pauli *et al.* 1987). Abnormal chondrogenesis seems to be a precursor of the abnormal ossification (Barr and Burdi 1976).

Heparin is the preferred anticoagulant during the first trimester (Ginsberg and Hirsch 1989; Ginsberg *et al.* 1989).

Drugs acting on the central nervous system

Centrally acting analgesics

There were 8 cases of respiratory malformations in the offspring of 563 women who were exposed to codeine during the first trimester, a statistically significant increase (Heinonen *et al.* 1977*b*). Other defects, including congenital heart defects and cleft lip and palate, were more common in babies born to women who took opiates during the first trimester (Saxén 1975; Bracken and Holford 1981).

Antiepileptic drugs

Children born to mothers with epilepsy have an increased risk of congenital malformation (Meadow 1970; Fedrick 1973). Major malformations, and total malformations, were significantly more common in the 305 children born to epileptic mothers in 50 282 mother–child pairs; intellectual development at 8 months and 4 years was slowed and mothers of children with craniofacial anomalies were more likely to have taken anticonvulsants, according to one case–control study (Shapiro *et al.* 1976). Craniofacial anomalies and congenital heart disease have been seen with increased frequency in several series (Speidel and Meadow 1972, Millar and Nevin 1973; Niswander and Wertlecki 1973; Nakane *et al.* 1980). Fetal and perinatal loss may also be increased (Speidel and Meadow 1972; Nakane *et al.* 1980; Akhtar and Millac 1987), and birth-weight, adjusted for sex and gestational age, may be reduced (Mastroiacovo *et al.* 1988).

There is evidence that all the commonly used antiepileptic drugs have some teratogenic potential (Dodson 1989). Folate deficiency, related to anticonvulsant therapy, may play a pathogenetic role (Hiilesmaa *et al.* 1983; Dansky *et al.* 1987), and there is some experimental evidence in animals that folic acid supplements are protective (Zhu and Zhou 1989).

It is uncertain whether maternal epilepsy itself, independent of drug usage, might predispose to malformations in the fetus (Gaily *et al.* 1989; Keller 1989). Annegers and others (1974) failed to find malformations in the 26 infants born to mothers with epilepsy 'in remission', or in the 61 babies born to mothers who subsequently developed epilepsy; there was one malformation amongst the 56 offspring of mothers with epilepsy who took no treatment during the first trimester, and 10 in 141 babies whose mothers had taken one or more antiepileptic drug during pregnancy. A Japanese study also found an increased malformation rate in the babies of treated, but not untreated, epileptic mothers (Nakane *et al.* 1980). The probable systematic differences between epileptic women who receive treatment and those who do not reduce the value of these studies.

Phenytoin

Phenytoin has been linked to a characteristic (but probably not specific) syndrome, the 'fetal hydantoin syndrome', with dysmorphic features: short nose with broad depressed bridge and inner epicanthic folds; mild hypertelorism; ptosis and strabismus; wide mouth and short webbed neck; cleft lip or palate, or both; and hypoplasia of the nails and distal phalanges. The syndrome usually comprises growth deficiency and developmental delay (Loughnan *et al.* 1973; Hanson and Smith 1977; Hanson 1986). The incidence of recognizable cases is probably 10 per cent of exposed children (Hanson *et al.* 1976).

The mechanism may require a genetically susceptible infant (Phelan *et al.* 1982), and it has been postulated that a genetic defect in the detoxification of a reactive arene oxide metabolite of phenytoin may increase the risk of the syndrome (Strickler *et al.* 1985). The gene for epoxide hydrolase may exist in two allelic forms, one coding for an enzyme of low activity. Buehler and others (1990) predicted the outcome of 19 pregnancies in women taking phenytoin on the basis of the enzyme activity in fetal fibroblast or amniocyte cultures. All four fetuses with epoxide hydrolase activity below 30 per cent developed the fetal hydantoin syndrome, but none of the 15 with activities above 30 per cent did so. The similarity of dysmorphic features related to maternal consumption of phenytoin, carbamazepine, primidone, ethanol, or toluene (Hersh *et al.* 1985) may, however, support a direct neurotoxic effect (Dodson 1989).

Sodium valproate

Use of sodium valproate by the mother is associated with a significantly increased risk of spina bifida in the infant, estimated to be 36 times the risk for the non-epileptic mothers and 4 times the risk of epileptic mothers on other therapy (*The Lancet* 1988). Retrospective assessment of risk from cases collected from registers is likely to be inaccurate (*The Lancet* 1988), so the findings are uncertain, but the association has been seen in France (Robert and Guibaud 1982), Italy (Mastroiacovo *et al.* 1983), and Spain (Martínez-Frías 1989), and in international studies (Bjerkedal *et al.* 1982; Lindhout and Schmidt 1986). Lumbar spina bifida occurs, but not anencephaly. It has also been suggested (Jäger-Roman *et al.* 1986; Winter *et al.* 1987; Chitayat *et al.* 1988) that sodium valproate causes a characteristic dysmorphic syndrome of epicanthic folds, a flat nasal bridge, a broad nasal base, anteverted nostrils, a shallow philtrum, a thin upper lip, and a thick lower lip.

Other anticonvulsant drugs

Primidone (Rudd and Freedom 1979; Myhre and Williams 1981; Krauss *et al.* 1984) and carbamazepine (Jones *et al.* 1989), in similar fashion, are associated with a dysmorphic facies, and also fingernail hypoplasia and developmental delay. Troxidone (trimethadione) also probably causes facial dysmorphogenesis, as well as central nervous system malformations, growth retardation, cardiac defects, and renal tract anomalies (German *et al.* 1970; Feldman *et al.* 1977).

There is evidence (Hiilsemaa *et al.* 1983; Lindhout *et al.* 1984, Kaneko *et al.* 1988) that the risks of teratogenesis are several times greater in mothers taking a combination of different antiepileptic drugs than in those treated with one agent. In the Japanese series (Kaneko *et al.* 1988), data were collected prospectively on 172 infants born to mothers who did not themselves have congenital anomalies but who received treatment for epilepsy during the first trimester. The malformation rate was 2 in 31 infants whose mother took a single agent, but 22 in 141 in those whose mothers received two or more antiepileptic drugs. Whenever possible, therefore, epilepsy in pregnant women should be controlled with a single agent. The relative risks of the different agents are not yet known (Bardy *et al.* 1981).

Psychotropic drugs

Benzodiazepines

Evidence that benzodiazepines are teratogenic comes from retrospective studies showing a higher risk of cleft lip and palate (Safra and Oakley 1975; Saxén and Saxén 1975) and from case reports of babies with dysmorphic features and growth retardation (Laegreid *et al.* 1987, 1989). The dysmorphic features resemble those ascribed to anticonvulsants and ethanol. This evidence has been criticized as insufficient to impute malformation to benzodiazepines (Jick 1988), and a case–control study of 611 infants with cleft lip or palate, or both, failed to demonstrate any increased risk (Rosenberg *et al.* 1983). A survey of 93 children born to mothers who had taken benzodiazepines during the first trimester failed to find any characteristic malformations (Bergman *et al.* 1990).

Haloperidol

Two case reports have suggested that haloperidol may be linked to limb malformation (Dieulangard *et al.* 1966; Kopelman *et al.* 1975), but none of the mothers of 38 infants with severe limb reduction deformities could recall taking haloperidol (Hanson and Oakley 1975), and no further evidence of the association has emerged.

Antidepressants

First-trimester exposure to antidepressants was linked with an odds ratio of 7.6 for the birth of an infant with congenital malformations, particularly anencephaly and transposition of the great arteries (Bracken and Holford 1981). Unfortunately, no details are given of which drugs were involved.

In the prospective Boston study (Heinonen *et al.* 1977*b*), the standardized relative risk for first-trimester exposure of antidepressants was 1.43 (4 of 59 malformed), but this was largely due to an excess of malformed infants in mothers treated with monoamine oxidase inhibitors (3 of 21 malformed, standardized relative risk 2.6).

Fewer than 1 in 500 of the mothers studied was taking an antidepressant.

Lithium

An International Register of Lithium Babies was set up in 1968 to record the outcome in pregnancies in the first trimester of which the mother took lithium (Schou *et al.* 1973; Schou 1976). An apparent increase in the incidence of cardiac defects, particularly of Ebstein's anomaly, has been noted (Nora *et al.* 1974; Weinstein and Goldfield 1975). Ebstein's anomaly, which consists of an abnormal tricuspid valve and right-sided heart defect, was found in 4 of 11 lithium babies with significant heart defects, out of a total of 180 infants; while in the general population the incidence is about 5 per 100 000 births. This surprisingly high incidence suggests that many patients with Ebstein's anomaly would have been exposed to lithium *in utero*, but the evidence is against this (Warkany 1988; Källén 1988). Only a prospective trial is likely to give a definitive answer. In the meantime, lithium treatment should be withdrawn or avoided during the first trimester if possible (Chapman 1989).

Antineoplastic agents

Cancer during pregnancy is fortunately rare, and when it occurs the risks of treatment to the fetus are usually of secondary importance. However, 'the risk appears to be significantly lower than is commonly appreciated probably because drug doses, frequency of administration and duration of exposure are important variables' (Doll et al. 1988, 1989).

Alkylating agents

Briggs and others (1986) recorded 6 malformed infants in 22 cases where the mother was exposed to busulphan. One of the 6 had renal tract abnormalities, and similar abnormalities have been reported after chlorambucil (Shotton and Monie 1963) and mustine hydrochloride (mecloethamine) (Mennuti et al. 1975). A mother given cyclophosphamide with prednisolone for systemic lupus erythematosus gave birth to a baby with multiple abnormalities, including a dysmorphic facies, dystrophic nails, absent thumbs, and ocular malformations (Kirshon et al. 1988). The alkylating agents may also increase the risk of spontaneous abortion (Nicholson 1968). Doll and colleagues (1989) report that the risk of fetal malformations after exposure to alkylating agents in the first trimester is 14 per cent, but there may have been inaccuracies in either the numerator (number of malformations) or the denominator (number of patients), which they obtained from case reports. It has also been suggested that use of single agents, as was previously the practice (Sokal and Lessmann 1960), may be less deleterious than the current clinical practice of giving combination chemotherapy (Garber 1989).

Antimetabolites

The folate antagonist aminopterin was at one time given during the first trimester as an abortifacient. When the pregnancy was continued, the fetus was at risk of severe multiple congenital abnormalities, including anencephaly, meningoencephalocoele, skull ossification defect, low-set ears, and abnormalities of the limbs (Goetsch 1962). Similar abnormalities have been seen after treatment with methotrexate, another folate antagonist (Milunsky et al. 1968; Powell and Ekert 1971). Babies with aminopterin embryopathy may acheive 'acceptably normal young-adult status' (Shaw and Rees 1980).

Babies with multiple congenital abnormalities have been born to mothers after fluorouracil (Stephens et al.

1980), busulphan, mercaptopurine (Diamond and Anderson 1960), and cytarabine (Wagner et al. 1980; Schafer 1981) during the first trimester.

The overall risk ascribed to antimetabolites by Doll and co-workers (1989) was 19 per cent, though this is weighted by the inclusion of aminopterin, which is not used as an antineoplastic agent.

Hormones and endocrine drugs

Drugs used to treat diabetes

Mothers with diabetes have a two-to-threefold increased risk of giving birth to infants with congenital malformations, particularly caudal regression (sacral or vertebral agenesis and hypoplasia or agenesis of the femora), renal tract abnormalities, situs inversus, and cardiac anomalies (Mills et al. 1979). These malformations depend on embryological events which occur in the first 6 weeks after conception. The high incidence of malformations makes it substantially more difficult to decide whether antidiabetic drugs are themselves teratogenic, and case reports of malformation in infants of mothers taking sulphonylureas (Soler et al. 1976) are difficult to evaluate.

Prostaglandins and prostaglandin analogues

Prostaglandins stimulate the contraction of uterine muscle, and are used as abortifacients, occasionally in the first trimester. Should the abortion fail, there is a risk that the baby will be malformed (Collins and Mahoney 1983). The synthetic prostaglandin analogue misoprostil, used in the treatment of peptic ulceration, may be expected to be abortifacient.

Sex hormones

Oestrogens and progestogens

The synthetic non-steroidal oestrogen diethylstilboestrol (also known as stilboestrol) was at one time given to women during pregnancy as treatment for threatened spontaneous abortion. If exposure occurred before the ninth week of pregnancy, most female fetuses developed the syndrome of vaginal adenosis, in which the vaginal wall contains histologically demonstrable glandular tissue in addition to the usual vaginal squamous epithelium (Ulfelder 1973, 1976; Herbst 1981). There may also be cervical erosions and malformations of the cervix and upper vagina. The relative prevalence of adenosis in a series of 43 exposed and 159 unexposed female stillbirths and neonates was 18 (95 per cent confidence limits 10–32) (Johnson et al. 1979). Clear-cell adenocarcinoma of the vagina or cervix, which is otherwise extremely rare, is associated with exposure to diethylstilboestrol *in utero* (Herbst *et al.* 1971). The cancer occurs between 7 and 29 years of age, in approximately 1 in 1000 women at risk (Herbst 1981; Melnick *et al.* 1987). A 7-year prospective study of 718 exposed and 710 control women showed a doubling of the incidence of cervical and vaginal dysplasia; but a history of genital herpes was also substantially more common in the women exposed to diethylstilboestrol (Robboy *et al.* 1984). A study of 186 cases of genital tract clear-cell adenocarcinoma and 1772 controls showed that a history of vaginal blood loss during pregnancy made only a small difference to the risk of cancer after exposure to diethylstilboestrol, making it clear that it is the drug and not the disease which is responsible for the increased incidence of this cancer (Sharp and Cole 1990). Primary infertility was significantly commoner in women whose mothers had received diethylstilboestrol as part of a double-blind controlled trial than in the daughters of unexposed controls, and the prognosis was poorer (Senekjian *et al.* 1988). The infertility was related to tubal abnormalities in over 40 per cent of the exposed women but none of the unexposed women.

Effects on sexual differentiation   Diethylstilboestrol exposure can also cause masculinization of a female fetus (Bongiovanni *et al.* 1959). Female infants may be born with partial masculinization of the external genitalia after first trimester exposure to synthetic progestogens, ethisterone and norethisterone, for example (Wilkins *et al.* 1958; Wilkins 1960; Voorhess 1967). Such exposure was common when progestogens were administered for threatened abortion, and as a test for pregnancy. Large doses of progestogens can result in labial ('labioscrotal') fusion before week 13, but clitoromegaly subsequently (Grumbach *et al.* 1959; Grumbach and Ducharme 1960). In male embryos, progestogens administered between 3 and 22 weeks of gestation may be feminizing, as shown by hypospadias. The position of the meatus has been correlated with the timing of the progestogen administration (Goldman 1980).

Female pseudohermaphroditism may also result from maternal treatment during the first trimester with danazol, a derivative of 17-α-ethyltestosterone (Duck and Katayama 1981; Rosa 1984), and testosterone (Resseguie *et al.* 1985).

Other malformations   Low doses of progestogens are widely used in combination with oestrogens in the oral contraceptive pill, and perhaps as many as 3 per cent of users will inadvertently start or continue the pill in the earliest stages of pregnancy (Gardner *et al.* 1971). None the less, no definite statement can yet be made about their teratogenicity. There have been suggestions of a syndrome of characteristic anomalies after embryonic exposure to female sex steroids, including the oral contraceptive pill. The acronym VACTERL, standing for vertebral, anorectal, cardiac, tracheo-[o]esophageal, renal, and limb defects, summarizes the clinical features (Nora and Nora 1975). A characteristic facial appearance, and other anomalies, has also been suggested to make up EFESSES, the embryo-fetal exogenous sex steroid exposure syndrome (Lorber *et al.* 1979). Components of VACTERL — the vertebral anomalies, resulting in neural tube defect (Kasan and Andrews 1980), the cardiac anomalies (Heinonen *et al.* 1977*a*), and tracheo-oesophageal atresia (Lammer and Cordero 1986) and limb defects (Janerich *et al.* 1974; McCredie *et al.* 1983; Kricker *et al.* 1986) — have been reported in case–control studies, but each of the positive studies identified only one significant association. There have been several negative studies (Goujard and Rumeau-Rouquette 1977; Savolainen *et al.* 1981; Cuckle and Wald 1982; Harlap *et al.* 1985; Katz *et al.* 1985; Resseguie *et al.* 1985). It seems unlikely that the risk of any major malformation for children born to women taking oral contraceptives in the first trimester differs by more than a few per cent from the risk of unexposed children (Savolainen *et al.* 1981; Smithells 1981; WHO 1981). The counsel of perfection is to stop the oral contraceptive for three or four cycles before conceiving.

Clomiphene citrate

This synthetic non-steroidal oestrogen, which stimulates the secretion of gonadotrophins by blocking hypothalamic oestrogen receptors, is used in the induction of ovulation. Neural tube defects, particularly anencephaly and spina bifida, may be more common in infants born after ovulation induction with clomiphene, perhaps by a factor of 2 (Cornel *et al.* 1989; Vollset 1990). Subfertility may itself be a risk factor for neural tube defect, according to James (1973). A case–control study examined 571 women whose fetus or infant had a neural tube defect, 546 women whose offspring had other abnormalities, and 573 women with normal children (Mills *et al.* 1990). It found that the odds ratio for maternal use of a fertility drug was 1.3 (95 per cent confidence interval 0.4–4.5) in the group with neural tube defects compared with women whose infants had other abnormalities, and 1.1 (0.56–2.0) when compared with the normal group. Only 24 of the 1680 women questioned had, however, been exposed to a fertility drug at the inception of the index pregnancy.

Corticosteroids

Corticosteroids in pharmacological doses do not appear to be teratogenic in man (Schardein 1985). Glucocorticoids such as cortisone do cause cleft palate in mice, as explained above. There are a few reports of a baby being born with this common defect after maternal corticosteroid ingestion.

Antithyroid drugs

Aplasia cutis congenita, the localized absence of skin at birth, as an isolated scalp defect, is rare (Kalb and Grossman 1986; van Dijke *et al.* 1987). It has occurred in the offspring of women treated with methimazole for hyperthyroidism in pregnancy (Milham and Elledge 1972; Kalb and Grossman 1986). Methimazole is the active metabolite of carbimazole. The risks for any individual patient are small (van Dijke *et al.* 1987).

Thyroid hormones do not cross the placenta, while antithyroid drugs do, so regimens in which the maternal thyroid is completely blocked by antithyroid drugs and the mother given thyroxine should not be used (Cooper 1984). Even doses of antithyroid drugs just sufficient to render the mother euthyroid may result in neonatal hypothyroidism (Cheron *et al.* 1981).

Prolonged iodine and iodide ingestion during pregnancy may cause neonatal hypothyroidism and congenital goitre which is sometimes sufficiently large to obstruct the trachea at birth and cause death by asphyxiation (Carswell *et al.* 1970; Mehta *et al.* 1983), and there is a possible association with bilateral cataract (Heinonen *et al.* 1977*b*). Povidone–iodine can be detected in neonatal blood after it has been used for perineal preparation prior to vaginal delivery (Bachrach *et al.* 1984). It was associated with hypothyroidism in the neonate when applied to a maternal surgical wound (Jackson and Sutherland 1981).

[131]I can be expected to cross the placenta and cause irreversible damage to the fetal thyroid, so pregnancy is an absolute contraindication to its use.

Drugs used in skin disorders

Vitamin A derivatives

Isotretinoin (13-cis-retinoic acid) is a potent teratogen in man, and causes facial dysmorphism with hypertelorism, microphthalmia, misplaced hair whorls and skull sutures, low-set abnormal ears, and complete cleft palate. Central nervous system anomalies, particularly hydrocephalus and agenesis of the cerebellar vermis; and cardiac malformations, including ventricular septal defect, often accompany the facial dysmorphism (Willhite *et al.* 1986). The risk is estimated at 20 per cent (Lammer *et al.* 1985). Interestingly, thymic hypoplasia may occur, perhaps because of a direct effect of the drug on the thymus (Lammer *et al.* 1985; Cohen *et al.* 1987). Etretinate, another vitamin A derivative, is also teratogenic (Hopf and Mathias 1988). Both drugs are very lipid-soluble and have long half-lives. As a result, maternal plasma etretinate and metabolite concentrations may be measurable many months after treatment ceases (Rinck *et al.* 1989). This implies that the teratogenic effects may also persist, and at least one case of embryopathy with craniofacial and dural anomalies, has been reported in a baby conceived one year after the cessation of etretinate treatment (Lammer 1988). The risks after discontinuing isotretinoin may be less (Dai *et al.* 1989), though there has been no formal case–control study or life-table analysis by time from exposure. Since these drugs are used to treat severe acne in women of childbearing age, their long-lasting and serious teratogenic effects are important. There is the added risk that if vitamin A analogues achieve their intended effect, they may make pregnancy more likely (C. Moss, personal communication). Consequently, they should only be prescribed to fecund women if contraception is assured.

Non-therapeutic drugs

Alcohol

Ethanol is teratogenic. Lemoine *et al.* (1968) described 127 cases of infants born to alcoholic parents (and particularly to alcoholic mothers) who showed a characteristic facies, considerable growth retardation, psychomotor perturbations, and an increased incidence of congenital malformations. The craniofacial abnormalities comprised mild to moderate microcephaly with short palpebral fissures, maxillary hypoplasia, a short nose, a smooth philtrum and a thin, smooth upper lip (Jones 1988). The picture is sufficiently characteristic to warrant the name 'fetal alcohol syndrome'.

The mechanism by which ethanol causes fetal damage is not known, though a number of rather incomplete explanations have been proposed (Hoyseth and Jones, 1989). Experiments in rats demonstrate that prenatal and early postnatal exposure to ethanol causes neuronal damage that resembles the damage caused by chronic ethanol administration in adult rats. This seems likely to be due either to disruption of the neural membrane lipids, or to changes in neural cell adhesion molecules, which are important in cell migration during embryogenesis.

The dose of ethanol needed to produce damage, and the period of susceptibility, remain undefined in human pregnancy. Most cases have been diagnosed in the offspring of alcoholic mothers. A recent prospective study of 650 women, most of whom did not drink heavily, showed a relative risk of low birth-weight ($<2500\,g$) of 1.46 ($p<0.05$, confidence intervals not stated) in drinkers (Day *et al.* 1989). In that study, there was a significant correlation between the consumption of ethanol and other 'abnormal substances', including tobacco and marijuana.

A previous study of 32 870 women had failed to find an increased risk for the offspring of women who took one or two drinks a day during the first trimester (Mills and Graubard, 1987). The risks of moderate drinking therefore remain undefined.

In Lemoine's description, 15 infants were born to normal mothers but had alcoholic fathers. Little attention seems to have been paid to this observation in subsequent studies.

Other abused substances

Tobacco usage has been associated with growth retardation and an increased incidence of intrauterine or neonatal death (Russell *et al.* 1966; Butler *et al.* 1972). This seems likely to be due either to vasoconstriction from nicotine (Manning and Feyerabend 1976) or reduced tissue oxygenation as an effect of carbon monoxide (Longo 1970).

Cocaine and perhaps amphetamines also cause growth retardation and neurobehavioural problems. It is unclear whether these are related to lack of perinatal care rather than direct toxicity (Dodson 1989).

The second and third trimesters

Following differentiation of tissues and organs, the fetus becomes progressively less susceptible to teratogenic insult. Drugs given after about the 56th day of gestation (70th day of pregnancy as conventionally calculated) are therefore unlikely to cause congenital defects, with the exception of the sex hormones which, because of the late development of the reproductive system, may cause urogenital defects up to and beyond 12 weeks' gestation. Maternal drug therapy in the second and third trimesters can, however, influence the growth or functional development of formed tissues and organs, or exert toxic effects on fetal tissues. Essentially, the fetus is subject to the spectrum of potential toxicity (usually Type A, predictable, adverse reactions) that the drug exhibits in the adult, but developing tissues are often more sensitive to drug effects, and adverse effects can occur at doses well within the therapeutic range for the mother. Mechan-

isms of biotransformation and excretion of many drugs are underdeveloped in the neonate, and drugs given at term may produce postpartum toxicity because maternal elimination can no longer occur. Many drugs are excreted in breast milk, and may be absorbed by the neonate in sufficient quantities to produce Type A adverse effects. This aspect has been comprehensively reviewed, with recommendations for advice to breastfeeding mothers (Bennett *et al.* 1988; Atkinson *et al.* 1988; American Academy of Pediatrics 1989), and will not be further considered here.

Gastrointestinal drugs

Antacids

Antacids are generally considered to be safe in the second and third trimesters, although few specific data are available on their effects on the fetus (Feeney 1982; Lewis *et al.* 1985; *Drug and Therapeutics Bulletin* 1990).

Histamine H_2-antagonists

Cimetidine and ranitidine are widely used in obstetric anaesthesia to prevent aspiration of acidic gastric contents during labour and delivery, and appear to cause few adverse effects on the fetus or neonate.

Neonatal Apgar scores and infant progress are reported to be unaffected by cimetidine (McGowan 1979; Ostheimer *et al.* 1982; Hodgkinson *et al.* 1983; McAuley *et al.* 1985). Cimetidine was undetectable in neonatal blood 19 hours after delivery (McGowan (1979), and it does not appear to affect the development of gastric acidity or to increase bacterial colonization of the gastrointestinal tract in the infant (McAuley *et al.* 1985). A case of transient hepatic impairment was, however, reported in an infant exposed to cimetidine in the final month of pregnancy (Glade *et al.* 1980) but there have been no confirmatory reports.

When used peripartum as prophylaxis against Mendelson's syndrome, ranitidine produced no adverse effects on fetal heart rate or rhythm, or on Apgar score and neonatal progress. Plasma levels in the neonate decline rapidly, and are virtually undetectable 12 hours after delivery (Gillet *et al.* 1984; McAuley *et al.* 1984; Boschi *et al.* 1984).

Antidiarrhoeal agents

Codeine may produce neonatal effects typical of narcotic analgesics (see below), including respiratory depression, dependence, and withdrawal effects (van Leeuwen *et al.* 1965; Mangurten and Benawra 1980). There are few data on the use of loperamide in pregnancy; only about 0.3

per cent of a standard 2 mg oral dose reaches the systemic circulation (Janssen Pharmaceuticals, personal communication), and pharmacological effects in late pregnancy would appear unlikely.

Laxatives

Senna preparations are generally believed to be safe in pregnancy (Fagan 1989). Castor oil, while obsolete as a cathartic agent, may occasionally be used for self-medication; Steingrub and colleagues (1988) report the case of a patient at full term who took castor oil to induce labour and suffered a cardiopulmonary arrest from amniotic fluid embolism within 60 minutes of taking it.

Sulphasalazine and related agents

Sulphasalazine appears to be well tolerated throughout pregnancy (Miller 1986; Esbjörner *et al.* 1987). It crosses the placenta and reaches a cord concentration about half that in maternal serum (Azad Khan and Truelove 1979). The sulphapyridine component may therefore displace bilirubin from its albumin-binding sites and, in theory, cause kernicterus. Esbjörner and colleagues (1987) found no displacing effect, however, in 15 children whose mothers had taken sulphasalazine throughout pregnancy. They concluded that sulphasalazine could be continued throughout pregnancy without risk of developing kernicterus in the child, although this conclusion may not be valid for premature infants or those with haemolytic disease.

One case of reversible congenital neutropenia has been reported in association with maternal sulphasalazine therapy (Levi *et al.* 1988).

In contrast to the substantial placental transfer of sulphapyridine, 5-aminosalicylic acid (mesalazine) reaches the fetus only in trace amounts (Christensen *et al.* 1987). While this pharmacokinetic finding is reassuring, the safety of mesalazine in pregnancy has yet to be confirmed by clinical studies.

Histamine H$_1$-antagonists

Antihistamines with anticholinergic activity might, in theory, cause neonatal anticholinergic effects if used in late pregnancy, but there is little clinical evidence of this to date. What evidence there is suggests that these agents should be avoided, if possible, in the last few weeks before delivery.

A patient who took clemastine in the last week of pregnancy delivered twins with thrombocytopenia and petechiae (Gadner 1979). Diphenhydramine has been associated with a withdrawal syndrome (restlessness and diarrhoea beginning on the 5th day postpartum) in an infant whose mother had taken 150 mg per day during pregnancy (Parkin 1974). In two early reports, intravenous dimenhydrinate was reported to exert an oxytocic effect on the full-term uterus (Rotter *et al.* 1958; Watt 1961). More recently, Kargas and others (1985) reported the unexpected stillbirth at term of a female infant less than 8 hours after her mother had taken a combination of diphenhydramine and temazepam; the authors proposed a synergistic effect.

A neonatal withdrawal syndrome of irritability, poor feeding, and clonic limb movements has also been described in a child whose mother took 600 mg hydroxyzine daily throughout pregnancy (Prenner 1977).

Promethazine is a phenothiazine antihistamine that has been used extensively as an antiemetic in pregnancy, and as an adjunct to obstetric analgesia. Briggs and colleagues (1986, p. 374) have reviewed the adverse effects of this drug in late pregnancy; significant respiratory depression has been reported in small numbers of neonates, but it was not confirmed in larger studies. Transient behavioural and EEG changes have been reported (Borgstedt and Rosen 1986), as has maternal (but not fetal) tachycardia (Riffel *et al.* 1973). Promethazine used in labour has been shown significantly to impair platelet aggregation in the neonate (Corby and Schulman 1971; Whaun *et al.* 1980). The clinical relevance of this finding is unknown, but the potential adverse effects of promethazine in labour have prompted one author to suggest that its use be discontinued, particularly when the fetus is at risk of hypoxia (Hall 1987).

Promotility agents

Metoclopramide is increasingly used to treat nausea and vomiting in late pregnancy, and to prevent gastro-oesophageal reflux during labour and during anaesthesia for Caesarean section. It appears to be well tolerated by both mother and neonate, although it equilibrates rapidly between the mother and fetus. Because it is a centrally acting dopamine antagonist, metoclopramide may affect levels of pituitary hormones, and it is known to cause hyperprolactinaemia and to promote lactation in the puerperium (Kauppila *et al.* 1983). Arvela and colleagues (1983) recorded a mean fetal : maternal ratio of 0.63, and found that metoclopramide increased maternal, but not fetal, plasma prolactin levels. They did, however, find a small but significant increase in TSH concentration in cord blood. Roti and others (1983) reported that metoclopramide had no effect on TSH levels in either maternal or cord blood. In a double-blind placebo-controlled study of metoclopramide in 23 patients undergoing general anaesthesia for Caesarean section, there were no marked differences in Apgar scores, cardiovascular variables, or neurobehavioural scores (Bylsma-Howell *et al.* 1983). Vella and others (1985) compared metoclopramide and promethazine in a double-blind study in 477 mothers in labour; they were equally effective antiemetics and there were no significant differences in neonatal outcome. Neonatal dystonic reactions have not been reported with maternal metoclopramide therapy, although these are theoretically possible. There is little documented experience of the use of domperidone or cisapride during pregnancy.

Anaesthetic agents

Most inhalational and intravenous anaesthetics are lipid-soluble and poorly ionized in maternal plasma, resulting in rapid and extensive placental transfer with consequent fetal central nervous system depression (Crawford 1982). Although it has been claimed that such exposure constitutes 'behavioural teratogenesis' (Butcher 1978), there is no evidence that perinatal exposure to CNS depressants produces other than short-term neurobehavioural impairment. The extent of such impairment will depend upon the depth and duration of maternal anaesthesia, and will also be influenced by changes in maternal ventilation, circulation, and uterine perfusion (Bryson 1986; James 1987; Finster 1988). Animal data suggest that deep surgical anaesthesia with halogenated agents such as isoflurane, halothane, or enflurane may produce significant falls in uterine blood flow, and cause fetal bradycardia and acidosis (Palahniuk and Shnider 1974; Biehl *et al.* 1983*a*,*b*). The substantial body of clinical evidence suggests, however, that anaesthetics are unlikely to present a significant risk to the fetus (Konieczko *et al.* 1987). On the other hand, several studies have shown an increased incidence of miscarriage, although this may have been due to factors unrelated to the anaesthetic, such as the stress of surgery or the underlying pathology.

Intravenous induction agents such as thiopentone also reach the fetus rapidly through the placenta. Thiopentone is detectable in cord blood within seconds of administration, reaching peak concentrations within 2–3 minutes and falling exponentially thereafter (Kosake *et al.* 1969). Concentrations decline rapidly due to redistribution and hepatic metabolism by both mother and fetus, and there is some evidence to suggest that a 'first-pass' effect in the fetal liver plays a role in preventing high concentrations from reaching the fetal systemic circulation and brain (Finster *et al.* 1972). If the interval between induction and delivery exceeds about 10 minutes, thiopentone concentrations are well below anaesthetic levels, although respiratory and neurological depression may still be seen in the neonate. With modern techniques, however, the outcomes of Caesarean section under general anaesthesia are similar to those achieved with epidural anaesthesia (Zagorzycki and Brinkman 1982).

Neuromuscular blocking agents

Muscle relaxants such as tubocurarine, gallamine, suxamethonium, pancuronium, and newer agents such as alcuronium, are highly ionized and poorly lipid-soluble. They therefore cross the placenta only to a limited degree and pose little or no hazard to the fetus when used in conventional dosages. Kivalo and Saarikoski (1976) reported a cord : maternal plasma ratio of 0.12 for tubocurarine. A comparable mean fetal : maternal ratio of 0.11 has also been reported for vecuronium, and 0.19 for pancuronium (Dailey *et al.* 1984). Neither drug adversely effected neonatal outcome as assessed by Apgar score. A slightly higher mean fetal : maternal concentration ratio of 0.26 has been reported for alcuronium, but no neonatal adverse effects were evident as judged by Apgar scores (Ho *et al.* 1981).

An early report that gallamine appeared to cross the placenta slightly more readily than tubocurarine but was unlikely to harm the neonate has been repeatedly misinterpreted by subsequent authors (Crawford 1982). Consequently, the unjustified view that gallamine is contraindicated in obstetric practice is widely held and has even, on occasion, been repeated in examination questions.

Local analgesics

Local analgesic agents of the amide group cross the placenta rapidly, although cord : maternal plasma ratios are usually low (e.g. 0.52–0.69 for lignocaine and 0.31–0.44 for bupivacaine) (Pederson *et al.* 1978). Pharmacokinetic data on obstetric analgesia were comprehensively reviewed by Krauer and others (1984).

Agents of the ester group, such as procaine (no longer widely used), are so rapidly hydrolysed by plasma esterase that they present little hazard to the fetus.

The fetal microsomal enzyme system for biotransformation of amide-type local analgesics is immature in the neonate (Zagorzycki and Brinkman 1982), but the neonate can nevertheless metabolise these drugs, albeit slowly. For example, high levels of lignocaine in the neonate following epidural anaesthesia fall slowly, as the drug is metabolised and excreted in the first few days of life (Kuhnert *et al.* 1979).

Local analgesics can indirectly affect the fetus through changes in utero-placental circulation, or by a direct action on the fetus. Fetal bradycardia, respiratory distress, seizures, and hyperirritability have all been reported (Hill and Stern 1979). Contributory factors to fetal bradycardia include maternal hypotension and fetal hypoxia, leading to metabolic acidosis, and a quinidine-like depressant action on fetal cardiac tissue. Central nervous system toxicity is manifested as respiratory and cardiovascular depression, low Apgar scores, episodes of apnoea, and convulsions (Guillozel 1975; Finster 1976).

Overall, up to 30 per cent of neonates who are exposed to amide-type local analgesics through maternal paracervical or epidural blocks are reported to display recognizable adverse effects at birth (Yaffe and Stern 1976). There are, however, significant pharmacokinetic differences within this group, and bupivacaine appears to be the drug of choice for continuous epidural analgesia in obstetrics (*Drug and Therapeutics Bulletin* 1983), since it has a relatively low fetal : maternal concentration ratio, probably due to extensive protein-binding of the drug in maternal plasma (Ralston and Shnider 1978). It has minimal effects on uterine function (Schellenberg 1977) and, in one study, neonates delivered under bupivacaine epidurals exhibited better muscle tone than those whose mothers had received lignocaine or mepivacaine (Scanlon *et al.* 1974).

Prilocaine is metabolised to toluidine and can produce neonatal methaemoglobinaemia with cyanosis when used in obstetric analgesia, particularly if large doses are used (Brindenbaugh *et al.* 1969). Crawford (1965) found, however, that 400 mg produced less than 1 per cent methaemoglobinaemia, which had disappeared within 2 hours. Unless the infant has suffered intrauterine hypoxia or is severely anaemic, the methaemoglobinaemia is unlikely to cause any serious harm (Crawford 1982). The manufacturers have not received any reports of problems arising from dental use of prilocaine in pregnancy during more than 20 years of world-wide usage of the drug (Watson 1988).

Anti-infective agents

Infections are relatively common during pregnancy, and need to be treated appropriately, but there are few reliable data confirming either the safety or efficacy of anti-infective agents in pregnancy. There is, however, an extensive body of clinical experience (albeit mainly empirical and anecdotal) which indicates that the older-established penicillins such as benzylpenicillin or ampicillin are safe in pregnancy. The treatment of infections in pregnancy has been reviewed by Landers and colleagues (1983) and, more recently, by Gilstrap and Faro (1990).

Because renal function is usually enhanced in pregnancy, the elimination of water-soluble antibiotics such as the penicillins may be increased. Thus the dose of ampicillin or pivampicillin may need to be doubled in pregnant women to achieve an adequate therapeutic response, particularly for severe infections (Jordheim and Hagen 1980).

Anthelmintics

Piperazine is potentially neurotoxic (Dukes 1980; Leach 1990), although there have been no reports of fetal or neonatal neurological effects.

Tetracyclines

Tetracyclines are potent chelating agents and form a complex with calcium that is incorporated in fetal bones and teeth. Calcification of the deciduous teeth begins towards the end of the first trimester, and the yellow-brown discolouration and enamel hypoplasia associated with maternal tetracycline therapy after this stage are now well-recognized (Porter *et al.* 1965; Kutscher *et al.* 1966; Genot *et al.* 1970). Because exchange of calcium does not occur after calcification of teeth is complete, the discolouration is permanent. In later pregnancy, the permanent teeth may be affected. All tetracyclines produce these effects, although Weyman (1965), in a study of 59 children with tetracycline staining of the teeth, showed that the colour varied depending on the drug used; the least objectionable staining (a creamy discolouration) was produced by oxytetracycline.

Tetracyclines are also incorporated into fetal bone, and can cause a reversible retardation of skeletal growth, particularly in premature infants (Cohlan *et al.* 1963; Greene 1976).

Tetracyclines may cause a dose-related acute fatty degeneration of the liver, especially in the presence of impaired renal function, characterized by azotaemia, jaundice, and pancreatitis (Whalley *et al.* 1964; Allen and Brown 1966). While the fetus may not be directly affected, the maternal disorder often leads to fetal morbidity and mortality.

Chloramphenicol

The fetus and neonate are deficient in the enzyme system which glucuronidates chloramphenicol. The drug is well known to cause the 'grey baby' syndrome of vomiting, hypothermia, and cardiovascular collapse when given directly to the neonate (Leitman 1979), but there are no reliable reports of this reaction arising from maternal exposure (Gilstrap and Faro 1990). Nevertheless, because of the theoretical risk, and because its haematological toxicity and effects on protein synthesis in dividing cells, chloramphenicol is best avoided throughout pregnancy.

Sulphonamides

Sulphonamides cross the placenta readily, achieving fetaly : maternal blood concentration ratios of up to 0.9 (Briggs *et al.* 1986, p. 418). They are highly protein-bound and compete with bilirubin for binding sites on plasma albumin, or they may compete with it for immature fetal glucuronyl transferase. In the neonate, when free bilirubin can no longer be cleared via the placenta, jaundice may occur (Dunn 1964), although this appears to be uncommon. Kernicterus is a theoretical possibility, but has not been reported in practice. The risk is likely to be greater in premature infants with immature hepatic function. Sulphonamides may also cause haemolytic anaemia, particularly in individuals deficient in glucose 6-phosphate dehydrogenase (Perkins 1971).

Quinolones

Ciprofloxacin, ofloxacin, and perfloxacin all cross the placenta readily (Giamarellou *et al.* 1989). These drugs are known to cause arthropathy in the weightbearing joints of immature animals (Schluter 1989) and, although there are no reports of arthropathy arising from exposure *in utero*, they should be avoided in pregnancy.

Aminoglycosides

The aminoglycosides can all produce dose-related eighth cranial nerve damage in adults, and must be regarded as potentially ototoxic or vestibulotoxic to the fetus. There are several reports of ototoxicity in the offspring of mothers treated with streptomycin (Snider *et al.* 1980; Donald and Sellars 1981). Kanamycin has also been reported to cause hearing loss (Good and Johnson 1971; Jones 1973). Fetal ototoxicity has not been reported with gentamicin or other aminoglycosides, but may potentially occur, particularly if plasma concentrations exceed the therapeutic range or if treatment is prolonged.

Antituberculous drugs

Ethambutol and isoniazid appear to be safe in pregnancy (Snider *et al.* 1980; de Swiet 1989a). Rifampicin, however, has been associated with two cases of neonatal hypoprothrombinaemia and haemorrhage, caused by maternal vitamin K deficiency (Chouraqui *et al.* 1982).

Anti-inflammatory agents

The use of non-steroidal anti-inflammatory drugs (NSAID) in pregnancy has been extensively reviewed (Rudolph 1981; Needs and Brooks 1985; Østensen and Husby 1985; Heymann 1986; Brooks and Needs 1989). Although these agents appear not to be teratogenic in man (Brooks and Needs 1989), their use in late pregnancy, either to treat arthritic disease or to delay premature labour, may be associated with a range of adverse effects.

Prostaglandins are important mediators of fetal function and development. Prostaglandin E_2 produces dilatation of both systemic and pulmonary blood vessels, and is involved in maintaining patency of the ductus arteriosus; prostaglandins may also influence blood flow in various organs, including the kidney. They have a major influence on platelet adhesion and aggregation, and they are also mediators of uterine contraction.

Inhibition of fetal cyclo-oxygenase by NSAID may therefore cause profound circulatory, renal, and haematological effects, and may delay the onset of, and prolong, labour.

Indomethacin has been widely used in the management of threatened premature labour, and its adverse effects are well documented. Manchester and co-workers (1976) reported primary pulmonary hypertension associated with maternal indomethacin therapy, and similar effects have been demonstrated in animal studies (Levin *et al.* 1979); and there have been several subsequent reports of this reaction with indomethacin (Truter *et al.* 1986; Demandt *et al.* 1990), naproxen (Wilkinson *et al.* 1979; Wilkinson 1980), and salicylate (Arcilla *et al.* 1969; Perkin *et al.* 1980). The increased pulmonary artery pressure is probably a direct consequence of constriction or premature closure of the fetal ductus arteriosus (Rudolph 1981; Moise *et al.* 1988a).

Levin and colleagues (1978) found increased smooth muscle development in the pulmonary vascular bed of infants exposed to NSAID and, in animal models, *in utero* exposure to indomethacin produces similar hypertrophy of pulmonary vascular smooth muscle (Levin *et al.* 1979).

It should be noted, however, that several studies have failed to confirm the association between NSAID and neonatal pulmonary hypertension (Kumor *et al.* 1979; Niebyl *et al.* 1980; Hendricks *et al.* 1990), and at least one study has been challenged (Ovadia 1988) and defended (Moise *et al.* 1988b) on methodological grounds. Many variables may influence whether an individual neonate suffers this adverse reaction, including the dose, timing, and duration of exposure to the NSAID, and possible differences in the sensitivity of the ductus arteriosus and pulmonary vasculature to changes in prostaglandin levels. Moreover, all the recorded cases have been associated with use in late pregnancy for threatened premature labour; it is not clear whether the use of NSAID at an earlier stage of pregnancy for non-obstetric indications carries similar risks. It would be prudent, however, to assume that all cyclo-oxygenase-inhibiting agents have the potential to cause cardiovascular complications, and to avoid them in pregnancy unless there is a clear and specific therapeutic indication.

Prostaglandins are synthesized in the kidney, and NSAID are known occasionally to cause acute renal insufficiency or renal tubular necrosis (see Chapter 12). It is therefore not surprising that renal problems in the neonate have been associated with maternal NSAID therapy. van der Heijden and others (1988) reported oedema, oliguria, and elevated serum creatinine in five of nine preterm neonates exposed to indomethacin. Simeoni and colleagues (1989) described severe acute renal failure in twins, and transient water and sodium retention with uraemia in a third infant. A case of anuria requiring peritoneal dialysis was associated with indomethacin therapy (Demandt et al. 1990).

Several cases of oligohydramnios have been associated with cyclo-oxygenase inhibitors, again in preterm labour (Kirshon 1988; Hickok et al. 1989; Goldenberg et al. 1989; Wiggins and Elliott 1990; Hendricks et al. 1990). Oligohydramnios, growth retardation, and anuria were reported in an infant whose mother had taken 150 mg indomethacin daily for juvenile arthritis, from weeks 27–37 of pregnancy (Cantor et al. 1980). A preterm infant developed severe hyponatraemia after fluid retention following the mother's taking an overdose of naproxen 8 hours before delivery (Alun-Jones and Williams 1986).

Neonatal ischaemic brain injury has been described in two pairs of twins, all of whom were exposed to indomethacin in utero (Simeoni et al. 1989; Haddad et al. 1990). Low urinary prostaglandin E_2 levels were recorded in two of the neonates, and cerebral vasoconstriction induced by indomethacin was postulated.

Aspirin inhibits platelet adhesion and aggregation and therefore impairs haemostasis. Maternal consumption of aspirin in late pregnancy consequently increases the risk of antepartum and postpartum haemorrhage, and of neonatal haemorrhage (Stuart et al. 1982). Bleyer and Breckenridge (1970) showed that neonatal haemostasis was sensitive to even small doses of aspirin taken by the mother in late pregnancy. Rumack and colleagues (1981) reported a significantly increased incidence of intracranial haemorrhage in premature infants exposed to aspirin in the last week of pregnancy.

Low-dose aspirin has been used successfully, however, and without neonatal haemorrhagic complications, in the management of women at risk of pregnancy-induced

hypertensive crises and pre-eclampsia (Benigni et al. 1989; Schiff et al. 1989); and Garrettson and others (1974) reported the case of a woman who took 6.5 g aspirin per day throughout pregnancy and was then delivered of a healthy female infant who had a plasma salicylate concentration of 250 mg per litre.

Cardiovascular drugs

Anticoagulants

Warfarin

This drug may cause abnormalities of the central nervous system such as hydrocephaly or microcephaly, optic atrophy, and developmental impairment; in contrast to warfarin embryopathy, there does not appear to be a critical period of exposure (Sherman and Hall 1976; Hall 1976; Holzgreve et al. 1976; Hall et al. 1980). Hall and colleagues (1980), in a review of published cases, concluded that about 3 per cent of liveborn infants exposed to warfarin demonstrated CNS abnormalities. The sequelae were more significant and debilitating than those of the embryopathy, and all had been exposed to warfarin in the second or third trimesters, or during both of these.

The microcephaly, optic atrophy, and mental retardation might be due to repeated small intracranial haemorrhages induced by warfarin (Sahul and Hall 1977). Chong and colleagues (1984), however, compared the physical and mental development of 22 children exposed to warfarin during pregnancy with matched controls. There were no significant differences between the exposed children and the controls, or within the study group according to the time of exposure to warfarin; none of the 18 children exposed in the second trimester showed CNS defects. In a study of 30 pregnancies during which the mothers took warfarin from week 13 onwards, there was one case of congenital hydrocephalus, but no case of microcephaly or eye defects (Chen et al. 1982). All except the infant with hydrocephalus subsequently showed normal developmental patterns. CNS defects arising from late exposure to warfarin therefore appear to be rare.

Warfarin can cause serious haemorrhagic complications in both mother and fetus towards the end of pregnancy (Villasanta 1965). The fetus and premature neonate have low levels of vitamin K-dependent clotting factors (II, VII, IX, and X) (Bonnar et al. 1971; Andrew et al. 1981). The fetus may therefore be receiving excessive anticoagulant while the mother's prothrombin time is within the normal range, and fetal or neonatal haemorrhage, sometimes fatal, may ensue. For this reason, a change to heparin is generally recommended in late pregnancy, between weeks 32 and 36, for the remainder of the pregnancy (Hirsh *et al.* 1970; *Drug and Therapeutics Bulletin* 1987; Ginsberg and Hirsh 1988, 1989).

Heparin

Heparin is a heterogeneous group of high-molecular-weight, polar compounds that do not cross the placenta in significant amounts. Heparin therapy is occasionally associated with maternal haemorrhage, but it is generally considered to be safe for the fetus, though Hall and others (1980) claimed that the fetal and neonatal morbidity and mortality associated with heparin was as high as with oral anticoagulants. They found that in 135 published cases of heparin exposure there were 19 stillbirths or abortions, 29 premature births (10 fatal), and normal outcomes in only 86.

This retrospective survey, however, included a large proportion of women with co-morbidity known to predispose to adverse fetal outcomes. Ginsberg and Hirsh (1989), in a careful review of the same reports, found that of the pregnancies in which heparin was used, 49 were associated with severe toxaemia, glomerulonephritis, or a history of recurrent abortions. There were 31 (63.3 per cent) adverse outcomes in this group. In an independent review of 186 published studies involving 1325 pregnancies exposed to anticoagulants, Ginsberg and others (1989) found adverse outcomes in 10.5 per cent of cases where heparin was used (after excluding co-morbidity). If prematurity with normal outcome was excluded, the incidence of adverse outcomes was only 3.6 per cent.

This analysis supported the findings of a small controlled trial in which 40 women were randomized to receive heparin or no treatment. There was no increased risk of antenatal or postnatal bleeding in the heparin group, and there was one abortion in each group, although more babies from the heparin group required neonatal intensive care (Howell *et al.* 1983). In a more recent, retrospective, study 100 pregnancies in 77 women treated with heparin were reviewed (Ginsberg *et al.* 1989). Rates of prematurity, abortion, stillbirth, neonatal death, and congenital defects were similar to those in the general population. The authors concluded that maternal heparin therapy was safe for the fetus, and carried an acceptable bleeding rate (there were only two episodes), and a low rate of thrombotic recurrence in the mother.

Heparin therefore appears to be effective and relatively safe in the prophylaxis and treatment of venous thromboembolic disease in pregnancy. Low-dose heparin is ineffective, however, in women with valvular heart disease and, while high-dose heparin may be effective, this has not been demonstrated in controlled clinical trials (Iturbe-Alessio *et al.* 1986; *Drug and Therapeutics Bulletin* 1987; Ginsberg and Hirsh 1988, 1989).

Heparin causes demineralization of bone, and osteoporosis may occur, usually in women treated for 6 months or more. In a study of 20 women given 20 000 units daily, heparin caused a dose-dependent osteopenia, although this was symptomatic in only one case (de Swiet *et al.* 1983). In a more recent study, 12 out of 70 women (17 per cent) given a mean dose of 31 000 units daily exhibited obvious osteopenia on X-rays of the spine and hip. Two suffered multiple fractures of the spine (Dahlman *et al.* 1990).

Antihypertensive agents

Methyldopa has been widely used to treat hypertension in pregnancy and most reports indicate that it presents little hazard to the fetus. A large, prospective, controlled study demonstrated the absence of any significant adverse effects, and the developmental progress of infants exposed to methyldopa has been followed up from periods of up to 7½ years (Mutch *et al.* 1977*a,b*; Ounsted *et al.* 1980; Cockburn *et al.* 1982; Redman and Ounsted 1982).

Fetuses exposed to methyldopa for the first time in mid-pregnancy (between 16–20 weeks) were found to have significantly smaller head circumferences at birth, but this did not affect development progress (Redman and Ounsted 1982) and the effect is considered to be of minor clinical significance (Redman 1989).

Methyldopa crosses the placenta freely, and may cause neonatal hypotension (Whitelaw 1981). Two cases of neonatal nasal obstruction have been reported recently (LeGras *et al.* 1990), and Shimohira and others (1986) described a child with abnormal sleep patterns that were attributed to maternal methyldopa administration. Low concentrations of noradrenaline in cerebrospinal fluid, associated with a marked tremor, were reported in three hypoxic neonates whose mothers had taken methyldopa (Bodis *et al.* 1982).

β-Adrenoceptor blocking agents

The use of β-blockers to treat hypertension in pregnancy is now well established, and they may replace methyldopa as the drug of choice for first-line therapy (Lubbe 1984; Myers 1990). Current evidence indicates that these agents are relatively safe in pregnancy (Frishman and Chesner 1990). Because β-adrenergic drive has, however, important effects on umbilical blood flow, uterine function, and fetal cardiovascular and metabolic functions, β-blockers may cause a range of pharmacological (Type A) adverse effects in the second and third trimesters. Many of these reactions may represent the consequences of fetal distress in severely hypertensive, high-risk, pregnancies but, until recently, the use of β-blockers in pregnancy has been controversial.

In an early study, intrauterine growth retardation was seen in 6 of 12 pregnancies in which propranolol was taken by the mother (Pruyn *et al.* 1979). The effect was attributed to impaired uterine blood flow secondary to β-blockade, but severe hypertension is itself known to be associated with placental insufficiency. At least two controlled clinical trials comparing β-blockers with methyldopa (Gallery *et al.* 1979; Rubin *et al.* 1983) have shown no excess incidence of growth retardation in babies exposed to β-blockers. A follow-up study of 55 infants who had been exposed to atenolol showed normal development at one year of age (Reynolds *et al.* 1984).

Other adverse effects occasionally reported with β-blockers are respiratory distress (Tunstall 1969), prolonged labour (Habib and McCarthy 1977), bradycardia and hypotension (Woods and Morrell 1982; Brosset *et al.* 1988), and hypoglycaemia (Brosset *et al.* 1988). With the exception of neonatal bradycardia, however, these effects have not been apparent in controlled clinical trials, and outcomes in pregnancies where β-blockers are used are generally favourable. To minimize effects on uterine contractility, and the risk of neonatal β-blockade, these agents should preferably be discontinued (gradually, to avoid withdrawal effects) a few days before the onset of labour (Frishman and Chesner 1990).

Labetalol is a unique agent that has both α-blocking and β-blocking activity, together with a direct vasodilator effect. Experience with this potent antihypertensive agent in pregnancy has been generally favourable, with few reports of clinically significant fetal hypoglycaemia, bradycardia, or respiratory depression. Macpherson and others (1986) made serial measurements of neonatal cardiovascular, metabolic, and thermoregulatory function for the first 72 hours of life in 11 infants exposed to labetalol and in 11 carefully matched controls. The former showed a mild transient hypotension (mean 4.5 mm Hg) which resolved within 24 hours; there were no other significant differences and the authors concluded that labetalol does not cause clinically important sympathetic blockade in the full-term neonate.

A more recent case report (Haraldsson and Geven 1989) suggests that maternal labetalol may be less well tolerated by the premature neonate; an infant born at 33 weeks' gestation had severe bradycardia, diminished femoral pulse, cyanosis, and respiratory depression after delivery by Caesarean section. In a randomized controlled trial against methyldopa in 176 women, however, cardiovascular, metabolic, and respiratory function findings were comparable, including those of a subgroup of 33 infants who were small-for-gestational-age or born before 37 weeks (Plouin *et al.* 1987).

Diuretics

Thiazides are best avoided in pregnancy. They may aggravate pre-eclampsia by increasing hypovolaemia, possibly precipitating renal failure (Palomaki and Lindheimer 1970). Maternal hypokalaemia (Pritchard and Walley 1961), pancreatitis (Minkowitz *et al.* 1964), and hyperuricaemia may occur, and neonatal thrombocytopenia has been reported (Rodriguez *et al.* 1974).

A recent report described metabolic acidosis, hypocalcaemia, and hypomagnesaemia in a preterm infant whose mother was treated with acetazolamide throughout pregnancy (Merlob *et al.* 1990). *In utero* exposure to ethacrynic acid throughout pregnancy has been implicated in a case of neonatal nephrolithiasis (Fischer *et al.* 1988). Ultrasonography at 30 weeks showed polyhydramnios, and massive neonatal diuresis occurred during the first day of life.

Calcium-channel blocking agents

These drugs are potentially useful in pregnancy-associated hypertension refractory to other agents, but clinical experience with this indication is limited, and their safety remains to be confirmed. Walters and Redman (1984) used nifedipine in 21 women with severe hypertension and, although maternal adverse effects (headache and flushing) were evident, no adverse effects on the fetuses were detected. More recently, Constantine and others (1987) reported on the use of nifedipine mainly in combination with atenolol in 23 pregnant women with severe hypertension. Blood pressure control was good, but there were high rates of Caesarean section, abnormal fetal ECGs, and premature or small-for-dates infants; whether this was due to the hypertension or the medication was uncertain.

Nifedipine is a potent uterine relaxant (Ulmsten *et al.* 1978; Andersson *et al.* 1979; Forman *et al.* 1982) that has been used in the management of preterm labour (Bult-Sarley and Lourwood 1988). Its use to treat hypertension in late pregnancy might therefore be expected to cause delayed or prolonged labour, although no cases have been reported to date.

Angiotensin-converting-enzyme (ACE) inhibitors

Although both captopril and enalapril have been used successfully in pregnancy (Fiocchi *et al.* 1984; Smith 1989; Baethge and Wolf 1989), both of these compounds are highly fetotoxic in animal studies, and there is considerable evidence from case reports and uncontrolled studies that their use in pregnancy carries a high risk of adverse fetal outcome.

The risk appears to be primarily associated with treatment in the second and third trimesters. When ACE inhibitors are stopped in the first trimester, the pregnancy is likely to continue to term with a normal outcome, whereas treatment throughout pregnancy leads to an increase in prematurity and low birth-weight (*The Lancet* 1989). ACE inhibitors are known to have adverse effects on the kidney in adults (see Chapter 12) and renal failure has been reported when captopril was used to treat severe neonatal hypertension (Tack and Perlman 1988). It is therefore not surprising that adverse renal effects and oligohydramnios feature prominently in reports of fetal and neonatal toxicity (Guignard *et al.* 1981; Rothberg and Lorenz 1984; Schubiger *et al.* 1988; Scott and Purohit 1989; Rosa *et al.* 1989; Cunniff *et al.* 1990). At least eight perinatal deaths associated with ACE-inhibitor therapy have been reported. Although the severity of the hypertension for which the ACE inhibitors were prescribed may be a confounding factor in many of these cases, the data clearly indicate that these drugs should be used in pregnancy with great caution, if at all.

Drugs affecting the endocrine system

Iodides and antithyroid agents

The fetal thyroid begins to secrete thyroxine by the twelfth week of gestation, and TSH becomes detectable in fetal blood. T_4 levels increase until, at full term, they are comparable to maternal levels (Fisher and Klein 1981; Ramsay 1990). The fetus is therefore vulnerable to drugs affecting thyroid function.

Maternal thyrotoxicosis during pregnancy needs to be treated, but the use of antithyroid drugs must be approached with caution. Radioactive iodine should never be used as it is concentrated avidly in the fetal thyroid in the second and third trimesters (Ramsay 1990), with a high risk of permanent damage to, or destruction of, the gland (Fisher *et al.* 1963).

Antithyroid drugs cross the placenta readily and can inhibit fetal thyroid function, leading to thyroid hypertrophy and goitre. Many cases of fetal goitre have been reported with the use of iodides (Carswell *et al.* 1970). The goitre can be large enough to obstruct the fetal trachea, and there have been several neonatal deaths. Chronic iodide therapy should therefore be avoided in pregnancy. While both propylthiouracil (Cheron *et al.* 1981) and carbimazole (Sugrue and Drury 1980) may depress fetal thyroid function, the risks are minimal if the lowest possible maintenance dose is used (Burrow 1985). Davis and others (1989) reported on 60 infants

whose gestation was complicated by overt maternal thyrotoxicosis. Propylthiouracil was given at doses of 300–800 mg daily, well above recommended maintenance doses in pregnancy (Ramsay 1990), with minimal adverse effects. In a study of 43 infants whose mothers had been taking propylthiouracil or methimazole for Graves' disease, 40 per cent had reduced levels of free T_4 in cord blood, but there were no signs or symptoms of hypothyroidism (Momotani *et al.* 1986). The authors concluded that the optimum dose regimen was one that maintained maternal T_4 levels in the upper normal to mildly thyrotoxic range. An alternative approach to the treatment of Graves' disease is to use a combination of antithyroid drugs and physiological replacement doses of thyroxine. Ramsay and others (1983) described 20 babies whose mothers had been treated in this way; all had normal T_4 concentrations in cord blood. Long-term follow-up of 25 children exposed *in utero* to carbimazole showed no developmental or endocrine abnormalities at 3–13 years of age (McCarroll *et al.* 1976).

Amiodarone is an antiarrhythmic agent with a high (39 per cent) iodine content. Both hyperthyroidism and hypothyroidism are well-recognized adverse reactions to the drug in adults, and similar effects have been reported in neonates. A case of severe congenital hypothyroidism and goitre was associated with the mother's taking 200 mg amiodarone daily from the thirteenth week of pregnancy (De Wolf *et al.* 1988), and elevated neonatal thyroxine levels have also been reported (Tubman *et al.* 1988).

Sex hormones

Because development of the urogenital system is not complete until the end of the first trimester, exposure to sex hormones relatively late in pregnancy can produce structural defects. Aarskog (1970, 1979) correlated the timing of exposure to oestrogens and progestogens with hypospadias in male infants; defects were associated with maternal medroxyprogesterone therapy initiated in the twelfth week.

Hypoglycaemic agents

Oral hypoglycaemic agents cross the placenta readily, achieving fetal plasma levels in the adult therapeutic range. They can therefore cause severe and prolonged neonatal hypoglycaemia (Zucker and Simon 1968; Kemball *et al.* 1970); in two cases, exchange transfusion was performed to remove the drug. These agents are therefore generally considered to be contraindicated in pregnancy.

Being a high-molecular-weight peptide, insulin does not cross the placenta, and therapeutic doses are devoid of any significant effects on the fetus. Most authorities therefore agree that pregnant diabetic women in whom dietary management alone is inadequate should be treated with insulin, both for the tighter diabetic control that can be achieved, and to avoid the problems associated with oral hypoglycaemic agents (Barss 1989; Beard and Maresh 1989).

Corticosteroids

Corticosteroids have two main indications in pregnancy; in the management of asthma and arthritic disease, and to accelerate lung maturity in cases of preterm labour. Available evidence indicates that they are relatively safe for these purposes. In an early study, the incidence of stillbirth and placental insufficiency was reported in 34 women receiving prednisolone for various disorders (Warrell and Taylor 1968). One study has reported an increased incidence (13.9 per cent) of low-birth-weight infants in mothers who took 10 mg prednisone daily throughout pregnancy (Reinisch et al. 1978). One case of severe intrauterine growth retardation has been associated with topical use of the potent fluorinated steroid triamcinolone from weeks 12–29 of gestation (Katz et al. 1990).

These findings have not been confirmed by other studies, however. Schatz and others (1975) found no increase in neonatal death or other adverse outcomes in a series of 70 pregnancies in which corticosteroids were used for asthma, apart from a slight excess of prematurity. Children treated in utero with corticosteroids to prevent the respiratory distress syndrome have been followed-up extensively, with no evidence of adverse effects on growth, on development, or on neurological function (MacArthur et al. 1982; Collaborative Group on Antenatal Steroid Therapy 1984; Smolders et al. 1990).

There have been occasional reports of neonatal pituitary–adrenal suppression, usually mild and transient, associated with maternal corticosteroid therapy (Grajwer et al. 1977; Ohrlander et al. 1977), but this appears not to be a serious or frequent problem. Corticosteroids are immunosuppressant and long-term therapy with these agents is known to increase the risk of infection in adults (see Chapter 23). There is also evidence of an increased incidence of neonatal infections when steroids are used in the antenatal period (Wong and Taeusch 1978; Kappy et al. 1979; Smolders et al. 1990).

Drugs acting on the central nervous system

Benzodiazepines

Benzodiazepines cross the placenta readily and may produce direct pharmacological effects in the fetus and neonate, or give rise to a perinatal withdrawal syndrome, or produce both of these effects. Diazepam equilibrates between the fetal and maternal circulations within 5–10 minutes, achieving concentrations in the fetal circulation equal to or greater than those in maternal blood (Erkkola et al. 1973; Mandelli et al. 1975; McAllister 1980).

A characteristic 'floppy infant syndrome' may therefore be seen, particularly after high or repeated maternal doses. The symptoms include lethargy and hypotonia, respiratory difficulties, thermoregulatory problems, and feeding difficulties (Cree et al. 1973; Rowlatt 1978), and the fetal heart rate may also be affected (Scher et al. 1972). The elimination half-lives of diazepam and its metabolite, desmethyldiazepam, are prolonged in the neonate, and these effects may therefore persist for several days (Mandelli et al. 1975). While the neonatal effects of diazepam have been most extensively documented, similar effects are seen with chlordiazepoxide (Stirrat et al. 1974), lorazepam (Whitelaw et al. 1981), and nitrazepam (Speight 1977) and should be anticipated with any agent in this group.

Published work has focused on the adverse effects of benzodiazepines when used as adjuncts to obstetric analgesia, but chronic maternal exposure to anxiolytic or hypnotic doses is likely to produce similar problems. A neonatal withdrawal syndrome may be seen, particularly if the maternal dosage has been high. The symptoms may take up to 2–3 weeks to appear and resemble those of opiate withdrawal; they include irritability, tremor, hypertonia, hyperactivity, tachypnoea, gastrointestinal disturbances, and vigorous sucking. Cases have been reported with diazepam (Rementeria and Bhatt 1977) and chlordiazepoxide (Athinarayanan et al. 1976), and similar effects may occur with any benzodiazepine, particularly those with long elimination half-lives and active metabolites.

Major tranquillizers

Phenothiazines given in single doses during labour do not appear to cause major adverse effects in the neonate, although chlorpromazine has been reported occasionally to produce marked maternal hypotension, which could be hazardous to the fetus (Briggs et al. 1986, p. 85). Chronic use of phenothiazines as psychotropic agents during pregnancy, particularly at high doses, may cause pharmacological effects in the fetus and neonate, including hypotonia, lethargy, and hyporeflexia (Hammond and Toseland 1970) and paralytic ileus due to anti-cholinergic activity (Falterman and Richardson 1980). These effects may be prolonged because of slow elimination of phenothiazines by the neonatal liver.

Third-trimester exposure to antipsychotic agents may also produce extrapyramidal effects in the neonate, characterized by agitation, hypertonicity, tremor, poor sucking and swallowing, and unusual movement patterns. This effect has been reported with chlorpromazine and thioridazine (Hill *et al.* 1966; Levy and Wisniewski 1974) and fluphenazine (O'Connor *et al.* 1981). The symptoms may take several months to resolve, but subsequent infant development appears to be satisfactory (Hill *et al.* 1966).

Withdrawal effects are not normally associated with neuroleptic agents, but Sexson and Barak (1989) have recently reported a case of withdrawal emergent syndrome, a subtype of tardive dyskinesia, in a neonate whose mother had taken haloperidol throughout pregnancy. The infant developed repeated tongue thrust, abnormal hand posturing, and tremor of all extremities. Most symptoms resolved within a few days, but tongue thrusting continued until 6 months of age.

Lithium

Use of lithium in pregnancy may produce severe neonatal toxicity; the features include hypotonia, cyanosis, arrhythmias, cardiomegaly, and diabetes insipidus (Mitzrahi *et al.* 1979; Wilson *et al.* 1983; Morrell *et al.* 1983). In many cases the neonatal toxicity is associated with inadequate control of maternal serum lithium concentrations, although fetal toxicity may occur even if maternal levels are in the normal range. The elimination half-life is greatly prolonged in neonates, values of up to 96 hours having been reported (Mackay *et al.* 1976), as against the usual adult value of about 20 hours. The symptoms of neonatal lithium intoxication may therefore take several weeks to resolve, and two cases of diabetes insipidus persisted for more than 2 months (Rane *et al.* 1978; Mitzrahi *et al.* 1979). Neonatal hypothyroidism has also been reported (Karlsson *et al.* 1975). More recently, two cases of maternal polyhydramnios, thought to be secondary to fetal diabetes insipidus, have been reported (Ang *et al.* 1990; Krause *et al.* 1990).

Antidepressants

Tricyclic antidepressants are slowly eliminated by the neonate, and may cause a range of adverse effects including tachyarrhythmias, irritability, tremor, urinary retention, tachypnoea, and muscle spasms (Shearer *et al.* 1972; Webster 1973; Prentice and Brown 1989). While many of these symptoms represent direct pharmaco-logical effects, for example, anticholinergic-induced tachycardia and urinary retention, it is clear that a neonatal withdrawal syndrome is sometimes seen, especially after chronic high-dose therapy, and particularly with clomipramine (Ben Musa and Smith 1979; Cowe and Lloyd 1982; Østergaard and Pederson 1982; Singh *et al.* 1990). Neonatal convulsions were a feature of the two cases reported by Cowe and colleagues (1982) and, in one infant, an intravenous infusion of clomipramine was needed for the first 17 days of life to control the convulsions.

Narcotic analgesics

Fetal exposure to narcotics in late pregnancy falls into two main categories: analgesia in labour or for Caesarean section, and abuse by dependent mothers.

The effects of peripartum narcotics on the neonate are well documented. Placental transfer of pethidine and other opioids is rapid and substantial. Pethidine is detectable in amniotic fluid within 30 minutes of a maternal intramuscular injection, and concentrations in cord blood are 80 to 130 per cent of maternal levels (Moore *et al.* 1973; Rothberg *et al.* 1978). The effect on the neonate is characterized by respiratory depression and a low Apgar score (Fishburn 1982), which is likely to be maximal about 3 hours after the intramuscular injection (Belfrage *et al.* 1981). The respiratory depressant effects can be reversed by naloxone.

Pethidine and its metabolite are only slowly eliminated by the neonate (Kuhnert *et al.* 1980), and neonatal neurobehavioural dysfunction may be evident for 2–3 days (Hodgkinson and Husain 1982). One study has attributed impaired behavioural patterns up to 6 weeks after birth to high cord blood levels of pethidine (Belsey *et al.* 1981). Follow-up studies have not demonstrated any long-term developmental effects from obstetric analgesia. Richards (1981) has reviewed studies in this area.

Narcotic dependency

Drug dependency in pregnant women is an increasing problem (de Swiet 1989b), and the incidence of neonatal complications is high. An American study in 830 women dependent on opiates and 400 matched controls found significantly increased risks of meconium staining, anaemia, haemorrhage, multiple pregnancy, prematurity, low birth-weight, low Apgar scores, and perinatal mortality. Children of addicts were 5.5 times more likely to be small for gestational age, and the relative risk of perinatal mortality was 2.7 (Ostrea and Chavez 1979).

The fetus may also develop dependence, and a high proportion of infants born to women dependent on narcotics will experience a withdrawal syndrome (de Swiet 1989*b*). The timing of the onset of withdrawal depends upon the rate of elimination of the narcotic; morphine and diamorphine withdrawal symptoms begin with 4–24 hours after delivery, whereas methadone withdrawal may be delayed for up to 1–2 weeks. The withdrawal syndrome is characterized by irritability, hypertonia, tremor, tachypnoea, and sometimes convulsions. It may be fatal, and withdrawal effects can occur *in utero* if the mother stops using narcotics or if narcotic antagonists are given.

The long-term effects of exposure to narcotics *in utero* are poorly understood. The results of follow-up studies are conflicting, and it is often difficult to differentiate the effect of narcotic exposure from that of confounding social and environmental factors (Kaltenbach and Finnegan 1989; Hans 1989). However, studies published to date indicate that prenatal narcotic exposure does not appear to have long-term developmental consequences (Strauss *et al.* 1979; Kaltenbach and Finnegan 1986, 1987).

References

Aarskog, D. (1970). Clinical and cytogenetic studies in hypospadias. *Acta Paediatr. Scand.* (suppl.) 303, 1.

Aarskog, D. (1979). Current concepts in cancer: Maternal progestins as a possible cause of hypospadias. *N. Engl. J. Med.* 300, 75.

Ad Hoc Committee. (1974). Occupational disease among operating-room personnel: a national study. *Anesthesiology* 41, 321.

Agapitos, M., Georgiou-Theodoropoulou, M., Koutselinis, A., and Papacharalampus, N. (1986). Cyclopia and maternal ingestion of salicylates. *Pediatr. Pathol.* 6, 309.

Akhtar, N. and Millac, P. (1987). Epilepsy and pregnancy: A study of 188 pregnancies in 92 patients. *Br. J. Clin Pract.* 41, 862.

Aldridge, L.M. and Tunstall, M.E. (1986). Nitrous oxide and the fetus. *Br. J. Anaesth.* 58. 1356.

Allen, E.S. and Brown, W.E. (1966). Hepatic toxicity of tetracycline in pregnancy. *Am. J. Obstet. Gynecol.* 95, 12.

Alun-Jones, E. and Williams, J. (1986). Hyponatremia and fluid retention in a neonate associated with maternal naproxen overdosage. *J. Toxicol. Clin. Toxicol.* 24, 257.

American Academy of Pediatrics, Committee on Drugs. (1989). Transfer of drugs and other chemicals into human milk. *Pediatrics* 84, 924.

Andersson, K.-E., Ingemarsson, I., Ulmsten, U., and Wingerup, L. (1979). Inhibition of prostaglandin-induced uterine activity by nifedipine. *Br. J. Obstet. Gynaecol.* 86, 175.

Andrew, M., Bhogal, M., and Karpatkin, M. (1981). Factors XI, XII and prekallikrein in sick and healthy premature infants. *N. Engl. J. Med.* 305, 1130.

Andrews, L.G. and Souma, J.A. (1989). Elevated serum alpha-fetoprotein in a pregnant woman with rheumatoid arthritis. *N. Engl. J. Med.* 321, 262.

Ang, M.S., Thorpe, J.A., and Parisi, V.M. (1990). Maternal lithium therapy and polyhydramnios. *Obstet. Gynecol.* 76, 517.

Annegers, J.F., Elveback, I,.R., Hauser, W.A., and Kurland, L.T. (1974). Do anticonvulsants have a teratogenic effect? *Arch. Neurol.* 31, 364.

Arcilla, R.A., Thilenius, O.G., and Ranniger, K. (1969). Congestive heart failure from suspected ductal closure in utero. *J. Pediatr.* 75, 74.

Armitage, P. and Berry G., (1987). *Statistical methods in medical research.* Blackwell Scientific, Oxford.

Arvela, P., Jouppila, R., Kauppila, A., Pakarinen, A., Pelkonen, O., and Tuimala, R. (1983). Placental transfer and hormonal effects of metoclopramide. *Eur. J. Clin. Pharmacol.* 24, 345.

Aselton, P.J. and Jick, H. (1983). Additional follow-up of congenital limb disorders in relation to Bendectin use. *JAMA* 250, 622.

Athinarayanan, P., Pierog, S.H., Nigam, S.K., and Glass, L. (1976). Chlordiazepoxide withdrawal in the neonate. *Am. J. Obstet. Gynecol.* 124, 212.

Atkinson, H.C., Begg, E.J., and Darlow, B.A. (1988). Drugs in human milk. Clinical pharmacokinetic considerations. *Clin. Pharmacokinet.* 14, 217.

Azad Khan, A.K. and Truelove, S.C. (1979). Placental and mammary transfer of sulphasalazine. *Br. Med. J.* ii, 1553.

Bachrach, L.K., Burrow, G.N., and Gare, D.J. (1984). Maternal–fetal absorption of povidone–iodine. *J. Pediatr.* 104, 158.

Baethge, B.A. and Wolf, R.E. (1989). Successful pregnancy with scleroderma renal disease and pulmonary hypertension in a patient using angiotensin converting enzyme inhibitors. *Ann. Rheum. Dis.* 48, 776.

Bardy, A.H., Hiilesmaa, V.K., Teramo, K., and Granstrom, M-L. (1981). Teratogenic risks of antiepileptic drugs. *Br. Med. J.* 283, 1405.

Barr, M. and Burdi, A.R. (1976). Warfarin-associated embryopathy in a 17-week-old abortus. *Teratology* 14, 129.

Barss, V.A. (1989). Diabetes and pregnancy. *Med. Clin. N. Am.* 73, 685.

Beard, R. and Maresh, M. (1989). Diabetes. In *Medical disorders in obstetric practice* (2nd edn) (ed. M. de Swiet), p. 584. Blackwell Scientific, Oxford.

Beck, F. and Lloyd, J.B. (1965). Embryological principles of teratogenesis. In *Embryopathic activity of drugs* (ed. J.M. Robson, F.M. Sullivan, and R.L. Smith), p. 1. Churchill, London.

Beckman D. A. and Brent, R.L. (1986). Mechanism of known environmental teratogens: drugs and chemicals. *Clin. Perinatol.* 13, 649.

Belfrage, P., Boreus, L.U., Hartvig, P., Jrestedt, L., and Raabe, N. (1981). Neonatal depression after obstetrical analgesia with pethidine. The role of the injection–delivery time interval and the plasma concentrations of pethidine and norpethidine. *Acta Obstet. Gynecol. Scand.* 60, 43.

Belsey, E.M., Rosenblatt, D.B., Lieberman, B.A., Redshaw, M., Caldwell, J., and Notorianni, L. (1981). The influence of maternal analgesia on neonatal behaviour. I. Pethidine. *Br. J. Obstet. Gynaecol.* 88, 398.

Ben Musa, A. and Smith, C.S. (1979). Neonatal effects of maternal clomipramine therapy. *Arch. Dis. Child.* 54, 405.

Benawra R., Mangurten, H.H., and Duffell, D.R. (1980). Cyclopia and other anomalies following maternal ingestion of salicylates. *J. Pediatr.* 96, 1069.

Benigni, A., Gregorini, G., Frusca, T., Chiabrando, C., Ballerini, S., Valcamonico, A., *et al.* (1989). Effect of low-dose aspirin on fetal and maternal generation of thromboxane by platelets in women at risk for pregnancy-induced hypertension. *N. Engl. J. Med.* 321, 357.

Bennett, P.N. (ed.) and members of the WHO Working Group (1988). *Drugs and human lactation*. Elsevier, Amsterdam.

Bergman, U., Boethius, G., Swartling, P.G., Isacson, D., and Smedby, B. (1990). Teratogenic effects of benzodiazepines use during pregnancy. *J. Pediatrics* 116, 490.

Biehl, D.R., Yarnell, R., Wade, J.G., and Sitar, D. (1983*a*). The uptake of isoflurane by the foetal lamb in utero: effect on regional blood flow. *Can. Anaesth. Soc. J.* 30, 581.

Biehl, D., Tweed, W.A., and Cote, J. (1983*b*). Effect of halothane on cardiac output and regional blood flow in the fetal lamb in utero. *Anesth. Analg.* 62, 489.

Binns, W., James, L.F., and Shupe, J.L. (1965). Embryopathic activity of a poisonous range plant, *Veratrum californicum*. In *Embryopathic activity of drugs* (ed. J.M. Robson, F.M. Sullivan, and R. L. Smith), p. 105. Churchill, London.

Bjerkedal, T., Czeizel, A., Goujard, J., Kallen, B., Mastroiacova, P., Nevin, N., *et al.* (1982). Valproic acid and spina bifida. *Lancet* ii, 1096.

Bleyer, W.A. and Breckenridge, R.T. (1970). The effects of prenatal aspirin on newborn haemostasis. *JAMA* 213, 2049.

Bodis, J., Sulyok, E., Ertl, T., Varga, L., Hartmann, G., and Csaba, I.F. (1982). Methyldopa in pregnancy hypertension and the newborn. *Lancet* ii, 498.

Bongiovanni, A.M., Di George, A.M., and Grumbach, M.M. (1959). Masculinization of the female infant associated with estrogenic therapy alone during gestation. *J. Clin. Endocrinol. Metab.* 19, 1004.

Bonnar, J., McNichol, G.P., and Douglas, A.S. (1971). The blood coagulation and fibrinolytic systems in the newborn and mother at birth. *J. Obstet. Gynaecol. Br. Commwlth* 78, 355.

Borgstedt, A.D. and Rosen, M.G. (1986). Medication during labor correlated with behavior and EEG of the newborn. *AJDC* 115, 21.

Boschi, S., Di Marco, M.G., Pigna, A., and Rossi, R. (1984). The effect of ranitidine on gastric pH and volume in patients undergoing Cesarean section: possible relationship to Mendelson's syndrome. *Curr. Ther. Res.* 35, 654.

Bracken, M.B. and Berg, A. (1983). Bendectin (Debendox) congenital diaphragmatic hernia. *Lancet* i, 586.

Bracken, M.B. and Holford, T.R. (1981). Exposure to prescribed drugs in pregnancy and association with congenital malformations. *Obstet. Gynecol.* 58, 336.

Brent, R.L. (1983). The Bendectin saga: another American tragedy. *Teratology* 27, 283.

Briggs, G.G., Freeman, R.K., and Yaffe, S.J. (1986). *Drugs in pregnancy and lactation* (2nd edn). Williams & Wilkins, Baltimore.

Brindenbaugh, P.O., Brindenbaugh, L.D., and Moore, D.C. (1969). Methaemoglobinaemia and infant-response to lidocaine and prilocaine in continuous caudal anaesthesia: a double blind study. *Anesth. Analg. Curr. Res.* 48, 824.

Brooks, P.U. and Needs, C.J. (1989). The use of antirheumatic medication during pregnancy and in puerperium. *Rheum. Dis. Clin. N. Am.* 15, 789.

Brosset, P., Roayette, D., Delhoume, B., Lacapeyre, F., Alain, J., Collet, D., *et al.* (1988). Effets métaboliques et cardiovasculaires chez le nouveau-né des bétabloquants pris par la mère. *Presse Med.* 17, 467.

Bryson, T.H.L. (1986). Anaesthesia during pregnancy. *Clin. Anaesth.* 4, 549.

Buehler, B.A., Delimont, D., van Waes, M., and Finnell, R.H. (1990). Prenatal prediction of risk of the fetal hydantoin syndrome. *N. Engl. J. Med.* 322, 1567.

Bult-Sarley, J. and Lourwood, D.L. (1988). Nifedipine for preterm labor. *Drug Intell. Clin. Pharm.* 22, 330.

Bunde, C.A. and Bowles, D.M. (1963). A technique for controlled survey of case records. *Curr. Ther. Res.* 5, 245.

Burrow, G.N. (1985). The management of thyrotoxicosis in pregnancy. *N. Engl. J. Med.* 313, 562.

Butcher, R.E. (1978). Halothane — a behavioral teratogen? *Anesthesiology* 49, 308.

Butler, N.R., Goldstein, H., and Ross, E.M. (1972). Cigarette smoking in pregnancy, its influence on birth weight and perinatal mortality. *Br. Med. J.* i, 127.

Bylsma-Howell, M., Riggs, K.W., McMorland, G.H., Rurak, D.W., McErlane, B., and Axelson, J.E. (1983). Placental transport of metoclopramide: Assessment of maternal and neonatal effects. *Can. Anaesth. Soc. J.* 30, 487.

Cantor, B., Tyler, T., and Nelson, R.M. (1980). Oligohydramnios and transient neonatal anuria. A possible association with the maternal use of prostaglandin synthetase inhibitors. *J. Reprod. Med.* 24, 220.

Carswell, F., Kerr, M.M., and Hutchison, J.H. (1970). Congenital goitre and hypothyroidism produced by ingestion of iodides. *Lancet* i, 1241.

Carter, M.P. and Wilson, F. (1962). Tetracycline and congenital limb abnormalities. *Br. Med. J.* iii, 407.

Carter, M.P. and Wilson, F. (1963). Antibiotics and congenital malformations. *Lancet* i, 1267.

Chapman, W.S. (1989). Lithium use during pregnancy. *J. FlaMed. Assoc.* 76, 454.

Check, W.A. (1979). CDC study: no evidence for teratogenicity of Bendectin. *JAMA* 242, 2518

Chen, W.W.C., Chan, C.S., Lee, P.K., Wang, R.Y., and Wong, V.C.W. (1982). Pregnancy in patients with prosthetic valves: an experience with 45 pregnancies. *Q. J. Med.* 203, 358.

Cheron, R.G., Kaplan, M.M., Larsen, P.R., Selenkow, H.A., and Crigler, J.F. (1981). Neonatal thyroid function after propylthiouracil therapy for maternal Graves' disease. *N. Engl. J. Med.* 304, 525.

Chitayat, D., Farrell, K., Anderson, L., and Hall, J.G. (1988). Congenital abnormalities in two sibs exposed to valproic acid in utero. *Am. J. Med. Genet.* 31, 369.

Chong, M.B., Harvey, D., and de Swiet, M. (1984). Follow-up study of children whose mothers were treated with warfarin during pregnancy. *Br. J. Obstet. Gynaecol.* 91, 1070.

Chouraqui, J.P., Bessard, G., Favier, M., Kolodie, L., and Rambaud, P. (1982). Haemorrhage due to vitamin K deficiency in pregnant women and newborn babies: relationship with rifampicin in 2 cases. *Therapie* 37, 447.

Christensen, L.A., Rasmussen, S.N., Hansen, S.H., Bondesen, S., and Hvidberg, E.F. (1987). Salazosulfapyridine and metabolites in fetal and maternal body fluids with special reference to 5-aminosalicylic acid. *Acta Obstet. Gynecol. Scand.* 66, 433.

Cipriani, S., Conti, R., and Vella, G. (1983). Ranitidina in gravidanza. *Clin. Europ.* 22, 86.

Cockburn, J., Moar, V.A., Ounsted, M., and Redman, C.W.G. (1982). Final report of study on hypertension during pregnancy: the effects of specific treatment on the growth and development of the children. *Lancet* i, 647.

Cohen, M., Rubinstein, A., Li, J.K., and Nathenson, G. (1987). Thymic hypoplasia associated with isotretinoin embryopathy. *AJDC* 141, 263.

Cohen, M.M. (1982). An update on the holoprosencephalic disorders. *J. Pediatr.* 101, 865.

Cohlan, S.Q., Bevelander, G., and Tiamsie, T. (1963). Growth inhibition of prematures receiving tetracyclines. A clinical and laboratory investigation of tetracycline-induced bone fluorescence. *AJDC* 105, 453.

Collaborative study on antenatal steroid therapy. (1984). Effects of antenatal dexamethasone administration in the infant: long term follow-up. *J. Pediatr.* 104, 259.

Collins, F.S. and Mahoney, M.J. (1983). Hydrocephalus and abnormal digits after failed first-trimester prostaglandin abortion attempt. *J. Pediatr.* 102, 620.

Constantine, G., Beevers, D.G., Reynolds, A.L., and Luesley, D.M. (1987). Nifedipine as a second line antihypertensive drug in pregnancy. *Br. J. Obstet. Gynecol.* 94, 1136.

Cooper, D.S. (1984). Antithyroid drugs. *N. Engl. J. Med.* 311,

Corazza, G.R., Gasbarrini, G., Di Nisio, Q., and Zulli, P. (1982). Cimetidine (Tagamet) in peptic ulcer therapy during pregnancy. *Clin. Trials J.* 19, 91.

Corby, D.G. and Schulman, I. (1971). The effects of antenatal drug administration on aggregation of platelets of newborn infants. *J. Pediatr.* 79, 307.

Corcoran, R. and Castles, J.M. (1977). Tetracycline for acne vulgaris and possible teratogenesis. *Br. Med. J.* ii, 807.

Cordero, J.F., Oakley, G.P., Greenberg, F., and James, L.M. (1981). Is Bendectin a teratogen? *JAMA* 245, 2307.

Cornel, M.C., Ten Kate, L.P., and Te Meerman, G.J. (1989). Ovulation induction, in-vitro fertilisation, and neural tube defects. *Lancet* ii, 1530.

Cowe, L. and Lloyd, D.J. (1982). Neonatal convulsions caused by withdrawal from maternal clomipramine. *Br. Med. J.* 184, 1837.

Crawford, J.S. (1982). Obstetric analgesia and anaesthesia. *Current reviews in obstetrics and gynaecology.* No. 1. Churchill Livingstone, Edinburgh.

Crawford, J.S. and Lewis, M. (1986). Nitrous oxide in early human pregnancy. *Anaesthesia* 41, 900.

Crawford, O.B. (1965). Methaemoglobinaemia following the use of prilocaine. *Acta Anaesthesiol. Scand.* (suppl.) 16, 183.

Craxi, A. and Pagliarello, F. (1980). Possible embryotoxicity of sulfasalazine. *Arch. Intern. Med.* 140, 1674.

Cree, J.E., Mexer, J., and Hailey, D.M. (1973). Diazepam in labour: its metabolism and effect on the clinical condition and thermogenesis of the newborn. *Br. Med. J.* iv, 251.

Cuckle, H.S. and Wald, N.J. (1982). Evidence against oral contraceptives as a cause of neural-tube defects. *Br J. Obstet. Gynecol.* 89, 547.

Cunniff C., Jones, K.L., Phillipson, J., Benirschke, K., Short, S., and Wujek, J. (1990). Oligohydramnios sequence and renal tubular malformation associated with maternal enalapril use. *Am. J. Obstet. Gynecol.* 162, 187.

Dahlman, T., Lindvall, N., and Hellgren, M. (1990). Osteopenia in pregnancy during long-term heparin treatment: a radiological study post partum. *Br. J. Obstet. Gynecol.* 97, 221.

Dai, W.S., Hsu, M-A., and Itri, L.M. (1989). Safety of pregnancy after discontinuation of isotretinoin. *Arch. Dermatol.* 125, 362.

Dailey, P.A., Fisher, D.M., Shnider, S.M., Baysinger, C.L., Shinohara, Y., Miller, R.D., *et al.* (1984). Pharmacokinetics, placental transfer, and neonatal effects of vecuronium and pancuronium administered during caesarean section. *Anesthesiology* 60, 569.

Dansky, L.V., Andermann, E., Rosenblatt, D., Sherwin, A.L., and Andermann, F. (1987). Anticonvulsants, folate levels, and pregnancy outcome: A prospective study. *Ann. Neurol.* 21, 176.

Davis, L.E., Lucas, M.J., Hankins, G.D., Roark, M.L., and Cunningham, F.G. (1989). Thyrotoxicosis complicating pregnancy. *Am. J. Obstet. Gynecol.* 160, 63.

Day, N.L., Jasperse, D., Richardson, G., Raboles, N., Sambamoorthi, U., Taylor, P., *et al.* (1989). Prenatal exposure to alcohol: effect on infant growth and morphologic characteristics. *Pediatrics* 84, 536.

de St Jorre, J. (1980*a*). New thalidomide-style drug fear. *Observer*, 20th January.

de St Jorre, J. (1980*b*). US Debendox ruling opens legal floodgate. *Observer*, 23rd March.

de Swiet, M., Dorrington Ward, P., Fidler, J., Horsman, A., Katz, D., Letsky, E., *et al.* (1983). Prolonged heparin therapy in pregnancy causes bone demineralization. *Br. J. Obstet. Gynecol.* 90, 1129.

de Swiet, M. (ed.) (1989*a*). Diseases of the respiratory system. In *Medical disorders in obstetric practice* (2nd edn), p. 19. Blackwell Scientific, Oxford.

de Swiet, M. (ed.) (1989*b*). Drug dependence. In *Medical disorders in obstetric practice* (2nd edn), p. 797. Blackwell Scientific, Oxford.

de Wolf, D., de Schepper, J., Verhaaren, H., Smitz, J., and Sacre-Smits, L. (1988). Hypothyroid goiter and amiodarone. *Acta Paediatr. Scand.* 77, 616.

Demandt, E., Legius, E., Devlieger, H., Lemmens, F., Proesmans, W., and Eggermont, E. (1990). Prenatal indomethacin toxicity in one member of monozygous twins; a case report. *Eur. J. Obstet. Gynecol. Reprod. Biol.* 35, 267.

Diamond, J. and Anderson, M.M. (1960). Transplacental transmission of busulfan (Myleran) in a mother with leukemia: production of fetal malformation and cytomegaly. *Pediatrics* 25, 85.

Dieulangard, P., Coignet, J., and Vidal, J.C. (1966). A case of ectro-phocomelia, possibly of drug-induced origin. *Soc. Nat. Gynecol. Obstet. Fr.* (Marseille) 18, 85.

Dodson, W.E. (1989). Deleterious effects of drugs on the developing nervous system. *Clin. Perinatol.* 16, 339.

Doll, D.C., Ringenberg, Q.S., and Yarbro, J.W. (1988). Management of cancer during pregnancy. *Arch. Intern. Med.* 148, 2058.

Doll, D.C., Ringenberg, Q.S., and Yarbro, J.W. (1989). Antineoplastic agents and pregnancy. *Sem. Oncol.* 16, 337.

Donald, P.R. and Sellars, S.L. (1981). Streptomycin ototoxicity in the unborn child. *S. Afr. Med. J.* 60, 316.

Drug and Therapeutics Bulletin (1983). Epidural anaesthesia in obstetrics. *Drug Ther. Bull.* 21, 29.

Drug and Therapeutics Bulletin (1987). Use of anticoagulants in pregnancy. *Drug Ther. Bull.* 25,1.

Drug and Therapeutics Bulletin (1990). Heartburn in pregnancy. *Drug Ther. Bull.* 28, 11.

Duck, S.C. and Katayama, K.P. (1981). Danazol may cause female pseudohermaphroditism. *Fertil. Steril.* 35, 230.

Dukes, M.N.G. (1980). Anthelmintic drugs. In *Meyler's side effects of drugs* (ed. M.N.G. Dukes), p. 538. Excerpta Medica, Amsterdam.

Duminy, P.C. and Burger, P.du.T. (1981). Fetal abnormality associated with the use of captopril during pregnancy. *S. Afr. Med. J.* 80, 805.

Duncan, P.G., Pope, W.D.B., Cohen, M.M., and Greer, N. (1986). Fetal risk of anesthesia and surgery during pregnancy. *Anesthesiology* 64, 790.

Dunn, P.M. (1964). The possible relationship between the maternal administration of sulphamethoxypyridazine and hyperbilirubinaemia in the newborn. *J. Obstet. Gynecol. Br. Cwlth* 71, 128.

Dunn, P.M., Stewart-Brown, S., and Peel, R. (1979). Metronidazole and the fetal alcohol syndrome. *Lancet* ii, 144.

Elder, H.A., Santamarina, B.A.G., Smith, S., and Kass, E.H. (1971). The natural history of asymptomatic bacteruria during pregnancy: The effect of tetracycline on the clinical course and the outcome of pregnancy. *Am. J. Obstet. Gynecol.* 111, 441.

Erkkola, R., Kangas, L., and Pekkarinen, A. (1973). The transfer of diazepam across the placenta during labour. *Acta Obstet. Gynecol. Scand.* 52, 167.

Esbjörner, E., Jarnerot, G., and Wranne, L. (1987). Sulphasalazine and sulphapyridine serum levels in children to mothers treated with sulphasalazine during pregnancy and lactation. *Acta Paediatr. Scand.* 76, 137.

Eskenazi, B. and Bracken, M.B. (1982). Maternal dicyclomine-doxylamine-pyridoxine use in pregnancy. *Am. J. Obstet. Gynecol.* 144, 919.

Fagan, E.A. (1989). Disorders of the gastrointestinal tract. In *Medical disorders in obstetric practice* (2nd edn) (ed. M. de Swiet), p. 562. Blackwell Scientific, Oxford.

Falterman, C.G. and Richardson, J. (1980). Small left colon syndrome associated with maternal ingestion of psychotropic drugs. *J. Pediatr.* 97, 308.

Fedrick, J. (1973). Epilepsy and pregnancy: a report from the Oxford record linkage study. *Br. Med. J.* ii, 442.

Feeney, J.G. (1982). Heartburn in pregnancy. *Br. Med. J.* 284, 1138.

Feldman, G.L., Weaver, D.D., and Lovrien, E.W. (1977). The fetal trimethadione syndrome. *AJDC* 131, 1389.

Finster, M. (1976). Toxicity of local anaesthetics in the foetus and the newborn. *Bull. N.Y. Acad. Med.* 52, 222.

Finster, M. (1988). Surgical anaesthesia for pregnant patient. *Can. J. Anaesth.* 35, 514.

Finster, M., Morishima, H.O., Mark, L.C., Perel, J.M., Dayton, P.G., and James, L.S. (1972). Tissue thiopental concentrations in the fetus and newborn. *Anesthesiology* 36, 155.

Fiocchi, R., Lijnen, P., Staessen, J., Fagard, R., Amery, A., van Assche, F., et al. (1984). Captopril during pregnancy. *Lancet* ii, 1153.

Fischer, A.F., Parker, B.R., and Stevenson, D.K. (1988). Nephrolithiasis following *in utero* diuretic exposure: an unusual case. *Pediatrics* 81, 712.

Fishburn, J.J. (1982). Systemic analgesia during labour. *Clin. Perinatol.* 9, 29.

Fisher, R.A. and Klein, A.H. (1981). Thyroid development and disorders of thyroid function in the newborn. *N. Engl. J. Med.* 304, 702.

Fisher, U.D., Voorhess, M.C., and Gardner, L.I. (1963). Congenital hypothyroidism in infant following maternal I^{131} therapy. *J. Pediatr.* 62, 132.

Forman, A., Gandrup, P., Andersson, K.-E., and Ulmsten, U. (1982). Effects of nifedipine on oxytocin and prostaglandin F$_{2\alpha}$-induced activity in the postpartum uterus. *Am. J. Obstet. Gynecol.* 144, 665.

Frishman, W.H. and Chesner, M. (1990). Use of beta-adrenergic blocking agents in pregnancy. In *Cardiac problems in pregnancy* (2nd edn) (ed. U. Elkayam and N. Gleicher), p. 351. Alan R. Liss, New York.

Gadner, H. (1979). Purpura bei neugeborenen Zwillingen nach Einnahme eines Antihistaminikums durch die Mutter. *Internist Praxis* 19, 542.

Gaily, E., Granström, M-L., Hiilesmaa, V., and Bardy, A. (1989). Minor anomalies in offspring of epileptic mothers. *J. Pediatr.* 112, 520.

Gallery, E.D.M., Saunders, D.M., Hunyer, S.M., and Gyory, A.Z. (1979). Randomized comparison of methyldopa and oxprenolol for treatment of hypertension in pregnancy. *Br. Med. J.* i, 1591.

Garber, J.E. (1989). Long-term follow-up of children exposed in utero to antineoplastic agents. *Sem. Oncol.* 16, 437.

Gardner, L.I., Assemany, S.R., and Neu, R.L. (1971). Syndrome of multiple osseous defects with pretibial dimples. *Lancet* ii, 98.

Garrettson, L.K., Procknal, J.A., and Levy, G. (1974). Fetal acquisition and neonatal elimination of a large amount of salicylate. *Clin. Pharmacol. Ther.* 17, 98.

Genot, M.T., Golan, H.P., Porter, P.J., and Kass, E.H. (1970). Effect of administration of tetracycline in pregnancy on the primary dentition of the offspring. *J. Oral Med.* 25, 75.

German, J., Ehlers, K.H., Kowal, A., de George, F.V., Engle. M.A., and Passarge, E. (1970). Possible teratogenicity of trimethadione and paramethadione. *Lancet* ii, 261.

Giamsarellou, H., Kolokythas, E., Petrikkos, G., Gazis, J., Aravantinos, D., and Sfikakis, P. (1989). Pharmacokinetics of three newer quinolones in pregnant and lactating women. *Am. J. Med.* 87, 495.

Gibson, G.T., Colley, D.P., McMichael, A.J., and Hartshorne, J.M. (1981). Congenital anomalies in relation to the use of doxylamine/dicyclomine and other antenatal factors. *Med. J. Aust.* i, 410.

Gillet, G.B., Watson, J.D., and Langford, R.M. (1984). Ranitidine and single-dose antacid therapy as prophylaxis against acid aspiration syndrome in obstetric practice. *Anaesthesia* 39, 638.

Gilstrap, L.C. and Faro, S. (ed.) (1990). *Infections in pregnancy*. Wiley-Liss, New York.

Ginsberg, J.S. and Hirsh, J. (1988). Optimum use of anticoagulants in pregnancy. *Drugs* 36, 505.

Ginsberg, J.S. and Hirsh, J. (1989). Anticoagulants during pregnancy. *Annu. Rev. Med.* 40, 79.

Ginsberg, J.S., Kowalchuk, G., Hirsh, J., Brill-Edwards, P., and Burrows, R. (1989). Heparin therapy during pregnancy. *Arch. Intern. Med.* 149, 2233.

Glade, G., Saccar, C.L., and Pereira, G.R. (1980). Cimetidine in pregnancy; apparent transient liver impairment in the newborn. *AJDC* 134, 87.

Goetsch, C. (1962). An evaluation of aminopterin as an abortifacient. *Am. J. Obstet. Gynecol.* 83, 1474.

Goldberg, J.D. and Golbus, M.S. (1986). The value of case reports in human teratology. *Am. J. Obstet. Gynecol.* 154, 479.

Goldenberg, R.L., Davis, R.O., and Baker, R.C. (1989). Indomethacin-induced oligohydramnios. *Am. J. Obstet. Gynecol.* 160, 1196.

Goldman, A.S. (1980). Critical periods of prenatal toxicological insults. In *Drug and chemical risks to the fetus and newborn* (ed. R.H. Schwarz and S.J. Yaffe), p. 26. Alan R. Liss, New York.

Goldman, A.S., Baker, M.K., Piddington, R., and Herold, R. (1983). Inhibition of programmed cell death in mouse embryonic palate in vitro by cortisol and phenytoin: receptor involvement and requirement of protein synthesis. *Proc. Soc. Exp. Biol. Med.* 174, 239.

Good, R. and Johnson, G. (1971). The placental transfer of kanamycin during late pregnancy. *Obstet. Gynecol.* 38, 60.

Goujard, J. and Rumeau-Rouquette, C. (1977). First-trimester exposure to progestagen/oestrogen and congenital malformations. *Lancet* i, 482.

Grajwer, L.A., Lilien, L.D., and Pildes, R.S. (1977). Neonatal subclinical adrenal insufficiency. Result of maternal steroid therapy. *JAMA* 238, 1279.

Greene, G.R. (1976). Tetracyclines in pregnancy. *N. Engl. J. Med.* 295, 512.

Grumbach, M.M. and Ducharme, J.R. (1960). The effects of androgens on fetal sexual development: androgen-induced female pseudohermaphroditism. *Fertil. Steril.* 11, 157.

Grumbach, M.M., Ducharme, J.R., and Moloshok, R.E. (1959). On the fetal masculinizing action of certain oral progestins. *J. Clin. Endocrinol. Metab.* 19, 1369.

Guignard, J-P., Burgener, F., and Calame, A. (1981). Persistent anuria in a neonate: a side-effect of captopril? *Int. J. Pediatr. Nephrol.* 2, 133.

Guillozel, N. (1975). The risk of paracervical anesthesia: intoxication and neurological injury of the newborn. *Pediatrics* 55, 533.

Habal, F.M. and Greenberg, G.R. (1987). Safety of oral 5-aminosalicylic acid in inflammatory bowel disease. *Clinical controversies in inflammatory bowel diseases. An international symposium.* Bologna. Sept 9–11.

Habib, A. and McCarthy J.S. (1977). Effects on the neonate of propranolol administered during pregnancy. *J. Pediatr.* 91, 808.

Haddad, J., Messer, J., Casanova, R., Simeoni, U., and Willard, D. (1990). Indomethacin and ischaemic brain injury in neonates. *J. Pediatr.* 116, 839.

Hall, J.G. (1976). Warfarin and fetal abnormality. *Lancet* i, 1127.

Hall, J.G., Pauli, R.M., and Wilson, K.M. (1980). Maternal and fetal sequelae of anticoagulation during pregnancy. *Am. J. Med.* 68, 122.

Hall, P.F. (1987). Use of promethazine (Phenergan) in labour. *Can. Med. Assoc. J.* 136, 690.

Hammond, J.E. and Toseland, P.A. (1970). Placental transfer of chlorpromazine. *Arch. Dis. Child.* 45, 139.

Hans, S.L. (1989). Developmental consequences of prenatal exposure to methadone. *Ann. N.Y. Acad. Sci.* 562, 195.

Hanson, J.W., (1986). Teratogen update: fetal hydantoin syndrome. *Teratology* 33, 349.

Hanson, J.W. and Oakley, G.P. (1975). Haloperidol and limb deformity. *JAMA* 231, 26.

Hanson, J.W. and Smith, D.W. (1977). Are hydantoins (phenytoins) human teratogens? *J. Pediatr.* 90, 674.

Hanson, J.W., Myrianthopoulos, N.C., Harvey, M.A.S., and Smith, D.W. (1976). Risks to the offspring of women treated with hydantoin anticonvulsants, with emphasis on the fetal hydantoin syndrome. *J. Pediatr.* 89, 662.

Haraldsson, A. and Geven, W. (1989). Severe adverse effects of maternal labetalol in a premature infant. *Acta Paediatr. Scand.* 78, 956.

Harlap, S., Shiono, P.H., and Ramcharan, S. (1985). Congenital abnormalities in the offspring of women who used oral and other contraceptives around the time of conception. *Int. J. Fertil.* 30, 39.

Harley, J.D., Farrar, J.F., Gray, J.B., and Dunlop, I.C. (1964). Aromatic drugs and congenital cataracts. *Lancet* i, 472.

Harpey, J-P., Jaudon, M-C., Clavel, J.-P., Galli, A., and Darbois, Y. (1983). Cutis laxa and low serum zinc after antenatal exposure to penicillamine. *Lancet* ii, 858.

Hart, C.W. and Naunton, R.F. (1964). The ototoxicity of chloroquine phosphate. *Arch. Otolaryngol.* 80, 407.

Hawkins, D.F. (ed.) (1987). *Drugs and pregnancy* (2nd edn). Churchill Livingstone, Edinburgh.

Heinonen, O.P., Slone, D., Monson, R.R., Hook, E.B., and Shapiro, S. (1977a). Cardiovascular birth defects and antenatal exposure to female sex hormones. *N. Engl. J. Med.* 296, 67.

Heinonen. O.P., Slone, D., and Shapiro, S. (1977b). *Birth defects and drugs in pregnancy.* Publishing Sciences Group, Acton, Mass.

Hendricks, S.K., Smith, J.R., Moore, D.E., and Brown, Z.A. (1990). Oligohydramnios associated with prostaglandin synthetase inhibitors in preterm labour. *Br. J. Obstet. Gynaecol.* 97, 312.

Herbst, A.L. (1981). Diethylstilbestrol and other sex hormones during pregnancy. *Obstet. Gynecol.* (suppl.) 58, 35S.

Herbst, A.L., Ulfelder, H., and Poskanzer, D.C. (1971). Adenocarcinoma of the vagina: association of maternal stilboestrol therapy with tumour appearance in young women. *N. Engl. J. Med.* 284, 878.

Hersh, J.H., Podruch, P.E., Rogers, G., and Weisskoft, B. (1985). Toluene embryopathy. *J. Pediatr.* 106, 922.

Heymann, M.A. (1986). Non-narcotic analgesics. Use in pregnancy and fetal and perinatal effects. *Drugs* 32 (suppl. 4), 164.

Hickok, D.E., Hollenbach, K.A., Reilley, S.F., and Nyberg, D.A. (1989). The association between decreased amniotic fluid volume and treatment with nonsteroidal anti-inflammatory agents for preterm labor. *Am. J. Obstet. Gynecol.* 160, 1525.

Hiilesmaa, V.K., Teramo, K., Granström, M-L., and Bardy, A.H. (1983). Serum folate concentrations during pregnancy in women with epilepsy: relation to antiepileptic drug concentrations, number of seizures, and fetal outcome. *Br. Med. J.* 287, 577.

Hill, R.M. and Stern, L. (1979). Drugs in pregnancy: effects on the fetus and newborn. *Drugs* 17, 182.

Hill, R.M., Desmond, M.M., and Kay, J.L. (1966). Extrapyramidal dysfunction in an infant of a schizophrenic mother. *J. Pediatr.* 69, 589.

Hirsh, J., Cade, J.F., and O'Sullivan, E.F. (1970). Clinical experience with anticoagulant therapy during pregnancy. *Br. Med. J.* i, 270.

Ho, P.C., Stephens, I.D., and Triggs, E.J. (1981). Caesarean section and placental transfer of alcuronium. *Anaesth. Intens. Care* 9, 113.

Hodgkinson, R. and Husain, F.J. (1982). The duration of effect of maternally administered meperidine on neonatal neurobehaviour. *Anesthesiology* 56, 51.

Hodgkinson, R., Glassenberg, R., Joyce, T.H., Coombs, D.W., Ostheimer, G.W., and Gibbs, C.P. (1983). Comparison of cimetidine (Tagamet) with antacid for safety and effectiveness in reducing gastric acidity before elective Cesarian section. *Anesthesiology* 59, 86.

Holmes, L.B. (1983). Teratogen update: Bendectin. *Teratology* 27, 277.

Holzgreve, W., Carey, J.C., and Hall, B.D. (1976). Warfarin-induced fetal abnormalities. *Lancet* ii, 914.

Hoo, J.J., Hadro, T.A., and Von Behren, P. (1988). Possible teratogenicity of sulfasalazine. *N. Engl. J. Med.* 318, 1128.

Hook, E.B. (1982). Incidence and prevalence as measures of the frequency of birth defects. *Am. J. Epidemiol.* 116, 743.

Hopf, G. and Mathias, B. (1988). Teratogenicity of isotretinoin and etretinate. *Lancet* ii, 1143.

Howell, R., Fidler, J., and Letsky, E. (1983). The risks of antenatal subcutaneous heparin prophylaxis: a controlled trial. *Br. J. Obstet. Gynecol.* 90, 1124.

Hoyseth, K.S. and Jones, P.J.H. (1989). Ethanol-induced teratogenesis: characterization, mechanisms and diagnostic approaches. *Life Sci.* 44, 643.

Iturbe-Alessio, I., del Carmen Fonseca, M., Mutchinik, O., Santos, M.A., Zajarias, A., and Salazar, E. (1986). Risks of anticoagulant therapy in pregnant women with artificial heart valves. *N. Engl. J. Med.* 315, 1390.

Jackson, H.J. and Sutherland, R.M. (1981). Effect of povidone–iodine on neonatal thyroid function. *Lancet* ii, 992.

Jäger-Roman, E., Deichl, A., Lakob, S., Hartmann, A-M., Koch, S., Rating, D., et al. (1986). Fetal growth, major malformations, and minor anomalies in infants born to women receiving valproic acid. *J. Pediatr.* 108, 997.

James, F.M. (1987). Anesthesia for nonobstetric surgery during pregnancy. *Clin. Obstet. Gynecol.* 30, 621.

James, W.H. (1973). Anencephaly, ovulation stimulation, subfertility and illegitimacy. *Lancet* ii, 916.

Janerich, D.T., Piper, J.M., and Glebatis, D.M. (1974). Oral contraceptives and congenital limb-reduction defects. *N. Engl. J. Med.* 291, 697.

Jick, H. (1988). Early pregnancy and benzodiazepines. *J. Clin. Psychopharmacol.* 8, 159.

Jick, H., Holmes, L.B., Hunter, J.R., Madsen, S., and Stergachis, A. (1981). First-trimester drug use and congenital disorders. *JAMA* 246, 343.

Johnson, L.D., Driscoll, S.G., Hertig, A.T., Cole, P.T., and Nickerson, R.J. (1979). Vaginal adenosis in stillborns and neonates exposed to diethylstilbestrol and steroidal estrogens and progestins. *J. Am. Coll. Obstet. Gynecol.* 53, 671.

Jones, D.G.C., Langman, M.J.S., Lawson, D.H., and Vessey, M.P. (1985). Post-marketing surveillance of the safety of cimetidine: twelve month morbidity report. *Q. J. Med.* 54, 253.

Jones, H.C. (1973). Intrauterine ototoxicity. *J. Nat. Med. Assoc.* 65, 201.

Jones, K.L. (1988). Fetal alcohol effects. In *Recognisable patterns of human malformation* (4th edn) (ed. K.L. Jones and D.W. Smith), p. 941. W.B. Saunders, Phildelphia.

Jones, K.L., Lacro, R.V., Johnson, X.A., and Adams, J. (1989). Pattern of malformations in the children of women treated with carbamazepine during pregnancy. *N. Engl. J. Med.* 320, 1661.

Jordheim, O. and Hagen, A.G. (1980). Study of ampicillin levels in maternal serum, umbilical cord serum and amniotic fluid following administration of pivampicillin. *Acta Obstet. Scand.* 59, 315.

Juchau, M.R. (1989). Bioactivation in chemical teratogenesis. *Annu. Rev. Pharmacol. Toxicol.* 29, 165.

Kalb, R.E. and Grossman, M.E. (1986). The association of aplasia cutis congenita with therapy of maternal thyroid disease. *Pediatr. Dermatol.* 3, 327.

Kaler, S.G., Patrinos, M.E., Lambert, G.H., Myers, T.F., Karlman, R., and Anderson, C.L. (1987). Hypertrichosis and congenital anomalies associated with maternal use of minoxidil. *Pediatrics* 79, 434.

Källén, B. (1988). Comments on teratogen update: Lithium. *Teratology* 38, 597.

Kaltenbach, K. and Finnegan, L.P. (1986). Developmental outcome of infants exposed to methadone in-utero: a longitudinal study. *Pediatr. Res.* 20, 57.

Kaltenbach, K. and Finnegan, L.P. (1987). Perinatal and developmental outcome of infants exposed to methadone in utero. *Neurotoxicol. Teratol.* 9, 311.

Kaltenbach K.A. and Finnegan, L.P. (1989). Prenatal narcotic exposure: perinatal and developmental effects. *Neurotoxicology* 10, 597.

Kaneko, S., Otani, K., Fukushima, Y., Ogawa, Y., Nomura, Y., Ono, T., *et al.* (1988). Teratogenicity of antiepileptic drugs: analysis of possible risk factors. *Epilepsia* 29, 459.

Kappy, K.A., Cetrulo, C.L., Knuppel, R.A., Ingardia, C.J., Sbarra, A.J., Scerbo, J.C., *et al.* (1979). Premature rupture of the membranes; a conservative approach. *Am. J. Obstet. Gynecol.* 134, 655.

Kargas, G.A., Kargas, S.A., Bruyere, H.J., Gilbert, E.F., and Opitz, J.M. (1985). Perinatal mortality due to interaction of diphenhydramine and temazepam. *N. Engl. J. Med.* 313, 1417.

Karlsson, K., Lindstedt, G., Lundberg, P.A., and Selstam, U. (1975). Tranplacental lithium poisoning: reversible inhibition of foetal thyroid. *Lancet* i, 1295.

Kasan, P.N. and Andrews, J. (1980). Oral contraception and congenital abnormalities. *Br. J. Obstet. Gynecol.* 87, 545.

Katz, V.L., Thorp, J.M., and Bowes, W.A. (1990). Severe symmetric intrauterine growth retardation associated with the topical use of triamcinolone. *Am. J. Obstet. Gynecol.* 162, 396.

Katz, Z., Lancet, M., Skornik, J., Chemke, J., Mogilner, B.M., and Klinberg, M. (1985). Teratogenicity of progestogens given during the first trimester of pregnancy. *J. Am. Coll. Obstet. Gynecol.* 65, 775.

Kauppila, A., Arvela, P., Koivisto, M., Kivinen, S., Ylikorkala, O., and Pelkonen, O. (1983). Metoclopramide and breast feeding: transfer into milk and the newborn. *Eur. J. Clin. Pharmacol.* 25, 819.

Keller, D.M. (1989). Teratogenic effects of carbamazepine. *N. Engl. J. Med.* 321, 1480.

Kemball, M.L., McIver, C., Milner, R.D.G., Nourse, C.H., Schiff, D., and Tiernan, J.R. (1970). Neonatal hypoglycaemia in infants of diabetic mothers given sulphonylurea drugs in pregnancy. *Arch. Dis. Child.* 45, 696.

Kerber, I.J., Warr, O.S., and Richardson, C. (1968). Pregnancy in a patient with a prosthetic mitral valve. *JAMA* 203, 157.

Khoury, M.J., Flanders, W.D., James, L.M., and Erickson, J.D. (1989). Human teratogens, prenatal mortality, and selection bias. *Am. J. Epidemiol.* 130, 361.

Kirshon, B. (1988). Prolonged maternal indomethacin therapy associated with oligohydramnios. *Br. J. Obstet. Gynecol.* 95, 956.

Kirshon, B., Wasserstrum, N., Willis, R., Herman, G.E., and McCabe, E.R.B. (1988). Teratogenic effects of first-trimester cyclophosphamide therapy. *Obstet. Gynecol.* 72, 462.

Kivalo, I. and Saarikoski, S. (1976). Placental transfer of ^{14}C-dimethyl-tubocurarine during caesarean section. *Br. J. Anaesth.* 48, 239.

Knott, P.D., Thorpe, S.S., and Lamont, C.A.R. (1989). Congenital renal dysgenesis possibly due to captopril. *Lancet* i, 451.

Knudsen, L.B. (1987). No association between griseofulvin and conjoined twinning. *Lancet* ii, 1097.

Konieczko, K.M., Chapple, J.C., and Nunn, J.F. (1987). Fetotoxic potential of general anaesthesia in relation to pregnancy. *Br. J. Anaesth.* 59, 449.

Kopelman, A.E., McCullar, F.W., and Heggeness, L. (1975). Limb malformations following maternal use of haloperidol. *JAMA* 231, 62.

Kosake, Y., Takanashi, T., and Mark, L.C. (1969). Intravenous thiobarbiturate anesthesia for caesarean section. *Anesthesiology* 31, 489.

Krauer, B., Krauer, F., and Hytten, F. (1984). *Drug prescribing in pregnancy*, p. 135. Churchill Livingstone, Edinburgh.

Krause, S., Ebbesen, F., and Lange, A.P. (1990). Polyhydramnios with maternal lithium treatment. *Obstet. Gynecol.* 75, 504.

Krauss, C.M., Holmes, L.B., VanLang, Q.N., and Keith, D.A. (1984). Four siblings with similar malformations after exposure to phenytoin and primidone. *J. Pediatr.* 105, 750.

Kreft-Jaïs, C., Plouin P-F., and Tchobrovtsky, C. (1988). Angiotensin converting enzyme inhibitors during pregnancy. *Br. J. Obstet. Gynecol.* 95, 420.

Krejčf, L. and Brettschneider, I. (1983). Congenital cataract due to tetracycline. *Ophthalmol. Paediatr. Genet.* 3, 59.

Kricker, A., Elliott, J.W., Forrest, J.M., and McCredie, J. (1986). Congenital limb reduction deformities and use of oral contraceptives. *Am. J. Obstet. Gynecol.* 155, 1072.

Kuhnert, B.R., Knapp, D.R., Kuhnert, P.M., and Prochaska, A.L. (1979). Maternal, fetal and neonatal metabolism of lidocaine. *Clin. Pharmacol. Ther.* 26, 213.

Kuhnert, B.R., Kuhnert, P.M., Prochaska, A.L., and Sokol, R.J. (1980). Meperidine disposition in mother, neonate, and nonpregnant females. *Clin. Pharmacol. Ther.* 27, 486.

Kumor, K.M., White, R.D., Blake, D.A., and Niebyl, J.R. (1979). Indomethacin as a treatment for premature labor. Neonatal outcome. *Pediatr. Res.* 13, 370.

Kutscher, A.H., Zegarelli, E.V., Tovell, H.M., Hochberg, B., and Hauptman, J. (1966). Discolouration of deciduous teeth induced by administration of tetracycline antepartum. *Am. J. Obstet. Gynecol.* 96, 291.

Laegreid, L., Olegård, R., Wahlström, J., and Conradi, N. (1987). Abnormalities in children exposed to benzodiazepines in utero. *Lancet* i, 108.

Laegreid, L., Olegård, R., Wahlström, J., and Conradi, N. (1989). Teratogenic effects of benzodiazepine use during pregnancy. *J. Pediatrics* 114, 126

Lammer, E.J. (1988). Embryopathy in infants conceived one year after termination of maternal etretinate. *Lancet* ii, 1080.

Lammer, E.J. and Cordero, J.F. (1986). Exogenous sex hormone exposure and the risk for major malformations. *JAMA* 255, 3128.

Lammer, E.J., Chen, D.T., Hoar, R.M., Agnish, N.D., Benke, P.J., Braun, J.T., *et al.* (1985). Retinoic acid embryopathy. *N. Engl. J. Med.* 313, 837.

The Lancet (1983a). Postcoital contraception. *Lancet* i, 855.

The Lancet (1983b). Malaria in pregnancy. *Lancet* ii, 84.

The Lancet (1983c). Pyrimethamine combinations in pregnancy. *Lancet* ii, 1005.

The Lancet (1988). Valproate, spina bifida, and birth defect registries. *Lancet* ii, 1404.

The Lancet (1989). Are ACE inhibitors safe in pregnancy? *Lancet* ii, 482.

Landers, D.U., Green, J.R., and Sweet, R.L. (1983). Antibiotic use during pregnancy and the post-partum period. *Clin. Obstet. Gynecol.* 26, 391.

Laver, M. and Fairley, X.F. (1971). D-Penicillamine treatment in pregnancy. *Lancet* i, 1019.

Leach, F.N. (1990). Management of threadworm infestation during pregnancy. *Arch. Dis. Child.* 65, 399.

LeGras, M.D., Seifert, B., and Casiro, O. (1990). Neonatal nasal obstruction associated with methyldopa treatment during pregnancy. *AJDC* 144, 143.

Leitman, P.S. (1979). Chloramphenicol and the neonate — 1979 view. *Clin. Perinatol.* 6, 151.

Lemoine, P., Harousseau, H., Borteyru, J-P., and Menuet, J-C. (1968). Les enfants de parents alcoöliques. Anomalies observées. *Ouest-Med.* 21, 476.

Lenz, W. and Knapp, K. (1962). Die Thalidomidembryopathie. *Dtsch. Med. Wochenschr.* 87. 1232.

Levi, S., Liberman, M., Levi, A., and Bjarnason, I. (1988). Reversible congenital neutropenia associated with maternal sulphasalazine therapy. *Eur. J. Pediatr.* 148, 174.

Levin, D.L., Fixler, D.E., Morriss, F.C., and Tyson, J. (1978). Morphologic analysis of the pulmonary vascular bed in infants exposed in utero to prostaglandin synthetase inhibitors, *J. Pediatr.* 92, 478.

Levin, D.L., Mills, L. J., and Weinberg, A.G. (1979). Hemodynamic, pulmonary vascular and myocardial abnormalities secondary to pharmacologic constriction of the fetal ductus arteriosus: a possible mechanism for persistent pulmonary hypertension and transient tricuspid insufficiency in the newborn infant. *Circulation* 60, 360.

Levy, W. and Wisniewski, K. (1974). Chlorpromazine causing extrapyramidal dysfunction in newborn infant of psychotic mother. *N.Y. State J. Med.* 74, 684

Lewis, H.L., Weingold, A.B., and the Committee on FDA-related Matters, American College of Gastroenterology. (1985). The use of gastrointestinal drugs during pregnancy and lactation. *Am. J. Gastroenterol.* 80, 912.

Linares, A., Zarranz, J.J., Rodriguez-Alarcon, J., and Diaz-Perez, J.L. (1979). Reversible cutis laxa due to maternal D-penicillamine treatment. *Lancet* ii, 43.

Lindhout, D. and Schmidt, D. (1986). In-utero exposure to valproate and neural tube defects. *Lancet* i, 1392.

Lindhout, D., Hoppener, J.E.A., and Meinardi, H. (1984). Teratogenicity of antiepileptic drug combinations with special emphasis on epoxidation (of carbamazepine). *Epilepsia* 25, 77.

Longo, L.D. (1970). Carbon monoxide in the pregnant mother and fetus and its exchange across the placenta. *Ann. N.Y. Acad. Sci.* 174, 313.

Lorber, C.A., Cassidy, S.B., and Engel, E. (1979). Is there an embryo-fetal exogenous sex steroid exposure syndrome (Efesses)? *Fertil. Steril.* 31, 21.

Loughnan, P.M., Gold, H., and Vance, J.C. (1973). Phenytoin teratogenicity in man. *Lancet* i, 70.

Lowe, C.R. (1964). Congenital defects among children born to women under supervision or treatment for pulmonary tuberculosis. *Br. J. Prev. Soc. Med.* 18, 14.

Lubbe, W.F. (1984). Hypertension in pregnancy. Pathophysiology and management. *Drugs* 28, 170.

Ludford, J., Dester, B., and Woolpert, S.F. (1973). Effect of isoniazid on reproduction. *Am. Rev. Respir. Dis.* 108, 1170.

Lyle, W.H. (1978). Penicillamine in pregnancy. *Lancet* i, 606.

McAllister, C.B. (1980). Placental transfer and neonatal effects of diazepam when administered to women just before delivery. *Br. J. Anaesth.* 52, 423.

MacArthur, B.A., Howie, R.N., de Zoete, J.A., and Elkins, J. (1982). School progress and cognitive development of six year old children whose mothers were treated antenatally with betamethasone. *Pediatrics* 70, 99.

McAuley, D.M., Moore, J., Dundee, J.W., and McCaughey, W. (1984). Oral ranitidine in labour. *Anaesthesia* 39, 433.

McAuley, D.M., Halliday, H.L., Johnston, J.R., Moore, J., and Dundee, J.W. (1985). Cimetidine in labour: absence of adverse effect on the high-risk fetus. *Br. J. Obstet. Gynecol.* 92, 350.

McBride, W.G. (1961). Thalidomide and congenital abnormalities. *Lancet* i, 271.

McCarroll, A.M., Hutchinson, M., McAuley, R., and Montgomery, D.A.D. (1976). Long-term assessment of children exposed in utero to carbimazole. *Arch. Dis. Child.* 51, 532.

McCredie, J., Kricker, A., Elliott, J., and Forrest, J. (1983). Congenital limb defects and the pill. *Lancet* ii, 623.

McCredie, J., Kricker, A., Elliott, J., and Forrest, J. (1984). The innocent bystander. *Med. J. Aust.* 140, 525.

McGowan, W.A.W. (1979). Safety of cimetidine in obstetric patients. *J. R. Soc. Med.* 72, 902.

Mackay, A.V.P., Loose, R., and Glen, A.I.M. (1976). Labour on lithium. *Br. Med. J.* i, 878.

McKinna, A.J. (1966). Quinine induced hypoplasia of the optic nerve. *Can. J. Ophthalmol.* 1, 261

McKusick, V.A. (1988). *Mendelian inheritance in man.* Johns Hopkins University Press, Baltimore.

MacMahon, B. (1981). More on Bendectin. *JAMA* 31, 371.

Macpherson, M., Pipkin, F.B., and Rutter, N. (1986). The effect of maternal labetalol on the newborn infant. *Br. J. Obstet. Gynecol.* 93, 539.

Manchester, D., Margolis, H.S., and Sheldon, R.E. (1976). Possible association between maternal indomethacin therapy and primary pulmonary hypertension of the newborn. *Am. J. Obstet. Gynecol.* 126, 467.

Mandelli, M., Morselli, P.L., Nordio, S., Pardi, G., Principi, N., Sereni, F., *et al.* (1975). Placental transfer of diazepam and its disposition in the newborn. *Clin. Pharmacol. Ther.* 17, 564.

Mangurten, H.H. and Benawra, R. (1980). Neonatal codeine withdrawal in infants of nonaddicted mothers. *Pediatrics* 65, 159.

Manning, F.A. and Feyerabend, C. (1976). Cigarette smoking and fetal breathing movements. *Br. J. Obstet. Gynecol.* 83, 262.

Martínez-Frías, M.L., Rodriguez-Pinilla, E., and Salvador, J. (1989). Valproate and spina bifida. *Lancet* i, 611.

Mastroiacovo, P., Bertolini, R., Morandini, S., and Segni, G. (1983). Maternal epilepsy, valproate exposure, and birth defects. *Lancet* ii, 1499.

Mastroiacovo, P., Bertollini, R., and Licata, D. (1988). Fetal growth in the offspring of epileptic women: results of an Italian multicentric cohort study. *Acta Neurol. Scand.* 78, 110 .

Meadow, S.R. (1970). Congenital abnormalities and anticonvulsant drugs. *Proc. R. Soc. Med.* 63, 48.

Meggs, W.J., Pescovitz, O.H., Metcalfe, D., Loriaux, D.L., Cutler, G., and Kaliner, M. (1984). Progesterone sensitivity as a cause of recurrent anaphylaxis. *N. Engl. J. Med.* 311, 1236.

Mehta, N. and Modi, N. (1989). ACE inhibitors in pregnancy. *Lancet* ii, 96.

Mehta, P.S., Mehta, S.J., and Vorherr, H. (1983). Congenital iodide goiter and hypothyroidism. *Obstet. Gynecol. Surv.* 38, 237.

Melnick, S., Cole, P., Anderson, D., and Herbst, A. (1987). Rates and risks of diethylstilbestrol-related clear-cell adenocarcinoma of the vagina and cervix. *N. Engl. J. Med.* 316, 514.

Mennuti, M.T., Shepard, T.H., and Mellman, W.J. (1975). Fetal renal malformation following treatment of Hodgkin's disease during pregnancy. *Obstet. Gynecol.* 46, 194.

Merlob, P., Litwin, A., and Mor, N. (1990). Possible association between acetazolamide administration during pregnancy and metabolic disorders in the newborn. *Eur. J. Obstet.* 35, 85

Métneki, J. and Czeizel, A. (1987). Griseofulvin teratology. *Lancet* i, 1042.

Meyer, H.H. and Brenner, P. (1988). Cleft hand and cleft foot malformation as a possible teratogenic side effect of the anthelmintic piperazine? *Internist* 29, 217.

Milham, S. and Elledge, W. (1972). Maternal methimazole and congenital defects in children. *Teratology* 5, 125.

Milkovich, L. and van den Berg, B. (1976). An evaluation of the teratogenicity of certain antinauseant drugs. *Am. J. Obstet. Gynecol.* 125, 244.

Millar, J.H.D. and Nevin, N.C. (1973). Congenital malformations and anticonvulsant drugs. *Lancet* i, 328.

Miller, J.P. (1986). Inflammatory bowel disease in pregnancy: a review. *J. R. Soc. Med.* 79, 221.

Mills, J.L. and Graubard, B.I. (1987). Is moderate drinking during pregnancy associated with an increased risk for malformations? *Pediatrics* 80, 309.

Mills, J.L., Baker, L., and Goldman, A.S. (1979). Malformations in infants of diabetic mothers occur before the seventh gestational week. *Diabetes* 28, 292.

Mills, J.L., Simpson, J.L., Rhoads, G.G., Graubard, B.I., Hoffman, H., Conley, M.R., *et al.* (1990). Risk of neural tube defects in relation to maternal fertility and fertility drug use. *Lancet* 336, 103.

Milunsky, A., Graef, J.W., and Gaynor, M.F. (1968). Methotrexate-induced congenital malformations. *J. Pediatr.* 72, 790.

Minkowitz, S., Soloway, H., Hall, E.J., and Yermakov, V. (1964). Fatal hemorrhagic pancreatitis following chlorothiazide administration in pregnancy. *Obstet. Gynecol.* 24, 337.

Mitchell, A.A., Rosenberg, L., Shapiro, S., and Slone, D. (1981). Birth defects related to Bendectin use in pregnancy. *JAMA* 245, 2311.

Mitzrahi, E.M., Hobbs, J.F., and Goldsmith, D.I. (1979). Nephrogenic diabetes insipidus in transplacental lithium intoxication. *J. Pediatr.* 94, 493.

Mjølnerød O.K., Dommerud, S.A., Rasmussen, K., and Gjeruldsen, S.T. (1971). Congenital connective-tissue defect probably due to D-penicillamine treatment in pregnancy. *Lancet* i, 673.

Moise, K.J. Jr., Huhta, J.C., Sharif, D.S., Ou, C.N., Kirshon, B., Wasserstrum, N., *et al.* (1988a). Indomethacin in the treatment of premature labor. Effects on the fetal ductus arteriosus. *N. Engl. J. Med.* 319, 327.

Moise, K.J. Jr, Huhta, J.C., and Mari, G. (1988b). Effects of indomethacin on the fetus. *N. Engl. J. Med.* 319, 1485.

Momotani, N., Noh, J., Oyanagi, H., Ishikawa, N., and Ito, K. (1986). Antithyroid drug therapy for Graves' disease during pregnancy. *N. Engl. J. Med.* 315, 24.

Moore, J., McNabb, T.G., and McGlynn, J.P. (1973). The placental transfer of pentazocine and pethidine *Br. J. Anaesth.* 45, (suppl.) 798.

Morelock, S., Hingson, R., Kayne, H., Dooling, E., Zuckerman, B., Day, N., *et al.* (1982). Bendectin and fetal development. *Am. J. Obstet. Gynecol.* 142, 209.

Morley, D., Woodland, M., and Cuthbertson, W.F.J. (1964). Controlled trial of pyrimethamine in pregnant women in an African village. *Br. Med. J.* i, 667.

Morrell, P., Sutherland, G.R., Buamah, P.K., Oo, M., and Bain, H.H. (1983). Lithium toxicity in a neonate. *Arch. Dis. Child.* 58, 539.

Mutch, L.M.M., Moar, V.A., Ounsted, M.K., and Redman, C.W.G. (1977a). Hypertension during pregnancy, with and without specific hypotensive treatment. *Early Hum. Dev.* 1, 47.

Mutch, L.M.M., Moar, V.A., Ounsted, M.K., and Redman, C.W.G. (1977b). Hypertension during pregnancy, with and without specific hypotensive treatment. II The growth and development of the infant in the first year of life. *Early Hum. Dev.* 1, 59.

Myers, S.A. (1990). Antihypertensive drug use during pregnancy. In *Cardiac problems in pregnancy* (2nd edn) (ed. U. Elkayam and N. Gleicher), p. 381. Alan R. Liss, New York.

Myhre, S.A. and Williams, R. (1981). Teratogenic effects associated with maternal primidone therapy. *J. Pediatr.* 99, 160.

Nakane, Y., Okuma, T., Takahashi, R., Sato, Y., Wada, T., Sato, T., *et al.* (1980). Multi-institutional study on the teratogenicity and fetal toxicity of antiepileptic drugs: a report of a collaborative study group in Japan. *Epilepsia* 21, 663.

Needs, C.J. and Brooks, P.M. (1985). Antirheumatic medication in pregnancy. *Br. J. Rheumatol.* 24, 282.

Nelson, M.M. and Forfar, J.O. (1971). Associations between drugs administered during pregnancy and congenital abnormalities of the fetus. *Br. Med. J.* i, 523.

Newman, N.M. and Dudgeon, G.I. (1977). A survey of congenital abnormalities and drugs in a private practice. *Aust. N.Z. J. Obstet. Gynecol.* 17, 156.

Newman, N.M. and Correy, J.F. (1983). Possible teratogenicity of sulphasalazine. *Med. J. Aust.* i, 528.

Nicholson, H.O. (1968). Cytotoxic drugs in pregnancy. *J. Obstet. Gynaec. Br. Cwlth* 75, 307.

Niebyl, J.R., Blake, D.A., White, R.D., Kumor, K.M., Dubin, N.H., Robinson, J.C., *et al.* (1980). The inhibition of premature labor with indomethacin. *Am. J. Obstet. Gynecol.* 136, 1014.

Nishimura, H. and Tanimura, T. (1976). *Clinical aspects of the teratogenicity of drugs.* Excerpta Medica, Amsterdam.

Niswander, J.D. and Wertelecki, W. (1973). Congenital malformation among offspring of epileptic women. *Lancet* i, 1062.

Nora, A.H. and Nora, J.J. (1975). A syndrome of multiple congenital anomalies associated with teratogenic exposure. *Arch. Environ. Health* 30, 17.

Nora, J.J., Nora, A.H., and Toews, W.H. (1974). Lithium, Ebstein's anomaly, and other congenital heart defects. *Lancet* ii, 594.

Normann, E.K. and Stray-Pedersen, B. (1989). Warfarin-induced fetal diaphragmatic hernia. *Br. J. Obstet. Gynecol.* 96, 729.

O'Connor, M., Johnson, G.H., and James, D.I. (1981). Intrauterine effects of phenothiazines. *Med. J. Aust.* i, 416.

Ohrlander, S., Gennser, G., Nilsson, K.O., and Eneroth, P. (1977). ACTH test to neonates after administration of corticosteroids during gestation. *Obstet. Gynecol.* 49, 691.

Orme, M.L'E. (1985). Debendox saga. *Br. Med. J.* 291, 918.

Østensen, M., and Husby, G. (1985). Antirheumatic drug treatment during pregnancy and lactation. *Scand. J. Rheumatology* 14, 1.

Østergaard, G. and Pedersen, S.E. (1982). Neonatal effects of maternal clomipramine treatment. *Pediatrics*, 69, 233.

Ostheimer, G.W., Morrison, J.A., Lavoie, C., Sepkoski, C., Hoffman, J., and Datta, S. (1982). The effect of cimetidine on mother, newborn and neonatal neurobehavior. *Anesthesiology* 57, A405 (abstract).

Ostrea, E.M. and Chavez, C.J. (1979). Perinatal problems (excluding neonatal withdrawal) in maternal drug addiction: a study of 830 cases. *J. Pediatr.* 94, 292.

Ounsted, M.K., Moar, V.A., Good. F.J., and Redman, C.W.G. (1980). Hypertension during pregnancy with and without specific treatment; the children at the age of 4 years. *Br. J. Obstet. Gynecol.* 87, 19.

Ovadia, M. (1988). Effects of indomethacin on the fetus. *N. Engl. J. Med.* 319, 1484.

Palahniuk, R.J. and Shnider, S.M. (1974). Maternal and fetal cardiovascular and acid-base changes during halothane and isoflurane anesthesia in the pregnant ewe. *Anesthesiology* 41, 462.

Palomaki, J.F. and Lindheimer, M.D. (1970). Sodium depletion simulating deterioration in a toxemic pregnancy. *N. Engl. J. Med.* 282, 88.

Parkin, D.E. (1974). Probable Benadryl withdrawal manifestations in a newborn infant. *J. Pediatr.* 85, 580.

Pauli, R.M., Lian, J.B., Mosher, D.F., and Suttie, J.W. (1987). Association of congenital deficiency of multiple vitamin K-dependent coagulation factors and the phenotype of the warfarin embryopathy: clues to the mechanism of teratogenicity of coumarin derivatives. *Am. J. Hum. Genet.* 41, 566.

Pederson, H., Morishima, H.O., and Finster, M. (1978). Uptake and effects of local anaesthetics in mother and foetus. In *International anesthesiology clinics* (Vol. 16). Regional anesthesia: advances and selected topics. p. 73. Little, Brown, Boston.

Perkin, R.M., Levin, D.L., and Clark, R. (1980). Serum salicylate levels and right-to-left ductal shunts in newborn infants with persistent pulmonary hypertension. *J. Pediatr.* 96, 721.

Perkins, R.P. (1971). Hydrops fetalis and stillbirth in a male glucose-6-phosphate dehydrogenase-deficient fetus possibly due to maternal ingestion of sulfisoxazole. *Am. J. Obstet. Gynecol.* 111, 379.

Pharoah, P.O.D., Alberman, E., Doyle, P., and Chamberlain, G. (1977). Outcome of pregnancy among women in anaesthetic practice. *Lancet* i, 34.

Phelan, M.C., Pellock, J.M., and Nance, W.E. (1982). Discordant expression of fetal hydantoin syndrome in heteropaternal dizygotic twins. *N. Engl. J. Med.* 307, 99.

Plouin, P.F., Breart, G., Maillard, F., Papiernik, E., and Relier, J.P. (1987). Maternal effects and perinatal safety of labetalol in the treatment of hypertension in pregnancy. Comparison with methyldopa in a randomized trial. *Arch. Mal. Coeur* 80, 952.

Porter, P.J., Sweeney, E.A., Golan, H., and Kass, E.H. (1965). Controlled study of the effect of prenatal tetracycline on primary dentition. *Antimicrob. Agents Chemother.* 668.

Powell, H.R. and Ekert, H. (1971). Methotrexate-induced congenital malformations. *Med. J. Aust.* ii, 1076.

Prenner, B.M. (1977). Neonatal withdrawal syndrome associated with hydroxyzine hydrochloride. *AJDC* 131, 529.

Prentice, A. and Brown, R. (1989). Fetal tachyarrhythmia and maternal antidepressant treatment. *Br. Med. J.* 298, 190.

Pritchard, J.A. and Walley, P.J. (1961). Severe hypokalemia due to prolonged administration of chlorothiazide during pregnancy. *Am. J. Obstet. Gynecol.* 81, 1241.

Pruyn, S.C., Phelan, J.P., and Buchanan, G.C. (1979). Long-term propranolol therapy in pregnancy: maternal and fetal outcome. *Am. J. Obstet. Gynecol.* 135, 485.

Ralston, D.H. and Shnider, S.M. (1978). The fetal and neonatal effects of regional anaesthesia in obstetrics. *Anesthesiology* 48, 34.

Ramsay, I., Kaur, S., and Krassas, G., (1983). Thyrotoxicosis in pregnancy: results of treatment by antithyroid drugs combined with T₄. *Clin. Endocrinol.* 18, 75.

Ramsay, I. (1990). Thyroid disease. In *Medical disorders in obstetric practice* (2nd edn) (ed. M. de Swiet), p. 633. Blackwell, Oxford.

Rane, A., Tomson, G., and Bjarke, B. (1978). Effects of maternal lithium therapy in a newborn infant. *J. Pediatr.* 93, 296.

RCGP (Royal College of General Practitioners) Oral Contraceptive Study (1976). The outcome of pregnancy in former oral contraceptive users. *Br. J. Obstet. Gynecol.* 83, 608.

Redman, C. (1989). Hypertension in pregnancy. In *Medical disorders in obstetric practice* (2nd edn) (ed. M. de Swiet), p. 285. Blackwell, Oxford.

Redman, C.W.G. and Ounsted, M.K. (1982). Safety for the child of drug treatment for hypertension in pregnancy. *Lancet* i, 1237.

Reinisch, J.M., Simon, N.G., Carow, W.G., and Gandelman, R. (1978). Prenatal exposure to prednisone in humans and animals retards intrauterine growth. *Science* 202, 436.

Rementeria, J.L. and Bhatt, K. (1977). Withdrawal symptoms in neonates from intrauterine exposure to diazepam. *J. Pediatr.* 90, 123.

Resseguie, L.J., Hick, J.F., Bruen, O'Fallon, W.M., and Kurland, L.T. (1985). Congenital malformations among offspring exposed in utero to progestins, Olmsted County, Minnesota, 1936–1974. *Fertil. Steril.* 43, 514.

Reynolds, B., Butters, L., Evans, J., Adams, J., and Rubin, P.C. (1984). First year of life after the use of atenolol in pregnancy associated hypertension. *Arch. Dis. Child.* 59, 1061.

Richards, M.P.M. (1981). Effect of analgesics and anaesthetics given in childbirth on child development. *Neuropharmacology* 20, 1259.

Riffel, H.D., Nochimson, D.J., Paul, R.H., and Hon, E.H. (1973). Effects of meperidine and promethazine during labor. *Obstet. Gynecol.* 42, 738.

Rinck, G., Gollnick, H., and Orfanos, C.E. (1989). Duration of contraception after etretinate. *Lancet* i, 845.

Robboy, S.J., Noller, K.L., O'Brien, P., Kaufman, R.H., Townsend, D., Barnes, A.B., et al. (1984). Increased incidence of cervical and vaginal dysplasia in 3980 diethylstilbestrol-exposed young women. *JAMA* 252, 2979.

Robert, E. and Guibaud, P. (1982). Maternal valproic acid and congenital neural tube defects. *Lancet* ii, 937.

Roberts, J.B. (1870) quoted in Taylor (1934). Does quinine, given a woman while pregnant, have any effect upon the fetus? *Richmond and Louisville Med. J.* 10, 238.

Rodriguez, S.U., Leiken, S.L., and Hiller, M.C. (1974). Neonatal administration of thiazide drugs. *N. Engl. J. Med.* 270, 881.

Rosa, F.W. (1984). Virilization of the female fetus with maternal danazol exposure. *Am. J. Obstet. Gynecol.* 149, 99.

Rosa, F.W., Hernandez, C., and Carlo, W.A. (1987a). Griseofulvin teratology, including two thoracopagus conjoined twins. *Lancet* i, 171.

Rosa, F.W., Idänpään-Heikkilä, J., and Asanti, R. (1987b). Fetal minoxidil exposure. *Pediatrics* 80, 120.

Rosa, F.W., Bosco, L.A., Graham. C.F., Milstien, J.B., Dreis, M., and Creamer, J. (1989). Neonatal anuria with maternal angiotensin-converting enzyme inhibition. *Obstet. Gynecol.* 74, 371.

Rosenberg, L., Mitchell, A.A., Parsells, J.L., Pashayan, H., Louik, C., and Shapiro, S. (1983). Lack of relation of oral clefts to diazepam use during pregnancy. *N. Engl. J. Med.* 309, 1282.

Rothberg, A.D. and Lorenz, R. (1984). Can captopril cause fetal and neonatal renal failure? *Lancet* ii, 482.

Rothberg, R.M., Rieger, C.H.L., and Hill, J.H. (1978). Cord and maternal serum meperidine concentrations and clinical status of the infant. *Biol. Neonate* 3, 80.

Rothman, K.J., Fyler, D.C., Goldblatt, A., and Kreidberg, M.B. (1979). Exogenous hormones and other drug exposures of children with congenital heart disease. *Am. J. Epidemiol.* 109, 433.

Roti, E., Robuschi, G., Emanuele, R., d'Amato, L., Gnudi, A., Fatone, M., et al. (1983). Failure of metoclopramide to affect thyrotropin concentration in the term human fetus. *J. Clin. Endocrinol. Metab.* 56, 1071.

Rotter, C.W., Whitaker, J.L., and Yared, J. (1958). The use of intravenous dramamine to shorten the time of labor and potentiate analgesia. *Am. J. Obstet. Gynecol.* 75, 1101.

Rowlatt, R.J. (1978). Effect of maternal diazepam on the newborn. *Br. Med. J.* i, 985.

Rubin, P.C. (1987). *Prescribing in pregnancy.* British Medical Journal, London.

Rubin, P.C., Clark, D.M., Sumner, D.J., Low, R.A., Butters, L., Reynolds, B., et al. (1983). Placebo-controlled trial of atenolol in treatment of pregnancy-associated hypertension. *Lancet* i, 431.

Rudd, N.L. and Freedom, R.M. (1979). A possible primidone embryopathy. *J. Pediatr.* 94, 835.

Rudolph, A.M. (1981). The effects of nonsteroidal antiinflammatory compounds on fetal circulation and pulmonary function. *Obstet. Gynecol.* 58, 635.

Rumack, C.M., Guggenheim, M.A., Rumack, B.H., Peterson, R.G., Johnson, M.L., and Braithwaite, W.R. (1981). Neonatal intracranial hemorrhage and maternal use of aspirin. *Obstet. Gynecol.* 58, 52S.

Russell, C.S., Taylor, R., and Maddison, R.N. (1966). Some effects of smoking in pregnancy. *J. Obstet. Gynecol. Br. Commonwlth* 73, 742.

Sackett, D.L. (1979). Bias in analytic research. *J. Chron. Dis.* 32, 51.

Safra, M.J. and Oakley, G.P. (1975). Association between cleft lip with or without cleft palate and prenatal exposure to diazepam. *Lancet* ii, 478.

Sahul, W.L. and Hall, J.G. (1977). Multiple congenital anomalies associated with oral anticoagulants. *Am. J. Obstet. Gynecol.* 127, 191.

Sareli, P., England, M.J., Berk, M.R., Marcus, R.H., Epstein, M., Driscoll, J., *et al.* (1989). Maternal and fetal sequelae of anticoagulation during pregnancy in patients with mechanical heart valve prostheses. *Am. J. Cardiol.* 63, 1462.

Savolainen, E., Saksela, E., and Saxén, L. (1981). Teratogenic hazards of oral contraceptives analyzed in a national malformation register. *Am. J. Obstet. Gynecol.* 140, 521.

Saxén, I. (1975). Epidemiology of cleft lip and palate. *Br. J. Prev. Soc. Med.* 29, 103.

Saxén, I. and Saxén, L. (1975). Association between maternal intake of diazepam and oral clefts. *Lancet* ii, 498.

Scanlon, J.W., Brown, W.V., Weiss, J.B., and Alper, M.H. (1974). Neurobehavioural response of newborn infants after maternal epidural anesthesia. *Anesthesiology* 40, 121.

Schafer, A.I. (1981). Teratogenic effects of antileukemic chemotherapy. *Arch. Intern. Med.* 141, 514.

Schardein, J.L. (1985). *Chemically induced birth defects.* Marcel Dekker, New York.

Schatz, M., Patterson, R., Zeitz, S., O'Rourke, J., and Melam, H. (1975). Corticosteroid therapy for the pregnant asthmatic patient. *JAMA* 233, 804.

Schellenberg, J.L. (1977). Uterine activity during lumbar epidural analgesia with bupivacaine. *Am. J. Obstet. Gynecol.* 127, 26.

Scher, J., Hailey, D.M., and Beard, R.W. (1972). The effects of diazepam on the foetus. *J. Obstet. Gynecol. Br. Commonwlth* 79, 635.

Schiff, E., Peleg, E., Goldenberg, M., Rosenthal, T., Ruppin, E., Tamarkin, M., *et al.* (1989). The use of aspirin to prevent pregnancy-induced hypertension and lower the ratio of thromboxane A_2 to prostacyclin in relatively high risk pregnancies. *N. Engl. J. Med.* 321, 351.

Schluter, G. (1989). Ciprofloxacin; toxicologic evaluation of additional safety data. *Am. J. Med.* 87, 375.

Schou, M. (1976). What happened later to the lithium babies? A follow-up study of children born without malformations. *Acta Psychiatr. Scand.* 54, 193.

Schou, M., Goldfield, M.D., Weinstein, M.R., and Villeneuve, A. (1973). Lithium and pregnancy — I. Report from the register of lithium babies. *Br. Med. J.* ii, 135.

Schubiger, G., Flury, G., and Nussberger, J. (1988). Enalapril for pregnancy-induced hypertension: acute renal failure in a neonate. *Ann. Intern. Med.* 108, 215.

Scott, A.A. and Purohit, D.M. (1989). Neonatal renal failure: a complication of maternal antihypertensive therapy. *Am. J. Obstet. Gynecol.* 160, 1223.

Senekjian, E.K., Potkul, R.K., Frey, K., and Herbst, A.L. (1988). Infertility among daughters either exposed or not exposed to diethylstilbestrol. *Am. J. Obstet. Gynecol.* 158, 493.

Sexson, W.R. and Barak, Y. (1989). Withdrawal emergent syndrome in an infatn associated with maternal haloperidol therapy. *J. Perinatol.* 9, 170.

Shapiro, S., Hartz, S.C., Siskind, V., Mitchell, A.A., Slone, D., Rosenberg, L., *et al.* (1976). Anticonvulsants and parental epilepsy in the development of birth defects. *Lancet* i, 272.

Shapiro, S., Heinonen, O.P., Siskind, V., Kaufman, D.W., Monson, R.R., and Slone, D. (1977). Antenatal exposure to doxylamine succinate and dicyclomine hydrochloride (Bendectin) in relation to congenital malformation, perinatal mortality rate, birth weight and intelligence quotient score. *Am. J. Obstet. Gynecol.* 128, 480.

Sharp, G.B. and Cole, P. (1990). Vaginal bleeding and diethylstilbestrol exposure during pregnancy: relationship to genital tract clear cell adenocarcinoma and vaginal adenosis in daughters. *Am. J. Obstet. Gynecol.* 162, 994.

Shaw, E.B. and Rees, E.L. (1980). Fetal damage due to aminopterin ingestion. *AJDC* 134, 1172.

Shearer, W.T., Schreiner, R.L., and Marshall, R.E. (1972). Urinary retention in a neonate secondary to maternal ingestion of nortriptyline. *J. Pediatr.* 81, 570.

Sherman, S. and Hall, B.D. (1976). Warfarin and foetal abnormality. *Lancet* i, 692.

Shimohira, M., Kohyama, J., Kawano, Y., Suzuki, H., Ogiso, M., and Iwakawa, Y. (1986). Effect of alpha-methyldopa administration during pregnancy on the development of a child's sleep. *Brain Dev.* 8, 416.

Shiono, P.H. and Klebanoff, M.A. (1989). Bendectin and human congenital malformations. *Teratology* 40, 151.

Shotton, D. and Monie, I.W. (1963). Possible teratogenic effect of chlorambucil on a human fetus. *JAMA* 186, 74.

Simeoni, U., Messer, J., Weisburd, P., Haddad, J., and Willard, D. (1989). Neonatal renal dysfunction and intrauterine exposure to prostaglandin synthesis inhibitors. *Eur. J. Pediatr.* 148, 371.

Singh, S., Gulati, S., Narang, A., and Bhakoo, O.N.M. (1990). Non-narcotic withdrawal syndrome in a neonate due to maternal clomipramine therapy. *J. Paediatr. Child Health* 26, 110.

Slone, D., Heinonen, O.P., Kaufman, D.W., Siskind, V., Monson, R.R., and Shapiro, S. (1976). Aspirin and congenital malformations. *Lancet* i, 1373.

Smith, A.M. (1989). Are ACE inhibitors safe in pregnancy? *Lancet* ii, 750.

Smithells, R.W. and Sheppard, S. (1983). Teratogenicity of Debendox and pyrimethamine. *Lancet* ii, 623.

Smithells, R.W. (1981). Oral contraceptives and birth defects. *Dev. Med. Child Neurol.* 23, 369.

Smolders, de H.H., Neuvel, J., Schmand, B., Treffers, P.E., Koppe, J.G., and Hoeks, J. (1990). Physical development and medical history of children who were treated antenatally with corticosteroids to prevent respiratory distress syndrome: a 10- to 12-year follow-up. *Pediatrics* 86, 65.

Snider, D.E., Layde, P.M., Johnson, M.W., and Lyle, M.A. (1980). Treatment of tuberculosis during pregnancy. *Am. Rev. Respir. Dis.* 122, 65.

Sokal, J.E. and Lessmann, E.M. (1960). Effects of cancer chemotherapeutic agents on the human fetus. *JAMA* 172, 1765.

Soler, N.G., Walsh, C.H., and Malins, J.M. (1976). Congenital malformations in infants of diabetic mothers. *Q. J. Med.* 45, 303.

Solomon, L., Abrams, G., Dinner, M., and Berman, L. (1977). Neonatal abnormalities associated with D-penicillamine treatment during pregnancy. *N. Engl. J. Med.* 296, 54.

Speidel, B.D. and Meadow, S.R. (1972). Maternal epilepsy and abnormalities of the fetus and newborn. *Lancet* ii, 839.

Speight, A.N.P. (1977). Floppy-infant syndrome and maternal diazepam and/or nitrazepam. *Lancet* ii, 878.

Steen, J.S.M. and Stainton-Ellis, D.M. (1977). Rifampicin in pregnancy. *Lancet* ii, 604.

Steingrub, J.S., Lopez, T., Teres, D., and Steingart, R. (1988). Amniotic fluid embolism associated with castor oil ingestion. *Crit. Care Med.* 16, 642.

Stephens, J.D., Globus, M.S., Miller, T.R., Wilber, R.R., and Epstein, C.J. (1980). Multiple congenital anomalies in a fetus exposed to 5-fluorouracil during the first trimester. *Am. J. Obstet. Gynecol.* 137, 747.

Stephens, T.D. (1988). Proposed mechanisms of action in thalidomide embryopathy. *Teratology* 38, 229.

Stirrat, G.M., Edington, P.T., and Berry, D.J. (1974). Transplacental passage of chlordiazepoxide. *Br. Med. J.* ii, 729.

Strauss, M.E., Lessen-Firestone, J.K., Chavez, C.J., and Stryker, J.C. (1979). Children of methadone treated women at five years of age. *Pharmacol. Biochem. Behav.* (suppl.) 11, 3.

Strickler, S.M., Miller, M.A., Andermann, E., Dansky, L.V., Seni, M.-H., and Spielberg, S.P. (1985). Genetic predisposition to phenytoin-induced birth defects. *Lancet* ii, 746.

Stuart, M.J., Gross, S.J., Eldrad, H., and Graeber, J.E. (1982). Effects of acetylsalicylic acid ingestion on maternal and neonatal haemostasis. *N. Engl. J. Med.* 307, 909 .

Sugrue, D. and Drury, M.I. (1980). Hyperthyroidism complicating pregnancy: results of treatment by antithyroid drugs in 77 pregnancies. *Br. J. Obstet. Gynecol.* 87, 970.

Sulik, K.R., Cook, C.S., and Webster, W.S. (1988). Teratogens and craniofacial malformations: relationships to cell death. *Development* 103 (suppl.), 213.

Tack, E.D. and Perlman, J.M. (1988). Renal failure in sick, hypertensive premature infants receiving captopril therapy. *J. Pediatr.* 112, 805.

Taylor, H.M. (1934). Prenatal medication as a possible etiologic factor of deafness in the newborn. *Arch. Otolaryngol.* 20, 790.

Teelmann, K. (1988). Retinoids: toxicology and teratogenicity to date. *Pharmacol. Ther.* 40, 29.

Truter, P.J., Franszen, S., van der Merwe, J.V., and Coetzee, M.J. (1986). Premature closure of the ductus arteriosus causing intra-uterine death. *S. Afr. Med. J.* 70, 557.

Tubman, R., Jenkins, J., and Lim. J. (1988). Neonatal hyperthyroxinaemia associated with maternal amiodarone therapy: case report. *Ir. J. Med. Sci.* 157, 243.

Tunstall, M.E. (1969). The effect of propranolol on breathing at birth. *Br. J. Anaesth.* 41, 792.

Tyl, R.W. (1988). Developmental toxicity in toxicologic research and testing. In *Perspectives in basic and applied toxicology* (ed. B. Ballantyne), p. 206. Wright, Bristol 1988.

Ulfelder, H. (1973). Stilboestrol, adenosis, adenocarcinoma. *Am. J. Obstet. Gynecol.* 117, 794.

Ulfelder, H. (1976). DES — Transplacental teratogen — and possibly also carcinogen. *Teratology* 13, 101.

Ulmsten, U., Anderson, K.E., and Forman, A. (1978). Relaxing effects of nifedipine on the non-pregnant uterus in vitro and in vivo. *Obstet. Gynecol.* 52, 436.

van Dijke, C.P., Heydendael, R.J., and De Kleine, M.J. (1987). Methimazole, carbimazole, and congenital skin defects. *Ann. Intern. Med.* 106, 60.

van der Heijden, A.J., Provoost, A.P., Nauta, J., Gross, W., Oranje, W.A., Wolff, E.D., *et al.* (1988). Renal function impairment in preterm neonates related to intrauterine indomethacin exposure. *Pediatr. Res.* 24, 644.

van Leeuwen, G., Guthrie, R., and Stange, F. (1965). Narcotic withdrawal reaction in a newborn infant due to codeine. *Pediatrics* 36, 635.

Vella, L., Francis, D., Houlton, P., and Reynolds, F. (1985). Comparison of the antiemetics metoclopramide and promethazine in labour. *Br. Med. J.* 290, 1173.

Vessey, M.P. and Nunn, J. F. (1980). Occupational hazards of anaesthesia. *Br. Med. J.* 281, 696.

Villasanta, V. (1965). Thromboembolic disease in pregnancy. *Am. J. Obstet. Gynecol.* 93, 142.

Vollset, S.E. (1990). Ovulation induction defects. *Lancet* 335, 178.

Voorhess, M.L. (1967). Masculinization of the female fetus associated with norethindrone-mestranol therapy during pregnancy. *J. Pediatr.* 71, 128.

Wagner, V.M., Hill, J.S., Weaver, D., and Baehner, R.L. (1980). Congenital abnormalities in baby born to cytarabine treated mother. *Lancet* ii, 98.

Walters, B.N.J. and Redman, C.W.G. (1984). Treatment of severe pregnancy-associated hypertension with the calcium antagonist nifedipine. *Br. J. Obstet. Gynaecol.* 91, 330.

Warkany, J. (1976). Warfarin embryopathy. *Teratology* 14, 205.

Warkany, J. (1988). Teratogen update: lithium. *Teratology* 38, 593.

Warrell, D.W. and Taylor, R. (1968). Outcome for the foetus of mothers receiving prednisolone during pregnancy. *Lancet* i, 117.

Watson, A.K. (1988). Local anaesthetics in pregnancy. *Br. Dent. J.* 165, 278.

Watson, G.I. (1962). Meclozine ('Ancoloxin') and foetal abnormalities. *Br. Med. J.* iv, 1446.

Watt, L.O. (1961). Oxytocic effect of dimenhydrinate in obstetrics. *Can. Med. Assoc. J.* 84, 533.

Webster, P.A.C. (1973). Withdrawal symptoms in neonates associated with maternal antidepressant therapy. *Lancet* ii, 318.

Webster, W.S., Lipson, A.H., and Sulik, K.K. (1988). Interference with gastrulation during the third week of pregnancy as a cause of some facial abnormalities and CNS defects. *Am. J. Med. Genet.* 31, 505.

Weinstein, L. and Dalton, A.C. (1968). Host determinants of response to antimicrobial agents (continued). *N. Engl. J. Med.* 279, 524.

Weinstein, M.R. and Goldfield, M.D. (1975). Cardiovascular malformations with lithium use during pregnancy. *Am. J. Psychiatry* 132, 529.

Werler, M.M., Mitchell, A.A., and Shapiro, S. (1989). The relation of aspirin use during the first trimester of pregnancy to congenital cardiac defects. *N. Engl. J. Med.* 321, 1639.

Weyman, J. (1965). Tetracyclines and the teeth. *Practitioner* 195, 661.

Whalley, P.J., Adams, R.H., and Combs, B. (1964). Tetracycline toxicity in pregnancy. *JAMA* 189, 357.

Whaun, J.M., Smith, G.R., and Sochor, V.A. (1980). Effect of prenatal drug administration on maternal and neonatal platelet aggregation and PF-4 release. *Haemostasis* 9, 226.

Whitelaw, A. (1981). Maternal methyldopa treatment and neonatal blood pressure. *Br. Med. J.* 283, 471.

Whitelaw, A.G.L., Gummings, A.J., and McFadyen, I.R. (1981). Effects of maternal lorazepam on the neonate. *Br. Med. J.* 282, 1106.

W.H.O. Scientific Group. (1981). *The effect of female sex hormones on fetal development and infant health.* WHO, Geneva.

Wiggins, D.A. and Elliott, J.P. (1990). Oligohydramnios in each sac of a triplet gestation caused by Motrin — fulfilling Koch's postulates. *Am. J. Obstet. Gynecol.* 162, 460.

Wilkins, L. (1960). Masculinization of female fetus due to use of orally given progestins. *JAMA* 172, 1028.

Wilkins, L., Jones, H.W., Holman, G.H., and Stempfel, R.S. (1958). Masculinization of the female fetus associated with administration of oral and intramuscular progestins during gestation: non-adrenal female pseudohermaphrodism. *J. Clin. Endocrinol. Metab.* 18, 559.

Wilkinson, A.R. (1980). Naproxen levels in preterm infants after maternal treatment. *Lancet* ii, 591.

Wilkinson, A.R., Aynsley-Green, A., and Mitchell, M.D. (1979). Persistent pulmonary hypertension and abnormal prostaglandin E levels in preterm infants after maternal treatment with naproxen. *Arch. Dis. Child.* 54, 942.

Willhite, C.C., Hill, R.M., and Irving, D.W. (1986). Isotretinoin-induced craniofacial malformations in humans and hamsters. *J. Craniofac. Genet. Dev. Biol.* (suppl.) 2, 193.

Willis, R.A. (1962). *The borderland of embryology and pathology* (2nd edn). Butterworths, London.

Wilson, J.G. (1977). Current status of teratology. In *Handbook of teratology* (ed. J.G. Wilson and F.C. Fraser), p. 47. Plenum Press, New York.

Wilson, N., Forfar, J.C., and Godman, M.J. (1983). Atrial flutter in the newborn resulting from maternal lithium ingestion. *Arch. Dis. Child.* 58, 538.

Winter, R.M., Donnai, D., Burn, J., and Tucker, S.M. (1987). Fetal valproate syndrome: is there a recognisable phenotype? *J. Med. Genet.* 24, 692.

Wolfe, M.S. and Cordero, J.F. (1985). Safety of chloroquine in chemosuppression of malaria during pregnancy. *Br. Med. J.* 290, 1466.

Wong, Y.L. and Taeutsch, H.W. (1978). White blood cell changes and incidence of fever after maternal treatment with glucocorticoids. *Pediatr. Res.* 12, 501.

Woods, D.L. and Morrell, D.F. (1982). Atenolol: side effects in a newborn infant. *Br. Med. J.* 285, 691.

Yaffe, S.J. and Stern, L. (1976). Clinical implications of perinatal pharmacology. In *Perinatal pharmacology and therapeutics* (ed. B.L. Mirkin), p. 355. Academic Press, New York.

Yakovlev, P.I. (1959). Pathoarchitectonic studies of cerebral malformations. *J. Neuropath. Exp. Neurol.* 18, 22.

Zagorzycki, M.T. and Brinkman, C.R. III (1982). The effect of general and epidural anesthesia upon neonatal Apgar scores in repeat caesarean section. *Surg. Gynecol. Obstet.* 155, 641.

Zhu, M-X. and Zhou, S-S. (1989). Reduction of the teratogenic effects of phenytoin by folic acid and a mixture of folic acid, vitamins, and amino acids. *Epilepsia* 30, 246.

Zierler, S. and Rothman, K.J. (1985). Congenital heart disease in relation to maternal use of bendectin and other drugs in early pregnancy. *N. Engl. J. Med.* 313, 347.

Zucker, P. and Simon, G. (1968). Prolonged symptomatic neonatal hypoglycaemia associated with maternal chlorpropamide therapy. *Pediatrics* 42, 824.

6. Disorders of the heart

J. C. COWAN, M. W. BAIG, and L-B. TAN

Introduction

It is an important truism that cardioactive drugs are used in patients with heart disease. Most adverse drug effects reflect both the properties of the drug concerned and the underlying disease state of the patient. Adverse reactions are frequently predictable on the basis of a drug's known pharmacological actions (Type A adverse reactions — see Chapter 3).

Sometimes it is the disease state which renders the patient susceptible to drug actions that might, in other circumstances, be therapeutic. Furthermore, actions that may be therapeutic in one disease state may be deleterious in another. Thus, drugs with negative inotropic effects may be beneficial in the treatment of ischaemic heart disease, but harmful in patients with reduced cardiac function. Similarly, antiarrhythmic drug therapy may be of value in patients with an established arrhythmia, but arrhythmogenic in others.

Adverse drug reactions on the heart are not confined to drugs primarily used in heart disease. Numerous agents used in the treatment of non-cardiac disorders may exhibit significant cardiotoxicity. For example, in the case of bronchodilator therapy, sympathomimetic effects may cause adverse cardiac effects, while neuroleptic medications may have Class I antiarrhythmic effects responsible for proarrhythmic adverse effects.

There are a myriad of case reports of adverse drug reactions involving the heart. In this chapter we have sought to emphasize the principles and mechanisms underlying these adverse effects, rather than to present an exhaustive catalogue of individual adverse reactions.

Drugs causing tachyarrhythmias

Antiarrhythmic drugs

Antiarrhythmic drug therapy is a two-edged sword, which can cause arrhythmias as well as prevent them.

The proarrhythmic actions of antiarrhythmic drugs are amongst the most serious adverse drug reactions, and may result in life-threatening arrhythmias or death (Ruskin et al. 1983; Cardiac Arrhythmia Suppression Trial Investigators 1989). They arise from a drug's primary pharmacological action. They are, therefore, Type A adverse reactions, though with antiarrhythmic drug therapy an equivalent electrophysiological effect may have an antiarrhythmic action in one patient and a proarrhythmic action in another.

In view of these different actions, the normal concepts of therapeutic and toxic ranges do not apply. Antiarrhythmic drug therapy is a prescribed risk. With judicious patient selection, the benefits of treatment can outweigh this, but with inadequate patient selection, the converse may apply and risks may exceed benefits. It is therefore of particular importance that physicians who prescribe these drugs should be aware of the serious adverse reactions that may arise and of the factors within an individual that may predispose him to increased risk.

Types of arrhythmogenesis

At the simplest level arrhythmogenesis can be divided into two categories, clinical and technical (Campbell 1987). Clinical arrhythmogenesis comprises all proarrhythmic effects that are of clinical significance. This includes worsening of an existing arrhythmia, which may accelerate, become more sustained, or become less well-tolerated haemodynamically. The appearance of a new arrhythmia, not seen prior to drug therapy, would also fall into this category. In many cases this new arrhythmia represents the unmasking of a latent susceptibility in a patient with a pre-existing predisposition.

Technical arrhythmogenesis refers to arrhythmogenesis detected by clinical investigations. It comprises an increased frequency of arrhythmias recorded on Holter monitoring or an increased susceptibility to arrhythmia detected by invasive electrophysiological investigation. In both instances the incidence of proarrhythmic events is dependent on the extent of increase in arrhythmia frequency or ease of inducibility which is considered significant. It is generally assumed that cases of technical arrhythmogenesis indicate an increased susceptibility to subsequent arrhythmias that would be of clinical significance. This assumption is, however, unproven, as few investigators would be prepared to take the risk of continuing antiarrhythmic drug therapy to determine whether technical arrhythmogenesis predicts clinical arrhythmogenesis.

Mechanisms of arrhythmogenesis

The electrophysiological actions of antiarrhythmic drugs that cause arrhythmias are the same as those which prevent them. This can be illustrated by considering mechanisms of arrhythmogenesis and the modulation of these mechanisms by antiarrhythmic drug therapy.

There are two basic mechanisms of arrhythmogenesis, re-entry and abnormal automaticity. Of these, re-entry mechanisms are thought to be more common. Re-entry is easily understood in the case of the Wolff–Parkinson–White syndrome, which involves a well-defined macro-re-entry circuit. In the majority of arrhythmias the re-entry circuit is less clearly defined, involving micro-re-entry within closely adjacent areas of myocardium.

For re-entry to occur there are several requirements (Figs 6.1 a–c). First, there must be an area of unidirectional conduction block. Secondly, there must be a slowing of conduction over the re-entry pathway such that the cycle length of the tachycardia is longer than the longest refractory period at any point over the pathway. Antiarrhythmic drugs can interrupt a re-entry circuit in a number of ways. Firstly, by slowing conduction they can change a zone of unidirectional block into a zone of

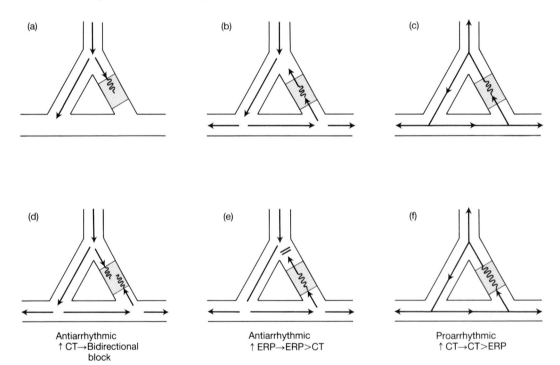

FIG. 6.1
(a)–(c) Mechanism of re-entrant arrhythmias. An impulse propagating anterogradely comes to a bifurcation in the Purkinje system; (a) the impulse is blocked in an area of slow conduction in one limb (shaded area) but continues to conduct through the other limb; (b) the latter impulse then enters the area of slow conduction retrogradely and is able to propagate in that direction; (c) provided the conduction time over the re-entry circuit exceeds the refractory period of the proximal fibres, re-entry can occur.

(d) and (e) Mechanisms of antiarrhythmic effects; (d) a Class II antiarrhythmic agent slows conduction time (CT) resulting in bidirectional block in the area of slow conduction preventing re-entry; (e) a Class III agent prolongs refractoriness so that the effective refractory period (ERP) now exceeds conduction time, preventing re-entry.

(f) Mechanism of proarrhythmic effect. A Class I agent acts on a latent re-entry circuit, which in its native state resembles (e), with refractory period exceeding conduction time. The drug slows conduction further, so that conduction time now exceeds the refractory period, thereby establishing criteria for re-entry.

bidirectional block (Fig. 6.1d). Secondly, they may prolong refractory periods, such that the longest refractory period exceeds the cycle length of tachycardia, which results in arrhythmia termination (Fig. 6.1e).

There is, however, another possibility. A patient may have potential re-entry circuits. These fail to fulfil requirements for re-entry in the drug-free state, because the longest refractory period in the pathway exceeds the conduction time over the re-entry pathway. When an antiarrhythmic drug is given, it may create the conditions for re-entry by slowing conduction over the re-entry pathway. The conduction time over the pathway may then exceed the maximum refractory period, resulting in re-entry and the initiation of tachycardia (Fig. 6.1f).

This principle of potential re-entry circuits is helpful in identifying patients at risk of provocation of arrhythmias by antiarrhythmic agents. Conduction slowing and areas of unidirectional block commonly arise because of fibrosis in the myocardium, resulting from previous infarction. Any patient with previous infarction is therefore at risk from an antiarrhythmic agent facilitating potential re-entry circuits. The likelihood of an antiarrhythmic drug meeting the critical requirements for re-entry will depend on the extent of the area of fibrosis. This is one reason why patients with severe impairment of left ventricular function are at increased risk from therapy with antiarrhythmic drugs (see below).

As regards the second mechanism of arrhythmogenesis, antiarrhythmic drugs can both suppress and increase automaticity (Levine *et al.* 1989). Once again, the electrophysiological mechanisms responsible for proarrhythmia are the same as those responsible for antiarrhythmic actions. Antiarrhythmic drugs in Classes Ia and Class III of the Vaughan-Williams classification prolong action potential duration. They achieve this effect by blocking the outward currents responsible for repolarization. It is now understood that the same effect in some individuals can result in after-depolarizations which can trigger arrhythmias (see below).

Identification of risk

Patient characteristics

A number of patient characteristics that indicate an increased susceptibility to arrhythmogenesis with antiarrhythmic drug therapy have been identified. First and foremost amongst these is the *severity of the rhythm disturbance* requiring treatment. In a series of 1330 patients treated for a mean of 292 days with flecainide, the incidence of proarrhythmic events was found to be zero in patients treated for ventricular premature beats, 0.9 per cent in patients treated for non-sustained tachy-

cardia, and 6.6 per cent in patients treated for sustained ventricular tachycardia (Morganroth *et al.* 1986).

Slater and others (1988) found that patients treated for either sustained ventricular tachycardia or ventricular fibrillation were 3.4 times more likely to demonstrate proarrhythmia than patients treated for non-sustained ventricular tachycardia or ventricular premature beats. It is easy to understand why this should be the case. If a patient already has a re-entry circuit responsible for a particular arrhythmia, he may well have other potential re-entry circuits that may be unmasked by the administration of an antiarrhythmic drug.

The second patient characteristic predictive of increased risk is *impaired left ventricular function*. Pratt and others (1989) observed a 15 per cent incidence of life-threatening proarrhythmic complications in patients with an ejection fraction less than 30 per cent, compared with an incidence of 2 per cent in patients with an ejection fraction greater than 30 per cent. Stanton and others (1989) demonstrated an association between left ventricular regional wall motion abnormalities and arrhythmogenesis. Slater and others (1988) found that patients with an ejection fraction less than 35 per cent were twice as likely to experience proarrhythmia as patients with an ejection fraction greater than 35 per cent.

There are several reasons why impairment of left ventricular function may lead to increased risk. First, increased susceptibility to proarrhythmia may simply be a reflection of an increased extent of fibrosis and an increased number of potential re-entry circuits which may be unmasked by antiarrhythmic drugs. Secondly, antiarrhythmic drugs have been shown to be less effective in suppressing arrhythmias in patients with heart failure (Pratt *et al.* 1989). This decreased efficacy may tilt the risk–balance equation in favour of risk. Thirdly, most antiarrhythmic drugs themselves have a depressant effect on cardiac function (see below). Fourthly, patients with impaired left ventricular function have increased sympathetic activity and the interaction between sympathetic activation and antiarrhythmic drug therapy may predispose to increased risk. Finally, patients with heart failure are likely to be receiving additional drug treatment for the management of the heart failure, creating the potential for drug interaction. In particular, diuretic-induced hypokalaemia may interact with antiarrhythmic drug therapy.

Structural heart disease is a further risk factor for proarrhythmic events. This is not an independent risk factor, as most patients with ventricular tachycardia and all patients with impaired left ventricular function will fall into a category of structural heart disease. None the less, it is a useful concept by virtue of exclusion. The risks of a proarrhythmic event in a patient without structural heart disease are relatively low.

There are, therefore, patient characteristics that will identify individuals at increased risk from proarrhythmic complications of antiarrhythmic drug therapy. The risks of arrhythmia aggravation are highest in patients who have already manifested sustained ventricular tachycardia and who have impaired left ventricular function. Knowledge of these predisposing factors is of value in determining the risk of a proarrhythmic event in individual patients. It has been suggested that, in particularly high-risk individuals, the risks of antiarrhythmic drug therapy may become too great for this treatment to be contemplated (Pratt *et al*. 1989). The situation, however, is more complex. As risks increase, potential benefits also increase. It is precisely the patient with malignant ventricular tachyarrhythmias and impaired left ventricular function who most needs successful arrhythmia prevention. Conversely, the patient with ventricular ectopic beats, in whom the risks of antiarrhythmic drug therapy may be remote, stands to benefit least from treatment. There is, therefore, a risk–benefit equation; risks and benefits increase in parallel. Potential benefits and risks need to be assessed individually in every patient in whom antiarrhythmic drug therapy is considered.

Prediction of arrhythmogenicity

Plasma concentrations

Proarrhythmic effects of antiarrhythmic drugs are more common when drug concentrations exceed the normal therapeutic range. This has been most clearly illustrated in the case of the Class Ic agent, flecainide (Morganroth and Horowitz 1984; Nathan *et al*. 1984). The minority of clinical reports of arrhythmogenesis, however, reflect drug toxicity. In the majority of cases arrhythmogenic effects arise within the normal therapeutic range (Rae *et al*. 1988; Velebit *et al*. 1982). Consequently, plasma drug concentrations, although important in detecting toxicity, are of very limited value as a screening test for the prediction of arrhythmogenic effects.

12-Lead electrocardiogram

Exaggeration of the normal therapeutic effect of an antiarrhythmic agent may result in changes in the 12-lead ECG that can be used as predictors of toxicity. An example is excessive prolongation of PR and QRS intervals induced by Class Ic agents such as flecainide (Morganroth and Horowitz 1984; Nathan *et al*. 1984). Once again, however, the majority of proarrhythmic effects occur in the normal therapeutic range, without any pronounced ECG changes. Consequently, ECG changes

are of limited predictive value and, in general, ECG criteria have not been predictive of proarrhythmia (Slater *et al*. 1988).

Arrhythmogenesis accompanying QT prolongation has been reported with many drugs (see below). QT prolongation is, however, a normal therapeutic effect of Class Ia and Class III antiarrhythmic drugs. The extent of QT prolongation after commencement of quinidine was not found to be predictive of arrhythmogenesis (Etvinssom and Orinius 1980). In general, therefore, QT prolongation has not been found to be a good predictor of arrhythmogenesis.

Dynamic electrocardiography

Holter monitoring can be of value in documenting clinically relevant arrhythmogenesis, as for example when ventricular tachycardia occurs for the first time in the patient receiving antiarrhythmic drug therapy for ventricular ectopic beats. More frequently, however, proarrhythmia is defined on technical grounds on the basis of an increased frequency or complexity of ventricular ectopic beats. The criteria for the recognition of such proarrhythmic events have been defined (Velebit *et al*. 1982) (Table 6.1). Based on these criteria, a proarrhythmic response has been reported to occur in 11 per cent of drug trials.

TABLE 6.1
Criteria for the Holter diagnosis of proarrhythmia

1.	Fourfold increase in the hourly frequency of ventricular extrasystoles compared with control recording
2.	Tenfold increase in the hourly frequency of repetitive forms (couplets of VT) compared with control recording
3.	First occurrence of sustained VT (lasting 1 minute or longer) not present during control studies.

Adapted from Velebit *et al*. (1982)

Invasive electrophysiological testing

Invasive electrophysiological testing has revolutionized the diagnosis and management of a wide range of supraventricular and ventricular tachycardias. Most of these tachycardias are re-entrant in nature and can hence be initiated by critically timed extrastimuli. These extrastimuli provide means of testing drug effects on the underlying re-entrant mechanism, sometimes termed the arrhythmic 'substrate'.

In some cases proarrhythmic effects are clear-cut, such as the appearance of a new sustained ventricular tachycardia when none could be initiated previously (Au *et al*. 1987). In other circumstances, however, the interpretation of electrophysiological findings is dependent on definitions. Rae and associates (1988) have shown that a difference in ease of induction of one extrastimulus is not meaningful, as this can arise from the spontaneous variability in the ease of induction in as many as 15 per cent of patients. In 40 patients in whom well-tolerated ventricular tachycardia was initiated with fewer extrastimuli during drug therapy than at baseline, the drug was continued during follow-up. The recurrence rate of tachycardia was no greater than in patients on regimens in which the number of extra stimuli required for initiation was not reduced. The authors concluded that a reduction in the initiating mode by one extrastimulus is not of sufficient predictive value to be used in clinical practice. In contrast, a difference in ease of induction of two extrastimuli is of value in detecting proarrhythmic effects. Four of five patients in whom this criterion was satisfied experienced sudden death or arrhythmia recurrence during follow-up. The authors suggested four criteria for the diagnosis of proarrhythmia in electrophysiological studies (Table 6.2). Based on these criteria, proarrhythmic effects were detected in 8 per cent of drug trials.

TABLE 6.2
Criteria for the diagnosis of proarrhythmia based on electrophysiological testing

---
1. Conversion of non-sustained to sustained VT
2. Conversion of haemodynamically stable VT to VT requiring cardioversion
3. Reduction by two extrastimuli of the number of extrastimuli required for arrhythmia induction
4. Spontaneous development of VT.

Adapted from Rae *et al.* (1988)

Exercise testing

Exercise testing is of value in detecting proarrhythmic effects of antiarrhythmic drug therapy. One-third of proarrhythmic responses can only be identified on exercise testing (Slater *et al.* 1988). Exercise testing is of particular importance in detecting proarrhythmic effects of Class Ic antiarrhythmic agents. The effects of Ic drugs on conduction are rate-dependent, the greater the heart rate the greater the depression of conduction. Increased QRS widening on exercise has been demonstrated with Class Ic agents (Ranger *et al.* 1989). The additional depressant effect on conduction during exercise may contribute to arrhythmogenesis (Anastasiou-Nana *et al.* 1987).

Time of occurrence of proarrhythmic events

Until very recently it was believed that proarrhythmic effects of antiarrhythmic drugs would arise early after starting treatment, within the first few days of commencing therapy. This belief was largely based on experience with quinidine. A small proportion of patients developed *torsade de pointes* within the first few days of commencing therapy (see below). These early arrhythmias on commencing quinidine became recognized as 'quinidine syncope'. Minardo and others (1988) considered 28 patients who developed ventricular fibrillation for the first time after commencing antiarrhythmic drug therapy. The median duration of therapy before the onset of ventricular fibrillation was 3 days. It has consequently been recommended that antiarrhythmic drug therapy should be commenced in hospital.

While there is certainly an increased incidence of proarrhythmia within the first few days of commencing treatment, it has now become clear that proarrhythmic effects are by no means confined to this time. The Cardiac Arrhythmia Suppression Trial (CAST) study randomized patients with an increased frequency of ventricular ectopic beats following myocardial infarction to treatment with flecainide, encainide, or placebo (CAST 1989). An increased mortality was observed in the two active treatment groups in comparison with placebo. This increased mortality was not confined to the first few days after commencing treatment but, rather, continued over weeks and months of treatment. Mortality in the active and placebo groups was still diverging on the premature termination of the study, after a mean treatment period of 10 months.

This finding has shown conclusively that proarrhythmia is not confined to the first few days of treatment. It still seems advisable to begin antiarrhythmic drug therapy in hospital, as there may well be an increased incidence of proarrhythmia in the first days of treatment. Continuing vigilance is, however, also necessary, and an awareness that any arrhythmia may have been caused by treatment rather than reflecting inefficacy of treatment.

Recommendations for the routine screening of a patient commencing antiarrhythmic drug therapy.

The empirical use of antiarrhythmic drug therapy, in patients with serious ventricular arrhythmias, is unsatisfactory. Patients should be screened for possible proarrhythmic effects.

There is no single technique or investigation that will detect all possible proarrhythmic effects. As a minimum requirement, a 12-lead ECG, Holter monitoring, and exercise testing should be undertaken. These investigations are relatively easily performed in most hospitals. Invasive electrophysiological testing is also of value, but may be confined to more specialized centres. In patients treated for malignant ventricular arrhythmias, particularly those with impaired left ventricular function, invasive electrophysiological testing is advisable, both to assess the efficacy of drug treatment and to guard against possible proarrhythmic effects. If appropriate means of testing are not available, it is questionable whether antiarrhythmic drug therapy should be commenced at all, as risks may exceed benefits.

Comparison of individual antiarrhythmic agents

With the possible exception of β-blockers, arrhythmia facilitation is a potential property of all antiarrhythmic drugs. Comparison of the relative incidence of proarrhythmic effects with different antiarrhythmic agents is difficult. Inevitably, different drugs have been used in different studies for different indications amongst different patient groups with different definitions of proarrhythmia. These factors alone will account for a varying incidence of proarrhythmic effects.

Consequently, comparisons of the relative incidence of proarrhythmia with different drugs are seldom meaningful. The reported incidence of proarrhythmia with different drugs varies between 1 and 12 per cent (Stanton *et al*. 1989).

Despite difficulties in comparison, certain patterns of proarrhythmia are emerging (Levine *et al*. 1989). Drugs that prolong the duration of action potentials (Vaughan Williams Class Ia and Class III) have a particular tendency to cause *torsade de pointes*. In contrast, Class Ic agents, whose most marked effect is slowing of conduction, give rise to monomorphic ventricular tachycardia. In each case, it is probable that the differing pattern of proarrhythmia reflects differences in the primary mechanism of antiarrhythmic action.

There is a general belief that the incidence of proarrhythmic effects is lower with amiodarone than with other antiarrhythmic drugs (Mattioni *et al*. 1989). An incidence of 4 per cent in antiarrhythmic drug trials has been reported (Fogoros *et al*. 1983). It is unclear why this should be the case, in particular why the incidence should be lower than with Class Ia agents, which also prolong action potential duration.

Management of proarrhythmic events

When a proarrhythmic event is suspected, the offending antiarrhythmic drug should be stopped. The possibility of drug or metabolic interactions should be considered, in particular the possibility of hypokalaemia or hypomagnesaemia, which might play a facilitatory role. Drug levels should be estimated to determine whether the arrhythmia might be due to toxicity. If an arrhythmia is

due to a drug, then the arrhythmogenic tendency should resolve as drug levels fall. This, however, poses a problem with amiodarone, as the half-life of this drug is measured in months.

If at all possible, addition of other antiarrhythmic drugs should be avoided, as potential drug interactions may further exacerbate the arrhythmia. In some cases, recurrence of arrhythmias can be prevented by ventricular pacing.

Torsade de pointes

The term '*torsade de pointes*' was coined by Dessertenne in 1966 to describe a distinct form of polymorphic ventricular tachycardia in which the QRS complexes appear to 'twist' around the isoelectric line. Over a period of 5–20 beats the amplitude of QRS complexes is seen gradually to increase and subsequently decrease. The pattern is then repeated.

The arrhythmia is important to recognize for a number of reasons. First, it is a serious and potentially fatal condition that is frequently due to drugs or toxins. Secondly, once recognized, it is relatively easily treated. If unrecognized, the arrhythmia can be exacerbated by inappropriate treatment.

The range of drugs that have been reported as causing *torsade de pointes* is extensive (Table 6.3). Antiarrhythmic agents are by far the most commonly reported class of drug associated with the arrhythmia. While any antiarrhythmic drug can cause *torsade*, it is most commonly associated with drugs that prolong action potential duration, that is, Class Ia and Class III agents. Amongst other drugs causing *torsade*, phenothiazines are the next commonest group. Significantly these drugs have electrophysiological properties that are similar to those of group Ia antiarrhythmic agents (see below).

Characteristically, when an ECG is available prior to the onset of arrhythmia, this shows QT prolongation. In many cases, giant U waves are evident. Indeed, it seems likely that QT prolongation is due to fusion of the U wave with the T wave. The value of QT prolongation as a predictor of arrhythmia occurrence, however, is unclear. Agents that predispose to *torsade* cause QT prolongation as part of their normal therapeutic action. It has not been possible to establish criteria for pathological degrees of QT prolongation that predict the development of the arrhythmia .

Stratmann and Kennedy (1987) reviewed 197 cases of drug-induced *torsade de pointes* in which information regarding QT intervals before and after drug administration was provided. In 35 per cent of cases QT prolongation was present even before administration of the drug

TABLE 6.3
Drugs associated with torsade de pointes

Antiarrhythmic drugs
Group Ia
Disopyramide
Procainamide
Quinidine
Group Ib
Lignocaine*
Mexiletine*
Group Ic
Encainide*
Group III
Amiodarone
Sotalol

Psychotropics
Amitriptyline*
Chlorpromazine*
Doxepin*
Maprotiline*
Thioridazine

Antihypertensives
Diuretics
Ketanserin

Calcium antagonists
Bepridil
Prenylamine

---

* Drugs marked with an asterisk are based on a relatively small number of case reports.

that was implicated. QT prolongation prior to drug administration may, therefore, constitute a risk factor.

The presence of pronounced U waves in many cases of *torsade de pointes* provides a clue to the electrophysiological mechanisms underlying this arrhythmia. Animal studies (Roden and Hoffman 1985, Levine *et al.* 1985) have shown that quinidine may cause after-depolarizations *in vitro*. This action is facilitated by bradycardia and hypokalaemia, conditions known to predispose to *torsade de pointes*. It is possible that the prominent U waves that frequently accompany the arrhythmia are manifestations in the surface ECG of after-depolarizations at the cellular level. It is now understood that these after-depolarizations are related to the same mechanisms that are responsible for prolongation of the plateau of the action potential (Sasyniuk *et al.* 1989), prolongation of which is due to inhibition of a slow outward potassium current responsible for repolarization. Inhibition of this outward current, combined with persisting inward current, gives rise to after-depolarizations. These result in accelerated automaticity and this is clinically manifest as polymorphic ventricular tachycardia of the *torsade de pointes* type.

A number of factors predispose to the occurrence of *torsade de pointes* during drug therapy. Hypokalaemia and bradycardia are particularly common contributory factors. A characteristic initiation sequence has been described. Kay and others (1983) reported that a long cycle (the compensatory pause following a premature ventricular contraction) followed by a short cycle (a second early premature ventricular contraction) immediately preceded the onset of arrhythmia in 41 of 44 episodes.

As for other proarrhythmic complications of antiarrhythmic drugs, toxic drug levels may be contributory, but the arrhythmia may also arise as an idiosyncratic reaction with drug levels in the normal therapeutic range. This is true of quinidine syncope; drug levels are not predictive of *torsade de pointes* (Selzer and Wray 1964; Bauman *et al.* 1984). With procainamide, by contrast, most cases of *torsade de pointes* are associated with excessive drug levels, which are particularly likely to occur following intravenous administration (Strasberg *et al.* 1981).

Management of torsade de pointes

Once an arrhythmia has been identified as *torsade de pointes*, drug therapy should be critically reviewed to determine the likely cause. Additional contributory factors, particularly hypokalaemia and hypomagnesaemia, should be considered and corrected. Sustained episodes of the arrhythmia causing haemodynamic deterioration should be terminated by DC cardioversion. Further antiarrhythmic drug therapy should be avoided. Once sinus rhythm has been restored, prophylaxis should be initiated against further episodes. As the initiation of episodes is bradycardia-related, this is accomplished by increasing heart rate. One way of achieving this is with an isoprenaline infusion, but this approach is hazardous, as excessive levels of catecholamines may exacerbate the arrhythmia. A much safer approach is to insert a temporary pacing wire to maintain heart rate in a target range of 100–120 beats per minute. Ventricular pacing is most commonly used and is the most reliable means of treatment, although in patients with marginal left ventricular function it may be necessary to use atrial pacing to preserve atrioventricular synchrony.

Following recovery, the need for continuing drug therapy should be critically evaluated. If the arrhythmia occurred with therapeutic or subtherapeutic levels of the implicated drug, then the drug must not be restarted. If, however, the arrhythmia occurred at markedly toxic levels, the drug could conceivably be restarted at a lower dose. If this option is selected, very careful monitoring of serum levels is necessary to prevent recurrence of toxicity.

In summary, *torsade de pointes* is a particularly distinctive form of ventricular tachycardia. It is a unique arrhythmia in that, in its acquired form, it is always related to drugs or toxins. Metabolic abnormalities frequently play a contributory role. Treatment is to discontinue the offending drug and correct any metabolic disturbance. In addition, temporary pacing is generally necessary to prevent recurrent attacks until aetiological factors have resolved.

Pacing and defibrillation thresholds

Class Ic antiarrhythmic agents cause a rise in pacing threshold, reflecting effects on ventricular conduction. At times this problem may be severe enough to interfere with ventricular capture (Hellestrand *et al.* 1983).

The advent of the automatic implantable cardioverter–defibrillator (AICD) has led to the discovery of a further adverse effect of antiarrhythmic drug therapy. A number of studies have shown that amiodarone therapy raises the threshold for defibrillation. As patients frequently require antiarrhythmic drug therapy concomitantly with an AICD, this is an important and potentially very serious interaction. Fogoros (1984) described a patient who became refractory to AICD cardioversion while taking amiodarone. Two studies have shown that the defibrillation threshold is significantly higher in AICD patients treated with amiodarone (Troup *et al.* 1985; Kelly *et al.* 1988).

For this reason it is advisable to undertake repeated testing of the defibrillation threshold in AICD patients receiving long-term amiodarone therapy.

Pharmacological causes of proarrythmia

Although the majority of proarrythmic complications of antiarrhythmic drug therapy arise with drug levels in the therapeutic range, a proportion of adverse reactions are related to drug toxicity. Pharmacological factors may contribute to these high levels.

In a number of reports, antiarrhythmic dosage protocols have been based on pharmacokinetic studies in normal volunteers or stable cardiac patients. These studies do not, however, adequately predict pharmacokinetics in patients with heart failure. This proved to be the case for flecainide. After satisfactory studies in stable cardiac patients, patients with severe disease developed higher than anticipated plasma concentrations of the drug and a high incidence of proarrhythmia (Nathan *et al.* 1984).

Decreased drug clearance may lead to increased plasma concentrations of antiarrhythmic drugs and thus cause exacerbation of arrhythmias. Antiarrhythmics

subject to extensive hepatic metabolism are particularly susceptible to interaction with drugs that induce or block hepatic enzymes. For example, cimetidine, which blocks some hepatic enzymes, can cause an increase in plasma levels of lignocaine (Feely *et al.* 1982). Similarly, in patients simultaneously receiving phenytoin and quinidine, withdrawal of phenytoin, which induces liver enzymes, has been shown to lead to toxic levels of quinidine (Data *et al.* 1976).

Genetic factors may also influence metabolism of antiarrhythmics. The classic example is acetylation of procainamide to *N*-acetylprocainamide. Patients fall into two phenotypes, slow acetylators and rapid acetylators. *N*-acetylprocainamide itself prolongs repolarization (Dangman and Hoffman 1981) and has antiarrhythmic and potential proarrhythmic properties. Some cases of *torsade de pointes* induced by procainamide may be due to accumulation of *N*-acetylprocainamide (Chow *et al.* 1984).

When antiarrhythmic drugs are used in combination, interactions may occur. A marked increase in digoxin levels may occur during quinidine (Holt *et al.* 1979) or amiodarone (Fenster *et al.* 1985) administration. Amiodarone has been shown to increase the plasma concentrations of both quinidine and procainamide (Saal *et al.* 1984).

Because of these pharmacokinetic interactions and the possibility of pharmacodynamic interactions, antiarrhythmic drug combinations should only be used with extreme caution.

Digitalis

Plasma levels in assessing toxicity

Unlike those caused by other antiarrhythmic agents, digitalis-induced arrhythmias are generally associated with drug toxicity. Therapeutic and toxic ranges, however, overlap: a digitalis level therapeutic in one patient may be toxic for another. Although the mean plasma digitalis level is elevated in patients with clinical features of toxicity, plasma digitalis levels are of limited predictive value in individual patients (G.A. Beller *et al.* 1971). Chamberlain and others (1970) found that 21 of 22 patients with signs of toxicity had levels above $2 \mu g$ per litre, but that 21 of 116 patients without signs of toxicity also achieved levels in this range.

Because of the limited value of digitalis estimations in diagnosing toxicity, assays should only be undertaken when there is a definite clinical indication. The fact that the patient is taking digitalis is not in itself sufficient justification for an assay, in the absence of other clinical indications. Appropriate indications include suspected toxicity, subtherapeutic clinical response, suspected poor compliance, changing renal function, potential drug interactions, and assessment of the need for continuing treatment (Aronson 1980).

As a generalization, provided the serum potassium is normal, toxicity is unlikely with digoxin concentrations below 2 μg per litre, and very likely with values greater than 4 μg per litre. It is, however, essential that samples be timed correctly. At least 6 hours should be allowed to elapse between the time of dosing and time of sampling. Samples drawn early after dosing give spuriously high digoxin levels and may lead to inappropriate clinical decisions (Gibb *et al.* 1986).

Factors influencing susceptibility to digitalis toxicity

Digoxin is excreted entirely by the kidney. The likelihood of toxicity therefore rises in patients with impaired renal function, particularly the elderly. Just as for other antiarrhythmic agents, the presence of heart disease influences susceptibility to proarrythmic effects. Thus patients with advanced heart disease are more likely to develop toxicity than less ill patients (G.A. Beller *et al.* 1971). Once again, therefore, the dangers of antiarrhythmic drug therapy are greatest in those patients most dependent on treatment.

The interaction of hypokalaemia with digitalis therapy has been recognized for many years. Hypokalaemia and hypomagnesaemia can provoke supraventricular arrhythmias, even in the presence of normal digitalis levels (Fisch 1973; Beller *et al.* 1974). As many patients receiving digitalis therapy will also be taking diuretics, there is a considerable potential for drug interaction.

Quinidine (Holt *et al.* 1979) and amiodarone (Fenster *et al.* 1985) increase plasma digitalis levels and increase susceptibility to digitalis toxicity (see above).

Features of digitalis toxicity

Digitalis toxicity has both cardiac and non-cardiac manifestations. The gastrointestinal, neurological, visual, and other non-cardiac manifestations of toxicity are discussed elsewhere in this book. Cardiac arrhythmias are common. The reported incidence of arrhythmias varies according to the clinical definition of toxicity. In some studies (e.g. G.A. Beller 1971) the presence of arrhythmias has been regarded as an essential prerequisite for the diagnosis of toxicity.

Digitalis toxicity may cause a wide variety of rhythm disturbances (Table 6.4). Digitalis can induce bradyarrhythmias. Increasing degrees of atrioventricular junctional block result from an exaggeration of the drug's normal therapeutic response. Bradycardia accompany

ing a regularization of ventricular response rate in atrial fibrillation strongly suggests complete heart block, with underlying digitalis toxicity. In patients in sinus rhythm, sinus bradycardia and sinoatrial block may be features of toxicity.

Supraventricular tachycardias are particularly common manifestations of digitalis toxicity. Two arrhythmias are so characteristic as to be pathognomonic — atrial tachycardia with atrioventricular block and non-paroxysmal atrioventricular nodal tachycardia (Bigger 1985). In atrial tachycardia with atrioventricular block, the ventricular rate is typically slower than in atrial flutter or paroxysmal atrioventricular nodal tachycardia, arrhythmias that would typically be considered in the differential diagnosis. The second pathognomonic arrhythmia is non-paroxysmal atrioventricular nodal tachycardia. The development of a regular tachycardia in a patient whose normal rhythm is atrial fibrillation, is suggestive of this arrhythmia. The ventricular rate is generally relatively slow. The arrhythmia may also be accompanied by atrioventricular dissociation, reflecting digitalis-induced inhibition of antidromic conduction into the atria.

Atrial fibrillation, the commonest indication for digitalis therapy, may itself be provoked by digitalis toxicity. This possibility should be considered when atrial fibrillation occurs in a patient treated with digitalis who was previously in sinus rhythm.

Digitalis may cause frequent or multifocal ventricular ectopic beats. The diagnosis of toxicity is more difficult than in cases of supraventricular arrhythmias, as many patients requiring digitalis therapy may already have frequent ventricular ectopic activity. The development of bigeminy in a patient with atrial fibrillation is strongly suggestive of digitalis toxicity.

Ventricular tachycardia and ventricular fibrillation are rare manifestations of toxicity. In both cases they indicate

TABLE 6.4
Arrhythmias due to digitalis toxicity

Bradycardia
  Sinus bradycardia
  Sinoatrial block
  A–V nodal block
  Marked slowing of ventricular response rate in AF

Supraventricular tachycardias
  Paroxysmal atrial tachycardia with A–V nodal block
  Non-paroxysmal A–V nodal tachycardia

Ventricular rhythms
  Frequent or multifocal ventricular extrasystoles
  Ventricular tachycardia/ventricular fibrillation

---

severe toxicity, and before the advent of digitalis antibodies carried a poor prognosis.

Management of digitalis toxicity

In patients with suspected digitalis toxicity, primary
treatment is, of course, to withdraw the drug. Resolution
of toxic effects will take several days, reflecting the long
half-life of digitalis preparations. In patients with impaired renal function, resolution will take even longer.
Hypokalaemia should be corrected. Magnesium deficiency should also be considered and corrected. A
search should be made for concurrent factors that may
have contributed to toxicity. Renal impairment due to
dehydration from excessive diuretic therapy is a particularly common precipitant. Any additional contributory
factors such as dehydration should be corrected.

In most cases of toxicity, these simple measures alone
will suffice. In cases of more severe toxicity, complicated
by rhythm disturbance, additional measures may be
necessary. Drug treatment of digitalis arrhythmias is
difficult and best avoided if possible. If treatment is
necessary, Class I agents such as lignocaine, procainamide, or phenytoin may be used with caution. Quinidine should be avoided because of its interaction with
digitalis. Cardioversion of supraventricular arrhythmias
is best avoided, because of risk of precipitating ventricular fibrillation. In general, if arrhythmias are so severe as
to necessitate consideration of antiarrhythmic drug therapy, treatment with digoxin immune antibody fragments
(Fab) may be preferable.

Digoxin immune antibody fragments are now established as the treatment of choice to achieve rapid reversal
of serious digitalis toxicity. They are prepared by injecting sheep with a digitalis–serum albumin complex over
several weeks and processing the digitalis-specific antibodies to yield antibody fragments. The fragments are
less immunogenic than the whole antibody and are
capable of being excreted by the kidneys. The antibody
has a greater drug affinity than the tissue receptors, and
binds the drug preferentially.

Digoxin immune antibody fragments have proved
highly successful in the treatment of digitalis overdosage
(Stolshek *et al.* 1988). They are indicated in patients with
serious or life-threatening arrhythmias as a result
of digitalis toxicity or in patients who have ingested
sufficient digitalis to cause concern that such arrhythmias may arise. Antman and others (1990) reported 150
cases of life-threatening digitalis intoxication treated
with Fab. Eighty per cent had complete resolution of all
signs and symptoms of toxicity, while another 10 per cent
showed improvement. Only 10 per cent failed to respond. Signs of toxicity generally resolve within a few

hours. Allergic reactions are surprisingly rare. Following
treatment, patients may experience hypokalaemia and
worsening of heart failure or a rise in ventricular rate,
because of withdrawal of the therapeutic effects of digitalis.

Digitalis and mortality

Digitalis has been a mainstay in the treatment of patients
with heart failure for many years. Although its efficacy in
patients with sinus rhythm has been questioned, recent
evidence has suggested that it may indeed have beneficial haemodynamic effects (DiBianco *et al.* 1989).

Doubts have been expressed, however, concerning the
safety of digitalis therapy. Moss and others (1981) reported a 30 per cent increase in morbidity at 4 months
associated with the use of digitalis in a high-risk group of
survivors of acute myocardial infarction who had congestive heart failure and complex ventricular extrasystoles.
Bigger and others (1985) reported a fivefold increase in
one-year mortality in post-infarction patients, associated with the use of digitalis. By contrast, Ryan and
others (1983), analysing data collected in the Coronary
Artery Surgery Study (CASS) register, failed to find any
increase in mortality in association with digitalis use.
Similarly, retrospective assessment of the MILIS (Multicentre Investigation of Limitation of Infarct Size) study
failed to demonstrate any excess mortality associated
with digoxin usage in patients following myocardial infarction (Muller *et al.* 1986).

The retrospective nature of these reports limits their
value. Patients treated with digitalis obviously have more
serious underlying heart disease, which may be reflected
in a poorer survival. Although multivariate analysis
techniques may purport to adjust for these differences in
morbidity, they do not necessarily compensate for clinical acumen and the ability of the physician to identify
patients with a poor prognosis, which may have led him
to prescribe a digitalis preparation. The question of the
effect of digitalis on mortality therefore remains open
and can only be answered by prospective randomized
studies (Cohn 1989).

Positive inotropic agents

The role of long-term inotropic therapy in the management of patients with heart failure remains uncertain.
Whereas the combination of hydralazine with isosorbide
dinitrate (Cohn *et al.* 1986) and the administration of
angiotensin-converting-enzyme inhibitors (Consensus
Trial Study Group 1987) have been shown to benefit
mortality, there is as yet no evidence that inotropic
agents improve survival. As discussed above, there are

fears, based on retrospective studies, that digitalis may increase mortality in this patient group. Similar concern has been expressed in relation to non-glycoside inotropic agents (Packer 1988).

Two groups of drugs are implicated. The phosphodiesterase inhibitors and β-adrenergic agonists. The myocardial actions of these agents are mediated through an elevation of intracellular cyclic-AMP levels. Animal studies have implicated cyclic-AMP elevation in the genesis of arrhythmias (Katz 1986). Patients with heart failure have a high incidence of serious arrhythmias (see above) and it is of obvious concern that administration of drugs with proarrhythmic adverse effects may increase these arrhythmias and adversely affect survival.

Phosphodiesterase inhibitors have been reported to increase the frequency of ventricular extrasystoles (Holmes *et al.* 1985; Anderson *et al.* 1986; Miles *et al.* 1989). As yet, there has been no trial of sufficient size to answer definitively whether these drugs influence mortality and it remains uncertain whether this increase in frequency of ventricular extrasystoles is significant. There are indications, however, of a possible adverse effect on survival. DiBianco and colleagues (1989) randomly assigned 230 patients in sinus rhythm to treatment with digitalis, milrinone, both, or placebo. The active treatments initially improved exercise times in comparison with placebo. Twenty per cent of patients receiving milrinone, however, deteriorated clinically within 2 weeks, compared with only 3 per cent of patients on digitalis. Eighteen per cent of the patients on milrinone fulfilled criteria of proarrhythmia, compared with only 4 per cent of the patients not receiving milrinone (p<0.03). Analysis of mortality on an intention-to-treat basis suggested an adverse effect of milrinone (p=0.064). An excess of patients with lower ejection fractions were, however, randomized to milrinone, and when this was taken into consideration the trend towards increased mortality was not significant. A recent study or oral enoximone has raised additional concerns that long-term use of phosphodiesterase inhibitors may have an adverse effect on mortality. Uretsky and colleagues (1990) demonstrated a statistically significant increase in mortality in patients treated with enoximone, in comparison with placebo.

As regards β-agonists, there are slightly stronger indications that these may be harmful, although again the issue is not clear-cut. Dies (1986) reported a double-blind controlled trial of intermittent intravenous dobutamine infusion in patients with heart failure. The drug was administered for 48 hours per week over a 24-week period. The trial was stopped prematurely after recruiting 60 patients. At this time 20 patients had died, and 15 of these had been assigned to or had crossed over to dobutamine. These findings did not achieve conventional statistical significance when analysed on either an intention-to-treat or treatment-received basis. Pre-existing ventricular tachycardia was predictive of death in the patients treated with dobutamine. Seven of the 15 deaths occurred during the weekly infusion of the drug. Taken together, these findings suggest the possibility of an increase in life-threatening arrhythmias during the dobutamine infusion. Although this report does not achieve statistical significance, it does raise serious concerns about the possible adverse effects of β-adrenergic stimulation in patients with heart failure.

Concerns have also been expressed in relation to the partial agonist xamoterol. An unpublished study reported to the Committee on Safety of Medicines in the UK has shown that patients with severe heart failure taking the drug are 2.5 times more likely to die than similar patients given placebo (CSM 1990).

In conclusion, it is as yet unclear whether positive inotropic agents influence survival. Fears have been expressed that they may have an adverse influence. These fears have neither been confirmed nor repudiated. The question will only be resolved by large-scale clinical trials designed specifically to address this issue (Cody *et al.* 1988).

β-Adrenoceptor blocking agents

Tachyarrhythmias induced by β-blockers are very rare. *Torsade de pointes* is a well-recognized complication of sotalol treatment (McKibbin *et al.* 1984). This proarrhythmic action, however, is related to the class III antiarrhythmic effects of sotalol rather than to its β-blocker activity. QT prolongation occurs with normal therapeutic doses of this drug. As with other antiarrhythmic agents, *torsade de pointes* may arise in the normal therapeutic range and does not imply drug toxicity.

Calcium antagonists

As a group, the calcium antagonists are relatively free of proarrhythmic actions. There are, however, two exceptions, prenylamine and bepridil, which are known to cause *torsade de pointes* (Perelman *et al.* 1987; Leclercq *et al.* 1983). It seems unlikely the proarrhythmic action is a reflection of calcium channel blockade, since other calcium antagonists do not share this proarrhythmic action. The reason why these two agents differ is uncertain. As far as prenylamine is concerned, a proposed explanation is that the drug may act as a calcium agonist at lower stimulation rates (Bayer *et al.* 1988), increasing transmembrane calcium current. The resultant action potential prolongation would predispose to early after-depolarizations and *torsade de pointes*. Bepridil is also an unusual calcium antagonist in that it has Class I antiarrhythmic properties (Kane and Winslow 1980). These additional properties may be related to its proarrhythmic potential.

Bronchodilators

In the late 1960s, mortality from asthma showed a sudden rise, in which circumstantial evidence implicated isoprenaline aerosols. Sales of this preparation were higher in countries that experienced increased mortality. In addition, mortality and isoprenaline sales fell in parallel once the problem had been recognized (Inman and Adelstein 1969). While the possibility cannot be excluded that the relationship was coincidental, both factors reflecting a changing pattern of asthma severity, it is widely believed isoprenaline aerosols directly caused the increase in deaths.

There are a number of possible mechanisms whereby an increase in mortality might have arisen. The introduction of inhalers may have given patients a false sense of security and delayed their seeking medical attention. Alternatively, the aerosols themselves may have had a direct toxic effect. In metered-dose aerosols, a β-agonist is combined with fluorinated hydrocarbons, which provide a liquid gas propellant. Excessive inhalation of fluorinated hydrocarbons has been associated with sudden death in solvent abuse (see below). It seems likely, however, that the risk from propellant alone is minimal, unless an aerosol is grossly overused (Dollery *et al.* 1970). The main concern has centred on the possibility that β-agonists may have caused arrhythmias. Patients with severe asthma would be expected to be vulnerable to arrhythmias as a result of hypoxia and endogenous catecholamine stimulation. The addition of exogenous catecholamines might increase this vulnerability. In addition, β-agonists cause hypokalaemia (Smith 1984), a further potential proarrhythmic factor. Hypokalaemia is due to β_2-mediated stimulation of the sodium–potassium exchange pump, which results in increased intracellular potassium uptake (Clausen and Flatman 1980).

Although selective β_2-agonists have a higher selectivity of bronchodilator over chronotropic effects than does isoprenaline, there continues to be concern that even selective β_2-agonists may contribute to arrhythmogenesis. At maximal therapeutic doses, the drugs increase heart rate (Crane *et al.* 1989). An increased frequency of arrhythmias has also been reported (Banner *et al.* 1979; Higgins *et al.* 1987). Fenoterol, in particular, has been noted to cause a more marked tachycardia and hypokal-

aemic response than salbutamol (Crane *et al.* 1989). This finding is of interest because of an over-representation of fenoterol amongst recent deaths of asthmatics in New Zealand (Sears *et al.* 1987). This observation is subject, however, to a number of interpretations and may simply represent physician preference for a newer drug in patients with more severe disease.

Theophylline similarly has the potential to induce arrhythmias, particularly when serum concentrations achieve toxic levels (Hendeles and Weinberger 1983). Concern has been expressed that combined therapy with theophylline and β_2-agonists may have additive proarrhythmic effects (Wilson *et al.* 1981). There is some evidence that the combination may be proarrhythmic. Laaban and others (1988) undertook Holter recordings during infusions of aminophylline and terbutaline in patients with status asthmaticus. Serious arrhythmias were surprisingly infrequent. Two of 29 patients developed sustained atrial tachycardia, and one developed non-sustained ventricular tachycardia. All the arrhythmias were well tolerated and resolved spontaneously.

The significance of proarrhythmia with bronchodilator therapy remains unresolved. It is generally impossible to establish whether patients dying from asthma have had an arrhythmia, since most deaths occur outside hospital. Even if an arrhythmia was established as the cause of death, it would be unclear whether this was related to the severity of an asthmatic attack or to the adverse effects of bronchodilator therapy. An international task force has recently recommended that 'further information is needed about the deleterious side-effects of antiasthma medications used alone and in combination' (Asthma Mortality Task Force 1987). Despite these concerns, undertreatment rather than overtreatment with drugs is probably the main cause of death from asthma (Johnson *et al.* 1984).

Diuretics, hypokalaemia, and arrhythmias

The efficacy of diuretic therapy in reducing the incidence of stroke in hypertensive patients is well established (Medical Research Council Working Party 1985). By contrast, diuretic treatment has not proved successful in preventing complications due to coronary heart disease. This paradox has raised the suspicion that unfavourable effects of diuretics in patients with ischaemic heart disease may offset the beneficial effects of pressure reduction.

It is well established that thiazides cause hypokalaemia. In the MRC trial of mild hypertension, mean serum potassium was 3.59 mmol per litre in patients receiving bendrofluazide 5 mg b.d., compared with 4.19

mmol per litre in a placebo group. Almost 50 per cent of patients on diuretics have been reported to have serum potassium values below 3.5 mmol per litre (Morgan and Davidson 1980). Diuretic therapy also causes hypomagnesaemia, which may be an additional contributory factor in the genesis of arrhythmias (Hollifield 1987).

There is no doubt that severe hypokalaemia, with a serum potassium value below 2.5 mmol per litre can cause arrhythmias (Davidson and Surawicz 1967). It is also clear that hypokalaemia can cause arrhythmias in patients on digitalis therapy and can interact with other drugs to cause *torsade de pointes* (see above). Whether moderate degrees of hypokalaemia, induced by diuretic therapy, cause arrhythmias, however, is controversial.

Many studies have assessed the effects of diuretics on the incidence of ventricular extrasystoles during 24-hour ECG recordings or on exercise testing. Some have found a relationship between diuretic-induced hypokalaemia and arrhythmias, while others have not (for review see Poole-Wilson 1987). The conflicting evidence may reflect the spontaneous variability of arrhythmias on Holter recording and the difficulty that this poses for demonstrating significant change in the incidence of arrhythmias.

Much the largest study was undertaken in conjunction with the Medical Research Council's mild hypertension trial (Medical Research Council Working Party 1983). In this study, patients on thiazide treatment had an increased incidence of ventricular extrasystoles. Although serum potassium correlated with the number of extrasystoles, serum urate correlated equally strongly. The authors concluded that hypokalaemia was a marker of thiazide intake, rather than causally related to the arrhythmias. These conclusions have been questioned (Poole-Wilson 1987). Since serum potassium is very variable and is measured at a single point in time, it is not surprising that the correlation with arrhythmias over a 24-hour period is low.

The balance of evidence favours the view that hypokalaemia induced by thiazides does cause an increased frequency of ventricular extrasystoles. The question then arises, does this matter and do diuretics place patients at risk? It is not possible to answer this question with any certainty. Some of the most suggestive observations are derived from subgroup analysis of the Multiple Risk Factor Intervention Trial (MRFIT). MRFIT (1982) was designed to determine the value of intervention directed at reducing multiple risk factors. The study recruited men with enhanced risk due to smoking, hypercholesterolaemia, or hypertension. Subjects were randomized to special intervention or usual care. Of over 12 000 participants, 8000 had hypertension at entry.

Special intervention for these individuals included a programme of stepped drug treatment, starting with a thiazide. In a subgroup of hypertensive men with abnormal ECGs, special intervention was associated with an increased mortality.

Retrospective subgroup analyses are, however, of limited value. They indicate possible effects, which serve to guide further research. It is of particular interest to examine similar subgroups in other studies. Unfortunately, the evidence is conflicting. Analysis of the Oslo Hypertension Study (Holme *et al.* 1984) supported the MRFIT conclusions. Analysis of the Hypertension Detection and Follow-up Programme study (HDFP 1984) and MRC trial (Miall and Greenberg 1987) failed, however, to show any increase in coronary heart disease mortality in the equivalent subgroup of patients treated with diuretics.

The link between diuretic-induced hypokalaemia and serious arrhythmias therefore remains unproven. To answer this question would require a much larger trial than any that has been conducted hitherto. The need for potassium conservation is therefore controversial. Although it is unproven that hypokalaemia matters, it is equally unproven that it does not. For this reason some suspicion must remain, so it seems reasonable to avoid hypokalaemia, where possible, through the addition of potassium supplements or the use of potassium-sparing diuretic combinations. It is interesting to note that the only trial hitherto that has demonstrated a reduction in coronary mortality in hypertensive patients was the EWPHE (European Working Party on High Blood Pressure in the Elderly) study, which used a potassium-sparing diuretic combination (hydrochlorothiazide + triamterene) (Amery *et al.* 1985). This may, of course, be coincidence.

Whatever the direct proarrhythmic effects of hypokalaemia, it is established that hypokalaemia can interact with other drug therapy to cause serious arrhythmias. The interaction of digitalis and hypokalaemia to cause digitalis toxicity is well known (Fisch 1973). Similarly, hypokalaemia is a common accompanying factor in many cases of *torsade de pointes* (Khan *et al.* 1981). A major interaction between potassium-losing diuretics and the serotonin antagonist ketanserin has recently been reported (Prevention of Atherosclerotic Complications with Ketanserin Trial Group 1989). A threefold increase in the incidence of sudden death was observed in patients treated with ketanserin who were taking a potassium-losing diuretic at randomization, in comparison with placebo. Ketanserin prolongs the QT interval of the ECG. Zehender and others (1989) reviewed eight patients who developed *torsade de pointes* or ventricular tachycardia during treatment with ketanserin. In most cases predisposing factors, particularly hypokalaemia or diuretic therapy, were evident. It seems possible, therefore, that the excess incidence of sudden death in hypertensive patients on a potassium-losing diuretic treated with ketanserin, is due to the occurrence of *torsade de pointes*. *Torsade de pointes* induced by ketanserin has also been reported in the absence of other predisposing factors (van Camp *et al.* 1989; Vandermotten *et al.* 1989).

Thrombolytic therapy

Reperfusion in animal models of myocardial infarction frequently causes ventricular fibrillation (Jewell *et al.* 1955). Early fears that thrombolytic therapy for myocardial infarction in man might similarly cause serious ventricular arrhythmias have proved unfounded. Reperfusion arrhythmias do occur, but are generally benign and of no haemodynamic consequence. The most common arrhythmia is accelerated idioventricular rhythm, which occurs in more than 50 per cent of patients with successful reperfusion (Goldberg *et al.* 1983). In addition, ventricular extrasystoles, sinus bradycardia, and atrioventricular block may occur. Ventricular tachycardia and ventricular fibrillation are rare.

Fears are none the less expressed that thrombolytic agents might cause ventricular fibrillation when used outside the coronary care unit. Experience is to the contrary. Simoons and co-workers (1985) reported an incidence of ventricular fibrillation of 14 per cent in patients receiving thrombolytic therapy compared with 23 per cent in a control group. These findings suggest that reduction in infarct size, consequent upon reperfusion, may in fact protect against ventricular fibrillation and more than offset any small incidence of ventricular fibrillation associated with reperfusion.

Antidepressants

Overdose of tricyclic antidepressants frequently results in ECG abnormalities, heart block, and arrhythmias (Pellinen *et al.* 1987). Similar problems can occasionally arise at therapeutic concentrations.

In the therapeutic range, tricyclic antidepressants frequently cause a slight increase in heart rate of up to 10 beats per minute. This effect is mainly due to anticholinergic actions, but in some patients orthostatic hypotension may be a contributory factor. The resulting sinus tachycardia is rarely of clinical consequence although an increase in oxygen consumption may be undesirable in patients with coronary artery disease.

Tricyclic drugs have Class Ia antiarrhythmic properties (Rawling and Fozzard 1978; Weld and Bigger

1980). In patients with heart disease, they have been shown to reduce the frequency of ventricular ectopic beats (Bigger *et al.* 1977; Veith *et al.* 1982). As with other antiarrhythmic agents, however, there is an accompanying proarrhythmic propensity. Fortunately, reports of serious proarrhythmic effects are rare. Amitriptyline and doxepin have been reported to cause *torsade de pointes* (Stratmann and Kennedy 1987).

As regards newer antidepressant drugs, maprotiline, a tetracyclic agent, has similar cardiovascular effects to the tricyclics. Its effects on conduction, and its antiarrhythmic and proarrhythmic properties are similar to those of the tricyclics. Like the tricyclics, it has been reported to cause *torsade de pointes* (Herrmann *et al.* 1983). Some of the newer antidepressant drugs appear to be less cardiotoxic than the tricyclics (Jackson *et al.* 1987; Halper and Mann 1988). The triazolopyridine derivative trazodone, which is unrelated to tricyclic and tetracyclic antidepressant agents, has no anticholinergic effects or depressant effects on conduction. Its proarrhythmic potential is low, although an increase in frequency of ventricular ectopic beats has been described (Janowsky *et al.* 1983). The selective 5-HT re-uptake blocker zimelidine is also considered to have low proarrhythmic potential. *Torsade de pointes* has, however, been reported during overdosage (Liljeqvist and Edvardsson 1989). Mianserin and fluoxetine have been reported to be devoid of proarrhythmic actions (Halper and Mann 1988).

It is important to recognize, when treating arrhythmias due to tricyclic overdose, that tricyclics have Class I antiarrhythmic properties. Treatment with additional Class I antiarrhythmic drugs is likely to be detrimental and these are best avoided.

Phenothiazines

Minor ECG changes are common in patients receiving normal therapeutic doses of phenothiazines. T wave changes, ST segment depression, and PQ and QT prolongation have been reported in up to 50 per cent of patients taking chlorpromazine (Huston and Bell 1966). These changes are not considered dangerous, and atrioventricular conduction disturbances are rare. Tachyarrhythmias are, however, a more serious problem. The drugs have a Class Ia antiarrhythmic action (Arita and Surawicz 1973). Antiarrhythmic effects are similar to those of quinidine (Madan and Pendse 1963), which may explain the small but definite incidence of serious ventricular arrhythmias. Phenothiazine therapy has been associated with syncope and sudden death. Ventricular tachycardia, ventricular fibrillation, and *torsade de pointes* have been identified as causes (Fowler *et al.* 1976; Kemper *et al.* 1983).

The antiarrhythmic properties of phenothiazines are a reason for caution when combining these agents with either conventional Class I antiarrhythmic drugs or tricyclic antidepressants. Such combinations are best avoided.

Alcohol

Alcohol is one of the commonest causes of atrial fibrillation, accounting for 15–35 per cent of hospital admissions with new-onset atrial fibrillation (Lowenstein *et al.* 1983; Koskinen *et al.* 1987). Amongst patients aged under 65, it has been reported to account for as many as two-thirds of cases of new-onset atrial fibrillation.

Some of these patients have an overt alcohol-related heart disease (see below). In others, however, there may be no overt chronic heart disease and it seems probable that the arrhythmia is due to acute intoxication. It is well established that alcoholic binges may induce episodes of atrial fibrillation. Attacks cluster at weekends and over holiday periods. Because of this, the arrhythmia has been termed the 'holiday heart syndrome' (Ettinger *et al.* 1978).

It is unclear why acute intoxication with alcohol should cause atrial fibrillation. There are a number of possibilities. These include electrolyte disturbances, such as hypokalaemia and hypomagnesaemia, which are often present in heavy drinkers, excess circulating catecholamines, and the effects of acetaldehyde, one of the metabolic products of alcohol. In addition, alcohol may have direct electrophysiological effects on the myocardium. Greenspon and Schaal (1983) studied 14 patients with a history of alcohol-related rhythm disturbances by invasive electrophysiological testing. In the baseline state, it was not possible to induce atrial tachyarrhythmias in any patient. After alcohol intake, repeated electrophysiological testing was able to induce a sustained atrial tachyarrhythmia in 5 of 14 patients.

Atrial fibrillation in patients with features of acute alcohol intoxication is generally of short duration, patients reverting spontaneously to sinus rhythm within 24 hours (Lowenstein *et al.* 1983). In the absence of haemodynamic compromise, additional treatment may not be necessary. Provided there is no overt cardiomyopathy, abstinence will generally prevent arrhythmia recurrence and additional prophylaxis is unnecessary.

Caffeine

Despite the widespread belief that coffee drinking is associated with palpitations, objective evidence that caffeine is arrhythmogenic in man is surprisingly sparse. Sutherland and colleagues (1985) found that coffee drinking did cause an increase in arrhythmias, but only in susceptible individuals. The evidence in relation to more serious ventricular arrhythmias is questionable. Two recent reports have assessed the effects of caffeine in high-risk patients. Myers and others (1987) studied 70 patients during the healing phase of myocardial infarction, and found that the double-blind, within-patient comparison showed no increase in either the frequency or the severity of ventricular arrhythmias; and Graboys and colleagues (1989) studied 50 patients with a history of malignant ventricular arrhythmias (ventricular tachycardia or ventricular fibrillation), also finding no evidence that caffeine was arrhythmogenic.

In conclusion, therefore, although susceptible individuals may experience caffeine-induced arrhythmias, there is no evidence that these place them at risk and no evidence that caffeine is contraindicated in patients with heart disease or a history of arrhythmias.

Drug and solvent abuse

The deliberate inhalation of volatile substances to obtain a 'high' is a relatively common cause of sudden death in young adolescents: 80 such deaths were recorded in Britain in 1983 (H.R. Anderson *et al.* 1985). Although solvent abuse may cause chronic toxicity and cardiomyopathy (McLeod *et al.* 1987), there is extensive evidence that these deaths are primarily arrhythmic, induced by acute drug toxicity (Boon 1987). Experimental evidence has shown that volatile substances can sensitize the heart to the action of catecholamines (Shepherd 1989). Sudden death in cases of solvent abuse is often associated with exercise (Bass 1970), so it has been suggested that volatile hydrocarbons may sensitize the heart to the arrhythmogenic effects of adrenergic stimulation (Boon 1987). Although in most instances the cause of death is not documented, ventricular fibrillation has been described (Gunn *et al.* 1989).

The 'recreational' use of cocaine carries a definite cardiac risk. Isner and colleagues (1986) reviewed 26 patients who had developed cardiovascular problems, directly related to cocaine. The adverse effects of cocaine in these cases included ventricular tachycardia, ventricular fibrillation, acute myocardial infarction, sudden death, or a combination of these events. The authors concluded that underlying heart disease was not a prerequisite and that serious cardiovascular events could arise in patients with normal hearts without predisposing factors. They further concluded that adverse cardiac consequences could occur with normal 'recreational' drug levels and that adverse effects were not confined to massive overdosage. Most patients who had experienced adverse cardiovascular effects took the drug intranasally. Adverse effects are therefore not confined to parenteral use of the drug. The effects of cocaine on myocardial perfusion are discussed below.

Sudden death has also been reported following abuse of the amphetamine analogues MDMA (3,4-methylenedioxymethamphetamine, 'Ecstasy') and MDEA (3,4,-methylenedioxyethamphetamine, 'Eve') (Dowling *et al.* 1987). Serious arrhythmias are well recognized as complicating amphetamine overdose (Benowitz *et al.* 1979) and it seems probable that at least some of these deaths are due to arrhythmias. Underlying heart disease is certainly one factor that predisposes individuals to sudden death while using these drugs. Whether individuals without cardiac disease are also at risk is unclear.

Drugs causing bradyarrhythmias

Drug-induced bradycardias are widely reported. Resultant conduction disturbances include sinus node dysfunction, progressive forms of atrioventricular block, and asystole. The mechanisms underlying these effects may be classified into:

(1) effects that are predictable from knowledge of a drug's electrophysiological properties. Examples of these include all antiarrhythmic agents, β-adrenoceptor antagonists, and calcium antagonists such as verapamil and diltiazem;

(2) indirect effects on cardiac impulse generation and conduction that are secondary to a drug's effects on the patient's metabolic status, including the induction of myocardial ischaemia (Reedy and Zwiren 1983; Richards *et al.* 1985; Martin *et al.* 1987; Nemer *et al.* 1988);

(3) indirect effects on cardiac impulse generation and conduction that are secondary to a drug's effects on haemodynamics. In response to these changes, activation of major reflex arcs, such as the Jarold–von Bezold reflex, occurs (Mark 1983). The efferent limb of this reflex comprises vasodilatation and an increase in vagal tone on the sinus and atrioventricular nodes resulting in significant bradycardia. Cardioinhibition induced through these mechanisms is exemplified by reports concerning nitrate-induced asystole (Rodger and Hyman 1932; Come and Pitt 1976; Lancaster and Fenster 1983);

(4) an idiopathic effect in which the mechanism has yet to be determined.

Unfortunately, in some reports of drug-induced cardiac arrest, the rhythm during the arrest is not given.

Many descriptions of drug-induced bradycardias appear in the form of isolated case reports in which essential details that would enable a reasonably firm cause-and-effect relationship to be derived are absent. In many instances the drug-induced bradycardia occurs when the offending agent is present in toxic doses (Sznajder *et al.* 1984; Brady and Horgan 1988). The compounding effects of pharmacokinetic and pharmacodynamic interactions are often not addressed (Durelli *et al.* 1985; Macnab *et al.* 1987).

The negative chronotropic and dromotropic effects of individual anaesthetic agents, either administered for a local effect or given systemically, are particularly difficult to assess. Many anaesthetic agents have well-defined effects on cardiac cellular electrophysiology, and bradycardia could be predicted from a knowledge of these effects. Serious bradycardia may occur after the induction of general anaesthesia, involving the administration of several drugs. Moreover, the induction of anaesthesia engenders complex changes in cardiovascular reflexes. Bradycardias may reflect a complex interplay between direct drug effects and reflex homoeostatic mechanisms. In the following review, only those agents that have been reported by several authors to cause pathological bradycardias when administered in recommended doses and for which a direct, causal relationship seems likely will be discussed.

β-Adrenoceptor blocking agents

As might be expected, β-blockers can cause an excessive bradycardia in some patients. This Type A adverse reaction is due to an excessive therapeutic effect. Often patients will have an underlying predisposition to bradycardia, such as sick sinus syndrome.

Excessive bradycardia may also arise from drug interactions. The interaction with verapamil is particularly well recognized, giving rise to sinus bradycardia and atrioventricular nodal block. Verapamil and β-blockers should not be administered together intravenously. Similarly, patients on oral treatment with one agent should not receive the other intravenously. Problems may also arise occasionally when the drugs are combined orally (Hutchison *et al.* 1984). Excessive bradycardia due to an interaction between oral verapamil and topical β-blockers, administered as eye drops, has been reported (Pringle and MacEwen 1987).

This interaction is not confined to verapamil. Although the combination of a β-blocker with diltiazem is widely used in the treatment of angina and is in general well tolerated, it may occasionally result in excessive bradycardia. Hassell and Creamer (1989) reported two cases of severe sinus bradycardia induced by the combination of diltiazem with a β-blocker.

Class I antiarrhythmics

It is rare for therapeutic doses of antiarrhythmic drugs to cause excessive bradycardia. By contrast, toxic doses can result in sinus bradycardia or arrest. When excessive sinus bradycardia does occur in the therapeutic range, this generally reflects pre-existing sinus node disease (Hellestrand *et al.* 1984; Goldberg 1982). Antiarrhythmic drugs may similarly result in sinoatrial block in patients with pre-existing sinus node dysfunction.

Class I antiarrhythmic drugs, particularly Ic agents (flecainide, encainide, and propafenone), frequently prolong the PR interval and QRS duration in the surface electrocardiogram. It is relatively rare, however, for higher degrees of block to arise within the therapeutic range. Higher degrees of block can arise with toxic drug levels, but once again block with therapeutic drug levels generally reflects pre-existing disease.

Antidepressants

Following the discovery of a causal link between lethal arrhythmias and the use of antidepressant drugs (Coull *et al.* 1970; Williams and Sherter 1971), especially amitriptyline, which is a member of the tricyclic group, there has been much debate about their safety in patients with cardiac disease (Halper and Mann 1988). Tricyclic agents may prolong the PR, QRS, and QT intervals of the surface ECG. The effects are dose-related and are more likely to arise with drug concentrations at the upper end of the therapeutic range (Glassman 1984). These electrocardiographic features are generally without consequence. Higher degrees of heart block are rare unless a patient has pre-existing conduction abnormalities.

Roose and colleagues (1987) conducted a prospective study in 196 patients with depression treated with tricyclic agents (imipramine or nortriptyline) over a period of 9 years; 155 patients had normal electrocardiograms on entry to the study, and the remainder had first-degree block or bundle branch block, or both. Plasma concentrations of the drugs were monitored in approximately half the patients. Nine per cent of those with bundle branch block progressed to second-degree heart block compared with only 0.7 per cent of those with normal cardiograms. In fact, the patient who developed heart block with a previously normal electrocardiogram was later shown to have abnormal His–Purkinje conduction and required permanent pacing. Of 11 patients with first-degree block, none showed progression. These findings

are consistent with the known electrophysiological actions of the tricyclics. These drugs act principally on the distal conduction system and hence are a particular risk in patients with bundle branch block.

In his review, Orme (1984) concluded that patients with severe heart disease, defined as heart failure, recent myocardial infarction, or electrocardiographic evidence of bundle branch block or high-degree atrioventricular block should not receive tricyclic agents. These recommendations appear to be well founded. Of the second-generation antidepressants, maprotiline (Hermann *et al.* 1983) and trazodone (Rausch *et al.* 1984) have similar effects to the tricyclics on conduction. The tetracyclic agent mianserin appears to be relatively safe in patients with cardiac disease (Burrows *et al.* 1979). The tachyarrhythmic complications of antidepressants are discussed above.

Carbamazepine

Carbamazepine has been used widely in the treatment of various forms of epilepsy and trigeminal neuralgia. Second and third-degree heart block, which resolved on withdrawing the drug, have been reported (Beermann *et al.* 1975; Ladefoged and Mogelvang 1982; Boesen *et al.* 1983; Benassi *et al.* 1987). Severe bradyarrhythmias generally occur within 7–10 days of commencing therapy. Most of the affected patients are elderly and have pre-existing abnormalities of the resting electrocardiogram. It is likely that carbamazepine unmasks latent conduction system disease. These effects are a consequence of its known Class I effects on mammalian cardiac electrophysiology (Steiner *et al.* 1970).

Methyldopa

Formal study of the electrophysiological properties of methyldopa has shown that it lengthens the functional and effective refractory periods of the atrioventricular node and significantly prolongs the atrio–His interval during atrial pacing (Gould *et al.* 1979). The drug has been reported to cause symptomatic sinus bradycardia (Davis *et al.* 1981), sinus pauses (Scheinmann *et al.* 1978) and carotid sinus reflex hypersensitivity (Bauerenfiend *et al.* 1978; Alfino *et al.* 1981). More recent reports have demonstrated reversible first (Sadjadi *et al.* 1984), second (Cregler and Mark 1987), and third-degree block (Rosen *et al.* 1988), respectively.

H₂-antagonists

Asystole and sinus arrest were reported by Cohen and colleagues (1979) in two patients given intravenous cimetidine. In both instances, the bradyarrhythmias occurred within 10 minutes of the injection. They were reinduced on later exposure to the drug by the same route. In later reports, Tordjman and others (1984) and Ishizaki and associates (1987) reported the development of reversible third-degree and first-degree heart block, respectively, in patients given oral cimetidine. Sinus bradycardia and sinus arrest have also been observed with both oral and intravenous cimetidine (Redding *et al.* 1977; Jefferys and Vale 1978).

Bradycardias are not confined to cimetidine. A significant reduction in sinus rate was observed in two patients who were given ranitidine by the oral and intravenous routes by Camarri and colleagues (1982). Interestingly, the bradycardia was abolished after the administration of atropine. Furthermore, it was not reinduced when the same patients were given cimetidine. In another report, asystole occurred after the fifth dose of intravenous ranitidine (Hart 1989) in a young man with no known cardiovascular disease.

The mechanism underlying these rare but dangerous bradycardias is unknown. It has been suggested that they may be manifestations of cardiac ischaemia induced by blockade of the H_2-receptors in the coronary vasculature, which leads to vasoconstriction (Baumann *et al.* 1982). Alternatively, there may be enhancement of parasympathetic tone by inhibition of cholinesterase (Hansen and Bertl 1983).

Drugs causing impairment of cardiac function

Drug effects on cardiac performance

The function of the heart as a pump may be adversely affected by drugs through changes in heart rhythm (as already discussed above) or through interference with the normal physiological contractile processes. Effects on the former have direct consequences on the latter, such as when the rate is too fast or too slow, or the rhythm too irregular, rendering cardiac chamber pumping activity ineffectual. The haemodynamic effects of cardiac arrhythmias have been well known for some time (Resnekov 1970). In addition, conduction defects may compromise cardiac pumping efficacy by inducing asynchronous ventricular contractions (Gibson *et al.* 1988). Asynchronous ventricular contraction induced by drugs is, however, of relatively minor importance in comparison with the ventricular asynchrony which may follow myocardial infarction. This issue will therefore not be discussed further in this chapter.

Drugs can adversely affect the contractile function of the myocardium by direct injury resulting in myocytolysis, which reduces the number of viable myocardial cells, or by direct effects on contractile force (inotropy) or ability to relax (compliance). In addition, drugs may influence contractile function indirectly by causing myocardial ischaemia, by altering preload or afterload, or by causing changes in the interstitial matrix of the myocardium (Caulfield and Bittner 1988). These drug effects may be desirable in certain circumstances but detrimental in others. For instance, β-adrenoceptor blockers and calcium antagonists are known to cause depression of myocardial excitability, conduction, and contraction, and these are put to good use in the treatment of angina, tachyarrhythmias, and hypertrophic obstructive cardiomyopathy, but they can be detrimental in heart failure. Any undesirable cardiac effects caused by these drugs can be regarded as pharmacologically predictable and avoidable by careful dose titration. Similarly, positive inotropic agents are very useful in severe heart failure, but when given to patients with obstructive cardiomyopathy, they can paradoxically induce or worsen the failure. Diuretics and nitrates are widely used in the treatment of patients with acute left ventricular failure following myocardial infarction, but their use in patients with right ventricular infarction may sometimes precipitate shock (due to relative hypovolaemia and hence underfilling of the left ventricle).

Unlike the diagnosis of arrhythmia, in which body surface and intracardiac electrocardiography can detect the abnormality clearly, the diagnosis of myocardial toxicity and depression cannot be made as readily *in vivo*, even with invasive techniques. Interpretation of the published results is therefore necessarily more complicated, and great care must be exercised before one can infer that myocardial toxicity or depression is directly due to the drug under investigation. Because of this, consideration of the methodology employed in studying these drug effects is warranted.

Cardiomyotoxic effects

Methods employed in studying cardiomyotoxic effects

The study of myocardial injury has traditionally relied on histological methods to identify morphological changes in the cellular structures that depict injury. The pattern of changes varies according to the initiating insult, the response to the injury, and the time of observation after the injury. The presence of late changes (e.g. fibrosis) would indicate that irreversible injury has occurred, but it is difficult to be categorical about which early changes signify the reversible or irreversible stages of injury. Furthermore, the sensitivity and specificity of these methods are usually adequate in the identification of large areas of damage, caused by such insults as myocardial infarction, but they may not be sensitive enough to detect single cell deaths, scattered throughout the myocardium. Such low-level changes are more typical of the injuries induced by drugs. Newer techniques, with greater sensitivity and specificity in identifying cell death, are required to study adverse drug reactions on the myocardium (Clark *et al.* 1989).

Many case reports have been published relating particular drugs to the development of cardiomyopathy. It is generally agreed that documentation of such observations is valuable, especially when the same observation is repeatedly made in different cases receiving the same medication. Otherwise, it is often difficult to establish the aetiological role of the drug. This is because of the fact that myocarditis and cardiomyopathy can often occur coincidentally during the course of drug therapy and the diagnosis of these conditions cannot be easily confirmed. It is therefore difficult to prove that a drug has caused a cardiomyopathy. It is equally difficult, however, to prove that a drug is innocent.

Positive inotropic agents

Sympathomimetic agents

By far the most cardiotoxic and the most extensively studied of all sympathomimetic agents is isoprenaline (isoproterenol). Other agents, however, such as adrenaline (epinephrine) and noradrenaline (norepinephrine), which are widely used in intensive care units, have also been shown to cause catecholamine cardiomyopathy. The analogous clinical condition is phaeochromocytoma (Alpert *et al.* 1972; Garcia and Jennings 1972; Cho *et al.* 1987). Whether other commonly used sympathomimetic agents, such as dopamine and dobutamine, can produce similar damage is unknown. The reason may well be that these agents are not as toxic as isoprenaline and noradrenaline. More sensitive methods of detecting small amounts of damage have only recently become available (Benjamin *et al.* 1989).

The characteristic features of the myocardial pathology induced by isoprenaline have been well described (Reichenbach and Benditt 1970; Todd *et al.* 1985a). Histological changes (contraction band lesions) can occur as early as 5 minutes after commencement of a high-dose isoprenaline infusion (Todd *et al.* 1985b) but these may not constitute irreversible cell damage. The earliest occurrence of cardiomyocyte death was noted 3 hours after subcutaneous injection of isoprenaline (Benjamin *et al.* 1989), and this reaches a peak at about 24 hours. Most of the necrosis occurs in the subendocardial region

(Benjamin *et al.* 1989). Unlike isoprenaline, noradrenaline has predominantly vasoconstrictive effects, but the pathological features of myocardial injury are similar to those induced by isoprenaline (Todd *et al.* 1985b).

Although catecholamine-induced cardiotoxicity has been known for over 30 years, the mechanisms responsible for the injury have not been fully elucidated. Rona (1985) has suggested that the injurious process is multifactorial, involving a combination of haemodynamic effects (myocardial hypoperfusion — especially in the subendocardial region, tachycardia, increased inotropy), free radical injury via catecholamine oxidative products, microvascular lesions, reperfusion injury, and intracellular calcium overload. The process is often exacerbated in the presence of pre-existing ischaemia secondary to coronary artery disease (Reichenbach and Benditt 1970).

Practical clinical guidelines

The question that arises from the above discussion is therefore whether one should refrain from using sympathomimetic agents to 'flog the tired horse', especially in post-myocardial infarction pump failure. There is an inevitable conflict between the need to 'rest' and preserve the myocardium and the need to stimulate cardiac performance to preserve life. The careful selection of patients who require inotropic support is necessary. Those with adequate cardiac output and systemic arterial pressure should receive vasodilators if support is indicated, rather than positive inotropic agents. Those with markedly impaired cardiac function, such that coronary perfusion pressure is compromised, would benefit from inotropic support, because improvement in coronary perfusion would allay further ischaemic injury. Those with a dilated ventricle may also benefit from inotropic support because a small reduction in ventricular volume may lead to reduction in one major component of myocardial oxygen consumption — the wall tension-related energy requirement (Gibbs *et al.* 1967).

Another practical question is: how long can one safely maintain the patient on catecholamine treatment? Obviously, if the cardiac status is such that inotropic support is no longer necessary, then a catecholamine infusion should be terminated. Not uncommonly, however, one finds that the patient is dependent on the inotropic support. Will the cumulative effect of a prolonged infusion be more detrimental? The answer is that, quite unlike doxorubicin cardiotoxicity, the injury is not proportional to the cumulative dose, provided a steady infusion is maintained. This is because, during prolonged steady infusion, there is gradual desensitization of β-adrenoceptors that renders the cardiac myocyte less susceptible to further catecholamine-induced injury (Tan and Clark 1990). In fact, prolonged infusion of dobuta-mine has been shown to produce beneficial functional effects (Liang *et al.* 1984). It is not uncommon to see some of the cardiogenic shock patients so treated able to walk out of hospital despite having very limited cardiac reserve. The mechanism of this beneficial effect is pre-sumably peripheral conditioning, similar to that ob-tained through exercise endurance training by athletes.

β-Adrenoceptor blocker withdrawal

Cardiac events such as unstable angina, acute myocar-dial infarction or exacerbation of arrhythmia, may follow abrupt β-blocker withdrawal (see below). Such rebound phenomena have been known for more than a decade (Slome 1973; Miller *et al.* 1975). Obviously, not all patients will suffer rebound phenomena on stopping β-blockers, but unfortunately there is no way of predict-ing which patients are susceptible. The mechanism is thought to be β-adrenoceptor up-regulation with pro-longed β-blockade (Heilbrunn *et al.* 1989; Glaubiger and Lefkowitz 1977). Sudden stoppage exposes these extra receptors to unopposed adrenergic stimulation and, in susceptible subjects, it may result in adverse cardiac events which include the cardiomyotoxic effects of endogenous catecholamines.

Other positive inotropic agents

As described above, the mechanism of a drug's ability to generate positive inotropic effects is closely linked to its ability to induce cardiotoxicity. The final common path-way may well be an increase in intracellular calcium, which, in the latter case, is excessive (Fleckenstein 1971; Katz and Reuter 1979; Auffermann *et al.* 1989). Inter-estingly, calcium excess is also one mode whereby these positive inotropic agents induce arrhythmias (see above). It has been proposed that calcium overload stimulates intracellular phospholipase activity, which in turn causes disintegration of the sarcolemmal membrane, which heralds cell death (Farber *et al.* 1981). It is therefore not surprising that other positive inotropic agents can also induce cardiomyotoxic effects.

Angiotensin has been shown to possess positive ino-tropic effects (Koch-Weser 1965; Freer *et al.* 1976), and also to cause myocardial necrosis (Gavras *et al.* 1971, 1975; Giacomelli *et al.* 1976; Bhan *et al.* 1982). Both exogenous and endogenous angiotensin II are capable of inducing cardiomyotoxicity (Tan *et al.* 1989).

Digoxin has been used in clinical practice for over 200 years, often as a positive inotropic agent although it is only a weak inotrope. It has a narrow therapeutic range, above which it can increase intracellular calcium (by inhibition of the sodium ATPase pump), but arrhythmo-genic effects are more prominent than any cardiomyo-lytic effects (see above).

Newer non-glycoside and non-catecholaminergic posi-tive inotropic agents, such as the phosphodiesterase inhibitors, amrinone, milrinone, and enoximone, have recently been introduced into clinical practice. Direct data on whether they cause cardiac myocyte necrosis is not yet available. Surveys on their effects on mortality in heart failure patients suggest that they may shorten patients' survival (Packer and Leier 1987), but whether this is due to cardiotoxic or proarrhythmic effects of the drugs, or due to the fact that patients receiving these agents are more severely ill, is unknown.

Chemotherapeutic agents

Anthracyclines

Doxorubicin (adriamycin) and daunorubicin (Rubido-mycin, Daunomycin) are the best known cardiotoxic antimitotic drugs of the anthracycline antibiotics class. Their antimitotic activity stems from binding to DNA and impairing DNA-polymerase activity and RNA syn-thesis (Galton 1983). They also interact with cellular enzymes, to generate free radicals which lead to damage of membrane lipids, and bind directly to the cytoskeletal protein spectrin and to cardiolipin, thereby disturbing ion transport. Unfortunately, cardiac myocytes may be susceptible to one or more of these mechanisms of action of the anthracyclines.

Prolonged administration causes cumulative irrevers-ible myocardial damage, culminating in dilated cardio-myopathy, congestive cardiac failure. and cardiogenic shock (Bonadonna and Monfardini 1969; Marmont *et al.* 1969; Kaduk and Seiler 1978). With daunorubicin the incidence of heart failure is dose-related, at 4 per cent in patients receiving cumulative doses up to 550 mg per m^2 and at 14 per cent in those receiving up to 1050 mg per m^2 (von Hoff and Layard 1981; von Hoff *et al.* 1979, 1982; Adams 1982). The risk is higher in children than adults. Overall, some 7–9 per cent of patients treated with doxorubicin may present with heart failure. This is also dose-related, occurring in 3 per cent of those receiving a cumulative dose of 400 mg per m^2 and 20 per cent of those receiving 700 mg per m^2 (Adams 1982; von Hoff *et al.* 1982). Moreover, one-fifth of asymptomatic patients had an abnormal resting left ventricular ejection fraction (Dresdale *et al.* 1983). Patients who have received radio-therapy to the chest or cyclophosphamide are more susceptible to anthracycline cardiotoxicity (Minow *et al.* 1977).

The development of heart failure in these patients depends on several factors. The occurrence of toxicity depends on the susceptibility not only of the individual patient but also of the individual myocytes. The reasons for variation in susceptibility are largely unknown. For some reason children are more susceptible. The elderly are also said to be more susceptible, but this may reflect diminished cardiac reserve before treatment in this age-group.

There have been several recommendations on how to institute anthracycline therapy so as to minimize cardiotoxicity (Minow et al. 1977; Legha et al. 1982). A rational approach is to assess cardiac function with whatever techniques are available locally (as a minimum, an ECG, chest radiograph, and an echocardiogram) before treatment, and to repeat the assessment at regular intervals during treatment. Changes indicative of significant cardiac myocyte loss (e.g. loss of R wave amplitude in the ECG, reduced systolic function in the echocardiogram), resulting in onset of compensatory mechanisms (e.g. resting tachycardia, ventricular and atrial dilatation), should indicate that the maximum advisable cumulative dose of anthracycline has been reached, even though the recommended maximum of 550 mg per m^2 may not have been exceeded. By the time patients present with symptoms and signs of heart failure, excessive myocardial damage must have occurred and the prognosis is very poor. Whether more invasive methods of monitoring cardiac effects, such as with regular endomyocardial biopsy (Billingham and Bristow 1984), would provide a more accurate aid in deciding when to discontinue treatment has not been established.

Alcohol

Although ethanol is no longer used in medical practice (except as a disinfectant and a solvent), it is a widely consumed sedative–hypnotic social drug. The syndrome of heart failure is common amongst patients who abuse alcohol. The genesis of the heart failure is multifactorial. Alcohol is a direct myocardial depressant; additionally, alcoholism may precipitate failure due to poor nutritional intake; and finally, alcohol abuse may cause cardiomyopathy, although evidence on this point is surprisingly poor.

There is still no scientifically rigorous evidence to support the hypothesis that alcohol induces dilated cardiomyopathy. To prove that a drug causes cardiomyopathy, it is essential to demonstrate that cardiac myocyte necrosis with its attendant fibrosis follows its administration. This has not been achieved in any animal experimental model with alcohol (Urbano-Marquez et al. 1989). The cumulative effect of necrosis eventually leads to the histological pattern of the myocardium seen in patients with dilated cardiomyopathy. The converse is not necessarily true: that is, the presence of histological evidence of dilated cardiomyopathy in a patient who has been abusing alcohol does not necessarily imply that alcohol is the cause. The histological features are indistinguishable from those of primary dilated cardiomyopathy and it is not possible to distinguish the two.

The questions whether those diagnosed as having 'alcoholic cardiomyopathy' would indeed have developed cardiomyopathy without alcohol, whether alcohol hastens the onset of heart failure in susceptible subjects, or whether it causes cardiomyopathy de novo, are as yet unsettled. It is worth noting that many long-term alcoholics do not develop dilated cardiomyopathy (Askanas et al. 1980; Kino et al. 1981; Kelbaek et al. 1984).

In vivo and in vitro administration of ethanol has been shown to depress myocardial function reversibly (Regan et al. 1965; Conway 1968; Nakano and Moere 1972; Timmis et al. 1975; Abel 1980; Thomas et al. 1980). They are associated with biochemical changes that are also reversible (Sarma et al. 1976; Rubin 1979). Alcoholics are notoriously unreliable in providing information about how much they drink (confabulation is not an unusual feature), but Urbano-Marquez and colleagues (1989) have recently claimed success in this attempt and showed dose-related left ventricular dysfunction in a group of alcoholics who have consumed the equivalent of 1200–3500 ml of wine per day for many years. Since alcohol directly depresses myocardial function, a practical point of vital importance is that all patients with dilated cardiomyopathy must abstain from further consumption of alcohol. Some improvement of cardiac function can be expected with abstinence.

There have been many reports of resolution of a cardiomyopathic picture on abstaining (Demakis et al. 1974; Kosinski 1989), but equally, in clinical practice, there are many more who remain in congestive heart failure despite abstinence and these cases are not published. Another reason why we need to keep an open mind is that it is not uncommon to see spontaneous normalization of cardiac function in patients with myocarditis. This condition can indeed occur coincidentally in some heavy drinkers, who are inevitably diagnosed as having alcoholic cardiomyopathy. If alcohol were truly toxic and produced histological features of fibrous tissue replacement of myocytes (Urbano-Marquez 1989), such cardiomyopathy would not be expected to resolve completely, unlike myocarditis.

That alcoholism can indirectly precipitate heart failure secondary to poor nutritional intake, resulting in beri-beri heart disease, is well known. In this condition, other manifestations of thiamine deficiency, such as peripheral neuropathy and myopathy, are often present. The treatment is abstinence, vitamin supplementation (including thiamine), and return to normal food intake. The prognosis is good and complete recovery can be expected. No doubt some alcoholics with heart failure may have subclinical levels of malnutrition, and may benefit from vitamin supplementation.

Cocaine

Abuse of cocaine has been associated with many hazards (Cregler and Mark 1986; Isner *et al.* 1986), including death (Mittleman and Wetli 1984; Schachne *et al.* 1984). In a canine model, it has been shown to produce dose-dependent ventricular systolic and diastolic depression (Abel *et al.* 1989). Direct cocaine cardiotoxicity has also been shown by endocardial biopsy (Peng *et al.* 1989). Cocaine is also known as a blocker of the noradrenaline uptake–1 process (Blinks 1966; Iversen 1967). It can therefore potentiate the effects of endogenous catecholamine and indirectly induce myocardial damage. More recently, Welder and colleagues (1988) have shown that it can induce necrosis directly in cardiac myocytes. The mechanism of this action has not been elucidated.

Myocardial depression

Methods used in studying drug-induced cardiodepression

Just as myotoxicity is often implicated when cardiomyopathy occurs during the use of certain drugs, there are abundant anecdotes of the onset of the syndrome of heart failure associated with drug therapy. This question is compounded by the fact that there is current confusion as to the most appropriate definition of heart failure (Poole Wilson 1989). It should be appreciated that the clinical syndrome of heart failure, as commonly understood, does not necessarily arise from myocardial depression. It can arise from undue loading of a non-failing heart, for example, with fluid overloading or with excessive vasoconstriction. Therefore, when perusing case reports that associate the onset of heart failure with drug therapy, caution has to be exercised to note whether the mechanism of failure is indeed myocardial depression, as opposed to contributions from arrhythmia, conduction defects, silent ischaemia per infarction, asynchronous ventricular contraction, heart rate alteration, or unsuitable preload or afterload. These factors, whether singly or in combination, can precipitate the clinical syndrome of heart failure.

The starting point in gathering information on inotropic effects of drugs is usually the study of cardiac muscle strips. Often, due to ease of isolation, atrial muscle is used, and this may behave differently from ventricular muscle. Results in isolated muscle do not necessarily correlate with *in vivo* haemodynamic results (see Procainamide section below). Similarly, *in vivo* animal experimental results cannot be automatically extrapolated and applied to clinical practice, owing to species differences and the greater complexity of clinical conditions. More recently, human cardiac muscle strips have been increasingly used to study drug inotropic effects. *In vitro* effects again, however, may not reflect clinical practice. For example, in a comparative study, nifedipine has been found to be more negatively inotropic in isolated human cardiac muscles than either verapamil or diltiazem (see below), which is quite contrary to clinical experience.

Unlike myotoxic effects of drugs, however, the negative inotropic effects are reversible. Myocardial depressant activity, therefore, can be studied by rechallenge under controlled conditions, in order to delineate the various factors influencing ventricular performance. Herein lies another problem: how does one evaluate cardiac function *in vivo*, especially in patients, to determine whether a drug directly depresses myocardial function? The most common methods of studying drug effects on myocardial function in the clinical context have been the use of non-invasive techniques, such as left ventricular ejection fraction, echocardiographic assessments, or systolic time intervals (Matos *et al.* 1977; Boudoulas *et al.* 1977a; Trimarco *et al.* 1983). It is well known that ejection fraction and systolic time intervals are highly dependent not only on inotropic states but also on the preload, afterload, heart rate, and the presence of valvular regurgitation. Even the absence of any changes in ejection fraction may be due to balanced effects from negative inotropism and vasodilation. Attempts to infer that a drug has directly depressed cardiac function because of an observed fall in ejection fraction (e.g. Kowey *et al.* 1982), without measuring effects on peripheral vascular resistance, are methodologically unjustifiable. Therefore, a large number of studies reporting drug inotropic effects using these methods need to be interpreted with care.

Various indices specific for inotropy have been proposed. The proponents of these indices derived them from studies of cardiac muscle mechanics, and made *a priori* claims that they are independent of other factors and solely reflect inotropy. Subsequently, however, when tested in intact hearts, especially in complex clinical cardiological situations, these indices have been found to be dependent on factors other than inotropy. Even the currently most widely accepted index of inotropy, the end-systolic ventricular elastance (E_{max}=end-systolic pressure/volume) has recently been shown to assess the pressure-generating capacity, leaving largely unassessed the flow-generating capacity (Shroff and Motz 1989). Because of these confounding factors, the use of these indices of contractility to identify direct myocardial depressant effects of drugs is often inconclusive.

The alternative to indices with *a priori* claims is to control the various factors individually and use analytical methods to arrive at the effects of the drug on a particular factor. For instance, heart rate and rhythm may be controlled by artificially pacing the right atrium. In the absence of changes in the morphology of surface electrocardiogram one can assume invariance of the conduction pattern. Preload can be controlled to some extent using physical means (e.g. by positive or negative lower-body pressure). The direct myocardial effect can then be measured by observing the haemodynamic changes brought about by intracoronary administration of the drug. This method is necessarily invasive and complex. Although it has been used in the study of certain positive inotropic agents (Colucci 1989), it has thus far not been used in the context of studying adverse drug effects on the myocardium. A less invasive and less complex analytical method has been proposed (Tan *et al*. 1987) that can in future be usefully applied to study drug reactions in patient populations, especially those with impaired ventricular function.

Antiarrhythmic agents

Apart from proarrhythmic effects, antiarrhythmic agents are also prone to depress myocardial function. Some, such as disopyramide, β-adrenoceptor blockers, and verapamil are more prone to precipitate cardiac failure than others. Antiarrhythmic agents that are thought to be least negatively inotropic are lignocaine, mexiletine, tocainide, and oral amiodarone.

Representative drugs from each of the Vaughan-Williams classes of antiarrhythmic agent are discussed below. Discussion on the mechanisms by which each drug induces negative inotropism is beyond the scope of this chapter. In general, drugs having direct myocardial depressant activity appear to decrease, by various pathways, the availability of calcium to the contractile elements (Silva Graça and van Zwieten 1972; Schlepper 1989). None of these antiarrhythmic agents is as yet known to induce cardiodepression by alteration in myofilament sensitivity to calcium (Blinks and Endoh 1986; Ruegg 1986).

Class Ia agents

Procainamide It may come as a surprise to some readers to learn that procainamide at high doses has been shown to exert significant positive inotropic effects on isolated cat right ventricular papillary muscle (Ham-

mermeister *et al*. 1972). This finding was later supported by observations of Williams and Mathew (1984). In the isolated Langendorff rat-heart preparation, however, there were mixed positive and negative inotropic effects of procainamide (Nahas *et al*. 1969).

In contrast, most *in vivo* animal studies have demonstrated a negative inotropic effect (Cote *et al*. 1973, 1975; Lertora *et al*. 1979) with doses above usual therapeutic levels. In conscious dogs, O'Rourke and co-workers (1969) did not observe any change in cardiac flow-generating capacity with procainamide infused at therapeutic doses. In a rare experiment, high-dose procainamide was injected into the left coronary artery, and this produced a transient decrease followed by a more sustained increase in left ventricular myocardial force (Folle and Aviado 1966).

The haemodynamic effects of procainamide in man are quite variable. Some studies show vasodilator effects (Burton *et al*. 1976; Block and Winkle 1983) while others show vasoconstriction (Karlsson and Sonnhag 1976) or no change (Miller *et al*. 1973). In most studies, some of them very elegantly performed, insufficient consideration has been given to the peripheral drug effects (e.g. Harrison *et al*. 1963; Jawad-Kanber and Sherrod 1974; Smitherman *et al*. 1979; Geleris *et al*. 1980), rendering the conclusions drawn on the direct inotropic effects of the drug rather questionable (MacAlpin 1975). Collating all the evidence, we may conclude that in man procainamide in therapeutic doses does not exert significant direct inotropic effects on the myocardium.

Quinidine There is no doubt that, at supratherapeutic doses, quinidine depresses the contraction of isolated cardiac muscle (Hammermeister *et al*. 1972; Tomoda *et al*. 1972). At therapeutic levels, however, some claimed that it was negatively inotropic (Hammermeister *et al*. 1972; Tomoda *et al*. 1972), while others disputed this (Kennedey and West 1969; Lameijer and van Zwieten 1974). Studies in intact animals were equally inconclusive, although they all show significant peripheral vasodilatation following intravenous quinidine (Angelakos and Hastings 1960; Folle and Aviado 1966; Walsh and Horwitz 1979). As discussed above, part of the reason for uncertainty is that investigators have found it difficult to separate the inotropic effects, secondary to reflex sympathetic stimulation, from the direct inotropic effects of the drug. One way of circumventing this problem is to study the drug effects in transplanted hearts, and this was done in five patients (Mason *et al*. 1977a). Unfortunately, although there was no change in peripheral vascular resistance, cardiac pump function was thought to be reduced by a decrease in preload, which was presumably secondary to the venodilating effect of quinidine — this leaves the question of direct inotropic effects of intravenous quinidine largely unanswered.

There appears to be a greater consensus on the myocardial effects of oral quinidine. In dogs, after 2 weeks of oral treatment, there was no obvious fall in blood pressure and myocardial contractility (O'Rourke and Horwitz 1981). Similar results have been reported in human volunteers and patients (Crawford *et al.* 1979). Most significantly, there was no apparent haemodynamic compromise in 652 patients (of whom 35 per cent had heart failure before treatment) treated with oral quinidine in the Boston Collaborative Drug Surveillance Program (Cohen *et al.* 1977).

Disopyramide There is general agreement that of all the Class I antiarrhythmic agents available disopyramide is the most negatively inotropic (Bourke *et al.* 1987; Honerjager *et al.* 1986). This detrimental effect is compounded by its vasoconstrictive effect, which also involves the coronary vasculature (Kötter *et al.* 1980). Studies on isolated cardiac muscle (Mokler and van Arman 1962; Naylor 1976), in intact animals (Walsh and Horwitz, 1979), and in man (Jensen *et al.* 1975; Befeler 1975; Willis 1975; Naqvi *et al.* 1979; Leach *et al.* 1980; Thadani *et al.* 1981; Bauman 1981) demonstrated the significant cardiac depressant property of the drug, which may culminate in progressive heart failure (Story *et al.* 1979; Podrid *et al.* 1980).

Class Ib agents

Lignocaine (lidocaine) The *in vitro* effects of lignocaine on isolated muscle strips are conflicting, with reports demonstrating both the presence of negative inotropism (Hammermeister *et al.* 1972; Sheu and Lederer 1985) and its absence (Tomoda *et al.* 1972; Tejerina *et al.* 1983). Evaluation in intact animal hearts showed no significant negative inotropic effects with lignocaine in the dose range used clinically (Lieberman *et al.* 1968; Nahas *et al.* 1969), but it became significantly negatively inotropic at doses above the therapeutic range (Austen and Moran 1965; Nahas *et al.* 1969; Cote *et al.* 1973). Clinical studies have confirmed this finding (Harrison *et al.* 1963; Kötter *et al.* 1980). Even in patients with significant left ventricular dysfunction (Miller *et al.* 1973; Burton *et al.* 1976) lignocaine is relatively free of negative inotropic effects, making it one of the safest antiarrhythmic agents for patients with ventricular arrhythmia. Interestingly, in the last groups of patients, therapeutic doses of lignocaine produced systemic vasoconstriction that may even raise the systemic arterial pressure (Miller *et al.* 1973; Burton *et al.* 1976), without direct myocardial depression.

Mexiletine Studies in animals (Banim *et al.* 1977; Kuhn *et al.* 1977; Pozenel 1977; Carlier 1980; Marshall *et al.* 1981) and man (Campbell *et al.* 1979; Chamberlain *et al.* 1980; Stein *et al.* 1984) have shown that the negative inotropic effect of intravenous and oral mexiletine is minimal and clinical problems are rare.

Tocainide Like mexiletine, tocainide has minimal negative inotropic effects. Few animal studies regarding its direct inotropic effects are available. There is a suggestion of cardiodepression when enormous doses are given (Coltart *et al.* 1974). Two studies in patients undergoing cardiac catheterization showed myocardial depression (Schwartz *et al.* 1979; Ikram 1980). In patients with ischaemic left ventricular dysfunction, however, tocainide produced only a slight and transient rise in peripheral vascular resistance with minimal inotropic changes (Winkle *et al.* 1978; MacMahon *et al.* 1985). During long-term oral treatment with tocainide, only 1.4 per cent of 369 patients developed exacerbation of heart failure (Horn *et al.* 1980).

Class Ic agents

Flecainide Animal studies have demonstrated a direct cardiodepressant effect of flecainide (Verdouw *et al.* 1979; Hoddess *et al.* 1979). Earlier studies on patients with coronary artery disease suggested negative inotropism (Legrand *et al.* 1983; Serruys *et al.* 1983). In a similar group of patients with left ventricular ejection fractions ranging from 20–80 per cent, Josephson and colleagues (1985) demonstrated that flecainide clearly exerted direct myocardial depression. This problem may be compounded by the fact that flecainide clearance from plasma is reduced in heart failure patients (Franciosa *et al.* 1983; Conard and Ober 1984).

Propafenone Pharmacological experiments indicate that propafenone can directly depress myocardial function, partly because it has mild β-blocking and weak calcium antagonist activities (Ledda *et al.* 1981; Dukes and Vaughan-Williams 1984; McLeod *et al.* 1984). In patients there are suggestions of negative inotropism (Shen *et al.* 1984; Brodsky *et al.* 1985; Baker *et al.* 1987), although categorical statements about whether the drug causes direct and clinically important cardiodepression must await more rigorous studies.

Class II agents

β-Blockers These agents have been used to treat arrhythmia for over 20 years (Gettes 1970). Their negative inotropic and chronotropic effects are also well known (Epstein *et al.* 1965; Sowton and Hamer 1966; Blinks 1967). Although these effects are desirable when treating, for example, myocardial ischaemia, hypertension,

atrial fibrillation, or hypertrophic cardiomyopathy, the danger of inducing cardiac failure should be borne in mind (Conway *et al.* 1968). These type A reactions (excessive myocardial depression and bradycardia) are generally dose-dependent, and may be avoided by dose reduction. Indeed, investigators have recently shown that low-dose β-blockade is not only safe but also beneficial in the treatment of dilated cardiomyopathy (J.L. Anderson *et al.* 1985; Engelmeier *et al.* 1985).

Treatment for adverse cardiac reaction to β-blockers depends on the haemodynamic status of the patient. If there is no significant haemodynamic compromise, the patient may be monitored on a coronary care unit until the β-blockade recedes. Bradycardia and conduction defects may be reversed by intravenous atropine (0.6 to 2.4 mg in an adult). If significant haemodynamic compromise occurs, and if the β-blocker is a competitive inhibitor (Blinks 1967; Dollery *et al.* 1969), then careful ECG and haemodynamic monitoring and infusion of an appropriate sympathomimetic agent should be instituted, with dosage titrated against response. High doses (e.g. 200 μg per kg per min of dobutamine) may be required. If there is insufficient response, or the β-blocker is non-competitive, then a phosphodiesterase inhibitor (e.g. milrinone or enoximone) with or without a vasoconstrictor agent may be needed.

β-Adrenoceptor down-regulation

After prolonged infusion of sympathomimetic agents as inotropic support, sudden stopping of the infusion sometimes results in precipitous circulatory collapse. This is secondary to adrenoceptor desensitization and uncoupling (Harden 1983; Karliner *et al.* 1986; Reithmann and Werdan, 1989), the consequences of which are similar to β-blockade. It is therefore advisable to tail off the infusion very gradually at a rate commensurate with the resensitization of the adrenoceptors, which may take a day or more (Karliner *et al.* 1986).

Class III agents

Amiodarone The most important issue surrounding the question 'does amiodarone induce myocardial depression?' is whether it is to the intravenous or the oral form of amiodarone that we are referring. Almost all reports on negative inotropism with amiodarone have been observed in the acute situation using the intravenous preparation of the drug (Singh *et al.* 1976; Installe *et al.* 1981; Schwartz *et al.* 1983). It is not clear how much of this is due to the solvent, polysorbate 80, which is known to be a vasodilator (Breithardt *et al.* 1980) and a cardiodepressant (Gough *et al.* 1982). Like other antiar-

rhythmic agents, the cardiodepressant activity of amiodarone is dose-dependent.

Clinical experience and careful follow-up of large numbers of patients taking oral amiodarone suggest that the oral preparation is devoid of negative inotropic effects (Leak and Eydt 1986; Cleland *et al.* 1987), so much so that if any patient develops heart failure during oral amiodarone therapy, it is important to look for other precipitating factors, such as silent myocardial infarction, before attributing the event to the drug. A haemodynamic study of oral amiodarone in dogs showed marked myocardial depression (Landymore *et al.* 1984), but the dose of 15 mg per kg per day was significantly in excess of the usual therapeutic dose, and the canine myocardial response may differ from the human. The animal result is also at variance with the results of a double-blind placebo-controlled trial in patients with congestive heart failure, in whom oral amiodarone not only increased the left ventricular ejection fraction but also improved exercise tolerance (Hamer *et al.* 1989).

The reason why acute and chronic antiarrhythmic and haemodynamic effects of amiodarone are different may lie in its mechanisms of action. Although the antiarrhythmic property of amiodarone is usually considered to be Class III (Singh and Vaughan Williams 1970), it has also been shown to have Class II (Charlier 1970) and Class I (Mason *et al.* 1984; Cobbe and Manley 1987) antiarrhythmic activities. The Class I and II effects are apparent with acute treatment, but the manifestation of Class III effects may be delayed (Singh and Vaughan Williams 1970), sometimes becoming obvious only after several weeks of oral treatment. It has been suggested that the mechanism by which amiodarone acts as a Class III agent is through selective inhibition of the effects of T_3 on the myocardium (Singh, 1983), perhaps through preferential peripheral conversion of T_4 to reverse-T_3 and inhibition of the binding of T_3 to cell nuclei (Franklyn *et al.* 1985). This explains why chronic treatment with amiodarone is required to convert the myocardium into a 'hypothyroid state' to realize the full benefit of its Class III antiarrhythmic activity. Once this state is reached, lower maintenance doses may be sufficient to achieve the antiarrhythmic goal, and therefore the cardiodepressant effect is minimized.

After prolonged therapy with oral amiodarone, there have been instances when it was difficult to wean patients undergoing cardiac surgery off cardiopulmonary bypass (Gallagher *et al.* 1981; MacKinnon *et al.* 1983), and sustained inotropic support with sympathomimetic agents may be necessary. While part of the explanation may be related to intraoperative loss of myocardium, decreased responsiveness to catecholamines is also contributory. Long-term use of amiodarone results in β-adrenoceptor down-regulation (Brevetti *et al.* 1986). Large doses of sympathomimetic agents, with or without phosphodiesterase inhibitors, may be required. The same treatment regimen described above for stopping inotropic support after prolonged infusion, may be necessary.

Class IV agents

Calcium antagonists Like β-adrenoceptor blockers, calcium antagonists possess negative inotropic and chronotropic effects that may be exploited for therapeutic purposes, but that may equally have detrimental consequences. The cardiodepressant effects of calcium antagonists are secondary to the uncoupling of excitation from contraction, by various mechanisms (Naylor 1980; Henry 1980; Capasso 1985). Their negative inotropic effect may be compounded by a decrease in velocity of myocardial relaxation (Vittone *et al.* 1985) to produce detrimental effects on cardiac function. In isolated cardiac muscle the *in vitro* negative inotropic effect was most marked with nifedipine, compared with verapamil and diltiazem (Henry 1980; Perez *et al.* 1982; Bohm *et al.* 1990), but in clinical practice experience suggests that verapamil is the most cardiodepressant, followed by nifedipine and diltiazem (Walsh 1987; Colucci 1987). It may be that the stronger vasodilator effect of nifedipine causes reflex sympathetic stimulation, obscuring the intrinsic negative inotropic effect that is nevertheless present (Clifton *et al.* 1990).

The treatment of cardiac pump failure induced by calcium antagonists is similar to that of excessive β-blockade, but sometimes an intravenous infusion of calcium may be required (Perkins 1978).

Newer calcium antagonists with a more selectively vasodilator than cardiodepressant action are now available, such as felodipine (Ljung 1985), nicardipine (Pepine 1989), and isradipine (Bohm *et al.* 1990). They may be used in patients who are unlikely to tolerate negative inotropism.

A practical clinical issue worth mentioning concerns the treatment of broad-complex tachycardia. In urgent situations, when no more sophisticated facilities are available, it is sometimes difficult to ascertain whether the tachycardia is ventricular, or supraventricular with aberrant conduction. A common pitfall is to assume the latter diagnosis and give intravenous verapamil. The consequence of this can be disastrous if the diagnosis is wrong, because a patient with ventricular tachycardia does not tolerate the negative inotropic effects of verapamil. In view of the fact that the majority of broad-complex tachycardias are ventricular, if the exact diagnosis is in doubt it is preferable from the point of view of probability and safety, to treat the tachycardia as ventricular and not to use verapamil.

Anaesthetic agents

During surgery there are many factors which can influence cardiac function (e.g. body temperature, level of ventilation and oxygenation, vasodilatation), and consequently it is difficult to isolate the direct effects of a single agent. Some degree of hypotension, for instance, from the cardiodepressant effect of anaesthetic agents, is sometimes considered desirable during surgery. Nevertheless, excessive negative inotropic effects, especially in patients with pre-existing cardiac failure, can become a problem.

Most volatile anaesthetic agents exert cardiodepressant effects. To study their relative potency, one needs to standardize and compare the negative inotropic effects at equivalent levels of anaesthesia. One way of achieving this is by using the same MAC (defined as the minimum alveolar concentration of an anaesthetic required to eliminate movement in response to surgical incision in 50 per cent of subjects). Shimosato and Etsten (1969) found that at equipotent anaesthetic concentrations halothane is about three times more cardiodepressant than cyclopropane, with methoxyflurane, enflurane, and ether (in descending order) lying in between. Paradise and Bibbins (1969) found that chloroform produced the most cardiac depression, with halothane > methoxyflurane > ether in decreasing rank order of depression. Brown and Crout (1971) found the following decreasing order of cardiodepression: enflurane > halothane > methoxyflurane > cyclopropane > ether. Kemmotsu and colleagues (1974) found that halothane, enflurane, isoflurane, and fluroxene showed equivalent cardiodepressant potency, about three to four times that of cyclopropane.

Drugs causing myocardial ischaemia

β-Adrenoceptor blocking agents

Effects of acute withdrawal

There are numerous reports from clinical trials of β-adrenoceptor blocking drugs showing that their abrupt withdrawal from patients with ischaemic heart disease may be associated with an exacerbation of symptoms and may lead to unstable angina, myocardial infarction, and sudden death (Wilson *et al.* 1969; Miller *et al.* 1975; Prichard and Walden 1982; Frishman 1987). Most of the reports have come from studies involving propranolol and most events have occurred during the phase of treatment withdrawal. The mechanisms underlying the syndrome of β-adrenoceptor blocker withdrawal are unknown but are thought to include an increased sensitivity of β-adrenoceptors (see above) (Boudoulas *et al.* 1977*b*; Nattel *et al.* 1979) and increased myocardial oxygen consumption caused by an increase in heart rate.

Walker and others (1985) studied the effect of abrupt cessation of atenolol therapy in twenty patients using exercise testing and ambulatory S–T-segment monitoring and found no evidence of rebound ischaemia with this long-acting drug although in a similar study Egstrup (1988) found evidence of a significant increase in silent ischaemia. Details of the β-blockers used in this investigation are not presented.

There appears to be evidence supporting the contention that abrupt removal of short-acting drugs such as propranolol may result in withdrawal symptoms in patients with angina. In contrast, withdrawal of long-acting agents such as atenolol does not appear to cause significant rebound angina. Review of the early reports of the β-blocker withdrawal syndrome, however, most of which involved propranolol, indicates that most patients who suffered adverse events had severe or unstable angina. Therefore, patient selection probably had a. major influence on the clinical syndrome that was initially described. Drugs with intrinsic sympathomimetic activity, such as pindolol, are not associated with problems of withdrawal. The presence of β-stimulant activity may therefore offset any increase in β-adrenoceptor sensitivity (Molinoff *et al.* 1982).

Effects on plasma lipid profile

Several large, much publicized studies of coronary risk factor intervention have reported a lack of reduction in mortality from coronary heart disease in treated hypertensives. A suggested explanation for this finding is that other coronary risk factors may be affected adversely by antihypertensive treatment (Leren 1987; Lardinois and Neuman 1988). In this regard, the deleterious effects of thiazide diuretics and some β-adrenoceptor antagonists on serum lipids have been examined extensively in recent studies. The effects of β-blockers on lipid metabolism have been reviewed (Kincaid-Smith 1984; Lehtonen 1985; Roberts 1989).

In general, β-blockers without intrinsic sympathomimetic activity tend to increase triglycerides and decrease high-density lipoprotein cholesterol but do not cause significant changes in total or low-density lipoprotein cholesterol levels. More specifically, the pooled results of the studies reviewed by van Brummelen (1983) showed that non-selective and β_1-selective agents raised plasma triglycerides by an average of 38 per cent and 21 per cent, respectively, compared with a mean 11 per cent rise for drugs with intrinsic sympathomimetic activity. The mean changes in serum high-density lipoprotein levels for the three groups of β-blockers were reductions of 19 per cent and 5 per cent for the non-selective and β_1-selective agents and an increase of 3 per cent for those compounds with intrinsic sympathomimetic activity. Sotalol is exceptional in that it causes significant elevations of both total and low-density lipoprotein cholesterol levels.

Catecholamines have complex effects on lipid metabolism and the exact mechanism whereby β-blockers affect serum lipid levels is unknown. Lipoprotein lipase, tissue lipase, and hepatic lipase are key enzyme systems involved in the catabolism of triglyceride-rich lipoproteins. The inhibition of these enzymes, either directly by β-blockers or by secondary, unopposed α-adrenoceptor stimulation, might account for the observed changes in the plasma lipid subfractions and triglycerides.

Although the adverse effects of β-blockade on plasma lipid profiles are a cause for concern, it must be stressed that there are no published data to confirm the clinical relevance of these effects.

Calcium antagonists

Calcium-channel blockers are a chemically heterogeneous group of drugs with potent cardiovascular effects. The main adverse effects of the group are dose-dependent and reflect their therapeutic actions, which include vasodilatation, negative inotropism (see above), and negative chronotropic and dromotropic effects (Hedner 1986). The principal classes of calcium antagonists are represented by nifedipine, verapamil, and diltiazem. Exacerbation of angina, whether judged by symptoms or by ambulatory ST-segment changes (Casolo *et al.* 1989), has been extensively reported with nifedipine. This phenomenon has been termed paradoxical angina.

The mechanism underlying the paradoxical angina seen with nifedipine involves reflex tachycardia secondary to vasodilatation (Stone *et al.* 1983) and increased myocardial oxygen consumption (Jariwalla and Anderson 1978; Rodger and Stewart 1978; Raftos 1980; Feldman *et al.* 1982). This may be further exacerbated by the coronary steal phenomenon (Boden *et al.* 1985). Paradoxical angina is more prevalent in patients with impaired left ventricular function and those with severe proximal coronary stenoses. An important hypotensive interaction between nifedipine and propranolol, manifesting as deterioration in angina, has been reported (Opie and White 1980).

Withdrawal or omission of calcium antagonists in patients with angina may result in worsening symptoms within 48 hours. This rebound phenomenon has been described for nifedipine (Kay *et al.* 1982, Nehring and Camm 1983; Myrhed and Wilhom 1986), and in isolated reports for verapamil and diltiazem (Bala Subramanian *et al.* 1983). The cause of rebound angina is unknown. Bala Subramanian and others (1983) have proposed that chronic treatment with calcium antagonists may deplete the intracellular pool of calcium ions. Withdrawal of the calcium-channel blockers may be accompanied by an increased flux of calcium ions into vascular smooth muscle cells resulting in an increased tendency to coronary vasospasm.

A recent study by Loaldi and colleagues (1989) offers information on the possible prevalence of paradoxical angina in patients prescribed nifedipine for angina. They compared angiographic, clinical, and electrocardiographic indices in patients with 'mixed' angina, occurring both on effort and at rest, and in patients with Prinzmetal angina. In the first group, 10 of the 22 patients showed evidence of increased ischaemia during treatment with nifedipine, whereas those with Prinzmetal angina had a uniformly favourable response during therapy with nifedipine. The exact mechanisms underlying the deleterious effects of nifedipine in some patients with mixed angina are unknown.

Nitrates

The benefits of a daily nitrate-free or nitrate-low interval in preventing nitrate tolerance are well established (Cowan 1986; Abrams 1989). Recent studies have suggested, however, that nitrate withdrawal may lead to rebound angina. In occasional patients, overnight removal of nitroglycerin patches has caused an exacerbation of anginal episodes (De Mots and Glasser 1989; Ferrantini *et al.* 1989). The extent to which these results can be extrapolated to other nitrate preparations is uncertain. It is possible that intermittent therapy with nitroglycerin patches is particularly prone to rebound, because of the rapid decline in nitroglycerin levels following patch removal. Certainly, previous studies of interval therapy, which have been based on oral preparations of isosorbide dinitrate and isosorbide mononitrate, have failed to find evidence of rebound. Oral preparations and regimens, however, have not undergone as close scrutiny as the patch and it is possible that the problems of nitrate withdrawal may have gone undetected. In view of these concerns, interval therapy should, where possible, be combined with other anti-anginal treatment, particularly β-blockers, to guard against the possibility of rebound (Cowan 1990).

β_2-Adrenoceptor agonists

β_2-Adrenoceptor agonists are administered intravenously for the inhibition of preterm labour (tocolysis). Ritodrine is used widely in the USA, from where most of the reports of its cardiovascular toxicity originate. Terbutaline and salbutamol are also used for this purpose (Tye *et al.* 1980; Katz *et al.* 1981). Retrosternal pain typical of angina pectoris and associated with electrocardiographic evidence of myocardial ischaemia has been reported by many authors and has been reviewed recently (Benedetti 1983; Ingemarsson *et al.* 1985). Myocardial infarction has been documented in some instances (Benedetti 1983), but in at least one case the patient was known to have coronary artery disease (Bass *et al.* 1979).

In a prospective study to determine the incidence of adverse cardiovascular effects during ritodrine infusion, Schneider and colleagues (1988) reported that 8 of their study group of 30 patients developed anginal pain. Certain clinical features were associated with an increased tendency to myocardial ischaemia. These included heart rate in excess of 130 beats per minute, hypokalaemia, hypotension, and anaemia. Anginal pain and the associated electrocardiographic abnormalities were readily reversed by discontinuation of the drug.

The pathophysiology of the myocardial ischaemia is thought to be multifactorial. Tachycardia will reduce the diastolic filling time of the coronary circulation and increase myocardial oxygen consumption. Other contributory factors are listed above. It has been suggested that the placental circulation resembles a large arteriovenous fistula, which reduces aortic diastolic blood pressure, thereby contributing to myocardial insufficiency (Benedetti 1983).

Amphetamines and cocaine

The abuse of the indirect sympathomimetic drugs cocaine and amphetamine has been documented as causing life-threatening cardiac arrhythmias (see above), angina, and myocardial infarction (Isner *et al.* 1986; Cregler and Mark 1986; Carson *et al.* 1987). Myocardial infarction may occur either in patients with known coronary artery disease or in those with normal coronary vasculature. Both agents cause an increase in systolic blood pressure and heart rate and thus myocardial oxygen demand. The exact pathophysiology of the coronary occlusion that causes myocardial infarction remains uncertain but it is thought to be a transient focal event. Both cocaine and amphetamine exert indirect pressor effects on the coronary circulation, potentiating the actions of noradrenaline and thereby causing vasospasm (Fiegl 1983). In addition, catecholamines are potent platelet aggregators and may cause thrombosis (Haft *et al.* 1982). Post-mortem studies of the hearts of patients who have died suddenly after taking amphetamines have found histological changes varying from no abnormality through a spectrum that includes arteriolar spasm (Carvey and Reed (1970) and interstitial and endocardial haemorrhage (Orrenius and Maehly 1970).

Dipyridamole

Dipyridamole is a potent coronary vasodilator (Kadatz 1959) that is used both therapeutically and, in conjunction with thallium scintigraphy, in the investigation of ischaemic heart disease. Its actions are mediated by its effects on the coronary and systemic circulations (Marchant *et al.* 1986). At the cellular level, dipyridamole increases the concentration of adenosine in the arterial wall of resistance vessels (Homback 1987). Although it has been used in the medical management of angina pectoris, it can cause coronary steal and may exacerbate anginal symptoms, particularly in patients with multivessel coronary disease (Feldman *et al.* 1981; Marchant *et al.* 1984).

Thyroxine

Previous reports of angina pectoris and myocardial infarction occurring in patients with thyrotoxicosis (Somerville and Levine 1949; Wei *et al.* 1979; Featherstone and Stewart 1983) have assumed that the ischaemic symptoms have been due to co-existing atheromatous coronary artery disease or coronary spasm (Kotler *et al.* 1973; Resnekov and Falicov 1977). Additionally, emboli from a fibrillating left atrium and primary *in situ* coronary thrombosis have been reported. These phenomena are thought to account for the permanent left ventricular segmental wall motion abnormalities that have been described in Graves' disease (Kotler *et al.* 1973; Proskey *et al.* 1977). These reports relate to patients with excessive amounts of endogenous thyroid hormones.

Bergeron and others (1988) have reported the case of a 68-year-old woman who deliberately took an excess of desiccated thyroid (260 mg per day) over a period of time and who presented with clinical thyrotoxicosis and a subendocardial anterior myocardial infarction associated with two large areas of ventricular dyskinesis. Subsequent cardiac catheterization and coronary angiography showed normal coronary artery anatomy and a normal pattern of left ventricular contraction. The authors suggest that coronary spasm with resultant reversible myocardial ischaemia was the most likely pathological mechanism, since all the abnormalities of left ventricular function resolved fully.

Encainide

Barron and Billhardt (1989) have reported a case of a 59-year-old man with dilated cardiomyopathy who developed angina pectoris after receiving 25 mg 8-hourly of the Class Ic antiarrhythmic agent encainide, which had been prescribed for high-grade ventricular ectopy. Previous coronary angiography had shown occlusion of a small diagonal branch of the left anterior descending artery as the only abnormality, although the subject did not have a history of prior angina. The patient complained of typical anginal pain that responded to sublingual nitrates and dyspnoea approximately 1–2 hours after each dose, which would equate with the time of peak plasma concentrations (Chase and Sloskey 1987). Encainide was withdrawn but subsequently restarted, when it resulted in identical symptoms. Patients with dilated cardiomyopathy are known to have reduced coronary flow reserve (Pasternac *et al.* 1982). The authors proposed that encainide might have caused vasoconstriction in the subendocardial vascular bed and thus ischaemia.

Fluorouracil

The antimetabolite fluorouracil has been used for over 30 years as a chemotherapeutic agent. Its adverse gastrointestinal and haematological effects are well known but recent case reports and reviews have indicated that it causes significant cardiotoxicity. This may take the form of myocardial depression (Chaudary *et al.* 1988) or the induction of angina pectoris (Dent and McColl 1975; Underwood *et al.* 1983; Blijham *et al.* 1986; Collins and Weiden 1987; Millward *et al.* 1988). Fatal myocardial infarction has also been described (Clavel *et al.* 1988; Ensley *et al.* 1989).

Collins and Weiden (1987) have estimated that 10 per cent of patients who receive fluorouracil will experience cardiotoxicity and that this is most usual when the drug is given by infusion rather than as an intravenous bolus. Myocardial ischaemia is manifest as anterior wall chest pain typical of angina, usually occurring after the second dose of the drug has been given. The symptoms are accompanied in 80 per cent of cases by significant ECG changes of ischaemia with ST-segment elevation and typical T wave abnormalities. It is probable that in the majority of cases fluorouracil exacerbates underlying heart disease, although it may also induce angina in patients with no previous history of ischaemic heart disease. The mechanism of the drug's cardiotoxicity has not been established. From the clinical observations of the reproducibility of the chest pain and associated ECG abnormalities following the administration of fluorouracil, it has been inferred that the drug may cause coronary spasm (Lang-Stevenson *et al.* 1977; Pottage *et al.* 1978; Labianca *et al.* 1982; Sanini *et al.* 1981; Kleinman *et al.* 1987). This seems possible, as several patients who have experienced anginal pain with this drug have been shown to have normal coronary angiograms (Collins and Weiden 1987).

Vincristine and vinblastine

Mandel and colleagues (1975) described the clinical course of a 58-year-old man with known but stable coronary artery disease who developed myocardial infarctions after the second and third doses of vincristine. Since this initial report, two other cases of myocardial infarction associated with the administration of vincristine (Warden *et al.* 1976; Somers *et al.* 1976) and one case after vinblastine therapy (Lejonc *et al.* 1980) have been published. Coronary angiography was undertaken in one patient and showed a normal coronary vasculature (Warden *et al.* 1976). To account for the changes, the authors speculated that coronary artery spasm had been induced by vincristine, and wondered if previous mantle irradiation might have facilitated this. Vinca alkaloids are toxic to myofibrils: a similar type of injury to vascular smooth muscle cells might induce coronary spasm and result in myocardial ischaemia and necrosis.

In a provocative report, Edwards and colleagues (1979) noted the post-mortem findings in two young men who had been treated unsuccessfully with a combination of vinblastine, bleomycin, and cisplatin for testicular teratomas. The subjects had none of the major risk factors for coronary disease. Neither of them had had symptoms of ischaemic heart disease in life and their ECGs were normal. Both, however, had advanced atherosclerotic disease of the major coronary arteries in the absence of atheromatous disease of other major vessels. The authors postulated that this combination of drugs may have accelerated the development of coronary atherosclerosis.

Adenosine and ATP

In recent years, considerable research has been undertaken into the physiological and pharmacological effects of the purine nucleoside adenosine and its phosphorylated derivatives. Adenosine is released from ischaemic cardiac cells into the coronary circulation following the breakdown of adenosine triphosphate (ATP) and adenosine monophosphate (AMP) (Arch and Newsholme 1978). It is thought to exert protective effects that include local vasodilatation and inhibition of platelet aggregation (Edlund *et al.* 1985). Sylven and others (1986, 1987) examined the hypothesis that adenosine causes angina pectoris and have cited evidence to this effect.

The potent negative dromotropic effects of adenosine and ATP on atrioventricular conduction coupled with its lack of significant negative inotropic effects have led to their use, by bolus injection, in the treatment of paroxysmal tachycardias (Di Marco *et al.* 1983). Several investigators have noted that, shortly after the intravenous administration of these agents, approximately one-third of patients complain of anginal-type chest pain but that this resolves within 60 seconds (Watt and Routledge 1985; Belhasen *et al.* 1988; Rankin *et al.* 1989). There are no concomitant ECG changes of ischaemia and no deleterious effects have been reported. It has therefore been postulated that adenosine and ATP cause angina by direct sensitization of autonomic nerves (Sylven *et al.* 1989).

Vasopressin

Vasopressin, or antidiuretic hormone, is a potent pressor agent affecting smooth muscle throughout the vasculature. The adverse cardiac effects of vasopressin are attributable to the induction of myocardial ischaemia. This is observed both in subjects with normal coronary arteries and those with atheromatous disease. Pressor effects are usually encountered at doses higher than those that cause a maximum antidiuretic effect. Vasopressin-induced myocardial infarction and death have been reported. The drug should not be used in patients known to have angina pectoris (B.M. Beller *et al.* 1971; Hays 1985). The synthetic analogue 1-desamino-8-D-arginine vasopressin (DDAVP) has full antidiuretic potency, but does not elevate blood pressure or contract smooth muscle. It is therefore more suitable for patients with ischaemic heart disease (Cobb *et al.* 1978).

Ergotamine

Ergotamine is an alkaloid derivative of ergot that has antagonistic actions at α-adrenergic and hydroxytryptamine receptors and is used in the treatment of migrainous disorders. It causes vasoconstriction and, in addition to its well-known effects on the peripheral vasculature, may cause angina (Scherf and Schlachman 1948; McNerney and Leedham 1950) and myocardial infarction (Goldfischer 1960; Klein *et al*. 1982; Rall and Schleifer 1985).

Methylxanthines

Theophylline and caffeine are the two most commonly encountered methylxanthines. Both have significant acute effects on the cardiovascular system. In addition, the possibility that coffee drinking may be a risk factor in the pathogenesis of coronary artery disease has been extensively investigated.

The results of earlier studies of coffee consumption and cardiovascular risk are conflicting. This may have been a consequence of suboptimal methodology in study design especially with regard to patient numbers and duration of follow-up (Dawber *et al*. 1974; La Croix *et al*. 1986; Rosenberg *et al*. 1988). Furthermore, some of these studies were retrospective (Jick *et al*. 1973; Klatsky *et al*. 1973). The apparently positive correlation between coffee drinking and cardiovascular morbidity has been attributed mainly to the adverse effects of coffee on serum low-density lipoprotein cholesterol levels.

Reports from Scandinavia indicate that the method of coffee brewing is a significant factor (Bonaa *et al*. 1988). The traditional method of preparation of coffee is by boiling in much of this region. Subjects who made coffee in this way were shown to have higher serum cholesterol levels than individuals who drank filtered coffee (Arnesen *et al*. 1984; Aro *et al*. 1987). These findings have been confirmed in a prospective, randomized, cross-over study comparing the effects of the two methods of brewing coffee (Bak and Grobbee 1989). Drinking four to six cups of boiled coffee per day over a 9-week period increased the total serum cholesterol level by a mean of 0.48 mmol per litre and the low-density lipoprotein cholesterol level by 0.39 mmol per litre from control values. In contrast, there was no significant change in these indices when the subjects consumed the same amount of filtered coffee over an identical period.

Methylxanthines have complex effects on several organ systems and those on the heart and circulation may be particularly significant. Their actions are mediated via several mechanisms including potentiation of the sympathetic nervous system, effects on adenosine and ATP, modulation of the renin–angiotensin system, and stimulation of the brainstem vagal and vasomotor centres (Rall 1985). The effects of methylxanthines on coronary blood flow in humans are controversial. Because of its vasodilator properties, theophylline has been used in the treatment of angina (Russek 1960), but it can

also cause myocardial ischaemia (McFadden and Ingram 1988). These reports reflect opposing effects on myocardial oxygen consumption, due to vasodilator properties on the one hand and chronotropic and inotropic effects on the other. The net effect will differ in different individuals and is therefore unpredictable.

The effects of caffeine, administered by drinking coffee, on the exercise tolerance and symptoms in a group of patients with chronic stable angina have been reported (Piters *et al*. 1985). Coffee drinking resulted in a significant increase in the duration of exercise before the onset of angina. The reasons underlying this effect are uncertain but the lack of any deleterious effect is reassuring.

Oestrogens and progestogens

There have been a number of case reports and series of unexpected myocardial infarction in young women without major risk factors for coronary disease (Dear and Jones 1961; Hartveit 1965; Waxler *et al*. 1971). Retrospective analysis of the early studies of the combined oral contraceptive pill had indicated an excess of thrombophlebitis and thromboembolism in patients taking these drugs (Inman and Vessey 1968; Mann and Inman 1975; Mann *et al*. 1975, 1976). This type of retrospective analysis has been criticized because cause-and-effect relationships are difficult to establish. The reports in fact present the prevalence of use of medication in those with complications versus those without.

Accordingly, prospective studies such as that of the Coronary Drug Project Research Group (1973) were conducted and confirmed that high-dose oestrogen preparations are associated with a threefold to fivefold increased risk of myocardial infarction (Beral 1976; Royal College of General Practitioners 1981; Slone *et al*. 1981). The relative risk of exogenous oestrogens contributing to the development of myocardial ischaemia in women increases with age and is most apparent in those aged over 35. Also, men with prostatic cancer given diethylstilboestrol have been shown to have an increased incidence of myocardial infarction and stroke (Veterans Administration 1967).

The risk of myocardial infarction associated with oral contraceptives is additive to other risk factors such as smoking, hypertension, and hyperlipidaemia. The introduction of combined oral contraceptive pills with a reduced oestrogen content has reduced the cardiovascular risk but has not abolished it (Speroff 1982). The exact mechanisms whereby oral contraceptives increase the thrombotic tendency are unknown but they are known to

have adverse effects on clotting factors, glucose tolerance, lipoproteins, and blood pressure. Coronary angiography in patients who have sustained a myocardial
infarction whilst taking the oral contraceptive pill shows
either normal coronary arteries or only minimal atheroma (Engel *et al.* 1977). A normal coronary angiogram
following myocardial infarction is a rare finding in
patients not taking oral contraceptives (Fox 1983). The
absence of atheroma supports the hypothesis that the
pathophysiological mechanism underlying infarction in
patients taking oral contraceptives is coronary thrombosis. It is likely that coronary thrombosis in the setting
of a normal coronary arterial system is brought about by
intense vasospasm (Legrand *et al.* 1982), with or without
an increased thrombotic tendency.

Hormone replacement therapy

In contrast to the relationship between thromboembolic
disorders and treatment with the relatively large doses of
oestrogens used for oral contraception, there is no good
evidence of an association between sex hormone replacement therapy and cardiovascular disease. Indeed,
it appears that oestrogens in low dosage exert a protective effect against ischaemic heart disease in postmenopausal women (Ross *et al.* 1981; Bush *et al.* 1983). The
postulated mechanism underlying this beneficial effect is
an elevation in the concentration of high-density lipoprotein cholesterol, accompanied by a reduction in low-
density lipoprotein cholesterol. These changes occur
when oestrogens are used in the very low doses appropriate to hormone replacement therapy.

Diuretics

Although neither thiazide nor loop diuretics are known
to cause myocardial ischaemia directly, concern has been
expressed regarding their effects on circulating lipid
levels and the possible atherogenic risks (Lasser *et al.*
1984). Increases in both serum triglyceride and low-
density lipoprotein cholesterol levels with a reduction or
no change in high-density lipoprotein cholesterol have
been demonstrated following prolonged administration
of both types of diuretics (Lant 1985; Weidmann *et al.*
1988). These effects are dose-dependent (Perez-Stable
and Caralis 1983). Although the pathogenesis of these
changes is unknown they may involve thiazide-induced
hyperinsulinaemia (Lardinois and Neuman 1988). As in
the case of β-blockers, there is no evidence at present
to confirm that the hyperlipidaemia associated with
chronic diuretic therapy results in accelerated coronary
atherosclerosis.

Drugs and myocardial healing

Non-steroidal anti-inflammatory drugs and corticosteroids

The development of a ventricular aneurysm in a patient
treated with high-dose corticosteroids for postmyo-
cardial infarction (Dressler's) syndrome alerted physicians to the possible deleterious effects of steroids on
myocardial healing (Bulkley and Roberts 1974). In a
later report, Owensby (1986) described the occurrence
of rupture of the right ventricular free wall after insertion
of a temporary pacing electrode. Four days after implantation, symptoms and signs of pleuropericarditis were
present together with echocardiographic evidence of a
small pericardial effusion. The pacing electrode was
removed and the effusion resolved over the following 9
days. The patient, however, developed cardiac tamponade 10 weeks later, requiring open drainage of a large
pericardial effusion. At operation, perforation of the
right ventricular apex was confirmed with evidence of
partially organized clot and adhesions, suggesting that
the perforation had occurred some time previously. The
development of the second effusion was attributed to
rupture of the right ventricular apex, the healing of
which had been impaired by chronic prednisone therapy
(10 mg per day) for steroid-dependent asthma.

More recently, there is a growing amount of evidence
to suggest that both corticosteroids and non-steroidal
anti-inflammatory drugs impair myocardial repair following myocardial infarction (Delborg *et al.* 1985; Silverman and Pfeifer 1987). In Silverman and Pfeifer's (1987)
series of 41 patients with left ventricular free wall rupture, 20 (49 per cent) had received an anti-inflammatory
agent. These patients were characterized by being elderly
with a mean age of 67 years, and a male preponderance.
Few had a history of previous myocardial infarction or
congestive cardiac failure and 60 per cent had sustained
large transmural anterior infarcts.

Eleven subjects had been given corticosteroids (prednisone, methylprednisone, or dexamethasone) alone,
seven had received corticosteroids and a non-steroidal
inflammatory agent, and two had had non-steroidal
agents only. Indomethacin was the non-steroidal agent
used in all but one instance. More than half the patients
who developed ventricular rupture had received three
doses of either type of anti-inflammatory drug and most
cases of ventricular rupture occurred within 3 days of
commencing therapy. It is possible, however, that the
pericarditis for which the anti-inflammatory agents were
prescribed was caused by a small extravasation of blood
into the pericardial space. This initial leak may have

occurred from a limited dehiscence of the ventricle that later extended to a full rupture.

A precursor stage to ventricular rupture is infarct expansion (Hutchins and Bulkley 1978), which begins within hours of the acute ischaemic event. Expansion is characterized by thinning and dilatation of the infarcted area that is not a consequence of further myocardial necrosis. Histologically, there is slippage between the sarcolemmal bundles, and during the healing process fibroblasts enter the myocyte compartment and lay down collagen which connects the disrupted myocytes. There are good experimental and human data to indicate that the administration of anti-inflammatory agents early after myocardial infarction results in enhanced infarct expansion and is a major contributory factor to the formation of ventricular aneurysms (Weisman and Healy 1987).

Infarct expansion ultimately results in ventricular dilatation and complex changes in ventricular architecture and function (Pfeffer and Braunwald 1990). Ventricular dilatation is associated with reduced survival, and clinical studies are in progress to assess the value of various pharmacological agents in preventing infarct expansion. Conversely, the avoidance of drugs that impair myocardial healing after acute infarction is desirable. The most commonly used agents in this regard are corticosteroids and non-steroidal anti-inflammatory drugs.

Drugs causing lesions of heart valves

Methysergide and ergotamine

Methysergide and ergotamine are both serotonin (5-hydroxytryptamine) antagonists used in the treatment of migrainous disorders. The cardiotoxic effects of methysergide are rare but were recognized over 20 years ago (Graham et al. 1966; Graham 1967; Bana et al. 1974; Misch 1974). Methysergide therapy is associated with both stenotic and regurgitant lesions of the mitral, aortic, and tricuspid valves, which occur after prolonged therapy. In addition, methysergide may cause myocardial fibrosis (Mason et al. 1977b). Spierings (1988) has reported the development of cardiac murmurs indicative of aortic valve disease in a patient with a history of chronic and excessive ergotamine intake. Hauck and others (1990) described two patients who had taken ergotamine tartrate (Cafergot) chronically for migraine, one of whom developed aortic regurgitation and the other mixed mitral valve disease. Both required valve replacement surgery. Neither subject had a history of rheumatic heart disease nor had they ever been given methysergide. Histological examination of the excised valves showed them to be involved by a proliferative process very similar to that seen in carcinoid heart disease and methysergide-associated valvular disease. Although methysergide and ergotamine are serotonin antagonists they also possess partial agonist activity. It is this property which may account for their cardiotoxic effects and provide a link with the similar pathological processes seen in the carcinoid syndrome.

Minocycline

Blue-black pigmentation of the aortic and mitral valves in an individual undergoing aortic valve replacement has been reported as a complication of chronic therapy with minocycline (Butler et al. 1985). Minocycline, a tetracycline derivative, had been prescribed at a dose of 200 mg per day for 5 years for chronic sinusitis and had resulted in cutaneous pigmentation. Valve replacement surgery was indicated for stenosis of a congenitally bicuspid aortic valve. At operation both the aortic and mitral valves were pigmented, but there was no evidence of any functional abnormality of the mitral valve. Microscopic examination of the excised aortic valve showed granular pigment distributed both within macrophages and free in the connective tissue and the appearances were identical to those found in the skin biopsies.

Drugs causing pericardial disease

Drugs causing pericardial disease can be classified into those that cause a drug-induced lupus syndrome and those that cause pericarditis as a direct toxic effect. In the latter group there is often evidence of myocarditis (Gold 1967), features of which may dominate the clinical problem (Smith 1966). In some cases of drug-induced lupus syndrome, acute pericarditis may be the first sign of the disease. Hydralazine (Anandadas and Simpson 1986), procainamide (Swarbrick and Gray 1972), and sulphasalazine (Clementz and Dolin 1988; Deboever et al. 1989) have been identified as causes of pericarditis in association with drug-induced lupus.

Pericarditis is a rare but well-documented adverse effect of chemotherapy. It has been described following treatment with anthracyclines (Harrison and Danders 1976; Bristow et al. 1978), actinomycin D (Corder and Flannery 1974), bleomycin (Durkin et al. 1976; Klein 1977), and when cisplatin and fluorouracil are used in combination (Jakubowski and Remeny 1983). Cyclophosphamide (Appelbaum et al. 1976; Buja et al. 1976; Steinherz et al. 1981) and cytarabine (Vaickus and Letendre 1984) may also cause pericarditis when used in high doses. Some authors have suggested that previous radiotherapy to the mediastinum, even if administered several months before chemotherapy is given, may predispose the patients to developing pericarditis but this is far from invariable (Corder and Flannery 1974; Durkin *et al.* 1976).

Pericarditis has been described as an idiosyncratic toxic reaction following the use of minoxidil (Krehlik *et et al.* al. 1985) and of phenylbutazone (Shafar 1965), and as part of penicillin hypersensitivity (Schoenwetter and Silber 1965). Fibrosis of the pericardium is associated with the oculomucocutaneous syndrome induced by practolol and may be seen in the fibrotic reaction seen with methysergide (see above).

An unusual complication of sclerotherapy of oesophageal varices was the accidental leakage of the sclerosant morrhuate sodium into the pericardial cavity after oesophageal perforation, resulting in acute pericarditis. Eight months later the patient presented with cardiac tamponade and constrictive pericarditis requiring operative intervention (Brown and Luchi 1987).

Haemopericardium with or without tamponade is described as a complication of anticoagulant therapy. This may occur spontaneously (Leung *et al.* 1990), or following instrumentation of the heart (Braunwald and Swan 1968). A recently recognized complication of thrombolytic therapy is its inappropriate use in acute aortic dissection that has been misdiagnosed as myocardial infarction (Blankenship and Almquist 1989; Butler *et al.* 1990; Curzen *et al.* 1990), resulting in fatal cardiac tamponade.

References

Abel, F.L. (1980). Direct effects of ethanol on myocardial performance and coronary resistance. *J. Pharmacol. Exp. Ther.* 212, 28.

Abel, F.L., Wilson, S.P., Zhao, R.R., and Fennell, W.H. (1989). Cocaine depresses the canine myocardium. *Circ. Shock* 28, 309.

Abrams, J. (1989). Interval therapy to avoid nitrate tolerance. Paradise regained? *Am. J. Cardiol.* 64, 931.

Adams, P.C. (1982). Drug-induced heart failure. *Adverse Drug React. Bull.* 92, 336.

Alfino, P.A., Thanavaro, S., Kleiger, R.E., Zeffren, B.F., Aronson, T.A., and Ruffy, R. (1981). Alpha-methyldopa and carotid sinus hypersensitivity. *N. Engl. J. Med.* 305, 344.

Alpert, L.I., Tanimura, A., and Wertheimer, S. (1972). Cardiomyopathy associated with pheochromocytoma. *Arch. Pathol.* 93, 544.

Amery, A., Birkenhager, W., and Brixko, P. (1985). Mortality and morbidity results from the European working party on high blood pressure in the elderly trial. *Lancet* i, 1349.

Anandadas, J.A. and Simpson, P. (1986). Cardiac tamponade, associated with hydralazine therapy, in a patient with rapid acetylator status. *Br. J. Clin. Pract.* 40, 305.

Anastasiou-Nana, M.I., Anderson, J.L., Stewart, J.R., Crevey, B.J., Yanowitz, F.G., Lutz, J.R., *et al.* (1987). Occurrence of exercise-induced and spontaneous wide-complex tachycardia during therapy with flecainide for complex ventricular arrhythmias: a probable proarrhythmic effect. *Am. Heart J.* 113, 1071.

Anderson, H.R., MacNair, R.S., and Ramsey, J.D. (1985). Deaths from abuse of volatile substances: a national epidemiological study. *Br. Med. J.* 290, 304.

Anderson, J.L., Lutz, J.R., Gilbert, E.M., Sorensen, S.G., Yanowitz, F.G., Menlove, R.L., *et al.* (1985). A randomized trial of low-dose beta-blockade therapy for idiopathic dilated cardiomyopathy. *Am. J. Cardiol.* 55, 471.

Anderson, J.L., Atkins, J.C., Gilbert, E.M., Menlove, R.L., and Lutz, J.R. (1986). Occurrence of ventricular arrhythmias in patients receiving acute and chronic infusions of milrinone. *Am. Heart J.* 111, 466.

Angelakos, E.T. and Hastings, E.P. (1960). The influence of quinidine and procaine amide on myocardial contractility *in vivo. Am. J. Cardiol.* 5, 791.

Antman, E.M., Wenger, T.L., Butler, V.P., Haber, E., and Smith, T.W. (1990). Treatment of 150 cases of life-threatening digitalis intoxication with digoxin-specific Fab antibody fragments. Final report of a multicentre study. *Circulation* 81, 1744.

Appelbaum, V.R., Strauchen, J.A., and Graw, G.R. (1976). Acute lethal carditis caused by high-dose combination chemotherapy. *Ann. Intern. Med.* 85, 339.

Arch, J.R.S. and Newsholme, E.A. (1978). The control of the metabolism of metabolism and hormonal role of adenosine. In *Essays in biochemistry*, Vol. 14 (ed. P.N. Campbell and W.N. Aldridge), p. 82. Academic Press, New York.

Arita, M. and Surawitz, B. (1973). Electrophysiological effects of phenothiazines on canine cardiac fibres. *J. Pharmacol. Exp. Ther.* 184, 619.

Arnesen, E., Forde, O.H., and Thelle, D.S. (1984). Coffee and serum cholesterol. *Br. Med. J.* 288, 1960.

Aro, A., Tuomilheto, J., Kostianinen, E., Usitalo, U., and Pietinen, P. (1987). Boiled coffee increases serum low density lipoprotein concentration. *Metabolism* 36, 1027.

Aronson, J.K. (1980). Indicators for the measurement of plasma digoxin. *Drugs* 26, 230.

Askanas, A., Udoshi, M., and Sadjadi, S.A. (1980). The heart in chronic alcoholism: a noninvasive study. *Am. Heart J.* 99, 9.

Asthma Mortality Task Force. (1987). Recommendations of the asthma mortality task force. *J. Allergy Clin. Immunol.* 80, 364.

Au, P.K., Bhandari, A.K., Bream, R., Schreck, D., Siddiqi, R., and Rahimtoola, S. (1987). Proarrhythmic effects of antiarrhythmic drugs during programmed stimulation in patients without ventricular tachycardia. *J. Am. Coll. Cardiol.* 9, 389.

Auffermann, W., Stefenelli, T., Wu, S.T., Parmley, W.W., Wikman-Coffelt, J., and Mason, D.T. (1989). Influence of positive inotropic agents on intracellular calcium transients. Part 1. Normal rat heart. *Am. Heart J.* 118, 1219.

Austen, W.G. and Moran, J.M. (1965). Cardiac and peripheral vascular effects of lidocaine and procainamide. *Am. J. Cardiol.* 16, 701.

Bak, A.A.A. and Grobbee, D.E. (1989). The effect on serum cholesterol levels of coffee brewed by filtering or boiling. *N. Engl. J. Med.* 321, 1432.

Baker, B.J., Brodsky, M.A., Dinh, H., Allen, B.J., Cotter, B., Luckett, C., *et al.* (1987). Hemodynamic effect of propafenone and the experience in patients with congestive heart failure. *J. Electrophysiol.* 1, 527.

Bala Subramanian, V., Bowles, M.J., Khurmi, N.S., Davies, A.S., O'Hara, M.J., and Raftery, E.B. (1983). Calcium antagonist withdrawal syndrome: objective demonstration with frequency modulated ST segment monitoring. *Br. Med. J.* 286, 520.

Bana, D.S., Macneal, P.S., Le Compte, P.M., Shah, Y., and Graham, J.R. (1974). Cardiac murmurs and fibrosis associated with methysergide therapy. *Am. Heart J.* 88, 640.

Banim, S.O., Da Silva, A., Stone, D., and Balcon, R. (1977). Observations of the haemodynamics of mexiletine. *Postgrad. Med. J.* 53, 74.

Banner, A.S., Sunderrajan, E.V., Agarwac, M.K., and Addington, W.W. (1979). Arrhythmogenic effects of orally administered bronchodilators. *Arch. Intern. Med.* 139, 434.

Barron, J.T. and Billhardt, R.A. (1989). Angina pectoris with encainide in dilated cardiomyopathy. *Am. Heart J.* 117, 701.

Bass, M. (1970). Sudden sniffing death. *JAMA* 212, 2075.

Bass, O., Friedemann, M., and Kuzil, M. (1979). A case of left myocardial insufficiency after tocolysis by means of beta stimulation. *Schweiz. Med. Wochenschr.* 109, 1427.

Bauerenfiend, R., Hall, C., Denes, P., and Rosen, K.M. (1978). Adverse effects of sympatholytic agents in patients with sinus node dysfunction. *Am. J. Med.* 64, 1013.

Bauman, D.J. (1981). Myocardial depression with disopyramide. *Ann. Intern. Med.* 94, 411.

Bauman, J.L., Bauernfeind, R.A., Hoff, J.V., Strasberg, B., Swiryn, S., and Rosen, K.M. (1984). Torsades de pointes due to quinidine: observations in 31 patients. *Am. Heart J.* 107, 425.

Baumann, G., Loher, U., and Felix, S.B. (1982). Deleterious effects of cimetidine in the presence of histamine on coronary circulation. *Res. Exp. Med.* 180, 209.

Bayer, R., Schwarzmaier, J., and Pernice, R. (1988). Basic mechanisms underlying prenylamine-induced 'torsade de pointes': differences between prenylamine and fenildine due to basic actions of the isomers. *Curr. Med. Res. Opin.* 11, 254.

Beermann, B., Edhag, O., and Vallin, H. (1975). Advanced heart block aggravated by carbamazepine. *Br. Heart J.* 37, 668.

Befeler, B. (1975). The hemodynamic effects of Norpace, Part 1. *Angiology* 26, 99.

Belhasen, B., Glick, A., and Laniado, S. (1988). Comparative clinical and electrophysiological effects of adenosine triphosphate and verapamil on paroxysmal reciprocating junctional tachycardia. *Circulation* 77, 795.

Beller, B.M., Trevino, A., and Urban, E. (1971). Pitressin-induced myocardial injury and depression in a young woman. *Am. J. Med.* 51, 675.

Beller, G.A., Smith, T.W., Abelmann, W.H., Haber, E., and Hood, W.B. (1971). Digitalis intoxication. A prospective clinical study with serum level correlations. *N. Engl. J. Med.* 184, 989.

Beller, G.A., Hood, W.B., Smith, T.W., Abelmann, W.H., and Wacker, W.E.C. (1974). Correlation of serum magnesium levels and cardiac digitalis intoxication. *Am. J. Cardiol.* 33, 225.

Benassi, E., Bo, G.P., Cocito, L., Maffini, M., and Loeb, C. (1987). Carbamazepine and cardiac conduction disturbances. *Ann. Neurol.* 22, 280.

Benedetti, T.J. (1983). Maternal complications of parenteral beta-mimetic therapy for preterm labour inhibition. *Am. J. Obstet. Gynecol.* 145, 1.

Benjamin, I.J., Jalil, J.E., Tan, L-B., Cho, K., Weber, K.T., and Clark, W.A. (1989). Isoproterenol-induced myocardial fibrosis in relation to myocyte necrosis. *Circ. Res.* 65, 657.

Benowitz, N.L., Rosenberg, J., and Becker, C.E. (1979). Cardiopulmonary catastrophe in drug-overdosed patients. *Med. Clin. North Am.* 83, 267.

Beral, V. (1976). Cardiovascular disease mortality trends and oral contraceptive use in young women. *Lancet* ii, 1047.

Bergeron, G.A., Goldsmith, R., and Schiller, N.B. (1988). Myocardial infarction, severe reversible ischaemia, and shock following excess thyroid administration in a woman with normal coronary arteries. *Arch. Intern. Med.* 148, 1450.

Bhan, R.D., Giacomelli, F., and Wiener, J. (1982). Adrenergic blockade in angiotensin-induced hypertension. Effect on rat coronary arteries and myocardium. *Am. J. Pathol.* 108, 60.

Bigger, J.T. (1985). Digitalis toxicity. *J. Clin. Pharmacol.* 25, 514.

Bigger, J.T., Fleiss, K.R., Rolnitsky, L.M., Merab, J.P., and Ferrick, K.J. (1985). Effect of digitalis treatment on survival after acute myocardial infarction. *Am. J. Cardiol.* 55, 623.

Bigger, J.T., Giardina, E.G.C., Perel, J.M., Kantor, S.J., and Glassman, A.H. (1977). Cardiac antiarrhythmic effect of imipramine hydrochloride. *N. Engl. J. Med.* 196, 206.

Billingham, M.E. and Bristow, M.R. (1984). Evaluation of anthracycline cardiotoxicity: predictive ability and function correlation of endomyocardial biopsy. *Cancer Treat. Symp.* 3, 71.

Blankenship, J.C. and Almquist, A.K. (1989). Cardiovascular complications of thrombolytic therapy in patients with a mistaken diagnosis of acute myocardial infarction. *J. Am. Coll. Cardiol.* 14, 1579.

Blijham, G.H., Fiolet, H.H., van Deijk, W.A., Hupperets, P.S.G.J., and Janssen, J.H.A. (1986). Angina pectoris associated with infusions of 5-FU and vindesine. *Cancer Treat. Rep.* 70, 314.

Blinks, J.R. (1966). Field stimulation as a means of effecting the graded release of autonomic transmitters in isolated heart muscle. *J. Pharmacol. Exp. Ther.* 151, 221.

Blinks, J.R. (1967). Evaluation of the cardiac effects of several beta-adrenergic blocking agents. *Ann. N.Y. Acad. Sci.* 139, 673.

Blinks, J.R. and Endoh, M. (1986). Modification of myofibrillar responsiveness to calcium as an inotropic mechanism. *Circulation* 73 (suppl. III), 85.

Block, P.J. and Winkle, R.A. (1983). Hemodynamic effects of antiarrhythmic drugs. *Am. J. Cardiol.* 52, 14.

Boden, W.E., Korr, K.S., and Bough, E.W. (1985). Nifedipine-induced hypotension and myocardial ischaemia in refractory angina pectoris. *JAMA* 253, 1131.

Boesen, F., Andersen, E.B., Jensen, E.K., and Ladefoged, S.D. (1983). Cardiac conduction disturbances during carbamazepine therapy. *Acta Neurol. Scand.* 68, 49.

Bohm, M., Schwinger, R.H.G., and Erdmann, E. (1990). Different cardiodepressant potency of various calcium antagonists in human myocardium. *Am. J. Cardiol.* 65, 1039.

Bonaa, K., Arnesen, E., Theele, D.S., and Forde, D.H. (1988). Coffee and cholesterol: is it all in the brewing? The Tromso study. *Br. Med. J.* 297, 1103.

Bonadonna, G. and Monfardini, S. (1969). Cardiac toxicity of daunorubicin. *Lancet* i, 837.

Boon, A. (1987). Solvent abuse and the heart. *Br. Med. J.* 794, 722.

Boudoulas, H., Schaal, S.F., Lewis, R.P., Welch, T.G., Degreen, P., and Kates, R.E. (1977a). Negative inotropic effects of lidocaine in patients with coronary arterial disease and normal subjects. *Chest* 71, 170.

Boudoulass, H., Lewis, R.P., Kates, R.E., and Dalmangas, G. (1977b). Hypersensitivity to adrenergic stimulation after propranolol in normal subjects. *Ann. Intern. Med.* 87, 433.

Bourke, J.P., Cowan, J.C., Tansuphaswadikul, S., and Campbell, R.W.F. (1987). Antiarrhymic drug effects on left ventricular performance. *Eur. Heart. J.* 8 (suppl. A), 105.

Brady, H.R. and Horgan, J.H. (1988). Lithium and the heart. Unanswered questions. *Chest* 93, 166.

Braunwald, E. and Swan, H.J.C. (1968). Cooperative study on cardiac catheterization. *Circulation* 37 (suppl. 1), 1.

Breithardt, G., Seipel, L., and Kuhn, H. (1980). Amiodarone. *Circulation* 61, 213.

Brevetti, G., Chiarello, M., Leone, R., Clemente, G., Caracciolo, G., and Condorelli, M. (1986). Amiodarone-induced decrease in lymphocyte beta-adrenergic receptor density. *Am. J. Cardiol.* 57, 698.

Bristow, M.R., Thompson, P.D., Martin, R.P., Mason, J.W., Billingham, B.E., and Harrison, D.C. (1978). Early anthrocycline cardiotoxicity. *Am. J. Med.* 65, 823.

Brodsky, M.A., Allen, B.J., Abate, D., and Henry, W.L. (1985). Propafenone therapy for ventricular tachycardia in the setting of congestive heart failure. *Am. Heart J.* 110, 794.

Brown, B.R. and Crout, J.R. (1971). A comparative study of the effects of five general anesthetics on myocardial contractility. *Anesthesiology* 34, 236.

Brown, D.L. and Luchi, R.J. (1987). Cardiac tamponade and constrictive pericarditis complicating endoscopic sclerotherapy. *Arch. Intern. Med.* 147, 2169.

Buja, L.M., Ferrans, V.J., and Graw, R.G. (1976). Cardiac pathologic findings in patients treated with bone marrow transplantation. *Hum. Pathol.* 7, 17.

Bulkley B.H. and Roberts, W.C. (1974). Steroid therapy during acute myocardial infarction. A cause of delayed healing and of ventricular aneurysm. *Am. J. Med.* 56, 244.

Burrows, G.D., Davies, B., Hamer, A., and Vohra, J. (1979). Effect of mianserin on cardiac conduction. *Med. J. Aust.* ii, 97.

Burton, J.R., Mathew, M.T., and Armstrong, P.W. (1976). Comparative effects of lidocaine and procainamide on acutely impaired hemodynamics. *Am. J. Med.* 61, 215.

Bush, T.L., Cowan, L.D., Barrett-Cooper, E., Criqui, M.H., Karon, J.M., Wallace, R.B., et al. (1983). Estrogen use and all-cause mortality. Preliminary results from the lipids research clinics program follow-up program. *JAMA* 249, 903.

Butler, J., Davies, A.H., and Westaby, S. (1990). Streptokinase in acute aortic dissection. *Br. Med. J.* 300, 517.

Butler, J.M., Marks, R., and Sutherland, R. (1985). Cutaneous and cardiac valvular pigmentation with minocycline. *Clin. Exp. Dermatol.* 10, 432.

Camarri, E., Chirone, E., Fanteria, G., and Zocchi, M. (1982). Ranitidine-induced bradycardia. *Lancet* ii, 160.

Campbell, N.P.S., Zaidi, S.A., Adgey, A.A.J., Patterson, G.C., and Pantridge, J.F. (1979). Observations on haemodynamic effects of mexiletine. *Br. Heart J.* 41, 182.

Campbell, R.W.F. (1987). Arrhythmogenesis—A European Perspective. *Am. J. Cardiol.* 59, 49E.

Capasso, J.M. (1985). Calcium-induced reversible alterations in excitation-contraction coupling in verapamil-treated rat myocardium. *J. Mol. Cell. Cardiol.* 17, 275.

Carlier, J. (1980). Hemodynamic, electrocardiographic and toxic effects of the intravenous administration of increasing doses of mexiletine in the dog. Comparison with similar effects produced by other antiarrhythmics. *Acta Cardiol.* 25 (suppl.), 81.

Carson, P., Oldroyd, K., and Phadke, K. (1987). Myocardial infarction due to amphetamine. *Br. Med. J.* 294, 1525.

Carvey, R.H. and Reed, D. (1970). Intravenous amphetamine poisoning. Report of three cases. *J. Forensic Sci. Soc.* 10, 109.

Casolo, G.C., Balli, E., Poggesi, L., and Gensini, G.F. (1989). Increase in number of myocardial ischemic episodes following nifedipine administration in two patients. Detection of silent episodes by Holter monitoring and role of heart rate. *Chest* 95, 541.

CAST (Cardiac Arrhythmia Suppression Trial Investigators) (1989). Increased morbidity due to encainide or flecainide in a randomized trial of arrhythmia suppression after myocardial infarction. *N. Engl. J. Med.* 321, 406.

Caulfield, J.B. and Bittner, V. (1988). Cardiac matrix alterations induced by adriamycin. *Am. J. Pathol.* 133, 298.

Chamberlain, D.A., White, R.J., Howard, M.R., and Smith, T.W. (1970). Plasma digoxin concentrations in patients with atrial fibrillation. *Br. Med. J.* iii, 429.

Chamberlain, D.A., Jewitt, D.E., Julian, D.G., Campbell, R.W.F., Boyle, D.McC., and Shanks, R.G. (1980). Oral mexiletine in high-risk patients after myocardial infarction. *Lancet* ii, 1324.

Charlier, R. (1970). Cardiac actions in the dog of a new antagonist of adrenergic excitation which does not produce competitive blockade of adrenoceptors. *Br. J. Pharmacol.* 39, 668.

Chase, S.L. and Sloskey, G.E. (1987). Encainide hydrochloride and flecainide acetate: two Class Ic antiarrhythmic agents. *Clin. Pharm.* 6, 839.

Chaudary, S., Song, S.Y., and Jaski, B.E. (1988). Profound, yet reversible, heart failure secondary to 5-fluorouracil. *Am. J. Med.* 85, 454.

Cho, T., Tanimura, A., and Saito, Y. (1987). Catecholamine-induced cardiopathy accompanied with pheochromocytoma. *Acta Pathol. Jpn* 37, 123.

Chow, M.J., Piergies, A.A., Bowsher, D.J., Murphy, J.J., Kushner, W., Ruo, T.I., et al. (1984). Torsades de pointes induced by N-acetylprocainamide. *J. Am. Coll. Cardiol.* 4, 621.

Clark, W.A., Tan, L-B., Jalil, J.E., and Weber, K.T. (1989). Assessment of non-ischemic myocardial necrosis with monoclonal antimyosin. *J. Mol. Cell. Cardiol.* 21 (suppl. II), S156.

Clausen, T. and Flatman, J.A. (1980). Beta-2 adrenoceptors mediate the stimulating effect of adrenaline on active electrogenic Na-K transport in rat soleus muscle. *Br. J. Pharmacol.* 68, 749.

Clavel, M., Simeone, P., and Grivet, B. (1988). Toxicité cardiaque du 5-fluorouracile. Revue de la littérature, cinq nouveau cas. *Presse Med.* 17, 1675.

Cleland, J.G.F., Dargie, H.J., Findlay, I.N., and Wilson, J.T. (1987). Clinical, haemodynamic, and antiarrhythmic effects of long-term treatment with amiodarone of patients in heart failure. *Br. Heart J.* 57, 436.

Clementz, G.L. and Dolin, B.J. (1988). Sulfasalazine-induced lupus erythematosus. *Am. J. Med.* 84, 535.

Clifton, G.D., Booth, D.C., Hobbs, S., Boucher, B.A., Foster, T.S., McAllister, R.G., et al. (1990). Negative inotropic effect of intravenous nifedipine in coronary artery disease: relation to plasma levels. *Am. Heart J.* 119, 283.

Cobb, W.E., Spare, S., and Reichlin, S. (1978). Neurogenic diabetes insipidus: management with DDAVP. *Ann. Intern. Med.* 88, 183.

Cobbe, S.M. and Manley, B.S. (1987). The influence of ischaemia on the electrophysiological properties of amiodarone in chronically treated rabbit hearts. *Eur. Heart J.* 8, 1241.

Cody, R.J. (1988). Do positive inotropic agents adversely affect the survival of patients with chronic congestive heart failure? *J. Am. Coll. Cardiol.* 12, 559.

Cohen, I.S., Jick, H., and Cohen, S.I. (1977). Adverse reactions to quinidine in hospitalized patients: findings based on data from the Boston Collaborative Drug Surveillance Program. *Prog. Cardiovasc. Dis.* 20, 151.

Cohen, J., Weetman, A.P., Dargie, H.J., and Krikler, D.M. (1979). Life-threatening arrhythmias and intravenous cimetidine. *Br. Med. J.* ii, 768.

Cohn, J.N. (1989). Inotropic therapy for heart failure. Paradise postponed. *N. Engl. J. Med.* 320, 729.

Cohn, J.N., Archibald, D.G., Ziesche, S., Franciosa, J.A., Harston, W.E., Tristani, F.E., et al. (1986). Efffect of vasodilator therapy on mortality in chronic congestive heart failure. Results of a Veterans Administration Co-operative study. *N. Engl. J. Med.* 314, 1547.

Collins, C. and Weiden, P.L. (1987). Cardiotoxicity of 5-fluorouracil. *Cancer Treat. Rep.* 71, 733.

Coltart, D.J., Berndt, T.D., Kernoff, R., and Harrison, D.C. (1974). Antiarrhythmic and circulatory effects of Astra W36095. A new lidocaine-like agent. *Am. J. Cardiol.* 34, 35.

Colucci, W.S. (1987). Usefulness of calcium antagonists for congestive heart failure. *Am. J. Cardiol.* 59, 52B.

Colucci, W.S. (1989). Observations on the intracoronary administration of milrinone and dobutamine to patients with congestive heart failure. *Am. J. Cardiol.* 63, 17A.

Come, P.C. and Pitt, B. (1976). Nitroglycerin-induced severe hypotension and bradycardias in patients with acute myocardial infarction. *Circulation* 54, 624.

Conard, G.J. and Ober, R.E. (1984). Metabolism of flecainide. *Am. J. Cardiol.* 53, 41B.

Consensus Trial Group. (1987). Effects of enalapril on mortality in severe congestive heart failure. *N. Engl. J. Med.* 316, 1429.

Conway, N. (1968). Haemodynamic effects of ethyl alcohol in coronary heart disease. *Am. Heart J.* 76, 581.

Conway, N., Seymour, J., and Gelson, A. (1968). Cardiac failure in patients with valvular heart disease after use of propranolol to control atrial fibrillation. *Br. Med. J.* ii, 213.

Corder, M.P. and Flannery, E.P. (1974). Possible radiation pericarditis precipitated by actinomycin D. *Oncology* 30, 81.

Coronary Drug Project Research Group (1973). The coronary drug project. Findings leading to discontinuation of the 2.5 mg/day oestrogen group. *JAMA* 226, 652.

Cote, P., Harrison, D.C., Basile, J., and Schroeder, J.S. (1973). Hemodynamic interaction of procainamide and lignocaine after experimental myocardial infarction. *Am. J. Cardiol.* 32, 937.

Cote, P., Schook, J., Harrison, D.C., and Schroeder, J.S. (1975). Hemodynamic effects of procainamide and quinidine and the influence of beta-blockade before and after experimental myocardial infarction (38935). *Proc. Soc. Exp. Biol. Med.* 149, 958.

Coull, D.C., Crooks, J., Dingwall-Fordyce, I., Scott, A.M., and Weir, R.D. (1970). Amitriptyline and cardiac disease: risk of sudden death identified by monitoring system. *Lancet* ii, 590.

Cowan, J.C. (1986). Nitrate tolerance. Editorial review. *Int. J. Cardiol.* 12, 1.

Cowan, J.C. (1990). Antianginal drug therapy. *Current Opinion in Cardiology* 5, 453.

Crane, J., Burgess, C., and Beasley, R. (1989). Cardiovascular and hypokalaemic effects of inhaled salbutamol, fenoterol and isoprenaline. *Thorax* 44, 136.

Crawford, M.H., White, D.H., and O'Rourke, R.A. (1979). Effects of oral quinidine on left ventricular performance in normal subjects and patients with congestive cardio-myopathy. *Am. J. Cardiol.* 44, 714.

Cregler, L.L. and Mark, H. (1986). Medical complications of cocaine abuse. *N. Engl. J. Med.* 315, 1495.

Cregler, L.L. and Mark, H. (1987). Second-degree atrio-ventricular block and alpha-methyldopa: a probable connection. *Mt Sinai J. Med.* 54, 168.

CSM (Committee on Safety of Medicines) (1990). *Current Problems*, No. 28.

Curzen, N.P., Clarke, B., and Gray, H.H. (1990). Intravenous thrombolysis for suspected myocardial infarction: a cautionary note. *Br. Med. J.* i, 513.

Dangman, K.H. and Hoffman, B.F. (1981). *In vivo* and *in vitro* antiarrhythmic and arrhythmogenic effects of *N*-acetyl procainamide. *J. Pharmacol. Exp. Ther.* 217, 851.

Data, J.L., Wilkinson, G.R., and Nies, A.S. (1976). Interaction of quinidine with anticonvulsant drugs. *N. Engl. J. Med.* 294, 699.

Davidson, S. and Surawicz, B. (1967). Ectopic beats and atrio-ventricular conduction disturbances in patients with hypopotassaemia. *Arch. Intern. Med.* 120, 280.

Davis, J.C., Reiffel, J.A., and Bigger, J.T. (1981). Sinus node dysfunction caused by methyldopa and digoxin. *JAMA* 245, 1241.

Dawber, T.R., Kannel, W.B., and Gordon, T. (1974). Coffee and cardiovascular disease: observations from the Framingham Study. *N. Engl. J. Med.* 291, 871.

Dear, H.D. and Jones, W.B. (1961). Myocardial infarction associated with the use of oral contraceptives. *Ann. Intern. Med.* 74, 236.

Deboever, G., Devogelaere, R., and Holvoet, G. (1989). Sulphasalazine-induced lupus-like syndrome with cardiac tamponade in a patient with ulcerative colitis. *Am. J. Gastroenterol.* 84, 85.

Delborg, M., Held, P., Swedberg, K., and Vedin, A. (1985). Rupture of myocardium, occurrence and risk factors. *Br. Heart J.* 54, 11.

Demakis, J.G., Proskey, A., Rahimtoola, S.H., Jamil, M., Sutton, G.C., Rosen, K.M., *et al.* (1974). The natural course of alcoholic cardiomyopathy. *Ann. Intern. Med.* 80, 293.

De Mots, H. and Glasser, S.P. (1989). Intermittent transdermal nitroglycerin therapy in the management of chronic stable angina. *J. Am. Coll. Cardiol.* 13, 786.

Dent, R.G. and McColl, I. (1975). 5-Fluorouracil and angina. *Lancet* i, 347.

Dessertenne, F. (1966). La tachycardie ventriculaire à deux foyers opposés variables. *Arch. Med. Coeur* 59, 263.

DiBianco, R., Shadetai, R., Rostuk, W., Moran, J., Schlant, R.C., and Wright, R. (1989). A comparison of milrinone, digoxin and their combination in the treatment of patients with chronic heart failure. *N. Engl. J. Med.* 320, 677.

Dies, F. (1986). Intermittent dobutamine in ambulatory patients with chronic cardiac failure. *Br. J. Clin. Pract.* (suppl. 45), 37.

Di Marco, J.P., Sellers, T., Berne, R.M., West, G.A., and Bellardinelli, L. (1983). Adenosine: electrophysiological effects and therapeutic use for terminating paroxysmal supraventricular tachycardia. *Circulation* 68, 1254.

Dollery, C.T., Patterson, J.W., and Conolly, M.E. (1969). Clinical pharmacology of beta-receptor-blocking drugs. *Clin. Pharmacol. Ther.* 10, 765.

Dollery, C.T., Draffman, G.H., Davies, D.S., Williams, F.M., and Conolly, M.E. (1970). Blood concentrations in man of fluorinated hydrocarbons after inhalation of pressurised aerosols. *Lancet* ii, 1164.

Dowling, G.P., McDonough, E.T., and Bost, R.O. (1987). 'Eve' and 'Ecstasy'. A report of five deaths associated with the use of MDEA and MDMA. *JAMA* 257, 1615.

Dresdale, A., Bonow, R.O., Wesley, T., Palmeri, S.T., Barr, L., Mathison, D., *et al.* (1983). Prospective evaluation of doxorubicin-induced cardiomyopathy resulting from postsurgical adjuvant treatment of patients with soft tissue sarcomas. *Cancer* 52, 51.

Dukes, I.D. and Vaughan Williams, E.M. (1984). The multiple modes of action of propafenone. *Eur. Heart J.* 5, 115.

Durelli, L., Mutani, R., Sechi, G.P., Monaco, F., Glorioso, N., and Gusmaroli, G. (1985). Cardiac side effects of phenytoin and carbamazepine. A dose-related phenomenon? *Arch. Neurol.* 42, 1067.

Durkin, W.J., Pugh, P.R., Solomon, J.T., Rosen, P., Pajak, Th. F., and Bateman, J.R. (1976). Treatment of advanced lymphomas with bleomycin (NSC-125066). *Oncology* 33, 140.

Edlund, A., Berglund, B., van Dorne, D., Kaijser, L., Nowak, J., Patrono, C., *et al.* (1985). Coronary flow regulation in patients with ischaemic heart disease: release of purines and prostacyclin and the effect of inhibitors of prostaglandin formation. *Circulation* 71, 1113.

Edwards, G.S., Lane, M., and Smith, P.E. (1979). Long-term treatment with *cis*-dichlorodiamineplatinum-vinblastine-bleomycin. Possible association with severe coronary artery disease. *Cancer Treat. Rep.* 63, 551.

Egstrup, K. (1988). Transient myocardial ischaemia after abrupt withdrawal of antianginal therapy in chronic stable angina. *Am. J. Cardiol.* 61, 1219.

Engel, H.J., Hundeshagen, H., and Lichtlen, P. (1977). Transmural myocardial infarction in young women taking oral contraceptives. Evidence of reduced regional coronary flow in spite of normal coronary arteries. *Br. Heart J.* 39, 477.

Engelmeier, R.S., O'Connell, J.B., Walsh, R., Rad, N., Scanlon, P.J., and Gunnar, R.M. (1985). Improvement in symptoms and exercise tolerance by metoprolol in patients with dilated cardiomyopathy: a double-blind, randomized, placebo-controlled trial. *Circulation* 72, 536.

Ensley, J.F., Patel, B., Kloner, R., Kish, J.A., Wynne, J., and Al-Sarraf, M. (1989). The clinical syndrome of 5-fluorouracil cardiotoxicity. *Invest. New Drugs* 7, 101.

Epstein, S.E., Robinson, B.F., Kahler, R.L., and Braunwald, E. (1965). Effects of beta-adrenergic blockade on the cardiac response to maximal and sub-maximal exercise in man. *J. Clin. Invest.* 44, 1745.

Ettinger, P.O., Wu, C.F., De La Gruz, C., Weisse, A.B., Ahmed, S.S., and Regan, T.J. (1978). Arrhythmias and the 'holiday heart'. *Am. Heart J.* 95, 555.

Etvinsson, G. and Orinius, E. (1980). Prodromal ventricular beats produced by a diastolic wave. *Acta Med. Scand.* 208, 445.

Farber, J.L., Chien, K.R., and Mittnacht, S. Jr (1981). The pathogenesis of irreversible cell injury in ischemia. *Am. J. Pathol.* 102, 271.

Featherstone, H.J. and Stewart, D.K. (1983). Angina in thyrotoxicosis: Thyroid-related coronary artery spasm. *Arch. Intern. Med.* 143, 554.

Feely, J., Wilkinson, G.R., McAllister, C.B., and Wood, A.J.J. (1982). Increased toxicity and reduced clearance of lignocaine by cimetidine. *Ann Intern. Med.* 96, 592.

Feldman, R.L., Nichols, W.M., Peppine, C.J., and Conti, C.R. (1981). Acute effect of intravenous dipyridamole on regional coronary haemodynamics and metabolism. *Circulation* 64, 333.

Feldman, R.L., Peppine, C.J., Whittle, J., and Conti, C.R. (1982). Short- and long-term responses to diltiazem in patients with variant angina. *Am. J. Cardiol.* 49, 554.

Fenster, P.A., White, N.W., and Hanson, C.D. (1985). Pharmacokinetic evaluation of the digoxin-amiodarone interaction. *J. Am. Coll. Cardiol.* 5, 108.

Ferrantini, M., Pirelli, S., Merlini, P., Silva, P., and Pollanini, G. (1989). Intermittent transdermal nitroglycerin monotherapy in stable exercise-induced angina: A comparison with continuous schedule. *Eur. Heart J.* 10, 998.

Fiegl, E.O. (1983). Coronary physiology. *Physiol. Rev.* 63, 1.

Fisch, C. (1973). Relation of electrolyte disturbances to cardiac arrhythmias. *Circulation* 47, 409.

Fleckenstein, A. (1971). Specific inhibitors and promoters of calcium action in the excitation-contraction coupling of heart muscle and their role in the prevention or production of myocardial cell lesion. In *Calcium and the heart* (ed. P. Harris and L. Opie), p. 135. Academic Press, London.

Fogoros, R.N. (1984). Amiodarone-induced refractoriness to cardioversion. *Ann. Intern. Med.* 100, 699.

Fogoros, R.N., Anderson, K.P., Winkle, R.A., Swerdlow, C.D., and Mason, J.T. (1983). Amiodarone: clinical efficacy and toxicity in 96 patients with recurrent, drug refractory arrhythmias. *Circulation* 68, 88.

Folle, L.E. and Aviado, D.M. (1966). The cardiopulmonary effects of quinidine and procainamide. *J. Pharmacol. Exp. Ther.* 154, 92.

Fowler, N.O., McCall, D., Chou, T.C., Holmes, J.C., and Hanewson, I.B. (1976). Electrocardiographic changes and cardiac arrhythmias in patients receiving psychotropic drugs. *Am. J. Cardiol.* 37, 223.

Fox, K.M. (1983). Myocardial infarction and the normal coronary arteriogram. *Br. Heart J.* 287, 446.

Franciosa, J.A., Wilen, M., Weeks, C.E., Tanenbaum, R., Kvam, D.C., and Miller, A.M. (1983). Pharmacokinetics and hemodynamic effects of flecainide in patients with chronic low output heart failure. *J. Am. Coll. Cardiol.* 1, 699.

Franklyn, J.A., Davis, J.R., Gammage, M.D., Littler, W.A., Ramsden, D.B., and Sheppard, M.C. (1985). Amiodarone and thyroid hormone action. *Clin. Endocrinol.* 22, 257.

Freer, R.J., Pappano, A.J., Peach, M.J., Bing, K.T., McLean, M.J., Vogel, S., *et al.* (1976). Mechanism for the positive inotropic effect of angiotensin II on isolated cardiac muscle. *Circ. Res.* 39, 178.

Frishman, W.H. (1987). Beta-adrenergic blocker withdrawal. *Am. J. Cardiol.* 59, 26F.

Gallagher, J.D., Lieberman, R.W., Meranze, J., Spielman, S.R., and Ellison, N. (1981). Amiodarone-induced complications during coronary artery surgery. *Anesthesiology* 55, 186.

Galton, D.A.G. (1983). Medical aspects of neoplasia. In *Oxford textbook of medicine* (ed. D.J. Weatherall, J.G.G. Ledingham, and D.A. Warrell), p. 473. Oxford University Press.

Garcia, R. and Jennings, J.M. (1972). Pheochromocytoma masquerading as a cardiomyopathy. *Am. J. Cardiol.* 29, 568.

Gavras, H., Brown, J.J., MacAdam, R.F., and Robertson, J.I.S. (1971). Acute renal failure, tubular necrosis, and myocardial infarction induced in the rabbit by intravenous angiotensin II. *Lancet* ii, 19.

Gavras, H., Kremer, D., Brown, J.J., Gray, B., Lever, A.F., MacAdam, R.F., *et al.* (1975). Angiotensin- and norepinephrine-induced myocardial lesions: experimental and clinical studies in rabbits and man. *Am. Heart J.* 89, 321.

Geleris, P., Boudoulas, H., Schaal, S.F., Lewis, R.P., and Lima, J.J. (1980). Effect of procainamide on left ventricular performance in patients with primary myocardial disease. *Eur. J. Clin. Pharmacol.* 18, 311.

Gettes, L.S. (1970). Beta-adrenergic blocking drugs in the treatment of cardiac arrhythmias. *Cardiovasc. Clin.* 2, 211.

Giacomelli, F., Anversa, P., and Wiener, J. (1976). Effects of angiotensin-induced hypertension on rat coronary arteries and myocardium. *Am. J. Pathol.* 84, 111.

Gibb, I., Cowan, J.C., Parnham, A.J., and Thomas, T.H. (1986). Use and misuse of a digoxin assay service. *Br. Med. J.* 293, 678.

Gibbs, C.L., Mommaerts, W.F.H.M., and Ricchiuti, N.V. (1967). Energetics of cardiac contractions. *J. Physiol. (Lond.)* 191, 25.

Gibson, D.G., Greenbaum, R.A., Pridie, R.B., and Yacoub, M.H. (1988). Correction of left ventricular asynchrony by coronary artery surgery. *Br. Heart J.* 59, 304.

Glassman, A.H. (1984). Cardiovascular effects of tricyclic antidepressants. *Annu. Rev. Med.* 35, 503.

Glaubiger, G. and Lefkowitz, R.J. (1977). Elevated beta-adrenergic receptor number after chronic propranolol treatment. *Biochem. Biophys. Res. Commun.* 78, 720.

Gold, R.G. (1967). Acute non-specific pericarditis. *Postgrad. Med. J.* 43, 534.

Goldberg, D., Reiffel, J.A., Davis, J.C., Gang, E., Livelli, F., and Bigger, J.T. (1982). Electrophysiologic effects of procainamide on sinus node function in patients with and without sinus node disease. *Am. Heart J.* 103, 75.

Goldberg, S., Greenspow, A.S., Urban, P.L., Muza, R.N., Berger, B., Walinsky, P., *et al.* (1983). Reperfusion arrhythmia: a marker of extraction of anterograde flow during intracoronary thrombolysis for acute myocardial infarction. *Circulation* 67, 796.

Goldfischer, J.D. (1960). Acute myocardial infarction secondary to ergot treatment. *N. Engl. J. Med.* 262, 860.

Gough, W.B., Zeiler, R.H., Barreca, P., and El-Sherif, N. (1982). Hypotensive action of commercial intravenous amiodarone and polysorbate 80 in dogs. *J. Cardiovasc. Pharmacol.* 4, 375.

Gould, L., Reddy, C.V.R., Singh, B.K., and Zen, B. (1979). Electrophysiologic properties of methyldopa in man. *Chest* 76, 310.

Graboys, T.B., Blatt, C.M., and Lown, B. (1989). The effect of caffeine on ventricular ectopic activity in patients with malignant ventricular arrythmia. *Arch. Intern. Med.* 149, 637.

Graham, J.R. (1967). Cardiac and pulmonary fibrosis during methysergide therapy for headache. *Trans. Am. Clin. Climatol. Assoc.* 78, 79.

Graham, J.R., Suby, H.L., Le Compte, P.R., and Jadowsky, N.L. (1966). Fibrotic disorders associated with methysergide treatment for headache. *N. Engl. J. Med.* 274, 359.

Greenspon, A.J. and Schaal, S.F. (1983). The 'holiday heart': Electrophysiological studies of alcohol effects in alcoholics. *Ann. Intern. Med.* 98, 135.

Gunn, J., Wilson, J., and Mackintosh, A.F. (1989). Butane sniffing causing ventricular fibrillation. *Lancet* i, 617.

Haft, J.I., Kranz, P.D., Albert, F.J., and Faoni, K. (1982). Intravascular platelet aggregation in the heart induced by norepinephrine: microscopic studies. *Circulation* 46, 698.

Halper, J.P. and Mann, J.J. (1988). Cardiovascular effects of antidepressant medications. *Br. J. Psychiatry* 153 (suppl. 3), 87.

Hamer, A.W.F., Arkles, L.B., and Johns, J.A. (1989). Beneficial effects of low dose amiodarone in patients with congestive cardiac failure: a placebo-controlled trial. *J. Am. Coll. Cardiol.* 14, 1768.

Hammermeister, K.E., Boerth, R.C., and Warbasse, J.R. (1972). The comparative inotropic effects of six clinically used antiarrhythmic agents. *Am. Heart J.* 81, 643.

Hansen, W.D. and Bertl, S. (1983). Inhibition of cholinesterase by ranitidine. *Lancet* i, 235.

Harden, T.K. (1983). Agonist-induced desensitisation of beta-adrenergic receptor linked adenylate cyclase. *Pharmacol. Rev.* 35, 5.

Harrison, D.C., Sprouse, J.H., and Morrow, A.G. (1963). The antiarrhythmic properties of lidocaine and procaine amide. Clinical and physiologic studies of their cardiovascular effects in man. *Circulation* 28, 486.

Harrison, D.T. and Danders, L.A. (1976). Pericarditis in a case of early daunorubicin cardiomyopathy. *Ann. Intern. Med.* 85, 339.

Hart, A. (1989). Cardiac arrest associated with ranitidine. *Br. Med. J.* 299, 519.

Hartveit, F. (1965). Complications of oral contraception. *Br. Med. J.* i, 60.

Hassell, A.B. and Creamer, J.E. (1989). Profound bradycardia after the addition of diltiazem to a beta-blocker. *Br. Med. J.* 198, 675.

Hauck, A.J., Edwards, W.D., Danielson, G.K., Mullany, C., and Bresnahan, D.R. (1990). Mitral and aortic valve disease associated with ergotamine therapy for migraine. Report of two cases and review of the literature. *Arch. Pathol. Lab. Med.* 114, 62.

Hays, R.M. (1985). Agents affecting the renal conservation of water. In *Goodman and Gilman's The pharmacological basis of therapeutics* (7th edn) (ed. A.G. Gilman, L.S. Goodman, T.W. Rall, and F. Murad), pp. 908. Macmillan, New York.

HDFP (Hypertension Detection and Follow-up Programme Co-operative Research Group) (1984). The effect of antihypertensive drug treatment on morbidity in the presence of resting electrocardiographic abnormalities at baseline: the HDFP experience. *Circulation* 70, 996.

Hedner T. (1986). Calcium channel blockers: spectrum of side effects and drug interactions. *Acta Pharmacol. Toxicol.* 58 (suppl. 2), 119.

Heilbrunn, S.M., Shah, P., Bristow, M.R., Valentine, H.A., Ginsburg, R., and Fowler, M.B. (1989). Increased β-receptor density and improved hemodynamic response to catecholamine stimulation during long-term metoprolol therapy in heart failure. *Circulation* 79, 483.

Hellestrand, K.J., Burnett, P.J., Milne J.R., Bexton, R.S., Nathan, A.W., and Camm, A.J. (1983). Effect of the antiarrhythmic agent flecainide acetate on acute and chronic pacing thresholds. *PACE* 6, 892.

Hellestrand, K., Nathan, A.W., Bexton, R.S., and Camm, A.J. (1984). Response of an abnormal sinus node to intravenous flecainide acetate. *PACE* 7, 436.

Hendeles, L. and Weinberger, M. (1983). Theophylline: a 'state of art' review. *Pharmacotherapy* 3, 2.

Hennekens, C.H. and Macmahon B. (1977). Oral contraceptives and myocardial infarction. *N. Engl. J. Med.* 296, 1116.

Henry, P.D. (1980). Comparative pharmacology of calcium antagonists: nifedipine, verapamil and diltiazem. *Am. J. Cardiol.* 46, 1047.

Herrmann, H.C., Kaplan, L.M., and Bierer, B.A. (1983). QT prolongation and torsades de pointes ventricular tachycardia produced by the tetracyclic antidepressant maprotiline. *Am. J. Cardiol.* 51, 904.

Higgins, R.M., Cookson, W.O.C.M., Lane, D.J., John, S.M., McCarthy, G.L., and McCarthy, S.T. (1987). Cardiac arrhythmias caused by nebulised beta-agonist therapy. *Lancet* ii, 863.

Hoddess, A.B., Follansby, W.P., Spear, J.F., and Moore, E.N. (1979). Electrophysiologic effects of a new antiarrhythmic agent, flecainide, on the intact canine heart. *J. Cardiovasc. Pharmacol.* 1, 427.

Hollifield, T.W. (1987). Magnesium depletion, diuretics and arrhythmias. *Am. J. Med.* 82 (suppl. 3A), 30.

Holme, I., Helgeland, A., Hjermann, I., Leren, P., and Lundlarsen, P.G. (1984). Treatment of mild hypertension with diuretics: the importance of ECG abnormalities in the Oslo study and in MRFIT. *JAMA* 251, 1298.

Holmes, J.R., Kubo, S.H., Cody, R.J., and Kligfield, P. (1985). Milrinone in congestive heart failure: observations on ambulatory ventricular arrhythmias. *Am. Heart J.* 110, 800.

Holt, D.W., Hayler, A.M., Edmonds, M.E., and Ashford, R.F.V. (1979). Clinically significant interaction between digoxin and quinidine. *Br. Med. J.* ii, 1401.

Homback, V., Behrenbeck, D.W., Tauchert, M.M., Gil-Sanchez, D., Jansen, W., Hotzel, J., *et al.* (1979). Myocardial metabolism of cyclic 3,5-adenosine monophosphate as influenced by dipyridamole and theophylline in patients with coronary artery disease. *Clin. Cardiol.* 2, 41.

Honerjager, P., Loibl, E., Steidl, I., Schonsteiner G., and Ulm, K. (1986).Negative inotropic effects of tetrodotoxin and seven Class I antiarrhythmic drugs in relation to sodium channel blockade. *Naunyn-Schmiedebergs Arch. Pharmacol.* 332, 184.

Horn, H.R., Hadidian, Z., Johnson, J.L., Vassallo, H.G., Williams, J.H., and Young, M.D. (1980). Safety evaluation of tocainide in the American Emergency Use Program. *Am. Heart J.* 100, 1037.

Hotzel, J., Niehues, B., and Hilger, H.H. (1979). Myocardial metabolism of cyclic 3,5 adenosine monophosphate as influenced by dipyridamole and theophylline in patients with coronary artery disease. *Clin. Cardiol.* 2, 41

Huston, J.R. and Bell, G.E. (1966). The effect of thioridazine chloride and chlorpromazine on the electrocardiogram. *JAMA* 198, 16.

Hutchins, G.M. and Bulkley, B.H. (1978). Infarct expansion versus extension: two different complications of acute myocardial infarction. *Am. J. Cardiol.* 41, 1127.

Hutchison, S.T., Lorimer, A.R., Larhdar, A., and McAlpine, S.G. (1984). Beta-blockers and verapamil: a cautionary tale. *Br. Med. J.* 289, 659.

Ikram, H. (1980). Hemodynamic and electrophysiologic interactions between antiarrhythmic drugs and beta blockers, with special reference to tocainide. *Am. Heart J.* 100, 1076.

Ingemarsson, I., Arulkumaran, S., and Kottegoda, S.R. (1985). Complications of beta-mimetic therapy in preterm labour. *Aust. N.Z. J. Obstet. Gynaecol.* 25, 182.

Inman, W.H.W. and Adelstein, A.M. (1969). Rise and fall of asthma mortality in England and Wales in relation to use of pressurised aerosols. *Lancet* ii, 279.

Inman, W.H.W. and Vessey, M.P. (1968). Investigation of deaths from pulmonary, coronary and cerebral thrombosis and embolism in women of childbearing age. *Br. Med. J.* ii, 203.

Installe, E., Schoevaerdts, J.C., Gadisseux, P., Charles, S., and Tremouroux, J. (1981). Intravenous amiodarone in the treatment of various arrhythmias following cardiac operations. *J. Thorac. Cardiovasc. Surg.* 81, 302.

Ishizaki, M., Yamada, Y., Kido, T., Yamaya, H., Nogawa, K., Matsu, S., *et al.* (1987). First-degree atrioventricular block induced by oral cimetidine. *Lancet* i, 225.

Isner, J.M., Estes, N.A., Thompson, P.D., Costanzo-Nordin, M.R., Subramanian, R., Miller, G., *et al.* (1986). Acute cardiac events temporally related to cocaine abuse. *N. Engl. J. Med.* 315, 1438.

Iversen, L.L. (1967). *The uptake and storage of noradrenaline in sympathetic nerves.* Cambridge University Press.

Jackson, W.K., Roose, S.P., and Glassman, A.H. (1987). Cardiovascular toxicity of antidepressant medications. *Psychopathology* 20 (suppl. 1), 64.

Jakubowski, A.A. and Remeny, N. (1983). Hypotension as a manifestation of cardiotoxicity in three patients receiving cisplatin and 5-fluorouracil. *Cancer* 62, 266.

Janowsky, D., Curtis, G., Zisook, S., Kuhn, K., Resovsky, K., and Le Winter, M. (1983). Ventricular arrhythmias possibly aggravated by trazodone. *Am. J. Psychiatry* 140, 796.

Jariwalla, A.G. and Anderson, E.G. (1978). Production of ischaemic cardiac pain by nifedipine. *Br. Med. J.* i, 1181.

Jawad-Kanber, G. and Sherrod, T.R. (1974). Effect of loading dose of procaine amide on left ventricular performance in man. *Chest* 66, 269.

Jefferys, D.B. and Vale, J.A. (1978). Cimetidine and bradycardia. *Lancet* i, 828.

Jensen, G., Sigurd, B., and Uhrenholt, A. (1975). Haemodynamic effects of intravenous disopyramide in heart failure. *Eur. J. Clin. Pharmacol.* 8, 167.

Jewell, W.H., Koth, D.R., and Huggins, C.E. (1955). Ventricular fibrillation in dogs after sudden return of flow to the coronary artery. *Surgery* 38, 1050.

Jick, H., Miettinen, D.S., Neff, R.K., Shapiro, S., Heinonen, O.P., and Slone, D. (1973). Coffee and myocardial infarction. *N. Engl. J. Med.* 289, 63.

Johnson, A.J., Nunn, A.J., Somner, A.R., Stableforth, D.E., and Stewart, C.J. (1984). Circumstances of death from asthma. *Br. Med. J.* 288, 1870.

Josephson, M.A., Kaul, S., Hopkins, J., Kvam, D., and Singh, B.N. (1985). Hemodynamic effects of intravenous flecainide relative to the level of ventricular function in patients with coronary artery disease. *Am. Heart J.* 109, 41.

Kadatz, R. (1959). The pharmacology of 2,6-bis-(diethanol-amino)-4,8-dipiperidinopyrimido (5,4-)-pyrimide, a new compound with coronary dilatory properties. *Arzneim.-Forsch.* 9, 39.

Kaduk, B. and Seiler, G. (1978). Congestive cardiomyopathy after doxorubicin (Adriamycin). *JAMA* 239, 2057.

Kane, K.A. and Winslow, E. (1980). Antidysrhythmic and electrophysiological effects of a new antianginal agent, bepridil. *J. Cardiovasc. Pharmacol.* 2, 193.

Karliner, J.S., Simpson, P.C., Honbo, N., and Woloszyn, W. (1986). Mechanisms and time course of beta-1 adrenoceptor desensitization in mammalian cardiac myocytes. *Cardiovasc. Res.* 20, 221.

Karlsson, E. and Sonnhag, C. (1976). Haemodynamic effects of procainamide and phenytoin at apparent therapeutic plasma levels. *Eur. J. Clin. Pharmacol.* 10, 305.

Katz, A.M. (1986). Potential deleterious effects of inotropic agents in the therapy of chronic heart failure. *Circulation* 73 (suppl. III), 184.

Katz, A.M. and Reuter, H. (1979). Cellular calcium and cardiac cell death. *Am. J. Cardiol.* 44, 188.

Katz, M., Robertson, P.A., and Creasy, R.K. (1981). Cardiovascular complications associated with terbutaline treatment for preterm labour. *Am. J. Obstet. Gynecol.* 139, 605.

Kay, G.N., Plumb, V.J., Arciniegas, J.G., Henthorn, R.W., and Waldo, A.L. (1983). Torsade de pointes: the long-short initiating sequence and other clinical features: observations in 32 patients. *J. Am. Coll. Cardiol.* 2, 806.

Kay, R., Blake, J., and Rubin, D. (1982). Possible coronary spasm rebound to abrupt nifedipine withdrawal. *Am. Heart J.* 103, 308.

Kelbaek, H., Eriksen, J., Brynjolf, I., Raboel, A., Lund, J.O., Munck, O., *et al.* (1984). Cardiac performance in patients with asymptomatic alcohol cirrhosis of the liver. *Am. J. Cardiol.* 54, 852.

Kelly, P.A., Cannom, D.W., Garan, H., Mirabal, G.S., Harthorne, J.W., Hurvitz, R.J., *et al.* (1988). The automatic implantable cardioverter-defibrillator: efficacy, complications and survival in patients with malignant ventricular arrhythmias. *J. Am. Coll. Cardiol.* 11, 1278.

Kemmotsu, O., Hashimoto, Y., and Shimosato, S. (1974). The effects of fluroxene and enflurane on contractile performance of isolated papillary muscles from failing hearts. *Anesthesiology* 40, 252.

Kemper, A.J., Duncap, R., and Pietro, D.A. (1983). Thioridazine-induced torsade de pointes. Successful therapy with isoproterol. *JAMA* 249, 2931.

Kennedy, B.L. and West, T.C. (1969). Factors influencing quinidine-induced changes in excitability and contractility. *J. Pharmacol. Exp. Ther.* 168, 47.

Khan, M.M., Logan, K.R., McComb, J.M., and Adgey, A.A.J. (1981). Management of recurrent ventricular tachyarrhythmias associated with QT prolongation. *Am. J. Cardiol.* 47, 1301.

Kincaid-Smith, P. (1984). Beta-adrenergic receptor blocking drugs in hypertension. *Am. J. Cardiol.* 53, 12A.

Kino, M., Imamitchi, H., Morigutchi, M., Kawamura, K., and Takatsu, T. (1981). Cardiovascular status in asymptomatic alcoholics, with reference to the level of ethanol consumption. *Br. Heart J.* 46, 545.

Klatsky, A.L., Friedman, G.D., and Siegelaub, A.B. (1973). Coffee drinking prior to acute myocardial infarction: results from the Kaiser-Permanente epidemiological study of myocardial infarction. *JAMA* 226, 540.

Klein, K. (1977). Complications of testicular treatment. *Int. J. Radiat. Oncol. Biol. Phys.* 2, 1049.

Klein, L.S., Simpson, R.J., Stern, R., Hayward, J.C., and Foster, J.R. (1982). Myocardial infarction following administration of sublingual ergotamine. *Chest* 82, 375.

Kleinman, N.S., Lehane, D.E., Geyer, C.Y., Pratt, C.M., and Young J.B. (1987). Prinzmetal's angina during 5-fluorouracil chemotherapy. *Am. J. Med.* 82, 566.

Koch-Weser, J. (1965). Nature of the inotropic action of angiotensin on ventricular myocardium. *Circ. Res.* 16, 230.

Kosinski, R.M. (1989). Alcoholic cardiomyopathy. *N.J. Med.* 86, 773.

Koskinen, P., Kupari, M., Leinonen, H., and Luomanmaki, K. (1987). Alcohol and new onset atrial fibrillation: a case-control study of a current series. *Br. Heart J.* 57, 468.

Kotler, M.N., Michaeides, K.M., Bouchard, R.J., and Warbasse, R. (1973). Myocardial infarction associated with thyrotoxicosis. *Arch. Intern. Med.* 132, 732.

Kötter, V., Linderer, T., and Schröder, R. (1980). Effects of disopyramide on systemic and coronary hemodynamics and myocardial metabolism in patients with coronary artery disease: Comparison with lidocaine. *Am. J. Cardiol.* 46, 469.

Kowey, P.R., Friedman, P.L., Podrid, P.J., Zielonka, J., Lown, B., Wynne, J., *et al.* (1982). Use of radionuclide ventriculography for assessment of changes in myocardial performance induced by disopyramide phosphate. *Am. Heart J.* 104, 769.

Krehlik, J.M., Hindson, D.A., Crowley, J.J., and Knight, L.L. (1985). Minoxidil-associated pericarditis and fatal cardiac tamponade. *West. J. Med.* 143, 527.

Kuhn, P., Klicpera, M., Kroiss, A., Zilcher, H., and Kaindl, F. (1977). Antiarrhythmic and haemodynamic effects of mexiletine. *Postgrad. Med. J.* 53, 81.

Laaban, J.P., Iung, B., Chauvet, J.P., Psychoyos, I., Proteau, J., and Rochemaure, J. (1988). Cardiac arrhythmias during the combined use of intravenous aminophylline and terbutaline in status asthmatics. *Chest* 94, 496.

Labianca, R., Beretta, G., Clerici, M., and Luporini, G. (1982). Cardiotoxicity of 5-fluorouracil: a study of 1083 patients. *Tumori* 68, 505.

La Croix, A.Z., Mead, L.A., Liang, K-Y., Thomas, C.B., and Pearson, T.A. (1986). Coffee consumption and the incidence of coronary heart disease. *N. Engl. J. Med.* 315, 977.

Ladefoged, S.D. and Mogelvang, J.C. (1982). Total atrio-ventricular block with syncope aggravated by carbamazepine. *Acta Med. Scand.* 212, 185.

Lameijer, W. and van Zwieten, P.A. (1974). The interaction between quinidine and propranolol on isolated heart muscle preparations. *Arch. Int. Pharmacodyn.* 209, 10.

Lancaster, L. and Fenster, P.E. (1983). Complete heart block after sublingual nitroglycerin. *Chest* 84, 111.

Landymore, R., Marble, A., Mackinnon, G., Leadon, R., and Gardner, M. (1984). Effects of oral amiodarone on left ventricular function in dogs: clinical implications for patients with life-threatening ventricular tachycardia. *Ann. Thorac. Surg.* 37, 141.

Lang-Stevenson, D., Mikhailidis, D.P., and Gillet, D.S. (1977). Cardiotoxicity of 5-fluorouracil. *Lancet* ii, 406.

Lant, A. (1985). Diuretics: clinical pharmacology and therapeutic use. Part I. *Drugs* 29, 57.

Lardinois, C.K. and Neuman, S.L. (1988). The effects of antihypertensive agents on serum lipids and lipoproteins. *Arch. Intern. Med.* 148, 1280.

Lasser, N.L., Ganditis, G., Cutler, J.A., Kuller, L.H., and Sherwin, R.W. (1984). Effect of antihypertensive therapy on serum lipids and lipoproteins in the Multiple Risk Factor Intervention Trial. *Am. J. Med.* 76 (2A), 52.

Leach, A.J., Brown, J.E., and Armstrong, P.W. (1980). Cardiac depression by intravenous disopyramide in patients with left ventricular dysfunction. *Am. J. Med.* 68, 839.

Leak, D. and Eydt, J.N. (1986). Amiodarone for refractory cardiac arrhythmias: 10-year study. Clinical and community studies. *Can. Med. Assoc. J.* 134, 495.

Leclercq, J.F., Ral, S., and Valere P. (1983). Bepridil et torsades de pointes. *Arch. Mal. Coeur* 76, 341.

Ledda, F., Mantelli, L., Manzini, L., Amerini, S., and Mugelli, A. (1981). Electrophysiological and antiarrhythmic properties of propafenone in isolated preparation. *J. Cardiovasc. Pharmacol.* 3, 1162.

Legha, S.S., Benjamin, R.S., Mackay, B., Ewer, M., Wallace, S., Valdivieso, M., *et al.* (1982). Reduction of doxorubicin cardiotoxicity by prolonged continuous intravenous infusion. *Ann. Intern. Med.* 96, 133.

Legrand, V., Deliege, M., Henrard, L., Boland, J., and Kulbertus, H. (1982). Patients with myocardial infarction and normal coronary arteriogram. *Chest* 82, 678.

Legrand, V., Vandormael, M., Collignon, P., and Kulbertus, H. (1983). Hemodynamic effects of a new antiarrhythmic agent, flecainide (R-818), in coronary heart disease. *Br. J. Clin. Pharmacol.* 51, 422.

Lehtonen, A. (1985). Effect of beta blockers on blood lipid profile. *Am. Heart J.* 109, 1192.

Lejonc, J.L., Vernant, J.P., Macquin, I., and Castaigne, A. (1980). Myocardial infarction following vinblastine treatment. *Lancet* ii, 692.

Leren, P. 1987. Effects of antihypertensive drugs on lipid metabolism. *Clin. Ther.* 9, 326.

Lertora, J.J.L., Glock, D., Stec, G.P., Atkinson, A.J., and Goldberg, L.I. (1979). Effects of *N*-acetylprocainamide and procainamide on myocardial contractile force, heart rate and blood pressure (40547). *Proc. Soc. Exp. Biol. Med.* 168, 332.

Leung, W.H., Lau, C.P., Wong, C.K., and Leung, C.Y. (1990). Fatal cardiac tamponade in systemic lupus erythematosus — a hazard of anticoagulation. *Am. Heart J.* 119, 422.

Levine, J.H., Spear, J.F., Guarnieri, T., Weisfeldt, M.L., De Langen, C.D.J., Becker, L.C., *et al.* (1985). Cesium chloride-induced long QT syndrome: demonstration of after depolarisations and triggered activity *in vivo*. *Circulation* 72, 1092.

Levine, J.H., Morganroth, J., and Kadish, A.H. (1989). Mechanisms and risk factors for proarrhythmia with type Ia compared with Ic antiarrhythmic drug therapy. *Circulation* 80, 1049.

Liang, C-S., Sherman, L.G., Doherty, J.U., Wellington, K., Lee, V.W., and Hood, W.B. (1984). Sustained improvement of cardiac function in patients with congestive heart failure after short-term infusion of dobutamine. *Circulation* 69, 113.

Lieberman, N.A., Harris, R.S., Katz, R.I., Lipschutz, H.M., Dolgin, M., and Fisher, V.J. (1968). The effects of lidocaine on the electrical and mechanical activity of the heart. *Am. J. Cardiol.* 22, 375.

Liljequist, J.A. and Eduardsson, N. (1989). Torsade de pointes tachycardias induced by overdosage of zimelidine. *J. Cardiovasc. Pharmacol.* 14, 666.

Ljung, B. (1985). Vascular selectivity of felodipine. *Drugs* 29 (suppl. 2), 46.

Loaldi, A., Fabbiocchi, F., Montorsi, P., De Cesare, N., Bartorelli, A., Polese, A., *et al.* (1989). Different coronary vasomotor effects of nifedipine and therapeutic correlates in angina with spontaneous and effort components versus Prinzmetal angina. *Am. Heart J.* 117, 315.

Lowenstein, S.R., Gabow, P.A., Cramer, J., Oliva, P.B., and Ratwer, K. (1983). The role of alcohol in new-onset atrial fibrillation. *Arch. Intern. Med.* 143, 1882.

MacAlpin, R. (1975). Intravenous procainamide and left ventricular performance. *Chest* 67, 737.

McFadden, E.R. and Ingram, R.H. (1988). Relationship between diseases of the heart and lungs. In *Heart disease. A textbook of cardiovascular medicine.* Vol. 2. (3rd edn) (ed. E. Braunwald), p. 1879. Saunders, Philadelphia.

McKibbin, J.K., Pocock, W.A., Barlow, J.B., Scott Millar, R.N., and Obel, I.W.P. (1984). Sotalol, hypokalaemia, syncope and torsade de pointes. *Br. Heart J.* 51, 157.

Mackinnon, G., Landymore, R., and Marble, A. (1983). Myocardial depressant effects of oral amiodarone and their significance in the surgical management of sustained ventricular tachycardia. *Can. J. Surg.* 26, 355.

McLeod, A.A., Stiles, G.L., and Shand, D.G. (1984). Demonstration of beta-adrenoceptor blockade by propafenone hydrochloride: clinical pharmacologic, radioligand binding and adenylate cyclase activation studies. *J. Pharmacol. Exp. Ther.* 228, 461.

McLeod, A.A., Martot, R., Monaghan, M.J., Hugh-Jones, P., and Jackson, G. (1987). Chronic cardiac toxicity after inhalation of 1,1,1-trichlorethane. *Br. Med. J.* 294, 727.

MacMahon, B., Bakshi, M., Branagan, P., Kelly, J.G., and Walsh, M.J. (1985). Pharmacokinetics and haemodynamic effects of tocainide in patients with acute myocardial infarction complicated by left ventricular failure. *Br. J. Clin. Pharmacol.* 19, 429.

Macnab, A.J., Robinson, J.L., Adderly, R.J., and D'Orsogna, L. (1987). Heart block secondary to erythromycin-induced carbamazepine toxicity. *Pediatrics* 80, 951.

McNerney, J.M. and Leedham, C.L. (1950). Acute coronary insufficiency pattern following intravenous ergotamine studies. *Am. Heart J.* 39, 629.

Madan, B.R. and Pendse, V.K. (1963). Antiarrhythmic activity of thioridazine hydrochloride. *Am. J. Cardiol.* 11, 78.

Magni, G. (1987). Mianserin in the treatment of elderly depressives. *J. Am. Geriatr. Soc.* 35, 707.

Mandel, E.M., Lelinski, N., and Djaldetti, M. (1975). Vincristine induced myocardial infarction. *Cancer* 36, 1979.

Mann, J.I. and Inman, W.H.W. (1975). Oral contraceptives and death from myocardial infarction. *Br. Med. J.* ii, 445.

Mann, J.I., Vessey, M.P., Thorogood, M., and Doll, R. (1975). Myocardial infarction in young women with special reference to oral contraceptive practice. *Br. Med. J.* ii, 241.

Mann, J.I., Inman, W.H.W., and Thorogood, M. (1976). Oral contraceptive use in older women and fatal myocardial infarction. *Br. Med. J.* ii, 445.

Marchant, E., Pichard, A.D., Casenegra, P., and Lindsay, J. (1984). Effect of intravenous dipyridamole on regional coronary blood flow with 1-vessel coronary artery disease: evidence against coronary steal. *Am. J. Cardiol.* 53, 718.

Marchant, E., Pichard, A., Rodriguez, J.A., and Casanegra, P. (1986). Acute effect of systemic versus intracoronary dipyridamole on coronary circulation. *Am. J. Cardiol.* 57, 1401.

Mark, A.L. (1983). The Bezold-Jarisch reflex revisited: clinical implications of inhibitory reflexes originating in the heart. *J. Am. Coll. Cardiol.* 1, 90.

Marmont, A.M., Damasio, E., and Rossi, F. (1969). Cardiac toxicity of daunorubicin. *Lancet* i, 837.

Marshall, R.J., Muir, A.W., and Winslow, E. (1981). Comparative antidysrrhythmic and haemodynamic effects of orally or intravenously administered mexiletine and org 6001 in the anaesthetised rat. *Br. J. Pharmacol.* 74, 381.

Martin, R.R., Lisehora, G.R., Braxton, M., and Barcia, P.J. (1987). Fatal poisoning from sodium phosphate enema. Case report and experimental study. *JAMA* 257, 2190.

Mason, J.W., Winkle, R.A., Ingels, N.B., Daughters, G.T., Harrison, D.C., and Stinson, E.B. (1977a). Hemodynamic effects of intravenously administered quinidine on the transplanted human heart. *Am. J. Cardiol.* 40, 99.

Mason, J.W., Billingham, M.E., and Friedman, J.R. (1977b). Methysergide-induced heart disease. A case of multivalvular and myocardial fibrosis. *Circulation* 56, 889.

Mason, J.W., Hondeghem, L.M., and Katzung, B.G. (1984). Block of inactivated sodium channels and of depolarization — induced automatically in guinea pig papillary muscle by amiodarone. *Circ. Res.* 55, 277.

Matos, L., Torok, E., and Hankoczy, J. (1977). Examinations on the inotropic effect of lidocaine. *Ther. Hung.* 25, 36.

Mattioni, T.A., Zheutlin, T.A., Dunnington, C., and Kehoe, R.F. (1989). The proarrhythmic effects of amiodarone. *Prog. Cardiovasc. Dis.* 31, 439.

Medical Research Council Working Party on Mild to Moderate Hypertension (1983). Ventricular extrasystoles during thiazide treatment: substudy of MRC mild hypertension trial. *Br. Med. J.* 287, 1249.

Medical Research Council Working Party. (1985). MRC trial of treatment of mild hypertension: principal results. *Br. Med. J.* 291, 97.

Miall, W.E. and Greenberg, G. (1987). *Mild hypertension: is there pressure to treat? An account of the MRC trial.* Cambridge University Press.

Miles, W.M., Heger, J.J., Minardo, J.D., Klein, L.S., Prystowsky, E.N., and Zipes, D.P. (1989). The electrophysiological effects of enoximone in patients with preexisting ventricular tachyarrhythmias. *Am. Heart J.* 117, 112.

Miller, R.R., Hilliard, G., Lies, J.E., Massumi, R.A., Zelis, R., Mason, D.T., *et al.* (1973). Hemodynamic effects of procainamide in patients with acute myocardial infarction and comparison with lidocaine. *Am. J. Med.* 55, 161.

Miller, R.R., Olson, H.G., Amsterdam, E.A., and Mason, D.T. (1975). Propranolol-withdrawal rebound phenomenon: exacerbation of coronary events after abrupt cessation of antianginal therapy. *N. Engl. J. Med.* 293, 416.

Millward, M.J., Ganju, V., and Buck, M. (1988). Cardiac arrest — a manifestation of 5-fluorouracil. *Aust. N.Z. J. Med.* 18, 693.

Minardo, J.D., Heger, J.J., Miles, W.M., Zipes, D.P., and Prystowsky, E.N. (1988). Clinical characteristics of patients with ventricular fibrillation during antiarrhythmic drug therapy. *N. Engl. J. Med.* 319, 257.

Minow, R.A., Benjamin, R.S., Lee, E.T., and Gottlieb, J.A. (1977). Adriamycin cardiomyopathy — risk factors. *Cancer* 39, 1397.

Misch, K.A. (1974). Developmment of heart valve lesions during methysergide therapy. *Br. Med. J.* ii, 365.

Mittleman, R.E. and Wetli, C.V. (1984). Death caused by recreational cocaine use. An update. *JAMA* 252, 1889.

Mokler, C.M. and van Arman, C.G. (1962). Pharmacology of a new antiarrhythmic agent, gamma-diisopropylamino-alpha-phenyl-alpha-(2-pyridyl)-butyramide (SC-7031). *J. Pharmacol. Exp. Ther.* 136, 114.

Molinoff, P.B., Aarons, R.D., Nies, A.S., Nies, A.S., Gerber J.G., Wolfe, B.B., *et al.* (1982). Effects of pindolol and propranolol on β-adrenergic receptors on human lymphocytes. *Br. J. Clin. Pharmacol.* 13, 365S.

Morgan, D.B. and Davidson, C. (1980). Hypokalaemia and diuretics: an analysis of publications. *Br. Med. J.* 280, 905.

Morganroth, J. and Horowitz, L.N. (1984). Flecainide: its proarrhythmic effect and expected changes on the surface electrocardiogram. *Am. J. Cardiol.* 53, 89B.

Morganroth, J., Anderson, J.L., and Gentzkow, G.D. (1986). Classification by type of ventricular arrhythmia predicts frequency of cardiac events from flecainide. *J. Am. Coll. Cardiol.* 8, 607.

Morganroth, J. (1987). Risk factors for the development of proarrhythmic events. *Am. J. Cardiol.* 59, 32E.

Moss, A.J., Davis, H.T., Coward, D.L., De Camilla, J.J., and Odoroff, C.L. (1981). Digitalis associated cardiac mortality after myocardial infarction. *Circulation* 64, 1150.

MRFIT (Multiple Risk Factor Intervention Trial Research Group) (1982). Multiple risk factor intervention trial. Risk factor changes and mortality results. *JAMA* 248, 1465.

Muller, J.E., Turpi, Z.G., Stone, P.H., Rude, R.E., Raabe, D.S., *et al.* (1986). Digoxin therapy and mortality after myocardial infarction. Experience in the MILIS study. *N. Engl. J. Med.* 314, 265.

Murphy, E., Jacob, R., and Lieberman, M. (1985). Cytosolic free calcium in chick heart cells. Its role in cell injury. *J. Mol. Cell. Cardiol.* 17, 221.

Myers, M.G., Harris, L., Leenen, F.H.H., and Grant, D.M. (1987). Caffeine as a possible cause of ventricular arrhythmias during the healing phase of acute myocardial infarction. *Am. J. Cardiol.* 59, 1024.

Myrhed, M. and Wiholm, B.E. (1986). Nifedipine — a survey of adverse effects. Four years' reporting in Sweden. *Acta Pharmacol. Toxicol. Copenh.* 58 (suppl. 2), 133.

Nahas, M., Lachapelle, J., and Tremblay, G. (1969). Comparative effect of procainamide and lidocaine on myocardial contractility. *Can. J. Physiol. Pharmacol.* 47, 1038.

Nakano, J. and Moere, S.E. (1972). Effect of different alcohols on the contractile force of the isolated guinea-pig myocardium. *Eur. J. Pharmacol.* 20, 266.

Naqvi, N., Thompson, D.S., Morgan, W.E., Williams, B.T., and Coltart, D.J. (1979). Haemodynamic effects of disopyramide in patients after open-heart surgery. *Br. Heart J.* 42, 587.

Nathan, A.W., Hellestrand, K.J., Bexton, R.S., Banim, S.O., Spurrell, R.A.J., and Camm, A.J. (1984). Proarrhythmic effects of the new antiarrhythmic agent flecainide acetate. *Am. Heart J.* 107, 222.

Nattell, S., Rangno, R.E., and Loon, G.V. (1979). Mechanism of propranolol withdrawal phenomena. *Circulation* 59, 1158.

Naylor, W.G. (1976). The pharmacology of disopyramide. *J. Int. Med. Res.* 4, 8.

Naylor, W.G. (1980). Calcium antagonists. *Eur. Heart J.* 1, 225.

Nehring, J. and Camm, A.J. (1983). Calcium antagonist withdrawal syndrome. *Br. Med. J.* 286, 1057.

Nemer, W.F., Teba, L., Schiebel, F., and Lazzell, V.A. (1988). Cardiac arrest after acute hyperphosphatemia. *South. Med. J.* 81, 1068.

Opie, L.H. and White, D.A. (1980). Adverse interaction between nifedipine and B-blockade. *Br. Med. J.* 281, 1462.

Orme, M.L'E. (1984). Antidepressants and heart disease. *Br. Med. J.* 289, 1.

O'Rourke, R.A., Bishop, V.S., Stone, H.L., and Rapaport, E. (1969). Lack of effect of procainamide on ventricular function of conscious dogs. *Am. J. Cardiol.* 23, 238.

O'Rourke, R.A. and Horwitz, L.D. (1981). Effect of chronic oral quinidine on left ventricular performance. *Am. Heart J.* 101, 769.

Orrenius, S. and Maehly, A.C. (1970). Lethal amphetamine intoxication. A report of three cases. *J. Legal Med.* 67, 184.

Owensby, D.A. (1986). Corticosteroid therapy and late right ventricular rupture after temporary pacing. *Am. J. Cardiol.* 58, 558.

Packer, M. (1988). Do positive inotropic agents adversely affect the survival of patients with chronic congestive heart failure? Protagonist's viewpoint. *J. Am. Coll. Cardiol.* 12, 562.

Packer, M. and Leier, C.V. (1987). Survival in congestive heart failure during treatment with drugs with positive inotropic actions. *Circulation* 75 (suppl. IV), 55.

Paradise, R.R. and Bibbins, F. (1969). Comparison of the effects of equi-effective concentrations of anesthetics on the force of contraction of isolated perfused rat hearts. *Anesthesiology* 31, 349.

Pasternac, A., Noble, J., Streulens, Y., Elie, R., Henscke, C., and Bourassa, M. (1982). Pathophysiology of chest pain in patients with cardiomyopathies and normal coronary arteries. *Circulation* 65, 778.

Pellinen, T.J., Farkkilae, M., Heikrila, J., and Luumanmaki, K. (1987). Electrocardiographic and clinical factors of tricyclic antidepressant intoxication. *Ann. Clin. Res.* 19, 12.

Peng, S.K., French, W.J., and Pelikan, P.C.D. (1989). Direct cocaine cardiotoxicity demonstrated by endomyocardial biopsy. *Arch. Pathol. Lab. Med.* 113, 842–5.

Pepine, C. (1989). Nicardipine, a new calcium channel blocker: role for vascular selectivity. *Clin. Cardiol.* 12, 240.

Perelman, M.S., McKenna, W.J., Rowland, E., and Krikler, D.M. (1987). A comparison of bepridil with amiodarone in the treatment of established atrial fibrillation. *Br. Heart J.* 58, 339.

Perez, J.E., Borda, L., Schuchleib, R., and Henry, P.D. (1982). Inotropic and chronotropic effects of vasodilators. *J. Pharmacol. Exp. Ther.* 221, 609.

Perez-Stable, E. and Caralis, P.V. (1983). Thiazide-induced disturbances in carbohydrate, lipid and potassium metabolism. *Am. Heart J.* 106, 245.

Perkins, C.M. (1978). Serious verapamil poisoning: treatment with intravenous calcium gluconate. *Br. Med. J.* ii, 1127.

Pfeffer, M.A. and Braunwald, E. (1990). Ventricular remodelling after myocardial infarction. Experimental observations and clinical implications. *Circulation* 81, 1161.

Piters, K.M., Colombo, A., Olson, H.G., and Butman, S.M. (1985). Effect of coffee on exercise-induced angina pectoris due to coronary artery disease in habitual coffee drinkers. *Am. J. Cardiol.* 55, 277.

Podrid, P.J., Schoeneberger, A., and Lown, B. (1980). Congestive heart failure caused by oral disopyramide. *N. Engl. J. Med.* 302, 614.

Poole-Wilson, P.A. (1987). Diuretics, hypokalaemia and arrhythmias in hypertensive patients: still an unsolved problem. *J. Hypertension* 5 (suppl. 3), 551.

Poole-Wilson, P.A. (1989). Chronic heart failure: causes, pathophysiology, prognosis, clinical manifestations, investigations. In *Diseases of the heart* (ed. D.G. Julian, A.J. Camm, K.M. Fox, R.J.C. Hall, and P.A. Poole-Wilson), p. 48. Baillière, London.

Pottage, A., Holt, S., Ludgate, S., and Langlands, A.O. (1978). Fluorouracil toxicity. *Br. Med. J.* i, 547.

Pozenel, H. (1977). Haemodynamic studies on mexiletine, a new antiarrhythmic agent. *Postgrad. Med. J.* 53, 78.

Pratt, C.M., Eaton, C., Francis, M., Woolbert, S., Mahmarian, J., Roberts, R., *et al.* (1989). The inverse relationship between baseline left ventricular ejection fraction and outcome of antiarrhythmic therapy: a dangerous imbalance in the risk-benefit ratio. *Am. Heart J.* 118, 433.

Prevention of Atherosclerotic Complications with Ketanserin Trial Group. (1989). Prevention of atherosclerotic complications: controlled trial of ketanserin. *Br. Med. J.* 298, 424.

Prichard, B.N.C. and Walden, R.J. (1982). The syndrome associated with the withdrawal of β-adrenergic receptor blocking drugs. *Br. J. Clin. Pharmacol.* 13 (suppl. 2), 337s.

Pringle, S.D. and MacEwen, C.J. (1987). Severe bradycardia due to interaction of timolol eye drops and verapamil. *Br. Med. J.* 294, 155.

Proskey, A.J., Saksena, F., and Towne, W.D. (1977). Myocardial infarction associated with thyrotoxicosis. *Chest* 72, 109.

Rae, A.P., Kay, H.R., Horowitz, L.N., Spielman, S.R., and Greenspan, A.M. (1988). Proarrhythmic effects of antiarrhythmic drugs in patients with malignant ventricular arrhythmias evaluated by electrophysiological testing. *J. Am. Coll. Cardiol.* 12, 131.

Raftos J. (1980). Verapamil in the long-term treatment of angina pectoris. *Med. J. Aust.* 2, 78.

Rall, T.W. (1985). Central nervous stimulants. The methylxanthines. In *Goodman and Gilman's The pharmacological basis of therapeutics* (7th edn) (ed. A.G. Gilman, L.S. Goodman, T.W. Rall, and F. Murad), p. 589. Macmillan, New York.

Rall, T.W. and Schleifer, L.S. (1985). Oxytocin, prostaglandins, ergot alkaloids, and other drugs; tocolytic agents. In

Goodman and Gilman's The pharmacological basis of thera-peutics (7th edn) (ed. A.G. Gilman, L.S. Goodman, T.W. Rall, and F. Murad), p. 926. Macmillan, New York.

Ranger, S., Talajie, M., Lemery, R., Roy, D., and Nattel, S. (1989). Amplification of flecainide-induced ventricular conduction slowing by exercise. *Circulation* 79, 1000.

Rankin, A.C., Oldroyd, K.G., Chong, E., Rae, A.P., and Cobbe S.M. (1989). Value and limitations of adenosine in the diagnosis and treatment of narrow and broad complex tachycardias. *Br. Heart J.* 62, 195.

Rausch, J.L., Pavlinac, D.M., and Newman, P.E. (1984). Complete heart block following a single dose of trazodone. *Am. J. Psych.* 141, 1472.

Rawling, D. and Fozzard, H.A. (1978). Electrophysiological effects of imipramine on cardiac Purkinje fibres. Abstract. *Am. J. Cardiol.* 41, 387.

Rawling, D.A. and Fozzard, H.A. (1979). Effects of imipramine on cellular electrophysiological properties of cardiac Purkinje fibers. *J. Pharmacol. Exp. Ther.* 209, 371.

Redding, P., Devroede, C., and Barbier, P. (1977). Bradycardia after cimetidine. *Lancet* ii, 1227.

Reedy, J.C. and Zwiren, G.T. (1983). Enema-induced hypocalcemia and hyperphosphatemia leading to cardiac arrest during induction of anesthesia in an outpatient surgery center. *Anesthesiology* 59, 578.

Regan, T.J., Weisse, A.B., Moschos, A.B., Lesnisk, L.J., Nadini, M., and Hellems, H.K. (1965). The myocardial effects of acute and chronic use of ethanol in man. *Trans. Assoc. Am. Physicians* 78, 282.

Reichenbach, D.D. and Benditt, E.P. (1970). Catecholamines and cardiomyopathy: the pathogenesis and potential importance of myofibrillar degeneration. *Hum. Pathol.* 1, 125.

Reithmann, C. and Werdan, K. (1989). Noradrenaline-induced desensitization in cultured heart cells as a model for the defects of the adenylate cyclase system in severe heart failure. *Naunyn-Schmiedebergs Arch. Pharmacol.* 339, 138.

Resnekov, L. (1970). Circulatory effects of cardiac dysrhythmias. *Cardiovasc. Clin.* 2, 49.

Resnekov, L. and Falicov, R.E. (1977). Thyrotoxicosis and lactate-producing angina pectoris with normal coronary arteries. *Br. Heart J.* 39, 1051.

Richards, A., Stather-Dunn, L., and Moodley, J. (1985). Cardiopulmonary arrest after the administration of magnesium sulphate. A case report. *S. Afr. Med J.* 67, 145.

Roberts, W.C. 1989. Recent studies on the effects of beta blockers on blood lipid levels. *Am. Heart J.* 117, 709.

Roden, D.M. and Hoffman, B.F. (1985). Action potential prolongation and induction of abnormal automaticity by low quinidine concentrations in canine Purkinje fibres. Relationship to potassium and cycle length. *Circ. Res.* 56, 857.

Rodger, C. and Stewart, A. (1978). Side effects of nifedipine. *Br. Med. J.* i, 1619.

Rodger, S.H. and Hyman, D. (1932). Harmful effects of nitroglycerin. *Am. J. Med. Sci.* 184, 480.

Rona, G. (1985). Catecholamine cardiotoxicity. *J. Mol. Cell. Cardiol.* 17, 291.

Roose, S.P., Glassman, A.H., Giardina, E.G.V., Walsh, T., Woodring, S., and Bigger, J.T. (1987). Tricyclic antidepress-ants in depressed patients with cardiac conduction disease. *Arch. Gen. Psychiatry* 44, 273.

Rosen, B., Ovsyshcher, I.A., and Zimlichman, R. (1988). Complete atrioventricular block induced by methyldopa. *PACE* 11, 1555.

Rosenberg, L., Palmer, J.R., Kelly, J.P., Kaufman, D.W., and Shapiro, S. (1988). Coffee drinking and non-fatal myocardial infarction in men under 55 years of age. *Am. J. Epidemiol.* 128, 570.

Ross, R.K., Paginini-Hill, A., Mack, T.M., Arthur, T.M., and Henderson, B.E. (1981). Menopausal oestrogen therapy and protection from death from ischaemic heart disease. *Lancet* i, 858.

Royal College of General Practitioners' Oral Contraceptive Study. (1981). Further analyses of mortality in oral contraceptive users. *Lancet* i, 541.

Rubin, E. (1979). Alcoholic myopathy in heart and skeletal muscle. *N. Engl. J. Med.* 301, 28.

Ruegg, J.C. (1986). *Calcium in muscle activation*. Springer-Verlag, Berlin.

Ruskin, J.N., McGovern, B., Garan, H., DiMarco, J.P., and Kelly, E. (1983). Antiarrhythmic drugs: a possible cause of out-of-hospital cardiac arrest. *N. Engl. J. Med.* 309, 1307.

Russek, H.I. (1960). Are the xanthines effective in angina pectoris? *Am. J. Med. Sci.* 239, 877.

Ryan, T.J., Bailey, K.R., McCabe, C.H., Luk, S., Fisher, L.D., Mock, M.B., *et al.* (1983). The effects of digitalis on survival in high-risk patients with coronary artery disease. The Coronary Artery Surgery Study (CASS). *Circulation* 67, 735.

Saal, A.K., Werner, J.A., Greene, H.L., Sears, G.K., and Graham, E.L. (1984). Effect of amiodarone on serum quinidine and procainamide levels. *Am. J. Cardiol.* 53, 1264.

Sadjadi, S.A., Leghari, R.U., and Berger, A.R. (1984). Prolongation of the PR interval induced by methyldopa. *Am. J. Cardiol.* 54, 675.

Sanini, S., Spaulding, M.B., Masud, A.R.Z., and Canty, R. (1981). 5-FU cardiotoxicity. *Cancer Treat. Rep.* 65, 1123.

Sarma, J.S., Ikeda, S., Fischer, R., Maruyama, Y., Weishaar, R., and Bing, R.J. (1976). Biochemical and contractile properties of heart muscle after prolonged alcohol administration. *J. Mol. Cell. Cardiol.* 8, 951.

Sasyniuk, B.I., Valdis, M., and Tioy, W. (1989). Recent advances in understanding the mechanisms of drug-induced torsade de pointes arrhythmias. *Am. J. Cardiol.* 64, 29J.

Schachne, J.S., Roberts, B.H., and Thompson, P.D. (1984). Coronary artery spasm and myocardial infarction associated with cocaine usage. *N. Engl. J. Med.* 310, 1665.

Scheinmann, M.M., Strauss, H.C., Evans, G.T., Ryan, C., Massie, B., and Wallis, A. (1978). Adverse effect of sympatholytic agent in patient with yhypertension and sinus node dysfunction. *Am. J. Med.* 64, 1013.

Scherf, D. and Schlachman, M. (1948). Electrocardiographic and clinical studies on action of ergotamine tartrate and dihydroergotamine 45. *Am. J. Med. Sci.* 216, 673.

Schlepper, M. (1989). Cardiodepressive effects of antiarrhythmic drugs. *Eur. Heart J.* 10 (suppl. E), 73.

Schneider, P.E., Jonas, E., and Tejani, N. (1988). Detection of cardiac events by continuous electrogram monitoring during ritodrine infusion. *Obstet. Gynecol.* 71, 361.

Schoenwetter, A.M. and Silber, E.N. (1965). Penicillin hypersensitivity, acute pericarditis and eosinophilia. *JAMA* 191, 672.

Schwartz, A., Shen, E., Morady, F., Gillespie, K., Scheinman, M., and Chatterjee, K. (1983). Hemodynamic effects of intravenous amiodarone in patients with depressed left ventricular function and recurrent ventricular tachycardia. *Am. Heart J.* 106, 848.

Schwartz, M., Covino, B., Duce, B., Narang, R., Fiore, J., Markelis, M., *et al.* (1979). Acute hemodynamic effects of tocainide in patients undergoing cardiac catheterization. *J. Clin. Pharmacol.* 19, 100.

Sears, M.R., Rea, H.H., Fenwick, J., Gillies, A.J.D., Holst, P.E., O'Donnell, T.V., *et al.* (1987). Seventy-five deaths in asthmatics prescribed home nebulisers. *Br. Med. J.* 294, 477.

Selzer, A. and Wray, H.W. (1964). Quinidine syncope. Paroxysmal ventricular fibrillation occurring during treatment of chronic atrial arrhythmias. *Circulation* 30, 17.

Serruys, P.W., Vanhaleweyk, G., van den Brand, M., Verdouw, P., Lubsen, J., and Hugenholtz, P. (1983). The hemodynamic effect of intravenous flecainide acetate in patients with coronary artery disease. *Br. J. Clin. Pharmacol.* 16, 51.

Shafar, J. (1965). Phenylbutazone-induced pericarditis. *Br. Med. J.* ii, 795.

Shen, E.N., Sung, R.J., Morady, F., Schwartz, A.B., Shineman, M.M., DiCarlo, L., *et al.* (1984). Electrophysiologic and hemodynamic effects of intravenous propafenone in patients with recurrent ventricular tachycardia. *J. Am. Coll. Cardiol.* 3, 1291.

Shepherd, R.T. (1989). Mechanism of sudden death associated with volatile substance abuse. *Hum. Toxicol.* 8, 287.

Sheu, S-S. and Lederer, W.J. (1985). Lidocaine's negative inotropic and antiarrhythmic actions. Dependence on shortening of action potential duration and reduction of intracellular sodium activity. *Circ. Res.* 57, 578.

Shimosato, S. and Etsten, B.E. (1969). Effects of anesthetic drugs on the heart: a critical review of myocardial contractility and its relationship to haemodynamics. *Clin. Anesthesia* 9, 17.

Shroff, S.G. and Motz, W. (1989). Left ventricular systolic resistance in rats with hypertension and hypertrophy. *Am. J. Physiol.* 257, 386.

Silva Graça, A. and van Zwieten, P.A. (1972). A comparison between the negative inotropic action of various antiarrhythmic drugs and their influence on calcium movements in heart muscle. *J. Pharm. Pharmacol.* 24, 367.

Silverman, H.S. and Pfeifer, M.P. (1987). Relation between use of anti-inflammatory agents and left ventricular free wall rupture during acute myocardial infarction. *Am. J. Cardiol.* 59, 363.

Simoons, M.L., Brand, M., Zwaan, C., Vermeugt, F.W.A., Reeme, W.J., Serruys, P.W., *et al.* (1985). Improved survival after early thrombolysis in acute myocardial infarction. *Lancet* ii, 578.

Singh, B.N. (1983). Amiodarone: historical development and pharmacologic profile. *Am. Heart J.* 106, 788.

Singh, B.N. and Vaughan Williams, E.M. (1970). The effect of amiodarone, a new anti-anginal drug, on cardiac muscle. *Br. J. Pharmacol.* 39, 657.

Singh, B.N., Jewitt, D.E., Downey, J.M., Kirk, E., and Sonnenblick, E.H. (1976). Effects of amiodarone and L 8040, novel antianginal and anti-arrhythmic drugs, on cardiac and coronary hemodynamic and on cardiac intracellular potentials. *Clin. Exp. Pharmacol. Physiol.* 3, 427.

Slater, W., Lampert, S., Podrid, P.T., and Lown, B. (1988). Clinical predictors of arrhythmic worsening by antiarrhythmic drugs. *Am. J. Cardiol.* 61, 349.

Slome, R. (1973). Withdrawal of propranolol and myocardial infarction. *Lancet* i, 156.

Slone, D., Shapiro, S., Kaufman, D.W., Rosenberg, L., Miettenen, O.S., and Stolley, P.D. (1981). Risk of myocardial infarction in relation to current and discontinued use of oral contraceptives. *N. Engl. J. Med.* 305, 420.

Smith, S.R. (1984). Metabolic responses to beta-2 stimulants. *J. R. Coll. Phys. Lond.* 18, 190.

Smith, W.G. (1966). Adult heart disease due to the coxsackie virus group B. *Br. Heart J.* 28, 204.

Smitherman, T.C., Gottlich, C.M., Narahara, K.A., Osborn, R.C., Platt, M., Rude, R.E., *et al.* (1979). Myocardial contractility in patients with ischemic heart disease during long-term administration of quinidine and procainamide. Direct measurement of segmental shortening with radiopaque epicardial markers. *Chest* 76, 552.

Somers, G., Abramov, M., Wittek, M., and Naets, J.P. (1976). Myocardial infarction: a complication of vincristine treatment. *Lancet* ii, 690.

Somerville, W. and Levine, S.A. (1949). Angina pectoris and thyrotoxicosis. *Br. Heart J.* 12, 245.

Sowton, E. and Hamer, J. (1966). Hemodynamic changes after beta adrenergic blockade. *Am. J. Cardiol.* 18, 317.

Speroff, L. (1982). The formulation of oral contraceptives: does the amount of oestrogen make any clinical difference? *Johns Hopkins Med. J.* 150, 170.

Spierings, E.L.H. (1988). Cardiac murmurs indicative of aortic valve disease with chronic and excessive intake of ergot. *Headache* 28, 278.

Stanton, M.S., Prystowsky, E.N., Fineberg, N.S., Miles, W.M., Zipes, D.P., and Heger, J.J. (1989). Arrhythmogenic effects of antiarrhythmic drugs. A study of 506 patients treated for ventricular tachycardia or fibrillation. *J. Am. Coll. Cardiol.* 14, 209.

Stein, J., Podrid, P., and Lown, B. (1984). Effects of oral mexiletine on left and right ventricular function. *Am. J. Cardiol.* 54, 575.

Steiner, C., Wit, A.L., Weiss, M.B., and Damato, A.R. (1970). The antiarrhythmic actions of carbamazepine (Tegretol). *J. Pharmacol. Exp. Ther.* 173, 323.

Steinherz, L.J., Steinherz, P.G., Mangiacasale, D., O'Reilly, R., Allen, J., Sorrell, M., *et al.* (1981). Cardiac changes with cyclophosphamide. *Med. Pediatr. Oncol.* 9, 417.

Stolshek, B.S., Osterhout, S.K., and Dunham, G. (1988). The role of digoxin-specific antibodies in the treatment of digitalis poisoning. *Med. Toxicol.* 3, 167.

Stone, P.H., Muller, J.E., Turi, Z.G., Geltman E., Jaffe, A.S., and Braunwald E. (1983). Efficacy of nifedipine therapy in patients with refractory angina pectoris: significance of the presence of coronary vasospasm. *Am. Heart J.* 106, 644.

Story, J.R., Abdulla, A.M., and Frank, M.J. (1979). Cardiogenic shock and disopyramide phosphate. *JAMA* 242, 654.

Strasberg, B., Sclarovsky, S., Erdberg, A., Duffy, C.E., Lam, W., Swiryns, S., *et al.* (1981). Procainamide-induced polymorphous ventricular tachycardia. *Am. J. Cardiol.* 47, 1309.

Stratmann, H.G. and Kennedy, H.L. (1987). Torsade de pointes associated with drugs and toxins: recognition and management. *Am. Heart J.* 113, 1471.

Sutherland, D.J., McPherson, D.D., Renton, K.W., Spencer, C.A., and Montague, T.J. (1985). The effect of caffeine on cardiac rate, rhythm and ventricular repolarization. *Chest* 87, 319.

Swarbrick, E.T. and Gray, I.R. (1972). Systemic lupus erythematosus during treatment with procainamide. *Br. Heart J.* 34, 288.

Sylven, C., Beermann, B., Jonzon, B., and Brandt, R.T.I. (1986). Angina pectoris-like pain provoked by intravenous adenosine in healthy volunteers. *Br. Med. J.* 293, 227.

Sylven, C., Jonzon, B., Brandt, R., and Beermann, B. (1987). Adenosine-provoked angina pectoris-like pain — time characteristics, influence of autonomic blockade and naloxone. *Eur. Heart J.* 8, 738.

Sylven, C., Beerman, B., Lagerquist, B., and Waldenstrom, A. (1989). Angina pectoris, adenosine and theophylline. *Lancet* i, 1328.

Sznajder, I., Bentur, Y., and Taitelman, U. (1984). First and second degree atrioventricular block in oxpentifylline overdose. *Br. Med. J.* 288, 26.

Tan, L-B. and Clark, W.A. (1990). Cardioprotective effects of homologous and heterologous beta-adrenergic receptor desensitization. *Eur. Heart J* 11, 212

Tan, L.B., Murray, R.G., and Littler, W.A. (1987). An analytical method to separate inotropic and vasodilatory drug effects in man. *Cardiovasc. Res.* 21, 625.

Tan, L.B., Jalil, J.E., Janicki, J.S., Weber, K.T., and Clark, W.A. (1989). Cardiotoxic effects of angiotensin II. *J. Am. Coll. Cardiol.* 13, 2A.

Tejerina, T., Barrigon, S., and Tamargo, J. (1983). Comparison of three β-amino anilides: IQB-M-81, lidocaine and tocainide, on isolated rat atria. *Eur. J. Pharmacol.* 95, 93.

Thadani, U., Manyari, D., Gregor, P., Olowoyeye, J., Leach, A., West, R.O., *et al.* (1981). Hemodynamic effects of disopyramide at rest and during exercise in normal subjects. *Cathet. Cardiovasc. Diagn.* 7, 27.

Thomas, G., Haider, B., Oldewurtel, H.A., Lyons, M.M., Yeh, C.K., and Regan, T.J. (1980). Progression of myocardial abnormalities in experimental alcoholism. *Am. J. Cardiol.* 46, 223.

Timmis, G.C., Ramor, R.C., Gordon, S., and Gangadharan, V. (1975). The basis for differences in ethanol-induced myocardial depression in normal subjects. *Circulation* 51, 1144.

Todd, G.L., Baroldi, G., Pieper, G.M., Clayton, F.C., and Eliot, R.S. (1985*a*). Experimental catecholamine-induced myocardial necrosis. I. Morphology, quantification and regional distribution of acute contraction band lesions. *J. Mol. Cell. Cardiol.* 17, 317.

Todd, G.L., Baroldi, G., Pieper, G.M., Clayton, F.C., and Eliot, R.S. (1985*b*). Experimental catecholamine-induced myocardial necrosis. II. Temporal development of isoproterenol-induced contraction band lesions correlated with ECG, hemodynamic and biochemical changes. *J. Mol. Cell. Cardiol.* 17, 647.

Tomoda, H., Chuck, L., and Parmley, W.W. (1972). Comparative myocardial depressant effects of lidocaine, ajmaline, propranolol and quinidine. *Jpn Circ. J.* 36, 433.

Tordjman, T., Korzets, A., Kotas, R., Manor, J., and Klajman, A. (1984). Complete atrioventricular block and long-term cimetidine therapy. *Arch. Intern. Med.* 144, 861.

Trimarco, B., Ricciardelli, B., de Luca, N., Volpe, M., Sacca, L., Rengo, F., *et al.* (1983). Disopyramide, mexiletine and procainamide in the long-term oral treatment of ventricular arrhythmias: antiarrhythmic efficacy and hemodynamic effects. *Curr. Ther. Res.* 33, 472.

Troup, P.J., Chapman, P.D., Olinger, G.N., and Kleinman, L.H. (1985). The implanted defibrillator: relation of defibrillating lead configuration and clinical variables to defibrillation threshold. *J. Am. Coll. Cardiol.* 6, 1315.

Tye, K.H., Deser, K.B., and Benchimol, A. (1980). Angina pectoris associated with terbutaline for premature labor. *JAMA* 244, 69.

Underwood, D.A., Groppe, C.W., Tsai, A.R., Yiannikas, J., and Heupfler, F. (1983). Coronary insufficiency and 5-fluorouracil therapy. *Cleve. Clin. J. Med.* 50, 29.

Urbano-Marquez, A., Estruch, R., Navarro-Lopez, F., Grau, J.M., Mont, L., and Rubin, E. (1989). The effects of alcoholism on skeletal and cardiac muscle. *N. Engl. J. Med.* 320, 409.

Uretsky, B.F., Jessup, M., Konstam, M.A., Dec, G.W., Leier, C.V., Benotti, J. *et al.* (1990). Multicenter trial of oral enoximone in patients with moderate to moderately severe congestive heart failure. Lack of benefit compared with placebo. *Circulation* 82, 774.

Vaickus, L. and Letendre, L. (1984). Pericarditis induced by high-dose cytarabine therapy. *Arch. Intern. Med.* 144, 1868.

van Brummelen, P. (1983). The relevance of intrinsic sympathomimetic activity for +-blocker induced changes in plasma lipids. *J. Cardiovasc. Pharmacol.* 5 (suppl. 1), S51.

van Camp, G., Dereppe, H., Renard, M., and Bernard R. (1989). Ketanserin and syncope. *Acta Cardiol.* 44, 429.

Vandermotten, M., Verhaeghe, R., and De Geest, H. (1989). Ventricular arrrhythmias and QT-prolongation during therapy with ketanserin: report of a case. *Acta Cardiol.* 44, 431.

Veith, R.C., Raskins, M.A., Caldwell, J.H., Barnes, R.F., Gumbrecht, G., and Ritchie, J.L. (1982). Cardiovascular effects of tricyclic antidepressants in depressed patients with chronic heart disease. *N. Engl. J. Med.* 306, 959.

Velebit, V., Podrid, P., Lown, B., Cohen, B.H., and Graboys, T.B. (1982). Aggravation and provocation of ventricular arrhythmias by antiarrhythmic drugs. *Circulation* 65, 886.

Verdouw, P.D., Deckers, J.W., and Conard, G.J. (1979). Antiarrhythmic and hemodynamic actions of flecainide acetate (R-818) in the ischemic porcine heart. *J. Cardiovasc. Pharmacol.* 1, 473.

Veterans Administration. (1967). The Veterans Administration co-operative urological research group; treatment and survival of patients with cancer of the prostate. *Surg. Gynecol. Obstet.* 124, 1011.

Vittone, L., Cingolani, H.E., and Mattiazzi, R.A. (1985). The link between myocardial contraction and relaxation: the effects of calcium antagonists. *J. Mol. Cell. Cardiol.* 17, 255.

von Hoff, D.D. and Layard, M.W. (1981). Risk factors for development of daunorubicin cardiotoxicity. *Cancer Treat. Rep.* 65 (suppl. 4), 19.

von Hoff, D.D., Layard, M.W., Basa, P., Davis, H.L.Jr, von Hoff, A.L., Rozencweig, M., *et al.* (1979). Risk factors for doxorubicin-induced congestive heart failure. *Ann. Intern. Med.* 91, 710.

von Hoff, D.D., Rozencweig, M., and Piccart, M. (1982). The cardiotoxicity of anticancer agents. *Semin. Oncol.* 9, 23.

Walker, P.R., Marshall, A.J., Farr, S., Bauminger, B., Walters, G., and Barritt, D.W. (1985). Abrupt withdrawal of atenolol in patients with severe angina. *Br. Heart J.* 53, 276.

Walsh, R.A. (1987). The effects of calcium-entry blockade on left ventricular systolic and diastolic function. *Circulation* 75 (suppl. V), 43.

Walsh, R.A. and Horwitz, L.D. (1979). Adverse hemodynamic effects of intravenous disopyramide compared with quinidine in conscious dogs. *Circulation* 60, 1053.

Warden, P., Greenwald, E.S., and Grossman, J. (1976). Unusual cardiac reaction to chemotherapy following medistinal irradiation in a patient with Hodgkin's disease. *Am. J. Med.* 60, 152.

Watt, A.H. and Routledge, P.A. (1985). Adenosine stimulates respiration in man. *Br. J. Clin. Pharm.* 20, 503.

Waxler, E.B., Kimbris, D., van den Broek, H., Segal, B.L., and Likoff, W. (1971). Myocardial infarction and oral contraceptive agents. *Am. J. Cardiol.* 28, 96.

Wei, J.Y., Genecin, A., Greene, H.L., and Achuff, S.C. (1979). Coronary spasm with ventricular fibrillation during thyrotoxicosis: response to attaining euthyroid state. *Am. J. Cardiol.* 43, 335.

Weidmann, P., Ferrier, C., Saxenhofer, H., Uelingher, D.E., and Trost, B.N. (1988). Serum lipoproteins during treatment with antihypertensive drugs. *Drugs* 35 (suppl. 6), 118.

Weisman, H.F. and Healy, B. (1987). Myocardial infarct expansion, infarct extension, and reinfarction: pathophysiologic concepts. *Prog. Cardiovasc. Dis.* 30, 73.

Weld, F.M. and Bigger, J.T. (1980). Electrophysiological effects of imipramine on bovine cardiac Purkinje's and muscle fibres. *Circ. Res.* 46, 167.

Welder, A.A., Smith, M.A., Ramos, K., and Acosta, D. (1988). Cocaine-induced cardiotoxicity *in vitro*. *Toxicology in Vitro* 2, 205.

Williams, J.F. and Mathew, B. (1984). Effect of procainamide on myocardial contractile function and digoxin inotropy. *J. Am. Coll. Cardiol.* 4, 1184.

Williams, R.B. and Sherter, C. (1971). Cardiac complications of tricyclic antidepressant therapy. *Ann. Intern. Med.* 74, 395.

Willis, P.W. (1975). The hemodynamic effects of Norpace (Part II). *Angiology* 26, 102.

Wilson, J.D., Sutherland, D.C., and Thomas, A.C. (1981). Has the change to beta agonists combined with oral theophylline increased cases of fatal asthma? *Lancet* i, 1235.

Wilson, D.F., Watson, O.F., Peel, J.S., and Turner, A.S. (1969). Trasicor in angina pectoris: a double-blind trial. *Br. Med. J.* ii, 155.

Winkle, R.A., Anderson, J.L., Peters, F., Meffin, P.J., Fowles, R.E., and Harrison, D.C. (1978). The hemodynamic effects of intravenous tocainide in patients with heart disease. *Circulation* 57, 787.

Zehender, M., Meinertz, T., Hohnloser, S., Geibel, A., Hartung, J., Seiler, K-U., *et al.* (1989). Incidence and clinical relevance of QT prolongation caused by the new selective serotonin antagonist ketanserin. *Am. J. Cardiol.* 63, 826.

7. Disorders of the peripheral vascular system

D. M. DAVIES

Drug-induced hypertension

Sympathomimetic drugs

The use of sympathomimetic drugs such as adrenaline, dobutamine, dopamine, metaraminol, noradrenaline, and phenylephrine by intravenous infusion to correct hypotension can obviously produce an excessive rise in blood pressure unless the dose and the rate of infusion are controlled by careful and continuous monitoring of the arterial pressure. Less likely to be recognized is the danger of systemic hypertension caused by such a drug when it is used for other purposes: as examples, adrenaline given subcutaneously for asthma has caused transient hypertension; a dramatic rise in blood pressure, accompanied by myocardial infarction, has occurred in a patient given the sympathomimetic vasoconstrictor levonordefrin together with mepivacaine for dental anaesthesia (Pearson *et al.* 1987); and the administration of 10% phenylephrine as eye-drops may be followed by systemic hypertension, especially in the neonate (Solosko and Smith 1972; Borromeo-McGrail *et al.* 1973; Matthews *et al.* 1977), and even 2.5% concentrations have had this effect (Lees and Cabal 1981). A significant rise in blood pressure was observed, experimentally, in some healthy young people given a single oral dose of one or other of two phenylpropanolamine-containing preparations, the first marketed as a nasal decongestant and the second as an appetite suppressant. The observers suggest that these drugs should not be available to patients, unless prescribed by a medical practitioner (Horowitz *et al.* 1979). Single doses have even caused hypertension severe enough to warrant admission to hospital (Horowitz *et al.* 1980; McEwen 1983). A severe hypertensive crisis with convulsions occurred in a 13-year-old girl who took a combination of phenylpropanolamine and caffeine daily for 2 weeks for weight reduction (Howrie and Wolfson 1983), and this interaction with coffee has been confirmed in a placebo-controlled study (Lake *et al.* 1989). Another crisis developed in a patient who took indomethacin shortly after phenylpropanolamine (Lee *et al.* 1979), and a third (Gibson and Warrell 1972) in a patient who took phenylpropanolamine after a meal of cheese. These drugs may also induce hypertension by interacting with other drugs (see below).

Antihypertensive drugs

Some of the antihypertensive agents mentioned here are now so little used as to be considered obsolescent, but they are discussed because they may still be prescribed on occasion for those patients who have been treated with them satisfactorily for long periods, in cases unresponsive to more modern drugs, or for disorders other than hypertension. All the drugs dealt with here are currently included in the *British National Formulary*. The most important, in the present context, are the β-adrenoceptor blockers.

Methyldopa, debrisoquine, and bethanidine can cause a rise in blood pressure when administered intravenously, the last two drugs by displacing noradrenaline from nerve endings. Consequently, these antihypertensives are best avoided in the treatment of serious hypertensive crises. Adrenergic-neurone-blocking drugs such as guanethidine, bretylium, bethanidine, and debrisoquine may render the patient unusually sensitive to the pressor effects of noradrenaline (Laurence and Nagle 1961; Muelheims *et al.* 1965), adrenaline, and metaraminol (Stevens 1966). They do this probably by competing with the sympathomimetic drugs for the 'amine pump', which normally helps to terminate the action of catecholamines on receptors by promoting their uptake into nerve endings. Transient hypertension has occurred when these sympathomimetics have been given to patients under treatment with adrenergic-neurone-blocking drugs.

Methyldopa and reserpine may also increase the effect of noradrenaline on the blood pressure, but to a lesser degree that is clinically insignificant (Stockley 1974). A pressor response to labetalol has been reported by Crofton and Gabriel (1977), and these authors suggest that intravenous boluses of this drug should be given with caution in patients who are already taking substantial amounts of a β-adrenoceptor blocker, methyldopa, or guanethidine (but see below and under *Effect of drugs in the presence of a phaeochromocytoma*). Hydralazine has caused a paradoxical rise in blood pressure in a patient with renal artery stenosis, the mechanism being obscure (Webb and White 1980).

Hypertension has also been caused by propranolol (Blum *et al.* 1975) and by acebutolol and sotalol (Gabriel 1976) when the dose of these drugs was increased rapidly. Gabriel (1976) also observed the same response when the dose of guanethidine was increased too quickly. The suggested explanation is that in the presence of high concentrations of circulating catecholamines β-blockade produces unopposed α-adrenoceptor stimulation (Imms *et al.* 1976).

It is now well recognized that the withdrawal of the antihypertensive drug clonidine may lead to a considerable, sometimes fatal, increase in blood pressure (Hökfelt and Dymling 1970; Hunyor *et al.* 1973; Hansson *et al.* 1973; Webster *et al.* 1974; Bailey and Neale 1976; Brodsky and Brave 1976; Brenner and Lieberman 1977; Vanholder *et al.* 1977; Reid *et al.* 1977; Stevens 1980; Ferguson and Alvino 1983; Stewart and Burris 1988), due to the massive release of catecholamines from the adrenal medulla (Hunyor *et al.* 1973). The rise in blood pressure may begin within a few hours or may be delayed for as long as 17 days (Stelzer *et al.* 1976) and hypertension may occasionally persist for about 2 weeks (Vanholder *et al.* 1977). Reid and others (1977) studied six patients in whom treatment with clonidine in doses of 0.45–5.4 mg daily was abruptly stopped. The blood pressures rose to pretreatment levels within 24–48 hours of withdrawal of the drug and this was accompanied by insomnia, headache, flushing, sweating, and apprehension. Symptoms began 18–24 hours after the last dose of clonidine had been given, and plasma noradrenaline levels and urinary catecholamine excretion increased 24–72 hours after withdrawal. Symptoms were most prominent in patients on higher doses (>1 mg per day) and in those who had previously been receiving other antihypertensive drugs. One patient on a very low dose (0.15 mg per day) had no symptoms and no significant change in blood pressure or catecholamine production after withdrawal. A patient whose oral tablets of clonidine were replaced by skin patches containing the drug

developed severe withdrawal hypertension after 6 days (Stewart and Burris 1988), and another patient had a similar reaction when short-term transdermal administration was terminated (Schmidt and Schuna 1988).

As for the treatment of hypertension following the withdrawal of clonidine, the risk involved in using the β-adrenoceptor-blocking drug propranolol has been stressed (Bailey and Neale 1976; Harris 1976) since hypertension may be made worse because of the high concentration of circulating catecholamines, a situation comparable to that present in patients with phaeochromocytoma (see below); but some authors (e.g. Brown *et al.* 1976; Agabiti-Rosei *et al.* 1976) have reported prompt reduction of blood pressure in such cases following the administration of labetalol, a compound which blocks both α-adrenoceptors and β-adrenoceptors, but the fact that this drug has provoked hypertension in the presence of high concentrations of catecholamines (in phaeochromocytoma — see below) should be borne in mind when the drug is used to treat clonidine-withdrawal hypertension.

Slow withdrawal of minoxidil over 4–12 weeks in three children caused rebound hypertension and encephalopathy. The occurrence of rebound hypertension correlated with the total cumulative dose of the drug in mg per kg per week given before withdrawal and the rapidity (4–8 weeks) with which minoxidil was withdrawn, but not with the total duration of therapy, duration at maximum dosage, or the amount of minoxidil in mg per kg on the day prior to withdrawal.

Rebound hypertension did not occur when minoxidil was withdrawn over 12 weeks or if a patient was receiving a small dose (2.5–5 mg per day). Pretreatment with an α-blocker (prazosin) or the discontinuation of the concomitantly administered β-blocker (propranolol) prior to withdrawal seemed to prevent rebound hypertension (Makker and Moorthy 1980). Rebound hypertension has rarely been encountered following the withdrawal of methyldopa (Burden and Alexander 1976; Scott and McDevitt 1976), or the withdrawal of propranolol or other β-adrenoceptor blockers, particularly those lacking sympathomimetic activity (Lewis *et al.* 1979).

Cyclosporin

Treatment with this immunosuppressive drug, to prevent rejection of transplanted organs or, less commonly, to treat primary autoimmune disorders has caused or aggravated hypertension in many cases. Affected patients have been recipients of transplanted kidneys (Hamilton *et al.* 1982; Canadian Multicentre Transplant Study Group 1983; Gordon *et al.* 1985; Ferguson and Sommer

1985; Krupp *et al.* 1986), heart (Hardesty *et al.* 1983; Thompson *et al.* 1986), heart and lungs (Dawkins *et al.* 1985; Burke *et al.* 1986), liver (Malatack *et al.* 1983; Williams *et al.* 1985), or bone marrow (Joss *et al.* 1982); or have been under treatment for rheumatoid arthritis (Berg *et al.* 1986; Dougados and Amor 1987; Weinblatt *et al.* 1987), uveitis, choroiditis, or cicatricial pemphigoid (Palestine *et al.* 1984), severe hypothyroidism (Sennesael *et al.* 1986), or insulin-dependent diabetes mellitus (Ribstein *et al.* 1989).

Hypertension appears to be most severe in cases of heart or heart and lung transplantation and in children (Weidle and Vlasses 1988), is not invariably accompanied by detectable impairment of renal excretory function (Loughran *et al.* 1985; Chapman *et al.* 1987), and cannot be correlated with the dose or serum concentrations of cyclosporin, previous renal disease or hypertension, or concurrent steroid therapy (Weidle and Vlasses 1988).

The precise mechanism by which cyclosporin causes or aggravates hypertension is still unclear, though it has been established that renal vascular resistance is increased by cyclosporin in experimental animals (Murray and Paller 1986) and in human subjects (Curtis *et al.* 1986) and that impaired sodium excretion occurs (Curtis *et al.* 1988). Experiments in animals have produced results that have conflicted with observations made in human subjects as regards the renin–angiotensin–aldosterone system and the production of vasodilatory prostaglandins, and clinical findings have themselves varied in different studies (Weidle and Vlasses 1988).

The subject is of great complexity, and readers should consult reviews by Weidle and Vlasses (1988), *The Lancet* (1988), Schachter (1988), and Tao *et al.* (1990) for detailed discussions of this and other aspects of cyclosporin toxicity.

Erythropoietin (EPO)

Many patients undergoing repeated haemodialysis for chronic renal failure have suffered a marked increase in blood pressure when given recombinant erythropoietin (EPO) for associated anaemia, this complication being more frequent (Eggert and Stick 1988) and most severe (Raine 1988) in those with pre-existing hypertension.

The mechanism involved is uncertain. Eggert and Stick (1988) concluded that the increase in blood pressure is due to the rise in haemoglobin concentration under the special circumstances obtaining in renal disease, rather than to some other effect of EPO, since the blood pressure in one of their patients rose regularly after transfusion of erythrocyte concentrates. Involvement of the renin–angiotensin system seems to have

been eliminated as a cause, as EPO has caused hypertension in anephric patients (Tomson *et al.* 1988; Edmunds and Walls 1988). Raine (1988) suggested that the sustained dose-dependent rise in haematocrit values leads to a greater whole-blood viscosity, with consequent increase in peripheral resistance, coupled with loss of hypoxic vasodilatation. Martin and Moncada (1988) postulated that the increased quantity of haemoglobin, resulting from EPO therapy, binds to nitric oxide, secreted by endothelial cells, thus negating its powerful vasodilator action, but Vallance and others (1988) opposed this view.

Thus the problem awaits further research for its solution.

Ketoconazole

This drug is used mainly for its antifungal properties, but it also inhibits steroid synthesis in the adrenal gland, ovary, and testes by blocking the activity of various enzyme systems and this has led to its use in conditions in which such effects are desirable (e.g. Cushing's syndrome; hyperaldosteronism; precocious puberty; hirsutism; and cancer of the prostate, male breast, and ovary).

A small number of patients have developed hypertension during long-term, high-dose treatment with the drug, and the mechanism is believed to be inhibition of 11β-hydroxylase, resulting in an increase in concentrations of 11-deoxycortisol and deoxycorticosterone (Aabo and De Coster 1987; Leal-Cerro *et al.* 1989), affected patients possibly being unusually sensitive to the mineralocorticoid effect of deoxycorticosterone (Aabo and De Coster 1987).

Alcohol (ethanol)

Several studies have shown a correlation between alcohol intake and a rise in blood pressure (Criqui *et al.* 1981; Saunders *et al.* 1981; Klatsky *et al.* 1986). The results of clinical experiments by Grassi and others (1989) suggest that this effect is mediated by activation of the sympathetic nervous system.

Salt

An excessive intake of salt can induce hypertension in susceptible people (Gavras and Gavras 1988). Salt-retaining drugs, particularly licorice and its derivative carbenoxolone, and mineralocorticoids also have this effect (Lai *et al.* 1991).

Drug interactions

In the past there has been uncertainty about the risks of

hypertensive crises due to possible interactions between antidepressant drugs and sympathomimetic substances contained in medicines and foods. The confusion has arisen mainly because it has sometimes been too readily assumed that drugs that have some actions in common are pharmacologically identical in all respects, which is not always the case.

This subject is also discussed in Chapter 30.

Monoamine oxidase inhibitor (MAOI) antidepressants

MAOI and directly acting sympathomimetics

The catecholamines adrenaline and noradrenaline are directly acting sympathomimetics, that is, they themselves directly stimulate adrenoceptors. Noradrenaline acts mainly on α-receptors, causing vasoconstriction and a rise in blood pressure, but usually no rise in pulse rate. Adrenaline acts on both α- and β-receptors causing tachycardia in addition to blood pressure changes. Inactivation of noradrenaline released at nerve endings and of injected noradrenaline and adrenaline is achieved mainly by uptake into sympathetic neurones and partly by the enzyme catechol-*o*-methyltransferase. Monoamine oxidase plays only a very minor part in the process, and that almost exclusively within cells. Consequently, on theoretical grounds it can be predicted that MAOI will not potentiate the effects of injected adrenaline and noradrenaline. With noradrenaline, experiments in man fulfil this prediction (Horwitz *et al.* 1960; Elis *et al.* 1967; Pettinger and Oates 1968; Barar *et al.* 1971), but with adrenaline they do not, for some actions of this drug are moderately potentiated by certain MAOI (tranylcypromine [Cuthbert and Vere 1971]), though not by others (phenelzine [Barar *et al.* 1971]). The vasoconstrictor felypressin is not potentiated by MAOI. Results of experiments with isoprenaline have been variable.

It is reasonable to conclude that any patient under treatment with an MAOI may safely be given either noradrenaline or felypressin in normal doses; that adrenaline may be given in normal doses if the patient is physically healthy; but that there is a risk involved in giving adrenaline to patients with cardiovascular disease.

In the present state of knowledge, isoprenaline should be given to patients under treatment with MAOI only when its use is absolutely essential.

MAOI and indirectly acting sympathomimetics

Amphetamine and tyramine are indirectly acting sympathomimetics, exerting their effect by releasing noradrenaline from stores in nerve endings. Ephedrine, metaraminol, phenylpropanolamine, and phenylephrine also have an indirect (as well as a direct) action. The noradrenaline released by nerve impulses is stored in vesicles, but the noradrenaline released by indirectly acting sympathomimetic drugs is 'free' within the cytoplasm (where its concentration is usually minimal due to the activity of monoamine oxidase). In the presence of MAOI, the concentration of 'free' cytoplasmic noradrenaline is markedly increased, so that the effects of indirectly acting sympathomimetic agents are enhanced. Hypertensive crises can therefore occur when an indirectly acting sympathomimetic is taken by a patient under treatment with an MAOI.

MAOI and food

Hypertensive crises in patients under treatment with MAOI antidepressants were first reported by Ogilvie (1955), who noted attacks of severe headaches associated with palpitations, flushing, sweating, and hypertension in 4 of 42 patients being treated with iproniazid. These symptoms did not occur in 47 patients treated with isoniazid which, although closely related chemically to iproniazid, is not a MAOI. The cause of this reaction remained obscure until Blackwell (1963) and Womack (1963) identified cheese as a precipitating factor. In the same year, Asatoor and others (1963) identified tyraine as the ingredient responsible. They showed that the ingestion of cheese was followed in normal subjects by the excretion of large amounts of *p*-hydroxyphenylacetic acid, a metabolic product of tyramine. In patients receiving MAOI, tyramine cannot be broken down and as it is an indirectly acting sympathomimetic agent it has the severe clinical effects described.

Since then a number of other foodstuffs have been identified as possible causes of hypertensive reactions in patients under treatment with MAOI. Yeast extract, which contains both tyramine and histamine, may produce such reactions (Blackwell *et al.* 1965). The oxidation of both of these substances is interfered with by the MAOI, and histamine is capable of releasing catecholamines from the adrenal medulla, a property of particular importance in patients with phaeochromocytoma (described below). Whole sliced broad beans, the pods of which contain significant amounts of dopa, may also produce hypertensive crises in patients taking MAOI (Hodge *et al.* 1964; Blomley 1964). Dopa is converted in the body to dopamine, the oxidation of which is impeded by MAOI.

Unfortunately, published lists of proscribed foods are inconsistent, and this has come about because some lists include items damned on the basis of their tyramine content or on the strength of poorly documented case reports. A critical review (Stewart 1976) concluded that a patient should be told to avoid matured cheese; hydrolysed protein extract (e.g. Marmite, Bovril, but not Bisto); other protein foods that are not fresh or that have been subjected to hydrolysis, fermentation, or 'hanging'; alcohol, except in *strict* moderation; broad bean pods; banana skins; raspberries; and any other food that the patient has previously had reason to suspect as a cause of unpleasant symptoms. As far as alcoholic drinks are concerned, Hannah and others (1988) have reassessed their risk to patients taking MAOI. They analysed the tyramine content of 9 types of beer, 12 of white wine, and 22 of red wine (including 12 of Chianti, which has previously achieved notoriety in this context), and concluded that a half litre of any of these beverages was unlikely to contain enough tyramine to be dangerous.

To this list the depressed gourmet should add caviar (Isaac *et al.* 1977), New Zealand prickly spinach (Comfort 1981), and over-ripe avocado (Generali 1981).

A single case of a hypertensive response to cheese in a patient taking the antihypertensive drug debrisoquine has been reported by Amery and Deloof (1970) who pointed out that this drug had been shown in animal experiments to have monoamine-oxidase-inhibiting properties.

The subject has been examined again in detail by Folks (1983).

Selegeline hydrocholoride is a selective type B monoamine oxidase, used mainly as an adjunct to levodopa therapy for Parkinson's disease, though it has also been used as an antidepressant. Because it inhibits only Type B monoamine oxidase (predominant in the striatum of the brain), leaving Type A active in the liver and gut, it has been believed on theoretical grounds not to produce the conditions necessary for the tyramine reaction, but a case has been described in which a patient under treatment with the drug developed transient hypertension and headache when he ate a meal with a high tyramine content (McGrath *et al.* 1989).

Tricyclic antidepressants

Tricyclics and directly acting sympathomimetics

These drugs inhibit the uptake of adrenaline and noradrenaline by nerve endings, so prolonging and intensifying their actions. Svedmyr (1968) observed that the effect of noradrenaline in man was increased ninefold and that of adrenaline threefold by concurrent treatment with a tricyclic antidepressant. Goldman and others (1971) confirmed those findings with noradrenaline, but not with adrenaline which, in their experiments, showed little or no potentiating effect. Felypressin was not potentiated by tricyclic drugs.

Tricyclics and indirectly acting sympathomimetics

It might be supposed that any sympathomimetic with an indirect action would be potentiated by tricyclic drugs because these could interfere with the uptake of catecholamines released by the sympathomimetic. Some sympathomimetics require, however, to be actively transported into the nerve ending before they can release noradrenaline, and tricyclics may prevent this method of uptake, in which case the effect of the sympathomimetic will be diminished rather than potentiated. Inhibition of this kind has been demonstrated (Svedmyr 1968). Nevertheless, it cannot safely be assumed that the effects of all indirectly acting sympathomimetics will be reduced in this way, for some do not require active transport and some have direct actions as well. Furthermore, there is experimental evidence suggesting that some tricyclic compounds may inhibit the metabolism of some indirectly acting sympathomimetics (Stockley 1974).

One may conclude that it is mandatory to avoid giving noradrenaline or adrenaline to patients taking tricyclic antidepressants, and probably best to avoid any sympathomimetic drug in such patients.

A case has been reported in which a patient under treatment with amitriptyline suffered a hypertensive crisis 34 hours after beginning treatment with levodopa, carbidopa, and metoclopramide (Rampton 1977); limited investigations for a phaeochromocytoma (in the presence of which metoclopramide has induced a hypertensive crisis—see below) were negative.

Other interacting drugs

Severe hypertension has occurred as the result of an interaction between phenylpropanolamine and methyldopa and oxprenolol (McLaren 1976).

Hypertensive effects of drugs in the presence of a phaeochromocytoma

Patients with phaeochromocytoma may be given drugs for a variety of reasons: in the unrecognized case for symptoms of the disease or during medical or surgical treatment of some unrelated condition; in the suspected case for diagnostic tests; and in the confirmed case for anaesthesia and adjuvant therapy at operation for removal of the tumour, or for long-term treatment when surgery is impracticable. Many of these drugs are believed to have caused hypertensive crises in these circumstances or thought, on theoretical grounds, to be capable of doing so.

Evaluating published reports is sometimes difficult. This is particularly true of reactions during the induction or maintenance of anaesthesia, because many of the drugs concerned, or closely related compounds, have been given to patients with phaeochromocytoma without ill effects; though it should be noted that in some of these cases drugs other than those suspected of having caused a reaction were administered to the patient concurrently (e.g. barbiturates, other than thiopentone; chloral hydrate; phenoxybenzamine) and these may have modified or prevented the hypertensive effects reported in other patients.

A number of 'explanations' for observed hypertensive crises induced by certain drugs in patients with phaeochromocytoma have been published, but many are simplistic and some conflict with available evidence. For example, in many published articles and in standard textbooks of pharmacology it has been tacitly assumed or even asserted that a number of different drugs release catecholamines either by direct or indirect stimulation via the autonomic nervous system. Thus, the effect of insulin on a phaeochromocytoma has been explained by the response of the sympathetic nervous system to hypoglycaemia, and that of tetraethylammonium to sympathetic discharge provoked by hypotension. These explanations presuppose that chromaffin tumours are innervated, but what little evidence is available on this point suggests that they are not. While literature on every other aspect of phaeochromocytoma is abundant, there is a quite extraordinary dearth of observations, surgical and pathological, on the presence or absence of nerves supplying phaeochromocytomata, and the very few authors who deal with this point state that the tumours do not have a normally developed nerve supply (Robinson and Williams 1956; Coupland 1965; Ratzenhofer 1968). Of course, findings in some phaeochromocytomata cannot confidently be extrapolated to all such tumours, but these pathological observations are supported pharmacologically by the fact that clonidine (which reduces central sympathetic discharge) fails to suppress catecholamine release in patients with phaeochromocytomata but does so in normal subjects — a phenomenon that forms the basis of a diagnostic test for the tumour (Bravo *et al.* 1981). Pentolinium, a ganglion-blocking drug that interrupts preganglionic nervous impulses to sympathetic nerves and the adrenal medulla, would be expected to cause a fall in catecholamine excretion from a phaeochromocytoma if the tumour were innervated but it fails to do so (Brown *et al.* 1980) and is therefore used in diagnosis.

One can reasonably conclude, therefore, that phaeochromocytomata have no functioning nerve supply and so cannot be stimulated or inhibited by drugs that affect the autonomic nervous system, either directly or indirectly.

Detailed examination of the pharmacological literature shows that the subject is of the greatest complexity (the more so when one takes into consideration the possible differences between man and the animals used in experiments, and the interspecies differences between the animal subjects) and that some drugs are theoretically capable of inducing hypertension in patients with phaeochromocytoma by more than one mechanism.

Postulated mechanisms for hypertensive reactions to drugs in the presence of a phaeochromocytoma are listed in Table 7.1. In Table 7.2 are listed the drugs reported to have caused hypertensive crises. Also included in this table are a few drugs (e.g. guanethidine and related compounds; monoamine oxidase inhibitors) believed on the strongest theoretical grounds to be capable of inducing hypertension in the presence of a phaeochromocytoma, and about which warnings to this effect have been

TABLE 7.1

Postulated mechanisms for hypertensive crises induced by drugs in the presence of a phaeochromocytoma

A Sudden release of large amounts of catecholamines

1 From the tumour

   1.1 by direct stimulation of phaeochromocytoma cells
   1.2 by release of histamine, which then stimulates phaeochromocytoma cells (histamine also causes release of catecholamines from nerve endings)
   1.3 by stimulation of phaeochromocytoma cells via the autonomic nerve system*

2 From accumulated excessive stores of catecholamines in nerve endings

   2.1 by direct action on nerve endings
   2.2 by indirect action via the autonomic system

B Interference with uptake of circulating catecholamines into nerve endings

C Induction of supersensitivity of catecholamine receptors

D Potentiation of effect of catecholamines on arterioles

E Non-selective β-blockade

F Other possible mechanisms

1 incomplete β-blockade resulting from inadequate doses of phenoxybenzamine preoperatively
2 blockade of presynaptic α_2-receptors without effect on α_1-receptors.

---

* This mechanism, postulated by several authors, presupposes that phaeochromocytomata are supplied by functioning nerves, but the surprisingly few relevant histological studies have found no evidence of a normally developed nerve supply to these tumours (see text).

TABLE 7.2

Drugs reported to have caused hypertensive crises in the presence of a phaeochromocytoma or believed on theoretical grounds to be capable of doing so

Drug	Known or postulated mechanism (as classified in Table 7.1)	References to clinical cases, experimental observations, or unsupported statements
Antihistamines	release histamine — see Histamine below	Paton 1957
Antiprotozoal diamidines	release histamine — see Histamine below	Webster 1985
Atropine	D	Swan 1949
β-Adrenoceptor blockers	E	Prichard 1964; Glover and Hutchinson 1964; Ross *et al.* 1967; Briggs *et al.* 1978; Wark and Larkins 1978; Sloand and Thompson 1984
Chlorpromazine	releases histamine — see Histamine below	Paton 1957
Corticosteroids	high concentrations produced by corticotrophin stimulation may reach the phaeochromocytoma via glandular veins and stimulate tumour cells — A 1.1	Yard and Kadowitz 1972; Critchley and Ungar 1974; Daggett and Franks 1977
Corticotrophin	increased secretion of corticosteroids — see Corticosteroids above	Ramsay and Langlands 1962; Moorhead *et al.* 1966; Critchley *et al.* 1974;
Curare/tubocurarine	release histamine — see Histamine below	Alam *et al.* 1939; Comroe and Dripps 1946; Westgate and van Bergen 1962; Koelle 1970
Dextran	releases histamine — see Histamine below	Lorenz *et al.* 1976
Droperidol	F 1	Bittar 1979; Maddern *et al.* 1976; Oh *et al.* 1978; Sumikawa and Amakata 1978
Ether	A 1.1	Bixby and Troncelliti 1952; Price and Dripps 1970
Gallamine (excessive doses)	releases histamine — see Histamine below	Mushin *et al.* 1949; Sniper 1952
Glucagon	A 1.1	Scian *et al.* 1960; Unger *et al.* 1962; Sarcione *et al.* 1963
Guanethidine and related compounds*	C	Emmelin and Enström 1961
Histamine	A 1.1 and A 2.1	Burn and Dale 1926; Szczygielski 1932; Siehe 1934; Athos *et al.* 1962; Engelman and Sjoerdsma 1964; Staszewska-Barczak and Vane 1965; Douglas *et al.* 1967; Douglas 1985; Euler 1966
Insulin	hypoglycaemia — A 2.2 and secretion of glucagon — A 1.1	Goldfein *et al.* 1958; Scian *et al.* 1960; Unger *et al.* 1962; Sarcione *et al.* 1963
Methacholine	hypotension — A 2.2 and (possibly) A 1.1	Volle and Koelle 1970
Metoclopramide/sulpiride	F 2	Corvol *et al.* 1974; Plouin *et al.* 1974; Agabiti-Rosei *et al.* 1977; Spedding 1980
Monoamine oxidase inhibitors*	permit tyramine (see Tyramine below) to enter via gut and liver	*The Lancet* 1965
Nicotine (cigarettes, snuff)	A 2.2 and (possibly) A 1.1	Burn *et al.* 1959; Stromblad 1960; Dugan 1967; Cryer *et al.* 1976; McPhaul *et al.* 1984
Opiates	release antihistamine — see Histamine above	Chaturvedi *et al.* 1974; Lawrence 1978; Fahmy *et al.* 1983
Plasma expanders	release histamine — see Histamine above	Lorenz *et al.* 1976
Saralasin	A 1.1 (possibly) directly and by increasing levels of angiotensin II	Feldberg and Lewis 1964; Peach 1971; Khairallah *et al.* 1971; Steel and Lowenstein 1975; Dunn *et al.* 1976; Peach *et al.* 1978
Sulpiride — see Metoclopramide		
Suxamethonium	releases histamine — see Histamine above	Smith 1957; Stoner and Urbach 1968

Table 7.2 continued

Drug	Known or postulated mechanism (as classified in Table 7.1)	References to clinical cases, experimental observations, or unsupported statements
Tetraethylammonium	hypotension — A 2.2 and (possibly) A 1.1	Wilkins *et al.* 1950; Volle and Koelle 1970
Thiopentone	releases histamine — see Histamine above	Lorenz and Doenicke 1978
Tricyclic antidepressants	B	Kaufmann 1974
Trimetaphan	releases histamine — see Histamine above	Volle and Koelle 1970
Tubocurarine —see Curare		
Tyramine	A 2.1	Weiner *et al.* 1962; Engelman and Sjoerdsma 1964
X-ray contrast media	release histamine — see Histamine above	Ansell 1970

* despite the theoretical possibility of such a reaction, no cases have been found in the literature.

published; but, interestingly, actual case reports of such reactions are hard to find and one can only surmise that the pharmacological *milieu* in a patient with phaeochromocytoma, in whom an excess of circulating catecholamines has been present continuously or intermittently for a long period, is unique and quite different from the situation in animal experiments on which predictions of adverse reactions are based.

The most important drugs in this context are the β-adrenoceptor blockers, because they are routinely used before and during operation for phaeochromocytoma. There is no doubt that non-selective β-adrenoceptor blockers (for a very full discussion of 'selectivity' see Kumana and Marlin 1978) may cause a significant rise in blood pressure in patients with phaeochromocytoma because they abolish the peripheral vasodilator effect of catecholamines while leaving the vasoconstrictor response of α-adrenoceptors unopposed. Consequently, treatment with non-selective β-adrenoceptor-blocking drugs in phaeochromocytoma should only be started *at the same time as* or *soon after* treatment with an α-adrenoceptor-blocking agent. This was pointed out some years ago by Ross *et al.* (1967), but adverse effects of β-blockers given alone in phaeochromocytoma continued to be reported (Wark and Larkins 1978; Sloand and Thompson 1984). The use of labetalol, a drug that blocks both β-adrenoceptors and α-adrenoceptors might seem to be one rational answer to this problem and, indeed, it has been used successfully for this purpose (Agabiti-Rosei *et al.* 1976). Other workers, however, have reported a case in which this drug provoked a hypertensive response in a patient with a predominantly adrenaline-secreting tumour (Briggs *et al.* 1978).

The subject of adverse reactions to drugs in the presence of a phaeochromocytoma has been reviewed in greater detail elsewhere (Davies 1987).

Other drugs causing hypertension

Treatment with corticotrophin (ACTH), adrenal corticosteroids, licorice preparations, and carbenoxolone; some anti-inflammatory drugs such as phenylbutazone and oxyphenbutazone; and sex hormones, including those contained in oral contraceptives, may cause a rise in blood pressure in previously normotensive patients or may aggravate established hypertension. The possible mechanisms are discussed fully in Chapter 15.

A wide variety of other drugs have occasionally caused transient hypertension by mechanisms that at the moment are not always clear. They include anticholinesterases used in eye-drops (Nelemans 1972); carbamazepine (Killian and Fromm 1968); chlormethiazole (Laurenson and Davis 1985); clomipramine (Hessov 1971; Collins 1971); dimercaprol (Brown and Kulkarni 1967); disulfiram (Supprian 1969); doxorubicin (Paterson 1978); ergometrine (Browning 1974), fat emulsions (Schindel 1972); fluorescein used for angiography (McAllister 1981); imipramine (Hessov 1970); indigo carmine used in renal function tests (Wu and Johnson 1969); ketamine (Knox *et al.* 1970); levodopa (*Drug and Therapeutics Bulletin* 1969); fluorometholone (Schroeder and Weeth 1967); naloxone (Tanaka 1974; Gremse *et al.* 1986; Schoenfeld *et al.* 1987); nalorphine (Otteni *et al.* 1969); pentazocine in large doses (Brown 1969); phentolamine (Marriott 1957); promethazine by intravenous injection (Adelman *et al.* 1959); sorbitol (Winter *et al.* 1973); sulpiride (Mayer and Montgomery 1989) (see also under *Phaeochromocytoma*); and tolazoline (Nickerson 1970).

Hypertension may also accompany analgesic nephropathy (Prescott 1972), and analgesic abuse may raise the blood pressure without evidence of nephropathy (Küster and Ritz 1989).

Peripheral vasoconstriction

Some drugs cause vasoconstriction; when this is of moderate degree the patient may experience coldness of the extremities which can at times mimic Raynaud's phenomenon (see below); when it is more severe it may produce intermittent claudication; and when intense it may cause tissue necrosis, particularly when the patient already has atheromatous narrowing of the arteries.

Drugs used for their vasoconstrictor effects

It is to be expected that drugs used for their vasoconstrictor effect (once popular in the treatment of shock) will at times cause ischaemia of peripheral tissues. Such complications appear, however, to be uncommon when the drugs are given intravenously unless there is leakage into the tissues surrounding the point of entry of the injection or infusion, when tissue necrosis may occur (noradrenaline [Close *et al.* 1956, 1958]; metaraminol [Dippy and Dorney 1959; Shaub 1960; Pelner and Waldman 1960]).

Dihydroergotamine has been used in combination with lignocaine and low-dose heparin to prevent postoperative thromboembolism, because of its action in constricting capacitance vessels thus promoting venous return; but unfortunately this form of treatment has occasionally been complicated by severe arterial spasm, sometimes resulting in gangrene (*SADRAC Bulletin* 1989).

Drugs used for migraine

Some of the drugs used in the treatment of migraine have vasoconstrictor properties which at times may be harmful. Thus, ergotamine has caused peripheral ischaemia, rarely resulting in gangrene, even when doses have not been excessive (Daimant-Berger *et al.* 1972; Hesson *et al.* 1972; Hirsch and Eger 1972; McLoughlin and Saunders 1972; Herlache *et al.* 1973; Imrie 1973; Rizk *et al.* 1973; Brinc and Hjeltrues 1974; Carliner *et al.* 1974; Husum *et al.* 1979).

There have been several reports of peripheral ischaemia in patients under treatment with either ergotamine or dihydroergotamine when they were also given the antibiotic triacetyloleandomycin. It has been suggested that in such cases the antibiotic may simply have inhibited the hepatic enzymes involved in the metabolism or the ergot alkaloid (a similar explanation has been proposed for the interaction between triacetyloleandomycin and carbamazepine [Dravet *et al.* 1977]), but actual hepatic damage caused by triacetyloleandomycin may have been present in some of the reported cases (Hayton 1969; Franco *et al.* 1978; Bacourt and Couffinhal 1978; Vayssairat *et al.* 1978). Methysergide has caused ischaemic pain (Leyton 1964) and coldness in the limbs, and even arterial occlusion (Raw and Gaylis 1976; Ameli *et al.* 1977).

Drugs used for other purposes

Ergometrine given intramuscularly has caused peripheral gangrene on rare occasions (Valentine *et al.* 1977).

Dopamine, used in the treatment of shock or acute cardiac failure may cause peripheral vasoconstriction and even tissue necrosis if the dose is excessive (Alexander *et al.* 1975; Julka and Nora 1976; Maggi *et al.* 1982).

Bromocriptine, a dopaminergic-receptor stimulant that has been used to inhibit the secretion of prolactin, to reduce circulating growth hormone levels, and to treat some cases of Parkinson's disease, may at times cause troublesome peripheral vasoconstriction (Sachdev *et al.* 1975; Wass *et al.* 1976; Wass *et al.* 1977).

Vasopressin, given by infusion in the treatment of portal hypertension, has caused cutaneous gangrene, even though there was no evidence of subcutaneous extravasation in several of the cases (Anderson and Johnston 1983).

β-Adrenoceptor blocking agents may induce vasoconstriction. This is usually mild and produces only coldness of the extremities but it has caused intermittent claudication in previously asymptomatic patients (Rodger *et al.* 1976) and even peripheral gangrene in rare instances (Vale and Jeffereys 1978). It has been suggested that the dominance of α-adrenergic sympathetic activity, resulting from β-adrenoceptor blockade, produces disturbances of the peripheral haemodynamics by eliminating the capacity of the blood vessels in muscle to respond to β_2-mediated vasodilatation (Dukes 1979).

A form of vasoconstriction with features suggestive of Raynaud's phenomenon has been induced by β-blockers (Marshall *et al.* 1966; Trash *et al.* 1976; Eliasson *et al.* 1978); bromocriptine (Quagliariello and Barakat 1987); cyclosporin (Deray *et al.* 1986); and combination cytotoxic therapy (Anderson *et al.* 1988; Werquin *et al.* 1987).

Drugs causing vasoconstriction only by local irritation

A variety of drugs that have no significant vasoconstrictor effects when given by mouth or by intravenous injection (without leakage from the site of injection) may cause intense arterial spasm, sometimes resulting in gangrene, if accidentally injected into or very near to an artery or if they reach an artery by spread from the site of an intramuscular or intravenous injection (e.g. barbiturates [Mindham 1975]; penicillin [Friederszick 1949]).

Methylmethacrylate, used in joint replacement surgery, has caused severe damage to arteries with which it has come into contact (Hirsh *et al.* 1976).

Acrocyanosis and erythromelalgia

Acrocyanosis is characterized by blueness and coldness of the hands and feet, sometimes accompanied by sweating of the affected parts, differing from Raynaud's disease in that it is not episodic. Erythromelalgia is a condition in which there is an unpleasant burning discomfort in the distal parts of the upper or lower limbs, with or without associated discolouration of the parts involved. In some cases described in the literature no clear distinction is made between the two conditions.

Acrocyanosis is usually idiopathic, but a case with similar features has been attributed to imipramine (Anderson and Morris 1988).

True erythromelalgia is probably due to thrombocythaemia, with intravenous activation of platelets leading to thromboses and arteriolar inflammation (Drenth 1989). A syndrome superficially resembling the disease has been associated with treatment with nifedipine (Brodmerkel 1983; Fisher and Padnick 1983) and nicardipine (Levesque *et al.* 1989); in the latter case a platelet count was made and was normal. An erythromelalgia-like eruption has also been attributed to treatment with bromocriptine (Eisler *et al.* 1981).

Drug-induced hypotension

Introduction

Drug-induced hypotension is difficult to categorize clearly and neatly, because the ways in which this adverse reaction may be produced are diverse and more than one

mechanism may operate in an individual reaction; and because published reports often provide too little information to enable one to do more than guess at the mechanism or mechanisms involved in the cases described. Furthermore, it is possible that some of the hypotensive reactions that have been attributed to injected drugs were due not to the drugs themselves but to a vasovagal response to anxiety in a nervous patient.

It should be noted that as the number of published reports of drug-induced hypotension is so large, references will not be given when the reaction is now firmly established as a complication of treatment with a widely used drug, but they will be provided when the reaction is considered to be an unusual response to the drug concerned.

Mechanisms

Drug-induced hypotension can be mediated by a fall in cardiac output due to direct myocardial depression or to reduced venous return (caused by either venodilatation or hypovolaemia), by a reduction in peripheral vascular resistance, or by a combination of these effects.

Reduced peripheral vascular resistance and venous dilatation

Hypotension due to reduction in peripheral vascular resistance can result from the effects of drugs on the neurological control of the vascular bed; from a direct effect on blood vessels by either the drug itself or by chemical mediators released by its action; or as a consequence of depletion of substances which normally help to maintain adequate vascular tone.

Antihypertensive drugs

Many antihypertensive drugs have an effect on the neurological control of the blood vessels. Some — the thiazides and hydralazine — appear to act principally by a direct effect on the vascular smooth muscle. The β-adrenoceptor blocking drugs have multiple and complex actions that still have not yet been completely elucidated. Irrespective of the site or sites of their primary action, however, in most cases their final effect is to reduce peripheral vascular resistance; and clearly all drugs with a very potent action of this kind can at times cause an excessive fall in blood pressure that may inconvenience or harm the patient. Such hypotension may occur acutely either during or soon after the giving of a drug or, when related to the posture of the patient, at any time during the period of action of the drug. Hypotension caused by drugs may also be of gradual onset and sustained, but it may still be acutely aggravated by changes in posture in some cases. Whether or not posture precipitates or aggravates drug-induced hypotension depends on the way in which a drug affects the control of peripheral resistance; when vascular reflexes are not greatly impaired then postural hypotension is not to be expected, but when they are lost then postural hypotension may be very severe.

Almost all antihypertensive drugs can at times cause severe hypotension (which may have very serious consequences, particularly in severe or malignant hypertension [*British Medical Journal* 1979]). This occurs most commonly during treatment with those agents that interfere with efferent sympathetic outflow; thus, the adrenergic-neurone blockers (e.g. bethanidine, bretylium, debrisoquine, guanethidine), and α-adrenoceptor blockers (e.g. prazosin) are particularly likely to cause postural hypotension. Most cases of severe postural hypotension caused by prazosin have occurred at the beginning of treatment (Bendall *et al.* 1975; Bloom *et al.* 1975; Committee on Safety of Medicines 1975; Curtis and Bateman 1975; Gabriel *et al.* 1975; Seedat *et al.* 1975; Turner 1976) and appear to be the result of α-blockade (Bateman *et al.* 1979), but tolerance develops rapidly (Graham *et al.* 1976).

This 'first-dose hypotension' is dose-related and usually occurs while the patient is standing, most often in those with depletion of extracellular fluid. It is characterized by a suddden change from tachycardia to bradycardia accompanied by a fall in blood pressure severe enough to cause syncope. The mechanism involved is said to be activation of the Bezold–Jarisch cardiovascular depressor reflex (Semple *et al.* 1988).

Other antihypertensive drugs that may have the first-dose effect are the other α-adrenoceptor blockers, indoramin (Gould *et al.* 1981) and terazosin (Sperzel *et al.* 1986); the 5-hydroxytryptamine antagonist ketanserin, which also has some α-blocking activity (Waller *et al.* 1987); angiotensin-converting-enzyme inhibitors (also used for heart failure) (Hodsman *et al.* 1983; Cleland *et al.* 1985; Wieland and Staübli 1988; Russell and Jones 1989); nifedipine (Bertel 1987; Wachter 1987); and some β-adrenoceptor blockers — acebutolol (Tirlapur *et al.* 1986) and atenolol (Kholeif and Isles 1989). The cases described by the latter authors were examples of the hyponatraemic–hypotensive syndrome — malignant hypertension accompanied by hyponatraemia and hyperkalaemia.

The thiazides, methyldopa, hydralazine, clonidine, and the β-adrenoceptor blockers appear to be less likely to cause severe postural hypotension, though clonidine has caused a severe hypotensive reaction when used as a diagnostic test in a patient with phaeochromocytoma (Given *et al.* 1983).

Drugs used for other purposes may also have this effect (see below). Saralasin, a drug given intravenously to detect angiotensin-mediated hypertension, may at times cause severe hypotension (Fagard *et al.* 1976; Pettinger and Keeton 1975) (this drug has also caused a hypertensive crisis in the presence of phaeochromocytoma — see earlier.) The α-adrenoceptor blockers benzodioxane and phentolamine were once widely used in tests for suspected phaeochromocytoma, with the object of reducing the blood pressure significantly, though not excessively, if the test proved positive. Unfortunately catastrophic hypotension occurred on occasion (Green and Grimsley 1953; Bierman and Partridge 1951) and was sometimes fatal (Emanuel *et al.* 1956; Roland 1959) and this was one reason why these tests fell into disuse. Haemorrhagic necrosis of phaeochromocytoma has been attributed to the use of such drugs, in particular phentolamine. The mechanism is unknown, but it is suggested that the lowering of the systolic blood pressure may cause the already precarious blood supply within the tumour to become inadequate or, alternatively, that the α-adrenoceptor blockers produce vasodilatation within the tumour, flooding an already necrotic area with blood and initiating a progressive interstitial haemorrhage within the tumour, ending in either haemorrhagic necrosis of the whole tumour or rupture of the capsule with retroperitoneal haematoma formation (Van Way *et al.* 1976).

Vasodilator drugs

Although all those antihypertensive drugs that reduce peripheral resistance could reasonably be called 'vasodilators', this term is more usually used for drugs commonly used for vasospastic disorders, such as Raynaud's phenomenon; for angina pectoris (see below); or (less rationally) for peripheral ischaemia caused by atheromatous narrowing of arteries. Some of these drugs act purely as α-adrenoceptor blocking agents; some act directly on vascular smooth muscle; a few have both these effects; and others enhance β-adrenergic activity. Many drugs of this kind (which indude thymoxamine, tolazoline, azapetine, inositol nicotinate, bemethan, kallidinogenase, nicotinyl tartate, isoxsuprine, and glyceryl trinitrate) may occasionally cause significant hypotension.

It is worth emphasizing that it is now accepted that glyceryl trinitrate, still regarded by some as a specific 'coronary artery vasodilator', produces its beneficial effect mainly by dilating the peripheral veins, causing an acute fall in venous return, a fall in cardiac output (reducing the cardiac workload), and systemic hypotension; first-dose hypotension (described earlier) has also been caused by this and other vasodilator organic nitrates (Semple *et al.* 1988). This hypotensive effect does not, however, cause symptoms unless aggravated by the hypotensive effect of a drug given concurrently. Thus, one of our patients who had been under treatment with glyceryl trinitrate for several years without any ill effect developed syncopal attacks that were attributed to epilepsy of late onset until it was realized that attacks had coincided with the taking of a glyceryl trinitrate tablet and had begun when the patient had started treatment with chlorpromazine (which also has a hypotensive effect), given for anxiety. A synergistic action of this kind may also be encountered when other combinations of drugs with hypotensive effects are used.

Vancomycin

Among the antibiotics, vancomycin appears to have a peculiar propensity to cause hypotension, sometimes severe, when given by intravenous infusion. This reaction is more likely when the infusion solution is too concentrated or administered too quickly, and it appears to be due to histamine release (Newfield and Roizen 1979), direct myocardial depression (Cohen *et al.* 1970), peripheral vasodilatation (Cohen *et al.* 1970), or a combination of these effects. Histamine release is probably responsible for the erythematous rash that has been an early feature of some of these cases (Lacouture *et al.* 1987; Best *et al.* 1989).

Fatal cardiac arrest has also followed intravenous administration of vancomycin in a 2-year-old girl after an operation (Mayhew and Deutsch 1985).

Endogenous vasodilator substances

Acute hypotension is one of the features of anaphylactic and anaphylactic-like reactions induced by drugs, when it is due to the effect on the blood vessels of one or more of a number of mediators, including histamine (see Chapter 25). Some drugs (e.g. dextrans, opiates) release histamine by a non-immunological mechanism, and such an action may be responsible for the hypotension that sometimes complicates the administration of radiographic contrast media (see Chapters 25 and 27).

Drugs used during anaesthesia

Almost all intravenously administered inducing agents and anaesthetic gases may cause hypotension by depressing the vasomotor centre. Some neuromuscular blocking agents can also cause a fall in blood pressure — probably by reducing venous return. Hypotension is a well-recognized feature of spinal or epidural anaesthesia.

Sedatives and tranquillizers

Most sedatives and tranquillizers can cause a fall in blood pressure, principally by an action on the vasomotor centre. When these drugs are given by mouth in normal therapeutic doses, the hypotensive response is minimal and usually of little clinical significance, but when administered by intravenous (or even intramuscular) injection the hypotensive effect is greater and can be severe if the injection is given too rapidly. This effect can be particularly pronounced in the elderly in whom cardiovascular reflex control may already be compromised. Great care should be taken with dosage.

Antidepressants

Antidepressants of the MAOI group or the tricyclic group may cause significant hypotension, particularly related to posture, in some patients. The mechanisms involved are complex and incompletely understood, but a decrease in peripheral vascular resistance, principally due to an effect on the vasomotor centre, is probably involved to some degree.

Oxytocin

Oxytocin is known to have a hypotensive effect, but usually this is mild and not clinically significant. Bolus injections, however, have caused a precipitous fall in blood pressure (*Journal of the American Medical Association* 1974).

Levodopa

Paradoxically, levodopa, a precursor of noradrenaline, is a well-recognized cause of troublesome postural hypotension (Calne *et al.* 1970; Hoehn 1975). It has been suggested that this effect is due to its breakdown to dopamine which is taken up by nerve endings and then released 'diluting' the effect of noradrenaline released concurrently (Burn 1970), and this hypothesis led to the use of propranolol to prevent levodopa-induced postural hypotension with the object of antagonizing the effect of the dopamine on peripheral resistance vessels, a treatment claimed to have been successful (Duvoison 1970). Shanks (1970) disputed these theories, however, and neither the reaction nor the prophylactic effect of propranolol can be said to have been satisfactorily explained.

Diuretics

Loop diuretics, such as frusemide, may induce first-dose hypotension, discussed above, when given intravenously (Semple *et al.* 1988).

Prostaglandins

Dinoprost (prostaglandin $F_{2\alpha}$), a prostaglandin used in obstetrics, has caused alarming, and sometimes fatal hypotension when injected into the myometrium (Douglas *et al.* 1989), extra-amniotically (Wein *et al.* 1989), or into the uterine cavity (Partridge *et al.* 1988). Such events may also be due to the first-dose effect (Semple *et al.* 1988).

Hypotension in peripheral neuropathy

Hypotension, particularly postural hypotension, may complicate drug-induced polyneuropathy, probably due to impairment of neurological control of peripheral vascular resistance and, when there is muscular paralysis, a fall in venous return.

Hypovolaemia

Hypovolaemia occurs in acute haemorrhage induced by drugs. It also complicates iatrogenic sodium and water depletion caused by diuretics, and is a feature of acute adrenal insufficiency which may occur in patients during adrenal corticosteroid therapy or following withdrawal of such therapy; during treatment with aminoglutethimide and metyrapone; or, very rarely, as a result of haemorrhage into the adrenals in patients taking anticoagulants (see Chapter 13). Hypovolaemia is also the mechanism by which hypotension is produced in drug-induced ketoacidosis and lactic acidosis (see Chapter 14).

Mixed or obscure mechanisms

A large number of isolated reports have attributed hypotensive reactions to a wide variety of drugs, particularly when given parenterally. The pharmacological mechanisms involved are at the moment incompletely understood. Of these reports, the most interesting relate to: acrylic bone cement (Newens and Volz 1972; Peebles *et al.* 1972; *The Lancet* 1974); atropine and propanidid (Clarke 1969); bromocriptine (Linch *et al.* 1978); cimetidine (Mahon and Kolton 1978); disulfiram and general anaesthesia (Diaz and Hill 1979); doxacuronium chloride (Reich 1989); ethamsylate (Watson 1972; Langdon 1977); lignocaine for retrobulbar block (Cardan *et al.* 1987); metoclopramide (Park 1978; Pegg 1980); paraldehyde (Sinal and Crowe 1976); pentagastrin (McCloy and Baron 1977); pentamidine (Western *et al.* 1976); phenoperidine with propranolol (Woods 1978); podophyllin (Montaldi *et al.* 1974); protamine sulphate (Fadali *et al.* 1974); salbutamol (Ng and Sen 1974); simvastatin (French and White 1989); soap enema (Egdell and Johnson 1973); terbutaline, by subcutaneous injection in patients with quadriplegia with autonomic dysfunction (Pingleton *et al.* 1982); thiothixene (Burnett *et al.* 1975); trazodone (Spivak *et al.* 1987); viloxazine (Pinder *et al.* 1977); and vitamin K_1 (Loeliger 1975).

Aortic dissection

The need for accuracy in the diagnosis of acute myocardial infarction before employing thrombolytic therapy has been stressed by Curzen and others (1990) and Butler and colleagues (1990), who have reported cases in which extension of aortic dissection was attributed to streptokinase given for presumed myocardial infarction.

Thromboembolic disease

Oral contraceptives

It is now well established that women taking oral contraceptives are more at risk of venous thrombosis than are women who do not take these drugs. The commonest sites for thrombosis are the veins of the lower legs, and the disorder may remain localized, ascend to involve other veins, including the vena cava and renal veins, or may give rise to emboli that may lodge in branches of the pulmonary artery or (in the rare case of paradoxical embolism) pass through an atrial or ventricular septal defect to reach a systemic artery. Thrombi may also form within arteries, leading to intermittent claudication (van V.roonhoven 1977), or cerebral, coronary, or mesenteric thrombosis.

Heparin and other antithrombotic drugs

Paradoxically, when heparin is used for preventing or treating thromboembolism it may sometimes cause venous or arterial thrombus formation as part of the 'thrombocytopenia and thrombosis' syndrome. First observed in animals (Copley and Robb, 1942; Fidlar and Jaques 1948; Quick *et al.* 1948), it has subsequently been recognized in human patients (Rhodes *et al.* 1973; Baird and Convery 1977; Kelton and Hirsh 1980; Carreras 1980; Godal 1980; Chong *et al.* 1982; Silver *et al.* 1983; Guay and Richard 1984; King and Kelton 1984; Ansell *et al.* 1985; Mandt *et al.* 1985; Barber *et al.* 1987). At least two types of heparin-induced thrombocytopenia have been described (Barber *et al.* 1987). One is common (incidence perhaps as high as 30 per cent), mild, of rapid onset (2nd–4th day), is not usually associated with haemorrhage or thrombosis, and therefore unlikely to be fatal, and is thought to be due to temporary sequestration of platelets (Gollub and Ulin 1962). Another is more severe; of delayed onset (7th–10th day), unless the patient has received heparin previously, in which case it may occur earlier; is accompanied by recurrent thrombotic episodes, with a mortality as high as 29 per cent (Barber *et al.* 1987); and appears to be associated with a heparin-dependent IgG antibody that is not directed against heparin but which induces synthesis of thromboxane and aggregation of platelets (Chong *et al.* 1982; Sandler *et al.* 1985). In both forms thrombocytopenia persists for as long as heparin is continued, but in the severe form thrombotic episodes may occur for a while after the platelet count has returned to normal. Recommended treatment is to withhold heparin and administer oral anticoagulants or aspirin and dipyridamole (Kelton and Hirsh 1980; Silver *et al.* 1983); and streptokinase, by intravenous or intra-arterial injection, has been used in some cases (Fiessinger *et al.* 1984). Transfusions of platelet concentrate have failed to raise the platelet count to normal (Babcock *et al.* 1976).

Thrombolytic therapy for acute myocardial infarction, with such drugs as streptokinase, anistreplase, and alteplase, carries the risk of disintegration of pre-existing clot with consequent microembolization, but Stafford and others (1989), who have reported such complications, concluded that the risks are outweighed by the potential benefits, a view with which some others concur (*Drug and Therapeutics Bulletin* 1990).

Diuretics

Thrombosis of the axillary vein is an uncommon condition usually caused by venous constriction by a cervical rib or fibrous band, malignant deposits, or subclavian venous catheters; or by excessive use of the arm in certain sports, or prolonged elevation of the limb during such household tasks as painting or papering of ceilings. An association with drug therapy must be excessively rare, but Green and colleagues (1988) have described a patient with severe congestive heart failure unresponsive to frusemide, ethacrynic acid, and spironolactone who, within 24 hours of being given the diuretic metolazone, had a profound diuresis and lost 4 kg in weight and then developed axillary vein thrombosis; this subsided within a few weeks of withdrawing the drug. The authors postulated that 'relative dehydration' of the intravascular compartment might have precipitated thrombosis. The patient was also under treatment for tuberculosis, though rifampicin (see below) was not part of the drug regimen. While the history is suggestive, one cannot draw a firm conclusion of a causal relationship from a single case but, if the authors are correct, presumably such an event could, rarely, follow the use of any potent diuretic.

Antituberculous therapy — rifampicin

A retrospective study comparing 7542 tuberculous patients with 252 controls with non-tuberculous lung abscesses was undertaken to determine whether there is an association between antituberculosis therapy and venous thrombosis (White 1989). A significantly greater number of the patients given rifampicin (2.7 per cent of 4391) than of patients not having the drug (0.5 per cent), or controls (0.4 per cent) developed venous thrombosis. The relative risk of venous thrombosis in patients treated with rifampicin was estimated to be 4.74, but the author concluded that the benefit of the drug in this disease outweighs its risks. He suggests that concurrent low-dose heparin therapy might be a useful prophylactic against this complication.

Cytotoxic drugs

Thromboembolic disease has been observed following anticancer therapy with various combinations of cytotoxic drugs (Hall *et al.* 1988; Levine *et al.* 1988; Milne *et al.* 1988).

ACE inhibitors

A single case of renal artery thrombosis following enalapril in a patient with atheroma of the artery has been reported (Main and Wilkinson 1989).

Vasculitis

Arteritis

Inflammatory changes in arteries may occur as a result of an adverse reaction to a drug, and although such changes are usually considered to be manifestations of a hypersensitivity reaction this has not been established beyond doubt. The subject is discussed in more detail in Chapters 17 and 25.

Phlebitis

Inflammatory changes in veins may be produced by drugs injected intravenously, or may be part of a widespread reaction of which arteritis may also be a feature; and an interesting case has been described in which phlebitis initially caused by an injection of diazepam recurred when the patient was later treated with penicillamine given orally (Brandstetter *et al.* 1981).

Cutaneous vasculitis

Lesions resulting from this disorder are described in Chapter 17.

Types of reactions

Of the adverse reactions affecting the peripheral vascular system, almost all of those in which the mechanism is known or suspected appear to be of Type A, though the reactions to intravenous radiographic contrast media and anaphylactic reactions are of Type B (see Chapter 3).

References

Aabo, K. and De Coster, R. (1987). Hypertension during high-dose ketoconazole treatment: a probable mineralocorticoid effect. *Lancet* ii, 637.

Adelman, M.H., Jacobson, E., Lief, A., and Miller, S.A. (1959). Promethazine hydrochloride in surgery and obstetrics. *JAMA* 169, 73.

Agabiti-Rosei, E., Brown, J.J., Lever, A.F., Robertson, A.S. Robertson, J.I.S., and Trust, P.M. (1976). Treatment of phaeochromocytoma and of clonidine withdrawal with labetalol. *Br. J. Clin. Pharmacol.* 3 (suppl. 3), 809.

Agabiti-Rosei, E., Alicandri, C.L., and Corea, L. (1977). Hypertensive crisis in patients with phaeochromocytoma given metoclopramide. *Lancet* i, 600.

Alam, M., Anrep, G.V., Barsoum, G.S., Talaat, M., and Wieninger, E. (1939). Liberation of histamine from the skeletal muscle. *J. Physiol.* (Lond.) 95,148.

Alexander, C.S., Sako, Y., and Mikulic, E. (1975). Pedal gangrene associated with the use of dopamine. *N. Engl. J. Med.* 293, 591.

Ameli, F.M., Nathanson, M., and Elkan, I. (1977). Methysergide therapy causing vascular insufficiency of the upper limb. *Can. J. Surg.* 20, 158.

Amery, A. and Deloof, W. (1970). Cheese reaction during debrisoquine treatment. *Lancet* ii, 613.

Anderson, J.R. and Johnston, G.W. (1983). Development of cutaneous gangrene during continuous peripheral infusion of vasopressin. *Br. Med. J.* 287, 1657.

Anderson, L.B., Thestrup-Pedersen, K., and Sell, A. (1988). Nifedipine treatment of Raynaud's phenomenon secondary to chemotherapy. *Dermatologica* 177, 19.

Anderson, R.P. and Morris B.A.P. (1988). Acrocyanosis due to imipramine. *Arch. Dis. Child.* 63, 204.

Ansell, G. (1970). Adverse reactions to contrast agents; scope of problem. *Invest. Radiol.* 5, 374.

Ansell, J.E., Price, J.M., Shah, S., and Beckner, R.R. (1985). Heparin-induced thrombocytopenia. What is its real frequency? *Chest* 88, 878.

Asatoor, A.M., Levi, A.J., and Milne, M.D. (1963). Tranylcypromine and cheese. *Lancet* ii, 733.

Athos, W.J., McHugh, B.P., Fineberg, S.E., and Hillon, J.G. (1962). The effect of guanethidine on the adrenal medulla. *J. Pharmacol. Exp. Ther.* 137, 229.

Babcock, R.B., Dumper, C.W., and Scharfman, W.B. (1976). Heparin-induced immune thrombocytopenia. *N. Engl. J. Med.* 295, 237.

Bacourt, F. and Couffinhal, J.H.C. (1978). Ischémie des membres par association déhydroergotamine triacétyloléandomycine. Nouvelle observation. *Nouv. Presse Med.* 7, 1561.

Bailey, R.R. and Neale, T.J. (1976). Rapid clonidine withdrawal with blood pressure overshoot exaggerated by beta-blockade. *Br. Med. J.* i, 943.

Baird, R.A. and Convery, F.R. (1977). Arterial thromboembolism in patients receiving systemic heparin therapy. A complication associated with heparin-induced thrombocytopenia. *J. Bone Joint Surg.* 59-A, 1061.

Barar, F.S.K., Boakes, A.J., Benedikter, L.B., Laurence, D.R., Prichard, B.N.C., Teoh, P.C. (1971). Interactions between catecholamines and tricyclic and monoamine oxidase inhibitor antidepressant agents in man. *Br. J. Pharmacol.* 43, 472P.

Barber, F.A., Burton, W.C., and Guyer, R. (1987). The heparin-induced thrombocytopenia and thrombosis syndrome. Report of a case. *J. Bone Joint Surg.* 68-A, 935.

Bateman, D.N., Hobbs, D.C., Twomey, T.M., Stevens, E. A., and Rawlins, M.D. (1979). Prazosin, pharmokinetics and concentration effect. *Eur. J. Clin. Pharmacol.* 16, 177.

Bendall, M.J., Baloch, K.H., and Wilson, P.R. (1975). Side effects due to treatment of hypertension with prazosin. *Br. Med. J.* ii, 727.

Berg, K.J., Forre, O., Bjerkhoel, F., Amundsen, E., Djøseland, O., Rugstad, H.E., *et al.* (1986). Side-effects of cyclosporin A treatment in patients with rheumatoid arthritis. *Kidney Int.* 29, 1180.

Bertel, O. (1987). Symptomatic hypotension induced by nifedipine. *Arch. Intern. Med.* 147, 1683.

Best, C.J., Ewart, M., and Summer, E. (1989). Perioperative complications following the use of vancomycin in children: a report of two cases. *Br. J. Anaesth.* 62, 576.

Bierman, H.R. and Partridge, J.W. (1951). Untoward reactions to tests for epinephrine-secreting tumours (pheochromocytoma). *N. Engl. J. Med.* 244, 582.

Bittar, D.A. (1979). Innovar-induced hypertensive crisis in patients with pheochromocytoma. *Anesthesiology* 50, 366.

Bixby, E.W. and Troncelliti, M.V. (1952). Anesthesia in operation for pheochromocytoma (abstract from correspondence). *JAMA* 148, 1443.

Blackwell, B. (1963). Tranylcypromine. *Lancet* ii, 414.

Blackwell, B., Marley, E., and Mabbit, L.A. (1965). Effects of yeast extract after monoamine oxidase inhibitors. *Lancet* i, 940.

Blomley, D.J. (1964). Monoamine oxidase inhibitors. *Lancet* ii, 1181.

Bloom, D.S., Rosendorff, C., and Kramer, R. (1975). Clinical evaluation of prazosin as the sole agent for the treatment of hypertension. A double-blind cross-over study with methyldopa. *Curr. Ther. Res.* 18, 144.

Blum, I., Atsmon, A., Steiner, M., and Wysenbeek, H. (1975). Paradoxical rise in blood pressure during propranolol treatment. *Br. Med. J.* iv, 623.

Borromeo-McGrail, V., Bordiuk, J.M., and Keitel, H. (1973). Systemic hypertension following ocular administration of 10% phenylephrine in the neonate. *Pediatrics* 51, 1032.

Brandstetter, R.D., Gotz, V.P., Mar, D.D., and Sachs, D. (1981). Exacerbation of diazepam-induced phlebitis by oral penicillamine. *Br. Med. J.* 283, 525.

Bravo, E.L., Tarazi, R.C., Fouad, F.M., Vidt, D.G., and Gifford, R. Jr (1981). Clonidine-suppression test. A useful aid in the diagnosis of pheochromocytoma. *N. Engl. J. Med.* 305, 623.

Brenner, W.I. and Lieberman, A.N. (1977). Acute clonidine withdrawal syndrome following open heart operation. *Ann Thor. Surg.* 24, 80.

Briggs, R.S.J., Birtwell, A.J., and Pohl, J.E.F. (1978). Hypertensive response in labetalol in phaeochromocytoma. *Lancet* i, 1045.

Brinc, L. and Hjeltrues, J. (1974). Ergotamin som årsak til arteriell insufisiens. *T. Norske Laegeforen* 94, 1906.

British Medical Journal (1979). Dangerous antihypertension treatment. *Br. Med. J.* ii, 228.

Brodmerkel, G.J. Jr (1983). Nifedipine and erythromelalgia. *Ann. Intern. Med.* 99, 415.

Brodsky, J.B. and Brave, J.A. (1976). Acute postoperative clonidine withdrawal syndrome. *Anesthesiology* 44, 519.

Brown, A.S. (1969). Pentazocine, a potent analgesic: evaluation for anaesthetic use. *Proc. R. Soc. Med.* 62, 805.

Brown, J.J., Robertson, A.S., Agabiti-Rosei, E., Robertson, J.I.S., Lever, A.F., and Trust, P.M. (1976). Emergency treatment of hypertensive crisis following clonidine withdrawal. *Br. Med. J.* i, 1341.

Brown, J.R. and Kulkarni, M.V. (1967). A review of the toxicity and metabolism of mercury and its compounds. *Med. Serv. J. Can.* 23, 786.

Brown, M.J., Lewis, P.J., and Dollery, C.T. (1980). Diagnosis of small phaeochromocytomas. *Lancet* i, 1185.

Browning, D.J. (1974). Serious side effects of ergometrine and its use in routine obstetric practice. *Med. J. Aust.* 1, 957.

Burden, A.X.C. and Alexander, C.P.T. (1976). Hypertension after acute methyldopa withdrawal. *Br. Med. J.* i, 1056.

Burke, C.M., Theodore, J., Baldwin, J.C., Tazelaar, H.D., Morris, A.J.. McGregor, C., et al. (1986). Twenty-eight cases of human heart-lung transplantation. *Lancet* i, 517.

Burn, J.H. (1970). Hypotension caused by L-dopa. *Br. Med. J.* i, 629.

Burn, J.H. and Dale H.H. (1926). The vasodilator action of histamine and its physiological significance. *J. Physiol.* (Lond.) 61, 185.

Burn, J.H., Leach, E.H., Rand, M.J., and Thompson, J.W. (1959). Peripheral effects of nicotine and acetylcholine resembling those of sympathetic stimulation. *J. Physiol.* (Lond.) 148, 332.

Burnett, G.B., Little, S.R.C.J., Graham, N., and Forrest, A.D. (1975). The assessment of thiothixene in chronic schizophrenia. A double-blind controlled trial. *Dis. Nerv. Syst.* 36, 625.

Butler, J., Davies, A.H., and Westaby, S. (1990). Streptokinase in acute aortic dissection. *Br. Med. J.* 300, 517.

Calne, D.B., Brennan, J., Spiers, A.S.D., and Stern, G.M. (1970). Hypotension caused by L-dopa. *Br. Med. J.* i, 474.

Canadian Multicentre Transplant Study Group (1983). A randomized clinical trial of cyclosporine in cadaveric renal transplantation. *N. Engl. J. Med.* 309, 809.

Cardan, E., Pop, R., and Neghutiu, S. (1987). Prolonged haemodynamic disturbance following attempted retrobulbar block. *Anaesthesia* 42, 668.

Carliner, N.A., Denune, D.P., Finch, C.S., and Goldberg, L.I. (1974). Sodium nitroprusside treatment of ergotamine-induced peripheral ischemia. *JAMA* 227, 308.

Carreras, L.O. (1980). Thrombosis and thrombocytopenia induced by heparin. *Scand. J. Haematol.* (suppl. 36), 64.

Chapman, J.R., Marcen, R., Arias, M., Raine, A.E.G., Dunnill, M.S., and Morris, P.L. (1987). Hypertension after renal transplantation. A comparison of cyclosporin and conventional immunosuppression. *Transplantation* 43, 860.

Chaturvedi, N.C., Walsh, M.J., Boyle, D. McC., and Barber, J.M. (1974). Diamorphine-induced attack of paroxysmal hypertension in phaeochromocytoma. *Br. Med. J.* ii, 538.

Chong, B.H., Pitney, W.R., and Castaldi, P.A. (1982). Heparin-induced thrombocytopenia. Association of thrombotic complications with heparin-dependent IgG antibody that induces thromboxane synthesis and platelet aggregation. *Lancet* ii, 1246.

Clarke, R.S.J. (1969). Hypotensive reaction after propanidid. *Br. Med. J.* iv, 369.

Cleland, J.G.F., Dargie, H.J., McAlpine, H., Ball, S.G., Morton, J.J., and Robertson, J.I.S. (1985). Severe hypotension after first dose of enalapril in heart failure. *Br. Med. J.* 291, 1309.

Close, A.S., Frackleton, W.H., and Cory, R.C. (1956). Cutaneous necrosis due to nor-epinephrine: mechanism and prevention. *Clin. Res. Proc.* 4, 241.

Close, A.S., Frackleton, W.H., and Cory, R.C. (1958). Cutaneous necrosis due to nor-epinephrine: analysis of reported cases and surgical treatment. *Wis. Med. J.* 57, 127.

Cohen, L.S., Weschler, A.S., and Mitchell, J.H. (1970). Depression of cardiac function by streptomycin and other antimicrobial agents. *Am. J. Cardiol.* 26, 505.

Collins, G.H. (1971). Hypertension during chlorimipramine therapy. *Br. Med. J.* ii, 170.

Comfort, A. (1981). Hypertensive reactions to New Zealand prickly spinach in woman taking phenelzine. *Lancet* ii, 472.

Committee on Safety of Medicines (1975). Prazosin and loss of consciousness. The present position. *Curr. Prob.* I.

Comroe, J.H. Jr and Dripps, R.D. (1946). The histamine-like action of curare and tubocurarine injected intracutaneously and intra-arterially in man. *Anesthesiology* 7, 260.

Copley, A.L. and Robb, T.P. (1942). Studies on platelets. III. The effect of heparin *in vivo* on the platelet count in mice and dogs. *Am. J. Clin. Pathol.* 12, 563.

Corvol, P., Bisseliches, F., Alexandre, J.M. (1974) Poussées hypertensives déclenchées par le sulpride. *Sem. Hop. Paris* 50, 1265.

Coupland, R.E. (1965). *The natural history of the chromaffin cell.* Longman, London.

Criqui, M.H., Wallace, R.B., Mishkel, M., Barret-Connor, E., and Heiss, G. (1981). Alcohol consumption and blood pressure: the Lipid Research Clinics Prevalence Study. *Hypertension* 3, 557.

Critchley, J.A.J.H. and Ungar, A. (1974). Do the anterior pituitary and adrenal cortex participate in the reflex response of the adrenal medulla to arterial hypoxia? *J. Physiol.* (Lond.) 239, 16.

Critchley, J.A.J.H., West, C.P., and Waite, J. (1974). Dangers of corticotrophin in phaeochromocytoma. *Lancet* ii, 782.

Crofton, M. and Gabriel, R. (1977). Pressor response after intravenous labetalol. *Br. Med. J.* ii, 737.

Cryer, P.E., Haymond, N.W., Santiago, J.V., and Sheh, S.D. (1976). Norepinephrine and epinephrine release and adrenergic mediation of smoking-associated hemodynamic and metabolic events. *N. Engl. J. Med.* 195, 573.

Curtis, J.J., Dubovsky, E., Welcher, J.D., Luke, E.G., Diethelm, A.G., and Jones, P. (1986). Cyclosporin in therapeutic doses increases renal allograft vascular resistance. *Lancet* ii, 477,

Curtis, J.J., Luke, E.G., Jones, O., and Diethelm, A.G. (1988). Hypertension in cyclosporin-treated renal transplant recipients is sodium-dependent. *Am. J. Med.* 85,134.

Curtis, J.R. and Bateman, F.J.A. (1975). Use of prazosin in the management of hypertension in patients with chronic renal failure and in renal transplant recipients. *Br. Med. J.* iv, 432.

Curzen, N.P., Clarke, B., and Gray, H.H. (1990). Intravenous thrombolysis for suspected myocardial infarction: a cautionary note. *Br. Med. J.* 300, 513.

Cuthbert, M.F. and Vere, D.W. (1971). Potentiation of the cardiovascular effects of some catecholamines by a monoamine oxidase inhibitor. *Br. J. Pharmacol.* 43, 471P.

Daggett, P. and Franks, S. (1977). Steroid responsiveness in a phaeochromocytoma. *Br. Med. J.* i, 84.

Daimant-Berger, F., Pasticier, A., Haas, C., Soyer, R., Ricordeau, G., and Dubosi, C. R. (1972). Intolérance vasculaire périphérique nécrosante à l'ergotamine thérapeutique. *Eur. J. Toxicol.* 5, 366.

Davies, D.M. (1987). Phaeochromocytoma and adverse drug reactions. *Adverse Drug React. Acute Poisoning Rev.* 6, 91.

Dawkins, K.D., Jamieson, S.W., Hunt, S.A., Baldwin, J.C., Burke, C.M., Morris, A., *et al.* (1985). Long-term results, hemodynamics, and complications after combined heart-lung transportation. *Circulation* 71, 919.

Deray, G., Hoang, P., Achour, L., Hornych, A., Landault, C., and Caraillon, A. (1986). Cyclosporin and Raynaud phenomenon. *Lancet* ii, 1092.

Diaz, J.H. and Hill, G.E. (1979). Hypotension with anesthesia in disulfiram-treated patients. *Anesthesiology,* 51, 366.

Dippy, W.E. and Dorney, E.P. (1959). Tissue necrosis and slough produced by metaraminol bitartrate. *JAMA* 170, 1647.

Dougados, M. and Amor, B. (1987). Cyclosporin in rheumatoid arthritis: preliminary clinical results of an open trial. *Arthritis Rheum.* 30, 83.

Douglas, M.J., Farquarson, D.F., Ross, P.L.E., and Renwick, J.E. (1989). Cardiovascular collapse following an overdose of prostaglandin F_2 alpha: a case report. *Can. J. Anaesth.* 36, 466.

Douglas, W.W. (1985). Autocoids: Histamine and 5-hydroxytryptamine (serotonin) and their antagonists. In *Goodman and Gilman's The physiological basis of therapeutics* (7th edn) (ed. A.G. Gilman, L.S. Goodman, T.W. Rall, and F. Murad), p. 609. Macmillan, New York.

Douglas, W.W., Kanno, T., and Sampson, S.R. (1967). Effects of acetylcholine and other medullary secretogogues and antagonists on the membrane potential of adrenal chromaffin cells: analysis employing techniques of tissue culture. *J. Physiol.* (Lond.) 188, 107.

Dravet, C.J., Mesdjian, E., Cenraud, B., and Roger, J. (1977). Interaction between carbamazepine and triacetyloleandomycin. *Lancet* i, 810.

Drenth, J.P.H. (1989). Erythromelalgia induced by nicardipine. *Br. Med. J.* 298, 1582.

Drug and Therapeutics Bulletin (1969). L-Dopa for Parkinsonism. *Drug Ther. Bull.* 7, 59.

Drug and Therapeutics Bulletin (1990). Thrombolytic therapy and pre-existing clots. *Drug Ther. Bull.* 28, 44.

Dugan, W.M. (1967). Pheochromocytoma and smoking. *Arch. Intern. Med.* 120, 365.

Dukes, M.N.G. (1979). Antianginal and beta-adrenoceptor blocking drugs. In *Side effects of drugs annual,* Vol. 3 (ed. M.N.G. Dukes), p. 164. Excerpta Medica, Amsterdam.

Dunn, F.G., De Carvalho, J.G.R., Kem, D.C., Higgins, J.R., and Frohlich, E.D. (1976). Pheochromocytoma crisis induced by saralasin. Relation of angiotensin analogue to catecholamine release. *N. Engl. J. Med.* 295, 605.

Duvoison, R.V. (1970). Hypotension caused by L-dopa. *Br. Med. J.* ii, 47.

Edmunds, M.E. and Walls, J. (1988). Blood pressure and erythropoietin. *Lancet* i, 352.

Egdell, R.W. and Johnson, W.D. (1973). Postpartum hypotension and erythema: an adverse reaction to soap enema. *Am. J. Obstet. Gynecol.* 117, 1146.

Eggert, P. and Stick, C. (1988). Blood pressure increase after erythrocyte transfusion in end-stage renal disease. *Lancet* i, 1343.

Eisler, T., Hall, R.P., Kalavar, K.A.R., and Calne, D.B. (1981). Erythromelalgia-like eruption in parkinsonian patients treated with bromocriptine. *Neurology* 31, 1368.

Eliasson, K., Johnsson, H., Kistner, S., Lins, L.E., Odar-Cederlof, I., and Sundqvist, K. (1978). Raynaud-fenomen efter terapi med beta-blockerare. *Lakartidningen* 75, 2118.

Elis, J., Laurence, D.R., Hattie, H., and Prichard B.N.C. (1967). Modification by monoamine oxidase inhibitors of the effect of some sympathomimetics on blood pressure. *Br. Med. J.* ii, 75.

Emanuel, D.A., Rowe, G.G., Musser, M.J., and Philpot, V.B. Jr (1956). Prolonged hypotension with fatal termination after phentolamine (Regitine) methanesulfonate test. *JAMA* 161, 436.

Emmelin, N. and Engström, J. (1961). Supersensitivity of salivary glands following treatment with bretylium or guanethidine. *Br. J. Pharmacol. Chemother.* 16, 315.

Engelman, K. and Sjoerdsma, A. (1964). A new test for pheochromocytoma: pressor responsiveness to tyramine. *JAMA* 189, 81.

Euler, U.S. von. (1966). Relationship between histamine and the autonomic nervous system. In *Histamine: its chemistry, metabolism and physiological and pharmacological actions* (ed. M. Rocha e Silva). Part 1. *Handbuch der experimentellen Pharmakologie*, Vol. 18, p. 318. Springer-Verlag, Berlin.

Fadali, M.A., Ledbetter, B.S., Papacostas, C.A., Duke, L.J., and Lemore, G. M. (1974). Mechanism responsible for the cardiovascular depressant effect of protamine sulphate. *Ann. Surg.* 180, 232.

Fagard, R., Amery, A., and Timmermans, U. (1976). Severe hypotension during infusion of saralasin. *Lancet* i, 1136.

Fahmy, N.R., Sunder, N., and Sojer, N.A. (1983). Role of histamine in the haemodynamic and plasma catecholamine responses of morphine. *Clin. Pharmacol. Ther.* 33, 615.

Feldberg, W. and Lewis, J. (1964). The action of peptides on the adrenal medulla and release of adrenaline by bradykines and angiotensin II. *J. Physiol.* (Lond.) 171, 98.

Ferguson, R.M. and Sommer, B.G. (1985). Cyclosporine in renal transplantation: a single institutional experience. *Am. J. Kidney Dis.* 5, 296.

Ferguson, R.P. and Alvino, E. (1983). Rebound hypertension after low-dose clonidine. *South. Med. J.* 76, 98.

Fidlar, E. and Jaques, L.B. (1948). The effect of commercial heparin on the platelet count. *J. Lab. Clin. Med.* 33, 1410.

Fiessinger, J.N., Aiach, M., Roncato, M., Debure, C., and Gaux, J.-C. (1984). Critical ischemia during herapin-induced thrombocytopenia: treatment by intra-arterial streptokinase. *Thromb. Res.* 33, 235.

Fisher, J.R. and Padnick, G. (1983). Nifedipine and erythromelalgia. *Ann. Intern. Med.* 98, 671.

Folks, D.G. (1983). Monoamine oxidase inhibitors: reappraisal of dietary considerations. *J. Clin. Psychopharmacol.* 3, 249.

Franco, A., Bourlard, P., Massot, C., Lecoer, J., Guidicelli, H. and Bessard, G. (1978). Ergotisme aigu par association dihydroergotamine-triacétyloléandomycine. *Nouv. Presse Med.* 7, 205.

French, J. and White, H. (1989). Transient symptomatic hypotension in a patient on simvastatin. *Lancet* ii, 807.

Friederszick, F.K. (1949). Embolien während intramuskulärer Penicillin Behandlung. *Klin. Wochenschr.* 27, 173.

Gabriel, R. (1976). Paradoxical rise in blood pressure during propranolol treatment. *Br. Med. J.* i, 219.

Gabriel, R., Meek, D., and Mamtora, H. (1975). Adverse reactions to prazosin. *Br. Med. J.* iv, 41.

Gavras, H. and Gavras, I. (1988). Salt-induced hypertension: the interactive role of vasopressin and of the sympathetic nervous system. *J. Hypertension* 7, 601.

Generali, J.A. (1981). Hypertensive crisis resulting from avocados and a MAO inhibitor. *Drug Intell. Clin. Pharmacol.* 15, 904.

Gibson, G.J. and Warrell, D.A. (1972). Hypertensive crises and phenylpropanolamine. *Lancet* ii, 492.

Given, B.D., Taylor, T., Lilly, L.S., and Dzau, V.J. (1983). Symptomatic hypotension following the clonidine suppression test for pheochromocytoma. *Arch. Intern. Med.* 143, 2195.

Glover, W.E. and Hutchinson, J.J. (1964). The effect of a beta-receptor antagonist (propranolol) on the cardiovascular response to intravenous infusion of noradrenaline in man. *J. Physiol.* (Lond.) 177, 59P.

Godal, H.C. (1980). Report of the International Committee on Thrombosis and Haemostasis. Thrombocytopenia and heparin. *Thromb. Haemost.* 43, 222.

Goldfien, A., Zileli, M.S., Despointes, L.H., and Bethune, J.E. (1958). The effect of hypoglycaemia on the adrenal secretion of epinephrine and norepinephrine in the dog. *Endocrinology* 62, 749.

Goldman, V., Astrøm, A., and Evers, H. (1971). The effect of a tricyclic antidepressant on the cardiovascular effects of local anaesthetic solutions containing different vasoconstrictors. *Anaesthesia* 26, 91.

Gollub, S. and Ulin, A.W. (1962). Heparin-induced thrombocytopenia in man. *J. Lab. Clin. Med.* 59, 430.

Gordon, R.D., Iwatsuki, S., Shaw, B.W., and Starzl, T.E. (1985). Cyclosporine–steroid combination therapy in 84 cadaveric renal transplants. *Am. J. Kidney Dis.* 5, 307.

Gould, B.A., Mann, S., Davies, A., Altman, D.G., and Raftery, E.B. (1981). Indoramin: 24-hour profile of intra-arterial ambulatory blood pressure: a double-blind placebo-controlled crossover study. *Br. J. Clin. Pharmacol.* 12, 675.

Graham, R.M., Thornell, I.R., Gain, J.M., Bagnoli, C., Oates, H.F., and Stokes, G.S. (1976). Prazosin: the first dose phenomenon. *Br. Med. J.* ii, 1293.

Grassi, G.M., Somers, V.K., Renk, W.S., Abboud, F.M., and Mark, A.L. (1989). Effects of alcohol on blood pressure and sympathetic nerve activity in normotensive humans: a preliminary report. *J. Hypertension* 7 (suppl. 6), S20.

Green, H.D. and Grimsley, W.T. (1953). Effect of Regitine (c-7337) in patients, particularly those with peripheral vascular disease. *Circulation* 7, 487.

Green, S.T., Ng, J.P., and Callaghan, M. (1988). Metolazone and axillary vein thrombosis. *Scott. Med. J.* 33, 211.

Gremse, D.A., Artman, M., and Boerth, R.C. (1986). Hypertension associated with naloxone treatment for clonidine poisoning. *Pediatrics* 108, 776.

Guay, D.R.P. and Richard, A. (1948). Heparin-induced thrombocytopenia. Association with a platelet aggregating factor and cross-sensitivity to bovine and porcine heparin. *Drug Intell. Clin. Pharm.* 18, 398.

Hall, M.R., Richards, M.A., and Harper, P.G. (1988). Thromboembolic events during combination chemotherapy for germ-cell malignancy. *Lancet* ii, 1259.

Hamilton, D.V., Carmichael, D.J.S., Evans, D.B., and Calne, R.Y. (1982). Hypertension in renal transplant recipients on cyclosporine A and corticosteroids and azathioprine. *Transplant Proc.* 14, 597.

Hannah, P., Glover, V., and Sandler, M. (1988). Tyramine in wine and beer. *Lancet* i, 879.

Hansson, L., Hunyor, S.N., Julius, S., and Hoobler, S.W. (1973). Blood pressure crisis following withdrawal of clonidine (Catapres, Catapressan) with special reference to arterial and urinary catecholamine levels, and suggestions for acute management. *Am. Heart J.* 85, 605.

Hardesty, R.L., Griffith, B.P., Debski, R.F., and Bahnson, H.T. (1983). Experience with cyclosporine in cardiac transplantation. *Transplant Proc.* 15 (suppl. 1), 2553.

Harris, A.L. (1976). Clonidine withdrawal and blockade. *Lancet* i, 596.

Hayton, A.C. (1969). Precipitation of acute ergotism by triacetyloleandomycin. *N.Z. Med. J.* 69, 42.

Herlache, J., Hoskins, P., and Schmidt, C.M. (1973). Unilateral brachial artery thrombosis secondary to ergotamine tartrate. *Angiology* 24, 369.

Hesson, H., Kromann-Andersen, C., and Madsen, B. (1972). Peripheral arterial insufficiency during ergotamine treatment. *Dan. Med. Bull.* 19, 236.

Hessov, I. (1970). Hypertension during imipramine treatment. *Lancet* i, 84.

Hessov, I. (1971). Hypertension during chlorimipramine therapy. *Br. Med. J.* i, 406.

Hirsch, M. and Eger, M. (1972). Angiography in diagnosis of ergotism. *Radiology* 103, 89.

Hirsh, S.A., Robertson, H., and Gorniowsky, M. (1976). Arterial occlusion secondary to methylmethacrylate use. *Arch. Surg.* 111, 204.

Hodge, J.V., Nye, E.R., and Emerson, G.W. (1964). Monoamine-oxidase inhibitors, broad beans, and hypertension. *Lancet* i, 1108.

Hodsman, G.P., Isles, C.G., Murray, G.D., Usherwood, T.P., Webb, D.J., and Robertson, J.I.S. (1983). Factors related to the first-dose hypotensive effect of captopril: prediction and treatment. *Br. Med. J.* 286, 832.

Hoehn, M.M. (1975). Levo-dopa-induced postural hypotension. *Arch. Neurol.* 32, 50.

Hökfelt, H.H. and Dymling, J.F. (1970). The influence of Catapres on catecholamines, renin and aldosterone in man. In *Catapres in hypertension* (ed. M. E. Connolly), p. 88. Butterworth, Sevenoaks.

Horowitz, J.D., McNeill, J.J., Sweet, B., Mendelsohn, F.A.D., and Louis, W.J. (1979). Hypertension and postural hypotension induced by phenylpropanolamine (Trimolets). *Med. J. Aust.* i, 175.

Horowitz, J.D., Lang, W.J., Howes, L.G., Fennessy, M.R., Christophides, N., Rand, M.J., et al. (1980). Hypertensive response induced by phenylpropanolamine in anorectic and decongestant preparations. *Lancet* i, 60.

Horwitz, D., Goldberg, L.I., and Sjoerdsma, A. (1960). Increased blood pressure responses to dopamine and norepinephrine produced by monoamine oxidase inhibitors in man. *J. Lab. Clin. Med.* 56, 747.

Howrie, D.L. and Wolfson, J.H. (1983). Phenylpropanolamine-induced hypertensive seizures. *J. Pediatrics* 102, 143.

Hunyor, S.N., Hansson, L., Harrison, T.S., and Hoobler, S.W. (1973). Effects of clonidine withdrawal: possible mechanisms and suggestions for management. *Br. Med. J.* ii, 209.

Husum, B., Metz, P., and Rasmussen, J.P. (1979). Nitroglycerin infusion for ergotism. *Lancet* ii, 794.

Imms, F.J., Neame, R.L.B., and Powis, D.A. (1976). Paradoxical rise in blood pressure during propranolol treatment. *Br. Med. J.* i, 218.

Imrie, C.W. (1973). Arterial spasm associated with oral ergotamine therapy. *Br. J. Clin. Pract.* 27, 457.

Isaac, T., Mitchell, B., and Grahame-Smith, D.G. (1977). Monoamine oxidase inhibitors and caviar. *Lancet* ii, 816.

Joss, D.V., Barrett, S.J., Kendra, J.R., Lucas, C.F., and Desai, S. (1982). Hypertension and convulsions in children receiving cyclosporin A. *Lancet* i, 906.

Journal of the American Medical Association (1974). Medical News — A warning about oxytocin in bolus form. *JAMA* 230, 1373.

Julka, N.K. and Nora, J.R. (1976). Gangrene aggravation after use of dopamine. *JAMA* 235, 2812.

Kaufmann, J.S. (1974). Pheochromocytoma and tricyclic antidepressants. *JAMA* 229, 1282.

Kelton, J.G. and Hirsh, J. (1980). Bleeding associated with antithrombotic therapy. *Sem. Hematol.* 17, 259.

Khairallah, P.A., Davila, D., and Papanicolaou, N. (1971). Effects of angiotensin infusion on catecholamine uptake and reactivity in blood vessels. *Circ. Res.* 28 (suppl. 2), 96.

Kholeif, M. and Isles, C. (1989). Profound hypotension after atenolol in severe hypertension. *Br. Med. J.* 298, 161.

Killian, J.M. and Fromm, G.A. (1968). Carbamazepine in the treatment of neuralgia. Use and side effects. *Arch. Neurol.* 19, 129.

King, D.J. and Kelton, J.G. (1984). Heparin-associated thrombocytopenia. *Ann. Intern. Med.* 100, 535.

Klatsky, A.L., Friedman, G.D., and Armstrong, M.A. (1986). The relationship between alcoholic beverage use and other traits to blood pressure: a new Kaiser Permanente Study. *Circulation* 73, 628.

Knox, J.W.D., Bovill, J.G., Clark, R.S.J., and Dundee, J.W. (1970). Clinical studies of induction agents, XXXVI: Ketamine. *Br. J. Anaesth.* 42, 875.

Koelle, G.B. (1970). Neuromuscular blocking agents. In *The pharmacological basis of therapeutics* (5th edn) (ed. L.S. Goodman and A. Gilman), p. 612. Collier Macmillan, London.

Krupp, P., Gulich, A., and Timonen, P. (1986). Treatment with cyclosporine combination therapy. *Transplant Proc.* 18, 991.

Kumana, C.P. and Marlin, G.E. (1978). Selectivity of beta-adrenoceptor agonists. In *Recent advances in clinical pharmacology* (ed. P. Turner and D.G. Shand), p. 31. Churchill, Edinburgh.

Küster, G. and Ritz, E. (1989). Analgesic abuse and hypertension. *Lancet* ii, 1105.

Lacouture, P.G., Epstein, M.F., and Mitchell, A.A. (1987). Vancomycin-associated shock and rash in infants. *J. Pediatr.* 111, 615.

Lai, K.N., Richards, A.M., and Nicholls, M.G. (1991). Drug-induced hypertension. *Adverse Drug React. Acute Toxicol. Rev.* 10, 1.

Lake, C.R., Zalaga, G., Bray, J., Rosenberg, D., and Chernow, B. (1989). Transient hypertension after two phenylpropanolamine diet aids and the effects of caffeine: a placebo-controlled follow-up study. *Am. J. Med.* 86, 427.

The Lancet (1965). Pressor attacks during treatment with monoamine oxidase inhibitors. *Lancet* i, 945.

The Lancet (1974). Acrylic cement and the cardiovascular system. *Lancet* ii, 1002.

The Lancet (1988). Cyclosporin hypertension. *Lancet* ii, 1234.

Langdon, L. (1977). Transient hypotension following intravenous ethamsylate (Dicynene). *Br. Med. J.* i, 1472.

Laurence, D.A. and Nagle, R.E. (1961). The interaction of bretylium with pressor agents. *Lancet* i, 593.

Laurenson, V.G. and Davis, F.M. (1985). An adverse reaction to clomethiazole. *Anaesth. Intens. Care* 13, 438.

Lawrence, C.A. (1978). Pethidine-induced hypertension in phaeochromocytoma. *Br. Med J.* i, 149.

Leal-Cerro, A., Garcia-Luna, P.P., Villar, J., Miranda, M.L., Pereira, J.L., Gomez-Pan, A., *et al.* (1989). Arterial hypertension as a complication of prolonged ketoconazole treatment. *J. Hypertension* 7 (suppl. 6), S 212.

Lee, K.Y., Beilin, L.J., and Vandongen, R. (1979). Severe hypertension after ingestion of an appetite suppressant (phenylpropanolamine) with indomethacin. *Lancet* i, 1110.

Lees, B.J. and Cabal, L.A. (1981). Increased blood pressure following pupillary dilatation with 2.5% phenylephrine hydrochloride in preterm infants. *Pediatrics* 68, 231.

Levesque, H., Moore, L.M., and Courtois, H. (1989). Erythromelalgia induced by nicardipine. *Br. Med. J.* 298, 1252.

Levine, M.N., Gent, M. Hirsh, J., Arnold, A., Goodyear, M.D., Hryniuk, W., *et al.* (1988). The thrombogenic effect of anticancer drug therapy in women with stage II breast cancer. *N. Engl. J. Med.* 318, 404.

Lewis, M.J., Ross, P.J., and Henderson, A.H. (1979). Rebound effect after stopping beta-blockers. *Br. Med. J.* ii, 606.

Leyton, N. (1964). Methysergide in the prophylaxis of migraine. *Lancet* i, 830.

Linch, D.C., Swan, K.M., Muttlemann, M.F., and Ross, E.J. (1978). Bromocriptine-induced postural hypotension in acromegaly. *Lancet* ii, 321.

Loeliger, E.A. (1975). Drugs affecting blood clotting and fibrinolysis. In *Meyler's side effects of drugs* (ed. M.N.G. Dukes), p. 777. Excerpta Medica, Amsterdam.

Lorenz, W. and Doenicke, A. (1978). Anaphylactoid reactions and histamine release by intravenous drugs used in surgery and anaesthesia. In *Adverse response to intravenous drugs* (ed. J. Watkins and A.M. Ward), p. 83. Academic Press, London.

Lorenz, W., Doenicke, A., Messmer, H.-J., Thermann, M., Lahn, W., Berr, J., *et al.* (1976). Histamine release in human subjects by modified gelatin (Haemaccel) and dextran: an explanation for anaphylactoid reactions observed under clinical conditions. *Br. J. Anaesth.* 48, 151.

Loughran, T.P., Deeg, H.J., Dahlberg, S., Kennedy, M.S., Storb, R., and Thomas, E.D. (1985). Incidence of hypertension after bone marrow transplantation among 112 patients randomized to either cyclosporin or methotrexate as graft-versus-host disease prophylaxis. *Br. J. Haematol.* 59, 547.

McAllister, R.G. Jr (1981). Hypertensive crisis and myocardial infarction after fluorescein angiography. *South. Med. J.* 74, 504.

McCloy, R.F. and Baron, J.H. (1977). Acute reaction to pentagastrin. *Lancet* i, 548.

McEwen, J. (1983). Phenylpropanolamine-associated hypertension after the use of over-the-counter appetite suppressant product. *Med. J. Aust.* ii, 71.

McGrath, P.J., Stewart, J.W., and Quitkin, F.M. (1989). A possible L-deprenyl-induced hypertensive reaction. *J. Psychopharmacol.* 9, 310.

McLaren, E.H. (1976). Severe hypertension produced by interaction of phenylpropanolamine with methyldopa and oxprenolol. *Br. Med. J.* ii, 283.

McLoughlin, M.G. and Saunders, R.J. (1972). Ergotism causing peripheral vascular ischaemia. *Rocky Mount. Med. J.* 69, 45.

McPhaul, M., Punzi, H.A., Sandy, A., Borganelli, M., Rude, R., and Kaplan, N.M. (1984). Snuff-induced hypertension in pheochromocytoma. *JAMA* 252, 2860.

Maddern, P.J., Davis, N.L. and McGlew, I. (1976). Case report: pheochromocytoma. Aspects of management. *Anaesth. Intens. Care* 4, 156.

Maggi, J.D., Angelots, J., and Scott, J.P. (1982). Gangrene in a neonate following dopamine therapy. *J. Pediatr.* 100, 323.

Mahon, W.A. and Kolton, N. (1978). Hypotension after intravenous cimetidine. *Lancet* i, 828.

Main, J. and Wilkinson, R. (1989). Early renal artery occlusion after enalapril in atheromatous renal artery stenosis. *Br. Med. J.* 229, 394.

Makker, S.P. and Moorthy, B. (1980). Rebound hypertension following minoxidil withdrawal. *J. Pediatr.* 96, 762.

Malatack, J.J., Zitelli, B.J., and Gartner, J.C. (1983). Pediatric liver transplantation under therapy with cyclosporin A and steroids. *Transplant Proc.* 15, 1292.

Mandt, P.R., Robinson, C.A., Sarnoff, R.B., and Colwell, C.W. Jr (1985). Heparin-associated thrombocytopenia with venous thrombosis. A case report. *J. Bone Joint Surg.* 67-A, 1123.

Marriott, H.J.L. (1957). An alarming pressor reaction to Regitine. *Ann. Intern. Med.* 44, 1001.

Marshall, A.J., Roberts, C.J.C., and Barritt, D.W. (1966). Raynaud's phenomenon as side-effect of beta-blocker in hypertension. *Br. Med. J.* i, 1498.

Martin, J. and Moncada, S. (1988). Blood pressure, erythropoietin, and nitric oxide. *Lancet* i, 644.

Matthews, T.G., Wilczek, Z.N., and Shennan, A.T. (1977). Eye-drop induced hypertension. *Lancet* ii, 827.

Mayer, R.D. and Montgomery, S.A. (1989). Acute hypertensive episode induced by sulpiride. *Hum. Psychopharmacol. Clin. Exp.* 4, 149.

Mayhew, J.F. and Deutsch, S. (1985). Cardiac arrest following administration of vancomycin. *Can. Anaesth. Soc. J.* 32, 65.

Milne, A., Talbot, S., Bevan, D. (1988). Thromboses during cytotoxic chemotherapy. *Br. Med. J.* 297, 624.

Mindham, R.H.S. (1975). Hypnotics and sedatives. In *Meyler's side effects of drugs* (ed. M.N.G. Dukes), p. 67. Excerpta Medica, Amsterdam.

Montaldi, D.H., Giambrone, J.P., Courey, N.G., and Taefi, P. (1974). Podophyllin poisoning associated with the treatment of condylomata acuminata: a case report. *Am. J. Obstet. Gynecol.* 119, 1130.

Moorhead, E.L.II., Caldwell, J.R., Kelly, A.R., and Morales, A.R. (1966). The diagnosis of pheochromocytoma: analysis of 26 cases. *JAMA* 196, 1107.

Muelheims, G.H., Entrup, R.W., Paiewonsky, D., and Mierzwiak, D.S. (1965). Increased sensitivity of the heart to catecholamine-induced arrhythmias following guanethidine. *Clin. Pharmacol. Ther.* 6, 757.

Murray, B.M. and Paller, M.S. (1986). Beneficial effects of renal denervation and prazosin on GFR and renal blood flow after cyclosporin in rats. *Clin. Nephrol.* 25 (suppl. 1), S37.

Mushin, W.W., Wien, R., Mason, D.F.J., and Langston. G.T. (1949). Curare-like actions of tri(diethylaminoethoxy)-benzine triethyliodide. *Lancet* i, 726.

Nelemans, F.A. (1972). Cholinomimetic drugs and anticholinesterases. In *Side effects of drugs* Vol. 7(ed. L. Meyler and A. Herxheimer), p. 240. Excerpta Medica, Amsterdam.

Newens, A.F. and Volz, R.G. (1972). Severe hypotension during prosthetic hip surgery with acrylic bone cement. *Anesthesiology* 36, 298.

Newfield, P. and Roizen, M.F. (1979). Hazards of rapid administration of vancomycin. *Ann. Intern. Med.* 91, 581.

Ng, K.H. and Sen, D.K. (1974). Hypotension with intravenous salbutamol in premature labour. *Br. Med. J.* iii, 211.

Nickerson, M. (1970). Drugs inhibiting adrenergic nerves and structures innervated by them. In *The pharmacological basis of therapeutics* (ed. L.S. Goodman and A. Gilman), p. 560. Collier Macmillan, London.

Ogilvie, C.M. (1955). The treatment of pulmonary tuberculosis with iproniazid (1-isonicotinyl-2-isopropyl hydrazine) and isoniazid (isonicotinyl hydrazine). *Q. J. Med.* 24, 175.

Oh, T.E., Turner, C.W., Ilett, K.F., Waterson, J.G., and Paterson, J.W. (1978). Mechanism of the hypertensive effects of droperidol in phaeochromocytoma. *Anaesth. Intens. Care* 6, 322.

Otteni, J.C., Sauvage, M.R., and Gauthier-Lafaye, J.P. (1969). Effets cardiovasculaires de la pentazocine. *Anaesth. Anal. Reanim.* 26, 271.

Palestine, A.G., Nussenblatt, B.B., and Chan, C.C (1984). Side-effects of systemic cyclosporine in a patient *not* undergoing transplantation. *Am. J. Med.* 77, 652.

Park, G.R. (1978). Hypotension following intravenous administration of metoclopramide during hypotensive anaesthesia for intracranial aneurysm. *Br. J. Anaesth.* 50, 1268.

Partridge, B.L., Key, T., and Reisner, L.S. (1988). Life-threatening effects of intravascular absorbtion of PGF_2 during therapeutic termination of pregnancy. *Anesth. Analg.* (Cleveland) 67, 111.

Paterson, A.H.G. (1978). Hypertensive reaction to adriamycin. *Cancer Treat. Rep.* 62, 1269.

Paton, W.D.M. (1957). Histamine release by compounds of simple chemical structure. *Pharmacol. Rev.* 9, 269.

Peach, M.J. (1971). Adrenal medullary stimulation induced by angiotensin, angiotensin II, and analogues. *Circ. Res.* 28 (suppl. 2), 107.

Peach, M.J., Cline, W.H.J.R., and Watts, D.T. (1978). Release of adrenal catecholamines by angiotensin II. *Circ. Res.* 35, 592.

Pearson, A.C., Labovitz, A.J., and Kern, M.J. (1987). Accelerated hypertension complicated by myocardial infarction after use of a local anesthetic/vasoconstrictor preparation. *Am. Heart J.* 114, 662.

Peebles, D.J., Ellis, R.H., Stride, S.D.K., and Simpson, B.R.J. (1972). Cardiovascular effects of methylmethacrylate cement. *Br. Med. J.* i, 349.

Pegg, M.S. (1980). Hypotension following metoclopramide injection. *Anaesthesia,* 35, 615.

Pelner, L. and Waldman, S. (1960). Tissue necrosis and metaraminol bitartrate. *JAMA* 172, 1196.

Pettinger, W.A. and Keeton, K. (1975). Hypotension during angiotensin blockade with saralasin. *Lancet,* i, 1387.

Pettinger, W.A., and Oates, J.A. (1968). Supersensitivity to tyramine during monoamine oxidase inhibition in man; mechanism at the level of adrenergic neuron. *Clin. Pharmacol. Ther.* 9, 341.

Pinder, R.M., Brogden, R.N., Speight, T.M., and Avery, G.S. (1977). Voloxazine: a review of its pharmacological properties and therapeutic efficacy in depressive illness. *Drugs* 13, 401.

Pingleton, S.K., Schwartz, O., Szymanski, D., and Epstein, M. (1982). Hypotension associated with terbutaline in acute quadriplegia. *Am. Rev. Resp. Dis.* 126, 723.

Plouin, P.F., Menard, J., and Corvol, P. (1976). Hypertensive crises in patient with phaeochromocytoma given metoclopramide. *Lancet* ii, 1357.

Prescott, L.F. (1972). Antipyretic analgesics and drugs used in rheumatic diseases and gout. In *Side effects of drugs*, Vol. 7 (ed. L. Meyler and A. Herxheimer), p. 156. Excerpta Medica, Amsterdam.

Price, H.L. and Dripps, R.D. (1970). General anaesthetics. In *The pharmacological basis of therapeutics* (ed. L.S. Goodman and A. Gilman), p. 81. Collier Macmillan, London.

Prichard, B.N.C. (1964). Some cardiovascular actions of adrenergic beta-receptor blocking drugs in man. *Pharmacologist* 6, 166.

Quagliarello, J. and Barakat, R. (1987). Raynaud's phenomenon in infertile women treated with bromocriptine. *Fertil. Steril.* 48, 877.

Quick, A.J., Schanberge, J.N., and Stefanini, M. (1948). The effect of heparin on platelets *in vivo. J. Lab. Clin. Med.* 33, 1424.

Raine, A.E.G. (1988). Hypertension, blood viscosity and cardiovascular morbidity in renal failure: implications of erythropoietin therapy. *Lancet* i, 97.

Rampton, D.S. (1977). Hypertensive crisis in a patient given Sinemet, metoclopramide, and amitriptyline. *Br. Med. J.* ii, 607.

Ramsay, I.D. and Langlands, J.H.M. (1962). Phaeochromocytoma with hypotension and polycythaemia. *Lancet* ii, 126.

Ratzenhofer, M. Personal communication to Winkler, H. and Smith, A.D. (1968). Catecholamines in phaeochromocytoma: normal storage but abnormal release? *Lancet* i, 793.

Raw, K. and Gaylis, H. (1976). Acute arterial spasm of the lower extremities after methysergide therapy. *S. Afr. Med. J.* 50, 1999.

Reich, D.L. (1989). Transient systemic arterial hypotension and cutaneous flushing in response to doxacuronium chloride. *Anesthesiology* 71, 783.

Reid, J.L., Wing, L.N.H., Dargie, H.J., Hamilton, C.A., Davies, D.S., and Dollery, C.T. (1977). Clonidine withdrawal in hypertension. Changes in blood pressure and plasma and urinary noradrenaline. *Lancet* i, 1171.

Rhodes, G.R., Dixon, R.H., and Silver, D. (1973). Heparin-induced thrombocytopenia with thrombotic and hemorrhagic manifestations. *Surg. Gynecol. Obstet.* 136, 409.

Ribstein, J., Rodier, M., and Mimran, A. (1989). Effect of cylosporin on blood pressure and renal function of recent type 1 diabetes mellitus. *J. Hypertension* 7 (suppl. 6), S198.

Rizk, G.K., El-Khoury, G.Y., and Deeb, Z.L. (1973). Peripheral arterial ischaemia due to ergotism. *J. Cardiovasc. Surg.* 14, 353.

Robinson, M.J. and Williams, A. (1956). Clinical and pathological details of two cases of phaeochromocytoma in childhood. *Arch. Dis. Child.* 31, 69.

Rodger, J.C., Sheldon, C.O., Lerski, R.A., and Livingston, W.R. (1976). Intermittent claudication complicating beta-blockade. *Br. Med. J.* i, 1125.

Roland, C.B. (1959). Pheochromocytoma in pregnancy. Report of a fatal reaction to phentolamine (Regitine) methanesulfonate. *JAMA* 171, 1806.

Ross, E.J., Prichard, B.N.C., Kaufman, L., Robertson, A.I.G., and Harries, B.J. (1967). Preoperative and operative management of patients with phaeochromocytoma. *Br. Med. J.* i, 191.

Russell, R.M. and Jones, R.M. (1989). Postoperative hypotension associated with enalapril. *Anaesthesia* 44, 837.

SADRAC Bulletin (1989). Dihydroergotamine + lidocaine — vasospasm. *Bulletin from the Swedish Adverse Drug Reactions Advisory Committee* 54, 1.

Sachdev, Y., Gomez-Pan, A., Tunbridge, W.M.G., Duns, A., Woigatman, D.R., and Hall, R. (1975). Bromocriptine therapy in acromegaly. *Lancet* ii, 1164.

Sandler, R.M., Seifer, D.B., Morgan, K., Pockros, P.J, Wypych, J., Weiss, L.M., *et al.* (1985). Heparin-induced thrombocytopenia and thrombosis. Detection and specificity of a platelet-aggregation IgG. *Am. J. Clin. Pathol.* 83, 760.

Sarcione, E.J., Back, N., Sokal, J.E., Mehlman, B., and Knoblock, E. (1963). Elevation of plasma epinephrine levels produced by glucagon *in vivo. Endocrinology* 72, 523.

Saunders, J.B., Beevers, D.G., and Paton, A. (1981). Alcohol-induced hypertension. *Lancet* ii, 856.

Schachter, M. (1988). Cyclosporin A and hypertension. *J. Hypertension* 6, 511.

Schindel, L. (1972). Intravenous infusion solutions and emulsions. In *Side effects of drugs* (ed. L. Meyler and A. Herxheimer), p. 479. Excerpta Medica, Amsterdam.

Schmidt, G.R. and Schuna, A.A. (1988). Rebound hypertension after discontinuation of transdermal clonidine. *Clin. Pharm.* 7, 772.

Schoenfeld, A., Friedman, S., Stein, L.B., Hirsch, M., and Ovadia, J. (1987). Severe hypertension reaction after naloxone injection during labor. *Arch. Gynecol.* 240, 45.

Schroeder, J.M. and Weeth, J.B. (1967). Phase II evaluation of fluorometholone (NSC-33001). *Cancer Chemother.* Abstr. 51, 525.

Scian, L.F., Westerman, C.D., Verdesca, A.S., and Hilton, J.G. (1960). Adrenocortical and medullary effects of glucagon in dogs. *Am. J. Physiol.* 199, 867.

Scott, J.N. and McDevitt, B.G. (1976). Rebound hypertension after acute methyldopa withdrawal. *Br. Med. J.* ii, 367.

Seedat, Y.K., Bhoola, R., and Rampono, J.G. (1975). Prazosin in treatment of hypertension. *Br. Med. J.* ii, 305.

Semple, P.F., Thoren, P., and Lever, A.F. (1988). Vasovagal reactions to cardiovascular drugs: the first dose effect. *J. Hypertension* 6, 601.

Sennesael, J., Dupont, A.G., Verbeeler, D.L., van Haelst, L., and Paul, L.C. (1986). Hypertension and cyclosporine. *Ann. Intern. Med.* 104, 729.

Shanks, R.G. (1970). Hypotension caused by L-dopa. *Br. Med. J.* iii, 403.

Shaub, R.O. (1960). Ischemic necrosis due to administration of metaraminol. *JAMA* 172, 154.

Siehe, H.J. (1934). Die Reaktion des denervierten Nebennierenmarkes auf humorale Sekretionsweise. *Arch. Ges. Physiol.* 234, 204.

Silver, D., Kapsch, D.N., and Tsoi, E.K.M. (1983). Heparin-induced thrombocytopenia, thrombosis, and hemorrhage. *Ann. Surg.* 198, 301.

Sinal S.H. and Crowe. J.E. (1976). Cyanosis and hypotension following administration of paraldehyde. *Pediatrics* 57, 158.

Sloand, E.M. and Thompson, B.T. (1984). Propranolol induced pulmonary edema and shock in a patient with pheochromocytoma. *Arch. Intern. Med.* 144, 173.

Smith, N.L. (1957). Histamine release by suxamethonium. *Anaesthesia* 12, 293.

Sniper, W. (1952). The estimation and comparison of histamine release by muscle relaxants. *Br. J. Anaesth.* 24, 232

Solosko, D. and Smith, R.B. (1972). Hypertension following 10 per cent phenylephrine ophthalmic. *Anesthesiology* 36, 187.

Spedding, M. (1980). Effects of metoclopramide and isoprenaline on the rat vas deferens: interaction with adrenoceptors. *Br. J. Pharmacol.* 71, 113.

Sperzel, W.D., Glassman, H.N., Jordan D.C., and Luther, R.R. (1986). Overall safety of terazosin as an antihypertensive agent. *Am. J. Med.* 80 (suppl. 5B), 77.

Spivak, B., Radvan, M., and Shine, M. (1987). Postural hypotension with syncope possibly precipitated by trazodone. *Am. J. Psychiatry* 144, 1512.

Stafford, P.J., Strachan, C.J.L., Vincent, R., and Chamberlain, D.A. (1989). Multiple microemboli after disintegration of clot during thrombolysis for acute myocardial infarction. *Br. Med. J.* 299, 1310.

Staszewska-Barczak, J. and Vane, J.R. (1965). The release of catecholamines from the adrenal medulla by histamine. *Br. J. Pharmacol.* 24, 728.

Steele, J.M. Jr, and Lowenstein, J. (1975). Differential effects of angiotensin II analogue on pressor and adrenal receptors in the rabbit. *Circ. Res.* 35, 592.

Stelzer, F.T., Stubenbord, J.J., Sreenivasan, V., and Venutto, R.C. (1976). Late toxicity of clonidine withdrawal. *N. Engl. J. Med.* 294, 1182.

Stevens, F.R.T. (1966). A danger of sympathomimetic drugs. *Med. J. Aust.* ii, 576.

Stevens, J.E. (1980). Rebound hypertension during anaesthesia. *Anaesthesia* 35, 490.

Stewart, M. (1976). MAOIs and food — fact and fiction. *Adverse Drug React. Bull.* 58, 196.

Stewart, M. and Burris, J.F. (1988). Clonidine: rebound hypertension. *Drug Intell. Clin. Pharm.* 22, 573.

Stockley, I. (1974). *Drug interactions and their mechanisms.* The Pharmaceutical Press, London.

Stoner, T.R. and Urbach, K.F. (1968). Cardiac arrhythmias associated with succinylcholine in a patient with pheochromocytoma. *Anesthesiology* 19, 1228.

Stromblad, B.C.R. (1960). Effect of denervation and of cocaine on action of sympathetic amines. *Br. J. Pharmacol.* 15, 328.

Sumikawa, K. and Amakata, Y. (1977). The pressor effect of droperidol on a patient with pheochromocytoma. *Anesthesiology* 46, 359.

Supprian, U. (1969). Ueber einen Fall von Antabusintoxikation. *Nervenarzt* 40, 276.

Svedmyr, N. (1968). The influence of a tricyclic antidepressant agent (protriptyline) on some of the circulatory effects of noradrenaline and adrenaline in man. *Life Sci.* 7, 77.

Swan, H.J.C. (1949). Effects of noradrenaline in the human circulation. *Lancet* ii, 508.

Szczygielski, J. (1932). Die adrenalinabsondernde Wirking des Histamins und ihre Beinflussung durch Nikotin. *Naunyn Schmiedebergs Arch. Exp. Pathol. Pharmakol.* 166, 319.

Tanaka, G.Y. (1974). Hypertensive reaction to naloxone. *JAMA* 228, 25.

Tao, P.K., Nicholls, M.G., and Lai, K.N. (1990). The complications of newer transplant antirejection drugs: treatment with cyclosporin A, OKT3, and FK506. *Adverse Drug React. Acute Poisoning Rev.* 9, 123.

Thompson, M.E., Shapiro, A.P., Johnsen, A.M., Itzkoff, J.M., Hardesty, R.L., Griffith, B.P., *et al.* (1986). The contrasting effects of cyclosporin A and azathioprine on arterial blood pressure and renal function following cardiac transplantation. *Int. J. Cardiol.* 11, 219.

Tirlapur, V.G., Evans, P.J., and Jones, M.K. (1986). Shock syndrome after acebutolol. *Br. J.Clin. Pract.* 40, 33.

Tomson, C.R.V., Venning, M.C., and Ward, M.K. (1988). Blood pressure and erythropoietin. *Lancet* i, 351.

Trash, D., Grundmann, M., Cargill, J., and Christopher, L., (1976). Cold extremities and beta-blockers. *Br. Med. J.* ii, 527.

Turner, A.S. (1976). Prazosin in hypertension. *Br. Med. J.* ii, 1257.

Unger, R.H., Eisentraut, A.M., McCall, M.S., and Maddison, L.L. (1962). Measurement of endogenous glucagon in plasma and the influence of blood glucose concentrations upon its secretion. *J. Clin. Invest.* 41, 682.

Vale, J.A. and Jeffereys, D.B. (1978). Peripheral gangrene complicating beta-blockade. *Lancet* i, 1216.

Valentine, B.H., Martin, M.A., and Phillips, N.V. (1977). Collapse during operation following intravenous ergotamine. *Br. J. Anaesth.* 49, 81.

Vallance, P., Benjamin, N., and Collier, J. (1988). Erythropoietin, haemoglobin, and hypertensive crises. *Lancet* i, 1107.

Vanholder, R., Carpenter, R.J., Schurgers, M., and Clemant, D.L. (1977). Rebound phenomenon during gradual withdrawal of clonidine. *Br. Med. J.* i, 1138.

van Vroonhoven, T.J.M.V. (1977). Intermittent claudication in premenopausal women. *J. Cardiovasc. Surg.* 18, 291.

van Way, C.W., Faraci, R.P., Cleveland, H.C., Foster, J.F., and Scott, H.W. (1976). Hemorrhagic necrosis of pheochromocytoma associated with phentolamine administration. *Ann. Surg.* 184, 26.

Vayssairat, M., Fiessinger, J.N., Becquemin, M.H., and Housset, E. (1978). Association déhydroergotamine et triacétyloléandomycine. Rôle dans une necrose digitale iatrogène. *Nouv. Presse Med.* 7, 2077.

Volle, R.L. and Koelle, G.B. (1970). Ganglionic stimulating and blocking agents. In *The pharmacological basis of therapeutics* (ed. L. S. Goodman and A. Gilman), pp. 596, 598. Collier Macmillan, London.

Wachter, R.M. (1987). Symptomatic hypertension induced by nifedipine in the acute treatment of severe hypertension. *Arch. Intern. Med.* 147, 556.

Waller, P.C., Cameron, H.A., and Ramsay, L.E. (1987). Profound hypotension after the first dose of ketanserin. *Postgrad. Med. J.* 63, 305.

Wark, J.D. and Larkins, R.G. (1978). Pulmonary oedema after propranolol therapy in two cases of phaeochromocytoma. *Br. Med. J.* i, 1395.

Wass, J.A.H., Thorner, M.O., and Besser, G.M. (1976). Digitalis vasospasm with bromocriptine. *Lancet* i, 1135.

Wass, J.A. H., Thorner, M.O., Morris, D.V., Rees, L.H., Mason, A.S., Jones, A.E., *et al.* (1977). Long-term treatment of acromegaly with bromocriptine. *Br. Med. J.* i, 875.

Watson, B. (1972). Transient hypotension following intravenous ethamsylate (Dicynene). *Br. Med. J.* i, 1664.

Webb, D.G. and White J.P. (1980). Hypertension after taking hydralazine. *Br. Med. J.* 280, 1582.

Webster, J., Jeffers, A., Galloway, D.B., and Petrie, J.C. (1974). Withdrawal of antihypertensive therapy. *Lancet* ii, 1381.

Webster, L.T. (1985). Drugs used in the chemotherapy of protozoal infections. In *Goodman and Gilman's The pharmacological basis of therapeutics* (7th edn) (ed. A.G. Gilman, L.S. Goodman, T.W. Rall, and F. Murad), p. 1062. Macmillan, New York.

Weidle, P.J. and Vlasses, P.H. (1988). Systemic hypertension associated with cyclosporine: a review. *Drug Intell. Clin. Pharm.* 22, 443.

Wein, P., Robertson, B., and Ratten, G.J. (1989). Cardiorespiratory collapse and pulmonary oedema due to intravascular absorption of prostaglandin $F_{2\alpha}$ administered intra-amniotically for midtrimester termination of pregnancy. *Aust. N.Z. J. Obstet. Gynaecol.* 29, 261.

Weinblatt, M.E., Coblyn, J.S., Fraser, P.A., Anderson, R.J., Spragg, J., Trentham, D.E., et al. (1987). Cyclosporin A treatment of refractory rheumatoid arthritis. *Arthritis Rheum.* 30, 11.

Weiner, N., Draskoczy, P.R., and Burack, W.R. (1962). Ability of tyramine to liberate catecholamines *in vivo*. *J. Pharmacol. Exp. Ther.* 137, 47.

Werquin, S., Kacet, S., Caron, J., Lacroix, D., Libersa, C., Cogeti, J.M., et al. (1987). Raynaud's phenomenon and finger necrosis after treatment of an ovarian seminoma with bleomycin, vinblastine, and 5-fluorouracil. *Ann. Cardiol. Angiol.* 36, 409.

Western, K.A., Perera, D.R., and Schultz, M.G. (1976). Pentamidine isethionate in the treatment of *Pneumocystis carinii* pneumonia. *Ann. Intern. Med.* 73, 695.

Westgate, H.D. and van Bergen, F.H. (1962). Changes in histamine blood levels following D-tubocurarine. *Can. Anesth. Soc. J.* 9, 497.

White, N.W. (1989). Venous thrombosis and rifampicin. *Lancet* ii, 434.

Wieland, T. and Staübli, M. (1988). Serious complications of enalapril therapy with cardiac failure. *Schweiz. Med. Wochenschr.* 118, 1789.

Wilkins, R.W., Geer, W.E.R., and Culbertson, J.W. (1950). Extensive laboratory studies of a patient with pheochromocytoma before and after successful operation. *Arch. Intern. Med.* 86, 51.

Williams, R., Blackburn, A., Neuberger, J., and Calne, R.Y. (1985). Long-term use of cyclosporin in liver grafting. *Q. J. Med.* 57, 897.

Winter, S., Frankle, H., Ribot, S., and Kirschner, M.A. (1973). Sorbitol-induced coma in uremic patients undergoing peritoneal dialysis. *J. Newark Beth Israel Med. Center* 23, 175.

Womack, A.M. (1963). Tranylcypromine. *Lancet* ii, 463.

Woods, K.L. (1978). Hypotensive effect of propranolol and phenoperidine in tetanus. *Br. Med. J.* ii, 1164.

Wu, C.C. and Johnson, A.J. (1969). The vasopressor effects of indigo carmine. *Henry Ford Hosp. Med. J.* 17, 131.

Yard, A.C. and Kadowitz, P.J. (1972). Studies on the mechanism of hydrocortisone potentiation of vasoconstrictor response to epinephrine in the anaesthetized animal. *Eur. J. Pharmacol.* 20, 1.

8. Respiratory disorders

N. P. KEANEY

Introduction

Pulmonary damage caused by undesired effects of drugs is being recognized with increasing frequency in clinical practice. The manner in which the lung responds to a toxic insult is limited. The symptoms and signs, and the radiological and laboratory features, are mainly non-specific. An adverse drug reaction (ADR) may therefore be readily confused with an exacerbation of a continuing disease process. This is especially true if the onset is subacute or chronic, and great vigilance is necessary if the correct diagnosis is to be made. Rechallenge is not usually undertaken to confirm a diagnosis of pulmonary adverse reactions — surprisingly in view of the widespread clinical use of challenge testing in the assessment of occupational asthma and extrinsic allergic alveolitis, for example, in pigeon fanciers.

In some instances the ADR is due to a known pharmacological effect of the drug (Type A reaction) and in others it is the result of totally aberrant and unpredictable effects (Type B reaction). In many, the underlying mechanism is obscure, but usually it is possible to identify the level in the respiratory tract at which the disorder is arising. Only the pulmonary vasculature, bronchi and lower airways, lung parenchyma, pleural space, mediastinum, and central ventilatory control and respiratory muscles will be discussed here; the upper airways and nose are discussed in Chapter 20.

Pulmonary vasculature

Pulmonary arteries

Pulmonary thromboembolism

Pharmacoepidemiological investigation was firmly established as a methodology in the 1960s with the convincing demonstration that the incidence of thromboembolic disease necessitating hospitalization was nine times higher in women who had taken oral contraceptives than in those who had not (Vessey and Doll 1968). The strong possibility of an association with the dose of oestrogen in combined preparations was subsequently shown (Inman *et al.* 1970), and Lehrman (1976), not surprisingly, found an increased risk of thromboembolism in transsexual males treated with high doses of oral oestrogen. More recently, Vessey and colleagues (1986) have confirmed the thromboembolic risk of oral contraceptives in a large prospective study of 17 000 married women, aged 25–39 years, in whom 105 episodes of venous thromboembolism occurred, 71 postoperatively. The incidence of certain or probable deep venous thrombosis or pulmonary embolism was 0.43 per thousand woman-years in users and 0.06 in non-users of oral contraceptives. The prevalence of postoperative problems was high, but the risk was confined to current users. Sue-Ling and Hughes (1988) believe the risk of pregnancy does not warrant discontinuing a combined oral contraceptive preoperatively but a progestogen-only pill is undoubtedly safer.

Other forms of embolism

Pulmonary embolization of particulate matter may occur during intravenous therapy and incorrect techniques may result in part of a cannula being sheared off. Intravenous illicit substance abuse may cause pulmonary thrombosis or granulomatous vasculitis or infections, for example, a staphylococcal abscess. Self-administration of crushed tablets is especially dangerous because of particulate fillers, which impact in pulmonary arterioles, and episodes with clinical features of pulmonary embolism may occur (Ali and Banks 1973). Progression to severe pulmonary hypertension and death may follow (Wendt *et al.* 1964). Foreign body granulomatosis due to corn starch (Hahn *et al.* 1969) or microcrystalline cellulose (Tomashefski *et al.* 1981) or talc (Heffner *et al.* 1990) is well recognized. Lysis and embolization of a right atrial clot infected with the cutaneous fungus *Malassezia furfur* followed urokinase administration, necessitating left pneumonectomy because of multiple pulmonary infarcts that had become infected with the fungus (Hassall *et al.* 1983). *M. furfur* pulmonary vasculitis has been reported following parenteral feeding with Intralipid (Redline and Dahms 1981) — the accumulation of lipid in pulmonary capillaries (well documented in neonates and infants) becoming the focus of the infection with this highly lipophilic fungus. Radiographic contrast media used in myelography (Todd and Gardner 1957) and in barium meal examinations (Mahboubi *et al.* 1974) have, astonishingly, been visualized in the lung fields by chest radiography.

Perfusion lung scans utilize embolized particles, for example, macroaggregated albumin labelled with the radioisotope ^{99m}technetium. The investigation has a remarkable safety record and is only risky in patients with severe pulmonary hypertension (Dworkin *et al.* 1966; Vincent *et al.* 1968; Williams 1974; Child *et al.* 1975).

Pulmonary hypertension

From 1967 to 1969 an increase in the incidence of pulmonary hypertension occurred. It was particularly noted in Switzerland and seems to have been confined to those countries in which the appetite-suppressant aminorex fumarate was marketed (Follath *et al.* 1971; Kay *et al.* 1971). The syndrome was characterized by progressive dyspnoea, cardiac failure, effort syncope, and sometimes sudden death. The evidence implicating aminorex fumarate is circumstantial but strong. Animal experiments failed, however, to reproduce the syndrome, even in primates (Kay 1974). Pulmonary hypertension has been reported in association with other anorectics including amphetamines (Malmquist *et al.* 1970) and fenfluramine (McMurray *et al.* 1986). It may follow use of an oral contraceptive (Kleiger *et al.* 1976) and, as mentioned above, may complicate intravenous substance abuse.

The eosinophilia–myalgia syndrome due to L-tryptophan: pulmonary hypertension

In 1989 a new syndrome typified by eosinophilia and myalgia was attributed to tryptophan used either as a health food supplement or as an antidepressant. It involves the skin, fascia, and muscle but breathlessness and cough are frequent (Medsger 1990). Surprisingly, even with severe respiratory distress the chest radiograph shows normal lung fields. Cardiomegaly may be present as in the patient described by MacLennan and Steward (1990) who presented with a 1-month history of increasing breathlessness 3 months after beginning treatment with tryptophan. The following investigations were

abnormal: eosinophil count 9.75×10^9 per litre; PaO_2 5.3 kPa; $PaCO_2$ 2.6 kPa; plasma sodium 111 mmol per litre; and vital capacity 60 per cent, and transfer factor for carbon monoxide 40 per cent, of the predicted values. Right heart catheterization showed pulmonary hypertension (pulmonary artery pressure 54/12 mm Hg) and the wedge pressure was normal. Treatment with 60 mg of prednisolone daily was begun and 4 days later the pulmonary artery pressure and the vital capacity had returned to normal and a pulmonary angiogram showed no abnormality. Another patient responded dramatically 2–3 days after 20 mg of prednisolone a day (and erythromycin) (Douglas *et al.* 1990). Belongia and colleagues (1990) identified the presence of a chemical constituent that was associated with specific conditions under which tryptophan was manufactured at one company that had been linked with the epidemic of the eosinophilia–myalgia syndrome in 1989. Medsger (1990) has also drawn attention to the many similarities of this syndrome to the toxic oil syndrome in Spain in 1981.

Pulmonary vasculitis

Pulmonary arteritis nodosa is usually idiopathic and not surprisingly, therefore, a number of drugs have been proposed as aetiological agents, for example, gold salts, iodides, penicillin, phenytoin, mercurials, and sulphonamides (Rich 1942; Knowles *et al.* 1953; Symmers 1958). The diagnosis of polyarteritis nodosa can be difficult in the absence of prominent typical systemic manifestations. The current view is that polyarteritis may be caused by widespread damage in the walls of medium-sized arteries due to the deposition of antigen–antibody–complement (immune) complexes such as occurs with Type III hypersensitivity reactions. The subsequent cascade of enzymatic processes and cellular interactions frequently results in necrosis of vessels. The ensuing extravasation of blood can be described as diffuse intrapulmonary (alveolar) haemorrhage (DIH). This phenomenon is best recognized in Goodpasture's syndrome, in which circulating antibodies to glomerular basement membrane (anti-GBM) can be detected, and glomerulonephritis (GN) is usual. Three fatal cases of DIH with GN due to penicillamine given for Wilson's disease have been described (Sternlieb *et al.* 1975). It has also occurred with penicillamine given for rheumatoid arthritis (Turner Warwick 1981) but, as anti-GBM was absent in the six patients in whom it was estimated, it is inappropriate to call the reaction Goodpasture's syndrome. The responses of the lung to a major vasculitic insult are limited, and recently a number of reports of DIH, with or without GN, have appeared implicating aminoglutethimide (Rodman *et al.* 1986); cocaine smoking (Murray *et al.* 1988); nitrofurantoin (Bucknall *et al.* 1987); febarbamate — a tranquillizer (Gali *et al.* 1986); and amphotericin (Haber *et al.* 1986). An interaction between amphotericin and leucocyte infusion in patients with leukaemia was reported by Wright and colleagues (1981). Fourteen of 22 patients receiving these therapies developed haemoptysis, and the chest X-rays showed widespread pulmonary infiltrates. Open lung biopsy in four showed DIH. Five of the 14 affected patients died from respiratory failure.

In DIH, haemoptysis is usual and may be profuse, and the decrease in haemoglobin level is proportional to the degree of pulmonary infiltration. The onset may be rapid and the clinical and radiological findings have been mistaken for left ventricular failure; the absence of cardiomegaly in DIH may be a helpful differentiating feature. At bronchoscopy, blood is seen throughout the bronchial tree and bronchoalveolar lavage will show haemosiderin-laden macrophages, as will transbronchial biopsy. Alveolar haemorrhage may also be seen on transbronchial biopsy but open lung biopsy or autopsy will show widespread bleeding into alveoli and alveolar walls. Very often the appearances obscure evidence of a pulmonary vasculitis. Smith (1990) has suggested that a capillaritis is the underlying pathological process in drug-related DIH, in contrast to the other diseases in which it has been described, for example, polyarteritis nodosa, rheumatoid arthritis (in the absence of penicillamine), Wegener's granulomatosis (positive anti-neutrophil cytoplasmic antibody), and a miscellany of other conditions, both infective and idiopathic. In view of the potential seriousness of DIH it is not surprising that rechallenge is rarely attempted, but Gali and colleagues (1986) reported eosinophilia and a skin rash when their patient was re-exposed to febarbamate.

Alveolar haemorrhage is not an inevitable consequence of pulmonary vasculitis. Two patients with a hypersensitivity reaction to phenytoin, manifesting as fever, breathlessness, hypoxaemia, maculopapular rash, lymphadenopathy, and bilateral pulmonary infiltrate on chest X-ray, were diagnosed as having hypersensitivity pneumonitis on transbronchial lung biopsy. Open lung biopsy, however, revealed histological evidence of a vasculitis (Michael and Rudin 1981).

Drug-related systemic lupus erythematosus (D-RSLE)

Pleuropulmonary manifestations are common in acute SLE, whether drug-induced or idiopathic. Cough, breathlessness, and pleuritic pain are usual presenting symptoms and radiologically there may be patchy pulmonary infiltrates or a pleural reaction, or both of these.

A small-lung syndrome is of unclear cause but does not seem to be due to pulmonary fibrosis. Withdrawal of the drug responsible and administration of corticosteroids usually results in complete resolution. A confounding feature, however, is the propensity with which patients with SLE react to drugs rather frequently. Procainamide is the most frequent cause of D-RSLE and a review of 17 cases (Byrd and Schanzer 1969) found that onset of SLE varied from 1–35 weeks from the start of treatment with this drug. Seven patients had pleurisy, sometimes with an effusion, but only one developed a pulmonary infiltrate. Hydralazine and isoniazid are also well recognized as causes of D-RSLE. A number of other drugs have been implicated and the subject is discussed further in Chapter 16.

Pulmonary capillaries: pulmonary oedema

Intravenous fluids

Excessive intravenous infusion of fluid is the most frequent cause of iatrogenic pulmonary oedema. Blood and plasma-expanding agents are a threat to patients with inadequate cardiac reserves, especially in the presence of renal impairment. In the presence of severe renal failure even solutions of glucose in water may be dangerous.

Adult respiratory distress syndrome (ARDS)

In severely ill patients, injury to the alveolar–capillary membrane can occur, with extravasation of a proteinacious fluid into the alveolar walls and alveoli resulting in stiff lungs and impaired gas exchange. Profound hypoxaemia follows and with multiple organ failure a mortality rate of 80–90 per cent is common. Thus, pulmonary oedema can follow replacement of major blood loss by electrolyte solutions (Roth *et al.* 1969; Schloerb *et al.* 1972) and the condition has been called the adult respiratory distress syndrome (ARDS), or non-cardiogenic pulmonary oedema. Measurement of pulmonary arterial and wedge pressure can help in the diagnosis.

Narcotics

Many cases of non-cardiogenic pulmonary oedema as a complication of heroin (diamorphine) abuse were encountered 20–25 years ago in the USA. (Steinberg and Karliner 1968; Frand *et al.* 1972). The condition was also described with methadone (Schaaf *et al.* 1973), of which as little as 60 mg orally was found to precipitate pulmonary oedema (Zyroff *et al.* 1974). Activation of neutrophils, which become sequestered in the pulmonary circulation and adhere to the pulmonary capillary endothelium thereby causing increasing leakiness of the basement membrane, has been proposed as the general mechanism underlying ARDS. There then follows the formation of intra-alveolar exudates that are rich in fibrin and other plasma proteins, including fibronectin. Incorporation of the intra-alveolar exudate into the alveolar wall will result in its organization and subsequent fibrosis, unless the insult is single and of short duration. With narcotics the problem is exacerbated by the possibility of continuing reactions to impurities in 'street' heroin injected by addicts, but it is well established that pulmonary oedema can be caused by pharmaceutically pure diamorphine. The syndrome is not like anaphylaxis, as the onset is commonly delayed, for more than 24 hours in some instances. The severity is variable, ranging from a few basal crackles to typical 'butterfly' infiltrative radiological changes, from mild dyspnoea to overwhelming respiratory failure with severe hypoxaemia necessitating mechanical ventilation. Improvement of clinical and blood gas states takes 1–2 days, and radiological changes clear after 1–4 days. Recovery of pulmonary function may be delayed for many days and may be incomplete. Transfer factor measurements may show impairment 3 months after an episode and may even be significantly reduced in addicts without pulmonary oedema or evidence of pulmonary disease (Karliner et al. 1969).

When a stuporose patient maintains a constant posture, unilateral oedema may occur, as was first described in 1880 by Osler. The mechanism of the oedema is not clear. The condition has been thought to be analogous to neurogenic pulmonary oedema, seen sometimes with raised intracranial pressure. Neither coma nor severe hypoxaemia are, however, prerequisites. Evidence of increased membrane permeability has been found in narcotic-related pulmonary oedema, in which oedema fluid with a higher protein content can be collected from the airways than in oedema due to raised pulmonary venous pressure in left ventricular failure (Katz et al. 1972). Intriguingly, naloxone has been reported to cause pulmonary oedema (Flacke et al. 1977; Schwartz and Koenigsberg 1987). Other reports implicate codeine (Sklar and Timms 1977) and dextropropoxyphene overdose (Bogartz and Miller 1971; Young 1972).

Other drugs

A reaction to hydrochlorothiazide, giving the appearances of pulmonary oedema in hypertensive patients without impaired left ventricular function, has been described in a number of patients (Steinberg 1968; Beaudry and Laplante 1973). Acute breathlessness, hypoxaemia, basal crackles, and radiological changes occurred within 45 minutes of ingestion. The response could be repeated on challenge with a single tablet. Administration of salicylates in high dosage may cause pulmonary oedema. This was initially described during treatment of rheumatic carditis (Reid et al. 1950) but has generally been due to overdosage (self-poisoning) (Granville-Grossman and Sergeant 1960; David and Burch 1974); one such patient was found to have a normal pulmonary wedge pressure (Hrnicek et al. 1974). Overdose of colchicine led to a fatal outcome in which pulmonary oedema was a feature (Hill et al. 1975). Phenylbutazone causes salt and water retention, and pulmonary oedema was seen in a few patients, some of whom had cardiac problems (Nevins et al. 1969). ARDS developing 4 days after overdosage with amitriptyline and progressing to death after 17 days has been described (Marshall and Moore 1973). Parenteral administration of β-adrenoceptor agonists, for example, terbutaline (Stubblefield 1978) or ritodrine (Elliott et al. 1978; Gentili et al. 1988), may cause pulmonary oedema. The mechanism is unclear, but a hyperdynamic circulation as in late pregnancy and premature labour seem to be predisposing factors. Adrenaline has produced fulminating pulmonary oedema when given during anaesthesia (Ersoz and Finestone 1971; Woldorf and Pastore 1972). Phenylephrine 10%, as eye drops, caused tachypnoea and hypertension in a premature infant with a ventricular septal defect (Matthews et al. 1977).

Intravenous urography has, rarely, caused pulmonary oedema (Cameron 1974; Chiu and Gambach 1974). Maxwell (1974) reported pulmonary oedema within 2 minutes of a second intravenous injection of cyclophosphamide and a female patient with lymphangitis carcinomatosa developed fatal ARDS 2 hours after intravenous chemotherapy with a combination of vinblastine and mitomycin (Ballen and Weiss 1988) (reactions to this combination are also discussed under Hypersensitivity pneumonitis). ARDS has also been reported after vinblastine alone (Israel and Olson 1987). McLeod and colleagues (1987) described a 54-year-old woman with chronic renal impairment given bleomycin in a dose of 20 units on three occasions over a 6-week period. Six weeks later ARDS developed, and at autopsy intra-alveolar fibroblast proliferation consistent with toxicity due to bleomycin was found.

Intravenous injection (illicit) of the sedative ethchlorvynol has caused non-cardiogenic pulmonary oedema (Glauser et al. 1976), and a similar problem arose in a 28-year-old woman who smoked crystals of methylamphetamine (Nestor et al. 1989). Biliary infusion of mono-octanoin to dissolve gallstones has been reported by Hine and co-workers (1988) to have caused pulmonary oedema in four individuals. They calculated a minimal incidence of 1 in 1000 cases. In a renal transplant recipient, Dean and colleagues (1987) reported ARDS following infusion of antilymphocytic globulin. Four litres of fluid had been given as well. Antithymocyte globulin led to ARDS after cardiac transplantation (Murdock *et al.* 1987). Pulmonary oedema occurring during blood transfusion is very likely to be attributed to circulatory overload, but some episodes occur in circumstances that preclude this explanation and sometimes the reaction is seen as part of a general anaphylactoid response. Antibodies to transfused IgA appear to underlie a proportion of reactions to otherwise compatible blood. Respiratory distress, overt pulmonary oedema, and even death may follow (Leikola *et al.* 1973; Pineda and Tazwell 1975). Reese and others (1975) have reported an adverse pulmonary reaction to cryoprecipitate in a haemophiliac in whom none of the above mechanisms seem applicable and who, in addition, had no antiplatelet or lymphocytotoxic antibodies. Pulmonary oedema following intravenous infusion of fresh frozen plasma, ascribed to an allergic reaction on the basis of systemic vasodilatation and a normal pulmonary capillary wedge pressure, has been described (O'Connor *et al.* 1981).

Pulmonary veins

Pulmonary veno-occlusive disease has been reported in three patients with malignancies who received cytotoxic chemotherapy (Lombard *et al.* 1987). One patient developed progressive breathlessness 10 years after MOPP (twice), COPP (four times), and radiotherapy for Hodgkin's disease. At autopsy there were multiple thromboemboli in the pulmonary arteries and in large and small pulmonary veins. No primary source of embolism was found. In two other patients with brain tumours, radiotherapy was followed by 6 months of treatment with carmustine. Four months later dyspnoea developed, progressing to death from respiratory failure within 6 weeks. At post-mortem examination, occlusive lesions were found in small pulmonary veins in both patients. The role of chemotherapy or radiotherapy in these cases is obscure, but the pathogenesis in the first case is clearly different from that in the other two. Joselson and Warnock (1983) also described this complication of cytotoxic chemotherapy.

Bronchi and lower airways

Foreign bodies

The true incidence of the inhalation of tablets and capsules is probably grossly underestimated, because most modern formulations are designed with rapid dissolution characteristics. Sustained-release preparations may possess wax matrices and persistence of these after inhalation of a salbutamol 'Spandet' and a terbutaline 'SA' tablet has been reported (Coppack *et al.* 1984). Considering the frailty of some recipients, especially the elderly, it is surprising that tablets and capsules are not incriminated as inhaled foreign bodies more frequently. Aspirin tablets, if inhaled, may cause respiratory crises in infants or very young children; Roden (1973) has reported death and mental retardation following such episodes.

Drug effects upon the sputum

Patients may perceive their sputum to have become more tenacious following effective antibiotic therapy, which eliminates purulence. Atropine and other drugs with anticholinergic properties, for example, tricyclic antidepressants (Baillie 1967), may cause unpleasant stickiness of bronchial secretions. Part of the clinical problem is due to drying of the mouth or pharynx, or both, so that sputum is more difficult to expectorate. In this regard, concern has arisen about the use of the quaternary atropine derivative ipratropium in patients with airflow obstruction due to chronic bronchitis. Crompton (1982) has reported anecdotally that sputum retention can be a problem with ipratropium. Because of its quaternary nature, however, little of the drug is distributed systemically, and bronchial mucus is not altered by it *in vitro* (Francis *et al.* 1975).

Following bronchography, oily contrast medium will be expectorated for several days. After lymphangiography, iodized oil can also appear in sputum for 6 weeks or more (Belin *et al.* 1966). Aspiration of oily medications from nose drops or oral medication may give rise to lipoid pneumonia, and sputum may contain globules of oil. Aspiration of cyclosporin solution into the airways has been reported as giving rise to a single pulmonary shadow from which fat globules were obtained by fine-needle aspiration and identified as the vehicle for cyclosporin (Gould *et al.* 1990).

Haemoptysis

This symptom may complicate thrombocytopenia due to cytotoxic drugs. Usually the blood produced appears only as streaks and is perhaps due to pharyngeal or laryngeal trauma, especially when there is ulceration. More dramatic haemoptysis may complicate intrapulmonary bleeding related to treatment with anticoagulants (Reussi *et al.* 1969; R.S. Bone *et al.* 1976), particularly where there are pulmonary infarcts or lung cysts (Kent 1965). (See also Pulmonary vasculitis — diffuse intrapulmonary haemorrhage).

Bronchial mucosa

Early clinical reports of the successful use of steroid aerosols in the long-term treatment of asthma commonly contained guarded reference to the theoretical possibility of atrophic changes, analogous to those produced in the skin by high doses of topical steroid preparations, developing in the bronchial wall. Histological studies of bronchial mucosa obtained by bronchoscopy (Andersson and Smidt 1974; Thiringer *et al.* 1975) have failed, however, to reveal any changes after over a year of continuous treatment and, after many years of very widespread long-term use of the preparations, there is no clinical evidence of such an effect. Infection with *Candida albicans* appears to be limited to the oropharynx and larynx, presumably because 80–90 per cent of inhaled particles are deposited at these sites.

Airflow obstruction

The calibre of small airways is dependent to a considerable extent upon the tone of bronchial smooth muscle. In normal individuals, changes in calibre are minor and barely appreciable; in the presence of chronic airflow obstruction, however, small differences can be important. In asthma, very large alterations of bronchial calibre can occur, owing partly to contraction of bronchial smooth muscle but also contributed to by mucosal oedema of airways and intraluminal inflammatory mucus. A multitude of humoral factors can influence bronchial tone either directly or via vagal cholinergic reflexes.

Allergic reactions (Type I hypersensitivity — immediate) (Gell and Coombs 1968) are characterized by IgE-linked release of pharmacologically active mediators from mast cells. This release may be modulated by physical, neural, humoral, and pharmacological factors. Non-specific release of mediators can also be effected, for example, by quaternary compounds or by surface-

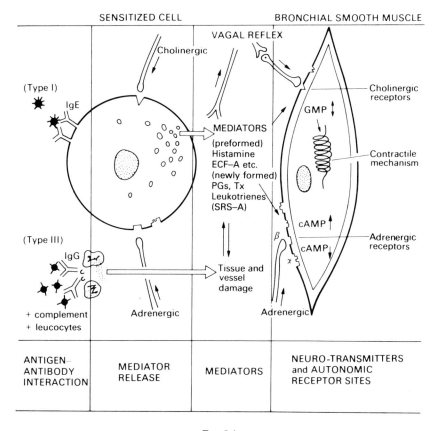

FIG. 8.1
The controlling factors in muscular tone. The action of drugs to cause airways obstruction may be at any of the four stages.

active agents. The mediators, some of which are preformed (e.g. histamine, eosinophilic chemotactic factor of anaphylaxis, various peptides), and others synthesized *de novo* (e.g. from the membrane-bound phospholipid arachidonic acid), determine the degree of bronchoconstriction and inflammation characteristic of local anaphylaxis in the airways. Immediate reactions may be followed hours later by delayed responses (Type III hypersensitivity), the effect of which can last hours to days. Drugs causing reversible airflow obstruction act through the mechanisms outlined above and the model shown in Figure 8.1 provides a basis for the classification of these drug reactions into:

1.   drugs that are antigenic;
2a. drugs that directly release mediators;
2b. drugs that affect the synthesis of mediators;
3a. drugs that stimulate reflex bronchoconstriction;
3b. drugs that are mediators or chemically related to mediators;
3c. drugs that inhibit mediator breakdown;
4.   drugs that act as agonists or antagonists at autonomic receptor sites;
5.   drugs that alter the disposition or metabolism of antiasthmatic drugs.

1. Drugs that are antigenic

Allergens used in tests and desensitization

Testing for allergy inevitably requires the administration of allergens topically or otherwise. Intradermal injection of such materials occasionally provokes dangerous asthmatic attacks that may be immediate or delayed. Such reactions are very much less frequent with the much smaller quantity of allergen introduced when skin prick testing is utilized, but in patients with eczema even this method can cause anaphylaxis. Courses of desensitizing injections used for the prophylaxis of hay fever may have to be curtailed because of the production of unacceptable asthma following each injection. The guidelines for the management of asthma produced by the British Thoracic Society (*British Medical Journal* 1990) advise against any attempts at desensitization.

Inhalation challenge testing using aerosols containing the suspected allergen has become more widely used in recent times, both for diagnosis and for the assessment of novel experimental antiallergic compounds. The dose–response methodology avoids the risk of immediate severe bronchospasm, but delayed reactions may occasionally be severe.

Drugs containing animal protein

Nasal insufflation of pituitary extract of porcine or bovine origin may induce asthma and parenchymal pulmonary reactions (Pepys 1969). A powdered pancreatic extract used by patients with cystic fibrosis may be inhaled while being added to food and Sakula (1977) has reported rhinitis and asthma in patients and relatives attributable to this cause. Enteric-coated formulations are now available.

Antibiotics

Anaphylaxis can follow administration of a variety of drugs, and asthma is a frequent accompaniment of such reactions. Penicillins are the most frequent cause of drug-induced anaphylaxis, and there is almost always a history of previous treatment with a course of penicillin which has usually been trouble-free. Dalgaard (1965) investigated 20 deaths due to penicillin in Denmark and found that 18 of the patients had previously received penicillin (6 with reactions, usually rashes). Of significance was the high incidence of a pre-existing allergic tendency, mostly asthma, in 11 of the dead. Similar findings have been reported in 151 fatal reactions (Idsøe *et al.* 1968). Penicillin sensitivity is complex and is due in some individuals to impurities. Prick and patch tests are unfortunately rather unreliable and deaths have resulted from intradermal tests of penicillin (Idsøe and Wang 1958). This topic is discussed in greater detail in Chapter 25.

Cross-reactions to cephalosporins in some patients allergic to penicillin have been a concern in view of the structural similarities (e.g. cephalothin) (Kabins *et al.* 1965). Sensitivity to cephalosporins is not an inevitable consequence of penicillin sensitivity (Rahal *et al.* 1968). Other antibiotics reported to have caused asthma are demeclocycline (Coles *et al.* 1967; Furey and Tan 1969), erythromycin (Abramov *et al.* 1978), nitrofurantoin (Walton 1966), griseofulvin, neomycin, streptomycin, and chloramphenicol (van Haeringen *et al.* 1972), but such reactions are rare when compared with those due to penicillin.

Dextran

Anaphylactic reactions to parenterally administered preparations of iron–dextran have been reported (Becker *et al.* 1966; Wallerstein 1968). Similar reactions can occur with intravenous solutions of dextran used in the treatment of hypovolaemia (Fanous *et al.* 1977; Furhoff 1977). The incidence is higher with the larger molecular-weight dextran 70 than with dextran 40 (Laxenaire *et al.* 1976a).

Other drugs have been reported to cause asthma in individual patients, for example, maprotiline (Dubovsky and Freed 1988), 8-methoxypsoralen (Ramsey and Marks 1988), and metoclopramide on two occasions in the same patient (Chung *et al.* 1985).

2a. Drugs that directly release mediators

Iodine-containing contrast media

Anaphylaxis occurring with these agents has an incidence of 1 in 14 000 and is accompanied in 12 per cent of cases by severe airflow obstruction (Ansell 1970), which may be fatal (Epstein 1977). The reactions are particularly likely to affect allergic individuals and the induced asthma may last for days. Small intravenous doses have been used to test 204 patients with a history of previous reactions, and the value of subsequent protection with an antihistamine is described by Yocum and others (1978). In those with only a vague history of previous hypersensitivity and negative pretests (untreated with an antihistamine), the incidence of reactions was 5 per cent. Amongst those with a clear history of a previous reaction but negative pretests, about 20 per cent had a second reaction, but this figure could be reduced to about 4 per cent by pretreatment with chlorpheniramine. Two-thirds of those with a positive pretest went on to have a second reaction despite pretreatment with chlorpheniramine. Pretreatment with corticosteroid drugs appears to offer some protection (Zweiman et al. 1975; Lasser et al. 1977); the dose may have to be moderately high. Mild bronchoconstriction (a mean decrease of 7.5 per cent in FEV_1) was observed in most patients receiving a high-osmolality agent, sodium iothalamate; allergic subjects were more likely to react (Dawson et al. 1983). The time-course of the reaction (onset after 4–5 minutes; recovery within 30 minutes) is compatible with mediator release, but whether a similar mechanism can be invoked for severe bronchospasm is unknown. Bronchography may markedly aggravate asthma and chronic bronchitis, perhaps partly from irritation and coughing and partly due to histamine release. Cough during pulmonary angiography is much more common with a high-osmolality agent (Smith et al. 1987).

Intravenous anaesthetic agents

Induction of anaesthesia can cause anaphylaxis, and cross-reactions occur — raising the possibility that a non-allergic mechanism is responsible. The reaction is usually rapid in onset but occasionally delayed for up to an hour (Laxenaire et al. 1976b). Death may ensue from circulatory failure or apparently complete airflow obstruction. A muscle relaxant is almost always given as well, and the relative importance of the two drugs is uncertain. The combination of thiopentone and suxamethonium is by far and away the most frequent cause of bronchoconstrictive reactions (Vignon et al. 1976), but it is unclear whether there is an explanation for this other than that this combination is that most often used. Clarke and others (1975, 1977) found that about a

quarter of those reacting to thiopentone were atopic and that previous exposure to thiopentone carried only a very slight increase in risk of an adverse reaction. A more clear-cut case for mediator release has been made for the poorly soluble steroid drugs alphaxalone and alphadolone (Althesin), which require a surface-active agent, polyoxyethylated castor oil (Cremophor EL) so that an adequate dose can be accommodated in a minimal volume (Kessel and Assem 1974; Jago and Restall 1978; CSM 1979).

Muscle relaxants

Anaphylaxis and marked bronchoconstriction may follow the intravenous administration of tubocurarine (Comroe and Dripps 1946), suxamethonium (Eustace 1967), pancuronium (Heath 1973), vecuronium (O'Callaghan et al. 1986), and atracurium and alcuronium (Beemer et al. 1988). The reaction is almost certainly due to histamine release by these quaternary ammonium compounds, a process demonstrable in vitro and by intradermal testing (Heath 1973; Buckland and Avery 1973).

Other drugs

Morphine administered parenterally is regularly found to cause bronchospasm and it can be shown to release histamine when given intradermally. Hydrocortisone as the sodium phosphate salt (Partridge and Gibson 1978) or the sodium succinate salt (Kounis 1976) may cause acute anaphylactic reactions. It seems unlikely that an endogenous corticosteroid would give rise to true allergy, and as the reaction is immediate and not delayed for many hours, a mechanism involving phospholipase A_2 is excluded. There is clinical evidence of systemic histamine release in such patients; and also with methylprednisolone (Mendelson et al. 1974). Quaternary preservatives such as benzalkonium are sometimes present in aerosol preparations (see below — ipratropium, beclomethasone) and probably act by causing mediator release rather than by an irritant action because, even when administered by injection as in a hepatitis B vaccine, thiomersal has caused asthma and urticaria (Lohiya 1987).

2b. Drugs that alter the synthesis of mediators

Aspirin and other non-steroidal anti-inflammatory drugs (NSAID)

Asthma usually develops in sensitive individuals about 30 minutes after ingestion of aspirin; it may be accompanied by flushing and rhinorrhoea. The severity of the reaction varies and does not seem to be proportional to the pre-existing airflow obstruction, as near-fatal attacks occur in patients with minimal or long-quiescent asthma. It is extremely important, therefore, that attention is paid to any patient acknowledging a previous history of 'allergy' to aspirin. Partial attacks involving rhinorrhea, angioedema, or urticaria, alone or in any combination, may occur. The phenomenon is particularly associated with late-onset intrinsic asthma and is often accompanied by nasal polyposis. The syndrome was first delineated by Samter and Beers (1967) and its incidence is estimated at 1 in 10 asthmatics (McDonald *et al.* 1972). Some patients may be unaware of their sensitivity, and 8 per cent of one group of patients developing some degree of bronchospasm after challenge with aspirin gave no such history (Spector *et al.* 1979).

Patients with aspirin sensitivity are almost invariably cross-reactive to NSAID (and to the food and drink colouring agent tartrazine [E102]). Numerous reports in the literature are to be found describing individuals who have reacted, sometimes fatally, to particular NSAID, for example, indomethacin, phenylbutazone, mefenamic acid, flufenamic acid, diclofenac, or naproxen. The structural heterogenicity of these compounds argues against an immune mechanism. There is some evidence, however, for a common property, namely inhibition of· the synthesis of prostanoids derived from arachidonic acid via cyclo-oxygenase activity. This inhibition was thought to result in an imbalance between the bronchoconstrictor prostaglandins (F, A, B, and D_2) and those that are bronchodilator (E series and epoprostenol [previously known as prostacyclin]). Arachidonic acid, released from membrane-bound phospholipid, is also available for conversion to the products of lipoxygenase activity, of which the most important are the leukotrienes, which together comprise the slow-reacting-substance of anaphylaxis. A shift from prostanoid to leukotriene synthesis is the currently favoured theory to account for asthma induced by aspirin and NSAID. Sodium cromoglycate has been shown to be protective in this condition (Martelli and Usandivaras 1977) and it is known to have no effect in preventing bronchoconstriction due to prostaglandin $F_{2\alpha}$ (Patel 1975), and aspirin-sensitive asthmatics are not more sensitive than other asthmatics to the bronchoconstrictor effects of this prostaglandin (Orehek *et al.* 1977; Szczeklik *et al.* 1977). The picture is far from complete and there is little positive evidence in favour of any hypothesis. A genetic predisposition seems likely — familial clustering (Miller 1971; von Maur *et al.* 1974) and an increased prevalence of the HLA-DQw2 antigen have been found (Mullarkey *et al.* 1986) — but modulation of bronchial reactivity also seems probable, as Spector and colleagues (1979) in their challenge studies found negative tests in about one-third of those reporting previous aspirin sensitivity. The

story is further complicated by occasional asthmatic reactions to paracetamol (acetaminophen), an analgesic without anti-inflammatory activity which inhibits intracerebral cyclo-oxygenase). Szczeklik and Gryglewski (1983) reported reactions to paracetamol and phenacetin in 4 per cent of aspirin-sensitive patients. It is of interest that some asthmatic patients are actually improved by aspirin (*British Medical Journal* 1973; Szczeklik and Nizankowska 1978).

Opiate derivatives such as codeine and dihydrocodeine are safe analgesics to use in patients of this group.

3a. Drugs that stimulate reflex bronchoconstriction

All therapeutic aerosols may reflexly trigger vagally mediated bronchoconstriction, preventable by prior administration of atropine or a bronchodilator. The effect is mediated by a non-specific physical or irritant action, for example, inhalation of sodium cromoglycate as a dry powder formulation may cause coughing and wheezing (Morrison Smith 1975). Beclomethasone dipropionate, even as a pressurized aerosol, not uncommonly initiates mild wheezing. There is indirect evidence against this being a specific hypersensitivity, as patients may respond to the propellant alone (Bryant and Pepys 1976; Shim and Williams 1987). It has become routine to recommend taking a bronchodilator before inhaling a steroid. Some surprise was caused when the anticholinergic drug ipratropium bromide was reported to cause bronchoconstriction in three patients using a metered-dose pressurized aerosol (Connolly 1982). Other workers reported bronchoconstriction when the drug was administered by nebulization (Patel and Tullet 1983; Howarth 1983). Altounyan showed that nebulized hypotonic solutions cause bronchoconstriction in asthmatics with hyperreactive airways (Schoeffed *et al.* 1981), and the manufacturers of ipratropium now market the drug in isotonic saline. Removal of the preservatives EDTA and benzalkonium has also been material in reducing the incidence of adverse reactions (Rafferty *et al.* 1988). Both ipratropium and benzalkonium are quaternary ammonium compounds (see above — Direct release of mediators), and benzalkonium has been proposed (Beasley *et al.* 1986) as the reason why an infant developed severe wheeze soon after receiving nebulized beclomethasone (Clark 1986). Unit-dose vials are to be encouraged; as they are sterile, no preservative is needed and cross-infection is less likely (Barclay *et al.* 1990).

Metabisulphite (E223) is used widely in food and drink as a preservative/antioxidant. It was also present in some bronchodilator aerosols; the bronchospasm it causes is likely to be due to the generation of sulphur dioxide (Meeker and Wiedemann 1990). Evidence against the degranulation of mast cells in the reaction has been reported by Sprenger and colleagues (1989) who challenged patients sensitive to metabisulphite; the circulating neutrophil chemotactic factor activity did not increase, in contrast to an increase observed following antigen challenge (Nagy *et al.* 1982). The phenomenon of metabisulphite sensitivity can be observed occasionally in hospital inpatients recovering from acute severe asthma, whose peak flow charts will show a dip at an unexpected time (e.g. afternoon). Examination of the labels on bottles (e.g. of Lucozade) on their bedside lockers will reveal the ingredients and appropriate advice can be given. Bronchial reactions to nebulized acetylcysteine (once used as a mucolytic aerosol in cystic fibrosis) usually occur in asthmatic subjects and seem to be related to the concentration of acetylcysteine used (Council on Drugs 1964). Aerosolized antibiotics regularly precipitate wheeze; examples are polymyxin (Marschke and Sarauw 1971), polymyxin with kanamycin (Dickie and de Groot 1973), gentamicin (Dally *et al.* 1978), and, more recently, pentamidine used in AIDS for the prophylaxis of *Pneumocystis carinii* pneumonia (Smith *et al.* 1988).

3b. Drugs that are mediators or pharmacologically related to mediators

Histamine used in test of gastric acid secretion may occasionally exacerbate airflow obstruction despite prior administration of an H_1-antagonist. Bronchial provocation tests with histamine may cause unexpectedly severe bronchospasm in asthmatic patients with marked bronchial hyperreactivity. As mentioned above, prostaglandin $F_{2\alpha}$ is bronchoconstrictive and severe asthma has been reported during its infusion to induce a therapeutic abortion in a patient with chronic eczema (Fishburn *et al.* 1972).

3c. Drugs that inhibit mediator breakdown

Anticholinesterases
Acetylcholine released from cholinergic nerves is rapidly hydrolysed by local acetylcholinesterase and exerts no activity remote from the site of release. An anticholinesterase would markedly increase local concentrations of acetylcholine, and neostigmine is given to reverse the action of long-acting competitive antagonist muscle relaxants, such as tubocurarine and pancuronium, used during anaesthesia and surgery. Atropine is usually used concomitantly with neostigmine to prevent the predictable bronchospasm and bradycardia. Interestingly, Pratt (1988) reported three patients in whom glycopyrronium did not prevent neostigmine inducing bronchospasm. Pyridostigmine and neostigmine are used in myasthenia gravis and may aggravate asthma. Ecothiopate, a long-

acting anticholinesterase used in eye drops for glaucoma, was reported to exacerbate airflow obstruction in a patient with emphysema (Fratto 1979).

Angiotensin-converting-enzyme (ACE) inhibitors
ACE inhibitors (e.g. captopril, enalapril) prevent the enzymatic activation of the peptide angiotensin I to angiotensin II. ACE also inactivates bradykinin and possibly other vasoactive peptides. Cough as an adverse effect of these drugs has been related to persistence of such peptides, and the incidence of this adverse reaction has varied from 0.2 per cent of 13 295 hypertensive patients taking part in postmarketing surveillance of captopril (Chalmers *et al.* 1987) to 1–3 per cent of individuals involved in prescription-event monitoring of a large population taking enalapril (Inman 1986; Inman *et al.* 1988). The cough is characteristically dry and unproductive and usually recurs when alternative ACE inhibitors are substituted. There seems to be a dose effect in some individuals. Experimental studies have shown that the cough reflex can be stimulated by capsaicin, a partial agonist at substance P receptors on non-myelinated sensory (C) nerve fibres, and sensitivity to capsaicin is increased by administration of an ACE inhibitor to patients known to have cough induced by the drug (Fuller and Choudry 1987). This is a complex area involving the modulatory interaction of many mediators, and, interestingly, the NSAID sulindac has been shown to prevent the induction of cough by ACE-inhibitors (Nicholis and Gilchrist 1987). Inhalation of bradykinin causes bronchoconstriction, and ACE inhibitors might therefore be expected to aggravate the asthma. There is little evidence of this, but Popa (1987) described a man whose FEV_1 fell when challenged with captopril but not when challenged with propranolol. More systematic investigation has shown an increase in bronchial hyperreactivity in symptomatic patients rechallenged with ACE inhibitors (Bucknall *et al.* 1988). In contrast, withdrawing captopril did not improve bronchial hyperreactivity in another study (Kaufman *et al.* 1989). Asthma seems to be a very much less likely adverse effect with ACE inhibitors than is cough.

4. Drugs that act as agonists or antagonists at autonomic receptor sites

Cholinergic agonists
Carbachol and related drugs are sometimes given to increase the contractility of the blood and may induce bronchoconstriction (Fig. 8.1). Aggravation of asthma has been reported with pilocarpine eye drops for glaucoma (Bruchhausen *et al.* 1969) and with deanol for severe dyskinesia (Nesse and Carroll 1976). Methacholine used in bronchial provocation testing can

occasionally cause unexpectedly severe bronchocon-striction even in individuals not regarded as asthmatic (Stenton *et al.* 1990).

β-Adrenoceptor agonists

Atypical responses to inhaled isoprenaline have been ascribed to overuse of this bronchodilator aerosol (Keighley 1966; Patterson *et al.* 1968). Bronchoconstric-tion is in general less marked with more recently devel-oped agents such as salbutamol and terbutaline. Two factors are relevant: dosage and selectivity. Isoprenaline has to be administered in high dosage to ensure an adequate duration of action because it is rapidly inacti-vated by catechol-*o*-methyltransferase (COMT). Unde-sirable systemic effects were frequently associated with high peak blood levels of isoprenaline. Of the modern β-agonist bronchodilators only rimiterol is a substrate for COMT. The duration of action of the others is therefore longer, and smaller doses (in terms of relative potency) need to be inhaled. $β_2$-Adrenoceptor selectiv-ity is an incidental advantage which followed from the design requirement of COMT resistance. When com-pared with the distributional selectivity achieved by administering these drugs by inhalation, rather than by the oral or parenteral routes, $β_2$-selectivity is relatively unimportant.

Lowering of arterial oxygen tension   Adrenergic and xanthine bronchodilators are also vasodilators and their administration will increase ventilation/perfusion (V/Q) mismatching and thereby lower arterial PO_2 in normal and asthmatic individuals (Haelmagyi and Cotes 1959; Chapman 1969). The observed changes are usually small and if nebulized bronchodilators are driven by oxygen then any changes will be clinically insignificant. The effect of intravenous salbutamol has been compared with that of the drug when inhaled and found to cause more V/Q imbalance in acute severe asthma (Ballester *et al.* 1989). A rise in cardiac output with intravenous salbut-amol can counterbalance the effect of pulmonary vas-odilatation, and in hypoxic patients with chronic bron-chitis the net effect can be no change in PO_2. Indeed, the manufacturers of pirbuterol have claimed that pulmon-ary vasodilatation is a positive advantage rather than an adverse effect!

Sudden death in asthma: role of pressurized aerosols
Between 1959 and 1966 the mortality from asthma in-creased dramatically in the UK (Speizer *et al.* 1968*a*), and overuse of isoprenaline inhalers was thought to be responsible (Speizer *et al.* 1968*b*; Fraser *et al.* 1971). Subsequently, caution was advised in the use of bron-chodilator aerosols and the mortality from asthma de-clined to previous levels (Inman and Adelstein 1969).

The mechanisms whereby isoprenaline might cause death have been widely discussed. Hypoxaemia is minor, as mentioned above. High doses can cause cardiac stimu-lation and possibly fatal arrhythmia. Resistance to β-adrenoceptor agonists can be demonstrated, for example, at cardiac chronotropic receptors, but the ob-servation that normal airways can become resistant to salbutamol (Holgate *et al.* 1977) could not be confirmed (Keaney *et al.* 1980; and unpublished observations). Resistance of asthmatic airways to oral adrenergic bronchodilators has not been found (Bhatan and Davis 1975; Larsson *et al.* 1977). The decline in mortality was sustained despite an ever-increasing prescription rate for $β_2$-selective bronchodilators. Inhaled prophylactic anti-asthmatic therapy with sodium cromoglycate and be-clomethasone became the norm in the early 1970s and was undoubtedly a very significant development. Never-theless, even at that time unacceptable deaths from asthma occurred and it seems that some patients, their families, and their doctors (both in the community and in hospital) are rather poor at recognizing the severity of an attack of acute asthma and at instituting early treatment with corticosteroids in sufficiently high doses (Ormerod and Stableforth 1980). Unfortunately, a small number of asthmatic deaths are due to severe immediate reactions and seem unavoidable.

Role of nebulized bronchodilators   In the light of the above discussion, there was a sense of *déjà vu* when the report of Jackson and colleagues (1982) appeared ident-ifying an increase in mortality from asthma in New Zealand not seen in other countries. Again it was prob-able that inadequate education of patients underlay the phenomenon (Clarke and Newman 1984). A new factor to be considered in the patients in New Zealand was excessive reliance on domiciliary aerosol treatment using nebulizers to deliver higher doses of bronchodilators. In a subsequent survey of 271 deaths from asthma between 1981 and 1983 in New Zealand, 75 individuals had home nebulizers (Sears *et al.* 1987). Poor patient compliance (36 per cent), delay in seeking help (35 per cent), and inadequate treatment or assessment (36 per cent) were identified in these patients; 81 per cent of deaths oc-curred 'during a witnessed attack of severe asthma unre-sponsive to usual treatment', which included nebulized high-dose β-agonists in two-thirds of cases. Of some concern was the observation that 45 per cent of patients with fatal asthma used fenoterol (49 per cent salbutamol) in their nebulizer, whereas the ratio of sales of fenoterol to those of salbutamol (in 20 ml units) was 13 800 to 35 000. The use of fenoterol in New Zealand was five times higher than in other countries and Crane and colleagues (1989) blamed fenoterol for the excess of asthma deaths. This conclusion has been disputed (O'Donnell *et al.* 1989; Buist *et al.* 1989) on the basis of inadequate assessment of the severity of the final attack. This criticism has been rejected as irrelevant and an extended analysis using different controls added further support to the hypothesis that inhaled fenoterol is associated with an increased risk of death in patients with severe asthma (Pearce *et al.* 1990*a*). The odds ratio of death from asthma was 1.99 (95 per cent confidence interval [CI] 1.12–3.55) in patients given fenoterol and rose to 9.82 (95 per cent CI 2.23– 43.4) for the group defined by admission for asthma in the previous year and by having had an oral corticosteroid prescribed at the time of admission. An alternative hypothesis that risk for death from asthma may simply be associated with a propensity for doctors to prescribe fenoterol (Spitzer and Buist 1990) has been rejected (Pearce *et al.* 1990*b*).

β-Adrenoceptor antagonists

This group of drugs will prevent adrenergic bronchodilators from exerting their therapeutic action. Asthmatic patients, however, are additionally susceptible to β- blockers, and even the small systemic concentrations that follow topical application of a β-blocker in eye drops for glaucoma, for example, timolol (Shoene *et al.* 1981), can provoke severe asthma. Timolol, like propranolol, is a non-selective β-blocker, but even highly cardioselective practolol may provoke bronchospasm (Macdonald and McNeill 1968; Bernecker and Roetscher 1970). Interestingly, propranolol has no effect on airway resistance in normal subjects (McNeill 1964) even in overdose (Frishman *et al.* 1979). The mechanism by which β-blockers cause bronchospasm in asthmatics is far from clear. It is not simply due to interference with the action of circulating adrenaline or released noradrenaline on bronchial smooth muscle, because anticholinergic drugs (Ind *et al.* 1989) and sodium cromoglycate (Koeter *et al.* 1982) prevent propranolol from inducing bronchoconstriction.

A β-blocking action may not be an obvious attribute of a drug marketed for treating mild cardiac failure, but xamoterol is an example of such a product which acts as a partial agonist at cardiac β-receptors and would· be expected to aggravate asthma (Waller 1990). Propafenone, used for treating cardiac arrhythmias, is primarily a Class 1c agent with some β-blocking activity (Dukes and Vaughan Williams 1984) and has recently been reported to precipitate asthma (Veale *et al.* 1990).

5. Interactions affecting the disposition or metabolism of antiasthmatic drugs

Induction of microsomal enzymes utilizing cytochrome P-450 increases the clearance of drugs that undergo oxidative metabolism, (e.g. prednisolone). Anticonvulsants such as carbamazepine, phenytoin, and phenobarbitone, and the antituberculous antibiotic rifampicin are the most commonly used drugs that cause enzyme induction. Asthma control was found to deteriorate in three patients on maintenance corticosteroid therapy following administration of phenobarbitone (Brooks *et al.* 1972). Evidence of increased steroid metabolism was observed, the elimination half-life of ingested dexamethasone being reduced.

The effect of bronchodilator drugs in masking the severity of asthma, so that treatment with inhaled or systemic corticosteroids is delayed, is a theme of much concern to respiratory physicians. New inhaled bronchodilators, such as salmeterol, have a duration of action of up to 12 hours and may in time raise issues similar to those involving isoprenaline in the 1960s and fenoterol currently.

Irreversible airflow obstruction

Bronchiolitis obliterans has been described in patients with rheumatoid arthritis and ulcerative colitis. Its occurrence in patients with these diseases has been attributed to penicillamine in rheumatoid disease (Scott *et al.* 1981) and to sulphasalazine in ulcerative colitis (Williams *et al.* 1982).

Lung parenchyma

The arrangement of topics in this section is arbitrary. Most approaches to classifying drug-related parenchymal damage have been pharmacopoeial in nature, which obviously necessitates much repetition. In order to keep repetition to a minimum parenchymal injury has been grouped into: (i) acute and (ii) subacute or chronic reactions. An alternative description would be of (i) reversible pneumonitis and (ii) fibrotic pulmonary disease. Inevitably some cases will overlap either with another category, or with ARDS, and attention will be drawn to this when appropriate. The clinical features of acute pneumonitis and pulmonary fibrosis are presented in general terms for each topic rather than with each drug mentioned; first, however, parenchymal complications of aspiration are discussed.

Inhalation

Sedative drugs, especially opiates, which obtund pharyngeal and laryngeal reflexes, permit inhalation of food, secretions, or vomitus, leading to the subsequent development of pneumonitis. Local anaesthesia of the glottis may also be followed by aspiration. Fatal respiratory failure has been caused by inhalation of activated charcoal, given to patients suffering from drug overdoses with lowered consciousness, when vomiting occurred (Rau *et al.* 1988). Liquid paraffin or oily nasal drops may lead to lipoid pneumonia from unrecognized aspiration. The clinical features are usually mild (Volk *et al.* 1951), and the diagnosis is confirmed by identifying globules of oil in sputum or lung biopsy material (Weill *et al.* 1964). Granuloma formation has been mistaken for bronchial carcinoma (Eyal *et al.* 1961; Borrie and Gwynne 1973). Inhalation of a capsule of cyclosporin, giving rise to a peripheral pulmonary mass, and the finding of the vehicle in which cyclosporin is dissolved on transthoracic fine-needle aspiration (Gould *et al.* 1990), have been mentioned earlier.

Drug-related infection of the lungs

Drugs may cause pneumonia (i) by being contaminated and inhaled (Barclay *et al.* 1990); (ii) by permitting aspiration of infected material (e.g. opiates); (iii) by suppressing host defences to pathogens (e.g. cytotoxic chemotherapy, high-dose corticosteroids); or (iv) by altering respiratory flora (e.g. alkalinization of gastric juice with antacids or cimetidine was associated with colonization of stomach and trachea by the same bacteria and a high incidence [60 per cent] of pneumonia in an intensive care unit) (DuMoulin *et al.* 1982), and Freeman (1980) has stated that prophylactic broad-spectrum antibiotics alter tracheal flora and cause increased mortality after cardiac surgery.

Opportunistic infections

Patients can become immunosuppressed owing to a number of factors and with a severity that varies, as does their susceptibility to different types of infection. Thus, even low-dosage corticosteroid therapy can reactivate pulmonary tuberculosis, but such an individual, like the patient being treated for leukaemia, who still has preserved immunoglobulin levels and an adequate neutrophil count, should not be regarded as immunodeficient. In general hospital clinical practice, cytotoxic chemotherapy is the most usual reason for immunodeficiency and the diagnostic approach to the problem of diffuse pulmonary infiltration in the immunocompromised host has been recently reviewed by Rosenow (1990). The presentation, physical examination, and chest X-ray are rarely diagnostic, and bronchoscopy with bronchial lavage and transbronchial biopsy may be needed to establish the cause. Rosenow describes the experience at the Mayo Clinic, where 75 per cent of immunocompromised patients with diffuse pulmonary disease have an opportunistic infection, sometimes with more than one unusual organism. Further investigation with open lung biopsy attributed the diffuse infiltration to adverse drug effects in 15 per cent of the total, and the remaining 10 per cent of cases were due to recurrence of underlying disease, idiopathic fibrosis (? from radiotherapy), or unrelated disease. The use of cyclosporin A as immunosuppressant agent has considerably reduced the problem of nosocomial infection in transplant patients. Nevertheless, cytomegalovirus and *Pneumocystis carinii* infections remain the most frequent problems; invasive aspergillosis and candidiasis are rather more difficult to diagnose without open lung biopsy. Drug-related infections are discussed further in Chapter 23.

Acute diffuse hypersensitivity pneumonitis

Drug-related hypersensitivity pneumonitis, with or without pulmonary eosinophilia, is characterized by a variety of radiological shadows evident on the chest X-ray, accompanied by eosinophilia of blood in many instances. More recently, eosinophilia or lymphocytosis, or both, of fluid obtained by bronchoalveolar lavage have been identified. The radiological shadowing may be of segmental appearance or irregularly fan-shaped, of medium density, and often of peripheral distribution. Occasionally a micronodular appearance is found. Pleural effusions are common. Gas transfer is impaired and airflow obstruction may occur. Symptoms are of cough, breathlessness, and occasionally wheezing. The prognosis with this type of reaction is good, principally because the acute presentation usually results in immediate withdrawal of the offending drug. Corticosteroid therapy speeds resolution and complete recovery is possible.

Antibacterial drugs

The first case of drug-related eosinophilia to be reported was due to penicillin (Reichlin *et al.* 1953). Acute pneumonitis due to ampicillin has also occurred with an eosinophilic alveolitis on transbronchial biopsy (Poe *et al.* 1980). Klinghoffer (1954) reported that even the lower doses of sulphonamide reaching the systemic circulation after vaginal administration could cause the syndrome. Oral sulphonamides (Feigenberg *et al.* 1967) and the sulphonamide derivatives chlorpropamide (Bell 1964) and sulphasalazine (Jones and Malone 1972; Thomas *et al.* 1974; Constantinidis 1976; Sigvaldson and Sorensen 1983) may also cause pulmonary eosinophilia.

Eosinophilia is not universal in pneumonitis due to sulphasalazine. Symptoms develop 2–5 months after the start of treatment. Occasionally the course of the pulmonary complication is fulminating, as in the case reported by Davis and MacFarlane (1974) in which pulmonary fibrosis was found at autopsy, even though the patient had been given steroid therapy prior to and, in higher dosage, during the month of the illness. Sodium aminosalicylate (PAS) has commonly caused allergic reactions, and lung involvement has been recorded (Wold and Zahn 1956). Metronidazole was administered on two occasions to a patient who developed hypersensitivity pneumonitis both times (Kristenson and Fryden 1988). Cephalexin (Smith and Weinstein 1987), tetracycline (Ho *et al.* 1979), nalidixic acid (Dan *et al.* 1986), and nitrofurantoin (Israel and Diamond 1962; Magee *et al.* 1986) may also give rise to an allergic pulmonary reaction.

The acute eosinophilic response to nitrofurantoin may become persistent (Vaughan-Jones and Goldman 1968), and the case reported by Magee and colleagues (1986) was of acute onset after 7 days' treatment. An open lung biopsy showed granulomata with giant cells, and rechallenge was positive. Subacute and chronic reactions to nitrofurantoin are discussed further below.

Non-steroidal anti-inflammatory drugs

With the high prescription rate for this group of drugs, some of which are available over the counter to the public, it is surprising that pulmonary eosinophilia is not more frequently reported, since the mode of action of NSAID involves inhibition of cyclo-oxygenase activity. Arachidonic acid is diverted to the synthesis of the products of lipoxygenase, many of which, like the leukotrienes, have eosinophilic chemotactic activity. Weber and Essigman (1986) briefly reviewed the literature regarding pulmonary alveolitis and NSAID. They also documented information obtained by the Committee on Safety of Medicines from the yellow-card reporting system. This adverse drug reactions register had recorded 29 reports of diffuse pneumonitis attributed to treatment with NSAID involving indomethacin, azapropazone, benoxaprofen, piroxicam, diclofenac, and ibuprofen. A positive rechallenge had been identified with indomethacin, and there was a cross-reaction between azapropazone and piroxicam. Only 12 of the 29 patients had rheumatoid arthritis (4 being seropositive), and patients with osteoarthritis are also susceptible (11 in this series). Cameron (1975) reported a patient with osteoarthritis who reacted to oxyphenylbutazone. She had a transiently positive LE test and on rechallenge had recurrence of the breathlessness despite concurrent diuretic

therapy to counteract the salt-retaining and water-retaining properties of the drug. The patient was well 5 years after the initial reaction. Phenylbutazone may have been responsible for a severe reaction in a 69-year-old hypothyroid woman (Thurston *et al.* 1976). Stromberg and others (1987) reported six cases of acute pulmonary infiltrates due to tolfenamic acid from Finland. Three occurred early in the course of treatment and three were delayed; the changes resolved in all cases when the drug was discontinued. Rechallenge was positive in three of the patients. Two chronic fibrotic reactions were also identified. Two similar reactions to fenbufen (Chuck *et al.* 1987; Swinburn 1988), three to azapropazone (Al-bazzad *et al.* 1986), and one to fenoprofen (Barbadi *et al.* 1986) have been described.

Cytotoxic drugs

Acute pulmonary reactions are relatively infrequent with cytotoxic drugs. Methotrexate accounts for most reports. Although the majority of the reported pulmonary complications of treatment with this folic acid antimetabolite have developed after many weeks of treatment, pulmonary reactions have been reported as early as 12 days after commencement. The reaction is not generally regarded as dose-related because the total dose received has varied from 40–6500 mg, but there may be a more subtle relationship with frequency of doses. There is a much higher incidence of pneumonitis in patients receiving daily methotrexate injections (Nesbit *et al.* 1976). Pulmonary reactions had not been reported in patients receiving less than 20 mg weekly until low-dose methotrexate (10 mg weekly) became established as a third-line treatment for rheumatoid arthritis. Of 23 cases of acute pneumonitis on low-dosage methotrexate, 3 were fatal and the prevalence has been established at 4 per cent (Searles and McKendry 1987; Green *et al.* 1988; Ridley *et al.* 1988; Zitnik and Cooper 1990). The main features in evolution of the pulmonary reactions to methotrexate have been described in three excellent reviews of the subject (Whitcomb *et al.* 1972; Nesbit *et al.* 1976; Sostman *et al.* 1976). Typically cough, fever, dyspnoea, and sometimes cyanosis are accompanied by diffuse pulmonary mottling evident on the chest X-ray. Other radiographic changes include alveolar filling pattern, especially in the lower zones, pleural effusion, and hilar lymphadenopathy (Everts *et al.* 1973). Occasionally, symptoms precede the radiological changes; in patients with leukaemia the disease is almost always in remission when the pulmonary complications develop. Eosinophilia is present in about half of the reported cases. Lung biopsies have revealed non-specific features resembling the changes seen in lung disease associated with other antineoplastic drugs with aggregates of inflammatory cells, including eosinophils, plasma cells, and lymphocytes in the interstitial tissue and, to a lesser extent, within alveolar spaces. In some cases symptoms and signs of pneumonitis have resolved spontaneously despite continuation of methotrexate treatment, usually with longer persistence of the X-ray changes. Resolution despite continued treatment is not a feature of other pulmonary reactions associated with eosinophilia (e.g. due to sulphasalazine). Rapid resolution of the pulmonary reaction is reported after administration of corticosteroid drugs. Of four deaths secondary to the pulmonary effects of methotrexate in higher dosage in one series, three were in individuals who did not receive corticosteroid treatment; the fourth was treated with a corticosteroid but succumbed to infection (Sostman *et al.* 1977). The pulmonary reaction to methotrexate can develop despite the concurrent administration of corticosteroid treatment. Relapse of pneumonitis on reintroduction of methotrexate has been recorded once (Goldman and Moschella 1971). Daunorubicin has been employed in the treatment of three cases (Pasquinucci *et al.* 1971) but spontaneous recovery was the probable reason for improvement (Cooper *et al.* 1986).

Procarbazine has been the subject of a number of reports of an allergic pneumonitis with prominent eosinophilia. Pleural effusions are common. The reaction may subside within a few days on withdrawal of the drug (Dohner *et al.* 1972; Lokich and Moloney 1972). Not surprisingly, steroids have been shown to be beneficial in this allergic reaction (Lewis 1984). Usually other drugs have been given, but prompt relapse has occurred on challenge with procarbazine (Jones *et al.* 1972; Ecker *et al.* 1978).

Azathioprine has been associated with an acute restrictive pulmonary reaction causing impairment of gas transfer and radiological signs of basal atelectasis or infiltration (Rubin *et al.* 1972; Weisenberger 1978; Carmichael *et al.* 1983). Withdrawal of the drug resulted in disappearance of the radiological abnormalities. There has been a single report of a similar reaction to mercaptopurine, the active metabolite of azathioprine (Sostman *et al.* 1977).

Mitomycin is an alkylating antibiotic and more than 50 cases of pulmonary toxicity associated with it have been recorded (Fielding *et al.* 1978; Gunstream *et al.* 1983; Twohig and Matthay 1990). There may be a fulminant fatal interstitial pneumonitis (Andrews *et al.* 1979). An incidence of approximately 5 per cent in a large series was reported by Buzdar and co-workers (1980), and interaction with *Vinca* alkaloids markedly increases the frequency of pneumonitis; for example Ozols and colleagues (1983) found this adverse reaction in 5 of 13 women (39 per cent) treated with mitomycin and vinblastine (with progesterone) for recurrence of ovarian carcinoma; 2 died of respiratory failure. Mitomycin alone occasionally causes a rapidly progressive interstitial pneumonitis, and an excellent response to corticosteroid therapy is to be expected (Buzdar *et al.* 1980). Despite the high incidence of the reaction there is little evidence to explain its pathogenesis. I have managed a patient with steroid-responsive mitomycin-related diffuse pneumonitis, who developed fatal thrombotic thrombocytopenic purpura (TTP) some months later. Mitomycin was the only cytotoxic drug given, and at autopsy there was minimal recurrence of colonic carcinoma a year after colectomy. A syndrome of renal insufficiency, thrombocytopenia, and microangiopathic haemolytic anaemia, very often aggravated by infusion of blood or blood products, has been linked with mitomycin, and some 40 patients with this problem (also labelled haemolytic–uraemic syndrome) have been described (Twohig and Matthay 1990). This mitomycin-related syndrome differs from idiopathic TTP in that neurological complications seem to be less prevalent. TTP is thought to be due to a defect in the capillary endothelium that affects its ability to release von Willebrand factor multimers enzymatically, and in experimental animals mitomycin injected into a platelet-free renal artery has caused local changes characteristic of TTP. The occurrence of pneumonitis and TTP in the same patient may be coincidental but the propensity for patients with the mitomycin-related TTP to develop non-cardiogenic pulmonary oedema argues for some relationship to pulmonary toxicity.

With bleomycin a chronic pulmonary fibrosis is recognized and this is discussed below, but there have been a couple of reports involving six patients with hypersensitivity pneumonitis and pulmonary eosinophilia due to bleomycin (Holyoye *et al.* 1978; Yousem *et al.* 1985).

Other drugs

Diffuse alveolitis has been attributed to penicillamine used in the treatment of rheumatoid arthritis (Eastmond 1976; Camus *et al.* 1982). Scott and colleagues (1981) described a syndrome of sudden onset of dyspnoea, crackles, and bilateral diffuse pulmonary shadowing on the chest X-ray beginning 5–16 weeks after the start of treatment in six patients who were being given gold injections. They also reviewed the literature, finding that of a total of 20 pulmonary reactions to gold, 9 had resolved. Gold treatment had been discontinued in all and 6 had received corticosteroid therapy. The total dose of sodium aurothiomalate given ranged from 350–

1000 mg. IgE levels rose after gold injection and an immune basis for the reaction is certain (Zitik and Cooper 1990) especially as Partenen and others (1987) showed that all but 3 of 17 patients with rheumatoid arthritis and gold-induced pneumonitis expressed at least one of two high-risk major histocompatibility-complex patterns. Lung biopsies have been taken in a number of cases and the histological changes are of septal thickening with infiltration by lymphocytes, plasma cells, and eosinophils (Autran et al. 1978), but the cellular reaction in one case was so dense as to resemble adenocarcinoma (James et al. 1978). In a further case the appearances were those of fibrosing alveolitis (Geddes and Brostoff 1976). Symptoms in this case recurred when gold was reintroduced and resolved completely when treatment stopped. This pattern seems fairly typical of other case reports. Impairment of pulmonary function may, however, prove to be permanent (Daymond and Griffiths 1980; Scott et al. 1981).

Pulmonary hypersensivity with perihilar infiltrates has been described following blood transfusion without hypervolaemia; the nature of the reaction is unclear (Ward et al. 1968). Pepys (1969) described pulmonary eosinophilia induced by pituitary snuff, and a similar reaction to inhaled cromoglycate has been described in two cases (Lobel et al. 1972; Repo and Nieminen 1976), although it is difficult to be certain of the aetiology in these latter instances as pulmonary eosinophilia occurs spontaneously in patients with asthma.

Intravesical BCG has been used for immunotherapy of recurrent transitional cell carcinoma, and three cases of hypersensitivity pneumonitis due to this method of treatment have been reported by Israel-Biet and colleagues (1987). An acute onset after multiple (3–8) treatments was characterized by lymphocytosis on bronchial alveolar lavage, with an increase in T_4/T_8 ratios compared with the patient's own circulating lymphocyte and control values. The chest X-ray showed no abnormality in one patient whereas bilateral micronodular shadowing was observed in the first two patients with the syndrome.

Individual cases of hypersensitivity pneumonitis have been reported with mephenesin (Rodman et al. 1958), imipramine (Wilson et al. 1963), phenytoin (Bayer 1976), metformin (Klapholz et al. 1986), and nomifensine (Patel et al. 1988).

Pulmonary oxygen toxicity

High concentrations of oxygen are toxic to the alveoli and pulmonary capillaries. Proliferative changes may develop in the walls of capillaries within a few hours of exposure to 100 per cent oxygen at atmospheric pressure. Normal subjects breathing pure oxygen at this pressure developed substernal distress which becomes unbearable after 48–72 hours (Clamanan and Becker-Freyseng 1939; Ohlsson 1947; Dolezal 1962). Bronchoscopic studies have shown reduced mucus velocity, and tracheitis developing during the first 6 hours (Sackner et al. 1975). Reduction in vital capacity and arterial desaturation accompany the exposure (Comroe et al. 1945; Ernsting 1961), but normality is restored within 48 hours. Shorter periods of exposure, up to 12 hours, do not appear to affect gas exchange or pulmonary circulation in normal subjects (van de Water et al. 1970). Patients undergoing intermittent positive pressure ventilation are prone to develop obscure pulmonary collapse and radiological shadowing; there are many potential causes of this (The Lancet 1967), but the use of a high concentration of inspired oxygen is probably important in some cases (Brewis 1969). Indirect evidence of the effect of oxygen has been provided at autopsy studies, and Nash and co-workers (1967) demonstrated a relationship between alveolar haemorrhage, thickening of the alveolar walls, and hyaline membrane formation, and the concentration of inspired oxygen employed before death. The molecular and clinical aspects of oxygen toxicity have been reviewed by Jackson (1990). A fraction of the oxygen consumed in aerobic metabolism is converted to superoxide and thence to hydrogen peroxide. The capacity of the normal scavenging mechanisms (e.g. superoxide dismutase [glutathione peroxidase], catalase, and the non-enzymatic antioxidants β-carotene, α-tocopherol, ascorbate, cysteine) may in some clinical circumstances be overwhelmed. Autocatalytic destructive peroxidation of membrane lipids then follows. In animal experiments, synthesis of surfactant is also impaired by hyperoxia. In man, the dose–duration response relationship between oxygen and toxicity is broad and inspired oxygen fractions below 0.45 are unlikely to be harmful except after an exceedingly long exposure (Comroe et al. 1945; Pratt 1974; Frank 1979). Short breaks in the exposure greatly improve tolerance, so that overt clinical evidence of oxygen toxicity tends to be limited to patients maintained on ventilators and higher oxygen concentrations without interruption (Hyde and Rawson 1969). Jackson (1990) has outlined toxic interactions between oxygen and various therapies (e.g. radiotherapy or bleomycin) with or without prophylactic corticosteroid therapy.

Drug-induced pulmonary fibrosis

Ganglion-blocking agents

Unexplained breathlessness and widespread radiological

shadowing that were not due to pulmonary oedema occurred in 3 of 54 patients being treated with the quaternary ganglion-blocker hexamethonium for severe hypertension (Doniach *et al.* 1954). This was the first instance of a report of drug-induced pulmonary fibrosis, and the histological features were further detailed by Heard (1962). The appearances were those of bronchiectasis and widespread fibrosis of the lungs with distortion and destruction of alveoli. A thorough postmortem study by Perry and colleagues (1957) found 'fibrinous pneumonitis' only in those patients who had received hexamethonium. Other ganglion-blockers, mecamylamine and pentolinium, were also found to be associated with the development of pulmonary fibrosis (Hildeen *et al.* 1958; Rokseth and Storstein 1960). While the above account is only of historical interest nowadays, it emphasizes the unexpected in pulmonary toxicology.

Cytotoxic drugs

That cytotoxic chemotherapy can cause chronic parenchymal lung damage is perhaps not surprising, and in this therapeutic area bleomycin has become a model drug in animal experimentation. Cytotoxic pulmonary toxicity has been recently reviewed very comprehensively by Jules-Elysee and White (1990), Twohig and Matthay (1990), Smith (1990), and Cooper and Matthay (1987), while Cooper and colleagues (1986) have given more detail about proposed mechanisms of toxicity. In general the factors predisposing to cytotoxic lung damage include (i) total cumulative dose; (ii) the age of the patient; (iii) prior or concurrent radiotherapy; (iv) (mainly subsequent) oxygen therapy; and (v) concomitant cytotoxic drug administration. Total cumulative dose seems to be important for bleomycin, busulphan, and carmustine. Older patients may be more sensitive to bleomycin toxicity. Synergistic toxicity between radiotherapy and bleomycin, busulphan, and mitomycin has been demonstrated. Postoperative oxygen therapy, for example, has been associated with enhanced bleomycin pulmonary toxicity, as have multidrug regimens that include carmustine, mitomycin (especially with vinblastine), cyclosphosphamide, bleomycin, and methotrexate.

Chronic pneumonitis/pulmonary fibrosis is the most common clinical presentation — a pattern associated with virtually all categories of cytotoxic drugs (except for procarbazine, with which only hypersensitivity has been described). The symptoms are of malaise, unproductive cough, and breathlessness progressing over several weeks or months. On examination there are usually crackles on auscultation of the chest. The chest X-ray is the principal screening test for detecting pulmonary fibrosis, although it is limited in sensitivity and speci-

ficity. The clinical application of diagnostic radiology in evaluating drug-induced pulmonary disease has been reviewed by Taylor (1990). Interstitial pulmonary fibrosis may present radiologically with a reticular or nodular pattern, or both, with many agents. Pleural effusions are uncommon in these reactions. Computed tomography is more sensitive in detecting bleomycin toxicity, the evolution of which can be studied as it progresses from an initially pleural-based to a basal reticulonodular pattern. Magnetic resonance imaging has not yet proved of value. It is very likely that monitoring of carbon monoxide transfer factor or vital capacity would detect changes earlier. In another context, the lesson from lung transplantation is that repeated transbronchial biopsy is the most sensitive technique available for detecting the early stages of the parenchymal reaction of rejection.

Diagnosis may be difficult if there has been previous radiotherapy and if opportunistic infection or progression of the primary disease cannot be excluded. By and large an invasive diagnostic effort will reduce uncertainty for both clinician and patient (Rosenow 1990). Rechallenge is seldom needed, as alternative therapy is almost always available. Transbronchial and open lung biopsies show typical features of damage to Type I pneumocytes with consequent proliferation of the cuboidal Type II pneumocytes that line part or all of the alveoli. Active reparative pneumocytes will also be affected by the cytotoxic drug initiating the damage, and the cytological consequences of interfering with synthesis of DNA will be apparent. These include large hyperchromatic nuclei, bizarre chromatin patterns, cell giantism, etc. Epithelial atypia is evident on cytological examination of sputum.

Bleomycin

Pulmonary toxicity with bleomycin was noted in the initial clinical studies and preclinical animal toxicology. The susceptibility of the lung partially relates to the high ambient PO_2, as bleomycin generates superoxide and also interacts with oxygen therapy and radiotherapy in augmenting pulmonary toxicity in man and experimental animals. Occasionally, as discussed earlier, acute hypersensitivity pneumonitis can develop, but the chronic reaction is much more frequent and is dose-related with patients varying in their susceptibility. Salem (1971) evaluated 56 patients aged 16–83 years by chest X-ray, lung biopsy, and pulmonary function testing, and found frank or suspected pulmonary fibrosis in 41 per cent of the 34 patients who were given a cumulative dose of more than 200 mg bleomycin per m^2 compared with 22 per cent of those given a lower dose. The older patients were more susceptible and 16 of the 19 reactions occurred in the 40 patients over 50 years of age. This influence of age seemed to be independent of a cumulative dose effect. Whether it related to renal dysfunction is unclear; bleomycin is excreted unchanged in urine but a proportion is inactivated enzymatically by a hydrolase. These early findings have been confirmed (Cooper *et al.* 1986) especially with regard to age and there seems to be a threshold at 450–500 units (450–500 mg) above which pulmonary toxicity is probable. There are well-documented cases of pulmonary fibrosis at lower doses, however, particularly in association with other risk factors. One patient of Salem (1971) had severe fibrotic changes at autopsy after 140 mg per m^2. The smallest reported dose associated with a pulmonary reaction was 60 units of bleomycin, which caused ARDS and alveolar fibroblast proliferation at autopsy in a patient with renal impairment (McLeod *et al.* 1987), and Iacovino and colleagues (1976) reported two fatal instances of interstitial pneumonitis in younger men given 105 and 165 units of bleomycin, respectively. A reversible reaction after 180 mg (15 mg weekly) has been described (Brown *et al.* 1978). Asymptomatic reactions without radiological changes have been detected by pulmonary function testing. This approach gave an overall incidence of pulmonary toxicity of between 33 per cent and 71 per cent (Pascual *et al.* 1973; Yagoda *et al.* 1972).

In younger age-groups, Lucraft and co-workers (1982) described 38 patients with testicular teratoma who received four doses of 90 mg of bleomycin and in whom the carbon monoxide transfer factor fell by 10 per cent after the first dose but not thereafter. An abnormal gallium scan, which reverted to normal after corticosteroid treatment, was seen in one patient whose lungs at autopsy were histologically normal (Rubery and Coakley 1980). Gallium is preferentially taken up by neutrophils, and the above report is of interest in view of the experimental finding that bleomycin can acutely increase the neutrophil count in fluid obtained by bronchoalveolar lavage in dogs (Fahey *et al.* 1982). A clinical correlate may be the increase in the percentage of neutrophils in the lavage fluid seen in four patients with bleomycin toxicity (Cooper *et al.* 1986). An increase in neutrophils is also found, however, in end-stage idiopathic pulmonary fibrosis and has been recognized as indicating a poor prognosis with little likelihood of a response to corticosteroid therapy. Another factor to be considered is whether bleomycin has been used in the past in a given patient. All previous regimens containing bleomycin should be included in calculating the total dose, as no period between doses adequate to abolish a possible increased risk of pulmonary dysfunction due to previous administration has yet been established (Cooper *et al.* 1986).

Alkylating agents

For many, busulphan lung is the archetype of drug-induced pulmonary toxicity, but other alkylating agents in common use, such as cyclophosphamide, chlorambucil, and melphalan, are also toxic to the lung.

Busulphan The incidence of pulmonary toxicity with this drug is 4 per cent (Cooper *et al.* 1986), but autopsy studies have shown subclinical damage in about half the cases. It is of interest that busulphan is chemically related to hexamethonium (see above). Almost always treatment will have been in progress for many months or even many years before symptoms develop, and there seems to be a threshold cumulative dose of 500 mg below which pulmonary toxicity has not occurred unless radiotherapy or other cytotoxic chemotherapy has been exhibited. The onset of toxicity is insidious. Fever is usual and is accompanied by cough and dyspnoea. The early histological features include proteinaceous alveolar oedema and dysplastic Type II pneumocytes, while advanced cases may have 'honeycomb lung' with alveoli replaced by masses of fibrous tissue (Heard and Cooke 1968). The condition is irreversible, and mean survival after diagnosis has been 5 months (Cooper *et al.* 1986). Pleural effusion has occurred in two cases. A complicating feature of pulmonary fibrosis due to busulphan has been the development of alveolar cell carcinoma (Min and Györkey 1968; Rosenow 1972). Busulphan should be withdrawn. There have been anecdotal reports of response to corticosteroid therapy, but awareness of the cumulative dose risk and monitoring of lung function at this threshold may help avoid clinical toxicity.

Chlorambucil and melphalan There have been fewer reports of pulmonary toxicity with these drugs but the clinical features are similar to other cases of drug-induced pulmonary fibrosis and the prognosis is poor (Twohig and Matthay 1990). One patient with chlorambucil toxicity, however, had a restrictive pulmonary defect (low transfer factor), a scattered interstitial mononuclear infiltrate on lung biopsy, and a dramatic response to withdrawal of the drug and corticosteroid therapy (Cole *et al.* 1978). Of seven patients reported with melphalan pulmonary toxicity, five died from progressive fibrosis (Major *et al.* 1980; Cooper *et al.* 1986). One patient who received 592 mg of melphalan over 8 months, even though the diagnosis of myeloma had not been established, developed a cough, progressive dyspnoea, and had a carbon monoxide transfer factor 30 per cent of the predicted value (Goucher *et al.* 1980). There was interstitial lung disease on an open lung biopsy. Corticosteroids were given but symptoms failed to improve despite radiological clearing. Westerfield and others (1980) described a patient whose recovery seemed complete. Major and colleagues (1980) reported one death, of a pharmacist who treated himself with melphalan apparently because myeloma had been mentioned in his differential diagnosis.

Cyclosphosphamide   This drug is very widely used as a cytotoxic agent and, in lower dosage, as an immunouppressant, yet Cooper and colleagues (1986) found only 20 cases of cyclophosphamide-induced pulmonary fibrosis recorded in the literature, in 8 of which the patients had also received vincristine. Its rarity makes it a diagnosis of exclusion, which may be difficult without lung biopsy, particularly in patients with systemic or pulmonary vasculitis or granulomatosis. Fever, cough, and progressive breathlessness are common. Interstitial pneumonitis has occurred after prolonged cyclophosphamide treatment for Hodgkin's disease (Topilow *et al.* 1973), whereas Patel and colleagues (1976) reported pulmonary fibrosis on open lung biopsy in a 72-year-old woman in whom the infiltrates cleared completely when cyclophosphamide (given concurrently with vincristine and prednisolone) was stopped and continuous treatment with high-dose prednisolone was instituted. Immunosuppressant doses have also caused two fatal pulmonary reactions (Burke *et al.* 1982). One patient had rapidly progressive glomerulonephritis (GN) and was given 100 mg per day for 7 weeks and the other had refractory nephrotic syndrome and received 200 mg per day for 13 weeks. Mark and colleagues (1978) also reported a patient with GN who developed a restrictive ventilatory defect with an 'extensive intra-alveolar histiocytic infiltrate and septal thickening'. Improvement after withdrawal of cyclophosphamide was slow in spite of the administration of prednisolone.

Carmustine   The nitrosoureas are particularly used as single agents in the treatment of intracranial tumours, and Twohig and Matthay (1990) identified more than 80 reports of pulmonary toxicity, the majority of which occurred with carmustine (BCNU). The first case was reported in 1976, more than 10 years after the introduction of this drug. A possible explanation for the delay is the variable survival of patients and also the slow development of the pulmonary fibrosis, which shows all the usual histological features of cytological dysplasia; uniquely, however, the fibroblast proliferation is not accompanied by an obvious degree of inflammatory cell infiltrate (Weiss *et al.* 1981). Indeed, many cases of

pulmonary toxicity developed quite late, for example, 3–4 years after treatment, and Cooper and others (1986) stated the incidence of this complication to be 20–30 per cent, while the mortality rate has varied from 45–55 per cent in different series. A recent report calls for a complete reappraisal of this brief summary of the scope of the problem, however. O'Driscoll and colleagues (1990) examined a cohort of survivors of carmustine chemotherapy in childhood. Of 31 children (aged 2–16 years) given carmustine for brain tumours, only 17 survived, and 6 of these died subsequently from pulmonary fibrosis, 2 within 3 years of treatment and 4 from 8–13 years after treatment. Eight of the remaining patients were available to be studied, 10–17 years after treatment. The findings were cough and dyspnoea in 4, and in 6 an abnormal chest X-ray with upper zone fibrotic changes with unique computed tomographic appearances; for the group, vital capacity was 54 per cent, and transfer factor ranged from 28–78 per cent, of the predicted values, whereas the transfer coefficient (K_{CO}) ranged from 93–151 per cent. Bronchoalveolar lavage showed an increase in the percentage of macrophages containing fibronectin. Transbronchial biopsy showed insterstitial fibrosis and elastosis. The recognition of an active pulmonary fibrotic process up to 17 years after treatment with carmustine emphasizes the need to follow up these patients and consider single lung transplantation as the pulmonary fibrosis progresses.

Nitrofurantoin

Pulmonary reactions to this drug are among the most frequently reported adverse effects on the lungs. A spectrum of reactions is seen in which acute, subacute, and chronic forms may be distinguished (Hailey *et al.* 1969; Sovijarvi *et al.* 1977). The acute reaction is discussed with other examples of hypersensitivity pneumonitis. Subacute reactions develop after about 4 weeks of continuous treatment, and fever and intense breathlessness occur. Eosinophilia is not universal and a raised antinuclear antibody can sometimes be detected (Selroos and Edgren 1975). Chronic reactions are of insidious onset and are associated with long-term prophylactic treatment lasting more than 6 months. Withdrawal of nitrofurantoin is the principal therapeutic approach. The majority of reactions are not severe, but persistent damage is common with the chronic reaction, in which lung biopsy will show vascular sclerosis with fibrosis and thickening of alveolar septa, together with interstitial inflammation. Interestingly, desquamative pneumonitis has been described with nitrofurantoin (R.D. Bone *et al.* 1976), and this type of reaction can be expected to respond reasonably satisfactorily to corticosteroid therapy with more complete resolution than if the drug were merely withdrawn.

Amiodarone

Amiodarone was used in Europe for some dozen or so years before it was employed more widely in the management of resistant ventricular and supraventricular arrhythmias in the 1980s. The doses used for this purpose were somewhat higher than previously needed, and the first report of amiodarone pulmonary toxicity was by Rotmensch and colleagues (1980). They described a 50-year-old man who developed lassitude and tachypnoea after 1 month of amiodarone in a dose of 400 mg daily. The chest X-ray showed diffuse pulmonary shadowing; FVC was 46 per cent of the predicted value; PaO_2 was 6.0 kPa, and pulmonary hypertension was found with a normal wedge pressure. Amiodarone was discontinued; prednisolone 60 mg per day was started; and within 2 weeks there was complete resolution. Many descriptions of individual cases and series followed but in most the speed of onset and resolution were not as rapid as this. Kennedy (1990) identifies two main clinical patterns. The more common is a subacute presentation with cough and increased breathlessness, sometimes with weight loss. A chest radiograph will show diffuse interstitial infiltrates bilaterally. The other mode of presentation resembles that of first patient described above and is a more acute illness. This group of patients are pyrexial and have chest X-ray changes with a more alveolar distribution of opacification. Pleural effusions are unusual but have been described (Sobol and Rakita 1982; Gonzales-Rothi et al. 1987). Eosinophilia is not a feature. Confluent opacities, which may be peripheral, apical, or pleurally based, have been described (Marchlinski et al. 1982; Gefter et al. 1983). Monitoring of the CO transfer factor as a method of early detection of amiodarone pulmonary toxicity was advocated in the third edition of this book. Kennedy (1990) has reviewed the evidence that has been presented in the interim and concludes that patients should have pulmonary function testing when they are in a stable condition before or soon after starting amiodarone. He states that testing should be repeated whenever the clinical picture suggests the possibility of pulmonary toxicity. A fall of 15–20 per cent in transfer factor is a certain predictor of amiodarone toxicity. Lesser degrees of impairment are not significant, especially if the patient is asymptomatic.

The histological features of pulmonary toxicity due to amiodarone are typical of this whole group of chronic fibrotic reactions with one exception, that is, the intra-alveolar accumulation of 'foamy' macrophages, which can also be detected after bronchoalveolar lavage. They are a marker of amiodarone accumulation and are present in patients who do not have pulmonary toxicity (Myers et al. 1987). Electron microscopy has shown that the 'foamy' appearance is due to dense lamellar cytoplasmic inclusions containing phospholipid (with amiodarone and desethylamiodarone). This phospholipidosis is probably central to the aetiology of amiodarone pulmonary toxicity and occurs because of the unique pharmacokinetic properties of the drug and its metabolite. They each have a huge volume of distribution (5000 litres) and this requires a very long elimination half-life ($t_{1/2}$) that is biphasic, representing clearance from well-diffused and poorly diffused tissues. The value of $t_{1/2}$ of 45–60 days is quoted (Martin 1990). It will be apparent therefore that stopping the drug in a patient with toxicity will not result in rapid clearing of the affected tissue or organ, particularly if the drug has accumulated significantly following administration for a prolonged period.

Both the parent drug and its major metabolite, desethylamiodarone, are concentrated in the lung up to 1000-fold compared with serum levels. Given this accumulation a direct toxic effect would be considered a likely mechanism, particularly as part of the damage seems to occur much more frequently in patients receiving higher doses (Marchlinski et al. 1982; Suarez et al. 1983; Gefter et al. 1983). Daily doses of amiodarone greater than 400 mg are associated with a 5–7 per cent incidence of interstitial pneumonitis. There are, however, two populations of patients, those with and those without evidence of inflammation and immunological reaction and it may be that these people also have different histological appearances on lung biopsy; for example, Myers and colleagues (1987) found 'organizing pneumonia' in a quarter of their patients with amiodarone toxicity. This type of histological picture is expected to respond to corticosteroid therapy, as did a patient who had features of fibrosing alveolitis associated with chronic amiodarone administration who continued to deteriorate when the drug was stopped (Butland and Millard 1984). One patient reported by Adams and colleagues (1986), however, developed frank toxicity despite receiving corticosteroid treatment incidentally. They also found that reduction or withdrawal of steroids was associated with clinical deterioration in two patients and with a decline in pulmonary function tests in four others. These were patients who received doses of 400–600 mg daily for 8 months or so and in whom the steroid therapy was reduced before one would expect clearance of amiodarone from tissues. In other patients improvement following reduction of the dose was greater than when steroids were given. Nevertheless, Kennedy (1990) recommends treating patients with amiodarone pulmonary toxicity with corticosteroids; a typical regimen consists of an initial dose of 40–60 mg with subsequent tapering based on the severity of the illness and the clinical response. Treatment continues for 4–6 months with close clinical follow-up. Some patients require continuous steroid therapy with the low, almost physiological, dose of 10 mg of prednisolone on alternate days. Given the life-threatening ventricular arrhythmias for which amiodarone therapy is usually instituted, it is understandable that doctors are reluctant to reduce the dose once a stable clinical situation has been achieved. Nevertheless, this would seem to be the best prophylactic means of reducing the incidence of amiodarone pulmonary toxicity.

Other drugs

Virtually all drug reactions that cause an acute hypersensitivity pneumonitis may lead to persistent sequelae, especially when the cause of the reaction is not recognized and the offending agent is not discontinued. This is likely if the onset is insidious or if respiratory disease is a recognized complicating feature of the underlying problem. With practolol, recognition was even more difficult as the fibrosis appeared as a delayed adverse effect (Erwteman et al. 1977). Six further cases were recorded (Marshall et al. 1977) and all had previously developed sclerosing peritonitis.

The antiarrhythmic drug tocainide has occasionally been associated with the development of pulmonary fibrosis, and a recent report described the computed tomographic appearances (Stein et al. 1988).

Other parenchymal problems

Carcinoma of the lung has been mentioned above in relation to busulphan lung, and theoretically it may complicate any chronic pulmonary fibrosis (cf. 'scar cancer' in healed fibrotic pulmonary tuberculosis). Pulmonary nodules have been described in patients receiving chemotherapy with cisplatin, bleomycin, and vinblastine (CBV) for germ-cell tumours (Zucker et al. 1987), and Trump and others (1988) saw new basal nodules on computed tomography after CBV in 11 patients with intrathoracic tumours. All of the patients recovered. Talcott and colleagues (1987) found cavitating granulomas on open lung biopsy following CBV. In 2.8 per cent of patients receiving an infusion of bleomycin, acute chest pain, which in some instances was thought to be due to myocardial ischaemia, developed; in others there was a pleuritic element. Six of the 10 patients had pulmonary metastases and pain developed on the second

or third day of therapy. The pain recurred in 2 of 7 patients. There were no long-term sequelae, and White and colleagues (1987) concluded that continuing the therapy was safe. An unusual consequence of intravenous drug abuse has been the development of severe bullous emphysema due to methylphenidate (Sherman et al. 1987), and this may follow other granulomatous reactions to other intravenous illicit substance abuse (Heffner et al. 1990).

Pleural space

Pleural effusion may complicate heart failure and the nephrotic syndrome and may be provoked by excessive intravenous infusion of colloid. Peritoneal dialysis has been associated with recurrent pleural effusions, presumably due to the passage of dialysis fluid through developmental transdiaphragmatic communications (Holm et al. 1971). Pleural effusions complicating ARDS may not be apparent if the chest X-ray is taken in the supine position. They may also occasionally occur as part of an acute or chronic parenchymal reaction to a drug, for example, with nitrofurantoin (Robinson 1964) or amiodarone (Sobol and Rakita 1982). Gonadotrophin has caused acute ascites and hydrothorax (Mrouch and Kase 1967).

Drugs affecting the pleura

Methysergide

Pleural thickening, fibrosis, and effusion can be produced by this drug. As a rule the patient has been taking the treatment for several months before the onset of the reaction is made apparent by the development of pleural pain, breathlessness, fever, and malaise. Examination may reveal signs of an effusion with a loud pleural rub. The chest X-ray usually shows a uniform hazy shadowing over the lower lung fields. A restrictive ventilatory defect is generally present. Occasionally there is nodular thickening of the pleura, which suggests tumour formation. Although the pleural lesion is usually described as fibrosis, improvement in symptoms and in the radiological appearance has been reported after cessation of treatment, and Kok-Jensen and Lindeneg (1970) found persisting severe disability in only 2 out of 12 cases in which treatment had been withdrawn because of pleuropulmonary complications. The mechanism underlying the development of the pleural changes is quite unknown and withdrawal of the drug is the only measure required to bring about improvement. Pulmonary mediastinal fibrosis and retroperitoneal fibrosis also occur with this drug.

Bromocriptine

Bromocriptine, like methysergide, is an ergot derivative and is used as a dopaminergic agonist in Parkinson's disease, particularly where 'on–off' phenomena occur with levodopa. Therapy therefore tends to be long-term, and Rinne (1981) drew attention to pleuropulmonary fibrosis with pleural effusion in 7 of 123 parkinsonian patients being treated with bromocriptine. Five of the 7 were also receiving levodopa. The manufacturer's cumulative experience from 1974 to 1981 amounted to 4000 patient-years and only a single report was on file (Krupp 1981); in the same correspondence LeWitt and Calne (1981) reported one patient. It is only with subsequent case reports and series and longer term treatment that convincing circumstantial evidence has accumulated of a very real problem in a minority of patients taking bromocriptine. Of 441 reports to the Committee on Safety of Medicines since 1971 mentioning bromocriptine, 2 are for pleural fibrosis and 2 for pulmonary fibrosis, but McElvaney and others (1988) found seven patients with pleuropulmonary fibrosis which they attributed to bromocriptine, in a survey based in British Columbia. The dose-range was 22–50 mg per day and all were men who were over 55 years of age and heavy cigarette smokers. The onset of symptoms occurred 9 months to 4 years after starting treatment. The patients complained of dyspnoea, pleuritic pain, and an unproductive cough. The chest X-ray showed unilateral or bilateral pleural thickening and basal pulmonary fibrosis. Lung function was impaired with reduced static and dynamic lung volumes, and the CO transfer factor was reduced in proportion to the change in lung volume, that is, the diffusion coefficient (K_{CO}) was normal or raised. Open pleural biopsy in two patients revealed an exudative effusion with eosinophilia and pleural fibrosis with occasional inflammatory cells. No cause other than bromocriptine was found after investigation and clinical benefit followed cessation of therapy in five patients. In two patients bromocriptine was continued and one deteriorated. Tornling and colleagues (1986) described four cases (three of them non-smokers) aged 61–65 years who developed their reactions 2–3 years after starting bromocriptine, the eventual doses being 20–50 mg per day. Corticosteroid therapy was used with some improvement but most benefit was seen after withdrawal of bromocriptine. I have managed a patient in whom symptoms began 7 years after the start of treatment with marked clinical improvement on stopping bromocriptine, especially with regard to his breathlessness and

cough that had been productive of mucoid sputum. His sense of well-being improved and weight gain was substantial, but radiological changes have been minor after 4 months. Having regard to this patient's late development of the reaction, one must suspect that many more cases of pleuropulmonary fibrosis will develop as time elapses and the duration of therapy increases. It is not surprising therefore that retroperitoneal fibrosis has also occurred with bromocriptine therapy (Bowler *et al.* 1986; Herzog *et al.* 1989), and Ward and others (1987) reported patients with both retroperitoneal and pleuropulmonary fibrosis. McElvaney and colleagues (1988) also described pleuropulmonary fibrosis in a patient treated with another ergot derivative, mesulergine, with clinical benefit following its withdrawal. The occurrence of progressive pulmonary fibrosis in patients taking methysergide, ergotamine, LSD, or bromocriptine seems to be dose-related. One theory of the aetiology suggests that antagonism at serotonin (5-HT) receptors is important, but further clarification is awaited, especially with regard to activity of these drugs at different 5-HT receptor subtypes.

Pleural fibrosis and effusion have been observed as a complication of practolol therapy (Hall *et al.* 1978).

Haemothorax

Haemothorax has occurred in patients on anticoagulant therapy who have fallen and fractured ribs (Hamaker *et al.* 1969; Diamond and Fell 1973) or who have developed haemorrhagic pulmonary infarction following pulmonary embolism (Simon *et al.* 1969; Millard 1971).

Pneumothorax and pneumomediastinum

Pneumothorax has been reported to complicate the chemotherapy of germ-cell tumours with pulmonary metastases (Schulman *et al.* 1979). Abusers of illicit substances may indulge in extraordinary measures to increase their 'high' (Heffner *et al.* 1990). As peripheral veins become thrombosed, jugular and subclavian access may be attempted, which may result in laceration of the apex of the lung and pneumothorax. Use of the inhalational route can be accompanied by attempts to maximize absorption from alveolar surfaces. A Valsalva manoeuvre after maximal inspiration is reasonably safe but abusers who get a partner to augment their total lung capacity may suffer barotrauma. Alkaloidal cocaine seems to be particularly associated with pneumomediastinum.

Respiratory muscles and their central nervous control

Drug-induced neuromuscular disorders

This subject is discussed in detail in Chapter 18 and there is little that applies exclusively to respiratory muscles. Prolonged apnoea after the administration of suxamethonium, due to pseudocholinesterase deficiency, is well recognized. The aminoglycoside antibiotics may also aggravate neuromuscular blockade, especially in the presence of renal impairment or myasthenia gravis. Neomycin is probably the most dangerous of the drugs in this regard. Spinal anaesthesia, accidentally produced by local anaesthetic agents, may cause dangerous respiratory depression, especially if the cervical spinal cord is affected.

An interesting reaction to levodopa in postencephalitic parkinsonism has been recognized (Granerus et al. 1974; De Keyser and Vincken 1985). Within 2 hours of taking levodopa, the rate and depth of respiration become irregular and symptomatic dyspnoea arises. The phenomenon is dose-related.

Tiapride, a substituted benzamide, effective in dyskinesia induced by levodopa, normalized the spirogram in one patient, who became free of dyspnoea (De Keyser and Vincken 1985). Hyperventilation is a well-recognized effect of salicylate overdose; the effect is sometimes quite striking and may be associated with tetany.

Depression of central ventilatory control

All sedative and anaesthetic agents are capable of depressing ventilation even in normal individuals, particularly if given in sufficiently high dosage. Patients with hepatic failure are particularly prone to respiratory depression when treated with agents that are largely detoxicated in the liver, for example, benzodiazepines; and patients with renal failure are vulnerable to morphine, as morphine-6-glucuronide has sedative activity and depends on renal excretion. Elderly individuals often show a surprising susceptibility to sedatives. Respiratory depression by drugs administered in standard doses is perhaps most often seen in patients with chronic bronchitis, long-standing airflow obstruction, and chronic compensated Type II respiratory failure. There is probably no drug capable of producing sedation with complete safety in such individuals. In severe asthma with exhaustion and retention of carbon dioxide, sedative drugs are particularly dangerous, and mechanical ventilation is the required treatment in this circumstance. Dangerous respiratory depression is most likely to arise from postoperative analgesia and during the intravenous sedation that is now commonly used to cover minor surgery, dental procedures, endoscopy, and various types of needle biopsy. Narcotic addiction in mothers has been associated with a fourfold increase in the sudden infant death. The defect in the chemical control of breathing persists in babies for several weeks, long after methadone, for example, has been cleared from their blood (Shannon and Kelly 1982).

Oxygen in respiratory failure with airflow obstruction

Patients with chronic respiratory failure and those who gradually develop respiratory failure are commonly insensitive to the ventilatory stimulus of carbon dioxide. During an acute infective exacerbation, worsening airflow obstruction causes further retention of carbon dioxide, and under these circumstances hypoxaemia is the main stimulus to breathing. If oxygen is administered, this hypoxic drive is removed and ventilation diminishes further, leading to still greater accumulation of carbon dioxide. Carbon dioxide exerts a narcotic effect at high partial pressures and stupor resulting from this will result in a failure to cough up secretions, leading in turn to further deterioration in ventilatory status and the likelihood of the development of bronchopneumonia. This sequence of events is now widely understood. Problems may be minimized by serial measurement of arterial blood gases and only giving sufficient oxygen to avoid progressive elevation of P_{CO_2}. Administration of an infusion of doxapram may be useful in the short term to stimulate ventilation and so permit adequate oxygen therapy. If deterioration occurs despite this therapy, mechanical ventilation may be necessary, especially in patients with bronchopneumonia.

References

Abramov, L.A., Yust, I.C., Fierstater, E.M., and Vardinon, N.E. (1978). Acute respiratory distress caused by erythromycin hypersensitivity. *Arch. Intern. Med.* 138, 1155.

Adams, P.G., Gibson, G.J., Morley, A.R., Wright, A.J., Corris, P.A., Reid, D.S., et al. (1986). Amiodarone pulmonary toxicity: Clinical and subclinical features. *Q. J. Med.* 59, 449.

Albazzaz, M.K., Harvey, J.E., Hoffman, J.N., and Siddorn, J.A. (1986). Alveolitis and haemolytic anaemia induced by azapropazone. *Br. Med. J.* 293, 1537.

Ali, N. and Banks, T. (1973). Pentazocine addiction causing bacterial endocarditis and pulmonary embolism. *Chest* 64, 762.

Andersson, L. and Smidt, C.M. (1974). An investigation of the bronchial mucous membrane after long-term treatment with beclomethasone diproprionate (Becotide). *Acta Allergol.* 29, 354.

Andrews, A.T., Bowman, H.S., Patel, S.B., and Anderson, W.M. (1979). Mitomycin and interstitial pneumonitis. *Ann. Intern. Med.* 90, 127.

Ansell, G. Adverse reactions to contrast agents — scope of problem. *Invest. Radiol.* 5, 374.

Autran, P., Garbe, L., Pommier De Santi, P., Baralis, G., and Charpin, J. (1978). Un cas d'accident rare de la chrysothérapie: une miliare pulmonaire allergique. *Rev. Fr. Mal. Respir.* 6, 183.

Baillie, R.M. (1967). Amitriptyline and sputum viscosity. *Lancet* ii, 369.

Ballen, K.K. and Weiss, S.T. (1988). Fatal acute respiratory failure following vinblastine and mitomycin administration for breast cancer. *Am. J. Med Sci.* 295, 558.

Ballester, E., Reyes, A., Roca, J., Guitard, R., Wagner, P.D., and Rodriguez-Roison, R. (1989). Ventilation–perfusion mismatching in acute severe asthma: effects of salbutamol and 100% oxygen. *Thorax* 44, 258.

Barbadi, F., Quenzer, F., and Rapp, K. (1986). Pulmonary sensitivity to Nalfon. *Ann. Allergy* 57, 205.

Barclay, K., Keaney, M.G.L., Glew, E., and Gray, J. (1990). Multiresistant *Haemophilus influenzae. Lancet* 335, 549.

Bayer, A.S. (1976). Dilantin toxicity, miliary pulmonary infiltrates and hypoxemia. *Ann. Intern. Med.* 85, 475.

Beasley, R., Rafferty, P., and Holgate, S. (1986). Benzalkonium chloride and bronchoconstriction. *Lancet* ii, 127.

Beaudry, C. and Laplante, L. (1973). Severe allergic pneumonitis from hydrochlorothiazide. *Ann. Intern. Med.* 78, 251.

Becker, C.E., MacGregor, R.R., Walker, K.S., and Jandy, J.H. (1966). Fatal anaphylaxis after intramuscular iron dextran. *Ann. Intern. Med.* 65, 745.

Beemer, G.H., Dennis, W.L., Platt, P.R., Bjorksten, A.R., and Carr A.B. (1988). Adverse reactions to atracurium and alcuronium. *Br. J. Anaesth.* 61, 680.

Belin, R.P., Shea, M.A., Stone, N.H., and Griffen, W.O. (1965). Iodolisposputosis following lymphangiography. Report of a case. *Dis. Chest* 48, 543.

Bell, R.J.M. (1964). Pulmonary infiltration with eosinophils caused by chlorpropamide. *Lancet* i, 1249.

Belongia, E.A., Hedberg, C.W., Gleich, G.J., White, K.E., Moyeno, A.N., Loegering, D.A., *et al.* (1990). An investigation of the cause of eosinophila–myalgia syndrome associated with tryptophan use. *N. Engl. J. Med.* 323, 357.

Bernecker, C. and Roetscher, I. (1970). The beta blocking effect of practolol in asthmatics. *Lancet* ii, 662.

Bertelsen, K. and Dalgaard, J.B. (1965). Death from penicillin; cases from Denmark with autopsies. *Nord. Med.* 73, 173.

Bhatia, SP.P. and Davies, H.J. (1975). Evaluation of tolerance after continuous oral administration of salbutamol to asthmatic patients. *Br. J. Clin. Pharmacol.* 2, 463.

Bogartz, L.J. and Miller, W.C. (1971). Pulmonary oedema associated with proproxyphene intoxication. *JAMA* 215, 259.

Bone, R.D., Wolfe, J., Sobonya, R.E., Kirby, G.R., Stechschulte, D., Ruth, W.E., *et al.* (1976). Desquamative interstitial pneumonia following chronic nitrofurantoin therapy. *Am. J. Med.* 60, 677.

Bone, R.S., Jay, S.J., Reynolds, R.C., and Johanson, W.G. (1976). Massive pulmonary haemorrhage: a rare complication of heparin therapy. *Am. J. Med. Sci.* 272, 197.

Borrie, J. and Gwynne, J.R. (1973). Paraffinoma of lung: lipoid pneumonia. *Thorax* 28, 214.

Bowler, J.V., Ormerod, I.E., and Legg, N.J. (1986). Retroperitoneal fibrosis and bromocriptine. *Lancet* ii, 466.

Brewis, R.A.L. (1969). Oxygen toxicity during artificial ventilation. *Thorax* 24, 656.

British Medical Journal (1973). Analgesics and asthma. *Br. Med. J.* iii, 419.

British Medical Journal. (1990). Guidelines for the management of asthma in adults. *Br. Med. J.* 301, 651.

Brooks, S.M., Werk, E.E., Ackerman, S.J., Sullivan, I., and Thrasher, K. (1972). Adverse effects of phenobarbital on corticosteroid metabolism in patients with bronchial asthma. *N. Engl. J. Med.* 286, 1125.

Brown, W.G., Hassan, F.M., and Barbee, R.A. (1978). Reversibility of severe bleomycin induced pneumonitis. *JAMA* 239, 2012.

Bruchhausen, D., Haschem, J., and Dardene, M.U. (1969). Effect of pilocarpine administered into the conjunctival sac on airway obstruction in asthmatics. *German Medical Monthly* 14, 587.

Bryant, D.H. and Pepys, J. (1976). Bronchial reactions to aerosol inhalant vehicle (beclomethasone dipropionate). *Br. Med. J.* i, 1319.

Buckland, R.W. and Avery, A.F. (1973). Histamine release following pancuronium: A case report. *Br. J. Anaesth.* 45, 518.

Bucknall, C.E., Adamson, M.R., and Banham, S.W. (1987). Non fatal pulmonary haemorrhage associated with nitrofurantoin. *Thorax* 42, 475.

Bucknall, C.E., Neilly, J.B., Carter, R., Stevenson, R.D., and Semple, P.F. (1988). Bronchial hyperreactivity in patients who cough after receiving angiotensin converting enzyme inhibitors. *Br. Med. J.* 296, 86.

Buist, A.S., Burney, P.G.J., Feinstein, A.R., Horwitz, R.I., Lanes, S.F., Rebuck, A.S., *et al.* (1989). Fenoterol and fatal asthma. *Lancet* i, 1071.

Burke, D.A., Stoddart, J.C., Ward, M.K., and Simpson, C.G. (1982). Fatal pulmonary fibrosis occurring during treatment with cyclophosphamide. *Br. Med. J.* 285, 696.

Butland, R.J.A. and Millard, F.J.C. (1984). Fibrosing alveolitis associated with amiodarone. *Eur. J. Respir. Dis.* 65, 616.

Buzdar, A.U., Legha, S.S., Luna, M.A., Tashima, C.K., Hortobagyi, G.N., and Blumenschein, G.R. (1980). Pulmonary toxicity of mitomycin. *Cancer* 45, 236.

Byrd, R.B. and Schanzer, B. (1969). Pulmonary sequelae in procainamide-induced lupus-like syndrome. *Dis. Chest* 55, 170.

Cameron, D.C. (1975). Diffuse pulmonary disorder caused by oxyphenbutazone. *Br. Med. J.* ii, 500.

Cameron, J.D. (1974). Pulmonary oedema following drip-infusion urography. Case report. *Radiology* 111, 89.

Camus, P., Reybet-Degat, O., Justrabo, E., and Jeannin, L. (1982). D-penicillamine-induced severe pneumonitis. *Chest* 81, 376.

Carmichael, D.J.S., Hamilton, D.V., Evans, D.B., Stovin, P.G.I., and Calne, R.Y. (1983). Interstitial pneumonitis associated with azathioprine in a renal transplant patient. *Thorax* 38, 951.

Chalmers, D., Dombey, S.L., and Lawson, D.H. (1987). Post marketing surveillance of captopril (for hypertension): a preliminary report. *Br. J. Clin. Pharmacol.* 24, 343.

Chapman, T.T. (1969). Bronchodilator aerosols. *Br. Med. J.* iv, 557.

Child, J.S., Wolfe, J.B., Tashkin, D., and Nakano, F. (1975). Fatal lung scan in case of pulmonary hypertension due to obliterative pulmonary vascular disease. *Chest* 67, 308.

Chiu, C.L. and Gambach, R.R. (1974). Hypaque pulmonary oedema, a case report. *Radiology* 111, 91.

Chuck, A.J., Wilcox, M., and Bossingham, D.H. (1987). Fenbufen-associated pneumonitis. *Br. J. Rheumatol.* 26, 475.

Chung, M.M., Chetty, K.G., and Jerome, D. (1985). Metoclopramide and asthma. *Ann. Intern. Med.* 103, 809.

Clamman, H.G. and Becker-Freyseng, H. (1939). Einwirkung des Sauerstoffs auf den Organismus bei hoherem als normalem Partialdruck unter besonderer Berucksichtigung des Menschen. *Luftfahrtmedizin* 4, 1.

Clark, R.J. (1986). Aggravation of asthma by beclomethasone in a thirty month old boy. *Lancet* ii, 574.

Clarke, R.S.J., Dundee, J.W., Garrett, R.T., Macardle, G.K., and Sutton, J.A. (1975). Adverse reactions to intravenous anaesthetics. A survey of 100 reports. *Br. J. Anaesth.* 47, 575.

Clarke, R.S.J., Fee, J.P.H., and Dundee, J.W. (1977). Factors predisposing to hypersentivity-reactions to intravenous anaesthetics. *Proc. R. Soc. Med.* 79, 782.

Clarke, S.W. and Newman, S.P. (1984). Therapeutic aerosols 2 — Drugs available by the inhaled route. *Thorax* 39, 1.

Cole, S.R., Myers, T.J., and Klatsky, A.U. (1978). Pulmonary disease with chlorambucil therapy. *Cancer* 41, 455.

Coles, R.B., Philips, J., and Nuttall, J.B. (1967). Anaphylactoid reaction to demethychlortetracycline (Ledermycin). *Br. Med. J.* ii, 313.

Comroe, J.H. Jr and Dripps, R.D. (1946). The histamine like action of curare and tubocurarine injected intra-cutaneously and intra-arterially in man. *Anaesthesiology* 7, 260.

Comroe, J.H. Jr, Dumke, P.R., and Deming, M. (1945). Oxygen toxicity. The effect of inhalation of high concentrations of oxygen for twenty-four hours on normal man at sea level and at a simulated altitude of 18,000 feet. *JAMA* 128, 710.

Connolly, K. (1982). Adverse reaction to ipratropium bromide. *Br. Med. J.* 285, 934.

Constantinidis. K.A. (1976). Eosinophilic pneumonia: an unusual side-effect of therapy with salicylazosulfapyridine. *Chest* 70, 315.

Cooper, J.A.D. Jr and Matthay, R.A. (1987). Drug induced pulmonary disease. *Disease-a-Month* 33, 61.

Cooper, J.A.D. Jr, White, D.A., and Matthay, R.A. (1986). Drug induced pulmonary disease Part 1: Cytotoxic drugs. *Am. Rev. Respir. Dis.* 133, 321.

Coppack, S.W., Gillett, M.K., and Snashall, P.D. (1984). Inappropriately inhaled bronchodilators. *Thorax* 39, 472.

Council on Drugs. (1964). A mucolytic agent; acetylcysteine (Mucomyst). *JAMA* 190, 147.

Crane, J., Pearce, N., Flatt, A., Burgess, C., Jackson, R., Kwong, T., *et al.* (1989). Prescribed fenoterol and death from asthma in New Zealand. 1981–1983: case control study. *Lancet* i, 917.

Crompton, G.K. (1982). Sputum viscosity and long-term ipratropium bromide nebuliser therapy. *Lancet* i, 1243.

CSM (Committee on Safety of Medicines) (1979). Alphaxalone/Alphadalone. *Current Problems* No. 4. HMSO, London.

Dalgaard, J.B. and Bertelsen, K. (1965). Penicillin dodsfald. 16 secerede danske tilfaelde. *Nord. Med.* 73, 173.

Dally, M.B., Kurrle, S., and Breslin, A.B.X. (1978). Ventilation effects of aerosol gentamicin. *Thorax* 33, 54.

Dan, M., Aderka, D., Topilsky, M., Livini, E., and Levo, Y. (1986). Hypersensitivity pneumonitis induced by nalidixic acid. *Arch. Intern. Med.* 146, 1423.

David, P.R. and Burch, R.E. (1974). Pulmonary oedema and salicylate intoxication. *Ann. Intern. Med.* 80, 553.

Davis, D. and Macfarlane, A. (1974). Fibrosing alveolitis and treatment with sulphasalazine. *Gut* 15, 185.

Dawson, P., Pitfield, J., and Brittan, J. (1983). Contrast media and bronchospasm: a study with iopamidol. *Clin. Radiol.* 34, 227.

Daymond, T.J. and Griffiths, I.D. (1980). Pulmonary disease due to gold in rheumatoid arthritis. *Rheumatol. Rehab.* 19, 120.

Dean, N.C., Amend, W.C., and Matthay, M.A. (1987). Adult respiratory distress syndrome related to antilymphocyte globulin therapy. *Chest* 91, 619.

De Keyser, J. and Vincken, W. (1985). L-dopa-induced respiratory disturbance in Parkinson's disease suppressed by tiapride. *Neurology* 35, 235.

Diamond, M.T. and Fell, S.C. (1973). Anticoagulant induced massive hemothorax. *N.Y. State J. Med.* 73, 691.

Dickie, K.J. and De Groot, W.J. (1973). Ventilatory effects of aerosolized kanamycin and polymyxin. *Chest* 63, 694.

Dohner, V.A., Ward, H.P., and Standord, R.E. (1972). Alveolitis during procarbazine, vincristine and cyclophosphamide therapy. *Chest* 62, 636.

Dolezal, V. (1962). Some humoral changes in man produced by continuous oxygen inhalations at normal barometric pressure. *Riv. Med. Aeronaut. Spaz.* 25, 219.

Doniach, I., Morrison, B., and Steiner, R.E. (1954). Lung changes during hexamethonium therapy for hypertension. *Br. Heart J.* 16, 101.

Douglas, A.S., Eagles, J.M., and Mowat, N.A.G. (1990). Eosinophilia–myalgia syndrome associated with tryptophan. *Br. Med. J.* 301, 387.

Dubovsky, S.L. and Freed, C. (1988). Exercise-induced bronchospasm caused by maprotiline. *Psychosomatics* 29, 104.

Dukes, I.D. and Vaughan Williams, E.M. (1984). The multiple modes of action of propafenone. *Eur. Heart J.*, 5, 115.

Du Moulin, G.C., Patterson, D.G., Hedley Whyte, J., and Lisbon, A. (1982). Aspiration of gastric bacteria in antacid treated patients; a frequent cause of post-operative colonisation of the airway. *Lancet* i, 242.

Dworkin, H.J., Smith, J.R., and Bull, F.E. (1966). A reaction following administration of macroaggregated albumin (MAA) for a lung scan. *Am. J. Roentgenol.* 98, 427.

Eastmond, C.J. (1976). Diffuse alveolitis as a complication of pencillamine treatment for rheumatoid arthritis. *Br. Med. J.* i, 1506.

Ecker, M.D., Jay, B., and Keohand, M.F. (1978). Procarbazine lung. *Am. J. Roentgenol.* 131, 527.

Elliott, H.R., Abdulla, V., and Hayes, P.J. (1978). Pulmonary oedema associated with ritodrine infusion and betamethasone administration in premature labour. *Br. Med. J.* ii, 799.

Epstein, N. (1977). Acute reactions to urographic contrast media. *Ann. Allergy* 39, 139.

Ernsting, J. (1961). The effect of breathing high concentrations of oxygen upon the diffusing capacity of the lung in man. *J. Physiol.* (Lond.) 155, 51P.

Ersoz, N. and Finestone, S.C. (1971). Adrenaline induced pulmonary oedema and its treatment: a report of two cases. *Br. J. Anaesth.* 43, 709.

Erwteman, T.M., Braat, M.C.P., and van Aken, W.G. (1977). Interstitial pulmonary fibrosis: a new side-effect of practolol. *Br. Med. J.* ii, 297.

Eustace, B.R. (1967). Suxamethonium-induced bronchospasm. *Anaesthesia* 22, 638.

Everts, C.S., Westcott, J.L., and Bragg, D.G. (1973). Methotrexate therapy and pulmonary disease. *Radiology* 107, 539.

Eyal, Z., Borman, J.B., and Milwidsky, H. (1961). Solitary oil granuloma of the lung: a report of three cases. *Br. J. Dis. Chest* 55, 43.

Fahey, P.J., Utell, M.J., Mayewski, R.J., Wandtke, J.D., and Hyde, R.W. (1982). Early diagnosis of bleomycin pulmonary toxicity using B.A.L. in dogs. *Am. Rev. Respir. Dis.* 126, 126.

Fanous, L.H., Gray, A., and Felmingham, J. (1977). Severe anaphylactoid reactions to dextran 70. *Br. Med. J.* ii, 1189.

Fiegenberg, D.S., Weiss, H., and Krishman, H. (1967). Migratory pneumonia with eosinophilia associated with sulphonamide administration. *Arch. Intern. Med.* 120, 85.

Fielding, J.W.I., Stockley, R.A., and Brookes, V.S. (1978). Interstitial lung disease in a patient treated with 5-fluorouracil–mitomycin C. *Br. Med. J.* ii, 602.

Fishburne. J.I. Jr, Brenner, W.E., Bracksma, J.T., and Hendricks, C.H. (1972). Bronchospasm complicating intravenous prostaglandin F for therapeutic abortion. *Obstet. Gynecol.* 39, 892.

Flacke, J.W., Flacke, W.E., and Williams, G.D. (1977). Acute pulmonary edema following naloxone reversal of high-dose morphine anaesthesia. *Anesthesiology* 47, 376.

Follath, F., Burkhart, F., and Schweitzer, W. (1971). Drug induced pulmonary hypertension? *Br. Med. J.* i, 265.

Francis, R.A., Thomson, M.L., Pavia, D., and Douglas, B. (1975). The effect of Sch 1000 MDI on the mucociliary clearance and lung function of healthy volunteers. *Postgrad. Med J.* 51 (suppl. 7), 110.

Frand, U.I., Shim, C.S., and Williams, M.H. (1972). Heroin induced pulmonary oedema; sequential studies of pulmonary function. *Ann. Intern. Med.* 77, 29.

Frank, L. (1979). The lung and oxygen toxicity. *Arch. Intern. Med.* 139, 347.

Fraser, P.M., Speizer, F.E., Waters, S.D.M., Dole, R., and Mann, N.M. (1971). The circumstances preceding death from asthma in young people in 1968–1969. *Br. J. Dis. Chest* 65, 71.

Fratto, C. (1979). Provocation of bronchospasm by eye drops. *Ann. Intern. Med.* 88, 362.

Freeman, R. (1980). Short term adverse effects of antibiotic prophylaxis for open heart surgery. *Thorax* 35, 941.

Frishman, W., Jacob, H., Eesenber, E., and Ribner, H. (1979). Clinical pharmacology of the new beta-adrenergic blocking drugs. Part 8. Self poisoning with beta-adrenoceptor blocking agents: recognition and management. *Am. Heart J.* 98, 798.

Fuller, R.W. and Choudry, N.B. (1987). Increased cough reflex associated with angiotensin converting enzyme inhibitor cough. *Br. Med. J.* 295, 1025.

Furey, W.W. and Tan, C. (1969). Anaphylactic shock due to oral demethychlortetracycline. *Ann. Intern. Med.* 70, 357.

Furhoff, A.K. (1977). Anaphylactoid reaction to dextran — a report of 133 cases. *Acta Anaesth. Scand.* 21, 161.

Gali, J.M., Vilanova, J.L., and Mayers, M. (1986). Pulmonary haemorrhage and eosinophilia due to febarbamate. *Respiration* 49, 231.

Geddes, D.M. and Brostoff, J. (1976). Pulmonary fibrosis associated with hypersensitivity to gold salts. *Br. Med. J.* i, 1444.

Gefter, W.B., Epstein, D.M., Pietra, G.G., and Miller, W.T. (1983). Lung diseases caused by amiodarone, a new antiarrhythmic agent. *Radiology* 147, 339.

Gell, P.G.H. and Coombs, R.R.A. (eds) (1968). *Clinical aspects of immunology*, p. 575. Blackwell, Oxford.

Gentili, D.R., Kelly, K.M., Benjamin, E., and Iberti, T.J. (1988). Ritodrine associated pulmonary oedema. *N.Y. State J. Med.* 88, 326.

Glauser, F.L., Smith, W.R., Caldwell, A., Hoshiko, M., Dolan, G.S., Baer, H., *et al.* (1976). Ethchlorvynol (Placidyl)-induced pulmonary oedema. *Ann. Intern. Med.* 84, 46.

Goldman, G.C. and Moschella, S.L. (1971) Severe pneumonitis occurring during methotrexate therapy. *Arch. Dermatol.* 103, 194.

Gonzalez-Rothi, R.J., Hannan, S.E., Hood, I., and Franzini, D.A. (1987). Amiodarone pulmonary toxicity presenting as bilateral exudative pleural effusions. *Chest* 92, 179.

Goucher, G., Rowland, V., and Hawkins, J. (1980). Melphalan-induced pulmonary interstitial fibrosis. *Chest* 77, 805.

Gould, F.K., McGregor, C.G., Freeeman, R., and Odom, N.J. (1990). Respiratory complications following cardiac surgery.

The role of microbiology in its evaluation. *Anaesthesia* 40, 1061.

Granerus, A.K., Jagenburg, R., Nilson, N.J., and Svanborg, A. (1974). Respiratory of disturbance during L-dopa treatment of Parkinson's syndrome. *Acta Med. Scand.* 195, 39.

Granville-Grossman, K.I. and Sergeant, H.G.S. (1960). Pulmonary oedema due to salicylate intoxication. *Lancet* i, 575.

Green, L., Shatner, A., and Birkinstat, H. (1988). Severe reversible interstitial pneumonitis induced by low dose methotrexate; report of a case and review of the literature. *J. Rheumatol.* 15, 110.

Gunstream, S.R., Seidenfeld, J.J., Sobonya, R.E., and McMahon, L.J. (1983). Mitomycin-associated lung disease. *Cancer Treat. Rep.* 67, 301.

Haber, R.H., Oddone, E.Z., Gurbels, P.A., and Stead, W.W. (1986). Acute pulmonary decompensation due to amphotericin B in the absence of granulocyte transfusions. *N. Engl. J. Med.* 315, 836.

Hahn, H.H., Schweid, A.I.D., and Beaty, H.N. (1969). Complications of injecting dissolved methylphenidate tablets. *Arch. Intern. Med.* 123, 656.

Hailey, F.J., Glasscock, H.W. Jr, and Hewitt, W.F. (1969). Pleuropneumonic reactions to nitrofurantoin. *N. Engl. J. Med.* 281, 1087.

Hall, D.R., Morrison, J.B., and Edwards, F.R. (1978). Pleural fibrosis after practolol therapy. *Thorax* 33, 822.

Halmagyi, D.F. and Cotes, J.E. (1959). Reduction in systemic blood oxygen as a result of procedures affecting the pulmonary circulation in patients with chronic pulmonary diseases. *Clin. Sci.* 18, 475.

Hamaker, W.R., Buchman, R.J., Cox, W.A., and Fisher, G.W. (1969). Hemothorax: a complication of anticoagulant therapy. *Ann. Thorac. Surg.* 8, 564.

Hassall, E., Vich, T., and Ament, M.E. (1983). Pulmonary embolus and *Malassezia* pulmonary infection related to urokinase therapy. *J. Pediatr.* 102, 722.

Heard, B.E. (1962). Fibrous healing of old iatrogenic pulmonary oedema (hexamethonium lung). *J. Pathol. Bacteriol.* 83, 159.

Heard, B.E. and Cooke, R.A. (1968). Busulphan lung. *Thorax* 23, 187.

Heath, M.L. (1973). Bronchospasm in an asthmatic patient following pancuronium. *Anaesthesia* 28, 437.

Heffner, J.E., Harkey, R.A., and Schabel, S.I. (1990). Pulmonary reactions from illicit substance abuse. *Clin. Chest Med.* 11, 151.

Herzog, H., Minne, H., and Ziegler, R. (1989). Retroperitoneal fibrosis in a patient with macroprolactinoma treated with bromocriptine. *Br. Med. J.* 298, 1315.

Hildeen, T., Krogsgaard, A.R., and Vimtrup, B.J. (1958). Fatal pulmonary changes during the medical treatment of malignant hypertension. *Lancet* ii, 830.

Hill, R.N., Spragg, R.G., Wedel, M.K., and Moser, K.M. (1975). Adult respiratory distress syndrome associated with colchicine intoxication. *Ann. Intern. Med.* 83, 523.

Hine, L.K., Arrowsmith, J.B., and Gallo-Torres, H.E. (1988). Mono-octanoin-associated pulmonary edema. *Am. J. Gastroenterol.* 83, 1128.

Ho, D., Tashkin, D.P., Bein, M., and Sharma, O. (1979). Pulmonary infiltrates with eosinophilia associated with tetracycline. *Chest* 76, 33.

Holgate, S.T., Baldwin, C.J., and Tattersfield, A.E. (1977). Beta-adrenergic agonist resistance in normal human airways. *Lancet* ii, 375.

Holm, J., Leiden, B., and Lindquist, B. (1971). Unilateral pleural effusion — a rare complication of peritoneal dialysis. *Scand. J. Urol. Nephrol.* 5, 84.

Holyoye, P.Y., Luna, M., Mackay, B., and Bedrossan, C.W.M. (1978). Bleomycin hypersensitivity pneumonitis. *Ann. Intern. Med.* 88, 47.

Howarth, P.H. (1983). Bronchoconstriction in response to ipratropium bromide. *Br. Med. J.* 286, 1825.

Hrnicek, G., Skelton, J., and Miller, W.C. (1974). Pulmonary oedema and salicylate intoxication. *JAMA* 230, 866.

Hyde, R.W. and Rawson, A.J. (1969). Unintentional iatrogenic oxygen pneumonitis: response to therapy. *Ann. Intern. Med.* 71, 517.

Iacovino, J.R., Leitner, J., Abbas, A.K., Lokich, J.L., and Snider, G.L. (1976). Fatal pulmonary reaction from low doses of bleomycin. An idiosyncratic tissue response. *JAMA* 235, 125.

Idsøe, O. and Wang, K.Y. (1958). Penicillin-sensitivity reactions in Taiwan. *Bull. WHO* 18, 323.

Idsøe, O., Guthe, T., Wilcox, R.R., and De Week, A.L. (1968). Nature and extent of penicillin side-reactions with particular reference to fatalities from anaphylactic shock. *Bull. WHO* 38, 159.

Ind, P.W., Dixon, C.M.S., Fuller, R.W., and Barnes, P.J. (1989). Anticholinergic blockade of beta-blocker-induced bronchoconstriction. *Am. Rev. Respir. Dis.* 139, 1390.

Inman, W.H.W. (1986). Enalapril-induced cough. *Lancet* ii, 1218.

Inman, W.H.W. and Adelstein, A. M. (1969). Rise and fall of asthma mortality in England and Wales in relation to use of pressurised aerosols. *Lancet* ii, 279.

Inman, W.H.W., Vessey, M.P., Westerholm, B., and Engelund, A. (1970). Thromboembolic disease and the steroidal content of oral contraception. A report to the Committee on Safety of Drugs. *Br. Med. J.* ii, 203.

Inman, W.H.W., Rawson, N.S.B., Wilton, L.V., Pearce, G.L., and Speirs, C.J. (1988). Post marketing surveillance of enalapril. 1: Results of prescription–event monitoring. *Br. Med. J.* 297, 826.

Israel, H.I. and Diamond. P. (1962). Recurrent pulmonary infiltration and pleural effusion due to nitrofurantoin sensitivity. *N. Engl. J. Med.* 266, 1024.

Israel, R.H. and Olson, J.P. (1978). Pulmonary edema associated with intravenous vinblastine. *JAMA* 240, 1585.

Israel-Biet, D., Venet, A., Sandron, J., Ziza, J.M., and Chrétien, J. (1987). Pulmonary complications of intravesical Bacille Calmette-Guérin immunotherapy. *Am. Rev. Respir. Dis.* 135, 763.

Jackson, R.M. (1990). Molecular pharmacologic and clinical aspects of oxygen-induced lung injury. *Clin. Chest Med.* 11, 73.

Jackson, R.T., Beaglehole, R., Rea, H.H., and Sutherland, D.C. (1982). Mortality from asthma: a new epidemic in New Zealand. *Br. Med. J.* 285, 771.

Jago, R.H. and Restall, J. (1978). Sensitivity testing for althesin. *Anaesthesia* 33, 644.

James, D.W., Winster, W.F., and Hamilton, E.B.D. (1978). Gold lung. *Br. Med. J.* i, 1523.

Jones, G.R. and Malone, D.N.S. (1972). Sulphasalazine-induced lung disease. *Thorax* 27, 713.

Jones, S.E., Moore, M., Blank, N., and Castellino, R.A. (1972). Hypersensivitity to procarbazine (Matulane) manifested by fever and pleuropulmonary reaction. *Cancer* 29, 498.

Joselson, R. and Warnock, M. (1983). Pulmonary venoocclusive disease after chemotherapy. *Hum. Pathol.* 14, 88.

Jules-Elysée, K. and White, D.A. (1990). Bleomycin-induced pulmonary toxicity. *Clin. Chest Med.* 11, 1.

Kabins, S.A., Einstein, B., and Cohen, S. (1965). Anaphylactoid reaction to an initial dose of sodium cephalothin. *JAMA* 193, 165.

Karliner, T.S., Steinberg, A.D., and Williams, M.H. Jr (1969). Lung function after pulmonary edema associated with heroin overdose. *Arch. Intern. Med.* 124, 350.

Katz, S., Aberman, A., Frand, U.I., Stein, I.M., and Fulop, M. (1972). Heroin pulmonary oedema. Evidence for increased pulmonary capillary permeability. *Am. Rev. Respir. Dis.* 106, 472.

Kaufman, J., Casanova, J.E., Riedl, P., and Schlueter, D.P. (1989). Bronchial hyperreactivity and cough due to angiotensin-converting enzyme inhibitors. *Chest* 95, 544.

Kay, J.J. (1974). The aminorex controversy. *Thorax* 29, 266.

Kay, J.M., Smith, P., and Heath, D. (1971). Aminorex and the pulmonary circulation. *Thorax* 26, 262.

Keaney, N.P., Churton, S., and Stretton, T.B. (1980). Failure to demonstrate tolerance to inhaled salbutamol in volunteers. In *Proceedings of the first world conference in clinical pharmacology and therapeutics* (ed. P. Turner), p. 165. Macmillan, London.

Keighley, J.F. (1966). Iatrogenic asthma associated with adrenergic aerosols. *Ann. Intern. Med.* 65, 985.

Kennedy, J.I. Jr (1990). Clinical aspects of amiodarone pulmonary toxicity. *Clin. Chest Med.* 11, 119.

Kent, D.G. (1965). Bleeding into pulmonary cyst associated with anticoagulant therapy. *Am. Rev. Respir. Dis.* 92, 108.

Kessel, J. and Assem, E-S.K. (1974). An adverse reaction to althesin. *Br. J. Anaesth.* 46, 209.

Klapholz. L., Leitersdorf, E., and Weinrauch, L. (1986). Pneumonitis and leucocytoclastic vasculitis due to metformin. *Br. Med. J.* 293, 483.

Kleiger, R.E., Boxer, M., Ingham, R.E., and Harrison, D.C. (1976). Pulmonary hypertension in patients using oral contraceptives. *Chest* 69, 143.

Klinghoffer, J.F. (1954). Loeffler's syndrome following use of a vaginal cream. *Ann. Intern. Med.* 40, 343.

Knowles, H.C., Zeek, P.M., and Blankenhorn, M.Aa. (1953). Studies on necrotizing angiitis; IV. Periarteritis nodosa and hypersensitivity angiitis. *Arch. Intern. Med.* 92, 789.

Koeter, G.H., Menrs, H., Manchy, J.G.R., and de Vries, K. (1982). Protective effect of disodium cromoglycate on propranolol challenge. *Allergy* 37, 587.

Kok-Jensen, A. and Lindeneg, O. (1970). Pleurisy and fibrosis of the pleura during methysergide treatment of hemicrania. *Scand. J. Respir. Dis.* 51, 218.

Kounis, N.G. (1976). Untoward reactions to corticosteroids: intolerance to hydrocortisone. *Ann. Allergy* 36, 203.

Kristenson, M. and Fryden, A. (1988). Pneumonitis caused by metronidazole. *JAMA* 260, 184.

Krupp, P. (1981). Pleuropulmonary changes during longer term bromocriptine treatment for Parkinson's disease. *Lancet* i, 44.

The Lancet (1967). Pulmonary respirator syndrome. *Lancet* i, 992.

Larsson, S., Svedmyr, N., and Thiringer, G. (1977). Lack of bronchial beta adrenoceptor resistance in asthmatics during long term treatment with terbutaline. *J. Allergy Clin. Immunol.* 59, 93.

Lasser, E.C., Lang, J., Sorak, M., Kolb, W., Lyon, S., and Hamlin, A.E. (1977). Steroids: theoretical and experimental basis for utilization in prevention of contrast media reactions. *Radiology* 125, 1.

Laxenaire, M.C., Jacob, F., and Noel, P. (1976*a*). Accidents anaphylactoïdes liées à l'emploi de dextran de poids moléculaire 40,000. *Ann. Anesth. Fr.* 17, 101.

Laxenaire, M.C., Monteret-Vautrin, D.A., Moeller, R., and Chastel, A. (1976*b*). Accidents anaphylactoïdes liées à l'emploi de produits anesthésiques et adjuvants à propos de 18 cas. *Ann. Anesth. Fr.* 17, 85.

Lehrman, K.L. (1976). Pulmonary embolism in a transexual man taking diethylstilbestrol. *JAMA* 235, 532.

Leikola, J., Koistinen, J., Lehtinen, J., and Virolainen, M. (1973). IgA-induced anaphylactic transfusion reactions: a report of four cases. *Blood* 42, 111.

Lewis, L.D. (1984). Procarbazine associated alveolitis. *Thorax* 39, 206.

LeWitt, P.A. and Calne, D.B. (1981). Pleuropulmonary changes during long-term bromocriptine treatment for Parkinson's disease. *Lancet* i, 44.

Lobel, H., Machtey, I., and Eldror, M.Y. (1972). Pulmonary infltrates with eosinophilia in asthmatic patient treated with disodium cromoglycate. *Lancet* ii, 1032.

Lohiya, G. (1987). Asthma and urticaria after hepatitis B. vaccination. *West. Med. J.* 147, 341.

Lokich, J.J. and Moloney, W.C. (1972). Allergic reaction to procarbazine. *Clin. Pharmacol. Ther.* 13, 573.

Lombard, C.M., Chung, A., and Winokur, S. (1987). Pulmonary veno-occlusive disease following therapy for malignant neoplasms. *Chest* 92, 871.

Lucraft, H.H., Wilkinson, P.M., Stretton, T.B., and Read, G. (1982). Role of pulmonary function tests in the prevention of bleomycin pulmonary toxicity during chemotherapy for metastatic testicular teratoma. *Eur. J. Cancer Clin. Oncol.* 18, 133.

Macdonald, A.G. and McNeill, R.S. (1968). A comparison of the effect on airway resistance of a new beta-blocking drug ICI 50172 and propranolol. *Br. J. Anaesth.* 40, 508.

MacDonald, J.R., Mathison, D.A., and Stevenson, D.D. (1972). Aspirin intolerance in asthma. *J. Allergy Clin. Immunol.* 50, 198.

McElvaney, N.G., Wilcox, P.G., Churg, A., and Fleetham, J.A. (1988). Pleuropulmonary disease during bromocriptine treatment for Parkinson's disease. *Arch. Intern. Med.* 148, 2231.

MacLennan, A.C. and Stewart, D.G. (1990). Eosinophilia-myalgia syndrome associated with tryptophan. *Br. Med. J.* 301, 387.

McLeod, B.F., Lawrence, H.J., Smith, D.W., Vogt, P.J., and Gandara, D.R. (1987). Fatal bleomycin toxicity from a low cumulative dose in a patient with renal insufficiency. *Cancer* 60, 2617.

McMurray, J., Bloomfield, P., and Miller, H.C. (1986). Irreversible pulmonary hypertension after treatment with fenfluramine. *Br. Med. J.* 292, 239.

McNeill, R.S. (1964). Effect of a beta-adrenergic blocking agent, propranolol, on asthmatics. *Lancet* ii, 1101.

Magee F., Wright, J.L., Chan, W., Currie, W., and Carr, G. (1986). Two unusual pathological reactions to nitrofurantoin: case reports. *Histopathology* 10, 701.

Mahboubi, S., Gohel, V.K., Dalinka, M.K., and Sang Yon Cho. (1974). Barium embolization following gastrointestinal examination. *Radiology* 11, 301.

Major, P.P., Laurin, S., and Bettez, P. (1980). Pulmonary fibrosis following therapy with melphalan: a report of two cases. *Can. Med. Assoc. J.* 123, 197.

Malmquist, J., Trell, E., Torp, A., and Lindstrom, C. (1970). A case of drug induced (?) pulmonary hypertension. *Acta Med. Scand.* 188, 265.

Marchlinski, F.E., Gansler, T.S., Waxman, H.L., and Josephson, M.E. (1982). Amiodarone pulmonary toxicity. *Ann. Intern. Med.* 97, 839.

Mark, G.J. Lehimgar-Zadeh, A., and Ragsdale, B.D. (1978). Cyclophosphamide pneumonitis. *Thorax* 33, 89.

Marschke, G. and Sarauw, A. (1971). Polymyxin inhalation: therapeutic hazard. *Ann. Intern. Med.* 74, 144.

Marshall, A. and Moore, K. (1973). Pulmonary disease after amitriptyline overdosage. *Br. Med. J.* i, 716.

Marshall, A.J., Eltringham, W.K., Barritt, D.W., Davies, J.D., Griffiths, D.A., Jackson, L.K., *et al.* (1977). Respiratory disease associated with practolol. *Lancet* ii, 1254.

Martelli, N.A. and Usandivaras, G. (1977). Inhibition of aspirin-induced bronchoconstriction by sodium cromoglycate inhalation. *Thorax* 32, 684.

Martin, W.J. (1990). Mechanisms of amiodarone pulmonary toxicity. *Clin. Chest Med.* ii, 131.

Matthews, T.G., Wilczek, Z.M., and Shennan, A.T. (1977). Eye-drops induced hypertension. *Lancet* ii, 827.

Maxwell, I. (1974). Reversible pulmonary edema following cyclophosphamide therapy. *JAMA* 229, 137.

Medsger, T.A. Jr (1990). Tryptophan-induced eosinophiliamyalgia syndrome. *N. Engl. J. Med.* 322, 926.

Meeker, D.P. and Wiedemann, H.P. (1990). Drug-induced bronchospasm. *Clin. Chest Med.* 11, 163.

Mendelson, L.M., Meltzer, E.O., and Hamburger, R.N. (1974). Anaphylaxis-like reactions to corticosteroid therapy. *J. Allergy Clin. Immunol.* 54, 125.

Michael, J.R. and Rudin, M.L. (1981). Acute pulmonary disease caused by phenytoin. *Ann. Intern. Med.* 95, 452.

Millard, C.E. (1971). Massive hemothorax complicating heparin therapy for pulmonary infarction. *Chest* 59, 235.

Miller, F.E. (1971). Aspirin-induced bronchial asthma in sisters. *Ann. Allergy* 29, 263.

Min, K.W. and Györkey, F. (1968). Interstitial pulmonary fibrosis, atypical epithelial changes and bronchiolar cell carcinoma following busulphan therapy. *Cancer* 22, 1027.

Morrison Smith, J. (1975). The value and safety of disodium cromoglycate. *Allergol. Immunopathol.* 3, 29.

Mrouch, A. and Kase, N. (1967). Acute ascites and hydrothorax after gonadotrophin therapy. *Obstet. Gynecol.* 30, 346.

Mullarkey, M.F., Thomas, P.S., Hansen, J.A., Webb, D.R., and Nisperos, B. (1986). Association of aspirin-sensitive asthma with HLA-DQW2. *Am. Rev. Respir. Dis.* 133, 261.

Murdock, D.K., Lawless, C.E., Collins, E., Hume, J.P., and Pifarne, R. (1987). ARDS following equine ATG therapy. *Chest* 92, 578.

Murray, R.J., Albin, R.J., Mergner, W., and Criner, G.J. (1988). Diffuse alveolar haemorrhage temporally related to cocaine smoking. *Chest* 93, 427.

Myers, J.L., Kennedy, J.I., and Plumb, V.J. (1987). Amiodarone lung: pathologic findings in clinically toxic patients. *Hum. Pathol.* 18, 349.

Nagy, L., Lee, T.H., and Kay, A.B. (1982). Neutrophil chemotactic activity in antigen-induced late asthmatic reactions. *N. Engl. J. Med.* 306, 497.

Nash, G., Blennerhasset, J.H., and Pontoppidan. H. (1967). Pulmonary lesions associated with oxygen therapy and artifical ventilation. *N. Engl. J. Med.* 276, 368.

Nesbit, M., Krivit, W., Heyn, R., and Sharp. H. (1976). Acute and chronic effects of methotrexate on hepatic, pulmonary and skeletal systems. *Cancer* 37, 1048.

Nesse, R. and Carroll. J. (1976). Cholinergic side-effects associated with deanol. *Lancet* ii, 50.

Nestor, T.A., Tamamoto, W.I., Kam, T.H., and Schultz, T. (1989). Acute pulmonary oedema caused by crystalline methamphetamine. *Lancet* ii, 1277.

Nevins, M., Berque, S., Corwin, N., and Lyon, L. (1969). Phenylbutazone and pulmonary oedema. *Lancet* ii, 1358.

Nicholis, M.G. and Gilchrist, N.L. (1987). Sulindac and cough induced by converting enzyme inhibitors. *Lancet* i, 21.

O'Callaghan, A.C., Scadding, G., and Watkins, J. (1986). Bronchospasm following the use of vecuronium. *Anaesthesia* 41, 940.

O'Connor, P.C., Erskine, J.G., and Pringle, T.H. (1981). Pulmonary oedema after transfusion with fresh frozen plasma. *Br. Med. J.* 379.

O'Donnell, T.V., Holst, P.E., Rea, H.H., and Sean, M.R. (1989). Fenoterol and fatal asthma. *Lancet* i, 1070.

O'Driscoll, B.R., Hasleton, P.S., Taylor, P.M., Poulter, L.W., Rao Gattemaneni, H., and Woodcock, A.A. (1990). Active lung fibrosis up to 17 years after chemotherapy with carmustine (BCNU) in childhood. *N. Engl. J. Med.* 323, 378.

Ohlsson, W.T.L. (1947). A study on oxygen toxicity at atmospheric pressure. *Acta Med. Scand.* (suppl. 190), 1.

Orehek, J., Gayrard, P., and Grimand, C. (1977). Bronchial response to inhaled prostaglandin F2 alpha in patients with common or aspirin-sensitive asthma. *J. Allergy Clin. Immunol.* 59, 414.

Ormerod, L.P. and Stableforth, D.E. (1980). Asthma mortality in Birmingham 1975–7. *Br. Med. J.* 280, 687.

Ozols, R.F., Hogan, W.M., Ostchega, Y., and Young, R.C. (1983). M.V.P. (mitomycin, vinblastine and progesterone): a second line regimen in ovarian cancer with a high incidence of pulmonary toxicity. *Cancer Treat. Rep.* 67, 721.

Partenen, J., Van Assendelft, A.H., Koskimies, S., Forsberg, S., Hakala, M., and Ilonen, J. (1987). Patients with rheumatoid arthritis and gold induced pneumonitis express two high-risk major histocompatibility complex patterns. *Chest* 92, 277.

Partridge, M.B. and Gibson, G.J. (1978). Adverse bronchial reactions to intravenous hydrocortisone in two aspirin-sensitive asthmatic patients. *Br. Med. J.* i, 1521.

Pascual, R.S., Mosher, M.B., Sikand, R.A., De Conti, R.C., and Bouhys, A. (1973). Effects of bleomycin on pulmonary function in man. *Am. Rev. Respir. Dis.* 108, 211.

Pasquinucci, G., Ferrar, P., and Castellari, R. (1971). Daunorubicin treatment of methotrexate pneumonia. *JAMA* 216, 2017.

Patel, A.R., Shah, P.C., Rhee, H.L., Sasson, H., and Rao, K.P. (1976). Cyclophosphamide therapy and interstitial pulmonary fibrosis. *Cancer* 38, 1542.

Patel, H., Keshavan, M.S., and Pitts, K.E. (1988). Adverse lung reactions to nomifensine: a posthumous note. *Clin. Neuropharmacol.* 10, 190.

Patel, K.R. (1975). Atropine, sodium cromoglycate and thymoxamine in PGF2 alpha-induced bronchoconstriction in extrinsic asthma. *Br. Med. J.* ii, 360.

Patel, K.R. and Tullett, W.M. (1983). Bronchoconstriction in response of ipratropium bromide. *Br. Med. J.* 286, 1318.

Paterson, J.W., Conolly, M.E., Davies, D.S., and Dollery, C.T. (1968). Isoprenaline resistance and the use of pressurised aerosols in asthma. *Lancet* ii, 426.

Pearce, N., Grainger, J., Atkinson, M., Crane, J., Burgess, C., Cutting, C., *et al.* (1990a). Case control study of prescribed fenoterol and death from asthma in New Zealand. *Thorax* 45, 170.

Pearce, N., Crane, J., Burgess, C., and Beasley, R. (1990b). Case-control study of prescribed fenoterol and death from asthma in New Zealand, 1977–81: authors' reply. *Thorax* 45, 745.

Pepys, J. (1969). *Hypersensitivity diseases of the lungs due to fungi and organic dusts*, p. 112. Karger, Basle.

Perry, H.M., O'Neil, R.M., and Thomas, W.A. (1957). Pulmonary disease following chronic chemical ganglionic blockade. *Am. J. Med.* 22, 37.

Pineda, A.A. and Taswell, H.F. (1975). Transfusion reactions associated with anti-IgA antibodies: report of four cases and review of the literature. *Transfusion* 15, 10.

Poe, R.H., Condemi, J.J., Weinstein, S.S., and Schuster, R.J. (1980). Adult respiratory distress syndrome related to ampicillin sensivity. *Chest* 77, 449.

Popa, V. (1987). Captopril-related (and induced?) asthma. *Am. Rev. Respir. Dis.* 136, 999.

Pratt, CI.I. (1988). Bronchospasm after neostigmine. *Anaesthesia* 43, 242.

Pratt, P.C. (1974). Pathology of pulmonary oxygen toxicity. *Am. Rev. Respir. Dis.* 110 (suppl.), 51.

Rafferty, P., Beasley, R., and Holgate, S.T. (1988). Comparison of the efficacy of preservative free ipratropium bromide and Atrovent nebuliser solution. *Thorax* 43, 446.

Rahal, J.J., Meyers, B.R., and Weinstein, L. (1968). Treatment of bacterial endocarditis with cephalothin. *N. Engl. J. Med.* 279, 1305.

Ramsey, B. and Marks, J.M. (1988). Bronchoconstriction due to 8-methoxypsoralen. *Br. J. Dermatol.* 119, 83.

Rau, N.R., Nagaraj, M.V., Prakash, P.S., and Nelli, P. (1988). Fatal pulmonary aspiration of oral activated charcoal. *Br. Med. J.* 297, 918.

Redline, R.W. and Dahms, B.B. (1981). *Malassezia* pulmonary vasculitis in an infant on long-term Intralipid therapy. *N. Engl. J. Med.* 305, 1395.

Reese, E.P. Jr, McCullough, J.J., and Craddock, P.R. (1975). An adverse pulmonary reaction to cryoprecipitate in a haemophiliac. *Transfusion* 15, 583.

Reichlin, S., Loveless, M.H., and Kane, E.G. (1953). Loeffler's syndrome following penicillin therapy. *Ann. Intern. Med.* 38, 113.

Reid, J., Watson, R.D., and Sproull, D.H. (1950). The mode of action of salicylates in acute rheumatic fever. *Q. J. Med.* 19, 1.

Repo, U.K. and Nieminen, P. (1976). Pulmonary infiltrates with eosinophilia and urinary symptoms during disodium cromoglycate treatment. A case report. *Scand. J. Respir. Dis.* 57, 1.

Reussi, C., Schiavi, J.E., Altman, R., Yussen, E.E., and Rouvier, J. (1969). Unusual complications in the course of *JAMA* 46, 460.

Rich, A.R. (1942). The role of hypersensitivity in periarteritis nodosa as indicated by seven cases developing during serum sickness and sulphonamide therapy. *Bull. Johns Hopkins Hosp.* 71, 123.

Ridley, M.G., Wolfe, C.S., and Mathews, J.A. (1988). Life threatening acute pneumonitis during low dose methotrexate treatment for rheumatoid arthritis: a case report and review of the literature. *Ann. Rheum. Dis.* 47, 784.

Rinne, U.K. (1981). Pleuropulmonary changes during long-term bromocriptine treatment for Parkinson's disease. *Lancet* i, 44.

Robinson, B.R. (1964). Pleuropulmonary reaction to nitrofurantoin. *JAMA* 189, 239.

Roden, N.J. (1973). Aspirin: a dangerous foreign body. *J. Pediatr.* 88, 266,8.

Rodman, D.M., Hanley, M., and Parsons, P. (1986). Aminoglutethimide, alveolar damage and haemorrhage. *Ann. Intern. Med.* 105, 633.

Rodman, T., Fraimow, W., and Myerson, R.M. (1958). Loeffler's syndrome: report of a case associated with administration of mephenesin carbamate (Tolseram). *Ann. Intern. Med.* 48, 668.

Rokseth, R. and Storstein, O. (1960). Pulmonary complication during mecamylamine therapy. *Acta Med. Scand.* 167, 23.

Rosenow, E.C. (1972). The spectrum of drug-induced pulmonary disease. *Ann. Intern. Med.* 77, 977.

Rosenow, E.C. (1990). Diffuse pulmonary infiltrates in the immunocompromised host. *Clin. Chest Med.* ii, 55.

Roth, E., Lax, L.C., and Maloney, J.V. (1969). Ringer's lactate solution and extracellular fluid volume in the surgical patient. *Ann. Surg.* 169, 149.

Rotmensch, H.H., Liron, M., Tupilski, M., and Lamedo, S. (1980). Possible association of pneumonia with amiodarone. *Am. Heart J.* 100, 412.

Rubery, E.D. and Coakley, A.J. (1980). Early detection of lung toxicity after bleomycin therapy. *Cancer Treat. Rep.* 64, 732.

Rubin, G., Baume, P., and Vandenberg, R. (1972). Azathioprine and acute restrictive lung disease. *Aust. N.Z. J. Med.* ii, 272.

Sackner, M.A., Lauda, J., Zapafa, A., Schapiro, J., and Schapiro, E. (1975). Pulmonary effects of oxygen breathing: a 6 hour study in normal men. *Ann. Intern. Med.* 82, 40.

Sakula, A. (1977). Bronchial asthma due to allergy to pancreatic extract: a hazard in the treatment of cystic disease. *Br. J. Dis. Chest* 71, 295.

Salem, P.A. (1971). Pulmonary changes and bleomycin. *Cancer Bull.* 23, 68.

Samter, M. and Beers, R.F. (1967). Concerning the nature of intolerance to aspirin. *J. Allergy* 40, 281.

Schaaf, J.T., Spivack, M.I., Rath, G.S., and Snider, G.L. (1973). Pulmonary oedema and adult respiratory distress syndrome following methadone abuse. *Am. Rev. Respir. Dis.* 107, 1047.

Schloerb, P.R., Hunt, P.T., Plummer, J.A., and Cage, G.K. (1972). Pulmonary edema after replacement of blood loss by electrolyte solutions. *Surg. Gynecol. Obstet.* 135, 893.

Schoeffed, R.E., Anderson, S.A., and Altounyan, R.E.C. (1981). Bronchial hyperreactivity in response to inhalation of ultrasonically nebulised solutions of distilled water and saline. *Br. Med. J.* 283, 1285.

Schoene, R.B., Martin, T.R., Charan, N.B., and French, C.L. (1981). Timolol-induced bronchospasm in asthmatic bronchitis. *JAMA* 206, 130.

Schulman, P., Cheng, E., Cvitkovic, E., and Golbey, R. (1979). Spontaneous pneumothorax as a result of intensive cytotoxic chemotherapy. *Chest* 75, 194.

Schwartz, J.A. and Koenigsberg, M.D. (1987). Naloxone-induced pulmonary edema. *Ann. Emerg. Med.* 16, 1294.

Scott, D.L., Bradby, G.V., Altman, T.J., Zaphiropoulos, G.C., and Hawkins, G.F. (1981). Relationship of gold and penicillamine therapy to diffuse interstitial lung disease. *Ann. Rheum. Dis.* 40, 136.

Searles, G. and McKendry, R.J.R. (1987). Methotrexate pneumonitis in rheumatoid arthritis: potential risk factors. Four case reports and a review of the literature. *J. Rheumatol.* 14, 1164.

Sears, M.R., Rea, H.H., Fenwick, J., Gillies, A.J.D., Holst, P.E., O'Donnell, T.V., *et al.* (1987). Seventy five deaths in asthmatics prescribed home nebulisers. *Br. Med. J.* 294, 477.

Selroos, O. and Edgren, J. (1975). Lupus-like syndrome associated with pulmonary reaction to nitrofurantoin. *Acta Med. Scand.* 197, 125.

Shannon, D.C. and Kelly, D.H. (1982). SIDS and near-SIDS. *N. Engl. J. Med.* 306, 959.

Sherman, C.B., Hudson, L.D., and Pierson, D.J. (1987). Severe precocious emphysema in intravenous methylphenidate (Ritalin) abusers. *Chest* 92, 1085.

Shim, C. and Williams, M.H. Jr (1987). Cough and wheezing from beclomethasone aerosol. *Chest* 91, 207.

Sigvaldson, A. and Sorenson, S. (1983). Interstitial pneumonia due to sulphasalazine. *Eur. J. Respir. Dis.* 64, 229.

Simon, H.B., Daggett, W., and De Sanctis, R.W. (1969). Hemothorax as a compliction of anticoagulant therapy in the presence of pulmonary infarction. *JAMA* 208, 1830.

Sklar, J. and Timms, R.M. (1977). Codeine-induced pulmonary edema. *Chest* 72, 230.

Smith, D.C., Lois, J.F., Gomes, A.S., Maloney, M.D., and Yahiken, P.Y. (1987). Pulmonary arteriography: Comparison of cough stimulation effects of diatrizoate and ioxaglate. *Radiology* 162, 617.

Smith, D.E., Herd, D., and Gazzard, B.G. (1988). Reversible bronchoconstriction with nebulised pentamidine. *Lancet* ii, 905.

Smith, G.J.W. (1990). The histopathology of pulmonary reactions to drugs. *Clin. Chest Med.* 11, 95.

Smith, J.H. and Weinstein, V.F. (1987). Cephalexin associated pulmonary infiltration with circulating eosinophilia. *Br. Med. J.* 294, 776.

Sobol, S.M. and Rakita, I. (1982). Pneumonitis and pulmonary fibrosis associated with amiodarone treatment: a possible complication of a new antiarrhythmic drug. *Circulation* 65, 819.

Sostman, H.D., Matthay, R.A., Putman, C.E., and Walker Smith, G.J. (1976). Methotrexate-induced pneumonitis. *Medicine* (Baltimore) 55, 371.

Sostman, H.D., Matthay, R.A., and Putman, C.E. (1977). Cytotoxic drug-induced disease. *Am. J. Med.* 62, 608.

Sovijarvi, A.R.A., Lemola, M., Stenius, B., and Idanpaan-Heikkila, J. (1977). Nitrofurantoin-induced acute, subacute and chronic pulmonary reactions. A report of 66 cases. *Scand. J. Respir. Dis.* 58, 41.

Spector, S.L., Wangarrd, C.H., and Farr, R.S. (1979). Aspirin and concomitant idiosyncrasies in adult and asthmatic patients. *J. Allergy Clin. Immunol.* 64, 500.

Speizer, F.E., Doll, R., and Heaf, P. (1968a). Observations on recent increase in mortality from asthma. *Br. Med. J.* i, 335.

Speizer, F.E., Doll, R., Heaf, P., and Strang, L.B. (1968b). Investigation into use of drugs preceding death from asthma. *Br. Med. J.* i, 339.

Spitzer, W.O. and Buist, A.S. (1990). Case-control study of prescribed fenoterol and death from asthma in New Zealand. *Thorax* 45, 645.

Sprenger, J.D., Altman, L.C., Marshall, S.G., Pierson, W.E., and Koenig, J.Q. (1989). Studies of neutrophil chemotactic factor of anaphylaxis in metabisulphite sensitivity. *Ann. Allergy* 62, 117.

Stein, M.G., Demarco, T., Gamsu, G., Finkbeiner, W., and Golen, J.A. (1988). Computed tomography: pathologic correlation in lung disease due to tocainide. *Am. Rev. Respir. Dis.* 137, 458.

Steinberg, A.D. (1968). Pulmonary oedema following ingestion of hydrochlorothiazide. *JAMA* 204, 825.

Steinberg, A.D. and Karliner, J.S. (1968). The clinical spectrum of heroin pulmonary oedema. *Arch. Intern. Med.* 122.

Stenton, S.C., Duddridge, M., Walters, E.H., and Hendrick, D.J. (1990). An unusual response to methacholine. *Thorax* 45, 819.

Sternlieb, L., Bennett, B., and Scheinberg, I.H. (1975). D-penicillamine-induced Goodpasture's syndrome in Wilson's disease. *Ann. Intern. Med.* 82, 673.

Stromberg, C., Palva, E., Alhova, E., Aranko, K., Idänpään Heikkila, J. (1987). Pulmonary infiltration induced by tolfenamic acid. *Lancet* ii, 685.

Stubblefield, P.G. (1978). Pulmonary oedema occurring after therapy with dexamethasone and terbutaline for premature labour: a case report. *Am. J. Obstet. Gynecol.* 132, 341.

Suarez, L.D., Poderoso, J.J., Elsner, B., Bunster, A.M., Esteva, H., and Bellotti, M. (1983). Subacute pneumopathy during amiodarone therapy. *Chest* 83, 566.

Sue-ling, H. and Hughes, L.E. (1988). Should the pill be stopped preoperatively? *Br. Med. J.* 296, 447.

Swinburn, C.R. (1988). Pulmonary infiltrations and lymphadenopathy in association with fenbufen. *Hum. Toxicol.* 35.

Symmers, W. St. C. (1958). The occurrence of so-called collagen diseases, and of other diseases systemically affecting the connective tissues as a manifestation of sensitivity to drugs. In *Sensitivity reactions to drugs* (ed. M.L. Rosenheim and R. Moulton), p. 209. Blackwell, Oxford.

Szczeklik, A. and Gryglewski, R.J. (1983). Asthma and antiinflammatory drugs. Mechanism and clinical patterns. *Drugs* 25, 533.

Szczeklik, A. and Nizankowska, E. (1978). Asthma relieved by aspirin and by other cyclo-oxygenase inhibitors. *Thorax* 33, 664.

Szczeklik, A., Gryglewski, R.J., Czerniawska-Mysik, G., and Pieton, R. (1977). Asthmatic attacks induced in aspirinsensitive patients by diclofenac and naproxen. *Br. Med. J.* ii, 231.

Talcott, J.A., Gernick, M.B., Stomper, P.C., Godleski, J.J., and Richie, J.P. (1987). Cavitary lung nodules associated with combination chemotherapy containing bleomycin. *J. Urol.* 138, 619.

Taylor, C.R. (1990). Diagnostic imaging techniques in the evaluation of drug induced pulmonary disease. *Clin. Chest Med.* 11, 87.

Thiringer, G., Eriksson, N., Nalmberg, R., Svedmyr, N., and Zettergren, O.L. (1975). Bronchoscopic biopsies of bronchial mucosa before and after beclomethasone dipropionate therapy. *Postgrad. Med. J.* 51 (suppl. 4), 30.

Thomas, P., Seaton, A., and Edwards, J. (1974). Respiratory disease due to sulphasalazine. *J. Clin. Allergy* 4, 41.

Thurston, J.G.B., Marks, P., and Trapnell, D. (1976). Lung changes associated with phenylbutazone treatment. *Br. Med. J.* ii, 1422.

Todd, E.M. and Gardner, W.J. (1957). Pantopaque intravasation (embolization) during myelography. *J. Neurosurg.* 14, 230.

Tomashefski, J.F. Jr, Hirsch, C.S., and Jolly, P.N. (1981). Microcrystalline cellulose pulmonary embolism and granulomatosis. A complication of illicit intravenous injections of pentazocine tablets. *Arch. Pathol. Lab. Med.* 105, 89.

Topilow, A.A., Rothenberg. S.P., and Cottrell, T.S. (1973). Interstitial pneumonia after prolonged treatment with cyclophosphamide. *Am. Rev. Respir. Dis.* 108, 114.

Tornling, G., Unge, G., Axelsson, G., Noring, L., and Granerus, A.K. (1986). Pleuropulmonary reactions in patients on bromocriptine treatment. *Eur. J. Respir. Dis.* 68, 35.

Trump, D.L., Bartel, E., and Pozniak, M. (1988). Nodular pneumonitis after chemotherapy for germ cell tumours. *Ann. Intern. Med.* 109, 431.

Turner-Warwick, M.E.H. (1981). Adverse reactions affecting the lung: possible association with D-penicillamine. *J. Rheumatol.* 8, 166.

Twohig, K.J. and Matthay, R.A. (1990). Pulmonary effects of cytotoxic agents other than bleomycin. *Clin. Chest Med.* 11, 31.

van de Water, J.M., Kagey, K.S., Miller, I.T., Parker, D.A., O'Connor, N.E., Jaen-Min Sheh, *et al.* (1970). Response of lung to 6 to 12 hours of 100 per cent oxygen inhalation in normal men. *N. Engl. J. Med.* 283, 621.

van Haeringen, J.R., Hilvering, C., and Sluiter, H.J. (1972). Disease of the respiratory tract due to drugs. In *Drug induced diseases*, vol. 4 (ed. L. Meyler and H.M. Peck), p. 498. Associated Scientific Publishers, Amsterdam.

Vaughan-Jones, R. and Goldman, L. (1968). Persistent eosinophilia after nitrofurantoin. *Lancet* i, 306.

Veale, D., McComb, J.M., and Gibson, G.J. (1990). Propafenone. *Lancet* 335, 979.

Vessey, M.P. and Doll, R. (1968). Investigation of relation between use of oral contraceptives and thromboembolic disease. *Br. Med. J.* ii, 199.

Vessey, M.P., Mant, D., Smith, A., and Yeates, D. (1986). Oral contraceptives and venous thromboembolism: findings in a large prospective study. *Br. Med. J.* 292, 526.

Vignon, H., Gay, R., and Laxenaire, M.C. (1976). Observations cliniques d'accidents anaphylactoïdes per et post anesthétiques. Résultat d'enquête a posteriori. *Ann. Anesth. Fr.* 17, 117.

Vincent, W.R., Goldberg, S.J., and Desilets, D. (1968). Fatality immediately following rapid infusion of macroaggregates of ^{99m}Tc albumin (MAA) for lung scan. *Radiology* 91, 1180.

Volk, B.W., Nathanson, L., Losner, S., Slade, W.R., and Jacoby, M. (1951). Incidence of lipoid pneumonia in a survey of 389 chronically ill patients. *Am. J. Med.* 10, 316.

von Maur, K., Adkinson, N.F., van Metre, T.E., Marsh, D.G., and Norman, P.S. (1974). Aspirin intolerance in a family. *J. Allergy Clin. Immunol.* 54, 380.

Waller, D.G. (1990). β-adrenoceptor partial agonists: a renaissance in cardiovascular therapy? *Br. J. Clin. Pharmacol.* 30, 157.

Wallerstein, R.A. (1968). Intravenous iron–dextran complex. *Blood* 32, 690.

Walton, C.H.A. (1966). Case report: asthma associated with use of nitrofurantoin. *Can. Med. Assoc. J.* 94, 40.

Ward, C.D., Thompson, J., and Humby, M.D. (1987). Pleuropulmonary and retroperitoneal fibrosis associated with bromocriptine treatment. *J. Neurol. Neurosurg. Psychiatry* 50, 1706.

Ward, H.N., Lipscomb, T.S., and Cawley, L.P. (1968). Pulmonary hypersensitivity reactions after blood transfusion. *Arch. Intern. Med.* 122, 362.

Weber, J.C.P. and Essigman, W.K. (1986). Pulmonary alveolitis and NSAIDs — fact or fiction? *Br. J. Rheumatol.* 25, 5.

Weill, H., Ferrans, V.J., and Gray, R.M. (1964). Early lipoid pneumonia: roentgenologic anatomic and physiologic characteristics. *Am. J. Med.* 36, 370.

Weisenberger, D.D. (1978). Interstitial pneumonitis associated with azathioprine therapy. *Am. J. Clin. Pathol.* 69, 181.

Weiss, R.B., Poster, D.S., and Penta, J.S. (1981). The nitrosoureas and pulmonary toxicity. *Cancer Treat. Rev.* 8, 111.

Wendt, V.E., Puro, H.E., Shapiro, J., Mathews, W., and Wolf, P.I. (1964). Angiothrombotic pulmonary hypertension in addicts with 'blue velvet' addiction. *JAMA* 188, 755.

Westerfield, B.T., Michalski, J.P., McCombs, C., and Light, R.W. (1980). Reversible melphalan-induced lung damage. *Am. J. Med.* 68, 767.

Whitcomb, M.E., Schwarz, M.I., and Tormey, D.C. (1972). Methotrexate pneumonitis: case report and review of the literature. *Thorax* 27, 636.

White, D.A., Schwartzberg, L.S., Kris, M.G., and Bose, G.J. (1987). Acute chest pain during bleomycin infusion. *Cancer* 59, 1582.

Williams, J.O. (1974). Death following injection of lung scanning agent in a case of pulmonary hypertension. *Br. J. Radiol.* 47, 61.

Williams, T., Eidns, L., and Thomas, P. (1982). Fibrosing alveolitis, bronchiolitis obliterans and sulfasalazine therapy. *Chest* 81, 766.

Wilson, I.C., Gambill, J.M., and Sandifer, M.G. (1963). Loeffler's syndrome occurring during imipramine therapy. *Am. J. Psychiatry* 119, 892.

Wold, D.E. and Zahn, D.W. (1956). Allergic (Loeffler's) pneumonitis occurring during antituberculous chemotherapy. *Am. Rev. Respir. Dis.* 74, 445.

Woldorf, N.M. and Pastore, P.N. (1972). Extreme epinephrine sensitivity with a general anaesthesia. *Arch. Otolaryngol.* 96, 272.

Wright, D.G., Robichard, K.J., Pizzo, P.A., and Deisseroth, A.B. (1981). Lethal pulmonary reactions associated with the combined use of amphotericin B and leukocyte transfusions. *N. Engl. J. Med.* 304, 1185.

Yagoda, A., Mukherji, B., Young, C., Etcubanas, E., Lamonte, C., Smith, J.R., *et al.* (1972). Bleomycin and antitumour antibiotic: clinical experience in 274 patients. *Ann. Intern. Med.* 77, 861.

Yocum, M.W., Heller, A.M., and Abels, R.I. (1978). Efficacy of intravenous pretesting and antihistamine prophylaxis in radiocontrast media-sensitive patients. *J. Allergy Clin. Immunol.* 62, 309.

Young, D.J. (1972). Propoxyphene suicides: report of nine cases. *Arch. Intern. Med.* 129, 62.

Yousem, S.A., Lifson, J.D., and Colby, T.V. (1985). Chemotherapy induced eosinophilic pneumonia: relation to bleomycin. *Chest* 88, 103.

Zitnik, R.J. and Cooper, J.A.D. (1990). Pulmonary disease due to antirheumatic agents. *Clin. Chest Med.* 11, 139.

Zucker, P.K., Khoun, N.F., Rosenshein, N.B. (1987). Bleomycin-induced pulmonary nodules: a variant of bleomycin pulmonary toxicity. *Gynecol. Oncol.* 28, 284.

Zweiman, B., Mishkin, M.M., and Hildreth, E.A. (1975). An approach to the performance of contrast studies in contrast material reactive persons. *Ann. Intern. Med.* 83, 159.

Zyroff, J., Slovis, T.L., and Nagler, J. (1974). Pulmonary edema induced by methadone. *Radiology* 112, 567.

9. Dental disorders

J. G. WALTON and R. A. SEYMOUR

'All the organ systems of the body play a role in the development of a clinical lesion in the mouth. The mouth serves as a mirror of systemic health and disease. Further, local lesions of the oral cavity have a direct effect on systemic health. There cannot be total health without oral health.' — Irwin W. Scopp (Clinical Professor of Periodontia and Oral Medicine, College of Dentistry, New York University)

Introduction

This chapter is about unwanted effects of drugs in the orofacial region. We have categorized them according to the structures involved, that is, the oral mucosa and tongue, periodontal tissues, dental structures, and salivary glands. Sections are included on drug-induced cleft lip and palate, muscular and neurological disturbances that affect the orofacial region, disturbances of taste and halitosis, oral infections, facial oedema, blood dyscrasias, and disturbances of haemostasis, though where a subject is dealt with in another chapter only brief mention of it is made here.

Some of the adverse drug reactions which affect the orofacial region are of the Type A category (see Chapter 3), for example, xerostomia caused by tricyclic antidepressants or oral ulceration by local irritants. Many adverse effects are associated, however, with an underlying hypersensitivity reaction and are thus of Type B.

Oral mucosa and tongue

Adverse drug reactions can produce a variety of disorders affecting the oral mucosa, including hypersensitivity reactions, oral ulceration, and lichenoid eruptions. In addition, systemic drug therapy can cause erythema multiforme and lupus erythematosus, which sometimes affect the mouth.

Hypersensitivity reactions

A wide variety of drugs may provoke hypersensitivity reactions in the oral cavity: these reactions range in severity from the slight to severe enough to interfere with oral function.

Essentially, there are two types of allergic reactions occurring in and around the mouth. The first (Type I of the Coombs and Gell classification) is the immediate or anaphylactic type reaction mediated by serum antibodies. Drugs that can cause Type I reactions and are of concern to the dental surgeon are penicillin, lignocaine, and aspirin.

The second (Type IV) is a delayed reaction mediated by sensitized T lymphocytes: this produces an eruption which is sometimes referred to as 'stomatitis medicamentosa' (fixed drug eruption) when it is due to systemic medication, and as 'stomatitis venenata' when due to contact hypersensitivity.

Stomatitis medicamentosa (fixed drug eruption)

Oral manifestations of drug hypersensitivity are considerably less common than skin reactions. The lesions vary greatly in appearance, from areas of erythema to areas of ulceration. In the early phase of the reaction, vesicles or bullae which quickly break down may be found on the palate, lips, or tongue. A fixed drug eruption is one that appears at the same site each time a particular drug is administered. The eruption may be a solitary lesion, particularly after the first attack, but after repeated attacks new lesions may appear together with lesions involving the original site. The time elapsing between ingestion of the drug and the appearance of the lesion varies from a few hours up to a day

Drugs commonly involved in fixed drug eruptions include phenacetin, phenazone, salicylates, meprobamate, sulphonamides, tetracyclines, dapsone, and oxyphenbutazone (Kay 1972). A common offender is phenolphthalein, which is often used as a laxative.

Fixed drug eruptions caused by tetracycline have been widely reported in the dermatology literature. Intraoral eruptions due to this drug are rare, but a case has been reported in which an oral lesion appeared when tetracycline was given and disappeared when the drug was withdrawn (Murray and Defco 1982).

Stomatitis with erythematous, bullous, or ulcerative lesions, in the absence of skin involvement, has been reported as an adverse reaction to barbiturates (Kennett 1968). Similarly, ulceration of the mouth caused by phenindione has been reported (Hollman and Wong 1964). Cases have been reported in which edentulous patients receiving indomethacin therapy developed ulceration of the oral mucosa (Guggenheimer and Ismail 1975). The lesions healed after reduction or withdrawal of the drug and may have resulted from an increased susceptibility to trauma following on a drug-induced suppression of the regenerative capabilities of the oral tissue.

Gold therapy has been used for many years in the treatment of rheumatoid arthritis. It has been reported that 30 per cent of patients on gold therapy developed an adverse reaction to the compound and 3.3 per cent developed a stomatitis and glossitis (Gordon *et al.* 1975). The use of gold may be associated with widespread oral ulceration which, on healing, may leave appearances suggestive of lichen planus. It has been suggested that the presence of Sjögren's syndrome is a contraindication to gold therapy, but in this survey reactions were not more common in patients with the syndrome than in those without.

Lignocaine is the most widely used local anaesthetic agent in dental practice. Adverse reactions to this drug are rare. A fixed drug eruption to lignocaine has been reported in a 7-year-old atopic child exposed to 2.2 ml of Xylonor 2% special (a solution containing lignocaine hydrochloride, noradrenaline, adrenaline, and saline) (Curley and Baxter 1987). A few hours after buccal and palatal infiltrations, an erythematous patch developed on the left side of the upper lip. This crusted over but left an area of pigmentation for 7 months. The clinical appearance was suggestive of a fixed drug eruption, and lignocaine was implicated by a process of exclusion.

Three cases of 'scalded mouth' that were caused by the angiotensin-converting-enzyme inhibitor captopril have been reported (Vlasses *et al.* 1982). These cases were not accompanied by an eosinophilia or by fever. The inclusion of these cases under this heading is doubtful, since the mechanism is unclear.

The mechanism involved in a fixed drug eruption is uncertain, but a humoral agent has been detected in serum during an exacerbation. An intradermal injection of the patient's serum produced an inflammatory response in previously affected areas of skin (Wyatt *et al.* 1972). Ultrastructural studies from lesions of fixed drug eruptions have demonstrated features similar to those in other bullous reactions (e.g. erythema multiforme and toxic epidermal necrolysis). Dyskeratotic bodies have been found in the epidermis which is indicative of severe epidermal injury (De Dobbeleer and Achten 1977).

Stomatitis venenata (contact stomatitis)

Contact hypersensitivity implies a local reaction of the mucosa after repeated contact with the causative agent. There are many substances that are capable of causing such a local reaction. Common allergens responsible for contact stomatitis include antibiotics, mouthwashes, toothpastes, topical anaesthetics, cosmetics, antiseptic lozenges, and chewing gum. The interval between contact with the allergen and the development of hypersensitivity may vary from days to years. The stomatitis may show erythematous lesions and there may be mucosal oedema. The patient may complain of a burning sensation in the mouth, together with xerostomia.

Allergic reactions to amalgam are rare, and when they occur are probably due to the mercury contained in the amalgam (Duxbury *et al.* 1982). In such cases, the intra-oral reaction consists of mucosal swelling accompanied by a burning sensation and blister formation (James *et al.* 1985).

A condition termed 'atypical gingivostomatitis' has been described (Perry *et al.* 1973). Affected patients complain of a 'burning mouth' and were found to have gingivitis, glossitis, and angular cheilitis. Histological findings in these cases included considerable plasma cell infiltration of the gingival tissues, and the term 'plasma cell gingivitis' is often used. Symptoms and signs abated in all patients when they avoided chewing gum and dentifrices, but recurred in most of them when they started using these substances again.

The constituents of various dentifrices are commonly implicated as a cause of contact sensitivity. Cinnamon and menthol were used as the main flavouring agent of 'Close Up'. Several reports of stomatitis occurred shortly after the introduction of this toothpaste (Millard 1973) and most patients showed a positive patch test to cinnamon oil (Kirton and Wilkinson 1973). Formalin is sometimes incorporated into toothpaste for the treatment of dentine sensitivity. One proprietary brand (Macleans Sensitive Teeth Formula Toothpaste) contained 1.3% formalin. After the introduction of this dentifrice, several reports appeared of burning sensation of the oral mucosa, redness and thickening of the oral mucosa and, in some, ulceration and sloughing (CSM 1984). The formalin has now been withdrawn from the toothpaste and replaced by strontium acetate hemihydrate 8% w/w.

Plasma cell gingivitis or contact stomatitis has also been reported to be caused by toothpaste containing cinnamonaldehyde (Thyne *et al.* 1989; Lamey *et al.* 1990), and herbal toothpaste (MacLeod and Ellis 1989).

Stainless steel wires are extensively used in dentistry — in orthodontics, in oral surgery, and in prosthodontics. The case of a patient who developed a reaction following immobilization of the jaws by stainless steel wires has been reported (Schriver *et al.* 1976). The patient complained of 'raw and sore' gums and later of swelling of the throat, palate, and gums. On removal of the wires, all the symptoms disappeared. The sensitivity appeared to be due to nickel, which is used in producing stainless steel alloys. Because of the escalating costs of precious metals, however, there is an increasing use of nickel–chromium alloys in dentistry. The alloys commonly available have a nickel content of between 60–80% by weight, so it is possible that adverse reactions to these alloys will become more common (Basker 1981).

A further case of a Type IV cell-mediated reaction to the nickel content of orthodontic wire has been described (Dunlop *et al.* 1989). Again, symptoms resolved when the wires were removed.

It is clear that contact stomatitis of the mouth to various substances does occur in some patients, possibly those with an allergic diathesis, and is simply relieved by removing the offending agent as soon as this has been identified. For instance, isolated cases have been reported of a localized allergic response to Scutan — an ethylene imine temporary crown material. The response is usually due to the unpolymerized material. Churgin and Payne (1981) reported that the incidence of allergic responses induced by Scutan may be in the order of 1:1000.

Iodoform, chlorhexidine, and stannous fluoride are three agents frequently used in dentistry. All compounds are applied topically. Three separate case reports have implicated these agents in causing contact stomatitis (Yaacob and Jalil 1986; Maurice *et al.* 1988; Razak and Latifah 1988). Clinical complaints in all three cases were similar, that of ulceration of the tongue and attached gingiva, and swelling of the lips. On withdrawal of the agent, the lesions resolved.

Erythema multiforme (Stevens–Johnson syndrome)

Erythema multiforme is a mucocutaneous disorder characterized by various clinical types of lesion including bullae, vesicles, papules, maculae, and wheals. The mucous membranes (oral, ocular, vaginal) are commonly involved, and at times the lesions are restricted to these membranes. Stevens–Johnson syndrome is a severe form of erythema multiforme. The aetiology of erythema multiforme varies from hypersensitivity to foods and drugs, to allergy secondary to viral, bacterial, or fungal infections. It has been estimated that drug therapy is the alleged trigger mechanism in 4 per cent of cases of erythema multiforme (Lozada and Silverman 1978), but in Stevens–Johnson syndrome drug association increases to 80 per cent (Cameron *et al.* 1966).

Drugs that have been frequently implicated in erythema multiforme are the long-acting sulphonamides, barbiturates, and penicillin (Cameron *et al.* 1966). Other drugs that have been associated with this condition are phenylbutazone and chlorpropamide (Tullett 1966; Kanefsky and Medoff 1980), phenytoin (Watts 1962), meprobamate and carbamazepine (Coombes 1965), salicylates and clindamycin (Fulghum and Catalano 1973), rifampicin (Nyirenda and Gill 1977), sulindac (Levitt and Pearson 1980), minoxidil (Di Santis and Flanagan 1981), ethambutol (Pegram *et al.* 1981), ampicillin (Konstantinidis *et al.* 1985), phenothiazines (Rees 1985), and doxycycline (Lewis-Jones *et al.* 1988). Erythema multiforme has also been attributed to the use of iodine containing mouthwashes (Tal and Dekel 1986), and to rosewood dust in a carpenter whose hobby was wood turning (Irvine *et al.* 1988). Rubin (1977) reported a case of Stevens-Johnson syndrome following the use of 30% sulphacetamide eye drops, the patient having been sensitized by previous sulphamethoxazole therapy. The Stevens–Johnson syndrome has also been caused by slow-release theophylline (Brook *et al.* 1989) and the antimalarial combination of chloroquine and sulphadoxine–pyrimethamine (Ortel *et al.* 1989).

The oral lesions of erythema multiforme should disappear within 14 days after cessation of the offending drug. Stevens–Johnson syndrome is much more serious, and potentially fatal. Local lesions are treated with topical steroids, but most cases require systemic steroid therapy and medical management.

Oral ulceration

Local irritants

A number of chemicals used by dental surgeons can cause 'burns' of the oral mucosa if injudiciously applied — for example, trichloracetic acid used in the treatment of pericoronitis. Drugs used for other purposes, however, may cause local irritation of the mouth; such drugs are discussed below.

Aspirin

Aspirin (acetylsalicylic acid) is a weak organic acid. Some patients attempt to relieve toothache by placing an aspirin tablet against the offending tooth. There is no evidence that this practice has any benefit in the manage-ment of toothache, and the corrosive action of the acidic aspirin may result in a fairly large area of ulceration. Surprisingly, the horrendous appearance which can be produced is not matched by equal discomfort. Aspirin has also been incorporated into chewing gum, and the use of this has been associated with oral ulceration (Claman 1967).

Toothache solutions

The active ingredients of toothache solution are men-thol, phenol, clove oil, camphor, and chloroform, in varying proportions. If the solution is injudiciously ap-plied, ulceration can occur on the adjacent mucosa and gingival tissues (Feaver 1982).

Hydrogen peroxide

Hydrogen peroxide is occasionally used in certain peri-odontal procedures and in the management of acute necrotizing ulcerative gingivitis. Oral ulceration has been reported when a 3% solution of hydrogen peroxide was used as a local irrigant (Rees and Orth 1986). The authors suggest that this concentration is too high, and its use in the management of periodontal problems is questionable.

Potassium

It is well known that high concentrations of potassium chloride may cause ulceration of mucosal surfaces, and slow-release preparations of this drug have been formu-lated in an attempt to overcome this problem. Such preparations should not be sucked, as this may cause ulceration (McAvoy 1974).

Isoprenaline

Isoprenaline tablets are often placed sublingually to relieve bronchospasm. Occasionally, such application may lead to ulceration of the floor of the mouth and undersurface of the tongue (Brown and Bolas 1973). It has also been suggested that prolonged symptomatic treatment of asthma with isoprenaline sulphate may lead to destruction of enamel if tablets of the drug are al-lowed to disintegrate slowly in contact with the teeth (Kay 1972).

Pancreatin

This drug is used for the treatment of fibrocystic disease of the pancreas. Pancreatin powder or tablets may cause severe mouth ulceration and angular cheilitis (Darby 1970). Three cases described were in children, and it was noticed that they held the preparations in their mouths for sometime before swallowing them. The oral ulcer-ation was thought to be due to digestion of the mucous

membrane by the pancreatin. Rapid improvement fol-lowed when the drug was withheld. Patients should be warned to swallow these extracts quickly to prevent damage to the mucous membranes of the mouth.

Emepronium bromide

Emepronium bromide possesses anticholinergic activity and was used in the management of urinary inconti-nence. In one series of cases, 17 per cent of patients treated with this drug developed mouth ulcers. One patient developed both mouth ulcers and a parotitis (Strouthidis *et al.* 1972). The lesions occurred in the first 3 weeks of treatment and were unilateral. They started as bullae, later ulcerating and involving the tongue and adjoining mucosa and occasionally the lower lip. The ulcers healed when the drug was withdrawn. The likely cause of the ulceration appeared to be local irritation, because of failure to swallow the tablets quickly. All the patients involved were mentally impaired. Duxbury and Turner (1982) reported on a further case of oral ulcer-ation induced by emepronium bromide. They suggested that the ulceration was due to an allergic reaction follow-ing repeated mucosal contact with the drug over pro-longed periods.

Emepronium bromide has now been withdrawn, mainly because of the high incidence of oesophageal ulceration, stricture, and perforation.

Cocaine

Cocaine abusers have been reported to suffer from extensive oral ulceration when the drug is applied top-ically (Dello-Russo and Temple 1982). The ulceration is probably due to the intense vasoconstrictive properties of the drug.

Paraquat

Paraquat is an ingredient of many proprietary weed-killers. Inadvertent contact between the compound and the oral mucosa can result in painful ulceration (Dobson and Smith 1987). The ulceration heals of its own accord, but topical application of benzydamine hydrochloride reduces the pain.

Other agents (acting systemically)

Oral ulceration, either primary or secondary to leuco-penia, may be caused by antineoplastic drugs such as methotrexate, fluorouracil, actinomycin D, doxorubi-cin, and bleomycin (Bottomley *et al.* 1977). Other drugs that can cause blood dyscrasias are discussed later.

Non-steroidal anti-inflammatory drugs (NSAID)

Oral ulceration may occur with virtually any of the NSAID. Those commonly implicated are phenylbuta-zone (Sperling 1969), indomethacin, and ibuprofen

(Guggenheimer and Ismail 1975). Naproxen, a propionic acid derivative, has also been reported as causing a severe neutropenia and oral ulceration (Kaziro 1980). In this case the ulceration was probably secondary to the neutropenia.

Proguanil hydrochloride

Proguanil is an effective and widely used antimalarial prophylactic. In one study it was reported that proguanil causes oral ulceration of sufficient severity to warrant a change in antimalarial prophylaxis. Of the 150 people taking part in the study, 7 had to be withdrawn because of oral ulceration (Daniels 1986).

Vesiculo-bullous lesions

Drug-induced vesiculo-bullous lesions affecting the orofacial region are rare. Corticosteroids may predispose the oral mucosa to bulla formation. Patients using steroid inhalers for more than 5 years are more prone to the development of oral blistering (High and Main 1989). The authors conclude that such use of corticosteroid inhalers may be one causal factor in the development of angina bullosa.

Naproxen has been implicated in the development of a bullous photodermatitis, with lesions affecting the hands and lips (Rivers and Barneston 1989). This unwanted effect may be dose-dependent.

Lupus erythematosus

Lupus erythematosus exists in two clinical forms; systemic lupus erythematosus (SLE), which affects various tissues and organs; and chronic discoid lupus erythematosus, which is basically a mucocutaneous disorder. The cause of the condition is unknown but genetic factors may play a part in the aetiology. It is now recognized that some cases of systemic lupus erythematosus are induced or precipitated by drugs. A characteristic immunological feature of systemic lupus erythematosus is the presence of antibodies to double-stranded DNA, although in the drug-related disease antibodies to DNA may be absent or low. The oral mucosa is involved in about 20 per cent of patients with SLE, and females are more often affected than males. The oral lesions may vary from erythematous areas to aphthous-like ulcerations or lesions resembling lichen planus.

Some common features of drug-related lupus include fever, polyarthritis, pleurisy, and lymphadenopathy. Renal and central nervous system involvement are rare and patients are unlikely to have the classic malar rash of systemic lupus erythematosus. On withdrawal of the offending drug, the condition resolves.

A wide variety of drugs has been implicated in causing drug-related systemic lupus erythematosus, including hydralazine and procainamide, which are amongst the most persistent offenders. This subject is discussed in some detail in Chapter 16, to which reference should be made.

Lichenoid eruptions

The term lichenoid drug eruptions can be used in two senses. First, drug eruptions similar to or identical with lichen planus; and, secondly, drug eruptions that do not necessarily resemble lichen planus clinically but have histological features very like this condition. β-Adrenoceptor blocking agents (e.g. propranolol, atenolol) are examples of drugs that cause lichenoid eruptions of the latter category.

Lichenoid eruptions have been reported in association with the oral hypoglycaemic drug chlorpropamide (Dinsdale *et al.* 1968). Eruptions occurred in a patient 8 months after starting antidiabetic therapy. Lesions started as 'white ulcerated sloughs' on the lips. A few days later these lesions had spread to the mucosa of the tongue and cheeks. Biopsy showed 'appearances suggestive of lichen planus'. Two weeks later, the patient's oral condition was worse, and chlropropamide therapy was stopped. Five days after this, the patient's oral symptoms had resolved. On reintroduction of the drug on another occasion, there was a recurrence of the ulceration. The condition, however, occurred only when the daily dose was raised to 250 mg.

NSAID are also commonly implicated in lichenoid eruptions (Hamburger and Potts 1983). The authors reported that 20 out of 75 patients with oral lichen planus were taking NSAID (ibuprofen, fenclofenac, diflunisal, and flurbiprofen) when first seen. They also described a case of erosive lichen planus induced by indomethacin, which healed on withdrawal of the drug but recurred when the drug was given by suppository. Ferguson and others (1984) have described a further case of an oral mucosal lichenoid eruption in a patient taking fenclofenac. The lesions resolved following withdrawal of the drug. It has subsequently been shown that there is significantly greater use of NSAID in patients with oral lichen planus than in control patients with other mucosal lesions (Potts *et al.* 1987).

Methyldopa is another drug that occasionally produces lesions of the oral mucosa resembling those of lichen planus. Hay and Reade (1978) described 17 patients, who presented over a period of 8 years, with oral lesions that were attributed to the drug. Five cases representative of the sample were described in some detail. The patients had been referred for the management of painful and persistent ulceration of the oral mucosa. The lesions in the mouth resembled erosive lichen planus or benign mucous membrane pemphigoid. The tongue and buccal mucosa were involved in most cases. The results of biopsies taken from eight of the patients varied: some histological features were strongly suggestive of oral lichen planus, whereas others were suggestive of benign mucous membrane pemphigoid (which was excluded in some doubtful instances by immunofluorescence investigations). The mechanism whereby methyldopa causes lichenoid reactions is uncertain. The patients in this series showed complete healing with relief of symptoms only on withdrawal of the drug. In some cases, the process of resolution took many months. One patient was further challenged with the drug and eruptions recurred. This finding may indicate a hypersensitivity type of reaction. The authors of this useful review stress the problem of diagnosis when a drug-induced disorder mimics a natural disease. An interesting observation in this study was the preponderance of females affected by drug-induced problems of the oral mucous membranes.

Other drugs that may cause lichenoid eruptions are amiphenazole (Dinsdale and Walker 1966), chloroquine, mepacrine, gold, arsenical compounds, bismuth, practolol (Felix *et al.* 1974), and captopril (Firth and Reade 1989). In addition, practolol has been reported as causing recurrent ulceration of the oral and nasal mucosa (Wright 1975). Lithium carbonate has also been reported to cause lichenoid eruptions (Hogan *et al.* 1985). The authors suggest that the effect of lithium on T cell function may be important in the pathogenesis of drug-induced lichenoid eruptions.

Unlike true lichen planus, which may last for 20 years or more, drug-induced lichenoid eruptions disappear once the drug has been stopped. It has been suggested that drugs associated with lichenoid reactions act as agents uncovering the latent disease of lichen planus or amplify a previous disorder, rather than inducing the disease *de novo* (Lacy *et al.* 1983).

Discolouration of the oral mucosa and the teeth

Oral mucosa

Discolouration of the tissues may be produced by direct contact with a drug or may follow the absorption of a drug after systemic administration. In the past, staining of the oral mucosa was often due to treatment involving metals such as silver, bismuth, gold, lead, mercury, zinc, and copper. These are now less used therapeutically, and if staining is found it may be a result of the person's occupation. For example, lead poisoning is an occupational hazard and chronic poisoning from ingestion,

inhalation, or skin absorption will produce a bluish line around the gingival margins. Cases of lead poisoning (from inadvertently eating 'old paint') tend to occur in children and the mentally retarded. Dentists working with such patients should be aware of the oral manifestations of lead poisoning (Lockhart 1981).

Stannous fluoride toothpastes sometimes produce blackish or greenish extrinsic stains on the teeth. This staining may be due to the combination of stannous ions with sulphides (released by bacterial action in the mouth), which produces insoluble stannous sulphide (Kay 1972). Animal experiments suggest that the low pH of stannous fluoride causes denaturation of the pellicle protein with subsequent exposure of the sulphydryl groups. The latter forms stannous sulphide with the stannous ions present in the preparation (Ellingsen *et al.* 1982).

Discolouration of the oral mucosa is often associated with some types of antimalarial therapy, chloroquine producing a bluish-grey pigmentation of the hard palate and mepacrine a yellowish mucosal pigmentation (Giansanti *et al.* 1971). McAllan and Adkins (1986) reported on four children with bluish-grey discolouration of their palates associated with amodiaquine treatment. The mechanism and localization (i.e. always in the palate) of quinoline-induced pigmentation is uncertain. Light and electron microscopy studies show that the pigment is either melanin or iron (Tuffanelli *et al.* 1963: Giansanti *et al.* 1971). Pigment is found in the epithelium and the macrophages of the underlying connective tissues (Watson and MacDonald 1974). The authors suggest the pathological pigment originates from the epithelial melanocytes, for they observed active melanocytes and compound melanosomes in keratocytes.

Other drugs that cause discolouration of the oral mucosa were reviewed by Vogel and Deasy (1977). They include long-term administration of phenothiazines, especially chlorpromazine, which causes a bluish-grey discolouration of the oral mucosa. The incidence of the discolouration is less than 1 per cent and it is suggested that the cause is an accumulation of a metabolite in the tissues. Pigmentation of the oral mucosa can also be caused by the use of oral contraceptives, the withdrawal of which does not produce complete regression of the abnormality. These drugs appear to have a stimulating effect on the secretion of pituitary melanocyte-stimulating hormone which is responsible for the discolouration. A further case report of epithelial melanosis of the gingival tissues from the use of the oral contraceptive supports this hypothesis (Hertz *et al.* 1980).

A bluish-grey band of pigmentation at the attached and free gingival junction has been reported to occur after systemic minocycline therapy (Beehner *et al.* 1986). In this case, the gingival discolouration arose from the underlying bone. When the gingival tissues were separated from the bone, they assumed their normal colour. The underlying bone, however, was grey, which suggests an interaction between the drug and bone during its formation.

Pigmented lesions of the tongue (dark macular patches) are reported to occur in heroin addicts who inhale the smoke (Westerhof *et al.* 1983). Histologically, the lesions are packed with melanocytes. The mechanism of these changes is uncertain.

A similar lesion secondary to methyldopa therapy has been described (Brody and Cohen 1986). Although biopsy material was not available, the authors suggested that the darkening of the tongue might have been due to a breakdown of methyldopa or its metabolites on exposure to air. The pigment produced is most likely to be melanin, a product of dopa metabolism.

The most common discolouration of the tongue is a condition known as black hairy tongue. This results from hypertrophy of the filiform papillae, which may grow to half-an-inch in length. The condition is usually asymptomatic, although the lengthened papillae may be a nuisance. The colour is usually black, but may be one of various shades of brown. Usually the filiform papillae are maintained at a functional length by normal physiological wear, but if the environment of the mouth is altered, the rate of desquamation of the filiform papillae may be reduced. The exact mechanism by which this condition is produced is unknown. Penicillin lozenges, oral penicillins, and other topical antimicrobials have caused black hairy tongue, as has sodium perborate used in mouthwashes. There is no really effective treatment for this condition.

Tetracycline staining of the teeth

Immediately after absorption, tetracyclines are incorporated in calcifying tissues and become a permanent feature of the teeth. In a clinical investigation of 59 children who had tetracycline staining of the teeth, it was found that the colour depended on the drug or drugs used (Weyman 1965): chlortetracycline produced a greyish-brown discolouration; yellow stains of varying intensity occurred in patients who had taken tetracycline, oxytetracycline, or demethylchlortetracycline; and a third type, a brownish-yellow discolouration, was of mixed origin. The degree of staining was variable: sometimes it was hardly noticeable. The least objectionable staining was produced by oxytetracycline. There is a clear linear relationship between the number of courses

of treatment with tetracyclines and the discolouration of developing teeth (Grossman *et al.* 1971).

If a tetracycline has to be prescribed during the period in which the crowns of the teeth are formed, then oxytetracycline is to be preferred. In a survey of the prevalence of tetracyclines in children's teeth, no evidence was found to suggest that prescribers were choosing oxytetracycline rather than another tetracycline (Stewart 1973). The study showed, however, that there had been a levelling-off in the proportion of children given tetracyclines during the first three years of life. This is an encouraging sign, but it is unfortunate that prescribers do not incline to oxytetracycline, which produces less objectionable staining than other tetracyclines, or, best of all, to alternative antimicrobial drugs.

Staining of the teeth in adults can also be induced by minocycline (Caro 1980; Poliak *et al.* 1985; Rosen and Hoffman 1989). In these cases, the teeth appeared grey and the discolouration was mainly confined to the middle portion of the teeth. The mechanism of the staining is uncertain, since no histological study has been carried out on extracted teeth. The drug has a strong avidity for iron and a diminished ability to bind to calcium and sulphur. These mechanisms may be important in tooth staining.

Periodontal tissues

Systemic drug therapy can have an adverse effect on the periodontal tissues. The most common example is drug-induced gingival hyperplasia (or overgrowth). Drugs implicated in this condition include phenytoin, cyclosporin, the calcium-channel-blocking drugs, and oral contraceptives. Additionally, certain types of systemic drug therapy can affect the inflammatory and immunological response of the periodontal tissues to bacterial plaque. Such drugs include immunosuppressives, corticosteroids, and NSAID. Patients on these drugs show a reduced response of their periodontal tissues to plaque (Seymour and Heasman 1988).

Gingival hyperplasia

Phenytoin

It is now well established that phenytoin therapy is associated with gingival overgrowth. Many studies reporting this unwanted effect have been reviewed by Hassell in 1981. The incidence of overgrowth due to phenytoin is approximately 50 per cent (Angelopoulos and Goaz 1972), but is higher in both teenagers (Kapur *et al.* 1973) and institutionalized epileptics (Hassell *et al.*

1984). The disorder does not appear to be related to the patient's age, sex, or race (Hassell 1981).

Gingival overgrowth usually becomes apparent in the first 3 months after starting phenytoin (Dummett 1954) and is most rapid in the first year (Aas 1963). Clinically the gingival overgrowth starts as a diffuse swelling of the interdental papillae which may then coalesce (Angelopoulos 1975). The gingival tissues may have a nodular appearance, but the colour (which ranges from coral pink to a deep bluish-red) depends upon the amount of inflammatory infiltrate present in the tissues (Esterberg and White 1945). In severe cases of gingival overgrowth, the clinical crowns may be covered (Dolin 1951). The incidence and severity are greatest on the labial aspects of the upper and lower anterior teeth (Esterberg and White 1945; Angelopoulos and Goaz 1972).

The relationship between the dose of phenytoin and the incidence and severity of gingival overgrowth is uncertain. A few studies have demonstrated a correlation between these variables (Panuska et al. 1961; Klar 1973), but most reports do not support this finding (Glickman and Lewitus 1941; Esterberg and White 1945; Dolin 1951; Angelopoulos and Goaz 1972; Conrad et al. 1974). There appears, however, to be a significant relationship between serum phenytoin levels and the severity of gingival overgrowth (Kapur et al. 1973; Little et al. 1975). There is marked interindividual variation between the dose of phenytoin and serum concentrations (Partington et al. 1974). Thus, serum concentrations of the drug, as opposed to dose, may provide more pertinent information on the incidence and the severity of gingival overgrowth.

Many studies have shown a clear relationship between patient's oral hygiene status and the incidence and extent of gingival overgrowth due to phenytoin, although some reports have contested this finding (for a review of studies see Hassell 1981). Mouth-breathing and other local factors, such as crowding of the teeth, significantly relate to the occurrence of gingival overgrowth (Glickman and Lewitus 1941).

It has been reported that patients receiving phenytoin have less bone loss than those taking sodium valproate (Seymour et al. 1985). Thus, patients on phenytoin appear to have a degree of 'resistance' to further periodontal destruction. This finding may also be attributable to the action of phenytoin on the immune system (see below).

Pathogenesis of gingival overgrowth due to phenytoin

Many theories have been suggested to explain why phenytoin causes gingival overgrowth. The most attractive theory at present is the direct effect of phenytoin or its metabolites on the gingival tissues (Conrad et al. 1972; Hassell 1981; Modeer et al. 1982). Although it would seem easy to confirm this hypothesis by tissue culture experiments, the results of such studies have shown marked variation, this probably arises because of differences in culture technique, concentration of drug employed, and degree of inflammation in the gingival tissues prior to harvesting (Hassell 1981).

It is suggested that there are different subpopulations of fibroblasts in the gingival tissues, some of which are capable of greater synthesis of protein and collagen (high-activity fibroblasts). Other fibroblasts are only capable of less protein synthesis (low-activity fibroblasts). The proportion of high-activity to low-activity fibroblasts appears genetically determined (Hassell and Gilbert 1983). Hassell has suggested that high-activity fibroblasts in the presence of certain predisposing factors (i.e. inflammation) become sensitive to phenytoin, with subsequent increase in collagen production. Phenytoin or its metabolites have no effect on other (low-activity) gingival fibroblasts. Alternatively, phenytoin or its metabolites may be cytotoxic to low-activity gingival fibroblasts thus facilitating an increase in the population of high activity fibroblasts.

For the drug or metabolites to act on the different subpopulations of fibroblasts, the substances have to be present in the gingival tissues at greater concentrations than in the systemic or peripheral circulation. It has been demonstrated that certain gingival fibroblasts have the ability to metabolise phenytoin and this metabolic activity may determine the susceptibility of a patient to phenytoin-induced gingival overgrowth (Fine et al. 1974; Hassell and Cooper 1980).

Other unwanted effects of phenytoin that may relate to gingival overgrowth

Immunosuppression Long-term phenytoin therapy is reported to cause immunosuppression (Sorrell et al. 1971; Seager et al. 1975; Fontana et al. 1976). Abnormalities in immune function include deficiency of circulating IgA; inability to develop antibody to various types of antigen challenge, for example, to *Salmonella typhi*; depression of the capacity to manifest delayed hypersensitivity reactions; and depression of lymphocyte transformation.

Attempts have been made to link the immunosuppressant properties of phenytoin with gingival overgrowth (Aarli 1976). In the gingival tissues, secretory IgA is one of the first lines of defence against bacterial plaque. A reduction in secretory IgA will render the tissues more susceptible to inflammation. Aarli

(1976) has suggested that it is the body's attempts to deal with this inflammation by its repair processes that causes gingival enlargement. A clear correlation between phenytoin-induced gingival overgrowth and crevicular fluid IgA levels would add support to this hypothesis.

The immunosuppressant properties of phenytoin may partly explain the lack of alveolar bone loss that occurs in patients treated with this drug (Seymour *et al.* 1985). Suppression of both the humoral and cell-mediated immune responses will result in a reduction of lymphokine production, formation of antibody-antigen complexes, and complement activation (MacKinney and Booker 1972; Church and Dolby 1978). All these factors, acting either directly or indirectly, are responsible for activating osteoclasts and hence causing bone resorption.

The action of phenytoin on the immune system may be a contributory (or predisposing) factor to gingival overgrowth, but it is unlikely to be the only cause. Other antiepileptic drugs (e.g. phenobarbitone and carbamazepine) also cause immunosuppression, but no other has been associated with gingival overgrowth.

Folic acid depletion Approximately 50 per cent of patients taking phenytoin have a low serum level of folic acid (Waxman *et al.* 1970). In such patients, the incidence of megaloblastic anaemia is of the order of 0.75 per cent (Flexner and Hartman 1960). The mechanism of folic acid depletion induced by phenytoin is uncertain. The drug may reduce absorption of folic acid from the gastrointestinal tract or block its transport across intestinal epithelium. Alternatively, phenytoin may inhibit folate reductase, an intestinal enzyme which hydrolyses dietary folate in polyglutamate form to the monoglutamate form, thus facilitating absorption (Mallek and Nakamoto 1981).

It has been suggested that phenytoin-induced gingival overgrowth is related to folic acid deficiency (Vogel 1977). Folic acid is essential for DNA synthesis; thus a deficiency will affect those cells with a high rate of turnover (e.g. bone marrow and oral epithelium). A deficiency of folic acid may result in impaired maturation of the gingival sulcular epithelium, thus rendering the underlying connective tissue more susceptible to inflammation (Dreizen *et al.* 1970). It has also been shown in animal studies that folic acid supplements reduce the incidence and severity of this gingival disorder (Vogel 1980). Some studies, however, have shown folic acid to be ineffective in reducing or eliminating gingival overgrowth in epileptics taking phenytoin (Mallek and Nakamoto 1981), but others have refuted this finding. Topical folate mouth rinses significantly inhibit gingival overgrowth from phenytoin (Drew *et al.* 1987). The efficacy of systemic folate in preventing such overgrowth appears to be related to plasma and red blood cell folate levels (Backman *et al.* 1989). The lower these baseline levels, the more beneficial systemic folate is in prevention.

Effect on the adrenal glands Phenytoin therapy is reported to cause an alteration in adrenal metabolism (Staple 1951, 1952) that results in impaired adrenocortical function, possibly due to suppression by the drug of corticotrophin (ACTH) production and consequently an alteration in pituitary–adrenal activity. Suppression of adrenocortical function results in a reduction of glucocorticoid synthesis and this has been suggested as an explanation for gingival overgrowth (Korff and Mutschelknauss 1963). When ACTH production is suppressed by phenytoin, there is a compensatory increase in the production of somatotrophic hormone (Nenning 1972). The latter hormone may cause fibroblast proliferation.

Phenytoin also stimulates the sodium pump (Bihler and Sawh 1971), which acts as a stimulus to fibroblasts.

Although these ideas are attractive, there is little experimental evidence to support an interaction between phenytoin and the adrenal glands for the mechanism of the gingival overgrowth. It may well be that suppression of adrenocortical function is yet another predisposing factor contributing to the sensitivity of gingival fibroblasts to phenytoin (Hassell 1981).

Cyclosporin

Cyclosporin is a selective immunosuppressant acting mainly on the T lymphocyte response. The drug is widely used in transplant surgery to prevent graft rejection.

It is now well recognized that one of the unwanted effects of cyclosporin therapy is gingival hyperplasia. Early studies evaluating the use of cyclosporin in transplant surgery reported gingival overgrowth as one of the unwanted effects associated with the drug (Starzl *et al.* 1981; Calne *et al.* 1981), and many further case reports have appeared in the dental literature (Rateitschak-Pluss *et al.* 1983; Wysocki *et al.* 1983; Adams and Davies 1984; Bennett and Christian 1985; Roystock *et al.* 1986). The disorder occurs in about 30 per cent of patients taking the drug (Wysocki *et al.* 1983; Seymour *et al.* 1987), the incidence being higher in children (Daley and Wysocki 1984) and slightly higher in female patients (Tyldesley and Rotter 1984); the incidence appears to be lower after bone marrow than after renal transplants (Beveridge 1983).

Clinically and histopathologically, gingival hyperplasia induced by cyclosporin resembles that caused by phenytoin, and hyperplasia occurs within 3 months of starting treatment. The epithelium covering the hyperplastic gingiva shows parakeratinization, and there are marked epithelial downgrowths into the underlying collagenous connective tissue. Inflammatory cells are present in the connective tissue in numbers dependent on the extent of oedema and inflammation present clinically before biopsy.

The pathogenesis of gingival hyperplasia from cyclosporin has not been fully determined. Furthermore, it is not established whether the hyperplasia is plaque-induced. Most studies recommend thorough oral hygiene to reduce the incidence of the condition. In a longitudinal study (Seymour *et al*. 1987) there was, however, no correlation between the extent of gingival hyperplasia and either gingival index or plaque scores. A further study has shown the presence of dental plaque to be related to the presence of gingival hyperplasia, but only a weak correlation between the abundance of plaque and the severity of gingival hyperplasia (Daley *et al*. 1986).

The efficacy of a plaque-control programme in preventing cyclosporin-induced gingival overgrowth has been evaluated in a group of adult renal transplant patients (Seymour and Smith 1990). Patients subjected to an intensive course of oral hygiene and removal of local gingival irritants showed better gingival health than controls. The oral hygiene measures did not, however, prevent the development of gingival overgrowth.

Obviously, comparisons have been made between gingival changes induced by phenytoin and those caused by cyclosporin. Histologically, the changes are similar. It is also interesting that both drugs cause hirsutism and immunosuppression, so perhaps there may be a common mechanism for induction of gingival hyperplasia.

It has been shown that the severity of the hyperplasia induced by cyclosporin is significantly related to the plasma concentration of the drug (Seymour *et al*. 1987); hyperplasia is more likely to develop if this exceeds 400 ng per ml. Other unwanted effects of cyclosporin are also dose-related and include nephrotoxicity, hepatotoxicity, and perioral hyperaesthesia (Laupacis *et al*. 1981; Daley and Wysocki 1984).

It seems likely that as cyclosporin usage increases so will the number of cases of gingival hyperplasia. Laboratory and clinical studies are required to elucidate the mechanism of this unwanted effect and possible ways of controlling it.

Calcium-channel blockers

Although nifedipine is the member of this group most often reported to have caused gingival overgrowth, all calcium-channel blockers are now believed to be capable of doing so.

Nifedipine

Gingival overgrowth associated with nifedipine therapy was first reported in 1984 (Lederman *et al*. 1984), and there have been several case reports since that time (Ramon *et al*. 1984; van der Wall *et al*. 1985; Lucas *et al*. 1985; Bencini *et al*. 1985; Jones, 1986; Puolijoki *et al*. 1988; Yusof 1989).

Clinically, gingival hyperplasia associated with nifedipine therapy resembles the disorder caused by phenytoin. It appears shortly after initiation of therapy and decreases on drug withdrawal (Lederman *et al*. 1984). Hyperplasia is most pronounced on the labial gingiva of the upper and lower anterior teeth, but does not occur in edentulous areas. The incidence of this problem may be of the order of 15 per cent, and its severity shows a weak correlation with the dose of nifedipine (Barak *et al*. 1987).

Histologically, the gingival epithelium shows parakeratinization with elongated rete pegs ('test tubes'). The underlying connective tissue consists of a diffuse mixture of dense collagen with a varying amount of ground substance. Inflammatory cells are present in the connective tissue and these are mainly plasma cells and lymphocytes. Histochemically, the hyperplasia seen with nifedipine also resembles that due to phenytoin. It is reported that gingival fibroblasts from both conditions contain strongly sulphated mucopolysaccharides and numerous secretory granules. Electron microscopy showed that nifedipine-induced gingival hyperplasia is due to an increase in ground substance (Lucas *et al*. 1985).

Animal studies have shown that gingival overgrowth is associated with two further dihydropyridines, oxodipine (Waner *et al*. 1988; Nyska *et al*. 1990) and nitrendipine (Heijl and Sundin 1988). In the oxodipine studies, gingival changes in both dogs and rats were dose-related. The histological findings consisted of purely fibroblastic proliferation without any infiltrate of inflammatory cells.

Nitrendipine administered to nine beagle dogs with established plaque and gingivitis caused the development of overgrowth as early as 10 weeks after dosage (Heijl and Sundin 1985). The principal histological change was that areas of non-infiltrated connective tissue in test specimens showed an increase in vascularity and appeared less dense. These vascular changes may be related to the vasodilatory properties of the drug.

Diltiazem

There have been fewer cases of gingival overgrowth associated with diltiazem therapy (Giustiniani *et al*. 1987; Bowman *et al*. 1988). The histological appearance of the gingival tissues is similar to that observed with nifedipine.

Verapamil

Again only a few cases of gingival overgrowth associated with verapamil have been reported in the literature (Cucchi *et al.* 1985; Smith and Glenert 1987; Pernu *et al.* 1989). One series of tissue culture studies has shown that the rates of proliferation and of protein and collagen production by fibroblasts harvested from overgrowth tissue were markedly lower than in control cells cultured from healthy gingiva. Incubation of fibroblasts in the presence of verapamil reduced protein and collagen synthesis (Pernu *et al.* 1989).

Oral contraceptives

The effects of oral contraceptives upon gingival and periodontal tissues are well documented. Several case reports have described a hyperplastic oedematous gingivitis following the use of oral contraceptives, resolving when the drugs are withdrawn (Lynn 1967; Kaufman 1969; Sperber 1969; Chevallier 1970). This response appears to be a secondary reaction to the presence of local irritants, especially dental plaque. The maintenance of adequate plaque control is conducive to gingival health, despite continued administration of oral contraceptives (Pearlman 1974). These reports have been confirmed by the results of studies that have shown clearly that hormonal contraceptives are associated with an increase in severity of gingival inflammation (El Ashiry *et al.* 1970; Das *et al.* 1971). Knight and Wade (1974) failed, however, to demonstrate significant differences in either plaque or gingivitis levels between a group of females taking oral contraceptives over a period of 18 months and age-matched controls. Subjects receiving the hormones for more than 18 months, however, exhibited greater periodontal destruction than either of the two previous groups and it was suggested that this was due to an altered host resistance seen in the long-term hormone group.

The effects of oestrogens and progestogens on the oral mucosa and periodontal tissues have been extensively studied. Oestrogens cause an increase in the acid mucopolysaccharide content of connective tissue in human oral mucosa (Schiff and Burn 1961). Progestogens increase the permeability of the gingival vasculature of rabbits by causing endothelial cell dysfunction and reversible gap formation (Mohamed *et al.* 1974).

Gingival exudate levels are also raised in females taking oral contraceptives (Lindhe and Bjorn 1967). The influence of the contraceptive is most marked during the menstrual phase when the production of ovarian oestrogen and progesterone is minimal (Lindhe *et al.* 1969). Sex hormones appear to have a more marked effect upon gingival exudate levels in the presence of chronic gingivitis (Lindhe *et al.* 1968*a*; Hugoson 1970). This effect may result from an increased vascularization of the chronically inflamed tissues (Lindhe and Branemark 1968) and an increase in the permeability of the gingival vessels (Lindhe *et al.* 1968*b*). These findings indicate that oestrogens and progestogens affect primarily the vascular response of irritated tissues, without necessarily aggravating the components of the classical inflammatory reaction.

The implication that oestrogens and progestogens are causal in producing or modifying the gingival response to dental plaque is dependent upon the demonstration of these hormones and their metabolic products within the tissues. There is now substantial evidence to suggest that there are oestrogen receptors in gingival tissues (Bashirelahi *et al.* 1977), and that the gingival tissues metabolise the sex hormones (El Attar and Hugoson 1974; El Attar 1974; Ojanotko and Harri 1978; Vittek *et al.* 1979). Chronically inflamed gingival tissue is twice as active as healthy tissue in metabolising progestogens and the chemical nature of progestogen metabolites differs in healthy and diseased tissues (El Attar 1971; El Attar *et al.* 1973; Harri and Ojanotko 1978). The metabolite 5-pregnanedione is a product of the conversion of progesterone in normal gingival tissue, whereas its isomer, 6-pregnanedione, is a metabolite in chronically inflamed tissue. In both instances, however, the major active metabolite of progesterone is 20-hydroxyprogesterone, which is increased fourfold in inflamed tissues (El Attar *et al.* 1973). This evidence suggests that the accumulation of metabolic products of the naturally occurring sex hormones is an important factor in the pathogenesis of chronic gingivitis. A positive correlation has been found between plasma levels of progesterone and its metabolites and the degree of gingival inflammation (Vittek *et al.* 1979). Although these biochemical analyses have been undertaken on naturally occurring hormones that are circulating at elevated levels in pregnancy, there is no evidence to suggest that different circumstances prevail in patients taking oral contraceptives.

Where there is an increase in circulating sex hormones either through pregnancy or taking an oral contraceptive, the patient's gingival tissues are more susceptible to plaque-induced inflammatory changes. It is therefore essential that such patients maintain optimal plaque control to reduce the risk of further periodontal damage.

Salivary glands

The salivary glands are under control of the autonomic nervous system, mainly the parasympathetic division.

Stimulation of the parasympathetic nerves causes glandular secretion. Because of their innervation, salivary gland function can be affected by a variety of drugs, producing either xerostomia or ptyalism. Certain systemic drug therapy can also produce pain and swelling of the salivary glands.

Xerostomia

Xerostomia (dryness of the mouth) can be caused by many drugs, and can be very troublesome to the patient. It can also cause a problem in denture retention, and dentists should be aware that drugs can be the cause. The only effective treatment is to stop the drug, but this is rarely necessary. Drugs that can cause dryness of the mouth by their parasympatholytic activity include the following.

Parasympatholytic drugs

(1) Drugs that compete with acetylcholine in parasympathetic (and sympathetic) ganglia. These include the ganglion-blocking antihypertensive drugs, such as pentolinium, mecamylamine, and pempidine, which have now been superseded by more selective agents;

(2) drugs that compete with acetylchloline release at parasympathetic effector junctions. Most drugs causing xerostomia do so in this way. They include atropine and atropine-like antispasmodics (e.g. poldine, and propantheline bromide), tricyclic antidepressants (e.g. amitriptyline), tetracyclic antidepressants (e.g. maprotiline hydrochloride), many antiparkinsonian drugs (e.g. benzhexol, benztropine mesylate, and orphenadrine), and histamine (H_1) blockers, some of which are phenothiazines. Somewhat weaker anticholinergic activity is exhibited by the phenothiazine derivatives, but this activity is sufficient to cause dryness of the mouth. Clonidine, which is used for the treatment of hypertension and of migraine, frequently produces xerostomia;

(3) drugs acting on the sympathetic effector function. Salivary flow is probably regulated to some extent by sympathetic as well as parasympathetic activity. Drugs acting at the sympathetic neuroeffector junction, such as amphetamine, may very slightly reduce salivary flow. A high incidence of caries has been observed in amphetamine abusers by Digugno and others (1981), who suggest that this is due to both the reduced salivary flow rate and a decrease in salivary calcium and phosphate concentration caused by this drug.

Other drugs

A number of other drugs, such as levodopa, have been reported to cause dryness of the mouth, and some of these have central actions. Antineoplastic drugs occasionally cause dryness of the mouth.

Ptyalism

Salivary secretion is increased by drugs that have a cholinergic effect, either by acting directly on parasympathetic receptors (e.g. pilocarpine) or by acting as cholinesterase inhibitors and so preventing the destruction of acetylcholine by cholinesterase (e.g. neostigmine).

Salivary secretion tends to be increased by mercurial salts, iodides, and bromides (drugs that are little used in modern therapeutics). Ketamine, an intravenous anaesthetic agent, may cause severe salivation. It has been suggested that all patients who are to receive ketamine should be premedicated with atropine (Davies 1972). Other drugs that occasionally cause excessive salivation include the antituberculous drug ethionamide and the anthelminthic niridazole.

Pain and swelling of the salivary glands

Salivary gland enlargement is associated with the use of a number of drugs, and sometimes the condition resembles mumps.

Anti-inflammatory drugs

The pyrazolone derivatives phenylbutazone and oxyphenbutazone may cause parotid swelling with or without submandibular swelling (O'Brien and Bagby 1985). Gross (1969) described the case of a 57-year-old woman taking 100 mg oxyphenbutazone four times daily for backache. On the third day of treatment she developed a temperature associated with dryness of the mouth; one day later, sudden, simultaneous, painless swelling of both parotid glands and, a day later, enlargement of the submandibular and sublingual glands. The condition was diagnosed as mumps, but on the following day her temperature had again risen and further enlargement of the salivary glands with profound xerostomia had developed. Oxyphenbutazone was stopped and steroid therapy initiated. The abnormal salivary glands shrank to normal size within 10 days. About a year later, a recurrence of backache led to further oxyphenbutazone therapy. After 24 hours, the patient noticed dryness of the mouth, and 48 hours later there was simultaneous swelling of both parotids accompanied by fever.

A further case of swelling of all salivary glands caused by oxyphenbutazone was described in a 52-year-old woman who had received treatment for 5 days (Chen et al. 1977). Although the mechanism for the acute enlargement is uncertain, in this case there was a transient eosinophilia, which suggests a possible allergic reaction. Oxyphenbutazone is no longer available for systemic administration, but is available as an ointment for ocular inflammation.

In a more extensive study on seven patients with the disorder, Speed and Spelman (1982) reported other disturbances such as fever, pericarditis, pleurisy, a rash, and disturbed hepatic function. They suggested that a hypersensitivity reaction to the drug was the most logical explanation for these findings. Phenylbutazone is a potent NSAID and its use is now restricted to hospitals, because of reported incidence of blood dyscrasias.

Anti-inflammatory drugs are extensively used in the treatment of rheumatoid arthritis. Sjögren's syndrome is quite common in patients with rheumatoid arthritis and parotid swelling may occur as part of it. It is important to remember, however, that in Sjögren syndrome the parotid swelling occurs relatively late in the course of the disease; the sudden appearance of salivary difficulties early in the course of rheumatoid arthritis may indicate an adverse reaction to an anti-inflammatory drug.

Iodides

Iodine compounds, including those used as radiographic contrast media, may cause painful swelling of the parotid and submandibular glands. The pain may radiate into the jaw and teeth. Imbur and Bourne (1972) reported a case of 'iodine mumps' in which bilateral swelling of the parotid and submandibular glands developed 3 hours after the injection of an iodinated contrast medium. The next day the salivary glands were greatly reduced in size, and after 48 hours the patient appeared normal. To confirm the cause of this reaction, another injection of the contrast medium was given, and 3 hours after the second injection the patient noticed recurrence of the bilateral parotid and submandibular swelling. The swelling was considerably less severe on the second occasion.

Such reactions to iodinated contrast media are rare and no case of sialadenitis was reported in a study of 2000 intravenous pyelograms (Tucker and Di Bagno 1956). Kohri and others (1977), however, described a case in which salivary gland swelling occurred as a sequel to excretory radiography with an organic iodide preparation. They also pointed out that parotid swelling is an infrequent manifestation of iodism and that only six cases had been reported previously.

Iodine mumps has also been reported to occur following parotid sialography (Katz et al. 1986). The authors described two cases of parotid swelling. One of the patients showed a positive skin allergy test to iodine, while in the other this test was negative.

The mechanism of iodine mumps is unknown. Salivary glands can concentrate iodide up to 100 times the plasma level (Talner et al. 1971). This high concentration of iodide in the glands and saliva may cause inflammation of the gland and oedema of the duct mucosa that, in turn, could obstruct the excretion of saliva, causing the salivary glands to swell. Reduction of the oedema would result in a reduction in swelling.

Antihypertensive drugs

Parotid swelling and tenderness can be caused by bretylium, and parotid pain or tenderness by bethanidine (Klein 1972). Three cases of sialadenitis have been reported following treatment with methyldopa (Mardh *et al.* 1974). In these cases, swelling of the salivary glands was accompanied by a raised temperature. Parotid pain has also been observed in patients treated with clonidine (Onesti *et al.* 1971), and with nifedipine (Bosch *et al.* 1986).

Warfarin sodium

A very unusual case in which submandibular gland haemorrhage occurred spontaneously in a patient receiving warfarin anticoagulant therapy was reported by De Castro and colleagues (1970). Clinically, the case presented with a swelling beneath the tongue. The ducts of the submandibular gland were engorged with clotted blood, and the submandibular glands themselves were enlarged and tender.

Other drugs

Parotid pain has been reported to occur in patients treated with the antimicrobial agent nitrofurantoin (Pellinen and Kalske 1982). The authors suggested that the pain might have arisen as a consequence of a Type III hypersensitivity reaction. Parotid swelling is also a rare unwanted effect of chlorhexidine mouth rinses.

H_2-receptor antagonists have been reported to cause an exacerbation of Sjögren's syndrome (Tomasko 1988). A patient with an intermittent history of the syndrome was treated with three different H_2-receptor antagonists (cimetidine, famotidine, and ranitidine) on separate occasions. Administration of any of these H_2-antagonists led to an abrupt increase of xerostomia and parotid gland enlargement.

Dental structures

Systemic drug therapy can affect the dental structures, although this is mainly an indirect effect mediated by a drug-induced alteration in the oral environment. The best example of this indirect effect is xerostomia and dental caries. Also considered in this section is the problem of sugar-based medicines and dental caries.

Xerostomia and dental caries

Prolonged treatment with a drug that reduces salivary flow can increase the risk of dental caries. Xerostomia and dental caries appear, however, to be a particular problem in patients treated with lithium and tricyclic antidepressants.

Lithium

Lithium salts are used in the prophylaxis of manic-depressive illness and in the treatment of mania. Dental caries is reported to be a complication of lithium treatment (Gillis 1978). In a review on lithium and dental caries (Rugg-Gunn 1979), the author referred to extensive surveys of natives of New Guinea (Schamschula *et al.* 1978) in which inverse correlations were found between caries experience and lithium levels in dental enamel, plaque, and saliva. No relation was found between caries experience and total lithium levels in the soil. This would suggest a possible cariostatic effect of lithium, and Rugg-Gunn (1979) postulated that the high caries increment reported was more likely to be due to impaired salivary secretion. Mason and others (1979) suggested that there were good reasons why patients on lithium therapy could have a high prevalence of dental caries, whether salivary gland function was impaired or not. Patients on lithium therapy can develop nephrogenic diabetes insipidus, as a consequence of which they become dehydrated and drink excessively. They may complain of dryness of the mouth, which might be accounted for in three ways: as a direct effect of the drug on salivary gland function; as a secondary effect of the dehydration; or as an effect of the the depressive illness. One patient reported by Mason and others (1979), who had been on lithium therapy for 5 years, had a high level of dental caries, the rate of which had increased since he began taking the drug. The patient had marked polyuria and drank about 5 litres of fluid a day. Although he complained of a dry mouth, there was nothing suggestive on the mucosa and his stimulated parotid salivary flow rates were within normal limits. The patient drank beverages with a high sugar content and sucked sweets regularly in an attempt to overcome the sensation of a dry mouth. The increase in consumption of refined carbohydrates undoubtedly contributed to his high caries incidence.

Tricyclic antidepressants

Most psychoactive drugs, especially the tricyclic antidepressants and the phenothiazines, have significant anticholinergic properties. This commonly results in dryness of the mouth which occasionally contributes to carious destruction of the teeth (Bassuk and Schoonover 1978). The tricyclics cause a marked decrease in salivary secretion during the first week of therapy, which then gradually improves.

More than one factor may be involved in the problem of caries induced by tricyclic antidepressants: the depressed patient may have a lower than normal rate of salivary flow, or the drug or drugs used in the treatment of the depression may cause a dryness of the mouth which, in the case of the tricyclics, may be severe. There is a clear relationship between salivary flow and the incidence of tooth decay. Because of the dryness of the mouth, the patient may eat a lot of sweets to try and ameliorate the condition. This in itself may contribute to the further carious destruction of the teeth.

Tricyclic antidepressants are sometimes used in children for the treatment of enuresis. It has been shown that children receiving such treatment also have a high incidence of dental caries (von Knorring and Wahlin 1986). Caries activity is only increased if the treatment period is longer than a month. The authors suggested that a drug-induced hyposecretion of saliva is the main cause of the increase in the dental caries. They also suggest, however, that enuretic children wake up more often in the night and often have some sugary drink or snack. It is thus not surprising that enuretic children not receiving treatment with antidepressants have a higher caries incidence than normal children (von Knorring and Wahlin 1986). They also suggest that physicians wishing to prescribe tricyclic antidepressants for a child should arrange an initial dental consultation for optimal caries prophylaxis.

Sugar-based medicines and dental disease

Sugar, whether as sucrose, fructose, or glucose, is widely used as a vehicle for medicines, especially to make paediatric formulations more palatable. It is now well established that long-term use of such medicines in children is associated with a high caries rate (Roberts and Roberts 1979), and the term 'medication caries' has been used to describe this condition (Hobson 1979). Plaque pH studies have shown that medicines sweetened with sucrose cause a prolonged pH depression (Feigal and Jensen 1982).

Sugar has many advantages as a constituent of medicines. It is cheap, non-toxic, and soluble. In 1984 nearly all paediatric preparations contained sugar (Hobson

1985). Various recommendations were put forward in 1985 to try and reduce the use of sugar in paediatric medicines and to encourage the pharmaceutical industry to produce sugar-free liquid preparations. Hobson and Fuller (1987) discussed the impact of these recommendations, and concluded that progress has been made in overcoming the problem of sugar-based medicines, but that there was still a need to omit sugar from those older preparations that still contain it.

Other drugs that can affect the dental structures

The anticonvulsant drug phenytoin is reported to cause abnormalities in the roots of teeth (Girgis *et al.* 1980). Defects include shortening of the root, root resorption, and an increased deposition of cementum. The mechanism of these abnormalities is uncertain, but may be related to the drug's inhibition of vitamin D metabolism or parathyroid hormone production (Harris and Goldhaber 1974; Robinson *et al.* 1978).

Increased sensitivity of the teeth and the gingivae may occasionally be caused by antineoplastic drugs (Bottomley *et al.* 1977).

Cleft lip and palate

From time to time a number of different drugs have been tentatively suggested as predisposing to the production of cleft lip, with or without cleft palate, in the offspring of mothers who have taken the drug during pregnancy. These include benzodiazepines, corticosteroids, sulphasalazine, tobacco (cigarette smoking), and the vitamin A analogue isotretinoin. Few drugs can be firmly categorized, however, as teratogenic in humans, except antineoplastic drugs and some hormones. These and other teratogenic disorders are discussed in detail in Chapter 5.

Muscular and neurological disorders

The muscles of facial expression and mastication can be affected by systemic drug therapy. Such effects will result in dyskinesia or dystonia (sometimes referred to as extrapyramidal reactions). Drug-induced dyskinesias can be acute or chronic (tardive). Drugs that have been implicated are predominantly the antipsychotic drugs (e.g. phenothiazines and butyrophenones). Other drugs that have produced orofacial dyskinesias include metoclopramide, tricyclic antidepressants, anticonvulsants, diazoxide, levodopa, and reserpine.

The extraordinary involuntary movements that can occur in the orofacial region include backward and forward movements of the tongue; sucking, pursing, and opening and closing of the lips; chewing and champing movements of the jaw; and facial grimacing. The strong uncontrollable movements of the jaws can lead to dislocation of the condyles (Kraak 1967; Abelson 1968; Bradshaw 1969; Smith 1973; Wood 1978). Salivation, dysphagia, and dysarthria may also be features of an extrapyramidal reaction. These reactions are discussed in detail in Chapter 18, to which reference should be made.

It is clearly important for the dental surgeon to appreciate that such bizarre reactions may be caused by drug therapy.

Facial pain and tardive dyskinesia

Tardive dyskinesia may possibly be an unrecognized cause of orofacial pain (Bassett *et al.* 1986). They stated that a dyskinesia is not a common cause of orofacial pain, but that the presenting complaints and symptoms are quite characteristic of this disorder. Two patients described had been taking antipsychotic drugs. As the authors point out, tardive dyskinesia is a painless syndrome in itself, but secondary orofacial pain can result from chronic mild trauma between a denture-bearing mucosa and dentures, which occurs with the abnormal movement. Not all patients taking antipsychotic drugs develop tardive dyskinesia. Furthermore, not all involuntary movements in a patient taking an antipsychotic drug are necessarily indicative of tardive dyskinesia. Many elderly people have a mild degree of involuntary dystonic-type movements to a mild degree. Ill-fitting dentures may also cause oral muscular activity (Sutcher *et al.* 1971). If the patient has clearly observable facial movements, however, and has also a history of taking antipsychotic drugs, it is not unreasonable to think of drug-induced tardive dyskinesia. There is no really satisfactory treatment for the disease other than cessation of drug therapy when, in some but not all instances, the condition will slowly improve. The management of such patients is for the supervising physician to undertake. The dental surgeon should be aware that such drug reactions exist and refer the patient when they are recognized. It is, of course, important to ensure that all dental work is satisfactory and that ill-fitting dentures are not adding to the problem, or the cause of the trouble.

Facial pain has also been reported following use of a controlled-release theophylline preparation (Townend 1989). The mechanism of this unwanted effect is uncertain.

Meige's syndrome

The blepharospasm–oromandibular dystonia syndrome (Meige's syndrome), has been related to long-term combination therapy with levodopa and carbidopa (Weiner and Nausieda 1982). The syndrome has also been associated with overuse of a self-prescribed nasal decongestant spray (Dristan), which contains phenylephrine hydrochloride 0.5%, chlorpheniramine maleate 0.2%, and benzalkonium chloride (Powers 1982).

Neuropathy

Many drugs are capable of causing a toxic neuritis of branches of the trigeminal nerves (Kay 1972). Drugs reported to have caused sensations of numbness, tingling, or burning in the face or mouth include the carbonic anhydrase inhibitor acetazolamide; the antibacterial drugs streptomycin, colistin, polymyxin B, isoniazid, nalidixic acid, and nitrofurantoin; several of the mono-amine-oxidase-inhibitor group of antidepressant drugs (e.g. phenelzine), and of the tricyclic group (e.g. amitriptyline); the β-adrenoceptor-blocking agent propranolol; the oral antidiabetic compounds tolbutamide and chlorpropamide; the migraine remedy ergotamine; the antihypertensive drug hydralazine; nicotinic acid in large doses; and the anaesthetic drug trichloroethylene. This subject is discussed in Chapter 18.

Taste disturbances and halitosis

Taste disturbances

Many drugs induce abnormalities of taste by processes not yet properly understood. The alteration in taste may be simply a blunting or decreased sensitivity in taste perception (hypogeusia), a total loss of the ability to taste (ageusia), or a distortion in perception of the correct taste of a substance (e.g. sour for sweet) — dysgeusia.

Sulphydryl compounds, especially penicillamine, are a common cause of taste disturbance.

Penicillamine

This drug is used to chelate copper in patients with Wilson's disease (hepatocellular degeneration). It is also used to treat rheumatoid arthritis, in which its mode of action is unknown.

In many patients, penicillamine causes partial or total loss of taste (Henkin et al. 1967). A decrease in taste acuity was reported to occur in 23 of 73 patients given penicillamine for conditions other than Wilson's disease (Scheinberg 1968). The incidence of taste disturbances in patients treated with penicillamine for Wilson's disease was much lower. About 25 per cent of patients with rheumatoid arthritis receiving penicillamine treatment experience taste disturbances (Jaffe 1968). It seems that there is a marked difference in the frequency of this unfortunate effect between patients being treated for Wilson's disease and those being treated for other conditions. It seems apparent that the loss of taste that may occur with penicillamine is directly related to the copper depletion that commonly follows the use of the drug. Penicillamine produces a negative copper balance, which is unlikely to occur in Wilson's disease, in which the total body copper is elevated. Administration of copper salts does not prevent this side effect, however, and taste abnormalities occur with other sulphydryl compounds that are not copper chelating agents (Jaffe 1983).

It has also been suggested that penicillamine-induced taste disturbance is due to a direct effect of the drug on the receptor cells (Lyle 1974). Furthermore, taste disturbances have been found to be dose-related (Day et al. 1974). If the dosage of penicillamine in patients with Wilson's disease is below 900 mg daily, there is a 25 per cent incidence of taste disturbance, but this increases to 50 per cent when the daily dose exceeds 900 mg. It would appear that taste disturbance is reversible within a period of 8–10 weeks, whether or not penicillamine is discontinued (Jaffe 1986).

Penicillamine has also been reported to cause a severe stomatitis (Lam 1980), and pemphigus-like mucosal lesions (Eisenberg et al. 1981). In both cases, resolution occurred after the drug was stopped.

Other drugs

Drugs reported as having caused disorders of taste, usually diminished taste acuity, include clofibrate, carbimazole, lithium carbonate, phenindione, imipramine, lincomycin, ethionamide, prothionamide, gold salts, levodopa, ethambutol, aspirin, and griseofulvin (Rollin 1978; Guerrier and Uziel 1979). Systemic griseofulvin can make certain foods seem profoundly tasteless, the effect gradually worsening as long as the patient takes the drug. Furthermore, the loss of taste may take some months to disappear after the drug is withdrawn (Griffiths 1976).

A metallic taste may be an unpleasant feature of treatment with the biguanide antidiabetic drug metformin. Similarly, a metallic taste is not uncommon in patients treated with metronidazole.

This subject is also discussed in Chapter 20.

Halitosis

One or two instances of drug-induced halitosis have been reported. Bauman (1975) reported that several patients taking the sublingual form of isosorbide dinitrate had complained of bad breath. This problem appeared with the onset of therapy, was reversible after discontinuing the medication, and recurred when therapy was resumed. Disulfiram is also reported to cause a slightly unpleasant breath odour (O'Reilly and Motley 1977). This is attributed to a metabolic product of the drug.

Oral infections induced or aggravated by drugs

Many types of systemic drug therapy can alter the oral flora and therefore predispose the mouth to infection. Drugs implicated include corticosteroids, antimicrobials, antimetabolites, immunosuppressive drugs, and oral contraceptives.

Corticosteroids

The glucocorticoids inhibit the inflammatory response of the body to injury, and may mask important diagnostic symptoms and signs. In one reported case, a patient on long-term steroid therapy developed spontaneously two large bilateral ulcerative necrotic lesions of the attached gingiva (Moskow et al. 1972). These worsened until eventually almost the entire surface of the maxilla was involved. Another patient on long-term steroid therapy for asthma, developed a severe and recurrent cellulitis following a tooth extraction (Mason 1970). The condition was refractory to antibiotic therapy and surgical treatment.

In a survey of 44 patients with oral thrush, it was found that 29 had received one or more antibiotics before the appearance of thrush. Corticosteroids had been used in 13 patients, and all but 2 of these had also been receiving antibiotic therapy. Two patients developed thrush after sucking hydrocortisone tablets for 6–10 days. Cytotoxic drugs had been used in 3 patients, who were also receiving corticosteroids or antibiotics. All patients in the survey were suffering from severe systemic disease, and it would seem evident that in most of them several factors capable of promoting thrush were present (Lehner 1964).

In a study of the use of steroid aerosols in asthma, no adverse effects other than fungal infections of the respiratory tract were encountered. The incidence of candidiasis of the pharynx was 13 per cent and of the larynx 5 per cent in patients who appeared to have no immunological disorders (McAllen et al. 1974). Children treated with steroid aerosols showed no clinical signs of candidiasis, however, and it was concluded that thrush does not occur in children as a result of aerosol steroid therapy (Godfrey et al. 1974).

It is generally agreed that treatment with corticosteroids in unphysiological amounts over a long period carries with it an increased risk of bacterial, fungal, or viral infections. Furthermore, the symptoms and signs of infection may be suppressed and the usual inflammatory response inhibited to such a degree that infection may assume unmanageable proportions. Fortunately, this is a rare event.

Antimicrobials

Antimicrobials, especially the broad-spectrum antibiotics, can alter the normal bacterial flora of the mouth, throat, and gut, so that resistant organisms may proliferate in the altered microbial environment. An overgrowth of Candida albicans may result, causing oral candidiasis (the so-called antibiotic stomatitis). Concurrent therapy with corticosteroids predisposes to such oral candidiasis. The condition is treated with lozenges or topical applications of an antifungal agent — nystatin, amphotericin B, or miconazole.

Antimetabolites

Topical fluorouracil has been associated with the activation of herpes labialis and the development of telangiectasia (Burnett 1982). It is suggested that these disorders occur as a result of the inflammatory reaction induced by this chemotherapeutic agent.

Immunosuppressive drugs

Infection commonly complicates renal transplantation, when it is mainly due to the use of immunosuppressive drugs to reduce the rejection phenomenon. Drugs that are often used for their immunosuppressive properties are azathioprine, prednisone, and cyclosporin. Although the infections are usually bacterial or fungal, fatal herpes simplex infection has been reported (Montgomerie et al. 1969).

Cytotoxic drugs

Drugs used for treatment of malignant disease are divided into groups, often depending on mode of action. They include alkylating agents (e.g. busulphan, carboplatin, carmustine, chlorambucil, cyclophosphamide, dacarbazine, ethoglucid, ifosfamide, lomustine, melphalan, and thiotepa); antimetabolites (e.g. cytarabine, mercaptopurine, methotrexate, and thioguanine); cytotoxic antibiotics (e.g. actinomycin D, epirubicin, idarubicin); vinca alkaloids (e.g. vinblastine, vincristine, vindesine) and etoposide; and other cytotoxic drugs (e.g. amsacrine, hydroxyurea, mitozantrone).

Many of the anticancer drugs cause bone marrow suppression (myelosuppression), although there are exceptions (e.g. vincristine). Infections in patients receiving myelosuppressive therapy are common and are important as they can have serious consequences. Additionally, such patients may experience oral pain, bleeding from the gingivae, and xerostomia. Oral ulceration is common in patients treated with cytotoxic drugs and these may occur early on in treatment and cause severe discomfort and pain. Oral bleeding is commonly a problem when drugs produce myelosuppression and can be very distressing as even soft toothbrushing may well be unacceptable.

Infection is a problem that may well occur with cancer chemotherapy. Ulcerated areas become infected and the organisms often involved are *Pseudomonas* spp., *Serratia* spp., klebsiellae, and *Escherichia coli*. *Candida* infections are common in such patients, who may also suffer from oral herpes.

Oral contraceptives

The use of oral contraceptives has been associated with a significant increase in the frequency of dry sockets (alveolar osteitis) after removal of impacted lower third molars (Catellani *et al.* 1980). The probability of dry sockets increases with the oestrogen dose in the oral contraceptive. The authors suggested that dry sockets can be minimized in patients taking these drugs by carrying out the extractions during days 23–28 of the tablet cycle.

Facial oedema

Facial oedema is often a manifestation of drug-induced hypersensitivity reactions. It has also been associated with administration of mianserin (Leibovitch *et al.* 1987), and secondarily to excessive use of an adrenaline bronchodilator (Loria and Wedner 1989). In the context of catecholamine use, this condition is believed to result from a sialadenotrophic effect of catecholamines that results in hypertrophy of the glands.

Drug-induced blood disorders

Blood dyscrasias frequently show oral manifestations.

The dental surgeon, who may be the first person to see such a patient, should be familiar with these manifestations. The oral manifestations of many of the blood disorders are similar to lesions occurring as a result of infection, and diagnosis on clinical grounds alone is not possible. Nevertheless, there are pointers that should alert to the possibility of a blood disorder, drug-induced or otherwise. The following signs and symptoms should arouse suspicion (Weiss 1973): unexplained spontaneous mucosal bleeding; numerous oral petechiae; excessive post-extraction haemorrhage; pallor of the oral mucosa; unresponsive oral infections; prolonged atrophy of lingual papillae; sore tongue or mouth without local irritation; ease of bruising; an ulcerated mucosa accompanied by pyrexia.

Drugs that interfere with haemostasis can present serious problems to the dental surgeon. It is now well recognized that aspirin inhibits platelet thromboxane and hence reduces platelet aggregation. There have been many cases of aspirin-induced bleeding after dental surgical procedures (Davis 1976; Foulke 1976; McGaul 1978).

Ibuprofen can induce thrombocytopenia and result in multiple oral petechiae and ecchymoses (Schelkun *et al.* 1987). This condition improves when the drug is discontinued and prednisone administered. The combination antimicrobial co-trimoxazole (trimethoprim and sulphamethoxazole) has also been implicated as a cause of thrombocytopenia. A case of a life-threatening sublingual haematoma arising after removal of a mandibular ameloblastoma has been reported (Barak *et al.* 1988). Prior to surgery, the patient had been taking trimethoprim 80 mg and sulphamethoxazole 400 mg for 5 days. The mechanism of this drug-induced thrombocytopenia is unclear.

Sublingual haematoma is also a serious complication of warfarin sodium therapy (Cohen and Warman 1989). Sore throat preceded the development of the haematoma and the authors stress that this early complaint must be taken seriously. Management of such cases is by prompt control of the airway and administration of vitamin K.

Blood disorders are discussed in detail in Chapter 22.

References

Aarli, J.A. (1976). Phenytoin-induced depression of salivary IgA and gingival hyperplasia. *Epilepsia* 17, 283.

Aas, E. (1963). Hyperplasia gingivae diphenylhydantoinea. *Acta Odont. Scand.* 21 (suppl. 34), 1.

Abelson, C.B. (1968). Phenothiazine-induced neck-face syndrome. *J. Oral Surg.* 26, 649.

Adams, D. and Davies, G. (1984). Gingival hyperplasia associated with cyclosporin. A report of two cases. *Br. Dent. J.* 157, 89.

Angelopoulos, A.P. (1975). Diphenylhydantoin gingival hyperplasia. A clinicopathological review. I. Incidence, clinical features and histopathology. *J. Can. Dent. Assoc.* 41, 103.

Angelopoulos, A.P. and Goaz, P.W. (1972). Incidence of diphenylhydantoin gingival hyperplasia. *Oral Surg.* 34, 898.

Backman, N., Holm, A-K., Hanstrom, L., Blomquist, H.K.S., Heikbel, J., and Safstrom, G. (1989). Folate treatment of diphenylhydantoin-induced gingival hyperplasia. *Scand. J. Dent. Res.* 97, 222.

Barak, S., Engelberg, I.S., and Hiss, J. (1987). Gingival hyperplasia caused by nifedipine. Histopathologic findings. *J. Periodontol.* 58, 639.

Barak, S., Shaked, Y., Bar, Z.G., and Samra, Y. (1988). Drug-induced post-surgical haemorrhage resulting from trimethoprim–sulphamethoxazole. *Int. J. Oral Maxillofac. Surg.* 17, 206.

Bashirelahi, N., Organ, R.J., and Bergquist, J.J. (1977). Steroid binding protein in human gingiva. *J. Dent. Res.* 56, 125.

Basker, R.M. (1981). Nickel sensitivity — some dental implications. *Br. Dent. J.* 151, 414.

Bassett, A., Remick, R.A., and Blasberg, B. (1986). Tardive dyskinesia: an unrecognised cause of orofacial pain. *Oral Surg.* 61, 570.

Bassuk, E. and Schoonover, S. (1978). Rampant dental caries in the treatment of depression. *J. Clin. Psychiatry* 39, 163.

Bauman, D. (1975). Halitosis from isosorbide dinitrate. *JAMA* 234, 482.

Beehner, M.E., Houston, G.D., and Young, J.D. (1986). Oral pigmentation secondary to minocycline therapy. *J. Oral Maxillofac. Surg.* 44, 582.

Bencini, P.L., Crosti, C., Sala, F., Montagnino, G., Tarantino, A., Menni, S., *et al.* (1985). Gingival hyperplasia by nifedipine: report of a case. *Acta Derm. Venereol.* (Stockh.) 64, 362.

Bennett, J.A. and Christian, J.M. (1985). Cyclosporin-induced gingival hyperplasia : case report and literature review. *J. Am. Dent. Assoc.* 111, 272.

Beveridge, T. (1983). Cyclosporin A : clinical results. *Transplant. Proc.* 15, 433.

Bihler, I. and Sawh, P.C. (1971). Effects of diphenylhydantoin on the transport of Na$^+$ and K$^+$ and the regulation of sugar transport in muscle in vitro. *Biochim. Biophys. Acta* 249, 240.

Bosch, X., Campistol, J.M., Botey, A., Cases, A., and Revert, L.L. (1986). Nifedipine-induced parotitis. *Lancet*, ii, 467.

Bottomley, W.K., Perlin, E., and Ross, G.R. (1977). Antineoplastic agents and their oral manifestations. *Oral Surg.* 44, 527.

Bowman, J.M., Levy, B.A., and Grubb, R.V. (1988). Gingival overgrowth — induced by diltiazem. *Oral Surg.* 65, 183.

Bradshaw, R.B. (1969). Perphenazine dystonia presenting as recurrent dislocation of the jaw. *J. Laryngol. Otol.* 83, 79.

British Medical Journal (1981). Teratogenic risks of antiepileptic drugs. *Br. Med. J..* 283, 515.

Brody, H.J. and Cohen, M. (1986). Black tongue secondary to methyldopa therapy. *Cutis* 38, 187.

Brook, U., Singer, L., and Fried, D. (1989). Development of severe Stevens–Johnson syndrome after administration of slow-release theophylline. *Pediatr. Dermatol.* 6, 126.

Brown, R.D. and Bolas, G. (1973). Isoprenaline ulceration of the tongue : a case report. *Br. Dent. J.* 134, 336.

Burnett, J.W. (1982). Further observations of two unusual complications of topical fluorouracil therapy. *Arch. Dermatol..* 118, 74.

Calne, R.Y., Rolles, K., and White, D.J.G., Thiru, S., Evans, D.B., Henderson, R., *et al.* (1981). Cyclosporin A in clinical organ grafting. *Transplant. Proc.* 13, 349.

Cameron, A.J., Baron, J.H., and Priestley, B.L. (1966). Erythema multiforme, drugs and ulcerative colitis. *Br. Med. J.* ii, 1174.

Caro, I. (1980). Discoloration of the teeth related to minocycline therapy for acne. *J. Am. Acad. Dermatol.* 3, 317.

Catellani, J.E., Harvey, S., Erikson, S.H., and Cherkind, D. (1980). Effect of oral contraceptive cycle on dry socket. *J. Am. Dent. Assoc.* 101, 777.

Chen, J.H., Ottolenghi, P., and Distenfeld, A. (1977). Oxyphenbutazone-induced sialadenitis. *JAMA* 238, 1399.

Chevallier, M.E. (1970). Mouth manifestations and oral contraceptives. *Rev. Odontol. Stomatol.* 28, 96.

Church, H.A. and Dolby, A.E. (1978). The effect of Dilantin on the cellular immune response to dento-gingival plaque extract. *J. Periodontol.* 49, 373.

Churgin, L.S. and Payne, J.C. (1981). Sensitised tissue response to an ethylene imine derivative transitional crown material. *J. Prosthet. Dent.* 46, 179.

Claman, H.N. (1967). Mouth ulcers associated with prolonged chewing of gum containing aspirin. *JAMA* 202, 651.

Cohen, A.F. and Warman, S.P. (1989). Upper airway obstruction secondary to warfarin-induced sublingual hematoma. *Arch. Otolaryngol. Head Neck Surg.* 115, 718.

Conrad, G.J., Haavik, C.O., and Finger, K.F. (1972). The relationship of 5,5-diphenylhydantoin metabolism to the species-specific induction of gingival hyperplasia in the rat. *Arch. Oral Biol.* 17, 311.

Conrad, G.J., Jeffay, H., Boshes, J., and Steinberg, A.D. (1974). Levels of 5,5-diphenyl-hydantoin and its major metabolite in human serum, saliva and hyperplastic gingiva. *J. Dent. Res.* 53, 1329.

Coombes, B.W. (1965). Stevens–Johnson syndrome associated with carbamazepine ('Tegretol'). *Med. J. Aust.* i, 895.

Craxi, A. and Pagliarello, F. (1980). Possible embryo-toxicity of sulfasalazine. *Arch. Intern. Med..* 140, 1674.

CSM (Committee on Safety of Medicines) (1984). Macleans Sensitive Teeth Formula Toothpaste. *Current problems* No. 13. HMSO, London.

Cucchi, G., Giustinian, S., and Robustelli, F. (1985). Gingival hyperplasia caused by verapamil. *Int. J. Cardiol.* 15, 556.

Curley, R.K. and Baxter, P.W. (1987). An unusual cutaneous reaction to lignocaine. *Br. Dent. J.* 162, 113.

Daley, T.D. and Wysocki, G.P. (1984). Cyclosporin therapy, its significance to the periodontist. *J. Periodontol.* 55, 708.

Daley, T.D., Wysocki, G.P., and Day, C. (1986). Clinical and pharmacological correlations in cyclosporin-induced gingival hyperplasia. *Oral Surg.* 62, 417.

Daniels, A.M. (1986). Mouth ulceration associated with proguanil. *Lancet* i, 269.

Darby, C.W. (1970). Pancreatic extracts. *Br. Med. J.*. ii, 299.

Das, A.K., Bhowmick, S., and Dutta, A. (1971). Oral contraceptives and periodontal disease. *J. Indian Dent. Assoc.* 43, 155.

Davies, C.K. (1972). Problems with ketamine anaesthesia. *Br. Med. J.*. iv, 178.

Davis, M.J. (1976). Aspirin-induced prolonged bleeding: report of a case. *J. Dent. Child.* 43, 350.

Day, A.T., Golding, J.R., Lee, P.N., and Butterworth, A.D. (1974). Penicillamine in rheumatoid disease : a long-term study. *Br. Med. J.* i, 180.

De Castro, C.M., Hall, R.J., and Glasser, S.P. (1970). Salivary gland haemorrhage — an unusual complication of Coumadin anticoagulation. *Am. Heart J.* 80, 675.

De Dobbeleer, G. and Achten, G. (1977). Fixed drug eruption : ultrastructural study of dyskeratotic cells. *Br. J. Dermatol.* 96, 239.

Dello-Russo, N.M. and Temple, H.V. (1982). Cocaine effects on the gingiva. *J. Am. Dent. Assoc.* 104, 13.

Digugno, F., Perec, C.J., and Tocci, A.A. (1981). Salivary secretion and dental caries experience in drug addicts. *Arch. Oral Biol.* 26, 363.

Dinsdale, R.C.W. and Walker, A.E. (1966). Amphiphenazole sensitivity with oral ulceration. *Br. Dent. J.* 121, 460.

Dinsdale, R.C.W., Ormerod, T.P., and Walker, A.E. (1968). Lichenoid eruption due to chlorpropamide. *Br. Med. J.* i, 100.

Di Santis, D.J. and Flanagan, T. (1981). Minoxidil-induced Stevens–Johnson syndrome. *Arch. Intern. Med.* 141, 1515.

Dobson, R.S. and Smith, A.C. (1987). Effect of paraquat on the oral mucosa. *Br. Dent. J.* 163, 160.

Dolin, H. (1951). Dilantin hyperplasia. *Milit. Surg.* 109, 134.

Dreizen, S., Levy, B.M., and Bernick, S. (1970). Studies on the biology of the periodontium of marmosets. VIII. The effect of folic acid deficiency on the marmoset's oral mucosa. *J. Dent. Res.* 49, 616.

Drew, H.J., Vogel, R.I., Molofsky, W., Baker, H., and Frank, O. (1987). Effect of folate on phenytoin hyperplasia. *J. Clin. Periodontol.* 14, 350.

Dummett, C.O. (1954). Oral tissue reactions from Dilantin medication in control of epileptic seizures. *J. Periodontol.* 25, 112.

Dunlap, C.L., Vincent, S.K., and Barker, B.F. (1989). Allergic reaction to orthodontic wire: report of a case. *J. Am. Dent. Assoc.* 118, 449.

Duxbury, A.J. and Turner, F.P. (1982). Oral ulceration induced by Cetiprin? *Br. Dent. J.* 152, 94.

Duxbury, A.J., Watts, D.C., and Eade, R.J. (1982). Allergy to dental amalgam. *Br. Dent. J.* 152, 344.

Eisenberg, E., Ballow, M., and Wolfe, S.H. (1981). Pemphigus-like mucosal lesions : a side effect of penicillamine therapy. *Oral Surg.* 51, 409.

El-Ashiry, G.M., El-Kafrawy, A.H., Nasr, M.F., and Younis, N. (1970). Comparative study of the influence of pregnancy and oral contraceptives on the gingivae. *Oral Surg.* 30, 472.

El-Attar, T.M.A. (1971). Metabolism of progesterone-7-^{3}H *in vitro* in human gingiva with periodontitis. *J. Periodontol.* 42, 721.

El-Attar, T.M.A. (1974). The *in vitro* conversion of male sex steroid 1,2-^{3}H-androstenedione in normal and inflamed human gingiva. *Arch. Oral Biol.* 19, 1185.

El-Attar, T.M.A. and Hugoson, A. (1974). Comparative metabolism of female sex steroids in normal and chronically inflamed gingiva of the dog. *J. Periodont. Res.* 9, 284.

El-Attar, T.M.A., Roth, G.D., and Hugoson, A. (1973). Comparative metabolism of 4-^{14}C-progesterone in normal and chronically inflamed human gingival tissue. *J. Periodont. Res.* 8, 79.

Ellingsen, J.E., Eriksen, H.M., and Rolla, G. (1982). Extrinsic staining caused by stannous fluoride. *Scand. J. Dent. Res.* 90, 9.

Ericson, A., Kallen, B., and Westerholm, P. (1979). Cigarette smoking as an aetiological agent in cleft-lip and palate. *Am. J. Obstet. Gynecol.* 135, 348.

Esterberg, H.L. and White, P.M. (1945). Sodium dilantin gingival hyperplasia. *J. Am. Dent. Assoc.* 32, 16.

Feaver, F. (1982). Action called for sale of toothache solutions. *Br. Dent. J.* 152, 3.

Fedrick, J. (1973). Epilepsy and pregnancy : a report from the Oxford record linkage study. *Br. Med. J.* ii, 442.

Feigal, R.J. and Jensen, M.E. (1982). The cariogenic potential of liquid medications : a concern for the handicapped patient. *Spec. Care Dent.* 2, 20.

Felix, R.H., Ive, F.A., and Dahl, M.G.C. (1974). Cutaneous and ocular reactions to practolol. *Br. Med. J.* iv, 321.

Ferguson, M.M., Wiesenfeld, D., and MacDonald, D.G. (1984). Oral mucosal lichenoid eruption due to fenclofenac. *J. Oral Med.* 39, 39.

Fine, A.S., Scopp, I.W., Egnor, R., Froum, S., Thaler, R., and Stahl, S.S. (1974). Subcellular distribution of oxidative enzymes in human inflamed and dilantin hyperplastic gingivae. *Arch. Oral Biol.* 19, 565.

Firth, N.A. and Reade, P.C. (1989). Angiotensin-converting enzyme inhibitors implicated in oral mucosal lichenoid eruptions. *Oral Surg.* 67, 41.

Flexner, J.M. and Hartman, R.C. (1960). Megaloblastic anaemia associated with anticonvulsant drugs. *Am. J. Med.* 28, 386.

Fontana, A., Grob, P.J., Sauter, R., and Joller, N. (1976). IgA deficiency, epilepsy and hydantoin medication. *Lancet* ii, 228.

Foulke, C.N. (1976). Gingival haemorrhage related to aspirin ingestion. A case report. *J. Periodontol.* 47, 355.

Fraser, F.C., Metrakos, J.D., and Zlatkin, M. (1978). Is the epileptic genotype teratogenic? *Lancet* i, 884.

Friis, M.L., Holm, N.V., Sindrup, E.H., Fogh-Andersen, P., and Hauge, M. (1986). Facial clefts in sibs and children of epileptic patients. *Neurology* 36, 346.

Fulghum, D.D. and Catalano, P.M. (1973). Stevens–Johnson syndrome from clindamycin. A case report. *JAMA* 223, 318.

Giansanti, J.S., Tillery, D.E., and Olansky, S. (1971). Oral mucosal pigmentation resulting from anti-malarial therapy. *J. Oral Surg.* 31, 66.

Gillis, A. (1978). Lithium carbonate and dental caries. *Br. Med. J.* ii, 1717.

Girgis, S.S., Staple, P.H., Miller, W.A., Sedransk, N., and Thompson, T. (1980). Dental root abnormalities and gingival overgrowth in epileptic patients receiving anticonvulsant therapy. *J. Periodontol.* 51, 474.

Giustiniani, S., Robustelli, D.C.F., and Marieni, M. (1987). Hyperplastic gingivitis during diltiazem therapy. *Int. J. Cardiol.* 15, 247.

Glickman, I. and Lewitus, M. (1941). Hyperplasia of the gingivae associated with Dilantin (sodium diphenylhydantoinate) therapy. *J. Am. Dent. Assoc.* 26, 199.

Godfrey, S., Hambleton, G., and Konig, P. (1974). Steroid aerosols and candidiasis. *Br. Med. J.* ii, 387.

Gordon, M.H., Tiger, L.H., and Ehrlich, M.D. (1975). Gold reactions are not more common in Sjögren's syndrome. *Ann. Intern. Med.* 82, 47.

Greenberg, G., Inman, W.H.W., Weatherall, J.A.C., Aldelstein, A.M., and Haskey, J.C. (1977). Maternal drug histories and congenital abnormalities. *Br. Med. J.* ii, 853.

Griffiths, I.P. (1976). Abnormalities of smell and taste. *Practitioner* 217, 907.

Gross, L. (1969). Oxyphenbutazone-induced parotitis. *Ann. Intern. Med.* 70, 1229.

Grossman, E.R., Walchek, A., and Freedman, H. (1971). Tetracyclines and permanent teeth. The relationship between dose and tooth colour. *Pediatrics* 47, 567.

Guerrier, Y. and Uziel, A. (1979). Clinical aspects of taste disorders. *Acta Otolaryngol.* 87, 232.

Guggenheimer, J. and Ismail, Y.H. (1975). Oral ulcerations associated with indomethacin therapy : report of 3 cases. *J. Am. Dent. Assoc.* 90, 632.

Hamburger, J. and Potts, A.J.C. (1983). Non-steroidal anti-inflammatory drugs and oral lichenoid reactions. *Br. Med. J.* 287, 1258.

Hanson, J.W., Myrianthopulos, N.C., and Harvey, M.A.S. (1976). Risks to the offspring of women treated with hydantoin anticonvulsants, with emphasis on the fetal hydantoin syndrome. *J. Pediatr.* 89, 662.

Harri, M-P. and Ojanotko, A.O. (1978). Progesterone metabolism in healthy and inflamed female gingiva. *J. Steroid Biochem.* 9, 826.

Harris, M. and Goldhaber, P. (1974). Root abnormalities in epileptics and the inhibition of parathyroid hormone-induced bone resorption by diphenylhydantoin in tissue cultures. *Arch. Oral Biol.* 19, 981.

Harrison, R.D. and Becker, B.A. (1969). Relation of dosage and time of administration of diphenylhydantoin to its teratogenic effects in mice. *Teratology* 2, 305.

Hassell, J.R., Greenberg, J.H., and Johnston, M.C. (1977). Inhibition of cranial neural crest cell development by vitamin A in the cultured chick embryo. *J. Embryol. Exp. Morphol.* 39, 267.

Hassell, T.M. (1981). *Epilepsy and the oral manifestations of phenytoin therapy*. Karger, Basel.

Hassell, T.M. and Cooper, C.G. (1980). Phenytoin gingival overgrowth: rate of drug metabolism by fibroblasts. *J. Dent. Res.* 59, 920.

Hassell, T.M. and Gilbert, G.M. (1983). Phenytoin sensitivity of fibroblasts as the basis for susceptibility to gingival enlargement. *Am. J. Pathol.* 112, 218.

Hassell, T.M., O'Donnell, J., Pearlman, J., Tesini, D., Murphy, T., and Best, H. (1984). Phenytoin-induced gingival overgrowth in institutionalised epileptics. *J. Clin. Periodontol.* 11, 242.

Hay, K.D. and Reade, P.C. (1978). Methyldopa as a cause of oral mucous membrane reactions. *Br. Dent. J.* 145, 195.

Heijl, L. and Sundin, Y. (1988). Nitrendipine-induced gingival overgrowth in dogs. *J. Periodontol.* 60, 104.

Henkin, R.I., Keiser, H.R., Jaffe, I.A., Sternlieb, I., and Scheinberg, I.H. (1967). Decreased taste sensitivity after D-penicillamine reversed by copper administration. *Lancet* ii, 1268.

Hertz, R.S., Beckstead, P.C., and Brown, W.J. (1980). Epithelial melanosis of the gingiva possibly resulting from the use of oral contraceptives. *J. Am. Dent. Assoc.* 100, 713.

High, A.S. and Main, D.M.G. (1989). Angina bullosa haemorrhagica: a complication of long-term steroid inhaler use. *Br. Dent. J.* 165, 176.

Hillesmaa, V.K., Teramo, K., Granstrom, M.L., and Bardy, A.H. (1981). Fetal head growth retardation associated with maternal antiepileptic drugs. *Lancet* ii, 165.

Hobson, P. (1979). Dietary control and prevention of dental disease in chronically sick children. *J. Hum. Nutr.* 33, 140.

Hobson, P. (1985). Sugar-based medicines and dental disease. *Community Dent. Health* 2, 57.

Hobson, P. and Fuller, S. (1987). Sugar-based medicines and dental disease — progress report. *Community Dent. Health* 4, 169.

Hogan, D.J., Burgess, W.R. Epstein, J.D., and Lane, P.R. (1985). Lichenoid stomatitis associated with lithium carbonate. *J. Am. Acad. Dermatol.* 13, 243.

Hollman, A. and Wong, H.O. (1964). Phenindione sensitivity. *Br. Med. J.* ii, 730.

Hugoson, A. (1970). Gingival inflammation and female sex hormones. *J. Periodont. Res.* (suppl. 5), 1.

Hurd, R.W., Wilder, B.J., and van Rinsvelt, H.A. (1983). Valproate, birth defects, and zinc. *Lancet* i, 181.

Imbur, D.J. and Bourne, R.B. (1972). Iodine mumps following excretory urography. *J. Urol.* 108, 629.

Irvine, C., Reynolds, A., and Finlay, A. (1988). Erythema multiforme-like reaction to 'rosewood'. *Contact Dermatol.* 19, 224.

Jaffe, I.A. (1968). Effects of penicillamine on the kidney and on taste. *Postgrad. Med. J.* 44 (suppl.), 15.

Jaffe, I.A. (1983). Thiol compounds with penicillamine-like activity and possible mode of action in rheumatoid arthritis. *Clin. Pharmacol. Ther.* 3, 555.

Jaffe, I.A. (1986). Adverse effects profile of sulphydryl compounds in man. *Am. J. Med.* 80, 471.

James, J., Ferguson, M.M., and Forsyth, A. (1985). Mercury allergy as a cause of burning mouth. *Br. Dent. J.* 159, 287.

Jones, C.M. (1986). Gingival hyperplasia associated with nifedipine. *Br. Dent. J.* 160, 416.

Kanefsky, T.M. and Medoff, S.J. (1980). Stevens–Johnson syndrome and neutropenia with chlorpropamide. *Arch. Intern. Med.*. 140, 1543.

Kapur, R.N., Girgis, S., Little, T.M., and Mosotti, R.E. (1973). Diphenylhydantoin-induced gingival hyperplasia; its relationship to dose and serum levels. *Dev. Med. Child Neurol.* 15, 483.

Karnofsky, D.A. (1965). Drugs as teratogens in animals and man. *Annu. Rev. Pharmacol.* 5, 447.

Katz, J., Marmary, Y., and Azaz, B. (1986). Iodine mumps following parotid sialography. *J. Oral Med.* 41, 149.

Kaufman, A.Y. (1969). An oral contraceptive as an aetiological factor in producing hyperplastic gingivitis and a neoplasm of the pregnancy tumour type. *Oral Surg.* 28, 666.

Kay, L.W. (1972). *Drugs in dentistry* (2nd edn). Wright, Bristol.

Kaziro, G.S. (1980). Oral ulceration and neutropenia associated with naproxen. *Aust. Dent. J.* 25, 333.

Keith, J. (1977). Effects of excess vitamin K on the cranial neural crest in the chick embryo. *Ann. R. Coll. Surg.* 59, 479.

Kennett, S. (1968). Stomatitis medicamentosa due to barbiturates. *Oral Surg.* 25, 351.

Kirton, V. and Wilkinson, D.S. (1973). Contact sensitivity to toothpaste. *Br. Med. J.* ii, 115.

Klar, L.A. (1973). Gingival hyperplasia during dilantin therapy; a survey of 312 patients. *J. Public Health Dent.* 33, 180.

Klein, F. (1972). Hypotensive drugs. In *Side effects of drugs*, Vol. 7 (ed. L. Meyler and A. Herxheimer), p. 298. Associated Scientific Publishers, Amsterdam.

Knight, G.M. and Wade, A.B. (1974). The effects of hormonal contraceptives on the human periodontium. *J. Periodont. Res.* 9, 18.

Kohri, K., Miyoshi, S., Nagahara, A., and Ohtani, M. (1977). Bilateral parotid enlargement ('iodine mumps') following excretory urography. *Radiology* 122, 654.

Konstantinidis, A.B., Markopoulos, A., and Trigonides, G. (1985). Ampicillin-induced erythema multiforme. *J. Oral Med.* 40, 168.

Korff, M. and Mutschelknauss, R. (1963). Die Hydantoin-Hyperplasie. *Dtsch. Zahnarztl. Z.* 28, 1157.

Kraak, J.G. (1967). A drug-initiated dislocation of the temporomandibular joint : report of a case. *J. Am. Dent. Assoc.* 74, 1247.

Lacy, M.F., Reade, P.C., and Hay, K.D. (1983). Lichen planus: theory of pathogenesis. *Oral Surg.* 56, 521.

Lam, P.P. (1980). Severe stomatitis caused by penicillamine. *Br. Dent. J.* 149, 180.

Lamey, P-J., Rees, T.D., and Forsyth, A. (1990). Sensitivity reaction to the cinnamonaldehyde component of toothpaste. *Br. Dent. J.* 168, 115.

Lammer, E.J., Chen. D.T., Hoar, R.M., Agnish, N.D., Benke, P.J., Braun, J.T., *et al.* (1985). Retinoic acid embryopathy. *N. Engl. J. Med.* 313, 837.

Laupacis, A., Keown, P.A., Ulan, R.A., Sinclair, N.R., and Stiller, C.R. (1981). Hyperbilirubinaemia and cyclosporin levels. *Lancet* ii, 1426.

Lederman, D., Lumerman, H., Reuben, S., and Freedman, P.D. (1984). Gingival hyperplasia associated with nifedipine therapy. Report of a case. *Oral Surg.* 57, 620.

Lehner, T. (1964). Oral thrush, or acute pseudo-membranous candidiasis. A clinicopathologic study of forty-four cases. *Oral Surg.* 18, 27.

Leibovitch, G., Maaravi, I., and Shalev, O. (1987). Severe facial oedema and glossitis associated with mianserin. *Lancet.* ii, 871.

Levitt, L. and Pearson, R.W. (1980). Sulindac-induced Stevens–Johnson syndrome. *JAMA* 243, 1262.

Lewis-Jones, M.S., Evans, S., and Thompson, C.M. (1988). Erythema multiforme occurring in association with lupus erythematosus during therapy with doxycycline. *Clin. Exp. Dermatol.* 13, 245-

Lindhe, J. and Bjorn, A.L. (1967). Influence of hormonal contraceptives on the gingiva of women. *J. Periodont. Res.* 2, 1.

Lindhe, J. and Branemark, P.I. (1968). The effect of sex hormones on vascularisation of granulation tissue. *J. Periodont. Res.* 3, 6.

Lindhe, J., Attstrom, R., and Bjorn, A.L. (1968a). Influence of sex hormones on gingival exudation in dogs with chronic gingivitis. *J. Periodont. Res.* 3, 279.

Lindhe, J., Birch, J., and Branemark, P.I. (1968b). Vascular proliferation in pseudo-pregnant rabbits. *J. Periodont. Res.* 3, 13.

Lindhe, J., Attstrom, R., and Bjorn, A.L. (1969). The influence of progestogen and gingival exudation during menstrual cycles. *J. Periodont. Res.* 4, 97.

Little, T.M., Girgis, S.S., and Masotti, R.E. (1975). Diphenylhydantoin-induced gingival hyperplasia : its response to changes in drug dosage. *Dev. Med. Child Neurol.* 17, 421.

Lockhart, P.B. (1981). Gingival pigmentation as the sole presenting sign of chronic lead poisoning. *Oral Surg.* 52, 143.

Loria, R.C. and Wedner, J.H. (1989). Facial swelling secondary to inhaled bronchodilator abuse: catecholamine-induced sialadenosis. *Ann. Allergy* 62, 289.

Loughnan, P.M., Gold, M., and Vance, J.C. (1973). Phenytoin teratogenicity in man. *Lancet* i, 70.

Lowe, C.R. (1973). Congenital malformations among infants born to epileptic women. *Lancet* i, 9.

Lozada, F. and Silverman, S. (1978). Erythema multiforme. Clinical characteristics and natural history in 50 patients. *Oral Surg.* 46, 628.

Lucas, R.M., Howell, L.P., and Wall, B.A. (1985). Nifedipine-induced gingival hyperplasia. A histochemical and ultrastructural study. *J. Periodontol.* 56, 211.

Lyle, W.H. (1974). Penicillamine and zinc. *Lancet* ii, 1140.

Lynn, B.D. (1967). 'The pill' as an etiological agent in hypertrophic gingivitis. *Oral Surg.* 24, 333.

McAllan, L.H. and Adkins, K.F. (1986). Drug induced palatal pigmentation. *Aust. Dent. J.* 31, 1.

McAllen, M.K., Kochanowski, S.J., and Shaw, K.M. (1974). Steroid aerosols in asthma : an assessment of betamethasone valerate and a 12-month study of patients on maintenance treatment. *Br. Med. J.* i, 171.

McAvoy, B.R. (1974). Mouth ulceration and slow-release potassium tablets. *Br. Med. J.* iv, 164.

McGaul, T. (1978). Postoperative bleeding caused by aspirin. *J.Dent.* 6, 207.

MacKinney, A.A. and Booker, H.E. (1972). Diphenylhydantoin effects on human lymphocytes in vitro and in vivo. *Arch. Intern. Med.* 129, 988.

MacLeod, R.I. and Ellis, J.E. (1989). Plasma cell gingivitis related to the use of herbal toothpaste. *Br. Dent. J.* 166, 375.

Mallek, H.M. and Nakamoto, T. (1981). Dilantin and folic acid status. Clinical implications for the periodontist. *J. Periodontol.* 52, 255.

Mardh, P.A., Belfrage, I., and Naversten, E. (1974). Sialadenitis following treatment with alphamethyldopa. *Acta Med. Scand.* 195, 333.

Mason, D.A. (1970). Steroid therapy and dental infection. Case Report. *Br. Dent. J.* 128, 271.

Mason, D.K., Ferguson, M.M., and Mason, W.N. (1979). Lithium treatment and dental caries. *Br. Dent. J.* 146, 136.

Maurice, P.D.L., Hopper, C., Punnia-Moorthy, A., and Rycroft, R.J.C. (1988). Allergic contact stomatitis and cheilitis from iodoform used in a dental dressing. *Contact Dermatitis* 18, 114.

Millard, L.G. (1973). Contact sensitivity to toothpaste. *Br. Med. J.* i, 676.

Modeer, T., Dahllof, G., and Otteskog, P. (1982). The effect of the phenytoin metabolite *p*-HPPH on proliferation of gingival fibroblasts in vitro. *Acta Odontol. Scand.* 40, 353.

Mohamed, A.M., Waterhouse, J.P., and Friederici, H.H.R. (1974). The microvasculature of the rabbit gingiva as affected by progesterone : an ultrastructural study. *J. Periodontol.* 45, 50.

Montgomerie, J.Z., Bedcroft, D.M.O., Croxson, M.C., Doak, P.B., and North, J.D.K. (1969). Herpes simplex virus infection after renal transplantation. *Lancet* ii, 867.

Moskow, B.S., Crikelair, G.F., and Wheaton, E.A. (1972). Severe oral infection associated with prolonged steroid therapy. Report of a case. *Oral Surg.* 34, 590.

Muniz, F., Houston, E., Schneider, R., and Nusyowitz, M. (1969). Chromosomal effects of diphenylhydantoins. *Clin. Res.* 17, 28.

Murray, V.K. and Defco, C.P. (1982). Intra-oral fixed drug eruptions following tetracycline administration. *J. Periodontol.* 53, 267.

Nenning, K. (1972). Erkronkungen durch Arzneimittel im Mund-und Kieferbereich. *Dtsch. Stomatol.* 22, 897.

Nyirenda, R. and Gill, G.V. (1977). Stevens–Johnson syndrome due to rifampicin. *Br. Med. J.* ii, 1189.

Nyska, A., Waner, T., Pirak, M., Galiano, A., and Zlotogorski, A. (1990). Gingival hyperplasia in rats induced by oxodipine — a calcium channel blocker. *J. Periodont. Res.* 25, 65.

O'Brien, W.M. and Bagby, G.F. (1985). Rare adverse reactions to NSAIDs. *J. Rheumatol.* 12, 562.

Ojanotko, A.O. and Harri, M.P. (1978). Testosterone metabolism in chronically inflamed male gingival tissue. *J. Steroid Biochem.* 9, 825.

Onesti, G., Bock, K.D., Heimsoth, V., Kim, K.E., and Merguet, P. (1971). Clonidine: a new antihypertensive agent. *Am. J. Cardiol.* 28, 74.

O'Reilly, R.A. and Motley, C.H. (1977). Breath odour after disulfiram. *JAMA* 238, 2600.

Ortel, B., Sivayathorn, A., and Honigsmann, H. (1989). An unusual combination of phototoxicity and Stevens–Johnson syndrome due to antimalarial therapy. *Dermatologica* 178, 39.

Panuska, H.J., Gorlin, R.J., Bearman, J.E., and Mitchell, D.F. (1961). The effect of anticonvulsant drugs upon the gingiva — a series of analysis of 1048 patients. Part I. *J. Periodontol.* 31, 15.

Partington, M.W., Reilly, D.M., Stewart, J.H., and Vickery, S.K. (1974). Serum disphenylhydantoin levels following a change in drug brand. *Can. J. Pharmacol. Sci.* 9, 31.

Pearlman, B.A. (1974). An oral contraceptive drug and gingival enlargement: the relationship between local and systemic factors. *J. Clin. Periodontol.* 1, 47.

Pegram, P.S., Mountz, J.D., and O'Bar, P.R. (1981). Ethambutol-induced toxic epidermal necrolysis. *Arch. Intern. Med.* 141, 1677.

Pellinen, T.J. and Kalske, J. (1982). Nitrofurantoin-induced parotitis. *Br. Med. J.* 285, 34.

Pernu, H.E., Oikarinen, K., Hietanen, J., and Knuuttila, M. (1989). Verapamil-induced gingival overgrowth; a clinical, histologic and biochemic approach. *J. Oral Pathol. Med.* 18, 422.

Perry, H.O., Deffner, N.F., and Sheridan, P.J. (1973). Atypical gingivostomatitis — nineteen cases. *Arch. Dermatol.*. 107, 872.

Poliak, S.C., DiGiovanna, J.J., and Gross, E.G. (1985). Minocycline-associated tooth discolouration in young adult. *JAMA* 254, 2930.

Potts, A.J.C., Hamburger, J., and Scully, C. (1987). The medication of patients with oral lichen planus and the association of non-steroidal anti-inflammatory drugs. *Oral Surg.* 64, 541.

Powers, J.M. (1982). Decongestant-induced blepharospasm and orofacial dystonia. *JAMA* 247, 3244.

Puolijoki, H., Siitonen, L., Saha, H., and Suojanen, I. (1988). Gingival hyperplasia caused by nifedipine. *Proc. Finn. Dent. Soc.* 84, 311.

Ramon, Y., Bemar, S., Kishon, Y., and Engelberg, I.S. (1984). Gingival hyperplasia caused by nifedipine — a preliminary report. *Int. J. Cardiol.* 5, 195.

Rateitschak-Pluss, E.M., Hefti, A., Lortscher, R., and Theil, G. (1983). Initial observations that cyclosporin-A induces gingival enlargement in man. *J. Clin. Periodontol.* 10, 237.

Razak, I.A. and Latifah, R.J. (1988). Unusual hypersensitivity reaction to stannous fluoride. *Ann. Dent.* 43, 37.

Rees, T.D. (1985). Phenothiazine : another possible aetiological agent in erythema multiforme. *J. Periodontol.* 56, 480.

Rees, T.D. and Orth, C.F. (1986). Oral ulcerations with the use of hydrogen peroxide. *J. Periodontol.* 57, 689.

Rivers, J.K. and Barneston, S.C.R. (1989). Naproxen-induced bullous photodermatitis. *Med. J. Aust.* 151, 167.

Roberts, E. and Rosa, F. (1983). Valproate and birth defects. *Lancet* ii, 1142.

Roberts, I.F. and Roberts, G.J. (1979). Relation between medicines sweetened with sucrose and dental disease. *Br. Med. J.* ii, 14.

Robinson, P.B., Rowe, D.J.F., and Harris, M. (1978). The effects of diphenylhydantoin and vitamin D deficiency on developing teeth in the rat. *Arch. Oral Biol.* 23, 137.

Rollin, H. (1978). Drug related gustatory disorders. *Ann. Otol. Rhinol. Laryngol.* 87, 1.

Rosen, T. and Hoffmann, T.J. (1989). Minocycline-induced discoloration of the permanent teeth. *J. Am. Acad. Dermatol.* 21, 569.

Rostock, M.H., Fry, H.R., and Turner, J.E. (1986). Severe gingival overgrowth associated with cyclosporin therapy. *J. Periodontol.* 57, 294.

Rubin, Z. (1977). Ophthalmic-sulphonamide-induced Stevens–Johnson syndrome. *Arch. Dermatol.* 113, 235.

Rugg-Gunn, A.J. (1979). Lithium treatment and dental caries. *Br. Dent. J.* 146, 136.

Safra, M.J., and Oakley, G.P. (1975). Association between cleft lip with or without cleft palate and prenatal exposure to diazepam. *Lancet* ii, 478.

Saxen, I. and Saxen, L. (1975). Association between maternal intake of diazepam and oral clefts. *Lancet* ii, 498.

Schamschula, R.G., Atkins, B.L., Barnes, D.E., Charlton, G., and Davey, B.G. (1978). *WHO study of dental caries aetiology in Papua, New Guinea*. WHO, Geneva.

Schardein, J.L. (1976). *Drugs as teratogens*. CRC press, Cleveland, Ohio.

Scheinberg, I.H. (1968). Toxicity of penicillamine. *Postgrad. Med. J.* 44 (suppl.) 11.

Schelkun, P.M., Bellome, J., Hiatt, W.R., and De Boom, G.W. (1987). Multiple oral petechiae and ecchymoses in a patient with osteoarthritis. *J. Am. Dent. Assoc.* 115, 735.

Schiff, M. and Burn, H.F. (1961). The effect of intravenous estrogens on ground substance. *Arch. Otolaryngol.* 71, 765.

Schriver, W.R., Shereff, R.H., Domnitz, J.M., Swintak, E.F., and Civjan, S. (1976). Allergic response to stainless steel wire. *Oral Surg.* 42, 578.

Seager, J., Jamison, D.L., Wilson, J., Hayward, A.R., and Soothill, J.F. (1975). IgA deficiency, epilepsy and phenytoin treatment. *Lancet* ii, 632.

Seymour, R.A. and Heasman, P.A. (1988). Drugs and the periodontium. A review. *J. Clin. Periodontol.* 15, 1.

Seymour, R.A. and Smith, D.G. (1990). The effect of a plaque control programme on the incidence and severity of cyclosporin-induced gingival changes. *J. Clin. Periodontol.* (In press).

Seymour, R.A., Smith, D.G., and Rogers, S.R. (1987). The comparative effects of azathioprine and cyclosporin on some gingival health parameters of renal transplant patients. *J. Clin. Periodontol.* 14, 610.

Seymour, R.A., Smith, D.G., and Turnbull, D.N. (1985). The effects of phenytoin and sodium valproate on the periodontal health of adult epileptic patients. *J. Clin. Periodontol.* 12, 413.

Shapiro, S., Hartz, S.C., Siskind, V., Mitchell, A.A., Slone, D., Rosenberg, L., *et al.* (1976). Anticonvulsants and parenteral epilepsy in the development of birth defects. *Lancet* i, 272.

Smith, A.J. (1973). Perphenazine side-effects presenting in oral surgical practice. *Br. J. Oral Surg.* 10, 349.

Smith, M. and Glenert, U. (1987). Gingival hyperplasi forarsaget af behandling med verapamil. *Tandlaegebladet* 91, 849.

Sorrell, T.R., Forbes, I.J., Burness, F.R., and Rischbieth, R.H.C. (1971). Depression of immunological function in patients treated with phenytoin (sodium diphenylhydantoin). *Lancet* ii, 1233.

Spain, K.M., Kisieleski, W., and Wood, N.K. (1975). Cleft palate induction: quantitative studies of ^{3}H-corticoid in A/Jax mouse tissues after maternal injections of ^{3}H-cortisol. *J. Dent. Res.* 54, 1069.

Speed, B.R. and Spelman, D.W. (1982). Sialadenitis and systemic reaction associated with phenylbutazone. *Aust. N.Z. J. Med.* 12, 261.

Sperber, G.H. (1969). Oral contraceptive hypertrophic gingivitis. *J. Dent. Assoc. S. Afr.* 24, 37.

Sperling, I.L. (1969). Adverse reactions with long-term use of phenylbutazone and oxyphenbutazone. *Lancet* ii, 535.

Staple, P.H. (1951). Action of diphenylhydantoin sodium on the adrenal gland. *Lancet* i, 1074.

Staple, P.H. (1952). Diphenylhydantoin, adrenal function and epilepsy. *J. Endocrinol.* 9, 18.

Starzl, T.E., Klintmalm, G.B.G., Porter, K.A., Iwatsuki, S., and Schroter, G.P.J. (1981). Liver transplantation with use of cyclosporin A and prednisone. *N. Engl. J. Med.* 395, 266.

Stewart, D.J. (1973). Prevalence of tetracycline staining in children's teeth. A resurvey after 5 years. *Br. Med. J.* iii, 320.

Strouthidis, T.M., Mankikar, G.D., and Irvine, R.E. (1972). Ulceration of the mouth due to emepronium bromide. *Lancet* i, 72.

Sutcher, H.D., Underwood, R.B., Beatty, R.A., and Sugar, O. (1971). Orofacial dyskinesia : a dental dimension. *JAMA* 216, 1459.

Tal, H. and Dekel, A. (1986). Oral mouthwash and erythema multiforme. *J. Oral Med.* 41, 147.

Talner, L.B., Lang, S.H., Brasch, R.C., and Lassen, E.C. (1971). Elevated salivary iodine and salivary gland enlargement due to iodinated contrast media. *Am. J. Roentgenol.* 112, 380.

Thyne, G., Young, D.W., and Ferguson, M.M. (1989). Contact stomatitis caused by toothpaste. *N.Z. Dent. J.* 85, 124.

Tomasko, M.A. (1988). Recurrent parotitis with H_2 receptor antagonist in a patient with Sjögren's syndrome. *Am. J. Med.* 85, 271.

Townend, J. (1989). Myofacial pain from theophylline. *Br. Dent. J.* 168, 438.

Tucker, A.S. and Di Bagno, G. (1956). Intravenous urography, a comparative study of Neo-Ipax and Urokon. *Am. J. Radiol.* 75, 855.

Tuffanelli, D., Abrahams, R.K., and Dubois, E.I. (1963). Pigmentation from anti-malarial therapy: its possible relationship to ocular lesions. *Arch. Dermatol.* 88, 419.

Tullet, G.L. (1966). Fatal case of toxic erythema after chlorpropamide (Diabinese). *Br. Med. J.* i, 148.

Tyldesley, W.R. and Rotter, E. (1984). Gingival hyperplasia induced by cyclosporin A. *Br. Dent. J.* 157, 305.

van der Wall, E.E., Tuinzing, D.B., and Hes, J. (1985). Gingival hyperplasia induced by nifedipine, an arterial vasodilating drug. *Oral Surg.* 60, 38.

Vittek, J., Rappaport, S.C., Gordon, G.G., Munnangi, P.R., and Southren, A.L. (1979). Concentration of circulating hormones and metabolism of androgens by human gingiva. *J. Periodontol.* 50, 254.

Vlasses, P.H., Rotmensch, H.H., Ferguson, R.K., and Sheaffer, S.L. (1982). 'Scalded mouth' caused by angiotensin-converting-enzyme inhibitors. *Br. Med. J.* 284, 1672.

Vogel, R.I. (1977). Gingival hyperplasia and folic acid deficiency from anticonvulsant therapy : a theoretical relationship. *J. Theor. Biol.* 67, 269.

Vogel, R.I. (1980). Relationship of folic acid to phenytoin-induced gingival overgrowth. In *Phenytoin-induced teratology and gingival pathology* (ed. T.M. Hassell, M.C. Johnson, and K.M. Dudley). Raven Press, New York.

Vogel, R.I. and Deasy, M.J. (1977). Extrinsic discoloration of the oral mucosa. *J. Oral Med.* 32, 14.

von Knorring, A.L. and Wahlin, Y.B. (1986). Tricyclic antidepressants and dental caries in children. *Neuropsychobiology* 15, 143.

Waner, T., Nyska, A., Nyska, M., Sela, M., Pirak, M., and Galiano, A. (1988). Gingival hyperplasia in dogs induced by oxodipine, a calcium channel blocker. *Toxicol. Pathol.* 16, 327.

Watson, I.B. and MacDonald, D.G. (1974). Amodiaquine-induced oral pigmentation — a light and electron-microscopic study. *J. Oral Pathol.* 3, 16.

Watts, J.C. (1962). Fatal case of erythema multiforme exudativum (Stevens–Johnson syndrome) following therapy with Dilantin. *Pediatrics* 30, 592.

Waxman, S., Corcino, J.J., and Herbert, V. (1970). Drugs, toxins and dietary amino acids affecting B_{12} and folic acid absorption on utilization. *Am. J. Med.* 48, 559.

Weiner, W.J. and Nausieda, P.A. (1982). Meige's syndrome during long-term dopaminergic therapy in Parkinson's disease. *Arch. Neurol.* 39, 451.

Weiss, J.I. (1973). Thrombocytopenic purpura : the dentist's responsibility. *J. Am. Dent. Assoc.* 87, 165.

Westerhof, W., Wolters, E.Ch., Brookbakker, J.T.W., Boelen, R.E., and Schipper, M.E.I. (1983). Pigmented lesions of the tongue in heroin addicts — fixed drug eruption. *Br. J. Dermatol.* 109, 605.

Weyman, J. (1965). The clinical appearances of tetracycline staining of the teeth. *Br. Dent. J.* 118, 289.

Wood, G.D. (1978). An adverse reaction to metoclopramide therapy. *Br. J. Oral Surg.* 15, 278.

Wright, P. (1975). Untoward effects associated with practolol administration: oculomucocutaneous syndrome. *Br. Med. J.* i, 595.

Wyatt, E., Greaves, M.W., and Sondergaard, J. (1972). Fixed drug eruption (phenolphthalein): evidence for a blood-borne mediator. *Arch. Dermatol.* 106, 671.

Wysocki, G.P., Gretzinger, H.A., Laupaus, A., Ulan, R.A., and Stiller, C.R. (1983). Fibrous hyperplasia of the gingiva : a side effect of cyclosporin A therapy. *Oral Surg.* 55, 274.

Yaacob, M. and Jalil, R. (1986). An unusual hypersensitivity reaction to chlorhexidine. *J. Oral Med.* 41, 145.

Yusof, W.Z.W. (1989). Nifedipine-induced gingival hyperplasia. *J. Can. Dent. Assoc.* 55, 389.

10. Gastrointestinal disorders

D. N. BATEMAN

Introduction

The gastrointestinal tract is a common site of adverse drug reactions, no doubt owing to the fact that most drug administration is by this route. Hurwitz and Wade (1969) reported over 20 years ago that the gut was the target site in between 20 and 40 per cent of well-documented adverse reactions in hospitals. Adverse reaction surveillance in the UK by 'yellow card' reporting continues to show that the gastrointestinal tract is prominent amongst organs reported as being involved, but this may reflect high reporting of adverse reactions to certain commonly used drugs, for example, non-steroidal anti-inflammatory agents. It is important to note that gastrointestinal adverse effects are a common cause of non-compliance in general practice (Martys 1979).

When addressing the issue of drug-induced gastrointestinal disorders, it should be borne in mind that virtually all drugs may cause disturbance of gastrointestinal function in some patients. It is important, therefore, to differentiate adverse reactions that involve a pathological change from those that do not, particularly when the symptoms are, for example, nausea and vomiting or change in bowel habit.

Symptoms of nausea and vomiting may have a psychological component, and it has been suggested that, as for some other adverse drug reactions, these are more likely to occur in women (Stewart and Cluff 1974).

Glossitis and stomatitis

These disorders are discussed in Chapters 9 and 20.

Oesophagus

Drug-induced changes in the oesophagus result from three principal causes: changes in motility, changes in mucosal integrity, and infection secondary to drugs. Rarely, the oesophagus may be the target organ of an effect whose primary site is another part of the body. Also rarely, drugs may obstruct the oesophagus by forming a mass of congealed material as in the case reported by Hart in which sucralfate prevented swallowing because it had formed such an obstruction (Hart *et al.* 1989).

Oesophageal motility

The tone of the lower oesophageal sphincter, and oesophageal motility are both important in swallowing and in ensuring that gastric acid is kept from the lower oesophagus. Drugs that impair the sphincter, such as opiates and anticholinergics are therefore to be expected to produce symptoms secondary to reflux of acid from the stomach.

Oesophageal spasm ('nutcracker oesophagus') has been caused by propranolol in therapeutic dosage (Bassoth *et al.* 1987) and in overdose (Panos *et al.* 1986). The presumed mechanism of this effect is β-adrenergic blockade. Interestingly, nifedipine, which reduces the amplitude of oesophageal contractions, was a successful substitute for propranolol in the management of hypertension in the case reported by Bassoth, mentioned above. Nifedipine itself is often associated with upper abdominal pain, which may be due in part to effects on oesophageal motility.

Chlormethiazole has been reported to cause dysphagia associated in one case with considerable (13 kg) weight loss (Dewis *et al.* 1982).

Ulceration and stricture

Oesophageal ulceration, with the possibility of resultant stricture, is recognized to occur with certain drug forms. Thus, doxycycline capsules (van Klingeren 1983; Al-Dujaili *et al.* 1983) seem particularly likely to cause this problem. Heller and colleagues (1982) reviewed 76 patients with benign oesophageal stricture and found more of them (22) had taken non-steroidal anti-inflammatory drugs (NSAID) than had members of a control group (10), but also found that emepromium bromide and potassium chloride were likely to be factors in 6 other patients. The latter two drugs are recognized causes of oesophageal ulceration (Al-Dujaili *et al.* 1983), and other case reports suggest that NSAID also cause oesophageal ulceration; this, however, may be more likely in patients with pre-existing oesophageal disease (Coates *et al.* 1986).

Ulcers of the oesophagus have been attributed to treatment with antibiotics other than doxycycline (see above), including tetracycline (Crowson *et al.* 1976), clindamycin (Sutton and Gosnold 1977), and phenoxymethylpenicillin tablets (Suissa *et al.* 1987). Ulceration of the oesophagus has also complicated treatment with clorazepate (Maroy and Moullot 1986). One common feature of many of these reports is the suggestion that posture may have been inappropriate, or that accompanying liquid drinks may have been inadequate to ensure passage of the tablet into the stomach. Experimental studies have shown that abnormal transit of tablets may be quite common and occur in up to 22 per cent of swallowing (Hey *et al.* 1982). Tablets should therefore be taken with the patient upright and with adequate fluid. Small, heavier tablets tend to pass more readily into the stomach. In one case report hiccups were believed to have caused impaired motility, leading to oesophageal injury by co-trimoxazole tablets (Seibert and Al-Kawas 1986).

Infection

Fungal infection of the oesophagus with *Candida* species is a well-recognized complication of broad-spectrum antibiotics. In one case, a child receiving erythromycin developed vomiting and haematemesis that was attributed to this complication (Hachiya *et al.* 1982). This type of infection is discussed further in Chapter 23.

Oesophageal injury in systemic disease

Rarely, oesophageal damage may result from other causes. Thus submucosal haematoma, causing retrosternal pain and haematemesis in a patient with polycythaemia rubra vera, was ascribed to the bleeding tendency caused by aspirin administration (Chapman *et al.* 1986). Oesophageal varices attributable to hepatic damage by busulphan and thioguanine, given to patients for treatment for chronic myeloid leukaemia, were reported by Key and colleagues (1987).

Nausea and vomiting

These are very common adverse reactions, and it is likely that most drugs will cause them under appropriate conditions. In practice, it is therefore necessary to differentiate drugs which almost always cause nausea and vomiting as do, for example, many cytotoxic drugs, from those that rarely do so. In addition, nausea and vomiting may be useful guides to toxicity from drugs for which plasma concentrations relate to pharmacological effects and when these symptoms are features of early toxicity. Examples are digitalis and theophylline (Mucklow 1978).

The pathophysiology of nausea and vomiting is poorly understood. In the brain the vestibular apparatus, the vomiting centre, the nucleus of the tractus solitarius, and higher centres are all possible sites of drug effects (Peroutka and Snyder 1982). That higher centres are important in inducing nausea is clear from the phenomenon of anticipatory vomiting seen in some patients receiving cytotoxic chemotherapy. The mechanisms by which cytotoxic drugs produce nausea and vomiting remain unclear (Harris 1982), but recent work on antiemetics for cancer chemotherapy suggests that for some cytotoxic drugs, particularly the highly emetic drug cisplatin, 5-hydroxytryptamine (5-HT) receptors are important, since ondansetron and other 5-HT$_3$-receptor antagonists are very effective in the management of vomiting induced by cancer chemotherapy. Interestingly, some of the newer antidepressants that block 5-HT uptake are prone to cause nausea as an adverse effect.

In animals, irritants that are instilled into the stomach can induce nausea and vomiting. Whether direct gastric irritation in man is a common cause of nausea and vomiting is unclear. Certainly, reflex pathways exist to carry stimuli from the gut to the relevant central centres in the nucleus of the tractus solitarius.

Most drugs that cause nausea and vomiting, including digitalis glycosides, opiates, oestrogens, and levodopa, all probably act on the chemoreceptor trigger zone, which is in the floor of the fourth ventricle and outside the blood–brain barrier. Tolerance develops to the nausea produced by some drugs, and this is seen with dopamine agonists, such as levodopa or bromocriptine (Wass *et al.* 1977), opiates, and oestrogens.

Nausea associated with the salts of potassium and iron is sometimes attributed to direct gastric irritation. The mechanisms by which antibiotics produce nausea are also unclear, though recent evidence suggests that erythromycin actually has effects on gut motility (Janssens *et al.* 1990). Exactly how this ties in with the nausea that seems to be associated more commonly with enteric-coated tablets (Carter *et al*. 1987) is unclear. Stang (1986) has suggested a possible association between erythromycin use and hypertrophic pyloric stenosis in a baby.

Stomach and duodenum

Altered gastric emptying

Drugs may either increase or reduce the rate of gastric emptying. Drugs that delay gastric emptying include those possessing anticholinergic activity, and opiates. Delay in gastric emptying may produce a sensation of fullness or nausea, but will also delay, and may impair, the absorption of concurrently administered compounds (Nimmo 1979). This effect needs to be remembered in patients receiving drugs with a narrow therapeutic index. Thus morphine has been shown to reduce the efficacy of mexilitine as an antiarrhythmic in patients following myocardial infarction (Pottage *et al*. 1978).

Drugs that increase gastric emptying, including metoclopramide, domperidone, and cisapride, may increase the absorption rate of other drugs. This may be particularly relevant for drugs producing central nervous sedative effects, including antihistamines, benzodiazepines, or alcohol. The sedative effects are more pronounced when these drugs are absorbed more quickly.

Drugs may occasionally form congealed masses (bezoars) in the stomach, and examples reported in the literature include potassium chloride (Antonescu 1989) and sustained-release theophylline tablets in overdosage. Smith (1987) reported the formation of bezoars in 4 of 11 patients admitted with an overdose of sustained-release theophylline tablets.

Peptic ulceration.

Non-steroidal anti-inflammatory drugs

The most common adverse drug reactions affecting the stomach and duodenum are those associated with NSAID. This is partly because these drugs are so widely prescribed. All these agents produce peptic ulceration in animals, and this, on occasions, makes interpretation of toxicological studies difficult. All NSAID are inhibitors of cyclo-oxygenase and this action results in impaired ability of the lining of the gut to resist acid attack (Horton 1979). That this is the mechanism is confirmed by the ability of prostaglandin analogues, for example, misoprostol, to inhibit ulcer formation in patients receiving NSAID.

The incidence of gastric erosions in patients taking NSAID has been studied in 249 patients with rheu-matoid arthritis or osteoarthritis by repeated endoscopies over a period of 12 months. In this study about 30 per cent of the patients developed gastric lesions and the incidence rose to 50 per cent in patients receiving more than one NSAID; some 10 per cent suffered frank peptic ulceration (Caruso and Bianchi Porro 1980). Approximately 6 per cent of patients receiving salicylates suffer upper gastrointestinal symptoms (Grigor *et al*. 1987).

The possible relationship between NSAID therapy and peptic ulcers has been extensively reviewed by Hawkey (1990). He emphasizes that a number of case–control and cohort studies have shown that both symptoms of gastric ulcers and the proportion of patients presenting with such complications as haematemesis, melaena, perforation, or death are higher in those who received NSAID. Looking at a number of published case–control studies, it is possible to calculate the relative risk of patients developing gastrointestinal disorders when taking aspirin or another NSAID, compared with controls. Hawkey reports that the relative risk for aspirin for upper gastrointestinal bleeding is of the order of 3.3, and for the non-aspirin NSAID 3.09. In contrast, the relative risk of perforation with NSAID is 5.93. When one considers death, the relative risk for non-aspirin NSAID use is even higher at 7.62.

Although paracetamol has been associated with gastrointestinal ulceration and upper gastrointestinal bleeding (Coggon *et al*. 1982), the usual interpretation of this association is that it is due to the use of paracetamol as symptomatic treatment for indigestion due to the ulcer rather than as cause of this. Observations showing an association between paracetamol use and previously diagnosed ulcers, and aspirin use and previously undiagnosed ulcers tend to support this hypothesis (McIntosh *et al*. 1988).

The evidence that aspirin and other NSAID are causative factors in duodenal ulcer is still controversial.

The issue is complicated further by the fact that cohort studies suggest that case–control studies exaggerate the likely risk of bleeding. A number of cohort studies all suggest that the relative risk of presentation with upper gastrointestinal bleeding or perforation is only 1.5, that is, a 50 per cent increase in risk as compared to the 300–500 per cent increase in risk suggested by the case–control studies. Even if the risk is only increased by 50 per cent, the wide use of these drugs still makes them an important problem. It should also be noted that this increase in risk of bleeding from NSAID occurs in the elderly (over 60 years) (Somerville *et al*. 1986). Bearing in mind that patients in this age group consume more of these drugs than young persons, it is not surprising that this condition is so common among older people.

Attempts to compare the relative risks of adverse events with different NSAID are fraught with difficulty. In the United Kingdom, the Committee on Safety of Medicines published a league table showing the numbers of serious gastrointestinal adverse reactions, and associated deaths, reported for the first 5 years of marketing of each of those drugs in the United Kingdom (CSM 1986). These data are used for regulatory purposes, and have resulted in a number of agents being withdrawn from the market. The data suggest that ibuprofen is associated with the lowest incidence of gastrointestinal bleeding and, of marketed drugs, aza-propazone and piroxicam with the highest. There is a problem, however, because when ibuprofen was first introduced the recommended dose was lower than that generally used in later times. These data are based on spontaneous reports, rather than on actual incidence. Nevertheless, they do provide the clinician with a useful starting point in determining which NSAID to choose.

Other drugs

A number of other agents have been associated with gastric damage. Bhasin and Singh (1988) reported four patients who developed haemorrhagic gastric erosions while being treated with chloroquine for malaria. A case of chronic gastritis associated with gold has been reported (Benfield et al. 1986). The largest survey of drug adverse effects on the upper gastrointestinal tract was reported by the Boston Collaborative Drug Surveillance Program (Jick 1981). Major gastrointestinal bleeding was reported in 4.5 per cent of patients receiving etha-crynic acid in this survey as compared with 1.2 per cent for heparin, 0.5 per cent for corticosteroids, 0.2 per cent for warfarin. There was an apparent summation effect when ethacrynic acid and steroids were combined, in that 2 out of 22 patients exposed to this combination developed gastrointestinal bleeding. Whether the etha-crynic acid is actually responsible for gastrointestinal bleeding has been debated, and Dargie and Dollery (1975) have suggested that the ethacrynic acid was started in some patients after bleeding had occurred.

When taken in overdose, theophylline and steroids have been reported to cause gastric perforation (Guss et al. 1986). This might be due to the increased acid production induced by theophylline and to the presence of corticosteroids.

The issue of corticosteroids and gastric ulceration remains controversial. As noted above, Jick (1981) reported an apparent increase in gastrointestinal haemor-rhage in patients receiving steroids. One problem is that corticosteroids may mask the symptoms of ulceration. An evaluation of data on 3064 patients in 71 clinical trials suggested a higher incidence of peptic ulcer disease (1.8 per cent) in patients receiving steroids than in controls (0.8 per cent). The incidence seemed to vary directly with the dose of steroids (Messer et al. 1983). Gastrointestinal haemorrhage was also more frequent in steroid-treated patients than in controls. Other workers have criticised this study on methodological grounds (Conn and Poynard 1984) but clinicians continue to report series of patients in whom steroid therapy seems to be a contributory factor in peptic ulceration. Thus, Dayton and colleagues (1987) reported that 25 out of 151 patients with perforated peptic ulcer had received corticosteroids within a week of the perforation.

Potassium salts, particularly if given in a wax-matrix formulation (McMahon et al. 1982), are associated with gastrointestinal lesions visible on gastroscopy. Delay in gastric emptying by an anticholinergic drug increases the effect of the potassium salt. Despite these data, a large prospective study from the Boston Collaborative Drug Surveillance Program did not associate potassium use and upper gastrointestinal bleeding in a group of 15 791 patients (Aselton and Jick 1983).

Rarely, very dramatic adverse effects on the stomach occur, such as the case of gastric rupture and death in a child who was given ipecacuanha syrup for treatment of poisoning (Knight and Doucet 1987), or the case reported by Ananth and colleagues (1988) in which lithium resulted in vomiting sufficient to cause a Mallory–Weiss tear.

Small intestine

Disordered motility

Drugs possessing anticholinergic or opiate activity will reduce small bowel motility, as well as gastric motility. On occasions this supression of activity may be sufficient to cause a paralytic ileus, and this has been reported with tricyclic antidepressants (Burkitt and Sutcliffe 1961; Gander and Devlin 1963; McNeill 1966; Clarke 1971) as well as with atropine (Beatson 1982). In patients suffering from poisoning with this type of drug, a clinical condition that simulates acute intestinal obstruction may occur (Figiel and Figiel 1973). Drug induced neuropathy can also effect the nerve supply to the gut, so producing a syndrome similar to paralytic ileus; this has been associated with vincristine (Mannes et al. 1976). Very rarely, obstruction of the small bowel lumen may occur from bezoar formation (Burruss et al. 1986).

Increased motility throughout the small bowel may result in diarrhoea, although clinically it is often difficult to tell whether the effects are principally on the large bowel or the small bowel. Thus, gold salts have been associated with diarrhoea and eosinophilia (Michet *et al.* 1987) and with terminal ileitis (Geltner *et al.* 1986), the latter case being of interest since the patient appeared to respond to chelation of the gold with dimercaprol. Purgatives increase the loss of duodenal mucosal cells and increase protein loss into the gut. In some patients this may be severe enough to present as steatorrhoea (Langman 1982). A patient has been described in whom diarrhoea and abdominal pain were associated with small intestinal biopsy changes that were attributed to sulindac (Freeman 1986).

Ulceration, haemorrhage, and infection

The small bowel is a site at which slow-release formulations have been demonstrated to cause local lesions, occasionally leading to stricture. Thus, potassium tablets are well recognized to cause this problem (Boley *et al.* 1965; Davies and Brightmore 1970). Lofgren and colleagues (1982) have described a case in which the use of slow-release potassium chloride was associated with jejunal perforation, and Brower (1986) reports this complication in a patient with Crohn's disease. Iron tablets have caused gangrene of a Meckel's diverticulum (Alaily 1974). Osmotic-pump delivery systems seem at particular risk of causing local ulceration or perforation of the small bowel, and for this reason a preparation of indomethacin (Osmosin) was withdrawn from the United Kingdom market (CSM 1983).

The vascular supply of the bowel may be damaged in a number of ways. Mesenteric venous thrombosis has been associated with oral contraceptive use (Greig 1989), and abuse of cocaine has resulted in gangrene in both an adult (Mizrahi *et al.* 1989) and in a neonate whose mother had taken the drug (Telsey *et al.* 1988). Mesenteric infarction may also result from the use of vasoconstrictor drugs, particularly in patients whose splanchnic circulation is already compromised (Brown *et al.* 1959; Alves *et al.* 1979). Mesenteric arterial occlusion has been reported in association with the oral contraceptive pill and may affect either the large or small bowel (Kilpatrick *et al.* 1968; Brennan *et al.* 1968; Cotton and Lea Thomas 1971; Nothmann *et al.* 1973). This adverse effect is likely to be associated with the use of oral contraceptives with higher oestrogen contents.

Jejunal haematomata have been reported in association with warfarin (Aziz Khan *et al.* 1982), and haemorrhagic necrosis of the small intestine has also been attributed to digitalis glycosides (Gazes *et al.* 1961; Muggia 1967), although this may have been in part due in

these patients to poor intestinal blood flow secondary to heart failure.

Ulceration and stricture of the small bowel have been reported with normal formulations of NSAID (Saverymuttu *et al.* 1986; Madhok *et al.* 1986). Gold, which one of the patients described by Madhok and colleagues (1986) was also receiving, may cause a panenteritis (Roe *et al.* 1972). Ischaemic damage to the small bowel has also been associated with vasculitis attributed to lithium therapy (Cannon 1982).

Flucytosine was reported to cause erosive enteritis affecting the small bowel of patients treated for *Cryptococcus neoformans* infections (White and Traube 1982). Omeprazole, which is very effective in reducing acid production in the stomach, may increase the risk of enteric infection and two authors have suggested this as a potential problem (Littman 1990; Wingate 1990), the latter author reporting a patient in whom this problem seemed to have occurred. The subject is discussed further in Chapter 23.

Malabsorption

Drug-induced malabsorption may occur because of an interaction between drugs and particular nutrients. Examples include chelation of tetracycline and calcium ions (Kuwin and Finland 1961), cholestyramine and iron (Thomas *et al.* 1972), cholestyramine and vitamin B_{12} (Coronato and Glass 1973). Cholestyramine also binds to bile salts and in this way causes steatorrhoea and malabsorption of fat-soluble vitamins (Zurier *et al.* 1965). This subject is discussed further in Chapters 23 and 30.

A single drug may also cause either specific malabsorption syndromes or a generalized malabsorption state. Thus, drugs that alter mitotic activity of the small intestinal wall may cause malabsorption, and examples of drugs that do this are colchicine (Race *et al.* 1970) and methotrexate (Trier 1962; Stebbins and Pearson 1967). Mild steatorrhoea is quite common with these drugs. Jejunal mucosal changes and steatorrhoea have also been associated with allopurinol (Chen *et al.* 1982), methyldopa (Schneerson and Gazzard 1977), and phenindione (Juel-Jensen 1959).

Some antibiotics have been associated with malabsorption, including neomycin, which in addition to binding bile salts (Hardison and Rosenberg 1969) probably also interferes with protein synthesis within the enterocyte causing damage to the brush border as shown by changes in disaccharidases (Reiner and Patterson 1966). Large doses of neomycin produce partial villous atrophy (Jacobson *et al.* 1960; Dobbins *et al.* 1968). Tetracyclines, in addition to impairing the absorption of ﬀtimescalcium, as mentioned above, may also cause steatorrhoea (Mitchell *et al*. 1982) and impair iron absorption (Greenberger *et al*. 1967). Malabsorption has also been demonstrated following treatment with kanamycin, polymyxin, or bacitracin (Steiner *et al*. 1961; Powell *et al*. 1962; Faloon *et al*. 1966).

Mefenamic acid causes a malabsorption syndrome and diarrhoea, associated in some patients with colitis (Hall *et al*. 1983). Of the adverse reaction reports to this drug received by the Committee on Safety of Medicines between 1963 and 1989, 18 per cent were for diarrhoea and colitis.

Cathartics may result in mild steatorrhoea, presumably due to intestinal hurry, particularly if taken in large amounts (Heizer *et al*. 1968).

Specific nutritional deficiencies affecting folate and B_{12} metabolism have been associated with drug therapy. Anticonvulsant therapy has been reported to cause a fall in red cell and serum folate in a high proportion of patients receiving these agents (Reynolds 1968). Some workers have suggested that these drugs impair folate absorption (Benn *et al*. 1971; Gerson *et al*. 1972). Other workers have suggested the principal problem in these patients is poor diet (Rose and Johnson 1978), or the enzyme-inducing effects of the anticonvulsants on folate metabolism (Labadarios *et al*. 1978).

Absorption of vitamin B_{12}, as mentioned above, is inhibited by neomycin and cholestyramine. Sodium aminosalicylate (PAS) interferes with the ileal transport of vitamin B_{12}, perhaps by inhibiting a folate-dependent enzyme system (Palva *et al*. 1966). Folic acid therapy seems to protect against this particular malabsorption syndrome (Paaby and Nervin 1966). Colchicine also seems capable of producing reversible impairment of vitamin B_{12} absorption (Webb *et al*. 1968), and the biguanides metformin and phenformin seem to impair it by an effect on mucosal transport (Berchtold *et al*. 1971; Tomkin *et al*. 1971; Tomkin 1973). Biguanides also have other effects on the brush border, including reduction in disaccharidase activity (Berchtold *et al*. 1971). An alteration in the pH of the ileal contents has been suggested as a cause of the impairment of the absorption of B_{12} seen with potassium chloride therapy (Palva *et al*. 1972), and one case of megaloblastic anaemia attributed to this cause has been reported (Salokannel *et al*. 1970).

Colon

Antibiotic-induced colitis

Antibiotics commonly produce diarrhoea as an adverse effect, this is particularly the case with broad-spectrum antibiotics and usually attributed to a change in normal intestinal flora. A far more serious complication of antibiotic use is pseudomembranous colitis, which is a specific form of colitis due to infection of the bowel with the organism *Clostridium difficile* and the production of a specific toxin that damages the gut mucosa (Simpson *et al*. 1978). Originally, this condition was believed to be particularly associated with treatment with lincomycin or clindamycin (Benner and Tellman 1970; Cohen *et al*. 1973), but virtually any antibacterial agent may be responsible. It may follow either oral or parenteral administration. It has been suggested that pseudomembranous colitis may be more common in patients with abnormally slow bowel motility (Schulze-Delrieu 1983) and it is interesting that some antibiotics may actually reduce colonic motility at plasma concentrations achieved clinically (Lees and Percy 1981).

This condition is also discussed in chapter 23.

Ischaemic colitis

Ischaemia of the colon has been reported as a complication of treatment with various drugs. Lambert and colleagues (1982) reported a patient who had received vasopressin for variceal haemorrhage and developed this syndrome. They felt that underlying atherosclerosis may have been a factor. Vasculitis has been associated with clindamycin therapy (Sweeny and Sheehan 1979), affecting the small vessels of the entire bowel wall. Colonic ischaemia has been attributed to treatment with cisplatin and fluorouracil for malignant disease, though the patient involved had also received radiation, another risk factor (Zilling and Ahren 1989). Ischaemic colitis has also been associated with hormonal therapy, in particular oral contraceptive steroids (Schneiderman and Cello 1986), and danazol (Miyata *et al*. 1988).

Other causes of colitis

NSAID, particularly mefenamic acid (Hall *et al*. 1983) but also fenbufen (Bunney 1989), flufenamic acid, naproxen, and ibuprofen (Ravi *et al*. 1986), have been reported to cause colitis. Penicillamine (Houghton *et al*. 1989) and gold (Kirkham *et al*. 1989) have also both been associated with colitis in patients suffering from rheumatoid arthritis.

Colitis has been reported in one patient in association with jaundice induced by methyldopa (Bonkowsky and Brisbane 1976), and Graham and co-workers (1981) have reported six cases of colitis with methyldopa which were positive on rechallenge. Martin and colleagues (1987) reported a patient in whom proctocolitis was associated with treatment with isotretinoin; they also commented on the fact that the manufacturers of this drug had data suggesting there might be other cases in which a similar association existed.

Other colonic disorders

Ulceration, bleeding, and perforation

Some authors suggest that NSAID may have precipitated a relapse of ulcerative colitis (Rampton and Sladen 1981), severe colonic bleeding (Schwartz 1981), or acute perforation of colonic diverticula (Coutrot *et al.* 1978).

Colonic cancer

The anthroquinone purgative danthron has been reported to cause tumours in animals, and a single case report has suggested such an association in an 18-year-old woman (Patel *et al.* 1989). There is also a report of colonic carcinoma after chemotherapy in a patient with Hodgkin's disease (Aggarwal *et al.* 1989).

Diarrhoea due to other causes

Diarrhoea may be due to drug effects on the small bowel, as mentioned above. It may be difficult to be precise about the particular site of action in an individual patient. Chronic diarrhoea can occur as a feature of purgative abuse (Cummings 1974), and this is particularly common in the United Kingdom where many elderly patients take purgatives regularly. Anthraquinones, such as senna, produce damage to the myenteric plexus of the large bowel in chronic use, and this may result in constipation for which the patient takes further doses of purgatives. The amount of watery diarrhoea produced by cathartics may be sufficient to cause electrolyte disturbance or weight loss.

Antacid salts, particularly magnesium, will produce osmotic diarrhoea, which is believed to be due to the presence of the poorly absorbed osmotically active compound in the gut lumen.

Digitalis overdose causes diarrhoea, and a number of other drugs acting on the cardiovascular system have been associated with diarrhoea. These include, particularly, the adrenergic-neurone blocking antihypertensives (e.g. guanethidine and debrisoquine) and, more rarely, methyldopa and β-adrenoceptor blocking agents (Bulpitt and Dollery 1973; Robinson and Burtner 1981).

Diarrhoea associated with bacterial overgrowth secondary to high-dose corticosteroids has been reported (Denison and Wallerstedt 1989). Chenodeoxycholic acid causes diarrhoea in a dose-related manner (Dowling 1977).

Diarrhoea in breast-fed infants

Single case reports associate the use of sulphasalazine or mesalazine with diarrhoea in the breast-fed infants of mothers receiving these drugs, suggesting excretion into breast milk (Branski *et al.* 1986; Nelis 1989).

Constipation

Constipation is commonly associated with drugs that delay gastrointestinal motility, such as opiates, antiparkinsonian drugs, or anticholinergics. Occasionally, this form of constipation may be particularly severe, and a case in which stercoral perforation of the bowel occurred in a patient receiving amitriptyline has been reported (Cass 1978). Faecal impaction has been caused by charcoal when used to treat a patient who had taken an amitriptyline overdose (Anderson and Ware 1987); such patients should therefore be given osmotic purgatives routinely.

Aluminium hydroxide and calcium carbonate antacids are constipating and iron salts are also a frequent cause of this complaint. Faecal impaction has been reported in an infant of low birth-weight who was given cholestyramine (Merten and Grossman 1980), and Swift and Thayer (1987) have reported a case of constipation associated with lithium in a patient who had scleroderma.

Proctitis

Proctitis is associated with the local application of irritant drugs in the form of suppositories. The NSAID indomethacin and phenylbutazone have both been reported to have caused proctitis and rectal ulceration (Cheli and Ciancamerla 1974; Levy and Gaspar 1975). Ergot suppositories have been associated with anal ulcers (Weinert and Grussenderf 1980). An unusual case of alcohol-induced proctitis, due to self-administration of whisky per rectum, was reported by Bhalotra (1988). The rare complication of rectovaginal fistula in a patient with granulocytopenia secondary to amidopyrine was reported by Garre and colleagues (1976). More recently, Hobbin and Champion (1986) reported a fistula between the vulva and the rectum associated with indomethacin suppositories, on this occasion presumably due to local damage to the rectal mucosa.

Anal burning has been associated with peppermint oil capsules (Weston 1987) and perineal irritation is well documented to occur after intravenous injection of dexamethasone (Baharav *et al.* 1986).

Pancreatitis

Although drug-induced pancreatic dysfunction is rarer than many other gastrointestinal adverse reactions, it is being increasingly recognized as a complication of treatment with a wide range of drugs. The mechanisms by which drugs produce pancreatic damage are not always clear. On occasions, however, it is obvious that a clear precipitant can be identified, as in the example of ergotamine-induced ischaemic pancreatitis reported after overdose of the drug (Deviere *et al.* 1987).

The largest group of drugs to be associated with pancreatitis are the sulphonamide antibacterials and their derivative diuretics. Block and colleagues (1970) described haemorrhagic pancreatitis associated with sulphamethizole and sulphasalazine. Many diuretics are derived from sulphonamides and pancreatitis has been associated with most of this group including chlorothiazide (Johnston and Cornish 1959; Cornish *et al.* 1961), chlorthalidone (Jones and Caldwell 1962), and frusemide (Wilson *et al.* 1967; Buchanan and Cane 1977). Drug-induced pancreatitis secondary to diuretics can be very severe and occasionally fatal (Eckhauser *et al.* 1987). Epidemiological studies suggest that thiazide diuretics are the drugs most commonly implicated in patients presenting with acute pancreatitis (Bourke *et al.* 1978; Pickleman *et al.* 1979). Kristensen and colleagues (1980) suggested that frusemide induced a rise of serum isoamylases in patients receiving the drug. This study is difficult to interpret, since frusemide could have an effect on the renal clearance of the enzyme.

The pancreatic dysfunction associated with sulphasalazine, which can be demonstrated on rechallenge (Suryapranata *et al.* 1986), was originally believed to be due to the sulphonamide component of the drug. Interestingly, more recent reports suggest that mesalazine (5-aminosalicylate), which is also used for treating ulcerative colitis, may cause pancreatitis (Deprez *et al.* 1989; Sachedina *et al.* 1989). This raises the possibility that the salicylate component of sulphasalazine was the agent responsible for pancreatic dysfunction in some of the earlier cases. Certainly, patients who are switched from sulphasalazine to a newer agent because of pancreatic dysfunction still need careful monitoring.

A number of other anti-infective agents have been associated with the pancreatitis. Pentamidine, which is structurally related to the biguanides (which have been implicated in pancreatitis in isolated cases [Bourke *et al.* 1978]), may cause diabetes, and has also been associated with acute pancreatitis (Murphy and Josephs 1981). The opportunistic infections that occur in patients suffering from AIDS have meant that pentamidine is being more

widely used. A case with potentially fatal pancreatitis was reported by Zuger and colleagues (1986) following intravenous pentamidine, and more recently Herer and colleagues (1989) reported two cases of abnormalities of serum amylase and lipase, compatible with pancreatitis, a diagnosis supported in one by CAT-scanning, associated with pentamidine administration by aerosol. Again, both patients were HIV-positive. A complicated case of pancreatitis, occurring in a patient who had undergone cadaver renal transplantation and developed *Nocardia* infection, has been described by Antonow (1986); in this patient initial administration of co-trimoxazole with subsequent rechallenge caused pancreatitis. This is perhaps not surprising in view of the fact that sulphonamides are known to cause pancreatic dysfunction. Other antibacterials associated with pancreatic dysfunction include metronidazole (in a case which was positive on a rechallenge [Celifarco *et al.* 1989]), and erythromycin, occurring at both standard therapeutic doses (Hawksworth 1989) and in overdose (Gumaste 1989). Nitrofurantoin has also been associated with pancreatitis, positive on rechallenge (Nelis 1983).

NSAID have been associated with pancreatic dysfunction. Sulindac caused pancreatitis on rechallenge (Siefkin 1980; Lilly 1981), and more recently a case has been described in which pancreatitis was associated with cholangitis in a patient who developed a high eosinophil count associated with the drug (Lerche *et al.* 1987). The authors considered that the bile duct injury was likely to have been caused by a hypersensitivity (allergic) reaction. In this patient rechallenge was positive, and the eosinophilic response was noted on more than one occasion. Haye (1986) has reported a case in which piroxicam was associated with clinical pancreatitis. A patient who developed pancreatitis while receiving mefenamic acid (van Walraven *et al.* 1982) was not rechallenged.

The anticonvulsant drugs sodium valproate and carbamazepine are also associated with pancreatic dysfunction. The evidence is far stronger with sodium valproate (Parker *et al.* 1981; CSM 1981; Ng 1982), and some deaths have been caused by this agent (Murphy and Lyon 1981; Williams *et al.* 1983). Soman and Swenson (1985) reported a case of pancreatitis induced by carbamazepine in an elderly lady of 73. They also noted that three other possible cases had been reported to the manufacturers of the drug.

The oral contraceptive pill has been associated with pancreatitis, and this is usually attributed to alteration in circulating lipids. Patients with existing hyperlipidaemias, particularly those of types IV and V in the Frederickson classification, seem to be particularly at risk. Parker (1983) has suggested that it is unlikely that patients with normal blood lipids are at risk of pancreatitis until they are aged over 40 years.

A number of cytotoxic agents used in the management of malignant disease, or as immunosuppressants, have been noted to cause pancreatic dysfunction. In one large study colaspase (asparaginase) caused acute pancreatitis in 2.5 per cent of 1400 patients treated (Greenstein *et al.* 1979), and azathioprine has also been associated with pancreatitis (Nakashima and Howard 1977). Since cytotoxic agents are often used in combination, it may be difficult to establish the true culprit. Thus, Puckett and colleagues (1982) reported a case of pancreatitis associated with a combination of cyclophosphamide, doxorubicin, and vincristine.

In two cases of pancreatitis suspected to have been caused by methyldopa (van der Heide *et al.* 1981; Ramsay *et al.* 1982) the diagnosis was supported by recurrence on rechallenge; but claims of an association between β-adrenoceptor blocking drugs and pancreatitis (Durrington and Cairns 1982) were not supported by such evidence.

It has been suggested that cimetidine prolongs the rise in serum amylase concentration when used in the management of pancreatitis, but whether this is due to increased pancreatic damage is uncertain (*British Medical Journal* 1981). A patient in whom pancreatic dysfunction was associated with taking cimetidine was reported by Nott and De Sousa (1989), but in view of its very widespread use cimetidine seems to carry a very low risk of causing pancreatic damage.

Pancreatic damage may also be a rare complication of therapy with gold, and cases associated with both intramuscular and oral administration of gold have been reported (Eisemann *et al.* 1989). Pancreatitis following administration of lovastatin, positive on rechallenge, has been reported from Germany in a patient with Gilbert's syndrome (Pluhar 1989). A case report from Canada noted overdose of amoxapine and procyclidine causing pancreatitis (Jeffries and Masson 1985). The fact that pancreatic dysfunction is associated with gallstones is relevant to the observation that the incidence of pancreatitis was increased in the treated group in the clofibrate study organized by the World Health Organization (ROCPI 1980), as clofibrate is known to cause gallstones.

More difficult is the issue of steroids and pancreatitis. Large doses of steroids have been reported to cause pancreatitis (Riemenschneider *et al.* 1968), and a high incidence of focal necrosis in the pancreas has been reported at autopsy in patients who had been treated with steroids (David *et al.* 1970). Steinberg and Lewis (1981) re-evaluated the evidence associating steroids and pancreatitis and noted that while there were many anec-

dotal reports of an association there were no consistent secretory or histological changes that could be attributed to the drugs. There were no rechallenge studies and their conclusions were that steroids probably did not cause this condition. Two-thirds of the reports identified by these authors involved children. Overall, it seems that steroids are not likely to be a significant contributory cause of pancreatitis in adults.

Peritonitis

Sclerosing peritonitis

This condition was recognized before the introduction of β-adrenergic antagonists (Meyboom 1975), but a large number of cases have been caused by treatment with one member of this group of drugs, practolol (Brown *et al.* 1974; Hensen *et al.* 1975; Dunstone and Ive 1975; Minton *et al.* 1975). There have been occasional reports of this disorder in association with treatment with other β-blockers, including oxprenolol (Kennedy and Ducrow 1977), timolol (Baxter-Smith *et al.* 1978), and metoprolol (Clark and Terris 1983); but detailed review by Castle (1985) has thrown doubt on the suggestion of a causal relationship in such cases.

Other types of peritonitis

Granulomatous peritonitis following surgery, as a result of the glove starch, is also well recognized and on occasions may be very severe, as in the case reported by Michowitz and Stavorovsky (1983), of a 52-year-old man who developed intestinal obstruction secondary to a mass of adhesions.

A case of infective peritonitis associated with methylprednisolone pulse therapy has been reported in a woman receiving this drug for rheumatoid arthritis (Oto *et al.* 1983).

Infective peritonitis may also complicate treatment of renal failure with peritoneal dialysis; it may then be fungal or bacterial.

Retroperitoneal fibrosis

This disorder is discussed in detail in Chapter 16.

Type A and Type B reactions

Most adverse effects of drugs on the gut represent Type A reactions. For other effects, for example pancreatitis, the mechanisms of the adverse reactions are not well understood and these reactions probably come into the category of Type B events.

References

Aggarwal, P., Sharma, S.K., Wali, J.P., and Sahani, P. (1989). Colonic carcinoma after chemotherapy of Hodgkin's disease. *J. Clin. Gastroenterol.* 1, 340.

Alaily , A.B. (1974). Gangrene of Meckel's diverticulum in pregnancy due to iron tablet. *Br. Med. J.* i, 103.

Al-Dujaili, M., Salole, E.G., and Florence, A.T. (1983). Drug formulation and oesophageal injury. *Adverse Drug React. Acute Poisoning Rev.* 2, 235.

Alves, M., Patel, V., Douglas, E., and Deutsch, E. (1979). Gastric infarction, a complication of selective vasopressin infusion. *Am. J. Dig. Dis.* 24, 409.

Ananth, J., Savodnik, I., and Yang, H. (1988). Lithium-associated Mallory–Weiss syndrome. *J. Clin. Psychiatry* 49, 412.

Anderson, I.M. and Ware, C. (1987). Syrup of ipecacuanha. *Br. Med. J.* 294, 578.

Antonescu, C.G. (1989). Potassium chloride and gastric outlet obstruction. *Ann. Intern. Med.* 111, 855.

Antonow, D.R. (1986). Acute pancreatitis associated with trimethoprim-sulphamethoxazole. *Ann. Intern. Med.* 104, 363.

Aselton, P.J. and Jick, H (1983). Short-term follow-up study of wax matrix potassium chloride in relation to gastrointestinal bleeding. *Lancet* i, 184.

Aziz Khan, R., Piepgrass, W., and Wilhelm, M.C. (1982). Anticoagulant-induced haematomas of the small intestine. *South. Med. J.* 75, 242.

Baharav, E., Harpaz, D., Mittelman, M., and Lewinski, U.H. (1986). Dexamethasone-induced perineal irritation. *N. Engl. J. Med.* 314, 515.

Bassoth, G., Gaburri, M., Pelli, M.A., and Morelli, A. (1987) Oesophageal pain exacerbated by propranolol. *Br. Med. J.* 294, 1655.

Baxter-Smith, D.C., Monypenny, I.J., and Dorricott, N.J. (1978). Sclerosing peritonitis in patients on timolol. *Lancet* ii, 149.

Beatson, N. (1982). Atropine and paralytic ileus. *Postgrad. Med. J.* 58, 451.

Benfield, G.F.A., Asquith, P., and Felix-Davies, D.D. (1986). Widespread gastric ulceration during auranofin therapy. *J. Rheumatol.* 13, 228.

Benn, A., Swan, C.H.J., Cooke, W.T., Blair, J.A., Matty, A.J., and Smith, M.E. (1971). Effect of intraluminal pH on the absorption of pteroylmonoglutamic acid. *Br. Med. J.* i, 148.

Benner, E.J. and Tellman, W.H. (1970). Pseudomembranous colitis as a sequel to oral lincomycin therapy. *Am. J Gastroenterol.* 54, 55.

Berchtold, P., Dahlqvist, A., Gustafson, A., and Asp, N.G. (1971). Effects of a biguanide (metformin) on vitamin B_{12} and folic acid absorption and intestinal enzyme activities. *Scand. J. Gastroenterol.* 6, 751.

Bhalotra, R. (1988). Alcohol-induced proctitis in a human. *J. Clin. Gastroenterol.* 10, 592.

Bhasin, D.K. and Singh, R. (1988). Chloroquine phosphate induced gastroduodenitis. *Gastrointest. Endosc.* 34, 488.

Block, M.B., Genant, H.K., and Kirsner, J.B. (1970). Pancreatitis as an adverse reaction to salicylazasulfapyridine. *N. Engl. J. Med.* 282, 380.

Boley, S.J., Allen, A.C., Schultz, L., and Schwartz, S. (1965). Potassium-induced lesions of the small bowel. I. Clinical aspects. *JAMA* 193, 997.

Bonkowsky, H.L. and Brisbane, J. (1976). Colitis and hepatitis caused by methyldopa. *JAMA* 236, 1602.

Bourke, J.B., McIllmurray, M.B., Mead, G.M., and Langman, M.J.S. (1978). Drug associated primary acute pancreatitis. *Lancet.* i, 706.

Branski, D., Kerem, E., Gross-Kieselstein, E., Hurvitz, H., Litt, R., and Abrabramov, A. (1986). Bloody diarrhoea — a possible complication of sulfasalazine transferred through human breast milk. *J. Pediatr. Gastroenterol. Nutr.* 5, 316.

Brennan, M.F., Clarke, A.M., and Macbeth, W.A.A.G. (1968). Infarction of the midgut associated with oral contraceptives. *N. Engl. J. Med.* 279, 1213.

British Medical Journal (1981). Non-ulcer uses of cimetidine. *Br. Med. J.* 283, 89.

Brower, R.A. (1986). Jejunal perforation possibly induced by slow-release potassium in a patient with Crohn's disease. *Dig. Dis. Sci.* 31, 1387.

Brown, P., Baddeley, H., Read, A.E., Davies, J.D., and McGarry, J. (1974). Sclerosing peritonitis, an unusual reaction to a beta-adrenergic-blocking drug (practolol). *Lancet* ii, 1477.

Brown, R.B., Rice, B.H., and Szakacs, J.E. (1959). Intestinal bleeding and perforation complicating treatment with vasoconstrictors. *Ann. Surg.* 150, 790.

Buchanan, N. and Cane, R.D. (1977). Frusemide-induced pancreatitis. *Br. Med. J.* iv, 1417.

Bulpitt, C.J. and Dollery, C.T. (1973). Side-effects of hypotensive agents evaluated by a self-administered questionnaire. *Br. Med. J.* iii, 485.

Bunney, R.G. (1989). Non-steroidal anti-inflammatory drugs and the bowel. *Lancet*, ii, 1047.

Burkitt, E.A. and Sutcliffe, C.K. (1961). Paralytic ileus after amitriptyline, *Br. Med. J.* ii, 1648.

Burruss, G.L., van Voarst, S.J., Crawford, A.J., and Bhattacharya, S.K. (1986). Small bowel obstruction from an antacid bezoar: a ranitidine antacid interaction. *South. Med. J.* 79, 917.

Cannon, S.R. (1982). Intestinal vasculitis and lithium carbonate- associated diarrhoea. *Postgrad. Med. J.* 58, 445.

Carter, B.L., Woodhead, J.C., Cole, K.S., and Milavety, G. (1987). Gastrointestinal side-effects of erythromycin preparations. *Drug Intell. Clin. Pharm.* 21, 734.

Caruso, I. and Bianchi Porro, G. (1980). Gastroscopic evaluation of anti-inflammatory agents. *Br. Med. J.* i, 75.

Cass, A.J. (1978). Stercoral perforation: case of drug-induced impaction. *Br. Med. J.* ii, 932.

Castle, W.M. (1985). Drugs and fibrotic reactions — Part I. *Adverse Drug React. Bull.* 113, 422.

Celifarco, A., Warschauer, C., and Burakoff, R. (1989). Metronidazole-induced pancreatitis. *Am. J. Gastroenterol.* 84, 958.

Chapman, C.S., Swart, S.S., and Wood, J.K. (1986). Oesophageal apoplexy associated with aspirin ingestion in polycythaemia rubra vera. *Clin. Lab. Haem.* 8, 265.

Cheli, R. and Ciancamerla, G. (1974). Proctiti emorragiche da medicamenti locali. *Minerva Gastroenterol.* 20, 56.

Chen, B., Shapira, J., Ravid, M., and Lang, R. (1982). Steatorrhoea induced by allopurinol. *Br. Med. J.* 284, 1914.

Clark, C.V. and Terris, R. (1983). Sclerosing peritonitis associated with metoprolol. *Lancet* i, 937.

Clarke, I.M.C. (1971). Adynamic ileus and amitriptyline. *Br. Med. J.* ii, 531.

Coates, A.G., Nostrant, T.T., Wilson, J.A.P., Elta, G.H., and Agha, F.P. (1986). Esophagitis caused by non-steroidal anti-inflammatory medication: case reports and reviews of the literature on pill-induced esophageal injury. *South. Med. J.* 79, 1094.

Coggon, D., Langman, M.J.S., and Speigelhalter, D. (1982). Aspirin, paracetamol, and haematemesis and melaena. *Gut* 23, 340.

Cohen, L.E., McNeill, C.J., and Wells, R.F. (1973). Clindamycin-associated colitis. *JAMA* 223, 1379.

Conn, H.O. and Poynard, T. (1984). Adrenocorticosteroid therapy and peptic ulcer disease. *N. Engl. J. Med.* 310, 201.

Cornish, A.L., McClellan, J.T., and Johnston, D.H. (1961). Effects of chlorothiazide on the pancreas. *N. Engl. J. Med.* 265, 673.

Coronato, A. and Glass, G.B.J. (1973). Depression of the intestinal uptake of radio-vitamin B_{12} by cholestyramine. *Proc. Soc. Exp. Biol. Med.* 142, 1341.

Cotton, P.B. and Lea Thomas, M. (1971). Ischaemic colitis and the contraceptive pill. *Br. Med. J.* iii, 27.

Coutrot, S., Roland, D., Barbier, J., van Der Marcq, P., Alcalay, M., and Matuchansky, C. (1978). Acute perforation of colonic diverticula associated with short-term indomethacin. *Lancet* ii, 1055.

Crowson, T.D., Head, L.H., and Ferrante, W.A. (1976). Esophageal ulcers associated with tetracycline therapy. *JAMA* 235, 2747.

CSM (Committee on Safety of Medicines) (1981). Sodium valproate (Epilim). *Current Problems No. 6.* HMSO, London.

CSM (Committee on Safety of Medicines) (1983). Osmosin (controlled-release indomethacin). *Current Problems No. 11.* HMSO, London.

CSM (Committee on Safety of Medcines) (1986). Non-steroidal anti-inflammatory drugs and serious gastrointestinal adverse reactions. *Br. Med. J.* 282, 1190.

Cummings, J.H. (1974). Laxative abuse. *Gut* 15, 758.

Dargie, H.J. and Dollery C.T. (1975). Adverse reactions to diuretic drugs. In *Meyler's side effects of drugs*, Vol. 8 (ed. M.N.G. Dukes), p. 483. Excerpta Medica, Amsterdam.

David, D.S., Grieco, M.H., and Cushman, P. (1970). Adrenal glucocorticoids after twenty years. A review of their clinically relevant consequences. *J. Chron. Dis.* 22, 637.

Davies, D.R. and Brightmore, T. (1970). Idiopathic and drug-induced ulceration of the small intestine. *Br. J. Surg.* 57, 134.

Dayton, M.T., Kleckner, S.C., and Brown, D.K. (1987). Peptic ulcer perforation associated with steroid use. *Arch. Surg.* 122, 376.

Denison, H. and Wallerstedt, S. (1989). Bacterial overgrowth after high-dose corticosteroid treatment. *Scand. J. Gastroenterol.* 24, 561.

Deprez, P., Descamps, Ch., and Fiasse, R. (1989). Pancreatitis induced by 5-aminosalicylic acid. *Lancet* ii, 445.

Deviere, J., Reuse, D., and Askenasi, R. (1987). Ischaemic pancreatitis and hepatitis secondary to ergotamine poisoning. *Clin. Gastroenterol.* 9, 350.

Dewis, P., Local, F., Anderson, D.C., and Bancewicz, J. (1982). Reversible oesophageal dysphagia and long-term ingestion of chlormethiazole. *Br. Med. J.* 284, 705.

Dobbins, W.O., Herrero, B.A., and Mansbach, C.M. (1968). Morphologic alterations associated with neomycin induced malabsorption. *Am. J. Med. Sci.* 255, 63.

Dowling, R.H. (1977). Chenodeoxycholic acid therapy of gallstones. In *Clinics in Gastroenterology, 6. Bile acids* (ed. G. Paumgartner), p. 141. W.B. Saunders, London.

Dunstone, G.H. and Ive, F.A. (1975). Sclerosing peritonitis and practolol. *Lancet* i, 275.

Durrington, P.N. and Cairns, S.A. (1982). Acute pancreatitis: a complication of beta-blockade. *Br. Med. J.* 284, 1016.

Eckhauser, M.L., Dokler, M.A., and Imbembo, A.L. (1987). Diuretic-associated pancreatitis: a collective review and illustrative cases. *Am. J. Gastroenterol.* 82, 865.

Eisemann, A.D., Becker, N.J., Miner, P.B., and Fleming, J. (1989). Pancreatitis and gold treatment of rheumatoid arthritis. *Ann. Intern. Med.* 111, 860.

Faloon, W.W., Paes, I.C., Woolfolk, D., Nankin, H., Wallace, K., and Haro, E.N. (1966). Effect of neomycin and kanamycin upon intestinal malabsorption. *Ann. N.Y. Acad. Sci.* 132, 879.

Figiel, L.S. and Figiel, S.J. (1973). Diphenoxylate hydrochloride intoxication simulating intestinal obstruction. *Am. J. Gastroenterol.* 59, 267.

Freeman, H.J. (1986). Sulindac associated. *J. Clin. Gastroenterol.* 8, 569.

Gander, D.R. and Devlin, H.B. (1963). Ileus after amitriptyline. *Br. Med. J.* i, 1160.

Garre, M., Campion, J.P., Bouget, J., and Thomas, R. (1976). Nécrose du rectum au cours d'une granulopénie due á l'amiodopyrine. *Nouv. Presse Med.* 5, 2633.

Gazes, P.C., Holmes, C.R., Moseley, V., and Pratt-Thomas, H.R. (1961). Acute haemorrhage and necrosis of the intestines associated with digitalization. *Circulation* 23, 358.

Geltner, D., Sternfield, M., Becker, S.A., and Kori, M. (1986). Gold-induced ileitis. *J. Clin. Gastroenterol.* 8, 184.

Gerson, C.D., Hepner, G.W., Browns, N., Cohen, N., Herbert, V., and Janowitz, H.D. (1972). Inhibition by diphenylhydantoin of folic acid absorption in man. *Gastroenterology* 63, 246.

Graham, C.F., Gallagher, K., and Jones, J.K. (1981). Acute colitis with methyldopa. *N. Engl. J. Med.* 304, 1044.

Greenberger, N.J., Ruppert, R.D., and Cuppage, F.E. (1967). Inhibition of intestinal iron transport induced by tetracycline. *Gastroenterology* 53, 590.

Greenstein, R., Nogeire, C., Ohnuma, T., and Greenstein, A. (1979). Management of asparaginase-induced hemorrhagic pancreatitis complicated by pseudocyst. *Cancer* 43, 718.

Greig, J.D. (1989). Oral contraceptives and intestinal ischaemia. *J. R. Coll. Gen. Pract.* 39, 76.

Grigor, R.R., Spitz, P.W., and Furst, D.E. (1987). Salicylate toxicity in elderly patients with rheumatoid arthritis. *J. Rheumatol.* 14, 60.

Gumaste, V.V. (1989). Erythromycin induced pancreatitis. *Am. J. Med.* 86, Part 1, 725.

Guss, D., Schneider, A.T., and Chigramonte, L.T. (1986). Perforated gastric ulcer in an asthmatic treated with theophylline and steroids: Case report and literature review. *Ann. Allergy* 56, 237.

Hachiya, K.A., Kobayashi, R.H., and Antonson, D.L. (1982). Candida esophagitis following antibiotic usage. *Pediatr. Infect. Dis.* 1, 168.

Hall, R.I., Petty, A.H., Cobden, I., and Lendrum, R. (1983). Enteritis and colitis associated with mefenamic acid. *Br. Med. J.* 287, 1182.

Hardison, W.G.M. and Rosenberg, I.H. (1969). The effect of neomycin on bile salt metabolism and fat digestion in man. *J. Lab. Clin. Med.* 74, 564.

Harris, A.L. (1982). Cytotoxic-therapy-induced vomiting is mediated via enkephalin pathways. *Lancet* i, 714.

Hart, R.S., Levin, B., and Gholson, C.F. (1989). Esophageal obstruction caused by sucralfate impaction. *Gastrointest. Endosc.* 35, 474.

Hawkey, C.J. (1990). Non-steroidal anti-inflammatory drugs and peptic ulcers. Facts and figures multiply, but do they add up? *Br. Med. J.* 300, 278.

Hawksworth, C.R.E. (1989). Acute pancreatitis associated with infusion of erythromycin lactobionate. *Br. Med. J.* 298, 190.

Haye, O.L. (1986). Piroxicam and pancreatitis. *Ann. Intern. Med.* 104, 895.

Heizer, W.D., Warshaw, A.L., Waldmann, T.A., and Laster, L. (1968). Protein-losing gastroenteropathy and malabsorption associated with factitious diarrhoea. *Ann. Intern. Med.* 68, 839.

Heller, S.R., Fellows, I.W., Ogilvie, A.L., and Atkinson, M. (1982). Non-steroidal anti-inflammatory drugs and benign oesophageal stricture. *Br. Med. J.* 285, 167.

Hensen, A., Rhemrev, P.E.R. and Kapteyn, J.T.L. O. (1975). Sclerosing peritonitis and practolol. *Lancet* i, 275.

Herer, B., Chinet, T., Labrune, S., Collignon, M.A., and Chretien, J. (1989). Pancreatitis associated with pentamidine by aerosol. *Br. Med. J.* 298, 605.

Hey, H., Jorgensen, F., Sorensen, K., Hasselbalch, JH., and Wamberg, T. (1982). Oesophageal transit of six commonly used tablets and capsules. *Br. Med. J.* 285, 1717.

Hobbin, E. and Champion, G. (1986). Indomethacin suppositories. *J. Am. Geriatr. Soc.* 34, 325.

Horton, E.W. (1979). Prostaglandin pharmacology. In *Topics in therapeutics 5* (ed. D.M. Davies and M.D. Rawlins), p. 3. Pitman Medical, London.

Houghton, A.D., Nadel, S., and Stringer, M.D. (1989). Penicillamine-associated total colitis. *Hepatogastroenterology* 36, 198.

Hurwitz, N. and Wade, O.L. (1969). Intensive hospital monitoring of adverse reactions to drugs. *Br. Med. J.* i, 531.

Jacobson, E.D., Prior, J.R., and Faloon, W.W. (1960). Malabsorptive syndrome induced by neomycin: morphologic alterations in the jejunal mucosa. *J. Lab. Clin Med.* 56, 245.

Janssens, J., Peeters, T.L., van Trappen, G., Tack, J., Urbain, J.L., De Roo, M., *et al.* (1990). Improvement of gastric emptying in diabetic gastroparesis by erythromycin: preliminary studies. *N. Engl. J. Med.* 322, 1028.

Jeffries, J.J. and Masson, J. (1985). Pancreatitis following overdose with amoxapine and procyclidine. *J. Psychiatry* 30, 546.

Jick, H. (1981). Effects of aspirin and acetaminophen in gastrointestinal hemorrhage. *Arch. Intern. Med.* 141, 316.

Johnston, D.H. and Cornish, A.L. (1959). Acute pancreatitis in patients receiving chlorothiazide. *JAMA* 170, 2054.

Jones, M.P. and Caldwell, J.R. (1962). Acute hemorrhagic pancreatitis associated with administration of chlorthalidone. *N. Engl. J. Med.* 267, 1029.

Juel-Jensen, B.E. (1959). Sensitivity to phenindione. Report of a case of severe diarrhoea. *Br. Med. J.* ii, 173.

Kennedy, S.C. and Ducrow, M. (1977). Fibrinous peritonitis. *Br. Med. J.* i, 1598.

Key, N.S., Emerson, P.M., Allan, N.C., Kelly, P.M.A., and Chapman, R.W.G. (1987). Oesophageal varices associated with busulphan-thioguanine combination therapy for chronic myeloid leukaemia. *Lancet* ii, 1050.

Kilpatrick, Z.M., Silverman, J.F., Betancourt, E., Faman, J., and Lawson, J.P. (1968). Vascular occlusion of the colon and oral contraceptives. *N. Engl. J. Med.* 278, 438.

Kirkham, B., Wedderburn, L., and Macfarlane, D.G. (1989). Gold-induced colitis. *Br. J. Rheumatol.* 28, 272.

Knight, K.M. and Doucet, J.H. (1987). Gastric rupture and death caused by ipecac syrup. *South. Med. J.* 80, 786.

Kristensen, B., Skov, J., and Pertslund, N. A (1980). Frusemide-induced increase in serum iso-amylases. *Br. Med. J.* ii, 978.

Kuwin, C.M. and Finland, D.M. (1961). Clinical pharmacology of the tetracycline antibiotics. *Clin. Pharm. Ther.* 2, 51.

Labadarios, D., Dickerson, J.W.T., Parke, E.B., Lucas, E. G., and Obuwa, G.H. (1978). The effects of chronic drug administration on hepatic enzyme induction and folate metabolism. *Br. J. Clin. Pharmacol.* 5, 167.

Lambert, M., de Peyer, R., and Muller, A.F. (1982). Reversible ischemic colitis after intravenous vasopressin therapy. *JAMA* 247, 666.

Langman, M.J.S. (1982). Gastrointestinal drugs. In *Side effects of drugs, Annual 6* (ed. M.N.G. Dukes), p. 315. Excerpta Medica, Amsterdam.

Lees, G.M. and Percy, W.M. (1981). Antibiotic-associated colitis: an in vitro investigation of the effects of antibiotics on intestinal motility. *Br. J. Clin. Pharmacol.* 73. 535.

Lerche, A., Vyberg, M., and Kirkegaard, E. (1987). Acute cholangitis and pancreatitis associated with sulindac (Clinoril). *Histopathology* 11, 647.

Levy, N. and Gaspar, E. (1975). Rectal bleeding and indomethacin suppositories. *Lancet* i, 577.

Lilly, E.L. (1981). Pancreatitis after administration of sulindac. *JAMA* 246, 2680.

Littman, A. (1990). Potent acid reduction and risk of enteric infection. *Lancet* i, 222.

Lofgren, R.P., Rothe, P.R., and Carlson, G.J. (1982). Jejunal perforation associated with slow release potassium chloride therapy. *South. Med. J.* 75, 1154.

McIntosh, J.H., Fung, C.S., Berry, G., and Piper, D.W. (1988). Smoking, non-steroidal anti-inflammatory drugs, and acetaminophen in gastric ulcer. *Am. J. Epidemiol.* 128, 761.

McMahon, F.G., Ryan, J.R., Akdamar, K., and Ertan, A. (1982). Upper gastrointestinal lesions after potassium chloride supplements: a controlled clinical trial. *Lancet* ii, 1059.

McNeill, D.C. (1966). Adynamic ileus and nortriptyline. *Br. Med. J.* i, 1360.

Madhok, R., MacKenzie, J.A., Lee, R.D., Bruckner, F.E., Terry, T.R., and Sturrock, R.D. (1986). Small bowel ulceration in patients receiving non-steroidal anti-inflammatory drugs for rheumatoid arthritis. *Q. J. Med.* 58, 53.

Mannes, P., Derriks, R., Moens, R., Laurent, C., and Dalcq, J.M. (1976). Multidisciplinary curative treatment for disseminated carcinoma of the breast. *Cancer Treat. Rep.* 60, 85.

Maroy, B. and Moullot, P. (1986). Oesophageal burn due to chlorazepate dipotassium (Tranxene). *Gastrointest. Endosc.* 32, 240.

Martin, P., Manley, P.N., Depew, W.T., and Blakeman, J.M. (1987). Isotretinoin-associated proctosigmoiditis. *Gastroenterology* 93, 606.

Martys, C.R. (1979). Adverse reactions to drugs in general practice. *Br. Med. J.* ii, 1194.

Merten, D.F. and Grossman, H. (1980). Intestinal obstruction associated with cholestyramine therapy. *AJR* 134, 827.

Messer, J., Reitman, D., Sacks, H.S., Smith, H. Jr, and Chalmers, T.C. (1983). Association of adrenocorticosteroid therapy and peptic-ulcer disease. *N. Engl. J. Med.* 309, 21.

Meyboom, R.H.B. (1975). Practolol and sclerosing peritonitis. *Lancet* i, 334.

Michet, C.J., Pakela, J., and Luthra, H. (1987). Auranofin-associated colitis and eosinophilia. *Mayo Clinic Proc.* 62, 142.

Michowitz, M. and Stavorovsky, M. (1983). Granulomatous peritonitis caused by glove starch. *Postgrad. Med. J.* 59, 593.

Minton, M., Newland, A., Knowles, G., and Turnbull, A. (1975). Sclerosing peritonitis and practolol. *Lancet* i, 276.

Mitchell, T.H., Stamp, T.C.B., and Jenkins, M.V. (1982). Steatorrhoea after tetracycline. *Br. Med. J.* 285, 780.

Miyata, T., Tamechika, Y., and Torisu, M. (1988). Ischaemic colitis in a 33-year-old woman on danazol treatment for endometriosis. *Am. J. Gastroenterol.* 83, 1420.

Mizrahi, s., Laor, D., Stamler, B. (1989). Intestinal ischaemia induced by cocaine abuse. *Arch. Surg.* 123, 394.

Mucklow, J.C. (1978). Plasma drug concentrations in the prevention and diagnosis of adverse drug reactions. *Adverse Drug React. Bull.* 73, 260.

Muggia, F.M. (1967). Haemorrhagic necrosis of the intestine: its occurrence with digitalis intoxication. *Am. J. Med. Sci.* 253, 263.

Murphy, S.A. and Josephs, A.S. (1981). Acute pancreatitis associated with pentamidine therapy. *Arch. Intern. Med.* 141, 56.

Murphy, M.J. and Lyon, L.W. (1981). Valproic acid associated pancreatitis in an adult. *Lancet* i, 41.

Nakashima, Y. and Howard, J.M. (1977). Drug induced acute pancreatitis. *Surg. Gynecol. Obstet.* 145, 105.

Nelis, G.F. (1983). Nitrofurantoin-induced pancreatitis: Report of a case. *Gastroenterology* 84, 1032.

Nelis, G.G. (1989). Diarrhoea due to 5-aminosalicylic acid in breast milk. *Lancet* i, 383.

Ng, J.Y.K. (1982). Acute pancreatitis and sodium valproate. *Med. J. Aust.* ii, 362.

Nimmo W. S. (1979). Gastric emptying and drug absorption. In *Drug absorption* (ed. L.F. Prescott and W.S. Nimmo), p. 11. Adis Press, Auckland.

Nothmann, B.J., Chittinand. S., and Schuster, M.M. (1973). Reversible mesenteric vascular occlusion associated with oral contraceptives. *Am. J. Dig. Dis.* 18, 361.

Nott, D.M. and De Sousa, B.A. (1989). Suspected cimetidine-induced acute pancreatitis. *Br. J. Clin. Pract.* 43, 264.

Oto, A., Oktay, A., and Sozen, T. (1983). Methylprednisolone pulse therapy and peritonitis. *Ann. Intern. Med.* 99, 282.

Paaby, P. and Nervin, E. (1966). The absorption of vitamin B_{12} during treatment with para-aminosalicyclic acid. *Acta Med. Scand.* 180, 561.

Palva, I.P., Heinivaara, O., and Mattila, M. (1966). Drug-induced malabsorption of vitamin B_{12}. 3. Interference of PAS and folic acid in the absorption of vitamin B_{12}. *Scand. J. Haematol.* 3, 149.

Palva, I.P., Salokannel, S.J., Timonen, T., and Palva, H.L.A. (1972). Drug-induced malabsorption of vitamin B_{12} during treatment with slow-release potassium chloride. *Acta Med. Scand.* 191, 335.

Panos, R.J., Tso, E., Barish, R.A., and Browne, B.J. (1986). Esophageal spasm following propranolol overdose relieved by glucagon. *Am. J. Emerg. Med.* 4, 227.

Parker, P.H., Helinek, G.L., Ghishan, F.K., and Greene, H. L., (1981). Recurrent pancreatitis induced by valproic acid: A case report and review of the literature. *Gastroenterology* 80, 826.

Parker, W.A. (1983). Estrogen-induced pancreatitis. *Clin. Pharm.* 2, 75.

Patel, P.M., Selby, P.J., Deacon, J., Chilvers, C., and McElwain, T.J. (1989). Anthraquinone laxatives and human cancer: an association in one case. *Postgrad. Med. J.* 65, 216.

Peroutka, S.J., and Snyder, S.H. (1982). Antiemetics: neurotransmitter receptor-binding predicts therapeutic actions. *Lancet* i, 658.

Pickleman J., Straus, F.H., and Paloyan, E. (1979). Pancreatitis associated with thiazide administration. *Arch. Surg.* 114, 1013.

Pluhar, W. (1989). A case of possibly lovastatin-induced pancreatitis in conjunction with Gilbert's syndrome. *Wien. Klin. Wochenschr.* 101, 551.

Pottage, A., Campbell, R.W.F., Achuff, S.C., Murray, A., Julian, D.G., and Prescott, L.F. (1978). The absorption of oral mexiletine in coronary care patients. *Eur. J. Clin. Pharmacol.* 13, 393.

Powell, R.C., Nunes, W.T., Harding, R.S., and Vacca, J.B. (1962). The influence of non-absorbable antibiotics on serum lipids and the excretion of neutral sterols and bile acids. *Am. J. Clin. Nutr.* 11, 156.

Puckett, J.B., Butler, W.M., and McFarland, J.A. (1982). Pancreatitis and cancer chemotherapy. *Ann. Intern. Med.* 97, 453.

Race, T.F., Paes, I.C., and Faloon, W.W. (1970). Intestinal malabsorption induced by oral colchicine. Comparison with neomycin and cathartic agents. *Am. J. Med. Sci.* 259, 32.

Rampton, D.S. and Sladen, G.E. (1981). Relapse of ulcerative proctocolitis during treatment with non-steroidal anti-inflammatory drugs. *Postgrad. Med. J.* 57, 297.

Ramsay, L.E., Wakefield, V.A., and Harris, E.E. (1982). Methyldopa-induced chronic pancreatitis. *Practitioner* 226, 1166.

Ravi, S., Keat, A.C., and Keat, E.C.B. (1986). Colitis caused by non-steroidal anti-inflammatory drugs. *Postgrad. Med. J.* 62, 773.

Reiner, E. and Patterson, M. (1966). The effect of neomycin on disaccharidase activity of the small bowel. *Clin. Res.* 14, 49.

Reynolds, E.H. (1968). Mental effects of anticonvulsants and folic acid metabolism. *Brain* 91, 197.

Riemenschneider, T.A., Wilson, J.E., and Vernier, R.L. (1968). Glucocorticoid-induced pancreatitis in children. *Pediatrics* 41, 428.

Robinson, J.D. and Burtner, D.E. (1981). Severe diarrhoea secondary to propranolol. *Drug Intell. Clin. Pharm.* 15, 49.

ROCPI (Report of the Committee of Principal Investigators) (1980). WHO co-operative trial on primary prevention of ischaemic heart disease using clofibrate to lower serum cholesterol: mortality follow-up. *Lancet* ii, 379.

Roe, M., Sears, A.D., and Arndt, J.H. (1972). Gold reaction panenteritis. A case report with radiodiagnostic findings. *Radiology* 104, 59.

Rose, M. and Johnson, I. (1978). Reinterpretation of the haematological effects of anticonvulsant treatment. *Lancet* i, 1349.

Sachedina, B., Saibil, F., Cohen, L.B., and Whittey, J. (1989). Acute pancreatitis due to 5-aminosalicylate. *Ann. Intern. Med.* 110, 490.

Salokannel, S.J., Palva, I.P., and Takkunen, J.T. (1970). Malabsorption of vitamin B_{12} during treatment with slow-release potassium chloride. *Acta Med. Scand.* 187, 431.

Saverymuttu, S.H., Thomas, A., Grundy, A., and Maxwell, J.P. (1986). Ileal stricturing after long-term indomethacin treatment. *Postgrad. Med. J.* 62, 967.

Schneiderman, D.J. and Cello, J.P. (1986). Intestinal ischaemia and infarction associated with oral contraceptives. *West. J. Med.* 145, 350.

Schulze-Delrieu, K. (1983). Pseudomembranous colitis and the neuromuscular actions of antibiotics. *Gastroenterology* 85, 1221.

Schwartz, H.A. (1981). Lower gastrointestinal side-effects of non-steroidal anti-inflammatory drugs. *J. Rheumatol.* 8, 952.

Seibert, D. and Al-Kawas, F. (1986). Trimethoprim–sulfamethoxazole, hiccups, and oesophageal ulcers. *Ann. Intern. Med* 105, 976.

Schneerson, J.M. and Gazzard, B.G. (1977). Reversible malabsorption syndrome caused by methyldopa. *Br. Med J.* ii, 1456.

Siefkin, A.D. (1980). Sulindac and pancreatitis. *Ann. Intern. Med.* 93, 932.

Simpson, R.W., Huang, C., and Grahame-Smith, D.G. (1978). Identification of *Clostridium difficile* as a cause of pseudomembranous colitis. *Br. Med. J.* i, 695.

Smith, W.D.F. (1987). Endoscopic removal of a pharmacobezoar of slow-release theophylline. *Br. Med. J.* 294, 125.

Soman, M. and Swenson, D. (1985). A possible case of carbamazepine-induced pancreatitis. *Drug. Intell. Clin. Pharm.* 19, 925.

Somerville, K., Faulkner, G., and Langman, M.J.S. (1986). Non-steroidal anti-inflammatory drugs and bleeding peptic ulcer. *Lancet* i, 462.

Stang, H. (1986). Pyloric stenosis revisited in St Paul. *Minn. Med.* 69, 661.

Stebbins, P.L. and Pearson, C.C. (1967). Methotrexate in treatment of psoriasis: case report of a severe reaction secondary to induced malabsorption. *Bull. Mason Clin.* 21, 20.

Steinberg, W.M. and Lewis, J.H. (1981). Steroid-induced pancreatitis: does it really exist? *Gastroenterology* 81, 799.

Steiner, A., Howard, E., and Akgun S. (1961). Effect of antibiotics on the serum cholesterol concentration of patients with atherosclerosis. *Circulation* 24, 729.

Stewart, R.B. and Cluff, L.E. (1974). Gastrointestinal manifestations of adverse drug reactions. *Am. J. Dig. Dis.* 19, 1.

Suissa, A., Parason, M., Lachter, J., and Eidelman, S. (1987). Penicillin VK-induced esophageal ulcerations. *Am. J. Gastroenterol.* 82, 482.

Suryapranata, H. and De Vries, H. (1986). Pancreatitis associated with sulphasalazine. *Br. Med. J.* 292, 732.

Sutton, D.R. and Gosnold, J.K. (1977). Oesophageal ulceration due to clindamycin. *Br. Med. J.* i, 1598.

Sweeney, E.C. and Sheehan, J.P. (1979). Clindamycin-associated colonic vasculitis. *Br. Med. J.* ii, 1188.

Swift, R.M. and Thayer, W. (1987). Increased obstipation in a patient with scleroderma following therapy with lithium. *J. Clin. Psychopharm.* 7, 358.

Telsey, A.M., Merrit, T.A., and Dixon, S.D. (1988). Cocaine exposure in a term neonate. *Clin. Pediatr.* 27, 547.

Thomas, F.B., Salaburey, D., and Greenberger, N.J. (1972). Inhibition of iron absorption by cholestyramine. *Am. J. Dig. Dis.* 17, 263.

Tomkin, G.H. (1973). Malabsorption of vitamin B_{12} in diabetic patients treated wtih phenformin: a comparison with metformin. *Br. Med. J.* iii, 673.

Tomkin G.H., Hadden, D.R., Weaver, J.A., and Montgomery, D.A.D. (1971). Vitamin B_{12} status of patients on long-term metformin therapy. *Br. Med. J.* ii, 685.

Trier, J.S. (1962). Morphologic alterations induced by methotrexate in the mucosa of the human proximal intestine. I. Serial observations by light microscopy. *Gastroenterology* 42, 297.

van der Heide, H., Ten Haaft, M.A., and Stricker, B.H. (1981). Pancreatitis caused by methyldopa. *Br. Med. J.* 282, 1930.

van Klingeren, B (1983). Penicillins, cephalosporins and tetracyclines. In *Side effects of drugs Annual 7* (ed. M.N.G. Dukes) p. 71. Excerpta Medica, Amsterdam.

van Walraven, A.A., Edels, M., and Fong, S. (1982). Pancreatitis caused by mefenamic acid. *Can. Med. Assoc. J.* 126, 894.

Wass, J.A.H., Thorner, M.O., Morris, D.V., Rees, L.H., Mason, A.S., Jones, A.E., *et al.* (1977). Long-term treatment of acromegaly with bromocriptine. *Br. Med. J.* i, 875.

Webb, D.I., Chodos, R.B., Mahar, C.Q., and Faloon, W. W. (1968). Mechanism of vitamin B_{12} malabsorption in patients receiving colchicine. *N. Engl. J. Med.* 279, 845.

Weinert, V. and Grussenderf, E.I. (1980). Anokutaner Ergotismus gangraenosus. *Hautarzt* 31, 668.

Weston, C.F. (1987). Anal burning and peppermint oil. *Postgrad. Med. J.* 63, 717.

White, C.A. and Traube, J. (1982). Ulcerating enteritis associated with flucytosine therapy. *Gastroenterology* 83, 1127.

Williams, L.H.P., Reynolds, R.P., and Emery, J.L. (1983). Pancreatitis during sodium valproate treatment. *Arch. Dis. Child.* 58, 543.

Wilson, A.E., Mehra, S.K., Gomersal, C.R., and Davies, D.M. (1967). Acute pancreatitis associated with frusemide therapy. *Lancet* i, 105.

Wingate, D.L. (1990). Potent acid reduction and risk of enteric infection. *Lancet* i, 222.

Zilling, T.L. and Ahren, B. (1989). Ischaemic pancolitis. A serious complication of chemotherapy in a previously irradiated patient. *Acta Chir. Scand.* 155, 77.

Zuger, A., Wolf, B.Z., El-Sadr, W., Simberkoff, M.S., and James, M.D. (1986). Pentamidine-associated fatal acute pancreatitis. *JAMA* 256, 2383.

Zurier, R.B., Hashim, S.A., and van Itallie, T.B. (1965). Effect of medium chain triglyceride on cholestyramine induced steatorrhoea in man. *Gastroenterology* 49, 490.

11. Hepatic disorders

M. DAVIS and R. WILLIAMS

Introduction

Most therapeutic agents are non-polar compounds that cannot readily be eliminated from the body, because they are avidly reabsorbed across renal tubular and bile-ductular epithelium. The drug-metabolising system converts these substances to polar, water-soluble derivatives that can be excreted efficiently in urine and bile. Some endogenous compounds (e.g. bilirubin and bile acids) are also handled in this way. Drug-metabolising enzymes are found in many tissues of the body, but because of its size the liver is quantitatively the most important. Reflecting this central role in drug biotransformation, the liver is a major target for adverse reactions to therapeutic agents (Benhamou 1988).

Spectrum of hepatotoxicity from drugs

The spectrum of liver lesions produced by drugs is broad and encompasses the whole range of hepatic abnormalities produced by other causes (Table 11.1). Clinically, it is convenient to classify these reactions according to whether they are:

Dose-dependent: arising in any individual who ingests a sufficient quantity of the drug.

Dose-independent: arising as a rare complication of therapeutic doses of drugs.

Drug metabolism and mechanisms of hepatotoxicity

Drug metabolism takes place in two stages. The first is Phase I metabolism, which involves the creation of a polar group by reactions such as oxidation, reduction, or demethylation. Generally these reactions lead to inacti-

TABLE 11.1
Spectrum of hepatic abnormalities from drugs

Metabolic
Interference with hepatic bilirubin uptake and
  excretion

Acute parenchymal
Hepatocellular necrosis – dose-dependent
                       – dose-independent

Fatty liver
Predominantly cholestatic lesions
Granulomatous infiltration

Chronic parenchymal
Active chronic hepatitis
Chronic cholestasis
Hepatic fibrosis and cirrhosis
Hepatic phospholipidosis and alcoholic hepatitis-like
  lesions

Biliary
Sclerosing cholangitis

Vascular
Budd–Chiari syndrome
Veno-occlusive disease
Sinusoidal lesions – dilatation
                   – peliosis hepatis
                   – perisinusoidal fibrosis
                   – non-cirrhotic portal hypertension
                   – nodular regenerative hyperplasia
                   – thrombosis of hepatic artery or
                       portal vein

Liver tumours
Benign adenomas
Focal nodular hyperplasia
Hepatocellular carcinoma
Angiosarcoma
Cholangiocarcinoma

vation of the drug. Occasionally, however, the products of Phase I reactions are more biologically active than the parent compound (e.g. the conversion of prednisone to

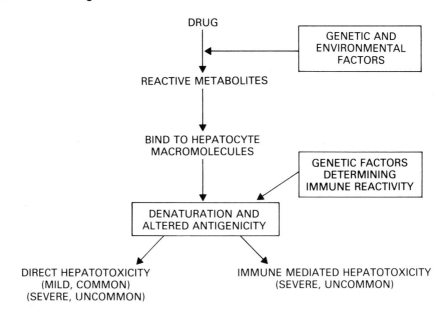

Fig. 11.1
Postulated relationship between direct toxicity and immunological mechanisms in the pathogenesis
of adverse hepatic drug reactions.

prednisolone). Some compounds are converted by such reactions to hepatotoxic derivatives, a process important in the pathogenesis of certain forms of drug-induced liver injury.

The most important site for Phase I reactions in the smooth endoplasmic reticulum of the hepatocyte, corresponding to the microsomal fraction on biochemical cell fractionation. The majority of these reactions are mediated by cytochrome P-450-containing mixed-function oxidases, so called because they catalyse the biotransformation of a wide variety of substrates. P-450 enzymes exist in multiple isoenzyme forms, with varying affinities for different substrates. There are individual variations in cytochrome P-450 isoenzyme profiles (Kalow 1987), which are probably important in determining rates of drug metabolism through different pathways.

The second stage is Phase II metabolism, which involves conjugation of the Phase I metabolite with a variety of substrates, notably glucuronide, sulphate, and glutathione. The resulting polar conjugate is then eliminated in urine or bile; the latter route assumes greater importance as the molecular weight of the conjugate increases over a threshold value of approximately 300.

As mentioned above, Phase I drug metabolism can result in the formation of hepatotoxic derivatives. Normally these products are formed in tiny quantities only and are rapidly detoxified, but if their rate of formation exceeds the liver's capacity for detoxification they will accumulate. Often liver damage is associated with the tight binding of such reactive drug metabolites to liver cell components (Fig. 11.1). This is the basis for the mechanism of hepatic damage following paracetamol overdose.

Some drugs associated with dose-independent hepatotoxicity probably also exert their deleterious effects indirectly through their metabolites (e.g. isoniazid, halothane, chlorpromazine). For these reactions, individual differences in metabolism to hepatotoxic derivatives are likely to determine susceptibility. Overt hepatotoxicity from dose-independent reactions is rare (0.1 per cent or less), but the incidence of minor hepatic dysfunction is 10 per cent or more for some drugs. The severity of liver involvement probably reflects the extent to which the drug is metabolised through hepatotoxic pathways. Both environmental and genetic factors are likely to be important in determining the balance between hepatotoxic and non-hepatotoxic pathways of drug metabolism. Thus the frequency and severity of hepatic damage from isoniazid is greater in patients treated concomitantly with the enzyme-inducing drug rifampicin (q.v.). Inherited individual differences in capacity for drug acetylation appear at least partially to determine susceptibility to liver damage from isoniazid (q.v.), whereas variations in hydroxylation capacity may be important in determining susceptibility to other reactions (e.g. perhexiline [q.v.]). These phenotypic differences probably reflect differences in cytochrome P-450 iso-enzyme profile (Kalow 1987; Oskiowska-Evers *et al.* 1987).

For some hepatic drug reactions, associated clinical and pathological abnormalities (e.g. fever, arthralgia, eosinophilia) suggest that immune mechanisms are involved in pathogenesis. There is evidence that certain reactions (e.g. hepatitis from halothane, methyldopa, or tienilic acid) are due to an immunological attack on drug metabolite-altered liver cells (Figure 11.1).

Type A or Type B? (see also Chapter 3)

Dose-dependent reactions, notably hepatocellular necrosis following overdose of paracetamol, arise as a result of exaggeration of normal properties of the drugs. These reactions can be classified as Type A.

Dose-independent reactions require the interaction of a host susceptibility factor for the reaction to appear, and these reactions can be classified as Type B.

Diagnosis and management of drug hepatotoxicity

Diagnosis of dose-dependent hepatotoxicity, notably hepatic necrosis from paracetamol overdose, is usually evident, but in occasional cases diagnosis can present a problem when a clear history of drug ingestion is not available, as for instance when a patient is admitted confused or unconscious in liver failure. Dose-independent reactions are much more difficult to pinpoint. The spectrum of histological liver injury is broad and the liver has a limited capacity to react to injurious stimuli, so the lesions produced by drugs are often indistinguishable from those due to other causes.

Diagnosis of these reactions is largely by exclusion of other causes. They are uncommon by comparison with other aetiologies, and alternative causes should always be sought, especially if symptoms develop 3 months or more after starting the drug. Underlying liver disease must be carefully excluded. A thorough history and a high index of suspicion are probably the most important aids to diagnosis.

Acute drug-induced diffuse liver damage resembles acute viral hepatitis, at times so closely that it is often impossible to differentiate it from that condition. Investigations should include serum titres of HBsAg, IgM antibodies to the hepatitis A virus, and exclusion of other causes of viral hepatitis, including hepatitis C, infectious mononucleosis, and cytomegalovirus.

Predominantly cholestatic drug-induced liver lesions have to be differentiated from other forms of obstructive jaundice, particularly extrahepatic biliary obstruction due to stones or carcinoma. This is especially true in cases involving drugs such as chlorpromazine, when recovery after withdrawal of the drug may be slow. Ultrasound and endoscopic or percutaneous cholangiography are helpful in such differentiation. Chronic drug-induced cholestasis (q.v.) can be difficult to differentiate from primary biliary cirrhosis.

Many systemic diseases are accompanied by disorders of hepatic function. These are reviewed in detail elsewhere (Holdstock *et al.* 1985). It is important to differentiate them from reactions to drugs given to treat these conditions.

Marked cholestatic jaundice may accompany severe sepsis and can also complicate the postoperative recovery of patients undergoing surgery for major trauma, who have usually received multiple blood transfusions. Differentiation from heptocellular injury is based on the demonstration of normal liver enzyme levels, although this may be difficult if there is major muscle or bone trauma, due to the lack of specificity of these enzymes for the liver (see below). Furthermore, severe prolonged hypotension can lead to hepatocellular necrosis, and patients with cardiac failure may become jaundiced, with elevations in serum transaminases from hepatic congestion as well as myocardial injury. Intrahepatic cholestasis can sometimes occur in lymphoma in the absence of mechanical obstruction, and gross elevations in hepatic alkaline phosphatase accompany diffuse infiltrative lesions of the liver, be they neoplastic, infective, or granulomatous.

Other conditions associated with abnormalities in hepatic function include inflammatory bowel disease, which is associated with a spectrum of lesions mainly involving the bile ductular system, manifested by elevations in hepatic alkaline phosphatase. Similarly, patients with rheumatoid arthritis often show such abnormalities, and other autoimmune diseases, including SLE and polyarteritis nodosa, can be complicated by liver lesions that could wrongfully be ascribed to drugs used in the treatment of these conditions.

Markedly elevated serum transaminases can occur in the first 24 hours after protracted seizures, reflecting centrilobular necrosis, presumably resulting from hypoxia (Ussery *et al.* 1989). They return to normal within 7 to 10 days and this pattern should help to distinguish hypoxic from anticonvulsant-induced liver injury.

There are no histological features specific for drug-induced liver lesions. On liver biopsy, suspicion of a hepatic drug reaction is aroused by a heavy eosinophilic infiltrate or the presence of granulomas. Marked fatty change is not usually a feature of viral hepatitis, but it can occur in drug-induced hepatitis (*The Lancet* 1974).

Identifying the agent responsible, especially if the patient is receiving several drugs, can pose problems. If alternative drugs can be used, they should be substituted. Occasionally, if no such alternative exists, it may be necessary to resort to diagnostic challenge, but this should not be undertaken lightly because it may precipitate a severe reaction. The mortality from hepatitic drug reactions that are clinically manifest (i.e. with jaundice) is approximately 10 per cent, while deaths from cholestatic reactions are less common, and challenge is safer. Diagnostic challenge should be carried out under inpatient supervision, starting with subtherapeutic doses of the drug. A patient should never be subjected to this procedure until liver function test abnormalities from the suspected reaction have returned completely to normal.

It is to be hoped that the development of techniques to demonstrate sensitization to drug-altered liver cell components in patients with some hepatic drug reactions (see Halothane hepatitis) will pave the way for the development of diagnostic tests which can be used clinically. Currently, metabolic screening (e.g. determination of hydroxylator, acetylator, or sulphoxidator status) does not provide information of sufficient specificity to differentiate drug induced liver damage from that due to other causes.

Monitoring liver function tests during drug therapy

Monitoring liver function tests in the first few weeks of therapy can give early warning of an impending reaction to some drugs (e.g. pyrazinamide, isoniazid), but is often logistically difficult under clinical conditions. It is advisable in patients taking drugs known to lead insidiously to chronic liver disease, although these tests often do not reflect the severity of hepatic disruption (e.g. methotrexate, dantrolene). Monitoring is of no value in predicting a hypersensitivity reaction. Minor abnormalities (AST ≤ twice normal) are often self-limiting and of little significance, while elevations greater than this should be taken seriously. There are pitfalls in the interpretation of abnormal liver function tests, which are outlined below.

Non-liver-specificity of transaminases and alkaline phosphatase

Although part of the battery of routine 'liver function tests', these enzymes do not measure liver function at all. They are simply markers of hepatocyte organelles or biliary ductules that leak out into the circulation in response to injury. They are found in many organs in the body, so abnormalities may reflect pathological changes other than those due to liver disease.

Aspartate aminotransferase (SGOT) is present in high concentrations in cardiac and skeletal muscle as well as liver, and damage to these organs can lead to elevated circulating levels of this enzyme. Large intramuscular injections, particularly of penicillin, are a frequently overlooked cause of this abnormality.

Alanine aminotransferase (SGPT) has the advantage of liver specificity, but many laboratories do not offer this assay. Other hepatocellular enzymes, including lactate dehydrogenase, isocitrate dehydrogenase, and ornithine carbamyl transferase, offer little diagnostic advantage clinically, either lacking specificity or sensitivity, or being difficult to measure (Price and Alberti 1985).

Alkaline phosphatase, because of its widespread distribution in the body, has poor specificity for liver disease. Gross elevations are seen in bone disorders in which osteoblastic activity is increased. Average normal values vary with age, being relatively high at puberty, then plateauing in middle age, to increase again in the elderly. Serum alkaline phosphatase activity may double in the late stages of normal pregnancy due to influx of the placental isoenzyme. Estimation of alkaline phosphatase isoenzymes or alternative biliary tract enzymes (e.g. gamma glutamyl transferase or 5-nucleotidase) can be helpful in localizing the abnormality to the liver.

Enzyme induction

A particular characteristic of gamma glutamyl transferase is its inducibility, and elevated circulating levels of this enzyme are found in patients taking enzyme-inducing agents such as rifampicin and many of the anticonvulsants (notably phenytoin, phenobarbitone, and carbamazepine). Enzyme induction may also produce modest elevations in alkaline phosphatase, and it is important to be aware of this effect, because it does not denote liver damage but rather an enhancement of hepatic metabolising capacity. It is not an indication for withdrawing a drug.

Interference by drugs with laboratory assays

Many therapeutic agents can interfere with laboratory assays of liver function tests (Sabath and Gerstein 1968; *Clinical Chemistry* 1972; Singh *et al.* 1972; Chan *et al.* 1978; Stone *et al.* 1979; Davis 1989). Such interactions are discussed further in Chapter 15.

Interference with hepatic bilirubin handling

Drugs can interfere with bilirubin metabolism at any point between its production in the reticuloendothelial system and its excretion into the bile. Depending upon the site of interference, the type of bilirubin responsible for the resulting hyperbilirubinaemia will either be unconjugated or conjugated.

Haemolysis

Drugs causing haemolysis are discussed in Chapter 22.

Interference with uptake and excretion of bilirubin

Although a number of compounds can interfere with the uptake, conjugation, and excretion of bilirubin by the hepatocyte, the only drugs of clinical significance to interact with bilirubin metabolism in this way are rifampicin and fusidic acid. Other agents having these properties, such as flavaspidic acid, are no longer used clinically. These reactions are characterized by isolated hyperbilirubinaemia, other liver function tests remaining normal.

Rifampicin

Unconjugated hyperbilirubinaemia is not uncommon during the first 1–2 weeks of therapy with rifampicin; the drug competes with bilirubin for uptake into the hepatocyte. Such an unconjugated hyperbilirubinaemia is often accompanied by a rise in the conjugated fraction, due to an interaction with the drug for excretion into the bile. These abnormalities usually clear within the first 2–3 weeks of treatment, reflecting the potent enzyme-inducing properties of rifampicin. If jaundice persists, underlying liver disease should be suspected (McConnell *et al.* 1981). This effect must be distinguished from the hepatocellular damage that can occur with combinations of rifampicin and isoniazid (see below).

Fusidic acid

This antibiotic competes with conjugated bilirubin at the biliary canaliculus for excretion into bile. Its use in patients with severe sepsis can be complicated by deep jaundice (Humble *et al.* 1980). This probably reflects an accentuation by the drug of the tendency to cholestasis produced by sepsis.

Acute dose-dependent liver disease

Analgesics

Paracetamol overdose

Overdose with the analgesic paracetamol is the most important cause of an acute toxic hepatitis in the United Kingdom, and its popularity as a means of attempted suicide is spreading to other parts of the world. Its mechanism of hepatotoxicity has been extensively studied, and this has led to the development of specific therapies. The topic will therefore be treated in detail.

Clinical features

These are now well known. The patient usually becomes nauseated and vomits in the early stages after overdose, and this is followed by a period of apparent recovery until signs of hepatic necrosis supervene, 48–72 hours after ingestion of tablets. Early loss of consciousness is not seen unless the patient has taken a mixed overdose with a sedative, or a combined preparation containing paracetamol and the narcotic analgesic propoxyphene (e.g. co-proxamol).

Hepatotoxicity almost invariably accompanies the ingestion of 15 g or more, and although the degree of liver damage produced by paracetamol is dose-related in experimental animals (Mitchell *et al.* 1973*a*), there appears to be considerable variation in susceptibility amongst humans (Davis *et al.* 1976). Individuals who abuse alcohol appear to be particularly at risk (see below).

The effects of paracetamol overdose vary widely from a trivial clinical illness with mild temporary abnormalities in liver function tests, to fulminant hepatic failure. The histological changes seen in the liver in man after paracetamol overdose are similar to those which can be produced experimentally in animals (Dixon *et al.* 1971). In less severely affected cases there is necrosis of hepatocytes in the centrilobular areas, while in those who progress to fulminant hepatic failure wide areas of confluent necrosis are seen, often with survival of only a few hepatocytes in the periportal areas. Survival after a paracetamol overdose is unlikely if more than 60 per cent of liver cells are necrotic (Portmann *et al.* 1975).

Abnormalities in the standard liver function tests are of some value in assessing the degree of hepatocellular necrosis, and the peak abnormalities in serum bilirubin and prothrombin time correlate well with the degree of hepatic damage as assessed histologically (Portmann *et al.* 1975).

Metabolism and hepatotoxicity of paracetamol

Following therapeutic doses of paracetamol, the majority of the drug is rapidly metabolised to glucuronide and sulphate conjugates, with a small proportion being converted by hepatic microsomal enzymes to an unstable and potentially hepatotoxic metabolite (Davis *et al.* 1976; Slattery and Levy 1979; Prescott 1980) (Fig. 11.2). This is probably *N*-acetyl-*p*-benzoquinoneimine (Miner and Kissinger 1979; Corcoran *et al.* 1980), and it is rapidly inactivated by conjugation with hepatic glutathione. The resulting paracetamol–glutathione conjugate is then excreted into bile and reabsorbed as the

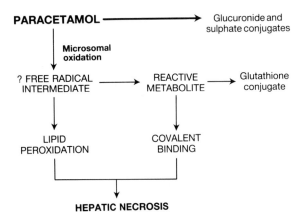

FIG. 11.2
Pathways of paracetamol metabolism
in relation to hepatotoxicity.

cysteine conjugate, after hydrolysis of the glutamyl and glycyl residues of glutathione in the gut (Grafstrom *et al.* 1979). Partial *N*-acetylation of paracetamol–cysteine in the kidney leads to the production of the *N*-acetyl-cysteine (mercapturic acid) conjugate (Jones *et al.* 1979), and following therapeutic doses of paracetamol approximately 5 per cent of the drug is excreted in the urine as these two glutathione-derived conjugates.

With increasing doses of the drug, the proportion excreted as the sulphate conjugate falls due to saturation of this metabolic pathway (Davis *et al.* 1976; Prescott 1980), and there is also evidence from clinical and experimental studies for a dose-dependent saturation of glucuronide conjugation (Davis *et al.* 1976; Hjelle and Klaassen 1984), although the relevance of the latter to human overdose has been questioned (Prescott 1983). In association with these changes there is a marked upswing in both the proportion and total quantity of the drug metabolised to the cysteine and mercapturic acid conjugates, reflecting an increased rate of formation of the reactive paracetamol metabolite. Depletion of hepatocellular glutathione occurs because hepatic synthesis of this nucleophile cannot keep pace with increased requirements for conjugation (Lauterburg and Mitchell 1981), a situation that is exacerbated by a suppression of glutathione synthesis in the first few hours after ingestion of hepatotoxic quantities of paracetamol (Lauterburg and Mitchell 1982). In consequence, the reactive paracetamol metabolite is free to bind to liver cell macro-molecules, although, as will be discussed below, the relationship between covalent binding and hepatocellular necrosis is far from clear.

Susceptibility to paracetamol overdose in man

Susceptibility to hepatotoxicity from paracetamol is governed mainly by a balance between the capacity for the formation of the reactive paracetamol metabolite and capacity for its detoxification. Alternative pathways for paracetamol metabolism (glucuronide and sulphate conjugation) are also theoretically important since they may determine how much of the drug is available for metabolic activation (Fig. 11.2).

Formation of the reactive paracetamol metabolite

Experimental studies have shown that the threshold for paracetamol hepatotoxicity is lowered by pretreatment with enzyme-inducing agents, while compounds that inhibit microsomal enzymes exert a protective effect (Mitchell *et al.* 1973a). Chronic ingestion of enzyme-inducing agents will theoretically increase susceptibility to liver damage from paracetamol. There is good evidence that this is the case for alcohol (see below) but the clinical importance of other drugs, particularly the anti-convulsants and the antibiotic rifampicin, is less certain. Phenytoin increases metabolic activation of paracetamol to its toxic derivative in man, but rifampicin does not (Bock *et al.* 1987).

Age-related differences in the metabolism of para-cetamol have been demonstrated in man (Miller *et al.* 1976; Alam *et al.* 1977), and it has been suggested that young children may be relatively resistant to para-cetamol hepatotoxicity (Peterson and Rumack 1981), although this has been disputed (Prescott 1983). The bulk of experimental evidence indicates, however, that neonatal and young animals are relatively resistant to liver damage from paracetamol. This is partly due to a relative inability of the immature mixed-function oxi-dase enzyme system to activate the drug metabolically (Hart and Timbrell 1979). It has been shown, however, that while 11-day-old rats developed less liver damage than their older counterparts, hepatic covalent binding and glutathione depletion were at least comparable and sometimes greater (Green *et al.* 1984; Green and Fischer 1984). This suggests that other factors, as yet unidenti-fied, must be important. One interesting suggestion is that covalent binding might be more diffusely distributed throughout the liver lobule in young animals. In conse-quence, the concentration of hepatotoxic metabolites in the centrilobular area would be relatively less, in spite of a similar total quantity being bound within the liver (Green and Fischer 1984). This implies that the centri-lobular localization of microsomal mixed-function oxi-dases, which produce the metabolite, might be an age-related phenomenon. Developmental changes have been observed in the distribution of another hepatic enzyme, glucose 6-phosphatase, within the liver lobule (Katz *et al.* 1976).

Constitutional factors, possibly genetically determined, may also be important in determining susceptibility. A small proportion of individuals convert an abnormally high proportion of a dose of paracetamol to glutathione-derived conjugates, implying a high rate of conversion to the toxic metabolite (Critchley *et al.* 1986). Whether such 'extensive metabolisers' of the drug are particularly at risk remains to be established.

Detoxification of the reactive paracetamol metabolite

A key factor regulating susceptibility to liver damage from paracetamol is the availability of reduced glutathione, which conjugates with and detoxifies the reactive metabolite (Mitchell *et al.* 1974). Pretreatment of experimental animals with diethylmaleate, which depletes hepatocellular glutathione, lowers the dose threshold, and potentiates paracetamol hepatotoxicity (Mitchell *et al.* 1973*b*). Starvation has a similar effect (Miller *et al.* 1986).

Synthesis of glutathione is mediated by glutathione synthetase, and there are individual variations in the activity of the enzyme. Lymphocytes from subjects deficient in glutathione synthetase are particularly susceptible to injury from paracetamol *in vitro* (Spielberg and Gordon 1984; Spielberg 1986). Whether there is a similar predisposition to hepatotoxicity is not known.

Glucuronide and sulphate conjugation

Inorganic sulphate exerts a small protective effect against paracetamol-induced liver damage in animals. This is probably because this substance increases stores of the co-factor phosphoadenosyl phosphosulphate (PAPS), and in consequence the capacity for sulphate conjugation (Slattery and Levy 1977; Galinsky *et al.* 1979). Similarly, measures to enhance glucuronide conjugation of paracetamol protect against liver damage (Hazelton *et al.* 1986). Conversely, hepatotoxicity from paracetamol is potentiated in rats by pretreating them with salicylate (Douidar *et al.* 1985). It appears that the latter drug impairs sulphate and glucuronide conjugation of paracetamol, causing more of the toxic metabolite to be formed. Gunn rats, which have a congenital deficiency of glucuronyl transferase, have increased susceptibility to liver damage from paracetamol (de Morais and Wells 1989). This suggests that humans with Gilbert's syndrome or the Crigler–Najjar syndrome might likewise be at risk, but the clinical relevance of this observation remains to be established.

Available evidence indicates that individual differences in sulphate conjugation have little impact on the metabolic activation of paracetamol (Lauterberg *et al.* 1983).

Hepatic necrosis from paracetamol in alcoholics

There is now a considerable body of clinical and experimental evidence that individuals who chronically abuse alcohol are particularly susceptible to hepatic damage from paracetamol. In such cases, doses within the therapeutic or high therapeutic range (1–6 g per day) have led to the development of centrilobular hepatic necrosis, identical to that seen after overdose (Kaysen *et al.* 1985; Black and Raucy 1986; Lesser *et al.* 1986; Rigas *et al.* 1986; Seef *et al.* 1986; Maddrey 1987*a*; Floren *et al.* 1987; Denison *et al.* 1987). In one patient, repeated episodes of toxic hepatitis led to the development of centrilobular fibrosis (O'Dell *et al.* 1986).

In experimental animals, chronic dosing with ethanol potentiates paracetamol-induced hepatic necrosis in association with increased intrahepatic binding of the reactive metabolite (Sato *et al.* 1981*a*; Carter 1987), owing to an increased rate of conversion of the drug to its hepatotoxic derivative. This is in keeping with the known stimulant effects of chronic alcohol consumption on drug metabolism (Rubin and Lieber 1968; Moldeus *et al.* 1980). Impaired detoxification of the reactive metabolite is probably also important. Chronic alcoholics have depressed circulating glutathione levels, reflecting subnormal hepatic stores of this nucleophile (Lauterburg and Velez 1988).

The possiblity of this interaction should be borne in mind when assessing abnormalities in liver function tests in alcoholics.

Hepatic necrosis from paracetamol in young children

Several reports in the paediatric literature emphasize the risks of repeated administration of compounds containing paracetamol to infants and young children, with the development of toxic levels of the drug and centrilobular hepatic necrosis. In all cases, the manufacturers' recommended dosage has been exceeded (Clark *et al.* 1983; Greene *et al.* 1983; Swetnam and Florman 1984; Smith *et al.* 1986).

Relationship between covalent binding and liver cell necrosis

Although the metabolic events leading to overproduction of the reactive paracetamol metabolite have been well characterized, there is little information on how this derivative causes liver damage. Because covalent binding and hepatic necrosis are closely correlated, it has been inferred that the two events are causally related and that liver damage is due to alkylation of vital macromolecules within the hepatocyte (Yamada 1983). Direct proof is lacking, however, and challenges to the theory have come from studies showing a dissociation between hepatic injury and covalent binding, particularly under the influence of certain protective agents (Labadarios *et al.* 1977; Devalia *et al.* 1982; Devalia and McLean 1983).

At present there is insufficient information to confirm or refute the covalent binding theory, but other potential mechanisms for liver injury must be considered.

Lipid peroxidation

There is now considerable evidence that peroxidative damage to lipids and proteins is important in the pathogenesis of liver injury from chemicals such as carbon tetrachloride and bromobenzene (Davis 1986; Clawson 1989). It has been shown that while both compounds can undergo metabolism to derivatives that bind covalently to liver cell macromolecules, hepatocyte disruption is mediated largely by lipid peroxidation (Rodgers *et al.* 1977; Casini *et al.* 1985). Furthermore, the latter process appears to be independent of covalent binding.

A number of studies have demonstrated that paracetamol can initiate such a chain of events. *In vivo*, the drug leads to increased generation of ethane, a marker of lipid peroxidation (Burk and Lane 1979; Wendel and Feuerstein 1981; Albano *et al.* 1983; Thelen and Wendel 1983), and more direct evidence for peroxidation has been obtained by spin-trapping experiments *in vitro* (Rosen *et al.* 1983). The fact that compounds such as promethazine (McLean and Nuttall 1978) and vitamin E (Walker *et al.* 1974) have been shown to protect against paracetamol-induced liver injury is additional evidence for a role for lipid peroxidation, because both are potent antioxidants and free radical scavengers.

Peroxidative damage by chemicals almost certainly arises from their metabolism by cytochrome P-450-dependent mixed function oxidases to free radicals; generation of superoxide and hydrogen peroxide during drug oxidation is well documented (Hildebrandt *et al.* 1973; Nordblom and Coon 1977). Free radicals are highly unstable and chemically reactive compounds because they contain an unpaired electron. Donation of this electron to oxygen leads to formation of highly reactive superoxide, and when a free radical comes into proximity to unsaturated lipids, as in cell membranes, it initiates a self-perpetuating peroxidative decomposition, with disruption of membrane structure and function (Slater 1984; Dormandy 1978).

Paracetamol is metabolised to a highly reactive and electrophilic free radical (Nelson *et al.* 1981), which can produce lipid peroxidation *in vitro* (Rosen *et al.* 1983; van-de-Straat *et al.* 1987) and *in vivo* in experimental animals (Wendel *et al.* 1989) (Fig. 11.2). It has been postulated that this compound is a precursor of the reactive metabolite *N*-acetyl-*p*-benzoquinoneimine (Rosen *et al.*

1983); the original theory that the latter is generated via an *N*-hydroxy metabolite has not found universal acceptance. Peroxidative damage by neutrophils, accumulating in response to hepatic necrosis, may compound hepatocellular injury (Jaeshke and Mitchell 1989).

The cell has a number of defence mechanisms for protection against lipid peroxidation (Slater 1984; Dormandy 1978).

Glutathione

Hepatic reduced glutathione plays just as vital a role in protecting against peroxidative damage as it does in detoxifying the reactive paracetamol metabolite, but its mode of action is different. In the latter situation, it acts primarily as a ligand to form a paracetamol–glutathione conjugate, and it may also function as a reducing agent to convert the reactive metabolite back to the parent compound. Its protective role against peroxidative injury is as a cofactor for the enzyme glutathione peroxidase, which reduces lipid hydroperoxides and hydrogen peroxide produced from oxygen-free radicals. As a result, glutathione becomes oxidized, and a decrease in the ratio of reduced to oxidised glutathione (GSH : GSSG) is a marker of peroxidative stress. Evidence for such a process following paracetamol has been obtained by some but not by others (Rosen *et al.* 1983; Lauterburg *et al.* 1984; Adams *et al.* 1983).

Selenium

Selenium is an important cofactor for glutathione peroxidase (Schwartz 1976), and deficiency of this element might be expected to enhance toxicity from paracetamol, as it does for other compounds producing tissue damage by lipid peroxidation (Burk *et al.* 1980). In fact, the reverse has been shown to be the case, and hepatotoxicity is attenuated in selenium-deficient animals (Devalia *et al.* 1982; Hill and Burk 1984). The reason for this apparent paradox is that selenium deficiency is associated with an increase in hepatic glutathione synthesis (Hill and Burk 1982, 1984), and this effect is presumably the overriding one.

Superoxide dismutase and catalase

Both these enzymes are important in minimizing exposure of cell components to oxidant stress. Superoxide dismutase catalyses the conversion of superoxide to hydrogen peroxide, and the latter compound is detoxified by catalase. There is little information on the role of either enzyme in modulating paracetamol-induced hepatotoxicity, although in one study increased levels of liver catalase appeared to exert a protective effect (Rosen *et al.* 1983).

Vitamin E

Deficiency of this important natural antioxidant is associated with enhanced susceptibility to liver damage from paracetamol (Walker *et al.* 1974). Interestingly, the viability of vitamin E-deficient hepatocytes is enhanced by low concentrations of paracetamol (Hill and Burk 1984). This is because the parent compound possesses antioxidant properties (Dubois *et al.* 1983).

The relative importance of covalent binding and lipid peroxidation in the pathogenesis of liver injury induced by paracetamol remains to be established and it is quite conceivable that both processes could be operative; under these circumstances they would be likely to potentiate each other. Thus, depletion of glutathione through conjugation with the reactive metabolite would diminish the efficacy of glutathione peroxidase in protecting against peroxidative damage. Conversely, the latter process would leave less reduced glutathione available for detoxification of the reactive metabolite.

Damage to cell membranes

Electron microscopic studies have demonstrated that, following exposure to paracetamol, abnormal weak areas appear in the hepatocyte membrane (Walker *et al.* 1983a,b). These are manifested *in vivo* as endocytic vacuoles, resulting from invagination of the affected areas of membrane by vascular pressure, while in isolated cells they appear as cellular protrusions. The functional significance of these and earlier changes is not known but there are two possibilities.

Disturbed calcium homoeostasis

Calcium ions are highly biologically active, and when present in excess will inhibit many processes vital for cellular viability. Although concentrations in extracellular fluid are high, the levels within the cell are low. This is due to a relative impermeability of the cell membrane to calcium coupled with an active transport system to facilitate its extrusion (Farber 1979). There is evidence that rapid influx of calcium ions accompanies covalent binding of paracetamol metabolites; this may be the event leading to cell death (Corcoran *et al.* 1988).

Hepatic sinusoidal congestion   In association with the changes in hepatocyte plasma membranes, hepatotoxic doses of paracetamol also lead to the appearance of pores in the sinusoidal epithelium, allowing the leakage of plasma and later erythrocytes (Walker *et al.* 1980; Walker *et al.* 1985). This has two important functional consequences. Firstly, in small animals up to 60 per cent of the blood volume can be transferred to the liver in the first few hours after ingestion of the drug, with resultant hypothermia and oligaemic shock (Walker *et al.* 1981).

Such a marked circulatory disturbance is not seen in man, because the liver makes a much smaller contribution to total body weight than in small animals. The second consequence, which is of potential importance to human overdose, is that sinusoidal congestion may lead to secondary hypoxic damage to liver cells, especially those in the centrilobular area where oxygen supply is normally lowest. Such abnormalities could well exacerbate toxic injury to hepatocytes caused by covalent binding or lipid peroxidation. This can be prevented by *N*-acetylcysteine (Walker *et al.* 1985).

Protective agents for paracetamol overdose

Antidotal therapy for paracetamol overdose centres around administration of agents to boost hepatic stores of glutathione, to expedite detoxification of the reactive metabolite. While glutathione itself would be the ideal antidote, it does not readily enter cells and it is of no practical value as a protective agent, because of the huge doses that are needed (Gazzard *et al.* 1974; Benedetti *et al.* 1975).

Cysteamine

This was the first antidote to be used in patients after it had been shown to protect animals against paracetamol-induced hepatic necrosis (Mitchell *et al.* 1974; Prescott *et al.* 1974). It appears to exert its effect by inhibiting formation of the reactive paracetamol metabolite (Buckpitt *et al.* 1979; Moldeus 1981; Tredger *et al.* 1981), and also possibly by converting it back to the parent compound (Harvey and Levitt 1976). A number of clinical studies have confirmed the beneficial effect of this compound when administered within 8–10 hours of overdose in man.

A disadvantage of cysteamine is that its use is associated with a high incidence of unacceptably severe gastrointestinal adverse effects, with abdominal pain, nausea, and vomiting (Douglas *et al.* 1976), and the compound is now of historical interest only.

Methionine

This is one of the agents commonly used in the treatment of paracetamol overdose. Its main mode of action appears to be via stimulation of hepatic glutathione synthesis following its conversion to cysteine (Buckpitt *et al.* 1979; Tredger *et al.* 1981). Given either orally or intravenously it appears effective in man, although it is perhaps not quite as potent a protective agent as *N*-acetylcysteine (Prescott *et al.* 1976; Vale *et al.* 1981; Prescott 1983). This is probably because methionine is generally given by mouth, and its absorption can be unpredictable in the face of nausea and vomiting, which occur early after paracetamol overdose. It has the advantage, however, of cheapness and ease of administration.

N-*acetylcysteine*

This compound is currently the treatment of choice, and its efficacy has been well demonstrated in animal studies (Piperno and Berssenbruegge 1976). It acts mainly through increasing hepatic synthesis of glutathione by acting as a source of cysteine (Lauterburg *et al.* 1983). Depletion of this amino acid, as a result of urinary losses of paracetamol–cysteine and mercapturate conjugates, becomes rate-limiting for glutathione synthesis following paracetamol overdose. The compound also reduces the reactive metabolite of paracetamol back to the parent drug (Tredger *et al.* 1981), and increases capacity for sulphate conjugation (Lin and Levy 1981; Lauterburg 1983), but the contribution of these pathways to the overall protective effect is probably small. Formation of adducts between the reactive paracetamol metabolite and *N*-acetylcysteine has been demonstrated using microsomal preparations *in vitro*, but this probably does not occur in the intact liver cell (Buckpitt *et al.* 1979; Moldeus 1981). The most likely reason for this discrepancy is that formation of these conjugates is nonenzymically mediated and proceeds less readily *in vivo* than glutathione conjugation, which is catalysed by specific glutathione S-transferases (Rollins and Buckpitt 1979). Studies using isolated hepatocytes have demonstrated that *N*-acetylcysteine may exert a hepatoprotective effect by restoring the capacity of the intracellular proteolytic system to degrade liver cell proteins denatured by paracetamol metabolites (Bruno *et al.* 1988). This provides a rationale for its use later after overdose (see below).

Agents of theoretical protective value

Cimetidine

Cimetidine is a potent inhibitor of microsomal mixed-function oxidase activity (Somogy and Gugler 1982; Knodell *et al.* 1982). The drug binds, probably by its imidazole ring, to the haem portion of cytochrome P-450 to cause both competitive and non-competitive inhibition of mono-oxygenation reactions (Rendic *et al.* 1983; Mitchell *et al.* 1984). Competitive inhibition is probably accentuated by the oxidative metabolism (sulphoxidation) that cimetidine itself undergoes (Taylor *et al.* 1978).

Cimetidine has been shown to protect against paracetamol-induced hepatic necrosis in rats given the drug 1 hour before and 6 hours after administration of the hepatotoxin (Speeg *et al.* 1983). Decreased covalent binding together with preservation of hepatic gluta-

thione levels indicate that the effect is mediated via inhibition of metabolic activation of the paracetamol (Mitchell *et al.* 1984). The mechanism is not entirely clear-cut, however: studies in mice have shown that while cimetidine inhibits covalent binding to microsomal proteins *in vitro*, it has no effect *in vivo* at doses that afford protection (Peterson *et al.* 1983). Hepatic glutathione levels were similarly unaffected. It is possible that the drug may exert a cytoprotective effect, preventing the deleterious effect of the bound metabolite. Further evidence in support of such an effect is the observation that cimetidine will still protect against paracetamol-induced hepatic necrosis if its administration is delayed for 4 hours (Mitchell *et al.* 1981; Speeg *et al.* 1983).

The dosage and route of administration of cimetidine are important determinants of its efficacy as a protective agent; at hepatotoxic doses the elimination of paracetamol is considerably slower than that of cimetidine, and to produce sustained inhibition of mixed-function oxidation more than one dose is necessary. Thus, in the two experimental studies in which the drug was found to be effective, two doses were given intraperitoneally (Peterson *et al.* 1983; Speeg *et al.* 1983), whereas a single oral dose given 30 minutes before administration of paracetamol had no effect on the development of hepatic necrosis (Leonard and Dent 1984).

Pharmacokinetic studies in humans have shown that for cimetidine to decrease the metabolic activation of paracetamol, pretreatment with the drug is necessary (Mitchell *et al.* 1984; Vendemiale *et al.* 1987). Acute dosing with cimetidine appears to have no effect on paracetamol activation (Critchley *et al.* 1983; Vendemiale *et al.* 1987).

The potential of cimetidine as a protective agent after paracetamol overdose remains to be established, although by extrapolation from animal studies, very large doses are likely to be needed. Experimental studies have shown that cimetidine and *N*-acetylcysteine exert an additive protective effect against paracetamol-induced hepatic necrosis (Speeg *et al.* 1983), and the possible role of cimetidine as an adjunct to treatment requires investigation.

The protective effect of cimetidine is related to its chemical structure, and is independent of its H_2-blocking action. The structurally similar compound metiamide is effective, whereas the chemically distinct ranitidine is not (Mitchell *et al.* 1981), except at very high doses (Speeg *et al.* 1984). This correlates with the observation that high concentrations of the latter drug inhibit oxidative drug metabolism *in vitro*, whereas low concentrations do not (Rendic *et al.* 1983). Interestingly, an experimental study has shown that while high doses of ranitidine (more than 100 mg per kg) protect, low doses (less than 50 mg per kg) actually potentiate hepatic necrosis from paracetamol in rats, with accentuation of covalent binding and glutathione depletion (Leonard et al. 1985). A possible explanation for these findings is that at low concentrations ranitidine selectively impairs glucuronide conjugation of paracetamol (Emery et al. 1985), thereby diverting more of the drug towards pathways for metabolic activation. At higher concentrations of ranitidine the drug binds sufficiently well to cytochrome P-450 to prevent oxidation of paracetamol to its hepatotoxic metabolite.

The relevance of these findings to man are not clear. Administration of ranitidine to human volunteers in a dose of 300 mg twice daily did not modify the metabolism of therapeutic doses of paracetamol, and in particular did not inhibit glucuronide conjugation (Jack et al. 1985).

Ethanol

Acute dosing with ethanol inhibits hepatic microsomal oxidation (Sato et al. 1981b). Rats given ethanol just before, or concurrently with a hepatotoxic dose of paracetamol are protected against hepatic necrosis. Covalent binding of the reactive paracetamol metabolite is inhibited, hepatic glutathione levels are preserved, and there is a decreased urinary excretion of the paracetamol–mercapturate conjugate (Sato et al. 1981a; Sato and Lieber 1981; Wong et al. 1980). All this indicates that ethanol inhibits the metabolic activation of the drug. It is possible that the common practice of taking a drug overdose with large quantities of alcohol may actually be beneficial in patients attempting suicide with paracetamol, although this could not be confirmed in a retrospective survey (R.B. Read et al. 1986).

There are no data on the use of ethanol as a protective agent in human paracetamol overdose. Critchley and colleagues (1983) administered ethanol (0.6 g per kg) to volunteers 30–60 minutes before a therapeutic dose of paracetamol, followed by hourly doses of 0.1–0.16 g per kg for 8 hours. This quantity of alcohol, which is equivalent to a total consumption (for a 70 kg man) of up to 8 pints of beer or approximately half a bottle of spirits, inhibited the urinary excretion of the paracetamol–cysteine and mercapturate conjugates, and by inference the production of the reactive metabolite.

Propylthiouracil

Oxidative drug metabolism decreases in hypothyroidism (Kato and Takahashi 1968) and hepatic levels of glutathione increase (Vuopio et al. 1970). Both these events should diminish hepatotoxicity from paracetamol and, indeed, pretreatment of rats with propylthiouracil exerts a protective effect (Linscheer et al. 1980; Raheja et al. 1987). Propylthiouracil, however, affords greater protection than thyroidectomy, despite comparable degrees of hypothyroidism. Furthermore the drug remains effective even if hypothyroidism is reversed by administration of thyroxine (Raheja et al. 1982) suggesting a mode of action independent of its effect on thyroid function. Current evidence suggests that it acts by conjugating with the reactive paracetamol metabolite, thereby acting as a surrogate glutathione (Yamada and Kaplowitz 1980; Yamada et al. 1979). It will protect against paracetamol-induced hepatic necrosis in animals pretreated with diethylmaleate to deplete hepatic glutathione stores (Raheja et al. 1983).

There is no information on the use of propylthiouracil in patients, but because of its different mode of action it has potential as an adjunct to treatment. More needs to be known about the efficacy of acute administration of the drug. In experimental studies so far, animals have been treated with propylthiouracil prior to dosing with paracetamol, a design which has little relevance to the clinical situation.

Miscellaneous compounds

Dimercaprol (Hughes et al. 1977) and penicillamine (Prescott et al. 1976) have both been tried in patients but found to be of little value, despite their theoretical potential as sulphydryl-group-containing compounds.

Mercaptopropionyl glycine has been shown to protect mice against hepatic necrosis from paracetamol (Labadarios et al. 1976). Interestingly, it has little effect on covalent binding of the reactive metabolite, suggesting that it may protect liver cells from the deleterious effects of such binding. There is no information on the use of the compound in man.

The antioxidant α-tocopherol (Vitamin E) has been shown to exert a weak protective effect in rats (Walker et al. 1974). Ascorbic acid inhibits covalent binding of the paracetamol metabolite to hepatic microsomes *in vitro* (Lake et al. 1981; Miller and Jollow 1984) and exerts a protective effect in mice in vivo (Raghuram et al. 1978). It is thought to act by converting the reactive metabolite back to the parent drug.

Clinical use of protective agents

A high proportion of patients presenting after a paracetamol overdose will not have absorbed enough of the drug to put them at risk, but a history is unreliable and the prognosis cannot be predicted from clinical features, because the onset of liver damage is delayed. A useful guide to the outcome can be obtained from an estimate of the plasma concentration of the parent drug at a known time after the overdose, and this has formed the basis for selection of patients for treatment with protective agents (Prescott *et al.* 1971; Gazzard *et al.* 1977). If the patient's plasma paracetamol concentration is plotted against time on a semilogarithmic graph, significant liver damage is likely if levels fall above a line joining a value of 200 mg per litre at 4 hours and 30 mg per litre at 15 hours after ingestion of tablets. In contrast, significant hepatic damage will not occur in patients with levels falling beneath this 'treatment line', and protective agents can safely be withheld. Plasma levels taken within 4 hours of overdose are unreliable because of continuing drug absorption. It is important that an appropriate analytical technique is used to measure paracetamol; older methods involving hydrolysis to *p*-aminophenol measure paracetamol conjugates as well as the parent drug.

Of practical importance is the fact that many patients do not present to hospital until 6–8 hours after overdose, when the potential efficacy of protective agents is beginning to diminish. Delay in administration of protective agents has been shown to be the single most important factor contributing to mortality from paracetamol overdose (Canalese *et al.* 1981; R.B. Read *et al.* 1986), so treatment should be started without delay; it can subsequently be withdrawn if the patient is shown not to be at risk (Table 11.2). Because of the expense of *N*-acetylcysteine, a reasonable compromise is to use the cheaper

TABLE 11.2
Dosage schedules for methionine and N-*acetylcysteine*

Methionine	2.5g orally 4 hourly for 16 hours
N-*acetylcysteine*	*intravenously:* 150 mg per kg in 5% dextrose over 15 minutes Followed by 50 mg per kg in 5% dextrose over 4 hours Followed by 100 mg per kg in 5% dextrose over 16 hours *orally* Loading dose of 140 mg per kg Followed by 70 mg per kg 4-hourly for 68 hours (total of 17 doses)

methionine for initial treatment and to substitute the former drug in patients requiring continuing therapy.

In the United Kingdom *N*-acetylcysteine is given intravenously, and has been shown to be effective if administered within 10–15 hours after overdose (Prescott *et al.* 1979). In the USA the drug is often given orally (Rumack 1981; Miller and Rumack 1983; Smilkstein *et al.* 1988), but it may be less effective by this route because vomiting may impair absorption.

Since its introduction as a protective agent in 1979, occasional adverse effects of *N*-acetylcysteine have been reported (Mant *et al.* 1984; Bateman *et al.* 1984). The commonest of these has been an urticarial rash, with occasional angioedema, bronchospasm, and hypotension. Reactions usually start 20–60 minutes after starting the infusion and are readily controlled by stopping the drug and giving symptomatic treatment with antihistamines. Similar but more severe reactions, which can be fatal, have accompanied accidental overdose with the compound as a result of incorrect calculations of the dosage.

The conventionally held view is that protective agents are only effective in preventing liver disease from paracetamol if given within the first 10–15 hours after overdose. This correlates with the results of experimental studies showing little efficacy once paracetamol metabolites have become covalently bound within the liver. A recent study has shown, however, that *N*-acetylcysteine can be beneficial even if administration is delayed for between 15–30 hours after overdose, with a lower mortality and a lower rate of progression to Grade III and IV encephalopathy (Harrison *et al.* 1990).

Salicylates

Elevations in serum transaminases have been reported in up to two-thirds of patients receiving high doses of salicylates for connective tissue disorders (Seaman *et al.* 1974; Prescott 1980). Patients with systemic lupus erythematosus appear especially susceptible to this complication, but it may also occur in individuals without underlying autoimmune disease (Garber *et al.* 1973). Most patients are young and females are affected more than males. Recovery is prompt if the drug is stopped, and clinically most patients are asymptomatic.

Hepatotoxicity from salicylates is dose-related and not seen unless the daily dose exceeds 2 g. Abnormalities in liver function tests correlate with plasma concentrations of the drug (Miller and Weissman 1976). Hepatic damage is not generally observed until levels are sustained at 250 mg per litre or over.

High doses of salicylates induce abnormalities in liver function in rabbits (Janota *et al.* 1960), and the drug exerts a dose-dependent toxicity on isolated hepatocytes at concentrations within the therapeutic range (Tolman *et al.* 1978).

Acute dose-independent liver disease

Anaesthetic agents

Halothane

In 1969, Klatskin and Kimberg reported the case of an anaesthetist with a previous history of asthma and hay fever who developed hepatitis seven times in 5 years. Each relapse coincided with his return to work and re-exposure to halothane, being acute in onset and heralded by fever, rigors, myalgia, nausea, and headache. Serial liver biopsies documented the development of postnecrotic cirrhosis. Because the nature of the patient's work made it imperative to know whether or not he was sensitive to halothane, he was deliberately given a subanaesthetic dose of the agent. Four hours later he developed myalgias and rigors, and biochemical signs of liver damage, with biopsy confirmation, were present 24 hours after exposure.

This and other similar reports of hepatitis resulting from occupational exposure to halothane (Belfrage *et al.* 1966; Klion *et al.* 1969; Johnston and Mendelsohn 1971; Keiding *et al.* 1984) leave little doubt that hepatitis can at least sometimes follow inhalation of this anaesthetic. There are numerous reports in the literature of liver damage in patients following anaesthesia (Neuberger and Williams 1984).

The clinical course is characteristic (Neuberger and Williams 1984). Sometimes the reaction begins with fever, and unexplained postoperative pyrexia may have been recorded after previous anaesthetics (Klatskin 1968; Trey *et al.* 1968; Reed and Williams 1972). This phenomenon has been interpreted as indicating sensitization to halothane, but it may occur after anaesthesia with other agents (Dykes 1971). Eosinophilia is seen in a variable proportion of cases (Barbior and Trey 1970; Reed and Williams 1972) and the transient appearance of microsomal antibodies occurs more frequently than in acute viral hepatitis (Williams *et al.* 1975; Walton *et al.* 1976). Obese females seem particularly prone to develop hepatitis after halothane anaesthesia and, in the series of Carney and Van Dyke (1972), 46 per cent of all patients gave a history of previous allergy.

A number of retrospective surveys of postoperative jaundice, including those by Mushin and others (1971), Inman and Mushin (1974), and the National Halothane Study (1966) in America, have shown that the majority of patients who developed jaundice after halothane had received the agent more than once within a period of 28 days. Furthermore, Inman and Mushin (1974) showed that the interval between exposure to halothane and development of jaundice was significantly shorter in patients who had had more than one halothane anaesthetic than in those who had been exposed just once.

Both minor and major hepatic dysfunction may occur after halothane exposure (Benjamin *et al.* 1985). The former, manifested by minor abnormalities in serum transaminases detected by screening otherwise asymptomatic patients, may be seen in up to 20 per cent of patients repeatedly anaesthetised with the agent (Wright *et al.* 1975; Trowell *et al.* 1975). Severe liver damage is so rare that accurate estimates of its frequency cannot be made; the incidence probably lies within 1 in 22 000 and 1 in 35 000 halothane anaesthetics (National Halothane Study 1966).

Traditionally, it is believed that children do not develop this complication, but there are a few well documented cases in the world literature (Kenna *et al.* 1987). In contrast to the adult cases, however, the number of reports implicating children is extremely small (Weis and Engelhardt 1989).

Although severe halothane hepatitis is extremely rare, the effects are devastating, and because of the clear association between this complication and repeated anaesthesia, particularly within a short period of time, it is generally considered that repeated administration of this agent to adults within 4 weeks constitutes malpractice (Weis and Engelhardt 1989). The Committee on Safety of Medicines strongly advised that the interval be extended to 6 months (CSM 1986). As with many other aspects of this syndrome, these recommendations attracted a good deal of controversy (Adams 1986; Rosen 1987; Mayhew 1987), and the relative risks of anaesthesia with other agents have been pointed out (Weis and Engelhardt 1989). Many anaesthetists now do not use halothane at all in adults, although the situation in children, who are clearly much less at risk, is less clear-cut.

Mechanisms

Direct toxicity Evidence that halothane might have the potential to produce direct hepatotoxicity comes from the studies of Cohen (1969) and subsequently others (van Dyke and Wood 1973; van Dyke and Gandolfi 1974; van Dyke and Wood 1975; Wood *et al.* 1986), who demonstrated that, following administration of radio-labelled halothane to rats and mice, a small amount of the drug could be found covalently bound to hepatocyte macromolecules. Pretreatment with enzyme-inducing agents increased the binding, which was mainly to microsomes, whereas enzyme inhibitors had the reverse effect. This indicated that the effect was due to an unstable metabolite produced by microsomal mixed-function oxidases, which reacted with cell constituents at its site of production.

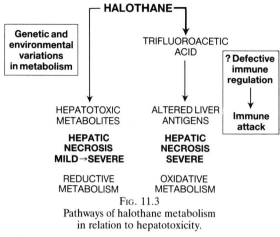

FIG. 11.3
Pathways of halothane metabolism
in relation to hepatotoxicity.

Chemically reactive metabolites of halothane are produced by two distinct metabolic pathways depending on the ambient oxygen concentration (Widger *et al.* 1976) (Fig. 11.3). It has been suggested that the compound produced by the oxidative pathway is a chemically reactive intermediate of the main halothane metabolite, trifluoroacetic acid (Brown and Sipes 1977), whereas the reductive pathway of halothane metabolism appears to involve removal of one of the fluorine atoms with the formation of a reactive difluoro intermediate. In keeping with this observation, Widger and others (1976) were able to demonstrate a rise in the plasma concentration of inorganic fluoride in rats anaesthetized with halothane in a hypoxic environment.

The potential importance of microsomal binding by halothane metabolites in the pathogenesis of liver injury has been demonstrated in animal models of halothane hepatitis. Brown and Sipes (1977) demonstrated centrilobular necrosis in rats pretreated with phenobarbitone 24 hours after halothane anaesthesia in a hypoxic environment. In this model, the specific involvement of reactive metabolites produced via the reductive pathway could be demonstrated by the failure of the drug to produce hepatic damage when given under high oxygen tensions (Jee *et al.* 1980).

The environmental manipulations required to produce this effect were more extreme than those encountered in clinical practice. Nevertheless, it has been shown that halothane undergoes reductive metabolism in man, albeit to a small degree, under normal oxygen tensions (Sharp *et al.* 1979).

Another animal model of halothane hepatitis, in which centrilobular necrosis can be induced by administration of 1% halothane in air for 2 hours to rats pretreated with tri-iodothyronine, adds a new dimension to controversy over the mechanisms of halothane hepato-toxicity (Uetrecht *et al.* 1983). Neither oxidative nor reductive metabolism appear to be involved in the pathogenesis of this lesion; circulating fluoride levels were not elevated, suggesting that reductive metabolism of the drug was not occurring, and inhibition of oxidative metabolism by deuteration of the molecule had no effect on the hepatotoxic potential of halothane in this model. Inhibition of drug metabolism prevents hepatotoxicity in the hypoxia model, but has no effect in the T_3 model (Smith *et al.* 1988). The underlying mechanisms are unknown, but hypoxia could be involved. There is an analagous model of alcohol toxicity in the rat, in which chronic administration of alcohol induces a hypermetabolic state in hepatocytes with increased requirement for oxygen. Induction of hyperthyroidism, which accentuates this, leads to centrilobular necrosis, possibly because oxygen demand exceeds supply in the relatively under-oxygenated centrilobular hepatocytes (Israel *et al.* 1975). The relevance of the hyperthyroid-rat model of halothane hepatotoxicity to humans is obscure; there is no evidence that hyperthyroid patients are particularly susceptible to liver damage from halothane or other halogenated anaesthetics (Seino *et al.* 1986), although all the thyrotoxic patients were on treatment for this condition when they underwent surgery.

Immunological mechanisms A high proportion of patients with halothane hepatitis have a circulating antibody reacting specifically with the hepatocyte surface membrane antigens of rabbits pretreated with halothane but not of control rabbits (Vergani *et al.* 1980; Kenna *et al.* 1984*a,b*). The demonstration in these patients of an antibody reacting with an altered antigenic determinant on rabbit hepatocytes indicated that a very similar, if not identical, determinant is generated in their own livers. The antibody is specific for severe halothane-associated hepatitis, and is not found in patients with postoperative viral hepatitis (Neuberger *et al.* 1982) or in patients with minor abnormalities only in liver function after halothane anaesthesia.

The altered antigenic determinant in these studies is generated by oxidative halothane metabolism (Neuberger *et al.* 1981; Kenna *et al.* 1984*a,b*); in contrast is the reductive pathway involved in direct toxicity from the drug (Fig. 11.3). The halothane metabolite responsible for antigenic alteration could be trifluoroacetic acid (Hubbard *et al.* 1988; Bird and Williams 1989).

Lastly there is the question of whether halothane acts by direct toxicity or by immunological mechanisms. Of patients with severe hepatic necrosis from halothane 20–30 per cent have no clinical or laboratory manifestations of hypersensitivity (Weis and Engelhardt 1989) and it is possible that these cases are due to an extreme case of overproduction of hepatotoxic reductive halothane metabolites (Fig. 11.3). Studies demonstrating wide variations in the binding of reductive halothane metabolites in liver biopsies taken from patients at the end of anaesthesia, support the concept that individual differences do exist for the metabolism of the drug to reactive derivatives (Sipes 1981).

In individuals in whom sensitization to halothane altered liver components has been demonstrated, variations in immune responsiveness, which are largely genetically determined, are probably the most important factor in determining susceptibility. It is probable that all subjects exposed to the drug produce altered hepatocyte membrane determinants but only a small minority react to them (Neuberger and Kenna 1988). The fact that many patients with this syndrome have circulating antibodies directed against other organs in the body (Walton et al. 1976), strongly suggests an underlying defect in immune regulation (Neuberger and Davis 1983).

Other factors, as yet unidentified, may also be important. Farrell and colleagues (1985) found that lymphocytes from patients with severe halothane hepatitis were uniquely susceptible to destruction by epoxide phenytoin metabolites generated in vitro in a rat hepatic microsomal system. Several family members of these individuals showed a similar abnormality. The identity of the factor, which could not be attributed to halothane anaesthesia per se, or to liver disease, remains quite unknown.

Isoflurane

Although a hepatotoxic potential for this drug has been demonstrated in rats (van Dyke 1982), there is little evidence that it causes liver damage in man. Metabolism in humans is extremely limited (Holaday et al. 1975). An expert committee (Stoelting 1987; Stoelting et al. 1987) reviewed 45 cases of suspected isoflurane hepatitis but could not positively exclude alternative aetiologies in any of them.

Enflurane

This anaesthetic agent undergoes minimal metabolism in man (Chase et al 1971) A review of 24 cases of suspected enflurane hepatitis suggested that the drug probably has a limited potential to produce hepatotoxicity with centrilobular hepatocyte necrosis (Lewis et al. 1983a; Eger et al. 1986), although it has been shown to be hepatotoxic in the rat T_3 model (Berman et al. 1983). It may, however, produce altered liver antigens that are recognized by antibodies from patients with previous halothane hepatitis (Christ et al. 1988; Hubbard et al.

1988). This suggests that changing from halothane to enflurane in susceptible individuals may not protect against the development of hepatic necrosis.

Antituberculous drugs

All of these compounds, with the exception of streptomycin (Sherlock 1972) and possibly ethambutol, cycloserine, and capreomycin (Segarra et al. 1968; Citron 1972), are liable to produce liver damage, although the spectrum of hepatic dysfunction is broad, ranging from slight elevations of serum aspartate aminotransferase in otherwise asymptomatic patients to severe hepatocellular necrosis.

Isoniazid

Asymptomatic elevation of serum alanine aminotransferase (SGOT) has been shown to occur in 10 to 20 per cent of patients receiving chemoprophylaxis with isoniazid (Smith and Scharer 1969; Kester 1971; AHCILD 1971; Byrd et al. 1972). These abnormalities generally appear within the first 2 months of therapy, and often revert spontaneously to normal despite continuing the drug (Bailey et al. 1973, 1974; Beaudry et al. 1974). In contrast, clinically overt hepatitis with jaundice is much less common in patients taking this drug, with an estimated incidence of about 0.1 per cent (Garibaldi et al. 1972; Maddrey and Boitnott 1973). The features of the illness are often indistinguishable from those of viral hepatitis (Garibaldi et al. 1972; Moss et al. 1972; Maddrey and Boitnott 1973), and manifestations of hypersensitivity, such as fever, arthralgia, rashes, and eosinophilia, are infrequent (Mitchell et al. 1976b). Most reported cases of florid isoniazid-related hepatitis have developed within the first 3 months of starting treatment, although there are a few well-documented cases in the literature of hepatitis developing at 4 and 5 months (Maddrey and Boitnott 1973). Black and others (1975) observed that the severity of hepatic damage was greater and the prognosis worse in patients developing symptoms within 2 months. While challenge with the drug may evoke a prompt relapse of the illness (Haber and Osborne 1959; Adriany 1960; Maddrey and Boitnott 1973), in other cases symptoms may reappear only after prolonged re-exposure (Maddrey and Boitnott 1973; Black et al. 1975).

A number of studies have shown that susceptibility to isoniazid-induced liver damage is age-related, being uncommon under the age of 35. The risks steadily increase thereafter to reach a peak between 50–65 years, with a decline in older patients (Black et al. 1975; Comstock and Edwards 1975; Riska 1976; Farer et al. 1977). In a more recent study, however, 40 per cent of deaths from isoniazid hepatotoxicity were in patients under the age of 35 (Moulding *et al.* 1989).

A combination of rifampicin and isoniazid is particularly prone to produce hepatic damage (Tsagaropoulou-Stinga *et al.* 1985). Lees and others (1971) found disturbed hepatic function in 35 per cent of cases receiving rifampicin and isoniazid, an incidence more than three times higher than in those on rifampicin and ethambutol.

Mechanisms

Isoniazid hepatotoxicity and the genetic and environmental factors that may predispose to it have been the subject of numerous studies over the past 15 years.

The initial and rate-limiting step in the detoxification of isoniazid involves acetylation of the molecule (Peters *et al.* 1965) with subsequent hydrolysis with the liberation of isonicotinic acid and acetylhydrazine. This derivative subsequently undergoes further acetylation to diacetylhydrazine (Fig. 11.4). Hepatotoxicity is mediated via a highly chemically reactive hydrazine metabolite of isoniazid which early studies suggested was derived exclusively from acetylhydrazine (Mitchell and Jollow 1975; Nelson *et al.* 1976). Since the rate of acetylation of isoniazid is genetically determined (Evans *et al.* 1960), it was proposed that individuals with the rapid acetylator phenotype would be more at risk from developing liver damage from the drug (Mitchell and Jollow 1975; Timbrell 1983; Woodward and Timbrell 1984), since a greater proportion of the drug would be available for conversion to the toxic metabolite. Some epidemiological studies (Mitchell *et al.* 1975; Yamamoto *et al.* 1986) suggested that this might be the case, but others could not confirm this, showing either no difference in prevalence between fast and slow acetylators (Riska

1976; Dickinson *et al.* 1977) or an increased prevalence amongst slow acetylators (Lal *et al.* 1972). Furthermore, pharmacokinetic studies in rapid acetylators showed that while they converted a greater proportion of isoniazid to acetylhydrazine, any propensity for accumulation of this potentially hepatotoxic precursor was offset by an increased rate of detoxification by conversion to diacetyl-isoniazid (Timbrell *et al.* 1978).

It was subsequently shown that acetylation of isoniazid was not a prerequisite for formation of a hydrazine derivative and that this could be produced from the parent molecule (Lauterberg *et al.* 1985), shifting the emphasis from rapid to slow acetylation status as being an important predisposing factor to liver damage from the drug. Thus a study of 3000 South Indian patients revealed a 1.4 per cent incidence of liver damage (clinical and subclinical) in slow, compared with 0.5 per cent in fast, acetylators (Gurumurthy *et al.* 1984). Circulating levels of free hydrazine are higher in slow than in fast acetylators (Beever *et al.* 1982).

Other factors are undoubtedly important in determining the incidence of hepatic reactions from isoniazid and probably the most important is concomitant therapy with rifampicin, which is a potent enzyme-inducing agent. This drug can stimulate the rate of hydrazine formation by microsomal oxidases from both isoniazid and acetylisoniazid. Pharmacokinetic and epidemiological studies suggest that the former pathway (i.e. conversion of isoniazid to hydrazine) via stimulation of the microsomal enzyme isoniazid hydroxylase, is the more important (Sarma *et al.* 1986; Gangadharam 1986). The incidence of hepatic dysfunction in both slow and fast acetylators of isoniazid receiving this drug in combination with rifampicin was approximately 3.5 per cent, in contrast with frequencies of 1.4 per cent and 0.5 per cent in slow and fast acetylators, respectively, receiving isoniazid alone (Gurumurthy *et al.* 1984). Pharmacokinetic studies indicate that rifampicin potentiates isoniazid toxicity by increasing conversion of the parent drug to a hydrazine derivative (Gangadharam 1986).

Other antituberculous drugs

Hypersensitivity reactions to sodium aminosalicylate (PAS) with fever, rashes, and lymphadenopathy occur in up to 5 per cent of patients receiving this drug (Simpson and Walker 1960), and in 40 per cent of these cases serum alanine aminotransferase (SGOT) becomes elevated (Smith and Springett 1966). If the drug is not withdrawn at an early stage in the reaction, a florid hepatitis may occur which has a reported mortality of 21 per cent (Simpson and Walker 1960). In contrast, such allergic manifestations are less commonly associated with hepa-

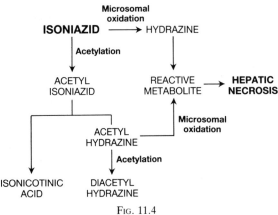

Fig. 11.4
Pathways of isoniazid metabolism
in relation to hepatoxicity

titis ascribed to ethionamide (Moulding and Goldstein 1962; Conn *et al.* 1964), pyrazinamide (Citron 1972), and rifampicin (Scheuer *et al.* 1974). Isoniazid and PAS are, however, commonly used together in the treatment of tuberculosis and it is often difficult to decide which, if either, of the two drugs to incriminate. Similarly, pyrazinamide and ethionamide are almost invariably used in combination with other antituberculous agents, which makes the 5–10 per cent incidence (Citron 1972) of overt and subclinical hepatitis reported for both of these drugs very difficult to interpret. In one large clinical trial, however, an 8 per cent incidence of abnormal liver function tests was noted on routine monitoring in patients receiving a combination of streptomycin, isoniazid, and pyrazinamide, but in no case did this occur when *p*-aminosalicylic acid was substituted for the latter drug (Girling 1978).

Hepatic reactions to pyrazinamide appear to be dose-related, with a 60 per cent incidence in patients taking 60 mg per kg daily (Fouquet *et al.* 1965), compared with 2 per cent receiving 20–40 mg per kg (East African/British Medical Research Council 1973). This drug, even in the lower doses now used, however, may produce hepatitis (Stricker and Spoelstra 1985).

Present evidence suggests that the combination of rifampicin and ethambutol has a low incidence of hepatotoxicity (Girling 1978).

Cross-hepatotoxicity may occur between drugs which are chemically related, as are isoniazid, pyrazinamide, and ethionamide (Weinstein and Hallet 1962; Phillips and Tashman 1963), and all of these agents should be avoided if a reaction occurs to one of them.

Antidepressants

Tricyclic and tetracyclic antidepressants

Whilst clinically manifest liver damage from tricyclic antidepressants is rare, more minor degrees of hepatic dysfunction, manifested by abnormalities in biochemical liver function tests in otherwise asymptomatic patients, are much more common (Pessayre and Larrey 1988). These abnormalities are often transient. Estimates of the incidence of this complication vary widely; figures of 0.08–10 per cent have been cited for amitriptyline (Dreyfus *et al.* 1989), while for imipramine and desipramine the estimated incidence varies between 0–24.7 per cent and 0–8.7 per cent respectively (Anderson and Kristiansen 1959; Kramp 1969; Price *et al.* 1984; Hoge and Biederman 1987).

Precise estimates of the incidence of severe hepatic damage from tricyclic antidepressants are difficult to obtain. A figure of 0.5–1 per cent is widely quoted, based on a paper published in 1965 (Klerman and Cole 1965); the true incidence is probably much lower. As might be predicted from their close structural similarities, cross-hepatotoxic reactions between different members of the group can occur (Klerman and Cole 1965; Kennedy 1983; Geneve *et al.* 1987).

Amitriptyline

Both acute hepatic necrosis and a predominantly cholestatic lesion have been reported with this drug (Anderson and Henrikson 1978; Dana *et al.* 1984; Geneve *et al.* 1987). Daily doses of the drug have ranged between 25–150 mg, with onset 25 days to 10 months after starting therapy. Prominent pyrexia and eosinophilia have been present in some cases. A prolonged cholestatic illness, initially associated with eosinophilia, has also been reported as a complication of amitriptyline therapy (Larrey *et al.* 1988*a*). The lesion resolved slowly over a 2-year period after discontinuing the drug.

Imipramine

Imipramine can produce acute hepatitis, often with a pronounced cholestatic component (Short *et al.* 1968; Weaver *et al.* 1977; Moskovitz *et al.* 1982;). As with amitriptyline, high fever and eosinophilia were often present. Chronic cholestasis with hepatic fibrosis has also been described (Horst *et al.* 1980).

Desipramine

This drug is the demethylated derivative of imipramine, to which the latter is metabolised *in vivo*. It has been implicated in the pathogenesis of acute hepatic necrosis in three reported cases (Powell *et al.* 1968; Price *et al.* 1983; Price *et al.* 1984). Doses between 125–150 mg had been taken for up to 3 weeks before onset of symptoms. One patient (Powell *et al.* 1968) had previously received imipramine, but it had been discontinued because of a rash; when desipramine was substituted the rash did not resolve and fatal hepatic necrosis supervened a few days later.

Amineptine

This tricyclic antidepressant is widely used in a number of countries, including France, where it accounts for 80 per cent of hepatitis caused by antidepressant drugs (Geneve *et al.* 1987; Pessayre and Larrey 1988). Both hepatic necrosis and pure cholestasis have been described. Liver damage characteristically occurs within 3 months of starting therapy and it is often associated with fever and eosinophilia. A quite different liver lesion, with prominent infiltration of liver cells by microvesicular fat droplets resembling alcoholic fatty liver, has also been described in association with this drug. The large number of cases of liver damage reported suggests that amineptine may have a greater hepatotoxic potential than the other tricyclic drugs.

Maprotiline

Two case reports (Moldawsky 1984; Aleem and Lingam 1987) have implicated this drug in the pathogenesis of acute hepatitis; in one patient, who was asymptomatic, the condition was detected on screening. The latent intervals were long (4 years and 288 days respectively), and although abnormalities resolved when the drug was discontinued, intercurrent non-A, non-B viral hepatitis could equally well have been the cause.

Dothiepin

A mixed cholestatic/hepatocellular pattern of injury has been reported with this drug (Stricker and Spoelstra 1985), but the reaction is obviously rare.

Lofepramine

Reports of cholestatic and hepatocellular injury have been received by the Committee on Safety of Medicines (CSM 1988). All occurred within 8 weeks of starting treatment and reversed on withdrawal of the drug. Nine patients developed jaundice.

Mianserin

Mianserin has been reported as causing both cholestasis and hepatocellular necrosis, with one case relapsing on reintroduction of the drug (Stricker and Spoelstra 1985).

Monoamine oxidase inhibitors

Iproniazid

Iproniazid was withdrawn from clinical use in Great Britain and the United States because of its propensity to cause liver damage, but it is still used in some countries, including France. The usual picture is one of hepatic necrosis, generally occurring in the first 3 months of treatment (Stricker and Spoelstra 1985).

Phenelzine

Phenelzine can also produce hepatic necrosis. Cross-toxicity has been described with different monoamine oxidase inhibitors which are chemically related (Davis and Williams 1985). The overall incidence of hepatotox-icicty is probably higher than with the tricyclic drugs, having been estimated at approximately 1 per cent.

Anticonvulsants and antispasmodics

Phenytoin

Hepatocellular necrosis is a well-documented complication of phenytoin therapy and is frequently accompanied by other manifestations of allergy (Robinson *et al.* 1965; Harney and Glasberg 1983; Olsson and Zettergren 1988; Smythe and Umstead 1989); with rashes, lymphaden-opathy, and eosinophilia. Anicteric hepatitis has also been described (Pezzimenti and Hahn 1970). Circulating antibodies to phenytoin have been described in association with hepatic damage (Kleckner *et al.* 1975); cell-mediated immunity to the drug has also been demonstrated in a patient who developed an allergic reaction to it with a rash, lymphadenopathy, hepatic necrosis, and eosinophilia. Sensitization was also demonstrated towards phenobarbitone in this patient, indicating cross-reactivity (Kahn *et al.* 1984).

Phenytoin is metabolised to a chemically reactive epoxide derivative (Pantarotto *et al.* 1982; Moustafa *et al.* 1983), and it has been suggested that individuals deficient in the enzyme epoxide hydrolase, might be at risk from hepatitis due to the drug (Spielberg *et al.* 1981; Spielberg 1986). Lymphocytes from patients with this deficiency were particularly susceptible to lysis by epoxide phenytoin metabolites generated *in vitro* by a murine hepatic microsomal system.

Phenobarbitone

Rarely, acute hepatitis may result from phenobarbitone, usually in the context of a generalized hypersensitivity illness (Pagliaro *et al.* 1969; Mockli *et al.* 1989).

Carbamazepine

Hepatitis from this drug usually occurs within the first 6–8 weeks of treatment and there may be a prominent cholestatic element (Horowitz *et al.* 1988). Granulomatous infiltration of the liver can also occur. The frequent concurrence of allergic manifestations suggests an immunological aetiology. Hepatic necrosis has been described after carbamazepine overdose, suggesting that the drug has a direct hepatotoxic potential (Luke *et al.* 1986).

Valproic acid

(see under Fatty liver)

Dantrolene

Dantrolene sodium, an agent chemically related to phenytoin and used in the treatment of spasticity, was associated with a 1.8 per cent incidence of abnormal liver function tests in one large series (Utili *et al.* 1977), in which one-third of the patients became jaundiced. Histologically, the liver lesions may resemble chronic active hepatitis, acute hepatic necrosis, or a non-specific portal tract infiltrate. In addition, Wilkinson and others (1979) described superimposed changes suggestive of ascending cholangitis in four patients with acute hepatitis associated with this drug. The cases reviewed by Utili and others (1977) had all been taking doses in excess of 200 mg daily, but three of the four patients in another series had been receiving 150 mg per day or less (Wilkinson et al. 1979). Rechallenge with a therapeutic dose of the drug can result in a prompt relapse of liver damage (Ogburn et al. 1976; Utili et al. 1977), although the reaction is not accompanied by the generalized hypersensitivity reaction which characterizes phenytoin hepatitis. (See also under Active chronic hepatitis.)

Anti-inflammatory drugs

Overt hepatic damage occurs in less than 0.1 per cent of patients taking phenylbutazone (Kuzell et al. 1953; Fowler et al. 1975). The commonest lesion is a hepatocellular necrosis, but cholestatic hepatitis occurs in up to one-third of cases. Patients usually present within 4 weeks of starting the drug, but in 20 per cent, the latent period is up to 1 year, or occasionally longer (Fowler et al. 1975). Fifty per cent of cases have associated manifestations of hypersensitivity, but the direct toxic potential of the drug is evidenced by the report by Juul (1965) of a patient who developed acute hepatocellular necrosis following overdose with phenylbutazone.

Indomethacin may produce hepatocellular necrosis, often accompanied by a generalized hypersensitivity reaction (Fenech et al. 1967; Opolon et al. 1969), and similar reactions have also been reported in association with probenecid (Reynolds et al. 1957), ibuprofen (Stempel and Miller 1977), allopurinol (Kantor 1970; Lang 1979; Al-Kawas et al. 1981; Raper et al. 1984; Tam and Carroll 1989), naproxen (Bass 1974), piroxicam (Hartmann et al. 1984; Lee et al. 1986), sulindac (Wood et al. 1985), and diclofenac (Iveson et al. 1990). The frequency of these adverse drug reactions has not been determined.

Antibiotics and antibacterial drugs

Penicillin

Acute hepatitis is a very rare complication of penicillin therapy and is associated with other manifestations of hypersensitivity (Valdivia-Barriga et al. 1963). Most of the penicillin derivatives in current use produce a predominantly cholestatic lesion (q.v.).

Sulphonamides

All sulphonamides may produce an acute hepatitic type of hypersensitivity reaction with or without involvement of other organs (Dujovne et al. 1967). There may be

sensitivity to one sulphonamide preparation but not to another (Konttinen 1972). Severe hepatocellular necrosis has been described as part of a generalized hypersensitivity reaction in a patient receiving sulphasalazine for inflammatory bowel disease (Sotolongo et al. 1978). Liver damage may be present as part of a multisystem reaction complicating prophylaxis with the sulphonamide-containing antimalarial Fansidar (Zitelli et al. 1987). A predominantly cholestatic jaundice may also occur in association with the use of sulphonamides (see below).

Ketoconazole

This antifungal drug can produce asymptomatic abnormalities in liver function tests in 5–10 per cent of individuals receiving it; the incidence of overt liver injury has been estimated at 1 in 15 000 (Janssen and Symoens 1983; Lewis et al. 1984). Females are affected twice as frequently as males and the timing of onset of liver injury is very variable, between 2–26 weeks of initiating therapy. Jaundice is usually hepatocellular in nature, although cholestatic lesions have also been described and, occasionally, fulminant hepatic failure may ensue. The reaction is not accompanied by signs of hypersensitivity and the drug has been shown to be directly hepatotoxic in animals (Lewis et al. 1984).

Cardiac and antihypertensive drugs

β-Adrenoceptor blockers

Hepatic reactions from these agents are extremely rare, but isolated reports have appeared of centrilobular hepatic necrosis associated with metoprolol with relapse on rechallenge (Larrey et al. 1988b). Metabolism of this drug is retarded in individuals with poor hydroxylator status, but hepatotoxicity from metoprolol is not associated with this phenotype (McGourty et al. 1985).

Fatal hepatic necrosis has been observed in a patient 2 months after starting labetalol (Douglas et al. 1989). There was no evidence of hypersensitivity in this reaction; the patient did not have circulating antimitochondrial antibodies or features of SLE, both of which have been associated with this drug. Hepatitis from acebutolol is accompanied by pyrexia, and some cases have relapsed promptly on rechallenge (Tanner et al. 1989). A mild cholestatic reaction has been reported with atenolol (Schwartz et al. 1989).

Calcium antagonists

Isolated instances of jaundice from hepatic necrosis have been described in association with diltiazem (Schroeder *et al.* 1985; Shallcross *et al.* 1987), verapamil (Hare and Horowitz 1986; Burgunder *et al.* 1988), and nifedipine. The incidence of these complications is very low.

Quinidine

Hepatic necrosis associated with this drug is usually associated with manifestations of hypersensitivity with rashes, fever, and eosinophilia (Knobler *et al.* 1986). The liver lesion is predominantly hepatitic with a variable element of cholestasis, and granulomatous infiltration can also occur. Relapse of the liver lesion on rechallenge is characteristic.

The chemically related compound quinine can produce a cholestatic hepatitis with granulomatous infiltration and other features of hypersensitivity; this is an extremely rare complication (Katz *et al.* 1983; Punukollu *et al.* 1990).

Anticoagulants

Hepatitis may develop in association with a generalized hypersensitivity reaction to phenindione (Perkins 1962; Mohamed 1965) and a cholestatic hepatitis has also been reported (Portal and Emanuel 1961).

Diuretics

Tienilic acid was withdrawn from use in the USA because of its high propensity to produce hepatic reactions (1 in 800), usually hepatocellular necrosis (Zimmerman *et al.* 1984). There is usually associated evidence of hypersensitivity, with eosinophilia and liver–kidney microsomal antibodies (LKM2 antibodies), which have a different specificity from those found in other liver diseases (Neuberger and Williams 1989). Detection of antibodies reacting with a liver antigen altered by a tienilic acid metabolite in some patients with this adverse reaction provides additional support for an immune-mediated pathogenesis.

Hepatitis has been described as an extremely rare complication of ethacrynic acid therapy (Datey *et al.* 1967). Frusemide is metabolised to a reactive intermediate in rodents and exhibits dose-related hepatotoxicity in mice (Mitchell *et al.* 1976*a*), but there is no evidence that it is hepatotoxic in man.

Antiulcer drugs

Cimetidine

Sharpe and Hawkins (1977), reviewing the results of treatment with cimetidine in 830 patients, found abnor-mal rises in transaminases of 3.8 per cent, although this incidence was not significantly different from a control group receiving a placebo. Subsequently, isolated reports of hepatitis due to this drug, with relapse on rechallenge, have appeared (Villeneuve and Warner 1979; van Steenbergen *et al.* 1985). The drug has also been implicated in the pathogenesis or relapse, or both, of active chronic hepatitis (Boyd *et al.* 1989).

Ranitidine

A few clinical reports implicate this drug as the cause of a predominantly cholestatic hepatitis, which may resemble ascending cholangitis with prominent fever and rigors (Black *et al.* 1984; Murphy *et al.* 1985; Hiesse *et al.* 1985). Eosinophilic infiltration within the liver, and a response to rechallenge in some cases, suggest that immunological mechanisms are involved in pathogenesis. A direct toxic action is also likely; H_2-blockers are toxic to isolated hepatocytes *in vitro* (Zimmerman *et al.* 1986) and also inhibit bile flow (Bassan *et al.* 1986).

Other drugs

Chenodeoxycholic acid and ursodeoxycholic acid

About one-third of patients treated with chenodeoxycholic acid (CDCA) show dose-related rises in serum transaminases (Schoenfield *et al.* 1981). These are asymptomatic, seldom exceed three times the upper limit of normal, are usually manifest in the first 3 months of treatment, and tend to resolve despite continuing the drug. It is questionable whether significant histological liver damage occurs. Light microscopy of liver biopsies from patients on CDCA has either been normal or has revealed minor non-specific changes (Fisher *et al.* 1985). In the National Co-operative Gallstone Study, electron microscopy of baseline liver biopsies showed some features of intrahepatic cholestasis, which became more prevalent after 9 and 24 months in both CDCA-treated groups (Phillips *et al.* 1983). Because none of the patients treated with placebo underwent liver biopsy, it is not clear whether the changes with time were drug-induced or reflected the natural history of gallstone disease.

Most orally administered CDCA is ultimately converted to lithocholic acid by enteric bacteria, and there was some concern that this bile acid might be the mediator of the CDCA-associated liver changes. Lithocholic acid is hepatotoxic in those animal species that are unable to sulphate it and excrete it (Gadacz *et al.* 1976). In man, however, sulphation and excretion are highly efficient and although in one study (Marks *et al.* 1981) a low measured lithocholic acid 'sulphation fraction' was associated with CDCA-induced hypertransaminasaemia, no relation between serum transaminase and biliary lithocholic acid levels has been demonstrated (Allan et al. 1976). The hypertransaminasaemia may result instead from a direct effect of CDCA on the hepatocyte plasma membrane (Miyazaki et al. 1984).

Ursodeoxycholic acid appears to have little or no potential for hepatotoxicity in man or experimentally in isolated liver cells (Miyazaki et al. 1984).

Cocaine

Cocaine is metabolised to hepatotoxic derivatives and produces centrilobular hepatic necrosis in mice (Thompson et al. 1979; Kloss et al. 1984). Similar liver lesions have been demonstrated at post-mortem in addicts dying after use of this drug, although hepatic failure was not the main cause of death (Perino et al. 1987; Porter et al. 1988; Kanel et al. 1990).

Disulfiram

An acute hepatitic reaction can occasionally complicate disulfiram therapy in alcoholics (Black and Richardson 1985; Wright et al. 1988). The reaction, which may be fatal, usually occurs within 2 to 8 weeks of starting therapy, and it is characterized by marked elevations in transaminases, unlike those seen with alcoholic liver disease.

Acute fatty infiltration of the liver

Hepatitic or cholestatic lesions produced by a number of drugs, including isoniazid, antithyroid drugs, methotrexate, phenothiazines, phenytoin, and sulphonamides may, in addition, be associated with some degree of lipid accumulation within hepatocytes (Thaler 1988), and if these combined abnormalities are present, a drug-induced abnormality should be strongly suspected. For other drugs, lipid accumulation is the major manifestation of hepatotoxicity.

Corticosteroids

Fatty infiltration of the liver, predominantly in the centrilobular region, is frequently found with corticosteroid therapy. The pathogenesis is imperfectly understood but probably relates both to increased lipid synthesis and reduced formation of VLDL lipoproteins with diminished export from hepatocytes (Thaler 1988).

Tetracyclines

Most of the reported cases of tetracycline-induced liver damage have been in pregnant women given large doses

intravenously for pyelonephritis (Whalley et al. 1970; Breitenbucher and Crowley 1970), although cases have also been reported in non-pregnant women (Damjanov et al. 1968) and in men (Robinson and Rywiin 1970). Tetracycline is excreted predominantly in the urine (Kunin et al. 1959a), and its plasma clearance is impaired in patients with renal failure (Kunin et al. 1959b). As a general rule, not more than 1 g of tetracycline should be given intravenously, nor more than 2 g orally in 24 hours, and if renal function is impaired lower doses should be given (Whalley et al. 1974).

The histological lesion is identical with the acute fatty liver of pregnancy (Davis and Kaufman 1966), with central and mid-zonal necrosis and prominent infiltration with fine intracytoplasmic fat droplets. An identical lesion can be reproduced in animals (Lepper et al. 1951). The fatty infiltration appears to be caused by impaired triglyceride excretion from the liver (Hansen et al. 1968), due to defective lipoprotein synthesis (Lewis et al. 1967); in addition it has been suggested that increased hepatic uptake of fatty acids together with their impaired mitochondrial oxidation may play an important role (Breen et al. 1975). In keeping with the latter mechanism is the observation that tetracycline accumulates in mitochondria and inhibits many enzyme systems in this organelle (Hoyumpa et al. 1975; Freneaux et al. 1988).

Reye-like syndrome

This condition is characterized by acute microvesicular hepatic steatosis and hyperammonaemia in infants and young children; it leads to fulminant hepatic failure, frequently with a fatal outcome. Numerous aetiologies have been proposed for it, but salicylates and the anticonvulsant, valproic acid, have fairly convincingly been causally incriminated.

Salicylates

Early reports implicating salicylates in the pathogenesis of Reye's syndrome were met with scepticism; it was thought that the drug could have been falsely implicated as a result of having been given as an antipyretic/analgesic in the prodromal phase of an illness due to other causes (Starko et al. 1980; Waldman et al. 1982; Halpin et al. 1982). More recent case–control studies have provided persuasive, albeit not completely conclusive, evidence that the drug is causally implicated (Hurwits et al. 1985, 1987; Hall et al. 1988; Forsyth et al. 1989). This has led to withdrawal of salicylate preparations designed specifically for paediatric use.

Valproic acid

This anticonvulsant is particularly prone to cause Reye's

syndrome in epileptic children under the age of 2. Concomitant therapy with anticonvulsant drugs greatly increases the risk (1 in 500 compared with 1 in 37000 receiving valproic acid alone) and mental retardation and other congenital abnormalities appear to be additional risk factors for reasons unknown (Powell-Jackson *et al.* 1984; Dreifuss *et al.* 1987). Recognition of these risk factors has led to a decline in the incidence of this complication from 1 in 10000 in 1978–84 to 1 in 49000 in 1985–86 (Dreifuss *et al.* 1989; Dreifuss 1989).

There are differences on electron microscopy between the liver lesion of Reye's syndrome and that produced by valproic acid (Partin 1989; Kimura *et al.* 1989). In Reye's syndrome there is generalized swelling of mitochondria throughout the liver lobule, whereas this is not seen in the lesion induced by valproic acid. A further difference is the presence of mitochondrial matrix granules in centrilobular hepatocytes of patients with valproic acid hepatotoxicity; these are not seen in classical Reye's syndrome.

Mechanisms The mechanism by which valproic acid causes liver damage is still not well understood. The subject has recently been well reviewed by Cotariu and Jaidman (1988). Hepatotoxicty is probably mediated by some of the metabolites of the parent drug, particularly 4-en-valproic acid. This metabolite is structurally similar to two other compounds that can produce illnesses with features of Reye's syndrome: methylenecyclopropylacetic acid is a metabolite of hypoglycin, a constituent of unripe akee fruits, which produce Jamaican vomiting sickness; 4-pentaenoic acid produces a Reye-like syndrome in rats. Valproic acid and its metabolites show dose-related toxicity in isolated rat hepatocytes and decrease fatty acid oxidation, as does 4-pentaenoic acid. There are several ways in which such inhibition of fatty acid oxidation could occur: valproic acid and its metabolites deplete acetyl co-enzyme A and also carnitine, and toxicity may occur via inhibition of metabolic pathways depending upon these cofactors. In man the drug has been shown to affect intermediary metabolism at several points (Bohles *et al.* 1982; Turnbull *et al.* 1986).

It might be expected that individuals forming increased quantities of the potentially hepatotoxic metabolite 4-en-valproic acid would be more at risk from liver damage, but in a single metabolic study this has not been shown to be the case (Tennison *et al.* 1988). Excretion of this metabolite, which is formed by microsomal enzymes, was greatly increased, however, in individuals receiving polytherapy with anticonvulsants. As discussed above, polytherapy is a major factor predisposing towards valproic acid hepatotoxicity in young children.

Predominantly cholestatic lesions

Phenothiazines

The estimated incidence of cholestatic hepatitis from phenothiazines lies between 0.1–0.5 per cent (Zimmerman 1978). Jaundice usually appears in the second to fourth week of treatment and the onset may be acute, with fever and abdominal pain, or insidious. Signs of hypersensitivity with fever and eosinophilia are seen in up to 70 per cent of subjects and associated rashes occur in up to 5 per cent (Zimmerman 1978).

Serum alkaline phosphatase levels are characteristically markedly elevated, while transaminase elevations are more modest. Typically, the histological picture includes cholestasis with relatively little hepatocellular injury. A portal inflammatory infiltrate is also characteristic with eosinophils in up to 50 per cent of cases. Neutrophil infiltration between portal areas and lobules is seen in approximately 25 per cent of cases (Ishak and Irey 1972).

Symptoms generally regress on drug withdrawal and two-thirds of patients will have recovered after 8 weeks. The remaining third may have a more prolonged course (see below under prolonged cholestasis).

Other phenothiazines have been reported to cause cholestasis. These include fluphenazine (Holt 1984), haloperidol (Dincsoy and Saelinger 1982), prochlorperazine (Ishak and Irey 1972), promazine and thioridazine (Barrancik *et al.* 1967), and trifluoperazine. Cross-sensitivity between chlorpromazine and other phenothiazines has been observed.

Mechanisms

Chlorpromazine and its metabolites can produce abnormalities in the hepatic cytoskeleton (Elias and Boyer 1979), and impair bile excretion (Ros *et al.* 1979; Tavoloni *et al.* 1979). The latter is associated with the disruption of cell membranes and impaired activities of the hepatocyte membrane enzymes $Na^+/K^+ATPase$ and $Mg^{2+}ATPase$, both of which are involved in secretion of bile (Seeman 1972; Ros *et al.* 1979; Boyer 1980). The extent of these toxic effects can be modified by metabolism of the drug. Thus, the dihydroxy metabolite of chlorpromazine impairs bile secretion at concentrations in which the parent compound has no effect and is 100 times more potent an inhibitor of hepatocyte membrane $Na^+/K^+ATPase$ (Boyer and Root 1976; Samuels and Carey 1978; Keefe *et al.* 1979; Plaa and Hewitt 1982). In contrast, the sulphoxide metabolite does not produce these effects. Those individuals who are poor metabolisers of chlorpromazine to the sulphoxide derivative or extensive metabolisers to the dihydroxy metabolite, or both, might thus be more susceptible to cholestatic liver damage from chlorpromazine (Elias *et al.* 1984).

The frequent association of hypersensitivity manifestations suggests the involvement of immune reactions directed against the drug or one of its metabolites. There are, however, few data on this.

Tricyclic antidepressants

These compounds can produce both an acute hepatitis and a predominantly cholestatic lesion. In this chapter they are discussed above under Acute hepatitis.

Benzodiazepines

Hepatic injury from this group of drugs is very uncommon. Occurrences of cholestatic jaundice attributed variously to chlordiazepoxide (Lo *et al.* 1967), diazepam (Tedesco and Mills 1982), and flurazepam (Reynolds *et al.* 1981) have been reported. The onset of liver disease occurs from a few days to several weeks after starting therapy and signs of hypersensitivity may be present.

Anticonvulsants

Cholestatic jaundice due to carbamazepine (Stricker and Spoelstra 1985) and also phenytoin (Speckler *et al.* 1981; Harney and Glasberg 1983) have been reported as variants from the predominantly hepatocellular jaundice usually produced by these drugs.

Antibacterial drugs

Erythromycin

Jaundice due to cholestatic hepatitis from erythromycin is most frequently associated with the estolate preparation (Robinson 1961; Bachman *et al.* 1982; Ginsburg 1986), although well-documented cases of jaundice complicating treatment with erythromycin ethylsuccinate (Keefe *et al.* 1982; Diehl *et al.* 1984), erythromycin propionate (Tolman *et al.* 1974) and the intravenous lactobionate formulation (Gholson and Warren 1990) have now been described. The latter, unusually, led to fulminant hepatic failure.

Jaundice usually appears on day 7–14 of treatment and is frequently accompanied by severe colicky abdominal pain which may mimic an acute abdomen (Oliver *et al.* 1972).

Pseudotumours of the liver simulating malignancy have been reported in a patient receiving erythromycin estolate. Histologically, eosinophilic infiltration and necrosis were the only abnormalities, and when the drug was stopped the abnormalities resolved (Rigauts *et al.* 1988).

A high (60 per cent) incidence of eosinophilia (*Australian Family Physician* 1973) and a prompt relapse of hepatitis on challenge with the drug are consistent with an allergic basis for erythromycin hepatitis (Robinson 1961; Gilbert 1962). On the other hand, a direct toxic potential for the drug has been shown by its capacity to produce a dose-related impairment in bile flow and BSP clearance in isolated rat liver preparations (Kendler *et al.* 1972). In addition, toxic effects can be seen in isolated hepatocytes incubated with therapeutic concentrations of erythromycin estolate, while unphysiological levels of other erythromycin preparations are needed to produce the same effect (Zimmerman *et al.* 1973).

Penicillins

Liver damage from penicillin itself is extremely rare (Valdivia Barriga *et al.* 1963), but cholestatic reactions to a number of penicillin derivatives have been well documented, including flucloxacillin (Lobatto *et al.* 1982; Bengtsson *et al.* 1985; Victorino *et al.* 1987; Turner *et al.* 1989), cloxacillin, and oxacillin. *In vitro* evidence of hypersensitivity to flucloxacillin (Victorino *et al.* 1987) and cloxacillin (Aderka *et al.* 1986) has been demonstrated in patients with cholestatic hepatitis from these drugs.

Amoxycillin does not cause liver damage but its combined preparation with clavulanic acid (Augmentin) has been the subject of several reports implicating it as a cause of cholestatic hepatitis (Stricker *et al.* 1989; Verhamme *et al.* 1989; Reddy *et al.* 1989). The clavulanic acid rather than the penicillin moiety appears to be responsible for the reaction (Stricker *et al.* 1989).

Cephalosporins

Hepatotoxicity from these antibacterial agents is extremely rare but occasional cases have been reported (Pessayre *et al.* 1985).

Sulphonamides

Cholestatic or hepatitic jaundice (q.v.) may complicate use of sulphonamides.

Trimethoprim–sulphamethoxazole (Bactrim, Septrin) characteristically produces cholestatic reactions (Thies and Dull 1984; Kaplowitz *et al.* 1986; Oliver *et al.* 1987). These are generally due to the sulphonamide component, although in one case trimethoprim may have been the cause (Tanner 1986; Kumar *et al.* 1989). Fulminant hepatic failure from the combination has also been described (Alberti-Flor *et al.* 1989).

Cholestatic hepatitis from sulphasalazine is usually associated with other manifestations of hypersensitivity and eosinophilic infiltration of the liver parenchyma (Holdsworth 1983; Farr *et al.* 1985; Haines 1986;

McGilchrist and Hunter 1986; Mitrane *et al.* 1986; Gremse *et al.* 1989). It can complicate therapy of both ulcerative colitis and rheumatoid arthritis with the drug. Neurotoxicity can be seen in association with the hepatotoxic reaction (Smith *et al.* 1982; Mitrane *et al.* 1986). One case report described the development of hepatic damage in a patient who had taken the drug without problems for 15 years (Lennard and Farndon 1983).

Nitrofurantoin

Cholestatic hepatitis, usually accompanied by systemic features of hypersensitivity, generally appears between 1–5 weeks after starting this drug (Goldstein *et al.* 1974). As with chronic active hepatitis produced by this drug, the reaction has a predilection for women. One unusual case reports the development of cholestatic hepatitis after drinking milk from a cow that was being treated with this drug (Berry *et al.* 1984).

Triacetyloleandomycin

This macrolide antibiotic has a well-defined potential to cause cholestasis (Larrey *et al.* 1987) and the incidence is particularly high when the drug is taken together with oral contraceptives (Fevery *et al.* 1983; Pessayre *et al.* 1985), probably due to the additive cholestatic effects of the two types of drug. Jaundice usually appears within the first week or two of treatment with the drug, in women who have used the Pill for years without previous problems. Jaundice has also been observed in a pregnant woman taking the antibiotic (Chaput *et al.* 1981).

Antifungal and anthelminthic drugs

Griseofulvin and ketoconazole

Griseofulvin has been reported to cause cholestasis (Chiprut *et al.* 1976), and ketoconazole may also occasionally produce a cholestatic lesion although the more usual pattern is one of hepatocellular injury (Lewis *et al.* 1984). Jaundice from actinomycin D has also been reported (D'Angio 1987).

Thiabendazole

This anthelminthic may cause cholestasis (Davidson *et al.* 1988), sometimes accompanied by the sicca syndrome (Rex *et al.* 1983) and progression to chronicity has been recorded (see below). Niclofolan, used for the treatment of fascioliasis, may also cause cholestatic jaundice (Reshef *et al.* 1982).

Analgesics and antirheumatic drugs

Non-steroidal anti-inflammatory drugs (NSAID)

These compounds can produce an acute hepatitis or a predominantly cholestatic reaction. They are dealt with under Acute hepatitis above.

Reports of jaundice from the NSAID benoxaprofen started to appear soon after its introduction in Great Britain (Taggart and Alderdice 1982; Goudie *et al.* 1982; Prescott *et al.* 1982). The histological liver lesion was one of cholestasis with little or no necrosis, and a most unusual feature of the reaction was its frequent association with renal failure. Other characteristics of the reaction included the long period of ingestion of the drug before development of jaundice (usually 3–6 months) and its high frequency in very elderly patients. The drug has now been withdrawn from the market.

Dextropropoxyphene

Cholestatic hepatitis from this drug is rare but well-documented (Bassendine *et al.* 1986). It characteristically presents with jaundice, abdominal pain, and rigors and may be mistaken for gallstone disease; a number of patients with this syndrome have undergone unnecessary laparotomies. Hypersensitivity to the drug appears to be involved with prompt relapse of the liver lesion on rechallenge.

Gold salts

These preparations have been associated with cholestatic jaundice in a number of cases (Schenker *et al.* 1973; Favreau *et al.* 1977; Edelman *et al.* 1983; Shaban *et al.* 1984; Harats *et al.* 1985). Jaundice usually appears after a second or subsequent dose and there is usually associated eosinophilia and other manifestations of hypersensitivity. The liver lesion characteristically improves on withdrawal of the drug, but the improvement may be slow.

Penicillamine

Accompanying penicillamine-associated cholestasis there are usually manifestations of hypersensitivity, and the liver lesion improves promptly on withdrawal of therapy (Rosenbaum *et al.* 1980; Langan and Thomas 1987).

Oral hypoglycaemic drugs

Chlorpropamide

This drug is reported to cause cholestatic hepatitis in 0.5 per cent of recipients (Zimmerman 1978; Gupta and Sachar 1985).

Tolbutamide

This antidiabetic agent may cause hepatic damage similar to that caused by chlorpropamide, but does so less commonly (Lo Indice and Lang 1978). Chronic cholestasis has been reported despite discontinuance of the drug (Nakao *et al.* 1985). Cross-sensitization between tolbutamide and chlorpropamide can occur.

Glibenclamide

Cross-sensitization between glibenclamide and chlor-propamide or tolbutamide does not seem to occur, and it has been given without incident to a patient who developed liver damage after both the latter two agents (Rumboldt and Bota 1984), although this drug does itself have a rare potential to cause a hypersensitivity cholestasis (R.C. Goodman *et al.* 1987).

Antithyroid drugs

Hepatic reactions to sulphonylureas are generally predominantly cholestatic, with the exception of propylthiouracil, which causes a predominantly hepatocellular lesion (Blom *et al.* 1985; Vitug and Goldman 1985; Schmidt *et al.* 1986; Limaye and Ruffolo 1987; Jonas and Eidson 1988). Clinical features suggest a hypersensitivity reaction; this is supported by immunological studies showing cell-mediated immunity to both carbimazole and propylthiouracil (Mihas *et al.* 1976; Blom *et al.* 1985) in patients with adverse hepatic reactions to these drugs.

Cardiovascular drugs

Several cases of cholestatic jaundice due to captopril have been reported (Parker 1984; Rahmat *et al.* 1985; Zimran *et al.* 1985; Bellary *et al.* 1989). The estimated incidence is 0.09 per 1000 patients. Liver damage is usually associated with fever, rashes, and eosinophilia, and most of the reported cases had involved much higher doses of the drug (up to 800 mg daily) than are currently used. The time to onset of the reaction is also variable, but in two-thirds of cases the reaction has developed 1–8 weeks after starting therapy. Acute hepatitis with eosinophilia has been described in association with enalapril (Rosellini *et al.* 1989).

Other cardiovascular drugs reported to cause cholestatic jaundice are disopyramide (Doody 1982; Bakris *et al.* 1983; Antonelli *et al.* 1984), flecainide (Hopmann and Surmann 1984), and the calcium-channel antagonists nifedipine and verapamil (Guarascio *et al.* 1984).

Immunosuppressive and antineoplastic drugs

Azathioprine

Azathioprine and the related drug mercaptopurine (MP) can occasionally cause pure cholestasis (Sparberg *et al.* 1969; De Pinho *et al.* 1984). Azathioprine differs from mercaptopurine in having an imidazole side-chain which undergoes hydrolysis *in vivo* with liberation of MP. Rechallenge studies in a patient with a hypersensitivity syndrome complicated by jaundice after azathioprine showed that the hypersensitivity syndrome was due to the imidazole side-chain and the jaundice to the MP moiety (Davis *et al.* 1980).

Cyclosporin

Cholestatic jaundice is now a rare but well-recognized complication of this immunosuppressant (Davis *et al.* 1980; Klintmalm *et al.* 1981; Pinto *et al.* 1984; Gulbis *et al.* 1988; Kassiandes *et al.* 1990). Its ability to produce liver damage in man probably correlates with its effects on inhibiting bile flow in experimental systems.

Other anticancer drugs causing hepatocellular injury include cyclophosphamide (Goldberg and Lidsky 1985) and etoposide (Johnson *et al.* 1983).

Oral contraceptives and anabolic steroids

Structural characteristics

Jaundice from this class of compounds is mainly associated with a 17-α-substituted 19-nor (no radical) configuration (Fig. 11.5). Substitution in the 17-α position with an alkyl or other other group greatly increases the cholestatic potential (Heaney and Whedon 1958; de Lorimer *et al.* 1965; Schreiber and Simon 1983). The incidence of steroid cholestasis in relation to other structural modifications has been investigated by Gallagher and others (1966), who found a phenolic configuration of the A ring of the molecule to be a particularly important determinant for this adverse effect. Jaundice has also been described in association with non-substituted steroids, particularly if these are used in high doses (Garrigues-Gil *et al.* 1986; Foitl *et al.* 1989; Fedorkow *et al.* 1989).

Oral contraceptives

Published figures for the incidence of jaundice from oral contraceptives (approximately 1 in 10 000 in Europe and North America but 1 in 4000 in Scandinavia and Chile) reflect use of the older preparations (Schaffner 1966), but see below for constitutional factors in Scandinavians and Chileans. The incidence is probably now much lower with the almost universal adoption of low-oestrogen formulations.

Symptoms and signs of liver damage usually occur within 4 weeks of starting the tablets (Ockner and Davidson 1967), with anorexia, malaise, pruritus, and jaundice: hepatic damage developing after the third month of usage is unlikely to be due to oral contraceptives. Systemic manifestations of hypersensitivity do not occur. Alkaline phosphatase levels are only modestly raised and may be normal (Metreau *et al.* 1972), and although transaminase elevation is not generally striking, severe hepatic necrosis has been reported (Stoll *et al.* 1966; Dooner *et al.* 1971). Recovery is usually prompt on discontinuing medication, although prolonged cholestasis has been reported in two sisters following treatment with the progestogen norethisterone (Somayaji *et*

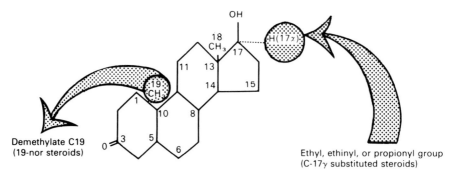

Fig. 11.5
Structural charateristics of steroids that cause jaundice.

al. 1968), and symptoms of active chronic hepatitis and primary biliary cirrhosis may be precipitated by the contraceptive pill. Relapse is likely to occur if the same agents or similar formulations are resumed (Thulin and Nermark 1966).

Long-term use of oral contraceptives has been shown to lead to abnormalities of hepatic ultrastructure involving particularly the mitochondria, which develop crystalline inclusions, together with hypertrophy of the smooth endoplasmic reticulum and changes in the biliary canaliculi (Larsson-Cohn and Stenram 1967; Perez *et al.* 1969).

Mechanisms Constitutional factors may be important in determining whether or not jaundice will develop, for it is especially prevalent in women whose pregnancies have been complicated by idiopathic recurrent cholestasis of pregnancy (Reyes 1982; Schreiber and Simon 1983), and their family members (Dalen and Westerholm 1974; Reyes *et al.* 1981). This explains the more frequent occurrence of jaundice in women taking oral contraceptives in Scandinavia (Adlercreutz and Ikonen 1964; Eisalo *et al.* 1965; Larsson-Cohn 1965) and Chile (Orrellana-Alcalde and Dominguez 1966), where the incidence of cholestasis of pregnancy is high. Individuals with Dubin–Johnson syndrome (Cohen *et al.* 1972) or benign recurrent cholestasis (De Pagler *et al.* 1976) may also be particularly susceptible.

Available evidence suggests that oestrogens are more potent cholestatic agents than progestogens (Adlercreutz and Tenhunen 1970). Challenge with mestranol provoked a relapse of pill jaundice in three patients, whereas administration of the progestogen component had no effect (Eisalo *et al.* 1964). Natural progestogens have no cholestatic action (Kappas 1968), although natural oestrogens may increase BSP retention (Urban *et al.* 1968), a phenomenon that occurs during normal pregnancy (Combes *et al.* 1963). Synthetic progestogens, however,

are partly converted to oestrogens *in vivo* (Brown and Blair 1960); in this way oestrogen jaundice can be potentiated by synthetic progestogens (Goldzieher 1964). That the two components of oral contraceptives may act synergistically to produce cholestasis has been demonstrated by clinical studies (Stoll *et al.* 1966).

The pathophysiology of oestrogen-induced cholestasis is not clear, but animal studies have shown that ethinyloestradiol inhibits bile flow (Gummucio and Valdivieso 1971) and also the biliary excretion of bilirubin and bile salts. Administration of ethinyloestradiol to experimental animals inhibits the activity of hepatocyte membrane $Na^+/K^+ATPase$, an enzyme intimately involved in the active transport and clearance of bile acids by the liver (Davis *et al.* 1978; Boyer 1980; Simon *et al.* 1980). The compound also induces a marked change in membrane lipid composition, with increases in cholesterol relative to lipid content. This is associated with an increase in membrane microviscosity with a consequent decrease in permeability to water (Simon *et al.* 1980). Oestrogens also increase the permeability of bile ductular cells to inert marker compounds (Forker 1969; Peterson and Fujimoto 1977) and this effect may play a role in pathogenesis by allowing increased back-diffusion of solutes once excreted into the bile.

Anabolic steroids

Pure cholestasis, with little or no parenchymal involvement, is said to occur in 1–2 per cent of all patients receiving orally active anabolic steroids, notably methyltestosterone and norethandrolone (Schaffner 1965). Methyltestosterone is an effective antipruritic, but its use in patients with primary biliary cirrhosis is invariably associated with a rise in serum conjugated bilirubin (Lloyd-Thomas and Sherlock 1952). Use of oxymetholone, a 17-substituted non-virilizing androgen, in the treatment of aplastic anaemia is associated with a high incidence of abnormal liver function tests, with elevation of serum alkaline phosphatase and conjugated bilirubin (Sanchez-Medal *et al.* 1969; Presant and Safdar 1973).

Clinically, jaundice due to anabolic steroids usually appears in the first few weeks of medication, preceded by symptoms of malaise, anorexia, nausea, and pruritus. The serum alkaline phosphatase is raised in two-thirds of cases, but rarely, in contrast with drugs causing cholestatic hepatitis, are values over three times normal (Zimmerman 1963). The transaminases may also be elevated, the effect apparently being dose-dependent (Ticktin and Zimmerman 1966). Histologically, the predominant lesion is bile stasis with little or no parenchymal damage (Schaffner *et al.* 1959), and the reason for the often disproportionate transaminase elevation is not clear.

Although frank cholestatic jaundice is a relatively uncommon complication of anabolic steroid therapy, bromsulphthalein (BSP) retention occurs frequently (Marquardt *et al.* 1961) and seems to be a dose-dependent phenomenon (Kory *et al.* 1959). The defect appears to lie in the excretion of BSP from the hepatocyte into the bile (Schoenfield and Foulk 1964), and a similar excretory defect has been demonstrated for bilirubin (Arias 1963). A major contributory factor appears to be a defect in bile secretion (Bassan *et al.* 1971; Despopoulos 1971; Paumgartner *et al.* 1976).

Cholestatic reactions to danazol have been reported (Silva *et al.* 1989; Xiol *et al.* 1989). In some patients, a positive lymphocyte transformation test to the drug suggests a hypersensitivity reaction (Silva *et al.* 1989).

Oestrogen and androgen antagonists

Abnormalities in liver function tests have been observed in patients taking cyproterone, and a case of fulminant hepatic failure due to this drug has also been reported (Levesque *et al.* 1989). Another antiandrogenic drug, flutamide, which is not chemically related to cyproterone, has also been described as causing acute hepatitis (Moller *et al.* 1990). Cholestatic jaundice has been reported occasionally in patients taking tamoxifen (Blackburn *et al.* 1984).

Granulomatous infiltration

Granulomatous infiltration of the liver can be due to a number of drugs (Table 11.3), sometimes without other hepatic abnormalities but more commonly accompanying an acute hepatitic or cholestatic reaction to a drug. Some of these reactions are accompanied by a generalized granulomatous reaction throughout the body (e.g. penicillin, some of the sulphonamides, phenylbutazone), whereas other reactions involve the liver exclusively (e.g. allopurinol, carbamazepine, quinidine).

TABLE 11.3
Drugs producing hepatic granulomata

Antibacterials	
Isoniazid	McMaster and Hennigar 1981
Nitrofurantoin	Sippel and Agger 1981
Penicillin	McMaster and Hennigar 1981
Sulphonamides	Stewart and Johnson 1980
Anticonvulsants	
Carbamazepine	Davion *et al.* 1984; Swinburn *et al.* 1986
Phenytoin	Mullick and Ishak 1980; Gaffey *et al.* 1986
Antirheumatic	
Allopurinol	Boyer *et al.* 1977; Vanderstigel 1986
Aspirin	McMaster and Hennigar 1981
Gold	Harats *et al.* 1985
Phenylbutazone	Benjamin *et al.* 1981; Ishak *et al.* 1977
Antiulcer	
Ranitidine	Offit and Sojka 1984
Cardiac/antihypertensive	
Diltiazem	Sarachek *et al.* 1985
Disopyramide	Koch *et al.* 1985
Hydralazine	Jori and Peschle 1973
Methyldopa	McMaster and Hennigar 1981
Procainamide	McMaster and Hennigar 1981
Quinidine	Katz *et al.* 1983
Oral hypoglycaemics	
Chlorpropamide	Rigberg *et al.* 1976
Tolbutamide	Bloodworth and Hamwei 1961
Others	
Chlorpromazine	Irani and Dobbins 1979

Diagnosis of a drug-induced granulomatous liver lesion depends on exclusion of other causes, because there are no features that are particularly specific for these lesions when they are produced by drugs. They are generally situated in the periportal areas and, with the exception of lesions induced by gold, do not contain particulate material. The concomitant presence of other liver lesions, particularly focal hepatocyte necrosis, cholestasis, and eosinophilic infiltration, is a pointer to a drug-induced aetiology.

Fibrin ring granulomata, previously considered to be unique for Q fever, are now known to complicate allopurinol therapy (Vanderstigel *et al.* 1986).

Chronic liver disease

Active chronic hepatitis

Active chronic hepatitis can be produced by many drugs (Maddrey and Boitnott 1977), all of which can also produce an acute hepatitis. The two agents now most commonly implicated are methyldopa and nitrofurantoin.

Methyldopa

This drug can produce an illness indistinguishable from autoimmune active chronic hepatitis with hyperglobulinemia and autoantibodies. The latter lesion usually develops after several months' methyldopa therapy, particularly if it is continued after the onset of signs of hepatocellular dysfunction (Goldstein *et al.* 1973; Hyer and Knell 1977; Balacz and Kovac 1981). In one reported case there was progression from acute to chronic liver damage after the drug had been stopped (Schweitzer and Peters 1974). A generalized systemic illness with fever and hepatic dysfunction has been attributed to methyldopa (Stanley and Mijch 1986). The illness resolved on drug withdrawal.

In vitro studies have demonstrated that the drug is converted by microsomal enzymes to an unstable metabolite which binds to its site of formation (Dybing *et al.* 1976). A direct toxic effect of the drug could form the basis for the high incidence of mild hepatic injury (up to 5 per cent) revealed by monitoring of liver function tests during drug administration (Elkington *et al.* 1969). An immunological basis for active chronic hepatitis from the drug is suggested by the observation that patients with this complication had antibodies directed against liver cell membrane antigens altered by a metabolite of the drug (Neuberger *et al.* 1985).

Nitrofurantoin

This urinary antibiotic has been reported as the cause of a condition resembling autoimmune active chronic hepatitis in a few patients who had mostly received the drug for periods of 6 months or longer (Sharp *et al.* 1980). The disease has a predilection for women and may be accompanied by a lupus-like syndrome. Pulmonary infiltrates have also been described in association with it.

Dantrolene

Histological changes typical of chronic active hepatitis have been reported in five of nine patients with hepatic reactions to dantrolene sodium, used for the management of spasticity (Utili *et al.* 1977). Three of these had cirrhosis and, in one, progression to cirrhosis was revealed by serial liver biopsies over a period of 2 years. Wilkinson and others (1979) noted a marked disparity between the severity of the hepatic lesions and the clinical symptoms; consequently, liver function tests should be routinely monitored to prevent insidious progression to cirrhosis.

Isoniazid

Active chronic hepatitis, which may progress to cirrhosis, has been recorded amongst the spectrum of hepatic complications produced by this antituberculous drug (Black *et al.* 1975). The lesion is not characteristically associated with mechanisms of hypersensitivity (Maddrey and Boitnott 1973; Mitchell *et al.* 1976*b*), suggesting that the lesion is due to a direct toxic effect of a metabolite of the drug.

Clometacin

This analgesic is widely used in France and is probably the major cause of drug-induced active chronic hepatitis in that country (Pessayre and Larrey 1988). The onset is often insidious and is frequently associated with manifestations of hypersensitivity; serum autoantibodies are frequently found. Histologically, giant multinucleated hepatocytes have been observed in a number of cases, and it is suggested that they may be a histological marker of the condition.

Oxyphenisatin

This laxative has now been withdrawn from many countries in the world because of its high propensity to cause active chronic hepatitis, but in countries where it is still available this complication continues to be seen (Teh *et al.* 1988). The latent period varies from 6 months to 2 years and rechallenge with the drug leads to a prompt return of symptoms (Reynolds *et al.* 1971).

The drug is toxic to hepatocytes in tissue culture and this toxicity is enhanced by docusate (Dioctyl), with which it is frequently combined medicinally (Dujovne and Shoeman 1972). The latter drug, which has detergent properties, may facilitate the passage of oxyphenisatin across hepatocyte membranes and, additionally, may interfere with its excretion into the bile (Dujovne and Shoeman 1972).

Other drugs

Two case reports (Johnson and Tolman 1977; Bonkowsky *et al.* 1978), have implicated paracetamol in doses between 3–4 g per day as a cause of active chronic hepatitis. The causative role of the drug was by no means proven, however, in either case. In a survey of patients with active chronic hepatitis, there was no evidence that paracetamol was an important factor either in the initiation or exacerbation of hepatic damage, although the doses taken were small (Neuberger et al. 1980a).

Other agents that have been implicated in the pathogenesis of active chronic hepatitis include benzarone (Babany et al. 1987), captopril (Bellary et al. 1989), diclofenac (Mazeika and Ford 1989), etretinate (Weiss et al. 1985), halothane (Thomas 1974), propylthiouracil (Fedotin and Lefer 1975), and sulphonamides (Tonder et al. 1974). Naturally occurring disease in patients who happened to be exposed to these drugs cannot be excluded in any of these cases, as with the reports associated with paracetamol (see above).

Management of drug-induced active chronic hepatitis

It is vitally important to take a careful drug history in all patients presenting with this lesion. If the offending agent is withdrawn, liver damage resolves, albeit slowly, over a period of weeks. Conversely, if the drug is continued, liver damage progresses even if the patient is treated with steroids or immunosuppressives or both of these (Maddrey and Boitnott 1977).

Hepatic fibrosis and cirrhosis

Methotrexate

This antimetabolite, which acts by inhibition of dihydrofolate reductase, has a well-established potential for hepatotoxicity. The early liver lesion comprises patchy hepatocellular necrosis with infiltration by large fat droplets and inflammation which is predominantly periportal in distribution (Lewis and Schiff 1988). Collagen deposition in the space of Disse and lysosomal abnormalities can be seen on electron microscopy in all patients receiving the drug (Bjorkmann et al. 1988), even if light microscopic appearances are normal (Aponte and Petrelli 1988). Progression of collagen deposition results in macroscopic fibrosis in periportal areas, and ultimately cirrhosis can develop (Nyfors 1977; Zachariae et al. 1980; Ashton et al. 1982). These abnormalities rarely result in symptoms and biochemical liver function tests usually show little or no abnormality (Shergy et al. 1988; Zachariae et al. 1987).

Development of methotrexate-induced liver damage is dose-related and the high (up to 25 per cent) incidence of hepatic fibrosis and cirrhosis reported in early studies with the drug reflected the use of high daily doses of the drug (up to 50 mg per week) (Dahl et al. 1971; Nyfors

1977; Zachariae et al. 1980). There is also good evidence that daily dosing is more hepatotoxic than giving the same cumulative amount in weekly doses (Dahl et al. 1971; Podurgiel et al. 1973; Weinstein et al. 1973). Current therapeutic regimens for psoriasis and rheumatoid arthritis comprise 15 mg per week or less, and with such doses the incidence of liver damage is minimal (Lanse et al. 1985; van de Kerkhof et al. 1985; Leonard et al. 1987; Szanto et al. 1987; Lewis and Schiff 1988).

In addition to total dose and the dosing regimen, other factors seem to be important in determining the susceptibility to methotrexate-induced liver injury. These include underlying liver disease, alcohol abuse, and the combination of obesity and diabetes mellitus (Nyfors 1986; Lewis and Schiff 1988). In most reported series, liver injury has been seen with cumulative doses in excess of 1.5–2 g (Tobias and Auerback 1973; Lewis and Schiff 1988) and there is some evidence that patients with psoriasis may be more susceptible to this complication than those with rheumatoid disease (Szanto et al. 1987; Kevat et al. 1988; Lewis and Schiff 1988; Bjorkman et al. 1988; Shergy et al. 1988). This may be because the prevalence of alcohol abuse is higher in psoriatic patients than those with rheumatoid arthritis. In most of the studies quoted, however, patients with the latter condition had received lower cumulative doses of methotrexate than those with psoriasis.

Current recommendations of the American College of Gastroenterology (Lewis and Schiff 1988) are that patients with psoriasis should undergo a liver biopsy before methotrexate is started; the presence of significant liver disease, particularly if the patient is actively drinking or has received prior hepatotoxic drugs (e.g. vitamin A), are relative contraindications (Lewis and Schiff 1988). While biochemical liver function tests do not give a particularly sensitive guide to the degree of underlying liver damage, it is recommended that these be monitored at 3–6 monthly intervals and that liver biopsy should be repeated after every 1.5–2 g cumulative dose of the drug.

Current recommendations for patients with rheumatoid arthritis are considerably more relaxed, and few rheumatologists in the United Kingdom would carry out liver biopsies on such patients, because of the very low risk of hepatotoxicity. In the USA, however, a more aggressive screening regimen has been advocated (Lewis and Schiff 1988).

Employment of hepatic ultrasound scanning may be useful in monitoring; a normal scan excludes pathological changes, whereas if it is abnormal, biopsy is needed to differentiate fatty change from fibrosis and cirrhosis (Miller et al. 1985; Coulson et al. 1987). Dynamic tests of liver function, such as galactose elimination (Lenler Peterson *et al.* 1982), and other biochemical tests, including measurement of antipyrine metabolism (Williams *et al.* 1987; Paramsothy *et al.* 1988) and procollagen peptide as an index of fibrogenesis (Mitchell *et al.* 1990), are of limited value because of their lack of specificity.

Serial histological studies have shown that cirrhosis induced by methotrexate does not progress in an aggressive fashion even if the drug is continued, although complications, particularly with portal hypertension, can occasionally be seen (Zachariae *et al.* 1987).

Acute liver damage from methotrexate can also occasionally occur after high doses. (Weber *et al.* 1987; Clegg *et al.* 1989).

Nicotinic acid

Isolated reports of portal fibrosis associated with long-term therapy with nicotinamide or nicotinic acid have appeared in the literature (Kohn and Montes 1969; Winter and Boyer 1973). At present it is not possible to estimate the frequency of this complication and the mechanism is unknown.

Acute hepatocellular necrosis from the drug has also been described (Clementz and Holmes 1987; Knopp 1989; Mullin *et al.* 1989).

Vitamin A

See under Vascular lesions

Phospholipidosis and alcoholic hepatitis-like liver lesions

These liver lesions can complicate therapy with three antianginal/antiarrhythmic drugs: diethylaminoethoxyhexoestrol, perhexiline maleate, and amiodarone (Thaler 1988). These three agents are all amphiphilic, and can enter lysosomes, where they become trapped due to the acidic environment within these organelles, forming a stable complex with phospholipids. The accumulations can be demonstrated histochemically and by electron microscopy. The lesions are similar to those seen with the congenital lipid storage diseases such as Tay–Sachs disease. The abnormalities are usually asymptomatic but progression, for reasons unknown, can occur to an alcoholic hepatitis-like lesion with polymorphonuclear cell infiltrates and Mallory bodies, resembling alcoholic hepatitis; fibrosis and cirrhosis can ensue.

Diethylaminoethoxyhexoestrol

The first reports of hepatic damage from this coronary vasodilator emanated from Japan, where abnormal phospholipid storage was also noted in lungs, myocardium, and spleen (Oda *et al.* 1970; Thaler 1988). Clinically, patients presented with hepatomegaly, pyrexia, oedema, and weight loss and some cases progressed to cirrhosis with a fatal outcome.

Perhexilene maleate

Liver damage from this drug appears after several months or even years of treatment and may be associated with other clinical manifestations of toxicity, including peripheral neuropathy due to accumulation of drug–phospholipid complexes (Pessayre *et al.* 1979; Hay and Gwynne 1983). The drug is metabolised by hydroxylation, and individuals of poor hydroxylator phenotype are particularly predisposed to both hepatic and neurological complications from this drug (Morgan *et al.* 1984) Cirrhosis can ensue (Pessayre *et al.* 1979; Pieterse *et al.* 1983).

Amiodarone

Mild elevations in serum transaminases occur in 25 per cent of patients receiving this drug (Geneve *et al.* 1989), although other causes could often be invoked. Hepatotoxicity appears to be dose-related, and other manifestations of amiodarone toxicity including corneal deposits, pulmonary fibrosis, neuropathy, and thyroid dysfunction may be associated (Rigas *et al.* 1986). Progression to cirrhosis can occur if the drug is not withdrawn (Simon *et al.* 1984; Babany *et al.* 1986*b*; Rigas *et al.* 1986; Rumessen 1986; Guigui *et al.* 1988; Lewis *et al.* 1990). Provided this stage has not been reached, the liver abnormality regresses on withdrawal of the drug, but this can take many months, presumably because of the slow rate at which intracellular drug-phospholipid complexes can be mobilized. Acute liver damage from amiodarone has also been reported (Yagupsky *et al.* 1985; Geneve *et al.* 1989).

It is not known whether the phospholipid inclusions are important in the pathogenesis of alcoholic hepatitis-like lesions. A morphological study of patients receiving the drug in doses of 200–400 mg per day for 4 months to 15 years, suggests that they are not. Lysosomal phospholipid inclusions were found in the livers of all patients receiving the drug, regardless of whether or not there was other evidence of liver damage (Guigui *et al.* 1988). The drug may, rarely, cause acute hepatic necrosis (Stevenson *et al.* 1989) or acute fatty infiltration resembling Reye's syndrome (Jones *et al.* 1988). These complications are almost certainly very rare.

Nifedipine

A similar spectrum of hepatic abnormalities has been described with nifedipine (Babany *et al.* 1989).

Chronic cholestasis

A syndrome that clinically and histologically resembles primary biliary cirrhosis (PBC) occurs in association with a number of drugs, all of which have been shown to produce acute cholestasis. Antimitochondrial antibodies are usually absent. The drugs most frequently implicated have been the phenothiazines, in particular chlorpromazine (Walker and Combes 1966; Ishak and Irey 1972). In up to 7 per cent of patients affected in this way, cholestasis may have a prolonged course. Chronic cholestasis has also been attributed to tolbutamide (Gregory *et al*. 1967; Bridges and Pittman 1980), thiabendazole (Manivel *et al*. 1987; Roy *et al*. 1989), imipramine (Horst *et al*. 1980), phenytoin (Taylor *et al*. 1984), and benoxaprofen (Babbs and Warnes 1986; Babani *et al*. 1986*a*).

The syndrome may be manifested either as chronic cholestatic jaundice with its attendant complications or just as persistently abnormal liver function tests (predominantly alkaline phosphatase) with no symptoms or signs. In either situation liver function usually returns to normal, although this may take several years (Read *et al*. 1961). In some cases, abnormalities can be permanent, albeit subclinical, as for imipramine (Horst *et al*. 1980). In others, the disease may progress; two reported cases of chronic cholestasis associated with treatment with thiabendazole required liver transplantation (Manivell *et al*. 1987; Roy *et al*. 1989). Prolonged cholestasis with progressive liver disease has been reported from a combination of chlorpropamide and erythromycin (Geubel *et al*. 1988) and chlorpromazine and valproic acid (Bach *et al*. 1989*a*). Mutual potentiation of the effects of two hepatotoxic drugs was presumably involved, but the mechanisms have not been identified.

Sclerosing cholangitis

Bile duct strictures resembling those seen in primary sclerosing cholangitis are frequently seen in patients treated by infusion of floxuridine into the common hepatic artery for treatment of hepatic metastases from colorectal carcinoma (Kemeny *et al*. 1985; Anderson *et al*. 1986). It generally develops several months after the start of the chemotherapy.

In some patients, bile duct strictures appear to be reversible (Kemeny *et al*. 1985) but in most they persist despite cessation of treatment (Hohn *et al*. 1985; Botet *et al*. 1985) and may progress (Schlangen and Wils 1984; Kemeny *et al*. 1985). Cirrhosis may develop (Pettavel *et al*. 1986). Strictures typically involve the upper part of the common bile duct and the confluence of the right and left hepatic ducts, sparing the distal common bile duct

(Anderson *et al*. 1986; Dikengil *et al*. 1986). This differs from the situation often seen in primary sclerosing cholangitis, in which the distal common bile duct is often involved.

The pathogenesis is unknown but ischaemic damage to the upper part of the common bile duct is currently thought to be the most likely explanation (Anderson *et al*. 1986; Dikengil *et al*. 1986). There is no established treatment, but steroid infusion has been proposed (Paquette *et al*. 1987).

Vascular lesions of the liver

Budd–Chiari syndrome

Oral contraceptives

Several case reports have suggested an association between use of oral contraceptives and hepatic vein thrombosis (Lalonde *et al*. 1982; Maddrey 1987*b*). Valla and colleagues (1986), in a case–control study of 33 women with Budd–Chiari syndrome, identified a relative risk of 2.37 for this complication in users of oral contraceptives, a figure very close to that for other vascular complications of 'the pill'. Current evidence suggests that, as with other vascular complications, oral contraceptives lead to hepatic vein thrombosis by exacerbating an underlying thrombogenic condition (Valla *et al*. 1986).

Dacarbazine

This alkylating agent usually produces thrombotic occlusion of small and medium-sized hepatic veins (see below), but cases of fulminant Budd–Chiari syndrome have also been described (Runne *et al*. 1980; Feaux de Lacroix *et al*. 1983).

Veno-occlusive disease

Veno-occlusive disease (VOD) is characterized by non-thrombotic concentric narrowing of the lumen of central hepatic veins by connective tissue. It occurs in the absence of obstruction of the large hepatic veins (Bras and Brandt 1979). Severe centrilobular congestion and necrosis reflects the venous blockage. Progression to extensive central fibrosis with nodular regeneration and ultimately cirrhosis may take place.

Pyrrolizidine alkaloids

These alkaloids are present in numerous plant species, but hepatotoxicity in man most commonly results from consumption of plants or extracts of plants belonging to the families Heliotropium, Crotalaria, and Senecio (Huxtable 1980).

Poisoning may present as an epidemic if it is due to contamination of food by alkaloid-containing plants (Wilmot and Robinson 1920; Mohabbat *et al.* 1976). Sporadic cases are generally due to inadvertent self-poisoning from consumption of alkaloid-containing plant extracts, with alleged health-giving properties (Ridker *et al.* 1985; Bach *et al.* 1989*b*; Ridker and McDermott 1989*a,b*; Katz and Saibil 1990). Particularly frequently implicated in this respect are infusions or tablets containing comfrey (Weston *et al.* 1987; Abbott 1988; Ridker and McDermott 1989*a,b*). A fatal case of VOD has been described in a baby whose mother took comfrey-containing herbal tea throughout pregnancy (Roulet *et al.* 1988). The mother suffered no ill effects.

Antineoplastic and immunosuppressive agents

Azathioprine

Numerous reports clearly implicate azathioprine and the chemically related drug mercaptopurine as a cause of VOD (Clark *et al.* 1960; A.E. Read *et al.* 1986; Katzka *et al.* 1986; Haboubi *et al.* 1988; Liano *et al.* 1989). Most patients have been renal transplant recipients receiving corticosteroids, and there is a striking preponderance of males. The onset is typically delayed for at least 6 months after starting the drug and may be much later than this. The mode of presentation is different from that associated with other causes of VOD, with prominent jaundice and histological features of both cholestasis and centrilobular necrosis. Sinusoidal and perivenular fibrosis, peliosis hepatis, and nodular regenerative hyperplasia can sometimes be seen as associated pathological lesions (Haboubi *et al.* 1988); it is possible that they are aetiologically linked (see below).

Rapid deterioration with death from hepatic failure and complications of portal hypertension may occur or the disease may take a more prolonged course. Mortality is high, but partial regression of the lesion after drug withdrawal, particularly in the less fulminant cases, has been reported (Katzka *et al.* 1986).

Although azathioprine-induced VOD is usually seen in renal transplant recipients, it has also been reported in a patient with rheumatoid arthritis after 3 months' treatment with the drug (Lemley *et al.* 1989).

Dacarbazine

Patients receiving this drug for melanoma seem particularly prone to develop injury to small and medium-sized hepatic veins. The reported incidence is between 1–3 per cent (Dancygier *et al.* 1983; Erichsen and Jonsson 1984; Ceci *et al.* 1988; Marsh 1989). The vascular lesion induced by dacarbazine differs from classical VOD in that it is thrombotic. Cases of Budd–Chiari syndrome (see above) probably represent retrograde extension of thrombus into the main hepatic veins.

The mechanism of this reaction may be direct toxicity to vascular endothelium, but the occurrence of eosinophilic infiltration in the liver and other organs in the reported cases and the fact that the reaction occurs during a second course of treatment, the first having been well tolerated, has led to speculation that a hypersensitivity mechanism is involved (McClay *et al.* 1987).

Thioguanine

This drug is chemically related to azathioprine and mercaptopurine. It has been implicated in the pathogenesis of VOD (Krivoy *et al.* 1982; Gill *et al.* 1982), but since it was generally used in association with other antineoplastic drugs a definite causal association cannot be proved. Liver histology may revert to normal on drug withdrawal (Krivoy *et al.* 1982).

Other antineoplastic drugs

A combination of cyclophosphamide and cyclosporin appears to be a potentially potent cause of this complication; in one series, 2 out of 10 patients receiving both drugs developed VOD, in contrast to none of 200 receiving the same dose of cyclophosphamide alone (Deeg *et al.* 1986).

Other drugs implicated include adriamycin (Kun and Camitta 1978; Craft and Pembrey 1987), vincristine (Hansen *et al.* 1982), carmustine (McIntyre *et al.* 1981), and mitomycin (Gottfried and Sulidowsky 1982; Craft and Pembrey 1987).

Irradiation and conditioning for bone marrow transplantation

Radiation damage to the liver is a common cause of VOD and is a dose-related complication, rarely being seen with doses below 30 Gy unless the patient is receiving concomitant chemotherapy (Ingold *et al.* 1965; Fajardo and Colby 1980). Damage is usually localized to the section of the liver that has been exposed (Lansing *et al.* 1968) and usually manifests itself within 2–5 weeks of irradiation. Anticoagulation has been proposed for prophylaxis (Lightdale *et al.* 1979) because there is evidence that activation of coagulation processes may play a role in pathogenesis (Fajardo and Colby 1980), but the value of this remains to be established.

Conditioning for bone marrow transplantation with irradiation and cytotoxic drugs, usually including cyclophosphamide, is the major cause of VOD. The condition usually presents within 4 weeks of transplantation with jaundice, right upper quadrant pain, and ascites. McDonald and colleagues (1986) reported an incidence of 21 per cent in 255 patients undergoing bone marrow transplantation for malignancy, and in their analysis significant risk factors for VOD were age over 15, an underlying malignancy other than acute lymphocytic leukaemia, and underlying chronic liver disease. The dose of irradiation associated with this complication (usually about 10 Gy) is lower than that required to cause VOD in patients not receiving antineoplastic drugs (Fajardo and Colby 1980), but the drug regimen does not appear to be important in determining susceptibility (McDonald *et al.* 1984). The condition does not seem to be a complication of bone marrow transplantation *per se* because the incidence of VOD in patients transplanted for aplastic anaemia is low (Rollins 1986).

Oestrogens

Although oestrogens can cause the Budd–Chiari syndrome, their role in producing VOD is controversial. In an interesting study, Setchell and colleagues (1987) found a high incidence of VOD amongst cheetahs in a zoo where there was also a high frequency of reproductive failure amongst this species. The latter was eventually traced to the fact that the animals' feeds contained plant-based oestrogens. When this was remedied, procreation resumed and there was a resolution of the hepatic abnormalities. Based on these observations, the authors suggested that oestrogens were the cause of VOD, although it has been pointed out that other dietary factors may also have been involved (Zimmerman and Ishak 1987). Synthetic oestrogens have also been implicated (Saint-Marc-Girardin *et al.* 1983).

Other agents

Cysteamine has been reported as the cause of VOD in a child treated with it for cystinosis (Avner *et al.* 1983) and the complication has also been reported following administration of an intravenous preparation of vitamin E in an infant (Bove *et al.* 1985).

Sinusoidal lesions

Sinusoidal dilatation

Dilatation of hepatic sinusoids has most frequently been associated with use of oral contraceptives; it is usually asymptomatic (Molleken *et al.* 1979) but, very rarely, it may be associated with right upper quadrant pain with jaundice and elevations in transaminases and alkaline phosphatase (Winkler and Poulsen 1975; Weinberger *et al.* 1985). The condition regresses after drug withdrawal.

A similar abnormality can be seen with azathioprine (Gerlag *et al.* 1985; Gerlag and van-Hooff 1987).

Peliosis hepatis

This liver lesion is characterized by dilated blood-filled cysts, bordered by hepatocytes. The condition is classically associated with chronic inflammatory conditions, particularly tuberculosis, and is usually an incidental finding at postmortem, having caused no symptoms during life. Occasionally, however, it may cause right upper quadrant abdominal pain due to liver enlargement or may rupture with haemoperitoneum (Yanoff and Rawson 1964).

Oral contraceptives

Peliosis hepatis has been reported in women taking oral contraceptives (Pliskin 1975; Kerlin *et al.* 1983), in whom it might represent an exaggerated form of the sinusoidal dilatation described above. In most cases, however, the vascular lesion was adjacent to a liver tumour and could well have been caused by localized venous obstruction.

Androgenic/anabolic steroids

Sinusoidal dilatation and peliosis hepatis in the absence of other liver lesions have been demonstrated in the livers of female-to-male transexuals receiving orally active anabolic steroids, which suggests that these compounds, which are chemically related to the synthetic steroids in oral contraceptives, have a true potential to produce these lesions (Westaby *et al.* 1976; Paradinas *et al.* 1977). Other reports have generally centred around patients with conditions such as rheumatoid arthritis or Hodgkin's disease, often accompanied by severe sepsis, and the vascular abnormality could have been caused by the disease rather than the drug (Naeim *et al.* 1973; Bagheri and Boyer 1974; Lyon *et al.* 1984; Wakabayashi *et al.* 1985).

Azathioprine

Azathioprine-associated peliosis hepatis has been reported mainly in renal transplant recipients, in whom it may occur alone or in combination with other abnormalities including veno-occlusive disease, perisinusoidal fibrosis, and nodular regenerative hyperplasia (Marrubio and Danielson 1975; Degott *et al.* 1978; Haboubi *et al.* 1988); portal hypertension with oesophageal varices and ascites can occur in association with it (Gerlag and van-Hooff 1987; Haboubi *et al.* 1988). The chemically related drug thioguanine can also produce peliosis (Larrey *et al.* 1988c).

Perisinusoidal fibrosis

This lesion is characterized by accumulation of collagen within the space of Disse and is seen most commonly in association with chronic alcohol abuse. The lesion has also been seen in association with azathioprine or mercaptopurine treatment of renal transplant recipients (Nataf *et al.* 1979), often in association with other pathological changes, including veno-occlusive disease, peliosis hepatis, and nodular regenerative hyperplasia (Haboubi *et al.* 1988).

Vitamin A

The recommended daily intake for this vitamin is 5000 IU for adult males and 4000 IU for non-pregnant adult females (Roenigk 1988). Ninety per cent of vitamin A is stored in the liver in Ito cells, which are modified fibroblasts lining the sinusoids. Supplements of vitamin A have been used in the treatment of psoriasis, in which the skin lesion bears some resemblance to that seen in vitamin A deficiency. Other less defined indications for vitamin A supplements include the prophylaxis of cancer and arthritis, and preparations containing this compound are readily available at some 'Health Food' shops (Olson 1983; Davidson 1984; Inkeles *et al.* 1986). When using such preparations, it is easy to exceed the recommended daily allowances by a factor of 10 or more, and it is at this level (around 50 000 IU per day for 2 years or more) that toxic symptoms may occur (Minuk *et al.* 1988). Patients with renal failure may be more susceptible, however, and there is a report of such a patient on dialysis who developed toxicity after supplementation of approximately 4000 units per day (Shmunes 1974).

Clinical manifestations of vitamin A toxicity include general malaise and weakness, alopecia, muscle wasting, pruritus, exfoliative dermatitis, and hepatotoxicity. The early liver lesion comprises fatty infiltration with large vesicles in Ito cells; subsequently perisinusoidal fibrosis may develop (Zafrani *et al.* 1984). This appears to occur as a result of Ito cells being transformed into fibroblasts with increased collagen production (Kent *et al.* 1976), a sequence of events which is also associated with alcohol-induced perisinusoidal fibrosis. Indeed, there is evidence that alcohol and vitamin A act synergistically to produce this lesion in experimental animals. Continuation of vitamin A eventually leads to cirrhosis (Jacques *et al.* 1979), whereas if it is stopped the liver lesion slowly regresses (Leo and Lieber 1983). Cases of non-cirrhotic portal hypertension have also been described as a consequence of obstruction to portal venules (Baadsgaard and Thomsen 1983; Guarascio *et al.* 1983).

Etretinate

This is an analogue of retinoic acid that does not accumulate in the liver in significant amounts. It has shown to be effective in the treatment of psoriasis. Because of the problems with vitamin A its effect on the liver have been carefully studied. The results obtained so far are a little difficult to interpret; some hepatic fibrosis has been observed, but in these cases the picture has been complicated either by alcohol abuse or by prior use of vitamin A or methotrexate (Glazer *et al.* 1982; Camuto *et al.* 1987; Roenigk 1988; Thirumoorthy and Shupack 1988; Roenigk 1989).

Non-cirrhotic portal hypertension

Obstruction of the portal venules in the absence of cirrhosis has been reported in association with a number of drugs, mainly those causing perisinusoidal fibrosis. These include vitamin A (Baadsgaard and Thomsen 1983; Guarascio *et al.* 1983), methotrexate (du Vivier *et al.* 1974), azathioprine (Podurgiel *et al.* 1973), and inorganic arsenicals (Datta *et al.* 1979).

Nodular regenerative hyperplasia

This condition is characterized by nodules of apparently regenerating hepatocytes scattered throughout the parenchyma. Intervening areas of atrophy are often seen, implying that the condition arises secondary to localized hepatocyte injury. It may be complicated by portal hypertension, presumably due to pressure effects, and it has mainly been described as a complication of azathioprine or mercaptopurine therapy in renal transplant recipients (Haboubi *et al.* 1988), but also in rheumatoid arthritis (Wanless *et al.* 1980; Stromeyer and Ishak 1981).

Abnormalities in liver function tests are seen in a high proportion of patients affected by the toxic-oil syndrome (Diaz de Rojas *et al.* 1985). In a few of these, nodular regenerative hyperplasia has been observed, with symptoms of mild jaundice, and sometimes signs of portal hypertension, appearing 19–37 months after exposure (Solis-Herrazo *et al.* 1986). Vascular lesions including centrizonal fibrosis, sinusoidal dilatation, and veno-occlusive disease may also coexist, suggesting a vascular aetiology for the hepatic nodules.

Relationship between peliosis hepatis, veno-occlusive disease, perisinusoidal fibrosis, and regenerative hyperplasia

Since these lesions can frequently coexist, it has been proposed that they may be aetiologically related. A recently proposed hypothesis (Haboubi *et al.* 1988) is that the primary damage is to sinusoidal endothelium;

when this affects the hepatic venules, it leads to fibrosis secondary to leakage of blood, and eventual obliteration of the vessels. When it affects sinusoidal cells, peliosis hepatis could result; an additional cause may be obstruction at sinusoid-central vein junctions from prolapsed hepatocytes, and there is electron microscope evidence to support this hypothesis in lesions associated with anabolic steroids (Paradinas *et al.* 1977). Nodular regenerative hyperplasia could result from liver cell regeneration consequent upon ischaemic damage. Additional factors may be compression from these nodules as well as increased sinusoidal pressure as a result of fibrosis and changes to endothelial cells.

Lesions of the hepatic artery

Hepatic infarction has been described in association with use of oral contraceptives (Jacobs 1984). This may be related to intimal hyperplasia in vessels throughout the body, which has been described in association with the agents, as well as in association with pregnancy.

Portal vein thrombosis

Along with other thrombotic complications of oral contraceptives, thrombosis of the portal vein has been the subject of a few case reports (Rose 1972; Capron *et al.* 1981).

Spontaneous rupture of the liver

This extremely rare complication of pregnancy has also been described following use of oestrogens and oral contraceptives (Frederick *et al.* 1974; Bell *et al.* 1977).

Liver tumours

Adenoma

Oral contraceptives

Since the first report by Baum and colleagues (1973) of hepatic adenomata in long-term users of oral contraceptives, a large number of reports confirming this association have appeared (Edmondson *et al.* 1976; Mays and Christoperson 1984; Greer 1989). The upsurge in the numbers of this previously extremely rare tumour indicated that its association with oral contraceptives was more than a matter of chance. Hormone dependence is further suggested by its occasional appearance in pregnancy and the puerperium, when levels of gonadal steroids are high (Christopherson and Mays 1977), and the

association of a virtually identical picture in association with synthetic anabolic steroids (see below).

A characteristic feature of these tumours is their extreme vascularity. Histologically they show collections of dilated thin-walled blood vessels resembling peliosis hepatis and similar to the lesions found in association with anabolic steroids. As a result of this extreme vascularity, haemorrhage into the tumour or rupture with haemoperitoneum are common modes of presentation (Klatskin 1977; Kerlin *et al.* 1983; Mays and Christopherson 1984). In many cases, however, tumours may present as an asymptomatic abdominal mass or with episodes of upper abdominal pain, probably due to small haemorrhages into the tumour. Neuberger and others (1980*b*) have drawn attention to the protean manifestations of these neoplasms, which have variously been diagnosed as cholecystitis, peptic ulcer, myocardial ischaemia, or epigastric hernia for periods of up to 8 years. Two of their cases presented with obstructive jaundice due to compression of the common bile duct by the tumour. Of interest is the fact that in many cases hepatomegaly had been documented in the clinical records but no account of this finding had been taken in arriving at the initial diagnosis. Elevated levels of serum alkaline phosphatase were frequently seen, as with any hepatic space-occupying lesion, and the erythrocyte sedimentation rate (ESR) was often elevated; serum α-fetoprotein levels were invariably normal.

Management

The behaviour of oral contraceptive-induced hepatic adenomata is unpredictable, which makes it difficult to give dogmatic guidelines on management. Progression is likely if oral contraceptives are not discontinued, and in many cases regression of the lesion has been reported if the pill is stopped (Edmondson *et al.* 1977; Steinbrecker *et al.* 1981; Buhler *et al.* 1982), but this is not invariable (Marks *et al.* 1988) and in others progress to hepatocellular carcinoma has been described (Davis *et al.* 1975; Gordon *et al.* 1986). Whether or not this will occur appears to be independent of the presence of oestrogen receptors within tumour cells (Porter *et al.* 1987). Association of hepatic adenoma with other malignancy has also been described (Grigsby *et al.* 1987).

Because of these problems, if tumour resection is not carried out the patient should be carefully monitored with serial ultrasound or CT scans of the liver, or both. Radioisotope scans can be misleading as, classically, adenomata and carcinomas of the liver do not contain Kuppfer cells and give 'cold spots' on Tecnetium liver scans, whereas these cells are present in focal nodular hyperplasia (see below) which give 'hot spots'. This is not invariable, however, because Kuppfer cells have been demonstrated in hepatic adenomata (Z.D. Goodman *et al.* 1987).

Anabolic steroids

Orally active anabolic steroids, which are chemically closely related to the synthetic steroids used in oral contraceptives, may produce hepatic adenomata (Anthony 1975; Paradinas *et al.* 1977). As with the pill-induced lesions, these tumours are often highly vascular with associated areas of peliosis hepatis (q.v.), and spontaneous rupture can occur. Athletes who use anabolic steroids in short bursts do not appear to develop this complication but one body-builder who took them for 3 years presented with a ruptured hepatic adenoma (Creagh *et al.* 1988).

These liver lesions have mostly been associated with 17-alkylated preparations, but multiple adenomata have been described in a renal transplant recipient who had been taking testosterone enanthrate, which is not a 17-alkylated compound (Carrasco *et al.* 1985). Hepatic adenomas have been reported in association with danazol (Fermand *et al.* 1990).

Focal nodular hyperplasia

Oral contraceptives

This lesion has also been frequently reported as complicating long-term use of oral contraceptives (Scott *et al.* 1984; Hagay *et al.* 1988). Histologically, adenoma and focal nodular hyperplasia are readily distinguishable in typical cases, but in many of the tumours associated with oral contraceptives there has been overlap, and classification has been difficult because the two lesions may coexist. Many of these abnormalities are discovered incidentally but may present with rupture and haemoperitoneum in association with long-term oral contraceptive use (Kerlin *et al.* 1983; Mays and Christopherson 1984).

Whether or not this lesion is aetiologically related to oral contraceptives is a matter of controversy but, overall, epidemiological evidence is against it (Moesner *et al.* 1977; Klatskin 1977; Nime *et al.* 1979; Mays and Christopherson 1984). It can occur in both sexes and at any age, and the overall incidence has not altered with the introduction of oral contraceptives as it has for adenoma. It is, however, highly likely that oral contraceptives increase the vascularity of these lesions and predispose to the haemorrhage and rupture, which bring them to clinical attention. Similar considerations apply to the association of this lesion with anabolic steroids (Sweeney and Evans 1976).

Hepatocellular carcinoma

Oral contraceptives

Because of the large number of women who use oral contraceptives, it is more difficult to ascribe a causal relationship to these agents in primary hepatocellular carcinoma, which is much more common than benign adenoma. Overall, however, current evidence suggests that use of the oral contraceptive pill is a risk factor for the development of this tumour; Neuberger and colleagues (1986) calculated a relative risk of 4.4 in women who had used the pill for 8 years or more, while others found a higher (29-fold) risk in this group of women (Forman *et al.* 1986). The absolute numbers involved were small, however, and both groups found no increase in incidence in women using the pill for less than 8 years. A study from Italy proposed a relative risk factor of 1.8 for use of oral contraceptives up to 5 years, rising to 8.3 after this period (La Vecchia *et al.* 1989). Studies in countries where hepatitis B is endemic have failed to demonstrate an increased risk, presumably because the oncogenic effect of the hepatitis B virus overrides that of synthetic gonadal steroids (Kew *et al.* 1990).

Hepatocellular carcinomas associated with oral contraceptives tend to present more frequently with rupture, haemorrhage, and pain than those not associated, and the survival is longer (Hromas *et al.* 1985). Some of these tumours are histologically identical to fibrolamellar hepatomas, which are characteristically seen in young people and have a better prognosis (Goodman and Ishak 1982). Patients suffering from hepatocellular carcinoma associated with oral contraceptives characteristically do not have elevated circulating levels of α-fetoprotein.

Anabolic steroids

Since the first report (Recant and Lacy 1965), approximately 25 cases of liver tumour in long-term users of synthetic anabolic and androgenic steroids have been recorded (Paradinas *et al.* 1977). In all cases, patients had been taking 17-α-alkylated steroids for the treatment of bone marrow aplasia, the correction of impotence, or for the maintenance of secondary sexual characteristics in female-to-male transsexuals and, in general, the doses taken were high. It appears that patients with Fanconi's anaemia are especially susceptible, developing liver tumours after a shorter period than patients taking androgens for other reasons (Westaby *et al.* 1984).

The majority of androgen-related tumours have been described as histologically indistinguishable from primary hepatocellular carcinoma. Elevated serum levels of α-fetoprotein, however, do not occur with these neoplasms (Paradinas *et al.* 1977), while, in contrast, high values are found in 50 per cent of patients with hepato-cellular carcinoma arising in a non-cirrhotic liver (Johnson *et al.* 1978). Furthermore, with one exception (Farrell *et al.* 1975), metastases have not been documented with androgen associated tumours and regression has been reported following withdrawal of these agents (Johnson *et al.* 1972; Farrell *et al.* 1975).

A characteristic feature of androgen-associated tumours is that they are frequently highly vascular (Paradinas *et al.* 1977), and the surrounding liver parenchyma may be infiltrated with dilated, blood-filled cysts, characteristic of peliosis hepatis (Yanoff and Rawson 1964; Bernstein *et al.* 1973; Naeim *et al.* 1973), which may rupture either into the liver parenchyma or the peritoneal cavity.

Hepatocellular carcinoma has also been demonstrated as a complication of treatment with danazol for 2–4 years (Buamah 1985; Weill *et al.* 1988).

Liver tumours following Thorotrast

Thorotrast, a colloidal suspension of thorium dioxide, was used as a radiological contrast medium between the late 1920s and mid-1950s. It accumulates in the reticulo-endothelial system, particularly in the liver, and since thorium is radioactive, with a half-life of approximately 400 years, the local radiation dose can be substantial. This is reflected in a high incidence of malignancies, particularly involving the liver, reported at varying intervals after exposure (Dejgaard *et al.* 1984; Morant and Ruttner 1987). The characteristic tumour associated with Thorotrast is angiosarcoma (Benjamin and Albukerk 1982; Kojiro *et al.* 1982; Roat *et al.* 1982; Morant and Ruttner 1987), but cholangiocarcinoma (Khan 1985; Morant and Ruttner 1987) and hepatocellular carcinoma (Morant and Ruttner 1987) have also been reported. Leiomyosarcoma associated with cholangio-carcinoma, has also been described (Shurbaji *et al.* 1987). Because of the long latent period between exposure and presentation (35 years or even longer), cases are still being reported.

Miscellaneous

Hepatic damage during parenteral nutrition

Abnormal liver function tests are not uncommon in patients receiving parenteral nutrition, and elevations in serum bilirubin, alkaline phosphatase, and transaminases are seen in approximately 25 per cent of patients in the first 2 weeks of treatment (Bengoa *et al.* 1985). Liver biopsy changes are often non-specific, although in mal-nourished infants a predominantly cholestatic picture is characteristic (Whitington 1985). Fatty infiltration is seen when excessive carbohydrate is given; rates of carbohydrate infusion above hepatic oxidative capacity promote fat deposition (Georgieff *et al.* 1985). Otherwise, the pathogenesis of hepatic abnormalities in patients receiving parenteral nutrition is unclear; postulated mechanisms include the increased production of the hepatotoxic bile acid, lithocholic acid (Fouin-Fortunet *et al.* 1982), a cholestatic effect of amino acids (Vileisis *et al.* 1980), and an adverse effect of intestinal bacteria (Capron *et al.* 1983). The exacerbation of underlying liver disease, especially sclerosing cholangitis in patients with inflammatory bowel disease, must also be considered.

Abnormalities in liver function tests during parenteral nutrition generally resolve promptly on cessation of therapy, and are usually not regarded as an indication for withdrawing nutritional support. There have, however, been reports of progression to chronic liver disease with hepatic fibrosis, and even death, in patients receiving long-term nutritional support; careful monitoring is therefore important in this group (Bowyer *et al.* 1985).

Hepatic damage from alternative medicines

A wide spectrum of liver damage can be seen after ingestion of herbal preparations, many of which contain hepatotoxic alkaloids. Other preparations, particularly vitamin A, can cause severe liver damage when taken in large quantities over a prolonged period as prophylaxis against various ailments.

Bush teas and other preparations containing pyrrolizidine alkaloids

See under Veno-occlusive disease.

Seatone

This preparation is derived from an extract of the New Zealand green-lipped mussel, and its use has been advocated in rheumatoid arthritis (Gibson and Gibson 1981). A granulomatous hepatitis presenting with severe abdominal pain has been reported after taking the compound for 3 weeks (Ahern *et al.* 1980).

Pennyroyal oil

Pennyroyal oil is a traditional abortifacient in some parts of the USA; it contains a high concentration of pulegone. Its use has been associated with centrilobular hepatic necrosis (Sullivan *et al.* 1979).

Mistletoe

Hepatitis from a herbal preparation containing mistletoe, a homoeopathic remedy for nervous tension, was associated with lymphocytic infiltration and focal necrosis on liver biopsy. Liver damage improved when the preparation was stopped and relapsed when it was restarted (Harvey and Colin-Jones 1981).

References

Abbott, P.J. (1988). Comfrey: assessing the low-dose health risk. *Med. J. Aust.* 149, 678.

Adams, A.P. (1986). Halothane and the liver. *Br. Med. J.* 293, 1023.

Adams, J.D., Lauterburg, B.H., and Mitchell, J.R. (1983). Plasma glutathione and glutathione disulphide in the rat. Regulation and response to oxidative stress. *J. Clin. Invest.* 73, 124.

Aderka, D., Livni, E., Salomon, F., Weinberger, A., and Pinkhas, J. (1986). Use of macrophage inhibition factor and mast cell degranulation test for diagnosis of cloxacillin induced cholestasis. *Am. J. Gastroenterol.* 81, 567.

Adlercreutz, H. and Ikonen, E. (1964). Oral contraceptives and liver damage. *Br. Med. J.* ii, 1133.

Adlercreutz, H. and Tenhunen, R. (1970). Some aspects of the interaction between natural and synthetic female sex hormones and the liver. *Am. J. Med.* 49, 630.

Adriany, J. (1960). Toxicity to para-amino salicylic acid and isoniazid. *Dis. Chest* 38, 107.

AHCILD (1971). Report of the Ad Hoc Committee on Isoniazid and Liver Disease. Centre for Disease Control, Department of Health, Education and Welfare. March 17–18. *Am. Rev. Respir. Dis.* 104, 454.

Ahern, M.J., Milazzo, S.C., and Dymock, R. (1980). Granulomatous hepatitis and seatone. *Med. J. Aust.* ii, 151.

Alam, S.N., Roberts, R.J., and Fischer, L.J. (1977). Age-related differences in salicylamide and acetaminophen conjugation in man. *J. Pediatr.* 90, 130.

Albano, E., Poli, G., Chiarpotto, E., and Biasi, F. (1983). Paracetamol-stimulated lipid peroxidation in isolated rat and mouse hepatocytes. *Chem. Biol. Interact.* 47, 249.

Alberti-Flor, J J., Hernandez, M.E., Ferrer, J.P., Howell, S., and Jeffers, L. (1989). Fulminant liver failure and pancreatitis associated with the use of sulfamethoxazole-trimethoprim. *Am. J. Gastroenterol.* 84, 1577.

Aleem, A. and Lingam, V. (1987). Hepatotoxicity following treatment with Maprotiline. *J. Clin. Psychopharmacol.* 7, 54.

Al-Kawas, F.H., Seef, L.B., Berendson, R.A., Zimmermann, H.J., and Ishak, K.G. (1981). Allopurinol hepatotoxicity. Report of two cases and review of the literature. *Ann. Intern. Med.* 95, 588.

Allan, R.N., Thistle, J.L., and Hofmann, A.F. (1976). Lithocholic metabolism during chenotherapy for gallstone dissolution. 2. Absorption and sulphation. *Gut* 17, 413.

Andersen, H. and Kristiansen, E.S. (1959). Tofranil treatment of endogenous depressions. *Acta Psychiatr. Neurol. Scand.* 34, 4387.

Anderson, B.N. and Henrikson, I.R. (1978). Jaundice and eosinophilia associated with amitryptiline. *J. Clin. Psychiatry* 39, 730.

Anderson, S.D., Holley, H.C., Berland, L.L., Van Dyke, J.A., and Stanley, R.J. (1986). Causes of jaundice during hepatic artery infusion chemotherapy. *Radiology* 161, 439.

Anthony, P.P. (1975). Hepatoma associated with androgenic steroids. *Lancet* i, 685.

Antonelli, D., Koltun, B., and Barzilay, J. (1984). Acute hepatotoxic effect of disopyramide. *Chest* 8, 274.

Aponte, J. and Petrelli, M. (1988). Histopathologic findings in the liver of rheumatoid arthritis patients treated with long-term bolus methotrexate. *Arthritis Rheum.* 31, 1457.

Arias, I.M. (1963). Effects of a plant acid (icterogenin) and certain anabolic steroids on the hepatic metabolism of bilirubin and sulfobromthalein (BSP). *Ann. N.Y. Acad. Sci.* 104, 1014.

Ashton, R.E., Millward-Sadler, G.H., and White, J.E. (1982). Complications in methotrexate treatment of psoriasis with particular reference to liver fibrosis. *J. Invest. Dermatol.* 79, 229.

Australian Family Physician. (1973). The erythromycins. A further report from the Australian Drug Evaluation Committee. *Aust. Fam. Physician* 2, 558.

Avner, E.D., Ellis, D., and Jaffe, R. (1983). Veno-occlusive disease of the liver associated with cysteamine treatment of nephropathic cystinosis. *J. Pediatr.* 102, 793.

Baadsgaard, O. and Thomsen, N.H. (1983). Chronic vitamin A intoxication. Portal hypertension without hepatic cirrhosis in a patient with chronic vitamin A intoxication. *Dan. Med. Bull.* 30, 51.

Babany, G., Uzzan, F., Larrey, D., Degott, C., Bourgeois, P., Rene, E., *et al.* (1986a). Primary biliary cirrhosis after benoxaprofen. *Br. Med. J.* 293, 241.

Babany, G., Mallat, A., Zafrani, E.S., Saint-Marc-Girardin, M.F., Carcone, B., and Dhumeaux, D. (1986b). Chronic liver disease after low daily doses of amiodarone. Report of three cases. *J. Hepatol.* 3, 228.

Babany, G., Larrey, D., Pessayre, D., Degott, C., Rueff, B., and Benhamou, J.P. (1987). Chronic active hepatitis caused by benzarone. *J. Hepatol* 5, 332.

Babany, G., Uzzan, F., Larrey, D., Degott, C., Bourgeois, P., Rene, E., *et al.* (1989). Alcoholic-like liver lesions induced by nifedipine. *J. Hepatol* 9, 252.

Babbs, C. and Warnes, T.W. (1986). Primary biliary cirrhosis after benoxaprofen. *Br. Med. J.* 293, 241.

Bach, N., Thung, S.N., Schaffner, F., and Tobias, H. (1989a). Exaggerated cholestasis and hepatic fibrosis following simultaneous administration of chlorpromazine and sodium valproate. *Dig. Dis. Sci.* 34, 1303.

Bach, N., Thung, S.N., and Schaffner, F. (1989b). Comfrey herb tea-induced hepatic veno-occlusive disease. *Am. J. Med.* 87, 97.

Bachman, B.A., Boyd, W.P. Jr, and Brady, P.G. (1982). Erythromycin ethylsuccinate-induced cholestasis. *Am. J. Gastroenterol.* 77, 397.

Bagheri, M.S. and Boyer, J.L. (1974). Peliosis hepatis associated with androgenic-anabolic steroid therapy. *Ann. Intern. Med.* 81, 610.

Bailey, W.C., Taylor, S.L., Dascomb, H.E., Greenberg, H.B., and Ziskind, M.M. (1973). Disturbed hepatic function during isoniazid chemoprophylaxis. *Am. Rev. Respir. Dis.* 107, 523.

Bailey, W.C., Weill, H., Dekoven, T.A., Ziskind, M.M., Jackson, H.A., and Greenberg, H.B. (1974). The effect of isoniazid on transaminase levels. *Ann. Intern. Med.* 81, 200.

Bakris, G.L., Cross, P.D., and Hammarsten, J.E. (1983). Disopyramide-associated liver dysfunction. *Mayo Clin. Proc.* 58, 265.

Balacz, M. and Kovach, G. (1981). Chronic aggressive hepatitis after methyldopa treatment. Case report with electron microscope study. *Hepatogastroenterology* 28, 199.

Barancik, M., Brandborg, L.L., and Albion, M.J. (1967). Thioridazine-induced cholestasis. *JAMA* 200, 69.

Barbior, B.M. and Trey, C. (1970). Drug hepatitis. *Int. Anesthesiol. Clin.* 8, 175.

Bass, B.H. (1974). Jaundice associated with naproxen. *Lancet* i, 998.

Bassan, H., Kendler, J., Harimasuta, U., and Zimmerman, H.J. (1971). Effects of an anabolic steroid (narbothelone) on the function of the isolated perfused rat liver. *Biochem. Pharmacol.* 20, 1429.

Bassan, H., Zimmerman, H.J., Jacob, L., Gillespie, J., and Lukacs, L. (1986). Effects of three H2 antagonists on the isolated perfused rat liver. Correlation of bile flow changes with potential for causing hepatic disease in patients. *Biochem. Pharmacol.* 35, 4519.

Bassendine, M.F., Woodhouse, K.W., Bennett, M., and James, O.F. (1986). Dextropropoxyphene induced hepatotoxicity mimicking biliary tract disease. *Gut* 27, 444.

Bateman, D.N., Woodhouse, K.W., and Rawlins, M.D. (1984). Adverse reactions to *N*-acetylcysteine. *Hum. Toxicol.* 3, 393.

Baum, J.K., Holtz, F., Bookstein, J.J., and Klein, E.W. (1973). Possible association between benign hepatomas and oral contraceptives. *Lancet* ii, 926.

Beaudry, H.P., Brickman, H.F., Wise, M.B., and MacDougall, D. (1974). Liver enzyme disturbances during isoniazid chemoprophylaxis in children. *Am. Rev. Respir. Dis.* 110, 581.

Beever, I.W., Blair., I.A., and Brodies, M.J. (1982). Circulating hydrazine during treatment with isoniazid rifampicin in man. *Br. J. Clin. Pharmacol.* 13, 599.

Belfrage, S., Ahlgren, I., and Axelsen, S. (1966). Halothane hepatitis in an anaesthetist. *Lancet* ii, 1466.

Bell, J.I., Bishop, M.C., and Britton, B.J. (1977). Haemoperitoneum in a transsexual. *Lancet* ii, 817.

Bellary, S.V., Isaacs, P.E., and Scott, A.W. (1989). Captopril and the liver. *Lancet* ii, 514.

Benedetti, M.S., Louis, S., Malnoe, A. (1975). Prevention of paracetamol-induced liver damage with glutathione. *J. Pharmacol.* 27, 629.

Bengoa, J.M., Hanauer, S.B., Sitrin, M.D., Baker, A.L., and Rosenberg, I.H. (1985). Pattern and prognosis of liver function test abnormalities during parenteral nutrition in inflammatory bowel disease. *Hepatology* 5, 79.

Bengtsson, F., Floren, C.H., Hagerstrand, I., Soderstrom, C., and Aberg, T. (1985). Flucloxacillin-induced cholestatic liver damage. *Scand. J. Infect. Dis.* 17, 125.

Benhamou, J.P. (1988). Drug-induced hepatitis: clinical aspects. In *Liver cells and drugs* vol. 164 (ed. A. Guillouzo), p. 3. Colloque INSERM/John Libby Eurotext Ltd, London/Paris.

Benjamin, A.G. and Albukerk, J.N. (1982). Thorotrast-induced angiosarcoma of liver. *N.Y. State J. Med.* 82, 751.

Benjamin, S.B., Goodman, Z.D., Ishak, K.G., Zimmerman, H.J., and Irey, N.S. (1985). The morphologic spectrum of halothane-induced hepatic injury: analysis of 77 cases. *Hepatology* 5, 1163.

Benjamin, S.E., Ishak, K.G., Zimmerman, H.J., and Grushka, A. (1981). Phenylbutazone liver injury: a clinical pathologic survey of 23 cases and review of the literature. *Hepatology* 1, 255.

Berman, M.L., Kuhnert, L., Phythyon, J.M., and Holaday, D.A. (1983). Isoflurane and enflurane induced hepatic necrosis in triiodothyronine pretreated rats. *Anesthesiology* 58, 1.

Bernstein, M.S., Hunter, R.L., and Yachnin, S. (1973). Hepatoma and peliosis hepatis developing in a patient with Fanconi's anaemia. *N. Engl. J. Med.* 284, 1135.

Berry, W.R., Warren, G.H., and Reichen, J. (1984). Nitrofurantoin-induced cholestatic hepatitis from cow's milk in a teenaged boy. *West. J. Med.* 140, 278.

Bird, G.L.A. and Williams, R. (1989). Detection of antibodies to a halothane metabolite hapten in sera from patients with halothane associated hepatitis. *J. Hepatol* 9, 366.

Bjorkman, D.J., Hammond, E.H., Lee, R.G., Clegg, D.O., and Tolman, K.G. (1988). Hepatic ultrastructure after methotrexate therapy for rheumatoid arthritis. *Arthritis Rheum.* 31, 1465.

Black, J.L.K. and Richardson, J.W. (1985). Disulfiram hepatotoxicity: case report. *J. Clin. Psychiatry* 46, 67.

Black, M. and Raucy, J. (1986). Acetaminophen, alcohol, and cytochrome P-450. *Ann. Intern. Med.* 104, 427.

Black, M., Mitchell, J.R., Zimmerman, H.J., Ishak, K.G., and Epler, G.R. (1975). Isoniazid-associated hepatitis in 114 patients. *Gastroenterology* 69, 289.

Black, M., Scott, W.E. Jr, and Kanter, R. (1984). Possible ranitidine hepatotoxicity. *Ann. Intern. Med.* 101, 208.

Blackburn, A.M., Amiel, S.A., Millis, R.R., and Rubens, R.D. (1984). Tamoxifen and liver damage. *Br. Med. J.* 289, 288.

Blom, H., Stolk, J., Schreuder, H.B., and von Blomberg van der Flier, M. (1985). A case of carbimazole-induced intrahepatic cholestasis. An immune-mediated reaction? *Arch. Intern. Med.* 145, 1513.

Bloodworth, J.M.B. and Hamwei, G.J. (1961). Histopathologic lesions associated with sulfonylurea administration. *Diabetes* 10, 90.

Bock, K.W., Wiltfang, J., Blume, R., Ullrich, D., and Bircher, J. (1987). Paracetamol as a test drug to determine glucuronide formation in man. Effects of inducers and of smoking. *Eur. J. Clin. Pharmacol.* 31, 677.

Bohles, H., Richter, K., Wagner-Thiessen, E., and Schafer, H. (1982). Decrease serum carnitine in valproate induced Reye syndrome. *Eur. J. Pediatr.* 139, 185.

Bonkowsky, H.L., Mudge, G.H., and McMurty, R.J. (1978). Chronic hepatic inflammation and fibrosis due to low doses of paracetamol. *Lancet* i, 1016.

Botet, J.F., Watson, R.C., Kemeny, N., Daly, J.M., and Yeh, S. (1985). Cholangitis complicating intra-arterial chemotherapy in liver metastases. *Radiology* 156, 335.

Bove, K.E., Kosmetatos, N., Wedig, K.E., Frank, D.J., Whitlatch, S., Saldivar, V., *et al.* (1985). Vasculopathic hepatotoxicity associated with E-Ferol syndrome in low-birth-weight infants. *JAMA* 254, 2422.

Bowyer, B.A., Fleming, C.R., Ludwig, J., Petz, J., and McGill, D.B. (1985). Does longterm home parenteral nutrition in adult patients cause chronic liver disease? *JPEN* 9, 11.

Boyd, P.T., Lepre, F., and Dickey, J.D. (1989). Chronic active hepatitis associated with cimetidine. *Br. Med. J.* 298, 324.

Boyer, J.L. (1980). New concepts of mechanisms of hepatocyte bile formation. *Physiol. Rev.* 60, 303.

Boyer, J.L. and Root, M. (1976). Chlorpromazine metabolites — inhibitors of Na+, K+ ATPase in liver plasm membranes. 'LPM' enriched in bile canaliculi. *Clin. Res.* 24, 281A

Boyer, T.D., Sun, N., and Reynolds, T.B. (1977). Allopurinol hypersensitivity vasculitis and liver damage. *West. J. Med.* 126, 143.

Bras, G. and Brandt, K.H. (1979). Vascular disorders. In *Pathology of the liver* (ed. N.M. MacSween, P.P. Anthony, and P.J. Scheuer), p. 316. Churchill Livingstone, Edinburgh.

Breen, K.J., Schenker, S., and Heimberg, M. (1975). Fatty liver induced by tetracycline in the rat. Dose-response relationship and the effect of sex. *Gastroenterology* 69, 714.

Breitenbucher, R.B. and Crowley, L.V. (1970). Hepatorenal toxicity of tetracycline. *Minn. Med.* 53, 949.

Bridges, M.E. and Pittman, F.E. (1980). Tolazamide-induced cholestasis. *South. Med. J.* 73. 1072.

Brown, B.R. and Sipes, I.G. (1977). Biotransformation and hepatotoxicity of halothane. *Biochem. Pharmacol.* 26, 2091.

Brown, J.B. and Blair, H.A.F. (1960). Urinary oestrogen metabolites of 17-norethisterone and esters. *Proc. R. Soc. Med.* 53, 433.

Bruno, M.K., Cohen, S.D., and Khairallah, E.A. (1988). Antidotal effectiveness of *N*-acetylcysteine in reversing acetaminophen-induced hepatotoxicity. Enhancement in the proteolysis of arylated proteins. *Biochem. Pharmacol.* 37, 4319.

Buamah, P.K. (1985). An apparent danazol-induced primary hepatocellular carcinoma. *J. Surg. Oncol.* 28, 114.

Buckpitt, A.R., Rollins, D.E., and Mitchell, J.R. (1979). Varying effects of sulphydryl nucleophiles on acetaminophen oxidation and sulphydryl adduct formation. *Biochem. Pharmacol.* 28, 2941.

Buhler, H., Pirovino, M., Akobiantz, A., Altorfer, J., Weitzel, M., Maranta, E., *et al.* (1982). Regression of liver cell adenoma. A follow-up study of three consecutive patients after discontinuation of oral contraceptive use. *Gastroenterology* 82, 775.

Burgunder, J.M., Abernethy, D.R., and Lauterburg, B.H. (1988). Liver injury due to verapamil. *Hepatogastroenterology* 35, 169.

Burk, R.F. and Lane, J.M. (1979). Ethane production and liver necrosis in rats after administration of drugs and other chemicals. *Toxicol. Appl. Pharmacol.* 50, 467.

Burk, R.F., Lawrence R.A., and Lane, J.M. (1980). Liver necrosis and lipid peroxidation in the rat as the result of paraquat and diquat administration. The effect of selenium deficiency. *J. Clin. Invest.* 65, 1024.

Byrd, R.B., Nelson, R., and Elliot, R.C. (1972). Isoniazid toxicity. *JAMA* 220, 1471.

Camuto, P., Shupack, J., Orbuch, P., Tobias, H., Sidhu, G., and Feiner, H. (1987). Long-term effects of etretinate on the liver in psoriasis. *Am. J. Surg. Pathol.* 11, 30.

Canalese, J., Gimson, A.E.S., Davis, M., and Williams, R. (1981). Factors contributing to mortality in paracetamol-induced hepatic failure. *Br. Med. J.* 282, 199.

Capron, J.P., Lemay, J.L., Muir, J.F., Dupas, J.L., Lebrec, D., and Gineston, J.L. (1981). Portal vein thrombosis and fatal pulmonary thromboembolism associated with oral contraceptive treatment. *J. Clin. Gastroenterol.* 3, 295.

Capron, J.P., Gineston, J.L., Herve, M.A., and Braillon, A. (1983). Metronidazole in prevention of cholestasis associated with total parenteral nutrition. *Lancet* i, 446.

Carney, F.M.T. and Van Dyke, R.A. (1972). Halothane hepatitis: a critical review. *Anesth. Analg. Curr. Res.* 51, 135.

Carrasco, D., Prieto, M., Pallardo, L., Moll, J.L., Cruz, J.M., Munoz, C., *et al.* (1985). Multiple hepatic adenomas after longterm therapy with testosterone enanthate. Review of the literature. *J. Hepatol.* 1, 573.

Carter, E.A. (1987). Enhanced acetaminophen toxicity associated with prior alcohol consumption in mice: prevention by cimetidine. *Alcohol* 4, 69.

Casini, A.F., Pompella, A., and Comporti, M. (1985). Liver glutathione depletion induced by bromobenzene, iodobenzene and diethylmaleate poisoning and its relation to lipid peroxidation and necrosis. *Am. J. Pathol.* 118, 225.

Ceci, G., Bella, M., Melissari, M., Gabrielli, M., Bocchi, P., and Cocconi, G. (1988). Fatal hepatic vascular toxicity of DTIC. Is it really a rare event? *Cancer* 61, 1988.

Chan, G., Merrills, K., and Schiff, D. (1978). Bilirubin quantitation with lipemic plasma. *Clin. Biochem.* 9, 96.

Chaput, J.C., Buffet, C., Labayle, D., Courpotin, G., and Etienne, J.P. (1981). Hépatite choléstatique due à la troléandomycine et grossesse. *Gastroenterol. Clin. Biol.* 5, 103.

Chase, R.E., Holaday, D.A., Fiserova-Bergerova, V., Saidman, L.J., and Mack F.E. (1971). The biotransformation of enflurane in man. *Anesthesiology* 35, 262.

Chiprut, R.D., Viteri, A., Jamroz, C., and Dyck, W.P. (1976). Intra-hepatic cholestasis after griseofulvin administration. *Gastroenterology* 70, 1141.

Christ, D.D., Kenna, J.G., Kammerer, W., Sahoh, H., and Pohl, L.R. (1988). Enflurane metabolism produces covalently bound liver adducts recognized by antibodies from patients with halothane hepatitis. *Anesthesiology* 69, 833.

Christopherson, W.M. and Mays, E.T. (1977). Liver tumours and contraceptive steroids: experience with the first hundred registry patients. *J. Natl Cancer Inst.* 58, 167.

Citron, K.M. (1972). Drugs used in the treatment of tuberculosis and leprosy. In *Side effects of drugs*, Vol 6 (ed. L. Meyler and A. Herxheimer), p. 423. Excerpta Medica, Amsterdam.

Clark, J.H., Russell, G.J., and Fitzgerald, J.F. (1983). Fatal acetaminophen toxicity in a 2-year old. *J. Indiana State Med. Assoc.* 76, 832.

Clark, P.A., Hsia, Y.E., and Huntsman, R.G. (1960). Toxic complications of treatment with 6-mercaptopurine. Two cases with hepatic necrosis and intestinal ulceration. *Br. Med. J.* i, 393.

Clawson, G.A. (1989). Mechanisms of carbon tetrachloride hepatotoxicity. *Pathol. Immunopathol. Res.* 8, 104.

Clegg, D.O., Furst, D.E., Tolman, K.G., and Pogue, R. (1989). Acute, reversible hepatic failure associated with methotrexate treatment of rheumatoid arthritis. *J. Rheumatol.* 16, 1123.

Clementz, G.L. and Holmes, A.W. (1987). Nicotinic acid-induced fulminant hepatic failure. *J. Clin. Gastroenterol.* 9, 582.

Clinical Chemistry (1972). Drug interferences with clinical laboratory tests. *Clin. Chem.* 18, 1041.

Cohen, E.N. (1969). Metabolism of halothane-2-(^{14}C) in the mouse. *Anesthesiology* 31, 560.

Cohen, L., Lewis, C., and Arias, I.M. (1972). Pregnancy, oral contraceptives and chronic familial jaundice with predominantly conjugated hyperbilirubinaemia (Dubin–Johnson syndrome). *Gastroenterology* 62, 1182.

Combes, B., Shibata, H., Adams, R., Mitchell, B.D., and Trammell, V. (1963). Alterations in sulphobromphthalein sodium removal mechanisms from blood during normal pregnancy. *J. Clin. Invest.* 42, 1431.

Comstock, G.W. and Edwards, P.Q. (1975). The competing risks of tuberculosis and hepatitis for adult tuberculin reactors. *Am. Rev. Respir. Dis.* 111, 573.

Conn, H.O., Binder, H.J., and Orr H.D. (1964). Ethionamide-induced hepatitis: a review with a report of an additional case. *Am. Rev. Respir. Dis.* 90, 542.

Corcoran, G.B., Mitchell, J.R., Vaishnav, Y.N., and Horning, E.C. (1980). Evidence that acetaminophen and N-hydroxy-acetaminophen form a common arylating intermediate N-acetyl-p-quinoneimine. *Mol. Pharmacol.* 18, 536.

Corcoran, G.B., Bauer, J.A., and Lau, T.W. (1988). Immediate rise in intracellular calcium and glycogen phosphorylase a activities upon acetaminophen covalent binding leading to hepatotoxicity in mice. *Toxicology* 50, 157.

Cotariu, D. and Jaidman, J.L. (1988). Valproic acid and the liver. *Clin. Chem.* 34, 890.

Coulson, I.H., McKenzie, J., and Neild, V.S. (1987). A comparison of liver ultrasound with liver biopsy histology in psoriatics receiving longterm methotrexate therapy. *Br. J. Dermatol.* 116, 491.

Craft, P.S. and Pembrey, R.G. (1987). Veno-occlusive disease of the liver following chemotherapy with mitomycin C and doxorubicin. *Aust. N.Z. J. Med.* 17, 449.

Creagh, T.M., Rubin, A., and Evans, D.J. (1988). Hepatic tumours induced by anabolic steroids in an athlete. *J. Clin. Pathol.* 41, 441.

Critchley, J.A.J.H., Dyson, E.H., Scott, A.W., Jarvie, D.R., and Prescott, L.F. (1983). Is there a place for cimetidine or ethanol in the treatment of paracetamol poisoning? *Lancet* i, 1375.

Critchley, J.A.J.H., Nimmo, G.R., Gregson, C.A., Woolhouse, N.M., and Prescott, L.F. (1986). Inter-subject and ethnic differences in paracetamol metabolism. *Br. J. Clin. Pharmacol.* 22, 649.

CSM (Committee on Safety of Medicines) (1986). Halothane hepatotoxicity. *Current Problems*, No. 18. HMSO, London.

CSM (Committee on Safety of Medicines) (1988). Loferramine (Gamanila) and abnormal tests of liver function. *Current Problems*, No. 23. HMSO, London.

Dahl, M.G.C., Gregory, M.M., and Scheuer, P.J. (1971). Liver damage due to methotrexate in patients with psoriasis. *Br. Med. J.* i, 625.

Dalen, E. and Westerholm, B. (1974). Occurrence of hepatic impairment in women jaundiced by oral contraceptives and their mothers and sisters. *Acta Med. Scand.* 195, 459.

Damjanov, I., Arnold, R., and Faour, M. (1968). Tetracycline toxicity in a non-pregnant woman. *JAMA* 204, 934.

Danan, G., Bernuau, J., Moullot, X., Degott, C., and Pessayre, D. (1984). Amitriptyline-induced fulminant hepatitis. *Digestion* 30, 179.

Dancygier, H., Runne, U., Leuschner, U., Milbradt, R., and Classen, M. (1983). Dacarbazine (DTIC)-induced human liver damage light and electron-microscope findings. *Hepatogastroenterology* 30, 93.

D'Angio, G.J. (1987). Hepatotoxicity with actinomycin D. *Lancet* ii, 104.

Datey, K.K., Deshmukh, S.N., Dalvi, C.P., and Purandare, N.M. (1967). Hepatocellular damage with ethacrynic acid. *Br. Med. J.* iii, 152.

Datta, D.V., Mitra, S.K., Chhutani, P.N., and Charkravarti, R.N. (1979). Chronic arsenical intoxication as a possible aetiological factor in idiopathic portal hypertension (non-cirrhotic portal fibrosis) in India. *Gut* 20, 378.

Davidson, R.A. (1984). Complications of megavitamin therapy. *South. Med. J.* 77, 200.

Davidson, R.N., Weir, W.R., Kaye, G.L., and McIntyre, N. (1988). Intrahepatic cholestasis after thiabendazole. *Trans. R. Soc. Trop. Med. Hyg.* 82, 620.

Davion, T., Capron, J.P., Andrejak, M., Geoffrey, P., Capron-Chivrac, D., and Quenum, C. (1984). Acute hepatitis due to carbamazepine (Tegretol). Study of a case and review of the literature. *Gastroenterol. Clin. Biol.* 8, 52.

Davis, J.S. and Kaufman, R.H. (1966). Tetracycline toxicity: a clinicopathologic study with special reference to liver damage and its relationship to pregnancy. *Am. J. Obstet. Gynaecol.* 95, 523.

Davis, M. (1986). Specific therapy for hepatotoxins. In *Liver failure* (ed. R. Williams), p. 171. Churchill Livingstone, Edinburgh.

Davis, M. (1989). Drugs and abnormal liver function tests. *Adverse Drug React. Bull.* 139, 522.

Davis, M. and Williams, R. (1985). Hepatic Disorders. In: *Textbook of adverse drug reactions* (3rd edn) (ed. D.M. Davies), p. 250. Oxford University Press.

Davis, M., Portmann, B., Searle, M., Wright, R., and Williams, R. (1975). Histological evidence of malignancy in a primary hepatic tumour associated with oral contraceptive. *Br. Med. J.* iv, 496.

Davis, M., Simmons, C.J., Harrison, N., and Williams, R. (1976). Paracetamol overdose in man: relationship between pattern of urinary metabolites and severity of liver damage. *Q. J. Med.* 45, 181.

Davis, R.A., Kern, F, Jr, Showalter, R., Sutherland, E., Sinensky, M., and Simon, F.R. (1978). Alterations of hepatic (Na+-K+) ATPase and bile flow by estrogen: effects on liver surface membrane lipid structure and function. *Proc. Natl Acad. Sci. (USA)* 75, 4130.

Davis, M., Eddleston, A.L., and Williams, R. (1980). Hypersensitivity and jaundice due to azathioprine. *Postgrad. Med. Journal* 56, 274.

Deeg, H.J., Shulman, H.M., Schmidt, E., Yee, G.C., Thomas, E.D., and Storb, R. (1986). Marrow graft rejection and veno-occlusive disease of the liver in patients with aplastic anemia conditioned with cyclophosphamide and cyclosporine. *Transplantation* 42, 497.

Degott, C., Rueff, B., Kreis, H., Duboust, A., Potet, F., and Benhamou, J.P. (1978). Peliosis hepatis in recipients of renal transplants. *Gut* 19, 748.

Dejgaard, A., Krogsgaard, K., and Jacobsen, M. (1984). Venoocclusive disease and peliosis of the liver after thorotrast administration. *Virchows Arch.* (A) 403, 87.

De Lorimer, A.A., Gordon, G.S., Lowe, R.C., and Carbone, J. (1965). Methyltestosterone related steroids and liver function. *Arch. Intern. Med.* 116, 289.

Demorais, S.M.F. and Wells, P.G. (1989). Enhanced acetaminophen toxicity in rats with bilirubin glucuronyl transferase deficiency. *Hepatology* 10, 163.

Denison, H., Kaczynski, J., and Wallerstedt, S. (1987). Paracetamol medication and alcohol abuse: a dangerous combination for the liver and the kidney. *Scand. J. Gastroenterol.* 22, 701.

De Pagler, A.G.F., van Berge Henegouwen, G.P., Ten Bokkel Huinink, J.A., and Brandt, K.H. (1976). Familial benign recurrent intrahepatic cholestasis. Interrelation with intrahepatic cholestasis of pregnancy and from oral contraceptives? *Gastroenterology* 71, 202.

DePinho, R.A., Goldberg, C.S., and Lefkowitch, J.H. (1984). Azathioprine and the liver. Evidence favoring idiosyncratic mixed cholestatic-hepatocellular injury in humans. *Gastroenterology* 86, 162.

Despopoulos, A. (1971). Hepatic and renal excretory metabolism of bile salts. A background for understanding steroid-induced cholestasis. *J. Pharmacol. Exp. Ther.* 176, 273.

Devalia, J.L. and McLean, A.E.M. (1983). Covalent binding and the mechanism of paracetamol toxicity. *Biochem. Pharmacol.* 32, 195.

Devalia, J.L., Ogilvie, R.C., and McLean, A.E.M. (1982). Dissociation of cell death from covalent binding of paracetamol by flavones in a hepatocyte system. *Biochem. Pharmacol.* 31, 3749.

Diaz de Rojas, F., Castro-Garcia, M., Abaitua-Borda, I., Posada de la Paz, M., and Tabuenca-Oliver, J.M. (1985). Hepatic injury in the toxic oil syndrome. *Hepatology* 5, 166.

Dickinson, R.G., Bassett, M.L., Searle, J., Tyrer, J.H., and Eadie, M.J. (1985). Valproate hepatotoxicity: a review and report of two instances in adults. *Clin. Exp. Neurol.* 21, 79.

Dickinson, R.G., Bassett, M.L., Searle, J., Tyrer, J.H., and Eadie, M.J. (1985). Valproate hepatotoxicity: a review and report of two instances in adults. *Clin. Exp. Neurol.* 21, 79.

Diehl, A.M., Latham, P., Boitnott, J.K., Mann, J., and Maddrey, W.C. (1984). Cholestatic hepatitis from erythromycin ethylsuccinate. Report of two cases. *Am. J. Med.* 76, 931.

Dikengil, A., Siskind, B.N., Morse, S.S., Swedlund, A., Bober-Sorcinelli, K.E., and Burrell, M.I. (1986). Sclerosing cholangitis from intra-arterial fluxuridine. *J. Clin. Gastroenterol.* 8, 690.

Dincsoy, H.P. and Saelinger, D.A. (1982). Haloperidol-induced chronic cholestatic liver disease. *Gastroenterology* 83, 694.

Dixon, M.F., Nimmo, J., and Prescott, L.F. (1971). Experimental paracetamol-induced necrosis: a histopathological study. *J. Pathol.* 103, 225.

Doody, P.T. (1982). Disopyramide hepatotoxicity and disseminated intravascular coagulation. *South. Med. J.* 75, 496.

Dooner, H.P., Hoyl, C., Aliaga, C., and Parada, J. (1971). Jaundice and oral contraceptives. *Acta Hepatosplenol.* 18, 84.

Dormandy, T. (1978). Free radical oxidation and antioxidants. *Lancet* i, 647.

Douglas, D.D., Young, R.D., Jensen, P., and Thiele, D.L. (1989). Fatal labetalol-induced hepatic injury. *Am. J. Med.* 87, 235.

Douidar, S.M., Boor, P.J., and Ahmed, A.E. (1985). Potentiation of the hepatotoxic effect of acetaminophen by prior administration of salicylate. *J. Pharmacol. Exp. Ther.* 233, 242.

Dreifuss, F.E. (1989). Valproic acid hepatic fatalities: revised table. *Neurology* 39, 1558.

Dreifuss, F.E., Santilis, N., Langer, D.H., Sweeney, K.P., Moline, K.A., and Menander, K.B. (1987). Valproic acid fatalities: a retrospective review. *Neurology* 37, 379.

Dreifuss, F.E., Langer, D.H., Moline, K.A., and Maxwell, J.E. (1989). Valproic acid hepatic fatalities. II. US experience since 1984. *Neurology* 39, 201.

Dreyfus, M., Jaeck, D., and Dreyfus, J. (1989). Adenomas of the liver and oral contraception. Clinical and therapeutic aspects apropos of a giant adenoma. *Rev. Fr. Gynecol. Obstet.* 84, 761.

Dubois, R.N., Hill, K.E., and Burk, R.F. (1983). Antioxidant effect of acetaminophen in rat liver. *Biochem. Pharmacol.* 17, 2621.

Dujovne, C.A. and Shoeman, D.W. (1972). Toxicity of a hepatotoxicity laxative preparation in tissue culture and excretion in bile in man. *Clin. Pharmacol. Ther.* 13, 602.

Dujovne, C.A., Chan, C.H., and Zimmerman, H.J. (1967). Sulphonamide hepatic injury. Review of the literature and report of a case due to sulphamethoxazole. *N. Engl. J. Med.* 277, 785.

Du Vivier, A., Munro, D.D., and Verbov, J. (1974). Treatment of psoriasis with azathioprine. *Br. Med. J.* i, 49.

Dybing, E., Nelson, S.D., Mitchell, J.R., Sasame, J.A., and Gillette, J.R. (1976). Oxidation of alpha-methyldopa and other catechols by cytochrome P-450 generated superoxide anion: possible mechanism of methyldopa hepatitis. *Molec. Pharmacol.* 12, 911.

Dykes, M.H.M. (1971). Unexplained postoperative fever. Its value as a sign of halothane sensitization. *JAMA* 216, 641.

East African/British Medical Research Council (1973). Retreatment Investigation Second Report. Streptomycin plus PAS plus pyrazinamide in the retreatment of pulmonary tuberculosis in East Africa. *Tubercle* 54, 283.

Edelman, J., Donnelly, R., Graham, D.N., and Percy, J.S. (1983). Liver dysfunction associated with gold therapy for rheumatoid arthritis. *J. Rheumatol.* 10, 510.

Edmondson, H.A., Henderson, B., and Benton, B. (1976). Liver cell adenomas associated with use of oral contraceptives. *N. Engl. J. Med.* 294, 470.

Edmondson, H.A., Reynolds, T.B., Henderson, B., and Benton, B. (1977). Regression of liver cell adenomas associated with oral contraceptives. *Ann. Intern. Med.* 86, 180.

Eger, E.I., Smuckler, E.A., Ferrell, L.D., Goldsmith, C.H., and Johnson, B.H. (1986). Is enflurane hepatotoxic? *Anesth. Analg.* 65, 21.

Eisalo, A., Jarvinen, P.A., Luukkainen, T. (1965). Hepatic impairment during the intake of contraceptive pills. *Br. Med. J.* ii, 426.

Eisalo, A., Jarvinen, P.A., and Lukkainen, T. (1964). Liver function tests during intake of contraceptive tablets in premenopausal women. *Br. Med. J.* i, 1416.

Elias, E. and Boyer, J.L. (1979). Chlorpromazine and its metabolites after polymerization and gelatin of actin. *Science* 206, 1404.

Elias, E., Waring, R.H., and Mitchell, S.C. (1984). Defective sulphoxidation combined with rapid carbon oxidation may predispose to chlorpromazine jaundice. *Gut* 25, A1130.

Elkington, S.G., Schreiber, W.M., and Conn, H.O. (1969). Hepatic injury caused by alpha methyldopa. *Circulation* 40, 589.

Emery, S., Oldham, H.G., Norman, S.J., and Chenergy, R.J. (1985). The effect of cimetidine and ranitidine on paracetamol glucuronidation an sulphation in cultured rat hepatocytes. *Biochem. Pharmacol.* 34, 1415.

Erichsen, C. and Jonsson, P.E. (1984). Veno-occlusive liver disease after dacarbazine therapy (DTIC) for melanoma. *J. Surg. Oncol.* 27, 268.

Evans, D.A.P., Manley, K.A., and McKusick, V.A. (1960). Genetic control of isoniazid metabolism in man. *Br. Med. J.* ii, 485.

Fajardo, L.F. and Colby, T.V. (1980). Pathogenesis of veno-occlusive liver disease after radiation. *Arch. Path. Lab. Med.* 104, 584.

Farber, E. (1979). Reactions of the liver to injury: necrosis. In *Toxic injury of the liver* (ed. E. Farber and M.M. Fisher). Marcel Dekker, New York.

Farer, L.S., Glassroth, J.L., and Snider, D.E. Jr (1977). Isoniazid related hepatotoxicity. *Ann. Intern. Med.* 86, 114.

Farr, M., Symmons, D.P., and Bacon, P.A. (1985). Raised serum alkaline phosphatase and aspartate transaminase levels in two rheumatoid patients treated with sulphasalazine. *Ann. Rheum. Dis.* 44, 798.

Farrell, G., Prendergast, D., and Murray, M. (1985). Halothane hepatitis. Detection of a constitutional susceptibility factor. *N. Engl. J. Med.* 313, 1310.

Farrell, G.C., Joshua, D.E., Uren, R.F., Baird, P.J., Perkins, K.W., and Kronenberg, H. (1975). Androgen induced hepatoma. *Lancet* i, 430.

Favreau, M., Tannerbaum, H., and Lough, J. (1977). Hepatic toxicity associated with gold therapy. *Ann. Intern. Med.* 87, 717.

Feaux-de-Lacroix, W., Runne, U., Hauk, H., Doepfmer, K., Groth, W., and Wacker, D. (1983). Acute liver dystrophy with thrombosis of hepatic veins: a fatal complication of dacarbazine treatment. *Cancer Treat. Rep.* 67, 779.

Fedorkow, D.M., Corenblum, B., and Shaffer, E.A. (1989). Cholestasis induced by oestrogen after liver transplantation. *Br. Med. J.* 299, 1080.

Fedotin, M.S. and Lefer, I.G. (1975). Liver disease caused by propylthiouracil. *Arch. Intern. Med.* 135, 319.

Fenech, F.F., Bannister, W.H., and Grech, J.L. (1967). Hepatitis with biliverdinaemia in association with indomethacin therapy. *Br. Med. J.* iii, 155.

Fermand, J.P., Levy, Y., Bouscary, D., D'Agay, M.F., Clot, P., Frija, J., *et al.* (1990). Danazol-induced hepatocellular adenoma. *Am. J. Med.* 88, 529.

Fevery, J., Van-Steenbergen, W., Desmet, V., Deruyttere, M., and De-Groote, J. (1983). Severe intrahepatic cholestasis due to the combined intake of oral contraceptives and triacetyloleandomycin. *Acta Clin. Belg.* 38, 242.

Fisher, M.M., Roberts, E.A., Rosen, I.F., Shapero, T.F., Sutherland, L.R., Davies, R.S., *et al.* (1985). The Sunnbrook Gallstone Study. A double-blind controlled trial of chenodeoxycholic acid for gallstone dissolution. *Hepatology* 5, 102.

Floren, C.H., Thesleff, P., and Nilsson, A. (1987). Severe liver damage caused by therapeutic doses of acetaminophen. *Acta Med. Scand.* 222, 285.

Foitl, D.R., Hyman, G., and Lefkowitch, J.H. (1989). Jaundice and intrahepatic cholestasis following high-dose megestrol acetate for breast cancer. *Cancer* 63, 438.

Forker, E.L. (1969). The effect of estrogen on bile formation in the rat. *J. Clin. Invest.* 48, 654.

Forman, D., Vincent, T.J., and Doll, R. (1986). Cancer of the liver and the use of oral contraceptives. *Br. Med. J.* 292, 1357.

Forsyth, B.W., Horwitz, R.I., Acampora, D., Shapiro, E.D., Viscoli, C.M., Feinstein, A.R., *et al.* (1989). New epidemiologic evidence confirming that bias does not explain the aspirin/Reye's syndrome association. *JAMA* 261, 2517.

Fouin-Fortunet, H., le Quernec, L., Erlinger, S., Lerebous, E., and Colin, R. (1982). Hepatic alterations with inflammatory bowel disease: a possible consequence of lithocholate toxicity. *Gastroenterology* 82, 932.

Fouquet, J., Teyssier, I., Bacle, Y., Bacle, F., Carrat, R., and Le Renard, J.L. (1965). L'action antibactillaire, l'usage thérapeutique et les dangers du pyrazinamide. *Rev. Tuberc.* 29, 930.

Fowler, P.D., Woolf, D., and Alexander, S. (1975). Phenylbutazone and hepatitis. *Rheum. Rehabil.* 14, 71.

Frederick, W.C., Howard, R.G., and Spatola, S. (1974). Spontaneous rupture of the liver in patient using contraceptive pills. *Arch. Surg.* 108, 93.

Freneaux, E., Labbe, G., Letteron, P., The-Le-Dinh, Degott, C., Geneve, J., *et al.* (1988). Inhibition of the mitochondrial oxidation of fatty acids by tetracycline in mice and in man: possible role in microvesicular steatosis induced by this antibiotic. *Hepatology* 8, 1056

Gadacz, T., Allan, R.N., Macke, E., and Hofmann, A.F. (1976). Impaired lithocholate sulfation in the Rhesus monkey: a possible mechanism for chenodeoxycholic toxicity. *Gastroenterology* 70, 1125.

Gaffey, C.M., Chun, B., Harvey, J.C., and Manz, H.J. (1986). Phenytoin-induced systemic granulomatous vasculitis. *Arch. Path. Lab. Med.* 110, 131.

Galinsky, R.E., Slattery, J.T., and Levy, G. (1979). Effect of sodium sulfate on acetaminophen elimination by rats. *J. Pharm. Sci.* 68, 803.

Gallagher, T.F., Mueller, M.W., and Kappas, A. (1966). Studies on the structural basis for estrogen-induced impairment of liver function. *Medicine (Baltimore)* 45, 471.

Gangadharam, P.R. (1986). Isoniazid, rifampin, and hepatotoxicity. *Am. Rev. Respir. Dis.* 133, 963.

Garber, E., Craig, R.M., and Bahn, R.M. (1973). Aspirin hepatotoxicity. *Ann. Intern. Med.* 82, 592.

Garibaldi, R.A., Drusin, R.E., Ferebeeh, S.H., and Gregg, M.B. (1972). Isoniazid-associated hepatitis. *Am. Rev. Respir. Dis.* 106, 357.

Garrigues-Gil, V., Berenguer-Lapuerta, J., Ponce-Garcia, J., and Rayon-Martin, M. (1986). A non-C17-alkylated steroid and longterm cholestasis. *Ann. Intern. Med.* 104, 135.

Gazzard, B.G., Hughes, R.D., Portmann, B., and Wiliams, R. (1974). Protection of rats against the hepatotoxic effect of paracetamol. *Br. J. Exp. Pathol.* 55, 601.

Gazzard, B.G., Hughes, R.D., Widdop, B., Goulding, R., Davis, M., and Williams, R. (1977). Early prediction of the outcome of a paracetamol overdose based on an analysis of 163 patients. *Postgrad. Med. J.* 53, 243.

Geneve, G., Larrey, D., Pessayre, D., Benhamou, J.P. (1987). Structure tricyclique des médicaments et hépatotoxicité. *Gastroenterol. Clin. Biol.* 11, 242.

Geneve, J., Zaffrani, E.S., and Dhumeaux, D. (1989). Amiodarone-induced liver disease. *J. Hepatol.* 9, 130.

Georgieff, M., Moldawer, L.L., Bistrain, B.R., and Blackburn, G.L. (1985). In *Metabolism and nutrition in liver disease* (ed. E. Holm and H. Kasper), p. 287. MTP Press, Lancaster.

Gerlag, P.G. and van-Hooff, J.P. (1987). Hepatic sinusoidal dilatation with portal hypertension during azathioprine treatment: a cause of chronic liver disease after kidney transplantation. *Transplant. Proc.* 19, 3699.

Gerlag, P.G., Lobatto, S., Driessen, W.M., Deckers, P.F., Van-Hooff, J.P., Schroder, E., *et al.* (1985). Hepatic sinusoidal dilatation with portal hypertension during azathioprine treatment after kidney transplantation. *J. Hepatol.* 1, 339.

Geubel, A.P., Nakad, A., Rahier, J., and Dive, C. (1988). Prolonged cholestasis and disappearance of interlobular bile ducts following chlorpropamide and erythromycin ethylsuccinate. Case of drug interaction? *Liver* 8, 350.

Gholson, C.F. and Warren, G.H. (1990). Fulminant hepatic failure associated with intravenous erythromycin lactobionate. *Arch. Intern. Med.* 150, 215.

Gibson, R.G. and Gibson, S.L. (1981). Seatone in arthritis. *Br. Med. J.* 282, 1785.

Gibson, R.G., Gibson, S.L., Conway, V., and Chappell, D. (1980). *Perna canaliculus* in the treatment of arthritis. *Practitioner* 224, 955.

Gilbert, F.I. (1962). Cholestatic hepatitis caused by esters of erythromycin and oleandomycin. *JAMA* 182, 1048.

Gill, R.A., Onstad, G.R., Cardamone, J.M., Maneval, D.C., and Summer, H.W. (1982). Hepatic veno-occlusive disease caused by 6-thioguanine. *Ann. Intern. Med.* 96, 58.

Ginsburg, C.M. (1986). A prospective study of the incidence of liver function abnormalities in children receiving erythromycin estolate, erythromycin ethylsuccinate or penicillin V for treatment of pneumonia. *Pediatr. Infect. Dis.* 5, 151.

Girling, D.J. (1978). The hepatic toxicity of anti-tuberculosis regimens containing isoniazid, rifampicin, and pyrazinamide. *Tubercle* 59, 13.

Glazer, S.D., Roenigk, H.H. Jr, Yokoo, H., and Sparberg, M. (1982). A study of potential hepatotoxicity of etretinate used in the treatment of psoriasis. *J. Am. Acad. Dermatol.* 6, 683.

Goldberg, J.W. and Lidsky, M.D. (1985). Cyclophosphamide-associated hepatotoxicity. *South. Med. J.* 78, 222.

Goldstein, G., Lam, K.C., and Mistilis, S.P. (1973). Drug-induced active chronic hepatitis. *Am. J. Dig. Dis.* 18, 177.

Goldstein, L.I., Ishak, K.G., and Burns, W. (1974). Hepatic injury associated with nitrofurantoin therapy. *Am. J. Dig. Dis.* 19, 987.

Goldzieher, J.W. (1964). Newer drugs in oral contraception. *Med. Clin. N. Am.* 48, 529.

Goodman, R.C., Dean, P.J., Radparvar, A., and Kitabelli, A.E. (1987). Glyburide-induced hepatitis. *Ann. Intern. Med.* 106, 837.

Goodman, Z.D. and Ishak, K.G. (1982). Hepatocellular carcinoma in women: probable lack of etiologic association with oral contraceptive steroids. *Hepatology* 2, 440.

Goodman, Z.D., Mikel, U.V., Lubbas, P.R., Ros, P.R., Langloss, J.M., and Ishak, K.M. (1987). Kupfer cells in hepatocellular adenomas. *Am. J. Surg. Pathol.* 11, 191.

Gordon, S.C., Reddy, K.R., Livingstone, A.S., Jeffers, L.J., and Schiff, E.R. (1986). Resolution of a contraceptive-steroid induced hepatic adenoma with subsequent evolution into hepatocellular carcinoma. *Ann. Intern. Med.* 105, 547.

Gottfried, M.R. and Sulidowsky, O. (1982). Hepatic veno-occlusive disease after high-dose mitomycine and autologous bone marrow transplantation therapy. *Hum. Pathol.* 13, 646.

Goudie, B.M., Birnie, G.F., Watkinson, G., MacSween, R.N.M., Kissen, L.H., and Cunningham, N.E. (1982). Jaundice associated with the use of benoxaprofen. *Lancet* i, 959.

Grafstrom, R., Ormstad, K., Moldeus, P., and Orrenius, S. (1979). Paracetamol metabolism in the isolated perfused rat liver with further metabolism of a biliary paracetamol conjugate by the small intestine. *Biochem. Pharmacol* 28, 3573.

Green, M.D. and Fischer, L.J. (1984). Hepatotoxicity of acetaminophen in neonatal and young rats II. Metabolic aspects. *Toxicol. Appl. Pharmacol.* 74, 125.

Green, M.D., Shires, T.K., and Fischer, L.J. (1984). Hepatotoxicity of acetaminophen in neonatal and young rats I: Age related changes in susceptibility. *Toxicol. Appl. Pharmacol.* 74, 116.

Greene, J.W., Craft, L., and Ghishan, F. (1983). Acetaminophen poisoning in infancy. *Am. J. Dis. Child.* 137, 386.

Greer, T. (1989). Hepatic adenoma and oral contraceptive use. *J. Fam. Pract.* 28, 322.

Gregory, D.H., Zaki, G.F., Sarcosi, G.A., and Carey, J.B. Jr (1967). Chronic cholestasis following prolonged tolbutamide administration, associated with obstructive cholangitis and cholangiolitis. *Arch. Pathol.* 84, 194.

Gremse, D.A., Bancroft, J., and Moyer, M.S. (1989). Sulfasalazine hypersensitivity with hepatotoxicity, thrombocytopenia, and erythroid hypoplasia. *J. Pediatr. Gastroenterol. Nutr.* 9, 261.

Grigsby, P., Meyer, J.S., Sicard, G.A., Huggins, M.B., Lamar, D.J., DeSchryver-Kecskermeti, K., et al. (1987). Hepatic adenoma within a spindle cell carcinoma in a woman with a long history of oral contraceptives. *J. Surg. Oncol.* 35, 173.

Guarascio, P., D'amato, C., and Sette, P. (1984). Liver damage from verapamil. *Br. Med. J.* 288, 362.

Guarascio, P., Portmann, B., Visco, G., and Williams, R. (1983). Liver damage with reversible portal hypertension from vitamin A intoxication: demonstration of Ito cells. *J. Clin. Pathol.* 36, 769.

Guigui, B., Perrot, S., Berry, J.P., Fleury-Feith, J., Martin, N., Metreau, J.M , *et al* (1988) Amiodarone-induced hepatic phospholipidosis: a morphological alteration independent of pseudoalcoholic liver disease. *Hepatology* 8, 1063.

Gulbis, B., Adler, M., Ooms, H.A., Desmet, J.M., Leclerc, J.L., and Primo, G. (1988). Liver function studies in heart-transplant recipients treated with cyclosporin A. *Clin. Chem.* 34, 1772.

Gummucio, J.J. and Valdivieso, V.D. (1971). Studies on the mechanism of the ethinylestradiol impairment of bile flow and bile salt excretion in rat. *Gastroenterology* 61, 339.

Gupta, R. and Sachar, D.B. (1985). Chlorpropamide-induced cholestatic jaundice and pseudomembranous colitis. *Am. J. Gastroenterol.* 80, 381.

Gurumurthy, P., Krishnamurthy, M.S., Nazareth, O., Parthasarathy, R., Sarma, G.R., Somasundaram, P.R., et al. (1984). Lack of relationship between hepatic toxicity and acetylator phenotype in three thousand South Indian patients during treatment with isoniazid for tuberculosis. *Am. Rev. Respir. Dis.* 129, 58.

Haber, E. and Osborne, R.K. (1959). Icterus and febrile reactions in response to isonicotinic acid hydrazine. *N. Engl. J. Med.* 260, 417.

Haboubi, N.Y., Ali, H.H., Whitwell, H.L., and Ackrill, P. (1988). Role of endothelial cell injury in the spectrum of azathioprine induced liver disease after renal transplant: light microscopy and ultrastructural observations. *Am. J. Gastroenterol.* 83, 256.

Hagay, Z.J., Leiberman, R.J., Katz, M., and Witznitzer, A. (1988). Oral contraceptives and focal nodular hyperplasia of the liver. *Arch. Gynecol. Obstet.* 243, 231.

Haines, J.D. Jr (1986). Hepatotoxicity after treatment with sulfasalazine. *Postgrad. Med.* 79, 193.

Hall, S.M., Plaster, P.A., Glasgow, J.F., and Hancock, P. (1988). Preadmission antipyretics in Reye's syndrome. *Arch. Dis. Child.* 63, 857.

Halpin, T.J., Holtzhauer, F.J., and Campbell, R.J. (1982). Reye's syndrome and medication use. *JAMA* 248, 687.

Hansen, C., Pearson, L.H., Shenker, S., and Combes, B. (1968). Impaired secretion of hepatic triglycerides—a cause of tetracycline-induced fatty liver. *Proc. Soc. Exp. Biol. Med.* 128, 143.

Hansen, M.M., Ranek, L., Walbom, S., and Nissen N.I. (1982). Fatal hepatitis following irradiation and vincristine. *Acta Med. Scand.* 212, 171.

Harats, N., Ehrenfeld, M., Shalit, M., and Lijovetzky, G. (1985). Gold induced granulomatous hepatitis. *Israel J. Med. Sci.* 21, 753.

Hare, D.L. and Horowitz, J.D. (1986). Verapamil hepatotoxicity: a hypersensitivity reaction. *Am. Heart. J.* 111, 610.

Harney, J. and Glasberg, M.R. (1983). Myopathy and hypersensitivity to phenytoin. *Neurology* 33, 790.

Harrison, P.M., Keays, R., Bray, G.P., Alexander, GJM, and Williams, R. (1990). Improved outcome of paracetamol-induced fulminant hepatic failure by late administration of acetylcysteine. *Lancet* 335, 1572.

Hart, J.G. and Timbrell, J.A. (1979). The effect of age on paracetamol hepatotoxicity in mice. *Biochem. Pharmacol.* 28, 3015.

Hartmann, H , Fischer, G , and Janning, G. (1984). Prolonged cholestatic jaundice and leukopenia associated with piroxicam. *Gastroenterology* 22, 343.

Harvey, F.D. and Levitt, T.E. (1976). Experimental evaluation of paracetamol antidotes. *J. Int. Med. Res.* 4 (suppl. 4), 130.

Harvey, J. and Colin-Jones, D.G. (1981). Mistletoe hepatitis. *Br. Med. J.* 282, 186.

Hay, D.R. and Gwynne, J.F. (1983). Cirrhosis of the liver following therapy with perhexilene maleate. *N.Z. J Med.* 96, 202.

Hazelton, G.A., Hjelle, J.J., and Klaassen, C.D. (1986). Effects of butylated hydroxyanisole on acetaminophen hepatotoxicity and glucuronidation in vivo. *Toxicol. Appl. Pharmacol.* 83, 474.

Heaney, R.P. and Whedon, G.D. (1958). Impairment of hepatic BSP clearance by two 17-substituted testosterones. *J. Lab. Clin. Invest.* 52, 169.

Hiesse, C., Cantarovich, M., Santelli, C., Francais, P., Charpentier, P., Fries, D., et al. (1985). Ranitidine hepatotoxicity in a renal transplant patient. *Lancet* i, 1280.

Hildebrandt, A.G., Speck, M., and Roots, I. (1973). Possible control of hydrogen peroxide production and degradation in microsomes during mixed function oxidation reaction. *Biochem. Biophys. Res. Commun.* 54, 968.

Hill, K.E. and Burk, R.F. (1982). Effect of selenium deficiency and vitamin E deficiency on glutathione metabolism in isolated rat hepatocytes. *J. Biol. Chem.* 257, 10668.

Hill, K.E. and Burk, R.F. (1984). Toxicity studies in isolated hepatocytes from selenium-deficient and vitamin E deficient rats. *Toxicol. Appl. Pharmacol.* 72, 32.

Hjelle, J.J. and Klaassen, C.D. (1984). Glucuronidation and biliary excretion of acetaminophen in rats. *J. Pharmacol. Exp. Ther.* 228, 407.

Hohn, D., Melnick, J., Stagg, R., Altman, D., Friedman, M., Ignotto, R., et al. (1985). Biliary sclerosis in patients receiving hepatic arterial infusions of floxuridine. *J. Clin. Oncol.* 3, 98.

Hoge, S.K. and Biederman, J. (1987). Liver function tests during treatment with desipramine in children and adolescents. *J. Clin. Psychopharmacol.* 7, 87.

Holaday, D.A., Fiserova Bererova, V., Latto, I.P., and Zumbiel, M.A. (1975). Resistance of isoflurane to biotransformation in man. *Anesthesiology* 43, 325.

Holdstock, G., Millward-Sadler, G.H., and Wright, R. (1985). Hepatic changes in systemic disease. In *Liver and biliary disease* (ed. R. Wright, G.W. Millward-Sadler, K.G.M.M. Alberti, and S. Karran). Baillière, London.

Holdsworth, C.D. (1983). Sulphasalazine hepatotoxicity after 15 years' treatment. *Br. Med. J.* 287, 759.

Holt, R.J. (1984). Fluphenazine decanoate-induced cholestatic jaundice and thrombocytopenia. *Pharmacotherapy* 4, 227.

Hopmann, G. and Surmann, T. (1984). Cholestatic jaundice during flecainide therapy. *Dtsch. Med. Wochenschr.* 109, 1863.

Horowitz S., Patwardhan, R., and Marcus, E. (1988). Hepatotoxic reactions associated with carbamazepine therapy. *Epilepsia* 29, 149.

Horst, D.A., Grace, N.D., and Lecompte, P.M. (1980). Prolonged cholestasis and progressive hepatic fibrosis following imipramine therapy. *Gastroenterology* 79, 550.

Hoyumpa, A.M., Greene, H.L., Dunn, G.D., and Schenker, S. (1975). Fatty liver: biochemical and clinical considerations. *Am. J. Dig. Dis.* 20, 1142.

Hromas, R.A., Srigley, J., and Murray, J.L. (1985). Clinical and pathological comparison of young adult women with hepatocellular carcinoma with and without exposure to oral contraceptives. *Am. J. Gastroenterol.* 80, 479.

Hubbard, A.K., Gandolfi, A.J., and Brown, B.R. (1988). Immunological basis of anaesthetic-induced hepatotoxicity. *Anesthesiology* 69, 814.

Hughes, R.D., Gazzard, B.G., Hanid, M.A., Trewsby, P.N., Murray-Lyon, I.M., Davis, M., et al. (1977). Controlled trial of cysteamine and dimercaprol after paracetamol overdose. *Br. Med. J.* ii, 1395.

Humble, M.W., Eykin, S.J., and Phillips. I. (1980). Staphylococcal bacteraemia, fusidic acid and jaundice. *Br. Med. J.* 280, 1495.

Hurwits, E.S., Barrett, M.J., Bregman, D., Gunn, W.J., Schonberger, L.B., Fairweather, W.R., et al. (1985). Public Health Service study on Reye's syndrome and medications. Report of the pilot phase. *N. Engl. J. Med.* 313, 849.

Hurwits, E.S., Barrett, M.J., and Bregman, D. (1987). Service study of Reye's syndrome and medications. *JAMA* 257, 1905.

Huxtable, R.J. (1980). Herbal teas and toxins: novel aspects of pyrrolizidine poisoning in the United States. *Perspect. Biol. Med.* 24, 1.

Hyer, S.L. and Knell, A.J. (1977). Cirrhosis and haemolysis complicating methyldopa treatment. *Br. Med. J.* i, 879.

Ingold, J.A., Reed, G.B., Kaplan, H.S., and Bagshaw, M.A. (1965). Radiation hepatitis. *Am. J. Roentgenol.* 93, 200.

Inkeles, S.B., Connor, W.E., and Illingworth, D.R. (1986). Hepatic and dermatologic manifestations of chronic hypervitaminosis A in adults. Report of two cases. *Am. J. Med.* 80, 491.

Inman, W.H.W. and Mushin, W.W. (1974). Jaundice after repeated exposure to halothane: an analysis of reports to the Committee on Safety of Medicines. *Br. Med. J.* i, 5.

Irani , S.K. and Dobbins, W.D. (1979). Hepatic granulomas; a survey of 73 patients from one hospital and survey of the literature. *J. Clin. Gastroenterol.* 1, 131.

Ishak, K.G. and Irey, N.S. (1972). Hepatic injury associated with the phenothiazines. Clinicopathologic and follow-up study of 36 patients. *Arch. Pathol.* 93, 283.

Ishak, K.G., Kirchner, J.P., and Dhar, J.K. (1977). Granulomas and cholestatic-hepatocellular injury associated with phenylbutazone. Report of two cases. *Am. J. Dig. Dis.* 22, 611.

Israel, Y., Kalant, H., Orrego, H., Khanna, J.M., Videla, L., and Phillips, J.M. (1975). Experimental alcohol-induced hepatic necrosis:suppression by propylthiouracil. *Proc. Natl Acad. Sci. (USA)* 72, 1137.

Iveson, T.J., Ryley, N.G., Kelly, P.M.A., Trowell, J.M., McGee, J.O.D., and Chapman, R.W.G. (1990). Diclofenac associated hepatitis. *J. Hepatol.* 10, 85.

Jack, D., Thomas, M., and Skidmore, I.F. (1985). Ranitidine and paracetamol metabolism. *Lancet* ii, 1067.

Jacobs, M.B. (1984). Hepatic infarction related to oral contraceptive use. *Arch. Intern. Med.* 144, 642.

Jacques, E.A., Buschmann, R.J., and Layden, T.J. (1979). The histopathologic progression of vitamin A induced hepatic injury. *Gastroenterology* 76, 599.

Jaeschke, H. and Mitchell, J.R. (1989). Neutrophil accumulation exacerbates acetaminophen-induced liver injury. *FASEBJ* 3, A920.

Janota, I., Wincey, C.W., Sandiford, M., and Smith, M.J.H. (1960). Effect of salicylate on the activity of plasma enzymes in the rabbit. *Nature* 185, 935.

Janssen, P.A. and Symoens, J.E. (1983). Hepatic reactions during ketoconazole treatment. *Am. J. Med.* 74, 80.

Jee, R.C., Sipes, I.T., Gandolfi, A.J., and Brown, B.R. (1980). Factors influencing halothane hepatotoxicity in the rat hypoxic model. *Toxicol. Appl. Pharmacol.* 52, 267.

Johnson, D.H., Greco, F.A., and Wolff, S.N. (1983). Etoposide-induced hepatic injury: a potential complication of high-dose therapy. *Cancer Treat. Rep.* 67, 1023.

Johnson, F.L., Feagler, J.R., Lerner, K.G., Majerus, P.W., Siegel, M., Hartman, J.R. et al. (1972). Association of androgenic-anabolic steroid therapy with development of hepatocellular carcinoma. *Lancet* ii, 1273.

Johnson, G.K. and Tolman, K.G. (1977). Chronic liver disease and acetaminophen. *Ann. Intern. Med.* 87, 302.

Johnson, P.J., Portmann, B., and Williams, R. (1978). Alpha-fetoprotein levels measured by radioimmunoassay in the diagnosis and exclusion of hepatocellular carcinoma in Great Britain. *Br. Med. J.* ii, 661.

Johnston, U. and Mendelsohn, F. (1971). Halothane hepatitis in a laboratory technician. *Aust. N.Z. J. Med.* 1, 511.

Jonas, M.M. and Eidson, M.S. (1988). Propylthiouracil hepatotoxicity: two pediatric cases and review of the literature. *J. Pediatr. Gastroenterol. Nutr.* 7, 776.

Jones, D.B., Mullick, F.G., Hoofnagle, J.H., and Baranski, B. (1988). Reye's syndrome-like illness in a patient receiving amiodarone. *Am. J. Gastroenterol.* 83, 967.

Jones, D.P., Sunby, G.B., Ormstad, K., and Orrenius, S. (1979). Use of isolated kidney cells for study of drug metabolism. *Biochem. Pharmacol.* 28, 929.

Jori, G.P. and Peschle, C. (1973). Hydralazine disease associated with transient granulomas in the liver. A case report. *Gastroenterology* 64, 1163.

Juul, J. (1965). Acute poisoning with Butazolidine (phenylbutazone). *Acta Pediatr. Scand.* 54, 503.

Kahn, H.D., Faguet, G.B., Agee, J.F., and Middleton, H.M. (1984). Drug induced liver injury. In vitro demonstration of hypersensitivity to both phenytoin and phenobarbital. *Arch. Intern. Med.* 144, 1677.

Kalow, W. (1987). Genetic variation in the human hepatic cytochrome P-450 system. *Eur. J. Clin. Pharmacol.* 31, 633.

Kanel, G.C., Cassidy, W., Shuster, L., and Reynolds, T.B. (1990). Cocaine induced liver cell injury: comparison of morphological features in man and in experimental animals. *Hepatology* 11, 646.

Kantor, G.L. (1970). Toxic epidermal necrolysis, azotemia and death after allopurinol therapy. *JAMA* 212, 478.

Kaplowitz, N., Aw, T.Y., Simon, F.R., and Stolz, A. (1986). Drug-induced hepatotoxicity (clinical conference). *Ann. Intern. Med.* 104, 826.

Kappas, A. (1968). Studies in endocrine pharmacology. *N. Engl. J. Med.* 278, 378.

Kassiandes, C., Nussenblatt, R., Palestine, A.G., Mellow, S.D., and Hoofnagle, J.H. (1990). Liver injury from cyclosporine A. *Dig. Dis. Sci.* 35, 693.

Kato, R. and Takahashi, A. (1968). Thyroid hormone and activities of drug-metabolism in enzymes and electron transport systems of rat liver microsomes. *Mol. Pharmacol.* 4, 109.

Katz, H., Weetch, M., and Chopra, S. (1983). Quinidine-induced granulomatous hepatitis. *Br. Med. J.* 286, 264.

Katz, M. and Saibil, F. (1990). Herbal hepatitis. Subacute hepatic necrosis secondary to chaparral leaf. *J. Clin. Gastroenterol.* 12, 203

Katz, N., Teutsch, H.F., Jungermann, K., and Sasse, D. (1976). Perinatal development of the metabolic zonation of hamster liver parenchyma. *FEBS Lett.* 69, 23.

Katzka, D.A., Saul, S.H., Jorkasky, D., Sigal, H., Reynolds, J.C., and Soloway, R.D. (1986). Azathioprine and hepatic venocclusive disease in renal transplant patients. *Gastroenterology* 90, 446.

Kaysen, G.A., Pond, S.M., Roper, M.H., Menke, D.J., and Marrama, M.A. (1985). Combined hepatic and renal injury in alcoholics during therapeutic use of acetaminophen. *Arch. Intern. Med.* 145, 2019.

Keefe, E.B., Blankenship, N.M., and Scharschmidt, B.S. (1979) Effect of chlorpromazine (CPZ) and its metabolites on liver plasma membrane (LPM) fluidity and ATPase activity. *Gastroenterology* 76, 1286.

Keefe, E.B., Reis, T.C., and Berland, J.E. (1982). Hepatotoxicity to both erythromycin estolate and erythromycin ethylsuccinate. *Dig. Dis. Sci.* 27, 701.

Keiding, S., Dossing, M., and Hardt, F. (1984). A nurse with liver injury associated with occupational exposure to halothane in a recovery unit. *Dan. Med. Bull.* 31, 255.

Kemeny, M.M., Battifora, H., Blayney, D.W., Cecci, G., Goldberg, D.A., Leong, L.A. et al. (1985). Sclerosing cholangitis after continuous hepatic artery infusion of FUDR. *Ann. Surg.* 202, 176.

Kendler, J., Anuras, S., Laborda, O., and Zimmerman, H.J. (1972). Perfusion of the isolated rat liver with erythromycin estolate and other derivates. *Proc. Soc. Exp. Biol. Med.* 139, 1272.

Kenna, J.G., Neuberger, J.M., and Williams, R. (1984a). An enzyme-linked immunosorbent assay for detection of antibodies against halothane-altered hepatocyte antigens. *J. Immunol. Methods* 75, 3.

Kenna, J.G., Neuberger, J.M., and Williams, R. (1984b). Characterisation of halothane-induced antigens by immunoblotting. *Biochem. Soc. Transact* 13, 910.

Kenna, J.G., Neuberger, J.M., Mieli Vergani, G., Mowat, A.P., and Williams, R. (1987). Halothane hepatitis in children. *Br. Med. J.* 249, 1209.

Kennedy, P. (1983) Liver cross-sensitivity to antipsychotic drugs. *Br. J. Psychiatry.* 143, 312.

Kent, G., Gay, S., Inouye, T., Bahu, R., Minick, O.T., and Popper, H. (1976). Vitamin A containing lipocytes and formation of type III collagen in liver injury. *Proc. Natl Acad. Sci. USA* 73, 3719.

Kerlin, P., Davis, L., McGill, D.G., Weiland, L.H., Adson, M.A., and Sheedy, P.G., (1983). Hepatic adenoma and focal nodular hyperplasia: clinical, pathologic and radiologic features. *Gastroenterology* 84, 994.

Kester, N.M. (1971). Isoniazid hepatotoxicity — fact or fantasy? *JAMA* 217, 699.

Kevat, S., Ahern, M., and Hall, P. (1988). Hepatotoxicity of methotrexate in rheumatic diseases. *Med. Toxicol. Adverse Drug Exp.* 3, 197.

Kew, M.C., Song, E., Mohammed, A., and Hodgkinson, J. (1990). Contraceptive steroids as a risk factor for hepatocellular carcinoma: a case control study in South African black women. *Hepatology* 11, 298.

Khan, A.A. (1985). Thorotrast-associated liver cancer. *Am. J. Gastroenterol.* 80, 699.

Kimura, A., Yoshida, I., Yamashita, F., Kuriya, N., Yamamoto, M., and Nagayama, K. (1989). The occurrence of intramitochondrial Ca2¢ granules in valproate-induced liver injury. *J. Pediatr. Gastroenterol. Nutr.* 8, 13.

Klatskin, G. (1968). Mechanisms of toxic and drug-induced hepatic injury. In *Toxicity of anaesthetics* (ed. B.R. Fink). Williams and Wilkins, Baltimore.

Klatskin, G. (1977). Hepatic tumours: possible relationship to use of oral contraceptives. *Gastroenterology* 73, 386.

Klatskin, G. and Kimberg, D.V. (1969). Recurrent hepatitis attributable to halothane sensitization in an anaesthetist. *N. Engl. J. Med.* 280, 515.

Kleckner, H.B., Yakulis, U., and Heller, P. (1975). Severe sensitivity to diphenylhydantoin with circulating antibodies to the drug. *Ann. Intern. Med.* 83, 522.

Klerman, G.L. and Cole, J.O. (1965). Clinical pharmacology of imipramine and related antidepressant compounds. *Pharmacol. Rev.* 17, 101.

Klintmalm, G.B.G., Iwatsuki, S., and Starzl, T.E. (1981). Cyclosporin A hepatotoxicity in 66 renal allograft recipients. *Transplantation* 32, 488.

Klion, F.M., Schaffner, F., and Popper, H. (1969). Hepatitis after exposure to halothane. *Ann. Intern. Med.* 71, 467.

Kloss, M.W., Rosen, G.M., and Rauckman, E.J. (1984). Cocaine-mediated hepatotoxicity. A critical review. *Biochem. Pharmacol.* 33, 169.

Knobler, H., Levi, I.S., Gavish, D., and Chajek-Shaul, T. (1986). Quinidine-induced hepatitis. *Arch. Intern. Med.* 146, 526.

Knodell, R.G., Holtzman, J.L., Crankshaw, D.L., Steele, M.M., and Stanley, L.N. (1982). Drug metabolism by rat and human hepatic microsomes in response to interaction with H₂ receptor antagonists. *Gastroenterology* 82, 84.

Knopp, R.H. (1989). Niacin and hepatic failure. *Ann. Intern. Med.* 111, 769.

Koch, H.K., Gropp, A., and Oehlert, W. (1985). Drug-induced liver injury in liver biopsies of the years 1981 and 1983, their prevalence and type of presentation. *Pathol. Res. Pract.* 179, 469.

Kohn, R.M. and Montes, M. (1969). Hepatic fibrosis following long acting nicotinic acid therapy. *Am. J. Med. Sci.* 258, 94.

Kojiro, M., Kawano, Y., Kawasaki, H., Nakashima, T., and Ikezaki, H. (1982). Thorotrast-induced hepatic angiosarcoma, and combined hepatocellular and cholangiocarcinoma in a single patient. *Cancer* 49, 2161.

Kojiro, M., Nakashima, T., Ito, Y., Ibezaki, H., Mori, T., and Kido, C. (1985). Thorium dioxide-related angiosarcoma of the liver: pathomorphologic study of 29 autopsy cases. *Arch. Pathol. Lab. Med.* 109, 853.

Konttinen, A. (1972). Hepatotoxicity of sulphamethoxypyridazine. *Br. Med. J.* ii, 168.

Kory, R.C., Bradley, M.H., Watson, R.N., Callahan, R., and Peters, B.J. (1959). A six month evaluation of an anabolic drug, norethandrolene, in underweight persons — II. Bromsulphthalein (BSP) retention and liver function. *Am. J. Med.* 26, 243.

Krivoy, N., Raz, R., Carter, A., and Alroy, G. (1982). Reversible hepatic veno-occlusive disease and 6-thioguanine. *Ann. Intern. Med.* 96, 788.

Kramp, J.L. (1965). Glutamic pyruvic acid transaminases during treatment with amitriptyline and imipramine. *Acta Psychiatr. Scand.* 43, 1.

Kumar, V.V., Mahesh, B.V., Raju, V.K., and Devi, K.R. (1989). Trimethoprim induced intrahepatic cholestasis. *Indian Paediatr.* 26, 181.

Kun, L.F. and Camitta, B.M. (1978). Hepatopathy following irradiation and adriamycin. *Cancer* 42, 81.

Kunin, C.M., Dornbush, A.C., and Finland, M. (1959a). Distribution and excretion of four tetracycline analogues in normal young men. *J. Clin. Invest.* 38, 1950.

Kunin, C.M., Rees, S.B., Merrill, J.P., and Finland, M. (1959b). Persistence of antibodies on blood of patients with acute renal failure — I: tetracycline and chlortetracycline. *J. Clin. Invest.* 38, 1487.

Kuzell, W.C., Schaffazick, R.W., Naugler, W.E., Gaudin, G., and Mankle, E.A. (1953). Phenylbutazone. Further clinical evaluation. *Arch. Intern. Med.* 92, 603.

Labadarios, D., Davis, M., and Williams, R. (1976). Paracetamol, alphamercaptopropionyl glycine and some observations on the toxicity of protective agents. *J. Int. Med. Res.* 4 (suppl. 4), 130.

Labadarios, D., Davis, M., Portmann, B., and Williams, R. (1977). Paracetamol-induced hepatic necrosis in the mouse — relationship between covalent binding, hepatic glutathione depletion and the protective effects of alphamercaptopropionyl glycine. *Biochem. Pharmacol.* 26, 31.

Lake, B.G., Harris, R.A., Phillips, J.C., and Gangolli, S.D. (1981). Studies on the effects of L-ascorbic acid on acetaminophen-induced hepatotoxicity I. Inhibition of the covalent binding of acetaminophen metabolites to hepatic microsomes in vitro. *Toxicol. Appl. Pharmacol.* 60, 229.

Lal, S., Singhal, S.N., Burley, D.M., and Crossley, G. (1972). Effect of rifampicin and isoniazid on liver function. *Br. Med. J.* i, 148.

Lalonde, G., Theoret, G., Daloze, P., Bettez, P., and Katz, S.S. (1982). Inferior vena cava stenosis and Budd–Chiari syndrome in a woman taking oral contraceptives. *Gastroenterology* 82, 1452.

The Lancet (1974). Guidelines for diagnosis of therapeutic drug-induced liver injury by liver biopsies, occasional survey. *Lancet* i, 854.

Lang, P.G. (1979). Severe hypersensitivity reactions to allopurinol. *South. Med. J.* 72, 1361.

Langan, M.N. and Thomas, P. (1987). Penicillamine-induced liver disease. *Am. J. Gastroenterol.* 82, 1318.

Lanse, S.B., Arnold, G.L., Gowans, J.D., and Kaplan, M.M. (1985). Low incidence of hepatotoxicity associated with long-term, low-dose oral methotrexate in treatment of refractory psoriasis, psoriatic arthritis, and rheumatoid arthritis. An acceptable risk/benefit ratio. *Dig. Dis. Sci.* 30, 104.

Lansing, A.M., Davis, W.M., and Brizel, H.E. (1968). Radiation hepatitis. *Arch. Surg.* 96, 878.

Larrey, D., Amouyal, G., Danan, G., Degott, C., Pessayre, D., and Benhamou, J.P. (1987). Prolonged cholestasis after troleandomycin-induced acute hepatitis. *J. Hepatol.* 4, 327.

Larrey, D., Amouyal, G., Pessayre, D., Degott, C., Danne, O., Machayekhi, J.P., *et al.* (1988*a*). Amitriptyline-induced prolonged cholestasis. *Gastroenterology* 94, 200.

Larrey, D., Henrion, J., Heller, F., Babani, G., Degott, C., Pessayre, D., *et al.* (1988*b*). Metoprolol induced hepatitis: rechallenge and drug oxidation phenotyping. *Ann. Intern. Med.* 108, 67.

Larrey, D., Freneaux, E., Berson, A., Babany, G., Degott, C., Valla, D., *et al.* (1988*c*). Peliosis hepatis induced by 6-thioguanine administration. *Gut* 29, 1265.

Larsson-Cohn, U. (1965). Oral contraceptives and liver function tests. *Br. Med. J.* i, 1414.

Larsson-Cohn, U. and Stenram, U. (1967). Liver ultrastructure and function in icteric and non-icteric women using oral contraceptive agents. *Acta Med. Scand.* 181, 257.

Lauterburg, B.H. and Mitchell, J.R. (1982). Toxic doses of acetaminophen suppress hepatic glutathione synthesis. *Hepatology* 2, 8.

Lauterburg, B.H. and Velez, M.E. (1988). Glutathione deficiency in alcoholics: risk factor for paracetamol hepatotoxicity. *Gut* 29, 1153.

Lauterburg, B.H., Corcoran, G.B., and Mitchell, J.R. (1983). Mechanism of action of *N*-acetylcysteine in the protection against the hepatotoxicity of acetaminophen in rats in vivo. *J. Clin. Invest.* 71, 980.

Lauterburg, B.H., Smith, C.V., Hughes, H., and Mitchell, J.R. (1984). Biliary excretion of glutathione and glutathione disulphide in the rat. Regulation and response to oxidative stress. *J. Clin. Invest.* 73, 124.

Lauterburg, B.H., Smith, C.V., Todd, E.L., and Mitchell, J.R. (1985). Pharmacokinetics of the toxic hydrazino metabolites formed from isoniazid in humans. *J. Pharmacol. Exp. Ther.* 235, 566.

La-Vecchia, C., Negri, E., and Parazzine, F. (1989). Oral contraceptives and primary liver cancer. *Br. J. Cancer* 59, 460.

Lee, S.M., O'Brien, C.J., Williams, R., Whitaker, S., and Gould, S.R. (1986). Subacute hepatic necrosis induced by piroxicam. *Br. Med. J.* 293, 540.

Lees, A.W., Allan, G.W., and Smith, T.J. (1971). Toxicity from rifampicin plus isoniazid and rifampicin plus ethambutol therapy. *Tubercle* 52, 182.

Lemley, D.E., Delacy, L.M., Seeff, L.B., Ishak, K.G., and Nashel, D.J. (1989). Azathioprine induced hepatic veno-occlusive disease in rheumatoid arthritis. *Ann. Rheum. Dis.* 48, 342.

Lenler-Petersen, P., Sogard, H., Thestrup-Pedersen, K., and Zachariae, H. (1982). Galactose tolerance test and methotrexate-induced liver fibrosis and cirrhosis in patients with psoriasis. *Acta Derm. Venereol.* 62, 448.

Lennard, T.W. and Farndon, J.R. (1983). Sulphasalazine hepatotoxicity after 15 years' successful treatment for ulcerative colitis. *Br. Med. J.* 287, 96.

Leo, M.A. and Lieber, C.S. (1983). Hepatic fibrosis after long-term administration of ethanol and moderate vitamin A supplementation in the rat. *Hepatology* 3, 1.

Leonard, P.A., Clegg, D.O., Carson, C.C., Cannon, G.W., Egger, M.J., and Ward, J.R. (1987). Low dose pulse methotrexate in rheumatoid arthritis: an 8 year experience with hepatotoxicity. *Clin. Rheumatol* 6, 575.

Leonard, T.B. and Dent, J.G. (1984). Effects of H2 receptor antagonists on the hepatotoxicity of various chemicals. *Res. Commun. Chem. Pathol. Pharmacol.* 44, 375.

Leonard, T.B., Morgan, D.G., and Dent, J.G. (1985). Ranitidine–acetaminophen interaction. Effects on acetaminophen-induced hepatotoxicity in Fischer 344 rats. *Hepatology* 5, 480.

Lepper, M.H., Zimmerman, H.J., Caroll, G., Caldwell, E.R., Spies, H.W., Wolfe, C.K., *et al.* (1951). Effect of large doses of aureomycin, terramycin and chloramphenicol on livers of mice and dogs. *Arch. Intern. Med.* 88, 284.

Lesser, P.B., Vietti, M.M., and Clark, W.D. (1986). Lethal enhancement of therapeutic doses of acetaminophen by alcohol. *Dig. Dis. Sci.* 31, 103.

Levesque, H., Trivalle, C., Manchou, N.D., Vinel, J.P., and Moore, N. (1989). Fulminant hepatitis due to cyproterone acetate. *Lancet* i, 215.

Lewis, J.H. and Schiff, E. (1988). Methotrexate-induced chronic liver injury: guidelines for detection and prevention. The ACG Committee on FDS-related matters. *Am. Coll. Dermatol.* 83, 1337.

Lewis, J H., Zimmermann, H.J., Ishak, K.G., and Mullick, F.D. (1983*a*). Enflurane hepatotoxicity. A clinicopathologic study of 24 cases. *Ann. Intern. Med.* 98, 984.

Lewis, J.H., Tice, H.L., and Zimmermann, H.J. (1983). Budd-Chiari syndrome associated with oral contraceptive steroids. Review of treatment of 47 cases. *Dig. Dis. Sci.* 28, 673.

Lewis, J.H., Zimmerman, H.J., Benson, G.D., and Ishak, K.G. (1984). Hepatic injury associated with ketoconazole therapy. Analysis of 33 cases. *Gastroenterology* 86, 503.

Lewis, J.H., Mullick, F., Ishak, K G., Ranard, R C., Ragsdale, B., Perse, R M., *et al.* (1990). Histopathologic analysis of suspected amiodarone hepatotoxicity. *Hum. Pathol.* 21, 59.

Lewis, M , Schenker, S., and S. Combes, B. (1967). Studies on the pathogenesis of tetracycline-induced fatty liver. *Am. J. Dig. Dis.* 12, 429.

Liano, F., Moreno, A., Matesanz, R., Teruel, J.L., Redondo, C., Garcia-Martin, F., *et al.* (1989). Veno-occlusive hepatic disease of the liver in renal transplantation: is azathioprine the cause? *Nephron* 51, 509.

Lightdale, C.J., Wasser, J., Coleman, M., Brower, M., Teft, M., and Pasmantier, M. (1979). Anticoagulation and high dose liver radiation. A preliminary report. *Cancer* 43, 174.

Limaye, A. and Ruffolo, P.R. (1987). Propylthiouracil-induced fatal hepatic necrosis. *Am. J. Gastroenterol.* 82, 152.

Lin, J.H. and Levy, G. (1981). Sulfate depletion after acetaminophen administration and replenishment by infusion of sodium sulfate or *N*-acetylcysteine in rats. *Biochem. Pharmacol.* 30, 2723.

Linscheer, W.G., Raheja, K.L., Cho, C., and Smith, N.J. (1980). Mechanisms of the protective effect of propylthiouracil against acetaminophen (Tylenol) hepatotoxicity in the rat. *Gastroenterology* 78, 100.

Lloyd-Thomas, H.G.L. and Sherlock, S. (1952). Testosterone therapy for the pruritus of obstructive jaundice. *Br. Med. J.* ii, 1289.

Lo, K.J., Eastwood, I.R., and Edelman, S. (1967). Cholestatic jaundice associated with chlordiazepoxide hydrochloride (Librium) therapy: report of a case and review of the literature. *Am. J. Dig. Dis.* 12, 845.

Lobatto, S., Dijkmans, B.A., Mattie, H., and van-Hooff, J.P. (1982). Flucloxacillin-associated liver damage. *Neth. J. Med.* 25, 47.

Lo Indice, T.A. and Lang, J.A. (1978). Tolazamide induced hepatic dysfunction. *Am. J. Gastroenterol.* 69, 81.

Luke, D.R., Rocci, M.L. Jr, Schaible, D.H., and Ferguson, R.K. (1986). Acute hepatotoxicity after excessively high doses of carbamazepine on two occasions. *Pharmacotherapy* 6, 108.

Lyon, J., Bookstein, J.J., Cartwright, C.A., Romano, A., and Heeney, D.J. (1984). Peliosis hepatis: diagnosis by magnification wedged hepatic venography. *Radiology* 150, 147.

McClay, E., Lusch, C.J., and Mastrangelo, M.J. (1987). Allergy-induced hepatic toxicity associated with dacarbazine. *Cancer Treat. Rep.* 71, 219.

McConnell, J.B., Powell-Jackson, P.R., Davis, M., and Williams, R. (1981). Use of liver function tests as predictors of rifampicin metabolism in patients with cirrhosis. *Q. J. Med.* 50, 77.

McDonald, G.B., Sharma, P., Matthews, D.E., Shulman, H.M., and Thomas, E.D. (1984). Veno-occlusive disease of the liver after bone marrow transplantation: diagnosis, incidence and predisposing factors. *Hepatology* 4, 116.

McDonald, G.B., Sulman, H.M., Sullivan, K.M., and Spencer, G.D. (1986). Intestinal and hepatic complications of human bone marrow transplantation. *Gastroenterology* 90, 460.

McGilchrist, A.J. and Hunter, J.A. (1986). Sulphasalazine hepatotoxicity: lack of a hypersensitivity response. *Ann. Rheum. Dis.* 45, 967.

McGourhy, J.M., Silas, J.H., Lennard, M.S., Tucker, G.T., and Woods, H.F. (1985). Metoprolol metabolism and debrisoquine oxidation polymorphism — population and family studies. *Br. J. Clin. Pharmacol.* 20, 555.

McIntyre, R.E., Magidson, J.G., Austin, G.E., and Gale, R.P. (1981). Fatal veno-occlusive disease of the liver following high-dose 1,3-bis (2-chloroethyl)-1-nitrosourea (BCNU) and autologous bone marrow transplantation. *Am. J. Clin. Path.* 75, 614.

McLean, A.E.M. and Nuttall, L. (1978). An *in vitro* model of liver injury using paracetamol treatment of liver slices and prevention of injury by some antioxidants. *Biochem. Pharmacol.* 27, 425.

McMaster, K.R. and Hennigar, G.R. (1981). Drug-induced granulomatous hepatitis. *Lab. Invest.* 44, 61.

Maddrey, W.C. (1987a). Hepatic effects of acetaminophen. Enhanced toxicity in alcoholics. *J. Clin. Gastroenterol.* 9, 180.

Maddrey, W.C. (1987b). Hepatic vein thrombosis (Budd–Chiari syndrome): possible association with the use of oral contraceptives. *Semin. Liver Dis.* 7, 32.

Maddrey, W.C. and Boitnott, J.K. (1973). Isoniazid hepatitis. *Ann. Intern. Med.* 79, 1.

Maddrey, W.C. and Boitnott, J.K. (1977). Drug-induced chronic liver disease. *Gastroenterology* 72, 1348.

Manivel, J.C., Bhomer, J.R., and Snover, D.C. (1987). Progressive bile duct injury after thiabendazole administration. *Gastroenterology* 93, 245.

Mant, T.K.G., Tempowske, J.H., Volans, G.N., and Talbot, J.C.C. (1984). Adverse reactions to acetylcysteine and the effects of overdose. *Br. Med. J.* 289, 217.

Marks, J.W., Sue, S.O., Perlman, B.J., Bonorris, G.G., Varady, P., Lachin J.M. *et al.* (1981). Sulfation of chenodeoxycholic acid-induced elevations of serum transaminase in patients with gallstones. *J. Clin. Invest.* 68, 1190.

Marks, W.H., Thompson, N., and Appleman, H. (1988). Failure of hepatic adenomas (HCA) to regress after discontinuance of oral contraceptives. An association with focal nodular hyperplasia (FNH) and uterine leiomyoma. *Ann. Surg.* 208, 190.

Marquardt, G.H., Fisher, C.I., Levy, P., and Dowben, R.M. (1961). Effect of anabolic steroids on liver function tests and creatinine excretion. *JAMA* 175, 851.

Marrubio, A.T. and Danielson, B. (1975). Hepatic veno-occlusive disease in a renal transplant patient receiving azathioprine. *Gastroenterology* 69, 739.

Marsh, J.C. (1989). Hepatic vascular toxicity of dacarbazine (DTIC): not a rare complication. *Hepatology* 9, 790.

Mayhew, J.F. (1987). Halothane hepatitis in children. *Br. Med. J.* 295, 392.

Mays, E.T. and Christopherson, W. (1984). Hepatic tumours induced by sex steroids. *Semin. Liver Dis.* 4, 147.

Mazeika, P K. and Ford, M J. (1989). Chronic active hepatitis associated with diclofenac sodium therapy. *Br. J. Clin. Pract.* 43, 125.

Metreau, J.M., Dhumeaux, D., and Berthelot, P. (1972). Oral contraceptives and the liver. *Digestion* 7, 318.

Mihas, A.A., Holley, P., and Koff, R.S. (1976). Fulminant hepatitis and lymphocyte transformation due to propylthiouracil. *Gastroenterology* 70, 770.

Miller, J.A., Dodd, H., and Rustin, M.H. (1985). Ultrasound as a screening procedure for methotrexate induced liver damage in severe psoriasis. *Br. J. Dermatol.* 113, 699.

Miller, J.J. and Weissman, D.B. (1976). Correlations between transaminase concentrations and serum salicylate concentration in juvenile rheumatoid arthritis. *Arthritis Rheum.* 19, 115.

Miller, L.F. and Rumack, B.H. (1983). Clinical safety of high oral doses of acetylcysteine. *Semin. Oncol.* 10, 76.

Miller, M.G. and Jollow, D.J. (1984). Effect of L-ascorbic acid on acetaminophen-induced hepatotoxicity and covalent binding in hamsters. Evidence that *in vitro* covalent binding differs from that in vivo. *Drug. Metab. Dispos.* 12, 271.

Miller, M.G., Price, V.F., and Jollow, D.J. (1986). Anomalous susceptibility of the fasted hamster to acetaminophen hepatotoxicity. *Biochem. Pharmacol.* 35, 817.

Miller, R.P., Roberts, R.J., and Fischer, L.J. (1976). Acetaminophen elimination kinetics in neonates, children and adults. *Clin. Pharmacol. Ther.* 19, 284.

Miner, D.J. and Kissinger, P.T. (1979). Evidence for the involvement of *N*-acetyl-p-quinoneimine in acetaminophen metabolism. *Biochem. Pharmacol.* 28, 3285.

Minuk, G.Y., Kelly, J.K., and Hwang, W.S. (1988). Vitamin A hepatotoxicity in multiple family members. *Hepatology* 8, 272.

Mitchell, D., Smith, A., Rowan, B., Warnes, T.W., Haboubi, N.Y., Lucas, S.B., *et al.* (1990). Serum type III procollagen peptide, dynamic liver function tests and hepatic fibrosis in psoriatic patients receiving methotrexate. *Br. J. Dermatol.* 122, 1.

Mitchell, J.R. and Jollow, D.J. (1975). Metabolic activation of drugs to toxic substances. *Gastroenterology* 68, 392.

Mitchell, J.R., Jollow, D.J., Potter, W.Z., Davis, D.C., Gillette, J.R., and Brodie, B.B. (1973a). Acetaminophen-induced hepatic necrosis — I. Role of drug metabolism. *J. Pharmacol. Exp. Ther.* 187, 211.

Mitchell, J.R., Jollow, D.J., Potter, W.Z., Gillette, J.R., and Brodie, B.B.(1973b). Acetaminophen induced hepatic necrosis IV. Protective role of glutathione. *J. Pharmacol. Exp. Ther.* 187, 217.

Mitchell, J.R., Thorgiersson, S.S., Potter, W.Z., Jollow, D.J., and Keiser, H.(1974). Acetaminophen-induced hepatic injury: Protective role of glutathione in man and rationale for therapy. *Clin. Pharmacol. Ther.* 16, 676.

Mitchell, J.R., Thorgiersson, U.P., Black, M., Timbrell, J.A., Snodgrass, W.R., Potter, W.Z., *et al.* (1975). Increase incidence of isoniazid hepatitis in rapid acetylators: possible relation to hydrazine metabolites. *Clin. Pharmacol. Ther.* 18, 70.

Mitchell, J.R., Nelson, W.L., Potter, W.Z., Sasame, H.A., and Jollow, D.J. (1976a). Metabolic activation of furosemide to a chemically reactive hepatotoxic metabolite. *J. Pharmacol. Exp. Ther.* 199, 41.

Mitchell, J.R., Zimmerman, H.J., Ishak, K.G., Thorgiersson, U.P., Timbrell, J.A., Snodgrass, W.R., et al. (1976b). Isoniazid liver injury: clinical spectrum, pathology and probable pathogenesis. *Ann. Intern. Med.* 84, 181.

Mitchell, M.C., Schenker, S., Avant, G.R., and Speeg, K.V. (1981). Cimetidine protects against acetaminophen hepatotoxicity in rats. *Gastroenterology* 81, 1052.

Mitchell, M.C., Schenker, S., and Speeg, K.V. (1984). Selective inhibition of acetaminophen oxidation and toxicity by cimetidine and other histamine H_2 receptor antagonists *in vivo* and *in vitro* in the rat and in man. *J. Clin. Invest.* 73, 383.

Mitrane, M.P., Singh, A., and Seibold, J.R. (1986). Cholestasis and fatal agranulocytosis complicating sulfasalazine therapy: case report. *J. Rheumatol.* 13, 969.

Miyazaki, K., Nakayama, F., and Koga, A. (1984). Effect of chenodeoxycholic and ursodeoxycholic acid on isolated adult human hepatocytes. *Dig. Dis. Sci.* 79, 1123.

Mockli, G., Crowley, M., Stern, R., and Warnock, M.L. (1989). Massive hepatic necrosis in a child after administration of phenobarbital. *Am. J. Gastroenterol.* 84, 820.

Moesner, J., Baunsgaard, P.,Starklint, H., and Thommesen, N. (1977). Focal nodular hyperplasia of the liver. *Acta Pathol. Microbiol. Scand.* 85, 113.

Mohabbat, O., Shafig Younos, M., Merzao, A.A., and Strivastava, R.N. (1976). An outbreak of hepatic veno-occlusive disease in Western Afghanistan. *Lancet* ii, 269.

Mohamed, S.D. (1965). Sensitivity reaction to phenindione with urticaria, hepatitis and pancytopenia. *Br. Med. J.* ii, 1475.

Moldawsky, R.J. (1984). Hepatotoxicity associated with maprotiline therapy: case report. *J. Clin. Psychiatry* 45, 178.

Moldeus, P. (1981). Capacity of conjugative pathways and glutathione homoeostasis: Use of isolated cells in the study of paracetamol metabolism an toxicity. In *Drug reactions and the liver* (ed. M. Davis, J.M. Tredger, and R. Williams). Pitman Medical, Tunbridge Wells.

Moldeus, P., Andersson, B., Norling, A., and Ormstad, K. (1980). Effect of chronic ethanol administration on drug metabolism in isolated hepatocytes with emphasis on paracetamol activation. *Biochem. Pharmacol.* 29, 1741.

Molleken, K., Stahl, E., and Bretzke, G. (1979). Morphologische und klinische Leberfunde nach Einnahme oraler Kontrazeptiva. *Z. Gesamte Inn. Med.* 2, 78.

Moller, S., Iversen, P., and Franzmann, M.B. (1990). Flutamide induced liver failure. *J. Hepatol.* 10, 346.

Morant, R. and Ruttner, J.R. (1987). Late complications of thorotrast. Experiences from Zurich. *Schweiz. Med. Wochenschr.* 117, 952.

Morgan, M.Y., Reshef, R., Shah, R.R., Oates, N.S., Smith, R.L., and Sherlock, S. (1984). Impaired oxidation of debrisoquine in patients with perhexiline liver injury. *Gut* 25, 1057.

Moskovitz, R., Devane, C.L., Harris, R., and Stewart, R.B. (1982). Toxic hepatitis and single daily dosage imipramine therapy. *J. Clin. Psychiatry* 43, 4165.

Moss, J.D., Lewis, J.E., and Knauer, C.M. (1972). Isoniazid-associated hepatitis. *Am. Rev. Respir. Dis.* 106, 849.

Moulding, T.S. Jr and Goldstein, S. (1962). Hepatotoxicity due to ethionamide. *Am. Rev. Respir. Dis.* 86, 252.

Moulding, T.S., Redeker, A.G., and Kanel, G.C. (1989). Twenty isoniazid-associated deaths in one state. *Am. Rev. Respir. Dis.* 140, 700.

Moustafa, M.A.A., Claesen, M., Adline, J., Vandervorst, D., and Poupaert, J.H. (1983). Evidence for an arene-3, 4-oxide as a metabolic intermediate in the *meta*- and *para*-hydroxylation of phenytoin in the dog. *Drug Metab. Dispos.* 11, 574.

Mullick, F.G. and Ishak, K.G. (1980). Hepatic injury associated with diphenylhydantoin therapy. A clinicopathological study of 20 cases. *Am. J. Clin. Pathol.* 74, 442.

Mullin, G.E., Greenson, J.K., and Mitchell, M.C. (1989). Fulminant hepatic failure after ingestion of sustained-release nicotinic acid. *Ann. Intern. Med.* 111, 253.

Murphy, J.V., Marquardt, K.M., and Shug, K.L. (1985). Valproic acid-associated abnormalities of carnitine metabolism. *Lancet* i, 820.

Mushin, W.W., Rosen, M., and Jones, E.V. (1971). Posthalothane jaundice in relation to previous administration of halothane. *Br. Med. J.* iii, 18.

Naeim, F., Copper, P.H., and Semion, A. (1973). Peliosis hepatis — possible etiologic role of anabolic steroids. *Arch. Pathol.* 98, 284.

Nakao, J.L., Gelb, A.M., Stenger, R.J., and Siegel, J.H. (1985). A case of chronic liver disease due to tolazamide. *Gastroenterology* 89, 192.

NAS/NRC Report (1966). Summary of the National Halothane Study. Possible association between halothane anaesthesia and postoperative hepatic necrosis. Report by Subcommittee on the National Halothane Study of the Committee on Anaesthesia, National Academy of Sciences — National Research Council. *JAMA* 197, 775.

Nataf, C., Feldman, G., Lebrec, D., Degott, C., Descamps, J.M., Rueft, B., *et al.* (1979). Idiopathic portal hypertension (perisinusoidal fibrosis) after renal transplantation. *Gut* 20, 531.

Nelson, S.D., Mitchell, J.R., Timbrell, J.A., Snodgrass, W.R., and Corcoran, G.B. (1976). Isoniazid and iproniazid: activation of metabolites to toxic intermediates in man and rat. *Science* 193, 901.

Nelson, S.D., Dahlin, E.J., Rauckman, E.J., and Rosen, G.M. (1981). Peroxidase-mediated formation of reactive metabolites of acetaminophen. *Mol. Pharmacol.* 20, 195.

Neuberger, J.M. and Davis, M. (1983). Immune mechanisms in drug induced liver injury. In *Recent advances in hepatology.* (ed. H.C. Thomas and R.N.M McSween), p. 89. Churchill Livingstone, Edinburgh.

Neuberger, J.M. and Kenna, J.G. (1988). Halothane hepatitis: a model of immunoallergic disease. In *Liver cells and drugs*, Vol. 164 (ed. A Guillouzo), p. 161. Colloque INSERM/John Libbey Eurotext Ltd, London/Paris.

Neuberger, J.M. and Williams, R. (1984). Halothane anaesthesia and liver damage. *Br. Med. J.* 289, 1136.

Neuberger, J.M. and Williams, R. (1989). Immune mechanisms in tienilic acid associated hepatotoxicity. *Gut* 30, 515.

Neuberger, J.M., Davis, M., and Williams, R. (1980a). Long-term ingestion of paracetamol and liver disease. *Proc. R. Soc. Med.* 73, 701.

Neuberger, J.M., Portmann, B., Nunnerley, H., Davis, M., and Williams, R. (1980b). Oral contraceptive-associated liver tumours: occurrence of malignancy and difficulties in diagnosis. *Lancet* i, 273.

Neuberger, J.M., Mieli-Vergani, G., Tredger, J.M., Davis, M., and Williams R. (1981). Oxidative metabolism of halothane in the production of altered hepatocyte membrane antigens in acute halothane-induced necrosis. *Gut* 22, 669.

Neuberger, J.M., Gimson, A.E.S., Davis, M., and Williams R. (1982). Specific serological markers in the diagnosis of fulminant hepatic failure associated with halothane anaesthesia. *Br. J. Anaesth.* 55, 15.

Neuberger, J.M., Kenna, J.G., Aria, K.N., and Williams, R. (1985). Antibody mediated hepatocyte injury in methyl dopa induced hepatotoxicity. *Gut* 26, 1233.

Neuberger, J.M., Forman, D., Doll, R., and Williams, R. (1986). Oral contraceptives and hepatocellular carcinoma. *Br. Med. J.* 292, 1355.

Nime, F., Pickren, J.W., and Vana, J. (1979). The histology of liver tumours in oral contraceptive users observed during a national survey by the American College of Surgeons Commission on Cancer. *Cancer* 44, 1481.

Nordblom, G.D. and Coon, M.J. (1977). Hydrogen peroxide formation and stoichiometry of hydroxylation reactions catalyzed by highly purified liver microsomal cytochrome. *Arch. Biochem. Biophys.* 180, 343.

Nyfors, A. (1977). Liver biopsies from psoriatics related to methotrexate therapy. Findings in post-methotrexate liver biopsies from 160 psoriatics. *Acta Pathol. Microbiol. Scand.* 85, 511.

Nyfors, A. (1986). Methotrexate hepatotoxicity in psoriasis and psoriatic arthritis. *Rheumatology* 9, 192.

Ockner, R.K. and Davidson, C.S. (1967). Hepatic side-effects of oral contraceptives. *N. Engl. J. Med.* 276, 331.

Oda, T., Shikata, T., and Naito, C. (1970). Phospholipid fatty liver: a report of three cases with a new type of fatty liver. *Jpn J. Exper. Med.* 40, 127.

O'Dell, J.R., Zetterman, R.K., and Burnett, D.A. (1986). Centrilobular hepatic fibrosis following acetaminophen-induced hepatic necrosis in an alcoholic. *JAMA* 255, 2636.

Offit, K. and Sojka, D.A. (1984). Ranitidine. *N. Engl. J. Med.* 310, 1603.

Ogburn, R.M., Myers, P.I., and Bundick, G.F. (1976). Hepatitis associated with dantrolene sodium. *Ann. Intern. Med.* 84, 53.

Oliver, L.E., Iser, J.A., Stenving, G.F., and Smallwood, R.A. (1972). Abdominal pain and erythromycin estolate. *Lancet* ii, 980.

Oliver, R.M., Rickenback, M.A., Thomas, M.R., and Neville, E. (1987). Intrahepatic cholestasis associated with co-trimoxazole. *Br. J. Clin. Pract.* 41, 975.

Olson, J.A. (1983). Adverse effects of large doses of vitamin A and retinoids. *Semin. Oncol.* 10, 290.

Olsson, R. and Zettergren, L. (1988). Anticonvulsant-induced liver damage. *Am. J. Gastroenterol.* 83, 576.

Opolon, P., Cartron, J., Chicot, D., and Caroli, J. (1969). Application of the lymphoblast transformation test to the diagnosis of drug-induced hepatitis. *Presse Med.* 77, 2041.

Orrellana-Alcalde, J.M. and Dominguez, J.P. (1966). Jaundice and oral contraceptive drugs. *Lancet* ii, 1278.

Oskiowska-Evers, B., Dayer, P., Meyer, U.A., Robertz, G.M., and Eichelbaum, M. (1987). Evidence for altered catalytic properties of the cytochrome P-450 involved in sparteine oxidation in poor metabolisers. *Clin. Pharmacol. Therap.* 41, 320.

Pagliaro, L., Camposi, G., and Aguglira, F. (1969). Barbiturate jaundice — report of a case due to barbital-containing drug with positive rechallenge to phenobarbital. *Gastroenterology* 56, 938.

Pantarotto, C., Arboix, M., Sezzana, P., and Abbruzzi, R. (1982). Studies on 5,5-diphenylhydantoin irreversible binding to rat liver microsomal proteins. *Biochem. Pharmacol.* 31, 1501.

Paquette, P., Campos, L.T., and Flax, I. (1987). Prevention and treatment of sclerosing cholangitis related to chemotherapy delivered by infusaid pump. *Proc Am. Soc. Clin. Oncol.* 6, 89.

Paradinas, F.J., Bull, T.B., Westaby, D., and Murray-Lyons, I.M. (1977). Hyperplasia and prolapse of hepatocytes into hepatic veins during long-term methyltestosterone therapy: possible relationships of these changes to the development of peliosis hepatis and liver tumours. *Histopathology* 1, 225.

Paramsothy, J., Strange, R., Sharif, H., Collins, M., Shaw, P., andLawrence, C.M.(1988). The use of antipyrine clearance to measure liver damage in psoriatic patients receiving methotrexate. *Br. J. Dermatol.* 119, 761.

Parker, W.A. (1984). Captopril-induced cholestatic jaundice. *Drug. Intell. Clin. Pharm.* 18, 234.

Partin, J.S. (1989). Valproic acid therapy and mitochondrial alterations. *J. Pediatr. Gastroenterol. Nutr.* 8, 5.

Paumgartner, G., Reichen, J., Von Bergmann, K., and Preisig, R. (1976). Elaboration of hepatocyte bile. *Bull. N.Y. Acad. Med.* 51, 455.

Perez, V., Gorodisch, S., De Martire, J., and Di Paola, G. (1969). Oral contraceptives: long-term use produces fine structural changes in liver mitochondria. *Science* 165, 805.

Perino, L.E., Warren, G.H., and Levine, J.S. (1987). Cocaine induced hepatotoxicity in humans. *Gastroenterology* 93, 176.

Perkins, J. (1962). Phenindione jaundice. *Lancet* i, 125.

Pessayre, D. and Larrey, D. (1988). Acute and chronic drug-induced hepatitis. In: *Baillière's Clin. Gastroenterol.* 2, 385.

Pessayre, D., Bichara, M., Feldmann, G., Degott, C., Potet, F., and Benhamou, J.P. (1979). Perhexiline maleate-induced cirrhosis. *Gastroenterology* 76, 170.

Pessayre, D., Larrey, D., Funck-Bretano, C., and Benhamou, J.P. (1985). Drug interactions and hepatitis produced by some macrolide antibiotics. *J. Antimicrob. Chemother.* 16, 181.

Peters, J.H., Miller, K.S., and Brown, P. (1965). Studies on the metabolic basis for the genetically determined capacities for isoniazid inactivation in man. *J. Pharmacol. Exp. Ther.* 150, 298.

Peterson, B.J. and Rumack, B.H. (1981). Age as a variable in acetaminophen overdose. *Arch. Intern. Med.* 141, 390.

Peterson, F.J., Knodell, R.G., Lindemann, N.J., and Steele, N.M. (1983). Prevention of acetaminophen and cocaine hepatotoxicity in mice by cimetidine treatment. *Gastroenterology* 85, 122.

Peterson, R.E. and Fujimoto, J.M. (1977). Increased biliary free permeability produced in rats by hepatoactive agents. *J. Pharmacol. Exp. Ther.* 202, 732.

Pettavel, J., Gardiol, D., Bergier, N., and Schnyder, P. (1986). Fatal liver cirrhosis associated with long-term arterial infusion of floxuridine. *Lancet* ii, 1162.

Pezzimenti, J.F. and Hahn, A.L. (1970). Anicteric hepatitis induced by diphenylhydantoin. *Arch. Intern. Med.* 125, 118.

Phillips, M.J., Fisher, R.L., Anderson, D.W., Lan, S.P., Lachin, J.M., and Boyer, J.L. (1983). Ultrastructural evidence of intrahepatic cholestasis before and after chenodeoxycholic acid therapy in patients with cholelithiasis: The National Co-operative Gallstone Study. *Hepatology* 3, 209.

Phillips, S. and Tashman, H. (1963). Ethionamide jaundice. *Am. Rev. Respir. Dis.* 87, 896.

Pieterse, A.S., Rowland, J., and Dunn, D. (1983). Perhexiline maleate induced cirrhosis. *Pathology* 15, 201.

Piperno, E. and Berssenbruegge, D.A. (1976). Reversal of experimental paracetamol toxicosis with *N*-acetylcysteine. *Lancet* ii, 738.

Plaa, G.L. and Hewitt, W.R. (1982). Biotransformation products and cholestasis. *Prog. Liver Dis.* 7, 179.

Pliskin, M. (1975). Peliosis hepatis. *Radiology* 114, 29.

Podurgiel, B.J., McGill, D.B., Ludwig, J., Taylor, W.F., and Muller, S.A. (1973). Liver injury associated with methotrexate therapy for psoriasis. *Mayo Clin. Proc.* 48, 787.

Portal, R.W. and Emanuel, R.W. (1961). Phenindione hepatitis complicating anticoagulant therapy. *Br. Med. J.* ii, 1318.

Porter, J.M., Sussman, M.S., and Rosen, G.M. (1988). Cocaine-induced hepatotoxicity. *Hepatology* 8, 1713.

Porter, L.E., Elm, M.S., Van Thiel, D.S., and Eagon, P.K. (1987). Hepatic estrogen receptor in human liver disease. *Gastroenterology* 92, 735.

Portmann, B., Talbot, I.C., Day, D.W., Davidson, A.R., Murray-Lion, I.M., and Williams, R. (1975). Histopathological changes in the liver following a paracetamol overdose: correlation with clinical and biochemical parameters. *J. Pathol.* 117, 169.

Powell, W.J., Koch-Weser, J., and Williams, R.A. (1968). Lethal hepatic necrosis after therapy with imipramine and desipramine. *JAMA* 206, 642.

Powell-Jackson, P.R., Tredger, J.M., and Williams, R. (1984). Progress report: Hepatotoxicity to sodium valproate, a review. *Gut* 25, 673.

Presant, G.A. and Safdar, S.H. (1973). Oxymetholone in myelofibrosis and chronic lymphocytic leukaemia. *Arch. Intern. Med.* 132, 175.

Prescott, L.F. (1980). Kinetics and metabolism of paracetamol and phenacetin. *Br. J. Clin. Pharmacol.* 10 (Suppl. 2), 291.

Prescott, L.F. (1983). Paracetamol overdosage. Pharmacological considerations and clinical management. *Drugs* 25, 290.

Prescott, L.F., Wright, N., Roscoe, P., and Brown, S.S. (1971). Plasma paracetamol half life and hepatic necrosis in patients with paracetamol overdosage. *Lancet* i, 519.

Prescott, L.F., Newton, R.W., Swainson, C.P., Wright, H., Forrest, A.R.W., and Matthew, H. (1974). Successful treatment of severe paracetamol overdosage with cysteamine. *Lancet* i, 588.

Prescott, L.F., Park, J., Sutherland, G.R., Smith, I.J., and Proudfoot, A.F. (1976). Cysteamine methionine and penicillamine in the treatment of paracetamol poisoning. *Lancet* ii, 109.

Prescott, L.F., Illingworth, R.N., Critchley, J.A.J.H., Stewart, M.J., Adam, R.D., Proudfoot, T., *et al.* (1979). Intravenous *N*-acetylcysteine: the treatment of choice for paracetamol poisoning. *Br. Med. J.* ii, 1097.

Prescott, L.F., Leslie, P.J., and Padfield, P. (1982). Side effects of benoxaprofen. *Br. Med. J.* 284, 1783.

Price, C.P. and Alberti, K.G.M.M. (1985). Biochemical assessment of liver function. In *Liver and biliary disease* (ed. R. Wright, G.H. Millward-Sadler, K.G.M.M. Alberti, and S. Karran). Baillière, London.

Price, L.H., Nelson, J.C., and Waltrip, R. (1983). Desipramine associated hepatitis. *J. Clin. Psychopharmacol.* 34, 243.

Price, L.H., Nelson, J.C., and Jatlow, P.I. (1984). Effect of desipramine on clinical liver function tests. *Am. J. Psychiatry* 141, 798.

Punukollu, R.C., Kumar, S., and Mullen, K.D. (1990). Quinine hepatotoxicity. An underrecognized or rare phenomenon? *Arch. Intern. Med.* 150, 1112.

Raghuram, T.C., Krishnamurthi, D., and Kalamegham, R. (1978). Effect of vitamin C on paracetamol hepatotoxicty. *Toxicol. Lett.* 2, 175.

Raheja, K.L., Linscheer, W.G., Cho, C., and Mahony, D. (1982). Protective effect of propylthiouracil independent of its hypothyroid effect on acetaminophen toxicity in the rat. *J. Pharmacol. Exp. Ther.* 220, 427.

Raheja, K.L., Linscheer, W.G., and Cho, C. (1983). Prevention of acetaminophen hepatotoxicity by propylthiouracil in the glutathione depleted rat. *Comp. Biochem. Physiol.* 76(C), 9.

Raheja, K.L., Cho, C.D., and Hirose, N. (1987). Effect of nutritional status on propylthiouracil-induced protection against acetaminophen hepatotoxicity in the rat. *Drug. Nutr. Interact.* 5, 21.

Rahmat, J., Gelfand, R.L., Gelfand, M.C., Winchester, J.F., Schreiner, G.E., and Zimmerman, H.J. (1985). Captopril-associated cholestatic jaundice. *Ann. Intern. Med.* 102, 56.

Raper, R., Ibels, L., Lauer, C., Barnes, P., and Lunzer, M. (1984). Fulminant hepatic failure due to allopurinol. *Aust. N.Z. J. Med.* 14, 63.

Read, A.E., Harrison, C.V., and Sherlock, S. (1961). Chronic chlorpromazine jaundice. *Am. J. Med.* 31, 249.

Read, A.E., Wiesner, R.H., La Brecque, D.R., Tisst, J.G., Mullen, K.D., Sheer, R.L. *et al.* (1986). Hepatic veno-occlusive disease associated with renal transplantation and azathioprine therapy. *Ann. Intern. Med.* 104, 651.

Read, R.B., Tredger, J.M., and Williams, R. (1986). Analysis of factors responsible for continuing mortality after paracetamol overdose. *Hum. Toxicol.* 5, 201.

Recant, L. and Lacy, P. (1965). Fanconi's anaemia and hepatic cirrhosis. *Am. J. Med.* 39, 464.

Reddy, K.R., Brillant, P., and Schiff, E.R. (1989). Amoxicillin–clavulanate potassium-associated cholestasis. *Gastroenterology* 96, 1135.

Reed, W.D. and Williams, R. (1972). Halothane hepatitis as seen by the physician. *Br. J. Anaesth.* 44, 935.

Rendic, S., Kajifez, F., and Ruf, H.H. (1983). Characterization of cimetidine, ranitidine and related structures' interaction with cytochrome P-450. *Drug Metab. Dispos.* 11, 137.

Reshef, R., Lok, A.S., and Sherlock, S. (1982). Cholestatic jaundice in fascioliasis treated with niclofolan. *Br. Med. J.* 285, 1243.

Rex, D., Lumeng, L., Eble, J., and Rex, L. (1983). Intrahepatic cholestasis and sicca complex after thiabendazole: report of a case and review of the literature. *Gastroenterology* 85, 718.

Reyes, H. (1982). The enigma of intrahepatic cholestasis of pregnancy: lessons from Chile. *Hepatology* 2, 87.

Reyes, H., Ribalta, J., Gonzales, M.C., Segovia, N., and Oberhauser, E. (1981). Sulfobromophthalein clearance tests before and after ethynyl estradiol administration in women and men with familial history of intrahepatic cholestasis of pregnancy. *Gastroenterology* 81, 226.

Reynolds, E.S., Schlant, R.C., Gonic, H.C., and Dammin, G.J. (1957). Fatal massive necrosis of the liver as a manifestation of hypersensitivity to probenecid. *N. Engl. J. Med.* 251, 592.

Reynolds, R., Lloyd, D.A., and Slinger, R.P. (1981). Cholestatic jaundice induced by flurazepam hydrochloride. *Can. Med. Assoc. J.* 124, 893.

Reynolds, T.B., Peters, R.L., and Yamada, S. (1971). Chronic active and lupoid hepatitis caused by a laxative — oxyphenisatin. *N. Engl. J. Med.* 285, 813.

Ridker, P.M. and McDermott, W.V. (1989a). Comfrey herb tea and hepatic veno-occlusive disease. *Lancet* i, 657.

Ridker, P.M. and McDermott, W.V. (1989b). Hepatotoxicity due to comfrey herb tea. *Am. J. Med.* 87, 701.

Ridker, P.M., Ohkuma, S., McDermott, W.V., Trey, C., and Huxtable, R.J. (1985). Hepatic venocclusive disease associated with the consumption of pyrrolizidine-containing dietary supplements. *Gastroenterology* 88, 1050.

Rigas, B., Rosenfeld, L.E., Barwick, K.W., Enriquez, R., Helzberg, J., Batsford, W.P., *et al.* (1986). Amiodarone hepatotoxicity. A clinicopathologic study of five patients. *Ann. Intern. Med.* 104, 348.

Rigauts, H.D., Selleslag, D.L., Van Eyken, P.L., Van Damme, F.J., Fevery, J.M., and Marchal, G.J. (1988). Erythromycin-induced hepatitis: simulator of malignancy. *Radiology* 169, 661.

Rigberg, L.A., Robison, M.J., and Espiritu, C.R. (1976). Chlorpropamide-induced granulomas. A probable hypersensitivity reaction in liver and bone marrow. *JAMA* 235, 409.

Riska, N. (1976). Hepatitis cases in isoniazid treated groups and in a control group. *Bull. Int. Union Tuberc.* 51, 203.

Roat, J.W., Wald, A., Mendelow, H., and Pataki, K.I. (1982). Hepatic angiosarcoma associated with short-term arsenic ingestion. *Am. J. Med.* 73, 933.

Robinson, D.S., MacDonald, G., and Hobin, F.P. (1965). Sodium diphenylhydantoin reaction with evidence of circulating antibodies. *JAMA* 192, 171.

Robinson, M.J. and Rywiin, A.M. (1970). Tetracycline associated fatty liver in the male: report of an autopsied case. *Am. J. Dig. Dis.* 15, 857.

Robinson, M.M. (1961). Antibiotics increase incidence of hepatotoxicity. *JAMA* 178, 89.

Rodgers, M.K., Glende, E.A., and Recknagel, R.O. (1977). Prelytic damage of red cells in filtrates from peroxidising microsomes. *Science* 196, 1221.

Roenigk, H.H. Jr (1988). Liver toxicity of retinoid therapy. *J. Am. Acad. Dermatol.* 19, 199.

Roenigk, H.H. Jr (1989). Liver toxicity of retinoid therapy. *Pharmacol. Ther.* 40, 145.

Rollins, B.J. (1986). Hepatic veno-occlusive disease. *Am. J. Med.* 81, 297.

Rollins, D.E. and Buckpitt, A.R. (1979). Liver cytosol catalysed conjugation of reduced glutathione with a reactive metabolite of acetaminophen. *Toxicol. Appl. Pharmacol.* 47, 331.

Ros, E., Small, D.M., and Carey, M.C. (1979). Effects of chlorpromazine hydrochloride on bile salt synthesis, bile formation and biliary lipid secretion in the rhesus monkey: a model for chlorpromazine-induced cholestasis. *Eur. J. Clin. Invest.* 9, 29.

Rose, M.B. (1972). Superior mesenteric vein thrombosis and oral contraceptives. *Postgrad. Med. J.* 48, 430.

Rosellini, S.R., Costa, P.L., Gaudio, M., Saragoni, A., and Miglio, F. (1989). Hepatic injury related to enalapril. *Gastroenterology* 97, 810.

Rosen, G.M., Singletary, W.V., Rauckman, E.J., and Killenberg, P.G. (1983). Acetaminophen hepatotoxicity. An alternative mechanism. *Biochem. Pharmacol.* 32, 2053.

Rosen, M. (1987). Guidelines on halothane. *Br. Med. J.* 294, 1229.

Rosenbaum, J., Katz, W.A., and Schumacher, H.R. (1980). Hepatotoxicity associated with use of D-penicillamine in rheumatoid arthritis. *Ann. Rheum. Dis.* 39, 152.

Roulet, M., Laurini, R., Rivier, L., and Calame, A. (1988). Hepatic veno-occlusive disease in new-born infant of a woman drinking herbal tea. *J. Pediatr.* 112, 433.

Roy, M.A., Nugent, F.W., and Aretz, H.T. (1989). Micronodular cirrhosis after thiabendazole. *Dig. Dis. Sci.* 34, 938.

Rubin, E. and Lieber, C.S. (1968). Microsomal enzymes in man and rats. Induction and inhibition by ethanol. *Science* 162, 690.

Rumack, B. (1981). Acetaminophen overdose. 662 cases with evaluation of oral acetylcysteine treatment. *Arch. Intern. Med.* 141, 380.

Rumboldt, Z. and Bota, B. (1984). Favorable effects of glibenclamide in a patient exhibiting idiosyncratic hepatotoxic reactions to both chlorpropamide and tolbutamide. *Acta Diabetol. Lat.* 21, 387.

Rumessen, J.J. (1986). Hepatotoxicity of amiodarone. *Acta Med. Scand.* 219, 235.

Runne, U., Doepfmer, K., Antz, H., Groth, W., and Feaux de Lacroix, W. (1980). Budd–Chiari Syndrom unter Dacarbazin. Todesfall während der adjuvanten Chemotherapie eines malignen Melanoms. *Dtsch. Med. Wochenschr.* 105, 230.

Sabath, L.D. and Gerstein, D.A. (1968). Serum glutamic oxalacetic transaminase. False elevations during administration of erythromycin. *N. Engl. J. Med.* 279, 1137.

Saint-Marc-Girardin, M.F., Zafrani, E.S., Prigent, A., Larde, D., Chauffour, J., and Dhumeaux, D. (1983). Unilobar small hepatic vein obstruction: possible role of progestogen given as oral contraceptive. *Gastroenterology* 84, 630.

Samuels, A.M. and Carey, M.C. (1978). Effects of chlorpromazine hydrochloride and its metabolites on Mg 2¢ and Na¢, K¢, ATPase activities of canalicular-enriched rat liver plasma. *Gastroenterology* 74, 1183.

Sanchez-Medal, L., Gomez-Leal, A., Duarte, L., and Rico, M.G. (1969). Anabolic androgenic steroids in the treatment of acquired aplastic anaemia. *Blood* 34, 283.

Sarachek, N.S., London, R.L., and Matulewicz, T.J. (1985). Diltiazem and granulomatous hepatitis. *Gastroenterology* 88, 1260.

Sarma, G.R., Immanuel, C., Kailasam, S., Narayana, A.S.L., and Venkateran, P. (1986). Rifampicin induced release of hydrazine from isoniazid. *Am. Rev. Respir. Dis.* 133, 1072.

Sato, C. and Lieber, C.S. (1981). Mechanism of the prevention effect of ethanol on acetaminophen-induced hepatotoxicity. *J. Pharmacol. Exp. Ther.* 218, 811.

Sato, C., Matsuda, Y., and Lieber, C.S. (1981a). Increased hepatotoxicity of acetaminophen after chronic ethanol consumption in the rat. *Gastroenterology* 80, 140.

Sato, C., Nakano, M., and Lieber, C.S. (1981b). Prevention of acetaminophen induced hepatotoxicity by acute ethanol administration in the rat: comparison with carbon tetrachloride hepatotoxicity. *J. Pharmacol. Exp. Ther.* 215, 805.

Schaffner, F. (1965). Effect of anabolic steroids in man. In *Symposium on therapeutic agents and the liver* (ed. N. MacIntyre and S. Sherlock), p. 99. Blackwell, Oxford.

Schaffner, F. (1966). The effect of oral contraceptives on the liver. *JAMA* 198, 1019.

Schaffner, F., Popper, H., and Chesrow, E. (1959). Cholestasis produced by the administration of norethandrolone. *Am. J. Med.* 26, 249.

Schenker, S., Olson, K.N., Dunn, D., Breen, K.J., and Combes, B. (1973). Intrahepatic cholestasis due to therapy of rheumatoid arthritis. *Gastroenterology* 64, 622.

Scheuer, P.J., Summerfield, J.A., Lal, S., and Sherlock, S. (1974). Rifampicin hepatitis. *Lancet* i, 421.

Schlangen, J. and Wils, J. (1984). Liver calcifications following hepatic artery infusion with 5-fluorouracil, adriamycin and mitomycin C (FAM). *ROFO* 140, 607.

Schmidt, G., Borsch, G., Muller, K.M., and Wegener, M. (1986). Methimazole-associated cholestatic liver injury: case report and brief literature review. *Hepatogastroenterology* 33, 244.

Schoenfield, L.J. and Foulk, W.T. (1964). Studies on sulphbromphthalein sodium (BSP) metabolism in man: (ii) the effect of artificially induced fever, norethandrolone (Nilevar) and iopanoic acid (Telepaque). *J. Clin. Invest.* 43, 1419.

Schoenfield, L.J. and Lachin, J.M. The Steering Committee and the National Co-operative Gallstone Study Group (1981). Chenodiol (Chenodeoxycholid Acid) for dissolution of gallstones: The National Co-operative Gallstone Study. *Ann. Intern. Med.* 95, 1257.

Schreiber, A.J. and Simon, F.R. (1983). Estrogen-induced cholestasis: clues to pathogenesis and treatment. *Hepatology* 3, 607.

Schroeder, J.S., Beier-Scott, L., Ginsburg, R., Bristow, M.R., and McAnley, B.J. (1985). Efficacy of diltiazem for medically refractory stable angina. Longterm follow up. *Clin. Cardiol.* 8, 480.

Schwartz, K. (1976). Essentiality and metabolic functions of selenium. *Med. Clin. North Am.* 60, 745.

Schwartz, M.S., Frank, M.S., Yanoff, A., and Morercki, R. (1989). Atenolol-associated cholestasis. *Am. J. Gastroenterol.* 84, 1084.

Schweitzer, I.I. and Peters, R.L. (1974). Acute submassive hepatic necrosis due to methyldopa. A case demonstrating possible initiation of chronic liver disease. *Gastroenterology* 66, 1203.

Scott, L.D., Katz, A.R., Duke, J.H., Cowan, D.F., and Maklad, N.F. (1984). Oral contraceptives, pregnancy, and focal nodular hyperplasia of the liver. *JAMA* 251, 1461.

Seaman, W.E., Ishak, K.G., and Plotz, P.H. (1974). Aspirin-induced hepatotoxicity in patients with systemic lupus erythematosus. *Ann. Intern. Med.* 80, 1.

Seeff, L.B., Cuccherini, B.A., Zimmerman, H.J., Adler, E., and Benjamin, S.B. (1986). Acetaminophen hepatotoxicity in alcoholics. A therapeutic misadventure. *Ann. Intern. Med.* 104, 399.

Seeman, P. (1972). The membrane actions of anesthetics and tranquilisers. *Pharmacol. Rev.* 24, 583.

Segarra, P.V., Lorain, V., and Sherman, D.S. (1968). Ethambutol treatment of tuberculosis in a controlled trial. *Scand. J. Respir. Dis.* 49, 202.

Seino, H., Dohi, S., Aiyoshi, Y., Mizutani, T., Nakamura, K., and Naito, H. (1986). Postoperative hepatic dysfunction after halothane or enflurane anesthesia in patients with hyperthyroidism. *Anesthesiology* 64, 122.

Setchell, K.D.R., Gosselin, S.J., Welsh, M.B., Johnston, J.O., Balisheri, W.F., Kramer, L.W., *et al.* (1987). Dietary estrogens — a probable cause of infertility and liver disease in captive cheetahs. *Gastroenterology* 93, 225.

Shaban, M.R., Golding, D.N., and Letcher, R.G. (1984). Fatal intraheptaic cholestasis and interstitial lung fibrosis following gold therapy for rheumatoid arthritis. *J. R. Soc. Med.* 77, 960.

Shallcross, H., Padley, S.P., Glynn, M.J., and Gibbs, D.D. (1987). Fatal renal and hepatic toxicity after treatment with diltiazem. *Br. Med. J.* 295, 1236.

Sharp, J.H., Trudell, J.M., and Cohen, E.N. (1979). Volatile metabolites and decomposition products of halothane in man. *Anesthesiology* 50, 2.

Sharp, J.R., Ishak, K.G., and Zimmerman, H.J. (1980). Chronic active hepatitis and severe hepatic necrosis associated with nitrofurantoin. *Ann. Intern. Med.* 92, 14.

Sharpe, P.C. and Hawkins, B.W. (1977). Efficacy and safety of cimetidine: long-term treatment with cimetidine. In *Cimetidine, Proceedings of the second symposium on histamine H₂-receptor antagonists* (ed. W.L. Burland and M. Allison), p. 358. Excerpta Medica, Amsterdam.

Shergy, W.J., Polisson, R.P., Caldwell, D.S., Rice, J.R., Pisetsky, D.S., and Allen, N.B. (1988). Methotrexate-associated hepatotoxicity: retrospective analysis of 210 patients with rheumatoid arthritis. *Am. J. Med.* 85, 771.

Sherlock, S. (1972). Liver disease due to drugs. In *Drug induced disease*, Vol. 4 (ed. L. Meyler and H.M. Peck), p. 241. Associated Scientific Publishers, Amsterdam.

Shmunes, E. (1974). Hypervitaminosis A in a patient with alopecia receiving renal dialysis. *Arch. Dermatol.* 115, 882.

Short, M.H., Burns, J.M., and Harris, M.E. (1968). Cholestatic jaundice and imipramine therapy. *JAMA* 206, 1791.

Shurbaji, M.S., Olson, J.L., and Kuhajda, F.P. (1987). Thorotrast-induced hepatic leiomyosarcoma and cholangiocarcinoma in a single patient. *Hum. Pathol.* 18, 524.

Silva, M.O., Reddy, K.R., McDonald, T., Jeffers, L.J., and Schiff, E.R. (1989). Danazol-induced cholestasis. *Am. J. Gastroenterol.* 84, 426.

Simon, F.R., Gonzales, M., Sutherland, E., and Accatino, L. (1980). Reversal of ethinyloestradiol-induced bile secretory failure with Triton WR-1339. *J. Clin. Invest.* 65, 851.

Simon, J.B., Manley, P.N., Prien, J.F., and Armstrong, P.W. (1984). Amiodarone hepatotoxicity simulating alcoholic liver disease. *N. Engl. J. Med.* 311, 167.

Simpson, D.G. and Walker, J.H. (1960). Hypersensitivity to para-aminosalicylic acid. *Am. J. Med.* 29, 297.

Singh, H.P., Hebert, M.A., and Gault, M.H. (1972). Effect of some drugs on clinical laboratory values as determined by the Technicon SMA 12/60. *Clin. Chem.* 18, 137.

Sipes, I.G. (1981). Halothane-associated hepatitis: evidence for direct toxicity. In *Drug reactions and the liver* (ed. M. Davis, J.M. Tredger and R. Williams), p. 157. Pitman Medical, Tunbridge Wells.

Sippel, S. and Agger, W.A. (1981). Nitrofurantoin-induced granulomatous hepatitis. *Urology* 18, 177.

Slater, T.F. (1984). Free radical mechanisms in tissue injury. *Biochem. J.* 222, 1.

Slattery, J.T. and Levy, G. (1977). Reduction of acetaminophen toxicity by sodium sulfate in mice. *Res. Commun. Chem. Pathol. Pharmacol.* 18, 167.

Slattery, J.T. and Levy, G. (1979). Acetaminophen kinetics in acutely poisoned patients. *Clin. Pharmacol. Therap.* 25, 184.

Smilkstein, M.J., Knapp, G.L., Kulig, K.W., and Rumack, B.H. (1988). Efficacy of oral *N*-acetylcystein in the treatment of acetaminophen overdose: analysis of the national multicenter study (1976-1985). *N. Engl. J. Med.* 319, 1557.

Smith, A.C., Roberts, S.M., Berman, L.M., Harbison, R.D., and James, R.C. (1988). Effects of piperonyl butoxide on halothane hepatotoxicity and metabolism in the hyperthyroid rat. *Toxicology* 50, 95.

Smith, D.W., Isakson, G., Frankel, L.R., and Kerner, J.A. Jr (1986). Hepatic failure following ingestion of multiple doses of acetaminophen in a young child. *J. Pediatr. Gastroenterol. Nutr.* 5, 822.

Smith, J.M. and Springett, V.H. (1966). Serum transaminase levels during treatment with isoniazid, streptomycin and *p*-aminosalicylic acid. *Tubercle* 47, 245.

Smith, J.P. and Scharer, L. (1969). Serum transaminase elevations and other hepatic abnormalities in patients receiving isoniazid. *Ann. Intern. Med.* 71, 1113.

Smith, M.D., Gibson, G.E., and Rowland, R. (1982). Combined hepatotoxicity and neurotoxicity following sulphasalazine administration. *Aust. N.Z. J. Med.* 12, 76.

Smythe, M.A. and Umstead, G.S. (1989). Phenytoin hepatotoxicity: a review of the literature. *Drug Invest.* 23, 13.

Sommer, M. (1989). Hepatic veno-occlusive disease and drinking of herbal teas. *J. Pediatr.* 115, 659.

Solis-Herrazo, J.A., Vidal, J.V., Colina, F., Santalla, F., and Castellano, G. (1986). Nodular regenerative hyperplasia of the liver associated with the toxic oil syndrome: report of five cases. *Hepatology* 6, 687.

Somayaji, B.N., Paton, A., Price, J.H., Harris, A.W., and Flewett, T.H. (1968). Norethisterone jaundice in two sisters. *Br. Med. J.* ii, 281.

Somogy, A. and Gugler, R. (1982). Drug interactions with cimetidine. *Clin. Pharmacokinet.* 7, 23.

Sotolongo, R.P., Neefe, L.I., Rudzki, C., and Ishak, K.G. (1978). Hypersensitivity reaction to sulfasalazine with severe hepatitis. *Gastroenterology* 75, 95.

Sparberg, M., Simon, N., and Del Greco, F. (1969). Intrahepatic cholestasis due to azathioprine. *Gastroenterology* 57, 439.

Speckler, S.J., Sperber, H., Doos, W.G., and Koff, R.S. (1981). Cholestasis and toxic epidermal necrolysis associated with phenytoin sodium ingestion: the role of bile duct injury. *Ann. Intern. Med.* 95, 455.

Speeg, K.V., Maldonado, A.L., and Mitchell, M.C. (1983). Additive protection by cimetidine and *N*-acetylcysteine against acetaminophen induced hepatotoxicity. (Abstr.) *Hepatology* 3, 860.

Speeg, K.V., Christian, D.C., and Mitchell, M.C. (1984). Ranitidine and acetaminophen hepatotoxicity. *Ann. Intern. Med.* 100, 315.

Spielberg, S.P. (1986). In vitro analysis of idiosyncratic drug reactions. *Clin. Biochem.* 19, 142.

Spielberg, S.P. and Gordon, G.B. (1984). Glutathione synthetase-deficient lymphocytes and acetaminophen toxicity. *Clin. Pharmacol. Ther.* 29, 51.

Spielberg, S.P., Gordon, G.B., Blake, D.A., Goldstein, D.A., and Herlong, H.F. (1981). Predisposition to phenytoin hepatotoxicity assessed in vitro. *N. Engl. J. Med.* 305, 722.

Stanley, P. and Mijch, A. (1986). Methyldopa: an often overlooked cause of fever and transient hepatocellular dysfunction. *Med. J. Aust.* 144, 603.

Starko, K.M., Ray, C.G., and Dominguez L.B. (1980). Reye's syndrome and salicylate use. *Pediatrics* 66, 859.

Steinbrecher, U.P., Lisbona, R., Huang, S.N., and Mishkin, S. (1981). Complete regression of hepatocellular adenoma after withdrawal of oral contraceptives. *Dig. Dis. Sci.* 26, 1045.

Stempel, D.A. and Miller, J.J. (1977). Lymphopenia and hepatic toxicity with ibuprofen. *J. Pediatr.* 90, 657.

Stevenson, R N., Nayani, T H., and Davies, J R. (1989). Acute hepatic dysfunction following parenteral amiodarone administration. *Postgrad. Med. J.* 65, 707.

Stewart, D.L. and Johnson, R.C. (1980). Acute hepatitis caused by sulfamethoxazole-trimethoprim. *Gastroenterology* 78, 1323A.

Stoelting, R.K. (1987). Isoflurane and postoperative hepatic dysfunction. *Can. J. Anaesth.* 34, 223.

Stoelting, R.K., Blitt, C.D., Cohen, P.J., and Merin, R.G. (1987). Hepatic dysfunction after isoflurane anaesthesia. *Anesth. Analg.* 66, 147.

Stoll, B.A., Andrews, J.T., and Motteram, R. (1966). Liver damage from oral contraceptives. *Br. Med. J.* i, 960.

Stone, W., McKinney, I., and Warnock, L. (1979). Spurious hyperbilirubinaemia in uraemic patients on propranolol therapy. *Clin. Chem.* 25, 1761.

Stricker, B.H.C. and Spoelstra, P. (1985). *Drug-induced hepatic injury.* Elsevier, Amsterdam.

Stricker, B.H., Van-den-Broek, J.W., Keuning, J., Eberhardt, W., Houben, H.G., Johnson, M., *et al.* (1989). Cholestatic hepatitis due to antibacterial combination of amoxicillin and clavulanic acid (Augmentin). *Dig. Dis. Sci.* 34, 1576.

Stromeyer, F.W. and Ishak, K.G. (1981). Nodular transformation (nodular 'regenerative' hyperplasia) of the liver. *Hum. Pathol.* 12, 60.

Sullivan, J.B., Rumarck, B.H., Thomas, H. Jr, Peterson, R.G., and Bryson, P. (1979). Pennyroyal oil poisoning and hepatotoxicity. *JAMA* 242, 2873.

Sweeney, E.C. and Evans, D.J. (1976). Hepatic lesions in patients treated with synthetic anabolic steroids. *J. Clin. Pathol.* 29, 626.

Swetnam, S.M. and Florman, A.L. (1984). Probable acetaminophen toxicity in an 18-month old infant due to repeated overdosing. *Clin. Pediatr.* 23, 104.

Swinburn, B.A., Croxson, M.S., Miller, M.V., and Crawford, K.B. (1986). Carbamazepine induced granulomatous hepatitis. *N.Z. Med. J.* 99, 167.

Szanto, E., Sandstedt, B., and Kollberg, B. (1987). Hepatotoxicity associated with low-dose, long-term methotrexate treatment of rheumatoid arthritis. *Scand. J. Rheumatol.* 16, 229.

Taggart, H.McA. and Alderdice, J.M. (1982). Fatal cholestatic jaundice in elderly patients taking benoxaprofen. *Br. Med. J.* 284, 1372.

Tam, S. and Carroll, W. (1989). Allopurinol hepatotoxicity. *Am. J. Med.* 86, 357.

Tanner, A.R. (1986). Hepatic cholestasis induced by trimethoprim. *Br. Med. J.* 293, 1072.

Tanner, L.A., Bosco, L.A., and Zimmerman, H.J. (1989). Hepatic toxicity after acebutolol therapy. *Ann. Intern. Med.* 111, 533.

Tavoloni, N., Reed, J.S., Hruban, Z., and Boyer, J.L. (1979). Effect of chlorpromazine on hepatic perfusion and bile secretory function in the isolated perfused rat liver. *J. Lab. Clin. Med.* 94, 726.

Taylor, D.C., Cresswell, P.R., and Bartlett, D.C. (1978). The metabolism and elimination of cimetidine, a histamine H2 receptor antagonist, in the rat, dog and man. *Drug Metab. Dispos.* 6, 21.

Taylor, J.W., Stein, M.N., Murphy, M.J., and Mitros, F.A. (1984). Cholestatic liver dysfunction after long-term phenytoin therapy. *Arch. Neurol.* 41, 500.

Tedesco, F.J. and Mills, L.R. (1982). Diazepam (Valium) hepatitis. *Dig. Dis. Sci.* 27, 470.

Teh, L.B., Chong, R., Ho, J.M., and Ong, Y.Y. (1988). Oxyphenisatin induced chronic active hepatitis — a potential health hazard in Singapore. *Singapore Med. J.* 29, 508.

Tennison, M.B., Miles, M.V., Pollack, G.M., Thorn, M.D., and Dupuis, R.E. (1988). Valproate metabolites and hepatotoxicity in an epileptic population. *Epilepsia* 29, 543.

Thaler, H. (1988). Fatty change. *Baillière's Clin. Gastroenterol.* 2, 453.

Thelen, M. and Wendel, A. (1983). Drug induced lipid peroxidation in mice V. Ethane production and glutathione release in the isolated liver upon perfusion with acetaminophen. *Biochem. Pharmacol.* 32, 1701.

Thies, P.W. and Dull, W.L. (1984). Trimethoprim-sulfamethoxazole-induced cholestatic hepatitis. Inadvertent rechallenge. *Arch. Intern. Med.* 144, 1691.

Thirumoorthy, T. and Shupack, J.L. (1988). Adverse hepatic reactions associated with etretinate in patients with psoriasis — analysis of 22 cases. *Ann. Acad. Med. Singapore* 17, 477.

Thomas, F.B. (1974). Chronic aggressive hepatitis induced by halothane. *Ann. Intern. Med.* 81, 487.

Thompson, M.L., Shuster, L., and Shaw, K. (1979). Cocaine induced hepatic necrosis in mice: the role of cocaine metabolism. *Biochem. Pharmacol.* 28, 2389.

Thulin, K.E. and Nermark, J. (1966). Seven cases of jaundice in women taking an oral contraceptive, Anovlar. *Br. Med. J.* i, 584.

Ticktin, H.E. and Zimmerman, H.J. (1966). Effects of a synthetic anabolic agent on hepatic function. *Am. J. Med. Sci.* 251, 674.

Timbrell, J.A. (1983). Drug hepatotoxicity. *Br. J. Clin. Pharmacol.* 15, 3.

Timbrell, J.A., Wright, J.M., and Baillie, T.A. (1978). Monoacetylhydrazine as a metabolite of isoniazid in man. *Clin. Pharmacol. Ther.* 22, 602.

Tobias, H. and Auerback, R. (1973). Hepatotoxicity of long-term methotrexate therapy for psoriasis. *Arch. Intern. Med.* 132, 391.

Tolman, K.F., Sannella, J.J., and Freston, J.W. (1974). Chemical structure of erythromycin and hepatotoxicity. *Ann. Intern. Med.* 81, 58.

Tolman, K.G., Peterson, P., Gray, P., and Hammar, S.P. (1978). Hepatotoxicity of salicylates in monolayer cell cultures. *Gastroenterology* 74, 205.

Tonder, M., Nordoy, E., and Egjo, K. (1974). Sulfonamide induced chronic liver disease. *Scand. J. Gastroenterol.* 9, 93.

Tredger, J.M., Smith, H.M., Davis, M., and Williams, R. (1981). In vitro interactions of sulfur-containing compounds with the hepatic mixed-function oxidase system in mice: Effects on paracetamol activation and covalent binding. *Toxicol. Appl. Pharmacol.* 59, 111.

Trey, C., Lipworth, L., Chalmers, T.C., Davison, C.S., Gottlieb, L.S., Popper, H., *et al.* (1968). Fulminant hepatic failure: presumed contribution of halothane. *N. Engl. J. Med.* 279, 798.

Trowell, J., Peto, R., and Crampton Smith, A. (1975). Controlled trial of repeated halothane anaesthetics in patients with carcinoma of the cervix treated with radium. *Lancet* i, 821.

Tsagaropoulou-Stinga, H., Mataki-Emmanouilidou, T., Karida-Kavalioti, S., and Manios, S. (1985). Hepatotoxic reactions in children with severe tuberculosis treated with isoniazid-rifampin. *Pediatr. Infect. Dis.* 4, 270.

Turnbull, D.M., Dick, D.J., Wilson, L., Sherratt, H.S., and Alberti, K.G. (1986). Valproate causes metabolic disturbance in normal man. *J. Neurol. Neurosurg. Psychiatry* 49, 405.

Turner, I.B., Eckstein, R.P., Riley, J.W., and Lunzer, M.R. (1989). Prolonged hepatic cholestasis after flucloxacillin therapy. *Med. J. Aust.* 137, 391.

Uetrecht, J., Wood, A.J., Phythyon, J.M., and Wood, M. (1983). Contrasting effects on halothane hepatotoxicity in the phenobarbital hypoxia and tri-iodothyronine model: mechanistic implications. *Anesthesiology* 59, 196.

Urban, E., Frank, B.W., and Kern, F., Jr (1968). Liver dysfunction with mestranol but not with norethynodrel in a patient with Enovid-induced jaundice. *Ann. Intern. Med.* 68, 598.

Ussery, X.T., Henar, E.L., Black, D.D., Berger, S., and Whittington, P.F. (1989). Acute liver injury after protracted seizures in children. *J. Pediatr. Gastroenterol. Nutr.* 9, 421.

Utili, R., Boitnolt, J.K., and Zimmerman, H.J. (1977). Dantrolene-associated hepatic injury. Incidence and character. *Gastroenterology* 62, 610.

Valdivia-Barriga, B., Feldman, A., and Orellana, J. (1963). Generalised hypersensitivity with hepatitis and jaundice after the use of penicillin and streptomycin. *Gastroenterology* 45, 114.

Vale, J.A., Meredith, T.J., and Goulding, R. (1981). Treatment of acetaminophen poisoning. The use of oral methionine. *Arch. Intern. Med.* 141, 394.

Valla, D., Le, M.G., Poynard, T., Zucman, N., Rueff, B., and Benhamou, J.P. (1986). Risk of hepatic vein thrombosis in relation to recent use of oral contraceptives. A case-control study. *Gastroenterology* 90, 807.

van-de-Kerkhof, P.C., Hoefnagels, W.H., van-Haelst, U.J., and Mali, J.W. (1985). Methotrexate maintenance therapy and liver damage in psoriasis. *Clin. Exp. Dermatol.* 10, 194.

Vanderstigel, M., Zafrani, E.S., Lejonc, J.L., Schaeffer, A., and Portos, J.L. (1986). Allopurinol hypersensitivity syndrome as a cause of hepatic fibrin ring granulomas. *Gastroenterology* 90, 188.

van de Straat, R., de-Vries, J., Debets, A.J., and Vermeulen, N.P. (1987). The mechanism of prevention of paracetamol-induced hepatotoxicity by 3,5-dialkyl substitution. The roles of glutathione depletion and oxidative stress. *Biochem. Pharmacol.* 36, 2065.

van Dyke, R.A. (1982). Hepatic centrilobular necrosis in rats after exposure to halothane, enflurane or isoflurane. *Anesth. Analg.* 61, 812.

van Dyke, R.A. and Gandolfi, A.J. (1974). Studies on irreversible binding of radioactivity from (14C)-halothane to rat hepatic microsomal lipids and protein. *Drug. Metab. Dispos.* 2, 469.

van Dyke, R.A. and Wood, C.L. (1973). Binding of radioactivity from (14C)-labelled halothane in isolated perfused rat livers. *Anesthesiology* 83, 328.

van Dyke, R.A. and Wood, C.L. (1975). *In vitro* studies on irreversible binding of halothane metabolite to microsomes. *Drug. Metab. Dispos.* 3, 51.

van Steenbergen, W., Vanstapel, M.J., Desmet, V., van Kerckvoorde, L., De-Keyzer, R., Brijs, R., *et al.* (1985). Cimetidine-induced liver injury. Report of three cases. *J. Hepatol.* 1, 359.

Vendemiale, G., Altomare, E., Trizio, T., Leandro, G., Manghisi, O.G., and Albano, O. (1987). Effect of acute and chronic cimetidine administration on acetaminophen metabolism in humans. *Am. J. Gastroenterol.* 82, 1031.

Vergani, D., Mieli- Vergani, G., Alberti, A., Neuberger, J., Eddleston, A.L.W.F., Davis, M., and Williams, R. (1980). Antibodies to the surface of halothane-altered rabbit hepatocytes in patients with severe halothane-associated hepatitis. *N. Engl. J. Med* 303, 66.

Verhamme, M., Ramboer, C., van de Bruaene, P., and Inderadjaja, N. (1989). Cholestatic hepatitis due to an amoxycillin/clavulanic acid preparation. *J. Hepatol.* 9, 260.

Victorino, R.M., Maria, V.A., Correia, A.P., and de-Moura, C. (1987). Floxacillin-induced cholestatic hepatitis with evidence of lymphocyte sensitization. *Arch. Intern. Med.* 147, 987.

Vileisis, R.A., Inwood, R.J., and Hung, C.E. (1980). Prospective controlled study of parenteral nutrition associated cholestatic jaundice: effect of protein intake. *J. Pediatr.* 96, 893.

Villeneuve, J.P. and Warner, H.A. (1979). Cimetidine hepatitis. *Gastroenterology* 77, 143.

Vitug, A.C. and Goldman, J.M. (1985). Hepatotoxicity from antithyroid drugs. *Horm. Res.* 21, 229.

Vuopio, P., Viherkoski, M., Nikkila, E., and Lamberg, B-N. (1970). The content of reduced glutathione (GSH) in the red blood cells in hypo and hyperthyroidism. *Ann. Clin. Res.* 2, 184.

Wakabayashi, T., Onda, H., Tada, T., Iijima, M., and Itoh, Y. (1984). High incidence of peliosis hepatis in autopsy cases of aplastic anemia with special reference to anabolic steroid therapy. *Acta Pathol. Jpn* 34, 1079.

Waldman, R.J., Hall, W.N., and McGee, H. (1982). Aspirin as a risk factor in Reye's syndrome. *JAMA* 247, 3089.

Walker, B.E., Kelleher, J., Dixon, M.F., and Losowsky, M.S. (1974). Vitamin E protection of the liver from paracetamol in the rat. *Clin. Sci. Mol. Med.* 47, 449.

Walker, C.O. and Combes, B. (1966). Biliary cirrhosis induced by chlorpromazine. *Gastroenterology* 51, 631.

Walker, R.M., Racz, W.J., and McElligott, T.F. (1980). Acetaminophen induced hepatotoxicity in mice. *Lab. Invest.* 42, 181.

Walker, R.M., Massey, T.E., McElligott, T.F., and Racz, W.I. (1981). Acetaminophen-induced hypothermia, hepatic congestion and modification by *N*-acetylcysteine in mice. *Toxicol. Appl. Pharmacol.* 59, 500.

Walker, R.M., McElligott, T.F., and Massey, T.E. (1983*a*). Ultrastructural effects of acetaminophen in isolated mouse hepatocytes. *Exp. Mol. Pathol.* 39, 163.

Walker, R.M., Racz, W.J., and McElligott, T.F. (1983*b*). Scanning electron microscopy of acetaminophen-induced hepatotoxicity in mice. *Am. J. Pathol.* 113, 321.

Walker, R.M., Racz, W.J., and McElligott, T.F. (1985). Acetaminophen induced hepatotoxic congestion in mice. *Hepatology* 5, 233.

Walton, B., Simpson, B.R., Strunin, L., Doniach, D., Perrin, J., and Appleyard, A.J. (1976). Unexplained hepatitis following halothane. *Br. Med. J.* i, 1171.

Wanless, I.R., Godwin, T.A., Allen, F., and Feder, A. (1980). Nodular regenerative disorders of the liver in haematologic disorders; a possible response to obliterative portal venopathy. A morphometric study of nine cases with an hypothesis on the pathogenesis. *Medicine (Baltimore)* 59, 367.

Weaver, G.A., Pavlinac, D., and Davis, J.S. (1977). Hepatic sensitivity to imipramine. *Dig. Dis.* 22, 551.

Weber, B.L., Tanyer, G., Poplack, D.G., Reaman, G.H., Feusner, J.H., Miser, J.S., and Bleyer, W.A. (1987). Transient acute hepatotoxicity of high-dose methotrexate therapy during childhood. *NCI-Monogr.* 5, 207.

Weill, B.J., Menkes, C.J., Cormier, C., Louvel, A., Dougados, M., and Houssin, D. (1988). Hepatocellular carcinoma after danazol therapy. *J. Rheumatol.* 15, 1447.

Weinberger, M., Garty, M., Cohen, M., Russo, Y., and Rosenfield, J.B. (1985). Ultrasonography in the diagnosis and follow up of hepatic sinusoidal dilatation. *Arch. Intern. Med.* 145, 927.

Weinstein, G., Roenigk, H., Maibach, H., Cosmides, J., Halprin, K., and Millard, M. (1973). Psoriasis–liver–methotrexate interactions. *Arch. Dermatol.* 198, 46.

Weinstein, H.J. and Hallett, W.Y. (1962). The absorption and toxicity of ethionamide. *Am. Rev. Respir. Dis.* 86, 576.

Weis, K.H. and Engelhardt, W. (1989). Is halothane obsolete? Two standards of judgement. *Anaesthesia* 44, 97.

Weiss, V.C., Layden, T., Spinowitz, A., Buys, C., Nemchausky, B.A., West, D., *et al.* (1985). Chronic active hepatitis associated with etretinate therapy. *Br. J. Dermatol.* 112, 591.

Wendel, A. and Feuerstein, S. (1981). Drug-induced lipid peroxidation in mice I. Modulation by monooxygenase activity, glutathione and selenium status. *Biochem. Pharmacol.* 30, 2513.

Wendel, A., Feuerstein, S., and Konz, K.H. (1989). Acute paracetamol intoxication of starved mice leads to lipid peroxidation in vivo. *Biochem. Pharmacol.* 32, 2053.

Westaby, D., Ogle, S.J., Swale, J., Randell, J., Paradinas, F.J., and Murray-Lyon, I.M. (1976). Prevalence of liver disease among androgen takers. *Gut* 17, 825.

Westaby, D.A., Portmann, B., and Williams, R. (1983). Androgen-associated liver tumours in non-Fanconi patients. *Cancer* 51, 1947.

Weston, C.F., Cooper, B.T., Davies, J.D., and Levine, D.F. (1987). Veno-occlusive disease of the liver secondary to ingestion of comfrey. *Br. Med. J.* 295, 183.

Whalley, P.J., Martin, F.G., Adams, R.H., and Combes, B. (1970). Disposition of tetracycline by pregnant women with acute pyelonephritis. *Obstet. Gynecol.* 36, 821.

Whalley, P.J., Adams, R.H., and Combes, B. (1974). Tetracycline toxicity in pregnancy. *JAMA* 189, 357.

Whitington, P.F. (1985). Cholestasis associated with total parenteral nutrition in infants. *Hepatology* 5, 693.

Widger, L.A., Gandolfi, A.J., and van Dyke, R.A. (1976). Hypoxia and halothane metabolism *in vivo*: release of inorganic fluoride and halothane metabolite binding to cellular constituents. *Anesthesiology* 44, 197.

Wilkinson, S.P., Portmann, B., and Williams, R. (1979). Hepatitis from dantrolene sodium. *Gut* 20, 33.

Williams, C.N., McCauley, D., Malatjalian, D.A., Turnbull, G.K., and Ross, J.B. (1987). The aminopyrine breath test, an inadequate early indicator of methotrexate-induced liver disease in patients with psoriasis. *Clin. Invest. Med.* 10, 54.

Williams, R., Davis, M., and Waldram, R. (1975). Postoperative jaundice. In *Eleventh symposium on advanced medicine* (ed. A. Lant), p. 45. Pitman Medical, Tunbridge Wells.

Wilmot, F.C. and Robinson, G.W. (1920). Senecio disease or cirrhosis of the liver due to senecio poisoning. *Lancet* ii, 848.

Winkler, K. and Poulsen, H. (1975). Liver disease with periportal sinusoidal dilatation. A possible complication to contraceptive steroids. *Scand. J. Gastroenterol.* 10, 699.

Winter, S.L. and Boyer, J.L. (1973). Hepatic toxicity from large doses of vitamin B$_3$ (nicotinamide). *N. Engl. J. Med.* 289, 1180.

Wong, L.T., Whitehouse, L.W., Solomonraj, G., and Paul, C.J. (1980). Effect of a concomitant single dose of ethanol on the hepatotoxicity and metabolism of acetaminophen in mice. *Toxicology* 17, 297.

Wood, L.J., Mundo, F., Searle, J., and Powell, L.W. (1985). Sulindac hepatotoxicity: effects of acute and chronic exposure. *Aust. N.Z. J. Med.* 15, 397.

Wood, M., Uetrecht, J., Phythyon, J.M., Shay, S., Sweetman, B.J., Shaheen, O., *et al.* (1986). The effect of cimetidine on anaesthetic metabolism and toxicity. *Anesth. Analg.* 65, 481.

Woodward, K.N. and Timbrell, J.A. (1984). Acetylhydrazine hepatotoxicity: the role of covalent binding. *Toxicology* 30, 65.

Wright, C.IV., Vafier, J.A., and Lake, C.R. (1988). Disulfiram-induced fulminating hepatis: guidelines for liver-panel monitoring. *J. Clin. Psychiatry* 49, 430.

Wright, R., Eade, O.E., Chisholm, M., Hawksley, M., Lloyd, B., Moles, T.M., *et al.* (1975). Controlled prospective study of the effect of liver function of multiple exposures to halothane. *Lancet* i, 817.

Xiol, X., Martinez-Lacasa, J., Pons, M., Marti, E., and Casais, L. (1989). Jaundice after danazol therapy for endometriosis. *Am. J. Gastroenterol.* 84, 834.

Yagupsky, P., Gazala, E., Sofer, S., Maor, E., and Abarbanel, J. (1985). Fatal hepatic failure and encephalopathy associated with amiodarone therapy. *J. Pediatr.* 107, 967.

Yamada, T. (1983). Covalent binding theory for acetaminophen hepatotoxicity. *Gastroenterology* 85, 202.

Yamada, T. and Kaplowitz, N. (1980). Propylthiouracil: A substrate for the glutathione S-transferases that compete with glutathione. *J. Biol. Chem.* 255, 3508.

Yamada, T., Ludwig, S., Kuhlenkamp, J., and Kaplowitz, N. (1979). Direct protection against acetaminophen hepatotoxicity by propylthiouracil. In vivo and *in vitro* studies in rats an mice. *J. Clin. Invest.* 67, 688.

Yamamoto, T., Suou, T., and Hirayama, C. (1986). Elevated serum aminotransferase induced by isoniazid in relation to isoniazid acetylator phenotype. *Hepatology* 6, 295.

Yanoff, M. and Rawson, A.J. (1964). Peliosis hepatis: an anatomic study with demonstration of two varieties. *Arch. Pathol.* 77, 159.

Zachariae, H., Krabkalle, K., and Sgaard, H. (1980). Methotrexate-induced liver cirrhosis. *Br. J. Dermatol.* 102, 407.

Zachariae, H., Schroder, H., Foged, E., and Sogard, H. (1987). Methotrexate hepatotoxicity and concentrations of methotrexate and folate in erythrocytes — relation to liver fibrosis and cirrhosis. *Acta Derm. Venereol.* (Stockh.) 67, 336.

Zafrani, E.S., Bernuau, D., and Feldmann, G. (1984). Peliosis-like ultrastructural changes of the hepatic sinusoids in human chronic hypervitaminosis A: report of three cases. *Hum. Pathol.* 15, 1166.

Zimmerman, H.J. (1963). Clinical and laboratory manifestations of hepatotoxicity. *Ann. N.Y. Acad. Sci.* 104, 954.

Zimmerman, H.J. (1978). *Hepatotoxicity: the adverse effects of drugs and other chemicals on the liver.* Appleton Century Crofts, New York.

Zimmerman, H.J. (1986). Effects of alcohol on other hepatotoxins. *Alcoholism* 10, 3.

Zimmerman, H.J. (1986). Hepatotoxic effects of oncotherapeutic agents. *Prog. Liver Dis.* 8, 621.

Zimmerman, H.J. and Ishak, K.G. (1987). Do estrogens cause venocclusive disease of the liver? *Gastroenterology* 93, 384.

Zimmerman, H.J., Kendler, J., and Libber, E. (1973). Studies on the *in vitro* cytotoxicity of erythromycin estolate. *Proc. Soc. Exp. Biol. Med.* 144, 759.

Zimmerman, H.J., Lewis, J.H., Ishak, K.G., and Maddrey, W.C. (1984). Ticrynafen-associated hepatic injury: analysis of 340 cases. *Hepatology* 4, 315.

Zimmerman, H.J., Jacob, L., Bassan, H., Gillespie, J., Lukacs, L., and Abernathy, C.O. (1986). Effects of H$_2$ blocking agents on hepatocytes in vitro: correlation with potential for causing hepatic disease in patients. *Proc. Soc. Exp. Biol. Med.* 182, 511.

Zimran, A., Abraham, A.S., and Hershko, C. (1985). Reversible cholestatic jaundice and hyperamylasaemia associated with captopril treatment. *Br. Med. J.* 287, 1676.

Zitelli, B.J., Alexander, J., Taylor, S., Miller, K.D., Howrie, D.L., Kuritsky, J.N., *et al.* (1987). Fatal hepatic necrosis due to pyrimethamine-sulfadoxine (Fansidar). *Ann. Intern. Med.* 106, 393.

12. Renal disorders

M. J. D. CASSIDY and D. N. S. KERR

Introduction

The kidneys receive 25 per cent of the cardiac output; they filter, concentrate, metabolise, and eliminate many different drugs and are particularly vulnerable to toxicity. A profile of drug metabolising enzymes in the human kidney was recently reviewed by Pacifici and colleagues (1989). Drug toxicity may occur through a variety of mechanisms, including direct and indirect biochemical effects as well as immunological effects. Pre-existing renal disease will potentiate the effects of renally metabolised and excreted drugs and will necessitate a change in drug dosage to avoid both renal and systemic toxicity; this problem is not addressed in this chapter.

The spectrum of drug-induced renal damage as we will discuss it is tabulated in table 12.1. Many drugs are capable of causing a variety of renal defects that may occur in isolation or in combination and are thus beyond the confines of artificial tabulation. These drugs are discussed in the sections we think they fit into best; for example, the aminoglycosides are discussed in the section on acute tubular necrosis (ATN), though before producing ATN they cause changes in tubular function. With other drugs such as the non-steroidal anti-inflammatory agents (NSAID) renal damage may take several forms; space is therefore given to these drugs in several sections, that is, in functional renal impairment, glomerulonephritis, and acute interstitial nephritis (AIN). One of the best reviews of the renal syndromes associated with the use of NSAID is provided by Clive and Stoff (1984).

Functional renal impairment

Under this heading we include those drugs that may acutely reduce glomerular filtration rate (GFR) by affecting the normal physiological mechanisms controlling

TABLE 12.1
The spectrum of drug-induced renal disease

1. Functional renal impairment
   affecting glomerular filtration
   affecting tubular secretion, reabsorption, or
     concentration

2. Acute renal failure
   tubular damage (acute tubular necrosis, osmotic
     nephrosis)
   vascular damage (acute vasculitis, haemolytic–uraemic
     syndrome)
   glomerular damage (rapidly progressive nephritis)
   interstitial damage (acute interstitial nephritis)
   obstruction (acute tubular blockage, retroperitoneal
     fibrosis, ureteric blockage, and acute retention

3. Glomerulonephritis
   nephrotic syndrome
   lupus nephritis

4. Crystalluria, renal calculi, and calcium nephropathy

5. Chronic interstitial nephritis and papillary necrosis
     (analgesic nephropathy)

6. Miscellaneous
   haematuria
   incontinence
   drugs affecting tests of renal function

glomerular filtration; we will also discuss those drugs that interfere with tubular function but which are not necessarily associated with structural change.

Glomerular effects

The NSAID have little effect on GFR in normal subjects but in salt-depleted patients, in those with congestive cardiac failure or cirrhosis, and in those with pre-existing renal failure GFR may fall significantly (Clive and Stoff 1984; Delaney and Segel 1985). Others at risk include premature infants, patients with systemic lupus erythematosus, and the elderly (Zipser and Henrich 1986).

Renal failure can be precipitated by the concomitant use of an NSAID and a diuretic (Lynn *et al.* 1985); triamterene appears to be a specific culprit (Weinberg *et al.* 1985) and it should not be used in combination with an NSAID.

The capacity to suppress renal prostaglandins (and thus exert this type of functional effect) may vary with different NSAID. It has been suggested, for example, that sulindac may have a 'renal sparing' effect (Ciabattoni *et al.* 1984), but not all reports agree (Riley *et al.* 1985); the discrepancies and arguments were reviewed by Weisman and colleagues (1985). Of the other NSAID that have been reported to have a better adverse reaction profile, diclofenac compares favourably (O'Brien 1986).

The commonest adverse effect of NSAID related to the kidney is hyperkalaemia; patients specifically at risk are diabetics, those with pre-existing renal disease, and patients receiving β-blockers, potassium-sparing diuretics, or angiotensin-converting-enzyme (ACE) inhibitors (Zipser and Henrich 1986). A combination of dehydration, an NSAID, and an ACE inhibitor is particularly hazardous as the under-perfused glomerulus normally relies on angiotensin II to maintain a pressure gradient across the glomerulus by its constrictor effect on mesangial cells and efferent arterioles (Blythe 1983).

Acute azotaemia may be due to other drugs that may functionally reduce GFR. In an illustrative case described by Reid and Muther (1987), acute oliguria developed in a patient with congestive cardiac failure and pneumonia who was given a nitroprusside infusion; the renal failure was rapidly reversible on tapering and discontinuing the infusion. They postulate a renal 'steal' with preferential dilatation of vascular beds as a cause. Hypotension and renal impairment of a functional nature have also been described during infusion of atrial natriuretic factor in patients with liver cirrhosis with ascites (Ferrier *et al.* 1989).

The metabolites of the tetracyclines (with the exception of doxycycline, which is metabolised by the liver) build up in renal failure and lead to vomiting and dehydration; this is in addition to their antianabolic effect, which causes a rise in blood urea, further aggravates the uraemic state, and can make dialysis necessary in some patients. Rarely, tetracyclines (minocycline) have been associated with interstitial nephritis (Walker *et al.* 1979; Wilkinson *et al.* 1989) and, as mentioned below, dimethylchlortetracycline can cause nephrogenic diabetes insipidus.

Interleukin 2 may also cause prerenal renal failure (Christiansen *et al.* 1988). By stimulating release of other cytokines, which cause endothelial cells to leak fluid, it can cause hypovolaemia and hypotension; as interleukin 2 also inhibits the release of renal prostaglandins, the normal compensatory mechanism for hypovolaemia is impaired and prerenal renal failure ensues (Hamblin 1990). As expected, the use of indomethacin compounds the problem. The effect on GFR can be partially reversed by noradrenaline (Allaouchiche *et al.* 1990).

The normal physiological mechanisms that autoregulate renal blood flow may be lost in the severely ill patient; in the intensive care unit, where urine output is measured hourly, it is well recognized that drugs which reduce blood pressure often reduce urine flow. With regard to the use of antihypertensive drugs in the clinic, β-blockers cause a mild reduction in GFR (Warren 1976), the relatively cardioselective agents causing less depression than propranolol (Wright *et al.* 1979, Wilkinson 1979, 1982). Clonidine, reserpine, minoxidil, and methyldopa (Pohl *et al.* 1974) have little effect on GFR, and the vasodilator prazosin may improve GFR in some cases, despite lowering blood pressure (Curtis and Bateman 1975). The calcium-channel blocker nifedipine probably has minimal clinical effect on renal function; similarly, nicardipine has no measurable effect on GFR or renal plasma flow but has a potent natriuretic effect (Lee *et al.* 1986). The importance of the control of blood pressure by the use of such agents, especially in chronic renal failure, far outweighs any minor fluctuation in GFR due to a functional effect. A particular caveat, however, applies to the use of ACE inhibitors in patients with generalized atherosclerosis. Hricik (1985) described 11 patients who developed acute renal failure while taking captopril; common to all was renal artery stenosis bilaterally or in a single kidney. The same has been reported in renal transplant recipients with graft artery stenosis (van-der-Woude *et al.* 1985). Though renal failure is often reversible after discontinuation of the drug, this is not always the case.

Acute azotaemia has also been described in patients with chronic heart failure treated with ACE inhibitors (Packer 1989) or with nifedipine (Eicher *et al.* 1988). Care should also be taken in prescribing potent diuretics to patients with congestive cardiac failure who are also taking captopril, as the natriuresis and fall in blood pressure may tip the balance in an already critically compromised renal perfusion (Hogg and Hillis 1986).

A rapid, reversible, acute renal failure, postulated to be due to functional disturbances, has also been described with amphotericin (Sacks and Fellner 1987).

Tubular effects

Proximal tubular damage may lead to a Fanconi syndrome (the features of which include amino-aciduria, phosphaturia, glycosuria, and renal tubular acidosis). This can be a feature of heavy metal toxicity. In the acute proximal tubular dysfunction that occurs with lead exposure, inclusion bodies consisting of lead–protein complexes are discernible in proximal tubular cells; toxicity can be reversed by treatment with chelating agents (Goyer 1989). Ingestion of outdated (of a formulation now obsolete) tetracyclines can also produce a Fanconi-type syndrome in addition to a concentrating defect (Mavromatis 1965; Cleveland et al. 1965); the effect has been attributed to the tetracycline degradation products anhydrotetracycline and epianhydrotetracycline (Benitz and Diermeier 1964; Lowe and Tapp 1966). Another report describes a case of lactic acidosis in association with a Fanconi syndrome after ingestion of tetracycline capsules that had been accidentally soaked, dried out, and stored (Montoliu et al. 1981).

Another tetracycline, demeclocycline, can produce a reversible, dose-dependent nephrogenic diabetes insipidus, which has nothing to do with the degradation of the drug; patients taking a high dose for prolonged periods, such as acne sufferers, are particularly at risk. The effect can be put to therapeutic use (in adults only) in the treatment of chronic hyponatraemia due to the syndrome of inappropriate ADH secretion. Treatment needs to be monitored closely to avoid dehydration and prerenal uraemia (Oster and Epstein 1977; Perks et al. 1979). This and other drugs that are associated with nephrogenic diabetes insipidus are listed in table 12.2.

TABLE 12.2
*Drugs associated with impaired
tubular response to ADH*

Amphotericin
Colchicine
Demeclocycline
Glibenclamide
Isofosfamide
Lithium
Methoxyflurane
Rifampicin
Vinblastine

The major renal adverse effect of lithium is a nephrogenic diabetes insipidus (Singer et al. 1972; Forrest et al. 1974; Singer 1981). It is dose-dependent (Penney et al. 1981; Vestergaard and Amdisen 1981), vasopressin resistant, and is usually reversible after discontinuation of the drug. A mild depression of GFR is not uncommon in some patients; this also tends to correlate with duration of treatment (Wallin et al. 1982).

Recovery of the concentrating defect usually takes place slowly over several months and may be incomplete in those that have taken the drug for years (Bucht and Wahlin 1980). The elderly are particularly at risk of toxicity. Mild and clinically unimportant polyuria is common; about half of patients taking lithium will demonstrate a concentrating defect (Wallin et al. 1982), but serious toxicity is infrequent provided plasma levels are maintained below about 0.6 mmol per litre. Constant levels are promoted by the use of sustained-release preparations (Wallin and Alling 1979). It is recommended by manufacturers that serum concentrations be measured once weekly until stabilization is achieved, then weekly for one month, and monthly thereafter. Massive diuresis may, however, be unpredictable and occur despite therapeutic levels of the drug, it may be further aggravated by hyperglycaemia (Martinez-Maldonado and Terrell 1973).

Salt and water depletion may precipitate toxicity, as lithium is avidly reabsorbed by the proximal tubule 'by mistake' for sodium. Common causes are diarrhoea and vomiting and stringent dieting; patients taking lithium should be warned of these hazards. The concomitant use of diuretics should also be avoided if possible.

Other drugs that may affect blood levels of lithium include NSAID (in particular indomethacin) and tetracyclines. Lithium is more likely to cause diabetes insipidus if combined with tricyclic antidepressants. As already indicated, with prolonged use or high doses the renal disorder progresses from a purely functional defect to one with structural changes within distal tubular cells and interstitium. Mitochondrial swelling and dilatation of the cisternae of endoplasmic reticulum progress to cell vacuolation, interstitial fibrosis (Aurell et al. 1981; Walker et al. 1982), tubular fall-out, and occasionally glomerular sclerosis (Bucht et al. 1980).

Lithium may also cause a nephrotic syndrome (Bear et al. 1985), usually due to a minimal change lesion and usually remitting on withdrawal of the drug (Alexander and Martin 1981; Singer 1981); it may also rarely be responsible for acute renal failure (Dias and Hocken 1972; Lavender et al. 1973) due to acute tubular necrosis. Other uncommon adverse effects of lithium that may have an indirect effect on renal function include hypercalcaemia and hypermagnesaemia; a rise in antinuclear antibodies occasionally occurs.

Methoxyflurane affects renal tubular function in several ways; it causes a nephrogenic diabetes insipidus (Crandell et al. 1966; Mazze et al. 1971; Merkle et al. 1971; Wong et al. 1974) which is associated with oxalate deposits in distal tubular cells (Panner et al. 1970; Bergstrand et al. 1972); whether these are causally related is unclear, as oxalosis is not generally associated with diabetes insipidus. Uric acid clearance is also reduced, and this may result in a rise in serum urate (Giler *et al.* 1977). The toxicity is dose-related, and the increase in plasma oxalate and fluoride, which is another possible culprit (methoxyflurane is metabolised in the liver to inorganic fluoride), correlates with the extent of functional and structural tubular damage, at least in rats (Mazze *et al.* 1973). The risk of toxicity increases with the dose and duration of anaesthesia and with obesity, which enhances methoxyflurane uptake (Samuelson *et al.* 1976), pre-existing renal disease, and the preceding or concomitant use of microsomal-enzyme-inducing drugs such as phenobarbitone (Churchill *et al.* 1976). Renal concentrating ability usually returns after several days or weeks, during which time attention to the prevention of ATN by adequate hydration is essential. In a few patients, chronic renal failure with progressive fibrosis ensues (Hollenberg *et al.* 1972; Halpren *et al.* 1973). The use of methoxyflurane has not been confined to general anaesthesia; Toomath and Morrison (1987) report two cases of fatal renal failure developing in elderly women taking repeated doses from a Penthrane Analgizer, an inhaler used for pain relief (the inhaler was withdrawn from the New Zealand market, from where the report emanates, in 1984). Enflurane anaesthesia can also cause a mild polyuria.

Rifampicin has also been reported to be associated with a nephrogenic diabetes insipidus but with structural tubulo-interstial damage (Quinn and Wall 1989).

Acute renal failure

Acute tubular necrosis

Tubular damage is inevitable with some drugs and develops *pari passu* with the beneficial effect of the drug. Examples are amphotericin, cisplatin, and the aminoglycosides; their efficacy in treating specific diseases, however, often precludes the substitution of alternatives and dictates their use. Acute tubular necrosis is characteristically polyuric with some of these drugs (e.g. aminoglycosides), though it can be oliguric. In the single nephron model activation of tubuloglomerular feedback mechanisms best explain the reduction in GFR in nephrotoxic forms of tubular injury (Peterson *et al.* 1989).

Amphotericin increases permeability of tubular cell membranes, and toxicity presents with hypokalaemia, hypomagnesaemia, impaired concentrating ability, and distal renal tubular acidosis. This is followed by a reduc-

tion in GFR and non-oliguric acute renal failure. Dehydration should be avoided at all costs; mannitol and sodium bicarbonate infusions may reduce toxicity, and a recent open prospective study evaluating the usefulness of sodium chloride loading to prevent toxicity showed it to be highly successful (Arning and Scharf 1989). In addition, reduction in dose and frequency of administration may contain the problem. When toxicity does occur the effects are not always reversible (Butler 1964) and nephrocalcinosis may develop later (Bhathena *et al.* 1978), though it rarely occurs nowadays.

Aminoglycoside antibiotics cause transient renal failure in up to 10–30 per cent of patients and are the cause of the largest proportion of acute drug-induced nephrotoxicity (Tulkens 1989). Typically, non-oliguric renal failure manifests about a week after treatment has started, is seldom severe enough to require dialysis and is usually reversible though recovery may be slow. Gentamicin is the most frequent offender, probably because of its regular use and efficacy.

An important caveat in drawing analogies from animal data to man and, indeed, in comparing different animal studies is illustrated by the aminoglycosides: for example, in the dog, gentamicin is nephrotoxic at two to three times the therapeutic dose, whereas, in the rat, up to 60 times the therapeutic dose may be tolerated (Falco *et al.* 1969); in addition Fischer Wistar rats appear more susceptible to toxicity than do Sprague-Dawley rats (Soberon *et al.* 1979).

Data from humans and animals indicate that aminoglycoside toxicity is directed predominantly against proximal tubular cells; the drug is concentrated in the renal cortex (Luft *et al.* 1977) and is taken up by proximal tubular cells. In rats and humans there is increased urinary excretion of proximal tubular enzymes before other noticeable changes in renal function; histological damage is initially only seen in proximal tubular cells, and electron microprobe analysis of non-necrotic proximal tubular cells demonstrates abnormalities in electrolyte concentrations not present in the distal tubules (Matsuda *et al.* 1988). Once taken up by the cells, gentamicin remains in a poorly exchangeable pool with tissue half-life of over 100 times that of blood. After binding to the proximal tubular membrane, it is incorporated into the cell in micro-vesicles and sequenced in lysosomes (an increased number of secondary lysosomes is a characteristic early sign of toxicity); subsequent lysosomal phospholipidosis results in cell death. There are various other alterations in the structure and function of subcellular components; for example gentamicin enhances renal cortical mitochondrial generation of reactive oxygen metabolites *in vitro* (Walker and Shah 1988).

A reduction in the risk of developing nephrotoxicity may be possible by an analysis of the patient and drug-related risk factors that have been reported. Excessive dose, or excessive duration of treatment, or both, are clearly the most important factors. The former is probably responsible for the increased frequency of toxicity in the elderly, in whom allowances for a reduced creatinine clearance in the presence of a normal serum creatinine may not be made in calculating dosage. Excessive dose is not the only factor; long-term subtherapeutic doses of gentamicin maintaining the serum aminoglycoside levels below the accepted therapeutic range for 6 months may produce renal failure in rats (Houghton *et al.* 1988). The uptake of aminoglycosides by the kidney is also saturable; thus multiple injections or a continuous infusion may increase the risk of toxicity. Monitoring several trough and peak levels may predict toxicity (Moore *et al.* 1984; Contreras *et al.* 1989).

Risk factors have been examined by Moore and others (1984), who found nephrotoxicity to be more common, with higher trough and peak levels, in women, and in patients with higher creatinine clearance and those with liver disease. The last observation confirmed data from Cabrera and colleagues (1982), who recognized an increased incidence of aminoglycoside toxicity in patients with advanced cirrhosis, and concur with more recent experimental evidence that gentamicin toxicity is enhanced after biliary obstruction in rats (Lucena *et al.* 1989).

The concomitant use of other drugs may augment or decrease the risk of toxicity. Animal models have shown that aminoglycoside toxicity may be augmented by protamine (Saito *et al.* 1987), diltiazem (Gomez *et al.* 1989), hydrocortisone (Beauchamp and Pettigrew 1988), potassium depletion, and captopril (Klotman *et al.* 1985), and volume depletion (Bennett *et al.* 1976); and it is ameliorated by a higher protein diet (Andrews and Bates 1987), oxygen radical scavengers (Walker and Shah 1988), bicarbonate, and acetazolamide (Aynedjian *et al.* 1988), magnesium supplements (Wong *et al.* 1989), calcium and thyroxine (Ernest 1989), and experimentally induced diabetes mellitus (Teixeria *et al.* 1982). Whether any of these factors are important in humans remains to be established. Drugs that have been associated with increased toxicity in humans include: frusemide, methoxyflurane, cisplatin, amphotericin, clindamycin, cephaloridine, and cephalothin.

The aminoglycoside prescribed is also important; unfortunately evaluation of comparative nephrotoxicity in humans from the literature is hampered by lack of consistent definition of toxicity, randomization of patients, and satisfactory control groups, and a paucity of double-blind studies. There is little to choose between tobramycin and gentamicin (Kahlmeter and Dahlager 1984; Moore *et al.* 1984), though Smith and colleagues (1980) have found tobramycin to be slightly less nephrotoxic. The toxicity of amikacin may be less still, but again the advantage is probably minimal (Holm *et al.* 1983), and there is little difference between tobramycin and netilmicin (Lerner *et al.* 1983). Netilmicin is associated with less cochlear and vestibular toxicity (Kahlmeter and Dahlager 1984; see also Chapter 20). When it comes to the choice of an aminoglycoside for the treatment of a Gram-negative infection, the evidence for one being less nephrotoxic than another is overshadowed by the results of culture and sensitivity of the organism, when available, and local unit policy in trying to reduce bacterial resistance. Recent studies have suggested that newer agents such as the third-generation cephalosporins and aztreonam may be as effective therapeutically as aminoglycosides but with less risk of toxicity (Appel 1990).

Considering the other aminoglycosides, neomycin is far more nephrotoxic than any other aminoglycoside, though as it is only given orally or topically little is absorbed; in chronic renal failure, however, accumulation may occur and renal damage has been described with oral therapy (De Beukelaer *et al.* 1971). Slight proteinuria is common with streptomycin but renal failure is rare (McDermott 1947). Similarly, kanamycin, though frequently producing changes in urine sediment, and proteinuria, seldom gives rise to renal failure except when given in doses above the therapeutic range or to patients with impaired renal function (Falco *et al.* 1969).

Other drugs that can cause acute tubular necrosis include some cytotoxic agents of which cisplatin is the chief offender. Used mainly in the treatment of testicular and ovarian tumours, it was nearly abandoned after phase 1 trials, because of severe gastrointestinal and renal adverse effects. It was subsequently demonstrated that its nephrotoxicity could be markedly reduced by keeping patients well hydrated before, during, and after its administration (Hayes *et al.* 1977). Chemotherapy emesis may exacerbate the nephrotoxicity (Cantwell *et al.* 1989), presumably by dehydration, but nausea and vomiting may be effectively controlled by administration of the selective antagonist to serotonin S_3 receptors ondansetron (Cubeddu *et al.* 1990). This is more effective than high-dose metoclopramide (Marty *et al.* 1990).

The principal route of excretion of cisplatin is via the kidney and accumulation occurs in the cortex. A decrease in renal plasma flow and increase in urinary enzymes is observed very early on in treatment, and hypomagnesaemia, hypocalcaemia, and hypokalaemia commonly occur (Fillastre and Raguenez-Viotte 1989).

The mechanism of toxicity remains unclear but it has been extensively investigated in rats. Certainly, the reduced GFR early on in renal failure due to cisplatin in rats results from reversible changes in renal blood flow and renal vascular resistance (Winston and Safirstein 1985). With 8 mg per kg administered intraperitoneally, damage to proximal, distal, and collecting tubules occurs in association with increased cell proliferation and DNA synthesis, and appearance of fibroblasts in the interstitium (Laurent et al. 1988); changes are more severe in the P3 segment of the proximal tubule (Jones et al. 1985). With a lower dose (5.5 mg per kg), reversible changes in renal function are accompanied by reversible changes in mitochondrial respiration and calcium accumulation (Gordon and Gattone 1986). In dogs and rats, acute proximal tubular changes precede any alterations in renal haemodynamics (Daugaard 1990).

In rats, protection against toxicity has been demonstrated with the free-radical scavenger o-(β-hydroxyethyl)-rutoside (Dobyan et al. 1986) and the calcium-channel blocker nifedipine (Deray et al. 1988). In patients given intrapleural or intraperitoneal cisplatin, intravenous thiosulphate has afforded clinically significant protection in some (Markman et al. 1985) and a phosphorylated sulphydryl compound, ethiofos, originally developed as a radioprotective agent, may protect the kidneys from toxicity (Mollman 1990). The ACTH (4-9) analogue Org 2766, which significantly prevents or attenuates cisplatin neuropathy, does not appear to affect renal toxicity (Gerritsen van der Hoop et al. 1990). Another way to avoid cisplatin toxicity would be to use carboplatin, which appears to have similar antineoplastic effects but fewer adverse effects (Fillastre and Raguenez-Viotte 1989). Acute tubular necrosis has also occurred with the use of the platinum compound TNO-6 (1,1-diaminomethyl cyclohexane sulphato platinum II) (Offerman et al. 1985).

Heavy metals may produce acute tubular necrosis or membranous glomerulonephritis (see below). In rats, mercury given intravenously accumulates in the proximal tubular cells of the kidney, preferentially in the S2 and S3 segments within lysosomes (Hultman and Enestrom 1986). The organic mercurial merthiolate has produced fatal acute tubular necrosis on a number of occasions when added in excess as a preservative for drugs given intramuscularly (Axton 1972).

Acute renal failure has also resulted from the absorption of copper sulphate (Holtzman et al. 1966) and boric acid (Baliah et al. 1969) from skin dressings, and from bismuth thiosulphate given intradermally for warts (Randall et al. 1972). Acute renal failure has been reported from Japan in a long-term user of a germanium preparation taken as an elixir. Postmortem examination of the kidney showed acute tubular necrosis, mild proliferation of mesangial matrix, foamy transformation of glomerular epithelial cells, red blood cell casts, and urate crystal deposition (Nagata et al. 1985). Chronic renal failure is a more common complication of germanium oxide; a characteristic clinical feature is the absence of proteinuria and haematuria. After discontinuation of the germanium, slow recovery may occur (Sanai et al. 1990).

Acute tubular necrosis can occur following paracetamol poisoning. Though usually complicating severe hepatic failure (Wilkinson et al. 1974) it may occur without hepatic failure (Cobden et al. 1982; Prescott et al. 1982; Dabbagh and Chesney 1985; Davenport and Finn 1988; Pillans and Hall 1985), and perhaps even after therapeutic doses in a few individuals (Gabriel et al. 1982); alcoholics are particularly susceptible (Kaysen et al. 1985; Keaton 1988). Renal and hepatic damage is prevented by the early administration of N-acetylcysteine (Prescott et al. 1979).

Osmotic nephrosis

Swelling and vacuolation of tubular cells can develop during and after filtration of mannitol and low-molecular-weight dextrans, though these histological changes may not be associated with alterations in tubular function (Engberg 1976). Whether or not the histological changes imply tubular damage has been disputed (Ericsson et al. 1967), and the exact mechanism whereby nephrotoxicity occurs is unclear. The patient with acute renal insufficiency associated with dextran-40 reported by Moran and Kapsner (1987), which was rapidly reversed by plasmapheresis argues the case for a hyperoncotic state where oncotic forces equal or exceed the hydraulic forces that determine GFR.

Mannitol is used predominantly to reduce cerebral oedema, to reduce intraocular pressure in glaucoma, and as a prophylactic agent in the prevention of acute renal failure. Nephrotoxicity is more likely to occur when the cumulative dose is high and there is chronic renal failure; diuretics may also have an additive effect (Horgan et al. 1989). The syndrome of mannitol toxicity is clinically manifested by intravascular fluid overload, hyponatraemia with a raised osmolar gap, and confusion as a result of its potent osmotic effect on the brain (Whelan et al. 1984; Horgan et al. 1989; Rello et al. 1989).

Though bizarre swelling of proximal tubular cells obliterating the lumen of the nephron has been described in patients developing acute renal failure after receiving dextran-40, many other reasons for developing renal failure were usually present (Wilkinson *et al.* 1965; Morgan *et al.* 1966; Mailloux *et al.* 1967). There are cases reported, however, in which no other cause of acute tubular necrosis was present (Fournier *et al.* 1969). More recently, the gelatin solution Gelofusine has been implicated in the development of renal failure (Hussain and Drew 1989), though other reasons for developing renal failure were present in the patient described. Hyperosmolality related to propylene glycol in an infant treated with enoximone infusion has also been reported (Huggon *et al.* 1990).

Vascular damage

Cyclosporin

There probably is no therapeutic window through which cyclosporin can shine. Though immunologically specific it has a number of non-immunological adverse effects including nephrotoxicity. These are predominantly dose-dependent and may take several different forms; we have divided toxicity initially into two major groups:
1. functional toxicity with minimal or no morphological change;
2. morphological forms of toxicity, which can be further subdivided clinically into acute, subacute, and chronic toxicity; and which morphologically include tubular, vascular, and interstitial change.

Functional toxicity of cyclosporin

Prospective serial renal function tests in patients treated with cyclosporin without renal disease show a sharp reduction in glomerular filtration and effective renal plasma flow, but without a change in filtration fraction, within the first week of treatment (Tegzess *et al.* 1988). This has been demonstrated non-invasively using engymetric radioisotope studies (Nowack *et al.* 1988). This functional disturbance is presumably due to intrarenal haemodynamic changes for which there may be several initiating mechanisms. We shall discuss five hypotheses, which are probably not mutually exclusive, concerning the renal vasoconstrictive effects of cyclosporin.

First, and most likely, cyclosporin interacts with the kallikrein–prostaglandin humoral system. Arguments for this include the changes that occur in the normal balance of arachidonic acid metabolites. Thromboxane A_2 (a powerful vasoconstrictor) synthesis is augmented by cyclosporin in rats (Coffman *et al.* 1987) and thromboxane A_2 inhibitors attenuate the nephrotoxicity; in addition urinary kallikrein excretion is reduced in humans receiving cyclosporin (Spragg *et al.* 1988). In other animal models, however, treatment with a prostaglandin

synthesis inhibitor (indomethacin) did not affect the renal response to cyclosporin, suggesting that prostaglandins may not play an important role in the functional haemodynamics of the renal toxicity (Barros *et al.* 1987).

Secondly, does the renin–angiotensin system play a role in these changes? Activation of the renin–angiotensin system in many disease states stimulates glomerular synthesis of prostacyclin and prostaglandin E_2, their vasodilator properties normally offset the vasoconstrictor effects of angiotensin II; this protective mechanism is lost in cyclosporin-treated animals (Perico *et al.* 1986). There is evidence from *in vivo* and *in vitro* animal experiments that there is activation of this humoral system and elevated plasma renin activity (PRA) but a variable response to captopril when it was used (Baxter *et al.* 1984; Murray *et al.* 1985; Dieperink *et al.* 1986; Barros *et al.* 1987; Kurtz *et al.* 1989). Not all agree, however: Gerkens and Smith (1985) were unable to detect changes in PRA in rats given cyclosporin and Whitworth and colleagues (1987) showed no rise in sheep given cyclosporin. Kahan (1989) in a review article on cyclosporin stated that the secretion of, and response to, renin–angiotensin is normal.

Thirdly, cyclosporin has been shown to enhance the release of intracellular free calcium from vascular smooth muscle and mesangial cells (Goldberg *et al.* 1989). A consequence of this may be an exaggerated contractile response by these cells to other stimuli, resulting in a reduction in renal blood flow and glomerular ultrafiltration. Calcium-channel blockers have been shown to exert a protective effect in rats (Barros *et al.* 1987) and may have similar effects in humans (Wagner *et al.* 1987).

Fourthly, cyclosporin has a direct sympathomimetic effect when infused into conscious rats (Murray *et al.* 1985), but as a renal allograft is denervated this is probably not relevant clinically.

Finally Kahan speculates that there may be a unifying hypothesis linking renal vasoconstriction with the immunosuppressive effects of cyclosporin, through inhibition of gene transcription of proteins concerned with normal vascular tone (Kahan 1989).

In patients with renal transplants, cyclosporin nephrotoxicity may have an additive effect to ischaemic injury in the kidney; this has been demonstrated in the rat (Chow *et al.* 1986; Jablonski *et al.* 1986; Kanazi *et al.* 1986) and may be the reason for the higher incidence of delayed function in human renal allograft recipients treated with cyclosporin (CMTSG 1986; Sheil *et al.* 1983; Hall *et al.* 1985).

In some patients toxicity is associated with hyperkalaemia that has been attributed to hypoaldosteronism, the additional use of β-blockers to treat hypertension, and a tubular defect of potassium secretion (Adu *et al.* 1983; Petersen *et al.* 1984).

Toxicity of cyclosporin with morphological changes

Acute toxicity may be due to an extension of functional change in that it is commonly seen in renal allografts when the allograft has been harvested under adverse conditions and renal ischaemia is already present. Less commonly, a thrombotic glomerular microangiopathy that clinically and histologically resembles the haemo-lytic–uraemic syndrome is found (Muirhead *et al.* 1987; Pahl *et al.* 1988). The aetiology of this drug reaction remains speculative; *in vitro* experiments suggest that cyclosporin is directly toxic to endothelial cells (Zoja *et al.* 1986) — a suggestion strengthened by *in vivo* animal (Benigni *et al.* 1988) and patient (Zaal *et al.* 1988) data — and endothelial damage may precipitate the acute angi-opathy (Remuzzi and Bertani 1989). This particular complication has been successfully treated by withdraw-ing cyclosporin and giving intra-arterial streptokinase (Muirhead *et al.* 1987) and FK506 (McCauley *et al.* 1989).

Subacute nephrotoxicity develops between weeks 1–8 of therapy and in the renal transplant patient is suggested by a rising creatinine without signs of graft rejection. Blood levels of cyclosporin are often high but not always so (Holt *et al.* 1986) and the toxicity is usually promptly reversible if the dose of cyclosporin is reduced. Renal biopsy and fine needle aspiration are valuable not so much in the diagnosis of cyclosporin toxicity (no mor-phological changes are diagnostic, though characteristic features are proximal tubular cell giant mitochondria, vacuolization, and microcalcification [Mihatsch *et al.* 1988*a*]) as in excluding rejection as a cause for deterio-rating renal function. Intrarenal pressure may help to distinguish the two (pressures in rejection >40 mmHg, pressures in cyclosporin toxicity <40 mmHg (Salaman and Griffin 1985). It has been suggested that this is less sensitive than fine-needle aspiration but useful in combi-nation in differentiating allograft rejection from cyclo-sporin toxicity (Ubhi *et al.* 1987).

Chronic nephrotoxicity occurs after a longer period of use, usually after one year; it may cause irreversible renal damage in heart transplant recipients (Myers *et al.* 1988). In patients with autoimmune uveitis treated with cyclosporin, a 50 per cent increase in serum creatinine was observed in 37 per cent of 73 patients (Austin *et al.* 1989). Though the elevation in serum creatinine was rapidly reversed by a reduction in dosage of withdrawal of the drug, after 3 months of treatment renal parenchy-mal injury did progress in a few patients, despite stable renal function and dose reduction (Austin *et al.* 1989). A

vascular basis for this type of toxicity is likely in view of increased renal resistance and hypertension that may precede a serum creatinine rise, illustrated in a patient being treated for chronic inflammatory demyelinating polyradiculopathy (Kolkin *et al.* 1987), and the promi-nent renal arteriolar changes seen in the biopsies of the patients studied by Austin and colleagues (1989).

Renal histology characteristically shows interstitial striped fibrosis, possibly as a result of tubular loss due to afferent arteriolar vasoconstriction (Palestine *et al.*. 1986; Remuzzi and Bertani 1989).

Acute cyclosporin nephrotoxicity has not emerged as a specific risk factor for the development of chronic toxicity in some studies (Greenberg *et al.* 1987) but has in others (Mihatsch *et al.* 1988*b*). Other risk factors for the development of chronic toxicity include high blood trough levels, concomitant use of nephrotoxic drugs,

TABLE 12.3
Drugs affecting cyclosporin toxicity

Enhancing toxicity

Acyclovir	additive toxicity	Bennett and Pulliam 1983
Aminoglycosides	additive toxicity	Hows *et al.* 1983
Amphotericin	additive toxicity	Kennedy *et al.* 1983
Ciprofloxacin	additive toxicity	Avent *et al.* 1988
Colchicine	additive toxicity	Menta *et al.* 1987
Co-trimoxazole	additive toxicity	Thompson *et al.* 1983
Corticosteroids	increase levels	Cockburn 1986
Diclofenac	additive toxicity	Deray *et al.* 1987
Diltiazem	increases levels	Wagner *et al.* 1986
Erythromycin	increases levels	Grino *et al.* 1986
Ethanol	increases levels	Paul *et al.* 1987
Frusemide	additive toxicity	Whiting *et al.* 1984
Ketoconazole	increases levels	Dieperink and Moller 1982
Melphalan	additive toxicity	Dale *et al.* 1985
NSAID	additive toxicity	Harris *et al.* 1988

Inhibiting toxicity (and efficacy if reducing blood levels)

Carbamazepine	reduces levels	Lele *et al.* 1985
Dopamine	inhibits toxicity	Kho *et al.* 1987
Enalapril	?inhibits toxicity	McAuley *et al.* 1987
Ethambutol	reduces levels	Leimenstoll *et al.* 1988
Fosfomycin	inhibits toxicity	Sack *et al.* 1987
Imipenem	reduces levels	Mraz *et al.* 1987
Isoniazid	reduces levels	Langhoff and Madsen 1983
Metoprolol	reduces levels	Chan 1986
Nafcillin	reduces levels	Veremis *et al.* 1987
Phenobarbitone	reduces levels	Carstenen *et al.* 1986
Phenytoin	reduces levels	Freeman *et al.* 1984
Prostaglandins	inhibit toxicity	Makowka *et al.* 1986
Rifampicin	reduces levels	Cassidy *et al.* 1985
Spironolactone	?inhibits toxicity	McAuley *et al.* 1987
Warfarin	reduces levels	Snyder 1988

more frequent rejection episodes, and primary poor renal function (Mihatsch *et al.* 1988*b*).

Various drugs can interfere with the metabolism and action of cyclosporin and these are listed in table 12.3. The nephrotoxicity of endotoxin may also be potentiated by cyclosporin (Cosio *et al.* 1987).

Other drugs causing vascular damage

Chronic glomerular microangiopathy may complicate metastatic carcinoma particularly when the latter is treated with mitomycin (Hostetter *et al.* 1987; Jain and Seymour 1987; Verweij *et al.* 1987; Mergenthaler *et al.* 1988). In a carefully monitored study of 44 patients treated with mitomycin, of whom 37 were evaluated, one patient developed a lethal haemolytic–uraemic syndrome after a high dose of mitomycin; the adverse effect was not predictable but based on this case and a review of the literature the authors concluded that renal toxicity was a dose-dependent adverse effect (Verwey *et al.* 1987). Plasmapheresis and antiplatelet agents have been used in its treatment (Murgo 1987).

The use of oral contraceptives (Brown *et al.* 1973) and that of metronidazole in children (Powell *et al.* 1988) have been implicated as causes of a haemolytic–uraemic syndrome. Postpartum renal failure associated with red cell fragmentation and arteriolar thrombosis may be caused by ergometrine (Robson *et al.* 1968; Williams and Hughes 1974).

Hypersensitivity angiitis due to thiazide diuretics may be associated with renal involvement (Björnberg and Gisslen 1965), though cutaneous vasculitis is much more common. Angiitis has also been attributed to sulphonamides (Berlyne 1972). Other drugs which have induced a granulomatous necrotizing angiitis include allopurinol (Jarzobski *et al.* 1970), carbamazepine (Imai *et al.* 1989), glibenclamide (Clarke *et al.* 1974), phenytoin (Yermakov *et al.* 1983; Gaffey *et al.* 1986), and quinidine (Quin *et al.* 1988). Skin eruption and eosinophilia are consistently found in addition to renal failure. The prognosis is generally poor but in the case reported by Quin and colleagues (1988) there was a prompt response to prednisone. Fatal renal vasculitis and minimal change glomerulonephritis have also complicated treatment with penicillamine (Falck *et al.* 1979).

Use of streptokinase has been associated with proteinuria and haematuria of glomerular origin (Argent and Adams 1990) and a serum sickness type reaction with vasculitis (Noel *et al.* 1987; Payne *et al.* 1989; Callan *et al.* 1990). Another thrombolytic agent, anistreplase (anisoylated plasminogen–streptokinase complex), has also been reported to cause a vasculitis (Ali *et al.* 1990).

The use of horse sera (De La Pava *et al.* 1962) and vaccines (Bishop *et al.* 1966) has also been described as causing an immune-complex nephritis and vasculitis. The abuse of amphetamines has also been associated with a classical polyarteritis-like syndrome (Citron *et al.* 1970; Bennett *et al.* 1977) and piroxicam has caused a Henoch–Schönlein syndrome with nephritis (Goebel and Mueller-Brodmann 1982).

Glomerular damage

Drug-induced glomerular damage resulting in a rapidly progressive glomerulonephritis is a rare cause of acute renal failure. More common are milder forms of nephritis, such as membranous glomerulonephritis and lupus nephritis, which are discussed later on in the chapter.

Devogelaer and co-workers (1987) provided a review of the literature as well as reporting a case of penicillamine-induced crescentic nephritis, and showed that treatment with withdrawal of the drug and immunosuppression is effective. Circulating antiglomerular basement membrane antibodies have been demonstrated in similar cases (Peces *et al.* 1987). Glue-sniffing has also been reported to cause Goodpasture's syndrome (Bonzel *et al.* 1987) and mesangiocapillary glomerulonephritis (Venkataraman 1981), as have other solvents (Lauwerys *et al.* 1985; Bernis *et al.* 1985); a proliferative glomerulonephritis with linear IgG deposition along glomerular capillary walls has occurred after exposure to paraquat (Stratta *et al.* 1988).

Rapidly progressive crescentic glomerulonephritis of the non-Goodpasture's type has been described with rifampicin (Murray *et al.* 1987) and hydralazine (Björck *et al.* 1983). We have treated two patients with systemic vasculitis, crescentic nephritis, and perinuclear cytoplasmic antibodies (p-ANCA) in which the antibody is directed against cytoplasmic myeloperoxidase related to penicillamine and hydralazine (unpublished data). Crescentic nephritis has also been described in a patient taking enalapril (Bailey and Lynn 1986).

Interstitial damage

Tubulointerstitial disease may occur as a component of nephritis where the primary insult is directed towards the glomerulus, such as in glomerulonephritis or systemic lupus erythematosus; or where the primary insult is vascular, as in vasculitis or the haemolytic–uraemic syndrome. It may also be the primary site of damage either through a direct dose-dependent toxicity (e.g. due to amphotericin) or as a result of a hypersensitivity reaction. The immunoallergic reactions causing interstitial nephritis may be induced by cellular and humoral mechanisms. There are no experimental models at present to substantiate the cellular mechanisms, but the characterization of inflammatory cells in the interstitium of the kidney in cases of drug-induced interstitial nephritis using monoclonal antibodies suggests a cellular basis for the condition (Gimenez and Mampaso 1986). There is also a considerable amount of data to support humoral mechanisms. Serum antitubular basement membrane antibodies have been detected in interstitial nephritis associated with methicillin (Border *et al.* 1974), and Joh and colleagues (1989) have demonstrated that experimental drug-induced acute interstitial nephritis (AIN) in mice is mediated by IgG antihapten antibodies. Other, probably less important, mechanisms include inoculation of Tamm–Horsfall protein into renal substance demonstrated in rabbits (Nagai and Nagai 1987) and tubular crystal deposition as in the case of acyclovir, both of which could spark off an immune reaction. As in drug-induced glomerulonephritis, the different immune reactions leading to AIN may produce a variety of histological and clinical pictures.

The classic type of AIN is best illustrated by the methicillin-induced disease. Methicillin, though not used nowadays, was the first semi-synthetic penicillin used clinically for treating infections caused by penicillinase-producing staphylococci. In one series of 80 children treated with the drug, 15 per cent developed features of AIN (Sanjad *et al.* 1974). Typically, the interstitial infiltrate on microscopy consists of mononuclear cells. Using monoclonal antibody techniques the majority of these cells are identified as T cells with varying numbers of CD4 and CD8 subtypes; these may vary with different drugs and may hint at different pathogeneses (Colvin and Fang 1989). Typically, eosinophils make up 2–10 per cent of the infiltrating cells. In addition, there is usually considerable interstitial oedema and secondary tubular necrosis. The former is in part responsible for the macroscopic swelling of the kidney (which can be picked up by ultrasound or on plain abdominal X-rays) and the loin discomfort frequently felt.

The clinical presentation is usually one of acute renal failure with very little else apart from exposure to the drug. On the other hand in seriously ill patients multiple-drug regimens are often used, other causes for renal failure are often present, and it is not possible to decide which, if any drug, is responsible. In Pusey's series, the time from exposure to the onset of symptoms ranged from 1–30 days (Pusey *et al.* 1983), but it may be far longer than this. In the case of rifampicin, renal failure is more common with intermittent therapy. A constellation of features suggesting a hypersensitivity reaction may be present, including; arthralgia, fever, skin rash, and evidence of abnormal liver function and eosinophilia on blood tests. The urine examination typically reveals mild to moderate proteinuria and haematuria. Eosinophiluria may also be present; Hansel's stain is a simple technique that is superior to Wright's stain for detecting urinary eosinophils (Nolan and Kelleher 1988). The test is sensitive, but it should be remembered that eosinophils may be found in the urine of patients suffering from other renal conditions such as glomerulonephritis. Though other less invasive techniques, such as gallium scanning (Linton *et al.* 1980), have been used in the diagnosis of interstitial nephritis, the diagnosis should be made by renal biopsy whenever possible.

In addition to the classic type of AIN, a histological subtype with a striking granulomatous reaction is well-recognized, acute granulomatous interstitial nephritis. In addition to those mentioned in the classic infiltrate, the cells in this condition include nodular aggregates of histiocytes, eosinophils and Langhans-type giant cells. Many of the drugs listed can cause this form of AIN, though less commonly than the classic form. Those most often implicated are the penicillins, co-trimoxazole, sulphonamides, allopurinol, and the thiazides. The clinical picture is frequently identical in the acute classical and the acute granulomatous types of interstitial nephritis. The response to withdrawal of the drug and corticosteroids is also similar and it is our policy to treat both these types of AIN with steroids (Pusey *et al.* 1983).

Assuming greater importance as it is becoming a better recognized and frequently diagnosed complication of the NSAID is AIN in association with a minimal change type of glomerular lesion (Finkelstein *et al.* 1982; Handa 1986; Marasco *et al.* 1987). As methicillin is the penicillin that has been most studied in classic AIN, so is fenoprofen for this type of renal injury. Usually, the glomerular lesions are non-specific and not severe enough to suggest that they contribute to the renal failure (Bender *et al.* 1984). The interstitial nephritis is often severe and is usually the cause (Ling *et al.* 1990).

Drugs other than the NSAID that have been associated with interstitial nephritis and a minimal change type of glomerular lesion include recombinant interferon-α, ampicillin, lithium, penicillamine, phenytoin (Colvin and Fang 1989), and rifampicin. In the reported cases implicating NSAID, the clinical picture is somewhat different from the classic AIN and granulomatous AIN. Most patients are over 60 years old; only rarely do they manifest the systemic features of an allergic reaction; oliguria is rare; and heavy proteinuria with a nephrotic syndrome is common. As with the other types of AIN, the drug may have been taken only for a short period or

TABLE 12.4
Drugs associated with acute interstitial nephritis

Antibacterials

Amoxycillin	Geller *et al.* 1986
Ampicillin	Maxwell *et al.* 1974; Ruley and Lisi 1974
Aztreonam	Pazmino 1988
Carbenicillin	Appel *et al.* 1978
Cefaclor	Pommer *et al.* 1986
Cefoxitin	Toll *et al.* 1987
Cephalexin	Verma and Kieff 1975
Cephalothin	Drago *et al.* 1976
Cephapirin	Lewis and Rindone 1987
Cephradine	Wiles *et al.* 1979
Ciprofloxacin	Ying and Johnson 1989
Cloxacillin	Grimm *et al.* 1989
Co-trimoxazole	Dry *et al.* 1975; Cryst and Hammer 1988
Gentamicin	Saltissi *et al.* 1979
Methicillin	Galpin *et al.* 1975; Mayaud *et al.* 1975
Mezlocillin	Cushner *et al.* 1985
Minocycline	Walker *et al.* 1979
Nafcillin	Parry *et al.* 1973
Oxacillin	Burton *et al.* 1974
Penicillin	Colvin *et al.* 1974; Orchard and Rooker 1974
Pyrazinamide	Sanwikarja *et al.* 1989
Rifampicin	Nessi *et al.* 1976; Katz and Lor 1986
Sulphonamides	Robson *et al.* 1970
Vancomycin	Bergman *et al.* 1988

Non-steroidal agents

Diclofenac	Cameron 1988
Diflunisal	Wharton *et al.* 1982
Fenoprofen	Finkelstein *et al.* 1982
Ibuprofen	Bender *et al.* 1984
Indomethacin	Gary *et al.* 1980
Ketoprofen	Cameron 1988
Mefenamate	Cameron 1988
Naproxen	Brezin *et al.* 1979
Phenylbutazone	Russell *et al.* 1978
Piroxicam	Cameron 1988
Pirprofen	Hurault de Ligny *et al.* 1986
Sulindac	Whelton *et al.* 1983
Tolmetin	Bender *et al.* 1984
Zomepirac	Bender *et al.* 1984

Miscellaneous

Allopurinol	Gelbart *et al.* 1977
Aspirin	McLeish *et al.* 1979
Azathioprine	Saway *et al.* 1988
Captopril	Hooke *et al.* 1982
Carbamazepine	Hogg *et al.* 1981
Cimetidine	Ozawa *et al.* 1987
Clofibrate	Cumming 1980
Contrast agents	Ihle *et al.* 1982
Diazepam	Sadjadi *et al.* 1987
Foscarnet	Nyberg *et al.* 1990

(Table 12.4 continued)

(Miscellaneous)

Frusemide	Jennings *et al.* 1986
Glafenine	Renier *et al.* 1975; Andrieu *et al.* 1976
Methyldopa	Wilson *et al.* 1974
Penicillamine	Feehally *et al.* 1987
Phenindione	Galea *et al.* 1963; Lee and Holden 1964
Phenytoin	Sheth *et al.* 1977; Hyman *et al.* 1978
Phenobarbitone	Faarup and Christensen 1974
Recombinant interferon-α	Averbuch *et al.* 1984
Sodium valproate	Lin and Chiang 1988
Sulphinpyrazone	Howard *et al.* 1981
Thiazides	Fuller *et al.* 1976; Goette and Beatrice 1988
Warfarin	Volpi *et al.* 1989

Drugs in bold type are those most commonly associated with AIN.

for years. Withdrawal of the drug usually results in resolution of both the renal failure and the nephrotic syndrome. Our impression is that steroids may hasten the recovery, though this has not been proved.

There is still much to be learnt; with advancements in immunohistochemistry and molecular biology the pathogenesis of drug-induced AIN should become clearer. A list of drugs that can cause AIN is given in table 12.4.

Obstruction

Drugs may cause obstruction to urine flow at the level of the nephron by tubular blockage from various proteins or by causing crystalluria and augmenting stone formation; other drugs may cause obstruction lower down in the urinary tract by producing ureteric obstruction from retroperitoneal fibrosis, blood clot and, rarely, tumours; they may also be responsible for bladder-neck obstruction. Drug-induced crystalluria, which may cause acute renal failure due to tubular blockage, is discussed in the section on renal stones and calcium nephropathy later in the chapter.

Tubular blockage

Light-chain casts

Light-chain proteinuria with and without acute renal failure, developing in patients with tuberculosis treated with rifampicin, has been reported by four groups (Graber *et al.* 1975; Kumar *et al.* 1976; Warrington *et al.* 1977; Soffer *et al.* 1987). This unique type of drug reaction was most recently reviewed by Soffer and co-workers in 1987. The cause is unclear but volume depletion may play a role in precipitation (Warrington *et al.*

1977). Renal histology is similar to that seen in the light-chain nephropathy of myeloma, though in the case described by Soffer and colleagues there was no giant-cell reaction to tubular casts. They speculate that this may have been due to the polyclonal origin of the light chains and the short duration of the disease process; light-chain proteinuria usually resolves within 10 days of discontinuing the drug.

Tubular blockage by light chains is also one of many mechanisms whereby myeloma may cause renal failure, and it has been suggested that the risk of precipitation may be aggravated by contrast media (Myers and Witten 1971). Baltzer and colleagues (1978), however, in a review of 89 pyelograms in patients with myeloma, did not find any patient who had suffered a decline in renal function after the procedure. The hazard that attends this investigation is probably dehydration rather than the contrast medium itself. Acute renal failure has also been described in a patient with primary macroglobulinaemia with small-molecule IgM κ-chain protein (Matsumoto et al. 1985) and in diffuse hypergammaglobulinaemia following intravenous urography (Antman et al. 1982).

Tamm–Horsfall protein

The pathophysiology of nephropathy induced by contrast media remains obscure; adverse effects on the kidney include direct tubular toxicity with enzymuria (Goldstein et al. 1976) and diuresis; albuminuria (Holtas 1978); changes in renal blood flow which may in part be due to vasopressin release (Trewhalla et al. 1990); and changes in glomerular filtration rate. Contrast media may also promote tubular obstruction. Tamm–Horsfall mucoprotein, predominantly secreted by the tubular cells of the thick ascending limb of Henle's loop (Kumar and Muchmore 1990), is the major constituent of casts and it can be precipitated in vitro by adding contrast media to the urine (Schwartz et al. 1970). It is possible that this may occur in vivo, although data from Dawnay and others (1985) show no increased rate in excretion of Tamm–Horsfall glycoprotein following routine intravenous urography.

The chance of an otherwise fit person developing acute renal failure after exposure to a contrast medium contrast is minuscule, but in the presence of risk factors, including diabetes (Harkonen and Kjellstrand 1979), advanced age (Weinrauch et al. 1978), dehydration (Swartz et al. 1978), pre-existing renal disease (Byrd and Sherman 1979), and severe cardiac failure (Taliercio et al. 1986) the chances are higher. The volume of contrast material used and the type of study performed also played a role in the cases studied retrospectively by Gomes and others (1985), involving 364 patients who

were undergoing major arteriography. The incidence of this contrast nephropathy is difficult to assess for various reasons, including variable definitions of nephrotoxicity, differing procedures and doses of contrast used in different studies and the retrospective, uncontrolled nature of many of these reports. There have been three more recent large controlled prospective studies (Cramer et al. 1985; Parfrey et al. 1989; Schwarb et al. 1989). Cramer and colleagues, defining nephrotoxicity as a rise in creatinine of greater than 1.2 mg per dl 2 days after administration of a contrast medium for computed tomography (CT) enhancement, in this study reported an incidence of 2.1 per cent, which was no different from that in controls. Parfrey and colleagues' definition was a rise of 50 per cent or more in baseline creatinine after contrast medium; differing procedures were not randomized, and the incidence of toxicity was 9 per cent in diabetics with pre-existing renal disease compared with 1.6 per cent in controls (who underwent CT scanning or abdominal imaging without contrast medium). Finally, Schwarb and others, defining toxicity as a rise in creatinine of greater than 44 μmol per litre above baseline within 48 hours, reported toxicity in 10.2 per cent of patients receiving ionic and 8.2 per cent of those receiving non-ionic contrast medium (difference not significant). In high-risk groups (diabetes, heart failure, and pre-existing renal failure) the corresponding figures were 17 per cent and 15 percent, again not a signficant difference.

The complication may be avoided by critically analysing the potential benefit-to-risk ratio in individual patients and by ensuring good hydration before giving a contrast medium. In addition, it has been shown that intravenous mannitol before or immediately after the medium is given may be beneficial (Snyder et al. 1968; Anto et al. 1981). Cigarroa and colleagues (1989), by adjusting the dose of contrast medium to the severity of azotaemia, found that limiting it reduced the incidence of acute renal dysfunction, particularly in diabetics. The low-osmolality non-ionic agents, in general, exhibit less toxicity, and on theoretical grounds the same should be true for nephrotoxicity (Dawson 1985). The two large clinical studies mentioned above (Parfrey et al. 1989; Schwarb et al. 1989), however, found no significant difference between groups receiving ionic and non-ionic contrast agents, and acute renal failure has been described following low-osmolality agents (Elliott and Reger 1988). It remains to be seen from the results of future controlled prospective studies if indeed nephrotoxicity is less with these than with conventional contrast agents. Calcium-channel blockers may exert a protective effect if given before administration of a contrast medium

(Neumayer *et al.* 1989), although not all agree (Cacoub *et al.* 1988). The toxic effects of contrast media are discussed in greater detail in Chapter 27.

Myoglobin

A consequence of drug-induced rhabdomyolysis is release of myoglobin into the circulation, and myoglobinuria. Myoglobin has a short half-life in the circulation and is probably not nephrotoxic *per se*, but within the renal tubule it is converted to ferrihaeme, which is a direct tubular cell toxin and causes tubular blockage.

Cocaine and 'crack' (cocaine base) have become the current popular recreational drugs in the affluent society; it has been estimated that 3 million Americans have tried cocaine and that a further 5 million use it on a regular basis. Although its life-threatening complications primarily affect the cardiovascular and neurological systems, there are increasingly frequent reports of the association of abuse with hyperpyrexia, rhabdomyolysis, and acute renal failure (Merigian and Roberts 1987; Menashe and Gottlieb 1988; Roth *et al.* 1988; Singhal *et al.* 1989; Anand *et al.* 1989; Cregler 1989; Jandreski *et al.* 1989; Ahijado *et al.* 1990). Though in many cases there are other predisposing factors causing rhabdomyolysis, as in the three cases reported by Singal and colleagues, namely, prolonged squatting; lying in an abnormal position, resulting in a compartmental syndrome; and violence. Of the 39 cases described by Roth and others (1988), 13 were hyperpyrexial. There are many cases where other predisposing factors are absent. Other recreational drugs that have caused rhabdomyolysis and renal failure include amphetamines (Kendrick *et al.* 1977; Terada *et al.* 1988), heroin (Richter *et al.* 1971; D'Agostino and Arnett 1979; Gibb and Shaw 1985), lysergide (Mercieca and Brown 1984), phencyclidine (Akmal *et al.* 1981), and toluene (Mizutani *et al.* 1989). It should be remembered that drug abuse may expose the user to other toxins that may contaminate the primary drug, for example, arsenic intoxication in cocaine abuse (Lombard *et al.* 1989). Arsenic is also a cause of renal failure (Muehrcke and Pirani 1968; Gerhardt *et al.* 1978).

In many instances, as in cases of alcohol abuse, rhabdomyolysis occurs after a prolonged period of stupor or coma during which limb ischaemia may occur due to compression; alcohol, however, also produces a myopathy that predisposes to this complication in the absence of such precipitants (Haapanen *et al.* 1984). Methanol poisoning has also been described as being complicated by myoglobinuric renal failure (Grufferman *et al.* 1985). Other drugs that have been associated with renal failure and myoglobinuria include pentamidine (Sensakovic *et al.* 1985); and there is evidence to suggest a particular susceptibility in patients with AIDS (Lachaal and Venuto 1989). Amphotericin (Drutz *et al.* 1970), carbenoxolone (Mitchell 1971), corticosteroids (Heitzman *et al.* 1962), diuretics (Oh *et al.* 1971), and a lotion containing 9-α-fluoroprednisolone (Mijares 1986) share a common pathway — via hypokalaemia — by which they induce rhabdomyolysis and renal failure; this is also the cause of the rhabdomyolysis associated with parenteral nutrition (Nadel *et al.* 1979).

The neuroleptic malignant syndrome (see Chapters 18 and 28), a complication of the use of major tranquillizers, the phenothiazines and haloperidol, may be further complicated by myoglobinuric renal failure (Eiser *et al.* 1982). Rhabdomyolysis and acute renal failure have also been induced by a combination of lovastatin and gemfibrozil (Marais and Larson 1990). The HMG-Co A reductase inhibitors may precipitate rhabdomyolysis, particularly in combination with other lipid-lowering agents (Kogan and Orenstein 1990). Though fibric acid derivatives such as clofibrate, bezafibrate, and fenofibrate have occasionally been associated with rhabdomyolysis, gemfibrozil used alone probably does not have this effect, but it may do so when given with lovastatin, as in 12 cases reported in the literature to date (Pierce *et al.* 1990); so this combination should be discouraged. The concomitant use of cyclosporin with HMG-Co A reductase inhibitors also increases the risk of developing rhabdomyolysis; the predicted odds ratio of developing rhabdomyolysis rises from 0.15 per cent with lovastatin alone to 5 per cent for patients taking lovastatin and gemfibrozil, and to 28 per cent with the combination of lovastatin, gemfibrozil, and cyclosporin (Kogan and Orenstein 1990).

Restoration of blood flow to an ischaemic limb or other tissue by the use of intra-arterial streptokinase can cause massive release of myoglobin into the circulation and cause renal failure (Lang 1985).

Other agents found guilty of causing renal damage by release of myoglobin into the circulation are listed in table 12.5.

Haemoglobin

An immune-mediated intravascular haemolysis caused by cianidanol has resulted in haemoglobinuria and renal impairment (Rotoli *et al.* 1985). Drug-induced red cell antibodies of IgG and IgM classes against the antidepressant nomifensine and its metabolites have been found in patients with acute intravascular haemolysis due to this drug, many of whom developed renal impairment (Salama and Mueller-Eckhardt 1985). Acute haemolysis may occur after a second exposure to a single

TABLE 12.5
Drugs causing rhabdomyolysis and acute renal failure

Recreational

Amphetamines	Terada *et al.* 1988
Cocaine and 'crack'	see text
Ethanol	Haapanen *et al.* 1984
Heroin	Gibb and Shaw 1985
Lysergide	Mercieca and Brown 1984
Methanol	Grufferman *et al.* 1985
Phencyclidine	Akmal *et al.* 1981
Toluene	Mizutani *et al.* 1989

Therapeutic

Amphotericin	Drutz *et al.* 1970
Bezafibrate	Yeshurun *et al.* 1989
Carbenoxolone	Mitchell 1971
Chlorthalidone	Oh *et al.* 1971
Clofibrate	Langer and Levy 1968
Corticosteroids	Heitzman *et al.* 1962
Cytarabine	Margolis *et al.* 1987
Fenofibrate	Giraud *et al.* 1982
9-α-fluoroprednisolone	Mijares 1986
Haloperidol and phenothiazines	Eiser *et al.* 1982
Halothane	Rubiano *et al.* 1987
Lovastatin	Pierce *et al.* 1990
Methylene chloride	Miller *et al.* 1985
Opiates	Blain *et al.* 1985
Pentamidine	Sensakovic *et al.* 1985
Streptokinase	Lang 1985
Suxamethonium	Hawker *et al.* 1985
Suxamethonium and enflurane	Lee *et al.* 1987

Overdosage

Amoxapine	Jennings *et al.* 1983
Diphenhydramine	Hampel *et al.* 1983
Doxylamine	Mendoza *et al.* 1987
Phenazopyridine	Gavish *et al.* 1986
Sodium valproate	Roodhooft *et al.* 1990
Terbutaline	Blake and Ryan 1989
Theophylline	Macdonald *et al.* 1985

capsule (Fulton *et al.* 1986), as can chronic haemolysis (Skinner and Ferner 1986). Acute haemolysis, and renal failure secondary to it, are also described with rifampicin (Tahan *et al.* 1985).

Retroperitoneal fibrosis

In most cases of retroperitoneal fibrosis no cause can be found, but a careful drug history may uncover one. The first drug to be implicated was methysergide (Graham 1964; Graham *et al.* 1966). This association was amply confirmed by other reports (Carr and Biswas 1966; Kerbel 1967; Gelford and Cromwell 1968; Bianchine and Freidman 1970; Watts 1973). Fibrosis may also occur around the rectum, sigmoid colon, scrotum, medias-

tinum, heart valves (Misch 1974), and pleura, causing pleural effusions (Hindle *et al.* 1970). Whereas methysergide is used in the prophylaxis of migraine, dihydroergotamine and ergotamine tartrate used in the treatment of the acute attack, have also been suspected, though the association is far more tenuous (Verin *et al.* 1974; Lepage-Savary and Vallières 1982; Malaquin *et al.* 1989). Other drugs under suspicion include the β-blockers propranolol (Pierce *et al.* 1981), atenolol (Doherty *et al.* 1978; Johnson and McFarland 1980), oxprenolol (McCluskey *et al.* 1980), timolol (Rimmer *et al.* 1983), metoprolol (Thompson and Julian 1982), and sotalol (Laakso *et al.* 1982). Since these reports are few in relation to the use of β-blockers it has been suggested that the association with these drugs may be coincidental (Pryor *et al.* 1983). Regression usually occurs following withdrawal of the drug, but progression may occur (Schwartz and Dunea 1966), requiring treatment with corticosteroids or by surgical ureterolysis.

Blood clot obstruction

Urinary tract bleeding may complicate over-anticoagulation, but acute renal failure due to bilateral ureteric clot obstruction is rare (Nade 1972; Rosen 1972). Bilateral ureteric obstruction due to retroperitoneal bleeding has also been described (Kaden and Friedman 1961). In massive haematuria due to other causes, such as haemophilia, the use of the antifibrinolytic agents tranexamic acid and aminocaproic acid has resulted in ureteric obstruction. Haemorrhagic cystitis with severe haemorrhage and clots was observed by Droller and colleagues (1982) in 8 of 97 patients receiving cyclophosphamide for malignancy, but this is unlikely to cause clot obstruction. The complication can largely be avoided by ensuring a good diuresis during treatment.

Urinary retention

This rarely causes acute renal failure. The complication is most frequently seen in elderly men with some degree of prostatic hypertrophy; confinement to bed makes things worse. It may also be the cause of confusion in the elderly. The drugs most commonly associated with this form of obstruction are sedatives, drugs with anticholinergic effects, and the opiates.

Glomerulonephritis and the nephrotic syndrome

Drugs may invoke an immune response that may in turn cause glomerulonephritis (Druet 1989) by a variety of mechanisms. Commonly they act as haptens; some may activate complement, possibly within glomeruli, to provoke an inflammatory response (Stark *et al.* 1985); and some (e.g. mercurials) may induce a polyclonal activation of B lymphocytes. Antibodies to glomerular basement membrane antigens can be detected within 8 days after administration of mercury to rats (Michaelson *et al.* 1985). That the T cell repertoire may be involved has been demonstrated by changes in T cell subpopulations before the appearance of such circulating antibodies (Bowman *et al.* 1987). Such drug reactions are largely dose-independent.

Less common is damage due to direct glomerular toxicity, which is largely dose-dependent. This has been well studied experimentally with the aminonucleoside of puromycin. The hypothesis of 'mesangial overloading' has been invoked as a prelude to glomerular sclerosis found in rats with aminonucleoside nephrosis (Grond *et al.* 1985); disruption of glomerular basement membrane anionic charge sites also occurs early on in this animal model of nephrosis (Mahan *et al.* 1986), and glomerular epithelial cell injury is probably a direct toxic effect of this drug (Diamond and Karnovsky 1986).

Those drugs that cause acute glomerular damage through a serum-sickness type reaction with vasculitis or a Goodpasture's syndrome with a rapidly progressive glomerulonephritis are described above in the section on vascular damage. Drug-induced lupus nephritis is discussed separately later in the chapter.

There are many more drugs that are associated with a more subtle perturbation of the immune system which can none the less produce profound disease in the form of more chronic glomerulonephritis. The most common form of this is a membranous glomerulonephritis, presenting clinically with a nephrotic syndrome. Of the drugs involved, perhaps the best known are gold salts and penicillamine. In common with captopril (also capable of causing a membranous glomerulonephritis [Case *et al.* 1980]), they have sulphydryl groups in their structure, which may be important as patients particularly at risk are poor sulphoxidators. The Class 2 major histocompatibility antigen DR3 confers susceptibility to toxicity from some of these agents (Druet 1989). The HLA major histocompatibility complex is also important in the strong association between Class 1 antigen B35-Cw4 and nephritis developing in patients with rheumatoid arthritis treated with tiopronin, a penicillamine-like compound (Ferraccioli *et al.* 1986). Genetic factors are therefore important in conferring susceptibility. This is further suggested by the fact that patients who develop proteinuria with penicillamine are more likely to do so with gold, and vice versa (Halla *et al.* 1982; Smith *et al.* 1982). Though it has been suggested that when pro-

teinuria is induced by penicillamine given after gold this may be due to mobilization of gold from tissue deposits by the penicillamine (Dodd *et al.* 1980), it could also be argued that it is more likely to be due to genetic susceptibility.

The incidence of proteinuria in patients being treated with gold for rheumatoid arthritis ranged from 1–7 per cent in the series reviewed by Sellars and Wilkinson (1983). It most commonly starts within the first 6 months of treatment but appears to be unrelated to the daily or cumulative dose. Microscopic haematuria and cylinduria may be present and the proteinuria may progress into the nephrotic range. In such cases, renal biopsy usually reveals a membranous glomerulonephritis (Tornroth and Skrivars 1974; Sellars and Wilkinson 1983; Francis *et al.* 1984). Gold is not found in the subepithelial immune deposits but has been detected in mesangial cells (Francis *et al.* 1984). Far less common is a minimal change lesion (Lee *et al.* 1965; Francis *et al.* 1984). Provided that the proteinuria remains less than about 1 g per day, and the gold is controlling the rheumatoid disease, it may be continued with close monitoring. Should the proteinuria be heavier, or if it is felt appropriate to withdraw the gold for other reasons, proteinuria usually diminishes within about 2 months although, rarely, this can take up to 3 years.

Tubular proteinuria and abnormal tubular function have also been described with gold therapy (Iesato *et al.* 1982), and gold deposits have been demonstrated in proximal tubular cells (Yarom *et al.* 1975). Renal tubular dysfunction can be induced in guinea-pigs by injection of sodium aurothiomalate, resulting in excretion of tubular basement membrane antigen and renal tubular epithelial antigen which is followed by an immune complex nephritis and tubulointerstitial change in the majority of animals (Ueda *et al.* 1986).

The nephrotic syndrome has also been described after oral gold (Atero *et al.* 1986), though it is less common than with the parenteral preparation. Three patients described by Tosi and others (1985), who had severe rheumatoid arthritis, were successfully treated with parenteral gold but developed membranous nephropathy; they were switched to oral gold and proteinuria ameliorated within 2 months.

As already stated, penicillamine can produce a more aggressive immunological mischief in the susceptible kidney. Not only is its use associated with a rapidly progressive nephritis and vasculitis (see above), but the incidence of membranous glomerulonephritis is approximately four times higher than with gold, averaging 12 per cent in four large series (Day and Golding 1974; Camus *et al.* 1976; Weiss *et al.* 1978; Stein *et al.* 1979). In addition to a membranous lesion, which is by far the most common, IgM nephropathy (Rehan and Johnson 1986) and minimal change nephropathy (Savill *et al.* 1988) have been reported. In contrast with gold, the incidence of most of the major adverse reactions with penicillamine increases with the dose (Day and Golding 1974). An important practical point illustrating this is that concurrent treatment with iron interferes with penicillamine absorption, and the sudden withdrawal of iron therapy has been described as precipitating renal toxicity (Harkness and Blake 1982). Proteinuria usually develops within 3–18 months of treatment and, as with gold, usually settles on withdrawal of the drug, usually over 4 to 24 months but it may be persistent (Camus *et al.* 1976).

It should be remembered that, although the majority of patients with rheumatoid arthritis and concomitant membranous glomerulonephritis are being treated with second-line agents, the nephritis is not always related to one of these drugs (Honkanen *et al.* 1987).

As already mentioned, in the animal model mercury induces a polyclonal activation of B cells that is related to the appearance of autoreactive T cells and causes a nephritis (Pelletier *et al.* 1987). In black Africans living in South Africa a nephrotic syndrome, which renal biopsy shows to be due to a membranous glomerulonephritis, secondary to the use of skin-lightening creams containing mercury, has been well-recognized for many years, although it was not reported in this country until 1987 (Oliveira *et al.* 1987). It has also been described as a hazard in dentistry (Smart 1985).

Other drugs that have caused a membranous glomerulonephritis include tiopronin (thiola, α-mercaptoproprionylglycine) used for the treatment of cystinuria; there may be an association here with the HLA-DR3 antigen (Salvarani *et al.* 1985).

A membranous glomerulonephritis has been described with the use of ketoprofen (Sennesael *et al.* 1986), but this is an unusual complication of an NSAID. A nephrotic syndrome on the other hand is a well-recognized complication of NSAID therapy, when it is usually due to minimal change glomerulonephritis in association with an interstitial infiltrate.

Minimal change glomerulonephritis is probably a T cell-mediated disease (Glassock *et al.* 1986); the mechanism whereby NSAID cause this is unknown. Withdrawal of the drug usually results in remission, though the lesion has progressed to focal glomerulosclerosis despite stopping the drug (e.g., fenoprofen — Artinano *et al.* 1986). The combination of interstitial nephritis and minimal change nephropathy has also been reported with some antibiotics (Baum *et al.* 1986).

Other drugs that have been associated with minimal change glomerulonephritis include captopril (Bailey and Lynn 1987), lithium (Richman *et al.* 1980; Wood *et al.* 1989), practolol (Farr *et al.* 1975), and probenecid (Hertz *et al.* 1972); lithium may also cause a focal segmental glomerulosclerosis (Santella *et al.* 1988) and aggravate proteinuria in diabetics (Pawel *et al.* 1989), but it is far better known for its adverse effect on tubular function discussed earlier in this chapter.

Diffuse and segmental glomerulosclerosis may be caused by intravenous abuse of heroin, pentazocine, or pyribenzamine (May *et al.* 1986). The nephrotic syndrome has also developed after treatment with interferon (Selby *et al.* 1985), mesalazine (5-aminosalicylic acid) (Novis *et al.* 1988), phenytoin (Orlandini and Garini 1989), and quinidine (Chisholm 1985).

Lupus nephritis

The earliest report of what may have been a drug-induced lupus-related syndrome appeared in 1945 (Hoffman 1945); subsequently hydralazine was implicated in 1953 (Morrow *et al.* 1953) and procainamide in 1962 (Ladd 1962). The number of drugs that have now been associated with either clinical lupus or serological abnormalities has increased to over 50 (Solinger 1988) and it is estimated that, in the United States, the disease is drug-related in about 10 per cent of the 500 000 patients suffering from systemic lupus erythematosus (Hess 1988). We shall confine this discussion to those drugs for which there is definite proof of the association and refer readers to Chapter 16 and the review on drug-related lupus by Solinger (1988) for details of the more tenuous associations. The drugs most commonly associated with lupus in clinical practice are chlorpromazine, hydralazine, and procainamide. The clinical syndrome may be indistinguishable from idiopathic lupus, although the usual age and sex criteria do not apply and renal involvement is said to be less common, though it most certainly does occur (Alarcón-Segovia *et al.* 1967). Renal and central nervous system involvement is distinctly uncommon as are the typical malar rash and the other skin manifestations. Fever, arthralgia, pleurisy, and pericarditis commonly occur (Hess 1988). The syndrome usually remits rapidly on withdrawal of the drug.

Genetic factors, which have been most extensively studied with hydralazine, play an important role in susceptibility to drug-related lupus. The syndrome is virtually confined to slow acetylators (Lunde *et al.* 1977), has a significant association with HLA-DR4 (Batchelor *et al.* 1980) and, like idiopathic lupus, is commoner in females, and is rare in blacks and carriers of C4 null alleles (Speirs *et al.* 1989).

Crystalluria, renal calculi, and calcium nephropathy

Nephrocalcinosis, stone formation, and hypercalcaemia are well known complications of pharmacological doses of vitamin D and its analogues. Even in normal doses vitamin D may produce nephrocalcinosis and renal failure in children who are excessively sensitive to the vitamin (Seelig 1969).

In some cases vitamin D is used as treatment for conditions in which its value is doubtful. Schwartzman and Franck in 1987 reported four patients with osteoporosis or osteomalacia who became hypercalcaemic and developed acute renal failure as a result of hypervitaminosis D; although the vitamin is indicated in many forms of osteomalacia, it has yet to be shown conclusively that it is of value in the treatment of osteoporosis. Other situations in which the use of vitamin D can be seriously questioned have resulted in renal failure; for example Todd and others (1987) reported a case of renal failure due to vitamin D used for the treatment of chilblains, and self-medication with preparations containing vitamin D and its analogues may be an important contributory cause of stone formation in the general population (Taylor 1972). Patients with impaired renal function and the elderly appear particularly at risk.

Other drugs that may cause hypercalcaemia and thus renal failure when taken in excess include vitamin A (Katz and Tzagournis 1972; Frame *et al.* 1974) and antacids taken with or without milk (Cameron and Spence 1967; Malone and Horn 1971). Thiazide diuretics, by reducing urinary calcium excretion, may also aggravate the hypercalcaemic effect of antacids (Hakim *et al.* 1979). Hypercalciuria can also be due to total parenteral nutrition (Adelman *et al.* 1977) or even the excipient contained in some tablets (Prati *et al.* 1972).

Nephrocalcinosis and calcium phosphate stone formation may also occur when urinary citrate excretion is reduced, as is the case with acetazolamide, which can cause a renal tubular acidosis (Persky *et al.* 1956; Parfitt 1969; Pepys 1970), and with other carbonic anhydrase inhibitors used to treat glaucoma, such as methazolamide (Shields and Simmons 1976).

Acute hyperphosphataemia from tumour lysis can produce nephrocalcinosis in the face of a normal serum calcium; anuria has occurred in patients with lymphosarcoma (Kanfer *et al.* 1979) and Burkitt's lymphoma (Monballyu *et al.* 1984). There are obvious parallels with hyperuricaemic acute renal failure in the treatment of conditions in which there is lysis of tumour mass and deposition of uric acid crystals in renal tubules, pelvis, and ureters (Lear and Oppenheimer 1950; Kravitz and Craver 1951; Greenbaum and Hope-Stone 1959; Kritzler 1958; Mitchell *et al.*. 1965; Maher *et al.* 1969); this should be largely preventable by pretreatment with allopurinol, a high fluid intake to promote diuresis, and alkalinization of the urine. Allopurinol, by inhibiting xanthine oxidase, blocks the transformation of xanthine to uric acid. Xanthine and hypoxanthine, though far more readily soluble than uric acid, may supersaturate the urine and, rarely, result in a xanthine nephropathy (Band *et al.* 1970) and acute renal failure (Ablin *et al.* 1972). When allopurinol has been used in conditions of chronic high production of urate, as in the Lesch–Nyhan syndrome, xanthine stones have occasionally been reported (Landgrebe *et al.* 1975).

Plasma urate levels also rise during weight reduction, and urate nephropathy can be precipitated by sudden reversion to a normal diet or by the inadvertent use of uricosuric agents (Zürcher *et al.* 1977).

Uric acid calculi are common in gout and may be precipitated by the use of uricosuric agents (Gutman and Yu 1968). Suprofen, an NSAID, deserves special mention as a noteworthy example of the value of spontaneous reporting of adverse drug reactions by physicians (Rossi *et al.* 1988). This drug was, within 6 months of marketing, clearly recognized as responsible for a flank-pain syndrome, usually associated with renal failure and haematuria that was reversible and probably due to intratubular precipitation of uric acid crystals with tubular obstruction (Wolfe 1987; Strom *et al.* 1989). Its uricosuric effects appeared no greater than those of other NSAID, yet the syndrome occurred in patients who did not have hyperuricaemia. The drug was similar structurally to ticrynafen, a diuretic that had also been reported to cause acute renal failure due to urate deposition in the kidney, though in those cases ticrynafen had been substituted for a thiazide and thus the patients were 'primed' to a certain extent, as they already had volume contraction and hyperuricaemia (Selby 1979). Phenylbutazone, before it was withdrawn, was also implicated in causing anuria by precipitating uric acid stones or crystals (Weisman and Bloom 1955).

Urinary oxalate excretion is increased by ingestion of large doses of vitamin C, possibly taken as a result of reports in the popular press that in such doses it can cure colds and cancer.

Acute renal failure due to crystallization of drugs in the kidney was a well-recognized complication of use of the sulphonamides in the 1930s, and sulphadiazine was the compound most frequently implicated, probably because it was the one most commonly used to treat infections before the advent of penicillin (Bull *et al.* 1958). In recent years, the use of sulfadiazine has increased, primarily to treat toxoplasmosis in patients with AIDS; two reports have highlighted the fact that it may still cause acute renal failure, though this can largely be prevented by maintaining an alkaline diuresis of at least 2 litres a day during treatment (Sahai *et al.* 1988; Christin *et al.* 1990).

Acyclovir may cause renal failure from crystalluria and obstructive nephropathy. Four patients with a chronic fatigue syndrome, described by Sawyer and others (1988), developed five episodes of acute renal failure when acyclovir was administered intravenously in high doses, despite precautions to avoid volume contraction. Three patients had birefringent needle-like crystals within leucocytes on urine microscopy; one patient underwent percutaneous renal biopsy revealing foci of interstitial inflammation. Acyclovir was subsequently given orally in all four patients with no demonstrable adverse effect on renal function. Provided the infusion is given over one hour and the patient is kept well hydrated, serious nephrotoxicity is unlikely to occur (Laskin 1984). Low-dose acyclovir, however, has also been reported as a cause of acute renal failure without recovery of function but, as no biopsy was performed, another cause cannot be ruled out; and if, indeed, the

acyclovir was to blame, another pathogenetic mechanism, possibly immunological or idiosyncratic, must be invoked (Giustina *et al.* 1988). In 2 patients (out of 23 given acyclovir) who developed a mild rise in blood urea, renal function improved in both with extra fluid administration, despite completing the course of acyclovir (Selby *et al.* 1979).

Other drugs causing crystalluria, dealt with more fully in the third edition of this book, include sulphonamides, acetazolamide (Glushien and Fisher 1956), mercaptopurine (Duttera *et al.* 1972), and high-dose methotrexate with citrovorum factor (Frei *et al.* 1975). Crystals of dihydroxyadenine have been found in the kidneys of patients dying after massive transfusion of stored blood; they were presumably derived from the acid–citrate–dextrose anticoagulant in banked blood (Falk *et al.* 1972). Triamterene can also crystallize out in urine and form stones (Dooley *et al.* 1989). A list of drugs associated with urinary crystals is given in table 12.6.

Papillary necrosis and chronic interstitial nephritis (analgesic nephropathy)

History

This subject was reviewed extensively by Winearls and Kerr (1985) in the third edition of this book. Analgesic nephropathy has been recognized as a clinical problem for the last three decades. One of the earliest references to potential dependence on analgesics, cited by Kincaid-Smith in a review of the subject (Kincaid-Smith 1988), is from a Sidney-based magazine called *The Lone Hand*, which in 1907 observed, 'What alcohol is for men in Australia the headache powder is for women'. It was not until 1953, however, when Spuhler and Zollinger described an association between chronic interstitial nephritis and heavy consumption of analgesics, notably of Saridone, which contained phenacetin, isopropyl antipyrine, and caffeine, that such an association was recognized.

Over the following 10 years, the incidence of renal papillary necrosis and chronic interstitial nephritis rose, in some countries at an alarming rate. For example, Gloor (1978) reported from Switzerland an increase in the autopsy rate of papillary necrosis from 2.7 per cent between 1938 and 1942 to 57 per cent between 1958 and 1962. A clinical picture was also forming: papillary necrosis was predominantly occurring in women who had consumed analgesic mixtures, whereas previously it had been an uncommon condition usually found in diabetics or patients with urinary obstruction. In most

TABLE 12.6
Drugs associated with crystalluria

Urate crystals

Cytotoxic drugs
Phenylbutazone
Probenecid
Salicylates
Zoxazolamine

Oxalate crystals

Ascorbic acid
Methoxyflurane
Warfarin

Drug crystals

Acyclovir
Dihydroxyadenine
Mercaptopurine
Sulphonamides
Triamterene

Other crystals

Magnesium trisilicate
Vitamin D

---

cases the mixtures were taken not for their analgesic properties but for their stimulant effects (both caffeine and phenacetin have mood-elevating properties), although in some instances they were used for accepted indications, such as rheumatoid arthritis (Moeschlin 1957; Rossi and Muhlethaler 1958; Larsen and Møller 1959; Lindeneg *et al.* 1959; Lindvall 1960; Clausen and Pedersen 1961; Hultengren 1961; Nordenfelt and Ringertz 1961; Bengtsson 1962; Harvald 1968). An exception to the female preponderance was found at Jønkøping (Nordenfelt and Ringertz 1961), where most of the patients were male. The anomaly was traced to the high consumption of Hjorton's powders by male workers at the small-arms factory at Huskvarna, in the belief that they improved work output.

For some time after the condition was first described, in many renal units throughout the world there was a certain amount of scepticism about its existence, but then the reported incidence naturally rose as it became generally recognized as a cause of chronic renal failure. It became clear that the prevalence varied markedly from country to country, and that within countries there was a marked geographical variation (Table 12.7); the reasons for this include the availability of the offending analgesic mixtures, the interest of the local renal unit in the condition, and under-reporting in some areas. Under-diagnosis is compounded by patients often concealing or grossly underestimating their intake of analgesics. It has also been suggested that the geographical variation is to some extent due to climate and dehydration. Bukalew and Schey (1986), by culling the literature on analgesic abuse and renal disease, demonstrated a highly significant linear relationship between the prevalence of nephropathy, when defined as an elevation

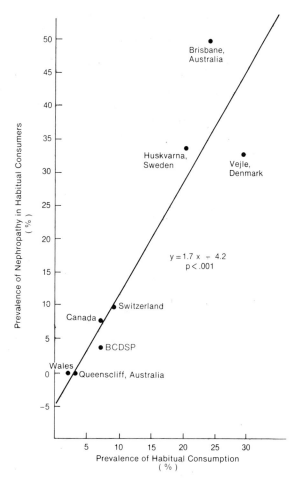

Fig. 12.1
The prevalence of analgesic nephropathy in habitual analgesic consumers against the prevalence of analgesic consumption in that population. BCDSP = Boston Cooperative Drug Surveillance Program. (Reproduced with permission from Buckalew, V.M., and Schey, H.M., Renal disease from habitual antipyretic analgesic consumption; an assessment of the epidemiologic evidence. *Medicine* **65**, 291. © Williams and Wilkins, 1986.)

with the highest prevalence of regular consumers in a manner analogous to alcohol-induced disease.

Causes

Phenacetin

The villain of the piece is commonly thought to be phenacetin, though it is not the only culprit. The epidemiological data in general, however, strongly implicate it. Nearly all patients reported up to 1975 had consumed mixtures that contained phenacetin. There has been a distinct fall in the incidence of analgesic nephropathy in

TABLE 12.7
Prevalence of analgesic nephropathy among patients with end-stage renal failure in different parts of the world

USA (overall) 1984	2%	NIH Consensus Conference
(North Carolina)	10%	Buckalew and Schey 1986
Federal Rep. of Germany	16.8%	Pommer *et al.* 1989
Australia	12%	Disney 1989
United Kingdom	1%	Wing *et al.* 1989
South Africa	9%	DuToit *et al.* 1988

in serum creatinine, in daily consumers of antipyretic analgesics and the prevalence of habitual consumption in the population from which the habitual consumers were derived (Fig. 12.1). This probably reflects an increase in the number of heavy consumers in those populations

Sweden (Bengtsson 1967; Nordenfelt 1972), Scotland (Murray 1972), Finland (Kasanen 1973), and Denmark (Mabeck and Wichmann 1979), occurring 3–8 years after sales of phenacetin were restricted by legislation or withdrawal from popular proprietaries. In Finland (Silanpaa *et al.* 1982) in the 1950s the total mortality from renal disease rose from about 500 to 1200 patients per year; the prevalence of papillary necrosis among medical patients at autopsy in a teaching hospital peaked at 30 per cent. Following the banning of phenacetin in 1965, both figures have fallen steadily back to their prewar level. In patients with end-stage renal failure in Michigan who were diagnosed between 1976 and 1984, the risk of end-stage renal failure was significantly related to phenacetin or paracetamol consumption (Steenland *et al.* 1990). In Australia, where the reported incidence was once the highest in the world, phenacetin was removed from one of the most popular over-the-counter compound analgesics in 1976, and analgesic legislation came into force in 1979. Although it has taken a long time, cases of analgesic nephropathy are now uncommon in Australian hospital wards, at least in Victoria, and there is a steady decline in the numbers of patients with analgesic nephropathy presenting for chronic dialysis (Kincaid Smith 1988). Though the global incidence is falling, it still remains an important cause of end-stage renal failure in many countries.

Other substances that have been implicated in the pathogenesis of analgesic nephropathy include *p*-chloracetanilide, a trace contaminant of commercial preparations of phenacetin (Harvald *et al.* 1960; Schnitzer and Smith 1966); the major metabolite of phenacetin, paracetamol (acetaminophen); and aspirin. In addition, renal papillary necrosis can develop from the use of the NSAID such as benoxaprofen (Erwin and Boulton-Jones 1982).

Paracetamol

Paracetamol is now the commonest ingredient of most compound analgesics and is also commonly used on its own for pain relief. It is concentrated in the renal papilla (Duggin and Mudge 1974) and is clearly a cause of acute tubular necrosis, both in acute poisoning, where it can occur without hepatic failure (Cobden *et al.* 1982; Dabbagh and Chesney 1985; Pillans and Hall 1985; Davenport and Finn 1988), and after therapeutic doses in a few individuals (Gabriel *et al.* 1982); alcoholics appear particularly vulnerable (Kaysen *et al.* 1985; Keaton 1988). Evidence for its being a cause of analgesic nephropathy is, however, tenuous. Very high doses of paracetamol can produce papillary necrosis in rats (Molland 1978); but in a study of 18 patients receiving high doses of

paracetamol, Edwards and colleagues (1971) found no significant damage after ingestion of 2–30 kg.

Furthermore, in only two cases published prior to 1980 was it considered to be the only culprit (Krikler 1967; Masters 1973). Nevertheless, in a retrospective study of dialysis patients and those who had undergone transplantation, Segasothy and others (1988) described five patients with papillary necrosis that they attributed to the consumption of paracetamol alone; these add to the 10 cases reported earlier by the same group (Segasothy *et al.* 1984, 1986).

Aspirin

Papillary necrosis can be caused experimentally in rats and rabbits by doses of aspirin equivalent to, or less than, the dosage of phenacetin that causes this disease (Clausen 1964; Nanra and Kincaid-Smith 1970). Rats have a particularly precarious blood supply to their renal papillae, however, and may not be the best model of human disease.

In humans, overdosage has been associated with acute renal failure (Campbell and Maclaurin 1958), and in lower dosage there is urinary wastage of proximal tubular cells (Kennedy and Saluga 1970), the excretion of which diminishes with continuation of the drug (Burry *et al.* 1976); the significance of this is unclear but it is unlikely to be related to the development of papillary necrosis. Papillary necrosis and analgesic nephropathy have occurred, however, in patients taking only aspirin.

Aspirin has been blamed by many for the high incidence of chronic interstitial nephritis in patients with rheumatoid arthritis. Prescott (1982) reported 151 cases of papillary necrosis in patients taking aspirin alone (88 cases) or combined with NSAID (63 cases). Conversely, there is considerable evidence for the lack of nephrotoxicity from aspirin given in therapeutic doses over many years. Studies of large numbers of patients (more than 1000) taking aspirin for rheumatoid arthritis have failed to find a single case of analgesic nephropathy (New Zealand Rheumatism Association 1974; Emkey and Mills 1982); and studies of smaller numbers but with heavier aspirin consumption, such as that by Akyol and colleagues (1982), could find no evidence of renal damage (including tests for concentrating defects) in 16 patients who had taken between 5–37 kg of aspirin over a long period for rheumatoid arthritis. These data are in accord with several other prospective studies that have failed to show any correlation between renal function and aspirin ingestion (Burry 1972; Burry *et al.* 1976; Wigley 1976; Emkey and Mills 1982). More recently Sandler and others (1989) could find no increased risk in in daily users of aspirin whereas there was with paracetamol. The debate still rages.

Many compound analgesics contain caffeine (e.g. Solpadeine tablets in the United Kingdom, Grand Pa powders in South Africa, Bex's and Vincent's in Australia). Caffeine promotes a diuresis and this could lead to subclinical dehydration and concentration of the other analgesics in the renal medulla. Headache, lasting 2–3 days, occurs when caffeine is withdrawn from coffee drinkers (mean caffeine intake 435 mg per day) (Dusseldorp and Katan 1990). Caffeine therefore probably contributes to the habit-forming properties of analgesic mixtures by causing withdrawal headache that is relieved by further doses.

In summary: though individual ingredients may be nephrotoxic, the combination of aspirin, phenacetin, and caffeine is particularly dangerous. It should also be stressed that prolonged abuse is required to produce renal failure; though minor defects in renal function, such as defects in concentrating ability, can be detected after a relatively small cumulative dose (<1 kg) it usually takes 2–3 kg of analgesic before clinically detectable renal disease occurs (Nanra et al. 1978). In six reports from around the world, summarized by Gault and others (1968), the average intake of phenacetin in patients with analgesic nephropathy varied from 6 to over 10 kg taken over 11–12 years.

Pathology

This has been reviewed by Gloor (1965, 1974, 1978) and by Nanra and others (1978). The earliest pathological changes are confined to the inner medulla and papillary tips. As the disease advances with continued use of analgesics, the ischaemia extends outwards to involve more of the medulla, and papillae become necrotic and detach. Patchy cortical changes occur initially overlying the necrotic papillae. Microscopically there is atrophy with a patchy interstitial infiltrate, tubular fall-out, and periglomerular fibrosis. Some glomeruli show varying degrees of sclerosis, while others are normal or show compensatory hypertrophy. A heavy deposition of golden-brown granules is a near-constant finding in the cells of the loops of Henle and collecting ducts. Brownish discolouration can also be seen around the ureteric orifices in the bladder at cystoscopy. Of particular interest are characteristic changes in blood vessels: arterial changes are frequently those of benign nephrosclerosis but capillaries, arterioles, and venules are strikingly thickened and stain heavily with periodic acid–Schiff and fat stains. The lumina are often completely obliterated. Such microangiopathy in the bladder is virtually pathognomonic of the condition (Mihatsch et al. 1983) but is found in only a minority of patients. Similar vessel changes have also been described in the skin of some patients (Abrahams et al. 1978).

Clinical feature

The clinical syndrome is usually characteristic and has been described by many authors, including Hultengren (1961), Bengtsson (1962), Duggan (1974), and Cove-Smith and Knapp (1978). It is predominantly a disease of females, presenting in their fourth or fifth decade. The patient is frequently asthenic, looks older than her years, and is neurotic and prone to other addictive pastimes, such as smoking and alcohol and purgative abuse. Analgesic use is often denied or minimized, so a history from other family members is often rewarding. Other features include anaemia disproportionate to the degree of renal failure. Factors contributing to this include occult gastrointestinal blood loss (there is a very high incidence of gastritis and peptic ulceration with mixtures containing aspirin) and haemolysis, reported with phenacetin (Moeschlin 1957). The latter may account for the splenomegaly that is occasionally present (Duggan 1974) and the increased incidence of gallstones (Maisel and Priest 1964; Bell et al. 1969). Other features of the clinical syndrome include symptoms of headache, dysmenorrhoea, and dyspepsia; accelerated atherosclerosis with all its attendant complications; often, increased skin pigmentation; and an increased incidence of urinary tract infection and urothelial malignancy.

Diagnosis

The diagnosis is dependent on obtaining a history of prolonged analgesic intake and is suspected from the clinical features mentioned above. Where suspicion is high but consumption is denied, measuring urinary salicylate levels or metabolites of other drugs may be helpful. The urine also often contains white cells without infection, protein, or blood. The characteristic radiographic features were reviewed by Lindvall (1978). Diagnostic features of renal papillary necrosis can be seen on intravenous urography, computerized tomographic scanning, and ultrasound appearances, the early findings may be highly variable, but as papillary necrosis appears distinctive radiological changes develop (Hartman et al. 1984). As already mentioned, typical features on bladder biopsy are diagnostic but inconsistent.

Prognosis and treatment

Analgesic nephropathy could be virtually abolished by

banning over-the-counter sales of analgesic mixtures. In patients with mild and moderate renal insufficiency, function usually stabilizes or improves if the patient can be persuaded to stop taking analgesics (Kincaid-Smith *et al.* 1971; Steele and Edwards 1971; Wilson 1972). Even when renal failure is advanced, stopping taking analgesics slows the rate of progression of renal failure, although Cove-Smith and Knapp (1978) suggest that patients with a plasma creatinine of above 400 μmol per litre usually progress to end-stage renal failure. Morbidity and mortality from other conditions related to the analgesic syndrome, such as ischaemic heart disease, are commoner than in other patients with other causes for renal failure; this is also the case in patients who are on dialysis (Schwarz *et al.* 1984; Balle and Schollmeyer 1990). Following transplantation, the graft may be lost from relapse to the addiction (Furman *et al.* 1976); there may also be a higher incidence of post-transplant malignant disease in this group (Hauser *et al.* 1990).

Management of such patients should include regular follow-up to ensure abstention from analgesics and NSAID, good control of hypertension, prompt treatment of urinary tract infection or obstruction, regular urinary tract imaging for evidence of progression of disease, and urine cytology in view of the increased incidence of urothelial malignancy in these patients. It is also beneficial to encourage a high fluid intake and to avoid dehydration.

Other urological complications of analgesic abuse

Carcinoma of the renal pelvis in association with analgesic nephropathy was initially noted by Hultengren (1961). It subsequently became clear that this was more than a chance association, and the incidence of carcinoma of the pelvis in patients with analgesic nephropathy has been reported as 1.5 per cent per annum (Bengtsson *et al.* 1968). Although carcinoma of the bladder has also been reported (Handa and Tewari 1981; Mihatsch and Knusli 1982), it is far less common than carcinoma of the renal pelvis; this and the close anatomical relationship between the tumours and necrotic papillae suggest that the latter may play a role in pathogenesis of the malignancy.

Ureteric strictures, typically in the region of the pelvic brim, also complicate analgesic nephropathy (Lindvall 1960; Hultengren 1961). Other renal complications such as acute interstitial nephritis and functional renal failure are mentioned under the relevant headings earlier in the chapter.

Miscellaneous

Haematuria

Urine dipsticks are very sensitive to blood; occasionally antiseptics used for the cleaning of urine receptacles may contaminate the urine to produce a false result. It is always essential therefore to examine the urine microscopically for red cells; this is also valuable in haemoglobinuria and myoglobinuria (mentioned above under rhabdomyolysis), in which the dipstick may record a large amount of blood with few or no red cells in the urine. Urine microscopy can also help to determine whether the source of the red cells is the glomerulus or the lower urinary tract; this can be done using fresh urine and an ordinary microscope, but is easier with a phase-contrast instrument (Fairley and Birch 1982).

Drugs that interfere with coagulation may cause haematuria. In addition, long-term anticoagulant therapy can cause gross haematuria with clot colic and, rarely, acute renal failure (Nade 1972; Rosen 1972). Bleeding into the retroperitoneal tissues may also obstruct the ureters (Kaden and Friedman 1961). It has also been suggested that warfarin may interfere with the structure of a urinary glycoprotein that normally inhibits crystallization of calcium oxalate, thus leading to an increased propensity for patients being treated with warfarin to form microscopic stones which can irritate the collecting system and cause haematuria (Fowler and Boyarsky 1986).

Cyclophosphamide may cause a haemorrhagic cystitis (Droller *et al.* 1982); characteristic changes are found on bladder biopsy. More sinister is the development of bladder cancer or of a leiomyosarcoma (Rowland and Elbe 1983). Haemorrhagic cystitis can be prevented by ensuring a good diuresis and by the use of mesna, which is excreted in the urine and reacts with acrolein and other metabolites of cyclophosphamide that are responsible for the urotoxic effects in the urine.

Drugs causing incontinence of urine

Drugs interfering with the normal α-adrenergic stimulation of the proximal urethra may cause incontinence (Kiruluta and Andrews 1983); this may be seen in patients treated with haloperidol, chlorpromazine, or thiohexane. The antihypertensives methyldopa (Raz 1974) and prazosin (Thien *et al.* 1978) have also been implicated.

Drugs affecting tests of renal function

The inhibition of tubular secretion of creatinine may

cause a rise in serum creatinine without a change in GFR, this has been described with trimethoprim (Berglund et al. 1975) and cimetidine (Larsson et al. 1980). As previously mentioned, both drugs can also cause interstitial nephritis.

References

Ablin, A., Stephens, B.G., Hirata, T., Wilson, K., and Williams, H.E. (1972). Nephropathy, xanthinuria and orotic aciduria complicating Burkitt's lymphoma treated with chemotherapy and allopurinol. *Metabolism* 21, 771.

Abrahams, C., Furman, K.I., and Salant, D. (1978). Dermal micro-angiopathy in patients with analgesic nephropathy. *S. Afr. Med. J.* 54, 393.

Adelman, R.D., Abern, S.B., Merten, D., and Halsted, C.H. (1977). Hypercalciuria with nephrolithiasis: a complication of total parenteral nutrition. *Pediatrics* 59, 473.

Adu, D., Turney, J., Michael, J., and McMaster, P. (1983). Hyperkalaemia in cyclosporin-treated renal allograft recipients. *Lancet* ii, 370.

Ahijado, F., Garcia de Vinuesa, S., and Luño, J. (1990). Acute renal failure and rhabdomyolysis following cocaine abuse. *Nephron* 54, 268.

Akmal, M., Valdin, J.R., McCarron, M.M., and Massry, S.G. (1981). Rhabdomyolysis with and without acute renal failure in patients with phencyclidine intoxication. *Am. J. Nephrol.* 1, 91.

Akyol, S.M., Thompson, M., and Kerr, D.N.S. (1982). Renal function after prolonged consumption of aspirin. *Br. Med. J.* 284, 631.

Alarcón-Segovia, D., Wakim, K.G., Worthington, J.W., and Ward, L.E. (1967). Clinical and experimental studies on the hydralazine syndrome and its relationship to systemic lupus erythematosus. *Medicine* (Baltimore), 46, 1.

Alexander, F. and Martin, J. (1981). Nephrotic syndrome associated with lithium therapy. *Clin. Nephrol.* 15, 267.

Ali, A., Barnes, J.N., Davison, A.J.W., Mostafid, E.H., and Sivathondan, Y. (1990). Proteinuria and thrombolytic agents. *Lancet* i, 106.

Allaouchiche, B., Mercatello, A., Tognet, E., Négrier, S., Moskovtchenko, J.F., Franks, C.R., et al. (1990). Prospective effect of norepinephrine infusion in acute renal insufficiency induced by interleukin 2 therapy. *Nephron* 55, 438.

Anand, V., Siami, G., and Stone, W.J. (1989). Cocaine-associated rhabdomyolysis and acute renal failure. *South. Med. J.* 82, 67.

Andrews, P.M. and Bates, S.B. (1987). Dietary protein as a risk factor in gentamicin nephrotoxicity. *Renal Failure* 10, 153.

Andrieu, J., Andebrand, C., Chassaigne, M., and Renier, E. (1976). Anémie hémolytique et insuffisance rénale imputables à la glafénine. *Nouv. Presse Med.* 5, 2394.

Antman, K.H., Parker, L.M., Goldstein, J.D., Skarin, A.T., and D'Orsi, C.J. (1982). Acute renal failure following intravenous pyelography (IVP) in a patient with diffuse hyper-

gammaglobulinemia: a case report. *Med. Pediatr. Oncol.* 10, 289.

Anto H.R., Chou, S.Y., Porush, J.G., and Shapiro, W.B. (1981). Infusion intravenous pyelography and renal function. Effect of hypertonic mannitol in patients with chronic renal insufficiency. *Arch. Intern. Med.* 141, 1652.

Appel, G.B. (1990). Aminoglycoside nephrotoxicity. *Am. J. Med.* 88, 16S.

Appel, G.B., Woda, B.A., Neu, H.C., Parry, M.F., Silva, F., and Pirani, C.L. (1978). Acute interstitial nephritis associated with carbenicillin therapy. *Arch. Intern. Med.* 138, 1265.

Argent, N. and Adams, P.C. (1990). Proteinuria and thrombolytic agents. *Lancet* i, 106.

Arning, M. and Scharf, R.E. (1989). Prevention of amphotericin B-induced nephrotoxicity by loading with sodium chloride: a report of 1291 days of treatment with amphotericin B without renal failure. *Klin. Wochenschr.* 67, 1020.

Artinano, M., Etheridge, W.B., Stroehlein, K.B., and Barcenas, C.G. (1986). Progression of minimal-change glomerulopathy to focal glomerulosclerosis in a patient with fenoprofen nephropathy. *Am. J. Nephrol.* 6, 353.

Atero, F., Rodriguez-Franco, R., Paramo, M.J., Baturone, M., Junquera, E., Esparrago, J., et al. (1986). Nephrotic syndrome after oral gold. *Br. J. Rheumatol.* 25, 315.

Aurell, M., Svalander, C., Wallin, L., and Alling, C. (1981). Renal function and biopsy findings in patients on long-term lithium treatment. *Kidney. Int.* 20, 663.

Austin, H.A., Palestine, A.G., Sabnis, S.G., Balow, J.E., Preuss, H.G., Nussenblatt, R.B., and Antonovych, T.T. (1989). Evolution of ciclosporin nephrotoxicity in patients treated for autoimmune uveitis. *Am. J. Nephrol.* 9, 392.

Avent, C.K., Krinsky, D., Kirklin, J.K., Bourge, R.C., and Figg, W.D. (1988). Synergistic nephrotoxicity due to ciprofloxacin and cyclosporine. *Am. J. Med.* 85, 452.

Averbuch, S.D., Austin, H.A. 3rd, Sherwin, S.A., Antonovych, T., Bun, P.A. Jr, and Longo, D.L. (1984). Acute interstitial nephritis with the nephrotic syndrome following recombinant leukocyte α-interferon therapy for mycosis fungoides. *N. Engl. J. Med.* 310, 32.

Axton, J.H.M. (1972). Six cases of poisoning after a parenteral organic mercurial compound (Merthiolate). *Postgrad. Med. J.* 48, 417.

Aynedjian, H.S., Nguyen, D., Lee, H.Y., Sablay, L.B., and Bank, N. (1988). Effects of dietary electrolyte supplementation on gentamicin nephrotoxicity. *Am. J. Med. Sci.* 295, 444.

Bailey, R.R. and Lynn, K.L. (1986). Crescentic glomerulonephritis developing in a patient taking enalapril. *N.Z. Med. J.* 99, 959.

Bailey, R.R. and Lynn, K.L. (1987). Steroid-responsive nephrotic syndrome due to minimal change nephropathy occurring while on captopril. *N.Z. Med. J.* 100, 187.

Baliah, T., MacLeish, H., and Drummond, K.N. (1969). Acute boric acid poisoning: report of an infant successfully treated by peritoneal dialysis. *Can. Med. Assoc. J.* 101, 166.

Balle, C. and Schollmeyer, P. (1990). Morbidity of patients with analgesic-associated nephropathy on regular dialysis treatment and after renal transplantation. *Klin. Wochenschr.* 68, 38.

Baltzer, V.G., Jacob, H., Esselborn, H., and Gassel, W.D. (1978). Uber den Einfluß jodhaltiger Konstrastmittel auf die Nierenfunktion bei Patienten mit multiplem Myelom. Eine retrospektive Studie. *Fortschr. Rontgenstr.* 129, 208.

Band, P.R., Silverberg, D.S., Henderson, J.F., Ulan, R.A., Wensel, R.H., Banjeree, T.K., *et al.* (1970). Xanthine nephropathy in a patient with lymphosarcoma treated with allopurinol. *N. Engl. J. Med.* 283, 354.

Barros, E.J., Boim, M.A., Ajzen, H., Ramos, O.L., and Schor, N. (1987). Glomerular hemodynamics and hormonal participation in cyclosporine nephrotoxicity. *Kidney Int.* 32, 19.

Batchelor, J.R., Welsh, K.I., Tinoco, R.M., Dollery, C.T., Hughes , G.R.V., Berstein, R., *et al.* (1980). Hydralazine-induced systemic lupus erythematosus: influence of HLA-DR and sex on susceptibility. *Lancet* i, 1107.

Baum, M., Piel, C.F., and Goodman, J.R. (1986). Antibiotic-associated interstitial nephritis and nephrotic syndrome. *Am. J. Nephrol.* 6, 149.

Baxter, C.R., Duggin, G.G., Hall, B.M., Horvarth, J.S., and Tiller, D.J. (1984). Stimulation of renin release from rat cortical slices by cyclosporin A. *Res. Commun. Chem. Pathol. Pharmacol.* 43, 417.

Bear, R.A., Sugar, L., and Paul, M. (1985). Nephrotic syndrome and renal failure secondary to lithium carbonate therapy. *Can. Med. Assoc. J.* 132, 735.

Beauchamp, D. and Pettigrew, M. (1988). Influence of hydrocortisone on gentamicin-induced nephrotoxicity in rats. *Antimicrob. Agents Chemother.* 32, 992.

Bell, D., Kerr, D.N.S., Swinney, J., and Yeates, W.K. (1969). Analgesic nephropathy. Clinical course after withdrawal of phenacetin. *Br. Med. J.* iii, 378.

Bender, W.L., Whelton, A., Beschorner, W.E., Darwish, M.O., Hall-Craggs, M., and Solez, K. (1984). Interstitial nephritis, proteinuria, and renal failure caused by nonsteroidal anti-inflammatory drugs. Immunologic characterization of the inflammatory infiltrate. *Am. J. Med.* 76, 1006.

Bengtsson, U. (1962). A comparative study of chronic non-obstructive pyelonephritis and renal papillary necrosis. *Acta Med. Scand.* (suppl. 338).

Bengtsson, U. (1967). Analgesic nephropathy — chronic pyelonephritis. In *Proceedings of 3rd International Congress on Nephrology*, Vol. 2. (ed. R.H. Heptinstall), p. 291. Karger, Basel.

Bengtsson, U., Angervall, L., Ekman, H., and Lehmann, L. (1968). Transitional cell tumors of the renal pelvis in analgesic abusers. *Scand. J. Urol. Nephrol.* 2, 145.

Benigni, A., Chiabrando, C., Piccinelli, A., Perico, N., Gavinelli, M., Furci, L., *et al.* (1988).Increased urinary excretion of thromboxane B2 and 2,3-dinor-TxB2 in cyclosporin A nephrotoxicity. *Kidney Int.* 34, 164.

Benitz, K.F. and Diermeier, H.F. (1964). Renal toxicity of tetracycline degradation products. *Proc. Soc. Exp. Biol. Med.* 115, 930.

Bennett, W.M. and Pulliam, J.P. (1983). Cyclosporine nephrotoxicity. *Ann. Intern. Med.* 99, 851.

Bennett, W.M., Hartnett, M.N., Gilbert, D., Houghton, D., and Porter, G.A. (1976). Effect of sodium intake on gentamicin nephrotoxicity in the rat. *Proc. Soc. Exp. Biol. Med.* 151, 736.

Bennett, W.M., Plamp, C., and Porter, G.A. (1977). Drug-related syndromes in clinical nephrology. *Ann. Intern. Med.* 87, 582.

Berglund, F., Killander, J., and Pompeius, R. (1975). Effect of trimethoprim-sulphamethoxazole on the renal excretion of creatinine in man. *J. Urol.* 114, 802.

Bergman, M.M., Glew, R.H., and Ebert, T.H. (1988). Acute interstitial nephritis associated with vancomycin therapy. *Arch. Intern. Med.* 148, 2139.

Bergstrand, A., Collste, L.G., Franksson, C., Glas, J.-E., Löfström, B., Magnusson, G., *et al.* (1972). Oxalosis in renal transplants following methoxyflurane anaesthesia. *Br. J. Anaesth.* 44, 569.

Berlyne, G.M. (1972). Renal involvement in the collagen diseases. In *Renal disease* (3rd edn) (ed. D.A.K. Black), p. 559. Blackwell, Oxford.

Bernis, P., Hamels, J., Quoidbach, A., Mahieu, Ph., and Bouvy, P. (1985). Remission of Goodpasture's syndrome after withdrawal of an unusual toxic. *Clin. Nephrol.* 23, 312.

Bhathena, D.B., Bullock, W.E., Nuttall, C.E., and Luke, R.G. (1978). The effects of amphotericin B therapy on the intrarenal vasculature and renal tubules in man. *Clin. Nephrol.* 9, 103.

Bianchine, J.R. and Freidman, A.P. (1970). Metabolism of methysergide and retroperitoneal fibrosis. *Arch. Intern. Med.* 126, 252.

Bishop, W.B., Carlton, R.F., and Sanders, L.L. (1966). Diffuse vasculitis and death after hyperimmunization with pertussis vaccine. *N. Engl. J. Med.* 274, 616.

Björck, S., Westberg, G., Svalander, C., and Mulec, H. (1983). Rapidly progressive glomerulonephritis after hydralazine. *Lancet* ii, 42.

Björnberg, A. and Gisslen, H. (1965). Thiazides: a cause of necrotising vasculitis? *Lancet* ii, 982.

Blain, P.G., Lane, R.J., Bateman, D.N., and Rawlins, M.D. (1985). Opiate-induced rhabdomyolysis. *Hum. Toxicol.* 4, 71.

Blake, P.G. and Ryan, F. (1989). Rhabdomyolysis and acute renal failure after terbutaline overdose. *Nephron* 53, 76.

Blythe, W.B. (1983). Captopril and renal autoregulation. *N. Engl. J. Med.* 308, 390.

Bonzel, K.E., Muller-Wiefel, D.E., Ruder, H., Wingen, A.M., Waldherr, R., and Weber, M. (1987). Anti-glomerular basement membrane antibody-mediated glomerulonephritis due to glue sniffing. *Eur. J. Pediatr.* 146, 296.

Border, W.A., Lehman, D.H., Egan, J.D., Sass, H.J., Glode, J.E., and Wilson, C.B. (1974). Antitubular basement-membrane antibodies in methicillin-associated interstitial nephritis. *N. Engl. J. Med.* 291, 381.

Bowman, C., Green, C., Borysiewicz, L., and Lockwood, C.M. (1987). Circulating T-cell populations during mercuric chloride-induced nephritis in the Brown Norway rat. *Immunology* 61, 515.

Brezin, J.H., Katz, S.M., Schwartz, A.B., and Chinitz, J.L. (1979). Reversible renal failure and nephrotic syndrome associated with non-steroidal anti-inflammatory drugs. *N. Engl. J. Med.* 301, 1271.

Brown, C.B., Robson, J.S., Thomson, D., Clarkson, A.R., Cameron, J.S., and Ogg, C.S. (1973). Haemolytic uraemic syndrome in women taking oral contraceptives. *Lancet* i, 1479.

Bucht, G. and Wahlin, A. (1980). Renal concentrating capacity in long-term lithium treatment and after withdrawal of lithium. *Acta Med. Scand.* 207, 309.

Bucht, G., Wahlin, A., Wentzel, T., and Winblad, B. (1980). Renal function and morphology in long-term lithium and combined lithium-neuroleptic treatment. *Acta Med. Scand.* 208, 381.

Buckalew, V.M. and Schey, H.M. (1986). Renal disease from habitual antipyretic analgesic consumption: an assessment of the epidemiologic evidence. *Medicine* (Baltimore) 65, 291.

Bull, G.M., Joekes, A.M., and Lowe, K.G. (1958). Acute renal failure due to poisons and drugs. *Lancet* i, 134.

Burry, H.C. (1972). Reduced glomerular function in rheumatoid arthritis. *Ann. Rheum. Dis.* 31, 65.

Burry, H.C., Dieppe, P.A., Bresnihan, F.B., and Brown, C. (1976). Salicylates and renal function in rheumatoid arthritis. *Br. Med. J.* i, 613.

Burton, J.R., Lichtenstein, N.S., Colvin, R.B., and Hyslop, N.E. (1974). Acute interstitial nephritis from oxacillin. *Johns Hopkins Med. J.* 134, 58.

Butler, W.T. (1964). Amphotericin B toxicity: changes in renal function. *Ann. Intern. Med.* 61, 344.

Byrd, L. and Sherman, R.L. (1979). Radiocontrast-induced acute renal failure: a clinical and physiologic review. *Medicine* (Baltimore) 58, 270.

Cabrera, J., Arroyo, V., Ballesta, A., Rimola, A., Gual, J., Elena, M., and Rodes, J. (1982). Aminoglycoside nephrotoxicity in cirrhosis. Value of urinary β_2-microglobulin to discriminate functional renal failure from acute tubular damage. *Gastroenterology* 82, 97.

Cacoub, P., Deray, G., Baumelou, A., and Jacobs, C. (1988). No evidence for protective effects of nifedipine against radiocontrast-induced acute renal failure. *Clin. Nephrol.* 29, 215.

Callan, M.F.C., Davies, K.A.A., Merrin, P.K., and Walport, M.J. (1990). Proteinuria and thrombolytic agents. *Lancet* i, 106.

Cameron, A.J. and Spence, M.P. (1967). Chronic milk–alkali syndrome after prolonged excessive intake of antacid tablets. *Br. Med. J.* iii, 656.

Cameron, J.S. (1988). Allergic interstitial nephritis: Clinical features and pathogenesis. *Q. J. Med.* 66, 97.

Campbell, E.J.M. and Maclaurin, R.E. (1958). Acute renal failure in salicylate poisoning. *Br. Med. J.* i, 503.

Camus, J-P., Crouzet, J., Prier, A., and Leca, A.P. (1976). Complications du traitement de la polyarthrite rheumatoïde par la D-pénicillamine. *Therapie* 31, 385.

Cantwell, B.M.J., Carmichael, J., Mannix, K.A., and Harris, A.L. (1989). Chemotherapy induced emesis may exacerbate the nephrotoxicity of combined ifosfamide/mesna and cisplatin chemotherapy. *Eur. J. Cancer Clin. Oncol.* 25, 917.

Carr, R.J. and Biswas, B.K. (1966). Methysergide and retroperitoneal fibrosis. *Br. Med. J.* ii, 1116.

Carstenen,H., Jacobsen, N., and Dieperink, H. (1986). Interaction between cyclosporin A and phenobarbitone. *Br. J. Clin. Pharmacol.* 21, 550.

Case, D.B., Atlas, S.A., Mouradian, J.A., Fishman, R.A., Sherman, R.L., and Laragh, J.H. (1980). Proteinuria during long-term captopril treatment. *JAMA* 244, 346.

Cassidy, M.J.D., van Zyl-Smit, R., Pascoe, M.D., Swanepoel, C.R., and Jacobson, J.E. (1985). Effect of rifampicin on cyclosporin A blood levels in a renal transplant recipient. *Nephron* 1985, 41, 207.

Chan, M.K. (1986). Cyclosporine pharmacokinetics in end-stage renal failure: the influence of heparin and metoprolol. In: *Proceedings of 2nd Asian Cyclosporine Workshop*, p. 38. Excerpta Medica, Amsterdam.

Chisholm, J.C., Jr (1985). Quinidine-induced nephrotic syndrome. *J. Natl Med. Assoc.* 77, 920.

Chow, S.S., Thorner, P., Baumal, R., and Wilson, D.R. (1986). Cyclosporine and experimental renal ischemic injury. *Transplantation* 41, 152.

Christiansen, N.P., Skubitz, K.M., Nath, K., Ochoa, A., and Kennedy, B.J. (1988). Nephrotoxicity of continuous intravenous infusion of recombinant interleukin-2. *Am. J. Med.* 84, 1072.

Christin, S., Baumelou, A., Bahri, S., Ben Hmida, M., Deray, G., and Jacobs, C. (1990). Acute renal failure due to sulfadiazine in patients with AIDS. *Nephron* 55, 233.

Churchill, D., Yacoub, J.M., Siu, K.P., Symes, A., and Gault, M.H (1976). Toxic nephropathy after low-dose methoxyflurane anesthesia: drug interaction with secobarbital? *Can. Med. Assoc. J.* 114, 326.

Ciabattoni, G., Cinotti, G.A., Pierucci, A., Simonetti, B.M., Manzi, M., Pugliese, F., *et al.* (1984). Effects of sulindac and ibuprofen in patients with chronic glomerular diseases: evidence for the dependence of renal function on prostacyclin. *N. Engl. J. Med.* 310, 279.

Cigarroa, R.G., Lange, R.A., Williams, R.H., and Hillis, L.D. (1989). Dosing of contrast material to prevent contrast nephropathy in patients with renal disease. *Am. J. Med.* 86, 649.

Citron, B.P., Halpern, M., McCarron, M., Lundberg, G.D., McCormick, R., Pincus, I.J., *et al.* (1970). Necrotizing angiitis associated with drug abuse. *N. Engl. J. Med.* 283, 1003.

Clarke, B.F., Campbell, I.W., Ewing, D.J., Beveridge, G.W., and MacDonald, M.K. (1974). Generalized hypersensitivity reaction and visceral arteritis with fatal outcome during glibenclamide therapy. *Diabetes* 23, 739.

Clausen, E. (1964). Histological changes in rabbit kidneys induced by phenacetin and acetylsalicylic acid. *Lancet* ii, 123.

Clausen, E. and Pedersen, J. (1961). Necrosis of the renal papillae in rheumatoid arthritis. *Acta Med. Scand.* 170, 631.

Cleveland, W.W., Adams, W.C., Mann, J.B., and Nyhan, W.L.

(1965). Aquired Fanconi syndrome following degraded tetracycline. *J. Pediatr.* 66, 333.

Clive D.M. and Stoff J.S. (1984). Renal syndromes associated with nonsteroidal antiinflammatory drugs. *N. Engl. J. Med.* 310, 563.

CMTSG (Canadian Multicentre Transplant Study Group) (1986). A randomised clinical trial of cyclosporine in cadaveric renal transplantation: analysis at three years. *N. Engl. J. Med.* 314, 1219.

Cobden, I., Record, C.O., Ward, M.K., and Kerr, D.N.S. (1982). Paracetamol-induced acute renal failure in the absence of fulminant liver damage. *Br. Med. J.* 284, 21.

Cockburn (1986). Cyclosporine A: a clinical evaluation of drug interactions. *Transplant. Proc.* 18 (suppl. 5), 50.

Coffman, T.M., Carr, D.R., Yarger, W.E., and Klotman, P.E. (1987). Evidence that renal prostaglandin and thromboxane production is stimulated in chronic cyclosporine nephrotoxicity. *Transplantation* 43, 282.

Colvin, R.B. and Fang, L.S.T. (1989). Interstitial nephritis. In *Renal pathology*, Vol. 1 (ed. C.C. Tisher and B.M. Brenner), p. 728. J.B. Lippincott, Philadelphia.

Colvin, R.B., Burton, J.R., Hyslop, N.E., Spitz, L., and Lichtenstein, N.S. (1974). Penicillin-associated interstitial nephritis. *Ann. Intern. Med.* 81, 404.

Contreras, A.M., Gamba, G., Cortes, J., Santiago, Y., Nares, F., Jimenez-Sanchez, G., *et al.* (1989). Serial trough and peak amikacin levels in plasma as predictors of nephrotoxicity. *Antimicrob. Agents Chemother.* 33, 973.

Cosio, F.G., Innes, J.T., Nahman, N.S. Jr, Mahan, J.D., and Ferguson, R.M. (1987). Combined nephrotoxic effects of cyclosporine and endotoxin. *Transplantation* 44, 425.

Cove-Smith, J.R. and Knapp, M.S. (1978). Analgesic nephropathy: an important cause of chronic renal failure. *Q. J. Med.* 47, 49.

Cramer, B.C., Parfrey, P.S., and Hutchinson, T.A. (1985). Renal function following infusion of radiologic contrast material: a prospective controlled study. *Arch. Intern. Med.* 145, 87.

Crandell, W.B., Pappas, S.G., and Macdonald, A. (1966). Nephrotoxicity associated with methoxyflurane anesthesia. *Anesthesiology* 27, 591.

Cregler, L.L. (1989). Cocaine-associated myoglobinuric renal failure. *Am. J. Med.* 86, 632.

Cryst, C. and Hammer, S.P. (1988). Acute granulomatous interstitial nephritis due to co-trimoxazole. *Am. J. Nephrol.* 8, 483.

Cubeddu, L.X., Hoffman, I.S., Fuenmayor, N.T., and Finn, A.L. (1990). Efficacy of Ondansetron (GR 38032F) and the role of serotonin in cisplatin-induced nausea and vomiting. *N. Engl. J. Med.* 322, 810.

Cumming, A. (1980). Acute renal failure and interstitial nephritis after clofibrate treatment. *Br. Med. J.* 281, 1529.

Curtis, J.R. and Bateman, F.J.A. (1975). Use of prazosin in management of hypertension in patients with chronic renal failure and in renal transplant recipients. *Br. Med. J.* iv, 432.

Cushner, H.M., Copley, J.B., Bauman, J., and Hill, S.C. (1985). Acute interstitial nephritis associated with mezlo-cillin, nafcillin, and gentamicin treatment for Pseudomonas infection. *Arch. Intern. Med.* 145, 1204.

D'Agostino, R.S. and Arnett, E.N. (1979). Acute myoglobinuria and heroin snorting. *JAMA* 241, 277.

Dabbagh, S. and Chesney, R.W. (1985). Acute renal failure related to acetaminophen (paracetamol) overdose without fulminant hepatic disease. *Int. J. Pediatr. Nephrol.* 6, 221.

Dale, B.M., Sage, R.E., Norman, J.E., Barber, S., and Kotasek, D. (1985). Bone marrow transplantation following treatment with high-dose melphalan. *Transplant. Proc.* 17, 1711.

Daugaard, G. (1990). Cisplatin nephrotoxicity: experimental and clinical studies. *Dan. Med. Bull.* 37, 1.

Davenport, A. and Finn, R. (1988). Paracetamol (acetaminophen) poisoning resulting in acute renal failure without hepatic coma. *Nephron* 50, 55.

Dawnay, A.B., Thornley, C., Nockler, I., Webb, J.A., and Cattell, W.R. (1985). Tamm–Horsfall glycoprotein excretion and aggregation during intravenous urography. Relevance to acute renal failure. *Invest. Radiol.* 20, 53.

Dawson, P. (1985). Contrast agent nephrotoxicity: an appraisal. *Br. J. Radiol.* 58, 121.

Day, A.T. and Golding, J.R. (1974). Hazards of penicillamine therapy in the treatment of rheumatoid arthritis. *Postgrad. Med. J.* 50 (suppl. 2), 71.

De Beukelaer, M.M., Travis, L.B., Dodge, W.F., and Guerra, F.A. (1971). Deafness and acute tubular necrosis following parenteral administration of neomycin. *Am. J. Dis. Child.* 121, 250.

De la Pava, S., Nigogosyan, G., and Pickren, J.W. (1962). Fatal glomerulonephritis after receiving horse anti-human-cancer serum. *Arch. Intern. Med.* 109, 67.

Delaney, V.B. and Segel, D.P. (1985). Indomethacin-induced renal insufficiency: recurrence on rechallenge. *South. Med. J.* 78, 1390.

Deray, G., Le-Hoang, P., Aupetit, B., Achour, A., Rottembourg, J., and Baumelou, A. (1987). Enhancement of cyclosporine A nephrotoxicity by diclofenac. *Clin. Nephrol.* 27, 213.

Deray, G., Dubois, M., Beaufils, H., Cacoub, P., Anouar, M., Jaudon, M.C., *et al.* (1988). Effects of nifedipine on cisplatinum-induced nephrotoxicity in rats. *Clin. Nephrol.* 30, 146.

Devogelaer, J.P., Pirson, Y., Vandenbroucke, J.M., Cosyns, J.P., Brichard, S., and Nagant-de-Deuxchaisnes, C. (1987). D-penicillamine induced crescentic glomerulonephritis: report and review of the literature. *J. Rheumatol.* 14, 1036.

Diamond, J.R. and Karnovsky, M.J. (1986). Focal and segmental glomerulosclerosis following a single intravenous dose of puromycin aminonucleoside. *Am. J. Pathol.* 122, 481.

Dias, N. and Hocken, A.G. (1972). Oliguric renal failure complicating lithium carbonate therapy. *Nephron* 10, 246.

Dieperink, H. and Moller, J. (1982). Ketoconazole and cyclosporin. *Lancet* ii, 1217.

Dieperink, H., Leyssac, P.P., Starklint, H., Jörgensen, K.A., and Kemp, E. (1986). Antagonist capacities of nifedipine, captopril, phenoxybenzamine, prostacyclin and indomethacin on cyclosporin A induced impairment of rat renal function. *Eur. J. Clin. Invest.* 16, 540.

Disney, A.P.S. (1989). *Twelfth Report of the Australia and New Zealand Dialysis and Transplant Registry.* The Queen Elizabeth Hospital, Woodville, South Australia.

Dobyan, D.C., Bull, J.M., Strebel, F.R., Sunderland, B.A., and Bulger, R.E. (1986). Protective effects of *o*-(beta-hydroxyethyl) rutoside on cisplatinum-induced acute renal failure in the rat. *Lab. Invest.* 55, 557.

Dodd, M.J., Griffiths, I.D., and Thompson, M. (1980). Adverse reactions to D-penicillamine after gold toxicity. *Br. Med. J.* ii, 1498.

Doherty, C.C., McGeown, M.G., and Donaldson, R.A. (1978). Retroperitoneal fibrosis after treatment with atenolol. *Br. Med. J.* 280, 1786.

Dooley, D.P., Callsen, M.E., and Geiling, J.A. (1989). Triamterene nephrolithiasis. *Milit. Med.* 154, 126.

Drago, J.R., Rohner, T.J., Sanford, E.J., Engle, J.E., and Schoolwerth, A. (1976). Acute interstitial nephritis. *J. Urol.* 115, 105.

Droller, M.J., Saral, R., and Santos, G. (1982). Prevention of cyclophosphamide-induced haemorrhagic cystitis. *Urology* 20, 256.

Druet, P. (1989). Contribution of immunological reactions to nephrotoxicity. *Toxicol. Lett.* 46, 55.

Drutz, D.J., Fan, J.H., Tai, T.Y., Cheng, J.T., and Hsieh, W.C. (1970). Hypokalemic rhabdomyolysis and myoglobinuria following amphotericin B therapy. *JAMA* 211, 824.

Dry, J., Leynadier, F., Herman, D., and Pradalier, A. (1975). L'association sulfaméthoxazole-triméthoprime (co-trimoxazole). Réaction immunoallergique inhabituelle. *Nouv. Presse Med.* 4, 36.

Duggan, J.M. (1974). The analgesic syndrome. *Aust. N.Z. J. Med.* 4, 365.

Duggin, G.G. and Mudge, G.H. (1974). Renal distribution of acetaminophen and its conjugates. *Kidney Int.* 6, 38A.

Dusseldorp, M.V. and Katan, M.B. (1990). Headache caused by caffeine withdrawal among moderate coffee drinkers switched from ordinary to decaffeinated coffee: a 12 week double blind trial. *Br. Med. J.* 300, 1558.

DuToit E.D., Pascoe M.D., MacGregor K.J., and Milne F.J. (1988). South African Dialysis and Transplant Registry. *Combined Report on Maintenance Dialysis and Transplantation in the Republic of South Africa.*

Duttera, M.J., Carolla, R.L., Gallelli, J.F., Gullion, D.S., Keim, D.E., and Henderson, E.S. (1972). Hematuria and crystalluria after high-dose 6-mercaptopurine administration. *N. Engl. J. Med.* 287, 292.

Edwards, O.M., Edwards, P., Huskisson, E.C., and Taylor, R.T. (1971). Paracetamol and renal damage. *Br. Med. J.* ii, 87.

Eicher, J.C., Morelon, P., Chalopin, J.M., Tanter, Y., Louis, P., and Rifle, G. (1988). Acute renal failure during nifedipine therapy in a patient with congestive heart failure. *Crit. Care Med.* 16, 1163.

Eiser, A.R., Neff, M.S., and Slifkin, R.F. (1982). Acute myoglobinuric renal failure. A consequence of the neuroleptic malignant syndrome. *Arch. Intern. Med.* 142, 601.

Elliott, C. and Reger, M. (1988). Acute renal failure following low osmolality radiocontrast dye. *Clin. Cardiol.* 11, 420.

Emkey, R.D. and Mills, J.A. (1982). Aspirin and analgesic nephropathy. *JAMA* 247, 55.

Engberg, A. (1976). Effects of dextran 40 on the proximal renal tubule. *Acta Chir. Scand.* 142, 172.

Ericsson, J.L.E., Andres, G., Bergstrand, A., Bucht, H., and Örsten, P-Å. (1967). Further studies on the fine structure of renal tubules in healthy humans. *Acta Pathol. Microbiol. Scand.* 69, 493.

Ernest, S. (1989). Model of gentamicin-induced nephrotoxicity and its amelioration by calcium and thyroxine. *Med. Hypotheses* 30, 195.

Erwin, L. and Boulton Jones, J.M. (1982). Benoxaprofen and papillary necrosis. *Br. Med. J.* 285, 694.

Faarup, P. and Christensen, E. (1974). IgE containing plasma cells in acute tubulo-interstitial nephropathy. *Lancet* ii, 718.

Fairley, K.F. and Birch, D.F. (1982). Hematuria: A simple method for identifying glomerular bleeding. *Kidney Int.* 21, 105.

Falck, H.M., Törnroth, T., Kock, B., and Wegelius, O. (1979). Fatal renal vasculitis and minimal change glomerulonephritis complicating treatment with penicillamine. *Acta Med. Scand.* 205, 133.

Falco, F.G., Smith, H.M., and Arcieri, G.M. (1969). Nephrotoxicity of aminoglycosides and gentamicin. *J. Infect. Dis.* 119, 406.

Falk, J.S., Lindblad, G.T.O., and Westman, B.J.M. (1972). Histopathological studies on kidneys from patients treated with large amounts of blood preserved with ACD-adenine. *Transfusion* 12, 376.

Farr, M.J., Wingate, J.P., and Shaw, J.N. (1975). Practolol and the nephrotic syndrome. *Br. Med. J.* ii, 68.

Feehally, J., Wheeler, D.C., Mackay, E.H., Oldham, R., and Walls, J. (1987). Recurrent acute renal failure with interstitial nephritis due to D-penicillamine. *Renal Failure* 10, 55.

Ferraccioli, G., Peri, F., Nervetti, A., Ambanelli, U., and Savi, M. (1986). Toxicity due to remission inducing drugs in rheumatoid arthritis. Association with HLA-B35 and Cw4 antigens. *J. Rheumatol.* 13, 65.

Ferrier, C., Beretta-Piccoli, C., Weidmann, P., Gnädinger, M.P., Shaw, S., Suchecka-Rachon, K., *et al.* (1989). Hypotension and renal impairment during infusion of atrial natriuretic factor in liver cirrhosis with ascites. *Am. J. Nephrol.* 9, 291.

Fillastre, J.P. and Raguenez-Viotte, G. (1989). Cisplatin nephrotoxicity. *Toxicol. Lett.* 46, 163.

Finkelstein, A., Fraley, D.S., Stachura, I., Feldman, H.A., Gandy, D.R., and Bourke, E. (1982). Fenoprofen nephropathy: lipoid nephrosis and interstitial nephritis. A possible T-lymphocyte disorder. *Am. J. Med.* 72, 81.

Forrest, J.N.Jr, Cohen, A.D., Torretti, J., Himmelhock, J.M., and Epstein, F.H. (1974). On the mechanisms of lithium induced diabetes insipidus in man and the rat. *J. Clin. Invest.* 53, 1115.

Fournier, A., Watchi, J-M., and Reveillaud, R-J. (1969). La néphrose dite osmotique ou vacuolisation hydropique des tubes proximaux. *Presse Med.* 77, 1987.

Fowler, W.E. and Boyarsky, S. (1986). A possible cause of hematuria in patients taking warfarin. *N. Engl. J. Med.* 315, 65.

Frame, B., Jackson, C.E., Reynolds, W.A., and Umphrey, J.E. (1974). Hypercalcemia and skeletal effects in chronic hypervitaminosis A. *Ann. Intern. Med.* 80, 44.

Francis, K.L., Jenis, E.H., Jensen, G.E., and Calcagno, P.L. (1984). Gold-associated nephropathy. *Arch. Pathol. Lab. Med.* 108, 234.

Freeman, D.J., Laupacis, A., Keown, P.A., Stiller, C.R., and Carruthers, G. (1984). Evaluation of cyclosporin-phenytoin interaction with observations on cyclosporin metabolites. *Br. J. Clin. Pharmacol.* 18, 887.

Frei, E., Jaffe, N., Tattersall, M.H.N., Pitman, S., and Parker, L. (1975). New approaches to cancer chemotherapy with methotrexate. *N. Engl. J. Med.* 292, 846.

Fuller, T.J., Barcenas, C.G., and White, M.G. (1976). Diuretic-induced interstitial nephritis. Occurence in a patient with membranous glomerulonephritis. *JAMA* 235, 1998.

Fulton, J.D., Briggs, J.D., Dominiczak, A.F., Junor, B.J., and Lucie, N.P. (1986). Intravascular haemolysis and acute renal failure induced by nomifensine. *Scott. Med. J.* 31, 242.

Furman, K.I., Galasko, G.T.F., Meyers, A.M., and Rabkin, R. (1976). Post-transplantation analgesic dependence in patients who formerly suffered from analgesic nephropathy. *Clin. Nephrol.* 5, 54.

Gabriel, R., Caldwell, J., and Hartley, R.B. (1982). Acute tubular necrosis, caused by therapeutic doses of paracetamol? *Clin. Nephrol.* 18, 269.

Gaffey, C.M., Chun, B., Harvey, J.C., and Manz, H.J. (1986). Phenytoin-induced systemic granulomatous vasculitis. *Arch. Pathol. Lab. Med.* 110, 131.

Galea, E.G., Young, L.N., and Bell, J.R. (1963). Fatal nephropathy due to phenindione sensitivity. *Lancet* i. 920.

Galpin, J.E., Friedman, G.S., Shinaberger, J.H., Shapiro, D.J., Blumenkrantz, M.J., Stanley, T.M., *et al.* (1975). Acute interstitial nephritis due to methicillin and similar drugs. *Kidney Int.* 8, 411.

Gary, N.E., Dodelson, R., and Eisinger R.P. (1980). Indomethacin-associated renal failure. *Am. J. Med.* 69, 135.

Gault, M.H., Rudwal, T.C., Engles, W.D., and Dossetor, J.B. (1968). Syndrome associated with the abuse of analgesics. *Ann. Intern. Med.* 68, 906.

Gavish, D., Knobler, H., Gottehrer, N., Israeli, A., and Kleinman, Y. (1986). Methemoglobinemia, muscle damage and renal failure complicating phenazopyridine overdose. *Isr. J. Med. Sci.* 22, 45.

Gelbart, D.R., Weinstein, A.B., and Fajardo, L.F. (1977). Allopurinol induced interstitial nephritis. *Ann. Intern. Med.* 86, 196.

Gelford, G.J. and Cromwell, D.K. (1968). Methysergide retroperitoneal fibrosis and retrosigmoid stricture. *Am. J. Roentgenol.* 104, 566.

Geller, R.J., Chevalier, R.L., and Spyker, D.A. (1986). Acute amoxicillin nephrotoxicity following an overdose. *Clin. Toxicol.* 24, 175.

Gerhardt, R.E., Hudson, J.B., Rao, R.N., and Sobel, R.E. (1978). Chronic renal insufficiency induced by arsenic poisoning. *Arch. Intern. Med.* 138, 1267.

Gerkens, J.F. and Smith, A.J. (1985). Effects of captopril and theophylline on cyclosporine-induced nephrotoxicity in rats. *Transplantation* 40, 213.

Gerritsen van der Hoop. R., Vecht, C.J., van der Burg, M.E.L., Elderson, A., Boogerd, W., Heimans, J.J., *et al.* (1990). Prevention of cisplatin neurotoxicity with an ACTH (4-9) analogue in patients with ovarian cancer. *N. Engl. J. Med.* 322, 89.

Gibb, W.R.G. and Shaw, I.C. (1985). Myoglobinuria due to heroin abuse. *J. R. Coll. Med.* 78, 862.

Giler, S., Sperling, O., Ventura, E., Levy, E., Urca, I., and de Vries, A. (1977). Effect of methoxyflurane anesthesia on serum uric acid in man. *Biomedicine* 27, 13.

Gimenez, A. and Mampaso, F. (1986). Characterization of inflammatory cells in drug-induced tubulointerstitial nephritis. *Nephron* 43, 239.

Giraud, P., Casson, M., Paul, R., and Guidet, M. (1982). Toxicité musculaire due au fénofibrate: à propos d'un cas. *Rev. Rheum.* 49, 162.

Giustina, A., Romanelli, G., Cimino, A., and Brunori, G. (1988). Low-dose acyclovir and acute renal failure. *Ann. Intern. Med.* 108, 312.

Glassock, R.J., Adler, S.G., Ward, H.J., and Cohen, A.H. (1986). Primary glomerular diseases. In *The kidney*, Vol. 1 (3rd edn) (ed. B.M. Brenner and F.C. Rector), p. 929. W.B. Saunders, Philadelphia.

Gloor, F.J. (1965). Some morphologic features of chronic interstitial nephritis (chronic pyelonephritis) in patients with analgesic abuse. In *Progress in pyelonephritis* (ed. E.H. Kass), p. 287. Davis, Philadelphia.

Gloor, F.J. (1974). Unsere heutigen Vorstellungen uber die Morphologie und Pathogenese der Analgetika-Nephropathie. *Schweiz. Med. Wochenschr.* 104, 785.

Gloor, F.J. (1978). Changing concepts in pathogenesis and morphology of analgesic nephropathy as seen in Europe. *Kidney Int.* 13, 27.

Glushien, A.S. and Fisher, E.R. (1956). Renal lesions of sulphonamide type after treatment with acetazolamide (Diamox). *JAMA* 160, 204.

Goebel, K.M. and Mueller-Brodmann, W. (1982). Reversible overt nephropathy with Henoch–Schönlein purpura due to piroxicam. *Br. Med. J.* 284, 311.

Goette, D.K. and Beatrice, E. (1988). Erythema annulare centrifugum caused by hydrochlorothiazide-induced interstitial nephritis. *Int. J. Dermatol.* 27, 129.

Goldberg, H.J., Wong, P.Y., Cole, E.H., Levy, G.A., and Skorecki, K.L. (1989). Dissociation between the immunosuppressive activity of cyclosporine derivatives and their effects on intracellular calcium signaling in mesangial cells. *Transplantation* 47, 731.

Goldstein, E.J., Feinfeld, D.A., Fleischner, G.M., and Elkin, M. (1976). Enzymatic evidence of renal tubular damage following renal angiography. *Radiology* 121, 617.

Gomes, A.S., Baker, J.D., Martin-Paredero, V., Dixon, S.M., Takif, F., H., Machleder, H.I., *et al.* (1985). Acute renal dysfunction after major arteriography. *AJR* 145, 1249.

Gomez, A., Martos, F., Garcia, R., Perez, B., and Sanchez-de-la-Cuesta, F. (1989). Diltiazem enhances gentamicin nephrotoxicity in rats. *Pharmacol. Toxicol.* 64, 190.

Gordon, J.A. and Gattone, V.H. (1986). Mitochondrial alterations in cisplatin-induced acute renal failure. *Am. J. Physiol.* 250, F991.

Goyer, R.A. (1989). Mechanisms of lead and cadmium nephrotoxicity. *Toxicol. Lett.* 46, 153.

Graber, C.D., Patrick, C.C., and Galphin, R.L. (1975). Light chain proteinuria and cellular mediated immunity in rifampin treated patients with tuberculosis. *Chest* 67, 408.

Graham, J.R. (1964). Methysergide for prevention of headache: experience in five hundred patients over three years. *N. Engl. J. Med.* 270, 67.

Graham, J.R., Sury, H.I., LeCompte, P.R., and Sadowsky, N.L. (1966). Fibrotic disorders associated with methysergide therapy for headache. *N. Engl. J. Med.* 274, 359.

Greenbaum, D. and Hope-Stone, H.F. (1959). Dangers of uric-acid excretion during treatment of leukaemia and lymphosarcoma. *Lancet* i, 73.

Greenberg, A., Egel, J.W., Thompson, M.E., Hardesty, R.L., Griffith, B.P., Bahnson, H.T., *et al.* (1987). Early and late forms of cyclosporine nephrotoxicity: studies in cardiac transplant recipients. *Am. J. Kidney Dis.* 9, 12.

Grimm, P.C., Ogborn, M.R., Larson, A.J., and Crocker, J.F. (1989). Interstitial nephritis induced by cloxacillin. *Nephron* 51, 285.

Grino, J.M., Sabate, I., Castelao, A.M., Guardia, M., Seron, D., and Alsina, J. (1986). Erythromycin and cyclosporine. *Ann. Intern. Med.* 105, 467.

Grond, J., Koudstaal, J., and Elema, J.D. (1985). Mesangial function and glomerular sclerosis in rats with aminonucleoside nephrosis. *Kidney Int.* 27, 405.

Grufferman, S., Morris, D., and Alvarez, J. (1985). Methanol poisoning complicated by myoglobinuric renal failure. *Am. J. Emerg. Med.* 3, 24.

Gutman, A.B. and Yu, T.F. (1968). Uric acid nephrolithiasis. *Am. J. Med.* 45, 756.

Haapanen, E., Pellinen, T.J., and Partanen, J. (1984). Acute renal failure caused by alcohol-induced rhabdomyolysis. *Nephron* 36, 191.

Hakim, R., Tolis, G., Goltzman, D., Meltzer, S., and Friedman, R. (1979). Severe hypercalcaemia associated with hydrochlorothiazide and calcium carbonate therapy. *Can. Med. Assoc. J.* 121, 591.

Hall, B.M., Tiller, D.J., Duggin, G.G., Horvath, J.S., Farnsworth, A., May, J., *et al.* (1985). Post-transplant acute renal failure in cadaver renal recipients treated with cyclosporine. *Kidney Int.* 28, 178.

Halla, J.T., Cassidy, J., and Hardin, J.G. (1982). Sequential gold and penicillamine therapy in rheumatoid arthritis. Comparative study of effectiveness and toxicity and review of the literature. *Am. J. Med.* 72, 423.

Halpren, B.A., Kempson, R.L., and Coplon, N.S. (1973). Interstitial fibrosis and chronic renal failure following methoxyflurane anesthesia. *JAMA* 223, 1239.

Hamblin, T.J. (1990). Interleukin 2. *Br. Med. J.* 300, 275.

Hampel, G., Horskotte, H., and Rumpf, K.W. (1983). Myoglobinuric renal failure due to drug-induced rhabdomyolysis. *Hum. Toxicol.* 2, 197.

Handa, S.P. and Tewari, H.D. (1981). Urinary tract carcinoma in patients with analgesic nephropathy. *Nephron* 28, 62.

Handa, S.P. (1986). Drug-induced acute interstitial nephritis: a report of 10 cases. *Can. Med. Assoc. J.* 135, 1278.

Harkness, J.A.L. and Blake, D.R. (1982). Penicillamine nephropathy and iron. *Lancet* ii, 1368.

Harkonen, S. and Kjellstrand, C.M. (1979). Intravenous pyelography in nonuremic diabetic patients. *Nephron* 24, 268.

Harris, K.P., Jenkins, D., and Walls, J. (1988). Nonsteroidal antiinflammatory drugs and cyclosporine: a potentially serious adverse interaction. *Transplantation* 46, 598.

Hartman, G.W., Torres, V.E., Leago, G.F., Williamson, B., and Hattery, R.R. (1984). Analgesic-associated nephropathy. *JAMA* 251, 1734.

Harvald, B. (1968). Renal papillary necrosis. A clinical survey of sixty-six cases. *Am. J. Med.* 35, 481.

Harvald, B., Valdorf-Hansen, F., and Nielsen, A. (1960). Effect on the kidney of drugs containing phenacetin. *Lancet* i, 303.

Hauser, A.C., Derfler, K., Stockenhuber, F., and Balcke, P. (1990). Post-transplantation malignant disease in patients with analgesic nephropathy. *Lancet* 335, 58.

Hawker, F., Pearson, I.Y., Soni, N., and Woods, P. (1985). Rhabdomyolytic renal failure and suxamethonium. *Anaesth. Intens. Care* 13, 208.

Hayes, D.M., Cvitkovic, E., Golbey, R.B., Scheiner, E., Helson, L., and Krakoff, I.H. (1977). High dose cis-platinum diammine dichloride: amelioration of renal toxicity by mannitol diuresis. *Cancer* 39, 1372.

Heitzman, E.J., Patterson, J.F., and Stanley, M.M. (1962). Myoglobinuria and hypokalemia in regional enteritis. *Arch. Intern. Med.* 110, 117.

Hertz, P., Yager, H., and Richardson, J.A. (1972). Probenecid-induced nephrotic syndrome. *Arch. Pathol.* 94, 241.

Hess, E. (1988). Drug-related lupus. *N. Engl. J. Med.* 318, 1460.

Hindle, W., Posner, E., Sweetnam, M.T., and Tan, R.S.H. (1970). Pleural effusion and fibrosis during treatment with methysergide. *Br. Med. J.* i, 605.

Hoffman, B.J. (1945). Sensitivity to sulfadiazine resembling acute disseminated lupus erythematosus. *Arch. Dermatol. Syph.* 51, 190.

Hogg, K.J. and Hillis, W.S. (1986). Captopril/metolazone induced renal failure. *Lancet* i, 501.

Hogg, R.J., Sawyer, M., Hecox, K., and Eigenbrodt, E. (1981). Carbamazepine-induced acute tubulointerstitial nephritis. *J. Pediatr.* 98, 830.

Hollenberg, N.K., McDonald, F.D., Cotran, R., Galvanek, E.G., Warhol, M., Vandam, L.D., and Merrill, J.P. (1972). Irreversible acute oliguric renal failure. *N. Engl. J. Med.* 286, 877.

Holm, S.E., Hill, B., Lowestad, R., Maller, R., and Vikerfors, T. (1983). A prospective randomised study of amikacin and gentamicin in serious infections with focus on efficacy, toxicity and duration of serum levels above the MIC. *J. Antimicrob. Chemother.* 12, 393.

Holt, D.W., Marsden, J.T., Johnston, A., Bewick, M., and Taube, D.H. (1986). Blood cyclosporin concentrations and renal allograft dysfunction. *Br. Med. J.* 293, 1057.

Holtas, S. (1978). Proteinuria following nephroangiography. Thesis. Malmo General Hospital, Malmo, Sweden.

Holtzman, N.A., Elliott, D.A., and Heller, R.H. (1966). Copper intoxication. *N. Engl. J. Med.* 275, 347.

Honkanen, E., Tornroth, T., Pettersson, E., and Skrifvars, B. (1987). Membranous glomerulonephritis in rheumatoid arthritis not related to gold or D-penicillamine therapy: a report of four cases and review of the literature. *Clin. Nephrol.* 27, 87.

Hooke, D., Walker, R.G., Walter, N.M.A., D'Apice, A.J.F., Whitworth, J.A., and Kincaid-Smith, P. (1982). Repeated renal failure with use of captopril in a cystinotic renal allograft recipient. *Br. Med. J.* 285, 1538.

Horgan, K.J., Ottaviano, Y.L., and Watson, A.J. (1989). Acute renal failure due to mannitol intoxication. *Am. J. Nephrol.* 9, 106.

Hostetter, A.L., Tubbs, R.R., Ziegler, T., Gephardt, G.N., McMahon, J.T., and Schreiber, M.J. Jr (1987). Chronic glomerular microangiopathy complicating metastatic carcinoma. *Hum. Pathol.* 18, 342.

Houghton, D.C., English, J., and Bennett, W.M. (1988). Chronic tubulointerstitial nephritis and renal insufficiency associated with long-term 'subtherapeutic' gentamicin. *J. Lab. Clin. Med.* 112, 694.

Howard, T., Hoy, R.H., Warren, S., Georgiev, M., and Selinger, H. (1981). Acute renal dysfunction due to sulfinpyrazone therapy in post myocardial infarction cardiomegaly: reversible hypersensitive interstitial nephritis. *Am. Heart J.* 102, 294.

Hows, J.M., Chipping, P.M., Fairhead, S., Smith, J., and Baughan, A. (1983). Nephrotoxicity in bone marrow transplant recipients treated with cyclosporin A. *Br. J. Haematol.* 54, 69.

Hricik, D.E. (1985). Captopril-induced renal insufficiency and the role of sodium balance. *Ann. Intern. Med.* 103, 222.

Huggon, I., James, I., and Macrae, D. (1990). Hyperosmolality related to propylene glycol in an infant treated with enoximone infusion. *Br. Med. J.* 301, 19.

Hultengren, N. (1961). Renal papillary necrosis. A clinical study of 103 cases. *Acta Chir. Scand.* (suppl. 277).

Hultman, P. and Enestrom, S. (1986). Localization of mercury in the kidney during experimental acute tubular necrosis studied by the cytochemical silver amplification method. *Br. J. Exp. Pathol.* 67, 493.

Hurault de Ligny, B., Ryckelynck, J.P., Levaltier, B., Gallet, B., and Trunet, P. (1986). Néphropathie interstitielle avec syndrome néphrotique induite par le pirprofène. *Rev. Med. Interne* 7, 525.

Hussain, S.P. and Drew, P.J.T. (1989). Acute renal failure after infusion of gelatins. *Br. Med. J.* 299, 1137.

Hyman, R.L., Ballow, M., and Knieser, M.R. (1978). Diphenylhydantoin interstitial nephritis. Roles of cellular and humoral immunological injury. *J. Pediatr.* 92, 915.

Iesato, K., Mori, Y., Ueda, S., Wakashin, Y.M., Matsui, N., Inoue, S., *et al.* (1982). Renal tubular dysfunction as a complication of gold therapy in patients with rheumatoid arthritis. *Clin. Nephrol.* 17, 46.

Ihle, B.U., Byrnes, C.A., and Simenhoff, M.L. (1982). Acute renal failure due to interstitial nephritis resulting from radio contrast agents. *Aust. N.Z. J. Med.* 12, 630.

Imai, H., Nakamoto, Y., Hirokawa, M., Akihama, T., and Miura, A.B. (1989). Carbamazepine-induced granulomatous necrotizing angiitis with acute renal failure. *Nephron* 51, 405.

Jain, S. and Seymour, A.E. (1987). Mitomycin C associated hemolytic uremic syndrome. *Pathology* 19, 58.

Jablonski, P., Harrison, C., Howden, B., Rae, D., Tavanlis, G., Marshall, V.C., *et al.* (1986). Cyclosporine and the ischemic rat kidney. *Transplantation* 41, 147.

Jandreski, M.A., Bermes, E.W., Leischner, R., and Kahn, S.E. (1989). Rhabdomyolysis in a case of free-base cocaine ('crack') overdose. *Clin. Chem.* 35, 1547.

Jarzobski, J., Ferry, J., Wombolt, D., Fitch, D.M., and Egan, J.D. (1970). Vasculitis with allopurinol therapy. *Am. Heart J.* 79, 116.

Jennings, A.E., Levy, A.S., and Harrington, J.T. (1983). Amoxapine-associated acute renal failure. *Arch. Intern. Med.* 143, 1525.

Jennings, M., Shortland, J.R., and Maddocks, J.L. (1986). Interstitial nephritis associated with frusemide. *J. R. Soc. Med.* 79, 239.

Joh, K., Shibasaki, T., Azuma, T., Kobayashi, A., Miyahara, T., Aizawa, S., *et al.* (1989). Experimental drug-induced allergic nephritis mediated by antihapten antibody. *Int. Arch. Allergy Appl. Immunol.* 88, 337.

Johnson, J.N. and McFarland, J.B. (1980). Retroperitoneal fibrosis associated with atenolol. *Br. Med. J.* 280, 864.

Jones, T.W., Chorpa, S., Kaufman, J.S., Flamenbaum, W., and Trump, B.F. (1985). Cis-diamminedichloroplatinum (II)-induced acute renal failure in the rat: enzyme histochemical studies. *Toxicol. Pathol.* 13, 296.

Kaden, W.S. and Friedman, E.A. (1961). Obstructive uropathy complicating anticoagulant therapy. *N. Engl. J. Med.* 265, 283.

Kahan, B.D. (1989). Drug therapy: Cyclosporine. *N. Engl. J. Med.* 321, 1725.

Kahlmeter, G. and Dahlager, J. (1984). Aminoglycoside toxicity — a review of clinical studies published between 1975 and 1982. *J. Antimicrob. Chemother.* 13, 9A.

Kanazi, G., Stowe, N., Steinmuller, D., Hwieh, H.H., and Novick, A.C. (1986). Effect of cyclosporine upon the function of ischemically damaged kidneys in the rat. *Transplantation* 41, 782.

Kanfer, A., Richet, G., Roland, J., and Chatelet, F. (1979). Extreme hyperphosphataemia causing acute anuric nephrocalcinosis in lymphosarcoma. *Br. Med. J.* i, 1320.

Kasanen, A. (1973). The effect of the restriction of the sale of phenacetin on the incidence of papillary necrosis established at autopsy. *Ann. Clin. Res.* 5, 369.

Katz, C.M. and Tzagournis, M. (1972). Chronic adult hypervitaminosis A with hypercalcaemia. *Metabolism* 21, 1171.

Katz, M.D. and Lor, E. (1986). Acute interstitial nephritis associated with intermittent rifampicin use. *Drug Intell. Clin. Pharm.* 20, 789.

Kaysen, G.A., Pond, S.M., Roper, M.H., Menke, D.J., and Marrama, M.A. (1985). Combined hepatic and renal injury in alcoholics during therapeutic use of acetaminophen. *Arch. Intern. Med.* 145, 2019.

Keaton, M.R. (1988). Acute renal failure in an alcoholic during therapeutic acetaminophen ingestion. *South. Med. J.* 81, 1163.

Kendrick, W.C., Hull, A.R., and Knochel, J.P. (1977). Rhabdomyolysis and shock after intravenous amphetamine administration. *Ann. Intern. Med.* 86, 381.

Kennedy, A. and Saluga, P.G. (1970). Urinary cytology in experimental toxic renal injury. *Ann. Rheum. Dis.* 29, 546.

Kennedy, M,S., Deeg, H.J., Siegel, M., Crowley, J.J., Storb, R., and Thomas E.D. (1983). Acute renal toxicity with combined use of amphotericin B and cyclosporin after marrow transplantation. *Transplantation* 35, 211.

Kerbel, N.C. (1967). Retroperitoneal fibrosis secondary to methysergide bimaleate. *Can. Med. Assoc. J.* 96, 1420.

Kho, T.L., Teule, J., Leunissen, K.M., Heidendal, G.A., Lijenen, P.J., Amery, A.K., *et al.* (1987). Nephrotoxic effect of cyclosporine A can be reversed by dopamine. *Transplant. Proc.* 19, 1749.

Kincaid-Smith, P. Analgesic nephropathy. (1988). *Aust. N.Z. J. Med.* 18, 251.

Kincaid-Smith, P., Nanra, R.S., and Fairley, K.F. (1971). Analgesic nephropathy: a recoverable form of chronic renal failure. In *Renal infection and renal scarring* (ed. P. Kincaid-Smith and K.F. Fairley), p. 385. Mercedes Publishing Services, Melbourne.

Kiruluta, H.G. and Andrews, K. (1983). Urinary incontinence secondary to drugs. *Urology* 22, 88.

Klotman, P.E., Boatman, J.E., Vlopp, B.D., Baker, J.D., and Yarger, W.E. (1985). Captopril enhances aminoglycoside toxicity in potassium-depleted rats. *Kidney Int.* 28, 118.

Kogan, A. and Orenstein, S. (1990). Lovastatin-induced acute rhabdomyolysis. *Postgrad. Med. J.* 66, 294.

Kolkin, S., Nahman, N.S., Jr, and Mendell, J.R. (1987). Chronic nephrotoxicity complicating cyclosporine treatment of chronic inflammatory demyelinating polyradiculoneuropathy. *Neurology* 37, 147.

Kravitz, S.C. and Craver, L.F. (1951). Uremia complicating leukemia chemotherapy. *JAMA* 146, 1595.

Krikler, D.M. (1967). Paracetamol and the kidney. *Br. Med. J.* ii, 615.

Kritzler, R.A. (1958). Anuria complicating the treatment of leukemia. *Am. J. Med.* 25, 532.

Kumar, S. and Muchmore, A. (1990). Tamm–Horsfall protein — uromodulin (1950–1990). *Kidney Int.* 37, 1395.

Kumar, S., Mehta, J.A., and Trivedi, H.L. (1976). Light chain proteinuria and reversible renal failure in rifampicin-treated patients with tuberculosis. *Chest* 70, 564.

Kurtz, A., Della Bruna, R., and Kühn, K. (1988). Cyclosporine A enhances renin secretion and production in isolated juxtaglomerular cells. *Kidney Int.* 33, 947.

Laakso, M., Arvala, I., Tervonen, S., and Sotarauta, M. (1982). Retroperitoneal fibrosis associated with sotalol. *Br. Med. J.* 285, 1085.

Lachaal, M. and Venuto, R.C. (1989). Nephrotoxicity and hyperkalemia in patients with acquired immunodeficiency syndrome treated with pentamidine. *Am. J. Med.* 87, 260.

Ladd, A.T. (1962). Procainamide-induced lupus erythematosus. *N. Engl. J. Med.* 267, 1357.

Landgrebe, A.R., Nyhan, W.L., and Coleman, M. (1975). Urinary tract stones resulting from the excretion of oxypurinol. *N. Engl. J. Med.* 292, 626.

Lang, E.K. (1985). Streptokinase therapy: complications of intra-arterial use. *Radiology* 154, 75.

Langer, T. and Levy, R.I. (1968). Acute muscular syndrome associated with administration of clofibrate. *N. Engl. J. Med.* 279, 856.

Langhoff, E. and Madsen, S. (1983). Rapid metabolism of cyclosporin and prednisone in kidney transplant patient receiving tuberculostatic treatment. *Lancet* ii, 1031.

Larsen, K. and Møller, C.E. (1959). A renal lesion caused by abuse of phenacetin. *Acta Med. Scand.* 164, 53.

Larsson, R., Bodemar, G., Kagedal, B., and Walan, A. (1980). The effects of cimetidine on renal function in patients with renal failure. *Acta Med. Scand.* 208, 27.

Laskin, O.L. (1984). Acyclovir. Pharmacology and clinical experience. *Arch. Intern. Med.* 144, 1241.

Laurent, G., Yernaux, V., Nonclercq, D., Toubeau, G., Maldague, P., Tulkens, P.M., *et al.* (1988). Tissue injury and proliferative response induced in rat kidney by cis-diamminedichloroplatinum (II). *Virchows Arch.* B. 55, 129.

Lauwerys, R., Bernard, A., Viau, C., and Buchet, J.P. (1985). Kidney disorders and hematotoxicity from organic solvent exposure. *Scand. J. Work Environ. Health.* 11 (suppl 1), 83.

Lavender, S., Brown, J.N., and Berrill, W.T. (1973). Acute renal failure and lithium intoxication. *Postgrad. Med. J.* 49, 277.

Lear, H. and Oppenheimer, G.D. (1950). Anuria following radiation therapy in leukemia. *JAMA* 143, 806.

Lee, H.A. and Holden, C.E.A. (1964). Phenindione nephropathy with recovery: studies of morphology and renal function. *Postgrad. Med. J.* 40, 326.

Lee, J.C., Dushkin, M., Eyring, E.J., Engleman, E.P., and Hopper, J. (1965). Renal lesions associated with gold therapy: light and electron microscopic studies. *Arthritis Rheum.* 8, 1.

Lee, S.C., Abe, T., and Sato, T. (1987). Rhabdomyolysis and acute renal failure following use of succinylcholine and enflurane: report of a case. *J. Oral Maxillofac. Surg.* 45, 789.

Lee, S.M., Williams, R., Warnock, D., Emmett, M., and Wolbach, R.A. (1986). The effects of nicardipine in hypertensive subjects with impaired renal function. *Br. J. Clin. Pharmacol.* 22, 297S.

Leimenstoll, G., Schlegelberger, T., Fulde, R., and Niedermayer, W. (1988). Interaction of cyclosporine and ethambutol–isoniazide. *Dtsch. Med. Wochenschr.* 113, 514.

Lele, P., Peterson, P., Yang, S., Jarrell, B., and Burke, J.F.. (1985). Cyclosporine and Tegretol — another drug interaction. *Kidney Int.* 27, 344.

Lepage-Savary, D. and Vallières, A. (1982). Ergotamine as a possible cause of retroperitoneal fibrosis. *Clin. Pharm.* 1, 179.

Lerner, A.M., Reyes, M.P., Cone, L.A., Blair, D.C., Jansen, W., Wright, G.E., *et al.* (1983). Randomised controlled trial of the comparative efficacy, auditory toxicity and nephrotoxicity of tobramycin and netilmicin. *Lancet* i, 1123.

Lewis, J.A. and Rindone, J.P. (1987). Acute interstitial nephritis associated with cephapirin [letter]. *Drug. Intell. Clin. Pharm.* 21, 380.

Lin, C.Y. and Chiang, H. (1988). Sodium valproate-induced interstitial nephritis. *Nephron* 48, 43.

Lindeneg, O., Fischer, S., Pedersen, J., and Nissen, N.I. (1959). Necrosis of the renal papillae and prolonged abuse of phenacetin. *Acta Med. Scand.* 165, 321.

Lindvall, N. (1960). Renal papillary necrosis. A roentgenographic study of 155 cases. *Acta Radiol.* (suppl. 192).

Lindvall, N. (1978). Radiological changes of renal papillary necrosis. *Kidney Int.* 13, 93.

Ling, B.N., Bourke, E., Campbell, W.G., Jr, and Delaney, V.B. (1990). Naproxen-induced nephropathy in systemic lupus erythematosus. *Nephron* 54, 249.

Linton, A.L., Clark, W.F., Driedger, A.A., Turnbull, D.I., and Lindsay, R.M. (1980). Acute interstitial nephritis due to drugs. Review of the literature with a report of nine cases. *Ann. Intern. Med.* 93, 735.

Lombard, J., Levin, I.H., and Weiner, W.J. (1989). Arsenic intoxication in a cocaine abuser. *N. Engl. J. Med.* 320, 869.

Lowe, M.B. and Tapp, E. (1966). Renal damage caused by anhydro 4-EPI-tetracycline. *Arch. Pathol.* 81, 362.

Lucena, M.I., Gonzalez-Correa, J.A., Andrade, R.J., Ibanez, J., Torres, D., and Sanchez-de-la-Cuesta, F. (1989). Enhanced gentamicin nephrotoxicity after experimental biliary obstruction in rats. *Pharmacol. Toxicol.* 65, 352.

Luft, F.C., Yum, M.N., Walker, P.D., and Kleit, S.A. (1977). Gentamicin gradient patterns and morphological changes in human kidneys. *Nephron* 18, 167.

Lunde, P.K.M., Frislid, K., and Hansteen, V. (1977). Disease and acetylation polymorphism. *Clin. Pharmacokinet.* 2, 182.

Lynn, K.L., Bailey, R.R., Swainson, C.P., Sainsbury, R., and Low, W.I. (1985). Renal failure with potassium-sparing diuretics. *N.Z. Med. J.* 98, 629.

Mabeck, C.E. and Wichmann, B. (1979). Mortality from chronic interstitial nephritis and phenacetin consumption in Denmark. *Acta Med. Scand.* 205, 599.

Macdonald, J.B., Jones, H.M., and Cowan, R.A. (1985). Rhabdomyolysis and acute renal failure after theophylline overdose. *Lancet* i, 932.

Mahan, J.D., Sisson-Ross, S., and Vernier, R.L. (1986). Glomerular basement membrane anionic charge site changes early in aminonucleoside nephrosis. *Am. J. Pathol.* 125, 393.

Maher, J.F., Raith, C.E., and Schreiner, G.E. (1969). Hyperuricemia complicating leukemia. Treatment with allopurinol and dialysis. *Arch. Intern. Med.* 123, 198.

Mailloux, L., Swartzschwarz, C.D., Capizzi, R., Kim, K.E., Onesti, G., Ramirez, O., *et al.* (1967). Acute renal failure after administration of low-molecular-weight dextran. *N. Engl. J. Med.* 277, 1113.

Maisel, J.C. and Priest, R.E. (1964). Fatal phenacetin nephritis. *Arch. Pathol.* 77, 646.

Makowka, L., Lopatin, W., Gilas, T., Falk, J., Phillips, M.J., and Falk, R. (1986). Prevention of cyclosporine (Cya) nephrotoxicity by synthetic prostaglandins. *Clin. Nephrol.* 25 (suppl. 1), S89.

Malaquin, F., Urban, T., Ostinelli, J., Ghedira, H., and Lacronique, J. (1989). Pleural and retroperitoneal fibrosis from dihydroergotamine. *N. Engl. J. Med.* 321, 1760.

Malone, D.N.S. and Horn, D.B. (1971). Acute hypercalcaemia and renal failure after antacid therapy. *Br. Med. J.* i, 709.

Marais, G.E. and Larson, K.K. (1990). Rhabdomyolysis and acute renal failure induced by combination lovastatin and gemfibrozil therapy. *Ann. Intern. Med.* 112, 228.

Marasco, W.A., Gikas, P.W., Azziz-Baumgartner, R., Hyzy, R., Eldredge, C.J., and Stross, J. (1987). Ibuprofen-associated renal dysfunction. Pathophysiologic mechanisms of acute renal failure, hyperkalemia, tubular necrosis, and proteinuria. *Arch. Intern. Med.* 147, 2107.

Margolis D., Ross, E., and Miller, K.B. (1987). Rhabdomyolysis associated with high-dose cytarabine. *Cancer Treat. Rep.* 71, 1325.

Markman, M., Cleary, S., and Howell, S.B. (1985). Nephrotoxicity of high-dose intracavitary cisplatin with intravenous thiosulfate protection. *Eur. J. Cancer Clin. Oncol.* 21, 1015.

Martinez-Maldonado, M. and Terrell, J. (1973). Lithium carbonate induced nephrogenic diabetes insipidus and glucose intolerance. *Arch. Intern. Med.* 132, 881.

Marty, M., Poullart, P., Scholl, S., Droz, J.P., Azab, M., Brion, N., *et al.* (1990). Comparison of the 5-hydroxytryptamine$_3$ (serotonin) antagonist ondansetron (GR 38032F) with high-dose metoclopramide in the control of cisplatin-induced emesis. *N. Engl. J. Med.* 322, 816.

Masters, D.R. (1973). Analgesic nephropathy associated with paracetamol. *Proc. R. Soc. Med.* 66, 36.

Matsuda, O., Beck, F.X., Dorge, A., and Thurau, K. (1988). Electrolyte composition of renal tubular cells in gentamicin nephrotoxicity. *Kidney Int.* 33, 1107.

Matsumoto, J., Yasaka, T., Ohya, I., and Ohtani, H. (1985). Acute renal failure in primary macroglobulinemia with small-molecule IgM. *Arch. Intern. Med.* 145, 929.

Mavromatis, F. (1965). Tetracycline nephropathy. *JAMA* 193, 191.

May, D.C., Helderman, J.H., Eigenbrodt, E.H., and Silva, F.G. (1986). Chronic sclerosing glomerulopathy (heroin-associated nephropathy) in intravenous T's and Blues abusers. *Am. J. Kidney Dis.* 8, 404.

Mayaud, C., Kourilsky, D., Kanfer, A., and Straer, J.D. (1975). Interstitial nephritis after methicillin. *N. Engl. J. Med.* 292, 1132.

Maxwell, D., Szwed, J.J., Wahle, W., and Kleit, S.A. (1974). Ampicillin nephropathy. *JAMA* 230, 585.

Mazze, R.I., Shue, G.L., and Jackson, S.H. (1971). Renal dysfunction associated with methoxyflurane anesthesia. *JAMA* 216, 278.

Mazze, R.I., Cousins, M.J., and Kosek, J.C. (1973). Dose related methoxyflurane nephrotoxicity in rats. *Anesthesiology* 36, 571.

McAuley, F.T., Whiting, P.H., Thomson, A.W., and Simpson, J.G. (1987). The influence of enalapril or spironolactone on experimental cyclosporin nephrotoxicity. *Biochem. Pharmacol.* 36, 699.

McCauley, J., Bronsther, O., Fung, J., Todo, S., and Starzl, T.E. (1989). Treatment of cyclosporin-induced haemolytic uraemic syndrome with FK506. *Lancet* ii, 1516.

McCluskey, D., Donaldson, R.A., and McGeown, M.G. (1980). Oxprenolol and retroperitoneal fibrosis. *Br. Med. J.* 281, 1459.

McDermott, W. (1947). Toxicity of streptomycin. *Am. J. Med.* 2, 491.

McLeish, K.R., Senitzer, D., and Gohara, A.F. (1979). Acute interstitial nephritis in a patient with aspirin hypersensitivity. *Clin. Immunol. Immunopathol.* 14, 64.

Menashe, P.I. and Gottlieb, J.E. (1988). Hyperthermia, rhabdomyolysis, and myoglobinuric renal failure after recreational use of cocaine. *South. Med. J.* 81, 379.

Mendoza, F., Atiba, J., Kreusky, A., and Scannell, L. (1987). Rhabdomyolysis complicating doxylamine overdose. *Clin. Pediatr.* 26, 595.

Menta, R., Rossi, E., Guariglia, A., David, S., and Cambi, V. (1987). Reversible acute cyclosporin nephrotoxicity induced by colchicine administration. *Nephrol. Dial. Transplant.* 2, 380.

Mercieca, J. and Brown, E.A. (1984). Acute renal failure due to rhabdomyolysis associated with the use of a straitjacket in lysergide intoxication. *Br. Med. J.* 288, 1949.

Mergenthaler, H.G., Binsack, T., and Wilmanns, W. (1988). Carcinoma-associated hemolytic-uremic syndrome in a patient receiving 5-fluorouraci–adriamycin–mitomycin C combination chemotherapy. *Oncology* 45, 11.

Merigian, K.S. and Roberts, J.R. (1987). Cocaine intoxication: hyperpyrexia, rhabdomyolysis and acute renal failure. *J. Toxicol. Clin. Toxicol.* 25, 135.

Merkle, R.B., McDonald, F.D., Waldman, J., Maynard, G.D., Petit, J., Fleming, P.J., *et al.* (1971). Human renal function following methoxyflurane anesthesia. *JAMA* 218, 841.

Michaelson, J.H., McCoy, J.P., Jr, Hirszel, P., and Bigazzi, P.E. (1985). Mercury-induced autoimmune glomerulonephritis in inbred rats. I. Kinetics and species specificity of autoimmune responses. *Surv. Synth. Pathol. Res.* 4, 401.

Mihatsch, M.J. and Knusli, C. (1982). Phenacetin abuse and malignant tumours. An autopsy study covering 25 years (1953–1977). *Klin. Wochenschr.* 60, 1339.

Mihatsch, M.J., Hoper, H.O., Gudat, F., Knusli, C., Torhorst, J., and Zollinger, H.U. (1983). Capillary sclerosis of the urinary tract and analgesic nephropathy. *Clin. Nephrol.* 20, 285.

Mihatsch, M.J., Thiel, G., and Ryffel, B. (1988*a*). Histopathology of cyclosporine nephrotoxicity. *Transplant. Proc.* 20, (suppl. 3), 759.

Mihatsch, M.J., Steiner, K., Abeywickrama, K.H., Landmann, J., and Thiel, G. (1988*b*). Risk factors for the development of chronic cyclosporine-nephrotoxicity. *Clin. Nephrol.* 29, 165.

Mijares, R.P. (1986). Hypokalemic rhabdomyolysis secondary to pseudohyperaldosteronism due to the use of a lotion containing 9-α-fluoroprednisolone. *Nephron* 43, 232.

Miller, L., Pateras, V., Friederici, H., and Engel, G. (1985). Acute tubular necrosis after inhalation exposure to methylene chloride. Report of a case. *Arch. Intern. Med.* 145, 145.

Misch, K.A. (1974). Development of heart valve lesions during methysergide therapy. *Br. Med. J.* ii, 365.

Mitchell, A.B.S. (1971). Duogastrone-induced hypokalaemic nephropathy and myopathy with myoglobinuria. *Postgrad. Med. J.* 47, 807.

Mitchell, G., Wilken, R.J., and Dixon, P. (1965). Acute renal failure complicating lymphosarcoma. *Br. Med. J.* i, 567.

Mizutani, T., Oohashi, N., and Naito, H. (1989). Myoglobinemia and renal failure in toluene poisoning: a case report. *Vet. Hum. Toxicol.* 31, 448.

Moeschlin, von S. (1957). Phenacetinsucht und-schaden Innenkorpernamien und interstitielle Nephritis. *Schweiz. Med. Wochenschr.* 87, 123.

Molland, E.A. (1978). Experimental renal papillary necrosis. *Kidney Int.* 13, 5.

Mollman, J.E. (1990). Cisplatin neurotoxicity (Editorial). *N. Engl. J. Med.* 322, 126.

Monballyu, J., Zachee, P., Verberckmoes, R., and Boogaerts, M.A. (1984). Transient acute renal failure due to tumour-lysis-induced severe phosphate load in a patient with Burkitt's lymphoma. *Clin. Nephrol.* 22, 47.

Montoliu, J., Carrera, M., Darnell, A., and Revert, L. (1981). Lactic acidosis and Fanconi's syndrome due to degraded tetracycline. *Br. Med. J.* 283, 1576.

Moore, R.D., Smith, C.R., Lipsky, J.J., Mellits, E.D., and Lietman, P.S. (1984). Risk factors for nephrotoxicity in patients treated with aminoglycosides. *Ann. Intern. Med.* 100, 352.

Moran, M. and Kapsner, C. (1987). Acute renal failure associated with elevated plasma oncotic pressure, *N. Engl. J. Med.* 317, 150.

Morgan, T.O., Little, J.M., and Evans, W.A. (1966). Renal failure associated with low-molecular-weight dextran infusion. *Br. Med. J.* iii, 737.

Morrow, J.D., Schroeder, H.A., and Perry, H.M. Jr (1953). Studies on the control of hypertension by Hyphex. II. Toxic reactions and side effects. *Circulation* 8, 829.

Mraz, W., Sido, B., Knedeo, M., and Hammer, C. (1987). Concomitant immunosuppressive and antibiotic therapy — reduction of cyclosporine A blood levels due to treatment with imipenem/cilastatin. *Transplant. Proc.* 19, 4017.

Muehrcke, R.C. and Pirani, C.L. (1968). Arsine-induced anuria. *Ann. Intern. Med.* 68, 853.

Muirhead, N., Hollomby, D.J., and Keown, P.A. (1987). Acute glomerular thrombosis with CsA treatment. *Renal Failure* 10, 135.

Murgo, A.J. (1987). Plasmapheresis and antiplatelet agents in the treatment of the hemolytic uremic syndrome secondary to mitomycin. *Am. J. Kidney Dis.* 9, 241.

Murray, A.N., Cassidy, M.J.D., and Templecamp, C. (1987). Rapidly progressive glomerulonephritis associated with rifampicin therapy for pulmonary tuberculosis. *Nephron* 46, 373.

Murray, B.M., Paller, M.S., and Ferris, T.F. (1985). Effect of cyclosporine administration on renal hemodynamics in conscious rats. *Kidney Int.* 28, 767.

Murray, R.M. (1972). Analgesic nephropathy: removal of phenacetin from proprietary analgesics. *Br. Med. J.* iv, 131.

Myers, B.D., Sibley, R., Newton, L., Tomlanovich, S.J., Boshkos, C., Stinson, E., *et al.* (1988). The long-term course of cyclosporine-associated chronic nephropathy. *Kidney Int.* 33, 590.

Myers, G.H. and Witten, D.N. (1971). Acute renal failure after excretory urography in multiple myeloma. *Am. J. Roentgenol.* 113, 583.

Nade, S. (1972). Acute urinary suppression presumed due to bilateral ureteric obstruction by blood clot. An unusual feature of anticoagulant therapy. *Med. J. Aust.* i, 378.

Nadel, S., Jackson, J., and Ploth, D. (1979). Hypokalemic rhabdomyolysis and acute renal failure. Occurrence following total parenteral nutrition. *JAMA* 241, 2294.

Nagai, T. and Nagai, T. (1987). Tubulointerstitial nephritis by Tamm–Horsfall glycoprotein or egg white component. *Nephron* 47, 134.

Nagata, N., Yoneyama, T., Yanagida, K., Ushio, K., Yanagihara, S., Matsubara, O., *et al.* (1985). Accumulation of germanium in the tissues of a long-term user of germanium preparation died of acute renal failure. *J. Toxicol. Sci.* 10, 333.

Nanra, R.S. and Kincaid-Smith, P. (1970). Papillary necrosis in rats caused by aspirin and aspirin-containing mixtures. *Br. Med. J.* iii, 559.

Nanra, R.S., Stuart-Taylor, J., de Leon, A.H., and White, K.H. (1978). Analgesic nephropathy: etiology, clinical syndrome and clinicopathologic correlations in Australia. *Kidney Int.* 13, 79.

Neumayer, H.-H., Junge, W., Küfner, A., and Wenning, A. (1989). Prevention of radiocontrast-media-induced nephrotoxicity by the calcium channel blocker nitrendipine: a prospective randomised clinical trial. *Nephrol. Dial. Transplant.* 4, 1030.

New Zealand Rheumatism Association Study. (1974). Aspirin and the kidney. *Br. Med. J.* i, 593.

Nessi , R., Bonoldi, G.L., Redaelli, B., and Di Fillipo, G. (1976). Acute renal failure after rifampicin: a case report and survey of the literature. *Nephron* 16, 148.

NIH Consensus Conference. (1984). Analgesic associated kidney disease. *JAMA* 251, 3123.

Noel, J., Rosenbaum, L.H., Gangadharan, V., Stewart, J., and Galeus, G. (1987). Serum sickness-like illness and leucocytoclastic vasculitis following intracoronary arterial streptokinase. *Am. Heart J.* 113, 395.

Nolan, C.R. and Kelleher, S.P. (1988). Eosinophiluria. *Clin. Lab. Med.* 8, 555.

Nordenfelt, O. (1972). Deaths from renal failure in abusers of phenacetin-containing drugs. *Acta Med. Scand.* 170, 385.

Nordenfelt, O. and Ringertz, N. (1961). Phenacetin takers dead with renal failure, 27 men and 3 women. *Acta Med. Scand.* 170, 385.

Novis, B.H., Korzets, Z., Chen, P., and Bernheim, J. (1988). Nephrotic syndrome after treatment with 5-aminosalicylic acid. *Br. Med. J.* 296, 1442.

Nowack, C., Garke-Nowack, F., Pretschner, D.P., Frei, U., Wonigeit, K., Pichlmayr, R., *et al.* (1988). The engymetric determination of acute functional impairment in kidney graft function caused by cyclosporine A. *Nucl. Med. Commun.* 9, 389.

Nyberg, G., Blohme, I., Persson, H., and Svalander, C. (1990). Forscarnet-induced tubulointerstitial nephritis in renal transplant patients. *Transplant. Proc.* 22, 241.

O'Brien, W.M. (1986). Adverse reactions to nonsteroidal anti-inflammatory drugs. Diclofenac compared with other nonsteroidal anti-inflammatory drugs. *Am. J. Med.* 80, 70.

Offerman, J.J., Hollema, H., Elema, J.D., Schraffordt-Koops, H., and de-Vries, E.G. (1985). TNO-6-induced acute renal failure. A case report. *Cancer* 56, 1511.

Oh, S.J., Douglas, J.E., and Brown, R.A. (1971). Hypokalemic vacuolar myopathy associated with chlorthalidone treatment. *JAMA* 216, 1858.

Oliveira, D.B., Foster, G., Savill, J., Syme, P.D., and Taylor, A. (1987). Membranous nephropathy caused by mercury-containing skin lightening cream. *Postgrad. Med. J.* 63, 303.

Orchard, R.T. and Rooker, G. (1974). Penicillin hypersensitivity nephritis. *Lancet* i, 689.

Orlandini, G. and Garini, G. (1989). Phenytoin-induced nephrotic syndrome. *Nephron* 52, 109.

Oster, J.R. and Epstein, M. (1977). Demeclocycline-induced renal failure. *Lancet* i, 52.

Ozawa, T.T., Smith, P.,Jr, Vance, D., Moore, N., and Lackey, L. (1987). Acute interstitial nephritis induced by cimetidine. *J. Tenn. Med. Assoc.* 80, 411.

Pacifici, G.M., Viani, A., Franchi, M., Gervasi, P.G., Longo, V., DiSimplicio, P., *et al.* (1989). Profile of drug-metabolizing enzymes in the cortex and medulla of the human kidney. *Pharmacology* 39, 299.

Packer, M. (1989). Identification of risk factors predisposing to the development of functional renal insufficiency during treatment with converting-enzyme inhibitors in chronic heart failure. *Cardiology* 76 (suppl. 2), 50.

Pahl, M.V., Barton, C.H., Ulich, T., Villalobos, R., and Kaupke, C.J. (1988). Renal dysfunction and micro-angiopathic changes in a renal transplant patient [clinical conference]. *Am. J. Nephrol.* 8, 72.

Palestine, A.G., Austin, H.A., and Nussenblatt, R.B. (1986). Renal tubular function in cyclosporine-treated patients. *Am. J. Med.* 81, 419.

Panner, B.J., Freeman, R.B., Roth-Mayo, L.A., and Marcowitch, W. (1970). Toxicity following methoxyflurane anesthesia. *JAMA* 214, 86.

Parfitt, A.M. (1969). Acetazolamide and sodium bicarbonate induced nephrocalcinosis and nephrolithiasis. *Arch. Intern. Med.* 124, 736.

Parfrey, P.S., Griffiths, S.M., Barrett, B.J., Paul, M.D., Genge, M., Withers, J., *et al.* (1989). Contrast material-induced renal failure in patients with diabetes mellitus, renal insufficiency, or both. A prospective controlled study. *N. Engl. J. Med.* 320, 143.

Parry, M.F., Ball, W., Conte, J.E., and Cohen, S.N. (1973). Nafcillin nephritis. *JAMA* 225, 178.

Paul, M.D., Parfrey, P.S., Smart, M., and Gault, H. (1987). The effect of ethanol on serum cyclosporine A levels in renal transplant recipients. *Am. J. Kidney Dis.* 10, 133.

Pawel, B.R., Kaye, W.A., Khan, M.Y., Fergusen, B.D., Federman, M., and Crosson, A.W. (1989). Aggravation of diabetic nephropathy by lithium: a case report and review of the literature. *J. Clin. Psychiatry* 50, 101.

Payne, S.T., Hosker, H.S.R., Allen, M.B., Bradbury, H., and Page, R.L. (1989). Transient impairment of renal function after streptokinase therapy. *Lancet* ii, 1398.

Pazmino, P. (1988). Acute renal failure, skin rash, and eosinophilia associated with aztreonam. *Am. J. Nephrol.* 8, 68.

Peces, R., Riera, J.R., Arboleya, L.R., Lopez-Larrea, C., and Alvarez, J. (1987). Goodpasture's syndrome in a patient receiving penicillamine and carbimazole. *Nephron* 45, 316.

Pelletier, L., Pasquier, R., Vial, M.C., Mandet, C., Moutier, R., Salomon, J.C., *et al.* (1987). Mercury-induced autoimmune glomerulonephritis: requirement for T-cells. *Nephrol. Dial. Transplant.* 1, 211.

Penney, M.D., Hullin, R.P., Srinivasan, D.P., and Morgan, D.B. (1981). The relationship between plasma lithium and the renal responsiveness to arginine vasopressin in man. *Clin. Sci.* 61, 793.

Pepys, M.B. (1970). Acetazolamide and renal stone formation. *Lancet* ii, 837.

Perico, N., Zoja, C., Benigni, A., Bosco, E., Rossini, M., Morelli, C., *et al.* (1986). Renin–angiotensin system and glomerular prostaglandins in early nephrotoxicity of ciclosporin. *Contrib. Nephrol.* 51, 120.

Perks, W.H., Walters, E.H., Tams, I.P., and Prowse, K. (1979). Demeclocycline in the treatment of the syndrome of inappropriate secretion of antidiuretic hormone. *Thorax* 34, 324.

Persky, L., Chambers, D., and Potts, A. (1956). Calculus formation and ureteral colic following acetazolamide (Diamox) therapy. *JAMA* 161, 1625.

Petersen, K.C., Silberman, H., and Berne, T.V. (1984). Hyperkalaemia after cyclosporin therapy. *Lancet* i, 1470.

Peterson, O.W., Gabbai, F.B., Myers, R.R., Mizisin, A.P., and Blantz, R.C. (1989). A single nephron model of acute tubular injury: role of tubuloglomerular feedback. *Kidney Int.* 36, 1037.

Pierce, J.R., Trostle, D.C., and Warner, J.J. (1981). Propranolol and retroperitoneal fibrosis. *Ann. Intern. Med.* 95, 244.

Pierce, L.R., Wysowski, D.K., and Gross, T.P. (1990). Myopathy and rhabdomyolysis associated with lovastatin–gemfibrozil combination therapy. *JAMA* 264, 71.

Pillans, P. and Hall, C. (1985). Paracetamol-induced acute renal failure in the absence of severe liver damage. *S. Afr. Med. J.* 67, 791.

Pohl, J.E.F., Thurston, H., and Swales, J.D. (1974). Hypertension with renal impairment: influence of intensive therapy. *Q. J. Med* 43, 569.

Pommer, W., Krause, P.H., Berg, P.A., Neumayer, H.H., Mihatsch, M.J., and Molzahn, M. (1986). Acute interstitial nephritis and non-oliguric renal failure after cefaclor treatment. *Klin. Wochenschr.* 64, 290.

Pommer, W., Bronder, E., Greiser, E., Helmert, U., Jesdinsky, H.J., Klimpel, A., *et al.* (1989). Regular analgesic intake and the risk of end-stage renal failure. *Am. J. Nephrol.* 9, 403.

Powell, H.R., Davidson, P.M., McCredie, D.A., Phair, P., and Walker, R.G. (1988). Haemolytic–uraemic syndrome after treatment with metronidazole. *Med. J. Aust.* 149, 222.

Prati, R.C., Alfrey, A.C., and Hull, A.R. (1972). Spironolactone-induced hypercalciuria. *J. Lab. Clin. Med.* 80, 224.

Prescott, L.F. (1982). Analgesic nephropathy: a reassessment of the role of phenacetin and other analgesics. *Drugs* 23, 75.

Prescott, L.F., Illingworth, R.N., Critchley, J.A.J.H., Stewart, M.J., Adam, R.D., and Proudfoot, A.T. (1979). Intravenous *N*-acetylcysteine: the treatment of choice for paracetamol poisoning. *Br. Med. J.* ii, 1097.

Prescott, L.F., Proudfoot, A.T., and Gregeen, R.J. (1982). Paracetamol-induced acute renal failure in the absence of fulminant liver damage. *Br. Med. J.* 284, 421.

Pryor, J.P., Castle, W.M., Dukes, D.C., Smith, J.C., Watson, M.E., and Williams, J.L. (1983). Do beta-adrenoceptor blocking drugs cause retroperitoneal fibrosis? *Br. Med. J.* 287, 639.

Pusey, C.D., Saltissi, D., Bloodworth, L., Rainford, D.J., and Christie, J.L. (1983). Drug associated acute interstitial nephritis: clinical and pathological features and response to high dose steroid therapy. *Q. J. Med.* 52, 194.

Quin, J., Adamski, M., Howlin, K., Jones, W., O'Neill, P., Stewart, G., *et al.* (1988). Quinidine-induced allergic granulomatous angiitis: an unusual cause of acute renal failure. *Med. J. Aust.* 148, 145.

Quinn, B.P. and Wall, B.M. (1989). Nephrogenic diabetes insipidus and tubulointerstitial nephritis during continuous therapy with rifampin. *Am. J. Kidney Dis.* 14, 217.

Randall, R.E., Osheroff, R.J., Bakerman, S., and Setter, J.G. (1972). Bismuth nephrotoxicity. *Ann. Intern. Med.* 77, 481.

Raz, S. (1974). Adrenergic influence on the internal sphincter. *Isr. J. Med.* 10, 608.

Rehan, A. and Johnson, K. (1986). IgM nephropathy associated with penicillamine. *Am. J. Nephrol.* 6, 71.

Reid, G.M. and Muther, R.S. (1987). Nitroprusside-induced acute azotemia. *Am. J. Nephrol.* 7, 313.

Rello, J., Triginer, C., Sànchez, J.M., and Net, A. (1989). Acute renal failure following massive mannitol infusion. *Nephron* 53, 377.

Remuzzi, G. and Bertani, T. (1989). Renal vascular and thrombotic effects of cyclosporine. *Am. J. Kidney Dis.* 13, 261.

Renier, J.C., Boasson, M., Pitois, M., and Alquier, P. (1975). Insuffisance rénale aiguë récidivante après ingestion de glafénine à dose thérapeutique. *Nouv. Presse Med.* 4, 670.

Richman, A.V., Masco, H.L., Rifkin, S.I., and Acharya, M.K. (1980). Minimal change disease and the nephrotic syndrome associated with lithium therapy. *Ann. Intern. Med.* 92, 70.

Richter, R.W., Challenor, Y.B., Pearson, J., Kagen, L.J., Hamilton, L.L., and Ramsey, W.H. (1971). Acute myoglobinuria associated with heroin addiction. *JAMA* 216, 1172.

Riley, L.J. Jr, Vlasses, P.H., Rotmensch, H.H., Swanson, B.N., Chremos, A.N., Johnson, C.L., *et al.* (1985). Sulindac and Ibuprofen inhibits furosemide-stimulated renin release but not natriuresis in men on a normal sodium diet. *Nephron* 41, 283.

Rimmer, E., Richens, A., Forster, M.E., and Ress, R.W.M. (1983). Retroperitoneal fibrosis associated with timolol. *Lancet* i, 300.

Robson, J.S., Martin, A.M., Ruckley, V.A., and MacDonald, M.K. (1968). Irreversible post-partum renal failure: a new syndrome. *Q. J. Med.* 37, 423.

Robson, M., Levi, J., Dolberg, L., and Rosenfeld, J.B. (1970). Acute tubulo-interstitial nephritis following sulfadiazine therapy. *Isr. J. Med. Sci.* 6, 561.

Roodhooft, A.M., Van-Dam, K., Haentjens, D., Verpooten, G.A., and Van-Acker, K.J. (1990). Acute sodium valproate intoxication: occurrence of renal failure and treatment with haemoperfusion-haemodialysis. *Eur. J. Pediatr.* 149, 363.

Rosen, M. (1972). Acute urinary suppression presumed due to bilateral ureteric obstruction by blood clot: an unusual feature of anticoagulant therapy. *Med. J. Aust.* i, 660.

Rossi, A.C., Bosco, L., Faich, G.A., Tanner, A., and Temple, R. (1988). The importance of adverse reaction reporting by physicians. Suprofen and the flank pain syndrome. *JAMA* 259, 1203.

Rossi, von G. and Muhlethaler, J.P. (1958). Phenacetin-abuses und chronische interstitielle Nephritis. *Helv. Med. Acta* 25, 510.

Roth, D., Alarcon, F.J., Fernandez, J.A., Preston, R.A., and Bourgoignie, J.J. (1988). Acute rhabdomyolysis associated with cocaine intoxication. *N. Engl. J. Med.* 319, 673.

Rotoli, B., Giglio, F., Bile, M., and Formisano, S. (1985). Immune-mediated acute intravascular hemolysis caused by cianidanol (catergen). *Haematologica Pavia* 70, 495.

Rowland, R.G. and Elbe, J.N. (1983). Bladder leiomyosarcoma and pelvic fibroblastic tumour following cyclophosphamide therapy. *J. Urol.* 130, 344.

Rubiano, R., Chang, J.L., Carroll, J., Sonbolian, N., and Larson, C. (1987). Acute rhabdomyolysis following halothane anesthesia without succinylcholine. *Anesthesiology* 67, 856.

Ruley, E.J. and Lisi, L.M. (1974). Interstitial nephritis and renal failure due to ampicillin. *J. Pediatr.* 84, 878.

Russell, G.I., Bing, R.F., Walls, J., and Pettigrew, N.M. (1978). Interstitial nephriitis in a case of phneylbutazone hypersensitivity. *Br. Med. J.* i, 1322.

Sack, K., Schulz, E., Marre, R., and Kreft, B. (1987). Fosfomycin protects against tubulotoxicity induced by cis-diaminedichloroplatin and cyclosporin A in the rat. *Klin. Wochenschr.* 65, 525.

Sacks, P. and Fellner, S.K. (1987). Recurrent reversible acute renal failure from amphotericin. *Arch. Intern. Med.* 147, 593.

Sadjadi, S.A., McLaughlin, K., and Shah, R.M. (1987). Allergic interstitial nephritis due to diazepam. *Arch. Intern. Med.* 147, 579.

Sahai, J., Heimberger, T., Collins, K., Kaplowitz, L., and Polk, R. (1988). Sulfadiazine-induced crystalluria in a patient with the aquired immunodeficiency syndrome: a reminder. *Am. J. Med.* 84, 791.

Saito, T., Sumithran, E., Glasgow, E.F., and Atkins, R.C. (1987). The enhancement of aminonucleoside nephrosis by the co-administration of protamine. *Kidney Int.* 32, 691.

Salama, A. and Mueller-Eckhardt, C. (1985). The role of metabolite-specific antibodies in nomifensine-dependent immune hemolytic anemia. *N. Engl. J. Med.* 313, 469.

Salaman, J.R. and Griffin, P.J.A. (1985). Fine needle intrarenal manometry in the management of renal transplant patients receiving cyclosporine. *Transplant. Proc.* 17, 1275.

Saltissi, D., Pusey, C.D., and Rainford, D. (1979). Recurrent acute renal failure due to antibiotic-induced interstitial nephritis. *Br. Med. J.* i, 1182.

Salvarani, C., Macchioni, P., Rossi, F., Iori, I., and Filippi, G. (1985). Nephrotic syndrome induced by tiopronin: association with the HLA-DR3 antigen. *Arthritis Rheum.* 28, 595.

Samuelson, P.N., Merin, R.G., Taves, D.R., Freeman, R.B., Calimlim, J.F., and Kumazawa, T. (1976). Toxicity following methoxyflurane anaesthesia. *Can. Anaesth. Soc. J.* 23, 465.

Sanai, T., Okuda, S., Onoyama, K., Oochi, N., Oh, Y., Kobayashi, K., *et al.* (1990). Germanium dioxide-induced nephropathy: a new type of renal disease. *Nephron* 54, 53.

Sandler, D.P., Smith, J.C., Weinberg, C.R., Buckalew, V.M., Jr, Dennis, V.W., Blythe, W.B., *et al.* (1989). Analgesic use and chronic renal disease. *N. Engl. J. Med.* 320, 1238.

Sanjad, S.A., Haddad, G.G., and Nassar, V.H. (1974). Nephropathy, an underestimated complication of methicillin therapy. *J. Pediatr.* 84, 873.

Santella, R.N., Rimmer, J.M., and MacPherson, B.R. (1988). Focal segmental glomerulosclerosis in patients receiving lithium carbonate. *Am. J. Med.* 84, 951.

Sanwikarja, S., Kauffmann, R.H., te-Velde, J., and Serlie, J. (1989). Tubulointerstitial nephritis associated with pyrazinamide. *Neth. J. Med.* 34, 40.

Savill, J.S., Chia, Y., and Pusey, C.D. (1988). Minimal change nephropathy and pemphigus vulgaris associated with penicillamine treatment of rheumatoid arthritis. *Clin. Nephrol.* 29, 267.

Saway, P.A., Heck, L.W., Bonner, J.R., and Kirklin, J.K. (1988). Azathioprine hypersensitivity. *Am. J. Med.* 84, 960.

Sawyer, M.H., Webb, D.E., Balow, J.E., and Straus, S.E. (1988). Acyclovir-induced renal failure. Clinical course and histology. *Am. J. Med.* 84, 1067.

Schnitzer, B. and Smith, E.B. (1966). Effects of the metabolites of phenacetin on the rat. *Arch. Pathol.* 81, 264.

Schwarb, S.J., Hlatky, M.A., Pieper, K.S., Davidson, C.J., Morris, K.G., Skelton, T.N., *et al.* (1989). Contrast nephrotoxicity: a randomised control trial of a non-ionic and an ionic radiographic contrast agent. *N. Engl. J. Med.* 320, 149.

Schwartz, F.D. and Dunea, G. (1966). Progression of retroperitoneal fibrosis despite cessation of treatment with methysergide. *Lancet* i, 955.

Schwartz, R.H., Berdon, W.E., Wagner, J., Becker, J., and Baker, D.H. (1970). Tamm–Horsfall urinary mucoprotein precipitation by urographic contrast agents: in vitro studies. *Am. J. Roentgenol.* 108, 698

Schwarz, A., Pommer, W., Keller, F., Kuehn-Freitag, G., Offermann, G., and Molzahn, M. (1984). Morbidity of patients with analgesic-associated nephropathy and end-stage renal failure. *Proc. Eur. Dial. Transplant Assoc. Eur. Ren. Assoc.* 21, 311.

Schwartzman, M.S. and Franck, W.A. (1987). Vitamin D toxicity complicating the treatment of senile, postmeno-pausal, and glucocorticoid-induced osteoporosis. *Am. J. Med.* 82, 224.

Seelig, M.S. (1969). Vitamin D and cardiovascular, renal, and brain damage in infancy and childhood. *Ann. N.Y. Acad. Sci.* 147, 537.

Segasothy, M., Kong, B.C.T., Kamal, A., Morad, Z., and Suleiman, A.B. (1984). Analgesic nephropathy associated with paracetamol. *Aust. N.Z. J. Med.* 14, 23.

Segasothy, M., Cheong, I., Kong, B.C.T., Suleiman, A.B., and Morad, Z. (1986). Further evidence of analgesic nephropathy in Malaysia. *Med. J. Malaysia* 41, 377.

Segasothy, M., Suleiman, A.B., Puvaneswary, M., and Rohana, A. (1988). Paracetamol: a cause for analgesic nephropathy and end-stage renal disease. *Nephron* 50, 50.

Selby, P., Kohn, J., Raymond, J., Judson, I., and McElwain, T. (1985). Nephrotic syndrome during treatment with interferon. *Br. Med. J.* 290, 1180.

Selby, P.J., Powles, R.L., Jameson, B., Kay, H.E.M., Watson, J.G., Thornton, R., et al. (1979). Parenteral acyclovir therapy for herpes virus infections in men. *Lancet* ii, 1267.

Selby, T. (1979). Acute renal failure from ticrynafen. *N. Engl. J. Med.* 301, 1180.

Sellars, L. and Wilkinson, R. (1983). Adverse effects of anti-rheumatic drugs on the kidney. *Adverse Drug React. Acute Poisoning Rev.* 2, 51.

Sennesael, J., van-den-Houte, K., and Verbeelen, D. (1986). Reversible membranous glomerulonephritis associated with ketoprofen. *Clin. Nephrol.* 26, 213.

Sensakovic, J.W., Suarez, M., Perez, G., Johnson, E.S., and Smith, L.G. (1985). Pentamidine treatment of *Pneumocystis carinii* pneumonia in the acquired immunodeficiency syndrome. Association with acute renal failure and myoglobinuria. *Arch. Intern. Med.* 145, 224.

Sheil, A.G.R., Hall, B.M., Tiller, D.J., Stephen, M.S., Harris, J.P., Duggin, G.C., et al. (1983). Australian trial of cyclosporine (CsA) in cadaveric donor renal transplantation. *Transplant. Proc.* 15 (suppl. 1), 2485

Sheilds, M.B. and Simmons, R.J. (1976). Urinary calculus during methazolamide therapy. *Am. J. Ophthalmol.* 81, 622.

Sheth, K.J., Casper, J.T., and Good, T.A. (1977). Interstitial nephritis due to phenytoin hypersensitivity. *J. Pediatr.* 91, 438.

Silanpaa, M., Kasanen, A., and Elonen, A. (1982). Changes of panorama in renal disease mortality in Finland after phenacetin restriction. *Acta Med. Scand.* 212, 313.

Singer, I. (1981). Lithium and the kidney. *Kidney Int.* 19, 374.

Singer, I., Rotenberg, D., and Puschett, J. B. (1972). Lithium induced nephrogenic diabetes insipidis: In vivo and in vitro studies. *J. Clin. Invest.* 51, 1081.

Singhal, P., Horowitz, B., Quinones, M.C., Sommer, M., Faulkner, M., and Grosser, M. (1989). Acute renal failure following cocaine abuse. *Nephron* 52, 76.

Skinner, R. and Ferner, R.E. (1986). Acute renal failure without acute intravascular haemolysis after nomifensine overdosage. *Hum. Toxicol.* 5, 279.

Smart, E.R. (1985). The hazards of mercury in dentistry. *Rev. Environ. Health.* 5, 59.

Smith, C.R., Lipsky, J.J., Laskin, O.L., Hellman, D.B., Mellits, E.D., Longstreth, J., et al. (1980). Double-blind comparison of the nephrotoxicity and auditory toxicity of gentamicin and tobramycin. *N. Engl. J. Med.* 302, 1106.

Smith, P.J., Swinburn, W.R., Swinson, D.R., and Stewart, I.M. (1982). Influence of previous gold toxicity on subsequent development of penicillamine toxicity. *Br. Med. J.* 285, 595.

Snyder, D.S. (1988). Interaction between cyclosporine and warfarin. *Ann. Intern. Med.* 108, 311.

Snyder, H.E., Killen, D.A., and Foster, J.H. (1968). The influence of mannitol on toxic reactions of contrast angiography. *Surgery* 64, 640.

Soberon, L., Bowman, R.L., Pasoriza-Munoz, E., and Kaloyanides, G.J. (1979). Comparative nephrotoxicities of gentamicin, netilmicin and tobramycin in the rat. *J. Pharmacol. Exp. Ther.* 210, 334.

Soffer, O., Nassar, V.H., Campbell, W.G., Jr, and Bourke, E. (1987). Light chain cast nephropathy and acute renal failure associated with rifampin therapy. Renal disease akin to myeloma kidney. *Am. J. Med.* 82, 1052.

Solinger, A.M. (1988). Drug-related lupus. Clinical and etiologic considerations. *Rheum. Dis. Clin. North Am.* 14, 187.

Speirs, C., Fielder, A.H.L., Chapel, H., Davey, N.J., and Batchelor, J.R. (1989). Complement system protein C4 and susceptibility to hydralazine-induced systemic lupus erythematosus. *Lancet* i, 922.

Spragg, J., Weinblatt, M.E., Coblyn, J., Fraser, P., and Austen, K.F. (1988). Effect of cyclosporine on urinary kallikrein excretion in patients with rheumatoid arthritis. *J. Lab. Clin. Med.* 112, 324.

Spuhler, O. and Zollinger, H.U. (1953). Die chronische interstitielle Nephritis. *Z. Klin. Med.* 151, 1.

Stark, H., Alkalay, A., Ben-Bassat, M., Hazaz, B., and Joshua, H. (1985). Levan-induced glomerulitis in rabbits: a possible role for direct complement activation in situ. *Br. J. Exp. Pathol.* 66, 165.

Steele, T.W. and Edwards, K.D.G. (1971). Analgesic nephropathy. Changes in various parameters of renal function following cessation of analgesic abuse. *Med. J. Aust.* i, 181.

Steenland, N.K., Thun M.J., Ferguson C.W., and Port F.K. (1990). Occupational and other exposures associated with male end-stage renal disease: a case control study. *Am. J. Public Health.* 80, 153.

Stein, H.B., Patterson, A.C., Offer, R.C., Atkins, C.J., Tuefel, A., and Robinson, H.S. (1979). Adverse effects of D-penicillamine in rheumatoid arthritis. *Ann. Intern. Med.* 91, 24.

Stratta, P., Mazzucco, G., Griva, S., Tetta, C., and Monga, G. (1988). Immune-mediated glomerulonephritis after exposure to paraquat. *Nephron* 48, 138.

Strom, B.L., West, S.L., Sim, E., and Carson, J.L. (1989). The epidemiology of the acute flank pain syndrome from suprofen. *Clin. Pharmacol. Ther.* 46, 693.

Swartz, R.D., Rubin, J.E., Leeming, B.W., and Silva, P. (1978). Renal failure following major angiography. *Am. J. Med.* 65, 31.

Tahan, S.R., Diamond, J.R., Blank, J.M., and Horan, R.F. (1985). Acute hemolysis and renal failure with rifampicin-dependent antibodies after discontinuous administration. *Transfusion* 25, 124.

Taliercio, C.P., Vlietstra, R.E., Fisher, L.D., and Burnett, J.C. (1986). Risks for renal dysfunction with cardiac angiography. *Ann. Intern. Med.* 104, 501.

Taylor, W.H. (1972). Renal calculi and self-medication with multi-vitamin preparations containing vitamin D. *Clin. Sci.* 42, 515.

Tegzess, A.M., Doorenbos, B.M., Minderhound, J.M., and Donker, A.J. (1988). Prospective serial renal function studies in patients with non-renal disease treated with cyclosporine A. *Transplant. Proc.* 20, (suppl 2), 390.

Teixeria, R.B., Kelly, J., Alpert, H., Pardo, V., and Vaamonde, C.A. (1982). Complete protection from gentamicin-induced acute renal failure in the diabetes mellitus rat. *Kidney Int.* 21, 600.

Terada, Y., Shinohara, S., Matui, N., and Ida, T. (1988). Amphetamine-induced myoglobinuric acute renal failure. *Jpn J. Med.* 27, 305.

Thien, T.H., Delaere, K.P.J., Debruyne, F.M.T., and Koene, R.A.P. (1978). Urinary incontinence caused by prazosin. *Br. Med. J.* i, 622.

Thompson, J. and Julian, D.G. (1982). Retroperitoneal fibrosis associated with metoprolol. *Br. Med. J.* 284, 83.

Thompson, J.F., Chalmers, D.H., Hunnisett, A.G., Wood, R.F., and Morris, P.J. (1983). Nephrotoxicity of trimethoprim and cotrimoxazole in renal allograft recipients treated with cyclosporine. *Transplantation* 36, 204.

Todd, M.A., Bailey, R.R., Espiner, E.A., and Lynn, K.I. (1987). Vitamin D2 for the treatment of chilblains — a cautionary tale. *N.Z. Med. J.* 100, 465.

Toll, L.L., Lee, M., and Sharifi, R. (1987). Cefoxitin-induced interstitial nephritis. *South. Med. J.* 80, 274.

Toomath, R.J. and Morrison, R.B. (1987). Renal failure following methoxyflurane analgesia. *N.Z. Med. J.* 100, 707.

Tornroth, T. and Skrivars, B. (1974). Gold nephropathy prototype of membranous glomerulonephritis. *Am. J. Pathol.* 75, 573.

Tosi, S., Cagnoli, M., Guidi, G., Murelli, M., Messina, K., and Colombo, B. (1985). Injectable gold dermatitis and proteinuria: retreatment with auranofin. *Int. J. Clin. Pharmacol. Res.* 5, 265.

Trewhalla, M., Dawson, P., Forsling, M., McCarthy, P., and O'Donnell, C. (1990). Vasopressin release in response to intravenously injected contrast media. *Br. J. Radiol.* 63, 97.

Tulkens, P.M. (1989). Nephrotoxicity of aminoglycoside antibiotics. *Toxicol. Lett.* 46, 107.

Ubhi, C.S., Guillou, P.J., Davison, A.M., and Giles, G.R. (1987). Combination fine-needle aspiration cytology and intrarenal manometry at the onset of renal dysfunction. *Br. J. Surg.* 74, 297.

Ueda, S., Wakashin, M., Wakashin, Y., Yoshida, H., Iesato, K., Mori, T., et al. (1986). Experimental gold nephropathy in guinea pigs: detection of autoantibodies to renal tubular antigens. *Kidney Int.* 29, 539.

van-der-Woude, F.J., van-Son, W.J., Tegzess, A.M., Donker, A.J., Slooff, M.J., van-der-Slikke, L.B., et al. (1985). Effect of captopril on blood pressure and renal function in patients with transplant renal artery stenosis. *Nephron* 39, 184.

Venkataraman, G. (1981). Renal damage and glue sniffing. *Br. Med. J.* 283, 1467.

Veremis, S.A., Maddux, M.S., Pollak, R., and Mozes, M.F. (1987). Subtherapeutic cyclosporine concentrations during nafcillin therapy. *Transplantation* 43, 913.

Verin, P., Bresque, E., Vizdy, A., and Lagoutte, F. (1974). Fibrose rétropéritonéale et dérivés de l'ergot. *Bull. Soc. Ophtalmol. Fr.* 31, 281.

Verma, S. and Kieff, E. (1975). Cephalexin-related nephropathy. *JAMA* 234, 618.

Verweij, J., van-der-Burg, M.E., and Pinedo, H.M. (1987). Mitomycin C-induced hemolytic uremic syndrome. Six case reports and review of the literature on renal, pulmonary and cardiac side effects of the drug. *Radiother. Oncol.* 8, 33.

Verwey, J., de-Vries, J., and Pinedo, H.M. (1987). Mitomycin C-induced renal toxicity, a dose-dependent side effect? *Eur. J. Cancer Clin. Oncol.* 23, 195.

Vestergaard, P. and Amdisen, A. (1981). Lithium treatment and kidney function. A follow-up study of 237 patients on long-term treatment. *Acta Psychiatr. Scand.* 63, 333.

Volpi, A., Ferrario, G.M., Giordano, F., Antiga, G., Battini, G., Fabbri, C., et al. (1989). Acute renal failure due to hypersensitivity interstitial nephritis induced by warfarin sodium. *Nephron* 52, 196.

Wagner, K., Albrecht, S., and Neumayer, H.H. (1986). Prevention of delayed graft function in cadaveric kidney transplantation by a calcium antagonist. *Transplant Proc.* 18, 510.

Wagner, K., Albrecht, S., and Neumayer, H.H. (1987). Prevention of posttransplant acute tubular necrosis by the calcium antagonist diltiazem: a prospective randomized study. *Am. J. Nephrol.* 7, 287.

Walker, P.D. and Shah, S.V. (1988). Evidence suggesting a role for hydroxyl radical in gentamicin-induced acute renal failure in rats. *J. Clin. Invest.* 81, 334.

Walker, R.G., Thomson, N.M., Dowling, J.P., and Ogg, C.S. (1979). Minocycline-induced acute interstitial nephritis. *Br. Med. J.* i, 524.

Walker, R.G., Bennet, W.M., Davies, B.M., and Kincaid-Smith, P. (1982). Structural and functional effects of long-term lithium therapy. *Kidney Int.* 21 (suppl. 11), S13.

Wallin, L. and Alling, C. (1979). Effect of sustained-release lithium tablets on renal function. *Br. Med. J.* ii, 1332.

Wallin, L., Alling, C., and Aurell, M. (1982). Impairment of renal function in patients on long-term lithium treatment. *Clin. Nephrol.* 18, 23.

Warren, D.J. (1976). Beta-adrenergic receptor blockade and renal function. *Am. Heart J.* 91, 265.

Warrington, R.J., Hogg, G.R., Paraskevas, F., and Tse, K.S. (1977). Insidious rifampin-associated renal failure with light-chain proteiunuria. *Arch. Intern. Med.* 137, 927.

Watts, H.G. (1973). Retroperitoneal fibrosis. *N.Z. Med. J.* 78, 247.

Weinberg, M.S., Quigg, R.J., Salant, D.J., and Bernard, D.B. (1985). Anuric renal failure precipitated by indomethacin and triamterene. *Nephron* 40, 216.

Weinrauch, L.A., Robertson, W.S., and D'Elia, J.A. (1978). Contrast media-induced acute renal failure. Use of creatinine clearance to determine risk in elderly diabetic patients. *JAMA* 239, 2018.

Weisman, J.I. and Bloom, B. (1955). Anuria following phenyl-butazone therapy. *N. Engl. J. Med.* 252, 1086.

Weisman, S.M., Felsen, D., and Vaughan, E.D., Jr (1985). Indications and contraindications for the use of nonsteroidal antiinflammatory drugs in urology. *Semin. Urol.* 3, 301.

Weiss, A.S., Markenson, J.A., Weiss, M.S., and Krammerer, W.H. (1978). Toxicity of D-penicillamine in rheumatoid arthritis. *Am. J. Med.* 64, 114.

Wharton, J.G., Oliver, D.O., and Dunnill, M.S. (1982). Acute renal failure associated with diflunisal. *Postgrad. Med. J.* 58, 104.

Whelan, T.V., Bacon, M.E., Madden, M., Patel, T.G., and Handy, R. (1984). Acute renal failure associated with mannitol intoxication. *Arch. Intern. Med.* 144, 2053.

Whelton, A., Bender, W., Vaghaiwalla, F., Hall-Craggs, M., and Solez, K. (1983). Sulindac and renal impairment. *JAMA* 249, 2892.

Whiting, P.H., Cunningham, C., Thomson, A.W., and Simpson, J.G. (1984). Enhancement of high dose cyclosporin A toxicity by frusemide. *Biochem. Pharmacol.* 33, 1075.

Whitworth, J.A., Mills, E.H., Coghlan, J.P., McDougall, J.G., Nelson, M.A., Spence, C.D., *et al.* (1987). The haemodynamic effects of cyclosporine A in sheep. *Clin. Exp. Pharmacol. Physiol.* 14, 573.

Wigley, R.A.D. (1976). The New Zealand experience. *Aust. N.Z. J. Med.* 6 (suppl. 1), 37.

Wiles, C.M., Assem, E.S.K., Cohen, S.L., and Fisher, C. (1979). Cephradine-induced interstitial nephritis. *Clin. Exp. Immunol.* 36, 342.

Wilkinson, R. (1979). Beta-blockers, blood sugar control, and renal function. *Br. Med. J.* i, 617.

Wilkinson, R. (1982). Beta-blockers and renal function. *Drugs* 23, 195.

Wilkinson, R., Muckle, T.J., and Kerr, D.N.S. (1965) Dextran nephrosis. *Proc. Eur. Dial. Transplant. Assoc.* 2, 320.

Wilkinson, S.P., Blendis, L.M., and Williams, R. (1974). Frequency and type of renal and electrolyte disorders in fulminant hepatic failure. *Br. Med. J.* i, 186.

Wilkinson, S.P., Stewart, W.K., Spiers, E.M., and Pears, J. (1989). Protracted systemic illness and interstitial nephritis

due to minocycline. *Postgrad. Med. J.* 65, 53.

Williams, G. and Hughes, M. (1974). Post-partum renal failure. *J. Pathol.* 114, 149.

Wilson, D.R. (1972). Analgesic nephropathy in Canada: a retrospective study of 351 cases. *Can. Med. Assoc. J.* 107, 752.

Wilson, M., Brown, D.J., Brown, R.W., and Agan, J.M. (1974). Renal failure from alpha-methyldopa therapy. *Aust. N.Z. J. Med.* 4, 415.

Winearls, C.G. and Kerr, D.N.S. (1985). In *Textbook of adverse drug reactions* (3rd edn) (ed. D.M. Davies), p. 291. Oxford University Press.

Wing, A.J., Brunner, F.P., Geerlings, W., Broyer, M., Brynger, H., Fassbinder, W., *et al.* (1989) Contribution of toxic nephropathies to end-stage renal failure in Europe: a report from EDTA–ERA registry. *Toxicol. Lett.* 46, 281.

Winston, J.A. and Safirstein, R. (1985). Reduced renal blood flow in early cisplatin-induced acute renal failure in the rat. *Am. J. Physiol.* 249, F490.

Wolfe, S.M. (1987). Suprofen-induced transient flank pain and renal failure. *N. Engl. J. Med.* 316, 1025.

Wong, E.G.C., Rowe, P.H., Blumenkrantz, M.J., and Coburn, J.W. (1974). Nephrotoxicity associated with use of methoxyflurane. *Nephron* 13, 174.

Wong, N.L., Magil, A.B., and Dirks, J.H. (1989). Effect of magnesium diet in gentamicin-induced acute renal failure in rats. *Nephron* 51, 84.

Wood, I.K., Parmelee, D.X., and Foreman, J.W. (1989). Lithium-induced nephrotic syndrome. *Am. J. Psychiatry* 146, 84.

Wright, A.D., Barber, S.G., Kendall, M.J., and Poole, P.H. (1979). Beta-adrenoceptor-blocking drugs and blood sugar control in diabetes mellitus. *Br. Med. J.* i, 159.

Yarom, R., Stein, H., Peters, P.D., Slavin, S., and Hall, T.A. (1975). Nephrotoxic effect of parenteral and intraarticular gold. *Arch. Pathol.* 99, 36.

Yermakov, V.M., Hitti, I.F., and Sutton, A.L. (1983). Necrotizing vasculitis associated with diphenylhydantoin: two fatal cases. *Hum. Pathol.* 14, 182.

Yeshurun, D., Dakak, N., Khoury, K., and Daher, E. (1989). Acute severe myositis due to bezafibrate treatment. *Harefuah* 116, 261.

Ying, L.S. and Johnson, C.A. (1989). Ciprofloxacin-induced interstitial nephritis. *Clin. Pharm.* 8, 518.

Zaal, M.J., de Vries, J., and Boen-Tan, Y.T. (1988). Is cyclosporin toxic to endothelial cells? *Lancet* ii, 956.

Zipser, R.D. and Henrich, W.L. (1986). Implications of nonsteroidal anti-inflammatory drug therapy. *Am. J. Med.* 80, 78.

Zoja, C., Furci, L., Ghilardi, F., Zilio, P, Benigni, A., and Remuzzi, G. (1986). Cyclosporin-induced endothelial cell injury. *Lab. Invest.* 55, 455.

Zürcher, H.U., Meier, H.R., Huber, M., Lammli, J., Wick, A., and Binswanger, U. (1977). Akutes Nierenversagen als Komplikation von Fastenkuren. *Schweiz. Med. Wochenschr.* 107, 1025.

13. Endocrine disorders

V. T. F. YEUNG and C. S. COCKRAM

Introduction

Drugs having actions on endocrine systems can be classified into two major categories: (1) those used primarily in the management of endocrine problems; and (2) those used primarily for other disorders but fortuitously affecting endocrine function.

The mechanisms of their actions are best understood in the light of their effects on control of hormone secretion and hormone action. Carbimazole and thyroxine, when given in excess, produce hypothyroidism and hyperthyroidism respectively. Amiodarone and lithium, however, may produce hypothyroidism or (less commonly) hyperthyroidism. Even these apparently contradictory effects can be explained by alterations in iodine metabolism and possibly also in immunomodulation. Excessive doses of glucocorticoids for a prolonged period will produce both Cushing's syndrome and suppression of the hypothalamic–pituitary–adrenal axis with a concomitant fall in endogenous glucocorticoid production. Ketoconazole, an antifungal agent acting on the fungal cytochrome P-450-dependent enzyme, induces adrenal crisis because of the concomitant and dose-dependent effect on the mammalian steroidogenic enzymes. Some psychotherapeutic agents, owing to their pharmacological effects on central dopaminergic or serotoninergic pathways, lead incidentally to hyperprolactinaemia and galactorrhoea. Even gynaecomastia, a superficially bizarre adverse effect of spironolactone, is in fact a dose-dependent oestrogen-like action of the drug. Thus, the adverse effects of drugs on endocrine function, although diverse, can mainly be explained as dose-related pharmacological reactions (augmented or Type A) rather than idiosyncratic (bizarre or Type B) reactions.

Drugs can also interfere with the investigation and diagnosis of endocrine disease by interfering with assay and measurement procedures. For example, certain medications can affect binding of hormone to binding proteins in blood, such as thyroxine-binding globulin. This can result in misdiagnosis of hyperthyroidism or hypothyroidism unless appropriate assay procedures are carried out. Other drugs can interfere with such hormonal assays as those for vanillylmandelic acid (VMA) or 5-hydroxyindole acetic acid (5-HIAA), either directly or by effects on the assayed metabolites, again potentially leading to erroneous diagnoses.

Knowledge of adverse effects of drugs is therefore essential to the diagnosis of drug-induced endocrine disorders and avoidance of misinterpretation of the results of endocrine investigations.

The hypothalamic–pituitary–thyroid axis

The thyroid gland synthesizes, stores, and secretes the thyroid hormones thyroxine and tri-iodothyronine. This function is controlled by pituitary thyroid-stimulating hormone (TSH), although there may be partial autoregulation by the thyroid itself. TSH is a glycoprotein hormone secreted under the control of hypothalamic neurohormones: stimulation by thyrotrophin-releasing hormone (TRH) and inhibition by dopamine and somatostatin. There is also evidence that noradrenaline, serotonin, and possibly other central neurotransmitters interact with the hypothalamic regulatory hormones in the control of thyrotrophin function. The thyroid hormones exert feedback control on the secretion of TSH at both the hypothalamic and pituitary levels. A reduced circulating thyroid hormone level stimulates the secretion of TSH. Conversely, an excess of the circulating thyroid hormones inhibits the release of TSH and probably TRH production. Other hormones, including sex hormones and corticosteroids, can also modulate TSH secretion.

More than 99 per cent of thyroxine (T_4) and tri-iodothyronine (T_3) in the blood are bound to proteins (mainly thyroxine-binding globulin, TBG), and only 1–2 per cent of circulating thyroid hormone is in the form of T_3. T_4 is converted peripherally, however, into T_3, which is three to four times as potent, and the inactive metabolite reverse T_3 (rT_3). It is believed that the small amounts of free T_4 (FT_4) and free T_3 (FT_3) mediate the biological actions, whereas the protein-bound fractions are inactive and serve as a storage pool of hormones.

Drugs affecting TRH and TSH production

Impaired TSH secretion

Therapeutic doses of thyroid hormones, particularly with T_4 greater than $200\,\mu g$ per day, can suppress TSH secretion (Evered et al. 1973; Erfurth and Hedner 1982). Pharmacological doses of glucocorticoids can impair basal and TRH-stimulated TSH concentrations (Wilber and Utiger 1969; Nicoloff et al. 1970; Otsuki et al. 1973). Dopamine and dopaminergic agents such as levodopa and bromocriptine inhibit basal TSH secretion and reduce the TSH response to TRH stimulation (Miyai et al. 1974; Refetoff et al. 1974; Kaptein et al. 1980), and some authors have questioned the safety of prolonged use of dopamine in critically ill patients because of the possibility of inducing secondary hypothyroidism and thus worsening the prognosis (Varl et al. 1988). Serotonin antagonists (metergoline, cyproheptadine), used for treatment of hyperprolactinaemia and for appetite stimulation, have been found to decrease TSH secretion (Ferrari et al. 1976; Delitala et al. 1978). Reserpine, a classic depletor of biogenic monoamines, and phentolamine, an α-blocking agent, reduce basal TSH and block the TSH response to cold stimulation (Tuomisto et al. 1973). Lowering of basal serum TSH concentration also occurs in patients with chronic renal failure treated with heparin. This was once attributed to increased FT_4 and FT_3 concentrations induced by heparin but is now regarded as an artefact (see section on Free thyroid hormone assays) (Mendel et al. 1987; Vagenakis 1988).

Enhanced TSH secretion

The neuroleptics chlorpromazine and haloperidol and other dopamine-receptor blocker drugs such as metoclopramide and sulpiride can raise basal TSH and enhance the TSH response to TRH (Kirkegaard et al. 1977, 1978; Massara et al. 1978; Scanlon et al. 1979). Theophylline increases TSH and T_4, possibly through β-adrenergic stimulation of the hypothalamus (Faglia et al. 1972; Hikita et al. 1989). Since TSH release is under feedback control by thyroid hormones, any goitrogenic medications that produce hypothyroidism can lead to compensatory increases in TSH concentrations.

Drugs affecting the thyroid

Iodine

Iodine preparations have diverse effects upon the thyroid. Acute administration of high doses of iodine inhibits the release of hormone from the thyroid. This effect is transient but has been used in the preparation of patients for thyroid surgery and in the management of thyroid crisis. Further, the iodine can suppress thyroid hormone formation, which is known as the Wolff–Chaikoff effect (Wolff and Chaikoff 1948). Prolonged exposure to iodide is accompanied by reduction in iodide trapping and inhibition of synthesis of thyroid hormones, leading to hypothyroidism and goitre formation in susceptible subjects (Wolff 1969; Vagenakis and Braverman 1975).

Iodide may exacerbate or cause relapse in patients with previous hyperthyroidism (Jod–Basedow phenomenon). In addition, iodide-induced thyrotoxicosis can occasionally occur in patients with no previous thyroid disease (Fradkin and Wolff 1983; Clark and Hutton 1985).

Hyperthyroidism

Inorganic iodide in the form of potassium iodide used as a cough expectorant can induce thyrotoxicosis, albeit uncommonly (Fradkin and Wolff 1983).

Organic iodine is more often incriminated in causing thyrotoxicosis. Drugs containing organic iodine include amiodarone, iodochlorhydroxyquinoline, the uricosuric benziodarone, and radiographic contrast media. Features of iodine-induced thyrotoxicosis include an absence of exophthalmos, a low incidence of antithyroid antibodies, and a low uptake of radioiodine, and a tendency for the hyperthyroidism to be self-limiting (1–6 months) on cessation of the medication.

Amiodarone is a widely used antiarrhythmic agent containing 37% iodine by weight. As much as 18 mg of iodine per day may be released from the usual maintenance dose (200–600 mg) of the drug, which is considerably in excess of the usual daily dietary intake of less than $200\,\mu g$ (Kennedy et al. 1989). The heavy iodine load is largely responsible for its profound effect on thyroid function, although the drug might also initiate an autoimmune process (Wiersinga and Trip 1986; Kennedy et al. 1988). Amiodarone causes increases in T_4 and rT_3 and a reduction of T_3 (Gammage and Franklyn 1987). The effect becomes evident a week after initiating therapy and is due to suppression of peripheral deiodination of T_4 to T_3 by inhibition of the enzyme 5′-monodeiodinase (Melmed et al. 1981; Aanderud et al. 1984). These changes are accompanied by an increase in the basal and

TRH-stimulated TSH levels, mostly within the normal range and in the first few weeks (Burger *et al.* 1976). Continuation of amiodarone is associated with a further rise in plasma T_4, free T_4, rT_3 and a fall in plasma T_3. TSH levels return gradually to pretreatment values and a steady state of thyroid hormone concentrations is reached by 3–4 months (Melmed *et al.* 1981). Clinically significant hyperthyroidism ranges from 1–23 per cent in different reports from different geographical areas. It tends to be higher in areas of iodine deficiency (Martino *et al.* 1984), and thyroid dysfunction is more common in subjects with a past history or family history of thyroid disease and in people with goitre (Amico *et al.* 1984). Autoimmunity does not, however, seem to play a significant role in the development of amiodarone-induced thyrotoxicosis (Martino *et al.* 1986a). Because of its non-specific adrenoceptor-blocking properties, amiodarone can mask many of the clinical features of hyperthyroidism. Weight loss and tiredness are often the presenting symptoms. Thyrotoxicosis should also be suspected if the heart rate exceeds the pretreatment value or when arrhythmia recurs or worsens during amiodarone therapy (Gammage and Franklyn 1987; Nademanee *et al.* 1989). No single hormonal test reliably predicts thyroid dysfunction associated with amiodarone therapy. If hyperthyroidism is suspected on clinical grounds, an increase in serum T_3, in addition to an increase in T_4, confirms the diagnosis, which is supported further by a suppressed TSH concentration or an absent TSH response to TRH. A normal T_3 does not, however, rule out hyperthyroidism since the value observed might be lowered by concomitant non-thyroidal illness. Further, many euthyroid patients on treatment with amiodarone can exhibit a blunted TSH response to TRH. Treatment of amiodarone-induced thyrotoxicosis may be difficult. Patients without goitre tend to remit spontaneously with discontinuation of medication (Martino *et al.* 1986b; Mechlis *et al.* 1987). Hyperthyroidism can be severe, however, and in some patients amiodarone may be the only effective drug for the underlying arrhythmia and therefore not able to be stopped. Treatment with radioactive iodine will not be effective, since its uptake is blocked; and thyroidectomy is contraindicated in patients with uncontrolled hyperthyroidism and underlying cardiac disease. In these cases, a combination of potassium perchlorate and thionamide, which prevents further iodine uptake and inhibits hormone synthesis, has been used with success (Martino *et al.* 1987a; Reichert and de Rooy 1989).

Lithium has been associated with thyrotoxicosis (Cubitt 1976; Reus *et al.* 1979) and there has been a report of hypothyroidism followed by hyperthyroidism during lithium treatment (McDermott *et al.* 1986). It is postulated that the underlying event is an iodide-induced thyrotoxicosis in susceptible patients due to blockade by lithium of thyroid iodine release and hence expansion of the intrathyroidal iodide pool.

Reversible hyperthyroxinaemia can be induced by heavy amphetamine abuse, which also produces clinical features resembling those of thyrotoxicosis (Morley *et al.* 1980). The elevation of T_4 concentration is apparently secondary to increased TSH secretion as a result of amphetamine effects on the hypothalamus or pituitary. One biochemical feature that may help to distinguish this from Graves' disease is that T_4 is inappropriately raised compared with T_3. Thyrotoxicosis with a similar thyroid hormone profile can also result from deliberate or accidental intake of exogenous thyroid hormones, as demonstrated by thyrotoxicosis due to consumption of hamburgers in the USA (Cohen III *et al.* 1989).

Hypothyroidism

Hypothyroidism can occur with prolonged administration of iodide. It can also be caused by over-treatment with antithyroid medications such as carbimazole and propylthiouracil. Many drugs not primarily employed for treatment of thyroid disorders can induce hypothyroidism and goitre by affecting the trapping of iodine or interfering with the synthesis or release of thyroid hormones. These are listed in Table 13.1.

Monovalent anions, such as perchlorate, block the uptake of iodine (Morgans and Trotter 1954). Amiodarone directly affects the trapping of iodine, but its dominant effect is inhibition of the synthesis and release of thyroid hormones (Wolff 1969). The incidence of hypothyroidism varies from 0.75–10 per cent (Borowski *et al.* 1985). In areas of iodine repletion, hypothyroidism is a more common complication than thyrotoxicosis (Martino *et al.* 1984). The presence of serum thyroid antibodies indicates a greater risk of development of amiodarone-induced hypothyroidism. About 50 per cent have circulating antithyroid antibodies at diagnosis. In patients without underlying thyroid disorders, the hypothyroidism remits spontaneously whereas it may persist in patients with underlying thyroid problems, particularly in those with positive thyroid antibodies (Martino *et al.* 1987b). On the other hand, amiodarone treatment does not seem to increase the incidence of antithyroid antibodies (Safran *et al.* 1988). Therefore, in some cases, hypothyroidism may represent unmasking of autoimmune thyroiditis in susceptible subjects, whereas in others the inhibitory effect of iodine on the thyroid may be the only factor. Classical hypothyroid symptoms may occur, but the hypothyroidism is often

TABLE 13.1
*Drugs inhibiting the synthesis and release
of thyroid hormones*

Inhibition of iodine trapping
Lithium (acute effect)
Potassium perchlorate

Inhibition of organification and iodotyrosine coupling

Adrenal suppressants	aminoglutethimide
	high-dose ketoconazole
Antiarrhythmic	amiodarone
Antirheumatic drugs	oxyphenbutazone
	phenylbutazone
Antithyroid drugs	carbimazole
	methimazole
	propylthiouracil
Antituberculous drugs	ethionamide
	p-aminosalicylic acid
	rifampicin
Sulphonamides	co-trimoxazole
	sulphadiazine
Miscellaneous	chlorpromazine
	pentazocine
	sulphonylureas

Inhibition of release
Amiodarone
Iodide (large doses)
Lithium (chronic effect)

relatively asymptomatic (subclinical) and detected by thyroid function tests in patients with minimal symptoms (Hawthorne *et al*. 1985). The diagnosis of amiodarone-induced hypothyroidism is confirmed by the demonstration of raised TSH levels and decreased thyroid hormones, although T_4 may remain within the normal range (Kennedy *et al*. 1989; Nademanee *et al*. 1989). Treatment is with T_4 replacement as guided by the clinical state, if amiodarone cannot be discontinued. Complete normalization of TSH levels may be unfavourable in some patients, because a dose sufficient to achieve this may lead to exacerbation of underlying cardiac problems.

Lithium is another goitrogenic agent commonly used in manic-depressive disorders. The reported prevalence of goitre in patients treated with this drug varies from 0–61.5 per cent (Lazarus 1982). Acutely, lithium blocks the uptake of iodine and release of thyroid hormones, possibly by inhibiting TSH-stimulated adenylate cyclase and blocking the effect of cyclic AMP on the biosynthetic pathway (Singer and Rotenberg 1973). During long-term administration, the uptake of iodine is enhanced but the release of thyroid hormones remains impaired.

In the past, hypothyroidism was considered to be a common complication of lithium treatment, the incidence ranging from 10–34 per cent in various lithium clinics (Hullin 1978). More recent long-term studies by Smigan and others (1984) and Maarbjerg and colleagues (1987) show, however, that although T_3 and T_4 tend to fall in the first few months of treatment, they return to pretreatment levels after 12 months and can exceed the pre-lithium values afterwards. Conversely, TSH tends to rise in the first few months but gradually returns to pretreatment levels after more than 12 months. Only about 2 per cent of patients develop clinical features of hypothyroidism and require thyroxine replacement. Single deviant thyroid hormone results during lithium treatment can, therefore, be transient and it now seems wise to subject the patient to re-examination at intervals before starting thyroxine, unless clinical features of hypothyroidism become overt.

Other agents that have antithyroid potential include the adrenal suppressants aminoglutethimide (Hughes and Burley 1970) and ketoconazole (Namer *et al*. 1986); the antituberculous drugs *p*-aminosalicylic acid (MacGregor and Somner 1954), ethionamide (Moulding and Fraser 1970), and possibly rifampicin (Isley 1987); sulphonamides (Milne and Greer 1962; Cohen *et al*. 1980); and the NSAID phenylbutazone (Morgans and Trotter 1955; Aboidun *et al*. 1973) and oxyphenbutazone (Lane *et al*. 1977). These agents apparently act through inhibition of thyroid hormone synthesis by blocking organic binding of iodine.

There have been isolated case reports of hypothyroidism following treatment with cyclophosphamide (Coffey 1971) and possible aggravation of hypothyroidism after pentazocine (Evans *et al*. 1972) and chlorpromazine (Mitchell *et al*. 1959).

Although sulphonylureas are known to lower circulating thyroid hormone concentrations, possibly by suppressing organification of iodine, no increased incidence of hypothyroidism with the use of these drugs has been demonstrated.

Drugs interfering with thyroid function tests

Interference with total hormone measurements due to effects on thyroid-hormone-binding proteins

Since more than 99 per cent of thyroid hormones are protein-bound (mainly as TBG), drug-induced changes in the concentration of transport proteins or inhibition of binding to these proteins can give rise to falsely high or low values, leading to misdiagnosis of hypothyroidism or hyperthyroidism. Table 13.2 provides a list of drugs with these effects.

TABLE 13.2
Drugs affecting thyroid-hormone-binding protein

Increase in TBG levels

Clofibrate
Fluorouracil
Oestrogens (including oral contraceptives)
Opiates (heroin, methadone)

Decrease in TBG levels

Androgens
Colaspase (asparaginase)
Colestipol/niacin (nicotinic acid)
Danazol
Glucocorticoids

Interference with hormone binding to transport proteins

Diazepam
Fenclofenac
Frusemide
o,p'-DDD
Phenylbutazone
Phenytoin
Salicylates
Sulphonylureas

The use of oestrogens and oral contraceptives is associated with an increase in serum T_4 and thyroxine-binding globulin concentration due to increased hepatic synthesis of TBG (Engbring and Engstrom 1959; Doe *et al.* 1967; Bockner and Roman 1967; Laurell *et al.* 1967; Walden *et al.* 1986). In heroin and methadone addicts, increases in TBG concentration and hence serum T_4 and T_3 levels may occur (Azizi *et al.* 1974). Similar phenomena have also been observed following therapy with the lipid-lowering agent clofibrate and the cytotoxic agent fluorouracil (McKerron *et al.* 1969; Beex *et al.* 1976).

Androgens (including danazol) and anabolic steroids reduce the TBG and serum T_4 concentrations despite an increase in TBPA capacity (Engbring and Engstrom 1959; Braverman and Ingbar 1967; Dickinson *et al.* 1969; Barbosa *et al.* 1971; Pannall and Maas 1977). Acute transient reduction in TBG and T_4 values occurs during treatment with colaspase (asparaginase) for acute leukaemia (Garnick and Larsen 1979; Heidemann *et al.* 1980). Combined colestipol (a bile acid sequestrant) and nicotinic acid therapy for hypercholesterolaemia has been reported to lower T_4 significantly, 19 per cent of patients having values in the hypothyroid range (Cashin-Hemphill *et al.* 1987). Large doses of glucocorticoids suppress TBG binding capacity but enhance that of the thyroxine-binding prealbumin. These effects tend to offset each other, and therefore the decrease in thyroid

hormones (Werner and Platman 1965; Oppenheimer and Werner 1966) could be due to other mechanisms, such as reduction in thyroid secretion (Chopra *et al.* 1975).

A number of drugs compete with thyroid hormones for TBG, and reduce total thyroid hormone levels. Such displacement often leads to increased metabolism and turnover of the free hormones. Salicylates compete with thyroid-hormone binding to transport proteins, resulting in a reduction of total T_4 and T_3 concentrations but elevation of the free hormones (Larsen 1972) that could account for the reduced basal and TRH-stimulated TSH concentrations as well as the hypermetabolic effects (Dussault *et al.* 1976; Langer *et al.* 1978). Both phenytoin and fenclofenac inhibit thyroid-hormone binding to TBG (Wolff *et al.* 1961; Chin and Schussler 1968; Taylor *et al.* 1980) and lead to alteration of hormone metabolism, although the displacement itself plays only a minor role in the reduction of serum concentrations of thyroid hormones (see below). o,p'-DDD, a compound that is chemically similar to phenytoin, also lowers the T_4 concentration by competitive binding to TBG (Marshall and Tompkins 1968). High concentrations of frusemide cause a dose-dependent inhibition of T_4 binding and may contribute to the low T_4 state in critically ill patients (Stockigt *et al.* 1984). Diazepam (Schussler 1971) and sulphonylureas (Hershman *et al.* 1968) also compete for thyroid-hormone binding proteins but the effects are not of clinical significance.

With the increasing availability of reliable assays for free T_4 and free T_3, and sensitive TSH assays, problems of interpretation of binding protein effects on thyroid function assessment have been lessened.

Interference due to alteration of thyroid hormone metabolism

Phenytoin increases the metabolism and clearance of thyroid hormones, presumably due to hepatic enzyme induction. This leads to reduction of both total and free thyroid hormone concentrations. The patients are clinically euthyroid, however, and TSH levels remain normal (Larsen *et al.* 1970; Liewendahl *et al.* 1978; Yeo *et al.* 1978; Cavalieri *et al.* 1979). This may be explained by achievement of a new steady state in which the increased rate of thyroid hormone clearance is balanced by a reduction in the free thyroid hormone pool or increased generation of T_3 from T_4 (Faber *et al.* 1985) or both.

Fenclofenac, an NSAID with structural similarity to thyroxine, is the most potent drug known to interfere with the binding of thyroid hormones to serum protein. It displaces T_4 and T_3 from TBG (Taylor *et al.* 1980), leading to transient reduction in TSH and a reduced TSH response to TRH (Kurtz *et al.* 1981). This gradually returns to normal after 2–4 weeks of treatment, as a new steady state is achieved between bound and free hormone pools. Free T_4 and T_3 concentrations tend to remain at low normal levels, however, presumably due to increased clearance with formation of a new steady state. Despite these biochemical changes there is no observable clinical disturbance.

β-Blockers such as propranolol and nadolol reduce the concentrations of T_3 relative to T_4 (Lotti et al. 1977; Peden et al. 1982). They appear to block 5'-deiodination and diminish the peripheral conversion of T_4 to T_3 (Heyma et al. 1980). Hyperthyroxinaemia has been reported in euthyroid patients taking high doses of propranolol (Cooper et al. 1982). Studies with other β-blockers (Nilsson et al. 1979; How et al. 1980) suggest that the benefits on control of thyrotoxic symptoms are more related to sympathetic inhibitory activity than to their action on peripheral T_4/T_3 metabolism.

As with amiodarone, the radiographic contrast agents ipodate and iopanoic acid block the T_4 conversion to T_3 in peripheral tissues and in the anterior pituitary (Kaplan and Utiger 1978; Larsen et al. 1979). Administration of these agents leads to decreased serum T_3 and increased rT_3. There is also enhancement of basal and TRH-stimulated TSH concentrations, possibly in response to the reduction in circulating and intrapituitary T_3 (Burgi et al. 1976; Suzuki et al. 1979). These hormonal changes return to normal after 2 weeks of exposure (Suzuki et al. 1981).

Propylthiouracil, though predominantly an inhibitor of synthesis of thyroid hormone, also suppresses the conversion of T_4 to T_3 and leads to preferential formation of the inactive metabolite reverse T_3 (rT_3) shortly after administration in high dosage. This may be an advantage, at least theoretically, in the treatment of thyrotoxicosis, particularly in severe cases (Westgren et al. 1977; Laurberg and Weeke 1978). High doses of glucocorticoids have a similar effect on T_4/T_3 metabolism (Chopra et al. 1975; Burr et al. 1976). This provides a rational basis for the use of propylthiouracil and steroids in the emergency management of thyroid storm.

Serum total T_4 and free T_4 may be decreased by rifampicin, presumably due to enhanced hepatic metabolism and biliary excretion. In contrast, the level of T_3 increases but the mechanism of this still awaits elucidation (Ohnhaus et al. 1981).

Interference of indirect methods of thyroid hormone measurement (*in vitro* uptake tests)

The *in vitro* uptake tests measure the unoccupied thyroid hormone binding sites on TBG. The tests involve the use of T_3 or T_4 labelled with [125]Iodine and some form of synthetic absorbent (usually an ion-exchange resin) to measure the proportion of radioactive hormone that is not tightly bound to serum proteins, and are accordingly named the resin T_3 or T_4 uptake tests. The uptake of the tracer is inversely proportional to the number of unsaturated binding sites. Thus, the uptake is increased when the amount of TBG decreases owing to excess thyroid hormone or reduction of TBG level. Conversely, an increase in the amount of unsaturated TBG due to a low serum thyroid hormone concentration or an increase of TBG results in a reduced uptake value. The techniques provide an indirect measure of total serum thyroxine, and the free thyroxine index thus derived corrects for changes in TBG levels induced by drugs. The uptake test results are still invalidated, however, by compounds that compete with thyroid hormone binding to TBG. The need for these tests in clinical practice has been reduced by the increased availability of assays that directly measure free T_4 and free T_3 concentrations.

Interference with free thyroid hormone assays

In the past, the direct measurement of free thyroid hormones in serum using equilibrium dialysis was limited to a few research laboratories. The advent of the simple free thyroid hormone assay employing labelled hormone tracers or, more commonly, labelled hormone analogues, has made the technique widely available and greatly obviated the problem of interference by drugs affecting the binding capacity of serum proteins (e.g. oral contraceptives, phenytoin). The labelled T_4 analogue binds to the hormone antibody and, theoretically, not to carrying proteins, thus competing only with the free hormones in the serum. It does bind to albumin (Pearce and Byfield 1986), however, and in one labelled-analogue radioimmunoassay heparin can produce low free T_4 results as an artefact (Mardell and Gamlen 1982). This is due to activation of lipoprotein lipase and production of free fatty acids that compete with the analogue for the binding sites on albumin. Interference by heparin also occurs with free T_4 measurement by equilibrium dialysis. Contrary to the analogue assay, however, the free fatty acids generated lead to falsely elevated free T_4 values (Mendel et al. 1987).

Effects on *in vivo* tests of thyroid gland activity

Thyroid radioiodine uptake, previously used for diagnosis of hypothyroidism and hyperthyroidism, has now been largely superseded by measurement of serum free hormones. It is still used in some centres, however, for estimating the dose of radioiodide to be delivered in the therapy of thyrotoxicosis and thyroid carcinoma and remains a valuable investigation in the diagnosis of thyrotoxicosis secondary to transient thyroiditis, iodine excess, exogenous thyroxine, or drugs such as lithium and amiodarone when radioiodine uptake is suppressed despite the presence of thyrotoxicosis. Uptake studies and thyroid scanning can be significantly affected by changes in the body iodine pool caused by intake of iodine-containing drugs and radiographic contrast media. The antithyroid or goitrogenic medications can also interfere with trapping and retention of iodide and thus the results of these investigations.

Hypothalamic–pituitary–adrenal axis

Synthesis and secretion of cortisol are controlled by ACTH (corticotrophin), a 39-aminoacid polypeptide derived from the precursor molecule pro-opiomelanocortin. Hypothalamic corticotrophin-releasing hormone (CRH) is the predominant regulator of ACTH formation and release by the pituitary. A parallel effect is seen with β-endorphin and with other pro-opiomelanocortin-related gene products. In man CRH is a 41-amino acid straight chain peptide (Vale *et al.* 1983). Among hormones of hypothalamic origin that can influence ACTH secretion (oxytocin, adrenaline, somatostatin, and vaso-active intestinal peptide), arginine vasopressin is most important in modulating pituitary ACTH release and it potentiates the action of CRH significantly (Gillies *et al.* 1982; De Bold *et al.* 1984). The cytokines interleukins 1 and 6 have been shown to enhance ACTH release, principally through stimulation of CRH (Uehara *et al.* 1987; Sapolsky *et al.* 1987; Naitoh *et al.* 1988). In this way they may act as an interface for communication between the endocrine and immune system.

Drugs affecting CRH and ACTH

Impaired CRH and ACTH secretion

CRH and ACTH secretion is impaired by negative feedback effects of glucocorticoids exerted at the hypothalamus and pituitary. Acute inhibition by corticosteroids occurs rapidly (within minutes) and is mediated via a membrane-dependent effect on the secretion of the hormones. Continued slow-onset feedback, however, involves suppression of hormone formation via an inhibitory effect on gene transcription (Taylor and Fishman 1988).

Physiological replacement doses of glucocorticoid hormones (hydrocortisone 20–30 mg, prednisone 7.5 mg or dexamethasone 0.5 mg daily) given for up to 18 months do not seem to cause suppression of ACTH secretion and cortisol levels (Livanou *et al.* 1967). High-

dose glucocorticoid administration of short duration, such as in the treatment of acute severe asthma, also produces only transient (<10 days) hypothalamic–pituitary–adrenal axis (HPA) suppression (Zora *et al.* 1986).

Marked suppression of the HPA axis can, however, occur with the prolonged use of supraphysiological doses of glucocorticoids. It may also follow chronic topical application of steroids, especially fluorinated preparations, because of systemic absorption (Sneddon 1976). Adrenal hypofunction can also develop with high doses of inhaled steroid (e.g. >1500 μg beclomethasone dipropionate) for treatment of asthma (Smith and Hodson 1983). The recovery of suppressed pituitary–adrenal function after cessation of therapy has been reported to take as long as 9 months (Graber *et al.* 1965), and our own experience suggests that much longer intervals are occasionally required. During this recovery period and for an additional 1–2 years, the patient will need steroid cover during periods of stress (Bayliss 1975).

Cyproterone acetate, an antiandrogen, may also reduce basal and stress-induced rises in ACTH if given for more than 3 months (Jeffcoate *et al.* 1976; Smals *et al.* 1978).

Increased ACTH production

The administration of amphetamines stimulates production of ACTH (Besser *et al.* 1969). Metoclopramide can cause increases in ACTH and cortisol secretion, possibly through an antidopaminergic action on the central pituitary dopamine receptors (Nishida *et al.* 1983a, 1987). Metyrapone and aminoglutethimide, by blocking the synthesis of cortisol, can stimulate secretion of ACTH by secondary reduction in negative feedback (Dexter *et al.* 1967). ACTH secretion also increases in response to an investigational drug RU 486, a glucocorticoid-receptor blocker used for the treatment of Cushing's syndrome, and can in turn stimulate further cortisol production, thus overcoming the effect of the drug in patients with pituitary-dependent Cushing's syndrome (Schteingart 1989). A feedback rise of ACTH secretion in this condition also occurs in response to metyrapone and may serve both to attenuate the effectiveness of the drug in treating Cushing's disease and to increase the likelihood of potentially troublesome adverse effects such as hirsutism.

Drugs affecting the adrenal cortex

Cushing's syndrome

Iatrogenic Cushing's syndrome can occur with the administration of pharmacological doses of glucocorticoids or ACTH. Prolonged and excessive alcohol ingestion can also lead to alcoholic pseudo-Cushing's syndrome (Lamberts *et al.* 1979) which improves rapidly following withdrawal of alcohol. The disorder is most likely to be due to a centrally mediated mechanism with hypersecretion of pituitary ACTH and secondary stimulation of the adrenals (Kapcala 1987; Kirkman and Nelson 1988).

Hypoadrenalism

Adrenocortical failure can develop in patients who have been previously treated with suppressive doses of glucocorticoids if appropriate steroid cover is not given following withdrawal. Hypoadrenalism can also occur in patients with Cushing's syndrome treated with aminoglutethimide, metyrapone, or *o,p'*-DDD, which block the steroid biosynthetic pathway. Both aminoglutethimide and *o,p'*-DDD inhibit the cholesterol side-chain-cleavage enzymes and 11-β-hydroxylase (Hughes and Burley 1970). In addition, *o,p'*-DDD, or more probably its metabolites, destroys cell mitochondria, leading to adrenocortical cell death (Sparagana 1987). Metyrapone inhibits 11-β-hydroxylase and blocks the final step of cortisol synthesis.

Ketoconazole is an imidazole derivative with a potent inhibitory effect on adrenal steroidogenesis. It interferes with the P-450-cytochrome enzymes, which include 17-20 desmolase (side-chain cleavage), 11- and 21-hydroxylase, 17-20 lyase, and 17- and 18-hydroxylase (Sonino 1987; Trachtenberg and Zadra 1988). Acute hypoadrenalism has been reported with both high-dose ketoconazole treatment in Cushing's syndrome and low-dose ketoconazole treatment of fungal infections (McCance *et al.* 1987; Best *et al.* 1987). Etomidate, a short-acting general anaesthetic, is another example of an imidazole derivative with significant inhibitory effects on 11-β-hydroxylase (Preziosi and Vacca 1988). Its use has also been associated with the development of adrenal insufficiency (Ledingham and Watt 1983).

Rifampicin, used in the treatment of mycobacterial infections, has been reported to precipitate acute adrenal insufficiency in patients with compromised adrenal reserve. This action is probably due to enhanced glucocorticoid metabolism, which presumably occurs through induction of microsomal enzymes (Kyriazopoulou *et al.* 1984). It is recommended that treatment with rifampicin in these patients be accompanied by doubling or tripling the dose of replacement steroids. Aminoglutethimide has also been reported to accelerate the degradation of some glucocorticoids, such as dexamethasone (but not hydrocortisone), and this may influence the decision regarding choice of replacement therapy in such patients (Santen *et al.* 1977).

Interference with biochemical tests

Spironolactone, monamine oxidase inhibitors, and minor tranquillizers such as hydroxyzine and chlordiazepoxide can interfere with the colour reaction of the Porter–Silber reactions for measurement of urinary 17-hydroxycorticosteroids (17-OHCS), giving rise to spuriously increased values (Borushek and Gold 1964). Interference with the β-glucuronidase employed in the assay (e.g. by high urinary acetylsalicylic acid concentrations) will lead to falsely low values. Likewise, the Zimmerman reaction for measurement of urinary 17-ketogenic steroids and 17-ketosteroids can be affected by acebutolol (Ooiwa *et al.* 1988), penicillin, and minor tranquillizers (Borsushek and Gold 1964).

Oestrogen, in the form of an oral contraceptive, is the most common drug to cause elevation of plasma cortisol concentrations secondary to change in the concentration of cortisol-binding globulin (CBG). Drugs that are inducers of hepatic mixed function oxidases (phenytoin, phenobarbitone, and *o,p'*-DDD) modify the metabolism of cortisol and related steroids, resulting in increased urinary excretion of 6-hydroxylated steroids and other multihydroxylated derivatives (Werk *et al.* 1964; Bledsoe *et al.* 1964; Burstein and Klaiber 1965). As a consequence, urinary 17-OHCS and 17-ketogenic steroid determinations may be falsely low. These agents also interfere with dexamethasone suppression and metyrapone stimulation tests by inducing enzymes that inactivate these compounds, thus rendering the tests ineffective and potentially leading to erroneous diagnoses of Cushing's syndrome (Meikle *et al.* 1969; Jubiz *et al.* 1970).

In general, radioimmunoassay and related tests on blood and urine show little clinically important cross-reactivity at usual doses with drugs such as dexamethasone and other steroid-based preparations. One important result is that drug-induced Cushing's syndrome secondary to administration of dexamethasone or prednisolone will usually be associated with lowered plasma and urine cortisol concentrations, which will not be the case if the exogenous steroid is hydrocortisone.

Aldosterone synthesis

Aldosterone production is regulated mainly by changes in blood volume, mediated through the renin–angiotensin system, although it can also be affected by changes in potassium and ACTH.

Secondary hyperaldosteronism occurs with the use of thiazide or loop diuretics (Vaughan *et al.* 1978; Griffing and Melby 1989). Lithium therapy has been associated with elevated aldosterone concentration and sodium retention (Murphy *et al.* 1969). Females taking oral contraceptives have raised plasma renin activity and aldosterone concentrations, which may account for the development of hypertension in some susceptible subjects (Beckerhoff *et al.* 1973). Metoclopramide stimulates the secretion of aldosterone through both an ACTH-dependent effect and an antidopaminergic adrenal action (Nishida *et al.* 1983*b*). Hyperaldosteronism with hypertension, relative hypernatraemia and hypokalaemia may be mimicked by the ingestion of large quantities of licorice (Conn *et al.* 1968) or injudicious use of mineralocorticoid agents such as 9-fludrocortisone (Armbruster *et al.* 1975; Whitworth *et al.* 1986) and it is a possible risk of carbenoxolone therapy (Pinder *et al.* 1976; Nicholls and Espiner 1983). Recent evidence suggests that the mineralocorticoid effect of licorice and carbenoxolone is primarily mediated through inhibition of the enzyme 11β-hydroxysteroid dehydrogenase, which catalyzes conversion of cortisol to cortisone, so leading to significant enhancement of the mineralocorticoid effect of cortisol (Stewart *et al.* 1987, 1990; MacKenzie *et al.* 1990).

Angiotensin-converting-enzyme (ACE) inhibitors such as captopril and enalapril can produce hyperreninaemic hypoaldosteronism which manifests as hyperkalaemia with a hyperchloraemic metabolic acidosis (Sakemi *et al.* 1988). Even at low doses, standard or low-molecular-weight heparins given for thromboembolic disorders can produce hypoaldosteronism, usually with a compensatory increase in renin concentration (Sherman and Ruddy 1986; Levesque *et al.* 1990). The effect is thought to occur by inhibition of the conversion of corticosterone to 18-hydroxycorticosterone (Conn *et al.* 1966). Thus, patients with a compromised renin–angiotensin–aldosterone system, as in diabetes mellitus or chronic renal insufficiency, are more prone to the development of hyperkalaemia with heparin administration (Edes and Sunderrajan 1985; Kutyrina *et al.* 1987).

Adrenal medulla

Adverse drug reactions in phaeochromocytoma

These are discussed fully in Chapter 7.

Drug interference with biochemical tests

Drug-induced alterations are perhaps the most common cause of erroneous interpretation of measurement of plasma or urinary catecholamines and their metabolites. Samples should preferably be collected under drug-free conditions. If this is not possible, a knowledge and avoidance of the principal offending medications is important. Drugs that alter sympathochromaffin physiology can affect the secretion of catecholamines or their metabolites, and certain other drugs can interfere with fluorimetric or non-specific chromatographic assays

TABLE 13.3
Drugs interfering with tests of adrenal medullary function

Catecholamines and metanephrines

Elevation	α-Adrenergic antagonists
	phenoxybenzamine, phentolamine,
	prazosin
	β-Adrenergic agonists
	isoprenaline, terbutaline
	β-Adrenoceptor blockers
	propranolol and related drugs
	Diuretics (if Na$^+$ depletion occurs)
	Indirectly acting sympathomimetics
	amphetamines, ephedrine
	Tricyclic antidepressants
	Vasodilators
	calcium-channel blockers (acutely)
	minoxidil, nitrates, phenothiazines,
	theophylline,
	Miscellaneous
	erythromycin
	labetalol, methyldopa, tetracycline
Reduction	ACE inhibitors
	α_2-Adrenergic agonist
	clonidine
	Monoamine oxidase inhibitors
	Miscellaneous
	bromocriptine, dexamethasone,
	α-methyl-paratyrosine

Urinary vanillylmandelic acid (VMA)

Elevation (due	Aspirin
to assay	Nalidixic acid
interference)	Penicillin
	Sulphonamides
Reduction	Clofibrate
	Methyldopa
	Monoamine oxidase inhibitors

N.B. Methyldopa characteristically produces elevated catecholamines, but not VMA, in some conventional chromatographic systems, owing to the production of *o*-methyl metabolites; the interference can be overcome with high-pressure liquid chromatography (HPLC).

(Rayfield *et al.* 1972; Cryer 1985; Feldman 1987; Sheps *et al.* 1988). These are summarized in Table 13.3.

Hypothalamic–pituitary–gonadal axis

In both sexes, the hypothalamus is the integrative centre of the reproductive axis. It receives messages from the central nervous system and from the gonads, which regulate the synthesis and release of gonadotrophin-releasing hormones (GnRH or LHRH). In addition, certain neurotransmitters (catecholamines, serotonin, acetylcholine) and endogenous opioid peptides have modulatory effects on GnRH release.

Episodic, pulsatile release of GnRH is essential for the synthesis and release of the gonadotrophins, namely luteinizing hormone (LH) and follicle-stimulating hormone (FSH), which are glycoproteins synthesized in the anterior pituitary. LH and FSH then bind to receptors at the target cells. In the male, LH stimulates synthesis of testosterone from Leydig cells and FSH promotes spermatogenesis in the germinal epithelium. In the female, FSH action leads to formation of the Graafian follicle which contains the ovum, and LH stimulates production of oestrogen from the follicle and subsequently progesterone from the corpus luteum following ovulation.

The secretion of GnRH and FSH/LH are under negative feedback control from testosterone and oestradiol. In addition, FSH secretion is inhibited by inhibin, a glycoprotein composed of interlinked α- and β-subunits, which is produced in the Sertoli cells of the testis and the granulosa cells of the ovary. In the female, there is also a positive feedback mechanism whereby LH and FSH surge in midcycle in response to increasing oestrogen secretion, and induce ovulation.

Drugs affecting gonadotrophin and gonadal sex hormone secretion

Gonadotrophin and sex hormone dysfunction

Pituitary gonadotrophin secretion can be inhibited by glucocorticoid excess, resulting in testicular or ovarian dysfunction with suppressed spermatogenesis and lowering of gonadal sex hormone levels (Sakakura et al. 1973; MacAdams et al. 1986; McClure 1987). Opiates such as heroin and methadone lower testosterone levels without concomitant elevation of gonadotrophin levels. The phenomenon could be due to direct central actions of the drugs and their effects on peripheral androgen metabolism (Mendelson et al. 1975). Ketoconazole decreases testicular production of testosterone by blocking 17,20-desmolase and 17-α-hydroxylase (Rajfer et al. 1986). Danazol, used in the treatment of endometriosis and angioedema, decreases the binding capacity of sex-hormone-binding globulin and increases free testosterone levels, which partially accounts for its adverse effects of hirsutism and virilization (Pugeat et al. 1987). A metabolite of danazol may also interfere with certain testosterone assays leading to falsely high results.

Drugs used in treatment of metastatic prostatic carcinoma tend to have significant effects on reproductive hormones. Prolonged oestrogen therapy may cause irreversible testicular damage and loss of the feedback response of the hypothalamic–pituitary–gonadal axis (Wortsman et al. 1989). The steroid antiandrogen cyproterone acetate, in addition to competitive antagonism at the target organ receptors, lowers LH, FSH and, consequently, testosterone levels and sperm count because of its strong progestational activity (Namer 1988). On the other hand, the non-steroid antiandrogens flutamide and anandron are specific androgen-receptor blockers without intrinsic activity. They can establish an effective peripheral androgen resistance despite increases in gonadotrophin and testosterone levels (Migliari et al. 1988).

Long-acting LHRH analogues used for treatment of such disorders as central precocious puberty, endometriosis, and prostatic and breast carcinoma act by abolishing the pulsatile nature of LHRH stimulation, thereby desensitizing the pituitary with reduction in gonadotrophin and hence gonadal sex hormone production, and producing 'medical castration'. The majority of women experience some degree of hot flushes, vaginal dryness, and loss of libido, with the potential long-term complication of osteoporosis; whereas in men decreased libido and impotence may be produced (Santen and Bourguignon 1987; Fraser and Baird 1987).

Oral contraceptives were once thought to increase the incidence of amenorrhoea. More recent studies have shown, however, that the incidence of post-pill amenorrhoea is similar to that of the development of spontaneous secondary amenorrhoea in the general population and that subsequent fertility is probably not impaired by previous use of oral contraceptives (Archer and Thomas 1981; Hull et al. 1981).

Drugs that induce hyperprolactinaemia, by various mechanisms (see section on Hyperprolactinaemia), can interfere with reproductive function at the level of hypothalamus, pituitary, or gonads.

Gonadal dysfunction after chemotherapy

In man, progressive dose-related depletion of germinal epithelium resulting in azoöspermia and infertility can occur with cytotoxic agents, particularly alkylating agents such as mustine hydrochloride, cyclophosphamide, chlorambucil, procarbazine, and busulphan (Miller 1971; Bajorunas 1980; Waxman et al. 1982). The Leydig cells remain morphologically intact, although they may be functionally abnormal. Other drugs that have been found to be toxic to the germinal epithelium include vinblastine, doxorubicin, ara-C, and o,p'-DDD.

The effects of newer agents such as ifosfamide, cisplatin and high-dose methotrexate are less clear and await further elucidation (Sparagana 1987; Aubier *et al.* 1989; Sherins and Mulvihill 1989). Ovarian failure also occurs in at least 50 per cent of female patients treated with single alkylating agents (Sherins and Mulvihill 1989). High-dose methotrexate is the only antimetabolite that has been assessed; it does not appear to have immediate ovarian toxicity (Shamberger *et al.* 1981).

Combination chemotherapy has a profound impact on spermatogenesis: 80 per cent of men who have received MOPP (mustine hydrochloride, vincristine, procarbazine, and prednisone) or a similar regimen for treatment of Hodgkin's lymphoma develop azoöspermia (Chapman *et al.* 1979a). This regimen also produces ovarian dysfunction in over 50 per cent of women (Chapman *et al.* 1979b; Horning *et al.* 1981; Waxman *et al.* 1982). In general, young patients (under age 30) tolerate the drug better and have higher chances of recovery from azoöspermia or amenorrhoea. A combination of adriamycin, bleomycin, vinblastine, and DTIC (ABVD) is cited as equally efficacious and less toxic to the gonads than the classical MOPP regimen, oligoazoöspermia being induced in only 54 per cent of patients and full recovery of spermatogenesis occurring in all patients within 18 months (Viviani *et al.* 1985).

Basal FSH rises as a result of germinal aplasia. Basal LH may either increase or, more commonly, remain normal (Waxman *et al.* 1982; Sherins and Mulvihill 1989). Booth and others (1987) have shown that, although still within the normal range, both levels and production of testosterone are in fact significantly reduced, signifying altered Leydig cell function and in line with the fact that challenge with LHRH usually results in excessive responses of both gonadotrophins.

Virilization

Anabolic steroids used in the treatment of aplastic anaemia, hereditary angioedema, and breast cancer have variable degrees of androgenic effect (Wynn and Path 1968). They can therefore cause virilization ranging from mild hirsutism to clitoromegaly, deepening of voice, and muscle development when given to women, and may produce precocious puberty or acceleration of bone age in young children. Furthermore, by suppressing endogenous gonadotrophin secretion, they can inhibit spermatogenesis, which provides a theoretical basis for clinical trials of androgens as male contraceptives (Swerdloff *et al.* 1978).

Most progestogens are weakly androgenic. They have been used for prevention of abortion, although this effect is controversial. Because of the enormous capacity of the placenta to aromatize the naturally occurring androgens to oestrogens, however, even high doses of progesterone and 17-α-hydroxyprogesterone have not been shown to be teratogenic (Chez 1978; Check *et al.* 1986). On the other hand, synthetic androgens and progestogens often cannot be aromatized, and norethisterone in doses of 10–20 mg daily can cause masculinization of the female fetus (Schardein 1980).

Cyproterone acetate, used in humans for the treatment of hirsutism, causes feminization in male fetal rats (Neumann 1978). Although feminization has not been reported in humans (Laudahn 1984), the drug should be avoided during pregnancy. Addition of oestrogen in a reversed sequential regimen can provide effective contraception and decrease the menstrual irregularity resulting from the strong progestational property and long elimination half-life of cyproterone acetate (Biffignandi and Molinatti 1987).

Gynaecomastia

A wide variety of drugs can produce gynaecomastia (Table 13.4), which arises mainly as a result of alteration of the balance between testosterone and oestradiol effects (Carlson 1980). Thus, conjugated oestrogens and oral contraceptives cause direct stimulation of the breasts, while hCG or LHRH used for induction of puberty and fertility in patients with hypogonadotrophic hypogonadism result in gynaecomastia by preferential stimulation of oestrogen production.

The major mechanism of production of gynaecomastia with cimetidine and spironolactone seems to be inhibition of dihydrotestosterone binding to its cellular receptor protein (Loriaux *et al.* 1976; Funder and Mercer 1979). In addition, cimetidine causes an increase in serum oestradiol concentration by inhibiting its 2-hydroxylation (Galbraith and Michnovicz 1989), and spironolactone has a partial suppressive effect on the 17-hydroxylation, which could explain its adverse effect of menstrual irregularity in females (Loriaux *et al.* 1976). Ketoconazole, through its suppressive effect on androgen and glucocorticoid synthesis, depresses serum testosterone concentrations more than serum oestradiol and produces an elevated oestradiol–testosterone ratio (Pont *et al.* 1985). Reduction in free testosterone concentration due to increased amount of sex-hormone-binding globulin and enhanced conversion of testosterone to oestradiol could explain the gynaecomastia due to phenytoin (Monson and Scott 1987).

Cytotoxic agents (Trump *et al.* 1982), antiandrogens such as cyproterone acetate (Geller *et al.* 1968) and flutamide (Caine *et al.* 1975), and the adrenal toxic agent *o,p'*-DDD (Luton *et al.* 1979; Slooten *et al.* 1984) can all cause gynaecomastia by damaging the testes or reducing the effect of testosterone.

TABLE 13.4
Drugs producing gynaecomastia

With oestrogenic activity
  Conjugated or synthetic oestrogens
  Digitoxin
  Oral contraceptives

Stimulating oestrogen secretion
  Human chorionic gonadotrophin (hCG)
  Luteinizing-hormone-releasing hormone (LHRH)

Reducing testosterone synthesis/effect
  Antiandrogens (cyproterone acetate, flutamide)
  Cimetidine
  Cytotoxic agents (busulfan, nitrosoureas, *o,p'*-DDD,
    vincristine)
  Ketoconazole
  Phenytoin
  Spironolactone

Unknown mechanisms
  Auranofin
  Calcium-channel blockers
  Captopril
  Diazepam
  Digoxin
  Ethionamide
  Etretinate
  Isoniazid
  Major tranquillizers (? prolactin effect)
  Marihuana
  Methadone
  Methyldopa
  Metronidazole
  Penicillamine
  Reserpine
  Thiacetazone

Although hyperprolactinaemia is not considered a direct cause of gynaecomastia, prolactin may contribute to breast enlargement through indirect effects on gonadal and possibly adrenal function. This may explain the effect of drugs such as methyldopa (*Journal of the American Medical Association* 1963), reserpine (Robinson 1957), phenothiazines (Margolis and Gross 1967), tricyclic antidepressants, and penicillamine (Reid *et al.* 1982; Kahl *et al.* 1985).

Digitoxin has inherent oestrogen-like properties (Le-Winn 1953), but digoxin probably produces gynaecomastia through a 'refeeding' mechanism in debilitated men. Isoniazid (Koang *et al.* 1955), ethionamide, and thiacetazone (Chunhaswasdikul 1974) may similarly act through a refeeding mechanism in men suffering from tuberculosis.

The mechanism of gynaecomastia remains unclear, a number of medications occasionally being reported to be associated with it. These include methadone (Thomas 1976), marihuana (Harmon and Aliapoulios 1972), captopril (Markusse and Meyboom 1988), calcium-channel blockers (Tanner and Bosco 1988), auranofin (Williams 1988), etretinate (Carmichael and Paul 1989), and metronidazole (Fagan *et al.* 1985).

Hypothalamic–pituitary–prolactin secretion

Prolactin is a polypeptide trophic hormone secreted from the anterior pituitary. Its secretion is primarily under the inhibitory control of hypothalamic dopamine, whereas the hypothalamic serotonergic system is stimulatory. A prolactin-releasing factor, probably regulated by serotonin, has been identified in hypothalamic extracts but not yet characterized. Thyrotrophin-releasing hormone is also a potent stimulator of prolactin release but is of uncertain physiological significance. Excessive secretion of prolactin may result in galactorrhoea, amenorrhoea, impotence, and infertility. Several possible mechanisms may be responsible for its effect on the menstrual cycle and fertility (Frantz 1978). First, prolactin could act at the hypothalamic level to interfere with either the tonic or the cyclic release of luteinizing-hormone-releasing hormone (LHRH). Secondly, high prolactin concentrations could desensitize the pituitary gland to the action of LHRH, leading to impaired gonadotrophin secretion. Thirdly, excessive prolactin could interfere with the steroidogenic action of gonadotrophin at the ovarian level. In addition, hyperprolactinaemia inhibits 5-α-reductase and hence peripheral conversion of testosterone to dihydrotestosterone, so interfering with spermatogenesis and other peripheral actions of testosterone (Carter *et al.* 1978).

Galactorrhoea has been associated with a wide variety of drugs that induce prolactin secretion (Table 13.5). Many of these substances act on the hypothalamus by either inhibiting the action of dopamine or enhancing the effect of serotonin. For instance, reserpine and methyldopa deplete catecholamine stores. The major tranquillizers, the phenothiazines and butyrophenones, block the dopamine receptors (Turkington 1972; Tolis *et al.* 1974). Metoclopramide and sulpiride are orthopramides that produce hyperprolactinaemia, presumably through their inhibitory effect on dopamine (McCallum *et al.* 1976; Aono *et al.* 1978). The tricyclics probably stimulate prolactin release by blocking the re-uptake of serotonin or enhancing the sensitivity of the postsynaptic serotonin receptors (Charney *et al.* 1984; Gadd *et al.* 1987). Monoamine oxidase inhibitors may shift the balance between dopaminergic inhibition and serotonergic

TABLE 13.5
Drugs causing galactorrhoea

Benzodiazepines	chlordiazepoxide
Butyrophenones	haloperidol
Cimetidine	
Dexamphetamine, fenfluramine	
Methyldopa	
Monoamine oxidase inhibitors	
Oestrogens and oral contraceptives	
Orthopramides	bromopiride
	metoclopramide
	sulpiride
Phenothiazines	chloropromazine
	perphenazine
	prochlorperazine
	promazine
	trifluoperazine
Rauwolfia alkaloids	reserpine
Tricyclic compounds	amitriptyline
	clomipramine
	imipramine
Verapamil	

stimulation of prolactin release (Slater *et al.* 1977). Prolactin concentrations also increase with fenfluramine, an anorexiant drug used in the treatment of obesity and capable of serotonergic stimulation (Barbieri *et al.* 1983).

Other drugs produce hyperprolactinaemia through less well-defined mechanisms. Oestrogens increase mean serum prolactin levels and also enhance responsiveness to prolactin-releasing stimuli (Frantz 1978). Administration of cimetidine has been reported rarely to increase prolactin secretion and produce galactorrhoea, suggesting that brain histamine could play a role in prolactin release (Bohnet *et al.* 1978; Ehrinpreis *et al.* 1989). Likewise, the possibility of opioid regulation is reflected by hyperprolactinaemia due to morphine and methadone (Frantz 1978). Verapamil has been found to elevate basal and TRH-stimulated prolactin concentrations, possibly via an inhibitory effect on dopaminergic tone (Gluskin *et al.* 1981; Nielsen-Kudsk *et al.* 1990). Galactorrhoea has also been associated with benzodiazepines,

though without hyperprolactinaemia (Kleinberg *et al.* 1977).

Treatment of troublesome drug-induced hyperprolactinaemia requires withdrawal of the offending medication if the clinical setting allows. The prolactin level and disturbed menstrual cycle should then return to normal within a few weeks, with restoration of fertility.

Drugs that inhibit prolactin release include levodopa; the ergot alkaloids (bromocriptine, pergolide), which act as dopamine agonists; and the serotonin-antagonist metergoline. These drugs are effective in reversing galactorrhoea and restoring ovulatory menses in patients with hyperprolactinaemia, whether due to a tumour or other causes (Vance *et al.* 1984; Bohnet *et al.* 1986). Further, the ergot derivatives can shrink prolactin-secreting pituitary tumours (Kleinberg *et al.* 1983; Vance *et al.* 1984) and are now a well-established means of treating such disorders.

Growth hormone

Growth hormone (GH) is synthesized in the somatotrophs of the pituitary. Its release is regulated by a balance between the actions of hypothalamic-growth-hormone-releasing hormone (GHRH) and somatostatin. These, in turn, are influenced by interactions between various neurotransmitters and neuropeptides at the hypothalamic or suprahypothalamic levels. Most of the growth-promoting effects of GH are mediated by somatomedins, principally insulin-like growth factor-1 (IGF 1) or somatomedin-C. Drugs may influence growth through their effects on GH secretion at the hypothalamic or pituitary level or through antagonism of its peripheral actions through effects on IGF 1. In addition, they may indirectly inhibit growth through interference with the metabolism of thyroid hormones or cortisol, which are also required for normal growth.

In children, prolonged treatment with corticosteroids, for example in asthma, has been associated with poor growth (Preece 1976; Chang *et al.* 1982). Although, however, large doses of glucocorticoids and Cushing's syndrome inhibit growth hormone secretion in adults, the suppression seems to be less significant in children (Strickland *et al.* 1972). Also, the administration of GH together with glucocorticoid does not reverse steroid-induced growth retardation in children (Solomon and Schoen 1976) and serum IGF 1 concentrations are not necessarily low in patients with glucocorticoid excess. These, together with other observations (Loeb 1976), suggest that the inhibitory effects of glucocorticoids on growth are due to direct actions on target tissue rather than alteration of GH secretion. The mechanisms are undoubtedly more complex than previously suspected.

Testosterone and its metabolite dihydrotestosterone are potent anabolic agents that enhance linear growth and weight gain. Androgen administration to prepubertal human children increases peak plasma GH levels after provocative stimuli but does not have consistent direct effects on plasma levels of IGF 1 (Craft and Underwood 1984). Therefore, the elevated plasma IGF 1 concentrations observed during puberty are probably secondary to sex-hormone-stimulated increases in GH secretion. Caution has to be exercised, however, in using androgens to stimulate growth, since they can lead to premature closure of epiphysial plates and a reduction in final adult height. Androgen replacement should not be commenced in young patients with hypopituitarism until other pituitary hormones have exerted their stimulatory effects on growth.

Although oestrogens increase basal plasma GH levels and enhance GH response to provocative stimuli, pharmacological doses of oestrogens reduce the concentrations of somatomedins (von Puttkamer et al. 1977) and enhance epiphysial maturation (Strickland and Sprinz 1973). This is the rationale for treating excessively tall girls with high-dose oestrogens (Wettenhall et al. 1975; Crawford 1978).

Thyroid hormones can influence growth by effects on the synthesis and secretion of GH by the pituitary gland, enhancement of the GH response to GHRH *in vitro* and *in vivo* (Wehrenberg et al. 1986) and possibly by an additional direct action on cartilage growth plates. Hypothyroid patients frequently have severely blunted GH responses to provocative stimuli, and they tend to have low serum Sm-C/IGF 1 levels (Chernausek et al. 1983). Hypothyroidism can be iatrogenic, and withdrawal of the offending medication, by correcting hypothyroidism, will lead to recovery of growth (Wilkinson et al. 1972).

A number of drugs that affect neurotransmitter (biogenic amines, GABA, and opioids) activity can influence growth hormone secretion. Drugs that stimulate GH secretion include levodopa (Huseman and Hassing 1984); apomorphine (Massara et al. 1985); bromocriptine and clonidine, which act via the dopaminergic or α-adrenergic pathways (Martin and Reichlin 1987); the serotonin precursors tryptophan and 5-OH-tryptophan, which increase central serotonin level (Martin et al. 1978); the GABA-ergic drugs muscimol, baclofen, and diazepam; some opiates such as methadone and nalorphine (Bercu and Diamond 1986); and β-blockers such as propranolol. The dopamine antagonist metoclopramide paradoxically stimulates GH secretion (Cohen et

al. 1979), which may be due to blockade of the presynaptic receptors leading to increased secretion of dopamine, or to its actions on other monoaminergic pathways. On the other hand, GH secretion, mostly that associated with sleep and insulin-induced hypoglycaemia, is inhibited by the α-blockers phenoxybenzamine and phentolamine; the dopamine-receptor blockers chlorpromazine and haloperidol; the amine depletor reserpine; the serotonin-receptor blocker cyproheptadine; and the β-agonists such as isoprenaline. The anticholinergic agents atropine and pirenzepine also block exercise-associated and drug-induced GH secretion (Casanueva et al. 1984; Chiodera et al. 1984). These drugs have been widely used for study of neuroendocrine control of GH secretion and sometimes applied clinically for screening tests of GH reserve (Cohen et al. 1979; Lanes and Hurtado 1982). Their long-term effects on GH secretion and growth, however, still remain unclear.

Posterior pituitary

Vasopressin

The posterior pituitary is principally made up of the axon terminals of the supraoptic and paraventricular nuclei in the hypothalamus. Vasopressin (antidiuretic hormone or ADH) and oxytocin are synthesized in both nuclei as parts of large precursor molecules and packaged with their respective neurophysins in neurosecretory granules that migrate along the axons to the posterior pituitary. A large number of stimuli, for example, emesis and hypoglycaemia, can cause release of vasopressin. Under physiological conditions, however, the major regulator is the plasma osmotic pressure, which is believed to exert its influence through specific osmoreceptor neurons situated at the anterior hypothalamus.

The syndrome of inappropriate secretion of ADH (SIADH)

The syndrome of inappropriate secretion of ADH has been associated with the use of a variety of antipsychotic medications, namely, phenothiazines (De Rivera 1975; Rao et al. 1975; Matuk and Kalyanaraman 1977; Hwang and Magraw 1989), tricyclic antidepressants (Luzecky 1974; Ajlouni et al. 1974; Dhar and Ramos 1978; Liskin et al. 1984; Mitsch and Lee 1986), and monoamine oxidase inhibitors (Peterson et al. 1978; Giese et al. 1989), presumably through increased secretion or potentiation of actions of vasopressin. Chlorpropamide causes antidiuresis, probably through enhancement of both the release and peripheral actions of ADH (Miller and Moses 1970; Moses *et al.* 1973*a*; Singer and Forrest 1976). Carbamazepine, structurally related to tricyclic

TABLE 13.6
Drugs affecting vasopressin release or function

I. Leading to SIADH

Chemotherapeutic agents	cisplatin
	cyclophosphamide
	melphalan
	vinblastine
	vincristine
Monoamine oxidase inhibitors	phenelzine
	tranylcypromine
Phenothiazines	fluphenazine
	thioridazine
Tricyclic antidepressants	amitriptyline
	desipramine
	imipramine
Miscellaneous	carbamazepine
	chlorpropamide
	fluoxetine
	haloperidol
	thiothixene
	vasopressin and its long-acting derivatives

II. Leading to diabetes insipidus (DI) (nephrogenic)

Demeclocycline
Ifosfamide
Lithium carbonate
  (short-term
   administration
   causes central DI)
Methoxyflurane

antidepressants, also induces water intoxication through stimulation of ADH release (Rado 1973; Kimura *et al.* 1974). Certain cytotoxic drugs also predispose to development of SIADH. They include cyclophosphamide (Defronzo *et al.* 1973), high-dose melphalan (Greenbaum- Lefkoe *et al.* 1985), vincristine (Robertson *et al.* 1973; Stuart *et al.* 1975), vinblastine (Antony *et al.* 1980), and cisplatin (Littlewood and Smith 1984; Ritch 1988). The water-retaining properties of these drugs are particularly noteworthy, since patients on cyclophosphamide or cisplatin require vigorous hydration to prevent the occurrence of cystitis or nephrotoxicity, and electrolyte disturbance can easily develop if the electrolytes are not monitored closely. Clofibrate enhances the release of

ADH, although clinically significant hyponatraemia has not been reported (Moses *et al.* 1973*b*).

Diabetes insipidus

Short-term lithium administration inhibits ADH secretion from the posterior pituitary, while prolonged use can lead to symptomatic nephrogenous diabetes insipidus in 10–30 per cent of patients (Forrest *et al.* 1974; Baylis and Heath 1978; Mannisto 1980). The disorder tends, however, to be mild and reversible in most patients on stopping the medication. Demeclocycline produces dose-dependent nephrogenic diabetes insipidus (Castell and Sparks 1965; Feldman and Singer 1974) and has been used for the treatment of SIADH. Nephrotoxicity with polyuria has also been associated with the general anaesthetic agent methoxyflurane, owing to the formation of inorganic fluoride from its metabolism (Mazze *et al.* 1971; Cousins *et al.* 1974). There has also been a case report of ifosfamide, a derivative of cyclophosphamide, causing diabetes insipidus in a patient treated for breast cancer. The underlying mechanism is, however, unclear (DeFronzo *et al.* 1974).

Oxytocin

The regulation of oxytocin secretion and its physiological role are still largely unknown, although breastfeeding is a recognized stimulus for oxytocin release in post-partum lactating women.

No clinical disorder due to deranged secretion of the hormone is known. Occasionally, however, high-dose oxytocin infusion has been associated with water intoxication, probably as a result of the antidiuretic potential of oxytocin together with simultaneous infusion of dextrose solution (Ahmad *et al.* 1975). Syntocinon infusion can occasionally lead to severe hyponatraemia during labour, particularly if labour is prolonged and dextrose is infused at the same time (personal observations).

Parathyroids and vitamin D

Several drugs have been reported to affect parathyroid function and vitamin D metabolism. Since drugs affecting vitamin D metabolism will be discussed in detail in Chapter 15, they are only briefly mentioned here.

Lithium treatment for manic-depressive illness is associated with mild hyperparathyroidism, apparently by interference with the normal negative feedback process whereby parathyroid hormone secretion is suppressed in response to elevation of the calcium level (Christiansen *et al.* 1980; McIntosh *et al.* 1987). The resulting chronic stimulation of the parathyroids has been found to cause an increase in gland size and may lead to hyperplasia or adenoma (Garfinkel *et al*. 1973; Mallette *et al*. 1989; Stancer and Forbath 1989).

Although thiazide diuretics (Christensson *et al*. 1977; Kohri *et al*. 1987) and diltiazem (Seely *et al*. 1989) have been reported to cause an increase of PTH concentrations, the clinical significance of this remains doubtful.

Ketoconazole lowers serum 1,25-dihydroxyvitamin D (1,25[OH]$_2$D) concentration by inhibition of renal 1-α-hydroxylase, a cytochrome-P-450-dependent enzyme (Glass and Eil 1986, 1988). It has recently been employed to treat a patient with sarcoidosis-associated hypercalcaemia (Adams *et al*. 1990). In theory, chronic administration of ketoconazole in high dosage may induce osteomalacia, but this remains unsubstantiated. Anticonvulsants such as phenytoin and phenobarbitone occasionally induce osteomalacia (Winnacker *et al*. 1977) by increasing hepatic conversion of vitamin D and 25-hydroxyvitamin D (25[OH]D) to more polar biologically inactive metabolites. Consequently the serum 25[OH]D is lowered. Serum 1,25[OH]$_2$D is usually normal (Hahn 1980), however. This, together with the fact that, in animals, phenytoin inhibits intestinal absorption of calcium and that phenytoin and phenobarbitone inhibit mobilization of calcium from bone *in vitro*, suggests that the drugs may cause bone disease by blocking the actions of 1,25[OH]$_2$D in target organs, rather than by a direct effect on 1,25[OH]$_2$D synthesis.

Gut hormones

Endocrine cells situated along the gastroenteropancreatic axis secrete hormones which not only regulate gastrointestinal functions (e.g. gastrin in stimulating gastric acid release, cholecystokinin in gall-bladder function) but also affect glucose control (insulin and glucagon). Many hormones originally isolated from the gut have also been identified as important neuropeptides in the nervous system, and vice versa (e.g. vasoactive intestinal polypeptide, cholecystokinin, and somatostatin). A major stimulus to exploration of this complex area of endocrinology is the existence of the relatively rare but intriguing gut-hormone-secreting tumours. Thus far there are relatively few reports on the effects of drugs on the secretion and measurement of these hormones.

Raised urinary 5-hydroxyindoleacetic acid (5-HIAA) derived from metabolism of serotonin is the classical finding for diagnosis of carcinoid tumours. The assay can, however, be influenced by a number of medications. The more commonly used drugs that may produce false positive results include paracetamol, fluorouracil, Lugol's iodine, melphalan, mephenesin, methocarbamol, reserpine, and glyceryl guaiacolate (in some cough syrups), whereas false negatives occur with heparin, imipramine, isoniazid, methyldopa, monoamine oxidase inhibitors, phenothiazines, and *p*-chlorophenylalanine, the latter two drugs often being employed for symptomatic treatment of carcinoid symptoms (Cryer 1988; Roberts 1988).

Radioimmunoassay of gastrin is essential for the diagnosis of the Zollinger–Ellison syndrome. Acid-reducing drugs such as H$_2$-receptor antagonists, anticholinergics, and the new proton-pump inhibitor omeprazole can, however, lead to elevation of gastrin levels owing to loss of acid inhibition (Debas 1987; Sharma *et al*. 1987; Gaginella *et al*. 1989). These medications should therefore be excluded when gastrin measurements are to be made. Tolbutamide has been found to suppress gastrin release in man, but the physiological significance of this is not clear (Chiba *et al*. 1988).

The long-acting somatostatin analogue Sandostatin has been used to treat a variety of gut-hormone-secreting tumours as well as acromegaly. Steatorrhoea is a recognized adverse effect, and inhibition of endocrine secretions could contribute to the pathogenesis (Lembcke *et al*. 1987). Gallstone formation due to suppression of cholecystokinin and hence of gall-bladder contractility is another potential problem (Comi 1989). Since Sandostatin inhibits the secretion of insulin, one would expect an impairment of glucose tolerance. This does not appear, however, to be a major problem (Ch'ng *et al*. 1986; Halse *et al*. 1990), probably because of its concomitant inhibitory effect on other counter-regulatory hormones, which oppose the action of insulin.

References

Aanderud, S., Sundsfjord, J., and Aarbakke, J. (1984). Amiodarone inhibits the conversion of thyroxine to triiodothyronine in isolated rat hepatocytes. *Endocrinology* 115, 1605.

Abiodun, M.O., Bird, R., Havard, C.W., and Sood, N.K. (1973). The effects of phenylbutazone on thyroid function. *Acta Endocrinol*. 72, 257.

Adams, J.S., Sharma, O.P., Diz, M.M., and Endres, D.B. (1990). Ketoconazole decreases the serum 1,25-dihydroxyvitamin D and calcium concentration in sarcoidosis-associated hypercalcemia. *J. Clin. Endocrinol. Metab*. 70, 1090.

Ahmad, A.J., Clark, E.H., and Jacobs, H.S. (1975). Water intoxication associated with oxytocin infusion. *Postgrad. Med. J*. 51, 249.

Ajlouni, K., Kern, M.W., Tures, J.F., Theil, G.B., and Hagen, T.C. (1974). Thiothixene-induced hyponatremia. *Arch. Intern. Med*. 134, 1103.

Amico, J.A., Richardson, V., Alpert, V., and Klein, I. (1984). Clinical and chemical assessment of thyroid function during therapy with amiodarone. *Arch. Intern. Med.* 144, 487.

Antony, A., Robinson, W.A., Roy, C., Pelander, W., and Donohue, R. (1980). Inappropriate antidiuretic hormone secretion after high dose vinblastine. *J. Urol.* 123, 783.

Aono, T., Shioji, T., Kinugasa, T., Onishi, T., and Kurachi, K. (1978). Clinical and endocrinological analyses of patients with galactorrhea and menstrual disorders due to sulpiride or metoclopramide. *J. Clin. Endocrinol. Metab.* 47, 675.

Archer, D.F. and Thomas, R.L. (1981). The fallacy of the postpill amenorrhea syndrome. *Clin. Obstet. Gynecol.* 24, 943.

Armbruster, H., Vetter, W., Reck, G., Beckerhoff, R., and Siegenthaler, W. (1975). Severe arterial hypertension caused by chronic abuse of a topical mineralocorticoid. *Int. J. Clin. Pharmacol.* 12, 170.

Aubier, F., Flamant, F., Brauner, R., Caillaud, J.M., Chaussain, J.M., and Lemerle, J. (1989). Male gonadal function after chemotherapy for solid tumors in childhood. *J. Clin. Oncol.* 7, 304.

Azizi, F., Vagenakis, A.G., Portnay, G.I., Braverman, L.E., and Ingbar, S.H. (1974). Thyroxine transport and metabolism in methadone and heroin addicts. *Ann. Intern. Med.* 80, 194.

Bajorunas, D.R. (1980). Disorders of endocrine function following cancer therapies. *Clin. Endocrinol. Metab.* 9, 405.

Barbieri, C., Magnoni, V., Rauhe, W.G., Zanasi, S., Caldara, R., and Ferrari, C. (1983). Effect of fenfluramine on prolactin secretion in obese patients: evidence for serotoninergic regulation of prolactin in man. *Clin. Endocrinol.* 19, 705.

Barbosa, J., Seal, U.S., and Doe, R.P. (1971). Effects of anabolic steroids on hormone-binding proteins, serum cortisol and serum nonprotein-bound cortisol. *J. Clin. Endocrinol. Metab.* 32, 232.

Baylis, P.H. and Heath, D.A. (1978). Water disturbances in patients treated with oral lithium carbonate. *Ann. Intern. Med.* 88, 607.

Bayliss, R.I.S. (1975). The use of corticosteroids and corticotrophins in non-endocrine diseases. *Prescribers' J.* 15, 46.

Beckerhoff, R., Vetter, W., Armbruster, H., and Luetscher, J.A. (1973). Plasma aldosterone during oral-contraceptive therapy. *Lancet* i, 1218.

Beex, L.V.A.M., Ross, A., Smals, A.G.H., and Kloppenborg, P.W.C. (1976). 5-Fluorouracil and the thyroid. *Lancet* i, 866.

Bercu, B.B. and Diamond, F.B. Jr (1986). Growth hormone neurosecretory dysfunction. *Clin. Endocrinol. Metab.* 15, 537.

Besser, G.M., Butler, P.W.P., Landon, J., and Rees, L. (1969). Influence of amphetamines on plasma corticosteroid and growth hormone levels in man. *Br. Med. J.* iv, 528.

Best, T.R., Jenkins, J.K., Murphy, F.Y., Nicks, S.A., Bussell, K.L., and Vesely, D.L. (1987). Persistent adrenal insufficiency secondary to low-dose ketoconazole therapy. *Am. J. Med.* 82, 676.

Biffignandi, P. and Molinatti, G.M. (1987). Antiandrogens and hirsutism. *Horm. Res.* 28, 242.

Bledsoe, T., Island, D.P., Ney, R.L., and Liddle, G.W. (1964). An effect of *o,p'*-DDD on the extra-adrenal metabolism of cortisol in man. *J. Clin. Endocrinol.* 24, 1303.

Bockner, V. and Roman, W. (1967). The influence of oral contraceptives on the binding capacity of serum proteins. *Med. J. Aust.* ii, 1187.

Bohnet, H.G., Greiwe, M., Hanker, J.P., Aragona, C., and Schneider, H.P.G. (1978). Effects of cimetidine on prolactin, LH, and sex steroid secretion in male and female volunteers. *Acta Endocrinol.* 88, 428.

Bohnet, H.G., Kato, K., and Wolf, A.S. (1986). Treatment of hyperprolactinemic amenorrhea with metergoline. *Obstet. Gynecol.* 67, 249.

Booth, J.D., Merriam, G.R., Clark, R.V., Loriaux, D.L., and Sherins, R.J. (1987). Evidence for Leydig cell dysfunction in infertile men with a selective increase in plasma follicle-stimulating hormone. *J. Clin. Endocrinol. Metab.* 64, 1194.

Borowski, G.D., Garofano, C.D., Rose, L.I., Spielman, S.R., Rotmensch, H.R., Greenspan, A.M., et al. (1985). Effect of long-term amiodarone therapy on thyroid hormone levels and thyroid function. *Am. J. Med.* 78, 443.

Borushek, S. and Gold, J.J. (1964). Commonly used medications that interfere with routine endocrine laboratory procedures. *Clin. Chem.* 10, 41.

Braverman, L.E. and Ingbar, S.H. (1967). Effects of norethandrolone on the transport in serum and peripheral turnover of thyroxine. *J. Clin. Endocrinol. Metab.* 27, 389.

Burger, A., Dinichert, D., Nicod, P., Jenny, M., Lemarchand-Beraud, T., and Vallotton, M.B. (1976). Effect of amiodarone on serum triiodothyronine, reverse triiodothyronine, thyroxin, and thyrotropin: a drug influencing peripheral metabolism of thyroid hormones. *J. Clin. Invest.* 58, 255.

Burgi, H.W., Wimpfheimer, C., Burger, A., Zaunbauer, W., Rosler, H., and Lemarchand-Beraud, T. (1976). Changes of circulating thyroxine, triiodothyronine and reverse triiodothyronine after radiographic contrast agents. *J. Clin. Endocrinol. Metab.* 43, 1203.

Burr, W.A., Ramsden, D.B., Griffiths, R.S., and Black, E.G. (1976). Effect of a single dose of dexamethasone on serum concentrations of thyroid hormones. *Lancet* ii, 58.

Burstein, S. and Klaiber, E.L. (1965). Phenobarbital-induced increase in 6 β-hydroxycortisol excretion: clue to its significance in human urine. *J. Clin. Endocrinol. Metab.* 25, 293.

Caine, M., Perlberg, S., and Gordon, R. (1975). The treatment of benign prostatic hypertrophy with flutamide (SCH 13521): a placebo-controlled study. *J. Urol.* 114, 564.

Carlson, H.E. (1980). Current concepts: gynecomastia. *N. Engl. J. Med.* 303, 795.

Carmichael, A.J. and Paul, C.J. (1989). Reversible gynaecomastia associated with etretinate. *Br. J. Dermatol.* 120, 317.

Carter, J.N., Tyson, J.E., Tolis, G., van Vliet, S., Faiman, C., and Friesen, H.G. (1978). Prolactin-secreting tumors and hypogonadism in 22 men. *N. Engl. J. Med.* 299, 847.

Casanueva, F.F., Villanueva, L., Cabranes, J.A., Cabezas-Cerrato, J., and Fernandez-Cruz, A. (1984). Cholinergic mediation of growth hormone secretion elicited by arginine, clonidine, and physical exercise in man. *J. Clin. Endocrinol. Metab.* 59, 526.

Cashin-Hemphill, L., Spencer, C.A., Nicoloff, J.T., Blanken-horn, D.H., Nessim, S.A., Chin, H.P., *et al.* (1987). Alterations in serum thyroid hormonal indices with colestipol-niacin therapy. *Ann. Intern. Med.* 107, 324.

Castell, L.D.O. and Sparks, C.H.A. (1965). Nephrogenic diabetes insipidus due to demethylchlortetracycline hydrochloride. *JAMA* 193, 137.

Cavalieri, R.R., Gavin, L.A., Wallace, A., Hammond, M.E., and Cruse, K. (1979). Serum thyroxine, free T$_4$, triiodothyronine, and reverse-T$_3$ in diphenylhydantoin treated patients. *Metabolism* 28, 1161.

Chang, K.C., Miklich, D.R., Barwise, G., Chai, H., and Miles-Lawrence, R. (1982). Linear growth of chronic asthmatic children: the effects of the disease and various forms of steroid therapy. *Clin. Allergy* 12, 369.

Chapman, R.M., Sutcliffe, S.B., Rees, L.H., Edwards, C.R.W., and Malpas, J.S. (1979*a*). Cyclical combination chemotherapy and gonadal function. *Lancet* i, 285.

Chapman, R.M., Sutcliffe, S.B., and Malpas, J.S. (1979*b*). Cytotoxic-induced ovarian failure in women with Hodgkin's disease. *JAMA* 242, 1877.

Charney, D.S., Heninger, G.R., and Sternberg, D.E. (1984). Serotonin function and mechanism of action of antidepressant treatment. *Arch. Gen. Psychiatry* 41, 359.

Check, J.H., Rankin, A., and Teichman, M. (1986). The risk of fetal anomalies as a result of progesterone therapy during pregnancy. *Fertil. Steril.* 45, 575.

Chernausek, S.D., Underwood, L.E., Utiger, R.D., and van Wyk, J.J. (1983). Growth hormone secretion and plasma somatomedin-C in primary hypothyroidism. *Clin. Endocrinol.* 19, 337.

Chez, R.A. (1978). Proceedings of the Symposium: Progesterone, progestins, and fetal development. *Fertil. Steril.* 30, 16.

Chiba, T., Okimura, Y., Kodama, H., Kadowaki, S., Chihara, K., and Fujita, T. (1988). Tolbutamide inhibits gastrin release in man. *Horm. Metabol. Res.* 20, 641.

Chin, W. and Schussler, G.C. (1968). Decreased serum free thyroxine concentration in patients treated with diphenylhydantoin. *J. Clin. Endocrinol.* 28, 181.

Chiodera, P., Coiro, V., Speroni, G., Capretti, L., Muzzetto, P., Volpi, R., *et al.* (1984). The growth hormone response to thyrotropin-releasing hormone in insulin-dependent diabetes involves a cholinergic mechanism. *J. Clin. Endocrinol. Metab.* 59, 794.

Ch'ng, J.L.C., Anderson, J.V., Williams, S.J., Carr, D.H., and Bloom, S.R. (1986). Remission of symptoms during long term treatment of metastatic pancreatic endocrine tumours with long acting somatostatin analogue. *Br. Med. J.* 292, 981.

Chopra, I.J., Williams, D.E., Orgiazzi, J., and Solomon, D.H. (1975). Opposite effects of dexamethasone on serum concentrations of 3,3′,5′-triiodothyronine (reverse T$_3$) and 3,3′,5-triiodothyronine (T$_3$). *J. Clin. Endocrinol. Metab.* 41, 911.

Christensson, T., Hellstrom, K., and Wengle, B. (1977). Hypercalcemia and primary hyperparathyroidism. Prevalence in patients receiving thiazides as detected in a health screen. *Arch. Intern. Med.* 137, 1138.

Christiansen, C., Baastrup, P.C., and Transbol, I. (1980). Development of 'primary' hyperparathyroidism during lithium therapy: longitudinal study. *Neuropsychobiology* 6, 280.

Chunhaswasdikul, B. (1974). Gynecomastia in association with administration of thiacetazone in the treatment of tuberculosis. *J. Med. Assoc. Thailand* 57, 323.

Clark, F. and Hutton, C.W. (1985). The effect of drugs upon the assessment of thyroid function. *Adverse Drug React. Acute Poisoning Rev.* 4, 59.

Coffey, V.J. (1971). Myxoedema during cyclophosphamide therapy. *Br. Med. J.* iv, 682.

Cohen, H.N., Hay, I.O., Thomson, J.A., Logue, F., Ratcliffe, W.A., and Beastall, G.H. (1979). Metoclopramide stimulation: a test of growth hormone reserve in adolescent males. *Clin. Endocrinol.* 11, 89.

Cohen, H.N., Beastall, G.H., Ratcliffe, W.A., Gray, C., Watson, I.D., and Thomson, J.A. (1980). Effect on human thyroid function of sulphonamide and trimethoprim combination drugs. *Br. Med. J.* 281, 646.

Cohen III, J.H., Ingbar, S.H., and Braverman, L.E. (1989). Thyrotoxicosis due to ingestion of excess thyroid hormone. *Endocrinol. Rev.* 10, 113.

Comi, R.J. (1989). Pharmacology and use in pituitary tumors. In: P. Gorden (moderator). Somatostatin and somatostatin analogue (SMS 201-995) in treatment of hormone-secreting tumors of the pituitary and gastrointestinal tract and non-neoplastic diseases of the gut. *Ann. Intern. Med.* 110, 35.

Conn, J.W., Rovner, D.R., Cohen, E.L., and Anderson, J.E. Jr (1966). Inhibition by heparinoid of aldosterone biosynthesis in man. *J. Clin. Endocrinol.* 26, 527.

Conn, J.W., Rovner, D.R., and Cohen, E.L. (1968). Licorice-induced pseudoaldosteronism: hypertension, hypokalemia, aldosteronopenia, and suppressed plasma renin activity. *JAMA* 205, 80.

Cooper, D.S., Daniels, G.H., Ladenson, P.W., and Ridgway, E.C. (1982). Hyperthyroxinemia in patients treated with high-dose propranolol. *Am. J. Med.* 73, 867.

Cousins, M.J., Mazze, R.I., Kosek, J.C., Hitt, B.A., and Love, F.V. (1974). The etiology of methoxyflurane nephrotoxicity. *J. Pharmacol. Exp. Ther.* 190, 530.

Craft, W.H. and Underwood, L.E. (1984). Effect of androgens on plasma somatomedin-C/insulin-like growth factor I responses to growth hormone. *Clin. Endocrinol.* 20, 549.

Crawford, J.D. (1978). Treatment of tall girls with estrogen. *J. Pediatr.* 62 (suppl.), 1189.

Cryer, P.F. (1985). Pheochromocytoma. *Clin. Endocrinol. Metab.* 14, 203.

Cryer, P.E. (1988). The carcinoid syndrome. In *Cecil Textbook of Medicine*, Vol. 2 (18th edn) (ed. J.B. Wyngaarden and L.H. Smith), p. 1467. W.B. Saunders, Philadelphia.

Cubitt, T. (1976). Lithium and thyrotoxicosis. *Lancet* i, 1247.

Debas, H.T. (1987). Gastrin. *Clin. Invest. Med.* 10, 222.

DeBold, C.R., Sheldon, W.R., DeCherney, G.S., Jackson, R.V., Alexander, A.N., Vale, W., *et al.* (1984). Arginine vasopressin potentiates adrenocorticotropin release induced by ovine corticotropin-releasing factor. *J. Clin. Invest.* 73, 533.

DeFronzo, R.A., Braine, H., Colvin, O.M., and Davis, P.J. (1973). Water intoxication in man after cyclophosphamide therapy. *Ann. Intern. Med.* 78, 861.

DeFronzo, R.A., Abeloff, M., Braine, H., Humphrey, R.L., and Davis, P.J. (1974). Renal dysfunction after treatment with isophosphamide (NSC-109724). *Cancer Chemother. Rep.* 58, 375.

Delitala, G., Rovasio, P.P., Masala, A., Alagna, S., and Devilla, L. (1978). Metergoline inhibition of thyrotropin and prolactin secretion in primary hypothyroidism. *Clin. Endocrinol.* 8, 69.

De Rivera, J.L.G. (1975). Inappropriate secretion of antidiuretic hormone from fluphenazine therapy. *Ann. Intern. Med.* 82, 811.

Dexter, R.N., Fishman, L.M., Ney, R.L., and Liddle, G.W. (1967). Inhibition of adrenal corticosteroid synthesis by amino-glutethimide: studies of the mechanism of action. *J. Clin. Endocrinol.* 27, 473.

Dhar, S.K. and Ramos, R.R. (1978). Inappropriate antidiuresis during desipramine therapy. *Arch. Intern. Med.* 138, 1750.

Dickinson, P., Zinneman, H.N., Swaim, W.R., Doe, R.P., and Seal, U.S. (1969). Effects of testosterone treatment on plasma proteins and aminoacids in man. *J. Clin. Endocrinol. Metab.* 29, 837.

Doe, R.P., Mellinger, G.T., Swaim, W.R., and Seal, U.S. (1967). Estrogen dosage effects on serum proteins: a longitudinal study. *J. Clin. Endocrinol.* 27, 1081.

Dussault, H.H., Turcotte, R., and Guyda H. (1976). The effect of acetylsalicylic acid on TSH and PRL secretion after TRH stimulation in the human. *J. Clin. Endocrinol. Metab.* 43, 232.

Edes, T.E. and Sunderrajan, E.V. (1985). Heparin-induced hyperkalemia. *Arch. Intern. Med.* 145, 1070.

Ehrinpreis, M.N., Dhar, R., and Narula, A. (1989). Cimetidine-induced galactorrhea. *Am. J. Gastroenterol.* 84, 563.

Engbring, N.H. and Engstrom, W.W. (1959). Effects of estrogen and testosterone on circulating thyroid hormone. *J. Clin. Endocrinol. Metab.* 19, 783.

Erfurth, E.M. and Hedner, P. (1982). Importance of thyroxine in suppressing secretion of thyroid-stimulating hormone after thyroidectomy. *Br. Med. J.* 284, 941.

Evans, B.M., Dunne, J., and Surveyor, I. (1972). Pentazocine in thyroid failure. *Br. Med. J.* ii, 716.

Evered, D., Young, E.T., Ormston, B.J., Menzies, R., Smith, P.A., and Hall, R. (1973). Treatment of hypothyroidism: a reappraisal of thyroxine therapy. *Br. Med. J.* iii, 131.

Faber, J., Lumholtz, I.B., and Kirkegaard, C. (1985). The effects of phenytoin (diphenylhydantoin) on the extrathyroidal turnover of thyroxine, 3,5,3'-triiodothyronine, 3,3',5'-triiodothyronine and 3',5'-triiodothyronine in man. *J. Clin. Endocrinol. Metab.* 61, 1093.

Fagan, T.C., Johnson, D.G., and Grosso, D.S. (1985). Metronidazole-induced gynecomastia. *JAMA* 254, 3217.

Faglia, G., Ambrosi, B., Beck-Peccoz P., Travaglini, P., and Ferrari, C. (1972). The effect of theophylline on plasma thyrotropin (HTSH) response to thyrotropin releasing factor (TRF) in man. *J. Clin. Endocrinol. Metab.* 34, 906.

Feldman, H.A. and Singer, I. (1974). Comparative effects of tetracyclines on water flow across toad urinary bladders. *J. Pharmacol. Exp. Ther.* 190, 358.

Feldman, J.M. (1987). Falsely elevated urinary excretion of catecholamines and metanephrines in patients receiving labetalol therapy. *J. Clin. Pharmacol.* 27, 288.

Ferrari, C., Paracchi, A., Rondena, M., Beck-Peccoz, P., and Faglia, G. (1976). Effect of two serotonin antagonists on prolactin and thyrotropin secretion in man. *Clin. Endocrinol.* 5, 575.

Forrest, J.N. Jr, Cohen, A.D., Torretti, J., Himmelhoch, J.M., and Epstein, F.H. (1974). On the mechanism of lithium-induced diabetes insipidus in man and the rat. *J. Clin. Invest.* 53, 1115.

Fradkin, J.E. and Wolff, J. (1983). Iodide-induced thyrotoxicosis. *Medicine* 62, 1.

Frantz, A.G. (1978). Prolactin. *N. Engl. J. Med.* 298, 201.

Fraser, H.M. and Baird, D.T. (1987). Clinical applications of LHRH analogues. *Baillière's Clin. Endocrinol. Metab.* 1, 43.

Funder, J.W. and Mercer, J.E. (1979). Cimetidine, a histamine H_2 receptor antagonist, occupies androgen receptors. *J. Clin. Endocrinol. Metab.* 48, 189.

Gadd, E.M., Norris, C.M., and Beeley, L. (1987). Antidepressants and galactorrhoea. *Int. Clin. Psychopharmacol.* 2, 361.

Gaginella, T.S., O'Dorisio, T.M., Mekhjian, H.S., O'Dorisio, M.S., and Woltering, E.A. (1989). Tumors of the gastroenteropancreatic axis. In *Sandostatin in the treatment of GEP endocrine tumors* (ed. T.M. O'Dorisio), p. 23. Springer-Verlag, Berlin.

Galbraith, R.A. and Michnovicz, J.J. (1989). The effect of cimetidine on the oxidative metabolism of estradiol. *N. Engl. J. Med.* 321, 269.

Gammage, M.D. and Franklyn, J.A. (1987). Amiodarone and the thyroid. *Q. J. Med.* 62, 83.

Garfinkel, P.E., Calvin, E., and Harvey, C.S. (1973). Hypothyroidism and hyperparathyroidism associated with lithium. *Lancet* ii, 331.

Garnick, M.B. and Larsen, P.R. (1979). Acute deficiency of thyroxine-binding globulin during L-asparaginase therapy. *N. Engl. J. Med.* 301, 252.

Geller, J., Vazakas, G., Fruchtman, B., Newman, H., Nakao, K., and Loh, A. (1968). The effect of cyproterone acetate on advanced carcinoma of the prostate. *Surg. Gynecol. Obstet.* 127, 748.

Giese, A.A., Leibenluft, E., Green, S., and Moricle, L.A. (1989). Phenelzine-associated inappropriate ADH secretion. *J. Clin. Psychopharmacol.* 9, 309.

Gillies, G.E., Linton, E.A., and Lowry, P.J. (1982). Corticotropin releasing activity of the new CRF is potentiated several times by vasopressin. *Nature* 299, 355.

Glass, A.R. and Eil, C. (1986). Ketoconazole-induced reduction in serum 1,25-dihydroxyvitamin D. *J. Clin. Endocrinol. Metab.* 63, 766.

Glass, A.R. and Eil, C. (1988). Ketoconazole-induced reduction in serum 1,25-dihydroxyvitamin D and total serum calcium in hypercalcemic patients. *J. Clin. Endocrinol. Metab.* 66, 934.

Gluskin, L.E., Strasberg, B., and Shah, J.H. (1981). Verapamil-induced hyperprolactinemia and galactorrhea. *Ann. Intern. Med.* 95, 66.

Graber, A.L., Ney, R.L., Nicholson, W.E., Island, D.P., and Liddle, G.W. (1965). Natural history of pituitary–adrenal recovery following long-term suppression with corticosteroids. *J. Clin. Endocrinol.* 25, 11.

Greenbaum-Lefkoe, B., Rosenstock, J.G., Belasco, J.B., Rohrbaugh, T.M., and Meadows, A.T. (1985). Syndrome of inappropriate antidiuretic hormone secretion: a complication of high-dose intravenous melphalan. *Cancer* 55, 44.

Griffing, G.T. and Melby, J.C. (1989). Reversal of diuretic-induced secondary hyperaldosteronism and hypokalemia by trilostane, an inhibitor of adrenal steroidogenesis. *Metabolism* 38, 353.

Hahn, T.J. (1980). Drug-induced disorders of vitamin D and mineral metabolism. *Clin. Endocrinol. Metab.* 9, 107.

Halse, J., Harris, A.G., Kvistborg, A., Kjartansson, O., Hanssen, E., Smiseth, O., *et al.* (1990). A randomized study of SMS 201-995 versus bromocriptine treatment in acromegaly: clinical and biochemical effects. *J. Clin. Endocrinol. Metab.* 70, 1254.

Harmon, J. and Aliapoulios, M.A. (1972). Gynecomastia in marihuana users. *N. Engl. J. Med.* 287, 936.

Hawthorne, G.C., Campbell, N.P.S., Geddes, J.S., Ferguson, W.R., Postlethwaite, W., Sheridan, B., *et al.* (1985). Amiodarone-induced hypothyroidism. A common complication of prolonged therapy: a report of eight cases. *Arch. Intern. Med.* 145, 1016.

Heidemann, P., Peters, H.H., and Stubbe, P. (1980). Influence of L-asparaginase and oxandrolone on serum thyroxine-binding globulin. *Acta Endocrinol.* 94 (suppl. 234) (Abstract 20), 19.

Hershman, J.M., Craane, T.J., and Colwell, J.A. (1968). Effect of sulfonylurea drugs on the binding of triiodothyronine and thyroxine to thyroxine-binding globulin. *J. Clin. Endocrinol. Metab.* 28, 1605.

Heyma, P., Larkins, R.G., and Campbell, D.G. (1980). Inhibition of propranolol of 3,5,3′-triiodothyronine formation from thyroxine in isolated rat renal tubules: an effect independent of β-adrenergic blockade. *Endocrinology* 106, 1437.

Hikita, T., Fukutani, K., Yamamoto, Y., Yoshimizu, N., and Sasaki, T. (1989). Effect of aminophylline injection on the pituitary thyroid axis in asthmatics. *Jpn J. Med.* 28, 303.

Horning, S.J., Hoppe, R.T., Kaplan, H.S., and Rosenberg, S.A. (1981). Female reproductive potential after treatment for Hodgkin's disease. *N. Engl. J. Med.* 304, 1377.

How, J., Khir, A.S.M., and Bewsher, P.D. (1980). The effect of atenolol on serum thyroid hormones in hyperthyroid patients. *Clin. Endocrinol.* 13, 299.

Hughes, S.W.M. and Burley, D.M. (1970). Aminoglutethimide: a 'side-effect' turned to therapeutic advantage. *Postgrad. Med. J.* 46, 409.

Hull, M.G.R., Bromham, D.R., Savage, P.E., and Jackson, J.A.M. (1981). Normal fertility in women with post-pill amenorrhoea. *Lancet* i, 1329.

Hullin, R.P. (1978). The place of lithium in biological psychiatry. In *Lithium in medical practice* (ed. F.N. Johnson and S. Johnson), p. 433. MTP Press, Lancaster.

Huseman, G.A. and Hassing, J.M. (1984). Evidence for dopaminergic stimulation of growth velocity in some hypopituitary children. *J. Clin. Endocrinol. Metab.* 58, 419.

Hwang, A.S. and Magraw, R.M. (1989). Syndrome of inappropriate secretion of antidiuretic hormone due to fluoxetine. *Am. J. Psychiatry* 146, 399.

Isley, W.L. (1987). Effect of rifampin therapy on thyroid function tests in a hypothyroid patient on replacement L-thyroxine. *Ann. Intern. Med.* 107, 517.

Jeffcoate, W.J., Edwards, C.R.W., Rees, L.H., and Besser, G.M. (1976). Cyproterone acetate. *Lancet* ii, 1140.

Journal of the American Medical Association. (1963). AMA Council on drugs: A new antihypertensive — methyldopa (aldomet). *JAMA* 186, 504.

Jubiz, W., Meikle, A.W., Levinson, R.A., Mizutani, S., West, C.D., and Tyler, F.H. (1970). Effect of diphenylhydantoin on the metabolism of dexamethasone: mechanism of the abnormal dexamethasone suppression in humans. *N. Engl. J. Med.* 283, 11.

Kahl, L.E., Medsger, T.A., and Klein, I. (1985). Massive breast enlargement in a patient receiving D-penicillamine for systemic sclerosis. *J. Rheumatol.* 12, 990.

Kapcala, L.P. (1987). Alcohol-induced pseudo-Cushing's syndrome mimicking Cushing's disease in a patient with an adrenal mass. *Am. J. Med.* 82, 849.

Kaplan, M.M. and Utiger, R.D. (1978). Iodothyronine metabolism in rat liver homogenates. *J. Clin. Invest.* 61, 459.

Kaptein, E.M., Spencer, C.A., Kamiel, M.B., and Nicoloff, J.T. (1980). Prolonged dopamine administration and thyroid hormone economy in normal and critically ill subjects. *J. Clin. Endocrinol. Metab.* 51, 387.

Kennedy, R.L., Jones, T.H., and Shaukat, H.N. (1988). Amiodarone and thyroid immunity. *Br. Med. J.* 297, 621.

Kennedy, R.L., Griffiths, H., and Gray, T.A. (1989). Amiodarone and the thyroid. *Clin. Chem.* 35, 1882.

Kimura, T., Matsui, K., Sato, T., and Yoshinaga, K. (1974). Mechanism of carbamazepine (Tegretol)-induced antidiuresis: evidence for release of antidiuretic hormone and impaired excretion of a water load. *J. Clin. Endocrinol. Metab.* 38, 356.

Kirkegaard, C., Bjoerum, C.N., Cohn, D., Faber, J., Lauridsen, U.B., and Nerup, J. (1977). Studies of the influence of biogenic amines and psychoactive drugs on the prognostic value of the TRH stimulation test in endogenous depression. *Psychoneuroendocrinology* 2, 131.

Kirkegaard, C., Bjoerum, N., Cohn, D., and Lauridsen, U.B. (1978). Thyrotrophin-releasing hormone (TRH) stimulation test in manic-depressive illness. *Arch. Gen. Psychiatry* 35, 1017.

Kirkman, S. and Nelson, D.H. (1988). Alcohol-induced pseudo-Cushing's disease: a study of prevalence with review of the literature. *Metabolism* 37, 390.

Kleinberg, D.L., Noel, G.L., and Frantz, A.G. (1977). Galactorrhea: a study of 235 cases, including 48 with pituitary tumors. *N. Engl. J. Med.* 296, 589.

Kleinberg, D.L., Boyd III, A.E., Wardlaw, S., Frantz, A.G., George, A., Bryan, N., *et al.* (1983). Pergolide for the treatment of pituitary tumors secreting prolactin or growth hormone. *N. Engl. J. Med.* 309, 704.

Koang, N.K., Hu, T.C., Tch'en K.L., and Chu, T.H. (1955). Gynecomastia during administration of INH (isonicotinic hydrazide) for pulmonary tuberculosis. *Chin. Med. J.* 73, 214.

Kohri, K., Takada, M., Katoh, Y., Kataoka, K., Iguchi, M., Yachiku, S., *et al.* (1987). Parathyroid hormone and electrolytes during long term treatment with allopurinol and thiazide. *Br. J. Urol.* 59, 503.

Kurtz, A.B., Capper, S.J., Clifford, J., Humphrey, M.J., and Lukinac, L. (1981). The effect of fenclofenac on thyroid function. *Clin. Endocrinol.* 15, 117.

Kutyrina, I.M., Nikishova, T.A., and Tareyeva, I.E. (1987). Effects of heparin-induced aldosterone deficiency on renal function in patients with chronic glomerulonephritis. *Nephrol. Dial. Transplant.* 2, 219.

Kyriazopoulou, V., Parparousi, O., and Vagenakis, A.G. (1984). Rifampicin-induced adrenal crisis in Addisonian patients receiving corticosteroid replacement therapy. *J. Clin. Endocrinol. Metab.* 59, 1204.

Lamberts, S.W.J., Klijn, J.G.M., de Jong, F.H., and Birkenhager, J.C. (1979). Hormone secretion in alcohol-induced pseudo-Cushing's syndrome. *JAMA* 242, 1640.

Lane, R.J.M., Clark, F., and McCollum, J.K. (1977). Oxyphenbutazone-induced goitre. *Postgrad. Med. J.* 53, 93.

Lanes, R. and Hurtado, E.J. (1982). Oral clonidine — an effective growth hormone releasing agent in prepubertal subjects. *J. Pediatr.* 100, 710.

Langer, P., Foldes, O., Michajlovskij, N., Jezova, D., Klimes, I., Michalko, J., *et al.* (1978). Short-term effect of acetylsalicylic acid analogue on pituitary–thyroid axis and plasma cortisol level in healthy human volunteers. *Acta Endocrinol.* 88, 698.

Larsen, P.R. (1972). Salicylate-induced increases in free triiodothyronine in human serum: evidence of inhibition of triiodothyronine binding to thyroxine-binding globulin and thyroxine-binding prealbumin. *J. Clin. Invest.* 51, 1125.

Larsen, P.R., Atkinson, A.J. Jr, Wellman, H.N., and Goldsmith, R.E. (1970). The effect of diphenylhydantoin on thyroxine metabolism in man. *J. Clin. Invest.* 49, 1266.

Larsen, P.R., Dick, T.E., Markovitz, B.P., Kaplan, M.M., and Gard, T.G. (1979). Inhibition of intrapituitary thyroxine to 3,5,3'-triiodothyronine conversion prevents the acute suppression of thyrotropin release by thyroxine in hypothyroid rats. *J. Clin. Invest.* 64, 117.

Laudahn, G. (1984). Sex hormones. In *Clinical Pharmacology in Pregnancy* (ed. H.P. Kuemmerle and K. Brendel), p. 294. Thieme-Stratton, New York.

Laurberg, P. and Weeke, J. (1978). Opposite variations in serum T$_3$ and reverse T$_3$ during propylthiouracil treatment of thyrotoxicosis. *Acta Endocrinol.* 87, 88.

Laurell, C.-B., Kullander, S., and Thorell, J. (1967). Effect of administration of a combined estrogen-progestin contraceptive on the level of individual plasma proteins. *Scand. J. Clin. Lab. Invest.* 22, 337.

Lazarus, J.H. (1982). Endocrine and metabolic effects of lithium. *Adverse Drug React. Acute Poisoning Rev.* 1, 181.

Ledingham, I.M. and Watt, I. (1983). Influence of sedation on mortality in critically ill multiple trauma patients. *Lancet* i, 1270.

Lembcke, B., Schleser, C.S., Schleser, S., Ebert, R., Shaw, C., and Koop, I. (1987). Effect of the somatostatin analogue sandostatin (SMS 201-995) on gastrointestinal, pancreatic and biliary function and hormone release in normal men. *Digestion* 36, 108.

Levesque, H., Verdier, S., Cailleux, N., Elie-Legrand, M.C., Gancel, A., Basuyau, J.P., *et al.* (1990). Low molecular weight heparins and hypoaldosteronism. *Br. Med. J.* 300, 1437.

LeWinn, E.B. (1953). Gynecomastia during digitalis therapy: Report of eight additional cases with liver-function studies. *N. Engl. J. Med.* 248, 316.

Liewendahl, K., Majuri, H., and Helenius, T. (1978). Thyroid function tests in patients on long-term treatment with various anticonvulsant drugs. *Clin. Endocrinol.* 8, 185.

Liskin, B., Walsh, B.T., Roose, S.P., and Jackson, W. (1984). Imipramine-induced inappropriate ADH secretion. *J. Clin. Psychopharmacol.* 4, 146.

Littlewood, T.J. and Smith, A.P. (1984). Syndrome of inappropriate antidiuretic hormone secretion due to treatment of lung cancer with cisplatin. *Thorax* 39, 636.

Livanou, T., Ferriman, D., and James, V.H.T. (1967). Recovery of hypothalamo–pituitary–adrenal function after corticosteroid therapy. *Lancet* ii, 856.

Loeb, J.N. (1976). Corticosteroids and growth. *N. Engl. J. Med.* 295, 547.

Loriaux, D.L., Menard, R., Taylor, A., Pita, J.C., and Santen, R. (1976). Spironolactone and endocrine dysfunction. *Ann. Intern. Med.* 85, 630.

Lotti, G., Delitala, G., Devilla, L., Alagna, S., and Masala, A. (1977). Reduction of plasma triiodothyronine (T$_3$) induced by propranolol. *Clin. Endocrinol.* 6, 405.

Luton, J.P., Mahoudeau, J.A., Bouchord, P., Thieblot, P., Hautecouverture, M., Simon, D., *et al.* (1979). Treatment of Cushing's syndrome by *o,p'*-DDD. Survey of 62 cases. *N. Engl. J. Med.* 300, 459.

Luzecky, M.H. (1974). The syndrome of inappropriate secretion of antidiuretic hormone associated with amitriptyline administration. *South. Med. J.* 67, 495.

Maarbjerg, K., Vestergaard, P., and Schou, M. (1987). Changes in serum thyroxine (T$_4$) and serum thyroid stimulating hormone (TSH) during prolonged lithium treatment. *Acta Psychiatr. Scand.* 75, 217.

MacAdams, M.R., White, R.H., and Chipps, B.E. (1986). Reduction of serum testosterone levels during chronic glucocorticoid therapy. *Ann. Intern. Med.* 104, 648.

McCallum, R.W., Sowers, J.R., Hershman, J.M., and Sturdevant, R.A.L. (1976). Metoclopramide stimulates prolactin secretion in man. *J. Clin. Endocrinol. Metab.* 42, 1148.

McCance, D.R., Hadden, D.R., Kennedy, L., Sheridan, B., and Atkinson, A.B. (1987). Clinical experience with keto-conazole as a therapy for patients with Cushing's syndrome. *Clin. Endocrinol.* 27, 593.

McClure, R.D. (1987). Endocrine investigation and therapy. *Urol. Clin. North Am.* 14, 471.

McDermott, M.T., Burman, K.D., Hofeldt, F.D., and Kidd, G.S. (1986). Lithium-associated thyrotoxicosis. *Am. J. Med.* 80, 1245.

MacGregor, A.G. and Somner, A.R. (1954). The anti-thyroid action of para-aminosalicylic acid. *Lancet* ii, 931.

McIntosh, W.B., Horn, E.H., Mathieson, L.M., and Sumner, D. (1987). The prevalence, mechanism and clinical significance of lithium-induced hypercalcaemia. *Med. Lab. Sci.* 44, 115.

MacKenzie, M.A., Hoefnagels, W.H.L., Jansen, R.W.M.M., Benraad, T.J., and Kloppenborg, P.W.C. (1990). The influence of glycyrrhetinic acid on plasma cortisol and cortisone in healthy young volunteers. *J. Clin. Endocrinol. Metab.* 70, 1637.

McKerron, C.G., Scott, R.L., Asper, S.P., and Levy, R.I. (1969). Effects of clofibrate (atromid S) on the thyroxine-binding capacity of thyroxine-binding globulin and free thyroxine. *J. Clin. Endocrinol.* 29, 957.

Mallette, L.E., Khouri, K., Zengotita, H., Hollis, B.W., and Malini, S. (1989). Lithium treatment increases intact and midregion parathyroid hormone and parathyroid volume. *J. Clin. Endocrinol. Metab.* 68, 654.

Mannisto, P.T. (1980). Endocrine side-effects of lithium. In *Handbook of lithium therapy* (ed. F.N. Johnson), p. 310. MTP Press, Lancaster.

Mardell, R. and Gamlen, T.R. (1982). Artifactual reduction in circulating free thyroxine concentration by radioimmuno-assay. *Lancet* i, 973.

Margolis, I.B. and Gross, C.G. (1967). Gynecomastia during phenothiazine therapy. *JAMA* 199, 942.

Markusse, H.M. and Meyboom R.H.B. (1988). Gynaeco-mastia associated with captropril. *Br. Med. J.* 296, 1262.

Marshall, J.S. and Tompkins, L.S. (1968). Effect of *o,p''*-DDD and similar compounds on thyroxine binding globulin. *J. Clin. Endocrinol.* 28, 386.

Martin, J.B. and Reichlin, S. (1987). Neuropharmacology of anterior pituitary regulation. In *Clinical Neuroendocrinol-ogy* (2nd edn), p. 45. F.A. Davis, Philadelphia.

Martin, J.B., Durand, D., Gurd, W., Faille, G., Audet, J., and Brazeau, P. (1978). Neuropharmacological regulation of episodic growth hormone and prolactin secretion in the rat. *Endocrinology* 102, 106.

Martino, E., Safran, M., Aghini-Lombardi, F., Rajatanavln, R., Lenziardi, M., Fay, M., *et al.* (1984). Environmental iodine intake and thyroid dysfunction during chronic ami-odarone therapy. *Ann. Intern. Med.* 101, 28.

Martino, E., Macchia, E., Aghini-Lombardi, F., Antonelli, A., Lenziardi, M., Concetti, R., *et al.* (1986a). Is humoral thyroid autoimmunity relevant in amiodarone iodine-induced thyrotoxicosis (AIIT)? *Clin. Endocrinol.* 24, 627.

Martino, E., Aghini-Lombardi, F., Mariotti, S., Lenziardi, M., Baschieri, L., Braverman, L.E., *et al.* (1986b). Treatment of amiodarone associated thyrotoxicosis by simultaneous ad-ministration of potassium perchlorate and methimazole. *J. Endocrinol. Invest.* 9, 201.

Martino, E., Aghini-Lombardi, F., Mariotti, S., Bartalena, L., Braverman, L., and Pinchera, A. (1987a). Amiodarone: a common source of iodine-induced thyrotoxicosis. *Horm. Res.* 26, 158.

Martino, E., Aghini-Lombardi, F., Mariotti, S., Bartalena L., Lenziardi, M., Ceccarelli, C., *et al.* (1987b). Amiodarone iodine-induced hypothyroidism: risk factors and follow-up in 28 cases. *Clin. Endocrinol.* 26, 227.

Massara, F., Camanni, F., Belforte, L., Vergano, V., and Molinatti, G.M. (1978). Increased thyrotrophin secretion induced by sulpiride in man. *Clin. Endocrinol.* 9, 419.

Massara, F., Tangolo, D., and Godano, A. (1985). The effect of metaclopramide, domperidone and apomorphine on GH secretion in children and adolescents. *Acta Endocrinol.* 108, 451.

Matuk, F. and Kalyanaraman, K. (1977). Syndrome of inappro-priate secretion of antidiuretic hormone in patients treated with psychotherapeutic drugs. *Arch. Neurol.* 34, 374.

Mazze, R.I., Shue, G.L., and Jackson, S.H. (1971). Renal dysfunction associated with methoxyflurane anesthesia: a randomized, prospective clinical evaluation. *JAMA* 216, 278.

Mechlis, S., Lubin, E., Laor, J., Margaliot, M., and Strasberg, B. (1987). Amiodarone-induced thyroid gland dysfunction. *Am. J. Cardiol.* 59, 833.

Meikle, A.W., Jubiz, W., Matsukura, S., West, C.G., and Tyler, F.H. (1969). Effect of diphenylhydantoin on the metabolism of metyrapone and release of ACTH in man. *J. Clin. Endocrinol.* 29, 1553.

Melmed, S., Nademanee, K., Reed, A.W., Hendrickson, J.A., Singh, B.N., and Hershman, J.M. (1981). Hyperthyrox-inemia with bradycardia and normal thyrotropin secretion after chronic amiodarone administration. *J. Clin. Endo-crinol. Metab.* 53, 997.

Mendel, C.M., Frost, P.H., Kunitakis, P.H., and Cavalieri, R.R. (1987). Mechanisms of heparin-induced increase in the concentration of free thyroxine in plasma. *J. Clin. Endocrinol. Metab.* 65, 1259.

Mendelson, J.H., Mendelson J.E., and Patch, V.D. (1975). Plasma testosterone levels in heroin addiction and during methadone maintenance. *J. Pharmacol. Exp. Ther.* 192, 211.

Migliari, R., Balzano, S., Scarpa, R.M., Campus, G., Pintus, C., and Usai, E. (1988). Short term effects of flutamide administration on hypothalamic–pituitary–testicular axis in man. *J. Urol.* 139, 637.

Miller, D.G. (1971) Alkylating agents and human spermato-genesis. *JAMA* 217, 1662.

Miller M. and Moses, A.M. (1970). Mechanism of chlor-propamide action in diabetes insipidus. *J. Clin. Endocrinol.* 30, 488.

Milne, K. and Greer, M.A. (1962). Comparison of the effects of propylthiouracil and sulfadiazine on thyroidal biosynthesis and the manner in which they are influenced by supplemen-tal iodide. *Endocrinology* 71, 580.

Mitchell, J.R.A., Surridge, D.H.C., and Wilson, R.G. (1959). Hypothermia after chlorpromazine in myxedematous psychosis. *Br. Med. J.* ii, 932.

Mitsch, R.A. and Lee, A.K. (1986). Syndrome of inappropriate antidiuretic hormone with imipramine. *Drug Intell. Clin. Pharm.* 20, 787.

Miyai, K., Onishi, T., Hosokawa, M., Ishibashi, K., and Kumahara, Y. (1974). Inhibition of thyrotropin and prolactin secretions in primary hypothyroidism by 2-Br-α-ergocryptine. *J. Clin. Endocrinol. Metab.* 39, 391.

Monson, J.P. and Scott, D.F. (1987). Gynaecomastia induced by phenytoin in men with epilepsy. *Br. Med. J.* 294, 612.

Morgans, M.E. and Trotter, W.R. (1954). Treatment of thyrotoxicosis with potassium perchlorate. *Lancet* i, 10, 749.

Morgans, M.E. and Trotter, W.R. (1955). The anti-thyroid effect of phenylbutazone. *Lancet* ii, 164.

Morley, J.E., Shafer, R.B., Elson, M.K., Slag, M.F., Raleigh, M.J., Brammer, G.L., *et al.* (1980). Amphetamine-induced hyperthyroxinemia. *Ann. Intern. Med.* 93, 707.

Moses, A.M., Numann, P., and Miller, M. (1973a). Mechanism of chlorpropamide-induced antidiuresis in man: evidence for release of ADH and enhancement of peripheral action. *Metabolism* 22, 59.

Moses, A.M., Howanitz, J., van Gemert, M., and Miller, M. (1973b). Clofibrate-induced antidiuresis. *J. Clin. Invest.* 52, 535.

Moulding, T. and Fraser, R. (1970). Hypothyroidism related to ethionamide. *Am. Rev. Respir. Dis.* 101, 90.

Murphy, D.L., Goodwin, F.K., and Bunney, W.E. Jr (1969). Aldosterone and sodium response to lithium administration in man. *Lancet* ii, 458.

Nademanee, K., Piwonka, R.W., Singh, B.N., and Hershman, J.M. (1989). Amiodarone and thyroid function. *Prog. Cardiovasc. Dis.* 31, 427.

Naitoh, Y., Fukato, J., Tominaga, T., Nakai, Y., Tamai, S., Mori, K., *et al.* (1988). Interleukin-6 stimulates the secretion of adrenocorticotropic hormone in conscious freely-moving rats. *Biochem. Biophys. Res. Commun.* 155, 1459.

Namer, M. (1988). Clinical applications of antiandrogens. *J Steroid. Biochem.* 31, 719.

Namer, M., Khater, R., Frenay, M., and Boublil, J.L. (1986). High dose of ketoconazole in the treatment of advanced breast cancers. *Bull. Cancer* 73, 89.

Neumann, F. (1978). Antiandrogens. In *Advances in gynaecological endocrinology* (ed. H.S. Jacobs). Proceedings of the 6th Study Group of the Royal College of Obstetricians and Gynaecologists, p. 335.

Nicholls, M.G. and Espiner, E.A. (1983). Liquorice, carbenoxolone and hypertension. In *Handbook of Hypertension, Vol. 2: Clinical aspects of secondary hypertension* (ed. J.I.S. Robertson), p. 189. Elsevier, Amsterdam.

Nicoloff, J.T., Fisher, D.A., and Appleman, M.D. Jr (1970). The role of glucocorticoids in the regulation of thyroid function in man. *J. Clin. Invest.* 49, 1922.

Nielsen-Kudsk, J.E., Bartels, P.D., and Dalby, J. (1990). Effects of verapamil on diurnal and thyrotropin-releasing hormone-stimulated prolactin levels in man. *J. Clin. Endocrinol. Metab.* 70, 1269.

Nilsson, O.R., Karlberg, B.E., Kagedal, B., Tegler, L., and Almqvist, S. (1979). Non-selective and selective β_1-adrenoceptor blocking agents in the treatment of hyperthyroidism. *Acta Med. Scand.* 206, 21.

Nishida, S., Matsuki, M., Nagase, Y., Horino, M., Endoh, M., Kakita, K., *et al.* (1983a). Stress-mediated effect of metoclopramide on cortisol secretion in man. *J. Clin. Endocrinol. Metab.* 56, 839.

Nishida, S., Matsuki, M., Nagase, Y., Horino, M., Endoh, M., Kakita, K., *et al.* (1983b). Adrenocorticotropin-mediated effect of metoclopramide on plasma aldosterone in man. *J. Clin. Endocrinol. Metab.* 57, 981.

Nishida, S., Matsuki, M., Adachi, N., Horino, M., Yoneda, M., Endoh, M., *et al.* (1987). Pituitary–adrenocortical response to metoclopramide in patients with acromegaly and prolactinoma: a clinical evaluation of catecholamine-mediated adrenocorticotropin secretion. *J. Clin. Endocrinol. Metab.* 64, 995.

Ohnhaus, E.E., Burgi, H., Burger, A., and Studer, H. (1981). The effect of antipyrine, phenobarbital and rifampicin on thyroid hormone metabolism in man. *Eur. J. Clin. Invest.* 11, 381.

Ooiwa, H., Shimamoto, K., Nakagawa, M. and Iimura, O. (1988). The interference of acebutolol administration in the measurement of urinary 17-ketosteroid by Zimmermann's method. *Endocrinol. Jpn* 35, 485.

Oppenheimer, J.H. and Werner, S.C. (1966). Effect of prednisone on thyroxine-binding proteins. *J. Clin. Endocrinol.* 26, 715.

Otsuki, M., Dakoda, M., and Baba, S. (1973). Influence of glucocorticoids on TRF-induced TSH response in man. *J. Clin. Endocrinol. Metab.* 36, 95.

Pannall, P.R. and Maas, D.A. (1977). Danazol and thyroid-function tests. *Lancet* i, 102.

Pearce, C.J. and Byfield, P.G.H. (1986). Free thyroid hormone assays and thyroid function. *Ann. Clin. Biochem.* 23, 230.

Peden, N.R., Isles, T.E., Stevenson, I.H., and Crooks, J. (1982). Nadolol in thyrotoxicosis. *Br. J. Clin. Pharmacol.* 13, 835.

Peterson, J.C., Pollack, W.R., and Mahoney, J.J. (1978). Inappropriate antidiuretic hormone secondary to a monoamine oxidase inhibitor. *JAMA* 239, 1422.

Pinder, R.M., Brogden, R.N., Sawyer, P.R., Speight, T.M., Spencer, R., and Avery, G.S. (1976). Carbenoxolone: a review of its pharmacological properties and therapeutic efficacy in peptic ulcer disease. *Drugs* 11, 245.

Pont, A., Goldman, E.S., Sugar, A.M., Siiteri, P.K., and Stevens, D.A. (1985). Ketoconazole-induced increase in estradiol-testosterone ratio. *Arch. Intern. Med.* 145, 1429.

Preece, M.A. (1976). The effect of administered corticosteroids on the growth of children. *Postgrad. Med. J.* 52, 625.

Preziosi, P. and Vacca, M. (1988). Adrenocortical suppression and other endocrine effects of etomidate. *Life Sci.* 42, 477.

Pugeat, M., Lejeune, H., Dechaud, H., Emptoz-Bonneton, A., Fleury, M.-C., Charrie, A., *et al.* (1987). Effects of drug administration on gonadotropins, sex steroid hormones and binding proteins in humans. *Horm. Res.* 28, 261.

Rado, J.P. (1973). Water intoxication during carbamazepine treatment. *Br. Med. J.* iii, 479.

Rajfer, J., Sikka, S.C., Rivera, F., and Handelsman, D.J. (1986). Mechanism of inhibition of human testicular steroidogenesis by oral ketoconazole. *J. Clin. Endocrinol. Metab.* 63, 1193.

Rao, K.J., Miller, M., and Moses, A. (1975). Water intoxication and thioridazine (Mellaril). *Ann. Intern. Med.* 82, 61.

Rayfield, E.J., Cain, J.P., Casey, M.P., Williams, G.H., and Sullivan, J.M. (1972). Influence of diet on urinary VMA excretion. *JAMA* 221, 704.

Refetoff, S., Fang, V.S., Rapoport, B., and Friesen, H.G. (1974). Interrelationships in the regulation of TSH and prolactin secretion in man: effects of L-dopa, TRH and thyroid hormone in various combinations. *J. Clin. Endocrinol. Metab.* 38, 450.

Reichert, L.J.M. and de Rooy, H.A.M. (1989). Treatment of amiodarone induced hyperthyroidism with potassium perchlorate and methimazole during amiodarone treatment. *Br. Med. J.* 298, 1547.

Reid, D.M., Martynoga, A.G., and Nuki, G. (1982). Reversible gynaecomastia associated with D-penicillamine in a man with rheumatoid arthritis. *Br. Med. J.* 285, 1083.

Reus, V.I., Gold, P., and Post, R. (1979). Lithium-induced thyrotoxicosis. *Am. J. Psychiatry* 136, 724.

Ritch, P.S. (1988). Cis-dichlorodiammineplatinum II-induced syndrome of inappropriate secretion of antidiuretic hormone. *Cancer* 61, 448.

Roberts II, L.J. (1988). Carcinoid syndrome and disorders of systemic mast-cell activation including systemic mastocytosis. *Endocrinol. Metab. Clin. North Am.* 17, 415.

Robertson, G.L., Bhoopalam, N., and Zelkowitz, L.J. (1973). Vincristine neurotoxicity and abnormal secretion of antidiuretic hormone. *Arch. Intern. Med.* 132, 717.

Robinson, B. (1957). Breast changes in the male and female with chlorpromazine or reserpine therapy. *Med. J. Aust.* ii, 239.

Safran, M., Martino, E., Aghini-Lombardi, F., Bartalena, L., Balzano, S., Pinchera, A., *et al.* (1988). Effect of amiodarone on circulating antithyroid antibodies. *Br. Med. J.* 297, 456.

Sakakura, M., Takebe, K., and Nakagawa, S. (1973). Inhibition of luteinizing hormone secretion induced by synthetic LRH by long-term treatment with glucocorticoids in human subjects. *J. Clin. Endocrinol. Metab.* 40, 774.

Sakemi, T., Ohchi, N., Sanai, T., Rikitake, O., and Maeda, T. (1988). Captopril-induced metabolic acidosis with hyperkalemia. *Am. J. Nephrol.* 8, 245.

Santen, R.J. and Bourguignon, J-P. (1987). Gonadotropin-releasing hormone: physiological and therapeutic aspects, agonists and antagonists. *Horm. Res.* 28, 88.

Santen, R.J., Wells, S.A., Runic, S., Gupta, C., Kendall, J., Rudy, E.B., *et al.* (1977). Adrenal suppression with aminoglutethimide. I: Differential effects of aminoglutethimide on glucocorticoid metabolism as a rationale for use of hydrocortisone. *J. Clin. Endocrinol. Metab.* 45, 469.

Sapolsky, R., Rivier, C., Yamamoto, G., Plotsky, P., and Vale, W. (1987). Interleukin-1 stimulates the secretion of hypothalamic corticotropin-releasing factor. *Science* 238, 522.

Scanlon, M.F., Weightman, D.R., Shale, D.J., Mora, B., Heath, M., Snow, M.H., *et al.* (1979). Dopamine is a physiological regulator of thyrotrophin (TSH) secretion in normal man. *Clin. Endocrinol.* 10, 7.

Schardein, J.L. (1980). Congenital abnormalities and hormones during pregnancy: a clinical review. *Teratology* 22, 251.

Schteingart, D.E. (1989). Cushing's syndrome. *Endocrinol. Metab. Clin. North Am.* 18, 311.

Schussler, G.C. (1971). Diazepam competes for thyroxine binding. *J. Pharmacol. Exp. Ther.* 178, 204.

Seely, E.W., LeBoff, M.S., Brown, E.M., Chen, C., Posillico, J.T., Hollenberg, N.K., *et al.* (1989). The calcium channel blocker diltiazem lowers serum parathyroid hormone levels in vivo and in vitro. *J. Clin. Endocrinol. Metab.* 68, 1007.

Shamberger, R.C., Rosenberg, S.A., Seipp, C.A., and Sherins, R.J. (1981). Effects of high-dose methotrexate and vincristine on ovarian and testicular functions in patients undergoing postoperative adjuvant treatment of osteosarcoma. *Cancer Treat. Rep.* 65, 739.

Sharma, B., Axelson, M., Pounder, R.P., Lundborg, P., Ohman, M., Santana, A., *et al.* (1987). Acid secretory capacity and plasma gastrin concentration after administration of omeprazole to normal subjects. *Aliment. Pharmacol. Ther.* 1, 67.

Sheps, S.G., Jiang, N.S., and Klee, G.G. (1988). Diagnostic evaluation of pheochromocytoma. *Endocrinol. Metab. Clin. North Am.* 17, 397.

Sherins, R.J. and Mulvihill, J.J. (1989). Gonadal dysfunction. In *Cancer: Principles and practice of oncology* (3rd edn) (ed. V.T. DeVita Jr, S. Hellman, and S.A. Rosenberg), p. 2170. J.B. Lippincott, Philadelphia.

Sherman, R.A. and Ruddy, M.C. (1986). Suppression of aldosterone production by low-dose heparin. *Am. J. Nephrol.* 6, 165.

Singer, I. and Forrest, J.N. Jr (1976). Drug-induced states of nephrogenic diabetes insipidus. *Kidney Int.* 10, 82.

Singer, I. and Rotenberg, D. (1973). Mechanisms of lithium action. *N. Engl. J. Med.* 289, 254.

Slater, S.L., Lipper, S., Shiling, D.J., and Murphy, D.L. (1977). Elevation of plasma-prolactin by monoamine-oxidase inhibitors. *Lancet* ii, 275.

Slooten, H.V., Moolenaar, A.J., van Seters, A.P., and Smeenk, D. (1984). The treatment of adrenocortical carcinoma with *o,p'*-DDD: prognostic simplifications of serum level monitoring. *Eur. J. Cancer. Clin. Oncol.* 20, 47.

Smals, A.G.H., Kloppenborg, P.W.C., Goverde, H.J.M., and Benraad, T.J. (1978). The effect of cyproterone acetate on the pituitary–adrenal axis in hirsute women. *Acta Endocrinol.* 87, 352.

Smigan, L., Wahlin, A., Jacobsson, L., and von Knorring, L. (1984). Lithium therapy and thyroid function tests: a prospective study. *Neuropsychobiology* 11, 39.

Smith, M.J. and Hodson, M.E. (1983). Effects of long term inhaled high dose beclomethasone dipropionate on adrenal function. *Thorax* 38, 676.

Sneddon, I.B. (1976). Clinical use of topical corticosteroids. *Drugs* 11, 193.

Solomon, I.L. and Schoen, E.J. (1976). Juvenile Cushing syndrome manifested primarily by growth failure. *Am. J. Dis. Child.* 130, 200.

Sonino, N. (1987). The use of ketoconazole as an inhibitor of steroid production. *N. Engl. J. Med.* 317, 812.

Sparagana, M. (1987). Primary hypogonadism associated with *o,p'*-DDD (mitotane) therapy. *Clin. Toxicol.* 25, 463.

Stancer, H.C. and Forbath, N. (1989). Hyperparathyroidism, hypothyroidism, and impaired renal function after 10 to 20 years of lithium treatment. *Arch. Intern. Med.* 149, 1042.

Stewart, P.M., Wallace, A.M., Valentino, R., Burt, D., Shackleton, C.H.L., and Edwards, C.R.W. (1987). Mineralocorticoid activity of liquorice: 11-β-hydroxysteroid dehydrogenase deficiency comes of age. *Lancet* ii, 821.

Stewart, P.M., Wallace, A.M., Atherden, S.M., Shearing, C.H., and Edwards, C.R.W. (1990). Mineralocorticoid activity of carbenoxolone: contrasting effects of carbenoxolone and liquorice on 11-β-hydroxysteroid dehydrogenase activity in man. *Clin. Sci.* 78, 49.

Stockigt, J.R., Lim, C.F., Barlow, J.W., Stevens, V., Topliss, D.J., and Wynne, K.N. (1984). High concentrations of furosemide inhibit serum binding of thyroxine. *J. Clin. Endocrinol. Metab.* 59, 62.

Strickland, A.L. and Sprinz, H. (1973). Studies of the influence of estradiol and growth hormone on the hypophysectomized immature rat epiphyseal cartilage growth plate. *Am. J. Obstet. Gynecol.* 115, 471.

Strickland, A.L., Underwood, L.E., Voina, S.J., French, F.S., Van Wyk, J.J., and Hill, C. (1972). Growth retardation in Cushing's syndrome. *Am. J. Dis. Child.* 123, 207.

Stuart, M.J., Cuaso, C., Miller, M., and Oski, F.A. (1975). Syndrome of recurrent increased secretion of antidiuretic hormone following multiple doses of vincristine. *Blood* 45, 315.

Suzuki, H., Kadena, N., Takeuchi, K., and Nakagawa, S. (1979). Effects of three-day oral cholecystography on serum iodothyronines and TSH concentrations: comparison of the effects among some cholecystographic agents and the effects of iopanoic acid on the pituitary–thyroid axis. *Acta Endocrinol.* 92, 477.

Suzuki, H., Noguchi, K., Nakahata, M., Nakagawa, S., and Kadena, N. (1981). Effect of iopanoic acid on the pituitary–thyroid axis: time sequence of changes in serum iodothyronines, thyrotropin, and prolactin concentrations and responses to thyroid hormones. *J. Clin. Endocrinol. Metab.* 53, 779.

Swerdloff, R.S., Palacios, A., McClure, R.D., Campfield, L.A., and Brosman, S.A. (1978). Male contraception: clinical assessment of chronic administration of testosterone enanthate. *Int. J. Androl.* 2, 731.

Tanner, L.A. and Bosco, L.A. (1988). Gynecomastia associated with calcium channel blocker therapy. *Arch. Intern. Med.* 148, 379.

Taylor, A.L. and Fishman, L.M. (1988). Corticotropin- releasing hormone. *N. Engl. J. Med.* 319, 213.

Taylor, R., Clark, F., and Griffiths, I.D. (1980). Prospective study of effect of fenclofenac on thyroid function tests. *Br. Med. J.* 281, 911.

Thomas, B.L. (1976). Methadone-associated gynecomastia. *N. Engl. J. Med.* 294, 169.

Tolis, G., Somma, M., Campenhout, J.V., and Friesen, H. (1974). Prolactin secretion in sixty-five patients with galactorrhea. *Am. J. Obstet. Gynecol.* 118, 91.

Trachtenberg, J. and Zadra, J. (1988). Steroid synthesis inhibition by ketoconazole: sites of action. *Clin. Invest. Med.* 11, 1.

Trump, D.L., Pavy, M.D., and Staal, S. (1982). Gynaecomastia in men following antineoplastic therapy. *Arch. Intern. Med.* 142, 511.

Tuomisto, J., Ranta, T., Saarinen, A., Mannisto, P., and Leppaluoto, J. (1973). Neurotransmission and secretion of thyroid stimulating hormones. *Lancet* ii, 510.

Turkington, R.W. (1972). Prolactin secretion in patients treated with various drugs. *Arch. Intern. Med.* 130, 349.

Uehara, A., Gottschall, P.E., Dahl, R.R., and Arimura, A. (1987). Interleukin-1 stimulates ACTH release by an indirect action which requires endogenous corticotropin releasing factor. *Endocrinology* 121, 1580.

Vagenakis, A.G. (1988). Pituitary–thyroid interaction: effects of thyroid hormone, non thyroidal illness and various agents on TSH secretion. *Acta Med. Austriaca* 15, 52.

Vagenakis, A. and Braverman, L. (1975). Adverse effects of iodides on thyroid function. *Med. Clin. North Am.* 59, 1075.

Vale, W., Rivier, C., Brown, M.R., Spiess, J., Koob, G., Swanson, L., *et al.* (1983). Chemical and biological characterization of corticotropin releasing factor. *Recent Prog. Horm. Res.* 39, 245.

Vance, M.L., Evans, W.S., and Thorner, M.O. (1984). Diagnosis and treatment: drugs five years later — bromocriptine. *Ann. Intern. Med.* 100, 78.

Varl, B., Tos, L., and Cokic, M. (1988). Influence of dopamine on the thyroid hormones and thyrotropin in acute respiratory distress syndrome. *Acta Med. Austriaca* 15, 59.

Vaughan, E.D. Jr, Carey, R.M., Peach, M.J., Ackerly, J.A., and Ayers, C.R. (1978). The renin response to diuretic therapy : a limitation of antihypertensive potential. *Circ. Res.* 42, 376.

Viviani, S., Santoro, A., Ragni, G., Bonfante, V., Bestetti, O., and Bonadonna, G. (1985). Gonadal toxicity after combination chemotherapy for Hodgkin's disease comparative results of MOPP vs ABVD. *Eur. J. Cancer Clin. Oncol.* 21, 601.

von Puttkamer, K., Bierich, J.R., Brugger, F., Hirche, W., and Schonberg, D. (1977). Oestrogen treatment of girls with increased growth. *Dtsch. Med. Wochenschr.* 102, 983.

Walden, C.E., Knopp, R.H., Johnson, J.L., Heiss, G., Wahl, P.W. and Hoover, J.J. (1986). Effect of estrogen/progestin potency on clinical chemistry measures. *Am. J. Epidemiol.* 123, 517.

Waxman, J.H.X., Terry, Y.A., Wrigley, P.F.M., Malpas, J.S., Rees, L.H., Besser, G.M., *et al.* (1982). Gonadal function in

Hodgkin's disease: long-term follow-up of chemotherapy. *Br. Med. J.* 285, 1612.

Wehrenberg, W.B., Esch, F., Baird, A., Ying, S-Y., Bolen, P., and Ling, N. (1986). Growth hormone-releasing factor: a new chapter in neuroendocrinology. *Horm. Res.* 24, 82.

Werk, E.E., MacGee, J., and Sholiton, L.J. (1964). Effect of diphenylhydantoin on cortisol metabolism in man. *J. Clin. Invest.* 43, 1824.

Werner, S.C. and Platman, S.R. (1965). Remission of hyperthyroidism (Graves' disease) and altered pattern of serum-thyroxine binding induced by prednisone. *Lancet* ii, 751.

Westgren, U., Melander, A., Wahlin, E., and Lindgren, J. (1977). Divergent effects of 6-propylthiouracil on 3,5,3′-triiodothyronine (T$_3$) and 3,3′,5′-triiodothyronine (rT$_3$) serum levels in man. *Acta Endocrinol.* 85, 345.

Wettenhall, H.N.B., Cahill, C., and Roche, A.F. (1975). Tall girls: a survey of 15 years of management and treatment. *J. Pediatr.* 86, 602.

Whitworth, J.A., Butkus, A., Coghlan, J.P., Denton, D.A., Mills, E.H., Spence, C.D., et al. (1986). 9-alpha-fluorocortisol-induced hypertension: a review. *J. Hypertens.* 4, 133.

Wiersinga, W.M. and Trip, M.D. (1986). Amiodarone and thyroid hormone metabolism. *Postgrad. Med. J.* 62, 909.

Wilber, J.F. and Utiger, R.D. (1969). The effect of glucocorticoids on thyrotropin secretion. *J. Clin. Invest.* 48, 2096.

Wilkinson, R., Anderson, M., and Smart, G.A. (1972). Growth-hormone deficiency in iatrogenic hypothyroidism. *Br. Med. J.* ii, 87.

Williams, H.J. (1988). Gynecomastia as a complication of auranofin therapy. *J. Rheumatol.* 15, 1863.

Winnacker, J.L., Yeager, H., Saunders, J.A., Russell, B., and Anast, C.S. (1977). Rickets in children receiving anticonvulsant drugs. *Am. J. Dis. Child.* 131, 286.

Wolff, J. (1969). Iodide goiter and the pharmacologic effects of excess iodide. *Am. J. Med.* 47, 101.

Wolff, J. and Chaikoff, I.L. (1948). Plasma inorganic iodide as a homeostatic regulator of thyroid function. *J. Biol. Chem.* 174, 555.

Wolff, J., Standaert, M.E., and Rall, J.E. (1961). Thyroxine displacement from serum proteins and depression of serum protein-bound iodine by certain drugs. *J. Clin. Invest.* 40, 1373.

Wortsman, J., Hamidinia, A., and Winters, S.J. (1989). Hypogonadism following long-term treatment with diethylstilbestrol. *Am. J. Med. Sci.* 297, 365.

Wynn, V. and Path, F.C. (1968). The anabolic steroids. *Practitioner* 200, 509.

Yeo, P.P.B., Bates, D., Howe, J.G., Ratcliffe, W.A., Schardt, C.W., Heath, A., et al. (1978). Anticonvulsants and thyroid function. *Br. Med. J.* i, 1581.

Zora, J.A., Zimmerman, D., Carey, T.L., O'Connell, E.J., and Yuninger, J.W. (1986). Hypothalamic–pituitary–adrenal axis suppression after long-term, high-dose glucocorticoid therapy in children with asthma. *J. Allergy Clin. Immunol.* 77, 9.

14. Disorders of metabolism 1

J. C. N. CHAN and C. S. COCKRAM

Carbohydrate metabolism

Diabetes mellitus

Diabetes mellitus is a clinical state characterized by hyperglycaemia and usually accompanied by glycosuria. This results from either an absolute or relative deficiency of insulin commonly combined with resistance to it. Presentation may either be acute, with diabetic keto-acidosis or hyperosmolar non-ketotic coma; or insidious, with polyuria, polydipsia, and weight loss. It may also be detected incidentally by screening or in the presence of concurrent illness. Elderly patients with less severe biochemical disturbance may present with one of the complications of diabetes mellitus.

Diagnostic criteria

In most clinical situations, oral glucose tolerance testing (OGTT) is not required to establish the diagnosis of diabetes mellitus. According to the recommendations of the World Health Organisation (WHO 1985), in the presence of symptoms indicative of diabetes mellitus, a fasting venous plasma glucose ≥7.8 mmol per litre or a postprandial or random venous plasma glucose ≥11.1 mmol per litre is sufficient to establish the diagnosis. On the other hand, a random venous plasma glucose <7.8 mmol per litre or a fasting value <6.0 mmol per litre excludes the diagnosis. When an OGTT with 75 g of glucose is used to establish the diagnosis in the absence of symptoms or when the metabolic abnormality is mild, then diabetes mellitus is defined on the basis of a fasting plasma glucose ≥7.8 mmol per litre and ≥11.1 mmol per litre at 2 hours. If only one of these two values is abnormal, then the plasma glucose of at least one of the intermediate (30-, 60-, or 90-minute) blood specimens has to be ≥11.1 mmol per litre in order to establish the diagnosis of diabetes mellitus; or, alternatively, a repeat OGTT is required. Impaired glucose tolerance (IGT) is defined in the presence of a fasting venous plasma glucose <7.8 mmol per litre and a venous plasma glucose ≥7.8 mmol per litre but <11.1 mmol per litre at 2 hours after a 75 g glucose load.

Classification

Diabetes mellitus is classically divided into Type I, insulin-dependent (IDDM), and Type II, non-insulin-dependent (NIDDM), though this categorization is far from precise. The classification into IDDM and NIDDM is made on clinical grounds, while that into Type I and II was originally based on the demonstration of genetic markers and immunological phenomena in the Type I patients. The latter classification has potentially aetiological implications. Since these markers can also, however, sometimes be found in patients with NIDDM or impaired glucose tolerance, the World Health Organization (WHO 1985) recommended that the terms Type I/Type II and IDDM/NIDDM should be used interchangeably and that any aetiological implications should be removed. Type I diabetes, which typically affects the young, is characterized by defective insulin secretion that is believed to be of autoimmune aetiology, since islet cell antibodies against β-cells have been demonstrated in many newly diagnosed patients. In addition, certain human leucocyte antigens (HLA) are associated with increased risk of development of Type I diabetes. Severe symptoms are usual at the time of presentation. The pathogenesis of Type II diabetes is not clear, and both young and old patients may be affected. The initial metabolic defect lies either in insulin deficiency, insulin resistance, or a combination of both. Ketosis is uncommon, although insulin may be required to achieve optimal metabolic control. Despite a strong familial tendency and racial differences in prevalence, there is no known association of NIDDM with HLA haplotype.

Malnutrition-related diabetes mellitus (MRDM)

MRDM as described in tropical countries has now been included within the WHO (1985) classification as a subtype of diabetes in its own right. The pathogenesis remains uncertain, but protein malnutrition and food toxins are thought to play a part. The true prevalence also remains uncertain, as overall diabetes prevalence rates tend to be low in countries where malnutrition is still a problem.

Secondary diabetes mellitus

Diabetes can develop secondarily to pancreatic disease, endocrine disorders (e.g. acromegaly, Cushing's disease), certain drugs, insulin-receptor defects, other rare genetic syndromes, and miscellaneous causes.

Impaired glucose tolerance (IGT)

Individuals with IGT have an increased risk of developing diabetes. The progression rate from IGT to diabetes is about 3 per cent per year without intervention and is higher in the presence of a family history of diabetes. This may be reducible to 1.3 per cent yearly with dietary advice. Periodic review is advisable in these patients.

Gestational diabetes

Glucose intolerance may first appear during pregnancy and is associated with increased fetal and perinatal mortality and morbidity. Glycosuria, which may be due to a low renal threshold in pregnancy, is usually present and is an indication for OGTT. The same WHO criteria as for non-pregnant individuals may be used but should encompass the criteria for IGT. Normoglycaemia must be restored and maintained in order to improve fetal outcome. Although the condition may revert to normal after delivery, it may recur during future pregnancies and the risk of NIDDM or IGT is considerably increased. About 50 per cent of these women develop permanent diabetes mellitus in later years. A further OGTT should be performed, not less than 6 weeks postpartum, to record glucose tolerance at this time.

Previous abnormality and potential abnormality

These subjects belong to the statistical risk class of diabetes mellitus, as distinct from the clinical classes above. They are subjects with normal glucose tolerance who are nevertheless at increased risk of developing diabetes. Individuals who exhibit glucose intolerance either spontaneously or in association with such stressful conditions as infection or in the presence of drugs that might affect glucose homoeostasis are usually known to have previous abnormalities of glucose tolerance.

The following individuals are considered as having a potential abnormality of glucose tolerance:

1. the identical non-diabetic twin of a diabetic;
2. an individual whose parents are both diabetic;
3. an individual with one diabetic parent and whose other parent has a diabetic parent, sibling, or offspring, or a sibling with a diabetic child;
4. a woman who has given birth to a live or stillborn child weighing 4.5 kg or more at birth, or to a stillborn child showing islet cell hyperplasia not related to rhesus incompatibility;
5. individuals whose histocompatibility haplotypes are identical to those of a diabetic sibling;
6. individuals with circulating pancreatic islet cell antibodies.

Drug-induced hyperglycaemia

There are a number of drugs that can precipitate diabetes mellitus in predisposed subjects or aggravate glycaemic control in diabetic patients. In general, these are Type A adverse reactions. The majority of patients receiving diabetogenic medication do not develop glucose intolerance. Individuals with a history of gestational diabetes mellitus or features that place them in the statistical risk group for development of diabetes mellitus are particularly at risk and should be kept under close observation while receiving these medications.

Drug-induced or drug-precipitated diabetes can present with classical symptoms as in idiopathic diabetes, but a significant number of patients with drug-induced glucose intolerance are asymptomatic, so that it is important to make regular checks for glycosuria or hyperglycaemia in patients receiving drugs known to have diabetogenic actions.

Plasma glucose homoeostasis

Plasma glucose concentration is normally maintained within a narrow range. This is dependent on a balance of actions between insulin, the only hormone known to have a glucose-lowering effect, and other counter-regulatory hormones, including glucagon, catecholamines, cortisol, and growth hormone, that tend to raise the glucose concentration.

Insulin

Insulin synthesized and secreted by the β-cells of the islets of Langerhans within the pancreas stimulates cellular glucose uptake and oxidation in many tissues. It increases the production of glycogen, protein, and lipids within liver, muscle, and adipose tissue. It inhibits glycogenolysis, gluconeogenesis, and lipolysis. Secretion of insulin is primarily stimulated by glucose, amino acids (e.g. arginine and leucine), ketones, and fatty acids in the presence of glucagon. Glucose-dependent insulinotrophic peptide (GIP), secretin, and pancreozymin potentiate the secretion of insulin. Other insulin secretagogues include prostaglandins and opioid neuropeptides. Sympathetic stimulation has a dual effect on insulin secretion: β-adrenoceptor stimulation increases insulin secretion while α-adrenoceptor stimulation has an inhibitory effect. Acetylcholine, cyclic-AMP, and calcium are all believed to play a stimulatory role in the secretion of insulin, while somatostatin inhibits its release.

Glucagon

This hormone, synthesized by the α-cells of the pancreatic islets, plays a direct role in insulin release. It also exerts direct actions on the liver resulting in glycogenolysis, and gluconeogenesis. These actions are particularly important during hypoglycaemic episodes, which are potent stimuli for glucagon secretion. It also causes lipolysis and ketogenesis. Glucagon is secreted in response to certain gut hormones, amino acids, stress, vagal stimulation, and β-adrenoceptor stimulation. On the other hand, release of glucagon is inhibited by insulin, somatostatin, and α-adrenoceptor agonists.

Catecholamines

Catecholamines released from the adrenal medulla and peripheral nerve endings have complex effects on carbohydrate metabolism. In addition to dual actions on the release of insulin, catecholamines directly enhance glycogenolysis, gluconeogenesis, and lipolysis with a tendency to increase plasma glucose and free fatty acid concentrations.

Glucocorticoids

Glucocorticoid secretion from the adrenal cortex, mediated by the adrenocorticotrophic hormone corticotrophin (ACTH), raises blood glucose by several mechanisms. Glucocorticoids stimulate pancreatic α-cells resulting in hyperglucagonaemia and hence increased glycogenolysis. They enhance gluconeogenesis by releasing certain gluconeogenic amino acids and lactate from peripheral tissues and increase the hepatic enzymes involved in gluconeogenesis, resulting in an increase in insulin resistance.

Growth hormone

Secretion of growth hormone by the anterior pituitary gland is also linked to carbohydrate metabolism. It is primarily stimulated by hypoglycaemia and inhibited by hyperglycaemia. Other pharmacological stimuli include glucagon, oestrogen, dopamine, and other neurotransmitters. Growth hormone secretion, on the other hand, is suppressed by somatostatin, β-adrenergic stimulation

and the actions of glucocorticoids, medroxyprogesterone, and fatty acids. The action of growth hormone is mediated by somatomedins (in particular, insulin-like growth factor 1), which inhibit its release by a negative feedback mechanism. The effect of growth hormone and somatomedins on carbohydrate metabolism is complex. Acute insulin-like activity results in a fall in blood glucose concentration and enhancement of glucose utilization, lipogenesis, and protein and glycogen synthesis. Growth hormone increases the blood glucose and free fatty acid concentrations, however, and reduces peripheral uptake of glucose during hypoglycaemia, and is potentially diabetogenic. Patients with acromegaly thus commonly have impaired glucose tolerance.

Glucose homoeostasis is therefore maintained by the interaction of these various hormones. Drugs that potentiate or inhibit the secretion or mimic or antagonize the actions of these hormones will lead to disturbances of carbohydrate metabolism. In addition, the liver and kidney play important roles in carbohydrate and drug metabolism, so that adverse effects of drugs on glucose homoeostasis are often enhanced in the presence of impaired liver or renal function, whether drug-related or intrinsic in nature.

Drugs causing hyperglycaemia

Antihypertensive agents

The association between hypertension and diabetes mellitus and their additive effects on both macrovascular and microvascular complications have received much attention during the last decade. Evidence is mounting that effective antihypertensive treatment may retard complications such as nephropathy and retinopathy. Consequently, diabetic patients are increasingly being treated with antihypertensive agents. Recently, hyperinsulinaemia has been postulated as a linking factor between hypertension and glucose intolerance. Antihypertensive treatment, however, particularly with diuretics and β-adrenoceptor blocking agents is also known to be associated with adverse effects on carbohydrate and lipid metabolism and to be able to interfere with the action or secretion of insulin. When choosing antihypertensive treatment in diabetic patients, these factors need to be taken into account. Deleterious effects upon carbohydrate and lipoprotein metabolism in hypertensive, non-diabetic patients may also offset some of the advantages of lowering the blood pressure.

Diuretics

Impaired glucose homoeostasis has been documented in both diabetic (Bloomgarden *et al.* 1984) and non-diabetic subjects (Lewis *et al.* 1976; Amery *et al.* 1986) receiving diuretic therapy. There have been reports of a return to normal glucose tolerance following discontinuation of thiazide therapy (Lowder et al. 1988). In a long-term study carried out by Amery and colleagues (1986), elderly patients treated with triamterene and hydrochlorothiazide had significantly higher fasting plasma glucose concentrations than patients receiving placebo. Bengtsson and colleagues (1984) showed that patients treated with diuretics had a higher risk of developing glucose intolerance than patients treated with other antihypertensive agents and the risk was comparable to that in patients receiving β-adrenoceptor blocking agents. Combination therapy with propranolol and hydrochlorothiazide has an additive deleterious effect on hyperglycaemia as shown by Dornhorst et al. (1985).

The adverse effect of thiazides on glucose metabolism has been found to result from both reduced insulin secretion (Fajans et al. 1966) and increased insulin resistance (Beardwood et al. 1965). The latter can be partly ameliorated by correction of hypokalaemia (Helderman et al 1983; Rowe et al. 1980). In a 6-year follow-up study, Berglund and Andersson (1981) failed to demonstrate a deleterious effect on glucose metabolism in patients treated with bendrofluazide and attributed this to unchanged potassium levels as well as a lower dosage of drug used.

Although Roux and Courtois (1981) reported that indapamide, an indoline diuretic structurally related to thiazide, did not adversely affect the glucose metabolism in a group of well-controlled diabetic subjects, a more recent study by Osei and colleagues (1986) showed a significant deterioration of glycaemic control in a group of diabetic patients who were treated with indapamide for 24 weeks, as confirmed by the increase in the mean glycosylated haemoglobin A_1.

Diuretics can precipitate hyperglycaemic hyperosmolar non-ketotic coma, particularly in the elderly patient who may or may not have a previous history of diabetes mellitus (Fonseca and Phear 1982). These include thiazides (Curtis et al. 1972) and thiazide-related diuretics, such as indapamide (Fonseca and Phear 1982); and metolazone, which is a sulphonamide diuretic related to quinethazone and chlorthalidone (Rowe and Mather 1985) (see Hyperglycaemic hyperosmolar non-ketotic coma).

In contrast to thiazides, loop diuretics in general appear to have less marked effects on glucose metabolism and their hyperglycaemic effect more closely parallels their hypokalaemic effect. Frusemide therapy has been associated with hyperglycaemia (Wilson 1966) ameliorated by correction of hypokalaemia (Toivonen and Mustala 1966; Lowe et al. 1979). Bumetanide has been shown to have minimal adverse effects on glucose metabolism in healthy volunteers and diabetic patients (Flamenbaum and Friedman 1982). Robinson and others (1981) showed that plasma insulin, glucagon, and growth hormone concentrations were unaffected by bumetanide. Chaudhuri and Catania (1988) reported that this drug was less likely to cause impaired glucose tolerance (14 per cent) when compared with frusemide (61 per cent) in a group of patients with heart failure. Both bumetanide (Hall 1982) and frusemide (Tasker and Mitchell-Heggs 1976) have been reported to precipitate hyperosmolar non-ketotic diabetic coma (see Hyperglycaemic hyperosmolar non-ketotic coma).

Existing data suggest that ethacrynic acid has no cross-sensitivity with the thiazides, unlike frusemide and bumetanide (Maclean and Tudhope 1983).

Diazoxide

Diazoxide, an antidiuretic benzothiadiazine and antihypertensive agent, causes hyperglycaemia via both pancreatic and extrapancreatic mechanisms. Its diabetogenic properties have been utilized in the treatment of severe hypoglycaemia associated with various islet cell tumours (Wright et al. 1980), growth hormone deficiency (Ventura et al. 1983), and leucine-sensitive hypoglycaemia (Roe and Kugut 1982). Diazoxide is known to inhibit insulin secretion (Howell and Taylor 1966). Direct stimulation of hepatic glucose production, increased adrenaline secretion, decreased tissue insulin sensitivity, and increased clearance of insulin have also been implicated as possible mechanisms for the hyperglycaemic action of diazoxide (Tamburrano et al. 1983; Skrka et al. 1989). Hyperglycaemia is more likely to occur with prolonged therapy, particularly if administered parenterally, and in patients with renal impairment (Pohl and Thurston 1971). Diuretics, often used concurrently to offset the adverse effect of fluid retention, can have an additive effect on hyperglycaemia. Normal glucose tolerance usually returns on cessation of therapy, and oral hypoglycaemic agents or insulin are only occasionally required. Both hyperosmolar non-ketotic hyperglycaemic coma (Charles and Danforth 1971; Harrison et al. 1972; Lancaster-Smith et al. 1974) and diabetic ketoacidosis have been observed, however, following the use of diazoxide (Updike and Harrington 1969; De Broe et al. 1972). Transplacental transfer of diazoxide given for severe maternal hypertension has resulted in neonatal hyperglycaemia with suppressed insulin secretion (Smith et al. 1982).

β-Adrenoceptor blocking agents

Several studies have confirmed the adverse effects of β-adrenoceptor blocking drugs on glucose and lipid metabolism (Otero *et al.* 1983; Greenberg *et al.* 1984). Mills and Horn (1985) recently reviewed the literature on the effects of β-adrenoceptor blocking drugs on carbohydrate metabolism. Glucose tolerance is usually unaffected by β-adrenoceptor blockers in normal subjects, although deterioration in glycaemic control has been observed in patients with Type II diabetes mellitus due to inhibition of insulin release (Wright *et al.* 1979; Holm *et al.* 1980). In Type I diabetics, hypoglycaemic symptoms can be masked particularly with non-selective β-adrenoceptor blocking drugs, and the hypoglycaemic episodes can be prolonged or enhanced due to inhibition of counter-regulatory hormone secretion.

Holm (1983) recently reviewed the autonomic stimulation of insulin secretion. Basal insulin secretion is under both central and peripheral regulatory control. Parasympathetic nervous system stimulation, mediated by the vagal nerve, results in hyperinsulinaemia. This is the primary central mechanism. α-Adrenergic stimulation results in inhibition of insulin release while β_2-adrenergic stimulation enhances both basal and glucose-stimulated insulin release. Since insulin secretion is mediated via β_2-receptors, β-adrenoceptor blocking agents or high-dose selective β_1-antagonists should be avoided in diabetic patients with limited insulin reserve. Propranolol has also been shown to augment exercise-induced release of growth hormone, which may have a diabetogenic effect (Maclaren *et al.* 1975). The inhibition of insulin release due to unopposed α-adrenergic stimulation, and lipolysis via blockade of the β-adrenoceptors have occasionally precipitated the development of severe hyperglycaemia when β-adrenoceptor blockers are used in combination with diuretics (Podolsky and Pattavina 1973; Rowe and Mather 1985), and other antihypertensive agents, such as clonidine (Josselson and Sadler 1986), that are also known to have an inhibitory effect on insulin secretion.

Calcium-channel blocking agents

The effects of calcium-channel antagonists on glucose metabolism remain inconclusive. Insulin release has been shown to be dependent on an increase in cytosolic calcium in *in vitro* studies (Wollheim *et al.* 1978). Deterioration in glycaemic control that improves after withdrawal of nifedipine has been reported in diabetic patients (Bhatnagar *et al.* 1984). Charles and colleagues (1981) reported an increase in fasting glucose concentrations in normal subjects treated with nifedipine. This was associated with a delayed insulin response and a rise in plasma glucagon concentration. Giugliano and his colleagues (1980) also undertook investigations into the actions of nifedipine and reported similar findings in

patients treated with this calcium-channel antagonist. Greenwood (1982), on the other hand, showed that low-dose nifedipine did not impair glucose tolerance, and Dante (1986) reported that the secretion of insulin and glucagon was not affected adversely by nifedipine in normal subjects. Abadie and others (1984) showed that nifedipine had no significant effect on the secretion of growth hormone and glycaemic control in diabetic patients.

Andersson and Rodjmark (1981) studied the effects of verapamil both orally and intravenously in non-insulin-dependent diabetic patients and reported that verapamil improved glucose tolerance in these patients without affecting insulin secretion. They proposed that verapamil might decrease glucagon release and enhance hepatic glucose uptake in these patients. Severe hyperglycaemia has, however, been reported following overdosage with verapamil in non-diabetic subjects (Enyeart *et al.* 1983). A. Roth and others (1989) reported a case of acute hyperglycaemia in a previously non-diabetic patient treated with slow-release verapamil for paroxysmal atrial fibrillation.

Most of the recent studies using diltiazem showed that glucose metabolism was not significantly affected in diabetic patients (Nagai *et al.* 1986; Andren *et al.* 1988; Jones *et al.* 1988), although Pershadsingh and colleagues (1987) reported an increase in insulin requirement in an insulin-dependent patient treated with diltiazem, suggesting increased insulin resistance.

Overall, the available evidence suggests an impairment of insulin secretion by high doses of calcium-channel blocking agents.

Other antihypertensive agents

Centrally acting drugs, α-adrenoceptor blocking agents, and vasodilators in general do not cause significant glucose intolerance (Holland and Pool 1988). Administration of clonidine to diabetic subjects has been shown to cause elevation of plasma glucose and a fall in insulin concentrations (Guthrie *et al.* 1983; Webster and McConnaughey 1982; Metz *et al.* 1978) via α_2-stimulation, but significant deterioration in glycaemic control is uncommon. Additive inhibitory effects on insulin release, following the combined use of metoprolol and clonidine, have, however, resulted in severe hyperglycaemia in a previously normoglycaemic subject. Glucose intolerance persisted despite discontinuation of therapy, perhaps indicating that the therapy had unmasked a preexisting β-cell defect (Josselson and Sadler 1986).

Most studies have shown that angiotensin-converting-enzyme inhibitors do not have adverse effects on glucose metabolism and could be associated with an improvement in glycaemic control, owing to enhanced insulin sensitivity (see under Hypoglycaemia).

β-Adrenoceptor agonists

These drugs are used with good effect in patients with asthma and in pregnant women in premature labour. Effects on glucose homoeostasis are complex, despite the underlying hyperglycaemic action of β-adrenoceptor agonists. While β-adrenoceptor stimulation increases insulin secretion (Gerich et al. 1976), activation of glycogenolysis and lipolysis can result in hyperglycaemia (Goldberg et al. 1975). These effects are modified by the prevailing glucose level (Pfeifer et al. 1980). Intravenous salbutamol infusion has been shown to cause a greater increase in plasma glucose, free fatty acids, ketones, and glycerol by increased cyclic-AMP production in diabetic patients than in normal individuals. The difference in the metabolic effects between normal subjects and diabetics could be explained by a greater increase in insulin response in the former. Significant hypokalaemia occurred in both groups of patients (Gündogdu et al. 1979). Leslie and Coats (1977) reported development of diabetic ketoacidosis in a woman treated with intravenous salbutamol for premature labour. Hyperglycaemia did not recur when the dosage was reduced. This accords with the findings of Huupponen and Pihlajamäki (1986), who studied the effects of intravenous salbutamol on glucose metabolism in normal volunteers after different glucose loads. When low-dose salbutamol was administered, there was no significant increase in plasma glucose concentration, owing to an intensified insulin response. At high doses, however, the hyperglycaemic effects of salbutamol predominated, resulting in relative insulinopenia and hyperglycaemia.

Prolonged oral terbutaline prophylaxis therapy against premature labour has been associated with significant impairment of glucose tolerance during pregnancy (Main et al. 1987). Although intravenous ritodrine therapy for inhibition of premature labour is associated with deterioration of maternal glucose tolerance (Spellacy et al. 1978; Kirkpatrick et al. 1980), oral ritodrine therapy has been reported to have either no effect (Main et al. 1985) or to cause less disturbance in glucose homoeostasis than terbutaline (Caritis et al. 1984); on the other hand, it was less effective in preventing premature labour in the latter study. Terbutaline is a less selective β₂-agonist and this may explain the difference in their effects on glucose tolerance. Paradoxically, ritodrine frequently causes hypoglycaemia in neonates exposed to the drug in utero (Musci et al. 1988), and a case of hyperinsulinaemic hypoglycaemia has been reported in a mother with a triple pregnancy treated with rito-

drine for premature labour (Caldwell et al. 1987) (see Hypoglycaemia).

Corticosteroids

Corticosteroids can cause impaired glucose tolerance in normal subjects and can worsen glycaemic control in diabetic patients. Several mechanisms may be involved, as discussed previously. Although glucose intolerance is usually mild, hyperosmolar non-ketotic hyperglycaemia has been reported following corticosteroid treatment (Spenney et al. 1969; Corcoran et al. 1971).

In non-diabetic subjects, there is no clear relationship between the dose of prednisone and the appearance of hyperglycaemia. In susceptible subjects, however, the degree of hyperglycaemia appears to be dose-related. Transient insulin therapy may be necessary to control plasma glucose, and high doses may occasionally be necessary to overcome the insulin resistance induced by corticosteroid therapy. Oxygenation in the 11- and 17-positions of the steroid molecule (e.g. as in hydrocortisone) as well as introduction of a 1,2 double bond in the A ring (e.g. as in prednisone and prednisolone) enhances the potency of corticosteroids upon carbohydrate metabolism. Although some authors advocate the use of alternate-day regimens to ameliorate the hyperglycaemic effect of corticosteroids (Walton et al. 1970), Greenstone and Shaw (1987) demonstrated alternate-day hyperglycaemia with this regimen.

Oral contraceptives

The oestrogen component of oral contraceptive steroids was previously believed to cause glucose intolerance by enhancing cortisol secretion and hence gluconeogenesis and insulin resistance. This appears, however, to have been related to the high dosage of oestrogen (50 μg or more) used in the older preparations. Since these have been replaced by the lower dosage (30 μg or less) oestrogen preparations, increasing evidence indicates that the progestogen component of oral contraceptive preparations also has an adverse effect on glucose homoeostasis (Spellacy et al. 1972). This appears to be related to dose and potency, with norethidrone having the least and norgestrel the greatest hyperglycaemic effect (Spellacy et al. 1981; Spellacy 1982; Perlman et al. 1985). In a 10-year prospective follow-up study, there was a higher incidence of impaired glucose tolerance in 'pill users' (16 per cent) than in non-users (8 per cent). Norgestrel was found to have the most potent adverse effect on carbohydrate metabolism, while synthetic oestrogens had no effect upon the indices of glucose intolerance (Perlman et al. 1985). In addition, there have been reports of hyperglycaemia following medroxyprogesterone therapy (Bottino and Tashima 1976) though Ansfield (1977) did not observe abnormal glucose tolerance in patients treated with megestrol.

The mechanism of hyperglycaemia induced by oral contraceptive steroids remains to be established with certainty. Progestational compounds alone or in combination with oestrogens can lead to insulin resistance (De Pirro *et al*. 1981; Spellacy 1982). De Pirro and colleagues (1978, 1981) postulated the underlying mechanism to be either a reduction in the number or affinity of insulin receptors on cell membranes. In addition, elevated cortisol concentration in contraceptive pill users can impair glucose tolerance by increasing hepatic glucose production and inhibition of peripheral glucose uptake (Munck 1971). van der Vange and others (1987) evaluated seven preparations of low-dose combined oral contraceptives (monophasic, biphasic, and triphasic) and failed to find any adverse effects on glucose metabolism in normal individuals, although a small but statistically insignificant rise in the insulin response to oral glucose loading was seen. Several risk factors have been associated with the development of abnormal glucose tolerance following the use of oral contraceptive pills. They include a positive family history, increased age, obesity, a past history of large babies or stillbirths, and a history of abnormal plasma glucose (Duffy and Ray 1984).

Skouby and colleagues (1985) compared the effect of a low-dose triphasic contraceptive pill (Triquilar) on glucose tolerance in normal women and women with a history of gestational diabetes mellitus and concluded that no adverse effect on glucose metabolism was seen in the latter group. Plasma cortisol, however, increased significantly and similarly in both groups of patients; insulin concentrations also rose significantly in the normal women during treatment. The basal insulin concentration was higher in women with a history of gestational diabetes mellitus and did not rise during the study period. Kung and colleagues (1987), however, reported that 4 out of 15 Chinese women with a history of gestational diabetes mellitus developed impaired glucose tolerance following the use of the same contraceptive preparation and suggested that even low-dose preparations could unmask defective β-cell function in these women.

Lithium

Lithium has an unpredictable effect on carbohydrate metabolism. The mechanisms of lithium action were reviewed by Singer and Rotenberg (1973). It has an insulin-like action and can cause hypoglycaemia (see Hypoglycaemia). In the presence of nephrogenic diabetes insipidus, the extracellular volume depletion can result in excessive reabsorption of glucose from the renal tubules. Hyperglycaemia has been reported to develop following the use of lithium (Craig *et al*. 1977; Waziri and Nelson 1978; Vendesborg 1979). Lee and others (1971) and Martinez-Maldonaldo and Terrell (1973) described cases of diabetic ketoacidosis occurring in association with nephrogenic diabetes insipidus following lithium therapy.

Antimicrobial agents

Fraser and Harrower (1977) reported a case of recurrent convulsions and hyperglycaemia in a patient treated with nalidixic acid. The glucuronides of nalidixic acid can also produce falsely positive glycosuria due to glucuronic acid, which acts as a reducing agent (Klumpp 1965). Isoniazid can produce falsely low plasma glucose measurements because hydrazine-containing compounds interfere with the glucose peroxidase assay. This does not occur if a hexokinase enzymatic process is used (Sharp 1972). Definite hyperglycaemia has also, however, been reported with isoniazid both in overdoses (Whitefield 1971) and in conventional dosage (Dickson 1962). Early-phase hyperglycaemia with exaggerated insulin response to glucose loading, similar to that seen in patients with thyrotoxicosis or after gastrectomy, was observed by Takasu and colleagues (1982) in patients treated with rifampicin, and was postulated to be related to enhanced intestinal absorption of glucose, although the effect was not considered to be diabetogenic.

Pentamidine, an antiprotozoal agent, has a multiphasic effect on glucose metabolism similar to streptozotocin, with acute hypoglycaemia due to a cytolytic effect on the pancreas followed by insulinopenia with hyperglycaemia (Bouchard *et al*. 1982). Diabetes mellitus has been reported to develop in patients treated with pentamidine for kala azar (Jha and Sharma 1984) or leishmaniasis (Belehu and Naafs 1982); it can persist despite discontinuation of pentamidine, and insulin therapy may be necessary (Bouchard *et al*. 1982; Jha and Sharma 1984; Shen *et al*. 1989). Pentamidine isethionate appears to be less toxic to the pancreas than pentamidine mesylate (Belehu and Naafs 1982).

Psychotropic agents

Zumoff and Hellman (1977) observed deterioration of glycaemic control in a patient with insulin-dependent diabetes mellitus when given chlordiazepoxide, and reviewed the literature on the effects of psychotropic drugs on carbohydrate metabolism. Tranquillizers, including dopamine blockers such as loxapine and amoxapine (Tollefson and Lesar 1983) and the phenothiazines (Arneson 1964), may cause hyperglycaemia, while some antidepressants (e.g. monoamine oxidase inhibitors [Cooper 1966]) may cause hypoglycaemia. This is probably not of major clinical significance, however, in view of the rarity of reported cases and the large number of patients who are treated with these drugs. The exact mechanism is unknown and may be related to their effects on the metabolism of various biogenic catecholamines in the brain.

Morphine has long been known to cause hyperglycaemia through a central effect and this may be mediated by the actions of encephalin and β-endorphin. Giugliano and colleagues (1982) showed that in Type II diabetic patients insulin secretion was enhanced by naloxone, and suggested that increased sensitivity to endogenous opiates might play a role in the pathogenesis of Type II diabetes.

Antiarrhythmic agents

Although Politi and others (1984) reported three cases of hyperglycaemia and hypertriglyceridaemia following the use of amiodarone, no adverse effect on carbohydrate metabolism was found in 10 non-diabetic subjects treated with amiodarone for 10 months (Lakhdar *et al*. 1988). Encainide, a new class IC antiarrhythmic drug, has been reported to cause deterioration in glucose tolerance. This occurred particularly in patients with pre-existing borderline hyperglycaemia and was not dose-related (Salerno *et al*. 1988).

Immunosuppressive and immunomodulating agents

Corticosteroids have frequently been used as an adjunctive agent both for chemotherapy in malignant conditions and immunosuppressive therapy following organ transplantation. Significant increases in plasma glucose and lipids in these patients have been reported (Ellis *et al*. 1986). Specific antineoplastic agents, however, including colaspase (asparaginase), which causes insulinopenia and relative hyperglucagonaemia (Pui *et al*. 1981; Turner *et al*. 1983), and homoharringtonine, which induces insulin resistance (Sylvester *et al*. 1989), have been reported to cause glucose intolerance. Cyclosporin therapy has been associated with diabetogenic effects in post-transplant patients, especially when combined with corticosteroids (Gunnarsson *et al*. 1983, D. Roth *et al*. 1989). Defective insulin secretion (D. Roth *et al*. 1989) and increased insulin resistance (Gunnarsson *et al*. 1983) have both been proposed as possible mechanisms.

Other drugs

Theophylline overdosage can lead to severe metabolic disturbance including hyperglycaemia and hypokalaemia. Hall and colleagues (1984) studied 22 cases of theophylline overdosage retrospectively and concluded that hyperinsulinaemia and increased catecholamine release mediated by elevated 2'5'-adenosine monophos-

phate concentrations are the underlying mechanisms for the hyperglycaemia. Phenytoin, in high dosage, has been reported to cause hyperglycaemia, particularly in the presence of diabetes mellitus and impaired renal function. The mechanism is uncertain, although inhibition of insulin release has been implicated (Fariss and Lutcher 1971).

High doses of aspirin can lead to hyperglycaemia, while hypoglycaemia can occur with normal doses (see Hypoglycaemia).

Hyperosmolar non-ketotic diabetic coma (HNC)

This condition is characterized by severe dehydration, hyperosmolality, and hyperglycaemia in the absence of ketosis. It typically occurs in elderly patients with or without NIDDM and is frequently precipitated by concurrent illness, such as infection or gastrointestinal upset. The disease presents insidiously over days or weeks with severe polydipsia (characteristically relieved by sweetened drinks), polyuria, and progressive deterioration of consciousness. It has a high mortality and morbidity and may be complicated by thromboembolic disease, such as myocardial infarction or cerebrovascular accident.

The pathogenesis is believed to be secondary to relative insulin deficiency, which fails to prevent hyperglycaemia but is not severe enough to provoke ketoacidosis. The osmotic diuresis leads to severe dehydration and renal insufficiency which further impairs urinary glucose excretion. A number of drugs have been implicated in precipitating HNC and these include diuretics (Fonseca and Phear 1982), dexamethasone (Spenney *et al*. 1969), phenytoin (Goldberg and Sanbar 1969), and glycerol (Sears 1976).

Diuretics are a particularly important group of drugs implicated in precipitating HNC due to their common use. Treatment with thiazide (Curtis *et al*. 1972) and thiazide-related compounds, including indapamide (Fonseca and Phear 1982), metolazone (Rowe and Mather 1985), and diazoxide (Lancaster-Smith *et al*. 1974), has been associated with the development of HNC. Loop diuretics such as frusemide (Tasker and Mitchell-Heggs 1976) and bumetanide (Hall 1982) have also been implicated. The underlying mechanism is not known with certainty, although deterioration in glucose tolerance with relative insulin deficiency is a well-recognized adverse effect of diuretic therapy. The hyperglycaemia in HNC does not correlate with the magnitude of dehydration or potassium loss. A few of these cases of HNC appeared to be precipitated by concomitant therapy with β-adrenoceptor blocking agents (Podolsky and Pattavina 1973; Fonseca and Phear 1982; Rowe and Mather

1985; Josselson and Sadler 1986). This may have been due to unopposed α-stimulation of gluconeogenesis and insulin inhibition secondary to β-blockade. When predisposed subjects under stressful situations are given β-adrenoceptor blocking agents and diuretics together, severe hyperglycaemia, which may progress to HNC, can occur.

Glycerol, used in the treatment of cerebral oedema and acute neovascular glaucoma, has been associated with hyperosmolar non-ketotic hyperglycaemic coma (Oakley and Ellis 1976; Sears 1976). Cases of fatal hyperosmolar non-ketotic diabetic coma have been reported in diabetic patients following overdosage with phenytoin (Goldberg and Sanbar 1969).

Lactic acidosis

Lactate homoeostasis is dependent upon a balance between production and utilization. Complete oxidation of carbohydrate to carbon dioxide and water during glycolysis occurs in the cellular mitochondria. Lactate, an end product of incomplete oxidation, is normally utilized by the liver and kidney for gluconeogenesis, and these organs play an important role in the homoeostasis of lactate metabolism. When there is inadequate tissue perfusion or mitochondrial dysfunction, increased anaerobic glycolysis results in overproduction of lactate from pyruvate. Lactate is a strong organic acid which rapidly dissociates forming hydrogen ions which can accumulate, leading to acidosis. Significant lactic acidosis is considered to be present when there is a systemic $pH \leqslant 7.25$ occurring in association with a lactate concentration $\geqslant 5$ mEq per litre and this is characterized by an increase in the anion gap $([Na^+]+[K^+])-([Cl^-]+[HCO_3^-])$ (Kreisberg 1984). Lactic acidosis typically occurs in the presence of poor tissue perfusion or oxygenation, such as during shock, sepsis, and cardiac failure (Type A lactic acidosis). Type B lactic acidosis occurs in association with certain drugs or toxins and disease states in which poor tissue oxygenation is not a typical feature except as a terminal event.

Many drugs or chemicals are known to be associated with lactic acidosis. Biguanides act on the mitochondrial membranes causing inhibition of gluconeogenesis with the resultant increase in gluconeogenic precursors of lactate, pyruvate, and alanine. This predisposes the patient to lactic acidosis, especially in the presence of impaired renal or hepatic function. Metformin, which is excreted by the kidney, has been reported to lead to lactic acidosis in 0.4 cases per 10 000 treatment years, with a mortality of 30 per cent. Mortality from phenformin-related lactic acidosis is higher at 70 per cent

(Berger 1985). In another review, by Campbell (1985), there were 18 deaths in 43 cases of metformin-associated lactic acidosis, and 40 had documented contraindications. Phenformin has now been withdrawn from the market in most countries. Metformin should be used with caution in the elderly, and in patients known to have renal, cardiac, or hepatic impairment.

Poisoning with methanol or ethylene glycol can lead to severe formate and lactic acidosis due to depression of the NAD/NADH$^+$ ratio, which enhances the conversion of pyruvate to lactate (*The Lancet* 1983). Ethanol is known to increase the lactate concentration in the blood, and both oral alcohol poisoning and intravenous therapy with alcohol for premature labour have resulted in severe lactic acidosis (Ott *et al*. 1976).

Lactic acidosis has been reported to occur in patients treated with nalidixic acid, and Phillips and colleagues (1979) suggested that nalidixic acid may cause both an increase in lactate production and reduction in hepatic uptake. Outdated tetracycline tablets degrade to form toxic chemicals of 4-epianhydrotetracycline and anhydrotetracycline that are known to cause Fanconi's syndrome. Montoliu and others (1981) reported a case of lactic acidosis associated with Fanconi's syndrome following the ingestion of degraded tetracycline tablets and both toxic chemicals were detectable on biochemical analysis of the tablets. Sodium nitroprusside therapy for severe hypertension can lead to accumulation of cyanmethaemoglobin and free cyanide ions, which are known to cause lactic acidosis (Humphrey and Nash 1978). Mann and others (1985) reported a case of lactic acidosis in a patient treated with lactulose for hepatic encephalopathy. Significant reabsorption of the lactic acid from the breakdown of lactulose in the presence of poor gut motility was proposed as a possible mechanism. Papaverine, which inhibits cellular oxidative pathways, was reported to cause severe lactic acidosis in a patient who took an overdose (Vaziri *et al*. 1981). Other agents known to be associated with lactic acidosis include salicylates, fructose, sorbitol, adrenaline, and isoniazid (Kreisberg 1984).

Hypoglycaemia

Hypoglycaemia is arbitrarily defined as a plasma glucose below 2.2 mmol per litre. The glucose level at which symptoms appear is, however, extremely variable. The neurohormonal response to hypoglycaemia results in a symptom complex which can be adrenergic or neuroglycopenic in nature. Adrenergic stimulation results in typical symptoms of sweating, tremor, tachycardia, and pallor, while neuroglycopenia may lead to diverse symptoms such as blurred vision, circumoral paraesthesia, poor concentration, ataxia, and hemiplegia and can progress to irrational behaviour, automatism, confusion, and coma. Adrenergic symptoms usually precede neuroglycopenic symptoms, except, notably, in diabetic patients with 'hypoglycaemic unawareness'.

In response to hypoglycaemia, glucagon and catecholamines are rapidly released to increase hepatic glucose production. Increased secretion of cortisol and growth hormone also occurs, and assists in restoring a normal plasma glucose concentration.

Hypoglycaemia resulting from drug therapy is seen in four types of situation: (1) when a hypoglycaemic agent is used therapeutically in diabetes; (2) when a deliberate or accidental overdose of a hypoglycaemic agent is taken; (3) when a hypoglycaemic agent interacts with other drugs taken by the patient, leading to enhancement or potentiation of the hypoglycaemic effect; (4) rarely, as a direct and unwanted effect of a drug that is not primarily a hypoglycaemic agent.

Risks of spontaneous and drug-induced hypoglycaemia are increased in the presence of renal and liver disease. The liver is the major site of glycogenesis, glycogenolysis, and gluconeogenesis and is vital for glucose homoeostasis. It is also an important site of drug metabolism. Hepatotoxic drugs can lead to hypoglycaemia through direct toxicity, though there is little correlation between the degree of liver damage and susceptibility to hypoglycaemia (Arky 1989). Patients with renal failure are predisposed to hypoglycaemia by several mechanisms. These include poor nutrition and calorie deprivation, impaired glycolysis and gluconeogenesis, reduced production of precursor of gluconeogenic substrate (e.g. alanine), defective counter-regulatory hormone secretion, and reduced insulin clearance. Such patients are also at increased risk of drug-induced hypoglycaemia due to impaired drug clearance, altered pharmacokinetics, and alterations in protein binding (Arem 1989).

Hypoglycaemic agents

Insulin is the only hormone known to lower plasma glucose directly, thus treatment with any type of insulin, or with drugs that augment secretion of insulin (e.g. sulphonylureas), can induce hypoglycaemia. Biguanides do not produce symptomatic hypoglycaemia under normal circumstances but do potentiate other hypoglycaemic agents. Defective secretion of counter-regulatory hormones is the other mechanism causing hypoglycaemia. There are numerous drugs that can affect the secretion of these hormones, leading to hypoglycaemia.

Interference with catecholamine release will delay the recovery from a hypoglycaemic episode and may distort the warning symptoms of hypoglycaemia, which arise mainly from adrenergic stimulation. Impairment of hepatic and renal function can both cause spontaneous hypoglycaemia and potentiate the hypoglycaemic effects of other agents.

Insulin

Hypoglycaemic coma commonly occurs in patients treated conventionally with insulin. Approximately 1 patient in 3 experiences coma at some time during insulin therapy; about 1 in 10 experiences coma in the course of an average year; and about 1 in 30 experiences recurrent problems with severe hypoglycaemia (Rees and Gale 1988). Insulin therapy is by far the commonest cause of hypoglycaemia seen in routine clinical practice.

Potter and others (1982) found in a prospective study that 200 of 204 patients admitted to an accident and emergency department because of hypoglycaemia were taking insulin, representing an incidence of hypoglycaemia of 9 per cent a year in their diabetic population. The incidence of hypoglycaemia treated at home was not known with certainty. Mismatch of food intake with insulin injection, over-zealous pursuit of good metabolic control, excessive insulin dosage, exercise, alcohol, and lack of warning were some contributing factors. No apparent precipitating cause was found in nearly 40 per cent of cases. Although major sequelae are uncommon, hypoglycaemic attacks can lead to disruption of the patients' life-styles, and it is possible that recurrent hypoglycaemia might lead to brain damage.

Absorption of insulin from injection sites can be erratic even in apparently well-controlled patients, typically before meals and in the early hours of the morning. Exercise enhances the absorption of insulin, and omission of meals frequently precipitates hypoglycaemic attacks. Glucagon secretion is progressively impaired with increasing duration of diabetes, and catecholamine secretion then asssmes increased importance in counter-regulation. Strict diabetic control has been shown to lower the glycaemic threshold at which counter-regulatory hormones, including catecholamines and growth hormone, are released (Amiel et al. 1988; Lager et al. 1988). In addition, frequent episodes of subclinical hypoglycaemia and fluctuating hyperglycaemia have been shown to blunt catecholamine responses (Gulan et al. 1988). All these factors contribute towards the defective counter-regulatory responses of diabetic patients. Failure of catecholamine secretion or autonomic neuropathy can lead to dangerous hypoglycaemic unaware-ness. Other risk factors include concurrent administration of alcohol, which inhibits gluconeogenesis, and β-adrenoceptor blocking agents, which may mask hypoglycaemic symptoms. Patients at the extremes of age are also more sensitive to hypoglycaemia. Insulin overdosage should be suspected if a hypoglycaemic episode is refractory to treatment and this can be confirmed by the detection of high circulating insulin concentrations in the presence of suppressed C peptide concentrations.

Long-acting protamine zinc insulin has no place in the modern management of diabetes, because of the risk of protracted and recurrent hypoglycaemia resulting from its long duration of action. The change from beef insulin to highly purified porcine insulin should be made with care, particularly when the insulin doses used are large, since hypoglycaemia occasionally occurs because of the lower antigenicity of the latter. There has been concern regarding the possibly increased incidence, and reduced awareness, of hypoglycaemic episodes in patients treated with human insulin. Pickup (1989), in a review article, found that most studies had failed to demonstrate either an increase in the number of hypoglycaemic episodes or an adverse effect on the release of counter-regulatory hormones when patients were changed from animal to human insulin, yet the incidence of 'hypoglycaemia unawareness' has been reported to vary from 6 per cent (Hepburn *et al.* 1988) to 36 per cent (Teuscher and Berger 1987) in patients treated with human insulin. In a double-blind, randomized crossover trial with human and porcine insulin, Berger and colleagues (1989) reported that hypoglycaemic symptoms were more often adrenergic (with sweating, palpitation, tremor) in patients treated with porcine insulin, but more often neuroglycopenic (with lack of concentration, visual disturbance, headache) in those treated with human insulin. Pickup (1989) discussed the possible mechanisms involved. Bovine insulin is known to be more antigenic than either porcine or human insulin (Peacock *et al.* 1983) and, in some patients, the reduced insulin antibody production following a change to human insulin therapy may result in increased sensitivity to human insulin. Stricter diabetic control following the change to human insulin therapy may impair the counter-regulatory response to hypoglycaemia (Gulan *et al.* 1988; Amiel *et al.* 1988; Lager *et al.* 1988).

At the present time, there is no definite indication that human insulin has intrinsic properties that render either hypoglycaemia or 'hypoglycaemic unawareness' more likely. Further study of the relative effects of human and porcine insulins upon counter-regulatory response is required, however, and until the matter is clarified physicians prescribing human insulin should be aware of the possibility. Differences in absorption rate, pharmaco-kinetics, antigenicity, or glycaemic control may lead to problems in a few patients transferred to human insulin from porcine or bovine insulin, but they can usually be dealt with by appropriate advice regarding dosage, timing, and adjustment.

Treatment   Insulin-induced hypoglycaemia usually responds to glucose therapy, which can be oral for mild cases. A bolus intravenous injection of 50% glucose should be given to the comatose patient or if the integrity of the gag reflex is in doubt. This should be followed by a continuous intravenous infusion of 10% or 20% glucose to prevent recurrence and until the patient is stable. Intramuscular glucagon and hydrocortisone are useful if intravenous glucose infusion fails to maintain the blood glucose level in the normal range.

Intentional massive insulin overdosage can usually be managed with relative ease using 10% glucose infusions despite grossly elevated plasma insulin concentrations, but if alcohol has also been taken, or if treatment is delayed, fatal brain damage can result (Critchley *et al.* 1984).

Sulphonylureas

Hypoglycaemia remains the most common and dangerous adverse effect associated with sulphonylurea therapy. Jennings and others (1989) reported that 20 per cent of patients treated with a sulphonylurea experienced hypoglycaemic symptoms. In a survey carried out in Sweden and Switzerland, there were 2 cases per 10 000 treatment-years of sulphonylurea-induced hypoglycaemia, with an associated mortality of 10 per cent (Berger 1985). In the review article by Ferner and Neil (1988), chlorpropamide and glibenclamide were found to be associated with higher incidences of severe hypoglycaemia, although this might occur with any sulphonylurea. Based on the incidence of hypoglycaemic episodes from various oral hypoglycaemic agents reported in another study by Berger and colleagues (1986), it was estimated that if the standardized incidence ratio for hypoglycaemia was 100 for chlorpropamide, that for glibenclamide would be 111, glipizide 46, and tolbutamide 21. The prolonged hypoglycaemic effect of glibenclamide, even at low doses, was discussed; this may result from an unidentified metabolite, accumulation of drug within the islets, or a persistent action at the β-cell membrane. Increased age, prolonged duration of treatment, concurrent medications, and impaired renal and liver function are risk factors for sulphonylurea-induced hypoglycaemia. Huminer and others (1989) reported two cases of severe hypoglycaemia due to inadvertent dispensing of sulphonylureas to non-diabetic subjects and reviewed 20 similar cases in the literature. This possibility should be considered in non-diabetic subjects with unexplained hypoglycaemic coma.

Treatment The treatment for sulphonylurea-induced hypoglycaemia is similar to that when it is due to insulin. Simultaneous administration of intramuscular glucagon and glucose has, however, been found to be of particular value in refractory cases (Davies *et al.* 1967; Dowell and Imrie 1972). Chlorpropamide-induced hypoglycaemia has been successfully treated with diazoxide (Johnson *et al.* 1977).

Drugs interacting with hypoglycaemic agents or causing hypoglycaemia spontaneously (see also Chapter 30)

Two main mechanisms underlie drug interactions with hypoglycaemic agents. First, interacting drugs can alter the pharmacokinetics of hypoglycaemic agents by enhancing or reducing drug absorption, accelerating or inhibiting drug metabolism and elimination, and affecting the balance of free and protein-bound drug; secondly, pharmocodynamic interactions involving direct effects of drugs on the control mechanisms of glucose homoeostasis can occur — these include the release of insulin, the responsiveness of peripheral tissues to insulin, the secretion of counter-regulatory hormones, and the peripheral production and uptake of glucose.

Ethanol, β-adrenoceptor blocking agents, phenylbutazone, monoamine oxidase inhibitors, sulphonamides, coumarin anticoagulants, and salicylates are well-recognized for their potentiating effects on hypoglycaemic agents. Drugs that reduce the efficacy of these agents include diuretics, glucocorticosteroids, oral contraceptives, phenobarbitone, β-adrenoceptor agonists, and glucagon (Hansen and Christensen 1977; Jackson and Bressler 1981). There have been reports on the interaction between sulphonylureas and tricyclic antidepressants (Shrivastava and Edwards 1983; Tollefson and Lesar 1983; True *et al.* 1987) resulting in hypoglycaemia, while histamine H_2-receptor antagonists (e.g. cimetidine) can enhance the actions of sulphonylureas by inhibiting hepatic microsomal enzymes (Feely and Peden 1983; MacWalter *et al.* 1985; Lee *et al.* 1987). Tables 14.1 and 14.2 list the drugs that can interact with sulphonylureas, and the underlying mechanisms involved.

Seltzer (1989) recently reviewed 1418 reported cases of drug-induced hypoglycaemia and reported that 63 per cent were due to sulphonylureas either alone or with a second hypoglycaemic or potentiating agent. Alcohol, salicylate, and propranolol, alone or with a hypoglycaemic drug, accounted for 19 per cent, while quinine, pentamidine, ritodrine, and disopyramide explained a further 7 per cent; 79 per cent of the hypoglycaemic deaths were due to a sulphonylurea and alcohol. Restricted calorie intake, and impaired renal and liver function were important contributing factors. Drug-induced hypoglycaemia in neonates can be the result of ritodrine, propranolol, or a sulphonylurea to mothers during pregnancy. Salicylate poisoning remains the most important cause of hypoglycaemia in the first 2 years of life, while alcohol predominates during the next 8 years. Between the ages of 11 and 50, insulin and oral hypoglycaemic agents alone, or in combination with alcohol, account for the majority of cases of hypoglycaemia, some of which are due to intentional overdosage. Alcohol and prior poor calorie intake appear to be key factors in deaths from insulin overdosage (Critchley *et al.* 1984). Over the age of 60, sulphonylureas are by far the most important cause of hypoglycaemia.

Ethanol

McDonald (1980) reviewed the effects of ethanol on carbohydrate metabolism and reported that in well-nourished subjects alcohol augments glycogenolysis and may cause elevation of plasma glucose, probably by increasing sympathetic activity. More importantly, however, prolonged hypoglycaemia can occur in the presence of ethanol taken alone or with other potentiating agents such as oral hypoglycaemic agents or insulin. Ethanol inhibits gluconeogenesis, which is a particularly important process for the maintenance of normal blood glucose concentration when there is insufficient glycogen reserve, as in the fasting state, in diabetic or malnourished subjects. In addition, alcohol enhances the plasma insulin response to a glucose load administered orally or intravenously in both normal and mildly diabetic subjects, and symptomatic reactive hypoglycaemia may occur.

In the presence of liver disease, alcohol can lead to severe hypoglycaemia due to disturbance of the intrahepatic pathways for maintenance of normal glucose metabolism. Inhibition of hepatic gluconeogenesis by ethanol occurs by several mechanisms: disruption of the gluconeogenic pathway by an increased NADH+/NAD ratio resulting from oxidation of ethanol, inhibition of release of alanine from muscle, and inhibition of hepatic uptake of lactate, glycerol, and alanine. Defective secretion of counter-regulatory hormones, including catecholamines and corticotrophin (ACTH), can occur in chronic alcoholism and further impair the recovery from hypoglycaemia (Arky 1989). This explains the lethal effect of insulin overdosage in association with excessive and prolonged alcohol ingestion. It is noteworthy that the cortical laminar necrosis and other features associated with hypoglycaemic brain damage seen at necropsy

TABLE 14.1
Interactions between sulphonylureas and potentiating drugs

Potentiating agent	Pharmocokinetic mechanisms	Pharmocodynamic mechanisms
Common interactions		
Antihypertensive agents, guanethidine, clonidine, reserpine		decrease peripheral glucose production increase 'hypoglycaemic unawareness'
β-Adrenoceptor blocking agents		decrease peripheral glucose production increase 'hypoglycaemic unawareness'
Chloramphenicol	inhibits hepatic metabolism	
Cibenozoline, disopyramide		increase insulin release
Cimetidine	inhibits hepatic metabolism	
Ethanol		decreases hepatic gluconeogenesis
Monoamine oxidase inhibitors		decrease insulin secretion decrease hepatic gluconeogenesis
Pentamidine		increases insulin release
Phenylbutazone	decreases protein binding inhibits hepatic metabolism	
Quinine, quinidine		increase insulin release
Ritodrine		increases insulin release
Salicylates		increase insulin release increase peripheral glucose production
Sulphonamides and related compounds	decrease protein binding inhibit hepatic metabolism	? increase insulin release
Less common interactions		
Clofibrate	decreased metabolism (?) decreased renal excretion (?)	
Cyclophosphamide		displaces of insulin from binding site
Oxytetracycline		increases responsiveness to insulin
Tricyclic antidepressants		uncertain
Possible interactions		
Allopurinol	decreases renal excretion	
Fenfluramine		increases glucose uptake
Methandrostenolone		uncertain
Methysergide		increases insulin release
Probenecid	decreases renal excretion	

following such combined poisoning are very similar to those seen after severe hypoxia (Critchley et al 1984).

Aspirin (acetylsalicylic acid)

The effects of aspirin and other non-steroidal anti-inflammatory agents on glucose homoeostasis have been studied by various workers (Newman and Brodows 1983;, Bratusch-Marrain *et al.* 1985, Giugliano *et al.* 1985). Although most workers confirmed the glucose-lowering effect of aspirin, the exact mechanism remains controversial. The effect of prostaglandin E_2 on insulin secretion remains uncertain. Elevation of plasma insu-

lin level following administration of aspirin has been demonstrated by Giugliano and others (1985). Although this insulinotropic effect could be blunted by infusion of prostaglandin E_2, it was not abolished by the simultaneous administration of prostaglandin synthetase inhibitors (Bratusch-Marrain *et al.* 1985). Newman and Brodows (1983) reported that aspirin ingestion resulted in a degree of peripheral insulin insensitivity despite the enhanced insulin response. Bratusch-Marrain and colleagues (1985) also showed that aspirin impaired tissue sensitivity to insulin and that this was counterbalanced by an increased plasma insulin response. Reduced clear

TABLE 14.2
Interactions between sulphonylureas and antagonizing drugs

Antagonizing agent	Pharmocokinetic mechanisms	Pharmocodynamic mechanisms
Common interactions		
β-Adrenoceptor agonists		increase peripheral glucose production
β-Adrenoceptor blocking agents		decrease insulin release
Calcium-channel blocking agents		decrease insulin release
Glucocorticosteroids		increase peripheral glucose production increase insulin resistance
Oral contraceptive steroids (progestogen components)		increase insulin resistance increase corticosteroid actions
Thiazides, loop diuretics, and diazoxide		decrease insulin release increase insulin resistance
Less common interactions		
Antiarrythmic agents (amiodarone, encainide)		uncertain
Ethanol		increases sympathetic activities
Glycerol		uncertain
Immunosuppressive/immunomodulating agents (cyclosporin, asparaginase, homoharringtonine)		decreased insulin secretion increased glucagon secretion
Lithium related to diabetes insipidus		increases glucose absorption
Methylxanthines (theophylline)		increase catecholamine release
Nalidixic acid		uncertain
Phenobarbitone	increases hepatic metabolism	
Phenytoin		inhibits insulin secretion
Psychotrophic agents (loxapine, amoxapine, morphine, phenothiazine)		increases glucose tolerance (?via effect on brain catecholamines)
Rifampicin	increases hepatic metabolism	
Streptozotocin		increases insulin due to pancreatic cytolysis

ance of insulin was suggested by an unaltered C peptide level. They also proposed that the hypoglycaemic effect of aspirin in NIDDM was due to a reduction in hepatic glucose production secondary to the increased availability of insulin. The authors further suggested that, since prostaglandin synthetase inhibitor treatment failed to reverse these aspirin-induced hormonal and metabolic events, an alternative, prostaglandin-independent mechanism was responsible for the hypoglycaemic effect.

Aspirin rarely produces hypoglycaemia in normal subjects. Symptomatic hypoglycaemia can occur, however, in combination therapy with other hypoglycaemic agents and in the presence of renal or hepatic impairment. Profound hypoglycaemia or hyperglycaemia can occur when large amounts of salicylate-containing compounds are ingested, and this is particularly important in children with accidental poisoning (Seltzer 1989).

β-Adrenoceptor blocking agents

Owing to the complex actions of β-adrenoceptor blocking agents on carbohydrate metabolism, both hyperglycaemia and hypoglycaemia can occur. In diabetic patients, β-blockade can delay recovery from hypoglycaemia and mask early hypoglycaemic symptoms by reduced awareness. Hypoglycaemia can occur in non-diabetic subjects after treatment with non-selective blocking agents such as propranolol (Holm *et al.* 1981; Arky 1989). Waal-Manning (1976) reviewed the mechanisms for the hypoglycaemic effects resulting from β-blockade. Hypoglycaemia results from a combination of enhanced activity of circulating insulin through inhibition of peripheral lipolysis, hepatic phosphorylation, and facilitation of peripheral glucose uptake. The effect is potentiated in the presence of liver disease or situations in which there is glycogen depletion or enhanced insulin sensitivity, such as fasting or exercise (Arky 1989). Warning signs of hypoglycaemia, particularly tachycardia, may be impaired by the reduction of β-sympathetic activity; this is particularly dangerous in insulin-dependent diabetes, in which the hypoglycaemic effects of β-blockade are most likely to occur. Cardioselective β-adrenoceptor blocking agents or those with intrinsic sympathomimetic activities may cause fewer problems (Lager et al. 1979). Sweating is, however, minimally affected.

Local ocular application of timolol for glaucoma has induced hypoglycaemia in a patient with insulin-dependent diabetes mellitus (Angelo-Nielson 1980).

Angiotensin-converting-enzyme inhibitors

Several studies have indicated that captopril has no hyperglycaemic effects in diabetic hypertensive subjects (Winocour et al. 1986; Shionoiri et al. 1987; Zanella et al. 1988; Pollare et al. 1989). Ferriere and colleagues (1985) reported cases of hypoglycaemia in both IDDM and NIDDM patients after introduction of captopril therapy and demonstrated enhanced insulin sensitivity with increased glucose disposal. Jauch and colleagues (1987) showed enhanced forearm glucose uptake in NIDDM patients treated with captopril and postulated that angiotensin-converting enzyme caused local accumulation of bradykinin, which has an insulin-like activity, due to kininase II inhibition. In a comparative study of captopril and hydrochlorothiazide, patients treated with captopril showed no change in basal insulin level, but an increase in the early, and decrease in the late, insulin peak suggestive of enhanced insulin sensitivity. This is in contrast to the increase of insulin level both at the basal level and in the late peak in the patients treated with hydrochlorothiazide (Pollare et al. 1989). Studies in dogs suggest that captopril and enalapril inhibit adrenaline secretion and thus will blunt counter-regulatory mechanisms (Critchley et al. 1988).

Antimalarial drugs

Spontaneous hypoglycaemia can occur in patients with severe malarial infection by *Plasmodium falciparum* due to depletion of hepatic glycogen reserves in the host and the parasites' metabolic demand for glucose. Hyperinsulinaemic hypoglycaemia, however, occurs not uncommonly in patients treated with quinine for *P. falciparum* infection (White et al. 1983) and particularly in children (Okitolonda et al. 1987) and pregnant women (Looaree-suwan et al. 1985). A stimulatory effect of quinine on insulin release from pancreatic β-cells has been postulated, but direct inhibition of hepatic gluconeogenesis and increased glucose utilization by the parasites may also play contributory roles (White et al. 1983). Quinine-induced hyperinsulinaemic hypoglycaemia can be profound and resistant to treatment. The long-acting synthetic somatostatin analogue Sandostatin has been found to be effective in reversing sustained hypoglycaemia secondary to quinine therapy in a patient with falciparum malaria (Phillips et al. 1986a).

Fatal hypoglycaemia has occurred following a chloroquine overdose (Bamber and Redpath 1987), though the mechanism is not known, and it remains controversial as to whether hypoglycaemia occurs with conventional dosages. In a study in healthy volunteers comparing quinine with other antimalarial agents, including chloroquine, amodiaquine, mefloquine, and halofantrine, hypoglycaemia was only found in association with quinine (Phillips et al. 1986b). Ogbuokiri (1987) also reported that chloroquine had no effect on glucose metabolism in healthy individuals. White and colleagues (1987) claimed that although chloroquine reduced insulin degradation and might improve glucose homoeostasis in diabetic subjects, there was no evidence that it caused hypoglycaemia in patients suffering from *P. falciparum* malaria.

Pentamidine

This is an antiprotozoal agent used in the treatment of trypanosomiasis, and also in *Pneumocystis carinii* pneumonia — which frequently occurs in immunosuppressed patients. Pentamidine is an aromatic diamide closely related to the biguanides (Sharpe 1983). Stahl-Bayliss and colleagues (1986) reported hypoglycaemia in 27 per cent of patients with the acquired immune deficiency syndrome (AIDS) who received pentamidine therapy, a sevenfold increase compared with other patients without AIDS receiving pentamidine. Nephrotoxicity was also present in all of these patients. Pentamidine has a multiphasic effect on blood glucose concentrations. Bouchard and others (1982) proposed that β-cell cytolysis results in hypoglycaemia due to acute release of insulin. This may be followed by persistent hyperglycaemia from destruction of the islet cells. Severe haemorrhagic pancreatitis associated with both hypoglycaemia (Salmeron et al. 1986) and hyperglycaemia (Zuger et al. 1986) have been reported following pentamidine therapy. Similar multiphasic effects on glucose metabolism have been seen with other β-cytotoxic drugs, such as streptozotocin and alloxan. Adverse effects on glucose metabolism are more likely to occur in the presence of renal impairment and when pentamidine is repeatedly administered in high dosage and for prolonged periods of time (Waskin *et al.* 1988). Hypoglycaemia has also been reported with the use of pentamidine by inhalation (Karboski and Godley 1988).

Antiarrythmic drugs

Disopyramide, a quinidine-like Class Ia antiarrythmic drug is known to be associated with hypoglycaemia. Croxson and others (1987) detected failure of suppression of insulin during hypoglycaemia in a patient treated with disopyramide and proposed that this drug might stimulate insulin release in the same way as quinidine and quinine. In a review of 14 cases of disopyramide-induced hypoglycaemia, 9 had significantly impaired renal function. Elderly and malnourished patients were also at particular risk, and toxicity could occur with normal therapeutic dosages (Cacoub *et al.* 1989). The action of other hypoglycaemic agents can be potentiated in the presence of disopyramide (Stapleton and Gillman 1983). Cibenzoline, a Class I drug, has been reported to cause hypoglycaemia with detectable insulin concentrations (Hilleman *et al.* 1987; Jeandel *et al.* 1988).

Ritodrine

Ritodrine, a β_2-agonist, has been used in the treatment of premature labour. Apart from its hyperglycaemic effect via gluconeogenesis, lipolysis, and glycogenolysis, β_2-stimulation can increase insulin release either directly or as a response to increased glucose production from the liver (Holm 1983). Administration of ritodrine to women with premature labour has been associated with an increased incidence of neonatal hypoglycaemia (Brazy and Pupkin 1979). Babies who were exposed to ritodrine up to the time of delivery were at greater risk than babies whose exposure was stopped at least one week before delivery (Musci *et al.* 1988). Caldwell and colleagues (1987) recently reported a case of hyperinsulinaemic hypoglycaemia in a woman with triple pregnancy treated with ritodrine for premature labour. They proposed that the hypoglycaemia had resulted from the enhancement of the hyperinsulinaemic state in pregnancy by the insulinotrophic effect of ritodrine (see also Hyperglycaemia).

Somatostatin

A long-acting analogue of somatostatin (Sandostatin) has been found to be effective in treating certain endocrine neoplasms. During treatment of acromegaly, suppresssion of insulin secretion can cause hyperglycaemia which tends to become less marked with progressive therapy, as the deleterious effect of growth hormone on carbohydrate metabolism is ameliorated by the treatment (Lamberts *et al.* 1985). Reduced glucose absorption and disturbance of counter-regulatory hormone

secretion with inappropriately suppressed growth hormone, glucagon, and catecholamines during hypoglycaemia has been reported, however, following the administration of Sandostatin for the treatment of insulinoma (Stehouwer *et al.* 1989), acromegaly (Popovic *et al.* 1989), and metastatic carcinoid tumours (Brunner *et al.* 1989).

Trimethoprim–sulphamethoxazole

The potentiating effect of sulphonamides in the presence of other hypoglycaemic agents is well-recognized (Hansen and Christensen 1977; Jackson and Bressler 1981). Trimethoprim–suphamethoxazole (co-trimoxazole) has been reported to potentiate the effect of chlorpropamide (Baciewicz and Swafford 1984). Hypoglycaemia induced by co-trimoxazole alone is a rare but recognized adverse effect (Poretsky and Moses 1984). Schattner and colleagues (1988) reported a case of hypoglycaemia with detectable circulating insulin in a patient suffering from AIDS who was treated with high-dose co-trimoxazole for *Pneumocystis carinii* pneumonia, and discussed the possible mechanisms. Sulphamethoxazole is known to displace sulphonylureas from binding proteins with enhancement of the hypoglycaemic effect. In addition, it may mimic sulphonylurea action by binding to pancreatic islet tissue and increasing insulin secretion.

Lithium

Lithium mimics the action of insulin by inhibiting adenyl cyclase activity and production of cyclic-AMP, which mediates the actions of many hormones (including epinephrine, ACTH, and glucagon), which are known to have an effect on glucose metabolism. This can lead to hypoglycaemia from increased glucose uptake by peripheral tissues and decreased lipogenesis and glucose production by the liver. Hunt (1987) reported a case of lithium-induced hypoglycaemia in a patient with non-insulin-dependent diabetes mellitus.

Other drugs

Propoxyphene used for the treatment of pain has been reported to cause hypoglycaemia, especially in the presence of renal impairment. The underlying mechanism for propoxyphene-induced hypoglycaemia is unknown, although the renal impairment could contribute to the disorder (Arem 1989). In their case report, Almirall and colleagues (1989) found adequate hormonal response with suppressed insulin and increased growth hormone and glucagon concentrations during hypoglycaemia.

Streptozotocin can cause profound hypoglycaemia by its cytolytic actions on the pancreas and it has been used in the treatment of malignant pancreatic tumours.

Fat metabolism

Cholesterol and triglycerides are hydrophobic compounds and their transport in plasma is facilitated by combination with phospholipids and a class of hydrophilic polypeptides, known as apoproteins, to form complexes called lipoproteins. Fatty acids on the other hand are transported in plasma bound to albumin.

Compositions of lipoproteins

There are several classes of apoproteins (apo A, consisting of apo A-I and apo A-II; apo B; apo C consisting of apoC-I, apoC-II, apoC-III; and apo E) which are mainly synthesized in the liver or intestinal mucosa. The various combinations of apolipoproteins with cholesterol and triglycerides result in the formation of five classes of lipoproteins which vary in their composition, functions, and other properties.

Chylomicrons consist mainly of dietary triglyceride with only a small amount of apoprotein. The very-low-density lipoproteins (VLDL) consist of endogenously synthesized triglycerides and are substantially smaller and denser than the chylomicrons, because of the incorporation of apoproteins, mainly of the apo B type. The VLDL is converted via intermediate-density lipoprotein (IDL) to low-density lipoprotein (LDL), which consists mainly of cholesterol and apo B. High-density lipoprotein (HDL) is the most dense form, with apo A as its major apoprotein and equal amounts of cholesterol and phospholipid. HDL has a major role in reverse transport of cholesterol from peripheral tissues to liver for the excretion of cholesterol. Apo E is mainly associated with VLDL and chylomicron remnants.

There are four enzymes involved in plasma lipid transport. Activity of lecithin cholesterol acyltransferase (LCAT) is stimulated by apo A-I and is involved in the synthesis of cholesterol ester. Lipoprotein lipase, found mainly in the liver and adipose tissue, splits triglycerides in chylomicrons and VLDL to glycerol and free fatty acids and its activity is stimulated by apo C-II. Hepatic lipase mainly hydrolyses triglycerides in the VLDL remnants. Mobilizing lipase releases free fatty acids from adipose tissue and is activated through the adenyl cyclase system by catecholamines, growth hormone, and glucocorticoids, and is inhibited by glucose and insulin.

Transport and metabolism of lipoproteins

Exogenous (dietary) lipid is transported by chylomicrons, which are resynthesized in the intestinal mucosa from the breakdown products of dietary triglyerides and cholesterol in the gastrointestinal tract. They consist principally of triglycerides and contain apo A and apo B. In the circulation, apo A is transferred to HDL, where the chylomicrons acquire apo C and apo E from HDL. Apo C-II then activates lipoprotein lipase in the peripheral tissues, mainly adipose tissue, muscle, and liver, where triglycerides are released from the chylomicrons. The fatty acids liberated from hydrolysis of triglycerides are then stored or used as a source of energy. The chylomicron remnants consisting of apo B, apo E, and cholesterol esters are taken up by the liver and catabolised. The sterol is then excreted in the bile.

In the fasting state, VLDL is synthesized in the liver and, to a lesser extent, the intestinal mucosa, and contains mainly triglycerides and some unesterified cholesterol with apo B and lesser amounts of apo E. Apo C is acquired from HDL and VLDL remnants in the plasma. Lipoprotein lipase, activated by apo C-II, removes triglycerides from VLDL in the adipose and other tissue. The apo C, unesterified cholesterol, and phospholipid are progressively transferred to HDL. The catabolism of VLDL results in the formation of IDL which is further hydrolysed to form LDL, consisting mainly of cholesterol and apo B. LDL either binds to apo B receptors in the liver, and is taken up when cholesterol esters are hydrolysed and apo B destroyed, or to receptors on peripheral tissues such as the adrenals where cholesterol is used for synthesis of steroids. A small proportion of LDL is taken up by the scavenger cells of the monocyte–macrophage system.

HDL is formed in the liver and intestinal mucosa and contains mainly apo C, apo E, equal amounts of cholesterol and phospholipid, and very little triglyceride. In the circulation, HDL acquires apo A-I mainly from chylomicrons, to which it transfers apo C and apo E. Apo A-I is a co-factor for LCAT, which esterifies free cholesterol on HDL. The more hydrophobic esterified cholesterol passes into the core of the HDL particle while the surface accepts more cholesterol and lipoproteins from other tissues for further esterification. The cholesterol ester is transferred from the HDL core to VLDL and LDL by a transfer protein (cholesteryl ester transfer protein) and is then taken up again by the liver and peripheral tissues through the recognition of apo B on LDL by apo B receptors.

Significance of dyslipoproteinaemia

The association of hypercholesterolaemia with coronary arterial disease has long been recognized. Most studies have now shown a positive association between elevated plasma LDL and remnant VLDL concentrations and ischaemic heart disease. On the other hand, HDL appears to confer a protective effect, and a high HDL cholesterol/total cholesterol ratio indicates low risk. An inverse relationship between HDL and LDL is frequently observed. In addition, the subfraction HDL_2 of HDL has recently been shown to be the specific component responsible for this protective role, while HDL_3 is associated with atherogenesis (Ballantyne et al. 1982; Ball and Mann 1986).

Although hypertriglyceridaemia itself is less clearly associated with increased risk of coronary arterial disease, very high levels of chylomicrons and VLDL are associated with recurrent pancreatitis.

Classification of dyslipoproteinaemia

Hyperlipidaemia may be defined as an elevation of cholesterol or triglyceride or both. The elucidation of the complex mechanism of lipid transport and metabolism, however, has allowed the recognition of the important roles played by apoproteins in the pathogenesis of disorders of lipid metabolism. Hyperlipoproteinaemia (dyslipoproteinaemia) is defined as an abnormality involving either the lipids or lipoproteins or both.

The World Health Organization classifies hyperlipoproteinaemia into five types (WHO 1985). Type I is characterized by gross hypertriglyceridaemia and hyperchylomicronaemia due to a deficiency of lipoprotein lipase or apo C-II, which activates lipoprotein lipase; pancreatitis is a well-recognized complication. Types IIa and IIb (familial hypercholesterolaemia) are characterized by elevation of LDL, and represent a result of defective cholesterol metabolism. In about 5 per cent of patients, defective expression or reduced activity of tissue apo B receptor for LDL, due to a genetic defect, has been identified. Patients with Type II hyperlipoproteinaemia are at increased risk of ischaemic heart disease. Type III is an uncommon disorder due to a defective catabolism of remnants of chylomicrons and VLDL resulting from an abnormality of apo E. LDL is characteristically depressed with abnormally high concentrations of VLDL remnants (IDL). These subjects are also at increased risk of arteriosclerosis. Types IV and V are due to defects in either the production or catabolism of VLDL, resulting in hypertriglyceridaemia with marked increase in VLDL and decrease in LDL and HDL. Some of these patients may have familial lipoprotein lipase deficiency, as with Type I; recurrent attacks of acute pancreatitis are a known complication of this form of dyslipoproteinaemia.

Although dyslipoproteinaemia can be genetically acquired, a large proportion is related to dietary intake. In addition, it may accompany disease states such as nephrotic syndrome, diabetes mellitus, and hypothyroidism. Drugs that alter the synthesis or clearance of apolipoproteins by actions on different enzymes may result in abnormal lipid metabolism. Such adverse effects can be particularly important in the presence of a pre-existing dyslipoproteinaemic state.

Drugs affecting lipid metabolism

Diuretics

Although thiazide diuretics are an effective form of antihypertensive therapy, adverse effects on lipid metabolism, at least in the short term, have been documented, and these may explain the failure of these drugs to lower the incidence of ischaemic heart disease in hypertensive subjects, despite their effectiveness in preventing cerebrovascular disease. A review by Ames (1986a) points out that, although most studies have demonstrated significant increases in total cholesterol (range 4–13 per cent), total triglyceride (range 14–37 per cent), LDL cholesterol (range 7–29 per cent), and VLDL cholesterol (7–56 per cent) in response to thiazides, both interindividual and intraindividual responses varied over time. In some studies in which control subjects were included, there was a tendency for lipid levels to fall in untreated subjects. Thus the improvement in lipid profiles in thiazide-treated patients reported in some studies may be more apparent than real. In addition, he concluded that examination of the lipoprotein fractions was necessary in order to document the adverse effects of diuretics on lipid metabolism fully.

The pathogenesis of diuretic-induced dyslipoproteinaemia is largely unkown. Again, Ames discussed the possible mechanisms in his review (1986a). Potassium-sparing diuretics have been reported to have no effect on lipid metabolism (Ames and Hill 1978; Amery et al. 1982), although a change of diuretic therapy to potassium sparing agents failed to improve existing lipid abnormalities (Ames and Peacock 1984). Dyslipoproteinaemia does not seem to occur in premenopausal women taking thiazides, which suggests a protective hormonal effect on lipid metabolism changes associated with thiazide therapy (Boehringer et al. 1982). Glycosylated lipoproteins are removed more slowly from the circulation (Steinbrecher and Witztum 1984), and Ames (1986a) suggested that this might provide a link between glucose intolerance and disturbances of lipid metabolism secondary to thiazide therapy and possibly other drugs such as β-adrenoceptor blocking agents.

It is noteworthy that hyperlipidaemia induced by thiazides or similar compounds may be dose-related, and low-dose antihypertensive treatment can be effective in lowering blood pressure while causing less unwanted effects on lipid metabolism (Tweeddale *et al.* 1977).

β-Adrenoceptor blocking agents

There is increasing evidence that β-adrenoceptor blocking agents have adverse effects on lipid metabolism, resulting in increased serum triglyceride and decreased high-density-lipoprotein (HDL) cholesterol levels (Gemma *et al.*1982; Otero *et al.* 1983; Lehren 1987). Most studies have shown that both selective (e.g. propranolol and timolol) and non-selective (e.g. metoprolol and atenolol) β-adrenoceptor blocking agents reduce HDL and increase triglyceride, resulting in an unfavourable reduction of the HDL/cholesterol ratio (Lehren 1987). β-Adrenoceptor blocking agents with intrinsic sympathomimetic activity (ISA) (e.g. pindolol and acebutolol) appear, however, to have no adverse effect on lipid metabolism. Durrington and others (1985) studied the effects of β-adrenoceptor blocking agents on lipoprotein metabolism and found a reduction in the cardioprotective HDL_2 subfraction of cholesterol, which is most apparent in patients treated with propranolol and atenolol. In patients with pre-existing hypertriglyceridaemia, there was a reduction in the clearance of triglycerides. This was not found in normolipidaemic patients, however, or in patients treated with β-adrenoceptor blocking agents with ISA. Increased hepatic synthesis of VLDL is the major determinant of the concentration of serum triglycerides, so that reduced hepatic production secondary to β-blockade may minimize the adverse effect on triglyceride clearance, which becomes important only in patients with pre-existing hypertriglyceridaemia.

Durrington and Cairns (1982) were the first to report cases of acute pancreatitis and massive hypertriglyceridaemia associated with the use of metoprolol and atenolol. They suggested that this was a result of reduced clearance of triglycerides due to unopposed α-adrenergic stimulation that reduced lipoprotein lipase activity. Since then, there have been similar reports of acute pancreatitis and hypertriglyceridaemia following treatment with atenolol (Haitas *et al.* 1988) and nadolol (O'Donoghue 1989). In some of these cases, genetic predisposition and alcoholism were probable contributory factors.

Other antihypertensive agents

Lehren (1987) and Ames (1986*b*) reviewed the effects of α-adrenergic blocking agents and concluded that most studies have shown prazosin to have a favourable effect

on lipid metabolism, with a reduction in triglyceride, cholesterol, and LDL, and elevation of HDL and HDL/cholesterol ratio. In his extensive review, Ames (1986*b*) examined the effects of other antihypertensive agents on lipid metabolism. The few studies on calcium-channel antagonists suggested either a neutral or favourable effect, while only limited information was available on centrally acting drugs. Methyldopa has been associated with an unfavourable reduction in the ratio of HDL to total cholesterol, although this is not conclusive. Angiotensin-converting-enzyme inhibitors do not appear to be associated with adverse effects on lipid metabolism, but more (and longer) studies are required. Pollare and colleagues (1989) recently reported little change in lipids or lipoproteins following captopril treatment as compared with hydrochlorothiazide.

Corticosteroids

Ibels and others (1975) reported that Type IV dyslipoproteinaemia with hypertriglyceridaemia was common among uraemic and dialysis patients. Their serum cholesterol levels were often normal although very variable. Following transplantation, however, hypercholesterolaemia was found more commonly in these patients than in uraemic or dialysis patients, and the pattern of dyslipoproteinaemia was more variable with Types IIa, IIb, and IV occurring equally frequently, suggesting a multifactorial aetiology attributable to obesity, prednisone therapy, and degree of residual uraemia. Transplant patients who were receiving prednisone and azathioprine had a significantly higher incidence of coronary arterial disease than uraemic patients and patients on haemodialysis. This was thought to be related to the hyperlipidaemic properties of the corticosteroids used for immunosuppression (Ibels *et al.* 1977).

The dyslipoproteinaemia associated with corticosteroid therapy includes elevations of triglycerides, cholesterol, VLDL, and LDL. This is often, though not always, accompanied by a low level of HDL-c. Although Jefferys and colleagues (1980) observed a lower level of HDL-c in females treated with corticosteroids, this gender difference was not found in corticosteroid-treated patients after renal transplantation (Ettinger *et al.* 1987*a*).

The pathogenesis of dyslipoproteinaemia associated with corticosteroid therapy is currently being investigated and appears multifactorial. Taskinen (1987) reported a correlation between plasma concentration of VLDL and HDL and enzymatic activities of lipoprotein lipase in both healthy subjects and patients with abnormal lipoprotein metabolism. Reduction of activity of lipoprotein lipase with impaired catabolism of VLDL following corticosteroid therapy has been demonstrated in *in vitro* studies (Krause *et al.* 1981; Bagdade *et al.* 1976). This abnormality was not found, however, in patients with systemic lupus erythematosus treated with corticosteroids (Ettinger and Hazzard 1988). The hyperinsulinaemic state associated with corticosteroid therapy can increase hepatic production of VLDL and HDL and impair receptor uptake of LDL (Henze *et al.* 1983; Hirsch and Mazzone 1986). Ettinger and Hazzard (1988) reported an elevation of plasma apo B in patients with systemic lupus erythematosus treated with corticosteroids, which might explain the increased synthesis of VLDL apo B. Patients with coronary arterial disease have been reported to have significantly lower Apo A-I and Apo-II and elevated Apo B with hypertriglyceridaemia, which are considered to be independent risk factors for arteriosclerosis (Kukita *et al.* 1985).

The effect of corticosteroids on HDL cholesterol is less well known. Ettinger and co-workers (1987*b*) reported a lack of correlation between the change in cholesterol level and that of HDL cholesterol. Irrespective of the HDL cholesterol level, abnormalities of the subfractions of HDL are probably of more important significance. Jung and others (1982) reported an abnormal composition of HDL-c with increased apo A/HDL cholesterol ratio and decreased apo A/HDL-triglyceride ratio that may impair the transport of cholesterol. Ettinger and colleagues (1987*a,b*) reported an increase in HDL_3 and decrease in the cardioprotective HDL_2 subfraction in patients treated with corticosteroids following renal transplantation and for systemic lupus erythematosus. The adverse effects of corticosteroids on lipid metabolism appear to be dose-related. Significantly higher levels of triglyceride and cholesterol were found in post-renal-transplant patients who required methylprednisolone (Ibels *et al.* 1975). A positive correlation between the prednisone dosage and severity of hyperlipidaemia has been observed (Ibels *et al.* 1978; Ponticelli *et al.* 1978; Cattran *et al.* 1979; Ettinger *et al.* 1987*b,c*) but this was ameliorated by the administration of an alternate day regimen (Cattran *et al.* 1979; Curtis 1982; Ettinger *et al.* 1987*b,c*).

Oral contraceptives

The Framingham Study (Castelli 1984) has shown that women under the age of 40 had a lower risk of arteriosclerosis, which was thought due to a protective effect of higher levels of HDL-c in females. With increasing age, the risk parallels that of males, with increasing levels of total and LDL cholesterol. The Lipid Research Clinics Program Prevalence Study (LaRosa *et al.* 1986) showed a 30 per cent prevalence of dyslipoproteinaemia

in women using gonadal hormones, compared with women who were non-users, although the HDL/LDL ratio was more favourable in the pill users. With increasing identification and understanding of the nature of various subfractions of HDL-c, interpretation of HDL becomes incomplete without analysis of these subfractions. It has been suggested that the HDL_2 subfraction confers protection against arteriosclerosis, while HDL_3 is associated with increased risk of coronary arterial disease (Ballantyne *et al.* 1982; Brensike *et al.* 1984; Levy *et al.* 1984).

Oestrogen and progestogen components of oral contraceptive steroids and postmenopausal replacement therapy have opposing effects on lipid metabolism. Oestrogens increase hepatic production of VLDL and HDL, reduce activity of lipoprotein lipase, and increase HDL and HDL_2 subfractions, while progestogens have opposite effects (Knopp 1986; Wahl *et al.* 1983). Hence, adverse effects on lipid metabolism are dependent on the relative potency and composition of the progestogen in the formulation. Miccoli and others (1989) compared the effects of three conventional formulations of lowdose oral contraceptives (two monophasic and one triphasic) on lipid and glucose metabolism. Plasma glucose remained unchanged, while triglycerides increased in all three groups of patients; total and LDL cholesterol were unaffected. HDL cholesterol was increased in the women taking the two monophasic formulations. The overall effect, however, was negligible. In another study, by Notelovitz and colleagues (1989), the effects of triphasic and monophasic pills on plasma lipid and lipoproteins were studied. Similar effects were seen in both groups: total, LDL, and HDL_3 cholesterols, apolipoproteins A-I and B, and triglyceride increased while HDL and HDL_2 cholesterols decreased. The changes were mild, however, and the authors concluded that they were unlikely to be of clinical significance.

Knopp (1986), in his review of the subject, concluded that the risk of arteriosclerosis and myocardial infarction in young women using oral contraceptive steroids is associated with increasing progestogen dose. Oestrogen therapy elevates HDL and HDL_2 cholesterol and confers a protective effect against myocardial infarction in postmenopausal women. The addition of a progestogen, however, may have a deleterious effect on lipoprotein metabolism, cancelling any benefit associated with oestrogen. Further long-term, detailed, prospective studies are required to characterize the effects of oral contraceptives on lipid metabolism and arteriosclerosis fully. Until such time, lipid profiles should be taken regularly in women who are contemplating the use of oral contraceptives, particularly in the presence of other risk factors, and their use is perhaps best avoided in patients with known dyslipoproteinaemic disorders.

Although oestrogen therapy selectively inhibits hepatic triglyceride lipase activity, the effect is only mild and rarely leads to clinically significant hypertriglyceridaemia (Applebaum *et al*. 1977). In patients with familial hyperlipidaemia, however, reduced clearance of plasma triglyceride secondary to oestrogen therapy has been reported to cause acute pancreatitis due to massive hypertriglyceridaemia (Glueck *et al*. 1972; Davidoff *et al*. 1973; Stuyt *et al*. 1986).

Tamoxifen

Tamoxifen, a non-steroidal oestrogen antagonist, is frequently used as adjuvant therapy for breast carcinoma. Rossner and Wallgren (1984) observed small changes in both lipid and lipoprotein concentrations following tamoxifen therapy. Concentrations of triglycerides and LDL triglyceride (VLDL) both increased, while cholesterol and LDL cholesterol (LDL) fell. This was accompanied by a reduction of orosomucoid and haptoglobin concentrations, and implied an oestrogen-like effect of tamoxifen on protein and lipoprotein metabolism. Brun and others (1986) reported a case of severe lipidaemia induced by tamoxifen with high plasma triglyceride, VLDL cholesterol, and VLDL apo B concentrations, and low levels of LDL cholesterol and LDL apo B. They demonstrated a reduction in the activities of lipoprotein lipase and hepatic triglyceride lipase, which impeded the conversion of VLDL to LDL. A fatal case of acute pancreatitis following tamoxifen has also been reported (Noguchi *et al*. 1987).

Ethanol

Chait and Brunzell (1990) reviewed the effects of alcohol intake on lipid metabolism. Alcohol increases HDL concentrations but appears to have little effect on LDL concentrations. Elevations of both HDL_3 and HDL_2 have been demonstrated. Dyslipoproteinaemia can also result from alcoholic liver disease. Ethanol competes with fatty acids in the liver for oxidation. The fatty acids are otherwise incorporated into triglycerides leading to an increased hepatic synthesis of VLDL. The increased production of VLDL is usually compensated for by increased clearance via the lipoprotein lipase system. If the secretion of VLDL is impaired, however, as in the case of liver disease or in the presence of pre-existing dyslipoproteinaemia, small increases in VLDL production may saturate the removal system, resulting in significant hypertriglyceridaemia and hyperchylomicronaemia.

Other drugs

Androgenic steroids, in particular anabolic steroids, can lower HDL levels. The mechanism probably involves impaired triglyceride clearance by lipoprotein lipase and accelerated HDL catabolism. Hypertriglyceridaemia with elevations of LDL and fall in HDL has been associated with the use of retinoids (isotretinoin and etretinate) but usually resolves on discontinuation of therapy (Chait and Brunzell 1990). Amiodarone has been reported to cause hypertriglyceridaemia, but the pattern of the lipoproteins was not examined in detail (Lakhdar *et al*. 1988).

References

Abadie, E., Gauville, C., and Brisson, C. (1984). Nifedipine and endocrine status in diabetic patients. *Br. J. Clin. Pharmacol*. 18, 648.

Almirall, J., Montoliu, J., Torras, A., and Revert, L. (1989). Propoxyphene induced hypoglycaemia in a patient with chronic renal failure. *Nephron* 53, 273.

Amery, A., Birkenhager, W., Bulpitt, C.P., Clement, D., and Duruytte, M. (1982). Influence of antihypertensive therapy on serum cholesterol in elderly hypertensive patients. *Acta Cardiologica* 37, 235.

Amery, A., Birkenhäger, W., Brixko, P., Clement, D., Duruytte, M., and De Schaepdryver, A., *et al*. (1986). Glucose intolerance during diuretic therapy in elderly hypertensive patients. A second report from the European Working Party on high blood pressure in the elderly (EWPHE). *Postgrad. Med. J*. 62, 919.

Ames, R.P. (1986*a*). The effects of antihypertensive drugs on serum lipids and lipoproteins. I. Diuretics. *Drugs* 32, 260.

Ames, R.P. (1986*b*). The effects of antihypertensive drugs on serum lipids and lipoproteins. II. Non diuretic drugs. *Drugs* 32, 335.

Ames, R.P. and Hill, P. (1978). Raised serum lipid concentrations during diuretic treatment of hypertension: a study of predictive indexes. *Clin. Sci. Mol. Med*. 55 (suppl. 4), 311S.

Ames, R.P. and Peacock, P. (1984). Serum cholesterol during treatment of hypertension with diuretic drugs. *Arch. Intern. Med*. 144, 710.

Amiel, S.A., Sherwin, R.S., Simonson, D.C., and Tamborlane, W.V. (1988). Effect of intensive insulin therapy on glycaemic threshold for counterregulatory hormone release. *Diabetes* 37, 901.

Andersson, D.E.H. and Rojdmark, S. (1981). Improvement of glucose tolerance by verapamil in patients with non-insulin-dependent diabetes mellitus. *Acta Med. Scand*. 210, 27.

Andren, L., Hoglund, P., Dotevall, A., Eggertsen R., Svensson A., Olson S., *et al*. (1988). Diltiazem in hypertensive patients with type II diabetes mellitus. *Am. J. Cardiol*. 62, 114G.

Angelo-Nielson K. (1980). Timolol topically and diabetes mellitus. *JAMA* 244, 2263.

Ansfield, F.J. (1977). Megace and no diabetes mellitus. *Ann. Intern. Med.* 86, 365.

Applebaum, D.M., Goldberg, A.P., Pykalisto, O.J., Brunzell, J.D., and Hazzard, W.R. (1977). Effect of estrogen on post-heparin lipolytic activity: Selective decline in hepatic triglyceride lipase. *J. Clin. Invest.* 59, 601.

Arem R. (1989). Hypoglycemia associated with renal failure. *Endocrinol. Metab. Clin. North. Am.* 18, 103.

Arky, R.A. (1989). Hypoglycaemia associated with liver disease and ethanol. *Endocrinol. Metab. Clin. North Am.* 18, 75.

Arneson, G.A. (1964). Phenothiazine derivatives and glucose metabolism. *J. Neuropsychiatry* 5, 181.

Baciewicz, A.M. and Swafford, W.B. Jr (1984). Hypoglycaemia induced by the interaction of chlorpropamide and co-trimoxazole. *Drug. Intell. Clin. Pharm.* 18, 309.

Bagdade, J.D., Yee, E., and Albers, J. (1976) Glucocorticoids and triglyceride transport; effects on secretion rates, lipoprotein lipase and plasma lipoproteins in rats. *Metabolism* 25, 253.

Ball, M. and Mann, J.I. (1986). Apoproteins: predictors of coronary heart disease? *Br. Med. J.* 293, 769.

Ballantyne, F.C., Clark, F.S., Simpson, H.S., and Ballantyne, D. (1982). High density and low density lipoprotein subfractions in survivors of myocardial infarction and in control subjects. *Metabolism* 31, 433.

Bamber, M.G. and Redpath, A. (1987). Chloroquine and hypoglycaemia. *Lancet* i, 1211.

Beardwood, D.M., Alden, J.S., Graham, C.A., Beardwood, J.T., and Marble, A. (1965). Evidence for a peripheral action of chlorothiazide in normal man. *Metabolism* 14, 561.

Belehu, A. and Naafs, B. (1982). Diabetes mellitus associated with pentamidine mesylate. *Lancet* i, 1463.

Bengtsson, C., Blohme, G., Lapidus, L., Lindquist, D., Lundgren, H., and Nyström, E., *et al.* (1984). Do antihypertensive drugs precipitate diabetes? *Br. Med. J.* 289, 1495.

Berger, W. (1985). Incidence of severe side effects during therapy with sulphonylureas and biguanides. *Horm. Metab. Res.* (suppl.), 15, 111.

Berger, W., Caduff, F., Pasquel, M., and Rump, A. (1986). The relatively frequent incidence of severe sulfonylurea-induced hypoglycaemia in the last 25 years in Switzerland. Results of 2 surveys in Switzerland in 1969 and 1984. *Schweiz. Med. Wochenschr.* 116, 145.

Berger, W., Keller, U., Honegger, B., and Jaeggi, E. (1989). Warning symptoms of hypoglycaemia during treatment with human and porcine insulin in diabetes mellitus. *Lancet* i, 1041.

Berglund, G. and Andersson, O. (1981). Beta-blockers or diuretics in hypertension? A six year follow-up of blood pressure and metabolic side effects. *Lancet* i, 744.

Bhatnagar, S.K., Amin, M.M.A., and Al-Yusuf, A.R. (1984). Diabetogenic effects of nifedipine. *Br. Med. J.* 289, 19.

Bloomgarden, Z.T., Ginsberg-Fellner, F., Rayfield, E.J., Bookman, J. and Brown, W.V. (1984). Elevated haemoglobin A_{1c} and low-density lipoprotein cholesterol levels in thiazide-treated diabetic patients. *Am. J. Med.* 77, 823.

Boehringer, K., Weidmann, P., Mordasini, R., Schiffl, H., and Bachmann, C. (1982). Menopause-dependent plasma lipoprotein alterations in diuretic treated women. *Ann. Intern. Med.* 91, 206.

Bottino, J.C. and Tashima, C.K. (1976). Medroxyprogesterone acetate and diabetes mellitus *Ann. Intern. Med.* 84, 341.

Bouchard, P., Sai, P., Reach, G., Caubarrère, I., Ganeval, D., and Assan, R. (1982). Diabetes mellitus following pentamidine-induced hypoglycaemia in humans. *Diabetes* 31, 40.

Bratusch-Marrain, P.R., Vierhapper, H., Komjati, M., and Waldhäusl, W.K. (1985) Acetyl-salicylic acid impairs insulin-mediated glucose utilization and reduces insulin clearance in healthy and non-insulin-dependent diabetic man. *Diabetologia* 28, 671.

Brazy, J.E. and Pupkin, M.J. (1979). Effects of maternal isoxsuprine administration on preterm infants. *J. Pediatr.* 94, 444.

Brensike, J.F., Levy, R.I., Kelsey, S.F., Passamani, E.R., Richardson, J.M., and Loh I.K. (1984) Effects of therapy with cholestyramine on progression of coronary arteriosclerosis: Results of the NHLBI Type II Coronary Intervention Study. *Circulation* 69, 313.

Brun, L.D., Gagne, C., Rousseau, C., Moorjani, S., and Lupien, P-J. (1986). Severe lipemia induced by tamoxifen. *Cancer* 57, 2123.

Brunner, J.E., Kruger, D.F., Basha, M.A., Meiri, E., and Kaatz, S.S. (1989). Hypoglycemia after administration of somatostatin analog (SMS 201-995) in metastatic carcinoid. *Henry Ford Hosp. Med. J.* 37, 60.

Cacoub, P., Deray, G., Baumelou, A., Grimaldi, A., Soubrie, C., and Jacobs, C. (1989). Disopyramide-induced hypoglycaemia case report and review of the literature. *Fundam. Clin. Pharmacol.* 3, 527.

Caldwell, G., Scougall, I., Boddy, K., and Toft, A.D. (1987). Fasting hyperinsulinemic hypoglycaemia after ritodrine therapy for premature labor. *Obstet. Gynaecol.* 70, 478.

Campbell, I.W. (1985). Metformin and the sulphonylureas : the comparative risk. *Horm. Metab. Res.* (suppl.), 15, 105.

Caritis, S.N., Toig, G., Heddinger, L.A., and Ashmead, G. (1984). A double-blind study comparing ritodrine and terbutaline in the treatment of preterm labor. *Am. J. Obstet. Gynecol.* 150, 7.

Castelli, W.P. (1984). Epidemiology of coronary heart disease: The Framingham study *Am. J. Med.* 76 (suppl. 2A), 4.

Cattran, D.C., Steiner, G., Wilson, D.R., and Fenton, S.S.A. (1979). Hyperlipidemia after renal transplantation: natural history and pathophysiology. *Ann. Intern. Med.* 91, 554.

Chait, A. and Brunzell, J.D. (1990). Acquired hyperlipidemia (secondary dyslipoproteinemias). *Endocrinol. Metab. Clin. North Am.* 2, 259.

Charles, M.A. and Danforth, E. Jr (1971). Non-ketotic hyperglycemia and coma during intravenous diazoxide therapy in uremia. *Diabetes* 20, 501.

Charles, S., Ketelslegers, J., Buysschaert, M., and Lambert, A.E. (1981). Hyperglycaemic effect of nifedipine. *Br. Med. J.* 283, 19.

Chaudhuri, M.L.D. and Catania, J, (1988). A comparison of the effects of bumetanide (Burinex) and frusemide on carbohydrate metabolism in the elderly. *Br. J. Clin. Pract.* 42, 427.

Cooper, A.J. (1966). The action of mebanazine, a monamine oxidase inhibitor antidepressant drug in diabetes, part II. *Int. J. Neuropsychiatry* 2, 342.

Corcoran, F.H., Granatir, R.F., and Schlang, H.A. (1971). Hyperglycemic hyperosmolar nonketotic coma associated with corticosteroid therapy. *J. Fla Med. Assoc.* 58, 38.

Craig, J., Abu-Saleh, M., Smith, B., and Evans, I. (1977). Diabetes mellitus in patients on lithium. *Lancet* ii, 1028.

Critchley, J.A.J.H., Proudfoot, A.T., Boyd, S.G., Campbell, I.W., Brown, N.S., and Gordon, A. (1984). Deaths and paradoxes after intentional insulin overdosage. *Br. Med. J.* 289, 225.

Critchley, J.A.J.H., MacLean, M.R., and Ungar, A. (1988). Inhibitory regulation by co-released peptides of catecholamine secretion by the canine adrenal medulla. *Br. J. Pharmacol.* 93, 383.

Croxson, M.S., Shaw, D.W., Henley, P.G., and Gabriel, H.D.L.L. (1987). Disopyramide-induced hypoglycaemia and increased serum insulin. *N.Z. Med. J.* 100, 407.

Curtis, J., Horrigan, F., and Ahearn, D. (1972). Chlorthalidone-induced hyperosmolar hyperglycaemic nonketotic coma. *JAMA* 220, 1592.

Curtis, J.J., Galla, J.H., Woodward, S.Y., Lucas, B.A., and Luke, R.G. (1982). Effect of alternate day prednisone on plasma lipids in renal transplant recipients. *Kidney Int.* 22, 42.

Dante, A. (1986). Nifedipine and fasting glycemia. *Ann. Intern. Med.* 104, 125.

Davidoff, F., Tishler, S., and Rosoff, C. (1973). Marked hyperlipidemia and pancreatitis associated with contraceptive therapy. *N. Engl. J. Med.* 289, 552.

Davies, D.M., MacIntyre, A., Millar, E.J., Bell, S.M., and Mehra, S.K. (1967). Need for glucagon in severe hypoglycaemia induced by sulphonylurea drugs. *Lancet* i, 363.

De Broe, M., Mussche, M., Ringoir, S., and Bosteels V. (1972). Oral diazoxide for malignant hypertension. *Lancet* i, 1397.

De Pirro, R., Fusco, A., Bertoli, A., Greco, A.V., and Lauro, R. (1978). Insulin receptors during the menstrual cycle in normal women. *J. Clin. Endocrinol. Metab.* 47, 1387.

De Pirro, R., Forte, F., Bertoli, A., Greco, A.V., and Lauro, R. (1981). Changes in insulin receptors during oral contraception. *J. Clin. Endocrinol. Metab.* 52, 29.

Dickson, I. (1962). Glycosuria and diabetes following INAH therapy. *Med. J. Aust.* i, 325.

Dornhorst, A., Powell, S.H., and Pensky, J. (1985). Aggravation by propranolol of hyperglycaemic effect of hydrochlorothiazide in type II diabetics without alteration of insulin secretion. *Lancet* i, 123.

Dowell, R.C. and Imrie, A. H. (1972). Chlorpropamide poisoning in non-diabetics. *Scott. Med. J.* 17, 337

Duffy, T.J. and Ray, R. (1984). Oral contraceptive use: Prospective follow-up of women with suspected glucose intolerance. *Contraception* 30, 197.

Durrington, P.N. and Cairns, S.A. (1982). Acute pancreatitis, a complication of beta-blockade. *Br. Med. J.* 284, 1016.

Durrington, P.N., Brownlee, W.C., and Large, D.M. (1985). Short term effects of beta-adrenoceptor blocking drugs with and without cardioselectivity and intrinsic sympathomimetic activity on lipoprotein metabolism in hypertriglyceridaemic patients and in normal men. *Clin. Sci.* 69, 713.

Ellis, M.E., Weiss, R.B., Korzun, A.H., Rice, M.A., Norton L, Perloff, M., *et al.* (1986). Hyperglycaemic complications associated with adjuvant chemotherapy of breast cancer. A cancer and leukemic group B (CALGB) study. *Am. J. Clin. Oncol.* 9, 53.

Enyeart, J.L., Price, W.A., Hoffman, D.A., and Woods, L. (1983). Profound hyperglycemia and metabolic acidosis after verapamil overdose. *J. Am. Coll. Cardiol.* 2, 1228.

Ettinger, W.H. Jr and Hazzard, W.R. (1988) Elevated apolipoprotein-B levels in corticosteroid-treated patients with systemic lupus erythematosus. *J. Clin. Endocrinol. Metab.* 67, 425.

Ettinger, W.H., Bender, W.L., Goldberg, A.P., and Hazzard, W.R. (1987a). Lipoprotein lipid abnormalities in healthy renal transplant recipients: persistance of low HDL$_2$ cholesterol. *Nephron* 47, 17.

Ettinger, W.H., Goldberg, A.P., Applebaum-Bowden, D., and Hazzard, W.R. (1987b). Dyslipoproteinemia in systemic lupus erythematosus: effect of corticosteroids. *Am. J. Med.* 83, 503.

Ettinger, W.H., Klinefelter, H.K., and Kwiterovich, P.O. (1987c). Effect of short term, low dose prednisone on plasma lipids. *Atherosclerosis* 63, 167.

Fajans, S.S., Floyd, J.C., Knopf, R.F., Rull, J., Guntsche, E.M., and Conn, J.W. (1966). Benzothiadiazine suppression of insulin release from normal and abnormal islet cell tissue in man. *J. Clin. Invest.* 45, 481.

Fariss, B.L. and Lutcher, C.L. (1971). Diphenylhydantoin-induced hyperglycaemia and impaired insulin release: effect of dosage. *Diabetes* 20, 177.

Feely, J. and Peden, N. (1983). Enhanced sulfonlyurea-induced hypoglycaemia with cimetidine. *Br. J. Clin. Pharmacol.* 16, 607P.

Ferner, R.E. and Neil, H.A.W. (1988). Sulphonylureas and hypoglycaemia. *Br. Med. J.* 296, 949.

Ferriere, M., Lachkar, H., Richard, J., Bringer, J., Orsetti, A., and Mirouze, J. (1985). Captopril and insulin sensitivity. *Ann. Intern. Med.* 102, 134.

Flamenbaum, W. and Friedman, R. (1982). Pharmacology, therapeutic efficacy and adverse effects of bumetanide, a new 'loop' diuretic. *Pharmacotherapy* 2, 213.

Fonseca, V. and Phear, D.N. (1982). Hyperosmolar non-ketotic diabetic syndrome precipitated by treatment with diuretics. *Br. Med. J.* 284, 36.

Fraser, A.G. and Harrower, A.D.B. (1977). Convulsions and hyperglycaemia associated with nalidixic acid. *Br. Med. J.* ii, 1518.

Gemma, G., Montanari, G., Suppa, G., Paralova, A., Franceschini, G., and Mantero, O. (1982). Plasma lipid and lipoprotein changes in hypertensive patients treated with propranolol and prazosin. *J. Cardiovasc. Pharmacol.* 4 (suppl. 2), S233.

Gerich, J.E., Charles, M.A., and Grodsky, G.M. (1976). Regulation of pancreatic insulin and glucagon secretion. *Annu. Rev. Physiol.* 38, 353.

Giugliano, D., Torrella, R., Cacciapuoti, F., Gentile, S., Verza, M., and Varricchio, M. (1980). Impairment of insulin secretion in man by nifedipine. *Eur. J. Clin. Pharmacol.* 18, 395.

Giugliano, D., Ceriello, A., di Pinto, P., Saccommanno, F., Gentile, S., and Cappiapuoti, F. (1982). Impaired insulin secretion in human diabetes mellitus. The effect of naloxone-induced opiate receptor blockade. *Diabetes* 31, 367.

Giugliano, D., Ceriello, A., Saccomanno, F., Quatraro, A., Paolisso, G., and D'Onofrio, F. (1985) Effects of salicylate, tolbutamide, and prostaglandin E_2 on insulin responses to glucose in noninsulin-dependent diabetes mellitus. *J. Clin. Endocrinol. Metab.* 61, 160.

Gleuck, C.J., Scheel, D., Fishback, J., and Steiner, P. (1972). Estrogen induced pancreatitis in patients with previous covert type V hyperlipoproteinemia. *Metabolism* 21, 657.

Goldberg, E.M. and Sanbar, S.S. (1969). Hyperglycaemic, nonketotic coma following administration of Dilantin (diphenylhydantoin). *Diabetes* 18, 101.

Goldberg, R., van As, M., Joffe, B.I., Krut, L., Bersohn, I., and Seftel, H.C. (1975). Metabolic responses to selective beta-adrenergic stimulation in man. *Postgrad. Med. J.* 51, 53.

Greenberg, G., Brennan, P.J., and Miall, W.E. (1984). Effects of diuretic and beta blocker therapy in the Medical Research Council Trial. *Am. J. Med.* 76, 45.

Greenstone, M.A. and Shaw AB. (1987). Alternate day corticosteroid causes alternate day hyperglycaemia. *Postgrad. Med. J.* 63, 761.

Greenwood, R.H. (1982). Hyperglycaemic effect of nifedipine. *Br. Med. J.* 284, 50.

Gulan, M., Perlman, K., Sole, M., Albisser, A.M., and Zinman, B. (1988). Counterregulatory hormone responses preserved after long-term intravenous insulin infusion compared to continuous subcutaneous insulin infusion. *Diabetes* 37, 526.

Gündogdu, A.S., Brown, P.M., Juul, S., Sachs, L., and Sönksen, P.H. (1979). Comparison of hormonal and metabolic effects of salbutamol infusion in normal subjects and insulin-requiring diabetics. *Lancet* ii, 1317.

Gunnarsson, R., Klintmalm, G., Lundgren, G., Wilczek H., Ostman, J., and Groth, C.G. (1983). Deterioration in glucose metabolism in pancreatic transplant recipients given cyclosporin. *Lancet* ii, 571.

Guthrie, G.P. Jr, Miller, R.E., Kotchen, T.A., and Koenig, S.H. (1983). Clonidine in patients with diabetes and mild hypertension. *Clin. Pharmacol. Ther.* 34, 713.

Haitas, B., Disler, L.J., Joffe, B.I., and Seftel, H.C. (1988). Massive hypertriglyceridemia associated with atenolol. *Am. J. Med.* 85, 586.

Hall, S. (1982). Hyperosmolar non-ketotic diabetic syndrome precipitated by treatment with diuretics. *Br. Med. J.* 284, 665.

Hall, K.W., Dobson, K.E., Dalton, J.G., Ghignone, M.C., and Penner, S.B. (1984). Metabolic abnormalities associated with intentional theophylline overdose. *Ann. Intern. Med.* 101, 457.

Hansen, J.M. and Christensen, L.K. (1977). Drug interactions with oral sulphonylurea hypoglycaemic drugs. *Drugs* 13, 24.

Harrison, B.D.W., Rutter, T.W., and Taylor, R.T. (1972). Severe non-ketotic hyperglycaemic precoma in a hypertensive patient receiving diazoxide. *Lancet* ii, 599.

Helderman, J.H., Elahi, D., Andersen, D.K., Raizes, G.S., Tobin, J.D., Shocken, D. et al. (1983). Prevention of the glucose tolerance of thiazide diuretics by maintenance of body potassium. *Diabetes* 32, 106.

Henze, K., Chait, A., Albers, J.J., and Bierman, E.L. (1983). Hydrocortisone decreases the internalization of low density lipoprotein in cultured human fibroblasts and arterial smooth muscle cells. *Eur. J. Clin. Invest.* 13, 171.

Hepburn, D.A., Patrick, A.W., Eadington, D.W., Colledge, N., and Frier, B.M. (1988). How common are changes in hypoglycaemic awareness after conversion from animal to human insulins? *Diabetic Med.* 5 (suppl. 2), 7.

Hilleman, D.E., Mohiuddin, S.M., Ahmed, T.S., and Dahl, J.M. (1987). Cibenzoline-induced hypoglycaemia. *Drug Intell. Clin. Pharm.* 21, 38.

Hirsch, L.J. and Mazzone, T. (1986). Dexamethasone-modulated lipoprotein metabolism in cultured human monocyte-derived macrophages: stimulation of scavenger receptor activity. *J. Clin. Invest.* 77, 485.

Holland, O.B. and Pool, P.E. (1988). Metabolic changes with antihypertensive therapy of the salt-sensitive patient. *Am. J. Cardiol.* 61, 53H.

Holm, G., Johansson, S., Vedin, A., Wilhelmsson, C., and Smith, U. (1980). The effect of beta-blockade on glucose tolerance and insulin release in adult diabetes. *Acta Med. Scand.* 208, 187.

Holm, G., Herlitz, J., and Smith, U. (1981). Severe hypoglycaemia during physical exercise and treatment with beta-blockers. *Br. Med. J.* 282, 1360.

Holm, G. (1983). Adrenergic regulation of insulin release. *Acta Med. Scand.* (suppl. 627), 21.

Howell, S.L. and Taylor, K.W. (1966). Effect of diazoxide on insulin secretion in vitro. *Lancet* i, 128.

Huminer, D., Shlomo, D., Rosenfeld, J.B., and Pitlik, S.D. (1989). Inadvertent sulfonylurea-induced hypoglycaemia. *Arch. Intern. Med.* 149, 1890.

Humphrey, S.H. and Nash, D.A. (1978). Lactic acidosis complicating sodium nitroprusside therapy. *Ann. Intern. Med.* 88, 58.

Hunt, N.J. (1987). Hypoglycaemic effect of lithium. *Biol. Psychiatry* 22, 798.

Huupponen, R. and Pihlajamäki, K. (1986). Effect of blood glucose level on the metabolic response of intravenous salbutamol. *Int. J. Clin. Pharmacol. Ther. Toxicol.* 24, 374.

Ibels, L.S., Simons, L.A., King, J.O., Williams, P.F., Neale, F.C., and Stewart, J.H. (1975). Studies on the nature and cause of hyperlipidemia in uraemia, maintanence dialysis and renal transplantation. *Q. J. Med.* 44, 601.

Ibels, L.S., Stewart, J.H., Mahoney, J.F., Neale, F.C., and Sheil, A.G.R. (1977). Occlusive arterial disease in uremic and hemodialysis patients and renal transplant recipients. A study of the incidence of arterial disease and of the prevalence of risk factors implicated in the pathogenesis of arteriosclerosis. *Q. J. Med.* 46, 197.

Ibels, L.S., Alfrey, A.C., and Weil, R. (1978). Hyperlipidemia in adult, pediatric and diabetic renal transplant recipients. *Am. J. Med.* 64, 634.

Jackson, J.E. and Bressler, R. (1981). Clinical pharmacology of sulphonylurea hypoglycaemic agents. 2. *Drugs* 22, 295.

Jauch, K-W., Hartl, W., Guenther, B., Wicklmayr, M., Rett, K., and Dietze, G. (1987). Captopril enhances insulin responsiveness of forearm muscle tissue in non-insulin-dependent diabetes mellitus. *Eur. J. Clin. Invest.* 17, 448.

Jeandel, C., Preiss, M.A., Pierson, H., Penin, F., Cuny, G., Bannwarth, B., et al. (1988). Hypoglycaemia induced by cibenzoline. *Lancet* i, 1232.

Jefferys, D.B., Lessof, M.H., and Mattock, M.B. (1980). Corticosteroid treatment, serum lipids and coronary artery disease. *Postgrad. Med. J.* 56, 491.

Jennings, A.M., Wilson, R.M., and Ward, J.D. (1989). Symptomatic hypoglycaemia in NIDDM patients treated with oral hypoglycaemic agents. *Diabetes Care* 12, 203.

Jha, T.K. and Sharma, V.K. (1984). Pentamidine-induced diabetes mellitus. *Trans. R. Soc Trop. Med. Hyg.* 78, 252.

Johnson, S.F., Schade. D.S., and Peake, G.T. (1977). Chlorpropamide-induced hypoglycaemia. Successful treatment with diazoxide. *Am. J. Med.* 63 799.

Jones, B.J., McKenney, J.M., Wright, J.T. Jr, and Goodman, R.P. (1988). Effects of diltiazem hydrochloride on glucose tolerance in persons at risk for diabetes mellitus. *Clin. Pharm.* 7, 235.

Josselson, J. and Sadler, J.H. (1986). Nephrotic-range proteinuria and hyperglycaemia associated with clonidine therapy. *Am. J. Med.* 80, 545.

Jung, K., Neumann, R., Scholz, D., and Nugel, E. (1982). Abnormalities in the composition of serum high density lipoprotein in renal transplant recipients. *Clin. Nephrol.* 17, 191.

Karboski, J.A. and Godley, P.J. (1988). Inhaled pentamidine and hypoglycemia. *Ann. Intern. Med.* 108, 490.

Kirkpatrick, C., Quenon, M., and Desir, D. (1980). Blood anions and electrolytes during ritodrine infusion in preterm labor. *Am. J. Obstet. Gynecol.* 138, 523.

Klumpp, T.G. (1965). Nalidixic acid — false-positive glycosuria and hyperglycaemia. *JAMA* 193, 746.

Knopp, R.H. (1986). Arteriosclerosis risk. The roles of oral contraceptives and postmenopausal estrogens. *J. Reprod. Med.* 31 (suppl.), 913.

Krause, I., Bar-on, H., and Shaffir, E. (1981). Origin and pattern of glucocorticoid-induced hyperlipidemia in rats. *Biochim. Biophys. Acta* 663, 69.

Kreisberg, R.A. (1984). Pathogenesis and management of lactic acidosis. *Annu. Rev. Med.* 35, 181.

Kukita, H., Hamada, H.M., Hiwada, K., and Kokubu, T. (1985). Clinical significance of measurements of serum apolipoprotein A-I, A-II and B in hypertriglyceridemic male patients with and without coronary heart disease. *Atherosclerosis* 55, 143.

Kung, A.W.C., Ma, J.T.C., Wong, V.C.W., Li, D.F.H., Ng, M.M.T., Wang, C.C.L., et al. (1987). Glucose and lipid metabolism with triphasic oral contraceptives in women with history of gestational diabetes. *Contraception* 35, 257.

Lager, I., Blohmé, G., and Smith, U. (1979). Effect of cardioselective and non-selective beta-blockade on the hypoglycaemic response in insulin-dependent diabetics. *Lancet* i, 458.

Lager, I., Attvall, W., Blohmé, G., and Smith, U. (1988). Altered recognition of hypoglycemic symptoms in type 1 diabetes during intensified control with continuous subcutaneous insulin infusion. *Diabetic Med.* 3, 322.

Lakhdar, A.A., Farish, E., Dunn, F.G., and Hillis, W.S. (1988). Amiodarone therapy and glucose tolerance — a prospective trial. *Eur. J. Clin. Pharmacol.* 34, 651.

Lamberts, S.W.J., Uitterlinden, P., Verschoor, L., van Dongen, K.J., and Del Pozo, E. (1985). Long-term treatment of acromegaly with the somatostatin analogue SMS 201-995. *N. Engl. J. Med.* 313, 1576.

Lancaster-Smith, M., Leigh, N.I., and Thompson, H.H. (1974). Death following non-ketotic hyperglycaemic coma during diazoxide therapy and peritoneal dialysis. *Postgrad. Med. J.* 50, 175.

The Lancet (1983). Methanol poisoning. *Lancet* i, 910.

LaRosa, J.C., Chambless, L.E., Criqui, M.H., Frantz, I.D., Glueck, J., Heiss, G., et al. (1986). Patterns of dyslipoproteinemia in selected North American populations. The Lipid Research Clinics Program Prevalence Study. *Circulation* 73 (suppl. I) I 12

Lee, K., Mize, R., and Lowenstein, S.R. (1987). Glyburide-induced hypoglycemia and ranitidine. *Ann. Intern. Med.* 107, 261.

Lee, R.V., Jampol, L.M., and Brown, W.V. (1971). Nephrogenic diabetes insipidus and lithium intoxication — complications of lithium carbonate therapy. *N. Engl. J. Med.* 284, 93.

Lehren, P. (1987). Comparison of effects on lipid metabolism of antihypertensive drugs with alpha- and beta- adrenergic antagonist propreties. *Am. J. Med.* 82 (suppl. 1A), 31.

Leslie, D. and Coats, P.M. (1977). Salbutamol-induced diabetic ketoacidosis. *Br. Med. J.* ii, 768.

Levy, R.I., Brensike, J.F., Epstein, S.E., Kelsey, S.F., Passamani, E.R., and Richardson, J.M. (1984). The influence of changes in lipid values induced by cholestyramine and diet on progression of coronary artery disease: Results of the NHLBI Tye II Coronary Intervention Study. *Circulation* 69, 325.

Lewis, P.J., Kohner, E.M., Petrie, A., and Dollery. C.T. (1976). Deterioration of glucose tolerance in hypertensive patients on prolonged diuretic treatment. *Lancet* i, 564.

Looareesuwan, S., Phillips, R.E., White, N.J., Kietinun, S., Karbwang, J., and Rackow, C. (1985) Quinine and severe falciparum malaria in late pregnancy. *Lancet* ii, 4.

Lowder, N.K., Bussey, H.I,, and Sugarek, N.J. (1988). Clinically significant diuretic-induced glucose intolerance. *Drug Intell. Clin. Pharm.* 22, 969.

Lowe, J., Gray, J., Henry, D.A., and Lawson, D.H. (1979). Adverse reactions to frusemide in hospital inpatients. *Br. Med. J.* ii, 360.

McDonald, J. (1980). Alcohol and diabetes. *Diabetes Care* 3, 629.

Maclaren, H.K., Taylor, G.E., and Raiti, S. (1975). Propranolol-augmented, exercise-induced human growth hormone release. *Pediatrics* 56, 804.

Maclean, D. and Tudhope, G.R. (1983). Modern diuretic treatment. *Br. Med. J.* 286, 1419.

MacWalter, R.S., El Debani, A.H., Feely, J., and Stevenson, I.H. (1985). Potentiation by ranitidine of the hypoglycaemic response to glypizide in diabetic patients. *Br. J. Clin. Pharmacol.* 19, 121P.

Main, D.M., Main, E.K., Strong, S.E., and Gabbe, S.G. (1985). The effect of oral ritodrine therapy on glucose tolerance in pregnancy. *Am. J. Obstet. Gynecol.* 152, 1031.

Main, E.K., Main, D.M., and Gabbe, S.G. (1987). Chronic oral terbutaline tocolytic therapy is associated with maternal glucose intolerance. *Am. J. Obstet. Gynecol.* 157, 644.

Mann, N.S., Russman, H.B., Mann, S.K., and Tsai, M.F. (1985). Lactulose and severe lactic acidosis. *Ann. Intern. Med.* 103, 637.

Martinez-Maldonaldo, M. and Terrell, J. (1973). Lithium carbonate-induced nephrogenic diabetes insipidus and glucose-intolerance. *Arch. Intern. Med.* 132, 881.

Metz, S.A., Halter, J.B., and Robertson, R.P. (1978). Induction of defective insulin secretion and impaired glucose tolerance by clonidine. *Diabetes* 27, 554.

Miccoli, R., Orlandi, M.C., Fruzzetti, F., Giampietro, O., Melis, G., and Ricci, C. (1989) Metabolic effects of three new low dose pills: a six month experience. *Contraception* 39, 643.

Mills, G.A. and Horn, J.R. (1985). Beta-blockers and glucose control. *Drug Intell. Clin. Pharm.* 19, 246.

Montoliu, J., Carrera, M., Darnell, A., and Revert, L. (1981). Lactic acidosis and Fanconi's syndrome due to degraded tetracycline. *Br. Med. J.* 283, 1576.

Munck, A. (1971). Glucocorticoid inhibition of glucose uptake by peripheral tisssues: old and new evidence, molecular mechanisms, and physiological significance. *Perspect. Biol. Med.* 14, 265.

Musci, M.N. Jr, Abbasi, S., Otis, C., and Bolognese, R.J. (1988). Prolonged fetal ritodrine exposure and immediate neonatal outcome. *J. Perinatol.* 8, 27.

Nagai, K., Takeda, N., Endo, Y., Kikuchi, M., Imai, T., Yasuda, K., *et al.* (1986). Effects of diltiazem hydrochloride in diabetics. *Int. J. Clin. Pharmacol. Ther. Toxicol.* 24, 602.

Newman, W.P. and Brodows, R.G. (1983). Aspirin causes tissue insensitivity to insulin in normal man. *J. Clin. Endocrinol. Metab.* 57, 1102.

Noguchi, M., Taniya, T., Tajiri, K., Miwa, K., Miyazaki, I., Koshino, H., *et al.* (1987). Fatal hyperlipaemia in a case of metastatic breast cancer treated by tamoxifen. *Br. J. Surg.* 74, 586.

Notelovitz, M., Feldman, E.B., and Gillespy, M. (1989). Lipid and lipoprotein changes in women taking low dose triphasic oral contraceptives: a controlled comparative 12-month clinical trial. *Am. J. Obstet. Gynecol.* 160, 1269.

Oakley, D.E. and Ellis, P.P. (1976). Glycerol and hyperosmolar nonketotic coma. *Am. J. Ophthalmol.* 81, 469.

O'Donoghue, D.J. (1989). Acute pancreatitis due to nadolol-induced hypertriglyceridaemia. *Br. J. Clin. Pract.* 43, 74.

Ogbuokiri, J.E. (1987). Does chloroquine cause hypoglycaemia in the absence of clinical malaria? *Lancet* ii, 281.

Okitolonda, W., Delacollette, C., Malengreau, M., and Henquin, J.C. (1987). High incidence of hypoglycaemia in African patients treated with intravenous quinine for severe malaria. *Br. Med. J.* 295, 716.

Osei, K., Holland, G., and Falko, J.M. (1986). Indapamide. Effects on apoproteins, lipoproteins and glucoregulation in ambulatory diabetic patients. *Arch. Intern. Med.* 146, 1973.

Otero, M.L., Pinilla, C.F., and Claros, N.M. (1983). The effect of long-term therapy of essential hypertension with atenolol and chlorthalidone on carbohydrate tolerance. *Primary Cardiology* 6 (suppl. 1), 193.

Ott, A., Hayes, J., and Polin, J. (1976). Severe lactic acidosis associated with intravenous alcohol for premature labor. *Obstet. Gynecol.* 48, 362.

Peacock, I., Tattersall, R.B., Taylor, A., Douglas, C.A., and Reeves, W.G. (1983). Effects of new insulins on insulin and C-peptide antibodies, insulin dose, and diabetic control. *Lancet* i, 149.

Perlman, J.A., Russell-Briefel, R., Ezzati, T., and Lieberknecht, G. (1985). Oral glucose tolerance and the potency of contraceptive progestins. *J. Chronic Dis.* 38, 857.

Pershadsingh, H.A., Grant, B., and McDonald, J.M. (1987). Association of diltiazem therapy with increased insulin resistance in a patient with type 1 diabetes mellitus. *JAMA* 257, 930.

Pfeifer, M.A., Halter, J.B., Graf, R., and Porte, D. Jr (1980). Potentiation of insulin secretion to nonglucose stimuli in normal man by tolbutamide. *Diabetes* 29, 335.

Phillips, P.J., Need, A.G., Thomas, D.W., Conyers, R.A.J., Edwards, J.B., and Lehmann, D. (1979). Nalidixic acid and lactic acidosis. *Aust. N.Z. J. Med.* 9, 694.

Phillips, R.E., Warrell, D.A., Looareesuwan, S., Turner, R.C., Bloom. S.R., Quantrill, D., *et al.* (1986a). Effectiveness of SMS 201-995, a synthetic, long-acting somatostatin analogue, in treatment of quinine-induced hyperinsulinaemia. *Lancet* i, 713.

Phillips, R.E., Looareesuwan, S., White, N.J., Chanthavanich, P., Karbwang, J., Supanarnond, W., *et al.* (1986b). Hyperglycaemia and antimalarial drugs: quinine and release of insulin. *Br. Med. J.* 292, 1319.

Pickup, J. (1989). Human insulin. Problems with hypogly-caemia in a few patients. *Br. Med. J.* 299, 991.

Podolsky, S. and Pattavina, C.G. (1973). Hyperosmolar non-ketotic diabetic coma: a complication of propranolol therapy. *Metabolism* 22, 685.

Pohl, J.E.F. and Thurston, H. (1971). Use of diazoxide in hypertension with renal failure. *Br. Med. J.* iv, 142.

Politi, A., Poggio, G., and Margiotta, A. (1984). Can amiodarone induce hyperglycaemia and hypertriglyceridaemia? *Br. Med. J.* 288, 285.

Pollare, T., Lithell, H., and Berne, C. (1989). A comparison of the effects of hydrochlorothiazide and captopril on glucose and lipid metabolism in patients with hypertension. *N. Engl. J. Med.* 28, 868.

Ponticelli, C., Barbi, G.L., Cantaluppi, A., De Vecchi, A., Annoni, G., and Donati, C. (1978). Lipid disorders in renal transplant recipients. *Nephron* 20, 189.

Popovic, V., Nesovic, M., Micic, D., Kendereski, A., Zarkovic, M., Djordjevic, P., *et al.* (1989). Hypoglycaemia in acromegalic patients with long acting somatostatin analogue (SMS 201-995). *Horm. Metab. Res.* 21, 282.

Poretsky, L. and Moses, A.C. (1984). Hypoglycaemia associated with trimethoprim/sulphamethoxazole therapy. *Diabetes Care* 7, 508.

Potter, J., Clarke, P., Gale, E.A.M., Dave, S.H., and Tattersall, R.B. (1982) Insulin-induced hypoglycaemia in an accident and emergency department: the tip of an iceberg? *Br. Med. J.* 285, 1180.

Pui, C.H., Burghen, G.A., Paul Bowman, W., and Aur, R.J.A. (1981). Risk factors for hyperglycemia in children with leukemia receiving L-asparaginase and prednisone. *J. Pediatr.* 99, 46.

Rees, A. and Gale E. (1988). Diabetic comas. In *Clinical diabetes an illustrated text* (ed. G.M. Besser, H.J. Bodansky, and A.G. Cudworth), p. 21.1. J.B. Lippincott, Philadelphia.

Robinson, D.S., Nilsson, C.M., Leonard, R.F., and Horton, E.S. (1981). Effects of loop diuretics on carbohydrate metabolism and electrolyte excretion. *J. Clin. Pharmacol.* 21, 637.

Roe, T.F. and Kugut, M.D. (1982). Idiopathic leucine-sensitive hypolycemia syndrome: insulin and glucagon responses and effects of diazoxide. *Pediatr. Res.* 16, 1.

Rossner, S. and Wallgren, A. (1984). Serum lipoproteins and proteins after breast cancer surgery and effects of tamoxifen. *Atherosclerosis* 52, 339.

Roth, A., Miller, H.I., Belhassen, B., and Laniado, S. (1989). Slow-release verapamil and hyperglycemic metabolic acidosis. *Ann. Intern. Med.* 110, 171.

Roth, D., Milgrom, M., Esquenazi, V., Fuller, L., Burke, G., and Miller, J. (1989). Posttransplant hyperglycaemia. Increased incidence in cyclosporine-treated renal allograft recipients. *Transplantation* 47 278.

Roux, P. and Courtois, H. (1981). Blood sugar regulation during treatment with indapamide in hypertensive diabetics. *Postgrad. Med. J.* 57 (suppl. 2), 70.

Rowe, P.A. and Mather, H.G. (1985). Hyperosmolar non-ketotic diabetes mellitus associated with metolazone. *Br. Med. J.* 291, 25.

Rowe, J.W., Tobin, J.D., Rosa, R.M., and Andres, R. (1980). Effects of experimental potassium deficiency on glucose and insulin metabolism. *Metabolism* 29, 498.

Salerno, D.M., Fifield, J., Krejci, J., and Hodges, M. (1988). Encainide-induced hyperglycaemia. *Am. J. Med.* 84, 39.

Salmeron, S., Petitpretz, P., Katalama, C., Herve, P., Brivet, F., Simmoneau, G., *et al.* (1986). Pentamidine and pancreatitis. *Ann. Intern. Med.* 105, 140.

Schattner, A., Rimon, E., Green, L., Coslovsky, R., and Bentwich, Z. (1988). Hypoglycaemia induced by co-trimoxazole in AIDS. *Br. Med J.* 297, 742.

Sears, E.S. (1976). Nonketotic hyperosmolar hyperglycemia during glycerol therapy for cerebral edema. *Neurology* 26, 89.

Seltzer, H.S. (1989). Drug-induced hypoglycaemia. A review of 1418 cases. *Endocrinol. Metab. Clin. North Am.* 18, 163.

Sharp, P. (1972). Interference in glucose oxidase-peroxidase blood glucose methods. *Clin. Chim. Acta.* 40, 115.

Sharpe, S.M. (1983). Pentamidine and hypoglycemia. *Ann. Intern. Med.* 99, 128.

Shen, M., Orwoll, E.S., Conte, J.E. Jr, and Prince, M.J. (1989). Pentamidine-induced pancreatic beta cell dysfunction. *Am. J. Med.* 86, 726.

Shionoiri, H., Miyakawa, T., Takasaki, I., Ishikawa Y., Hiroto, S., Kaneko, Y. et al. (1987). Glucose tolerance during chronic captopril therapy in patients with essential hypertension. *J. Cardiovasc. Pharmacol.* 9, 160.

Shrivastava, R.K., and Edwards, D. (1983). Hypoglycemia associated with imipramine. *Biol. Psychiatry* 18, 1509.

Singer, I. and Rotenberg, D. (1973). Mechanisms of lithium action. *N. Engl. J. Med.* 289, 254.

Skouby, S.O., Kühl, C., Molsted-Pedersen, L., Peterson, K., and Christensen, M.S. (1985). Triphasic oral contraception: metabolic effects in normal women and those with previous gestational diabetes. *Am. J. Obstet. Gynecol.* 153, 495.

Skrha, J., Svacina, S., Sramkova, J., and Pav. J. (1989). Use of euglycaemic clamping in evaluation of diazoxide treatment of insulinoma. *Eur. J. Pharmacol.* 36, 199.

Smith, M.J., Aynsley-Green, A., and Redman, C.W.G. (1982). Neonatal hyperglycemia after prolonged treatment with diazoxide. *Br. Med. J.* 284, 1234.

Spellacy, W.N. (1982). Carbohydrate metabolism during treatment with estrogen, progestogen and low-dose oral contraceptives. *Am. J. Obstet. Gynecol.* 142, 732.

Spellacy, W.N., Buhi, W.C., and Birk, S.A. (1972). The effect of estrogens on carbohydrate metabolism: glucose, insulin and growth hormone studies on one hundred and seventy-one women ingesting Premarin, mestranol and ethinyl-estradiol for six months. *Am. J. Obstet. Gynecol.* 114, 378.

Spellacy, W.N., Cruz, A.C., Buhi, W.C., and Birk, S.A. (1978). The acute effects of ritodrine infusion on maternal metabolism: measurements of levels of glucose, insulin, glucagon, triglycerides, cholesterol, placental lactogen, and chorionic gonadotrophin. *Am. J. Obstet. Gynecol.* 131, 637.

Spellacy, W.N., Buhi, W.C., and Birk, S.A. (1981). Prospective studies of carbohydrate metabolism in 'normal' women using norgestrel for eighteen months. *Fertil. Steril.* 35, 167.

Spenney, J.G., Eure, C.A., and Kreisberg, R.A. (1969). Hyperglycemic, hyperosmolar, non-ketoacidotic diabetes: a complication of steroid and immunosuppressive therapy. *Diabetes* 18, 107.

Stahl-Bayliss, C.M., Kalman, C.M., and Laskin, O.L. (1986). Pentamidine-induced hypoglycaemia in patients with the acquired immune deficiency syndrome. *Clin. Pharmacol. Ther.* 39, 271.

Stapleton, J.T. and Gillman, M.W. (1983). Hypoglycemic coma due to disopyramide toxicity. *South. Med. J.* 76, 1453.

Stehouwer, C.D., Lems, W.F., Fischer, H.R., Hackeng, W.H., and Naafs, M.A. (1989). Aggravation of hypoglycaemia in insulinoma patients by the long-acting somatostatin analogue octreotide (Sandostatin). *Acta Endocrinol.* 21, 34.

Steinbrecher, U.P. and Witztum, J.L. (1984). Glycosylation of low-density lipoproteins to an extent comparable to that seen in diabetes slows their metabolism. *Diabetes* 33, 130.

Stuyt, P.M.J., Demacker, P.N.M, and Stalenhoef, A.F.H. (1986). Pancreatitis induced by oestrogen in a patient with type I hyperlipoproteinaemia. *Br. Med. J.* 293, 734.

Sylvester, R.K., Lobell, M., Ogden, W., and Stewart, J.A. (1989). Homoharringtonine-induced hyperglycaemia. *J. Clin. Oncol.* 7, 392.

Takasu, N., Yamada, T., Miura, H, Sakamoto, S., Korenaga, M., Nakajima, K., *et al.* (1982). Rifampicin-induced early phase hyperglycemia in humans. *Am. Rev. Respir. Dis.* 125, 23.

Tamburrano, G., Lala, A., Mauceri, M., Leonetti, F., Libianchi, S., and Andreani, D. (1983). Diazoxide infusion test in patients with single benign insulinoma. *Horm. Res.* 17, 141.

Tasker, P.R.W. and Mitchell-Heggs, P.F. (1976). Non-ketotic diabetic precoma associated with high dose frusemide therapy. *Br. Med. J.* i, 626.

Taskinen, M.R. (1987). Lipoprotein lipase in hypertriglyceridemias. In *Lipoprotein lipase* (ed. J. Borensztajn), p. 201. Evener, Chicago.

Teuscher, A. and Berger, W.G. (1987). Hypoglycaemia unawareness in diabetics transferred from beef/porcine insulin to human insulin. *Lancet* ii, 382.

Toivonen, S. and Mustala, O. (1966). Diabetogenic action of frusemide. *Br. Med. J.* i, 920.

Tollefson, G. and Lesar, T. (1983). Non-ketotic hyperglycemia associated with loxapine and amoxapine: case report. *J. Clin. Psychiatry* 44, 347.

True, B.L., Perry, P.J., and Burns, E.A. (1987). Profound hypoglycaemia with the addition of a tricyclic antidepressant to maintenance sulfonylurea therapy. *Am. J. Psychiatry* 144, 1220.

Turner, G.R., Marks, J.F., and Buchanan, G.R. (1983). Relative hyperglucagonemia in L-asparaginase and prednisone-induced glucose intolerance in management of acute lymphocytic leukemia. *Clin. Pediatr.* 22, 363.

Tweeddale, M.G., Ogilvie, R.I., and Roedy, J. (1977). Antihypertensive and biochemical effects of chlorthalidone. *Clin. Pharmacol. Ther.* 22, 519.

Updike, S.J. and Harrington, A.R. (1969). Acute diabetic ketoacidosis, a complication of intravenous diazoxide treatment for refractory hypertension. *N. Engl. J. Med.* 280, 768.

van der Vange, N., Kloosterboer, H.J., and Haspels, A.A. (1987). Effect of seven low-dose combined oral contraceptive preparations on carbohydrate metabolism. *Am. J. Obstet. Gynecol.* 156, 918.

Vaziri, N.D., Stokes, J., and Treadwell, T.R. (1981). Lactic acidosis, a complication of papaverine overdose. *Clin. Toxicol.* 18, 417.

Vendesborg, P.B. (1979). Lithium treatment and glucose tolerance in manic melancholic patients. *Acta Psychiatr. Scand.* 59, 306.

Ventura, A., Canciani, M., and Tamaro, P. (1983). Efficacy of diazoxide in preventing hypoglycemia in a child affected by hypopituitary dwarfism. *Acta Pediatr. Scand.* 72, 309.

Waal-Manning, H.J. (1976). Hypertension: which β-blocker? *Drugs* 12, 412.

Wahl, P., Walden, C., Knopp, R., Hoover, J., Wallace, R., Heiss, G., *et al.* (1983). Effect of estrogen/progestin potency on lipid/lipoprotein cholesterol. *N. Engl. J. Med.* 308, 862.

Walton, J., Watson, B.S., and Ney, R.L. (1970). Alternate day or shorter interval steroid administration. *Arch. Intern. Med.* 126, 601.

Waskin, H., Stehr-Green, J.K., Helmick, C.G., and Sattler, F.R. (1988). Risk factors for hypoglycaemia associated with pentamidine therapy for pneumocystis pneumonia. *JAMA* 260, 345.

Waziri, R. and Nelson, J. (1978). Lithium in diabetes mellitus: A paradoxical response. *J. Clin. Psychiatry* 39, 623.

Webster, W.B. and McConnaughey, M.M. (1982). Clonidine and glucose intolerance. *Drug Intell. Clin. Pharm.* 16, 325.

White, N.J., Warrell, D.A., Chanthavanich, P., Looareesuwan, S., Warrell, M.J., Krishna, S. et al. (1983). Severe hypoglycaemia and hyperinsulinemia in falciparum malaria. *N. Engl. J. Med.* 309, 61.

White, N.J., Miller, K.D., and Marsh, K., Berry, C.D., Turner, R.C., Williamson, D.H. et al. (1987). Does chloroquine cause hypoglycaemia in the absence of clinical malaria? *Lancet* ii, 281.

Whitefield, C.L. (1971). Isoniazid overdose: report of 40 patients, with a critical analysis of treatment and suggestions for prevention. *Am. Rev. Resp. Dis.* 103, 887.

World Health Organisation (WHO) (1985). Technical report series No. 727, p. 10.

Wilson, A.T. (1966). Diabetogenic action of frusemide. *Br. Med. J.* ii, 290.

Winocour, P., Waldek, S., and Anderson, D.C. (1986). Captopril and blood glucose. *Lancet* ii, 461.

Wollheim, C.B., Kikuchi, M., Renold, A.E., and Sharp, C.W.G. (1978). The roles of intracellular and extracellular

Ca^{ee} in glucose-stimulated biphasic insulin release by rat islets. *J. Clin. Invest.* 62, 451.

Wright, A.D., Barber, S.G., Kendall, M.J., and Poole, P.H. (1979). Beta-adrenoreceptor-blocking drugs and blood sugar control in diabetes mellitus. *Br. Med. J.* i, 159.

Wright, J., Abolfathi, A., Penman, E., and Marks, V. (1980). Pancreatic somatostatinoma presenting with hypoglycemia. *Clin. Endocrinol.* 12, 603.

Wynn, V., Adams, P.W., Godsland, I., Melrose, J., Niththyananthan, R. Okely, N.W., and Seed, M. (1979). Comparison of effects of different combined oral-contraceptive formulations on carbohydrate and lipid metabolism. *Lancet* i, 1045.

Zanella, M.T., Santiago, R.C.M., de Sa, J.R., Salgado, B.T., de Faria, S.F., and Peres, R.B. (1988). Hypertension and diabetes: clinical problems. *Drugs* 35 (suppl. 6), 135.

Zuger, A., Wolf, B.Z., El-Sadr, W., Simberkoff, M.S., and Rahal, J.J. (1986). Pentamidine associated fatal acute pancreatitis. *JAMA* 256, 2383.

Zumoff, B. and Hellman, L. (1977). Aggravation of diabetic hyperglycemia by chlordiazepoxide. *JAMA* 237, 1960.

15. Disorders of metabolism 2

R. SWAMINATHAN

Acid–base balance

Acidosis

Respiratory acidosis

In respiratory acidosis, the blood pH is reduced and pCO_2 is elevated. The bicarbonate concentration is normal in acute respiratory acidosis and becomes elevated in chronic respiratory acidosis. Drugs may cause respiratory acidosis by reducing ventilation either by depressing the respiratory centre or by interfering with the neuromuscular transmission.

Any drug that causes coma or reduces consciousness may depress the respiratory centre and lead to respiratory acidosis. This is most commonly seen with overdose, but respiratory depression may also occur with some drugs in therapeutic doses. Such drugs include narcotics, barbiturates, benzodiazepines, non-barbiturate hypnotics, and alcohols (Cohn 1983). Morphine and heroin reduce the hypoxic and hypercapnic ventilatory drives in normal subjects when given in therapeutic doses, and in overdose there is respiratory depression. The respiratory acidosis in heroin overdose is often complicated by pulmonary oedema, which further reduces gas exchange. Narcotic analgesics given to the mother during labour can cause respiratory depression and acidosis in the neonate. Buprenorphine and meperidine used in the postoperative period have been reported to cause respiratory acidosis severe enough to require mechanical ventilation (Carl et al. 1987). The degree of depression by barbiturates is directly related to the level of drug within the nervous system. In patients with underlying lung disease barbiturates may cause acute respiratory acidosis. Acute respiratory failure and respiratory acidosis are universally seen with severe overdoses of barbiturates. Benzodiazepines, in therapeutic doses, will depress respiration in patients with chronic obstructive airways disease and produce CO_2 retention (Molony and Jacobson 1986); in higher doses respiratory depression is

seen even in normal subjects, but it is not as severe as that with barbiturates unless other depressants such as alcohol are taken. The muscle-relaxant property of benzodiazepines further aggravates the respiratory depression in patients with chronic obstructive airways disease, in whom the work of respiration is increased (Sybrecht 1983). Other non-barbiturate hypnotic sedatives, especially when taken in combination with alcohol or other depressants, can cause severe depression of respiration in cases of overdose. Alcohol, both ethanol and methanol, can cause significant respiratory depression in acute intoxication (Cohn 1983). Anaesthetic agents such as fentanyl may cause delayed respiratory depression (Adams and Pybus 1978; Lehot 1989).

Respiratory acidosis can also be caused by an effect on the respiratory muscles. Such events are seen with muscle relaxants, drug-induced hypokalaemia (Molony and Jacobson 1986), and hypophosphataemia (Newmann et al. 1977). A similar effect is seen with some antibiotics which block the neuromuscular junction and cause a peripheral myopathy (Lippmann et al. 1982). This effect is seen at high dosage and the antibiotics that have been implicated include the aminoglycosides, polymyxins A, B, and E, bacitracin, clindamycin, lincomycin, colistin, and the tetracyclines (Rutten et al. 1980).

Treatment

Respiratory acidosis can be treated by discontinuing the drug concerned and increasing the removal of the drug from the body in cases of overdose. Specific antidotes, if available, such as in the case of morphine poisoning, should also be given. Artificial ventilation may be required in severe cases.

Metabolic acidosis

Metabolic acidosis is characterized by a low arterial pH, a reduced plasma bicarbonate, and a compensatory decrease in pCO_2. Drugs can cause metabolic acidosis by increasing the acid load, by increasing the loss of bicarbonate, or by interfering with hydrogen ion excretion. Metabolic acidosis can be classified according to whether there is an increased anion gap or normal anion gap (hyperchloraemic acidosis) (Table 15.1).

TABLE 15.1
Drug-induced metabolic acidosis

Increased anion-gap acidosis

　Alcohols — benzyl alcohol, ethanol, ethylene
　　　　　　glycol, methanol, propylene glycol

　Biguanides

　Paracetamol

　Polyhydric sugars — fructose, sorbitol, xylitol

　Salicylate

　Miscellaneous—β-agonists and catecholamines,
　　　　　　folk remedies (sulphur), isoniazid,
　　　　　　Lugol's iodine, nalidixic acid,
　　　　　　nitroprusside, paraldehyde,
　　　　　　pentamidine, povidone–iodine,
　　　　　　streptozotocin, verapamil

Normal anion-gap acidosis

　1.　Gastrointestinal loss of bicarbonate
　　　cholestyramine, purgatives

　2.　Renal loss of bicarbonate (Type 2 renal tubular
　　　acidosis)
　　　arginine hydrochloride, carbonic anhydrase
　　　　inhibitors, gentamicin, heavy metals
　　　　(cadmium, lead, mercury),
　　　　mercaptopurine, methyl-3-chrome, outdated
　　　　tetracyclines, streptozotocin, sulphanilamide,
　　　　valproic acid

　3.　Decreased hydrogen ion secretion (Type 1 RTA)
　　　amiloride, amphotericin, analgesic abuse,
　　　cyclamate, lithium, non-steroidal anti-
　　　inflammatory drugs, toluene

　4.　Ingestions
　　　ammonium chloride, hydrochloric acid,
　　　L-arginine and L-lysine

Increased anion-gap acidosis

Biguanide administration is well recognized as a cause of lactic acidosis, and since the first case report in 1959 large numbers of cases have been reported (Paterson *et al.* 1984). The frequency of lactic acidosis in biguanide treatment has not been accurately assessed: the estimate varies from 1 in 1500 to 1 in 5700 patients (Kreisberg and Wood 1983; Paterson *et al.* 1984). In addition to the lactic acidosis seen with therapeutic dosage, it has been reported in cases of frank overdose. It is most frequently seen with

phenformin and least frequently with metformin. When the hyperlactataemic effects of phenformin and metformin were compared in a double-blind study, phenformin was found to produce significantly the higher blood lactate level and greater impairment of the intracellular redox state (Cavallo-Perin *et al.* 1989). The frequency of metformin-induced lactic acidosis was estimated to be 0.4 cases per 10 000 treatment years with a mortality of 30 per cent, which was lower than the 70 per cent mortality seen with phenformin (Berger 1985). Although some patients develop lactic acidosis when the blood levels of the drug are high, in others the levels are within the therapeutic range (Lambert *et al.* 1987). Factors that influence the development of lactic acidosis during biguanide therapy are impaired renal function, the presence of cardiovascular (Luft *et al.* 1978) or hepatic disease (Assan *et al.* 1975), increasing age (Kreisberg and Wood 1983), and concomitant drug therapy such as ethanol and tetracyclines (Luft *et al.* 1978; Paterson *et al.* 1984). Some authors have suggested that lactic acidosis is unlikely to occur if metformin is properly used. Others have suggested, however, that biguanide-induced lactic acidosis occurs in those individuals who have inborn errors of hepatic hydroxylating enzymes (Kreisberg and Wood 1983). In a review of the 42 cases of metformin-induced lactic acidosis reported in the literature to December 1982, there were contraindications to the use of metformin in 40, and 2 cases were due to overdosage (Campbell 1985). More recently, however, a case of lactic acidosis was reported in a patient who had no known risk factors (Tymms and Leatherdale 1988). Despite intensive study, the mechanism of biguanide-induced lactic acidosis is not clear. There is evidence to suggest that biguanide increases lactate production from the splanchnic bed and inhibits lactate utilization by the liver (Arieff *et al.* 1980).

Treatment of biguanide-induced lactic acidosis is unsatisfactory and mortality is relatively high. Treatment with insulin and glucose has been recommended (Kreisberg and Wood 1983) together with bicarbonate (Ryder 1987). Dichloroacetate has also been proposed as an alternative in the treatment of the lactic acidosis (Stacpoole *et al.* 1983), and some have used bicarbonate haemodialysis with some success (Lalau *et al.* 1984). Others have suggested sodium carbonate as the most effective treatment (Bersin and Arieff 1988).

Ethanol may cause a metabolic acidosis that is mainly due to ketoacids (Narins *et al.* 1985). Factors contributing to the acidosis include increased mobilization of free fatty acids, relative or absolute deficiency of insulin, and changes in the ketogenic capacity of the liver (Lefevre *et al.* 1970).

Methanol is metabolised to formaldehyde and then to formic acid, and severe high anion-gap metabolic acidosis follows its ingestion, usually after a delay, reaching a peak at 12 hours. The acidosis is mainly due to formic acid although other metabolites may contribute (Guillaume *et al.* 1987). Treatment involves the use of ethanol and dialysis.

Ethylene glycol has many metabolites and of these glycolic and oxalic acids are the most toxic and responsible for the high anion-gap metabolic acidosis which follows ingestion (Gabow *et al.* 1986; Jacobsen *et al.* 1988*a*; Garella 1988). The acidosis is further complicated by renal failure. Lactate levels are only slightly elevated (Jacobsen *et al.* 1988*a*), except when there is circulatory failure. An unusual case of ethylene glycol poisoning with normal anion gap, due to occult bromide intoxication, has been reported (Heckerling 1987). The treatment of ethylene glycol poisoning consists of ethanol infusion to reduce the metabolism of ethylene glycol to toxic metabolites together with dialysis to eliminate toxic metabolites.

Propylene glycol (1,2-propanediol) is a clear, colourless, odourless, and viscous liquid with a sweet taste that is used as a vehicle for a large number of drugs that are insufficiently soluble or are unstable in water (Reynolds 1989). Although a large proportion (up to 45 per cent) of propylene glycol is excreted unchanged in the urine, a significant amount is metabolised to lactate and pyruvate in the liver, and when large amounts are administered as a vehicle, lactic acidosis may result, especially in the presence of renal impairment (Cate and Hedrick 1980; Kelner and Bailey 1985). In a study of 28 patients receiving nitroglycerin (containing propylene glycol) intravenously 6 patients (21 per cent) had high lactate levels (Demey *et al.* 1988); the authors, however, dismissed the elevation as being of minor clinical significance. Kelner and Bailey (1985), on the other hand, found elevated lactate levels (up to 24 mmol per litre) in patients receiving intravenously solutions containing propylene glycol and they suggested that it may be an important cause of lactic acidosis in hospitalized patients.

Benzyl alcohol is used in subcutaneous or intramuscular injections for its disinfectant and anaesthetic action (Reynolds 1989). Menon and co-workers (1984) reported that the use of benzyl alcohol in neonatal intensive care units was associated with metabolic acidosis and they observed an improvement in survival after its use was discontinued.

In the above situations the presence of an osmolar gap (difference between measured and calculated osmolality) usually gives a clue to the presence of unidentified osmoles such as alcohols (Gabow 1988).

Polyhydric sugars, fructose, xylitol, and sorbitol, have been used as substitutes for glucose in parenteral nutrition and have been associated with lactic acidosis (Krebs *et al.* 1975). Metabolism of fructose causes depletion of hepatic adenosine triphosphate levels, which leads to an increase in glycolysis and lactate levels. Sorbitol and xylitol act in the same way in that they cause depletion of adenine nucleotides (Krebs *et al.* 1975). Fructose can cause a striking dose-related renal tubular acidosis in the very occasional patient with the rare disease hereditary fructose intolerance (Morris *et al.* 1972).

Salicylate intoxication, in addition to causing respiratory alkalosis by direct stimulation of the respiratory centre, can also cause metabolic acidosis. The toxicity of salicylate is in part due to uncoupling of oxidative phosphorylation in mitochondria (Emmett and Seldin 1989), when the resulting disturbance in carbohydrate metabolism leads to increased lactate as well as ketoacids. The increased anion gap seen in salicylate overdose is therefore due to accumulation of lactate, ketoacids, salicylate and other organic acids (Arena *et al.* 1978; Gabow *et al.* 1978; Gabow 1988). Salicylate intoxication in adults usually causes respiratory alkalosis or mixed metabolic acidosis and respiratory alkalosis, whereas in children and infants metabolic acidosis is more prominent. Treatment of salicylate intoxication involves increasing the elimination of the drug by forced alkaline diuresis or haemodialysis.

Although the major manifestation of paracetamol toxicity is liver failure, metabolic acidosis has been described in paracetamol overdose (Zabrodski and Schnurr 1984; Flanagan and Mant 1986; Gray *et al.* 1987; Kritharides *et al.* 1988). In these cases the anion gap is increased. High lactate levels are found in those with toxic plasma levels of paracetamol (Gray *et al.* 1987) and metabolic acidosis was more common in those presenting too late (more than 15 hours after overdose) for treatment with *N*-acetylcysteine. Metabolic acidosis may be found in as many as 20 per cent of patients with paracetamol toxicity (Gray *et al.* 1987).

Paraldehyde has been reported to cause high anion-gap metabolic acidosis (Hayward and Boshell 1957; Beier *et al.* 1963; Linter and Linter 1986). It is usually seen in chronic alcoholics who ingest large amounts of paraldehyde. Although paraldehyde is metabolised to acetic acid, the metabolic acidosis is due to accumulation of multiple organic acids (Beier *et al.* 1963). Severe lactic acidosis following paraldehyde administration has also been reported (Linter and Linter 1986).

Isoniazid poisoning has been associated with lactic acidosis (Coyer and Nicholson 1976) which is usually secondary to the grand mal fits. The acidosis can be very severe (Hankins *et al.* 1987) but usually disappears within several hours of control of the fits (Chin *et al.* 1979). Acute metabolic acidosis due to β-hydroxy-butyrate, however, has been reported in isoniazid toxicity (Pahl *et al.* 1984). Several cases of isoniazid toxicity associated with metabolic acidosis have been reported in Cambodian refugees (Blanchard *et al.* 1986); whether this high incidence represents a racial difference is not clear. Patients with isoniazid poisoning have been successfully treated with large doses of intravenous pyridoxine hydrochloride (Wason *et al.* 1981; Blanchard *et al.* 1986).

Cyanide poisoning resulting from the use of sodium nitroprusside (Aitken *et al.* 1977; Humphrey and Nash 1978) causes lactic acidosis due to inhibition of oxidative phosphorylation, electron transport, and cellular respiration by the cyanide. Nitroprusside is converted to cyanide through a chemical reaction with haemoglobin, and poisoning is usually seen after the use of large doses of nitroprusside over a prolonged period; several deaths have been attributed to nitroprusside (Greiss *et al.* 1976). Sodium azide may be converted endogenously to cyanide and cause poisoning (Brater 1986), and severe metabolic acidosis has been described in a case of fatal sodium azide ingestion (Albertson *et al.* 1986).

Catecholamines may rarely produce lactic acidosis as a result of increased glycogenolysis, glycolysis, reduced tissue blood flow, and reduced oxygenation (Kolendrof and Moller 1974; Hardaway 1980; Guerin *et al.* 1988). In patients with vascular collapse, catecholamines may exaggerate an already present lactic acidosis (Relman 1978). β-Adrenergic drugs such as ritodrine (Gross and Sokol 1980; Richards *et al.* 1983; Braden *et al.* 1985*a*) and theophylline in therapeutic doses (Braden *et al.* 1985*b*; Assadi 1989) or in toxic doses (Kearney *et al.* 1985; Sawyer *et al.* 1985) can cause metabolic acidosis. In most cases lactic acidosis was found, although keto-acidosis has also been reported (Richards and Klingel-berger 1987; Halpren *et al.* 1988; Ryan *et al.* 1989).

Streptozotocin (Brater 1986), Lugol's iodine (Dyck *et al.* 1979), and nalidixic acid (Phillips *et al.* 1979; Leslie *et al.* 1984; Gustafson 1985) have all been reported to cause lactic acidosis. It has also been reported with the use of papaverine (Vaziri *et al.* 1981), which inhibits cellular respiration, and with the use of povidone–iodine in burns as ointment (Pietsch and Meakins 1976) or as irrigation fluid (Glick *et al.* 1985).

Pentamidine, a drug used in treatment of patients with AIDS complicated by *Pneumocystis carinii*, or in some cases of trypanosomiasis and leishmaniasis, has been reported to cause ketoacidosis (Lambertus *et al.* 1988). Verapamil, a potent calcium antagonist, caused hyper-glycaemia and metabolic acidosis following an overdose (Enyeart *et al.* 1983) and this was attributed to the inhibitory effect of verapamil on insulin secretion. Similar hyperglycaemic metabolic acidosis has been reported with slow-release verapamil (Roth *et al.* 1989).

Ingestion of folk remedies containing sulphur is associated with generation of sulphuric acid (Blum and Coe 1977) and the sulphate is normally excreted rapidly in the urine. In the presence of renal failure, ingestion of sulphur may result in severe metabolic acidosis (Schwartz *et al.* 1986). Administration of prednisolone to two boys with Kearns–Sayre syndrome (progressive external ophthalmoplegia, heart block, elevated CSF protein, and ragged muscle fibres) was associated with acidosis — in one lactic acidosis and in the other ketoacidosis (Bachynski *et al.* 1986; Curless *et al.* 1986). The use of cetrimonium bromide to sterilize a hydatid cyst during surgery was reported to cause high anion-gap metabolic acidosis (Momblano *et al.* 1984), probably due to the absorption of the cetrimonium bromide. Use of pethidine in labour has been associated with metabolic acidosis in the newborn (Kariniemi and Rosti 1986).

Normal anion-gap acidosis

Gastrointestinal loss of bicarbonate can give rise to metabolic acidosis with normal anion gap and high plasma chloride; this is seen in laxative abuse (Schwartz and Relman 1953; Harris 1983; Batlle *et al.* 1987, 1988*b*). Cholestyramine, used in the treatment of hypercholesterolaemia, acts as an anion exchange resin and exchanges chloride for endogenous bicarbonate, leading to metabolic acidosis (Kleinman 1974).

Bicarbonate reabsorption in the tubules is mediated by carbonic anhydrase, and carbonic anhydrase inhibitors such as acetazolamide will cause normal anion-gap metabolic acidosis (Coudon and Block 1976). As acetazolamide is cleared by the kidney, the blood levels are related to creatinine clearance and the risk of acidosis is greater in patients with renal impairment (Chapron *et al.* 1989). Heller and colleagues (1985) reported that in elderly patients severe acidosis occurred in 3.7 per cent, moderate acidosis in 37 per cent, and mild acidosis in 14.8 per cent. Concomitant treatment with salicylates increased the risk of acidosis (Cowan *et al.* 1984). Streptozotocin and sulphanilamide produce acidosis by a similar mechanism (Fennell and Fall 1981; Kreisberg and Wood 1983). Mafenide acetate, used topically in treating burns, is absorbed and inhibits carbonic anhydrase, causing metabolic acidosis (Asch *et al.* 1970).

Drugs may also cause acidosis by inducing a Fanconi syndrome. Drugs thus implicated are: outdated tetracyclines; methyl-3-chrome; 6-mercaptopurine; toluene (glue sniffing); valproate; and heavy metals such as lead, mercury, and cadmium (Gross 1963; Moss *et al.* 1980; Cogan 1982; Batlle 1989*a*). The offending agents with tetracycline were the degradation products rather than the parent drug (Benitz and Diermeier 1964); this syndrome is now rarely seen as the formulation of tetracycline has been changed. Renal tubular acidosis following the use of methoxyflurane has been reported (Zeana *et al.* 1982).

Distal acidification defects will give rise to metabolic acidosis and are seen with amphotericin (Finn *et al.* 1977), lithium (Batlle *et al.* 1982), toluene (Streicher *et al.* 1981; Batlle *et al.* 1988*a*), cyclamate (Sebastian *et al.* 1982), and analgesic nephropathy. Amphotericin interacts with the tubular membrane and causes increased permeability, allowing back-diffusion of hydrogen ions (Steinmetz and Lawson 1970). Toluene (Narins *et al.* 1985) and lithium (Brater 1986) have been thought to act in a similar fashion, though in the case of lithium some studies do not support this (Arruda *et al.* 1980). Although a renal acidification defect is seen in patients treated with lithium, metabolic acidosis is not often seen (Boton *et al.* 1987). An unusual case of toluene-induced metabolic acidosis in which ketoacids were found has recently been described (Jone and Wu 1988).

Impairment in hydrogen ion secretion is also seen in Type 4 renal tubular acidosis, which is due to aldosterone deficiency or aldosterone resistance. This is associated with hyperkalaemia. Type 4 renal tubular acidosis has been reported with indomethacin (Goldszer *et al.* 1981), amiloride (Wan and Lye 1980), triamterene (Sebastian *et al.* 1982), captopril (Sakemi *et al.* 1988) and spironolactone (Gabow *et al.* 1979; Rado 1988). Patients with intrinsic renal disease are more susceptible (Brater 1986). Severe metabolic acidosis associated with overdose of ibuprofen (Lee and Finkler 1986; Linden and Townsend 1987; Primos *et al.* 1987) and naproxen (Martinez *et al.* 1989) has been described. Other analgesics, particularly phenacetin, may also cause Type 4 renal tubular acidosis. Phenacetin metabolites damage the renal medulla to cause a chronic tubulointerstitial nephritis, generalized dysfunction of distal tubules, and aldosterone insensitivity (Kreisberg and Wood 1983).

Ingestion of acids can also cause normal anion gap acidosis. This is seen following administration of ammonium chloride (Bushinsky and Coe 1985), hydrochloric acid (Batlle 1989*b*), and the cationic amino acids arginine, lysine, and histidine, which are used in parenteral nutrition as the chlorides (Kaplan *et al.* 1969). The acid load of total parenteral nutrition can be reduced by supplementation with acetate (Montorsi *et al.* 1984; Berkelhammer *et al.* 1988). Concurrent administration

of potassium-sparing diuretics to patients receiving total parenteral nutrition caused metabolic acidosis which disappeared on discontinuing the diuretic (Kushner and Sitrin 1986). Severe metabolic acidosis may follow the ingestion of household bleach (NaOCl) owing to the formation of hypochlorous acid in the stomach (Ward and Routledge 1988). Metabolic acidosis with hyperglycaemia, after ingestion of large quantities of cough mixture (Benylin) containing diphenhydramine, ammonium chloride, and sodium citrate (MacRury *et al.* 1987), and metabolic acidosis with renal salt wasting and hyperkalaemia following trimethoprim–sulphamethoxazole therapy (Kaufman *et al.* 1983) have been described.

Cyclosporin caused hyperchloraemic metabolic acidosis in about 17 per cent of renal transplant recipients (Stahl *et al.* 1986). Metabolic acidosis developed in seriously ill children who received chloramphenicol intravenously (Evans and Kleiman 1986), but the cause of the acidosis was not clear. Cisplatin treatment was reported to cause a renal acidification defect in 4 of 12 patients, but there was no clinical metabolic acidosis (Swainson *et al.* 1985). Cocaine poisoning has been associated with respiratory and metabolic acidosis (Jonsson *et al.* 1983).

Treatment

In the treatment of metabolic acidosis the offending drug should be withdrawn and in severe cases bicarbonate may be infused to correct the acidosis; enough bicarbonate should be infused to raise the pH to about 7.2 (Riley *et al.* 1989). Correction of pH to 7.4 with bicarbonate is not recommended (Rose 1989, p. 543). In lactic acidosis, administration of sodium bicarbonate seems to be the most effective treatment (Bersin and Arieff 1988).

Alkalosis

Respiratory alkalosis

In respiratory alkalosis there is a primary decrease in pCO_2 owing to an increase in ventilation, and the pH is increased. Bicarbonate concentration will be low in chronic respiratory alkalosis. Any drug that stimulates respiration may cause respiratory alkalosis.

Salicylate in high doses causes hyperventilation, and respiratory alkalosis is a common feature of salicylate intoxication, the hyperventilation being characterized by an increase in rate rather than depth. The respiratory stimulation is due to a direct effect on the respiratory centre; the mechanism is not known, but possibly involves uncoupling of oxidative phosphorylation and local changes in pH within the central nervous system.

Salicylate also causes a metabolic acidosis due to its effect on metabolism, and the acid–base picture can therefore be variable. Gabow and colleagues (1978) have reported that 78 per cent of patients with salicylate intoxication show respiratory alkalosis. Other pharmacological agents, such as nikethamide and xanthines in high doses, can cause respiratory alkalosis. Leson and co-workers (1988) described the disorder in a case of caffeine overdose in a 16-year-old male who ingested 6–8 g of caffeine. Nortriptyline has been reported to cause severe respiratory alkalosis that required mechanical ventilation to correct (Sunderrajan *et al.* 1985).

Treatment

Withdrawal of the offending drug may be the only treatment required. In cases of overdose, efforts to accelerate the elimination of the drug may be necessary. Very rarely, mechanical ventilation may be required.

Metabolic alkalosis

Metabolic alkalosis is characterized by an elevation of pH and plasma bicarbonate with a compensatory decrease in pCO_2. It can be induced by increased retention of bicarbonate or increased loss of acid. The causes of drug-induced metabolic alkalosis are listed in Table 15.2.

It is important to note that in most situations of metabolic alkalosis the mechanism not only generates the alkalosis but also maintains it (Rose 1989, p. 480).

Loss of hydrogen ions

Drugs that cause protracted vomiting can cause sufficient loss of acid to cause metabolic alkalosis. Occasionally, anticancer agents such as cisplatin can cause severe vomiting that cannot be controlled by antiemetics. Severe hypochloraemic metabolic alkalosis has been described in an infant as a result of increased gastric acid secretion induced by tolazoline (Adams *et al.* 1980). Chronic intake of antacids such as magnesium hydroxide has been reported to cause metabolic alkalosis, especially in combination with cation-exchange resins (sodium polystyrene sulphonate), which are used in the treatment of hyperkalaemia. When magnesium hydroxide is ingested alone, the hydrogen ions of the gastric juice are buffered by the hydroxyl component of the compound leaving the magnesium to form insoluble complexes with bicarbonate, fats, and phosphates. This leaves only a small amount of bicarbonate to be absorbed and this does not cause alkalosis as long as renal function is normal. In the presence of the cation-exchange resin some of the magnesium binds to the resin leaving free bicarbonate to be absorbed. The net result is a gain of alkali and metabolic alkalosis. This is further aggravated by the presence of renal impairment, which reduces the ability to excrete the excess bicarbonate (Schroeder 1968). Inadvertent administration of antacids included as 'fillers' or buffers in tablets as, for example, in 'Panadol soluble' may cause alkalosis (Acomb *et al.* 1985).

TABLE 15.2
Drug-induced metabolic alkalosis

Loss of hydrogen ions
Gastrointestinal loss
antacid therapy — especially in combination with cation exchange resins
drug-induced vomiting
Renal loss
carbenicillin and other penicillin derivatives
diuretics
mineralocorticoid administration
Retention of bicarbonate
administration of bicarbonate or its precursors
massive blood transfusion and plasma protein infusion
milk–alkali syndrome
Shift of hydrogen ions into cells
hypokalaemia
refeeding

Diuretics — both loop and thiazide types — are common causes of metabolic alkalosis, the severity of which varies with the degree of diuresis and the extent of depletion of extracellular fluid (Gyory and Lissner 1977). The factors contributing to the alkalosis are volume contraction and increased urinary loss of hydrogen ions. The latter is due to increased secretion as a result of three factors: secondary hyperaldosteronism, increased distal flow, and the associated hypokalaemia (Garella *et al.* 1975; Gyory and Lissner 1977; Hropot *et al.* 1985; Rose 1989, p. 486). Metabolic alkalosis is a significant problem in neonates and infants treated with diuretics (Laudignon *et al.* 1989), and in adults from surreptitious ingestion of diuretics (Katz *et al.* 1972; Rosenblum *et al.* 1977). Diuretic-induced alkalosis can be severe enough to mask coexisting metabolic acidosis as, for example, in a diabetic patient with ketosis who presented initially with alkalosis (Cronin *et al.* 1984).

Excess mineralocorticoids or mineralocorticoid-like activity will cause metabolic alkalosis and hypokalaemia. The alkalosis results from a direct effect of these agents on hydrogen ion secretion in the distal tubules concurrently with increasing sodium reabsorption (Harrington *et al.* 1986), and the hypokalaemia they cause maintains the alkalosis (Rose 1989, p. 486). The causes are further discussed under Hypokalaemia.

Carbenicillin and other penicillins, when given in high doses, can cause metabolic alkalosis and hypokalaemia owing to the presence of carbenicillin in the renal tubular fluid as a non-reabsorbable anion (see Hypokalaemia) (Brunner and Frick 1968).

Retention of bicarbonate

Sodium bicarbonate administered in the treatment of metabolic acidosis may result in metabolic alkalosis if large amounts are given. This is typically seen in situations where the cause of the acidosis, for example, diabetic ketoacidosis (Narins and Gardner 1981) or the lactic acidosis of cardiac arrest (Mattar *et al.* 1974), is treated. Severe overshoot alkalosis (pH 7.90 and a bicarbonate concentration of 60–70 mmol per litre) has been reported following the indiscriminate use of sodium bicarbonate during cardiopulmonary resuscitation (Mattar *et al.* 1974). Ingestion of large quantities of sodium bicarbonate, accidentally or otherwise, is associated with severe metabolic alkalosis (Linford and James 1986; Mennen and Slovis 1988). Topical application of baking soda for the treatment of a diaper rash has caused the disorder (Gonzalez and Hogg 1981).

Administration of precursors such as lactate, acetate, citrate, or gluconate, which are rapidly metabolised to bicarbonate in the body, may lead to metabolic alkalosis. Preserved blood contains about 17 mmol of citrate per unit and transfusion of large quantities of blood may lead to alkalosis (Litwin *et al.* 1959). Administration of human plasma protein fraction, which contains 40–50 mmol per litre of acetate, may have a similar result (Rahilly and Berl 1979). Citrate is used as an anticoagulant in haemodialysis and alkalosis may follow its use (Kelleher and Schulman 1987). Use of acetate and bicarbonate in regular haemodialysis will cause elevation of the bicarbonate concentration of plasma, although the rise in plasma bicarbonate is lower in the case of acetate (Scheppach *et al.* 1988). The milk–alkali syndrome, in which the alkalosis is due to ingestion of large amounts of alkali, is discussed under Calcium.

Shift of hydrogen ions into cells

Alkalosis may also result from a shift of hydrogen ions into cells. This, in addition to other mechanisms, occurs in hypokalaemia, and the pH of extracellular fluid rises (Rose 1989, p. 487). Refeeding after a prolonged fast can also raise the pH acutely, probably from intracellular shift of hydrogen ions as there is no volume depletion nor any or abnormal increase in hydrogen ion excretion (Stinebaugh and Schloeder 1972).

Treatment

Withdrawal of the drug concerned and correction of any volume depletion and potassium depletion (if present) are enough to correct the metabolic alkalosis. Rarely, treatment with hydrochloric acid or ammonium chloride may be necessary. In situations such as diuretic-induced alkalosis it is important to correct the chloride depletion as well (Rosen *et al.* 1988).

Sodium and water balance

In an adult weighing 70 kg, there are approximately 4000 mmol of sodium and 42 litres of water. Sodium is mainly present in the extracellular fluid (ECF) and 60 per cent of the body water is intracellular. Sodium ion and its accompanying anions are the major determinants of ECF osmolality, which in turn is responsible for movement of water between ECF and intracellular fluid (ICF) (Rose 1986). Changes in body sodium are therefore usually accompanied by changes in water, and thus loss of body sodium will cause depletion of ECF volume and increase in body sodium will lead to expansion of ECF, and oedema. Volume depletion may be present without any change in plasma sodium concentration, or it may give rise to a low plasma osmolality and hyponatraemia (see below). Changes in water content lead to changes in plasma osmolality and plasma sodium concentration.

Hypernatraemia

An increase in plasma sodium concentration can arise either due to administration of sodium (without water) or due to loss of water. The latter, water depletion, is the commonest cause of hypernatraemia in clinical practice.

Rapid infusion of hypertonic saline or sodium bicarbonate may lead to sodium overload and hypernatraemia. In infants, hypernatraemia may result from incorrect use of oral rehydration (glucose–electrolyte) solutions (Kahn and Blum 1980; Kahn *et al.* 1981), from high-salt feeds (Miller and Finberg 1960; Finberg *et al.* 1963) or from administration of sodium bicarbonate (Simmons *et al.* 1974). In adults, sodium bicarbonate infusion during cardiopulmonary resuscitation (Mattar *et al.* 1974), accidental administration of hypertonic saline (Walter and Maresch 1987), or massive salt ingestion (Addleman *et al.* 1985) may cause hypernatraemia. Severe hypernatraemia may also follow the absorption of sodium from wound packs soaked in antiseptic containing buffered sodium hypochlorite solution in hypertonic saline (Thorp *et al.* 1987). Hypernatraemia can also result from infusion of sodium sulphate (Heckman and Walsh 1967), sodium phosphate enemas (Martin *et al.* 1987), sodium citrate tablets (Shannon and Barclay 1974), and sodium emetics (Ward 1963). Intra-amniotic administration of saline can cause a rise in plasma sodium concentration (Wong *et al.* 1972). The use of cation-exchange resin in the sodium phase may lead to excessive intake of sodium and hypernatraemia (Reynolds 1989). Overdose or excessive use of baking soda as an antacid can lead to hypernatraemia, especially in children (Fachs and Listernick 1987; Schindler and Hiner 1988). Some antacids can contribute substantial amounts of sodium, and can lead to hypernatraemia when given in large doses. Severe hypernatraemia (plasma sodium concentration 171 mmol per litre), hyperosmolality (400 mosmol per kg), cerebral dehydration and coma as a result of administration of large doses of the antacid magnesium trisilicate, which contains 600 mmol of sodium, have been reported (Faraj 1989). A moderate rise in plasma sodium concentration follows the administration of mineralocorticoids, or other steroids, or drugs like carbenoxolone that have mineralocorticoid-like activity (see Hypokalaemia). Hypernatraemia and acidosis can result from topical treatment of burns with povidone–iodine (Scoggin *et al.* 1977) and after valproate intoxication (Schnabel *et al.* 1984).

Hypernatraemia as a result of excessive loss of water may arise from loss of water either from the gastrointestinal tract or by the kidney. Therapeutic administration of lactulose (Nanji and Lauener 1984) or sorbitol (in the form of activated charcoal–sorbitol suspension) has caused severe hypernatraemic dehydration (Farley 1986; Moore 1988). The mechanism of hypernatraemia is a shift of water into the gut lumen as a result of the osmotic load (Farley 1986). Cathartics, when used in the management of overdose (Caldwell *et al.* 1987) or when abused (Alvis *et al.* 1985), can cause hypernatraemia.

Loss of water in the urine results from inability to concentrate urine and conserve water. This may arise either as a result of inhibition of antidiuretic hormone (ADH) or owing to inhibition of action of ADH on the renal tubules (nephrogenic diabetic insipidus). Ethanol and phenytoin inhibit ADH secretion (Moses *et al.* 1985) and ethanol ingestion may lead to a small increase in plasma sodium concentration (Leppanen and Grasbeck 1987), and severe hypernatraemic coma is seen in phenytoin intoxication (Luscher *et al.* 1983). Lithium, demeclocycline, and methoxyflurane can cause nephrogenic diabetes insipidus (Robertson 1988): 20–25 per cent of patients on lithium therapy are reported to have polyuria and polydipsia due to inhibition of the interaction between ADH and adenylate cyclase in the distal renal tubules (Boton *et al.* 1987; Salata and Klein 1987). Impaired concentrating ability has been found in 54 per cent of patients on lithium therapy (Boton *et al.* 1987). Hypernatraemia arises in patients treated with lithium, because of intoxication with the drug (ter Wee *et al.* 1985) or as a result of failure to maintain water intake. Demeclocycline can also cause reversible nephrogenic diabetes insipidus (Singer and Rotenberg 1973; Robertson 1988).

Hypernatraemia may be seen in osmotic diuresis induced by high-protein infant feeding, intravenous hyperalimentation, and mannitol administration (Alvis *et al.* 1985). Impairment in concentrating ability, and consequently hypernatraemia, occurs in hypokalaemia and hypercalcaemia (Cox *et al.* 1985). For causes of drug-induced hypokalaemia and hypercalcaemia see the relevant sections.

It is important to note that hypernatraemia develops in all the above instances as a result of failure to maintain adequate water intake.

Treatment

Therapy for hypernatraemia depends on whether there is excess sodium or a true water depletion (Marsden and Halperin 1985). In absolute water depletion the deficit should be corrected slowly with water by mouth or with intravenous dextrose solution. It is important to correct the water depletion slowly over a 48-hour period, as too rapid correction may lead to cerebral oedema (Pollock and Arieff 1980; Rose, 1989, p. 662). In cases of hypernatraemia due to sodium excess, in addition to giving sodium-free solutions, attempts should be made to encourage the excretion of sodium (e.g. by administration of a loop diuretic) in order to prevent volume overload. In patients with poor renal function, dialysis may be necessary.

Hyponatraemia

Hyponatraemia may arise either from volume depletion or from impaired ability to excrete (Table 15.3). It should be pointed out that volume depletion may occur without hyponatraemia.

Volume depletion

Volume depletion without hyponatraemia may arise as a result of loss of sodium and water — either from the gastrointestinal tract or the kidney. Drugs that cause persistent vomiting or diarrhoea (cathartic agents) will lead to volume depletion. Volume depletion due to renal loss of sodium and water may arise due to agents which cause negative sodium balance such as diuretics.

TABLE 15.3
*Drugs causing hyponatraemia classified according to
their mechanism of action*

A. Volume depletion
  1. Gastrointestinal loss
  2. Renal salt loss — carboplatin, cisplatin,
     diuretics, ketoconazole

B. Increased production of ADH
   carbamazepine
   cyclophosphamide
   psychotropic drugs
     antidepressants — tricyclic antidepressants,
     amitryptiline, imipramine, monamine oxidase
       inhibitors
     antipsychotic drugs — haloperidol,
     phenothiazines, thioridazine, thiothixene,
     trifluoperazine
     Others
       bromocriptine, clofibrate, lorcainide,
       vincristine or vinblastine

C. Drugs which potentiate the action of ADH
   carbamazepine and oxycarbazine,
   chlorpropamide, tolbutamide,
   cyclophosphamide
   somatostatin, sulphonylureas
   NSAID — ibuprofen, indomethacin, naproxen,
   propafenone

D. Exogenous ADH
   oxytocin, vasopressin desmopressin

E. Shift of water out of the cell
   glycerol, mannitol

F. Miscellaneous
   ACE inhibitors, captopril, enalapril, irrigation
   fluids (1.5% glycine)

Drugs may induce volume depletion with hypo-natraemia. Some drugs cause volume depletion by their toxic effects on the kidney causing salt wasting. Cisplatin (Lammers *et al.* 1984) and carboplatin (Welborn *et al.* 1988) have been reported to cause renal salt loss and hyponatraemia. Giaccone and others (1985) reported hyponatraemia in 4 per cent of patients receiving cisplatin, but others have noted a significant decrease in plasma sodium concentration in all patients (Jones, personal communication). In one report inappropriate antidiuretic hormone secretion rather than renal salt loss was suggested to be the mechanism (Ritch 1988).

Hyponatraemia is a common complication of diuretic therapy, but until recently the magnitude of this problem was not well recognized. In the Medical Research Council trial concerning the treatment of mild to moderate hypertension, hyponatraemia was not mentioned as a complication; indeed, the plasma sodium concentration after 3 years of treatment was reported to be the same as

at entry to the study (MRC Working Party Report 1981). Since then, however, numerous reports have appeared on the frequency of hyponatraemia and on the morbidity and mortality associated with it (Sunderam and Manikkar 1983; Rozkovec and Marshall 1983). It is usually mild (Ayus 1986; Bayer *et al.* 1986) but may be severe (Ashouri 1986; Friedman *et al.* 1989), particularly in patients who drink large volumes of water (Kennedy and Earley 1970) and in elderly females (Ashouri 1986; Friedman *et al.* 1989). The factors contributing to the hyponatraemia are increased ADH release due to volume depletion (Johnson and Wright 1983; Ghose 1985), potassium depletion, and direct inhibition of urinary dilution (Kennedy and Earley 1970; Rose 1989, p. 607). The latter mechanism applies particularly to thiazides, which act on the distal tubule in the renal cortex and do not interfere with the ability of ADH to increase water retention (Szatalowicz *et al.* 1982). Loop diuretics, by virtue of their action on the medullary thick ascending limb, diminish the interstitial osmolality, and thus the ADH released in response to volume depletion is not effective in increasing water reabsorption (Szatalowicz *et al.* 1982). Hyponatraemia induced by diuretics occurs within a few weeks of therapy, after which there is a new steady state when intake and excretion are equal (Maronde *et al.* 1983). If hyponatraemia develops in a patient who is receiving long-term diuretics, it is usually because of an additional problem such as vomiting, diarrhoea, or increased water intake (Kone *et al.* 1986), or an increase in drug dosage. The incidence of hyponatraemia following diuretic usage has been reported to be 3.4 per cent in newborns and infants (Laudignon *et al.* 1989), and 0.08 per cent to 12.2 per cent in adults (Borland *et al.* 1986; Walters *et al.* 1987). The effect of diuretics is potentiated by some drugs, such as aminoglutethimide, that block the synthesis of aldosterone (Bork and Hansen 1986), and non-steroidal anti-inflammatory drugs such as ibuprofen that block prostaglandin synthesis (Goodenough and Lutz 1988).

Ketoconazole, a drug that blocks adrenal steroidogenesis, has been reported to cause hyponatraemia (Pillans *et al.* 1985), probably by a mechanism similar to that operating in Addison's disease.

Increased total body water

Some drugs, either by increasing ADH (AVP) secretion or by increasing the sensitivity to ADH (Table 15.3), increase the total body water content and cause hyponatraemia.

Carbamazepine and oxycarbamazepine can cause a decrease in plasma sodium concentration and in some cases give rise to symptomatic or severe hyponatraemia

(Pendlebury *et al*. 1989). The incidence of hyponatraemia has been reported to be between 21.7 per cent and 25 per cent (Lahr 1985; Yassa *et al*. 1988) and the risk is higher in the elderly (Nielsen *et al*. 1988) and in those with a higher serum carbamazepine level (>6 mg per litre). Occasionally, hyponatraemia has occurred with low-dose carbamazepine therapy (Appleby 1984; Taliani *et al*. 1988). In the case of oxycarbamazepine (Johannessen and Nielsen 1987), hyponatraemia was found in 51.2 per cent of patients, with a tendency for increased frequency in the elderly and in those on higher doses.

The mechanism of the hyponatraemia induced by carbamazepine is probably multifactorial. Although carbamazepine inhibits the excretion of a water load (Kimura *et al*. 1974) it has no intrinsic antidiuretic action (Moses *et al*. 1985). Several studies have shown that it increases the plasma ADH concentration (Kimura *et al*. 1974; Smith and Espir 1977) by an unknown mechanism. Other studies, however, have not confirmed this (Stephens *et al*. 1977; Thomas *et al*. 1978), and this has led to the suggestion that carbamazepine potentiates the effect of ADH. Thomas and co-workers (1978), however, in a study in normal subjects, failed to show either an increase in ADH secretion or increased sensitivity to ADH as assessed by the slope of the relationship between ADH and urine osmolality and they suggested that carbamazepine modifies the threshold of the hypothalamic osmoreceptors.

Cyclophosphamide, especially when administered intravenously in high doses, can cause hyponatraemia (DeFronzo *et al*. 1973; Bressler and Huston 1985). To avoid renal toxicity during such therapy, a high fluid intake is recommended and this, together with the increased ADH secretion, can lead to severe and occasionally fatal hyponatraemia (DeFronzo *et al*. 1973; Harlow *et al*. 1979). It has also been suggested that cyclophosphamide increases the action of ADH (Brater 1986).

Vincristine and vinblastine have been reported to cause hyponatraemia by an inappropriate elevation of ADH (Robertson *et al*. 1973; Zavagli *et al*. 1988). Renal loss of sodium as a result of tubular damage has been suggested as a contributing factor (Zavagli *et al*. 1988).

Many psychotropic drugs are known to cause hyponatraemia (Table 15.3) (O'Sullivan and Oyebode 1987) but in spite of their widespread use the incidence of hyponatraemia is unknown. Patients receiving phenothiazines were noted to have a significantly lower plasma sodium concentration (Kimelman and Albert 1984) and severe hyponatraemia developed when there was an added stimulus to ADH secretion such as volume depletion (Kimelman and Albert 1984). In a patient with the syndrome of inappropriate secretion of antidiuretic

hormone (SIADH), due to carcinoma of the lung, trifluoperazine therapy worsened the hyponatraemia (Kennedy *et al*. 1987), suggesting that these drugs may potentiate the release of ADH even from the tumour.

Clofibrate (chlorphenoxyisobutyrate) has a well-documented antidiuretic effect (Bonnici 1973) due to stimulation of ADH secretion (Moses *et al*. 1973); it does not affect the renal response to ADH (Moses *et al*. 1985). It seldom causes significant hyponatraemia when used in therapeutic doses, three to four times the therapeutic dose being required to produce hyponatraemia (Rado *et al*. 1975).

Lorcainide, an antiarrhythmic drug, has been reported to cause a decrease in plasma sodium concentration which in the majority of patients returned to normal within 3–12 months of treatment (Somani *et al*. 1984). In one patient, severe hyponatraemia developed when hydrochlorothiazide was given in addition. The mechanism was suggested to be inappropriate ADH secretion. One case of hyponatraemia associated with methyldopa has been reported (Varkel *et al*. 1988).

Chlorpropamide, a sulphonylurea used in the treatment of diabetes mellitus, is the most common cause of drug-induced SIADH-like syndrome. The incidence of hyponatraemia in patients taking chlorpropamide has been estimated to vary from 4–16 per cent (Kadowaki *et al*. 1983). In a recent survey, 21 per cent of patients treated with sulphonylurea were found to have reduced plasma sodium concentrations, although in only 8 per cent was this less than 129 mmol per litre, and the levels returned to normal when the drug was discontinued. A decrease in plasma sodium concentration was observed with all sulphonylureas (Gin *et al*. 1988), but hyponatraemia is less frequent with tolbutamide or glibenclamide (Hagen and Frawley 1970; Darlow 1977; Kadowaki *et al*. 1983). Significant risk factors for the development of hyponatraemia following chlorpropamide are increasing age and concurrent administration of diuretics (Kadowaki *et al*. 1983; Zalin *et al*. 1984). The mechanism of action of chlorpropamide in producing hyponatraemia is thought to be due to a direct effect on the ADH receptor and potentiation of the effect of ADH on the renal tubules (Moses *et al*. 1985). Medullary hypertonicity is increased (Kusano *et al*. 1983; Welch *et al*. 1986), and there is increased cyclic AMP production as well as inhibition of prostaglandin synthesis (Moses *et al*. 1985). In addition to the direct action on tubules there is some evidence to suggest that chlorpropamide may also increase ADH release, although this report has not been confirmed (Moses *et al*. 1985).

Non-steroidal anti-inflammatory drugs (NSAID) potentiate the action of ADH by inhibiting the synthesis of prostaglandins, which normally antagonize the action of ADH (Patrono and Dunn 1987); hyponatraemia rarely develops, as ADH secretion is inhibited following initial retention of water (Ishikawa *et al.* 1981). These drugs may, however, increase the risk of the disorder in patients with volume depletion or who have SIADH (Goodenough and Lutz 1988). Symptomatic hyponatraemia has been occasionally reported with the use of indomethacin (Hammerman *et al.* 1985), ibuprofen (Blum and Aviram 1980; Dunn and Buckley 1986), naproxen (Alun-Jones and Williams 1986), and propafenone (Dirix *et al.* 1988), and it was seen in an infant born to a mother who had taken an overdose of naproxen 8 hours before delivery. NSAID have also been reported to potentiate the effect of low-dose cyclophosphamide (Webberley and Murray 1989).

Somatostatin and its analogues, which are being increasingly used therapeutically, cause a reduction in free-water clearance (Walker *et al.* 1985) and severe hyponatraemia developed in two patients after 2–3 weeks of continuous intravenous infusion (Halma *et al.* 1987). The authors suggested that somatostatin increases the sensitivity of the collecting tubules to ADH.

Bromocriptine, a dopaminergic agonist, was reported to cause hyponatraemia which reappeared when the patient was rechallenged with bromocriptine (Marshall *et al.* 1982). The mechanism of action is not understood.

Two cases of hyponatraemia during treatment with co-trimoxazole have been reported (Eastell and Edmonds 1984; Ahn and Goldman 1985), one in association with diuretics. It was suggested that co-trimoxazole may have an effect similar to that of chlorpropamide, and hyponatraemia seems to occur when there is an added factor, such as the use of a diuretic or increased fluid load, as in the case reported by Ahn and Goldman (1985).

Antidiuretic hormone (ADH), or its synthetic analogue desmopressin (DDAVP), and oxytocin, which has significant antidiuretic effect, will cause hyponatraemia, especially when accompanied by administration of large amounts of fluid (without sodium). DDAVP used for haemostasis was reported to cause hyponatraemia and seizures in children (Shepherd *et al.* 1989; Smith *et al.* 1989) and in adults (Weinstein *et al.* 1989). Infusion of oxytocin with 5% dextrose to induce labour has caused severe hyponatraemia and seizures in both mothers and the newborn (Pittman 1963; Schwartz and Jones 1978). More recently the use of oxytocin nasal spray to facilitate breast-emptying, or in the treatment of obsessive–compulsive disorders and nocturnal enuresis, has been reported to produce hyponatraemia (Bamford and Cruickshank 1989). Hyponatraemia that followed the infusion of ACTH (in 5% dextrose) over 12–45 hours

(Baumann 1979) was probably due to contamination of the ACTH with ADH (Baumann *et al.* 1972).

The use of 1.5% glycine solution for irrigation before or during surgery such as transurethral prostatectomy (Osborn *et al.* 1980; Sunderrajan *et al.* 1984; Malone *et al.* 1986), percutaneous lithotripsy (Schultz *et al.* 1983), or transcervical resection of endometrium (Baumann *et al.* 1990) has been shown to lower the plasma sodium concentration. In a few patients, severe symptomatic and sometimes fatal hyponatraemia develops (Rao 1987).

Angiotensin-converting-enzyme (ACE) inhibitors used in the treatment of hypertension and heart failure have variable effects on plasma sodium concentration. They increase the plasma sodium concentration when the pretreatment levels are low (Nicholls 1987), but when the initial plasma sodium concentration is normal there may be a fall (Nicholls *et al.* 1980) and it is suggested that this is due to stimulation of thirst (Nicholls 1987). Although the plasma sodium concentration decreases in these patients, symptomatic or severe hyponatraemia is seldom seen. Collier and Webb (1987) have described a patient who developed mild hyponatraemia when treated with bendrofluazide, but developed severe hyponatraemia (plasma sodium concentration 115 mmol per litre) when enalapril was added. Al-Mufti and Arieff (1985) have described a patient with congestive heart failure who developed severe hyponatraemia (Na 114 mmol per litre) after administration of captopril. This patient developed marked thirst and consumed 6–7 litres of water prior to admission. In summary, the effect of ACE inhibitors on plasma sodium concentration is variable and more study is required to identify those patients who are likely to become hyponatraemic.

Infusion of hypertonic solutions of mannitol, glycerol, or glucose can cause hyponatraemia by shifting water from the intracellular space (Borges *et al.* 1982; Feig and McCurdy 1977). The decrease in plasma sodium concentration is profound and prolonged if the agent is not eliminated or metabolised. Mannitol, often used in patients with reduced renal function, can cause severe hyponatraemia (Borges *et al.* 1982).

Treatment

Treatment of hyponatraemia involves treatment of the underlying cause, discontinuing the offending drug, and correcting any abnormality in ECF volume. Once the offending drug is removed and the volume abnormality is corrected (i.e. by volume replacement in the case of depletion or water restriction in the case of water overload) plasma sodium will eventually return to normal. There is controversy as to whether the low plasma sodium itself should be reversed (*The Lancet* 1990). In general, it is agreed that the plasma sodium should be corrected actively when the hyponatraemia is symptomatic or if the hyponatraemia is severe (i.e. plasma Na<110 mmol per litre) (Arieff 1986). The correction of low plasma sodium involves the use of hypertonic saline. A loop diuretic is added in cases in which there is water overload (Hantmann *et al.* 1973); the latter is required to prevent fluid overload, especially in the elderly.

Despite the dangers of hyponatraemia, rapid correction has been shown to cause more harm than good (Ayus *et al.* 1985), causing a central demyelinating lesion of the pons, central pontine myelinolysis (Laureno 1983; Laureno and Karp 1988). There is now general agreement that serum sodium should be corrected slowly, probably by no more than 0.5 mmol per litre per hour (Laureno and Karp 1988) until a level of 120 mmol per litre is reached, when the patient is likely to be out of danger. Further correction of hyponatraemia is carried out slowly over several days. It may, however, be necessary to raise plasma sodium more quickly (i.e. >0.5 mmol per litre per hour) if the patient has seizures. The importance of correction of hyponatraemia was recently highlighted by Fraser and Arieff (1990), who reported the course of 11 patients with severe hyponatraemia for which no specific treatment was given. All these patients died and at postmortem there was evidence of tentorial herniation.

Potassium

Total potassium content in an adult is 3000–4000 mmol (50–55 mmol per kg body-weight) and 98 per cent of this is found in the cells, in contrast to sodium, which is mainly an extracellular cation. This difference in distribution of potassium is reflected in the concentration difference between the two compartments, 4–5 mmol per litre in extracellular fluid and 140 mmol per litre in intracellular cell water. This concentration gradient is maintained by the active sodium pump in the cell membrane, which pumps sodium out of and potassium into the cell in a ratio of 3:2. Drugs may cause disturbances in plasma potassium concentration either by altering the distribution between intracellular and extracellular compartments or by altering external potassium balance.

Hyperkalaemia

Drugs may cause hyperkalaemia by one of three mechanisms: a shift from the intracellular compartments, increased intake, or reduced renal excretion (Table 15.4). Chronic hyperkalaemia is always associated with impaired renal excretion.

TABLE 15.4
Drug-induced hyperkalaemia

---

1. Transcellular shift
   arginine, β-blockers, cardiac glycosides, chemotherapeutic agents, drug-induced acidosis, suxamethonium

2. Increased potassium intake
   potassium penicillin, potassium supplements, salt substitutes

3. Decreased renal excretion
   decreased delivery of sodium to distal tubules— any drug that causes volume depletion, drug-induced renal failure
   hypoaldosteronism
       angiotensin-converting-enzyme blockers, cyclosporin, heparin, non-steroidal anti-inflammatory drugs
   decreased tubular secretion of potassium, potassium-sparing diuretics, triamterene

---

Transcellular shift

Shift of potassium out of cells is a relatively common cause of acute hyperkalaemia in clinical practice. The transcellular gradient is maintained by the active sodium pump, which is specifically modified by cardiac glycosides (Smith 1988), administration of which can lead to an increase in plasma potassium concentration. In therapeutic concentrations digitalis causes only a small increase (Seller *et al.* 1975) and this may be accompanied by some impairment in the ability to handle a potassium load (Lown *et al.* 1960). Severe hyperkalaemia has been reported with accidental or suicidal taking of an overdose of digitalis (Smith and Willerson 1971).

Catecholamines promote potassium entry into cells by activation of the sodium pump (Clausen and Flatman 1980, 1987) mediated by the β_2-adrenergic receptors (DeFronzo *et al.* 1981), and β-adrenergic blockers interfere with this β_2-adrenergic-stimulated potassium entry into cells (Rosa *et al.* 1980). Hyperkalaemia with the use of β-adrenergic blockers is rare and in most instances the rise in plasma potassium concentration is less than 0.5 mmol per litre (Sterns *et al.* 1981), as the potassium entering the extracellular compartment is rapidly excreted by the kidney. Hyperkalaemia can occur, however, if there is increased potassium to dispose of, as in severe exercise (Carlsson *et al.* 1978), increased potassium load (Swenson 1986), hypoaldosteronism, or cardiac surgery (Bethune and McKay 1978).

Suxamethonium, a muscle relaxant, causes depolarization of cell membranes resulting in movement of potassium out of cells. In healthy subjects this causes a small transient increase in plasma potassium concentration (Birch *et al.* 1969). In a minority of patients severe hyperkalaemia and cardiac arrhythmias may follow (Cooperman 1970); patients with burns, trauma, tetanus, or neuromuscular disease seem to be more susceptible than others.

Infusion of arginine hydrochloride can cause hyperkalaemia (Hertz and Richardson 1972; Bushinsky and Gennari 1978), probably due to the movement of potassium out of cells associated with the entry of cationic arginine. Risk of hyperkalaemia is higher in those with impaired ability to metabolise or eliminate arginine (patients with liver and renal disease) and in those with impaired ability to excrete potassium. Infusion of 0.5 g arginine per kg increased the plasma potassium by 1.02 ($\pm$0.14) mmol per litre in healthy subjects and by 1.42 ($\pm$0.15) mmol per litre in diabetic subjects (Massara *et al.* 1979). Several patients with hepatic or renal disease who developed life-threatening hyperkalaemia after infusion of arginine have been described (Bushinsky and Gennari 1978).

Increased catabolism or necrosis of tissues will cause rapid release of potassium from cells and may cause hyperkalaemia even when renal failure is absent. Treatment of malignant lymphomas, leukaemia, and Hodgkin's disease with cytotoxic drugs (Arseneau *et al.* 1973), and massive haemolysis (Fortner *et al.* 1970) have all been reported to cause hyperkalaemia.

Drug-induced metabolic acidosis can lead to hyperkalaemia due to the shift of potassium out of cells in exchange for movement of hydrogen ions into the cells (see Metabolic acidosis). The degree of hyperkalaemia depends on the severity and nature of the metabolic acidosis (Magner *et al.* 1988).

Increased intake

When renal function is normal, increased potassium intake is not a frequent cause of hyperkalaemia. With increased oral intake its excretion will increase with only a small increase in plasma potassium concentration (Nicolis *et al.* 1981). Severe hyperkalaemia may occur if the intake is greater than 160 mmol (Illingworth and Proudfoot 1980) or if potassium is infused rapidly. Severe hyperkalaemia and cardiac arrest were reported after bolus injection of potassium penicillin (Moss and Rasen 1962; Mercer and Logic 1973) and following high-dose glucose–insulin–potassium for inotropic support (Böhrer *et al.* 1988). The most frequent sources of exogenous potassium are the various potassium supplements (Brater 1986). Hyperkalaemia can follow the ingestion of large amounts of 'salt substitutes' (Kallen *et al.* 1976).

The use of potassium supplements or salt substitutes is more likely to cause hyperkalaemia when there is increased proximal tubular reabsorption of sodium, as with salt restriction. Salt restriction will limit sodium delivery to distal tubules and therefore limit potassium secretion. Hyperkalaemia as a result of accidental poisoning with a sustained release potassium preparation has been reported (Steedman 1988); it is also likely to occur with the use of stored blood for exchange transfusion (Scanlon and Krakaur 1980), owing to the leakage of potassium from red cells during storage. In any of the above situations of increased potassium intake, hyperkalaemia is more common if there is impairment of potassium excretion. Several cases of hyperkalaemia during dialysis due to inadvertent use of a high-potassium dialysate have been described (Brady *et al.* 1988).

Decreased renal excretion

Renal handling of potassium involves filtration, reabsorption, and distal tubular secretion; the amount of potassium excreted depends on the amount of potassium secreted. A drug may cause hyperkalaemia by decreasing the functional renal mass, by reducing sodium delivery to distal tubules, by causing hypoaldosteronism, or by interfering with tubular secretion of potassium.

In states of volume depletion the proximal tubular reabsorption of sodium is increased, leading to decreased delivery of sodium to the distal tubules and this limits the capacity to secrete potassium in exchange for sodium. Drugs that cause volume depletion (see section on Sodium) may lead to hyperkalaemia, especially if potassium supplements are being given at the same time.

Drugs that interfere with the renin–angiotensin–aldosterone axis or that block the action of aldosterone cause hyperkalaemia. The best examples are ACE inhibitors, which block the conversion of angiotensin I to II and thereby decrease the synthesis of aldosterone. Decrease in potassium secretion follows and plasma potassium concentration rises, but if renal function is normal usually by not more than 0.5 mmol per litre (Veterans Administration Co-operative Study 1984). Severe hyperkalaemia has, however, been reported in patients who have renal insufficiency (Sakemi *et al.* 1988), in patients who are also taking potassium-sparing diuretics, and in those taking potassium supplements (Consensus Trial Study Group 1987). The ACE inhibitors, enalapril (Abraham *et al.* 1988), ramipril (Kindler *et al.* 1989), and cilazapril (Swainson *et al.* 1989), when used in the treatment of hypertensive patients with renal disease, caused significant elevation of plasma potassium concentrations. The risk of hyperkalaemia is particularly high when ACE inhibitors are the cause of renal failure (Speires *et al.* 1988) and with long-acting preparations (DiBianco 1986). Hyperkalaemia was the cause of withdrawal of enalapril therapy in 0.3 per cent of patients. The rapid rise in serum potassium concentration seen in patients with chronic renal failure treated with ACE inhibitors was shown to be due to their inability to increase aldosterone secretion in response to the hyperkalaemia (Zanella *et al.* 1985).

Prostaglandins promote renin secretion and facilitate aldosterone release. Hence, NSAID that inhibit prostaglandin synthesis cause hyporeninaemic hypoaldosteronism and may cause hyperkalaemia (Norby *et al.* 1978). The increase in plasma potassium concentration seen with NSAID is usually small or negligible in patients with normal renal function, even in the elderly (Allred *et al.* 1989). Significant hyperkalaemia has been reported with indomethacin (Beroniade *et al.* 1979; Mactier and Khanna 1988), ibuprofen (Marasco *et al.* 1987), and sulindac (Horowitz *et al.* 1988). The incidence of hyperkalaemia can be as high as 26 per cent in the presence of pre-existing mild to moderate renal failure (Zimran *et al.* 1985) and it is less with sulindac (Nesher *et al.* 1988), which does not interfere with prostaglandin synthesis. Overdose with ibuprofen in a young healthy adult caused fulminant hyperkalaemia (8.3 mmol per litre) and cardiac arrhythmias (Menzies *et al.* 1989).

Heparin decreases the synthesis of aldosterone by direct action on the adrenal gland (O'Kelly *et al.* 1983), but it is not clear whether this is due to heparin itself or is due to chlorobutol used as a preservative (Sequeira and McKenna 1986). Plasma aldosterone levels decrease by 75 per cent within 4–7 days of commencing heparin therapy (Sherman and Ruddy 1986), and there is a significant increase in plasma potassium (Monreal *et al.* 1989). Hyperkalaemia, however, is not seen unless there is an additional problem such as increased potassium load or reduced renal function (Kutyrina *et al.* 1987; Busch *et al.* 1987), and the frequency of hyperkalaemia was found to be less than 1 per cent (Monreal *et al.* 1989) in patients treated with heparin.

Cyclosporin, used as an immunosuppressive agent in renal transplantation, causes hyperkalaemia. In a multicentre trial the mean plasma potassium concentration in patients treated with cyclosporin was found to be significantly raised (European Multicentre Trial 1982). Adu and co-workers (1983) reported sustained hyperkalaemia inappropriate for the degree of impairment of renal function in 16 per cent of patients, all of whom had hyperchloraemic acidosis with defective renal tubular

secretion of potassium. The hyperkalaemia is due to hypoaldosteronism and renal tubular damage (Bantle *et al.* 1985; Zazgornik *et al.* 1988). The use of β-blockers, which blunt the aldosterone response to hyperkalaemia, further worsens it.

The potassium-sparing diuretics amiloride, triamterene, and spironolactone reduce the secretion of potassium and hydrogen ions in the collecting tubules and, as a result, hyperkalaemia and metabolic acidosis may follow (Greenblatt and Koch-Weser 1973; Tormey *et al.* 1989). This is more likely to occur in the presence of a potassium load, such as potassium supplements, or if there is reduced renal function or simultaneous administration of ACE inhibitors (Burnakis and Mioduch 1984). As many as 9 per cent of hospitalized patients taking spironolactone have hyperkalaemia (Whang 1976).

Increase in plasma potassium concentration follows treatment with erythropoietin (Eschbach *et al.* 1989; Moynot *et al.* 1990). Frank hyperkalaemia has not been reported, however. Aminoglutethimide, a drug that inhibits adrenal hormone synthesis, has been reported to cause severe hyperkalaemia (Davies *et al.* 1989), but this complication is very rare. Pentamidine, used for the treatment of *Pneumocystis carinii* pneumonia in patients with acquired immunodeficiency syndrome (AIDS), has caused life-threatening hyperkalaemia (Peltz and Hashmi 1989; Lachaal and Venuto 1989) due to its nephrotoxic effect. Lovastatin, an inhibitor of HMG-CoA reductase, caused hyperkalaemia in diabetic patients with renal impairment taking ACE inhibitors (Edelman and Witztum 1989). The authors suggested that the myopathy induced by lovastatin and the resulting release of potassium, combined with renal insufficiency and the use of ACE inhibitors, caused the hyperkalaemia.

Prolonged infusion of ACTH for infantile spasm has been associated with hyperkalaemia (Zeharia *et al.* 1987) shortly after cessation of the infusion. The exact mechanism of this hyperkalaemia is not well understood. Hyperkalaemia is seen in acute fluoride toxicity (McIvor 1987; Cummings and McIvor 1988) and in malignant hyperthermia induced by anaesthetic agents, such as isoflurane, in susceptible subjects (Simons and Goldman 1988). Hetastarch, a colloidal plasma-volume expander, has caused hyperkalaemia when used as a pump-priming fluid during cardiopulmonary bypass (Schmidt and Sesin 1987).

Hypokalaemia

Drugs may cause hypokalaemia without potassium depletion as a result of transcellular shift or they may cause

TABLE 15.5
Drug-induced hypokalaemia

1. Increased entry into cells (redistribution)
   β-adrenergic agonists, drug-induced metabolic
   alkalosis, insulin

2. Increased gastrointestinal losses
   laxative/purgative abuse, vomiting

3. Increased renal loss
   amphotericin, carbenoxolone, diuretics, drug-
   induced renal tubular acidosis, gossypol,
   hypomagnesaemia, increased mineralocorticoid
   activity, steroids, levodopa, licorice, penicillin

4. Miscellaneous
   fluconazole, haloperidol, ifosfamide/mesna,
   mithramycin, zimeldine

hypokalaemia and potassium depletion by increasing the loss of potassium (Table 15.5).

Transcellular shift

In alkalosis hydrogen ions move from the ICF to ECF to minimize the elevation of ECF pH. To preserve electroneutrality, potassium ions enter the cells. The hypokalaemia in alkalosis is usually mild and the fall in plasma potassium usually less than 0.4 mmol per litre for each 0.1 unit of pH increase. Administration of sodium bicarbonate to correct metabolic acidosis can cause hypokalaemia due to a rapid shift of potassium into the cells (Fraley and Adler 1977). It is important to note that hypokalaemia and metabolic· alkalosis are commonly found together, either because the causative agent, such as a diuretic, induces both low potassium and high pH, or because the alkalosis may be the result of hypokalaemia due to increased tubular secretion of hydrogen ions (Sabatini and Kurtzman 1984; Capasso et al. 1987).

Insulin increases potassium uptake into cells by stimulating the Na^+,K^+ pump. The effect is maximal 60–90 min after an injection of insulin and persists for more than 3 hours. Hypokalaemia can occur during the treatment of diabetic ketoacidosis when there is potassium depletion. A decrease in plasma potassium is also seen after a glucose load or administration of insulin as, for example, in the performance of an insulin tolerance test. Spuriously low potassium concentrations may also be found in specimens from patients given insulin, if blood samples are left standing for several hours before separation of plasma from red cells (Kalsheker and Hales 1985). The mechanism of this effect is not fully understood but it is thought to be due to a shift of potassium into red cells *in vitro* during storage, somehow triggered by insulin administration *in vivo* (Kalsheker and Hales 1985).

$β_2$-Agonists promote potassium uptake into liver as well as peripheral tissues — muscle being the major site (Tannen 1986). Hypokalaemia has been reported after administration of β-adrenergic agonists including adrenaline (DeFronzo et al. 1981), salbutamol, terbutaline, fenoterol (Siebers et al. 1989; Burgess et al. 1989), and ritodrine (Shin and Kim 1988). Infusion of terbutaline in therapeutic doses decreases plasma potassium below the reference range in all patients, the decrease in potassium being largely reversed within 30 minutes after the drug is discontinued. Intravenous administration (Rey et al. 1989), as well as inhalation of $β_2$-agonists, decreases the plasma potassium concentration (Siebers et al. 1989; Lipworth et al. 1989a; DaCruz and Holburn 1989). The effect of fenoterol and terbutaline lasts longer than salbutamol (4 hours vs 2 hours) (Burgess et al. 1989). The most potent hypokalaemic $β_2$-agonist is fenoterol, followed by terbutaline and salbutamol (Deenstra et al. 1988; Burgess et al. 1989). Prior administration of thiazide diuretics aggravated the hypokalaemia and ECG effects of the $β_2$-agonist albuterol (Lipworth et al. 1989b) and this interaction may increase the risk of arrhythmias, especially if there is concomitant hypoxaemia, ischaemic heart disease, or acidosis (Crane et al. 1987; Lipworth et al. 1989b). The hypokalaemic effect of intravenous salbutamol was potentiated by theophylline (Whyte et al. 1988a), and theophylline in therapeutic doses significantly decreased plasma potassium (Zantvoort et al. 1986). Hypokalaemia is more frequent and severe in poisoning or overdose. In one study 85 per cent of patients admitted with acute theophylline poisoning had plasma potassium concentrations less than 3.5 mmol per litre and 45 per cent had levels below 3.0 mmol per litre and the degree of hypokalaemia was correlated with the peak serum theophylline concentration (Amitai and Lovejoy 1988). The frequency of hypokalaemia in chronic theophylline poisoning was 32 per cent (Shannon and Lovejoy 1989). The reason why the frequency of hypokalaemia in chronic theophylline intoxication is lower has not been fully explained. Theophylline-induced hypokalaemia may contribute to the sudden respiratory arrest seen in asthmatic subjects (Kolski et al. 1988; Epelbaum et al. 1989). Hypokalaemia has also been reported in an individual who took an overdose (6–8g) of caffeine (Leson et al. 1988). The hypokalaemia induced by $β_2$-agonists could be prevented by the administration of β-blockers (J. Reid et al. 1986).

Severe hypokalaemia (K<1.5 mmol per litre) was reported after a massive acute chloroquine overdosage; this was probably due to an intracellular shift (Lofaso et al. 1987).

Gastrointestinal losses

Drugs that cause vomiting may lead to hypokalaemia through a combination of factors: loss of potassium in gastric juice, metabolic acidosis due to loss of acid, and increased renal losses.

Loss of potassium in stools due to chronic laxative abuse will lead to hypokalaemia. Potassium loss in the stools can amount to 50–60 mmol per litre and together with this there may be renal loss of potassium due to secondary hyperaldosteronism.

Renal losses

Diuretics of the loop and thiazide types are one of the commonest causes of hypokalaemia and accounted for 3.4 per cent of all admissions to an acute medical unit (Fitzgerald *et al.* 1989). The loss of potassium induced by diuretics is due to increased flow to the distal tubules as a result of inhibition of sodium chloride reabsorption in the proximal segments. The relative dilution of potassium in the tubular fluid allows more potassium to be secreted, as the secretion of potassium is normally limited by the concentration gradient between distal tubular fluid and cells. In addition to the increased flow rate there may be secondary hyperaldosteronism due to the induction of volume depletion (Hropot *et al.* 1985). Hypomagnesaemia induced by diuretics may further aggravate the renal loss of potassium (Rose 1989, p. 722).

The magnitude, frequency, and extent of hypokalaemia have been studied extensively. The incidence of hypokalaemia (plasma K<3.5 mmol per litre) is dose-related, and increases from 25 per cent with 50 mg hydrochlorothiazide per day to 40–50 per cent with 100 mg per day (Morgan and Davidson 1980; Knochel 1984; Dyckner and Wester 1984; Hollifield 1984) and is higher with longer acting diuretics such as chlorthalidone (Morgan and Davidson 1980). The incidence of hypokalaemia with frusemide was 5 per cent (Morgan and Davidson 1980). The question whether potassium-depletion accompanies this hypokalaemia has been debated, as plasma potassium concentration does not reflect total body potassium status (Linderman 1976; Morgan *et al.* 1981). Measurement of total body potassium in patients treated with diuretics for prolonged periods showed a deficit of about 200 mmol or 5 per cent of total body potassium (Kassirer and Harrington 1977; Morgan and Davidson 1980), and muscle potassium was also found to be low (Dorup *et al.* 1988).

There has been intense debate as to whether diuretic-induced hypokalaemia may cause ill effects. It is well known that hypokalaemia will increase the risk of digoxin toxicity (Shapiro and Taubert 1975), and diuretics may also aggravate the hypokalaemia induced by catecholamines (in response to stress); both together may cause ventricular arrhythmias and possibly sudden death (Poole-Wilson 1987; Whyte *et al.* 1988*b*). The incidence of ventricular arrhythmias after acute myocardial infarction was positively correlated with hypokalaemia (Clausen *et al.* 1988), and the occurrence of premature ventricular contractions correlated with the decrease in plasma potassium (Hollifield 1984). On reviewing the evidence Hollifield (1989*a*) concluded that diuretics increase the risk of ventricular ectopic activity; Freis (1989), on the other hand, concluded that there is not enough evidence to support this.

Increased mineralocorticoid activity will lead to hypokalaemia and potassium depletion. Ingestion of licorice or licorice-containing tobacco can cause hypokalaemia (Conn *et al.* 1968; Blachley and Knochel 1980; Sunderam and Swaminathan 1981; Achar *et al.* 1989). Glycyrrhizic acid present in licorice inhibits the enzyme 11β-hydroxysteroid dehydrogenase and thereby inhibits the conversion of cortisol to cortisone in the kidney (Stewart *et al.* 1987, 1990; Funder *et al.* 1988) leading to marked increase in mineralocorticoid activity and hypokalaemia. The administration of a thiazide diuretic (Sunderam and Swaminathan 1981) or sodium bicarbonate (Kirkham *et al.* 1987) aggravates the hypokalaemia or precipitates symptoms. Carbenoxolone, which is synthesized from glycyrrhetinic acid, can also cause hypokalaemia by a similar mechanism (Dickinson and Swaminathan 1978; Armanini *et al.* 1982; Metcalfe and Entrican 1987) in 43 per cent of patients (Ganguli and Mohamed 1980). The effect was dose-dependent and the elderly were more susceptible to the development of hypokalaemia. The use of 9α-fluoroprednisolone in nasal sprays (Foresti *et al.* 1987; Wu *et al.* 1989), in antihaemorrhoid ointments (Marin *et al.* 1989), and other topical preparations (Lauzurica *et al.* 1988) has been reported to be able to cause severe hypokalaemia.

Penicillins are frequently used as sodium salts and, especially when given in large doses, may give rise to increased potassium secretion in the distal tubules. The presence of the penicillin anion, which cannot be reabsorbed, leads to increased secretion of potassium and hydrogen ions, giving rise to hypokalaemia and metabolic alkalosis (Lipner *et al.* 1975). Hypokalaemia has been reported with the use of amoxycillin (Appel and Neu 1977), ampicillin (Gill *et al.* 1977), carbenicillin (Lipner *et al.* 1975), cephalexin (Young *et al.* 1973), nafcillin (Mohar *et al.* 1979; Andreoli *et al.* 1980), oxacillin (Schlaeffer 1988), penicillin (Brunner and Frick 1968; Kovnat *et al.* 1973), and ticarcillin (Parry and Neu 1978). It is more common with carbenicillin because of the large doses used and high sodium content (Brunner and Frick 1968; Klastersky *et al.* 1973).

Amphotericin causes hypokalaemia (Koren *et al.* 1988) by increasing urinary losses as a result of renal tubular acidosis (discussed under Acidosis). Increased urinary loss of potassium is due to increased potassium permeability of the luminal membrane because of an interaction of the drug with the membrane (Cheng *et al.* 1982). Hypokalaemia is seen in up to 50 per cent of patients (Douglas and Healy 1969); it can be prevented by administration of amiloride (Smith *et al.* 1988).

Hypomagnesaemia and hypokalaemia are commonly seen together in up to 40 per cent of cases (Whang *et al.* 1981). In some instances this is due to impairment of reabsorption of potassium and magnesium by a common causative factor as, for example, in cisplatin toxicity (Schilsky and Anderson 1979; Rodriguez *et al.* 1989). In addition, hypomagnesaemia can lead to hypokalaemia by a poorly understood mechanism (Shils 1969). An important role has been attributed to increased aldosterone secretion (Francisco *et al.* 1982). In the presence of hypomagnesaemia, the hypokalaemia is refractory to potassium replacement (Whang *et al.* 1985; Rodriguez *et al.* 1989).

Increased loss of potassium in the urine occurs in metabolic acidosis. In proximal renal tubular acidosis induced by drugs, the reduction in bicarbonate reabsorption leads to increased delivery of sodium and bicarbonate to the distal tubules, causing potassium loss (Sebastian *et al.* 1971). In distal renal tubular acidosis, the reduction in hydrogen ion secretion enhances the exchange of potassium for sodium and results in loss of potassium. Gossypol, which has been used as a male contraceptive, causes hypokalaemia by increasing loss of potassium in the urine (Liu *et al.* 1987; Duo *et al.* 1988; Liu *et al.* 1988a).

Levodopa increases potassium loss in the urine by an unknown mechanism and can cause hypokalaemia in up to 10 per cent of patients (Granerus *et al.* 1977).

Miscellaneous

Zimeldine, a selective blocker of serotonin uptake, was associated with hypokalaemia in a case of overdose (Lilijeqvist and Edvardsson 1989). Chemotherapy with ifosfamide with mesna was associated with hypokalaemia, and a fatal case has been described (Husband and Watkin 1988).

Treatment with nisoldipine has been reported to cause a significant decrease in plasma potassium concentration — although within the reference range (Takahashi *et al.*

1989). This effect is presumably due to the increase in plasma catecholamines. Treatment with nifedipine did not cause a significant change in plasma potassium concentration (Yurtkuran *et al.* 1989).

Hypokalaemia has been described in haloperidol overdosage (Aunsholt 1989), in patients with acute myeloid leukaemia treated with fluconazole (Kidd *et al.* 1989), and in a patient receiving mithramycin for Paget's disease (Bashir and Tomson 1988).

Non-ionic radiographic contrast media have been reported to cause a small (5.1 per cent) decrease in plasma potassium concentration, probably due to the high osmolality of the contrast medium and consequent haemodilution (Brunet *et al.* 1989).

ACE inhibitors are recognized to cause hyperkalaemia, but some patients taking diuretics and ACE inhibitors have developed hypokalaemia (D'costa *et al.* 1990). The mechanism and the significance of this observation are not clear.

Calcium

Most of the calcium in the body is in the skeleton and the extracellular fluid calcium accounts for only a small percentage of the total body calcium. However, the concentration of calcium in plasma (2.25–2.60 mmol per litre) is kept within narrow limits by homoeostatic mechanisms. In plasma the calcium is present in three forms: ionized (about 45 per cent); protein-bound, mainly to albumin (about 40 per cent); and complexed (about 15 per cent). It is the ionized calcium concentration that is physiologically important. In clinical laboratories, however, it is the total plasma calcium concentration that is measured and therefore an awareness of the changes in total calcium concentration caused by changes in protein concentration is important.

The plasma ionized calcium concentration is regulated by parathyroid hormone (PTH) and vitamin D. Calcitonin, the third calcium-regulating hormone, does not play an important role. In addition to PTH and vitamin D, several other factors such as thyroid hormones, growth hormone, and glucocorticoids influence the plasma calcium concentration. The effects of all these factors are mediated by their action on one or more of the three main organs: kidney, bone, and intestine. Of these three organs, the kidney plays an important role because of the large amount of calcium it handles (240 mmol per day compared with intestinal absorption of about 1–2 mmol per day) (Nordin 1990). Drugs may affect one or more of the organs involved in calcium regulation. The causes of drug-induced hypercalcaemia and hypocalcaemia are listed in Tables 15.6 and 15.7.

TABLE 15.6
Drug-induced hypercalcaemia

Increased absorption from the intestine
    milk–alkali syndrome
    vitamin D and its metabolites

Increased mobilization from bone
    vitamin A
    vitamin D and its metabolites

Decreased renal excretion
    calcium-channel blockers
    lithium
    thiazides

TABLE 15.7
Drug-induced hypocalcaemia

Decreased absorption from the intestine
    alteration in vitamin D metabolism—alcohol,
    anticonvulsants, and glutethimide

Decreased bone mobilization
    calcitonin, diphosphonates, drug-induced
    hypomagnesaemia, gallium nitrate, mithramycin

Increased renal excretion
    loop diuretics, magnesium sulphate

Complexing of calcium
    EDTA, neomycin, phosphate

Hypercalcaemia

Increased intestinal absorption

Ingestion of large quantities of milk and antacids for prolonged periods of time in the management of peptic ulcer can cause hypercalcaemia. The mechanism of hypercalcaemia in this milk–alkali syndrome is unclear and multifactorial. The absorption of large amounts of alkali leads to alkalosis, which promotes renal tubular reabsorption of calcium (Agus and Goldfarb 1985; Pak 1986). This is accompanied by increased calcium absorption leading to hypercalcaemia. In some patients, renal failure further limits calcium excretion. The importance of increased renal tubular absorption in the pathogenesis of hypercalcaemia (Nordin 1990) in the milk–alkali syndrome is illustrated by the absence of hypercalcaemia in absorptive hypercalciuria (Pak 1986). The milk–alkali syndrome, however, is now uncommon (Shek *et al.* 1990). Calcium carbonate has also been used as a substitute for aluminium hydroxide in the control of plasma phosphate in haemodialysed patients, and plasma calcium concentration has been shown to increase with the use of calcium carbonate (Okada *et al.* 1989a; Anelli *et al.* 1989) and hypercalcaemia has been reported. Calcium ion-exchange resins used in the management of

hyperkalaemia in renal failure patients may precipitate hypercalcaemia (Sevitt and Wrong 1968). Hypercalcaemia has also been reported following the use of haemostatic compresses (Sorbacal) containing 4.6–6.8% w/w calcium acetate (Texier *et al.* 1982).

Vitamin D and its metabolites, 25-hydroxycholecalciferol (25-OHD$_3$) and 1,25-dihydroxycholecalciferol (1,25-DHCC), and alphacalcidol (1α-hydroxycholecalciferol [1α-OHD$_3$]), when taken in large doses can cause hypercalcaemia from increased intestinal absorption of calcium and increased bone resorption (Heath 1984). Hypercalcaemia may also arise as a result of overdosage with these preparations following self-medication or in the treatment of hypocalcaemic states (Pak 1986; Okada *et al.* 1989b). The duration of hypercalcaemia after withdrawal of the drug depends on the preparation used, with vitamin D > dihydrotachysterol > 25-OHD$_3$ > 1α-OHD$_3$ > 1,25-DHCC (Kanis and Russell 1977). The duration of hypercalcaemia is usually much longer than the serum half-lives of the metabolites, because of the persistence of its physiological action, for example, the serum half-life of 1,25-DHCC is in hours but the hypercalcaemia following 1,25-DHCC may persist for 1–2 days. A recent case report suggests that danazol may potentiate the effect of 1α-OHD$_3$ (Hepburn *et al.* 1989).

Increased mobilization from bone

Vitamin A in toxic doses causes hypercalcaemia due to increased bone resorption. Hypercalcaemia following vitamin A intoxication has been reported in haemodialysed patients (Farrington *et al.* 1981) and in those taking 50–100 000 units of vitamin A per day (Kartz and Tzagourins 1972).

Decreased renal excretion

The use of thiazide diuretics is associated with an increase in serum calcium concentration An increased total calcium concentration was reported in 2 per cent of patients receiving thiazide diuretics (Christensson *et al.* 1977). The degree of hypercalcaemia is mild (usually <2.75 mmol per litre) and is mostly due to haemoconcentration (Yendt and Cohanim 1978). The plasma calcium returns to normal within 2 weeks of withdrawing the thiazides (Mohamedi *et al.* 1979). True hypercalcaemia, however, may develop during thiazide therapy under conditions of high bone turnover such as primary hyperparathyroidism (Brickman *et al.* 1972) and secondary hyperparathyroidism (Koppfel *et al.* 1970). In the series of Christensson and co-workers (1977), of the patients with hypercalcaemia due to thiazide diuretics 75 per cent had primary hyperparathyroidism. Based on this and similar findings, thiazides are occasionally used as provocative agents in the diagnosis of primary hyperparathyroidism.

The mechanism of true hypercalcaemia in thiazide therapy is not fully understood (Pak 1986). Thiazides reduce the urinary excretion of calcium by increasing its tubular absorption (Steiniche et al. 1989), which is attributed to volume depletion and the accompanying increased proximal tubular reabsorption of sodium and calcium (Porter et al. 1978), as well as to an increase in distal tubular reabsorption of calcium (Costanzo and Windhager 1978).

Lithium therapy has been reported to increase plasma calcium concentration and decrease serum phosphate concentration and urinary calcium excretion (Christiansen et al. 1978; Davies et al. 1981; Mallette and Eichhorn 1986). Hyperparathyroidism has occasionally been reported (Ananth and Dubin 1983) in patients treated with lithium and there is still controversy as to whether lithium can cause hyperparathyroidism (Salata and Klein 1987). Mallette and Eichhorn (1986) noted that plasma calcium and parathyroid hormone PTH levels increase within the normal range in 80 per cent of patients during the first 4 weeks of lithium therapy and rise above normal in 10 per cent of patients after long-term therapy. Lithium treatment is known to cause hypocalciuria due to increased renal tubular reabsorption of calcium (Brater 1986). Several investigators have reported increases in serum PTH levels after a few weeks or months of lithium treatment (Davies et al. 1981; Rosenblatt et al. 1989; Seely et al. 1989a). As these increases may be due to renal retention of inactive PTH fragments, Mallette and co-workers (1989), using an immunoradiometric assay to measure intact PTH, have found that in those treated with lithium for less than 6 months the PTH was normal in spite of an increased serum ionized calcium. This was interpreted as a shift in the set point of PTH secretion, as suggested by Marel and others (1982). In those on long-term lithium treatment (over 3 years), serum intact PTH was high, serum phosphate was lower, and serum chloride and 1,25-DHCC were higher. This was accompanied by enlargement of the parathyroid glands. It still remains to be determined whether this chronic stimulation of the parathyroid will lead to the development of adenoma (Mallette et al. 1989).

Hypercalcaemia has also been reported in association with hormonal therapy in 5–10 per cent of breast cancer patients (Cornbleet et al. 1977; Legha et al. 1981). It is often difficult to differentiate hormone-induced hypercalcaemia from spontaneous hypercalcaemia. Hypercalcaemia following hormonal therapy tends to develop rapidly and is associated with increased urinary excretion of hydroxyproline, indicating increased bone resorption (O'Connell 1981). Tamoxifen treatment has been reported to cause hypercalcaemia in a small proportion of patients (Legha et al. 1981), and patients with osteolytic bone metastasis appear to be at greater risk.

Hypercalcaemia following exposure to manganese has been reported (Roels et al. 1987). It has been suggested that the high ionized calcium concentration found in infants born to mothers receiving magnesium sulphate therapy is caused by displacement of calcium from albumin by the magnesium (Liu et al. 1988b).

Calcium-channel blockers have been reported to cause abnormalities in plasma calcium concentration and PTH levels. Studies reported up to now, however, have produced conflicting results and, so far, frank hypercalcaemia with the use of calcium-channel blockers has not been reported. Verapamil (Resnick et al. 1989), nifidepine (Resnick et al. 1987), felodipine (Hespel et al. 1987) and nisoldipine (Odigwe et al. 1986) have been reported to increase ionized calcium concentration. Other studies, however, have not been able to show an increase (Sjoden et al. 1987; Benjamin et al. 1988; Graves et al. 1988). Diltiazem lowered serum PTH, increased urinary calcium, and decreased phosphate excretion (Seely et al. 1989b).

Treatment

Plasma calcium concentrations raised by drugs usually return to normal once the drug is withdrawn. If the plasma calcium is very high or is associated with ill effects, then active treatment may be required. The first step is rehydration and treatment with frusemide. Other measures are administration of a glucocorticoid, calcitonin, or sodium phosphate or diphosphonates (for review see Pak 1986). Very rarely, haemodialysis may be required to lower serum calcium when other methods fail.

Hypocalcaemia

As 40 per cent of plasma calcium is bound to plasma proteins, mainly albumin, hypoalbuminaemia is the commonest cause of apparent hypocalcaemia in clinical practice. Wrong conclusions can be avoided by correcting the plasma total calcium concentration for low albumin using one of the many available formulae (e.g. Payne et al. 1973).

Decreased intestinal absorption

Hypocalcaemia has been reported to occur in up to 48 per cent of epileptic patients on anticonvulsant therapy (Richens and Rowe 1970; Agus et al. 1982; Weinstein et *al.* 1984) and this is thought to be due to altered metabolism of vitamin D (see Vitamin D for further details). A syndrome similar to that seen with anticonvulsant treatment is also seen with chronic abuse of alcohol (Fink 1984) and in association with long-term administration of glutethimide (Brater 1986), probably produced by similar mechanisms.

Corticosteroids used in the treatment of hypercalcaemia lower plasma calcium concentration at least partly by reducing intestinal calcium absorption (Fox *et al.* 1978). Frank hypocalcaemia, however, is not likely to be seen with the use of steroids.

Decreased mobilization from bone

Hypomagnesaemia of any aetiology causes hypocalcaemia and it is due to a combination of decreased release of PTH and decreased response of bone to PTH (Agus and Goldfarb 1985) (see section on Hypomagnesaemia). In these situations, administration of calcium alone does not correct the hypocalcaemia. Hypomagnesaemia due to cisplatin or gentamicin treatment (Nanji and Denegri 1984) is one such example of treatment causing severe hypocalcaemia. Blom and colleagues (1985), however, have reported that, in cisplatin treatment, serum calcium levels decrease in spite of magnesium supplementation but the serum calcium returns spontaneously to normal some months after the last course of cisplatin.

Drugs used in the treatment of severe hypercalcaemia such as mithramycin, calcitonin, clodronate, gallium nitrate (Warrell *et al.* 1986, 1987, 1988) and diphosphonates (Raisz 1980) may cause hypocalcaemia by reducing bone resorption.

Increased renal excretion

Loop diuretics increase the urinary excretion of calcium and together with saline infusion are used widely in the treatment of hypercalcaemia (Suki *et al.* 1970; Agus and Goldfarb 1985). Frusemide has been reported to cause hypocalcaemia (Toft and Roin 1971; Clasen *et al.* 1988). Fujita and co-workers (1984), however, found that in normal subjects, in spite of the excessive loss of calcium in urine, serum total and ionized calcium concentrations were unchanged. This was accompanied by increased renal cyclic-AMP excretion and the authors suggested that the calciuric effect of frusemide is compensated by secondary hyperparathyroidism. On the other hand, Ogawa and others (1984) reported an increase in serum total calcium (corrected for changes in serum protein) after frusemide treatment. Further studies with measurement of ionized calcium concentration are required to clarify these conflicting results.

Magnesium sulphate used in the treatment of pre-eclampsia has been found to lower the plasma calcium concentration (Lamm *et al.* 1988; Ramanathan *et al.* 1988). Suzuki and colleagues (1986) showed that infusion of magnesium sulphate is associated with a progressive decrease in serum calcium concentration, an increase in urinary calcium excretion, and a decrease in renal cyclic-AMP excretion. The increased renal loss of calcium induced by magnesium is the main factor in lowering the plasma calcium (Lau 1985).

Radioactive iodine (I^{131}), used in the management of thyroid cancer has been reported to cause a significant decrease in plasma calcium concentration. In one study, 58 per cent of patients who received I^{131} had hypocalcaemia and this was not related to age, sex, or the amount of I^{131} uptake by the thyroid (Glazebrook 1987). The hypocalcaemia is due to PTH deficiency and is related to pretreatment plasma calcium concentration, which was lower in those who subsequently developed hypocalcaemia.

Sodium phosphate, used in the treatment of severe hypercalcaemia, can cause hypocalcaemia by precipitation of calcium salts in the soft issue when given in large doses or too rapidly (Heyburn 1984). Phosphate absorption from sodium phosphate enemas or after phosphate taken by mouth may cause hypocalcaemia and hypernatraemia (Martin *et al.* 1987).

Disodium edetate (EDTA) chelates divalent cations and can be used to lower the plasma calcium concentration in hypercalcaemic states. The complexed calcium (EDTA–calcium complex) is excreted by the kidney. The rate and amount of administration of EDTA determines the fall in plasma calcium. Hypocalcaemia may be caused by too rapid infusion of EDTA (Brater 1986), but the hypocalcaemia is short-lived. By complexing calcium, neomycin may cause hypocalcaemia (Yao *et al.* 1980). Hypocalcaemia was found in an infant treated with desferrioxamine for aluminium overload associated with parenteral nutrition. The mechanism was probably rapid uptake of calcium by the bone (Klein *et al.* 1989).

Infusion of adrenaline or administration of the sympathomimetic agent ritodrine lowers plasma ionized calcium concentration (Kawarabayashi *et al.* 1989; Joborn *et al.* 1990). The mechanism and significance of these findings are not clear.

Neuroleptics used in psychiatric patients are associated with low serum ionized calcium levels, together with neuroleptic-induced extrapyramidal symptoms (Kuny and Binswanger 1988, 1989).

When large amounts of blood are transfused, hypocalcaemia may follow (Linko and Saxelin 1986; Wilson *et al.* 1987). In one study of patients receiving 20 or more units of blood within 24 hours, the ionized calcium level was less than 0.70 mmol per litre in 53 per cent (Wilson *et al.* 1987). The hypocalcaemia is caused by complexing of calcium by citrate. Significant hypocalcaemia may also occur during therapeutic plasma exchange (Bongiovanni *et al.* 1983).

Oestrogen replacement therapy in the menopause will cause a significant decrease in plasma calcium concentration (Herbai and Ljunghall 1984), the mechanism being thought to be resetting of the threshold for secretion of PTH (Selby and Peacock 1986*a*).

Fluorescein used in angiography was found to cause a significant decrease in ionized calcium concentration, probably due to complexing of calcium by the fluorescein (Turetta *et al.* 1985). Cysteamine, used in the treatment of paracetamol intoxication, reduced serum calcium level when administered to normal subjects (Copeland *et al.* 1986).

Treatment

Treatment of hypocalcaemia consists of withdrawal of the offending drug and the administration of calcium supplements.

Bone disease

Drugs may interfere with metabolism of calcium, phosphate, vitamin D, or bone to cause metabolic bone disease ranging from osteoporosis, in which there is a reduction in volume of bone tissue, to osteomalacia or rickets, characterized by increased osteoid tissue. In some instances of drug-induced metabolic bone disease, the bone morphology is more complicated.

Corticosteroid-induced osteoporosis

The adverse effects of therapeutic doses of glucocorticoids on bone are well recognized. Exposure to high doses of glucocorticoids will lead to loss of bone mass and pathological fractures. Although glucocorticoids have been used for nearly 40 years glucocorticoid-induced osteoporosis still remains a serious medical problem. The pathogenesis of this osteoporosis is not fully understood and there are no established methods of preventing or treating this condition (Hodgson 1990). Longitudinal studies of patients receiving glucocorticoids show that the bone loss occurs rapidly during the early part of treatment and the rate of bone loss subsequently stabilizes; the early loss was observed to be 27 per cent (Lo Cascio *et al.* 1984). The bone loss is dependent on the cumulative amount of glucocorticoid used

(Varanos *et al.* 1987) and risk factors such as age, sex, race, and menopausal status, which are important in involutional osteoporosis, are relatively less important in the glucocorticoid-induced disorder (Nordin *et al.* 1984; Hodgson 1990). The incidence of pathological fractures in glucocorticoid-induced osteoporosis has been reported to be as high as 42 per cent in asthmatic patients treated with glucocorticoids (Adinoff and Hollister 1983). In contrast to oral steroids, high-dose inhalation of budesonide did not cause adverse effects on calcium metabolism although the dose was high enough to suppress the hypothalamic–pituitary–adrenal axis (Toogood *et al.* 1988). This was a short-term study (7 days) and long-term studies with bone density measurements are required to confirm that inhaled steroids do not cause osteoporosis.

The mechanism of glucocorticoid-induced osteoporosis is not fully understood (see Hodgson 1990 for a review). Several factors seem to contribute, in that glucocorticoids (a) reduce calcium absorption by a direct effect on the intestine (Fox *et al.* 1978); (b) decrease the tubular reabsorption and increase the excretion of calcium (Suzuki *et al.* 1983); and (c) suppress osteoblastic activity. *In vitro* studies show that glucocorticoids inhibit osteoblast growth, and synthesis of several proteins. The serum levels of osteocalcin, a marker of osteoblastic activity, are low in patients treated with glucocorticoids for either short or long periods (I. Reid *et al.* 1986; Peretz *et al.* 1989*a*). In addition to these direct effects, there is increased PTH secretion and increased sensitivity of bone cells to PTH.

In the treatment of glucocorticoid-induced osteoporosis, calcium supplements, vitamin D (Nuti *et al.* 1984), fluoride, oestrogens, anabolic steroids, and calcitonin have all been used. In women with glucocorticoid-induced osteoporosis, oestrogen implants have been shown to increase bone density (Studd *et al.* 1989).

Anticonvulsant-induced bone disease

Long-term administration of anticonvulsants has been reported to cause bone disease with features of osteomalacia (Dent *et al.* 1970). Weinstein and colleagues (1984) showed, however, by histomorphometric studies of bone that the features are those of increased skeletal turnover, rather than of osteomalacia. Furthermore, there is controversy as to the incidence of bone disease associated with anticonvulsants. Some studies show that in epileptics treated with anticonvulsants the incidence of pathological fracture rates is 10 per cent (Nilsson *et al.* 1986), and other studies show biochemical evidence of bone disease in 40 per cent of patients (Krause *et al.*

1988). On the other hand, there are studies that show very little or no evidence of bone disease (biochemical or radiological) (Williams *et al.* 1984; Ala-Houhala *et al.* 1986; Harrington and Hodgkinson 1987). These differences are attributed to physical activity, diet, and exposure to sunlight (Nishiyama *et al.* 1986). The possible mechanism of action of anticonvulsants is discussed under vitamin D. Briefly, anticonvulsants may have an effect on vitamin D metabolism and a direct effect on intestine and bone. The final manifestation of disease depends on, among other things, the factors mentioned above.

Anticoagulant-induced osteoporosis

Osteoporosis and pathological fractures were found in patients treated with large doses of heparin for over 6 months (Griffith *et al.* 1965), but this is an uncommon problem, although several cases of symptomatic osteoporosis have been described in pregnant women (see review by Amerena *et al.* 1990). The risk of osteoporosis is related to the dose and duration of treatment. The mechanism of action of heparin is not clear; it has been suggested that heparin may increase bone resorption (Nordin *et al.* 1984) although reduced 1,25-DHCC levels have been reported in one patient (Aarskog *et al.* 1980).

Osteocalcin is an α-carboxyl-glutamyl protein that may have a regulatory role in bone metabolism. Serum levels of osteocalcin reflect osteoblastic activity (Epstein 1988). It is a vitamin K-dependent protein and therefore administration of vitamin K antagonists may inhibit its formation and so affect bone. Decrease in serum osteocalcin levels was found in patients treated with phenprocoumon (Pietschmann *et al.* 1988), but not in others given warfarin (Menon *et al.* 1987). It remains to be seen whether long-term oral anticoagulant therapy will cause osteoporosis.

Aluminium and bone disease

It is now generally recognized that aluminium is an aetiological factor in the pathogenesis of one form of bone disease seen in dialysis patients (Wills 1990). This form is less common since the introduction of water purification. The sources of aluminium are discussed under Aluminium. The bone disease associated with aluminium is resistant to vitamin D and its biologically active metabolites (Gruskin 1988). Its mechanism is not fully understood. Aluminium impairs the mineralization of bone (Wills and Savory 1989) and it also directly affects the numbers or function of osteoblasts (Hurley and MacMahon 1990). In addition, it has complex effects

on PTH secretion and vitamin D metabolites (for review see Gruskin 1988; Wills and Savory 1989; Wills 1990).

Aluminium-related bone disease can be prevented by using purified water and phosphate binders containing no aluminium. Aluminium can be removed by desferrioxamine (Gruskin 1988).

Bone disease of total parenteral nutrition

Metabolic bone disease is a relatively common complication of long-term parenteral nutrition. In patients receiving this treatment at home, incidences ranging from 42–100 per cent have been reported (Hurley and McMahon 1990). Neonates fed intravenously for long periods develop rickets with histological features similar to those of the rickets of phosphate deficiency (Oppenheimer and Snodgrass 1980). The metabolic bone disease seen in home parenteral nutrition is much more complex (for review see Hurley and McMahon 1990). Many factors contribute to the development of metabolic bone disease, including inadequate calcium, inadequate phosphate, hypercalciuria (induced by factors such as high protein intake, acidosis, high sodium content, hypertonic dextrose, and insulin), and aluminium toxicity (see section on Aluminium). As patients on long-term parenteral nutrition are at high risk of developing metabolic bone disease they should be carefully monitored.

Bone disease associated with other drugs

Loss of oestrogens is well known to be associated with accelerated loss of bone (Nordin *et al.* 1984), and low oestrogen levels may result from treatment with long-acting gonadotrophin-releasing hormone (GnRH) agonists (Waibel-Traber *et al.* 1989) or neuroleptics. The latter suppress oestrogen levels as a result of inducing hyperprolactinaemia (Ataya *et al.* 1988). The anti-oestrogenic drug tamoxifen did not cause significant reduction in bone density in a patient with mastalgia treated for 3–6 months (Fentiman *et al.* 1989).

Hypermagnesaemia causes hypercalciuria and hypocalcaemia (see Magnesium) and long-term infusion (up to 13 weeks) of magnesium sulphate for prolongation of labour can cause congenital rickets (Lamm *et al.* 1988).

Chemotherapy for malignant conditions may cause abnormalities in calcium, magnesium, and vitamin D metabolism. In children treated for acute lymphoblastic leukaemia, bone mineral content was found to be low 6 months after the end of treatment (Atkinson *et al.* 1989).

Phosphate

Like potassium, phosphorus is mainly intracellular and only a small fraction is present in plasma. In plasma, phosphate exists in two main forms: organic (ester and lipid phosphates) and inorganic (orthophosphate). Fifteen per cent of plasma inorganic phosphate is bound to protein and the rest is dialysable. The concentration of plasma inorganic phosphate in health varies with age, sex, and time of day (Young 1990). Drugs may cause changes in plasma phosphate concentration by affecting the distribution between the intracellular and extracellular compartments, or by altering the intestinal absorption or renal excretion (Conner 1984; Brater 1986) (Table 15.8).

Hypophosphataemia

Intracellular shift

Acute shift of phosphate from the extracellular to the intracellular compartment is frequently responsible for hypophosphataemia (Stoff 1982). The most frequent cause of this redistribution is the intravenous administration of carbohydrates with or without insulin (Lau 1986). When glucose or other carbohydrates enter cells

TABLE 15.8
Drug-induced hypophosphataemia

A. Distribution into cells
    β-adrenoceptor agonists—adrenaline, bronchodilators, carbohydrate administration (e.g. total parenteral nutrition), respiratory alkalosis induced by drugs

B. Reduced intestinal absorption
    antacids, sucralfate

C. Increased excretion
    diuretics, glucocorticoids, ifosfamide, metabolic alkalosis, paracetamol

D. Miscellaneous mechanisms
    anticonvulsants, diphosphonates and gallium nitrate, oestrogens

---

they are accompanied by phosphate, because of phosphorylation of hexose intermediates within the cell. One mole of glucose uses 4 moles of phosphate in the glycolytic process. In hospital patients, infusion of carbohydrates accounted for 43–73 per cent of all the cases of hypophosphataemia (Swaminathan *et al.* 1979; Juan and Elrazak 1979; Stoff 1982; King *et al.* 1987). Administration of 5% dextrose or dextrose saline causes a moderate decrease in plasma phosphate (0.25–0.35 mmol per litre) (Guillou *et al.* 1976). Severe, sometimes symptomatic, hyposphosphataemia is caused by glucose–insulin–potassium therapy (Swaminathan *et al.* 1978; Marwick and Woodhouse 1988) and by intravenous feeding regimens containing high concentrations of glucose without phosphate supplements (Travis *et al.* 1971). The degree of hypophosphataemia is related to the number of calories infused and the nutritional state, being severe in starving, malnourished individuals (Silvis and Paragas 1972) and alcoholics (Brater 1986; Lau 1986). Severe hypophosphataemia (0.16–0.39 mmol per litre) has also been reported following enteral feeding of carbohydrates (Hayek and Eisenberg 1989). Insulin administration without glucose has similar hypophosphataemic effects (Heine *et al.* 1984), and profound hypophosphataemia is not uncommon during treatment of diabetic ketoacidosis and hyperosmolar coma with insulin (Ditzel 1973; Bohannon 1989).

Administration of carbohydrates other than glucose, such as fructose, xylitol, or sorbitol, causes hypophosphataemia that is more severe than that seen after glucose (Ritz 1982; Brater 1986).

Respiratory alkalosis caused by drugs such as salicylates can lower plasma phosphate by transcellular shift of phosphates and stimulation of glycolysis (Lau 1986).

Administration of adrenaline causes hypophosphataemia (Body *et al.* 1983; Joborn *et al.* 1990) and this effect of adrenaline is mediated by effects on β-adrenoceptors (Massara and Cammani 1970; Ljunghall *et al.* 1984) and is believed to be caused by a shift of phosphate into cells due to increased glycogenolytic activity (Massara and Cammani 1970). Similar mechanisms account for the hypophosphataemia complicating bronchodilator therapy of acute severe asthma (Brady *et al.* 1989). Hypophosphataemia developed in 54 per cent of patients admitted for emergency bronchodilator therapy, and serum phosphate and serum theophylline concentrations were negatively correlated (Brady *et al.* 1989).

Acetate in concentrations ranging from 2–140 mmol per litre is used in dialysis fluids and the fluids used in surgery. The use of acetate may lower plasma phosphate concentration, probably because of a transcellular shift (Cardoso *et al.* 1988; Veech and Gitomer 1988).

Reduced intestinal absorption

Decreased absorption of phosphate from the intestine accounts for the hypophosphataemia induced by chronic use of phosphate binders (Lau 1986; Roxe *et al.* 1989). These agents not only reduce the absorption of dietary phosphate, but also that of secreted phosphate and cause a net negative balance (Shields 1978). Prolonged use of antacids may lead to osteomalacia (Baker *et al.* 1974).

The use of antacids accounted for about 2 per cent of the hypophosphataemia in one survey (Juan and Elrazak 1979).

Increased excretion

Metabolic alkalosis causes an increased loss of phosphate in the urine and thereby causes hypophosphataemia (Mostellar and Tuttle 1964).

Diuretics, especially those that inhibit sodium reabsorption in segments of the nephron that also transport phosphate, may cause hypophosphataemia (Lau 1986). Thus, diuretics such as acetazolamide frequently cause phosphaturia and hypophosphataemia, whereas those thatact on the loop of Henle, such as frusemide, bumetanide, or ethacrynic acid do not produce phosphaturia. Distally acting diuretics such as thiazides and chlorthalidone rarely produce significant hypophosphataemia, despite the fact that 10–15 per cent of phosphate is reabsorbed in the distal segments, because there is a compensatory increase in phosphate transport in the proximal segment in response to a mild depletion (Lau 1986). Other diuretics, such as metolazone and osmotic diuretics, also reduce proximal tubular reabsorption and can cause increased phosphate excretion and thus lower plasma phosphate (Brater 1986).

Glucocorticoids in pharmacological doses have been shown to cause increased phosphate excretion (Lau 1986), and this may account for the low phosphate levels seen during steroid therapy (Nuti *et al.* 1984) and ACTH infusions for infantile spasm (Riikonen *et al.* 1986).

Hypophosphataemia is a feature of paracetamol poisoning and this was demonstrated to be due to phosphaturia (Jones *et al.* 1989). Estramustine has been reported to cause significant hypophosphataemia during the first 6 weeks of treatment of metastatic prostatic cancer. The cause of hypophosphataemia is increased phosphate excretion as shown by a reduced renal tubular threshold for phosphate reabsorption ($TmPO_4/GFR$) (Citrin *et al.* 1986). It was also suggested that this is probably an oestrogenic effect of estramustine.

Miscellaneous

Oestrogen administered orally (Christiansen *et al.* 1982; Marshall *et al.* 1984) or intradermally (Selby and Peacock 1986*b*) lowers plasma phosphate. The exact mechanism of this oestrogen effect is not clear, although it has been suggested to be due to increased bone formation. Ifosfamide, a drug used for the treatment of solid tumours, produces hypophosphataemia and phosphaturia because of its renal toxicity (DeFronzo *et al.* 1974; Sangster *et al.* 1984). In children this results in hypophosphataemic rickets (Skinner *et al.* 1989; Newbury-Ecob

and Barbor 1989). Anticonvulsant therapy has been reported to cause a lower plasma phosphate concentration (Bogliun *et al.* 1986; Nishiyama *et al.* 1986), probably through its effect on vitamin D metabolism (see section on Calcium, Bone, and Vitamin D). Urine phosphate excretion, however, was reported to be lower in a study of 155 institutionalized epileptics (Nilsson *et al.* 1986).

Patients treated for malignant hypercalcaemia with pamidronic acid (amino hydroxypropylidine bisphosphonate), a potent inhibitor of osteoclast-mediated bone resorption, were reported to show a significant decrease in plasma phosphate (Thiebaud *et al.* 1986). Gallium nitrate, another hypocalcaemic drug, was found to reduce plasma phosphate concentration by 27 per cent (Warrell *et al.* 1986, 1988).

Treatment

Hypophosphataemia, especially when it is severe and prolonged, requires treatment with phosphate supplements either orally or parenterally, as it has been shown that the disorder can have adverse effects (Swaminathan *et al.* 1979).

Hyperphosphataemia

Increased plasma phosphate concentration can arise from increased absorption or reduced excretion of phosphate. Increase in phosphate intake only produces mild elevation of serum phosphate, as the renal excretion is efficient. If the amount administered is large, plasma phosphate will increase (Smith and Nordin 1964). Hyperphosphataemia may occur in infants fed unadapted cows' milk (Oppe and Redstone 1968). Severe hyperphosphataemia with hypocalcaemia has been reported after phosphate enemas (Reedy and Zwiren 1983), or laxatives containing phosphate (McConnell 1971; Ilberg *et al.* 1978). Over-treatment of hypophosphataemia or hypercalcaemia by intravenous phosphate infusion may lead to hyperphosphataemia, especially if the renal function is poor.

Drugs that cause renal failure (see Chapter 12) will cause hyperphosphataemia. Rhabdomyolysis causes release of intracellular phosphate and hence hyperphosphataemia, particularly if renal function is impaired. For instance, opiate overdosage has been reported to cause rhabdomyolysis and hyperphosphataemia which lasted for 7–10 days (Blain *et al.* 1985).

Hyperphosphataemia may also result from hypervitaminosis D and hypervitaminosis A. In hypervitaminosis D there is increased intestinal absorption and, in addition, reduced renal excretion due to suppression of PTH (Kurokawa *et al.* 1985). A neonate who ingested 60 times the recommended daily dose of vitamin A for 11 days developed hyperphosphataemia; this was probably due to accelerated bone resorption (Bush and Dahms 1984).

Administration of recombinant human erythropoietin to patients with renal failure on regular haemodialysis caused a small but significant increase in plasma phosphate (Eschbach *et al.* 1989). Treatment with gonadotrophin-releasing hormone analogues for 6 months caused a pronounced increase in serum phosphate concentration probably by increasing bone resorption (Gudmundsson *et al.* 1987). Diphosphonate administration has been associated with hyperphosphataemia (Russell *et al.* 1974); this effect is not seen until 2 weeks after the start of treatment and is due partly to reduced renal clearance of phosphate and partly to a shift of intracellular phosphate (Walton *et al.* 1975).

Severe hyperphosphataemia and hypocalcaemia may also occur following chemotherapy of certain malignant diseases, especially lymphomas, because of rapid release of phosphate from lysing cells (Ettinger *et al.* 1978). Growth hormone administration is known to cause increased tubular reabsorption of phosphate and an increase in plasma phosphate, although severe hyperphosphataemia is rare (Corvilain and Abramour 1962).

Propranolol and metoprolol caused an increase in plasma phosphate levels in hyperthyroid patients, probably because of a shift of phosphate from cells as a result of β-blockade (Murchison *et al.* 1979; Feely 1981).

Treatment

Treatment of hyperphosphataemia is the treatment of the underlying cause and the renal failure (if present). Occasionally, additional measures may be required and administration of phosphate binders is suggested. Intravenous sodium bicarbonate or actazolamide, or both, will increase phosphate excretion, but in severe cases dialysis may be required (Lau 1986).

Magnesium

After potassium, magnesium is the most abundant intracellular cation. Less than 1 per cent of the body magnesium is in the ECF and, consequently, plasma magnesium is not a good indicator of whole-body magnesium status. The plasma magnesium concentration ranges from 0.68–1.00 mmol per litre in healthy subjects and of this 60 per cent is ionized, 25 per cent protein-bound, and 15 per cent complexed. As intracellular magnesium plays a critical role in many metabolic processes, intracellular magnesium concentration is maintained at the expense of ECF and bone magnesium. Approximately 30–40 per cent of ingested magnesium is absorbed; factors controlling its absorption are not well understood, but vitamin D metabolites and parathyroid hormone (PTH) are known to be involved. Magnesium absorption can be reduced by intraluminal complexing agents such as phytate. The major organ regulating magnesium homoeostasis is the kidney, in which magnesium is filtered and reabsorbed. Factors that influence reabsorption by the tubules include PTH, changes in plasma magnesium concentration, and ECF volume (Lau 1985; Cronin 1986).

Hypermagnesaemia

As the kidney can excrete large loads of magnesium, it is unusual to encounter hypermagnesaemia, which tends to occur with the use of magnesium-containing preparations in the presence of renal impairment (Wilson *et al.* 1986). Even in the absence of renal impairment hypermagnesaemia may occur if the intake of magnesium is very high. The use of antacids containing magnesium caused hypermagnesaemia, hypotension, respiratory depression, and coma in an adult (Ferdinandus *et al.* 1981) and hypermagnesaemia and intestinal perforation were described in a premature infant following antacid administration (Brand and Greer 1990). The magnesium content of antacid preparations can be as high as 7.0 mmol in 5 ml (Brater 1986). Intravenous or intramuscular administration of magnesium sulphate may cause hypermagnesaemia (Sibai *et al.* 1984; Rogiers *et al.* 1989). Abuse of laxatives containing magnesium can lead to high magnesium levels (Smilkstein *et al.* 1988; Castelbaum *et al.* 1989), and in one patient hypermagnesaemia, quadriparesis, and a defect in neuromuscular function followed (Castelbaum *et al.* 1989). The use of magnesium salts in the treatment of pre-eclampsia can cause hypermagnesaemia in both mother and infant (Brady and Williams 1967; Hill *et al.* 1985). Magnesium intoxication may follow the use of magnesium sulphate in rectal enemas (Stevens and Wolff 1950); urological irrigation solutions containing magnesium salts (Fassler *et al.* 1985); Renacidin, a proprietary urinary stone-dissolving agent containing magnesium salts as well as citric acid (Wilson *et al.* 1986); and Epsom salts for bowel preparation (Aucamp *et al.* 1981).

Treatment

Treatment of magnesium intoxication involves removal or withdrawal of the drug concerned and, if the patient is symptomatic, supportive therapy such as rehydration, intravenous calcium, and ventilation (Fassler *et al.* 1985). Occasionally, dialysis may be required to remove the magnesium, especially in those with renal insufficiency (Lau 1985).

Hypomagnesaemia

Drugs that cause hypomagnesaemia are classified according to their possible mechanisms of action, which are listed in Table 15.9.

Redistribution

Redistribution of magnesium into ICF can cause hypomagnesaemia; it occurs in situations which are similar to those for redistribution of potassium. Hypomagnesaemia occurs in malnourished or starving children during refeeding (Montgomery 1960) and in patients fed intravenously with glucose and aminoacids but without an adequate amount of magnesium (Dyckner and Wester 1981). Insulin administration decreased plasma magnesium concentration by 15–20 per cent (Ratzmann 1985), probably as a result of the shift of magnesium into ICF. Furthermore, hypomagnesaemia has been reported

TABLE 15.9
Causes of drug-induced hypomagnesaemia

1. Redistribution between ECF and ICF
   metabolic alkalosis, catecholamines and
   β-agonists, insulin, oral or intravenous nutrition

2. Decreased gastrointestinal absorption
   drug-induced malabsorption, laxative abuse

3. Increased renal loss
   aminoglycosides, diuretics, cisplatin, cyclosporin

4. Others
   anticonvulsants, cytotoxic drugs, lithium,
   pentamidine

in 47 per cent of children undergoing an insulin hypoglycaemia test (Ratzmann and Zollner 1985). Adrenaline infusion has been shown to cause a decrease in plasma magnesium concentration (Joborn *et al.* 1990), as has also been reported following the administration of ritodrine (Kawarabayashi *et al.* 1989), terbutaline (Bremme *et al.* 1986), albuterol or other β-agonists (Whyte *et al.* 1987; Rolla and Bucca 1988; Lipworth *et al.* 1989*b*). This effect is due to β-adrenoreceptor-stimulated magnesium transport (Flatman 1984). Robertson (1985) has reported a fatal overdose of theophylline due to ingestion of approximately 9 g of sustained-release theophylline preparation (Theo-Dur); this patient had generalized

seizures, hypomagnesaemia, hypokalaemia, hypophosphataemia, and hyperglycaemia. Shift of magnesium into the cells is also responsible for the decrease in plasma magnesium concentration during acute metabolic alkalosis (Lau 1985).

Decreased gastrointestinal absorption

Hypomagnesaemia, with reduced urinary magnesium, may be seen in any drug-induced malabsorption syndrome, such as those due to cholestyramine, neomycin, or chronic abuse of laxatives (Brautbar and Massry 1987).

Increased renal loss

Magnesium depletion is a relatively common finding following diuretic treatment, from renal loss of magnesium (Swales 1982; Ryan 1987; Dorup *et al.* 1988). Loop diuretics directly inhibit the reabsorption of magnesium (Ryan 1987), and in one study hypomagnesaemia was present in all of 33 patients treated with loop diuretics (Dyckner and Wester 1984) and there was marked reduction in muscle potassium content. Thiazides, on the other hand, have little acute effect on renal magnesium handling, but are associated with chronic magnesium depletion, probably due to secondary hyperparathyroidism. The use of potassium-sparing diuretics or ACE inhibitors prevents this magnesium loss (Widman *et al.* 1982; Ryan 1986; Dyckner *et al.* 1988). Although magnesium depletion is relatively common after diuretics, plasma magnesium may very often be normal (Dorup *et al.* 1988; Dyckner *et al.* 1988). Muscle magnesium content is reduced in as many as 50 per cent of patients (Dorup and Skajaa 1989). Magnesium deficiency increases potassium loss and in the presence of magnesium deficiency it is difficult to correct the potassium depletion. The loss of magnesium and potassium from muscle is accompanied by reduction in sodium–potassium pumps (Dorup *et al.* 1988). The use of diuretics in hypertension and heart failure has consistently been associated with low serum magnesium and magnesium depletion in at least a proportion of subjects (Hollifield 1989*b*), and elderly subjects seem to be more at risk (Halawa 1989; Hollifield 1989*a*). The importance of the low serum magnesium, and magnesium depletion, lies in the inability to correct the potassium deficit by potassium supplements alone. Furthermore, there is an increased risk of digoxin toxicity (Martin *et al.* 1988) and a potential risk of ventricular arrhythmias and sudden death (Ryan 1987). A relationship between the occurrence of premature ventricular contractions and the decrease in potassium and magnesium has been demonstrated (Hollifield 1986). It is also suggested that the low potassium and magnesium states induced by diuretics may potentiate the effect of catecholamines in further lowering magnesium and potassium concentrations. In one study, long-continued thiazide or frusemide therapy increased the severity of hypokalaemia during short-term infusion of adrenaline but had no effect on adrenaline-induced hypomagnesaemia (Whyte *et al.* 1988*b*). Thus the use of diuretics should be accompanied by careful monitoring of magnesium status, and magnesium supplementation if necessary. Although magnesium depletion is common with the use of diuretics in cardiovascular disease, no evidence of magnesium depletion has been found (Cohen *et al.* 1985) in those taking thiazides for renal stones.

Cisplatin is an effective chemotherapeutic agent for the treatment of certain tumours, but the use of the drug is associated with nephrotoxicity and hypomagnesaemia secondary to renal magnesium wasting (Schilsky and Anderson 1979). The incidence of hypomagnesaemia has been reported to be as high as 50–100 per cent (Bell *et al.* 1985; Stewart *et al.* 1985; Swainson *et al.* 1985; Trump and Hortvet 1985; Vogelzang *et al.* 1985; Hartmann *et al.* 1988). Symptomatic hypomagnesaemia was seen in fewer patients (Ashraf *et al.* 1983), up to 10 per cent in one study (Salem *et al.* 1984). The hypomagnesaemia is dose-related (Lam and Adelstein 1986), cumulative in sequential therapy with repeated courses (Swainson *et al.* 1985), and more common with continuous infusion than with intermittent bolus injections (Forastiere *et al.* 1988), suggesting that the total exposure to free platinum contributes to the toxicity. It is well documented that the hypomagnesaemia of cisplatin treatment is due to renal magnesium loss (Lam and Adelstein 1986; Mavichak *et al.* 1988). The exact mechanism of this effect is not known, but a lesion in the distal tubules has been suggested (Mavichak *et al.* 1988). Carboplatin, a newer drug, is associated with a lower incidence of hypomagnesaemia: only 2 of 30 patients developed a low magnesium concentration in one study (Leyvraz *et al.* 1985). In an uncontrolled study in which intravenous thiosulphate was administered with cisplatin, hypomagnesaemia was only seen in 8 per cent of patients (Markman *et al.* 1986). Whether this is a protective effect of thiosulphate needs to be established in control trials.

Aminoglycosides are associated with excessive renal losses of magnesium, and hypomagnesaemia is common in patients on prolonged treatment with, or high doses of, an aminoglycoside (Bar *et al.* 1975). Hypomagnesaemia has been reported with gentamicin (Watson *et al.* 1983; Beatty *et al.* 1989), tobramycin (Watson *et al.* 1984), and other members of this group. Symptomatic hypomagnesaemia with tetany has been reported in

some patients (Vithayasai *et al.* 1989; Wilkinson *et al.* 1986). Zaloga and others (1984) reported that even with therapeutic dosages hypomagnesaemia may occur in more than one-third of patients. Hypomagnesaemia is more common in those who have poor magnesium intake. The nephrotoxic effect of aminoglycosides is mainly on the proximal tubules, and it is possible that aminoglycosides inhibit proximal tubular transport of magnesium.

Cyclosporin and cyclophosphamide, used for immunosuppression, are associated with renal toxicity and hypomagnesaemia. Hypomagnesaemia due to renal wasting of magnesium developed in 88 per cent of bone marrow transplant recipients given one of these drugs (Kone *et al.* 1988). The incidence of the disorder was higher with cyclosporin and it was suggested that this agent aggravates its severity. In another study of renal transplant recipients, in which cyclosporin was associated with reduction in serum magnesium concentration and inappropriately increased urinary excretion of magnesium, nearly all patients required magnesium supplements (Barton *et al.* 1987). Severe hypomagnesaemia and neurotoxicity following cyclosporin therapy resolved or did not recur with adequate magnesium replacement (Thompson *et al.* 1984; June *et al.* 1986).

Mild hypomagnesaemia has been reported in a case of accidental overdose with lithium (Corbett *et al.* 1989); hypomagnesaemia and hypocalcaemia were reported after treatment with mitoxantrone, an antineoplastic drug (Griffiths and Parry 1988), and other cytotoxic drugs (Matzen and Martin 1985; Wandrup and Kancir 1986). Chronic anticonvulsant treatment is associated with deficiency of magnesium, the incidence of which increases with duration of treatment (Steidl *et al.* 1987). This effect may be related to the effect of anticonvulsants on vitamin D metabolism (Christiansen *et al.* 1974). Hypomagnesaemia was also observed during pentamidine treatment of parasitic diseases (Wharton *et al.* 1987). Neonatal hypomagnesaemia from excessive use of the stool softener docusate sodium by the mother has been reported (Schindler 1984).

Trace elements

Copper

Copper is an essential trace element, and several important enzymes such as cytochrome C oxidase contain it (Aggett 1985). Adult man has about 80 mg of copper and about 50 per cent of this is found in muscle and bone, but the highest concentration being in liver (Jacob 1986). The dietary intake of copper is approximately 2 mg per day and about 50 per cent of this is absorbed (Aggett 1985). In plasma, 90–95 per cent of copper is bound to the α_2-globulin caeruloplasmin; 10 per cent is associated or loosely bound to albumin; and a small fraction is complexed with low-molecular-weight compounds such as amino acids (Delves 1985).

A copper-deficiency syndrome, with low red cell and plasma copper concentrations, is seen in patients receiving total parenteral nutrition with no copper (Karpel and Peden 1972). In some infants receiving total parenteral nutrition, an unusual skeletal disorder resembling that seen in scurvy has also been described (Sivasubramanian *et al.* 1978). Copper deficiency has also been associated with oral zinc therapy for sickle cell disease (Porter *et al.* 1977; Prasad *et al.* 1978; Abdulla 1979) because of the effect of zinc on copper absorption. Deficiency of copper may occur during treatment with chelating agents such as penicillamine, used in the treatment of Wilson's disease, as well as in other diseases such as rheumatoid arthritis (Jacob 1986).

Thiamazole, which forms complexes with copper, may also lead to loss of taste (Hanlon 1975), a disorder that may also occasionally follow treatment with captopril, for which copper or zinc deficiency has been held to blame, although serum copper levels have been unaltered in patients treated with captopril (O'Connor *et al.* 1987).

Copper toxicity has been reported as a complication of long-term haemodialysis (Blomfield *et al.* 1971), and with the use of copper-containing intrauterine contraceptive devices (Jacob 1986). Plasma copper levels increase after treatment with oral contraceptives (Tovey and Lathe 1968), and after oral ethinyloestradiol treatment in postmenopausal women (Chilvers *et al.* 1985), as a result of increased synthesis of caeruloplasmin by the liver. Chilvers and associates (1985) showed that 80 per cent of the increase in plasma copper is due to a rise in caeruloplasmin-bound copper and 20 per cent was due to an increase in the amount of copper bound to albumin.

Zinc

Zinc is an essential element and is a co-factor in many metalloenzymes; over 200 zinc-dependent enzymes have been described (Aggett 1985). Total body-zinc content in adult man is 1.4–2.3 g, of which 70–80 per cent is in bone, skin, and muscle. The zinc concentration of red cells is about 10 times that of plasma, because of their high content of carbonic anhydrase. The average intake of zinc is about 15 mg per day, of which approximately 20–30 per cent is absorbed (Prasad 1985). About 98 per cent of the zinc in plasma is protein bound, 80–85 per

cent to albumin, 15 per cent to α_2-macroglobulin, less than 2 per cent to retinal-binding protein, and less than 1–2 per cent 'free' or ultrafiltrable (Foote and Delves 1984; Delves 1985). Although it is plasma zinc that is usually measured, this is not a good measure of zinc status (Delves 1985).

When zinc is not added during total parenteral nutrition, plasma and red cell zinc fall progressively (Kay *et al.* 1976) and the zinc deficiency syndrome develops (Kay *et al.* 1976). The risk of zinc deficiency is greater in those with hypercatabolic states (Jeejeebhoy 1984), and it is recommended that adults be given at least 2.5 mg of zinc daily during total parenteral nutrition (Prasad 1985).

Zinc deficiency has been reported in patients receiving penicillamine therapy (Klinberg *et al.* 1976; de Virgiliis *et al.* 1988). Diuretic treatment increases urinary excretion of zinc, but the plasma zinc levels are normal (Wester 1975). Long-term diuretic therapy is associated with zinc deficiency (Wester 1975). Low plasma zinc levels are seen after treatment with oestrogens (Chilvers *et al.* 1985) as a result of decreased albumin concentration leading to a decrease in the amount of albumin-bound zinc. Reduced taste acuity seen after captopril treatment resembles that accompanying zinc deficiency. Abu-Hamdan and co-workers (1988) found increased urinary zinc excretion and low plasma zinc concentration to be associated with hypogeusia. There was no effect in short-term treatment. No change in serum zinc levels was found by O'Connor and colleagues (1987) in patients treated with captopril for 5–6 months, or by Neil-Dwyer and Marus (1989) in those treated with captopril or lisinopril for 8 weeks. Nevertheless, long-term ACE inhibitor treatment may reduce plasma zinc concentration.

Foote and Hinks (1988) have reported that the intestinal absorption of zinc is defective in chronic haemodialysis patients. Reduced zinc absorption is observed with the use of high-fibre diets (e.g. containing bran) which contain phytate (Hall *et al.* 1989), or the administration of ferrous sulphate, aluminium hydroxide (Abu-Hamdan *et al.* 1986), or subtances with a high inorganic iron content (Valberg *et al.* 1984). Folic acid supplements, commonly used in pregnancy, are thought to reduce intestinal absorption of zinc. This is especially important, as zinc deficiency has been associated with low-birth-weight babies (Arumanayagam *et al.* 1986). Milne and co-workers (1984) found that faecal excretion of zinc was increased significantly and urinary zinc was reduced by folate supplementation in normal men, especially when the dietary zinc was low, and they suggested that folate may form insoluble complexes and thereby reduce absorption. Simmer and colleagues

(1987) also found reduced zinc absorption during folate supplementation. On the other hand, Keating and others (1987) failed to show any effect of folate on a 25 mg oral zinc absorption test. Butterworth and colleagues (1988) found that plasma and red cell zinc levels were not altered by folate supplementation for 4 months, but they did not measure zinc absorption or urinary zinc excretion. Thus it is likely that folate has a deleterious effect on zinc absorption and may be potentially harmful during pregnancy, especially if the intake of zinc is marginal or low. The use of oral contraceptives is associated with a decrease in plasma zinc and an increase in red cell zinc (Jacob 1986). Corticosteroid therapy causes a rapid decrease in plasma zinc and a marked increase in urinary zinc (Peretz et al. 1989b). Treatment with cisplatin (Sweeney et al. 1989) and anabolic steroids may cause zinc deficiency (Jacob 1986). Treatment with antiepileptics did not cause any significant zinc depletion (Yuen et al. 1988).

Marked increases in serum zinc concentration have been reported in patients receiving total parenteral nutrition, from inadvertent administration of excessive doses of zinc (Brocks et al. 1977). The diuretic chlorthalidone has been associated with raised plasma and hair zinc levels (Geissler et al. 1986). The significance of this effect is not clear. Glucose polymers used as an energy source were found to increase the absorption of zinc (Bei et al. 1986). Acute zinc toxicity has been reported in patients undergoing haemodialysis (Gallery et al. 1972). Oral zinc treatment is increasingly used in the treatment of subfertile men (Kynaston et al. 1988), to improve cellular immunity (Allen et al. 1985; Labadie et al. 1986), and for tropical ulcers (Lin et al. 1985; Watkinson et al. 1985). Zinc toxicity may occur in these patients.

Aluminium

Aluminium toxicity has been described in patients undergoing dialysis for chronic renal failure. The manifestations of toxicity include encephalopathy, osteomalacic dialysis osteodystrophy, and microcytic anaemia (Gruskin 1988; Wills 1990). These manifestations correlate with serum aluminium concentrations (Rovelli et al. 1988), brain aluminium content (Fraser and Arieff 1988), and bone aluminium content (Goodman et al. 1984; de Broe et al. 1984). The microcytic anaemia of aluminium toxicity has been used as a reversible marker of aluminium toxicity (Swartz et al. 1987), being reversed when the aluminium concentration in the dialysate is reduced (Kaiser and Schwartz 1985; Abreo et al. 1989). The sources of aluminium are the tap water used in the preparation of the dialysate (Platts et al. 1977; Nordberg

et al. 1985), aluminium-containing phosphate-binding agents (Salusky et al. 1984), and aluminium cookware (Mendis 1988). The tissue accumulation of aluminium occurs mainly in chronic renal failure patients having haemodialysis or peritoneal dialysis (Wills 1990), owing to their inability to excrete the aluminium. Aluminium toxicity has been described in renal failure patients not being treated by dialysis, however, from the use of aluminium-containing phosphate binders (Baluarte et al. 1977; Kaye 1983). Two patients with chronic liver disease were found to have aluminium-associated osteodystrophy and elevated serum aluminium concentrations. This was attributed to the long-term use of aluminium-containing antacids; the authors suggested that biliary excretion is an important route of elimination of aluminium and that the reduced biliary excretion in these patients was responsible for the aluminium toxicity (Williams et al. 1986). Evidence of raised aluminium intake, as shown by increased concentration of plasma, urine, and bone aluminium content has been found in infants receiving intravenous therapy contaminated with aluminium (Sedman et al. 1985). Contamination of casein (used in long-term total parenteral nutrition) with aluminium has led to aluminium toxicity in adults (Klein et al. 1980, 1982; Ott et al. 1983).

Treatment involves the use of aluminium-free antacids and water, and desferrioxamine to remove the aluminium (Ackrill and Day 1985; Sprague et al. 1986).

Lead

Lead poisoning from ingestion of traditional remedies (kushtas) (Haq and Asghar 1989) or oriental cosmetics (surma) is seen in Asian communities in Britain (Healy and Aslam 1986), North America (MMWR 1984; Pontifex and Garg 1985), in Middle Eastern countries (Rahman et al. 1986; Abu Melha et al. 1987), and in the Mexican community in the USA (MMWR 1983). Lead content of these preparations is high and the levels may be as high as 82.5 per cent in some (Rahman et al. 1986). Lead poisoning has been reported in association with the use of illicit methamphetamine (Allcott et al. 1987; MMWR 1989), contaminated heroin (Parras et al. 1987; Antonini et al. 1989), and the use of contaminated water to reconstitute milk feeds for infants (Shannon and Graef 1989).

Mercury

Mercury poisoning or increased blood mercury levels may be found in patients given normal human IgG, which contains the organic mercurial thiomersal as preservative. Over 70 per cent of hypogammaglobulinaemic patients given IgG have increased urinary excretion of mercury (Haeney *et al.* 1979). Increased blood mercury levels and increased mercury levels in brain and kidney are also found in subjects with dental fillings (amalgam) containing the metal (Abraham *et al.* 1984; Nylander *et al.* 1987; Snapp *et al.* 1989). Mercury concentrations may reach toxic levels following postoperative wound treatment with the antiseptic mebromine (mercurochrome), because of absorption from the wound surface (Kloppel and Weiler 1985).

Silver

Increased intake of silver and possibly poisoning may occur after ingestion of traditional medicines (*kushtas*) used by the Indo-Pakistan community. These remedies have been reported to contain mercury and silver in addition to lead (Haq and Asghar 1989). The use of anti-smoking lozenges containing silver acetate may cause silver poisoning (MacIntyre *et al.* 1978; Shelton and Goulding 1979) and the use of anti-smoking chewing gum containing silver acetate increases the levels of silver in serum and skin biopsies (Jensen *et al.* 1988). The use of silver sulphadiazine as a topical antimicrobial agent in burns patients is associated with absorption of silver from the raw skin surface, resulting in high serum silver levels and raised urinary silver excretion. In burns patients with involvement of more than 60 per cent of the skin, urinary excretion of silver was 1000-fold greater on treatment with silver sulphadiazine (Boosalis *et al.* 1987). It has been recommended that yellow-phosphorus skin burns should be treated with silver nitrate solution instead of copper sulphate solution (Song *et al.* 1985). This is likely to cause increased silver absorption but this has not been reported so far.

Fluoride

Fluoride is used in the treatment of osteoporosis (Budden *et al.* 1988), as it stimulates bone formation and increases cancellous bone mass. Accidental fluoride overdosage may occur due to the use of excess hydrofluorosilicic acid in the water supply (Petersen *et al.* 1988).

When the fluorinated anaesthetics halothane, methoxyflurane, enflurane, and isoflurane are metabolised, fluoride is released into the circulation, resulting in an increase in plasma fluoride concentration (Crowhurst and Rosen 1984; Oikkonen and Meretoja 1989). Peak levels of serum fluoride were seen 3 days after anaesthesia with methoxyflurane, 24 hours after halothane, and soon after the end of anaesthesia in the cases of enflurane and isoflurane (Cousins *et al.* 1987). This difference is accounted for by the high lipid-solubility of methoxyflurane. The peak level was also considerably higher with methoxyflurane than with enflurane or isoflurane, and the high fluoride levels may account for the nephrotoxicity of methoxyflurane (Mazze 1984). When isoflurane is compared with enflurane, the serum fluoride was higher with enflurane (Oikkonen 1984). The urinary excretion of fluoride is increased after isoflurane and enflurane but not after halothane (Cousins *et al.* 1987; Davidkova *et al.* 1988; Kofke *et al.* 1989). Ethanol affects defluorination of enflurane (Pantuck *et al.* 1985).

Administration of aluminium hydroxide decreases plasma fluoride levels by 50 per cent, by reducing net absorption (Spencer *et al.* 1985).

Porphyrins

Porphyrins are a group of cyclic tetrapyrroles that are red in colour. They are intermediates in the synthesis of haem and cytochromes. Porphyrias are a group of metabolic disorders of haem biosynthesis in which there is increased formation of porphyrins and their precursors (Goldberg *et al.* 1987; Bloomer and Bonkovsky 1989). Porphyrias are classified as either hepatic or erythroid, depending on the principal site of expression of the specific enzyme defect (Table 15.10). In addition to these inherited disorders, several different diseases, particularly anaemias and hepatobiliary diseases, or toxins may cause secondary porphyrinuria.

The erythropoietic porphyrias do not appear to be affected or aggravated by drugs or toxins. On the other hand, a wide variety of drugs can affect the hepatic porphyrias. The porphyrias can also be divided into acute and non-acute, both of which can be affected by drugs. The acute porphyrias are disorders in which patients may present with 'acute attacks'. These acute porphyrias include acute intermittent porphyria, variegate porphyria, hereditary coproporphyria, and plumboporphyria (ALA dehydratase deficiency porphyria).

Acute porphyrias

Patients with acute porphyrias may present with acute abdominal pain, mental dysfunction, and peripheral neuropathy. During an attack the urine develops a dark red-brown colour, deepening with exposure to light. Acute attacks are precipitated by various factors, including alcohol, infection, hormones, reduced calorie intake (as in fasting or dieting), and drugs. Comprehensive lists of drugs that have been reported to precipitate acute attacks, and drugs that have been shown to be porphyrinogenic in experimental animals or in cell culture systems have been published (Moore and Disler 1988). A

TABLE 15.10
Classification of porphyrias

Erythropoietic

Congenital erythropoietic porphyria	++	Uroporphyrin and coproporphyrin in urine
Erythropoietic protoporphyria	++	Protoporphyrin in stool

Hepatic

ALA dehydratase deficiency porphyria (plumboporphyria)	—	ALA in urine
Acute intermittent porphyria	—	ALA and PBG in urine
Hereditary coproporphyria	+	ALA, PBG and coproporphyrin
Variegate porphyria	+	ALA, PBG, and coproporphyrin
Porphyria cutanea tarda	++	Uroporphyrin
Hepatoerythropoietic porphyria	+	Uroporphyrin

+ Photosensitivity may be present
++ Photosensitivity predominant
ALA—Delta amino laevulinic acid
PBG—Porphobilinogen

selected list of drugs reported to have caused with acute attacks of porphyria is given in Table 15.11; it includes drugs, such as barbiturates and phenytoin, that induce hepatic microsomal enzymes. It has been pointed out by Moore and Disler (1988) that there is no property common to all these drugs, and it is difficult to predict whether or not a drug will precipitate an acute attack. The possible mechanism of action of some drugs is discussed by DeMatteis (1988). Fuller lists of drugs, including those which are thought to be safe in porphyrias, have been published by Moore and Disler (1988) and Moore and McColl (1989).

The common form of acute porphyria, acute intermittent porphyria (AIP), is diagnosed by the presence of reduced erythrocyte PBG deaminase activity (Bottomley and Muller-Eberhard 1988). In 7 per cent of patients with AIP, however, the erythrocyte enzyme value is normal, because of the molecular heterogenicity of the defective enzyme protein. Herrick and others (1989a) have reported two patients who developed AIP on anticonvulsant therapy, but had normal erythrocyte PBG deaminase activity.

Treatment of acute porphyrias consists of symptomatic and specific therapy (Moore and Disler 1988).

TABLE 15.11
Drugs that have been reported to be associated with acute attacks of porphyria

Antibacterial, antifungal, and antimalarial agents
  chloramphenicol, griseofulvin, pivampicillin, pyrazinamide, sulphonamides

Anticonvulsants
  barbiturates (phenobarbitone), carbamazepine, deoxybarbiturates (primidone) hydantoins (phenytoin)

Hormones and antidiabetic drugs
  chlorpropamide, oral contraceptives, progesterone

Hypnotics, sedatives, and tranquillizers
  barbiturates, carbromal, carisoprodol, chlordiazepoxide, dichloralphenazone, ethchlorvynol, glutethimide, meprobamate, methylprylon

Miscellaneous
  Alphaxalone : Alphadolone, bemegride, dimenhydrinate, ergot compounds (dihydro-ergotamine), ethanol, flufenamic acid, halothane, hyoscine butylbromide, imipramine, methyldopa, methylsulphonal, nikethamide, orphenadrine, pentazocine, pentylenetetrazol, thiopentone sodium, theophylline

(Adapted from Moore and McColl 1989)

Specific therapies are few and include high carbohydrate intake and haem arginate (haematin) therapy. Herrick and others (1989b) reported that haem arginate therapy reduced the excretion of PBG and the clinical abnormalities. In women with AIP who develop frequent exacerbations related to the menstrual cycle, luteinizing hormone releasing factor (LHRH) analogues have been used to prevent the cyclical attacks by hormonal manipulation (Anderson 1989). Although LHRH analogues prevent the cyclical attacks they do not normalize abnormal porphyrin precursor excretion and do not prevent acute attacks precipitated by other factors (Anderson 1989).

Non-acute porphyria (cutaneous porphyrias)

Porphyria cutanea tarda (PCT), the most common form of porphyria, is characterized by a deficiency of hepatic uroporphyrinogen decarboxylase activity. PCT can be inherited or acquired (sporadic). In the acquired form, the enzyme defect is confined to the liver and is often triggered by environmental agents, amongst which alcohol is a well-recognized precipitating factor (Grossman *et al.* 1979), though its mechanism of action is not well understood (Kappas *et al.* 1989). Oestrogen administration for prostatic carcinoma (Weimar *et al.* 1978; Coulson and Misch 1989), or for postmenopausal symptoms and signs, or in the form of the contraceptive pill (Behm and Unger 1974) has aggravated or precipitated PCT. Iron has been shown to be another important factor in its pathogenesis (Magnus 1984). Other compounds that have been implicated in this way include polychlorinated hydrocarbons (Schmid 1960), diazinon, an organophosphorus insecticide (Bleakley *et al.* 1979), rifampicin (Millar 1980), cyclophosphamide (Manzione *et al.* 1988), and zidovudine (azidothymidine) (Ong *et al.* 1988).

Several drugs have been reported to cause skin lesions similar to PCT but without disturbances in porphyrin metabolism. This is described as 'pseudoporphyria'; it has been described in association with amiodarone (Parodi *et al.* 1988), chlorthalidone (Baker *et al.* 1989), cyclophosphamide (Sola *et al.* 1987), etretinate (McDonagh and Harrington 1989), naproxen (Judd *et al.* 1986; Rivers and Barnetson 1989) and other NSAID agents (Shelley *et al.* 1987; Taylor and Duffill 1987), and tetracycline and frusemide (Kappas *et al.* 1989).

Apart from removing the offending agent, chloroquine in low doses has been reported to be an effective therapy in PCT (Ashton *et al.* 1984). It forms a water-soluble complex with uroporphyrin, which is excreted (Bloomer and Bonkovsky 1989). Some authors advocate a short course of high-dose chloroquine (Tsega 1987).

Erythropoietic protoporphyria

Erythropoietic protoporphyria is an inherited porphyria associated with decreased activity of ferrochelatase and is characterized by cutaneous photosensitivity (Kappas *et al.* 1989). There appear to be no known precipitating agents for this condition (Kappas *et al.* 1989), but four patients with this disorder in whom oral iron produced clinical and biochemical exacerbation have been described (Milligan *et al.* 1988). The authors suggested that there are two biochemically and genetically distinct subgroups with different responses to oral iron therapy.

Secondary porphyrinuria

Moderate elevation of porphyrin excretion is associated with several diseases (such as anaemias and hepatobiliary diseases), drugs, and toxins (Bloomer and Bonkovsky 1989). Lead poisoning is a well-recognized cause of secondary porphyrinuria, the metal inhibiting ALA dehydratase and causing increased excretion of ALA and

coproporphyrin (McColl and Goldberg 1980; Henderson and Toothill 1983). Other heavy metals such as mercury, bismuth, copper, silver, gold, and arsenic cause coproporphyrinuria but without elevation of urinary ALA (Tephly *et al.* 1977; Labbe and Lamon 1986). Alcohol, especially in large amounts, can cause secondary porphyrinuria (McColl and Goldberg 1980), and other agents thought to have been responsible are hexachlorobenzene, sedatives, hypnotics such as chloral hydrate, morphine, ether, and nitrous oxide.

Uric acid

Uric acid is the end-product of metabolism of purines of endogenous and dietary origin. Dietary purines may contribute up to 50 per cent of uric acid production (Emmerson 1983). About 25 per cent of the uric acid produced is excreted through the intestines and this proportion increases in chronic renal failure (Wills 1990). In plasma, uric acid is present almost entirely as a monovalent anion, there is very little protein-binding and more than 95 per cent of plasma urate is freely filtered by the glomeruli (Fuiano *et al.* 1989). The amount of urate excreted is about 10 per cent of the filtered load. During the passage through the tubules filtered urate is almost entirely reabsorbed in the proximal tubules. An amount equivalent to about 50 per cent of the filtered load is secreted in the mid-proximal tubule and most of this is reabsorbed in the late proximal tubule (Kahn and Weinman 1985; Levinson and Sorensen 1980), leaving an amount equivalent to about 10 per cent of the filtered load to be excreted. Drugs may influence the production or excretion of uric acid, or both of these processes (German and Holmes 1986) (Table 15.12).

TABLE 15.12
Drugs causing hyperuricaemia and hypouricaemia

Hyperuricaemia
  Over-production
    alcohol, cytotoxic drugs, fructose, nitroglycerine, theophylline (?)

  Decreased excretion
    cyclosporin, drug-induced acidosis—lactic or keto acidosis, drug-induced ECF volume contraction, low-dose aspirin, nicotinic acid, pyrazinamide, thiazide diuretics, vasopressin

Hypouricaemia
  Reduced production
    allopurinol, azathioprine

  Increased excretion
    anticonvulsants, aspirin, oral anticoagulants, radiographic contrast media, urocosuric agents

---

Hyperuricaemia and gout

Increased production of urate

Apart from genetic causes, several acquired factors can increase the production of uric acid. Hyperuricaemia and gout are well-recognized complications of myeloproliferative and haemolytic disorders, in which there is increased turnover of uric acid (German and Holmes 1986; Palella and Fox 1989). This is further aggravated by treatment with cytotoxic agents. Hyperuricaemia is also seen during treatment of other malignant disorders with cytotoxic drugs (Batist et al. 1985; Stewart et al. 1986).

Hyperuricaemia and gout are more common in alcoholics (German and Holmes 1986). Beer contains sufficient purines to increase the purine load in beer drinkers, and alcohol itself is thought to increase uric acid production (Faller and Fox 1982). Furthermore, the increased lactate levels found in alcoholics may further reduce uric acid excretion (Palella and Fox 1989).

Rapid intravenous administration of fructose causes an increased uric acid level. The rapid phosphorylation of fructose leads to dephosphorylation of adenine nucleotides, which are subsequently degraded to uric acid (Fox 1981). The rate of administration of fructose is important in determining hyperuricaemia (Emmerson 1983). Lactic acidosis caused by fructose further increases serum uric acid levels by reducing renal excretion (Woods and Alberti 1972).

Serum uric acid levels are about 50 per cent higher in asthmatics treated with theophylline and there is a significant correlation between serum theophylline and uric acid levels. As intravenous theophylline failed to affect the renal clearance of urate and in vitro studies showed that theophylline inhibited the enzyme hypoxanthine guanine phosphoribosyl transferase, it has been suggested that the effect of theophylline is on production of urate (Morita et al. 1984).

In patients receiving intravenous nitroglycerin for unstable angina, acute gout developed and serum uric acid increased. This was attributed to the alcohol content of the intravenous nitroglycerin preparation (Shergy et al. 1988).

Decreased excretion

In volume depletion there is increased reabsorption of urate, leading to an increased plasma uric acid concentration (Weinman et al. 1975; Feinstein et al. 1984). Thus, any drug causing volume depletion may lead to hyperuricaemia. Hyperuricaemia is also a feature of renal failure induced by drugs (see Chapter 12).

Salicylate at all doses inhibits uric acid secretion but at high doses it reduces tubular reabsorption. Thus, low dose salicylate causes hyperuricaemia and high concentrations lead to hypouricaemia (Emmerson 1983; Palella and Fox 1989).

Diuretics are the most common cause of drug-induced hyperuricaemia (Langford et al. 1987). In most patients the increase in serum urate is small but in some it is greater (Emmerson 1983). Main mechanisms contributing to the reduced renal excretion of urate are volume depletion induced by diuretics, and reduced filtration rate (Steele and Oppenheimer 1969). It has been suggested that the increased reabsorption of urate is mediated by angiotensin II, which is released in response to hypovolaemia. Angiotensin II may play a part in enhancing the activity of Na^+–H^+ exchange, which leads to a parallel increase in urate–OH^- exchange (Rose 1989, p. 401). The majority of patients with hyperuricaemia induced by diuretics are asymptomatic and do not require treatment (Liang and Fries 1978), and gouty arthritis occurs mainly in those with a predisposition to gout (e.g. family history). Frusemide, in addition to volume depletion, inhibits secretion of urate due to increased lactic acid levels (Holmes 1985), and the risk of gout is higher with loop diuretics than thiazides (Waller and Ramsay 1989). All diuretics, apart from amiloride, triamterene, spironolactone (Jeunemaitre et al. 1987), and the uricosuric group of diuretics, will cause an increase in serum uric acid concentration. Elderly women are particularly prone to diuretic-induced tophaceous gout (MacFarlane and Dieppe 1985; Wordsworth and Mowat 1985). Administration of cicletanine, a less commonly used diuretic, to healthy volunteers was reported to increase serum urate acutely but not during long-term treatment (Bippi and Guinot 1988).

The antituberculous drug pyrazinamide has a dose-related effect on uric acid levels (Sanwikarja et al. 1989) and it increases the risk of gout (Auvergne et al. 1988) through inhibition of urate secretion (Steele and Rieselback 1967) by pyrazionic acid, its main metabolite. Allopurinol, a hypouricaemic agent that reduces uric acid synthesis, has no effect on the hyperuricaemia induced by pyrazionic acid (Lacroix et al. 1988).

Cyclosporin treatment is associated with hyperuricaemia in both renal transplant recipients (Chapman et al. 1985; Palestine et al. 1986) and patients not undergoing transplantation (Helgeland 1983). Hyperuricaemia occurs in about 30–55 per cent of renal transplant recipients during the first 2 years (Kahan et al. 1987) and was associated with gout in 11.8 per cent of patients (West et al. 1987). Others have reported higher incidences of hyperuricaemia (Gores et al. 1988; Lin et al. 1989). Detailed studies of urate metabolism showed that the hyperuricaemia is due to decreased urate clearance (Lin et al. 1989).

Nicotinic acid at a dose of 1.5 g thrice daily (Gershon and Fox 1974) and the antituberculous drug ethambutol (German and Holmes 1986) have been found to reduce uric acid excretion and cause hyperuricaemia.

Suprofen, an NSAID, has been reported to cause a syndrome with acute flank pain, postulated to be due to diffuse crystallization of uric acid in the renal tubules (Strom *et al.* 1989). The NSAID azapropazone, diflunisal, and indomethacin decrease renal clearance of urate (Tiitinen *et al.* 1983). Lead poisoning is also associated with hyperuricaemia and gout (Goyer 1989; Poor and Mituszova 1989), probably owing to the effects of lead on the kidney (Cameron and Simmonds 1981; Kelly *et al.* 1989), the mechanism of which is not known.

Ramipril, an ACE inhibitor, increased serum uric acid in hypertensive subjects (Walter *et al.* 1987).

Renal impairment may be responsible for the hyperuricaemia seen in some patients receiving azapropazone and that seen in amoxapine overdose (Thompson and Dempsey 1983; Sipila *et al.* 1986). The anticoagulant warfarin was reported to increase uric acid levels significantly, probably as a result of increased production (Menon *et al.* 1986), but this was not confirmed by others (Walker *et al.* 1988). In those treated with the β-adrenoceptor blocker propranolol, there was a tendency for serum uric acid concentration to increase (Helgeland 1983; Sugino *et al.* 1984). Treatment with the H_2-receptor antagonists cimetidine and ranitidine (Einarson *et al.* 1985), or with levodopa (Honda and Gindin 1972) was reported to cause gouty arthritis. The use of the anaesthetic agent methoxyflurane was associated with increased serum uric acid levels probably due to the nephrotoxic effect of fluoride on distal tubular function (Hamilton and Robertson 1974).

Hypouricaemia

Hypouricaemia due to decreased production is seen with the use of xanthine oxidase inhibitors such as allopurinol and azathioprine (Emmerson 1983).

Increased urate excretion is seen in volume expansion and this has been suggested as the mechanism of the hypouricaemia and hyponatraemia in the syndrome of inappropriate secretion of antidiuretic hormone (SIADH) (Beck 1979; DeCaux *et al.* 1985). Uricosuric drugs such as probenecid, sulphinpyrazone, benzbromarone, and benziodarone all reduce serum urate by increasing urate clearance. High doses of aspirin and phenylbutazone have a similar effect (Palella and Fox 1989).

Many radiographic contrast media (such as iopanoic acid, sodium diatrizoate, and meglumine iodipamide) are uricosuric and cause a decrease in the serum urate

level (Postlethwaite and Kelley 1971). Serum uric acid levels were found to be lowered in epileptic patients on long-term antiepileptic drugs, especially with phenytoin (Krause *et al.* 1987). A number of anticoagulants, such as ethylbiscoumacetate, phenindione, and dicoumarol cause hypouricaemia (Holmes 1985; Palella and Fox 1989). Other drugs that have been shown to cause a low serum urate are Etofibrate (a derivative of clofibrate with nicotinic acid) (Degenring *et al.* 1983), the anticholinergic agent glycopyrrolate, glyceryl guaiacolate (a common component of cough mixtures), the antipsychotic drug chlorprothixene (Shalev *et al.* 1987*a*), and prednisone and other adrenal steroids (Emmerson 1983).

Urinastatin, a proteinase inhibitor, reduces serum uric acid levels in patients treated with cisplatin (Umeki *et al.* 1989). Traxanox and tienilic acid reduce serum uric acid and increase uric acid excretion in hypertensive patients (Lau *et al.* 1977; Bolli *et al.* 1978; Fujimura *et al.* 1989). Oxaprozin, a propionic acid analogue, was reported to cause a fall in serum uric acid and increased excretion of uric acid in healthy volunteers (Goldfarb *et al.* 1985). Indacrinone, a loop diuretic, has a uricosuric effect and causes hypouricaemia (Vlasses *et al.* 1984). Any drug or agent that causes a Fanconi-like syndrome will cause hypouricaemia (see section on Acidosis and Chapter 12).

Oxalate

Healthy subjects excrete less than 0.45 mmol of oxalate per 24 hours (Kasidas 1988; Williams and Wandzilak 1989). Approximately 10–20 per cent of urinary oxalate comes from dietary sources such as cocoa, tea, rhubarb, and spinach while the rest comes from endogenous metabolism of precursors, mainly glyoxylate and ascorbic acid. About 35–50 per cent of the total oxalate comes from ascorbic acid (Hillman 1989); the major sources of glyoxylate include glycine, glycolic acid, and serine (Willams and Wandzilak 1989). Oxalate is excreted almost exclusively in the urine, and renal tubular secretion plays an important role (Hillman 1989). Hyperoxaluria can arise as a result of primary genetic disorders, of which there are two types. Type I is due to a defect in the (peroxisomal) enzyme alanine glyoxylate aminotransferase and Type II, which is rare, is due to a defect in hydroxypyruvate metabolism (Hillman 1989). Secondary hyperoxaluria can result from excessive production of oxalate, due either to an increase in endogenous synthesis or increased intake of oxalate precursors.

Increased excretion of oxalate

Hyperoxaluria and renal failure may follow administration of the anaesthetic agent methoxyflurane, which is metabolised to oxalate (Frascino *et al.* 1970; Taves *et al.* 1970; McIntyre *et al.* 1973). Abuse of methoxyflurane was reported to cause hyperoxaluria and widespread retinal crystalline deposits (Novak *et al.* 1988). Xylitol, which has been used in parenteral nutrition as a source of calories, may also lead to hyperoxaluria (Thomas *et al.* 1972; Rofe *et al.* 1979). It may follow the use of glycine-rich fluid during prostatectomy (Fitzpatrick *et al.* 1981; Arvieux *et al.* 1984, 1985) and of ascorbic acid during total parenteral nutrition (Swartz *et al.* 1984). Increased intake of ascorbic acid by mouth can lead to hyperox-aluria (Briggs *et al.* 1973; Schmidt *et al.* 1981), which is a potential adverse effect of 'megadoses' of ascorbic acid (Sestili 1983).

Hyperoxaluria due to increased intestinal absorption follows oral phosphate administration in the treatment of hypophosphataemic rickets (Reusz *et al.* 1990). Long-term administration (for 6 months) of the somatostatin analogue octreotide to a patient with carcinoid tumour caused hyperoxaluria and renal stones, probably due to increased intestinal absorption of oxalate (Ranft and Eibl-Eibesfeldt 1990). Pyridoxilate, used in the treatment of angina pectoris or arterial insufficiency, contains an equimolar combination of glyoxylate and pyridoxine and causes increased excretion of oxalate and renal stones (Daudon *et al.* 1987). Ingestion of 250 g of sucrose daily for 7 days increased oxalate excretion (Li *et al.* 1986).

Decreased excretion of oxalate

Administration of magnesium (Berg *et al.* 1986) or calcium (Caspray *et al.* 1977; Barilla *et al.* 1978) reduces the excretion of oxalate, presumably by precipitating oxalate in the intestinal lumen. Cholestyramine binds to oxalate in the intestine and reduces its excretion (Caspray *et al.* 1977). Aluminium hydroxide has similar actions (Nordenvall *et al.* 1983). Allopurinol, in addition to reducing uric acid excretion, also reduces oxalate excretion (Ettinger *et al.* 1986; Hesse *et al.* 1987). Pyridoxine administration to recurrent stone-formers (Harrison *et al.* 1981) was reported to lower the excretion of oxalate.

Proteins

Protein metabolism can be affected by many drugs and hormones. Of the hormones, glucocorticoids and thyroxine are catabolic and cause a net negative balance. Oestrogens stimulate androgens and tend to decrease the synthesis of several plasma proteins by the liver (see below). Androgens are anabolic at the tissue level and increase the tissue protein content and this is accompanied by a positive nitrogen balance.

Total plasma protein

Increase in total plasma protein

Agents or drugs that produce volume depletion will cause an increase in plasma total protein concentration (see section on Sodium and Water). Vasopressor drugs, like adrenaline, noradrenaline, and angiotensin will raise the plasma protein concentration due to vasoconstriction and loss of protein-free fluid to the extravascular space (Young 1990). Drugs (e.g. growth hormone) that increase hepatic protein synthesis will cause an increase in plasma total protein concentration. Plasma protein concentrations are reported to be raised in heroin and cocaine addicts (Marks and Chapple 1967). Felodipine infusion caused a small but significant increase in total protein concentration (Sluiter *et al.* 1984).

Decreased plasma protein concentration

The concentration of total protein will decrease in all situations in which there is an increase in ECF volume or total body water (see section on Sodium and Water). Oestrogens and oestrogen-containing contraceptives can decrease total protein concentration (Sadik *et al.* 1985). Significant (13.7 per cent) decrease in total protein was produced by non-ionic radiographic contrast medium (Brunet *et al.* 1989) and this could not be explained by dilution. Exposure to lead caused a significant decrease in plasma total protein concentration (Wagnerova *et al.* 1986).

Artefacts

Many drugs or agents can interfere with total protein determination and cause spuriously low or high results. Drugs that have been reported as causing an apparent increase in total protein concentration are aspirin (Jelic-Ivanovic *et al.* 1985*a*), carbenicillin (Letellier and Desjarlais 1985) and other penicillins, cephalothin, chloramphenicol (Young 1990), dextrans (Barnes *et al.* 1985; Flack and Woolen 1984), and radiographic contrast media. Drugs that cause an apparent decrease are aspirin (Jelic-Ivanovic *et al.* 1985*b*), caproxamine (Jaden-Starodoubsky *et al.* 1973), cefotaxime (Baer *et al.* 1983), dextran 40, and sulphasalazine (Moriarty *et al.* 1983). The effect depends on the method of determination of total protein. For example, aspirin decreases the total protein concentration measured by the biuret method and increases it by the spectrophotometric method (Jelic-Ivanovic *et al.* 1985*a*).

Albumin

Albumin, which has a molecular weight of about 68 000 is synthesized by the liver and accounts for 40–60 per cent of the total protein concentration in plasma.

Increase in plasma albumin

Plasma albumin concentration will be high in situations similar to that for plasma total protein.

Decrease in plasma albumin

The plasma albumin concentrations will decrease in hepatocellular disease caused by drugs (see Chapter 11) and in drug-induced malabsorption syndromes (see Chapter 10). Decreased albumin synthesis is probably responsible for the decrease in albumin concentration seen after administration of oestrogen and the contraceptive pill (Adlercreutz et al. 1968; Cavalieri et al. 1979; Sadik et al. 1985). Contraceptive pills with low oestrogen content or steroids with an oestrogenic effect do not affect plasma albumin concentration (Hawkins and Benster 1977). Phenytoin has been reported by some to cause a decrease in plasma albumin concentration (Andreasen et al. 1973; Haruda 1979), whereas others failed to find any effect (Jacobsen et al. 1976; Parker and Shearer 1979). Valproate decreased plasma albumin levels (Sussman and McLain 1979; Le Bihan et al. 1980; Itoh et al. 1982), but other anticonvulsants had no effect (Salway 1989). Other drugs that have been reported to cause a decrease in plasma albumin concentration in a single case or few cases include gold salts (Griffin 1979; Pessayre et al. 1979a), flurbiprofen (Kotowski and Grayson 1982), indomethacin (Fenech et al. 1967), propylthiouracil (Mihas et al. 1976), perhexiline maleate (Paliard et al. 1978), oxyphenisatin (Goldstein et al. 1973), and nitrofurantoin (Klemola et al. 1975; Bouchard et al. 1982). The clinical significance of these findings remains to be established. Ibuprofen decreased plasma albumin by 20 per cent in rheumatoid patients (Jelic-Ivanovic et al. 1985b).

Artefacts

Pencillin, heparin (Hardy and Bjurstrom 1984), salicylate (Notrica et al. 1972), and clofibrate (Calvo et al. 1985) interfere with some methods of albumin measurement and cause an apparent decrease in albumin level.

Prealbumin

Prealbumin, which has a molecular weight of 54 000, is synthesized by the liver, and because of its short half-life serves as a sensitive marker of protein malnutrition. It acts as a carrier protein for thyroid hormone and for vitamin A in association with retinol-binding protein.

Increase in plasma prealbumin

The prealbumin concentration is increased by androgens and anabolic steroids (Barbosa et al. 1971; Culberg 1984) owing to increased hepatic synthesis. Prednisolone, betamethasone (Gamstedt et al. 1979, 1981), propranolol (Franklyn et al. 1985a), and intravenous nutrition (Young et al. 1979) increase prealbumin concentrations. Ornithine α-ketoglutarate, given in addition to intravenous nutrition, further improved nitrogen balance and prealbumin levels (Demarcq et al. 1984).

Decrease in plasma prealbumin

Plasma concentrations of prealbumin decrease during pregnancy (Franklyn et al. 1983) and after administration of oestrogens or oral contraceptives (Schatz et al. 1968; Barbosa et al. 1971). Amiodarone decreases prealbumin levels by about 20 per cent (Franklyn et al. 1985b).

Retinol-binding protein (RBP)

Retinol-binding protein is a low-molecular-weight protein (21 000) and is synthesized by the liver. In association with prealbumin it transports vitamin A. Plasma RBP level is a useful indicator of protein nutritional status.

Increase in plasma RBP

Like other plasma proteins (SHBG, TBG), RBP levels are increased by oestrogens and oral contraceptives (Cumming and Briggs 1983; Gleeson et al. 1987). The anticonvulsants phenobarbitone, phenytoin, and carbamazepine increase the levels (Olsson et al. 1983; Kozlowski et al. 1987). Cord-blood RBP levels are increased in babies born to mothers who had been given betamethasone before delivery (Georgieff et al. 1988). As with prealbumin, plasma RBP levels are increased by intravenous nutrition (Young et al. 1979).

Decrease in plasma RBP

Administration of growth hormone (GH) to GH-deficient children caused a significant reduction in RBP (Kemp and Canfield 1983).

Cortisol-binding globulin (CBG)

Cortisol-binding globulin is an α-globulin which carries about 90 per cent of circulating cortisol. It is increased by oestrogens (Barbosa *et al.* 1971) and oestrogen-containing contraceptive pills and decreased by androgens (Barbosa *et al.* 1971).

Thyroxine-binding globulin (TBG)

Thyroxine-binding globulin binds and transports the thyroid hormones T_4 and T_3.

Increase in plasma TBG

Oestrogens and oral contraceptives increase TBG levels (Carey 1971), an effect similar to that in pregnancy (Franklyn *et al.* 1983; Swaminathan *et al.* 1989). The increase in TBG is dose-dependent. Tamoxifen, with its weak oestrogen effect, has been reported by some to increase TBG (Gordon *et al.* 1986), whereas others did not find any effect (Jensen 1985). Carbamazepine increased TBG in hypothyroid patients (Aanderud *et al.* 1981) but had no effect in euthyroid volunteers (Connell *et al.* 1984*a*) or epileptics (De Luca *et al.* 1986) during short-term treatment, but a decrease in TBG level was reported with longer term treatment (Strandjord *et al.* 1981). Clofibrate (Young 1990), long-term methadone treatment (Bastomsky *et al.* 1977), clomipramine (Schlienger *et al.* 1980), perphenazine (Chattoraj and Watts 1986), and phenothiazines (Young 1990) are some of the other drugs reported to increase plasma TBG concentration.

Decrease in plasma TBG

Androgens and steroids with androgenic properties such as danazol and stanozolol decrease TBG concentration (Pannall and Maas 1977). Glucocorticoids (Gamstedt *et al.* 1979, 1981) decrease TBG levels. Other drugs reported to decrease plasma TBG concentration are propranolol (Wilkinson *et al.* 1983; Wilkins *et al.* 1985; Franklyn *et al.* 1985*a*), nadolol (Wilkinson *et al.* 1983), colaspase (asparaginase) (Garnick and Larson 1979; Heidemann *et al.* 1980, 1981), co-trimoxazole (Cohen *et al.* 1981), fenclofenac (Ratcliffe *et al.* 1980), fluoxymesterone (Morley *et al.* 1981), colestipol, oxandrolone (Heidemann *et al.* 1980), and phenytoin (Suzuki *et al.* 1984); this last has also been reported to have no effect on TBG (Larsen *et al.* 1970), but this may have been due to the short duration of treatment. TBG levels were within the reference range in eight subjects treated with fenclofenac (John *et al.* 1983).

Sex-hormone-binding globulin (SHBG)

Sex-hormone-binding globulin (SHBG) is a glycoprotein with a high affinity for sex steroid hormones, in particular 5α-dihydrotestosterone and testosterone. The affinity for oestradiol is lower (Lindstedt *et al.* 1985).

Increase in serum SHBG

Sex-hormone-binding globulin levels are increased by oestrogens and oral contraceptives (Lindstedt *et al.* 1985; Ottosson *et al.* 1986). Of the oestrogens, ethinyl-oestradiol was more potent than oestradiol valerate (Mall-Haefeli *et al.* 1983). Furthermore, oestrogen was less effective when administered percutaneously than when given orally (Nilsson *et al.* 1984). The increase in SHBG induced by oestrogens is sometimes used as a sensitive index of oestrogen effect (Ottosson *et al.* 1986). Oestrogen-containing oral contraceptive pills increase the SHBG level by 46–213 per cent (Bergink *et al.* 1981; Vermeulen and Thiery 1982; Murphy *et al.* 1990). Dexamethasone increased SHBG levels by 35.5 per cent in hirsute women (Cunningham *et al.* 1985), whereas large doses of glucocorticoids decreased the levels (Lindstedt *et al.* 1985). Administration of excess thyroid hormone (Ruder *et al.* 1971), and the anticonvulsants phenobarbitone, phenytoin, valproate, primidone, and carbamazepine increase SHBG levels (Barragry *et al.* 1978; Dana-Haeri *et al.* 1982; Beastall *et al.* 1985). The increase induced by carbamazepine was seen within 7 days of starting the drug (Connell *et al.* 1984*b*) and the levels increased by 110 per cent in epileptics treated with phenytoin (Toone *et al.* 1980; Dana-Haeri *et al.* 1982). Rifampicin, the antituberculous drug, caused 47–75 per cent increase in SHBG levels (Back *et al.* 1980; Brodie *et al.* 1981; Lonning *et al.* 1989). The synthetic anti-oestrogen clomiphene citrate produces a moderate rise in serum SHBG levels (Marshall *et al.* 1972). The antifungal agent ketoconazole, which affects steroidogenesis, increases the serum SHBG level (Heyns *et al.* 1985). Fluconazole, a novel antifungal agent, produced no significant rise in SHBG (Devenport *et al.* 1989).

Decrease in serum SHBG

A fall in serum SHBG concentration occurs during treatment with androgens (Lindstedt *et al.* 1985) or androgenic steroids such as danazol (Wynn 1977) and stanozolol (Small *et al.* 1984). Progestogens such as medroxyprogesterone acetate (Tomic *et al.* 1988), levonorgestrel (Ruokonen and Kaar 1985; Song *et al.* 1989), lynoestrenol (Ruokonen and Kaar 1985), megestrol (Alexieva-Figusch *et al.* 1984), and desogestrel (Cullberg 1984) cause a decrease in SHBG levels. Cyproterone acetate, which has some progestogenic activity, decreases SHBG levels in hirsute women (Vincens *et al.* 1989).

Haptoglobin

Haptoglobin, which binds free haemoglobin in plasma, is an acute-phase reactant and is a glycoprotein which moves in the α_2 region.

Increase in plasma haptoglobin

Androgens and steroids with androgenic activity increase plasma haptoglobin levels (Barbosa *et al.* 1971). High doses of medroxyprogesterone acetate used in the treatment of prostatic and renal carcinoma caused a significant increase in haptoglobin levels (Nilsson *et al.* 1989).

Decrease in plasma haptoglobin

Haptoglobin levels decrease whenever there is free haemoglobin in the circulation, and drugs like dapsone, that cause haemolytic anaemia (see Chapter 22), will cause a decrease in plasma haptoglobin (Young 1990). Oestrogens and oestrogen-containing contraceptives decrease the plasma haptoglobin level, probably by reducing hepatic synthesis (Briggs and Briggs 1971; Lipsett *et al.* 1971). Colaspase (asparaginase) decreases haptoglobin levels, possibly by decreasing hepatic synthesis (Menard *et al.* 1980). Dextrose, given intravenously, decreases haptoglobin, possibly by forming a complex (Skrede *et al.* 1973). Treatment of rheumatoid arthritis patients with adrenal steroids decreased plasma haptoglobin (McConkey *et al.* 1973), possibly due to a decrease in acute-phase response.

Caeruloplasmin

Caeruloplasmin is the principal copper-containing protein of plasma and is a late acute-phase reactant. Its possible function is as an antioxidant.

Increase in plasma caeruloplasmin

Oestrogens increase the synthesis of caeruloplasmin and elevated levels are seen in patients taking oestrogens and oestrogen-containing contraceptive pills (Meani and Cartei 1970). Norethindrone and tamoxifen, because of their oestrogen effects, increase caeruloplasmin levels (Rossner and Wallgren 1984; Song *et al.* 1989). The anticonvulsant drugs phenobarbitone, phenytoin, and carbamazepine, either alone or in combination, increase caeruloplasmin levels (Olsson *et al.* 1983; Werther *et al.* 1986). In copper poisoning, higher levels of serum caeruloplasmin are found (Young 1990). As caeruloplasmin is an acute-phase protein, it is increased in many conditions, e.g. rheumatoid arthritis (Peretz *et al.* 1989*b*). Exposure to vinyl chloride, once commonly employed as an aerosol propellant and in cosmetics, but now banned for this use in many countries (Bencko *et al.* 1988; Wagnerova *et al.* 1988), and lead (Wagnerova *et al.* 1986) causes an increase in caeruloplasmin levels.

Decrease in plasma caeruloplasmin

Colaspase (asparaginase) decreases the synthesis and plasma levels of caeruloplasmin (Oettgen *et al.* 1970; Menard *et al.* 1980). Levonorgestrel, used as a contraceptive implant or as a contraceptive pill, caused a significant fall in caeruloplasmin levels (Shaaban *et al.* 1984). Plasma caeruloplasmin levels are also low in malnutrition, malabsorption, the nephrotic syndrome, and severe liver disease (Silverman *et al.* 1986).

Transferrin (TRF)

Transferrin is the principal transporter of iron in plasma. It is a negative acute-phase reactant and is a β-globulin with a molecular weight of 77 000.

Increase in serum TRF

A progressive increase in TRF is seen in pregnancy (Rosenmund *et al.* 1986). Oestrogens and oral contraceptives have a similar effect but not to the same degree as pregnancy (Horne *et al.* 1970). Low-oestrogen oral contraceptives have no effect on TRF levels (Rosenmund *et al.* 1986). Increased plasma TRF levels were found in the cord blood of infants whose mothers had betamethasone treatment prior to delivery (Georgieff *et al.* 1988). Transferrin in plasma exists in different isoforms differing in their carbohydrate content. Alcohol abuse increases one of these transferrins (carbohydrate-deficient transferrin) (Crabb 1990). Exposure to organic solvents caused a similar increase in this isotransferrin (Petren and Vesterberg 1987). Serum TRF is increased by GH administration to GH-deficient children (Kemp and Canfield 1983).

Decrease in plasma TRF

Testosterone (Barbosa *et al.* 1971), colaspase (asparaginase) (Oettgen *et al.* 1970; Menard *et al.* 1980), and cortisone cause a reduction in plasma TRF by decreasing synthesis. High-molecular-weight dextran (dextran 70) decreases plasma TRF, while low-molecular-weight dextran (dextran 40) does not (Skrede *et al.* 1973).

Fibrinogen

Fibrinogen, a large dimeric protein, is converted to fibrin by thrombin and polymerizes to form an insoluble gel.

Increase in plasma fibrinogen

Plasma fibrinogen concentrations are increased by oestrogens and oestrogen-containing oral contraceptives (Simpson 1971; Lipsett et al. 1971) because of increased synthesis by the liver. Pyrazinamide, xanthine, and aspirin raise fibrinogen levels in some patients (Young 1990).

Decrease in plasma fibrinogen

Androgens and anabolic steroids decrease the plasma fibrinogen (Barbosa et al. 1971; Nugent et al. 1986), as do clofibrate (Chakrabarti et al. 1968), dextrans (Skrede et al. 1973), fluroxene (Johnston et al. 1973), kanamycin, and valproic acid (Sussman and McLain 1979). Celiprolol, an antihypertensive drug, caused an unexpected decrease in serum fibrinogen level (Herrmann and Mayer 1988).

Immunoglobulins (α-globulin)

Increase in plasma immunoglobulins

An increase in γ-globulin due to stimulation of antibody production followed treatment with aminopyrine, hydantoin derivatives, methimazole, propylthiouracil (Wing and Fantus 1987), and tubocurarine (Stovner et al. 1972). Colaspase (asparaginase) (Oettgen et al. 1970), nitrofurantoin (Holmberg et al. 1980), and tolazamide (Young 1990) have also been reported to increase immunoglobulins. Serum concentrations of immunoglobulins A, G, and M are increased by administration of colaspase (Oettgen et al. 1970), methyldopa (Delpre et al. 1979), and nitrofurantoin (Miller et al. 1982). Oxyphenisatin increased IgG and IgM by causing chronic active hepatitis (Dietrichson 1975). Chlorpromazine treatment in schizophrenic patients increases IgM levels in a dose-dependent manner (Zarrabi et al. 1979).

Decrease in plasma immunoglobulins

A fall in plasma immunoglobulins follows the administration of gold, methotrexate, and prednisone (Christensen et al. 1985). Decrease in immunoglobulins A, G, and M follows administration of aurothioglucose (van Riel et al. 1984), glucocorticoids (Butler and Rossen 1973; Bond 1977) and phenytoin (Sorrell et al. 1971; Bardana et al. 1984). Dextrans (Skrede et al. 1973) and carbamazepine (Gilhus et al. 1982) decrease plasma IgA and IgM. Administration of T_4 to infants with hypothyroidism decreased serum IgA levels (Seager 1984).

Serum enzymes

Enzymes found in the blood can be classified according to their site of function: (a) enzymes that act or function in plasma (plasma-specific enzymes, e.g. those involved in the blood-clotting mechanism or fibrinolysis); (b) enzymes that are secreted — enzymes of the gastrointestinal tract exemplify this group; (c) cellular enzymes that function intracellularly — most clinically relevant enzymes fall into this category. This section is mainly concerned with cellular enzymes. These are present in various compartments of the cell such as cytoplasm, mitochondria, and lysosomes. They are present in small amounts in the serum of normal subjects, and the amount increases in various disease processes. This increase is used diagnostically. The pathophysiological mechanisms involved in changes in serum enzymes are, however, not fully understood (Pappas 1989). Some of the factors thought to influence the concentration of serum enzymes in health and disease are: the rate of release of the enzyme (due to cell death or injury and increased synthesis), rate of clearance of the enzyme, and leakage of the enzyme from the cells (for review see Pappas 1989).

Drugs may cause changes in serum enzymes due to injury or damage to an organ (e.g. large doses of paracetamol cause elevation of AST) or due to increased synthesis (e.g. increased synthesis of GGT by alcohol or barbiturates).

Creatine kinase

Creatine kinase (ATP: creatine N-phosphotransferase; EC2.7.3.2, CK) is widely distributed throughout the human body but is particularly concentrated in muscle tissues. Three cytosolic isoenzymes (CK-MM, CK-MB, CK-BB) and one mitochondrial isoenzyme of CK have been identified (Apple 1989). The tissue sources are primarily skeletal muscle for CK-MM, heart for CK-MB, and brain for CK-BB (Lott and Stang 1989). In the circulation the tissue forms of the enzyme are converted to serum forms by loss of the c-terminal residue. The resulting serum isoforms are termed MM_1, MM_2, MM_3, MB_1 and MB_2 (for review see Jones and Swaminathan 1990).

Increase in serum CK

Increase in serum CK may follow strenuous exercise (Nicholson et al. 1985; Lott and Wolf 1986a) or intramuscular injections (Konikoff et al. 1985; Jones and Swaminathan 1990). Several drugs can cause elevation of CK (Lott and Landesman 1984), some by causing rhabdomyolysis. The mechanism by which other drugs cause an elevation in CK may be a disturbance in membrane function or an actual toxic effect on the cells (Lott and

Wolf 1986*a*). A classification of drug-induced muscle damage is given by Blain and Lane (1983) (and see Chapter 18).

Aminocaproic acid therapy in a few patients causes acute muscle cell injury and elevation of CK (see Blain and Lane 1983). Clofibrate treatment causes a mild increase in serum CK in some patients (Langer and Levy 1968; Dujovne *et al.* 1976), but a more pronounced rise is seen in obese (Belaiche *et al.* 1977) and renal failure patients (Pierides and Alvasez-Ude 1975). Some of these patients have myalgia or acute muscle cramps or weakness which disappears on stopping clofibrate treatment (Schneider *et al.* 1980).

In alcoholics, elevated CK levels may be seen due to alcoholic rhabdomyolysis (DiSilvio 1978). A direct toxic effect of alcohol on skeletal muscle causing loss of cellular integrity has also been suggested (Spargo 1984). Drugs such as thiazide diuretics, carbenoxolone, licorice, purgatives, and amphotericin cause skeletal muscle damage and a moderate rise in CK due to hypokalaemia (Sunderam and Swaminathan 1981; Argov and Mastaglia 1988).

Other drugs or agents that cause rhabdomyolysis are drugs of abuse such as opiates and heroin (Lott and Wolf 1986*a*), drugs which cause hypophosphataemia (see section on Phosphate), phencyclidine (Lott and Wolf 1986*a*), amphetamines (Blain and Lane 1983), and phenylpropanolamine (Swenson *et al.* 1982).

The phenothiazines prochloperazine, perphenazine, and thioridazine, and the butyrophenone haloperidol have been shown to increase CK levels in some patients (Lui 1979; Pearlman *et al.* 1988), and in others withdrawal of the drugs caused elevation of CK (Malas and van Kammen 1982) and sometimes a malignant neuroleptic syndrome (Gibb and Lees 1985; Goldwasser *et al.* 1989).

Elevated CK levels were observed in overdose with the tricyclic antidepressants imipramine (Sueblinvong and Wilson 1969) and amitriptyline (Guthrie and Lott 1986), and the β-blockers pindolol (Saruta *et al.* 1985), propranolol (Forfar *et al.* 1979), labetalol (Teicher *et al.* 1981), bucindolol (Reid *et al.* 1985), and carteolol (Saruta *et al.* 1985) caused elevation of serum CK. Increase in CK is more common and more marked with pindolol, and isoenzyme studies show the elevation to be due mainly to the MM type (Saruta *et al.* 1985).

The β-adrenoreceptor agonist salbutamol has been associated with muscle cramps and elevated CK (Lisi 1989). Elevated CK-MB levels observed in children with status asthmaticus treated with isoprenaline are suggested to be an indication of myocardial injury associated with this treatment (Maguire *et al.* 1986). Theophylline over-

dosage is associated with gross elevation of total CK and the MM isoenzyme (Modi *et al.* 1985). The elevation is partly due to hypokalaemia-induced muscle damage and partly to CK release from muscle as a result of grand mal seizures. Quinidine therapy was reported to cause gross elevation in CK and CK-MM isoenzyme in one patient (Weiss *et al.* 1979), levels returning to normal once the drug was stopped and increasing again when the drug was restarted. Elevation of CK and mild myopathy have been found in patients treated with bumetanide, metolazone (Blain and Lane 1983), danazol (Spaulding 1979), stanozolol (Sheffer *et al.* 1981), lithium (Ghose 1977), emetine and vincristine (Argov and Mastaglia 1988). In overdosage with such drugs as barbiturates (Sabiniewicz and Szajewski 1979), gluthethimide (Henderson *et al.* 1970), and amoxapine (Abero *et al.* 1982), CK levels are elevated probably as a result of crush injury (Lott and Wolf 1986*a*). Elevated total CK, CK-MB, and BB levels were found in a case of salicylate overdose (Vladutiu and Reitz 1980). Isotretinoin, a retinoid used in the treatment of acne, caused a marked increase in CK (McBurney and Rosen 1984).

Radiographic contrast agents caused an elevation of serum CK after 24 hours (Carlsson *et al.* 1985) and isoenzyme studies showed that there is elevation of B subunits, probably due to breakdown of the blood–brain barrier (Pfeiffer *et al.* 1987).

Intramuscular injections of ampicillin, carbenicillin, chlordiazepoxide, digoxin, fluphenazine, lignocaine, pentazocine, and pethidine have been reported to cause elevation of CK (Salway 1989). In many cases the degree of elevation was greater than expected from the injection, suggesting that the drugs caused muscle damage in some manner.

A small increase in CK followed long-term administration of captopril (Katayama *et al.* 1987); halofenate, a hypolipidaemic agent (Dujovne *et al.* 1976); and HMG co-reductase inhibitors (Walker 1988).

Steroids cause a myopathy and can cause an elevation of CK in some patients and a decrease in others (Lott and Wolf 1986*a*). In subjects who are susceptible to malignant hyperthermia, halothane, suxamethonium, and lignocaine can cause gross elevation of CK (Paasuke and Brownell 1986; Rosenberg and Fletcher 1986; Argov and Mastaglia 1988), and suxamethonium can also cause an elevation of serum CK in patients without this disorder (Umino *et al.* 1985; Lott and Wolf 1986*a*).

Decrease in serum CK

A decrease from initially high values is seen in schizophrenic patients treated with a phenothiazine (Young 1990). Decreased CK values are also seen in women during the luteal phase of menstruation, in women taking alcohol (Paterson and Lawrence 1972), in pregnancy (King *et al.* 1972), and in some patients given prednisolone (Lott and Wolf 1986*a*).

Artefacts

A decrease in serum CK levels is seen due to *in vitro* effects of acetylsalicylic acid, clothiapine, EDTA, heparin, and pindolol (Young 1990). Freezing and thawing of samples decreases the activity by 50 per cent. Thiols such as cysteine and cystine increase the measured CK activity (Young 1990).

Lactate dehydrogenase

Lactate dehydrogenase (LD), a zinc-containing enzyme that catalyses the oxidation of lactate to pyruvate, is present in the cytoplasm of all cells (Wolf 1989). Highest levels are found in skeletal muscle, liver, heart, kidney, and red blood cells. LD is a tetramer composed of two subunits, H and M, and five isoenzymes can be demonstrated. Recently a sixth isoenzyme of LD has been described (Wolf 1989).

Increase in serum LD

Since LD is present in high concentrations in muscle, heart, liver, and red blood cells, drugs that cause damage to these organs or cells can be expected to cause elevation of serum LD.

Hepatic necrosis or injury caused by drugs such as paracetamol, halothane (Sherlock 1971), xylitol (Schumer 1971), and drugs that cause cholestasis, such as imipramine (Karkalas and Lal 1971), will lead to an elevation of LD. Drugs that cause muscle damage and release CK will also cause an elevation of LD (e.g. in rhabdomyolysis induced by alcohol).

Decrease in serum LD

Serum LD tends to decrease with age, and fluoride and clofibrate cause a decrease in serum LD by an *in vivo* effect (Young 1990).

Artefacts

Drugs or chemicals that have been shown to decrease serum LD by analytical interference are oxalate, aspirin, ascorbic acid, cefotaxime, ketoprofen, methotrexate, and theophylline. Paracetamol, caffeine, phenobarbitone, rifampicin, and triamterene have been reported to increase the activity of LD (Young 1990).

Aminotransferases (transaminases)

These are a group of enzymes that catalyse the reversible transfer of the amino group from an α-amino group to an oxo acid. Although there are over 50 such enzymes, only 2, aspartate aminotransferase (AST, SGOT, EC 2.6.1.1) and alanine aminotransferase (ALT, SGPT, EC 2.6.1.2) are used widely in clinical practice. Both enzymes are widely distributed in tissues, high concentrations of AST being found in liver, heart, skeletal muscle, and kidney, but high concentrations of ALT being found mainly in the liver. Isoenzymes of AST and ALT exist in both mitochondria and cytoplasm (Rej 1989).

Asparate aminotransferase (AST, SGOT)

AST is a dimer of two identical subunits, and two isoenzymes have been identified: a mitochondrial form of AST and a cytoplasmic form of AST.

Increase in AST

An increased serum AST may originate from liver, heart, or skeletal muscle. Serum AST is elevated in any type of hepatocellular injury, and over 300 drugs are reported to cause a rise in AST levels in this way (Young 1990) (see also Chapter 11).

Anticonvulsant treatment with phenytoin, carbamazepine, or valproate causes a significant increase in AST activity (Deutsch *et al.* 1986; Aldenhovel 1988), as do sulphasalazine (Farr *et al.* 1985; Dougados *et al.* 1987), ritodrine, and fenoterol (Rej 1989), this last being seen in cord blood of neonates born to mothers being treated with it (Kovacs *et al.* 1985). Heparin therapy causes elevation of AST (Dukes *et al.* 1984; Monreal *et al.* 1989) and this is more common with conventional heparin than with the low-molecular-weight form (Monreal *et al.* 1989). The exact mechanism of this increase is not known but may involve induction of enzymes. In patients treated with the HMG-CoA reductase inhibitors lovastatin and simvastatin, increases in AST were seen (Walker 1988). Another hypocholesterolaemic agent, nicotinyl alcohol (pyridylcarbinol), has also been reported to cause increased AST (Keller *et al.* 1988). The antimicrobial agents teicoplanin (Bibler *et al.* 1987) and aztreonam (Miller *et al.* 1983) are known to cause elevation of AST. The NSAID fenbufen (Crossley 1983) and suprofen (Michos *et al.* 1985) cause elevation of AST by their hepatotoxic effects (Prescott 1986*a,b*). Diethylcarbamazine (Awadzi *et al.* 1986) and the antimetabolite 5-fluoro-2-deoxyceridine (Doria *et al.* 1986) have been reported to cause significant but reversible elevation of AST.

Serum AST is increased in drug-induced disorders of muscle. All drugs mentioned in the section on CK will therefore cause elevation of AST.

Decrease in serum AST

Drugs affecting vitamin B_6 status or which react with pyridoxal phosphate reduce serum AST (Rej 1989). The effect of cefazolin in decreasing AST levels in experimental animals may be due to the reaction of the drug with pyridoxal phosphate (Dhami *et al.* 1979). Haemodialysis may decrease AST levels, owing to loss of pyridoxal phosphate (Wolf *et al.* 1972). In haemophiliacs, treatment with stanozolol caused a decrease in AST levels abnormal at the start of the treatment (Greer *et al.* 1985). A significant decrease in AST was reported in users of one high-oestrogen oral contraceptive (Walden *et al.* 1986).

Artefacts

Drugs may interfere with the analytical method of measurement of AST and cause an artefactual increase or decrease (Young 1990). Drugs that have been reported to cause a decrease in AST include metronidazole (Dennis and Ericksen 1980; Rosenblatt and Edson 1987), rifampicin (Ball *et al.* 1987), pindolol (Inloes *et al.* 1987), and ibuprofen (Jelic-Ivanovic *et al.* 1984). Drugs like chlordiazepoxide (Letellier and Desjarlais 1985), fluorescein (Inloes *et al.* 1987), and isoniazid (Singh *et al.* 1972) cause an apparent elevation of AST by analytical interference.

Alanine aminotransferase (ALT, SGPT)

Serum ALT is increased by drugs that affect the liver (see section on AST).

Alkaline phosphatase

Alkaline phosphatase (ALP, E.C. 3.1.3.1) refers to a group of non-specific phosphomonoesterases that hydrolyse phosphate monoesters (Kim and Wyckoff 1989). The natural substrate and the specific function of ALP are not known, but it is ubiquitous and is found attached to plasma membranes, indicating that it is involved in fundamental biological processes (Kim and Wyckoff 1989). The ALP are glycoproteins and there are at least four genes that code for the main groups of ALP isoenzymes (Harris 1989): the intestinal, placental, placental-like, and hepatic/renal/bone (or tissue non-specific) isoenzyme groups. Of the four groups, the hepatic/renal/bone isoenzyme has received most attention in clinical practice. Changes in plasma ALP activity occur most frequently from hepatic or skeletal causes. A variety of methods are available for the identification and quantitation of the different isoenzymes, but none fully separates the bone and hepatic isoenzymes satisfactorily.

Increase in serum ALP

In clinical practice, increases in serum ALP are most often seen in liver or bone disease.

Hepatic origin

The liver isoenzyme is located in the exterior surface of the bile canalicular membrane and serum ALP rises when there is bile duct obstruction. This forms the basis of its clinical usefulness. An increase in serum ALP is seen in many types of liver disease, including hepatitis, cholestasis, and space-occupying lesions (Nemesanszky 1986). ALP values are usually higher in biliary tract obstruction than in hepatocellular lesions (Nemesanszky 1986). A large number of drugs can cause elevation of serum ALP of hepatic origin (Young 1990). The mechanism of the increase is either a hepatocellular effect as with paracetamol, or cholestasis as with anabolic steroids (see Chapter 11 and also Davis 1982, 1989).

Skeletal origin

Increase in osteoblastic activity will cause an elevation of serum ALP. Drugs that cause metabolic bone disease, such as anticonvulsants, will cause an elevation of serum ALP (see section on Bone disease).

An ALP isoenzyme with unusual mobility found in a patient who had taken an overdose of colchichine was identified as being of renal origin (Rosalki *et al.* 1989).

Decrease in serum ALP

A decrease in serum ALP has been reported with the use of fluoride (Ferguson 1971), clofibrate (Schade *et al.* 1977; Whitaker *et al.* 1979; Probstfield *et al.* 1983), sulphonamides (Schiele *et al.* 1983), stanozolol (Couch *et al.* 1986), danazol (Purdie *et al.* 1987), contraceptives (Herbeth *et al.* 1981), and oestrogens (Christiansen *et al.* 1984; Marshall *et al.* 1984; Stock *et al.* 1985).

Artefacts

A number of drugs and compounds cause an apparent decrease in serum ALP by interference with analytical methods (Young 1990). These include fluorides, oxalate, zinc, EDTA (Young 1990), theophylline (Letellier and Desjarlais 1985), detergents (Schwartz 1973), cystine, and cysteine (Letellier and Desjarlair 1985). It is important to note that these interferences are method-dependent and not all methods of ALP determination are affected to the same extent.

γ-Glutamyltransferase

γ-Glutamyltransferase (GGT) is a membrane-bound enzyme found in cells that show high secretory or absorptive capacity, such as the epithelial cells lining the biliary tract, hepatic canaliculi, renal tubules, and intestinal brush borders. High activity is found in kidney, liver, pancreas, and intestine. Most of the GGT found in serum comes from liver.

Increase in serum GGT

Serum GGT is elevated in all types of hepatobiliary disease, including hepatocellular damage, cholestasis, and space-occupying lesions. Examples of drugs that elevate GGT by causing hepatocellular damage include paracetamol, captopril (Vandenburg et al. 1981), halothane (Shah and Brandt 1983), enflurane (Fee et al. 1979), methyldopa (Balazs and Kovach 1981), and streptokinase (Sallen et al. 1983). Haloperidol (Dinscoy and Saelinger 1982), warfarin (Adler et al. 1986; Amerena et al. 1990), sulindac (McIndoe et al. 1981), and phenothiazine (Kennedy 1983) are examples of drugs that elevate GGT by causing cholestasis. Thyroxine replacement in hypothyroidism may cause elevation of GGT, due to liver damage (Gow et al. 1989).

Serum GGT is also elevated by drugs that cause induction of microsomal enzymes as a result of enhanced synthesis of GGT and release of membrane-bound GGT. Alcohol and anticonvulsant drugs are well known to cause elevation of serum GGT by this mechanism. Excess alcohol intake causes significant elevation of GGT and elevated levels are seen in 75 per cent of alcoholics (Rosalki 1984). Anticonvulsants elevate GGT in a variable proportion of patients (Aldenhovel 1988), depending on the age and sex of the patient, the choice of drug, and duration of treatment (Braide and Davies 1987). The serum GGT activity was higher in patients treated with phenytoin than in those given phenobarbitone; elevation occurred 6 months after starting the treatment.

Bone cement used in joint replacement has been shown to cause elevation in serum GGT (Ritter et al. 1984; Pople and Phillips 1988) and the degree of elevation was dose-related. Anabolic steroids caused a small but significant increase in GGT in healthy subjects (Alen 1985); and oral contraceptives have the same effect (Arnesen et al. 1986; Calic et al. 1989), the extent varying with their composition (Hajos et al. 1981; Herbeth et al. 1981; Calic et al. 1989).

Decrease in serum GGT

A decrease in GGT is reported with clofibrate (Ferrari et al. 1976; Whitaker et al. 1979; Probstfield et al. 1983).

Artefacts

Cefotaxime and heparin cause an apparent reduction in GGT measured by some methods (Baer et al. 1983; Weber and van Zanten 1987).

Amylase

Amylases are calcium-containing metallo-enzymes and hydrolyse α-1,4-glycosidic bonds in glucose polymers such as starch, glycogen, and dextrin. The amylase molecule consists of a single peptide chain. Although pancreatic and salivary amylases are secretory enzymes, some amylase is found in the serum.

Increase in serum amylase

Drugs that cause spasm of the sphincter of Oddi, such as cholinergics and narcotics, may cause elevation of serum amylase (Lott and Wolf 1986b). The commonest cause of an elevated amylase is pancreatitis, and the drugs most often associated with this disease are discussed in Chapter 10. In smokers, basal serum amylase activity is 100 per cent higher than in non-smokers (Dubick et al. 1987) and this is further increased after injection of secretin (but there was no increase in non-smokers). A herbal tea used in Brazil was found to increase amylase (Leite et al. 1986). The plasma volume expander Letastarch (hydroxyethyl starch solution) significantly increased serum amylase activity (Korttila et al. 1984).

Decrease in serum amylase

During administration of 20% glucose and 8% amino acid solution, serum pancreatic isoamylase decreased and the decrease was proportional to the plasma glucose concentration (Skrha et al. 1986). Decreased serum amylase was also found with propylthiouracil and anabolic steroids (Tuzhilin et al. 1982).

Cholinesterase

Serum cholinesterase, or pseudocholinesterase, is synthesized by the liver and hydrolyses acylcholine esters. It is a large mucoprotein and there are several variants (Evans 1986). Its function is still not fully understood.

Low cholinesterase activity may be genetically determined, or acquired secondarily to liver disease, malnutrition, or recent infection (Evans 1986; Sawhney and Lott 1986). Drugs may lower the activity of serum cholinesterase either by inhibiting the enzyme directly or by reducing the hepatic synthesis of the enzyme. Serum cholinesterase can be inhibited by a variety of chemicals, including organophosphorus compounds and cholinergic drugs such as physostigmine, neostigmine, isofluophate, and ecothiopate (Sawhney and Lott 1986).

Very low or undetectable serum cholinesterase activity is seen in poisoning with organophosphorus insecticides such as parathion (Sawhney and Lott 1986; Besser *et al.* 1989). Metriphonate, an organophosphorus compound used in the treatment and control of urinary schistosomiasis, causes a marked fall in serum cholinesterase activity. Workers in the insecticide industry also have low serum cholinesterase activity from chronic exposure to insecticides (Sawhney and Lott 1986; Misra *et al.* 1988).

Low levels of serum cholinesterase, accounted for by reduced hepatic synthesis, are seen after paracetamol poisoning (Stewart and Simpson 1973) and after treatment with streptokinase (Schmidt *et al.* 1972) or colaspase (asparaginase) (Cucuianu *et al.* 1972). Oestrogens, contraceptive pills (Lepage *et al.* 1985; Calic *et al.* 1989), and anabolic steroids (Barbosa *et al.* 1971) reduce the levels by altering hepatic metabolism. Anticancer compounds such as cyclophosphamide (Zsigmond and Robins 1972) inhibit the enzyme activity. Other drugs that have been reported to cause reversible inhibition of serum cholinesterase include antimalarial drugs, barbiturates, caffeine, chlorpromazine and other phenothiazines, ether, folic acid, quinine, quinidine, theophylline, sulphonamides, and vitamin K (Sawhney and Lott 1986; Young 1990). Irreversible inhibition of the enzyme is seen with alkyl fluorophosphates.

Acid phosphatase

Acid phosphatase (ACP, EC 3.1.3.2) refers to a group of non-specific phosphatases that show maximal activity near pH 5.0. It exists in multimolecular form and is distributed widely in the body. Highest ACP activity is found in the prostate.

Increase in serum ACP

Administration of androgens to females increases serum ACP. In patients with prostatic carcinoma treated with GnRH analogue buserelin, there was an initial increase in ACP associated with an increase in testosterone, followed by a fall of both ACP and testosterone (Huhtaniemi *et al.* 1985). Clofibrate has been reported to increase ACP (Young 1990). Digital examination of the prostate leads to an elevation of serum ACP during the 24 hours following the examination (Pearson *et al.* 1983).

Decrease in serum ACP

Fluoride is said to decrease serum ACP (Young 1990). Treatment of prostatic carcinoma with oestrogen will reduce the raised ACP levels (Grayhack 1984; Maatman *et al.* 1984). Treatment with GnRH analogue for 2–3 weeks reduced the raised ACP levels seen in patients

with prostatic carcinoma (Huhtaniemi *et al.* 1985). Ketoconazole, an oral antimycotic agent with potent inhibitory effects on adrenal and gonadal steroids, has been successfully used in the treatment of prostatic carcinoma with reduction in serum ACP (Trachtenberg and Pont 1984; Sonino 1987).

Artefacts

Haemolysis can increase, and inappropriate storage of samples can decrease, the serum ACP activity (Young 1990). Fluoride, oxalate, copper, alcohol, and detergent decrease the activity of ACP (Young 1990). In certain immunoassay procedures sodium azide falsely elevates ACP (Cobbledick and Hinberg 1984).

Angiotensin-converting-enzyme (ACE)

Angiotensin-converting-enzyme (EC 3.4.15.1) converts angiotensin I to angiotensin II by cleavage of a dipeptide. It also inactivates bradykinins.

Increase in serum ACE

Administration of tri-iodiothyronine has been observed to increase serum ACE (Graninger *et al.* 1986).

Decrease in serum ACE

Decrease in serum ACE is seen with the use of ACE inhibitors captopril (Kamoun *et al.* 1982), enalapril (Jackson and Johnston 1984; Fouad *et al.* 1984), ramipril (Crozier *et al.* 1987), and perindopril (Bussien *et al.* 1986). The effects of the two major ACE inhibitors captopril and enalapril differ. Captopril has a more rapid onset of ACE inhibition (30 minutes) than enalapril (1–4 hours). The inhibitory effect of captopril is markedly reduced with storage of the serum and, furthermore, it is reversed by dilution of the sample or following dialysis. Enalapril, on the other hand, does not lose its inhibitory effect during storage or dilution (Lieberman 1989). Administration of magnesium sulphate in the treatment of pregnancy-induced hypertension caused a decrease in serum ACE (Fuentes and Goldkrand 1987). Prednisone reduced serum ACE in those who had an elevated value initially (Romer and Jacobsen 1982).

Artefacts

Freezing and thawing of serum increases ACE activity by 15 per cent (Schweisfurth and Schioberg-Schiegnitz 1984). Uric acid at high concentrations can increase activity (Pietila and Koivula 1984) and EDTA, hydroxyquinoline, methylprednisolone, and phenanthroline can decrease the activity of ACE measured by some methods (Young 1990).

Vitamins

Water-soluble vitamins

The vitamin B complex

Vitamin B₁ (thiamine)

Thiamine, in its coenzyme form thiamine pyrophosphate (TPP), is essential for decarboxylation and transketolase reactions. Thiamine deficiency leads to neurological effects — peripheral neuropathy (dry beriberi), encephalopathy (cerebral beriberi) — or cardiac effects (wet beriberi). Thiamine deficiency can be detected by the *in vitro* activation of erythrocyte transketolase by thiamine pyrophosphate, or by direct measurement of thiamine levels by microbiological, enzymatic, or HPLC methods (Ryle and Thomson 1984).

Biochemical and clinical evidence of thiamine deficiency is commonly found in alcoholics. The thiamine deficiency is due to a combination of poor intake, increased metabolic demands from the alcohol consumption, and decreased intestinal absorption. Alcohol has been shown to interfere with the transport of thiamine due to inhibition of the Na^+K^+-ATPase (Thomson and Majumdar 1981). Similar mechanisms may interfere with the transport of thiamine across the blood–brain barrier. Furthermore, the folate deficiency and the general malnutrition seen in alcoholics may further aggravate the malabsorption of thiamine (Ryle and Thomson 1984).

Increased demands due to prolonged intravenous feeding with high-carbohydrate fluids can also lead to thiamine deficiency (Bozzetti 1979). A syndrome resembling Wernicke–Korsakoff's syndrome has been described in patients with colorectal carcinoma treated with high doses of the antitumour drugs doxifluridine and fluorouracil (Heier and Fossa 1986). This toxic effect was dose-related.

Wernicke's encephalopathy has also been described in a patient with AIDS treated with zidovudine (azidothymidine) (Davtyan and Vinters 1987). A diabetic patient treated with tolazamide developed Wernicke's encephalopathy, and fibroblasts from these patients had abnormal transketolase (as shown by a high K_m for TPP) (Mukherjee *et al.* 1986). Wernicke's encephalopathy has also been described following lithium-induced diarrhoea (Epstein 1989); and after high doses of nitroglycerin (Shorey *et al.* 1984), possibly because of its high alcohol content. Sulphates, which are added to some infusion solutions to prevent non-enzymic browning and decomposition during sterilization, have been suspected of causing destruction of thiamine, which may have clinical consequences (Bassler and Heidenreich 1984). Thiamine status was reported not to be affected by long-term anticonvulsant treatment (Krause *et al.* 1988).

Vitamin B₂ (riboflavine)

Riboflavine in the form of flavine nucleotides is required for the electron transport system, and deficiency causes rough scaly skin, angular stomatitis, cheilosis, glossitis, and stomatitis. Riboflavine deficiency can be detected by the measurement of erythrocyte glutathione reductase and its activation by *in vitro* addition of flavine adenine dinucleotide (FAD) (Bates *et al.* 1982).

Many drugs such as chlorpromazine, imipramine, amitriptyline, and adriamycin have been shown to cause riboflavine deficiency or depletion under experimental conditions (Pinto *et al.* 1981), but no clinical or biochemical riboflavine deficiency due to such drugs has been demonstrated. Alcoholics have been shown to have biochemical evidence of riboflavine deficiency as shown by low erythrocyte glutathione reductase and increased *in vitro* activation by FAD (Ryle and Thomson 1984). Reduced intake, reduced absorption, and increased requirement contribute to the deficiency. Oral contraceptive users have biochemical evidence of riboflavine deficiency (Sanpitak and Chayutimonkul 1974; Tyrer 1984). This could be important in areas of the world where riboflavine deficiency is common due to poor nutrition. In a more recent study, however, riboflavine was not found to be affected by the use of oral contraceptives (Amatayakul *et al.* 1984). Riboflavine deficiency has been reported in 17 per cent (Cimino *et al.* 1985) and 30–40 per cent (Krause *et al.* 1988) of patients on long-term anticonvulsant therapy. The deficiency disappeared when the diet was changed, in spite of continued drug therapy. Thus the deficiency is probably a direct effect of poor nutrition rather than an effect of the anticonvulsants.

Nicotinic acid

Nicotinamide, formed from nicotinic acid, is the active constituent of important co-factors (NAD and NADP) in oxidation–reduction reactions. Nicotinic acid deficiency leads to the syndrome of pellagra, which comprises dermatitis, diarrhoea, and dementia. Nicotinic acid status is assessed by the measurement of 24-hour excretion of the metabolites $N(1)$-methylnicotinamide and $N(1)$-methyl-3-carboxamide-6-pyridone (McCormick 1986) or by measurement of fasting plasma tryptophan and other amino acids.

Nicotinic acid deficiency with pellagra-like features has been described in patients with tuberculosis undergoing treatment with isoniazid (Meyrick *et al.* 1981); the symptoms disappeared after treatment with niacin and pyridoxine. Isoniazid is a pyridoxine antagonist (see below) and pyridoxine is necessary for the synthesis of nicotinic acid from tryptophan. The extent of nicotinic acid deficiency in isoniazid treatment is illustrated by the diagnosis of 8 cases of pellagra at postmortem examination of 106 cases of tuberculosis (Ishii and Nishihara 1985). Pellagroid erythema caused by isoniazid has been reported (Schmutz *et al.* 1987). Sodium valproate (Gillman and Sandyk 1984), abuse of morazone (an analgesic) (Kingreen and Breger 1984), and glibenclamide (Berova and Lazarova 1988) have all been reported to cause nicotinic acid deficiency. Pellagra-like encephalopathy following treatment of *Mycobacterium avium intracellulare* with several drugs has been reported (Brooks-Hill *et al.* 1985).

Vitamin B_6 (pyridoxine)

The vitamin pyridoxine exists in three forms, pyridoxal, pyridoxine, and pyridoxamine, which are converted to the active phosphate form. This vitamin is a co-factor for the transaminases and for decarboxylation of amino acids. Deficiency of pyridoxine leads to roughness of the skin, peripheral neuropathy, and sore tongue. Pyridoxine status can be assessed by the excretion of xanthuric acid after a tryptophan load or by the measurement of erythrocyte aspartate aminotransferase and its activation by pyridoxal phosphate. It can also be assessed by direct measurement of pyridoxine phosphate by an enzymatic or HPLC method (Barnard *et al.* 1987).

Isoniazid is an antagonist of pyridoxine that forms hydrazones with pyridoxal and pyridoxal phosphate which are lost in the urine. These compounds inhibit pyridoxal kinase and pyridoxal phosphate-dependent enzymes (Snider 1980; McCormick 1986).

Measurement of erythrocyte aspartate aminotransferase activity showed evidence of pyridoxine deficiency in patients receiving isoniazid (Standal *et al.* 1974; Pellock *et al.* 1985). The incidence was dose-related, and prophylactic pyridoxine was recommended. Hydralazine and phenelzine have been shown to reduce pyridoxine levels in experimental animals. Pyridoxine deficiency and peripheral neuropathy associated with phenelzine therapy have been described (Heller and Friedman 1983; Demers *et al.* 1984; Stewart *et al.* 1984).

A number of studies have demonstrated abnormalities of tryptophan metabolism (as shown by the tryptophan load test) in women receiving oestrogens as oral contraceptives or menopausal hormone replacement therapy (Prasad *et al.* 1975; Adams *et al.* 1976; Tyrer 1984; Amatayakul *et al.* 1984). Some have even suggested that women using oral contraceptives should be given pyridoxine supplements (Applegate *et al.* 1979), but others

have found no difference in vitamin B_6 status between users and non-users of oral contraceptives (Brown *et al.* 1975; Smith *et al.* 1975). Some studies have shown that the tryptophan load test used in many studies may not be a valid index of pyridoxine status, as the oestrogen conjugates inhibit kynureminase independently of the pyridoxine status, thereby causing an abnormal result (Bender 1983). Using the erythrocyte aspartate aminotransferase activation index, however, evidence of pyridoxine deficiency was found in 35 per cent of Sudanese women taking oral contraceptives (Salih *et al.* 1986). The evidence for pyridoxine deficiency in oral contraceptive users is not strong and may only be present in some groups, especially those who have marginal dietary deficiency to start with. Although Adams and others (1976) suggested that oral contraceptives increase the metabolism of tryptophan through the nicotinic acid pathway, leading to an increase in the requirement of pyridoxine, Bender and colleagues (Bender 1983; Bender *et al.* 1983) have not been able to demonstrate an increase in the activity of tryptophan oxygenase.

Penicillamine may also cause symptoms of pyridoxine deficiency by inactivating it, forming a thiazolidine derivative (Jaffe 1972; Bhagavan 1985).

Alcoholics often show biochemical evidence of pyridoxine deficiency due to the effect of ethanol on the utilization of pyridoxine and from decreased intake (Ryle and Thomson 1984).

Reynolds and Natta (1985) found reduced plasma and erythrocyte pyridoxal phosphate levels in asthmatic patients. On the other hand, Hall and co-workers (1981) could not find any evidence of pyridoxine deficiency using the erythrocyte AST activation test. Recently Delport and others (1988) confirmed that plasma pyridoxal phosphate levels are low and plasma pyridoxal levels are normal in asthmatic patients, thus suggesting that the depression of plasma pyridoxal phosphate levels was not of nutritional origin. Ubbink and co-workers (1990) found that administration of theophylline to volunteers caused a reduction in plasma and erythrocyte pyridoxal phosphate without a reduction in pyridoxal levels (Delport *et al.* 1988), and the decrease in pyridoxal phosphate was correlated with plasma theophylline levels. They found that this decrease was due to noncompetitive inhibition of pyridoxal kinase activity by theophylline. The authors concluded that long-term theophylline therapy in asthmatics will lead to chronic depression of vitamin B_6 status, and deficiency of vitamin B_6 may contribute to the toxicity of theophylline (Ubbink *et al.* 1989).

A number of studies have shown that the vitamin B_6 status in patients taking anticonvulsants was poor (Davis *et al.* 1975; Majumdar 1981; Krause *et al.* 1988). Krause and co-workers (1988) showed lower pyridoxal phosphate levels and higher activation of erythrocyte AST in epileptics. The plasma level of pyridoxal phosphate correlated with the dose and duration of treatment.

Vitamin B_{12}

A number of drugs are known to affect the absorption and utilization of vitamin B_{12} in man (Davis 1985) and malabsorption may be induced by para-aminosalicylic acid (PAS), metformin, slow-release potassium iodide, colchicine, trifluoperazine, cholestyramine, and ethanol (Dickerson 1988). The malabsorption of vitamin B_{12} seen with cholestyramine is thought to be due to binding to intrinsic factor and interference with the formation of intrinsic factor–B_{12} complex (Coronato and Glass 1973). A similar mechanism has been proposed for neomycin (Jacobson et al. 1960). Colchicine interferes with absorption of vitamin B_{12} by altering the function of the ileal mucosa (Webb *et al.* 1968). In the case of PAS, studies on patients with tuberculosis have confirmed that the drug does not interfere with intrinsic factor, but probably acts by inhibiting some folate-dependent enzyme system in the gut (Dickerson 1988).

The biguanides metformin and phenformin cause malabsorption of vitamin B_{12} (Tomkin 1973), as shown by an abnormal Schilling test, and the malabsorption did not improve with addition of intrinsic factor; it is reversible within 2–8 weeks of stopping treatment (Davis 1985). Megalobastic anaemia from long-term treatment with metformin has been reported (Callaghan *et al.* 1980).

Malabsorption of B_{12} has been reported with methyldopa (Shneerson and Gazzard 1977); cimetidine, which inhibits the secretion of intrinsic factor (Fielding *et al.* 1978); and allopurinol (Chen *et al.* 1982).

Ascorbic acid in high doses was associated with low serum B_{12} levels (Herbert *et al.* 1978), which were thought to be due to the destruction of B_{12} by the ascorbate (Herbert 1981), but this has not been confirmed (Rivers 1987). It is likely that only some forms of cobalamins not found in food are destroyed by ascorbic acid (Hogenkamp 1980).

Serum vitamin B_{12} concentrations were found to be significantly lowered in women taking oral contraceptives, but B_{12}-binding protein was not found to be altered (Costanzi *et al.* 1978). Hjelt and others (1985), however, found reduced B_{12}-binding capacity in oral contraceptive users. Oral contraceptives had no effect on B_{12} absorption or excretion of labelled cobalamin (Hjelt *et al.* 1985). It is worth noting that these authors found a low haemoglobin concentration in those who had low serum B_{12} levels.

Malabsorption of B_{12} due to interference with binding of the intrinsic factor–B_{12} complex to the intestine can be demonstrated in up to 50 per cent of alcoholics (Ryle and Thomson 1984). Serum B_{12} levels in the majority of alcoholics, however, are normal, probably due to the presence of liver damage. Any frank deficiency of vitamin B_{12} is relatively uncommon in alcoholics (Davis 1985).

A high incidence of megaloblastic change was noted in patients receiving nitrous oxide (Amess *et al.* 1978); it was thought to be due to an acute B_{12} deficiency (Cullen *et al.* 1979). The serum B_{12} levels measured by biological assay were normal (Amess *et al.* 1978), but the deoxyuridine test was abnormal (Amos *et al.* 1985). Nitrous oxide was shown to change reduced cobalamin to the oxidized form which is inactive (Chanarin 1980), and reduced cobalamin is required in the methionine synthetase pathway. Serum B_{12} levels were apparently normal, because the organism used in the assay utilized both the reduced and oxidized forms (Davis 1985).

Folate

Folate coenzymes are essential for the transfer of single carbon units and one of the important examples of this is the synthesis of DNA. Drugs may cause folate deficiency in a number of different ways. They may interfere with the absorption of the vitamin by inhibiting the intestinal conjugase enzyme which reduces dietary polyglutamate to the monoglutamate form before absorption. Drugs like methotrexate may inhibit the enzyme dihydrofolate reductase which catalyses the conversion of dihydrofolate to tetrahydrofolate, which is a co-factor necessary for the synthesis of DNA. Drugs which cause B_{12} deficiency will affect the demethylation of methylfolate. Those which induce pyridoxine deficiency can also act on folate metabolism, as pyridoxine is involved in the demethylation of methylfolate (Dickerson 1988).

Co-trimoxazole, a combination of sulphamethoxazole and trimethoprim, is an effective antibacterial agent. The sulphonamide blocks the utilization of *p*-aminobenzoic acid and thereby blocks the synthesis of folate, while trimethoprin acts as a spurious substrate for the bacterial dihydrofolate reductase, preventing the reduction of any folate that may be formed (Davis 1986). Treatment with co-trimoxazole might therefore be expected to cause folate deficiency, but in early studies no evidence of folate deficiency was found with conventional assays. Marginal deficiency was found using a sensitive deoxyuridine suppression test (Davis, 1986). Furthermore, several case reports of folate deficiency and megaloblastic anaemia have appeared in the literature (Rooney and Housley 1972; Chan *et al.* 1980).

Considering the widespread use of co-trimoxazole, the incidence of folate deficiency is very low (Salter 1973; Davis 1986) and folate status of some of those developing deficiency may have already been low before treatment (Rooney and Housley 1972; Davis 1986). Another sulphonamide, sulphasalazine, has been reported to cause folate deficiency (Kane and Boots 1977; Schneider and Beeley 1977). In patients with colitis treated with sulphasalazine, a dose-related decrease in red cell folate level was reported, and although the levels were not in the clinically significant range there may be subclinical tissue depletion (Longstretch and Green 1983). Sulphasalazine treatment in rheumatoid arthritis was not associated with any change in red cell or serum folate levels. The observed increase in mean corpuscular volume was probably due to the reticulocytosis (Grindulis and McConkey 1985). The differing effects of this drug in rheumatoid arthritis and chronic colitis are not explained. Nevertheless, macrocytic anaemia and folate deficiency have been reported in ulcerative colitis (Grieco et al. 1986) and rheumatoid arthritis (Prouse et al. 1987). Some authors have advocated supplementation with folic acid or folinic acid to prevent folate deficiency in these patients and folinic acid was found to be more effective (Pironi et al. 1988). Megaloblastic anaemia may develop in patients treated with pyrimethamine, an antimalarial agent (Davis 1986; Reynolds 1989).

Methotrexate (4-amino-10-methyl-L-pteroylglutamic acid), which binds to dihydrofolate reductase, is used in the treatment of malignant disorders and psoriasis, and for immunosuppression. The use of methotrexate has been associated with megaloblastic anaemia (Dodd et al. 1985; Fulton 1986; Reynolds 1989) and reduced red cell folate levels (Kamen et al. 1984; Hendel and Nyfords 1985). Even with low-dose methotrexate therapy, as is used in psoriasis, Refsum and others (1989) showed abnormality in the fasting plasma homocysteine concentration, which is used as a sensitive parameter of antifolate effect.

The association between anticonvulsant therapy and reduced concentration of serum and red cell folate is well recognized (Reynolds 1974, 1983), and occasionally overt megaloblastic anaemia has been reported (Reynolds 1974; Rivey et al. 1984; Pereira et al. 1985; Davis 1986; Shalev et al. 1987b). Phenytoin is the most studied in this respect, but folate deficiency has also been reported with phenobarbitone (Flexner and Hartmann 1960), phensuximide (Doig and Stanton 1961), and primidone (Davis 1986). Biochemical evidence of folate deficiency is also seen with other drugs, such as phenothiazines and tricyclic antidepressants (Labadarios et al.

1978). Reduction in serum folate (Krause et al. 1982) and red cell folate was found in a large proportion of patients taking anticonvulsants (Maxwell et al. 1972). In a more recent study, low red cell folate was found in 17 per cent of those taking carbamazepine, 13 per cent of those taking phenytoin, and 22 per cent of those taking more than one drug. The serum folate was negatively correlated with the plasma phenytoin level (Goggin et al. 1987; Krause et al. 1988).

The mechanism of action of anticonvulsants in reducing folate status is not fully understood. Some authors have suggested that anticonvulsants may inhibit the intestinal absorption of folate (Elsborg 1974; Hendel et al. 1984), while others do not support this (Fehling et al. 1973). Anticonvulsants may stimulate the induction of hepatic enzymes that require folate, and this may lead to folate deficiency (Maxwell et al. 1972; Labadarios et al. 1978). Krause and others (1988) have suggested that anticonvulsants may disturb the conversion of folic acid to 5-methyltetrahydrofolate. Goggin and co-workers (1987) found a correlation between red cell folate and dietary folate in patients receiving anticonvulsant therapy and, furthermore, Cimino and colleagues (1985) showed that the folate deficiency seen in patients on anticonvulsant therapy disappeared with a good dietary regimen. These studies suggest that low dietary intake of folate may be an exacerbating factor.

Although anaemia due to folate deficiency is uncommon, it has been suggested that folate deficiency may cause other adverse effects such as neuropsychiatric effects (Reynolds and Trimble 1985), congenital malformations, and an increased spontaneous abortion (Dansky et al. 1985, 1987).

Treatment of folate deficiency induced by anticonvulsants remains controversial. It has been suggested that folate supplements may reduce serum levels of the drug and increase the frequency of fits (Reynolds 1967; Dennis and Taylor 1969; Rivey et al. 1984). A good diet adequate in folate has been reported, however, to eliminate folate deficiency (Eastham et al. 1975; Cimino et al. 1985).

Oral contraceptive agents are reported to cause folate deficiency, although the incidence may be low (Shojania et al. 1971; Tyrer 1984). Low serum folate levels were found in subjects taking oral contraceptives (Hettiarachchy et al. 1983; Davis 1986), and occasional cases of megaloblastic anaemia have been described (Green 1975; Korenberg et al. 1989). A case of folate deficiency in the breast-fed infant of a mother who was taking oral contraceptives has also been described (Mandel and Berant 1985). Haemoglobin concentrations in women taking oral contraceptives are not low, but some studies show a significant increase in the mean corpuscular volume (Chalmers *et al.* 1979). The exact mechanism of folate deficiency is not clear, but decreased absorption has been suggested as a possible mechanism (Toghill and Smith 1971; Dickerson 1988), or there may be increased clearance of the absorbed folate. From the available evidence it appears that oral contraceptives may marginally depress the body folate pool, but this is of little consequence in most women. It is of importance, however, in the event that pregnancy should take place shortly after stopping an oral contraceptive, as folate deficiency can lead to congenital malformations (Smithells *et al.* 1976).

Folate deficiency may be seen in a large proportion of alcoholics (Chanarin 1982; Ryle and Thomson 1984). Factors contributing to this deficiency are poor diet, reduced absorption, decreased body stores due to liver damage, reduced enterohepatic circulation (Halsted 1980), and an antagonistic effect of alcohol on the haematopoietic effects of folic acid (Larkin and Watson-Williams 1984). Ethanol in combination with folate deficiency depresses the absorption of folate (Cook 1976; Ryle and Thomson 1984). Nutritional deficiency seems to be a major determinant in the development of folate deficiency, as megaloblastosis with folate deficiency is rare in alcoholics whose diet is adequate (Ryle and Thomson 1984).

Acute folate deficiency has also been found in patients in an intensive care unit receiving intravenous nutrition (Wardrop *et al.* 1977; Tennant *et al.* 1981*a,b*); it may be due to the amino acid composition of the fluids used, as certain amino acids such as methionine may cause a decrease in serum folate (Connor *et al.* 1978).

Nitrous oxide was reported to cause folate deficiency 3 days after its use in anaesthesia, as shown by the deoxyuridine suppression test. Urinary folate was increased at this time (Amos *et al.* 1985). Other drugs associated with folate deficiency are methyldopa (Shneerson and Gazzard 1977), cholestyramine (West and Lloyd 1975), cycloserine, and allopurinol (Davis 1986).

Other water-soluble vitamins

Ascorbic acid (vitamin C)

Ascorbic acid is essential for man but its function is not fully understood. Vitamin C is involved in hormone and neurotransmitter synthesis, is required for collagen synthesis, and acts as an antioxidant (Burns 1987). Deficiency of ascorbate causes scurvy, which is now rare. Low levels of ascorbate, however, may be harmful in other ways, such as affording poor protection against free radicals (Anderson and Lukey 1987). Ascorbate

status is assessed by the measurement of ascorbate level in plasma or leucocytes by a chemical method or by HPLC (Jacob et al. 1987; Omaye *et al.* 1987). There is still controversy, however, as to whether plasma, platelet, or leucocyte ascorbate gives the best assessment of vitamin C status (Omaye *et al.* 1987).

Reduced levels of ascorbate have been observed in the plasma, leucocytes, platelets, and urine of users of oral contraceptives when compared with levels in non-users (Harris *et al.* 1973; Horwitt *et al.* 1975; Tyrer 1984). Possible explanations for the reduced levels include the stimulation by oral contraceptives of caeruloplasmin (which has ascorbate oxidase activity), decreased absorption, changes in tissue distribution, increased excretion, and reduced levels of reducing compounds such as reduced glutathione (Tyrer 1984).

Low levels of ascorbate in leucocytes have been found in alcoholics (Devgun *et al.* 1981), in whom reduced intake and malabsorption contribute, and low levels of ascorbate have been reported with the use of corticosteroids (Chretien and Garagusi 1973; *The Lancet* 1979), tetracycline (Windsor *et al.* 1972), and cholestyramine (Beattie and Sherlock 1976; *British Medical Journal* 1977). Smokers have a lower intake of vitamin C and lower serum ascorbate levels than non-smokers, and even after adjustment for intake their serum levels are lower than those of non-smokers, suggesting an increased requirement (Smith and Hodges 1987). Deficiency of vitamin C, and of other vitamins, was reported in patients on long-term anticonvulsant therapy (Klein *et al.* 1977), though Krause and others (1988) found normal vitamin C levels in male patients and low levels in female patients taking these drugs. The low levels could not be attributed to drug treatment. Low vitamin C levels and increased urinary excretion were observed in women taking oral contraceptives (Harris *et al.* 1973; Horwitt *et al.* 1975).

The relationship between intake of vitamin C and the plasma concentration of vitamin C is sigmoidal (Newton *et al.* 1983), and when large amounts of vitamin C are taken high plasma levels are seen. 'Megadoses' of vitamin C are sometimes taken, as it has been suggested that vitamin C is effective in the treatment or prevention of a wide array of conditions including the common cold and acetaldehyde toxicity. A high intake of ascorbate can lead to increased excretion of urinary oxalate (Schmidt *et al.* 1981; Rivers 1987) and it increases the requirement for some vitamins such as vitamin E (Chen 1981). People who are susceptible to iron overload may be adversely affected by excess vitamin C (Rivers 1987). Recent evidence has failed to confirm the suggestion that vitamin C may cause destruction of vitamin B_{12} in food, or that vitamin C affects plasma uric acid levels (Rivers 1987).

Fat-soluble vitamins

Vitamin A

Vitamin A plays an important role in vision, stabilization of cellular and intracellular membranes, maintenance of the integrity of epithelial tissue, synthesis of glycoproteins, and spermatogenesis. Deficiency of vitamin A can lead to failure of normal growth, poor dark adaptation, keratomalacia, xerophthalmia, and follicular hyperkeratosis of the skin. Vitamin A has also been linked with cancer (Willett and MacMohon 1984) and with immunity (Tomkins and Hussey 1989). There are three main forms of vitamin A: retinol, retinal, and retinoic acid and each has a characteristic action on individual target organs. Vitamin A status is usually assessed by measurement of plasma retinol levels, although these only decrease when liver stores are depleted and increase when these are saturated. Vitamin A content of liver gives the best estimate of vitamin A status (Tomkins and Hussey 1989).

Malabsorption of vitamin A can occur whenever there is drug-induced malabsorption such as that seen with cholestyramine, neomycin, and allopurinol. Low serum vitamin A and carotene levels and symptoms of vitamin A deficiency associated with steatorrhoea were reported with the use of methyltestosterone (Nisbeth *et al.* 1985). The symptoms and biochemical abnormalities reversed within 9 months of discontinuation of the drug. Alcoholics may have lower plasma retinal levels (Russell 1980; Devgun *et al.* 1981). It must be pointed out, however, that an apparently low plasma retinol may result from changes in RBP, which is the specific transport protein of retinol. Plasma vitamin A levels may also be high in alcoholics, owing to hepatocellular damage (Ryle and Thomson 1984). In a large series of patients receiving anticonvulsant therapy, a significantly lowered vitamin A level was reported (Krause *et al.* 1988), but the level did not correlate with variables in the anticonvulsant therapy and none of the patients had very low levels.

In women taking oral contraceptives, plasma levels of vitamin A are 30–80 per cent higher than in controls (Horwitt *et al.* 1975; Amatayakul *et al.* 1984; Tyrer 1984; Bamji *et al.* 1985). The increased plasma level is due to an increase in the binding protein, RBP, and the levels of free vitamin A are unchanged (Briggs 1974) but hepatic stores may be depleted. Hypervitaminosis A can occur if there is excessive intake of the vitamin (Bollag 1983) or as an adverse effect of inappropriate therapy (Korner and Vollun 1975).

Vitamin D

Most of the vitamin D_3 (cholecalciferol) present in the body is formed in the skin by the action of ultraviolet light. Vitamin D_3 is transported in the plasma bound to a specific carrier protein and metabolised to its active form, 1,25-dihydroxycholecalciferol (1,25-DHCC) (DeLuca 1988). Deficiency of vitamin D leads to osteomalacia and rickets. Marginal vitamin D deficiency may increase the risk of osteoporosis (Heaney 1988). Vitamin D status is usually assessed by the measurement of plasma 25-hydroxyvitamin D (25-OHD), the major circulating form of vitamin D. Methods are also available to measure the active metabolite 1,25-DHCC (Porteous *et al.* 1987). Drugs may induce vitamin D deficiency by causing malabsorption or by interfering with the metabolism of vitamin D.

Drug-induced malabsorption (see Chapter 10) will lead to vitamin D deficiency together with deficiency of other fat-soluble vitamins. Neomycin and cholestyramine cause malabsorption by binding to bile salts in the intestinal lumen. Low plasma 25-OHD has been reported in alcoholics (Devgun *et al.* 1981; Ryle and Thomson 1984), probably due to a combination of malabsorption, poor intake, reduced exposure to sunlight, and reduced storage. As a significant amount of the daily requirement of vitamin D comes from *in vivo* synthesis by the effect of sunlight, use of sunscreening agents may reduce vitamin D levels. Matsuoka and colleagues (1988) observed that in chronic users of the sunscreening agent *p*-aminobenzoic acid, plasma 25-OHD levels were low and in one subject the level was in the vitamin D deficiency range.

Anticonvulsants cause biochemical, radiological, and clinical features of vitamin D deficiency (Richens and Rowe 1970; Dent *et al.* 1970). Although there are many reports of anticonvulsant-induced osteomalacia (Doriguzzi *et al.* 1984; Duus 1986), there is some confusion as to the extent of the problem and the possible mechanism. In institutionalized patients, 10 per cent were found to have fractures, and bone biopsy revealed a mixture of osteomalacia, osteoporosis, and hyperparathyroidism (Nilsson *et al.* 1986). The reported incidence of abnormal biochemical findings varies from 5 per cent (Harrington and Hodkinson 1987) to 40 per cent (Krause *et al.* 1988). Most of these studies have been done in institutionalized subjects or in northern Europe. Thus other factors like lack of exposure to sunlight, diet poor in vitamin D, and lack of physical activity may have contributed (Beghi and Di Mascio 1986). In active adolescent subjects on anticonvulsants, there was no biochemical evidence of vitamin D deficiency (Ala-

Houhala *et al.* 1986). In a study from Florida, USA, on subjects on anticonvulsant therapy, marginal biochemical changes were found but there was no radiological evidence of rickets or osteomalacia (Williams *et al.* 1984). Thus the available evidence suggests that in patients treated with anticonvulsants (phenytoin, phenobarbitone, carbamazepine), if they are institutionalized or have poor exposure to sunlight, up to 25 per cent may have evidence of osteomalacia or rickets.

It has been suggested that anticonvulsants increase the degradation of 25-OHD to inactive metabolites due to induction of hepatic microsomal enzymes (Dent *et al.* 1970). Plasma 25-OHD levels were reported to be low (Krause *et al.* 1988) and were related to the dose and duration of the treatment (Gascon-Barre *et al.* 1984). Interestingly, it was also reported that low doses of phenytoin increased the plasma 25-OHD levels, further supporting the enzyme-induction hypothesis. Furthermore, Maislos and co-workers (1985) reported reduction in serum 25-OHD and 1,25-DHCC levels in a hypercalcaemic patient treated with phenytoin and phenobarbitone. Treatment with vitamin D (Rajantie *et al.* 1984), or 1,25-DHCC (Beghi and Di Mascio 1986; Comair *et al.* 1988) was reported to improve the biochemical and radiological features of osteomalacia. Plasma 1,25-DHCC levels were, however, found to be normal by others (Gascon-Barre *et al.* 1984; Weinstein *et al.* 1984). Thus there is no conclusive evidence that anticonvulsants alter the metabolism of vitamin D. Phenytoin has also been shown to have a direct effect on the skeleton, and on the intestine to reduce calcium absorption (Hahn 1980). Thus, the effect of anticonvulsants on calcium and bone metabolism is a result of the vitamin D status of the individual, the effect of the drugs on vitamin D metabolism, and the direct effect of these drugs on skeleton and intestine.

Rifampicin has also been reported to accelerate the rate of degradation of vitamin D and its metabolites (Brodie *et al.* 1980, 1982).

Diphosphonate, clodronate, and etidronate cause a picture similar to that of osteomalacia (Gibbs *et al.* 1986; Chestnut 1988), but this is due to the direct effect of the drugs on bone rather than to an effect on vitamin D metabolism.

Increased levels of vitamin D or its metabolites will occur when the intake of either is excessive (see Hypercalcaemia). Toxic effects include hypercalcaemia, renal impairment, mental change, and ectopic calcification. The commonest cause of increased intake of vitamin D or its metabolites is overtreatment (Paterson 1980). Vitamin D intoxication due to high concentrations in cooking oil has been reported (Down *et al.* 1979).

Treatment of hypovitaminosis D is by supplementation with vitamin D or its analogues and, if practicable, withdrawal of the offending drug. Treatment of hypervitaminosis consists of withdrawal of the offending drug and treatment of the hypercalcaemia (see Hypercalcaemia section).

Vitamin E

Vitamin E plays an important role in maintaining the integrity of plasma membranes and is an antioxidant preventing lipid peroxidation and modulating the metabolism of the arachidonic acid cascade. It has been thought to play a role in the prevention of free-radical damage in many diseases, including cancer, arthritis, cataract (Packer and Landvik 1989), and cardiovascular disease (Duthie *et al.* 1989*a*). Vitamin E status is usually assessed by the measurement of plasma vitamin E levels. It is now recognized, however, that vitamin E levels fluctuate in relation to plasma lipids, and vitamin E is best expressed as a ratio in relation to total lipids (Lehmann *et al.* 1988; Mino *et al.* 1989). Vitamin E status can also be assessed by red cell vitamin E levels (Mino *et al.* 1983) and on the basis of peroxidizability of red cell ghosts and lipoprotein fractions exposed to oxidant stress (Mino *et al.* 1989). Features of vitamin E deficiency include haemolytic anaemia, increased erythrocyte fragility, and creatinuria. Vitamin E deficiency has also been associated with many other clinical entities (Aranda *et al.* 1986).

Low vitamin E levels are found in malabsorption induced by drugs such as cholestyramine. Levels are normal in smokers, although erythrocytes from smokers had a greater tendency to peroxidize (Duthie *et al.* 1989*b*). Plasma α-tocopherol (the predominant form in plasma) was reported to be reduced in patients taking anticonvulsant drugs (Kataoka *et al.* 1990). Reduced vitamin E levels were reported in children receiving anticonvulsant treatment (Ogunmekan 1979), but consistent results were not found in a more recent study of over 500 epileptics (Krause *et al.* 1988). Experimental studies have shown a significant reduction in plasma α-tocopherol, as a result of contraceptives. Others, however, found the use of oral contraceptives was not associated with any change (Horwitt *et al.* 1975; Tyrer 1984).

Vitamin E is used commonly in paediatric practice and possible toxic effects associated with high plasma levels have been reported. These include inhibition of wound healing, fibrinolysis, and platelet aggregation, and a reduction in vitamin K-dependent coagulation, necrotizing enterocolitis, and sepsis (Johnson *et al.* 1985; Aranda *et al.* 1986). Intravenous use of tocopherol was associated with several deaths and with hepatic, renal, and haematopoietic toxicity (Lorch *et al.* 1985). The exact cause of the toxicity is not known, but it has been suggested to be due to a contaminant. In the newborn, potentially toxic levels of vitamin E can arise with oral preparations due to variation in intestinal absorption (Lemons and Maisels 1985).

Vitamin K

Vitamin K is necessary for the synthesis of plasma clotting factors, prothrombin, (factor II), VII, IX, and X by the liver. It cannot be synthesized by man but is synthesized by bacterial flora in the colon and absorbed from this site. The reduced form of vitamin K (hydroxyquinone) takes part in the incorporation of CO_2 into $\geq$-methylene of specific L-glutamyl residues of prothrombin and other proteins (Olson 1984). The protein oestocalcin in bone is a vitamin K-dependent $\geq$-carboxy glutamyl (Gla) protein and it may serve a regulatory function in mineralization (Olson 1987). Vitamin K deficiency leads to a bleeding tendency, and vitamin K status is readily assessed indirectly by the measurement of prothrombin time. Recently, two new methods of assessing vitamin K status have been introduced. One is an HPLC method for the measurement of vitamin K (Suttie *et al.* 1988) and the other is the measurement of an under-carboxylated prothrombin precursor (PIVKA II) induced by absence of vitamin K (Motohara *et al.* 1985).

Vitamin K deficiency can arise as a result of reduction in intake, absorption, or utilization. As bacterial synthesis of vitamin K contributes significantly to the daily requirement, drugs that inhibit the bacterial flora, such as sulphonamides and broad-spectrum antibiotics, can reduce the vitamin K status leading to prolonged prothrombin time (Olson 1987).

Malabsorption induced by drugs such as neomycin and cholestyramine (Gross and Brotman 1970) will lead to deficiency. In alcoholics, vitamin K deficiency is common, as demonstrated by a prolonged prothrombin time that is rapidly correctable by vitamin K supplementation, showing that it is due to reduced intake or malabsorption, or both. In severe alcoholic liver disease vitamin K supplementation cannot correct the abnormal prothrombin time as there is a decrease in hepatic synthesis of coagulation factors (Ryle and Thomson 1984). Drugs that cause cholestasis will lead to reduced vitamin K absorption together with malabsorption of fat and other fat-soluble vitamins (see Chapter 11).

Drugs that cause destruction of hepatic parenchymal cells, such as paracetamol (see Chapter 11), will lead to reduced synthesis of vitamin K-dependent clotting factors, and a prolonged prothrombin time will result.

Large amounts of vitamin A and E are known to antagonize vitamin K. In experimental animals, a close relationship between dietary vitamin A (when it is high) and prothrombin levels has been shown. As the effect was not seen when vitamin A was given parenterally, it was thought that vitamin A prevents the absorption of vitamin K (Olson 1987). Prolongation of prothrombin time as a result of large doses of vitamin E has been reported (Corrigan and Marcus 1974; Korsan-Bengsten *et al.* 1974). It is not fully clear whether vitamin E affects the intestinal absorption or the metabolism of vitamin K. It is likely that the effect of vitamin E is due to inhibition of vitamin K-dependent carboxylase activity by α-tocopherol quinone (Olson 1987).

In newborns the plasma levels of prothrombin and other vitamin K-dependent proteins may decrease to as low as 30 per cent of those in later life. This is due to poor transfer of vitamin K by the placenta and absence of synthesis of vitamin K in the gut, which is sterile during the first few days of life. Infants born to mothers treated with anticonvulsants are more prone to vitamin K deficiency (Evans *et al.* 1970), and to neonatal bleeding, which can be fatal (Bleyer and Skinner 1976). The anticonvulsants involved include phenytoin, barbiturates, or a combination of these. Anticonvulsants may also cause subclinical vitamin K deficiency in adults as shown by raised serum levels of PIVKA II (Davies *et al.* 1985).

The anticoagulants bishydroxycoumarin (dicoumarol) and ethylbiscoumacetate, when given to pregnant women, may cause stillbirths and neonatal haemorrhages (Hall *et al.* 1980).

Patients on long-term parenteral nutrition may develop deficiency of vitamin K if supplements are not given (Ryan 1976).

Antagonism

The coumarin group of drugs, of which warfarin is the most popular, induces a reduction in vitamin K-dependent clotting factors (Olson 1984). Surreptitious abuse of anticoagulants is not infrequent among medical and paramedical personnel (O'Reilley and Aggeler 1976; Olson 1984), and this will cause prolonged prothrombin time. Such abuse can be detected by the accumulation of vitamin K 2,3-epoxide (Bechtold *et al.* 1983). A bleeding tendency due to surreptitious administration of anticoagulant by a psychiatrically disturbed mother was noted in a child (White *et al.* 1985).

In spite of close monitoring of the prothrombin time, there is still wide variation between individuals in the response to these anticoagulants, and as many as 25 per cent may develop haemorrhagic complications. Apart from covert warfarin abuse, drug interaction is a common problem. One of the factors which may be responsible for the increased sensitivity may be variation in the availability of vitamin K, from variations in intake, absorption, or utilization. Several drugs are known to alter warfarin action by different mechanisms (see Chapter 30).

Cephalosporins, especially the second-generation and third-generation drugs, may cause hypoprothrombinaemia which could be reversed by vitamin K administration (Hooper *et al.* 1980; Weitekamp and Aber 1983). These antibiotics cause a direct inhibition of γ-carboxylation by their *N*-methyl-thio-tetrazole (NMTT) side-chain or metabolites. Inhibition of vitamin K-dependent factors by cephalosporins appears to be unrelated to their bactericidal effects. It is unlikely, however, that the NMTT side chain *per se* has any hypoprothrombinaemic effect, as the amount required to inhibit the γ-carboxylase reaction *in vitro* is several-fold higher than the plasma levels achieved after therapeutic doses (Bang *et al.* 1982; Lipsky *et al.* 1984).

References

Aanderud, S., Myking, O.L., and Strandjord, R.E. (1981). The influence of carbamazepine on thyroid hormones and thyroxine binding globulin in hypothyroid patients substituted with thyroxine. *Clin. Endocrinol.* 15, 247.

Aarskog, D., Aksnes, L., and Lehmann, V. (1980). Low 1,25-dihydroxyvitamin D in heparin-induced osteopenia. *Lancet* ii, 650.

Abdulla, M. (1979). Copper levels after oral zinc. *Lancet* i, 616.

Abero, K., Shelp, W.D., Kosseff, A., and Thomas, S. (1982). Amoxapine-associated rhabdomyolysis and acute renal failure: case report. *J. Clin. Psychiatry* 43, 426.

Abraham, J.E., Svare, C.W., and Frank, C.W. (1984). The effect of dental amalgam restorations on blood mercury levels. *J. Dent. Res.* 63, 71.

Abraham, P.A., Opsahl, J.A., Halstenson, C.E., and Keane, W.F. (1988). Efficacy and renal effects of enalapril therapy for hypertensive patients with chronic renal insufficiency. *Arch. Intern. Med.* 148, 2358.

Abreo, K., Brown, S.T., and Sella, M. (1989). Correction of microcytosis following elimination of an occult source of aluminum contamination of dialysate. *Am. J. Kidney Dis.* 13, 465.

Abu Melha, A., Ahmed, N.A., and el Hassan, A.Y. (1987). Traditional remedies and lead intoxication. *Trop. Geogr. Med.* 39, 100.

Abu-Hamdan, D.K., Mahajan, S.K., Migdal, S.D., Prasad, A.S., and McDonald, F.D. (1986). Zinc tolerance test in uremia. Effect of ferrous sulfate and aluminum hydroxide. *Ann. Intern. Med.* 104, 50.

Abu-Hamdan, D.K., Desai, H., Sondheimer, J., Felicetta, J., Mahajan, S., and McDonald, F. (1988). Taste acuity and zinc metabolism in captopril-treated hypertensive male patients. *Am. J. Hypertens.* 1, 303s.

Achar, K.N., Abduo, T.J., and Menon, N.K. (1989). Severe hypokalemic rhabdomyolysis due to ingestion of liquorice during Ramadan. *Aust. N.Z. J. Med.* 19, 365.

Ackrill, P. and Day, J.P. (1985). Desferrioxamine in the treatment of aluminum overload. *Clin. Nephrol.* 24, S94.

Acomb, C., Hordon, L.D., Judd, A.T., and Turney, J.H. (1985). Metabolic alkalosis induced by 'Panadol Soluble'. *Lancet* ii, 614.

Adams, A.P. and Pybus, D.A. (1978). Delayed respiratory depression after use of fentanyl during anaesthesia. *Br. Med. J.* i, 278.

Adams, J.M., Hyde, W.H., Procianoy, R.S., and Rudolph, A.J. (1980). Hypochloremic metabolic alkalosis following tolazoline-induced gastric hypersecretion. *Pediatrics* 65, 298.

Adams, P.W., Wynn, V., Folkard, J., and Seed, M. (1976). Influence of oral contraceptives: pyridoxine, vitamin B_6 and tryptophan on carbohydrate metabolism. *Lancet* i, 759.

Addleman, M., Pollard, A., and Grossman, R.F. (1985). Survival after severe hypernatremia due to salt ingestion by an adult. *Am. J. Med.* 78, 176.

Adinoff, A.D. and Hollister, J.R. (1983). Steroid-induced fractures and bone loss in patients with asthma. *N. Engl. J. Med.* 309, 265.

Adler, E., Benjamin, S.B., and Zimmerman, H.J. (1986). Cholestatic hepatic injury related to warfarin therapy. *Arch. Intern. Med.* 146, 1837.

Adlercreutz, H., Eisalo, A., Heino, A., Luukkainen, T., Pentila, I., Saukkonen, H., *et al.* (1968). Investigations on the effect of an oral contraceptive and its components on liver function, serum proteins, copper, caeruloplasmin and gamma-glutamyl peptidase in postmenopausal women. *Scand. J. Gastroenterol.* 3, 273.

Adu, D., Turney, J., Michael, J., and McMaster, P. (1983). Hyperkalaemia in cyclosporin-treated renal allograft recipients. *Lancet* ii, 370.

Aggett, P.J. (1985). Physiology and metabolism of essential trace elements: an outline. *Clin. Endocrinol. Metab.* 14, 513.

Agus, Z.S. and Goldfarb, S. (1985). Calcium metabolism: Normal and abnormal. In *Fluid electrolyte and acid-base disorders* (ed. A.I. Arieff and R.A. DeFronzo), p. 511. Churchill Livingstone, Edinburgh.

Agus, Z.S., Wasserstein, A., and Goldfarb, S. (1982). Disorders of calcium and magnesium homeostasis. *Am. J. Med.* 72, 473.

Ahn, Y-H. and Goldman, J.M. (1985). Trimethoprim–sulfamethoxazole and hyponatremia. *Ann. Intern. Med.* 103, 161.

Aitken, D., West, D., Smith, F., Poznanski, W., Cowman, J., Hurting, J., *et al.* (1977). Cyanide toxicity following nitroprusside induced hypotension. *Can. Anaesth. Soc. J.* 24, 651.

Al-Mufti, H.I. and Arieff, A.I. (1985). Captopril-induced hyponatremia with irreversible neurologic damage. *Am. J. Med.* 79, 769.

Ala-Houhala, M., Korpela, R., Koivikko, M., Koskinen, T., Koskinen, M., and Koivula, T. (1986). Long-term anticonvulsant therapy and vitamin D metabolism in ambulatory pubertal children. *Neuropediatrics* 17, 212.

Albertson, T.E., Reed, S., and Siefkin, A. (1986). A case of fatal sodium azide ingestion. *J. Toxicol. Clin. Toxicol.* 24, 339.

Aldenhovel, H.G. (1988). The influence of long-term anticonvulsant therapy with diphenylhydantoin and carbamazepine on serum gamma-glutamyl transferase, aspartate aminotransferase, alanine aminotransferase and alkaline phosphatase. *Eur. Arch. Psychiatry Neurol. Sci.* 237, 312.

Alen, M. (1985). Androgenic steroid effects on liver and red cells. *Br. J. Sports Med.* 19, 15.

Alexieva-Figusch, J., Blankenstein, H.A., Hop, W.C.J., Klijn, J.G.M., Lamberts, S.W.J., De Jong, F.H., *et al.* (1984). Treatment of metastatic breast cancer patients with different doses of megesterol acetate: Dose, relations, metabolic and endocrine effect. *Eur. J. Cancer. Clin. Oncol.* 20, 33.

Allcott, J.V. III, Barnhart, R.A., and Mooney, L.A. (1987). Acute lead poisoning in two users of illicit methamphetamine. *JAMA* 258, 510.

Allen, J.I., Bell, E., Boosalis, M.G., Oken, M.M., McClain, C.J., Levine, A.S., and Morley, J.E. (1985). Association between urinary zinc excretion and lymphocyte dysfunction in patients with lung cancer. *Am. J. Med.* 79, 209.

Allred, J., Wong, W., and Kafetz, K. (1989). Elderly people taking non-steroidal anti-inflammatory drugs are unlikely to have excess renal impairment. *Postgrad. Med. J.* 65, 735.

Alun-Jones, E. and Williams, J. (1986). Hyponatremia and fluid retention in a neonate associated with maternal naproxen overdosage. *J. Toxicol. Clin. Toxicol* 24, 257.

Alvis, R., Geheb, M., and Cox, M. (1985). Hypo and hyperosmolar states: Diagnostic approaches. In *Fluid electrolyte and acid-base disorders* (ed. A.I. Arieff and R.A. De-Fronzo), p. 185. Churchill Livingstone, Edinburgh.

Amatayakul, K., Uttaravichai, C., Singkamani, R., and Ruckphaopunt, S. (1984). Vitamin metabolism and the effects of multivitamin supplementation in oral contraceptive users. *Contraception* 30, 179.

Amerena, J., Mashford, M.L., and Wallace, S. (1990). Adverse effects of anticoagulants. *Adverse Drug React. Acute Poisoning Rev.* 9, 1.

Amess, J.A., Burman, J.F., Rees, G.M., Nancekievill, D.G., and Mollin, D.L. (1978). Megaloblastic haemopoiesis in patients receiving nitrous oxide. *Lancet* ii, 339.

Amitai, Y. and Lovejoy, F.H. Jr (1988). Hypokalemia in acute theophylline poisoning. *Am. J. Emerg. Med.* 6, 214.

Amos, R.J., Amess, J.A., Hinds, C.J., and Mollin, D.C. (1985). Investigations into the effect of nitrous oxide anaesthesia on folate metabolism in patients receiving intensive care. *Chemotherapia* 4, 393.

Ananth, J. and Dubin, S.E. (1983). Lithium and symptomatic hyperparathyroidism. *J. R. Soc. Med.* 76, 1026.

Anderson, K.E. (1989). LHRH analogues for hormonal manipulation in acute intermittent porphyria. *Semin. Haematol.* 26, 10.

Anderson, R. and Lukey, R.J. (1987). A biological role for ascorbate in the selective neutralisation of extracellular phagocyte-derived oxidants. *Ann. N.Y. Acad. Sci.* 498, 229.

Andreasen, P.B., Lyngbye, J., and Trolle, E. (1973). Abnormalities in diphenylhydantoin therapy in epileptic outpatients. *Acta Med. Scand.* 194, 261.

Andreoli, S.P., Kleiman, M.B., Glick, M.R., and Bergstein, J.M. (1980). Naficillin, pseudo-proteinuria, and hypokalemic alkalosis. *J. Pediatr.* 97, 841.

Anelli, A., Brancaccio, D., Damasso, R., Padovese, P., Gallieni, M., and Garella, S. (1989). Substitution of calcium carbonate for aluminum hydroxide in patients on hemodialysis. Effects on acidosis, on parathyroid function, and on calcemia. *Nephron* 52, 125.

Antonini, G., Palmieri, G., Millefiorini, E., Spagnoli, L.G., and Millefiorini, M. (1989). Lead poisoning during heroin addiction. *Ital. J. Neurol. Sci.* 10, 105.

Appel, G.B. and Neu, H.C. (1977). The nephrotoxicity of antimicrobial agents. *N. Engl. J. Med.* 296, 663-70, 722.

Apple, F.S. (1989). Diagnostic use of CK-MM, and CK-MB isoforms for detecting myocardial infarction. *Clin. Lab. Med.* 9, 643.

Appleby, L. (1984). Rapid development of hyponatraemia during low-dose carbamazepine therapy. *J. Neurol. Neurosurg. Psychiatry* 47, 1138.

Applegate, W.V., Forsythe, A., and Bauernfeind, J.B. (1979). Physiological and psychological effects of vitamins E and B_6 on women taking oral contraceptives. *Int. J. Vitam. Nutr. Res.* 49, 43.

Aranda, J.V., Chemtob, S., Laudiganon, W., and Sasyniuk, B.I. (1986). Frusemide and vitamin E. Two problem drugs in neonatology. *Pediatr. Clin. N. Am.* 33, 583.

Arena, F.P., Dugowson, C., and Saudek, C.D. (1978). Salicylate-induced hypoglycemia and ketoacidosis in a nondiabetic adult. *Arch. Intern. Med.* 138, 1153.

Argov, Z. and Mastaglia, F.L. (1988). Drug-induced neuromuscular disorders in man. In *Disorders of voluntary muscle* (5th edn) (ed. J.N. Walton), p. 981. Churchill Livingstone, Edinburgh.

Arieff, A., Park, R., Leach, W.J., and Lazarowitz, V.C. (1980). Pathophysiology of experimental lactic acidosis in dogs. *Am. J. Phsyiol.* 8, F315.

Arieff, A.I. (1986). Hyponatremia, convulsions, respiratory arrest, and permanent brain damage after elective surgery in healthy woman. *N. Engl. J. Med.* 314, 1529.

Armanini, D., Karbowiak, I., Krozowski, Z., Funder, J.W., and Adam, W.R. (1982). The mechanism of mineralocorticoid action of carbenoxolone. *Endocrinology* 111, 1683.

Arnesen, E., Huseby, N.E., Brenn, T., and Try, K. (1986). The Tromsø heart study: Distribution of, and determinants for, gamma-glutamyltransferase in a free-living population. *Scand. J. Clin. Lab. Invest.* 46, 63.

Arruda, J.A.L., Dytko, G., Mola, R., and Kurtzman, N.A. (1980). On the mechanism of lithium-induced renal tubular acidosis. Studies in the turtle bladder. *Kidney Int.* 17, 196.

Arseneau, J.C., Bagley, C.M., Anderson, T., and Canellos, G.P. (1973). Hyperkalaemia, a sequel to chemotherapy of Burkitt's lymphoma. *Lancet* i, 10.

Arumanayagam, M., Wong, F.W., Chang, A.M., and Swaminathan, R. (1986). Zinc concentration in umbilical cord tissue and cord plasma in appropriate for gestational age babies. *Eur. J. Obstet. Gynecol. Reprod. Biol.* 23, 121.

Arvieux, C., Peyrin, J.C., Dechelette, E., Davin, J.L., Naud, G., and Faure, G. (1984). Insuffisance rénale aiguë au décours de la chirurgie endo-uréthrale sous irrigation de glycocolle. *J. Urol.* 90, 107.

Arvieux, C.C., Rambaud, J.J., Alibeu, J.P., Davin, J.L., Combes, P., and Faure, G. (1985). Etude du catabolisme du glycocolle utilisé dans les solutions de lavage en chirurgie urologique. A propos d'une étude prospective de 20 patients soumis à une résection endourétrale de prostate. *J. Urol.* 91, 417.

Asch, M.J., White, M.G., and Pruitt, B.A. (1970). Acid base changes associated with topical sulfamylon therapy: retrospective study of 100 burn patients. *Ann. Surg.* 172, 946.

Ashouri, O.S. (1986). Severe diuretic-induced hyponatremia in the elderly. *Arch. Intern. Med.* 146, 1355.

Ashraf, M., Scotchel, P.L., Krall, J.M., and Flink, E.B. (1983). cis-Platinum-induced hypomagnesemia and peripheral neuropathy. *Gynecol. Oncol.* 16, 309.

Ashton, R.E., Hawk, J.L., and Magnus, I.A. (1984). Low dose oral chloroquine in the treatment of porphyria cutanea tarda. *Br. J. Dermatol.* 111, 609.

Assadi, F.K. (1989). Therapy of acute bronchospasm. Complicated by lactic acidosis and hypokalemia. *Clin. Pediatr.* 28, 258.

Assan, R. Heuchin, C., Girard, J.R., LeMaire, F., and Altali, J.R. (1975). Phenformin-induced lactic acidosis in diabetic patients. *Diabetes* 24, 791.

Ataya, K., Abbasi, A., Mercado, A., Moghissi, K.S., and Kartaginer, J. (1988). Bone density and reproductive hormones in patients with neuroleptic-induced hyperprolactinemia. *Fertil. Steril.* 50 876.

Atkinson, S.A., Fraher, L., Gundberg, C.M., Andrew, M., Pai, M., and Bar, R.D. (1989). Mineral homeostasis and bone mass in children treated for acute lymphoblastic leukaemia. *J. Pediatr.* 114, 793.

Aucamp, A.K., Van Achtebergh, S.M., and Theron, E. (1981). Potential hazard of magnesium sulphate administration. *Lancet* ii, 1057.

Aunsholt, N.A. (1989). Prolonged Q-T interval and hypokalaemia caused by haloperidol. *Acta Psychiatr. Scand.* 79, 411.

Auvergne, B., Liote, R., Roucoules, J., and Kuntz, D. (1988). Pyrazinamide, hyperuricémie et arthrite goutteuse. *Rev. Rhum. Mal. Osteoartic.* 55, 797.

Awadzi, K., Adjepon-Yamoah, K.K., Edwards, G., Orme, M.L., Breckenridge, A.M., and Gilles, H.M. (1986). The effect of moderate urine alkalinisation on low dose diethylcarbamazine therapy in patients with onchocerciasis. *Br. J. Clin. Pharmacol.* 21, 669.

Ayus, J.C. (1986). Diuretic-induced hyponatremia. *Arch. Intern. Med.* 146, 1295.

Ayus, J.C., Krothapalli, R.K., and Arieff, A.I. (1985). Changing concepts in treatment of severe symptomatic hyponatremia. *Am. J. Med.* 78, 897.

Bachynski, B.N., Flynn, J.T., Rodrigues, M.M., Rosenthal, S., Cullen, R., and Curless, R.G. (1986). Hyperglycemic acidotic coma and death in Kearns-Sayre syndrome. *Ophthalmology* 93, 391.

Back, D.J., Breckenridge, A.M., Crawford, F.E., MacIver, M., Orme, M.L.E., Perucca, E., et al. (1980). The effect of oral contraceptive steroids and enzyme inducing drugs on sex hormone binding globulin capacity in women. *Br. J. Clin. Pharmacol.* 9, 115p.

Baer, D.M., Jones, R.N., Mullooly, J.P., and Horner, W. (1983). Protocol for the study of drug interferences in laboratory tests: Cefotaxime interference in 24 clinical tests. *Clin. Chem.* 29, 1736.

Baker, E.J., Reed, K.D., and Dixon, S.L. (1989). Chlorthalidone-induced pseudoporphyria: clinical and microscopic findings of a case. *J. Am. Acad. Dermatol.* 21, 1026.

Baker, L.R.I., Ackrill, P., Cattell, W.R., Stamp, T.C.B., and Watson, L. (1974). Iatrogenic oesteomalacia and myopathy due to phosphate depletion. *Br. Med. J.* iii, 150.

Balazs, M. and Kovach, G. (1981). Chronic aggressive hepatitis after methyldopa treatment: case report with electron microscopic study. *Hepatogastroenterology* 28, 199.

Ball, M.J., Paul, J., and Kay, J.D.S. (1987). Analytical interference by rifampacin with tests of liver function. *Ann. Clin. Biochem.* 24 (suppl. S1), 75.

Baluarte, H.J., Gruskin, A.B., Hiner, L.B., Foley, C.M., and Grover, W.D. (1977). Encephalopathy in children with chronic renal failure. *Proc. Clin. Dial. Transplant Forum* 7, 95.

Bamford, M.F. and Cruickshank, G. (1989). Dangers of intranasal desmopressin for nocturnal enuresis. *J. R. Coll. Gen. Pract.* 39, 345.

Bamji, M.S., Prema, K., Jacob, C.M., Rani, M., and Samyakta, D. (1985). Vitamin supplements to Indian women using low dosage oral contraceptives. *Contraception* 32, 405.

Bang, N.U., Tessler, S.S., Heidenreich, R.O., Marks, C.A. and Mattler, L.E. (1982). Effects of moxalactane on blood coagulation and platelet function. *Rev. Infect. Dis.* 4 (suppl. 1), S546.

Bantle, J.P., Nath, K.A., Sutherland, D.E.R., Najarian, J.S., and Ferris, T.F. (1985). Effects of cyclosporine on the renin–angiotensin–aldosterone system and potassium excretion in renal transplant recipients. *Ann. Intern. Med.* 145, 505.

Bar, R.S., Wilson, H.E., and Mazzaferri, E.L. (1975). Hypomagnesemic hypocalcemia secondary to renal magnesium wasting: a possible consequence of high dose gentamicin therapy. *Ann. Intern. Med.* 82, 646.

Barbosa, J., Seal, U.S., and Doe, R.P. (1971). Effects of anabolic steroids on haptoglobin, orosomucoid, plasminogen, fibrinogen, transferrin, ceruloplasmin. α-1-antitrypsin, β-glucuronidase and total serum proteins. *J. Clin. Endocrinol. Metab.* 33, 388.

Bardana, E.J. Jr, Gabourel, J.D., Davies, G.H., and Craig, S. (1984). Effects of phenytoin on man's immunity: Evaluation of changes in serum immunoglobulins, complement and antinuclear antibody. *Am. J. Med.* 74, 289.

Barilla, D.E., Notz, C., Kennedy, D., and Pak, C.Y.C. (1978). Renal oxalate excretion following oral oxalate loads in patients with ileal disease and with renal and absorptive hypercalciuria. Effect of calcium and magnesium. *Am. J. Med.* 64, 579.

Barnard, H.C., de Kock, J.J., Vermaak, W.J., and Potgieter, G.M. (1987). A new perspective in the assessment of vitamin B_6 nutritional status during pregnancy in human. *J. Nutr.* 117, 1303.

Barnes, D.B., Pierce, G.F., Lichtl, D., Landt, M., Koenig, J., and Chan, K.M. (1985). Effects of dextran on five biuret-based procedures for total protein in serum. *Clin. Chem.* 31, 2018.

Barragry, J.M., Makin, H.L.J., Trafford, D.J.H., and Scott, D.F. (1978). Effect of anticonvulsants on plasma testosterone and sex hormone binding globulin levels. *J. Neurol. Neurosurg. Psychiatry* 41, 913.

Barton, C.H., Vaziri, N.D., Martin, D.C., Choi, S., and Alikhani, S. (1987). Hypomagnesemia and renal magnesium wasting in renal transplant recipients receiving cyclosporine. *Am. J. Med.* 83, 693.

Bashir, Y. and Tomson, C.R. (1988). Cardiac arrest associated with hypokalaemia in a patient receiving mithramycin. *Postgrad. Med. J.* 64, 228.

Bassler, K.H. and Heidenreich, O. (1984). Zur Problematik von Sulfitzusatz zu Infusionslosungen. *Infusionsther. Klin. Ernahr.* 11, 31.

Bastomsky, C.H., Dent, R.R., and Tolis, G. (1977). Elevated serum concentrations of thyroxine-binding globulin and caeruloplasmin in methadone-maintained patients. *Clin. Biochem.* 10, 124.

Bates, C.J., Prentice, A.M., Watkinson, M., Morrell, P., Sutcliffe, B.A., Foord, F.A., *et al.* (1982). Riboflavin requirements of lactating Gambian woman: a controlled supplementation trial. *Am. J. Clin. Nutr.* 35, 701.

Batist, G., Klecker, R.W. Jr, Jayaram, H.N., Jenkins, J.F., Grygiel, J., Ihde, D.C., *et al.* (1985). Phase I and pharmacokinetic study of tiazofurin (TCAR, NSC 286193) administered by continuous infusion. *Invest. New Drugs* 3, 349.

Batlle, D.C. (1989a). Renal tubular acidosis. In *The regulation of acid–base balance* (ed. D.W. Seldin and G. Giebisch), p. 353. Raven Press, New York.

Batlle. D.C. (1989b). Hyperchloremic metabolic acidosis. In *The regulation of acid–base balance* (ed. D.W. Seldin and G. Giebisch), p. 319. Raven Press, New York.

Batlle, D.C., Gaviria, M., Grupp, M., Arruda, J.A.L., Wynn, J., and Kurtzman, N.A. (1982). Distal nephron function in patients receiving chronic lithium therapy. *Kidney Int.* 21, 477.

Batlle, D.C., von Riotte A., and Schlueter, W. (1987). Urinary sodium in the evaluation of hyperchloremic metabolic acidosis. *N. Engl. J. Med.* 316, 140.

Batlle, D.C., Sabatini, S., and Kurtzman, N.A. (1988a). On the mechanism of toluene-induced renal tubular acidosis. *Nephron* 49, 210.

Batlle, D.C., Hizon, M., Cohen, E., Gutterman, C., and Gupta, R. (1988b). The use of the urinary anion gap in the diagnosis of hyperchloremic metabolic acidosis. *N. Engl. J. Med.* 318, 594.

Baumann, G. (1979). Hyponatremia during adrenocorticotropin (ACTH) infusions. *Ann. Intern. Med.* 91, 499.

Baumann, G., Rayfield, E.J., Rose, L.T., Williams, G.H., and Dingman, J.F. (1972). 'Trace' contamination of cortico-trophin and human growth hormone with vasopressin: clinical significance. *J. Clin. Endocrinol. Metab.* 34, 801.

Baumann, R., Magos, A.L., Kay, J.D.S., and Turnbull, A.C. (1990). Absorption of glycine irrigating solution during transcervical resection of endometrium. *Br. Med. J.* 300, 304.

Bayer, A.J., Farag, R., Browne, S., and Pathy, M.S.J. (1986). Plasma electrolytes in elderly patients taking fixed combination diuretics. *Postgrad. Med. J.* 62, 159.

Beastall, G.H., Cowan, R.A., Gray, J.M., and Fogelman, I. (1985). Hormone binding globulins and anticonvulsant therapy. *Scott. Med. J.* 30, 101.

Beattie, A.D. and Sherlock, S. (1976). Ascorbic acid deficiency in liver disease. *Gut* 17, 571.

Beatty, O.L., Campbell, N.P., and Neely, R.D. (1989). Tetany in association with gentamicin therapy. *Ulster Med. J.* 58, 108.

Bechtold, H., Trenk, D., Jähnchen, E., and Meinertz, T. (1983). Plasma vitamin K_1-2,3-epoxide as diagnostic aid to detect surreptitious ingestion of oral anticoagulant drug. *Lancet* i, 596.

Beck, L.H. (1979). Hypouricemia in the syndrome of inappropriate secretion of antidiuretic hormone. *N. Engl. J. Med.* 301, 528.

Beghi, E. and Di Mascio, R. (1986). Antiepileptic drug toxicity: definition and mechanism of action. *Ital. J. Neurol. Sci.* 7, 209.

Beghi, E., Di Mascio, R., and Tognoni, G. (1986). Adverse effects of anticonvulsant drugs — a critical review. *Adverse Drug React. Acute Poisoning Rev.* 2, 63.

Behm, A.R. and Unger, W.P. (1974). Oral contraceptives and porphyria cutanea tarda. *Can. Med. Assoc. J.* 110, 1052.

Bei, L., Wood, R.J., and Rosenberg, I.H. (1986). Glucose polymer increases jejunal calcium, magnesium, and zinc absorption in humans. *Am. J. Clin. Nutr.* 44, 244.

Beier, L.S., Pits, W.H., and Gonick, H.C. (1963). Metabolic acidosis occurring during paraldehyde intoxication. *Ann. Intern. Med.* 58, 155.

Belaiche, J., Le Carrer, M., Krainik, F., and Cattan, D. (1977). Clofibrate-induced increase in serum creatine-phosphokinase level. *Lancet* i, 149.

Bell, D.R., Woods, R.L., and Levi, J.A. (1985). cis-Diamminedichloroplatinum-induced hypomagnesemia and renal magnesium wasting. *Eur. J. Cancer. Clin. Oncol.* 21, 287.

Bencko, V., Wagner, V., Wagnerova, M., Batora, J., and Hrebacka, J. (1988). Immunobiochemical profiles of workers differing in the degree of occupational exposure to vinyl chloride. *J. Hyg. Epidemiol. Microbiol. Immunol.* 32, 375 (P56).

Bender, D.A. (1983). Effects of oestradiol and vitamin B_6 on tryptophan metabolism in the rat: implications for the interpretation of the tryptophan load test for vitamin B_6 nutritional status. *Br. J. Nutr.* 50, 33.

Bender, D.A., Laing, A.E., Vale, J.A., Papadaki, L., and Pugh, M. (1983). The effects of oestrogen administration on tryptophan metabolism in rats and in menopausal women receiving hormone replacement therapy. *Biochem. Pharmacol.* 32, 843.

Benitz, K-F. and Diermeier, H.F. (1964). Renal toxicity of tetracycline degradation products. *Proc. Soc. Exp. Biol. Med.* 115, 930.

Benjamin, N., Phillips, R.J., and Robinson, B.F. (1988). Verapamil and bendrofluazide in the treatment of hypertension: a controlled study of effectiveness alone and in combination. *Eur. J. Clin. Pharmacol.* 34, 249.

Berg, W., Bothor, C., Pirlich, W., and Janitzky, V. (1986). Influence of magnesium on the absorption and excretion of calcium and oxalate ions. *Eur. Urol.* 12, 274.

Berger, W. (1985). Incidence of severe side effects during therapy with sulfonylureas and biguanides. *Horm. Metab. Res.* (suppl. 15), 111.

Bergink, E.W., Holma, P., and Pyorala, T. (1981). Effect of oral contraceptive combinations containing levonorgestrel or desogestrel on serum proteins and androgen binding. *Scand. J. Clin. Lab. Invest.* 41, 663.

Berkelhammer, C.H., Wood, R.J., and Sitrin, M.D. (1988). Acetate and hypercalciuria during total parenteral nutrition. *Am. J. Clin. Nutr.* 48, 1482.

Beroniade, V., Corneille, L., and Haraoui, B. (1979). Indomethacin-induced inhibition of prostaglandin with hyperkalemia. *Ann. Intern. Med.* 91, 499.

Berova, N. and Lazarova, A. (1988). Pellagra-ähnliche Veranderungen nach Glibenklamid-Behandlung bei einer Patientin mit Diabetes mellitus und Vitiligo. *Dermatol. Monatsschr.* 174, 50.

Bersin, R.M. and Arieff, A.I. (1988). Improved hemodynamic function during hypoxia with carbicarib: A new agent for the management of acidosis. *Circulation* 77, 227.

Besser, R., Gutman, L., and Weilemann, L.S. (1989). Inactivation of end-plate acetylcholinesterase during the course of organophosphate intoxications. *Arch. Toxicol.* 63, 412.

Bethune, D.W. and McKay, R. (1978). Paradoxical changes in serum potassium during cardiopulmonary bypass in association with non-cardioselective beta blockade. *Lancet* ii, 380.

Bhagavan, H.N. (1985). Interaction between vitamin B_6 and drugs. In *Current topics in nutrition and disease. Vitamin B_6: its role in health and disease*, Vol. 13 (ed. R.D. Reynolds and J.E. Leklem), p. 401. Alan R. Liss, New York.

Bibler, M.R., Frame, P.T., Hagler, D.N., Bode, R.B., Staneck, J.L., Thamlikitkul, V., *et al* (1987). Clinical evaluation of efficacy, pharmacokinetics, and safety of teicoplanin for serious gram-positive infections. *Amtimicrob. Agents Chemother.* 31, 207.

Bippi, H. and Guinot, P. (1988). Study of the effects of cicletanine on the renin-angiotensin-aldosterone system. *Drugs Exp. Clin. Res.* 14, 215.

Birch, A.A., Mitchell, G.D., Playford, G.A., and Lang, C.A. (1969). Changes in serum potassium response to succinylcholine following trauma. *JAMA* 210, 490.

Blachley, J.D. and Knochel, J.P. (1980). Tobacco chewer's hypokalemia: licorice revisited. *N. Engl. J. Med.* 302, 784.

Blain P.G. and Lane, P.J.M. (1983). Drugs and muscle. *Adverse Drug React. Acute Poisoning Rev.* 2, 1.

Blain, P.G., Lane, R.J., Bateman, D.N., and Rawlins, M.D. (1985). Opiate- induced rhabdomyolysis. *Hum. Toxicol.* 4, 71.

Blanchard, P.D., Yao, J.D., McAlpine, D.E., and Hurt, R.D. (1986). Isoniazid overdose in the Cambodian population of Olmsted County, Minnesota. *JAMA* 256, 3131.

Bleakley, P., Nichol, A.W., and Collins, A.G. (1979). Diazinon and porphyria cutanea tarda. *Med. J. Aust.* i, 314.

Bleyer, W.A. and Skinner, A.L. (1976). Fatal neonatal hemorrhage after maternal anticonvulsant therapy. *JAMA* 235, 626.

Blom, J.H., Kurth, K.H., and Splinter, T.A. (1985). Renal function, serum calcium and magnesium during treatment of advanced bladder carcinoma with cis-dichlorodiamminoplatinum: impact of tumour site, patient age and magnesium suppletion. *Int. Urol. Nephrol.* 17, 331.

Blomfield, J., Dixon, S.R., and McCredie, D.A. (1971). Potential hepatotoxicity of copper in recurrent hemodialysis. *Arch. Intern. Med.* 128, 555.

Bloomer, J.R. and Bonkovsky, H.L. (1989). The porphyrias. *Disease-a-month* 35, 1.

Blum, J.E. and Coe, F.L. (1977). Metabolic acidosis after sulfur ingestion. *N. Engl. J. Med.* 297, 869.

Blum, M. and Aviram, A. (1980). Ibuprofen induced hyponatraemia. *Rheumatol. Rehabil.* 19, 258.

Body, J.J., Cryer, P.E., Offord, K.P., and Heath, H. III. (1983). Epinephrine is a hypophosphatemic hormone in man. *J. Clin. Invest.* 71, 572.

Bogliun, G., Beghi, E., Crespi, V., Delodovici, L., and d'Amico, P. (1986). Anticonvulsant drugs and bone metabolism. *Acta Neurol. Scand.* 74, 284.

Bohannon, N.J.V. (1989). Large phosphate shifts with treatment for hyperglycemia. *Arch. Intern. Med.* 149, 1423.

Böhrer, H., Fleischer, F., and Krier, C. (1988). Hyperkalemic cardiac arrest after cardiac surgery following high-dose glucose–insulin–potassium infusion for inotropic support. *Anesthesiology* 69, 949.

Bollag, W. (1983). Vitamin A and retinoids: from nutrition to pharmacotherapy in dermatology and oncology. *Lancet* i, 860.

Bolli, P., Simpson, F.O., and Waal-Manning, H.J. (1978). Comparison of tienilic acid with cyclopenthiazide in hyperuricaemic hypertensive patient. *Lancet* ii, 595.

Bond, W.S. (1977). Toxic reactions and side effects of glucocorticoids in man. *Am. J. Hosp. Pharm.* 34, 479.

Bongiovanni, M.B., Strauss, J.E., Ziselman, E.M., and Wurzel, H.A. (1983). Parathyroid response during therapeutic plasma exchange. *Transfusion* 23, 535.

Bonnici, F. (1973). Antidiuretic effects of clofibrate and carbamazepine in diabetes insipidus: studies on free water clearance and response to a water load. *Clin. Endocrinol. Metab.* 2, 265.

Boosalis, M.G., McCall, J.T., Ahrenholz, D.H., Solem, L.D., and McClain, C.J. (1987). Serum and urinary silver levels in thermal injury patients. *Surgery* 101, 40.

Borges, H.F., Hocks, J., and Kjellstrand, C.M. (1982). Mannitol intoxication in patients with renal failure. *Arch. Intern. Med.* 142, 63.

Bork, E. and Hansen, M. (1986). Severe hyponatremia following simultaneous administration of aminoglutethimide and diuretics. *Cancer Treat. Rep.* 70, 689.

Borland, C., Amadi, A., Murphy, P., and Shallcross, T. (1986). Biochemical and clinical correlates of diuretic therapy in the elderly. *Age Ageing* 15, 357.

Boton, R., Gaviria, M., and Batlle, D.C. (1987). Prevalence, pathogenesis and treatment of renal dysfunction associated with chronic lithium therapy. *Am. J. Kidney Dis.* 10, 329.

Bottomley, S.S. and Muller-Eberhard, U. (1988). Pathophysiology of heme synthesis. *Semin. Haematol.* 25, 282.

Bouchard, P.H., Sai, P., Reach, G., Caubarrere, I., Ganeval, D., and Assan, R. (1982). Diabetes mellitus following pentamidine-induced hypoglycemia in humans. *Diabetes* 31, 40.

Bozzetti, F. (1979). Parenteral nutrition related beri-beri in patients on long-term parenteral nutrition. *Br. Med. J.* i, 487.

Braden, G., von Oeyen, P., Smith, M., Gingras, D., Germain, M., and Fitzgibbons, J. (1985a). Mechanism of ritodrine and terbutaline-induced hypokalemia and pulmonary edema. *Kidney Int.* 27, 304.

Braden, G.L., Johnston, S.S., Germain, M.J., Fitzgibbons, J.P., and Dawson, J.A. (1985b). Lactic acidosis associated with the therapy of acute bronchospasm. *N. Engl. J. Med.* 313, 890.

Brady, H.R., Goldberg, H., Lunski, C., and Uldalll, P.R. (1988). Dialysis-induced hyperkalaemia presenting as profound muscle weakness. *Int. J. Artif. Org.* 11, 43.

Brady, H.R., Ryan, F., Cunningham, J., Tormey, W., Ryan, M.P., and O'Neill, S. (1989). Hypophosphatemia complicating bronchodilator therapy for acute severe asthma. *Arch. Intern. Med.* 149, 2367.

Brady, J.P. and Williams, H.C. (1967). Magnesium intoxication in a premature infant. *Pediatrics* 40, 100.

Braide, S.A. and Davies, T.J. (1987). Factors that affect the induction of gammaglutamyltransferase in epileptic patients receiving anti-convulsant drugs. *Ann. Clin. Biochem.* 24, 391.

Brand, J.M. and Greer, F.R. (1990). Hypermagnesemia and intestinal perforation following antacid administration in a premature infant. *Pediatrics* 85, 121.

Brater, D.C. (1986). Drug-induced electrolyte disorders. In *Fluids and electrolytes.* (ed. J.P. Kokko and R.L. Tannen), p. 760. W.B. Saunders, Philadelphia.

Brautbar, N. and Massry, S.G. (1987). Hypomagnesemia and hypermagnesemia. In *Clinical disorders of fluids and electrolyte metabolism* (ed. M.H. Maxwell, C.R. Kleman, R.G. Narins), p. 831. McGraw-Hill, New York.

Bremme, K., Eneroth, P., Nordstrom, L., and Nilsson, B. (1986). Effects of infusion of the beta-adrenoceptor agonist terbutaline on serum magnesium in pregnant women. *Magnesium* 5, 85.

Bressler, R.B. and Huston, D.P. (1985). Water intoxication following moderate-dose intravenous cyclophosphamide. *Arch. Intern. Med.* 145, 548.

Brickman, A.S., Massry, S.G., and Coburn, J.W. (1972). Changes in serum and urinary calcium during treatment with hydrochlorothiazide: studies on mechanism. *J. Clin. Invest.* 51, 945.

Briggs, M.H. (1974). Vitamin A and the teratogenic risks of oral contraceptives. *Br. Med. J.* iii, 170.

Briggs, M.H. and Briggs, M. (1971). Effects of oral ethinylestradiol on serum proteins in normal women. *Contraception* 3, 381.

Briggs, M.H., Garcia-Webb, P., and Davies, P. (1973). Urinary oxalate and vitamin C supplements. *Lancet* ii, 201.

British Medical Journal (1977). Liver disease and vitamin C. *Br. Med. J.* i, 735.

Brocks, A.S., Reid, H., and Glazer, G. (1977). Acute intravenous zinc poisoning. *Br. Med. J.* i, 1390.

Brodie, M.J., Boobis, A.R., Dollery, C.T., Hillyard, C.J., Brown, D.J., MacIntyre, I., et al. (1980). Rifampicin and vitamin D metabolism. *Clin. Pharmacol. Ther.* 27, 810.

Brodie, M.J., Boobis, A.R., Gill, M., and Mashiter, K. (1981). Does rifampicin increase serum levels of testosterone and oestradiol by inducing sex hormone binding globulin capacity? *Br. J. Clin. Pharmacol.* 12, 431.

Brodie, M.J., Boobis, A.R., Hillyard, C.J., Abeyasekera, G., Stevenson, J.C., MacIntyre, I., et al. (1982). Effect of rifampicin and isoniazid on vitamin D metabolism. *Clin. Pharmacol. Ther.* 32, 525.

Brooks-Hill, P.W., Bishop, B.E., and Vellend, H. (1985). Pellagra-like encephalopathy complicating a multiple drug regimen for the treatment of pulmonary infection due to mycobacterium avium-intracellular. *Am. Rev. Respir. Dis.* 131, 476.

Brown, R.R., Rose, D.P., Leklem, J.E., Linkswiler, H., and Anard, R. (1975). Urinary 4-pyridoxic acid, plasma pyridoxal phosphate, and erythrocyte aminotransferase levels in oral contraceptive users receiving controlled intakes of vitamin B_6. *Am. J. Clin. Nutr.* 28, 10.

Brunet, W.G., Hutton, L.C., and Henderson, A.R. (1989). The effect of nonionic radiographic contrast medium on serum electrolytes and proteins during intravenous urography. *Can. Assoc. Radiol. J.* 40, 139.

Brunner, F.P. and Frick, P.G. (1968). Hypokalaemia, metabolic alkalosis, and hypernatraemia due to 'massive' sodium penicillin therapy. *Br. Med. J.* iv, 550.

Budden, F.H., Bayley, T.A., Harrison, J.E., Josse, R.G., Murray, T.M., Sturtridge, W.C., et al. (1988). The effect of fluoride on bone histology in postmenopausal osteoporosis depends on adequate fluoride absorption and retention. *J. Bone Miner. Res.* 3 127.

Burgess, C.D., Flatt, A., Siebers, R., Crane, J., Beasley, R. and Purdie, G. (1989). A comparison of the extent and duration of hypokalaemia following three nebulized beta 2-adrenoceptor agonists. *Eur. J. Clin. Pharmacol.* 36, 415.

Burnakis, T.G. and Mioduch, H,J. (1984). Combined therapy with captopril and potassium supplementation. A potential for hyperkalemia. *Arch. Intern. Med.* 144, 2371.

Burns, J.T. (1987). Concluding remarks. Third conference on vitamin C. *Ann. N.Y. Acad. Sci.* 498, 534.

Busch, E.H., Ventura, H.O., and Lavie, C.J. (1987). Heparin-induced hyperkalemia. *South. Med. J.* 80, 1450.

Bush, M.E. and Dahms, B.B. (1984). Fatal hypervitaminosis A in a neonate. *Arch. Pathol. Lab. Med.* 108, 838.

Bushinsky, D.A. and Coe, F.L. (1985). Hyperkalemia during acute ammonium chloride acidosis in man. *Nephron* 40, 38.

Bushinsky, D.A. and Gennari, F.J. (1978). Life-threatening hyperkalemia induced by arginine. *Ann. Intern. Med.* 89, 632.

Bussien, J.P., d'More, T.F., Perret, L., Porchet, M.O., Nussberger, J., Waeber, B., et al. (1986). Single and repeated dosing of the converting enzyme inhibitor perindopril to normal subjects. *Clin. Pharmacol. Ther.* 39, 554.

Butler, W.T. and Rossen, R.D. (1973). Effect of corticosteroids on immunity in man. I. Decreased serum IgGconcentration caused by 3 or 5 days of high doses of methylprednisolone. *J. Clin. Invest.* 52, 2629.

Butterworth, C.E., Hatch, K., Cole, P., Sauberlich, H.E., Tamura, T., Cornwell, P.E., et al. (1988). Zinc concentration in plasma and erythrocytes of subjects receiving folic acid supplementation. *Am. J. Clin. Nutr.* 47, 484.

Caldwell, J.W., Nava, A.J., and de Haas D.D. (1987). Hypernatremia associated with cathartics in overdose management. *West. J. Med.* 147, 593.

Calic, R., Straus, B., and Cepelak, I. (1989). Changes of activities of some transferases, alkaline phosphatase and cholinesterase in the blood of women using oral contraceptives and in vitro influence of these agents on tissular enzyme levels in rat liver. *Z. Med. Lab. Diagn.* 30, 375.

Callaghan, T.S., Hadden, D.R., and Tomkin, G.H. (1980). Megaloblastic anaemia due to vitamin B_{12} malabsorption associated with long-term metformin treatment. *Br. Med. J.* 280, 1214.

Calvo, R., Carlos, R., and Erill, S. (1985). Underestimation of albumin content by bromocresol green, induced by drug displacers and uremia. *Int. J. Clin. Pharmacol. Ther. Toxicol.* 23, 76.

Cameron, J.S. and Simmonds, H.A. (1981). Uric acid gout and the kidney. *J. Clin. Path.* 34, 1245.

Campbell, I.W. (1985). Metformin and the sulphonylureas: the comparative risk. *Horm. Metab. Res.* (suppl. 15), 105.

Capasso, G., Jaeger, P., Giebisch, G., Guckian, V., and Malnic, G. (1987). Renal bicarbonate reabsorption in the rat. II. Distal tubule load dependence and effect of hypokalemia. *J. Clin. Invest.* 80, 409.

Cardoso, M., Shoubridge, E., Arnold, D., Leveille, M., Prud'Homme, M., St- Louis, G., et al. (1988). NMR monitoring of the energy status of skeletal muscle during hemodialysis using acetate. *Clin. Invest. Med.* 11, 292.

Carey, H.M. (1971). Principles of oral contraception: 2 side effects of oral contraceptives. *Med. J. Aust.* ii, 1242.

Carl, P., Crawford, M.E., Madsen, N.B., Ravlo, O., Bach, V., and Larsen, A.I. (1987). Pain relief after major abdominal surgery: a double-blind controlled comparison of sublingual buprenorphine, intramuscular buprenorphine, and intramuscular meperidine. *Anesth. Analg.* 66, 142.

Carlsson, E., Fellenius, E., Lundborg, P., and Svensson, L. (1978). β-Adrenoceptor blockers, plasma potassium and exercise. *Lancet* ii, 424.

Carlsson, E.C., Rudolph, A., Stanger, P., Teitel, D., Weber, W., and Yoshida, H. (1985). Pediatric angiocardiography with iohexol. *Invest. Radiol.* 20, (suppl. 1), S75.

Caspray, W.F., Tonissen, J., and Lankisch, P.G. (1977). 'Enteral' hyperoxaluria. Effect of cholestyramine, calcium, neomycin and bile acids on intestinal oxalate absorption in man. *Acta Hepatol. Gastroenterol.* 24, 193.

Castelbaum, A.R., Donofrio, P.D., Walker, F.O., and Troost, B.T. (1989). Laxative abuse causing hypermagnesemia, quadriparesis, and neuromuscular junction defect. *Neurology* 39, 746.

Cate, J.C. and Hedrick, R. (1980). Propylene glycol intoxication and lactic acidosis. *N. Engl. J. Med.* 303, 1237.

Cavalieri, R.R., Gavin, L.A., Wallace, A., Hammond, M.E., and Cruse, K. (1979). Serum thyroxine free T_4, triiodothyronine and reverse-T_3 in diphenylhydantoin-treated patients. *Metabolism* 28, 1161.

Cavallo-Perin, P., Aluffi, E., Estivi, P., Bruno, A., Carta, Q., Pagano, G., et al. (1989). The hyperlactaemic effect of biguanides: a comparison between phenformin and metformin during a 6-month treatment. *Riv. Eur. Sci. Med. Farmacol.* 11, 45.

Chakrabarti, R., Fearnley, G.R., and Evans, J.F. (1968). Effects of clofibrate on fibrinolysis, platelet stickiness, plasmafibrinogen, and serum cholesterol. *Lancet* ii, 1007.

Chalmers, D.M., Levi, A.J., Chanarin, I., North, W.R.S., and Meade, T.W. (1979). Mean cell volume in a working population: the effects of age, smoking, alcohol and oral contraception. *Br. J. Haematol.* 43, 631.

Chan, M.K., Beale, D., and Moorhead, J.F. (1980). Acute megaloblastosis due to cotrimoxazole. *Br. J. Clin. Pract.* 34, 187.

Chanarin, I. (1980). Cobalamins and nitrous oxide: a review. *J. Clin. Pathol.* 33, 909.

Chanarin, I. (1982). Haemopoiesis and alcohol. *Br. Med. Bull.* 38, 81.

Chapman, J.R., Griffiths, D., Harding, N.G., and Morris, P.J. (1985). Reversibility of cyclosporin nephrotoxicity after three months' treatment. *Lancet* i, 128.

Chapron, D.L., Gomolin, I.H., and Sweeney, K.R. (1989). Acetazolamide blood concentrations are excessive in the elderly: propensity for acidosis and relationship to renal function. *J. Clin. Pharmacol.* 29, 348.

Chattoraj, S.C. and Watts, N.B. (1986). Endocrinology. In *Textbook of Clinical Chemistry* (ed. N.W. Tietz), p. 997. W.B. Saunders, Philadelphia.

Chen, B., Shapira, J., Ravid, M., and Lang, R. (1982). Steatorrhoea induced by allopurinol. *Br. Med. J.* i, 1914.

Chen, L.H. (1981). An increase in vitamin E requirement induced by high supplementation of vitamin C in rats. *Am. J. Clin. Nutr.* 34, 1036.

Cheng, J.T., Witty, R.T., Robinson, R.R., and Yarger, W.E. (1982). Amphotericin B nephrotoxicity: increased renal resistance and tubule permeability. *Kidney Int.* 22, 626.

Chestnut, C.H. III (1988). Drug therapy: Calcitonin, biphosphonates, anabolic steroids, and hPTH (1-34). In *Osteoporosis, etiology, diagnosis, and management* (ed. B.L. Riggs and L.J. Melton III), p. 403. Raven Press, New York.

Chilvers, D.C., Jones, M.M., Selby, P.L., Dawson, J.B., and Hodgkinson, A. (1985). Effects of oral ethinyl oestradiol and norethisterone on plasma copper and zinc complexes in post-menopausal women. *Horm. Metab. Res.* 17, 532.

Chin, L., Sievers, M.L., Herrier, R.N., and Picchioni, A.L. (1979). Convulsion as the etiology of lactic acidosis in acute isoniazid toxicity in dogs. *Toxicol. Appl. Pharmacol.* 49, 377.

Chretien, J.H. and Garagusi, V.F. (1973). Correction of corticosteroid-induced defects of polymorphonuclear neutrophil function by ascorbic acid. *J. Reticuloendothel. Soc.* 14, 280.

Christensen, E., Schlichting, P., Fauerholdt, L., Juhl, E., Poulsen, H., and Tygstrup, N. (1985). Changes of laboratory variables with time in cirrhosis: prognostic and therapeutic significance. *Hepatology* 5, 843.

Christensson, T., Hellstrom, K., and Wengle, B. (1977). Hypercalcemia and primary hyperparathyroidism. Prevalence in patients receiving thiazides as detected in health screen. *Arch. Intern. Med.* 137, 1138.

Christiansen, C., Nielsen, S.P., and Rodbro, P. (1974). Anticonvulsant hypomagnesaemia. *Br. Med. J.* i, 198.

Christiansen, C., Baastrup, P.C., Lindgreen, P., and Transbol, I. (1978). Endocrine effects of lithium: II primary hyperparathyroidism. *Acta Endocrinol.* 88, 528.

Christiansen, C., Christensen, M.S., Larsen, N.E., and Transbol, I.B. (1982). Pathophysiological mechanisms of oestrogen effect on bone metabolism: Dose-response relationships in early postmenopausal women. *J. Clin. Endocrinol. Metab.* 55, 1124.

Christiansen, C., Rodbro, P., and Tjellesen, L. (1984). Serum alkaline phosphatase during hormone treatment in early post-menopausal women. A model for establishing optimal prophylaxis and treatment in postmenopausal osteoporosis. *Acta Med. Scand.* 216, 11.

Cimino, J.A., Epel, R., and Cooperman, J.M. (1985). Effect of diet on vitamin deficiencies in retarded individuals receiving drugs. *Drug Nutr. Interact.* 3, 201.

Citrin, D.L., Wallemark, C.B., Nadler, R., Geiger, C., Tuttle, K., Kaplan, E.H., *et al.* (1986). Estramustine affects bone mineral metabolism in metastatic prostate cancer. *Cancer* 58, 2208.

Clasen, W., Khartabil, T., Imm, S., and Kindler, J. (1988). Torasemide for diuretic treatment of advanced chronic renal failure. *Arzneimittelforschung* 38, 209.

Clausen, T. and Flatman, J.A. (1980). Beta$_2$-adrenoceptors mediate the stimulating effect of adrenaline on active elec-trogenic Na–K transport in rat soleus muscle. *Br. J. Pharmacol.* 68, 749.

Clausen, T. and Flatman, J.A. (1987). Effect of insulin and epinephrine on Na$^+$,K$^+$-ATPase and glucose transport in soleus muscle. *Am. J. Physiol.* 252, E492.

Clausen, T.G., Brocks, K., and Ibsen, H. (1988). Hypokalemia and ventricular arrhythmias in acute myocardial infarction. *Acta Med. Scand.* 224, 531.

Cobbledick, R.E. and Hinberg, I.H. (1984). Sodium azide interference with a radioimmunoassay for prostatic acid phosphatase. *Clin. Chem.* 30, 1264.

Cogan, M.G. (1982). Disorders of proximal nephron function. *Am. J. Med.* 72, 275.

Cohen, H.N., Pearson, D.W.M., Thomson, J.A., Patclief, W.A. and Beastall, G.H. (1981). Trimethoprim and thyroid function. *Lancet* i, 676.

Cohen, L., Kitzes, R., and Shnaider, H. (1985). The myth of long-term thiazide-induced magnesium deficiency. *Magnesium* 4, 176.

Cohn, M.A. (1983). Hypnotics and the control of breathing. A review. *Br. J. Clin. Pharmacol.* 16 (suppl.), 245S.

Collier, J.G. and Webb, D.J. (1987). Severe thiazide-induced hyponatraemia during treatment with enalapril. *Postgrad. Med. J.*, 63, 1105.

Comair, A., Bogino, V., Cougoule, J.P., and Bernadet, R. (1988). Ostéomalacie et traitements anticonvulsants chez des sujets grabataires. A propos de deux observations. *Encephale* 14, 33.

Conn, J.W., Roune, D.R., and Cohen, E.L. (1968). Licorice-induced pseudoaldosteronism. Hypertension, hypokalemia, aldosteronopenia, and suppressed plasma renin. *JAMA* 205, 492.

Connell, J.M., Rapeport, W.G., Gordon, S., and Brodie, M.J. (1984*a*). Changes in circulating thyroid hormones during short-term hepatic enzyme induction with carbamazepine. *Eur. J. Clin. Pharmacol.* 26, 453.

Connell, J.M., Rapeport, W.G., Beastall, G.H., and Brodie, M.J. (1984*b*). Changes in circulating androgens during short term carbamazepine therapy. *Br. J. Clin. Pharmacol.* 17, 347.

Conner, C.S. (1984). Hypophosphatemia. *Drug Intell. Clin. Pharm.* 18, 594.

Connor, H., Newton, D.J., Preston, F.E., and Woods, H.F. (1978). Oral methionine loading as a cause of serum folate deficiency: its relevance to parenteral nutrition. *Postgrad. Med. J.* 54, 318.

The Consensus Trial Study Group (1987). Effects of enalapril on mortality in severe congestive heart failure. Results of the Cooperative North Scandinavian Enalapril Survival Study (CONSENSUS). *N. Engl. J. Med.* 316, 1429.

Cook, G.C. (1976). Absorption of xylose, glucose, glycine, and folic (pteroglutamic) acid in Zambian Africans with anaemia. *Gut.* 17, 604.

Cooperman, L.H. (1970). Succinylcholine-induced hyperkalemia in neuromuscular disease. *JAMA* 213, 1867.

Copeland, P.M., Martin, J.B., and Ridgway, E.C. (1986). Cysteamine decreases prolactin responsiveness to thyrotropin-releasing hormone in normal men. *Am. J. Med. Sci.* 291, 16.

Corbett, J.J., Jacobson, D.M., Thompson, H.S., Hart, M.N., and Albert, D.W. (1989). Downbeating nystagmus and other ocular motor defects caused by lithium toxicity. *Neurology* 39, 481.

Cornbleet, M., Bondy, P.K., and Powles, T.J. (1977). Fatal irreversible hypercalcaemia in breast cancer. *Br. Med. J.* i, 145.

Coronato, A. and Glass, G.B. (1973). Depression of the intestinal uptake of radio-vitamin B$_{12}$ by cholestyramine. *Proc. Soc. Exp. Biol. Med.* 142, 1341.

Corrigan, J.J. and Marcus, F.I. (1974). Coagulopathy associated with vitamin E ingestion. *JAMA* 230, 1300.

Corvilain, J. and Abramour, M. (1962). Some effects of human growth hormone on renal haemodynamics and on tubular phosphate transport in man. *J. Clin. Invest.* 41, 1230.

Costanzi, J.J., Young, B.K., and Carmel, R. (1978). Serum vitamin B$_{12}$ and B$_{12}$ binding protein levels associated with oral contraceptives. *Tex. Rep. Biol. Med.* 36, 69.

Costanzo, L.S. and Windhager, E.E. (1978). Calcium and sodium transport by the distal convoluted tubules of the rat. *Am. J. Physiol.* 235, F492.

Couch, M., Preston, F.E., Malia, R.G., Graham, R., and Russell, G. (1986). Changes in plasma osteocalcin contentration following treatment with stanozolol. *Clin. Chim. Acta* 158, 43.

Coudon, W.L. and Block, A.J. (1976). Acute respiratory failure precipitated by a carbonic anhydrase inhibitor. *Chest* 69, 112.

Coulson, I.H. and Misch, K. (1989). Fosfestrol-induced porphyria cutanea tarda. *Br. J. Urol.* 63, 648.

Cousins, M.J., Gourlay, G.K., Knights, K.M., Hall, P.D., Lunam, C.A., and O'Brien, P. (1987). A randomized prospective controlled study of the metabolism and hepatotoxicity of halothane in humans. *Anesth. Analg.* 66, 299.

Cowan, R.A., Hartnell, G.G., Lowdell C.P., Baird, I.M., and Leak, A.M. (1984). Metabolic acidosis induced by carbonic anhydrase inhibitors and salicylates in patients with normal renal function. *Br. Med. J.* 289, 347.

Cox, M., Geheb, M., and Singer, I. (1985). Disorders of thirst and renal water excretion. In *Fluid electrolyte and acid-base disorders* (ed. A.I. Arieff and R.A. DeFronzo), p. 119. Churchill Livingstone, Edinburgh.

Coyer, J.R. and Nicholson, D.P. (1976). Isoniazid-induced convulsion: part I — clinical. *South. Med. J.* 69, 294.

Crabb, D.W. (1990). Biological markers for increased risk of alcoholism and for quantitation of alcohol consumption. *J. Clin. Invest.* 85, 311.

Crane, J., Burgess, C.D., Graham, A.N. and Maling, T.J. (1987). Hypokalaemic and electrocardiographic effects of aminophylline and salbutamol in obstructive airways disease. *N.Z. Med. J.* 100, 309.

Cronin, J.W., Kroop, S.F., Diamond, J., and Rolla, A.R. (1984). Alkalemia in diabetic ketoacidosis. *Am. J. Med.* 77, 192.

Cronin, R.E. (1986). Magnesium disorders. In *Fluids and electrolytes* (ed. J.P. Kokko and R.L. Tannen), p. 472. W.B. Saunders, Philadelphia.

Crossley, R.J. (1983). Side effect and safety data for fenbufen. *Am. J. Med.* 75, 84.

Crowhurst, J.A. and Rosen, M. (1984). General anaesthesia for caesarean section in severe pre-eclampsia. Comparison of the renal and hepatic effects of enflurane and halothane. *Br. J. Anaesth.* 56, 587.

Crozier, I.G., Ikram, H., Nicholls, M.G., and Jans, S. (1987). Acute hemodynamic, hormoral and electrolyte effects of ramipril in severe congestive heart failure. *Am. J. Cardiol.* 59, 155D.

Cucuianu, M., Bornuz, F., and Macavei, I. (1972). Effect of L-asparaginase therapy upon serum pseudocholinesterase and ceruloplasmin levels in patients with acute leukemia. *Clin. Chim. Acta* 38, 97.

Cullberg, C. (1984). Androgenic, anabolic, estrogenic and antiestrogenic effects of desogestrel and lynestrenol: effects on serum proteins and vaginal cytology. *Contraception* 30, 73.

Cullen, M.H., Rees, G.M., Nancekievill, D.G., and Amess, J.A. (1979). The effect of nitrous oxide on the cell cycle in human bone marrow. *Br. J. Haematol.* 42, 527.

Cumming, F.J. and Briggs, M.H. (1983). Changes in plasma vitamin A in lactating and nonlactating oral contraceptive users. *Br. J. Obstet. Gynaecol.* 90, 73.

Cummings, C.C. and McIvor, M.E. (1988). Fluoride-induced hyperkalemia: the role of Ca^{2+}-dependent K$^+$ channels. *Am. J. Emerg. Med.* 6, 1.

Cunningham, S.K., Loughlint, T., Culliton, M., and McKenna, T.J. (1985). The relationship between sex steroids and sex hormone-binding globulin in plasma in physiological and pathological conditions. *Ann. Clin. Biochem.* 22, 489.

Curless, R.G., Flynn, J., Bachynski, B., Gregorios, J.B., Benke, P., and Cullen, R. (1986). Fatal metabolic acidosis, hyperglycemia, and coma after steroid therapy for Kearns-Sayre syndrome. *Neurology* 36, 872.

DaCruz, D. and Holburn, C. (1989). Serum potassium responses to nebulized salbutamol administered during an acute asthmatic attack. *Arch. Emerg. Med.* 6, 22.

Dam, M. (1988). Side-effects of drug treatment in epilepsy. *Acta Neurol. Scand.* (suppl. 117), 34.

Dana-Haeri, J., Oxley, J., and Richens, A. (1982). Reduction of free testosterone by antiepileptic drugs. *Br. Med. J.* 284, 85.

Dansky, L., Andermann, E., Andermann, F., Sherwin, A.L., Rosenblatt, D., Remillard, G., *et al.* (1985). Pregnancy outcome in relation to maternal plasma antiepileptic (AED) levels and folate (abstract). *Can. J. Neurol. Sci* 12, 182.

Dansky, L.V., Andermann, E., Rosenblatt, D., Sherwin, A.L., and Andermann, F. (1987). Anticonvulsants, folate levels, and pregnancy outcome: a prospective study. *Ann. Neurol.* 21, 176.

Darlow, B.A. (1977). Symptomatic hyponatraemia associated with tolbutamide therapy. *Postgrad. Med. J.* 53, 223.

Daudon, M., Reveillaud, R.J., Normand, M., Petit, C., and Jungers, P. (1987). Piridoxilate-induced calcium oxalate calculi: a new drug-induced metabolic nephrolithiasis. *J. Urol.* 138, 258.

Davidkova, T., Kikuchi, H., Fujii, K., Mukaida, K., Sato, N., Kawachi, S., *et al.* (1988). Biotransformation of isoflurane: Urinary and serum fluoride ion and organic fluorine. *Anesthesiology* 69, 218.

Davies, B.M., Pfefferbaum, A., Krutzik, S., and Davis, K.L. (1981). Lithium's effect on parathyroid hormone. *Am. J. Psychiatry* 138, 489.

Davies, J.P., Bentley, P., and Ghose, R.R. (1989). Aminoglutethimide-induced hyperkalaemia. *Br. J. Clin. Pract.* 43, 263.

Davies, V.A., Rothberg, A.D., Argent, A.C., Atkinson, P.M., Staub, H., and Pienaar, N.L. (1985). Precursor prothrombin status in patients receiving anticonvulsant drugs. *Lancet* i, 126.

Davis, M. (1982). Drug reactions and the liver. *Adverse Drug React. Acute Poisoning. Rev.* 1, 1.

Davis, M. (1989). Drugs and abnormal 'liver function tests'. *Adverse Drug React. Bull.* 139, 520.

Davis, R.E. (1985). Clinical chemistry of vitamin B$_{12}$. *Adv. Clin. Chem.* 24, 163.

Davis, R.E. (1986). Clinical chemistry of folic acid. *Adv. Clin. Chem.* 25, 234.

Davis, R.E., Reed, P.A., and Smith, B.K. (1975). Serum pyridoxal, folate, and vitamin B$_{12}$ levels in institutionalized epileptics. *Epilepsia* 16, 463.

Davtyan, D.G. and Vinters H.V. (1987). Wernicke's encephalopathy in AIDS patient treated with zidovudine. *Lancet* i, 919.

D'costa, D.F., Basu, S.K., and Gunasekera, N.P.R. (1990). ACE inhibitors and diuretics causing hypokalaemia. *Br. J. Clin. Pract.* 44, 26.

De Broe, M.E., van de Vyver, F.L., Bekaert, A.B., D'Haese, P., Paulus, G.J., Visser, W.J., *et al.* (1984). Correlation of serum aluminum values with tissue aluminum concentration. *Contrib. Nephrol.* 38, 37.

DeCaux, G., Dumont, I., Waterlot, Y., and Hanson, B. (1985). Mechanism of hypouricemia in the syndrome of inappropriate secretion of antidiuretic hormone. *Nephron* 39, 164.

De Luca, F., Arrigo, T., Pandullo, E., Siracusano, M.F., Benvenga, S., and Trimarchi, F. (1986). Changes in thyroid function tests induced by 2 month carbamazepine treatment in L-thyroxine-substituted hypothyroid children. *Eur. J. Pediatr.* 145, 77.

DeLuca, H.F. (1988). The vitamin D story: a collaboration effort of basic science and clinical medicine. *FASEB J* 2, 224.

Deenstra, M., Haalboom, J.R., and Struyvenberg, A. (1988). Decrease of plasma potassium due to inhalation of beta-2-agonists: absence of an additional effect of intravenous theophylline. *Eur. J. Clin. Invest.* 18, 162.

DeFronzo, R.A., Braine, H., Calvin, O.M., and Davis, P.J. (1973). Water intoxication in man after cyclophosphamide therapy: time course and relation to drug activation. *Ann. Intern. Med.* 78, 861.

DeFronzo, R.A., Abeloff, M., Braine, H., Humphrey, R.L., and Davis, A.J. (1974). Renal dysfunction after treatment with isophosphamide (NSC-109724). *Cancer Chemother Rep.* 58, 375.

DeFronzo, R.A., Bia, M., and Birkhead, G. (1981). Epinephrine and potassium homeostasis. *Kidney Int.* 20, 83.

Degenring, F.H., Schatton, W., and Hotz, W. (1983). Atherosklerose-Behandlung mit Etofibrat retard. Neue Perspektiven. *Fortschr. Med.* 101, 1391.

Delport, R., Ubbink, J.B., Serfontein, W.J., Becker, P.J., and Walters, L. (1988). Vitamin B$_6$ nutritional status in asthma. The effect of theophylline therapy on plasma pyridoxal 5-phosphate and pyridoxal levels. *Int. J. Vit. Nutr. Res.* 58, 67.

Delpre, G., Grinblat J., Kadish, U., Livini, E., Shohat, B., Lewitus, Z., *et al.* (1979). Immunological studies in a case of hepatitis following methyldopa administration. *Am. J. Med. Sci.* 277, 207.

Delves, H.T. (1985). Assessment of trace metal status. *Clin. Endocrinol. Metab.* 14, 725.

Demarcq, J.M., Delbar, M., Trochu, G., and Crignon, J.J. (1984). Effets de l'alpha cétoglutarate d'ornithine sur l'état nutritionnel des malades de réanimation. *Cah. Anesthesiol.* 32, 229.

DeMatteis, F. (1988). Toxicological aspects of liver heme biosynthesis. *Semin. Haematol.* 25, 321.

Demers, R.G., McDonagh, P.H., and Moore, R.J. (1984). Pyridoxine deficiency with phenelzine. *South. Med. J.* 77, 641.

Demey, H.E., Daelemans, R.A., Verpooten, G.A., De Broe, M.E., Van Campenhout, C.M., Lakiere, F.V., *et al.* (1988). Propylene-glycol induced side effects during intravenous nitroglycerin therapy. *Intens. Care Med.* 14, 221.

Dennis, J. and Taylor, D.C. (1969). Epilepsy and folate deficiency. *Br. Med. J.* iv, 807.

Dennis, P.M. and Ericksen, C.M. (1980). Interference of metronidazole (Flagyl) with serum aspartate aminotransferase (AST) assays. *Med. J. Aust.* ii, 343.

Dent, C.E., Richens, A., Rowe, D.J.F., and Stamp, T.C.B. (1970). Osteomalacia with long-term anticonvulsant therapy in epilepsy. *Br. Med. J.* iv, 69.

Deutsch, J., Fritsch, G., Golles, J., and Semmelrock, H.J. (1986). Effects of anticonvulsive drugs on the activity of gammaglutamyltransferase and aminotransferases in serum. *J. Pediatr. Gastroenterol. Nutr.* 5, 542.

Devenport, M.H., Crook, D., Wynn, V., and Lees, L.J. (1989). Metabolic effects of low-dose fluconazole in healthy female users and non-users of oral contraceptives. *Br. J. Clin. Pharmacol.* 27, 851.

Devgun, M.S., Fiabane, A., Paterson, C.R., Zarembski, P., and Guthrie, A. (1981). Vitamin and mineral nutrition in chronic alcoholics including patients with Korsakoff's psychosis. *Br. J. Nutr.* 45, 469.

De Virgiliis, S., Congia, M., Turco, M.P., Frau, F., Dessi, C., Argiolu, F., *et al.* (1988). Depletion of trace elements and acute ocular toxicity induced by desferrioxamine in patients with thalassaemia. *Arch. Dis. Child.* 63, 250.

Dhami, M.S., Drangova, R., Farkas, R., Balazs, T., and Fever, G. (1979). Decreased aminotransferase activity of serum and various tissues in the rat after cefazolin treatment. *Clin. Chem.* 25, 1263.

DiBianco, R. (1986). Adverse reactions with angiotensin converting enzyme (ACE) inhibitors. *Med. Toxicol.* 1, 122.

Dickerson, J.W.T. (1988). The interrelationships of nutrition and drugs. In *Nutrition in the clinical management of disease* (2nd edn) (ed. J.W.T. Dickerson and H.A. Lee), p. 392. Edward Arnold, London.

Dickinson, R.J. and Swaminathan, R. (1978). Total body potassium depletion and renal tubular dysfunction following carbenoxolone therapy. *Postgrad. Med. J.* 54, 836.

Dietrichson, O. (1975). Chronic active hepatitis: aetiological considerations based on clinical and serological studies. *Scand. J. Gastroenterol.* 10, 617.

Dinscoy, H.P. and Saelinger, D.A. (1982). Haloperidol-induced chronic cholestatic liver disease. *Gastroenterology* 83, 694.

Dirix, L.Y., Moeremans, C., Fierens, H., Dielen, D., Vrints, C., Van Agt, E., *et al.* (1988). Symptomatic hyponatremia related to the use of propafenone. *Acta Clin. Belg.* 43, 143.

DiSilvio, T.V. (1978). Alcoholic myopathy and changes in serum enzyme activity. *Clin. Chem.* 24, 1653.

Ditzel, J. (1973). Importance of plasma inorganic phosphate on tissue oxygenation during recovery from diabetic ketoacidosis. *Horm. Metab. Res.* 5, 471.

Dodd, H.J., Kirby, J.D.T., and Munro, D.D. (1985). Megaloblastic anaemia in psoriatic patients treated with methotrexate. *Br. J. Dermatol.* 112, 630.

Doig, A. and Stanton, J.B. (1961). Megaloblastic anaemia during combined phensuximide and phenobarbitone therapy. *Br. Med. J.* ii, 998.

Doria, M.I. Jr, Shepard, K.V., Levin, B., and Riddell, R.H. (1986). Liver pathology following hepatic arterial infusion chemotherapy. Hepatic toxicity with FUDR. *Cancer* 58, 855.

Doriguzzi, C., Mongini, T., Jeantet, A., and Monga, G. (1984). Tubular aggregates in a case of osteomalacic myopathy due to anticonvulsant drugs. *Clin. Neuropathol.* 3, 42.

Dorup, I. and Skajaa, K. (1989). Magnesium og langvarig diuretikabehandling. *Ugeskr. Laeger.* 151, 759.

Dorup, I., Skajaa, K., Clausen, T., and Kjeldsen, K. (1988). Reduced concentrations of potassium, magnesium, and sodium-potassium pumps in human skeletal muscle during treatment with diuretics. *Br. Med. J.* 296, 455.

Dougados, M., Boumier, P., and Amor, B. (1987). Traitement de la spondylarthrite ankylosante par la salazosulfapyridine. Une étude en double aveugle controlée chez 60 malades. *Rev. Rhum. Mal. Osteoartic* 54, 255.

Douglas, J.B. and Healy, J.K. (1969). Nephrotoxic effects of amphotericin B, including renal tubular acidosis. *Am. J. Med.* 46, 154.

Down, P.F., Polak, A., and Regan, R.J. (1979). A family with massive acute vitamin D intoxication. *Postgrad. Med. J.* 55, 897.

Dubick, M.A., Conteas, C.N., Billy, H.T., Majumdar, A.P., and Geokas, M.C. (1987). Raised serum concentrations of pancreatic enzymes in cigarette smokers. *Gut* 28, 330.

Dujovne, C.A., Azarnoff, D.L., Huffman, D.H., Pentikainen, P., Hurwitz, A., and Shoeman, D.W. (1976). One-year trials with halofenate, clofibrate and placebo. *Clin. Pharmacol. Ther.* 19, 352.

Dukes, G.E., Sanders, S.W., Russo J.J., Swenson, E., Burnakis, T.G., Saffle, J.R., *et al.* (1984). Transaminase elevations in patients receiving bovine or porcine heparin. *Ann. Intern. Med.* 100, 646.

Dunn, A.M. and Buckley, D.M. (1986). Non-steroidal anti-inflammatory drugs and the kidney. *Br. Med. J.* 293, 202.

Duo, X., Cai, W.J., Zhu, B.H., Dong, C.J., Zheng, Z.C., and Gao, Z.Q. (1988). Clinical safety of long-term administration of gossypol in 32 cases. *Contraception* 37, 129.

Duthie, G.G., Wahle, K.W.J., and James, W.P.T. (1989a). Oxidants, antioxidants and cardiovascular disease. *Nutr. Res. Rev.* 2, 51.

Duthie, G.G., Arthur, J.R., James, W.P.T., and Vint, H.M. (1989b). Antioxidant status of smokers and non smokers. *Ann. N.Y. Acad. Sci.* 570, 435.

Duus, B.R. (1986). Fractures caused by epileptic seizures and epileptic osteomalacia. *Injury* 17, 31.

Dyck, R.F., Bear, R.A., Goldstein, M.B., and Halperin, M.L. (1979). Iodine–iodide toxic reaction: case report with emphasis on the nature of metabolic acidosis. *Can. Med. Assoc. J.* 120, 704.

Dyckner, T., and Wester, P.O. (1981). Magnesium deficiency: guidelines for diagnosis and substitution therapy. *Acta Med. Scand.* 661 (suppl.), 37.

Dyckner, T., and Wester, P.O. (1984). Intracellular magnesium loss after diuretic administration. *Drugs* 28 (suppl. 1), 161.

Dyckner, T., Wester, P.O., and Widman, L. (1988). Amiloride prevents thiazide-induced intracellular potassium and magnesium losses. *Acta Med. Scand.* 224, 25.

Eastell, R. and Edmonds, C.J. (1984). Hyponatraemia associated with trimethoprim and a diuretic. *Br. Med. J.* 289, 1658.

Eastham, R.D., Jancar, J., and Cameron, J.D. (1975). Red cell folate and macrocytosis during long-term anticonvulsant therapy in non-anaemia mentally retarded epileptics. *Br. J. Psychiatry* 126, 263.

Edelman, S., and Witztum, J.L. (1989). Hyperkalemia during treatment with HMG-CoA reductase inhibitor. *N. Engl. J. Med.* 320, 1219.

Einarson, T.R., Turchet, E.N., Goldstein, J.E., and MacNay, K.R. (1985). Gout-like arthritis following cimetidine and ranitidine. *Drug Intell. Clin. Pharm.* 19, 201.

Elsborg, L. (1974). Inhibition of intestinal absorption of folic acid by phenytoin. *Acta Hematol.* 52, 24.

Emmerson, B.T. (1983). *Hyperuricaemia and gout in clinical practice.* ADIS Health Science Press, Sydney.

Enyeart, J.J., Price, W.A., Hoffman, D.A., and Woods, L. (1983). Profound hyperglycemia and metabolic acidosis after verapamil overdose. *J. Am. Coll. Cardiol.* 2, 1228.

Epelbaum, S., Benhamou, P.H., Pautard, J.C., Devoldere, C., Kremp, O., and Piussan, C. (1989). Arrêt respiratoire chez une enfant asthmatique traitée par β-2-mimétiques et théophylline. Rôle possible de l'hypokaliémie dans les décès subits des asthmatiques. *Ann. Pediatr.* 36, 473.

Epstein, R.S. (1989). Wernicke's encephalopathy following lithium-induced diarrhea. *Am. J. Psychiatry* 146, 806.

Epstein, S. (1988). Serum and urinary markers of bone remodelling: assessment of bone turnover. *Endocrinol. Rev.* 9, 437.

Eschbach, J.W., Abdulhadi, M.H., Browne, J.K., Delano, B.G., Downing, M.R., Egrie, J.C., *et al.* (1989). Recombinant human erythropoietin in anemic patients with end-stage renal disease. Results of a phase III multicenter clinical trial. *Ann. Intern. Med.* 111, 992.

Ettinger, B., Tang, A., Citron, J.T., Livermore, B., and Williams, T. (1986). Randomized trial of allopurinol in the prevention of calcium oxalate calculi. *N. Engl. J. Med.* 315, 1386.

Ettinger, D.S., Harker, W.G., Gerry, H.W., Sanders, R.C., and Saral, R. (1978). Hyperphosphataemia, hypocalcaemia and transient renal failure. Results of cytotoxic treatment of acute lymphoblastic leukemia. *JAMA* 239, 2472.

European Multicentre Trial. (1982). Cyclosporin A as sole immunosuppressive agent in recipients of kidney allografts from cadaver donors. *Lancet* ii, 57.

Evans, A.R., Forrester, R.M., and Discombe, C. (1970). Neonatal haemorrhage following maternal anticonvulsant therapy. *Lancet* i, 517.

Evans, L.S. and Kleiman, M.B. (1986). Acidosis as a presenting feature of chloramphenicol toxicity. *J. Pediatr.* 108, 475.

Evans, R.T. (1986). Cholinesterase phenotyping: clinical aspects and laboratory applications. *CRC Crit. Rev. Clin. Lab. Sci.* 23, 35.

Fachs, S. and Listernick, R. (1987). Hypernatremia and metabolic alkalosis as a consequence of the therapeutic misuse of baking soda. *Pediatr. Emerg. Care* 3, 242.

Faller, J. and Fox, I.H. (1982). Ethanol induced hyperuricemia: evidence for increased urate production by activation of adenine nucleotide turn over. *N. Engl. J. Med.* 307, 1598.

Faraj, J.H. (1989). Hyperosmolality due to antacid treatment. *Anaesthesia* 44, 911.

Farley, T.A. (1986). Severe hypernatremic dehydration after use of an activated charcoal-sorbitol suspension. *J. Pediatr.* 109, 719.

Farr, M., Symmons, D.P., and Bacon, P.A. (1985). Raised serum alkaline phosphatase and aspartate transaminase levels in two rheumatoid patients treated with sulphasalazine. *Ann. Rheum. Dis.* 44, 798.

Farrington, K., Miller, P., Varghese, Z., Baillod, R.A., and Moorhead, J.F. (1981). Vitamin A toxicity and hypercalcaemia in chronic renal failure. *Br. Med. J.* 282, 1999.

Fassler, C.A., Rodriguez, R.M., Badesch, D.B., Stone, W.J., and Marini, J.J. (1985). Magnesium toxicity as a cause of hypotension and hypoventilation. Occurrence in patients with normal renal function. *Arch. Intern. Med.* 145, 1604.

Fee, J.P.H., Black, G.W., Dundee, J.W., McIlroy, P.D.A., Johnson, H.M.L., Johnston, S.B., *et al.* (1979). A prospective study of liver enzyme and other changes following repeat administration of halothane and enflurane. *Br. J. Anaesth.* 51, 1133.

Feely, J. (1981). Propranolol and the hypercalcaemia of thyrotoxicosis. *Acta Endocrinol.* 98, 528.

Fehling, C., Jagerstad, M., Lindstrand, K., and Westesson A-K. (1973). The effect of anticonvulsant therapy upon the absorption of folates. *Clin. Sci.* 44, 595.

Feig, P.U., and McCurdy, D.K. (1977). The hypertonic state. *N. Engl. J. Med.* 297, 1444.

Feinstein, E.I., Quion, V.H., Kaptein, E.M., and Massry, S.G. (1984). Severe hyperuricemia in patients with volume depletion. *Am. J. Nephrol.* 48, 77.

Fenech, F.F., Bannister, W.H., and Grech, J.L. (1967). Hepatitis with biliverdinaemia in association with indomethacin therapy. *Br Med. J.* iii, 155.

Fennell, J.S. and Fall, W.F. (1981). Steptozotocin nephrotoxicity: studies on the defect in renal tubular acidification. *Clin. Nephrol.* 15, 97.

Fentiman, I.S., Caleffi, M., Rodin, A., Murby, B., and Fogelman, I. (1989). Bone mineral content of women receiving tamoxifen for mastalgia. *Br. J. Cancer* 60, 262.

Ferdinandus, J., Pederson, J.A., and Whang, R. Hypermagnesemia as a cause of refractory hypotension, respiratory depression, and coma. *Arch. Intern. Med.* 141, 669.

Ferguson, D.B. (1971). Effects of low doses of fluoride on serum proteins and a serum enzyme in man. *Nature* 231, 159.

Ferrari, C., Testori, G., Scanni, A., Frezzati, S., Bertazzoni, A., Romussi, M., *et al.* (1976). Reduction of serum alkaline phosphatase and gamma-glutamyl transpeptidase activities by short-term clofibrate. *N. Engl. J. Med.* 295, 449.

Fielding, L.P., Chalmers, D.M., Chanarin, I., and Levi, A.J. (1978). Inhibition of intrinsic factor secretion by cimetidine. *Br. Med. J.* i, 818.

Finberg, L., Kiley, J., and Luttrell, C.N. (1963). Mass accidental salt poisoning in infancy. A study of a hospital disaster. *JAMA* 184, 187.

Fink, R. (1984). The effects of alcohol on endocrine function. In *Clinical biochemistry of alcoholism* (ed. S.B. Rosalki), p. 271. Churchill Livingstone, Edinburgh.

Finn, J.T., Cohen, L.H., and Steinmetz, P.R. (1977). Acidifying defect induced by amphotericin B: comparison of bicarbonate and hydrogen ion permeability. *Kidney Int.* 11, 261.

Fitzgerald, G.R., Delaney, E., Cushen, M., and Fitzgerald, M.G. (1989). Diuretic-associated hypokalaemia in hospital admissions. *Res. Clin. For.* 11, 49.

Fitzpatrick, J.M., Kasidas, G.P., and Rose, G.A. (1981). Hyperoxaluria following glycine irrigation for transurethral prostatectomy. *Br. J. Urol.* 53, 250.

Flack, C.P. and Woolen, J.W. (1984). Prevention of interference by dextran with biuret-type assay of serum proteins. *Clin. Chem.* 30, 559.

Flanagan, R.J. and Mant, T.G. (1986). Coma and metabolic acidosis early in severe acute paracetamol poisoning. *Hum. Toxicol.* 5, 179.

Flatman, P.W. (1984). Magnesium transport across cell membranes. *J. Membr. Biol.* 80, 1.

Flexner, J.M. and Hartmann, R.C. (1960). Megaloblastic anemia associated with anticonvulsant drugs. *Am. J. Med.* 28, 386.

Foote, J.W. and Delves, H.T. (1984). Albumin bound and α_2-macroglobulin bound zinc concentrations in the sera of healthy adults. *J. Clin. Path.* 37, 1050.

Foote, J.W. and Hinks, L.J. (1988). Zinc absorption in haemodialysis patients. *Ann. Clin. Biochem.* 25, 398.

Forastiere, A.A., Belliveau, J.F., Goren, M.P., Vogel, W.C., Posner, M.R., and O'Leary, G.P. Jr (1988). Pharmacokinetic and toxicity evaluation of five-day continuous infusion versus intermittent bolus cis-diamminedichloroplatinum (II) in head and neck cancer patients. *Cancer Res.* 48, 3869.

Foresti, V., Parisio, E., and Ricci, G. (1987). Sindrome da eccesso di mineralcorticoidi secondaria a spray nasali contenenti 9-alpha-fluoroprednisolone. *Minerva. Med.* 78, 1305.

Forfar, J.C., Brown, G.J., and Cull, R.E. (1979). Proximal myopathy during beta-blockade. *Br. Med. J.* ii, 1331.

Fortner, R.W., Nowakowski, A., and Carter, C.B. (1970). Death due to overheated dialysate during dialysis. *Ann. Intern. Med.* 73, 443.

Fouad, F.M., Tarazi, R.C., Bravo, E.L., and Textor, S.C. (1984). Hemodynamic and antihypertensive effects of the new oral angiotensin-converting-enzyme inhibitor MK-421 (enalapril). *Hypertension* 6, 167.

Fox, I.H. (1981). Metabolic basis for disorders of purine nucleotide degradation. *Metabolism* 30, 616.

Fox, J., Care, A.D., and Marshall, D.H. (1978). Reversal of betamethasone-induced inhibition of intestinal calcium absorption by 1-alpha-hydroxycholecalciferol. *J. Endocrinol.* 78, 187.

Fraley, D.S. and Adler, S. (1977). Correction of hyperkalemia by bicarbonate despite constant blood pH. *Kidney Int.* 12, 354.

Francisco, L.L., Sawin, L.L., and DiBona, G.F. (1982). Mechanism of negative potassium balance in the magnesium-deficient rat. *Proc. Soc. Exp. Biol. Med.* 168, 382.

Franklyn, J.A., Sheppard, M.C., Ramsden, D.B., and Hoffenberg, R. (1983). Free triiodothyronine and free thyroxin, in sera of pregnant women and subjects with congenitally increased or decreased thyroxin-binding globulin. *Clin. Chem.* 29, 1527.

Franklyn, J.A., Wilkins, M.R., Wilkinson, R., Ramsden, D.B., and Sheppard, M.C. (1985a). The effect of propranolol on circulating thyroid hormone measurements in thyrotoxic and euthyroid subjects. *Acta Endocrinol.* 108, 351.

Franklyn, J.A., Davis, J.R., Gammage, M.D., Littler, W.A., Ramsden, D.B., and Sheppard, M.C. (1985b). Amiodarone and thyroid hormone action. *Clin. Endocrinol.* 22, 257.

Frascino, J.A., Vanamee, P., and Rosen, P.P. (1970). Renal oxalosis and azotemia after methoxyflurane anaesthesia. *N. Engl. J. Med.* 283, 676.

Fraser, A.D. (1980). Chemotherapy as a cause of low serum creatine kinase activity. *Clin. Chem.* 26, 1629.

Fraser, C.L. and Arieff, A.I. (1988). Nervous system complications in uremia. *Ann. Intern. Med.* 109, 143.

Fraser, C.L. and Arieff, A.I. (1990). Fatal central diabetes mellitus and insipidus resulting from untreated hyponatremia: a new syndrome. *Ann. Intern. Med.* 112, 113.

Freis, E.D. (1989). Critique of the clinical importance of diuretic-induced hypokalemia and elevated cholesterol level. *Ann. Intern. Med.* 149, 2640.

Friedman, E., Shadel, M., Halkin, H., and Farfel, Z. (1989). Thiazide-induced hyponatremia. Reproducibility by single dose rechallenge and an analysis of pathogenesis. *Ann. Intern. Med.* 110, 24.

Fuentes, A. and Goldkrand, J.W. (1987). Angiotensin-converting enzyme activity in hypertensive subjects after magnesium sulfate therapy. *Am. J. Obstet. Gynecol.* 156, 1375.

Fuiano, G., Federico, S., Conte, G., and Andreucci, V.E. (1989). Uric acid and kidney. *Adv. Exp. Med. Biol.* 252, 107.

Fujimura, A., Ebihara, A., Hino, N., and Koike, Y. (1989). Effects of traxanox sodium on blood pressure and serum uric acid in hypertensive patients: a preliminary study. *J. Clin. Pharmacol.* 29, 327.

Fujita, T., Chan, J.C., and Bartter, F.C. (1984). Effects of oral fruosemide and salt loading on parathyroid function in normal subjects. Physiological basis for renal hypercalciuria. *Nephron* 38, 109.

Fulton, R.A. (1986). Megaloblastic anaemia and methotrexate treatment. *Br. J. Dermatol.* 114, 267.

Funder, J.W., Pearce, P.T., Smith, R., and Smith, A.I. (1988). Mineralocorticoid action: Target tissue specificity is enzyme, not receptor, mediated. *Science* 242, 583.

Gabow, P.A. (1985). Disorders associated with an altered anion gap. *Kidney Int.* 27, 472.

Gabow, P.A. (1988). Ethylene glycol intoxication. *Am. J. Kidney Dis.* 11, 277.

Gabow, P.A., Anderson, R.J., Potts, D.E., and Schrier, R.W. (1978). Acid-base disturbances in the salicylate-intoxicated adult. *Arch. Intern. Med.* 138, 1481.

Gabow, P.A., Moore, S., and Schrier, R.W. (1979). Spironolactone-induced hyperchloremic acidosis in cirrhosis. *Ann. Intern. Med.* 90, 338.

Gabow, P.A., Clay, K., Sullivan, J.B., and Lepoff, R. (1986). Organic acids in ethylene glycol intoxication. *Ann. Intern. Med.* 105, 16.

Gallery, E.D., Blomfield, J., and Dixon, S.R. (1972). Acute zinc toxicity in haemodialysis. *Br. Med. J.* iv, 331.

Gamstedt, A., Jarnerot, G., Kagodal, B., and Soderholm, B. (1979). Corticosteroids and thyroid function. *Acta Med. Scand.* 205, 379.

Gamstedt, A., Jarnerot, G., and Kagedal, B. (1981). Dose related effects of betamethasone on iodothyronines and thyroid hormone-binding protein. *Acta Endocrinol.* 96, 484.

Ganguli, P.C. and Mohamed, S.D. (1980). Long-term therapy with carbenoxolone in the prevention of recurrence of gastric ulcer. Natural history and evolution of important side-effects and measures to avoid them. *Scand. J. Gastroenterol.* 15 (suppl. 65), 63.

Garella, S. (1988). Extracorporeal techniques in the treatment of exogeneous intoxications. *Kidney Int.* 33, 735.

Garella, S., Chang, B.S., and Kahn, S.I. (1975). Dilution acidosis and contraction alkalosis: review of a concept. *Kidney Int.* 8, 279.

Garnick, M.B. and Larsen, P.R. (1979). Acute deficiency of thyroxine-binding globulin during L-asparaginase therapy. *N. Engl. J. Med.* 301, 252.

Gascon-Barre, M., Villeneuve, J.P., and Lebrun, L.H. (1984). Effect of increasing doses of phenytoin on the plasma 25-hydroxyvitamin D and 1,25-dihydroxyvitamin D concentrations. *J. Am. Coll. Nutr.* 3, 45.

Geissler, A.H., Turnlund, J.R., and Cohen, R.D. (1986). Effect of chlorthalidone on zinc levels, testosterone, and sexual function in man. *Drug Nutr. Interact.* 4, 275.

Georgieff, M.K., Chockalingam, U.M., Sasanow, S.R., Gunter, E.W., Murphy, E., and Ophoven, J.J. (1988). The effect of antenatal betamethasone on cord blood concentrations of retinol-binding protein, transthyretin, transferrin, retinol, and vitamin E. *J. Pediatr. Gastroenterol. Nutr.* 7, 713.

German, D.C. and Holmes, E.W. (1986). Hyperuricemia and gout. *Med. Clin. North Am.* 70, 419.

Gershon, S.L. and Fox, I.H. (1974). Pharmacological effects of nicotinic acid on human purine metabolism. *J. Lab. Clin. Med.* 84, 179.

Ghose, K. (1977). Lithium salts: therapeutic and unwanted effects. *Br. J. Hosp. Med.* 18, 578.

Ghose, R.R. (1985). Plasma arginine vasopressin in hyponatraemic patients receiving diuretics. *Postgrad. Med. J.* 61, 1043.

Giaccone, G., Donadio, M., Ferrati, P., Ciuffreda, L., Bagatella, M., Gaddi, M., *et al.* (1985). Disorders of serum electrolytes and renal function in patients treated with cis-platinum on an outpatient basis. *Eur. J. Cancer Clin. Oncol.* 21, 433.

Gibb, W.R.G. and Lees, A.J. (1985). The neuroleptic malignant syndrome — a review. *Q. J. Med.* 220, 421.

Gibbs, C.J., Aaron, J.E., and Peacock, M. (1986). Osteomalacia in Paget's disease treated with short term, high dose sodium etidronate. *Br. Med. J.* 292, 1227.

Gilhus, N.E., Strandjord, R.E., and Aarli, J.A. (1982). The effect of carbamazepine on serum immunoglobulin concentrations. *Acta Neurol. Scand.* 66, 172.

Gill, M.A., DuBe, J.E., and Young, W.W. (1977). Hypokalaemia, metabolic alkalosis induced by high-dose ampicillin sodium. *Am. J. Hosp. Pharm.* 34, 528.

Gillman, M.A. and Sandyk, R. (1984). Nicotinic acid deficiency induced by sodium valproate. *S. Afr. Med. J.* 65, 986.

Gin, H., Lars, I., Morlat, P., Beauvieux, J.M., and Aubertin, J. (1988). Hyponatrémie induite par les sulfamides hypoglycémiants: étude chez 70 patients. *Ann. Med. Interne* 139, 455.

Glazebrook, G.A. (1987). Effect of decicurie doses of radioactive iodine 131 on parathyroid function. *Am. J. Surg.* 154, 368.

Gleeson, J.M., Dukes, C.S., Elstad, N.L., Chan, I.F., and Wilson, D.E. (1987). Effects of estrogen/progestin agents on plasma retinoids and chylomicron remnant metabolism. *Contraception* 35, 69.

Glick, P.L., Guglielmo, B.J., Tranbaugh, R.F., and Turley, K. (1985). Iodine toxicity in a patient treated by continuous povidone–iodine mediastinal irrigation. *Ann. Thorac. Surg.* 39, 478.

Glimp, R.A., Wingert, T.D., and Rodas, A.G. (1980). Hypocalcemia associated with oral phosphate replacement therapy. *JAMA* 243, 731.

Gocmen, A., Peters, H.A., Cripps, D.J., Bryan, G.T., and Morris, C.R. (1989). Hexachlorobenzene episode in Turkey. *Biomed. Environ. Sci.* 2, 36.

Goggin, T., Gough, H., Bissessar, A., Crowley, M., Baker, M., and Callaghan, N. (1987). A comparative study of the relative effects of anticonvulsant drugs and dietary folate on the red cell folate status of patients with epilepsy. *Q. J. Med.* 65, 911.

Goldberg, A., Moore, M.R., McColl, K.E.L., and Brodie, M.J. (1987). Porphyrin metabolism and the porphyrias. In *Oxford textbook of medicine* (2nd edn) (ed. D.J. Weatherall, J.G.C. Ledingham, and D.A. Warrell), p. 136. Oxford University Press.

Goldfarb, S., Walker, B.R., and Agus, Z.S. (1985). The uricosuric effect of oxaprozin in humans. *J. Clin. Pharmacol.* 25, 144.

Goldstein, G.B., Lam, K.C., and Mistilis, S.P. (1973). Drug-induced active chronic hepatitis. *Dig. Dis.* 18, 177.

Goldszer, R.C., Coodley, E.L., Rosner, M.J., Simons, W.M., and Schwartz, A.R. (1981). Hyperkalemia associated with indomethacin. *Arch. Intern. Med.* 141, 802.

Goldwasser, H.D., Hooper, J.F., and Spears, N.M. (1989). Concomitant treatment of neuroleptic malignant syndrome and psychosis. *Br. J. Psychiatry* 154, 102.

Gonzalez, J. and Hogg, R.J. (1981). Metabolic alkalosis secondary to baking soda treatment of a diaper rash. *Pediatrics* 67, 820.

Goodenough, G.K. and Lutz, L.J. (1988). Hyponatremic hypervolemia caused by a drug–drug interaction mistaken for syndrome of inappropriate ADH. *J. Am. Geriatr. Soc.* 36, 285.

Goodman, W.G., Henry, D.A., Horst, R., Nudelman, R.K., Alfrey, A.C., and Coburn, J.W. (1984). Parenteral aluminum administration in the dog; II. induction of osteomalacia and effect on vitamin D metabolism. *Kidney Int.* 25, 370.

Gordon, D., Beastall, G.H., McArdle, C.S., and Thomson, J.A. (1986). The effect of tamoxifen therapy on thyroid function tests. *Cancer* 58, 1422.

Gores, P.F., Fryd, D.S., Sutherland, D.E., Najarian, J.S., and Simmons, R.L. (1988). Hyperuricemia after renal transplantation. *Am. J. Surg.* 156, 397.

Gow, S.M., Caldwell, G., Toft, A.D., and Beckett, G.J. (1989). Different hepatic responses to thyroxine replacement in spontaneous and ^{131}I-induced primary hypothyroidism. *Clin. Endocrinol.* 30, 505.

Goyer, R.A. (1989). Mechanisms of lead and cadmium nephrotoxicity. *Toxicol. Lett.* 46, 153.

Granerus, A.K., Jagenburg, R., and Svanborg, A. (1977). Kaliuretic effect of L-dopa treatment in Parkinsonian patients. *Acta Med. Scand.* 201, 291.

Graninger, W., Pirich, K.R., Speiser, W., Deutsch, E., and Waldhausl, W.K. (1986). Effect of thyroid hormones on plasma protein concentrations in man. *J. Clin. Endocrinol. Metab.* 63, 407.

Graves, J., Kenamond, T.G., and Whittier, F.C. (1988). Acute effects of nifedipine on renal electrolyte excretion in normal and hypertensive subjects. *Am. J. Med. Sci.* 296, 114.

Gray, T.A., Buckley, B.M., and Vale, J.A. (1987). Hyperlactataemia and metabolic acidosis following paracetamol overdose. *Q. J. Med.* 65, 811.

Grayhack, J.T. (1984). Prostatic carcinoma: management. *J. Urol.* 132, 92.

Green, J.D. (1975). Megaloblastic anaemia in a vegetarian taking oral contraceptives. *South. Med. J.* 68, 249.

Greenblatt, D.J. and Koch-Weser, J. (1973). Adverse reactions to spironolactone. A Report From the Boston Collaborative Drug Surveillance Program. *JAMA* 225, 40.

Greer, I.A., Greaves, M., Madhok, R., McLoughlin, K., Porter, N., Lowe, G.D., *et al.* (1985). Effect of stanozolol on factors VIII and IX and serum aminotransferases in haemophilia. *Thromb. Haemost.* 53, 386.

Greiss, L., Tremblay, N.A.G., and Davies, D.W. (1976). The toxicity of sodium nitroprusside. *Can. Anaesth. Soc. J.* 23, 480.

Grieco, A., Caputo, S., Bertoli, A., Caradonna, P., and Greco, A.V. (1986). Megaloblastic anaemia due to sulphasalazine responding to drug withdrawal alone. *Postgrad. Med. J.* 62, 307.

Griffin, A.J. (1979). Cholestatic hepatitis induced by gold. *Rheumatol. Rehab.* 18, 174.

Griffith, G.C., Nichols, G. Jr, Asher, J.D., and Flanagan, B. (1965). Heparin osteoporosis. *JAMA* 193, 91.

Griffiths, K.D. and Parry, D.H. (1988). Hypomagnesaemia and hypocalcaemia after treatment with mitoxantrone. *Br. Med. J.* 297, 488.

Grindulis, K.A. and McConkey B. (1985). Does sulphasalazine cause folate deficiency in rheumatoid arthritis? *Scand. J. Rheumatol.* 14, 265.

Gross, J.M. (1963). Fanconi syndrome (adult type) developing secondary to the ingestion of outdated tetracycline. *Ann. Intern. Med.* 58, 523.

Gross, L. and Brotman, M. (1970). Hypoprothrombinemia and hemorrhage associated with cholestyramine therapy. *Ann. Intern. Med.* 72, 95.

Gross, T.L. and Sokol, R.J. (1980). Severe hypokalemia and acidosis: a potential complication of beta-adrenergic treatment. *Am. J. Obstet. Gynecol.* 138, 1225.

Grossman, M.E., Bickers, D.R., Poh-Fitzpatrick, M.B., De-Leo, V.A., and Harber, L.C. (1979). Porphyria cutanea tarda. Clinical features and laboratory findings in 40 patients. *Am. J. Med.* 67, 277.

Gruskin, A.B. (1988). Aluminum: a pediatric overview. *Adv. Pediatr.* 35, 281.

Gudmundsson, J.A., Ljunghall, S., Bergquist, C., Wide, L., and Nillius, S.J. (1987). Increased bone turnover during gonadotropin-releasing hormone superagonist-induced ovulation inhibition. *J. Clin. Endocrinol. Metab.* 65, 159.

Guerin, J.M., Meyer, P., and Habib, Y. (1988). Is there a direct relationship between lactic acidosis and epinephrine administration? *Arch. Intern. Med.* 148, 980.

Guillaume, C., Perrot, D., Bouffard, Y., Delafosse, B., and Motin, J. (1987). Intoxication au méthanol. *Ann. Fr. Anesth. Reanim.* 6, 17.

Guillou, P.J., Morgan, D.B., and Hill, G.L. (1976). Hypophosphataemia: a complication of 'innocuous dextrose saline'. *Lancet* ii, 710.

Gustafson, P.R. (1985). Profound lactic acidosis in a young woman treated with nalidixic acid. *Tex. Med.* 81, 53.

Guthrie, R.M. and Lott, J.A. (1986). Abnormal serum CK-MB following an aminotriptyline overdose. A case report and review of the literature. *J. Fam. Pract.* 22, 550.

Gyory, A.Z. and Lissner, D. (1977). Independence of ethacrynic acid-induced renal hydrogen ion excretion of sodium — volume depletion in man. *Clin. Sci. Mol. Med.* 53, 125.

Haeney, M.R., Carter, G.F., Yeoman, W.B., and Thompson, R.A. (1979). Long-term parenteral exposure to mercury in patients with hypogammmaglobulinaemia. *Br. Med. J.* ii, 12.

Hagen, G.A. and Frawley, T.F. (1970). Hyponatremia due to sulfonylurea compounds. *J. Clin. Endocrinol. Metab.* 31, 570.

Hahn, T.J. (1980). Drug-induced disorders of vitamin D and mineral metabolism. *Clin. Endocrinol. Metab.* 9, 107.

Hajos, P., Berlin, I., Intody, Z., Tornyossy, M., and Kaldor, A. (1981). The effect of oral contraceptives on serum lipids, gamma-glutamyl transpeptidase, and excretion of D-glucaric acid. *Int. J. Clin. Pharm. Ther. Toxicol.* 19, 117.

Halawa, B. (1989). Hipotensyjne i metaboliczne działanie małych dawek hydrochlorotiazydu stosowanego przewlekle u osób wieku podeszłym, chorych na nadciśnienie tętnicze skurczowe. *Wiad. Lek.* 42, 210.

Hall, J.G., Pauli, R.M., and Wilson, K.M. (1980). Maternal and fetal sequelae of anticoagulation during pregnancy. *Am. J. Med.* 68, 122.

Hall, M.A., Thom, H., and Russell, G. (1981). Erythrocyte aspartate aminotransferase activity in asthmatic and non-asthmatic children and its enhancement by vitamin B_6. *Ann. Allergy* 47, 464.

Hall, M.J., Downs, L., Ene, M.D., and Farah, D. (1989). Effect of reduced phytate wheat bran on zinc absorption. *Eur. J. Clin. Nutr.* 43, 431.

Halma, C., Jansen, J.B., Janssens, A.R., Griffioen, G., and Lamers, C.B. (1987). Life-threatening water intoxication during somatostatin therapy. *Ann. Intern. Med.*, 107, 518.

Halpren, E.W., Soifer, N.E., Haenel, L.C., Manara, L.R., and Belsky, D.H. (1988). Ketoacidosis secondary to oral ritodrine use in a gestational diabetic patient; report of a case. *J. Am. Osteopath. Assoc.* 88, 241.

Halsted, C.H. (1980). Folate deficiency in alcoholism. *Am. J. Clin. Nutr.* 33, 2736.

Hamilton, W.F.D. and Robertson, G.S. (1974). Changes in serum uric acid related to the dose of methoxyflurane. *Br. J. Anaesth.* 46, 54.

Hammerman, C., Zaia, W., and Wu, H.H. (1985). Severe hyponatremia with indomethacin — a more serious toxicity than previously realized? *Dev. Pharmacol. Ther.* 8, 260.

Hankins, D.G., Saxena, K., Faville, R.J. Jr, and Warren, B.J. (1987). Profound acidosis caused by isoniazid ingestion. *Am. J. Emerg. Med.* 5, 165.

Hanlon, D.P. (1975). Interaction of thiamazole with zinc copper. *Lancet* i, 929.

Hantman, D., Rossier, B., Zohlman, R., and Schrier, R. (1973). Rapid correction of hyponatremia in the syndrome of inappropriate secretion of antidiuretic hormone: an alternative treatment to hypertonic saline. *Ann. Intern. Med.* 78, 870.

Haq, I. and Asghar, M. (1989). Lead content of some traditional preparations — 'Kushtas'. *J. Ethnopharmacol.* 26, 287.

Hardaway, R.M. (1980). Metabolic acidosis produced by vasopressors. *Surg. Gynecol. Obstet.* 151, 203.

Hardy, M.J. and Bjurstrom, C.H. (1984). Effect of heparin in determination of plasma albumin by Beckmen Astra 8 (CG) and Du Pont ACA II (BCP) autoanalyzers. *Ann. Clin. Biochem.* 21, 387.

Harlow, P.J., DeClerck, Y.A., Shore, N.A., Ortega, J.A., Carranza, A., and Heuser, E. (1979). A fatal case of inappropriate ADH secretion induced by cyclophosphamide therapy. *Cancer* 44, 896.

Harrington, M.G. and Hodgkinson, H.M. (1987). Anticonvulsant drugs and bone disease in the elderly. *J. R. Soc. Med.* 80, 425.

Harrington, J.T., Hulter, H.N., Cohen, J.J., and Madias, N.E. (1986). Mineralocorticoid-stimulated renal acidification. The critical role of dietary sodium. *Kidney Int.* 30, 43.

Harris, H. (1989). The human alkaline phosphatases: what we know and what we don't know. *Clin. Chim. Acta* 186, 133.

Harris, R.T. (1983). Bulimarexia and related serious eating disorders with medical complications. *Ann. Intern. Med.* 99, 800.

Harris, A.B., Hartley, J., and Moor, A. (1973). Reduced ascorbic acid excretion and oral contraceptives. *Lancet* ii, 201.

Harrison, A.R., Kasidas, G.P., and Rose, G.A. (1981). Hyperoxaluria and recurrent stone formation apparently cured by short courses of pyridoxine. *Br. Med. J.* 282, 2097.

Hartmann, O., Pinkerton, C.R., Philip, T., Zucker, J.M., and Breatnach, F. (1988). Very-high-dose cisplatin and etoposide in children with untreated advanced neuroblastoma. *J. Clin. Oncol.* 6, 44.

Haruda, F. (1979). Phenytoin hypersensitivity : 38 cases. *Neurology* 29, 1480.

Hawkins, D.F. and Benster, B. (1977). A comparative study of three low dose progestogens, chlormadinone acetate, megestrol acetate, and norethisterone, as oral contraceptives. *Br. J. Obstet. Gynaecol.* 84, 708.

Hayek, M.E. and Eisenberg, P.G. (1989). Severe hypophosphatemia following the institution of enteral feedings. *Arch. Surg.* 124, 1325.

Hayward, J.N. and Boshell, B.R. (1957). Paraldehyde intoxication with metabolic acidosis. Report of two cases, experimental data and a critical review of the literature. *Am. J. Med.* 23, 965.

Healy, M.A. and Aslam, M. (1986). Lead-containing preparations in the Asian community: a retrospective survey. *Public Health* 100, 149.

Heaney, R.P. (1988). Nutritional factors in bone health. In *Osteoporosis: aetiology, diagnosis and management* (ed. B.L. Riggs and L.J. Melton III), p. 369. Raven Press, New York.

Heath, D.A. (1984). Other hypercalcaemias. In *Metabolic bone disease* (ed. B.E.C. Nordin), p. 143. Churchill Livingstone, Edinburgh.

Heckerling, P.S. (1987). Ethylene glycol poisoning with a normal anion gap due to occult bromide intoxication. *Ann. Emerg. Med.* 16, 1384.

Heckman, B.A. and Walsh, J.H. (1967). Hypernatraemia complicating sodium sulphate therapy for hypercalcemic crisis. *N. Engl. J. Med.* 276, 1082.

Heidemann, P., Peters, H-H., and Stubbe, P. (1980). Influence of L-asparaginase and oxandrolone on serum thyroxine-binding globulin. *Acta Endocrinol.* 94 (suppl. 234), 19.

Heidemann, P.H., Stubbe, P., and Beck, W. (1981). Transient secondary hypothyroidism and thyroxine binding globulin deficiency in leukemic children during polychemotherapy: An effect of L-asparaginase. *Eur. J. Pediatr* 14, 291.

Heier, M.S. and Fossa, S.D. (1986). Wernicke–Korsakoff-like syndrome in patients with colorectal carcinoma treated with high-dose doxifluridine (5'd-FUrd). *Acta Neurol. Scand.* 73, 449.

Heine, R.J., Ponchner, M., Hanning, I., Home, P.D., Brown, M., Williams, D., et al. (1984). A comparison of the effects of semisynthetic human insulin and porcine insulin on transmembrane ion shifts and glucose metabolism during euglycaemic clamping. *Acta Endocrinol.* 106, 241.

Helgeland, A. (1983). Double-blind comparison of trimazosin and propranolol in essential hypertension. *Am. Heart J.* 106, 1253.

Heller, C.A. and Friedman, P.A. (1983). Pyridoxine deficiency and peripheral neuropathy associated with long-term phenelzine therapy. *Am. J. Med.* 75, 887.

Heller, I., Halevy, J., Cohen, S., and Theodor, E. (1985). Significant metabolic acidosis induced by acetazolamide. Not a rare complication. *Arch. Intern. Med.* 145, 1815.

Hendel, J., Dam, M., Gram, L., Winkel, P., Jogensen, I. (1984). The effects of carbamazepine and valproate in folate metabolism in man. *Acta Neurol. Scand.* 69, 226.

Hendel, J. and Nyfords, A. (1985). Impact of methotrexate therapy on the folate status of psoriatic patients. *Clin. Exp. Dermat.* 10, 30.

Henderson, M.J. and Toothill, C. (1983). Urinary coproporphyrin in lead intoxication — a study in the rabbit. *Clin. Sci.* 65, 527.

Henderson, L.W., Metz, M., and Wilkinson, J.H. (1970). Serum enzyme elevation in glutethimide intoxication. *Br. Med. J.* iii, 751.

Hepburn, W.C., Abdul-Aziz, L.A.S., and Whiteoak, R. (1989). Danazol-induced hypercalcaemia in alphacalcidol-treated hypoparathyroidism. *Postgrad. Med. J.* 65, 849.

Herbai, G. and Ljunghall, S. (1984). Treatment of primary hyperparathyroidism with cyclofenil — a synthetic stilbestrol derivative with minimal feminizing effects. *Horm. Metab. Res.* 16, 374.

Herbert, V. (1981). Vitamin B₁₂. *Am. J. Clin. Nutr.* 34, 971.

Herbert, V., Jacob, E., Wong, K.T., Scott, J., and Pfeffer, R.D. (1978). Low serum vitamin B₁₂ levels in patients receiving ascorbic acid in megadoses: studies concerning the effect of ascorbate on radioisotope vitamin B₁₂ assay. *Am. J. Clin. Nutr.* 31, 253.

Herbeth, B., Bangrel., A., Dalo, B., Siest, G., Leclerc, J., and Rauber, G. (1981). Influence of oral contraceptives of differing dosages on alpha-1-antitrypsin, gamma-glutamyltransferase and alkaline phosphatase. *Clin. Chim. Acta* 112, 293.

Herrick, A.L., McColl, K.E., Moore, M.R., Brodie, M.J., Adamson, A.R., and Goldberg, A. (1989a). Acute intermittent porphyria in two patients on anticonvulsant therapy and with normal erythrocyte porphobilinogen deaminase activity. *Br. J. Clin. Pharmacol.* 27, 491.

Herrick, A.L., Moore, M.R., McColl, K.E.L., Cook, A., and Goldberg, A. (1989b). Controlled trial of haem arginate in acute hepatic porphyria. *Lancet* ii, 1295.

Herrmann, J.M. and Mayer, E.O. (1988). A long-term study of the effects of celiprolol on blood pressure and lipid-associated risk factors. *Am. Heart J.* 116, 1416.

Hertz, P. and Richardson, J.A. (1972). Arginine-induced hyperkalemia in renal failure patients. *Arch. Intern. Med.* 130, 778.

Hespel, P., Lijnen, P., Fiocchi, R., Lissens, W., Moerman, E., and Amery, A. (1987). Effects of calcium antagonism on the resting and exercise-stimulated renin-aldosterone axis. *Methods Find. Exp. Clin. Pharmacol.* 9, 461.

Hesse, A., Schneeberger, W., and Vahlensieck, W. (1987). Untersuchungen zur Wirkung eines Allopurinol/Benzbromaron-Praparates auf die Harnzusammensetzung im zirkakianen Verlauf. *Klin. Wochenschr.* 65, 218.

Hettiarachchy, N.S., Sri Kantha, S.S., and Corea, S.M. (1983). The effect of oral contraceptive therapy and of pregnancy on serum folate levels of rural Sri Lankan women. *Br. J. Nutr.* 50, 495.

Heyburn, P.J. (1984). Hypocalcaemia. In *Metabolic bone disease* (ed. B.E.C. Nordin), p. 159. Churchill Livingstone, Edinburgh.

Heyns, W., Drochmans, A., van der Schueren, E., and Verhoeren, G. (1985). Endocrine effects of high-dose ketoconazole therapy in advanced prostatic cancer. *Acta Endocrinol.* 110, 276.

Hill, W.C., Gill, P.J., and Katz, M. (1985). Maternal paralytic ileus as a complication of magnesium sulfate tocolysis. *Am. J. Perinatol.* 2, 47.

Hillman, R.E. (1989). Primary hyperoxalurias. In *The metabolic basis of inherited disease* (6th edn) (ed. C.R. Scriver, A.L. Beaudet, W.S. Sly, and D. Valle), p. 933. McGraw-Hill, New York.

Hjelt, K., Brynskov, J., Hippe, E., Lundstrom, P., and Munck, O. (1985). Oral contraceptives and the cobalamin (vitamin B₁₂) metabolism. *Acta Obstet. Gynecol. Scand.* 64, 59.

Hodgson, S.F. (1990). Corticosteroid-induced osteoporosis. *Endocrinol. Metab. Clin. N. Am.* 19, 65.

Hogenkamp, H.P. (1980). The interaction between vitamin B₁₂ and vitamin C. *Am. J. Clin. Nutr.* 33, 1.

Hollifield, J.W. (1984). Potassium and magnesium abnormalities: diuretics and arrhythmias in hypertension. *Am. J. Med.* 77 (suppl. 5A), 28.

Hollifield, J.W. (1986). Thiazide treatment of hypertension. Effects of thiazide diuretics on serum potassium, magnesium, and ventricular ectopy. *Am. J. Med.* 80, 8.

Hollifield, J.W. (1989a). Electrolyte disarray and cardiovascular disease. *Am. J. Cardiol.* 63, 21B.

Hollifield, J.W. (1989b). Thiazide treatment of systemic hypertension: effects on serum magnesium and ventricular ectopic activity. *Am. J. Cardiol.* 63, 22G.

Holmberg, L., Boman, G., and Bottiger, L.E. (1980). Adverse reactions to nitrofurantoin: analysis of 921 reports. *Am. J. Med.* 69, 733.

Holmes, E.W. (1985). Clinical gout and the pathogenesis of hyperuricemia. In *Arthritis and allied conditions* (10th edn) (ed. D.J. McCarty), p. 1445. Lea and Febiger, Philadelphia.

Honda, H. and Gindin, R.A. (1972). Gout while receiving levodopa for Parkinsonism. *JAMA* 219, 55.

Hooper, C.A., Haney, B.B., and Stone, H.H. (1980). Gastrointestinal bleeding due to vitamin K deficiency in patients on parenteral cefamandole. *Lancet* i, 39.

Horne, C.H.W., Howie, P.W., Weir, R.J., and Goudie, R.B. (1970). Effect of estrogen–progestogen oral contraceptives on serum levels of alpha₂ macroglobulin, transferrin and IgG. *Lancet* i, 49.

Horowitz, J., Sukenik, S., and Altz-Smith, M. (1988). Recurrent hyperkalemia and acute renal failure following sulindac therapy. *Isr. J. Med. Sci.* 24, 433.

Horwitt, M.K., Harvey, C.C., and Dahm, C.H. Jr (1975). Relationship between levels of blood lipids, vitamin C, A, and E, serum copper compounds, and urinary excretion of tryptophan metabolites in women taking oral contraceptive therapy. *Am. J. Clin. Nutr.* 28, 403.

Hropot, M., Fowler, N., Karlmark, B., and Giebisch, G. (1985). Tubular action of diuretics: Distal effects on electrolyte transport and acidification. *Kidney Int.* 28, 477.

Huhtaniemi, I., Nikula, H., and Rannikko, S. (1985). Treatment of prostatic cancer with a gonadotrophin-releasing hormone agonist analog: acute and long term effects on endocrine functions of testis tissue. *J. Clin. Endocrinol. Metab.* 61, 698.

Humphrey, S.H. and Nash, D.A. (1978). Lactic acidosis complicating sodium nitroprusside therapy. *Ann. Intern. Med.* 88, 58.

Hurley, D.L. and McMahon, H.M. (1990). Long-term parenteral nutrition and metabolic bone disease. *Endocrinol. Metab. Clin. N. Am.* 19, 113.

Husband, D.J. and Watkin, S.W. (1988). Fatal hypokalaemia associated with ifosfamide/mesna chemotherapy. *Lancet* i, 1116.

Ilberg, J.J., Turner, G.G., and Nultall, F.Q. (1978). Effect of phosphate or magnesium cathartics on serum calcium. *Arch. Intern. Med.* 138, 1114.

Illingworth, R.N. and Proudfoot, A.T. (1980). Rapid poisoning with slow-release potassium. *Br. Med. J.* ii, 485.

Inloes, R., Clark, D., and Drobnies, A. (1987). Interference of fluorescein, used in retinol angiography, with certain clinical laboratory tests. *Clin. Chem.* 33, 2126.

Ishii, N. and Nishihara, Y. (1985). Pellagra encephalopathy among tuberculous patients: its relation to isoniazid therapy. *J. Neurol. Neurosurg. Psychiatry* 48, 628.

Ishikawa, S-E., Saito, T., and Yoshida, S. (1981). The effect of prostaglandins on the release of arginine vasopressin from the guinea pig hypothalamo-neurohypophyseal complex in organ culture. *Endocrinology* 108, 193.

Itoh, S., Yamaba, Y., Matsuo, S., Saka, M., and Ichinoe, A. (1982). Sodium valproate-induced liver injury. *Am. J. Gastroenterol.* 77, 875.

Jackson, B. and Johnston, C.I. (1984). Angiotensin converting enzyme during acute and chronic enalapril therapy in essential hypertension. *Clin. Exp. Pharmacol. Physiol.* 11, 355.

Jacob, R.A. (1986). Trace elements. In *Textbook of clinical chemistry* (ed. N.W. Tietz), p. 965. W.B. Saunders, Philadelphia.

Jacob, R.A., Skala, J.H., and Omaye, S.T. (1987). Biochemical indices of human vitamin C status. *Am. J. Clin. Nutr.* 46, 818.

Jacobsen, N.O., Mosekilde, L., Myhre-Jensen, D., Redersen, E., and Wildenhoff, K.E. (1976). Liver biopsies in epileptics during anticonvulsant therapy. *Acta Med. Scand.* 199, 345.

Jacobson, E.D., Chodos, R.B., and Faloon, W.W. (1960). An experimental malabsorption syndrome induced by neomycin. *Am. J. Med.* 28, 524.

Jaden-Starodoubsky, A., Delwaide, P.A., Penders, C., Collard, J., and Heusghem (1973). Psychotropic drug interferences with clinical chemistry determination. In *Reference values in Human Chemistry* (ed. Ci. Siest), pp. 299. Karger, Basel.

Jaffe, I.A. (1972). The antivitamin B$_6$ effect of penicillamine: clinical and immunological implications. *Adv. Biochem. Psychopharmacol.* 4, 217.

Jeejeebhoy, K.N. (1984). Zinc and chromium in parenteral nutrition. *Bull. N.Y. Acad. Med.* 60, 118.

Jelic-Ivanovic, Z., Majkic-Singh, N., Spasic, S., Todorovic, P., and Stakic, D.Z. (1984). Effect of analgesic and anti-rheumatic drugs on SMA II procedures. *Clin. Chem.* 29, 1859.

Jelic-Ivanovic, Z., Majkic-Singh, N., Spasic, S., Todorovic, P., and Zivanov-Stakic, D. (1985a). Interference by analgesic and antirheumatic drugs in 25 common laboratory assays. *J. Clin. Chem. Clin. Biochem.* 23, 287.

Jelic-Ivanovic, Z., Spasic, S., Majkic-Singh, N., and Todorovic, P. (1985b). Effects of some anti-inflammatory drugs on 12 blood constituents: protocol for the study of *in vivo* effects of drugs. *Clin. Chem.* 31, 1141.

Jensen, I.W., (1985). Oestrogen-like effect of tamoxifen on concentration of thyroxin-binding globulin. *Lancet* ii, 1020.

Jensen, E.J., Rungby, J., Hansen, J.C., Schmidt, E., Pedersen, B., and Dahl, R. (1988). Serum concentrations and accumulation of silver in skin during three months treatment with an anti-smoking chewing gum containing silver acetate. *Hum. Toxicol.* 7, 535.

Jeunemaitre, X., Chatellier, G., Kreft-Jais, C., Charru, A., DeVries, C., Plouin, P.F., Corvol, P., and Menard, J. (1987). Efficacy and tolerance of spironolactone in essential hypertension. *Am. J. Cardiol.* 60, 820.

Joborn, H., Hjemdahl, P., Larsson, P.T., Lithell, H., Olsson, G., Wide, L., et al. (1990). Effects of prolonged adrenaline infusion and of mental stress on plasma minerals and parathyroid hormone. *Clin. Physiol.* 10, 37.

Johannessen, A.C. and Nielsen, O.A. (1987). Hyponatremia induced by oxcarbazepine. *Epilepsy Res.* 1, 155.

John, R., Kadury, S., Woodhead, J.S., and Pritchard, M.H. (1983). Fenclofenac and thyroid function tests. *Ann. Clin. Biochem.* 20, 381.

Johnson, J.E. and Wright, L.F. (1983). Thiazide-induced hyponatremia. *South. Med. J.* 76, 1363.

Johnson, L., Bowen, F.W., Abbasi, S., Horrmann, N., Weston, M., Sacks, L., et al. (1985). Relationship of prolonged pharmacologic serum levels of vitamin E to incidence of sepsis and necrotizing enterocolitis in infants with birth weight 1500 grams or less. *Pediatrics* 75, 619.

Johnston, R.R., Cromwell, T.H., Eger, E.I. II, Cullen, D., Stevens, W.C., and Joas, T. (1973). The toxicity of fluroxene in animals and man. *Anesthesiology* 38, 313.

Jone, C.M. and Wu, A.H. (1988). An unusual case of toluene-induced metabolic acidosis. *Clin. Chem.* 34, 2596.

Jones, A.F., Harvey, J.M., and Vale J.A. (1989). Hypophosphataemia and phosphaturia in paracetamol poisoning. *Lancet* ii, 608.

Jones, M.G. and Swaminathan, R. (1990). The clinical biochemistry of creatine kinase. *IFCCJ* 2, 108.

Jonsson, S., O'Meara, M., and Young, J.B. (1983). Acute cocaine poisoning. Importance of treating seizures and acidosis. *Am. J. Med.* 75, 1061.

Juan, D. and Elrazak, M.A. (1979). Hypophosphataemia in hospitalized patients. *JAMA* 242, 163.

Judd, L.E., Henderson, D.W., and Hill, D.C. (1986). Naproxen-induced pseudoporphyria. A clinical and ultrastructural study. *Arch. Dermatol.* 122, 451.

June, C.H., Thompson, C.B., Kennedy, M.S., Loughran, T.P. Jr, and Deeg, H.J. (1986). Correlation of hypomagnesemia with the onset of cyclosporine-associated hypertension in marrow transplant patients. *Transplantation* 41, 47.

Kadowaki, T., Hagura, R., Kajinuma, H., Kuzuya, N., and Yoshida, S. (1983). Chlorpropamide-induced hyponatremia: incidence and risk factors. *Diabetes Care* 6, 468.

Kahan, B.D., Flechner, S.M., Lorber, M.I., Golden, D., Conley, S., and Van Buren, C.T. (1987). Complications of cyclosporine-prednisone immunosuppression in 402 renal allograft recipients exclusively followed at a single center for from one to five years. *Transplantation* 43, 197.

Kahn, A. and Blum, D. (1980). Hyperkalaemia and UNICEF type rehydration solution. *Lancet* i, 1082.

Kahn, A.M. and Weinman, E.J. (1985). Urate transport in the proximal tubule: in vivo and vesicle studies. *Am. J. Physiol.* 249, F789.

Kahn, A., Blum, D., Mozin, M.J., and Vis, H.L. (1981). Glucose electrolyte solutions in a European context. *Lancet* ii, 361.

Kaiser, L. and Schwartz, K.A. (1985). Aluminum-induced anemia. *Am. J. Kidney Dis.* 6, 348.

Kallen, R.J., Rieger, C.H.L., Cohen, H.S., Sutter, M.A., and Ong, K.J. (1976). Near-fatal hyperkalemia due to ingestion of salt substitute by an infant. *JAMA* 235, 2125.

Kalsheker, N.A. and Hales, C.N. (1985). Insulin *in vivo* increases the *in vitro* fall of plasma potassium concentration in human venous blood. *Eur. J. Clin. Invest.* 15, 113.

Kamen, B.A., Holcenberg, J.S., Turo, K., and Whitehead, V.M. (1984). Methotrexate and folate content of erythrocytes in patients receiving oral vs intramuscular therapy with methotrexate. *J. Pediatr.* 104, 131.

Kamoun, P.P., Bardet, J.I., Di Giulio, S., and Grunfield, J.P. (1982). Measurements of angiotensin converting enzyme in captopril-treated patients. *Clin. Chim. Acta* 118, 333.

Kane, S.P. and Boots, M.A. (1977). Megaloblastic anaemia associated with sulphasalazine treatment. *Br. Med. J.* ii, 1287.

Kanis, J.A. and Russell, R.G.G. (1977). Rate of reversal of hypercalcaemia and hypercalcuria induced by vitamin D and its 1-α-hydroxylated derivatives. *Br. Med. J.* i, 78.

Kaplan, M.S., Mares, A., Quintana, P., Strauss, J., Haxtable, R.F., Brennan, P., *et al.* (1969). High caloric glucose-nitrogen infusions. *Arch. Surg.*, 99, 567.

Kappas, A., Sassa, S., Galbraeth, R.A., and Nordmann, Y. (1989). The porphyrias. In *The metabolic basis of inherited disease* (6th edn) (ed. C.R. Scriver, A.L. Beaudet, W.S. Sly, and D. Valle), p. 1305. McGraw-Hill, New York.

Kariniemi, V. and Rosti, J. (1986). Intramuscular pethidine (meperidine) during labor associated with metabolic acidosis in the newborn. *J. Perinat. Med.* 14, 131.

Karkalas, Y. and Lal, H. (1971). Jaundice following therapy with imipramine and cyproheptadine. *Clin. Toxicol.* 4, 47.

Karpel, J.T. and Peden, V.H. (1972). Copper deficiency in long-term parenteral nutrition. *J. Pediatr.* 80, 32.

Kartz, C.M. and Tzagourins, M. (1972). Chronic adult hypervitaminosis A with hypercalcaemia. *Metabolism* 21, 117.

Kasidas, G.F. (1988). Assay of oxalate and glycollate in urine. In *Oxalate metabolism in relation to urinary stone* (ed. G.A. Rose), p. 7. Springer-Verlag, Berlin.

Kassirer, J.P. and Harrington, J.T. (1977). Diuretic and potassium metabolism: A reassessment of the need, effectiveness and safety of potassium therapy. *Kidney Int.* 11, 505.

Kataoka, K., Kanamori, N., Oishi, M., Yamaji, A., Tagawa, T., and Miwaki, T. (1990). Vitamin E status in pediatric patients receiving antiepileptic drugs. *Dev. Pharmacol. Ther.* 14, 96.

Katayama, S., Inaba, M., Maruno, Y., Omoto, A., Itabashi, A., Kawazu, S., *et al.* (1987). Captopril induced creatine kinase elevations: a possible role of the sulfhydryl group. *Hypertension* 10, 234.

Katz, F.H., Eckert, R.C., and Gebott, M.D. (1972). Hypokalemia caused by surreptitious self-administration of diuretics. *Ann. Intern. Med.* 76, 85.

Kaufman, A.M., Hellman, G., and Abramson, R.G. (1983). Renal salt wasting and metabolic acidosis with trimethoprim–sulfamethoxazole therapy. *Mt Sinai J. Med.* 50, 238.

Kawarabayashi, T., Tsukamoto, T., Kishikawa, T., and Sugimori, H. (1989). Changes in serum calcium, magnesium, cyclic AMP and monoamine oxidase levels during pregnancy and under prolonged ritodrine treatment for preterm labor. *Gynecol. Obstet. Invest.* 28, 132.

Kay, R.G., Tasman-Jones, C., Pybus, J., Whiting, R., and Black, H. (1976). A syndrome of acute zinc deficiency during total parenteral alimentation in man. *Ann. Surg.* 183, 331.

Kaye, M. (1983). Oral aluminum toxicity in a non-dialyzed patient with renal failure. *Clin. Nephrol.* 20, 208.

Kearney, T.E., Manoguerra, A.S., Curtis, G.P., and Ziegler, M.G. (1985). Theophylline toxicity and the beta-adrenergic system. *Ann. Intern. Med.* 102, 766.

Keating, J.N., Wada, L., Stokstad, E.L., and King, J.C. (1987). Folic acid: effect on zinc absorption in humans and in the rat. *Am. J. Clin. Nutr.* 46, 835.

Kelleher, S.P. and Schulman, G. (1987). Severe metabolic alkalosis complicating regional citrate hemodialysis. *Am. J. Kidney Dis.* 9, 235.

Keller, C., Zoller, W., Wolfram, G., and Zollner, N. (1988). Unusual but reversible hepatic lesions following long-term treatment with pyridylcarbinol for familial hypercholesterolemia. *Klin. Wochenschr.* 66, 647.

Kelly, W.N., Fox, I.H., and Palella, T.D. (1989). Gout and related disorders of purine metabolism. In *Textbook of rheumatology* (3rd edn) (ed. W.N. Kelly, E.D. Harris Jr, S. Ruddy, and C.B. Sledge), p. 1395. W.B. Saunders, Philadephia.

Kelner, M.J. and Bailey, D.N. (1985). Propylene glycol as a cause of lactic acidosis. *J. Anal. Toxicol.* 9, 40.

Kemp, S.F. and Canfield, M.E. (1983). Acute effects of growth hormone administration: vitamin A and visceral protein concentrations. *Acta Endocrinol.* 104, 390.

Kennedy, P. (1983). Liver cross-sensitivity to antipsychotic drugs. *Br. J. Psychiatry* 143, 312.

Kennedy, R.M. and Earley, L. (1970). Profound hyponatremia resulting from a thiazide-induced decrease in urinary diluting capacity in a patient with primary polydipsia. *N. Engl. J. Med.* 282, 1185.

Kennedy, M.J., Shelley, R.K., and Daly, P.A. (1987). Potentiation of small cell lung cancer-related SIADH by trifluoperazine. *Eur. J. Respir. Dis.* 71, 450.

Kidd, D., Ranaghan, E.A., and Morris, T.C. (1989). Hypokalaemia in patients with acute myeloid leukaemia after treatment with fluconazole. *Lancet* i, 1017.

Kim, E.E. and Wyckoff, H.W. (1989). Structure of alkaline phosphatases. *Clin. Chim. Acta* 186, 175.

Kimelman, N. and Albert, S.G. (1984). Phenothiazine-induced hyponatremia in the elderly. *Gerontology* 30, 132.

Kimura, T., Matsui, K., Sato, T., and Yoshinaga, K. (1974). Mechanism of carbamazepine (Tegretol)-induced antidiuresis: evidence for release of antidiuretic hormone and impaired excretion of a water load. *J. Clin. Endocrinol. Metab.* 38, 356.

Kindler, J., Schunkert, H., Gassmann, M., Lahn, W., Irmisch, R., Debusmann, E.R., *et al.* (1989). Therapeutic efficacy and tolerance of ramipril in hypertensive patients with renal failure. *J. Cardiovasc. Pharmacol.* 13 (suppl. 3), S55.

King, B., Spikesman, A., and Emery, A.E. (1972). The effect of pregnancy on serum levels of creatine kinase. *Clin. Chim. Acta* 36, 267.

King, A.L., Sica, D.A., Miller, G., and Pierpaoli, S. (1987). Severe hypophosphatemia in a general hospital population. *South. Med. J.* 80, 831.

Kingreen, J.C. and Breger, G. (1984). Pellagra bei 'Morazon'-Abusus. *Z. Hautkr.* 59, 573.

Kirkham, B., Cowell, R., and Rees, J. (1987). Severe hypokalaemia from kaolin and morphine abuse. *Postgrad. Med. J.* 63, 589.

Klastersky, J., Vanderkelen, B., Daneau, D., and Mathieu, M. (1973). Carbenicillin and hypokalemia. *Ann. Intern. Med.* 78, 774.

Klein, G.L., Florey, J.B., Goller, V.L., Larese, R.J., and van Meter, Q.L. (1977). Multiple vitamin deficiencies in association with chronic anticonvulsant therapy. *Pediatrics* 60, 767.

Klein, G.L., Ament, M.E., Bluestone, R., Norman, A.W., Targoff, C.M., Sherrard, D.J., *et al.* (1980). Bone disease associated with total parenteral nutrition. *Lancet* ii, 1041.

Klein, G.L., Alfrey, A.C., Miller, N.L., Sherrard, D.J., Hazlet, T.K., Ament, M.E., *et al.* (1982). Aluminum loading during total parenteral nutrition. *Am. J. Clin. Nutr.* 35, 1425.

Klein, G.L., Snodgrass, W.R., Griffin, M.P., Miller, N.C., and Alfrey, A.C. (1989). Hypocalcemia complicating deferoxamine therapy in an infant with parenteral nutrition-associated aluminium overload. Evidence for a role of aluminium in the bone disease of infants. *J. Pediatr. Gastroenterol. Nutr.* 9, 400.

Kleinman, P.K. (1974). Cholestyramine and metabolic acidosis. *N. Engl. J. Med.* 290, 861.

Klemola, H., Penttila, O., Runeberg, L., and Tallqvist, G. (1975). Anicteric liver damage during nitrofurantoin medication. *Scand. J. Gastroenterol.* 10, 501.

Klinberg, W.G., Parsad, A.S., and Oberleas, D. (1976). Zinc deficiency following penicillamine therapy. In *Trace elements in human health and disease*, Vol. 1 (ed. A.S. Prasad), p. 51. Academic Press, New York.

Kloppel, A. and Weiler, G. (1985). Erhohte bis toxische Quecksilberkonzentrationen nach post-operativer Wundehandlung mit Merbromin. *Beitr. Gerichtl. Med.* 43, 169.

Knochel, J.P. (1984). Diuretic-induced hypokalemia. *Am. J. Med.* 77 (suppl. 5A), 18.

Kofke, W.A., Young, R.S., Davis, P., Woelfel, S.K., Gray, L., Johnson, D., *et al.* (1989). Isoflurane for refractory status epilepticus: a clinical series. *Anesthesiology* 71, 653.

Kolendrof, K. and Moller, B.B. (1974). Lactic acidosis in epinephrine poisoning. *Acta Med. Scand.* 196, 465.

Kolski, G.B., Cunningham, A.S., Niemec, P.W. Jr, Davignon, G.F. Jr, and Freehafer, J.G. (1988). Hypokalemia and respiratory arrest in an infant with status asthmaticus. *J. Pediatr.* 112, 304.

Kone, B., Gimenez, L., and Watson, A.J. (1986). Thiazide-induced hyponatremia. *South. Med. J.* 79, 1456.

Kone, B.C., Whelton, A., Santos, G., Saral, R., and Watson, A.J. (1988). Hypertension and renal dysfunction in bone marrow transplant recipients. *Q. J. Med.* 69, 985.

Konikoff, F., Halevy, J., and Theodor, E. (1985). Serum creatine kinase after intramuscular injections. *Postgrad. Med. J.* 61, 595.

Koppel, M.H., Massry, S.G., Shinaberger, J.H., Hartenbower, D.L., and Coburn, J.W. (1970). Thiazide induced rise in serum calcium and magnesium in patients on maintenance hemodialysis. *Ann. Intern. Med.* 72, 895.

Koren, G., Lau, A., Klein, J., Golas, C., Bologa-Campeanu, M., Soldin, S., *et al.* (1988). Pharmacokinetics and adverse effects of amphotericin B in infants and children. *J. Pediatr.* 113, 559.

Korenberg, A., Segal, R., Theitler, J., Yona, R., and Kaufman, S. (1989). Folic acid deficiency, megaloblastic anaemia and peripheral polyneuropathy due to oral contraceptives. *Isr. J. Med. Sci.* 25, 142.

Korner, W.F. and Vollun, J. (1975). New aspects of the tolerance of retinol in humans. *Int. J. Vit. Nutr. Res.* 45, 363.

Korsan-Bengsten, K., Elmfeldt, D., and Holm, T. (1974). Prolonged plasma clotting time and decreased fibrinolysis after long term treatment with alpha-tocopherol. *Thromb. Diath. Haemorr.* 31, 505.

Korttila, K., Grohn, P., Gordin, A., Sundberg, S., Salo, H., Nissinen, E., *et al.* (1984). Effect of hydroxyethyl starch and dextran on plasma volume and blood hemostasis and coagulation. *J. Clin. Pharmacol.* 24, 273.

Kotowski, K.E. and Grayson, M.F. (1982). Side effect of non-steroidal anti-inflammatory drugs. *Br. Med. J.* 285, 377.

Kovacs, L., Pal, A., and Horvath, K. (1985). The effect of fenoterol on fetal metabolism: cord blood studies. *Acta Paediatr. Hung.* 26, 41.

Kovnat, P., Labovitz, E., and Levison, S.P. (1973). Antibiotics and the kidney. *Med. Clin. North Am.* R57, 1045.

Kozlowski, B.W., Taylor, M.L., Baer, M.T., Blyler, E.M., and Trahms, C. (1987). Anticonvulsant medication use and circulating levels of total thyroxine, retinol binding protein and vitamin A in children with delayed cognitive development. *Am. J. Clin. Nutr.* 46, 360.

Krause, K-H., Berlit, P., Bonjour, J.P., Schmidt-Gayk, H., Schellenberg, B., and Gillen, J. (1982). Vitamin status in patients on chronic anticonvulsant therpay. *Int. J. Vitam. Nutr.* 52, 375.

Krause, K.H., Berlit, P., Schmidt-Gayk, H., and Schellenberg, B. (1987). Antiepileptic drugs reduce serum uric acid. *Epilepsy Res.* 1, 306.

Krause, K-H., Bonjour, J-P., Berlit, P., Kynast, G., Schmidt-Gayk, H., and Schellenberg, B. (1988). Effects of long-term treatment with antiepileptic drugs on the vitamin status. *Drug Nutr. Interact.* 5, 317.

Krebs, H.A., Woods, H.F., and Alberti, K.G.M.M. (1975). Hyperlactaemia and lactic acidosis. *Essays Med. Biochem.* 1, 81.

Kreisberg, R.A. and Wood, B.C. (1983). Drugs and chemical-induced metabolic acidosis. *Clin. Endocrinol. Metab.* 12, 391.

Kritharides, L., Fassett, R., and Singh, B. (1988). Paracetamol-associated coma, metabolic acidosis, renal and hepatic failure. *Intens. Care Med.* 14, 439.

Kuny, S. and Binswanger, U. (1988). Ionized calcium and neuroleptic-induced extrapyramidal symptoms. *Pharmacopsychiatry* 21, 300.

Kuny, S. and Binswanger, U. (1989). Neuroleptic-induced extrapyramidal symptoms and serum calcium levels. Results of a pilot study. *Neuropsychobiology* 21, 67.

Kurokawa, K., Levine, B.S., Lee, D.B.N., and Massry, S.G. (1985). Physiology of phosphorus metabolism and pathophysiology of hypophosphatemia and hyperphosphatemia. In *Fluid electrolyte and acid-base disorders* (ed. A.I. Arieff and R.A. DeFronzo), p. 625. Churchill Livingstone, Edinburgh.

Kusano, E., Braun-Werness, J.L., Vick, D.J., Keller, M.J., and Dousa, T.P. (1983). Chlorpropamide action on renal concentrating mechanism in rats with hypothalamic diabetes insipidus. *J. Clin. Invest.* 72, 1298.

Kushner, R.F. and Sitrin, M.D. (1986). Metabolic acidosis. Development in two patients receiving a potassium-sparing diuretic and total parenteral nutrition. *Arch. Intern. Med.* 146, 343.

Kutyrina, I.M., Nikishova, T.A., and Tareyeva, I.E. (1987). Effect of heparin-induced aldosterone deficiency on renal function in patients with chronic glomerulonephritis. *Nephrol. Dial. Transplant.* 2, 219.

Kynaston, H.G., Lewis-Jones, D.I., Lynch, R.V., and Desmond, A.D. (1988). Changes in seminal quality following oral zinc therapy. *Andrologia* 20, 21.

Labadarios, D., Obuwa, G.H., Lucas, E.G., Dickerson, J.W.T., and Parke, D.V. (1978). The effects of chronic drug administration on hepatic enzyme induction and folate metabolism. *Br. J. Clin. Pharmacol.* 5, 167.

Labadie, H., Verneau, A., Trinchet, J.C., and Beaugrand, M. (1986). L'apport oral de zinc améliore-t-il l'immunité cellulaire des malades atteints de cirrhose alcoölique? *Gastroenterol. Clin. Biol.* 10, 799.

Labbe, R.F. and Lamon, J.M. (1986). Porphyrins and disorders of porphyrin metabolism. In *Textbook of clinical chemistry* (ed. V.W. Tietz), p. 1589. W.B. Saunders, Philadephia.

Lachaal, M. and Venuto, R.C. (1989). Nephrotoxicity and hyperkalemia in patients with acquired immunodeficiency syndrome treated with pentamidine. *Am. J. Med.* 87, 260.

Lacroix, C., Guyonnaud, C., Chaou, M., Duwoos, H., and Lafont, O. (1988). Interaction between allopurinol and pyrazinamide. *Eur. Respir. J.* 1, 807.

Lahr, M.B. (1985). Hyponatremia during carbamazepine therapy. *Clin. Pharmacol. Ther.* 37, 693.

Lalau, J.D., Debussche, X., Tolani, M., Arlot, S., and Quichaud, J. (1984). Acidose lactique chez les diabètiques traités par metformine. Intérêt de l'hémodialyse avec bain au bicarbonate de sodium. *Presse Med.* 13, 2581.

Lam, M. and Adelstein, D.J. (1986). Hypomagnesemia and renal magnesium wasting in patients treated with cisplatin. *Am. J. Kidney Dis.* 8, 164.

Lambert, H., Isnard, F., Delorme, N., Claude, D., Bollaert, P.E., Straczek, J., *et al.* (1987). Approche physiopathologique des hyperlactatémies pathologiques chez le diabètique. Intérêt de la metforminémie. *Ann. Fr. Anesth. Reanim.* 6, 88.

Lambertus, M., Murthy, A.R., Nagami, P., and Goetz, M.B. (1988). Diabetic keto-acidosis following pentamidine therapy in a patient with the acquired immunodeficiency syndrome. *West. J. Med.* 149, 602.

Lamm, C.I., Norton, K.I., Murphy, R.J.C., Wilkins, I.A., and Rabinowitz, J.G. (1988). Congenital rickets associated with magnesium sulfate infusion for tocolysis. *J. Pediatr.* 113, 1078.

Lammers, P.J., White, L., and Ettinger, L.J. (1984). Cisplatinum-induced renal sodium wasting. *Med. Pediatr. Oncol.*, 12, 343.

The Lancet (1979). Ascorbic acid: immunological effects and hazards. *Lancet* i, 308.

The Lancet (1990). Severe symptomatic hyponatraemia: dangers in lack of therapy. *Lancet* 335, 825.

Langer, T. and Levy, R.I. (1968). Acute muscular syndrome associated with administration of clofibrate. *N. Engl. J. Med.* 279, 856.

Langford, H.G., Blaufox, M.D., Borhani, N.O., Curb, J.O., Molteni, A., Schneider, K.A., *et al.* (1987). Analysis of data from the hypertension detection and follow-up program. *Arch. Intern. Med.* 147, 645.

Larkin, E.C. and Watson-Williams, E.J. (1984). Alcohol and the blood. *Med. Clin. N. Am.* 68, 105.

Larsen, P.R., Atkinson, A.J., and Wellman, H.N. (1970). The effect of diphenylhydantoin on thyroxine metabolism in man. *J. Clin. Invest.* 49, 1266.

Lau, K. (1985). Magnesium metabolism: normal and abnormal. In *Fluid, electrolyte and acid–base disorders* (ed. A.I. Arieff and R.A. DeFronzo), p. 575. Churchill Livingstone, Edinburgh.

Lau, K. (1986). Phosphate disorders. In *Fluids and electrolytes* (ed. J.P. Kokko and R.L. Tannen), p. 398. W.B. Saunders, Philadelphia.

Lau, K., Stote, R.M., Goldberg, M., and Agus, Z.S. (1977). Mechanism of the urocosuric effect of the diuretic tienilic acid (ticrynafen) in man. *Clin. Sci. Molec. Med.* 53, 379.

Laudignon, N., Ciampi, A., Coupal, L., Chemtob, S., and Aranda, J.V. (1989). Frusemide and ethacrynic acid. Risk factors for the occurrence of serum electrolyte abnormalities and metabolic alkalosis in newborns and infant. *Acta Pediatr. Scand.* 78, 133.

Laureno, R. (1983). Central pontine myelinolysis following rapid correction of hyponatremia. *Ann. Neurol.* 13, 232.

Laureno, R. and Karp, B.I. (1988). Pontine and extrapontine myelinolysis following rapid correction of hyponatremia. *Lancet* i, 1439.

Lauzurica, R., Bonal, J., Bonet, J., Romero, R., Teixido, J., Serra, A., *et al.* (1988). Rhabdomyolysis, oedema and arterial hypertension: different syndromes related to topical use of 9-alpha-fluoroprednisolone. *J. Hum. Hypertens.* 2, 183.

Le Bihan, G., Bourreille, J., Sampson, M., Leroy, J., Szekely, A.M., and Coquerel, A. (1980). Fetal hepatic failure and sodium valproate. *Lancet* ii, 1298.

Lee, C.Y. and Finkler, A. (1986). Acute intoxication due to ibuprofen overdose. *Arch. Pathol. Lab. Med.* 110, 747.

Lefevre, A.L., Adler, H., and Lieber, C.S. (1970). Effect of ethanol on ketone metabolism. *J. Clin. Invest.* 49, 1775.

Legha, S.S., Powell, K., Buzdar, A.U., and Blumenschein, G.R. (1981). Tamoxifen-induced hypercalcemia in breast cancer. *Cancer* 47, 2803.

Lehmann, J., Rao, D.D., Canary, J.J., and Judd, J.T. (1988). Vitamin E and relationships among tocopherols in human plasma, platelet, lymphocytes and red blood cells. *Am. J. Clin. Nutr.* 47, 470.

Lehot, J.J. (1989). Delayed respiratory depression following fentanyl anesthesia for cardiac surgery. *Crit. Care Med.* 17, 299.

Leite, J.R., Seabra, M. de L., Maluf, E., Assolant, K., Suchecki, D., Tufik, S., *et al.* (1986). Pharmacology of lemongrass (*Cymbopogon citratus* Stapf). III. Assessment of eventual toxic, hypnotic and anxiolytic effects on humans. *J. Ethnopharmacol.* 17, 75.

Lemons, J.A. and Maisels, M.J. (1985). Vitamin E — how much is too much? *Pediatrics* 76, 625.

Lepage, L., Schiele, F., Gueguen, R., and Siest, G. (1985). Total cholinesterase in plasma: biological variations and reference limits. *Clin. Chem.* 31, 546.

Leppanen, E.A. and Grasbeck, R. (1987). Experimental basis of standardized specimen collection. The effect of moderate ethanol consumption on some serum components (K, Na, ASAT, ALT, CK, LD, total protein). *Scand. J. Clin. Lab. Invest.* 47, 337.

Leslie, P.J., Cregeen, R.J., and Proudfoot, A.T. (1984). Lactic acidosis, hyperglycaemia and convulsions following nalidixic acid overdosage. *Hum. Toxicol.* 3, 239.

Leson, C.L., McGuigan, M.A., and Bryson, S.M. (1988). Caffeine overdose in an adolescent male. *J. Toxicol. Clin. Toxicol.* 26, 407.

Letellier, G. and Desjarlais, F. (1985). Analytical interference of drugs in clinical chemistry: Study of twenty drugs on seven different instruments. *Clin. Biochem.* 18, 345.

Levinson, D.J. and Sorensen, L.B. (1980). Renal handling of uric acid in normal and gouty subjects: evidence for a 4-component system. *Ann. Rheum. Dis.* 39, 173.

Leyvraz, S., Ohnuma, T., Lassus, M., and Holland, J.F. (1985). Phase 1 study of carboplatin in patients with advanced cancer, intermittent intravenous bolus, and 24-hour infusion. *J. Clin. Oncol.* 3, 1385.

Li, M.K., Kavanagh, J.P., Prendiville, V., Buxton, A., Moss, D.G., and Blacklock, N.J. (1986). Does sucrose damage kidneys? *Br. J. Urol.* 58, 353.

Liang, M.H. and Fries, J.F. (1978). Asymptomatic hyperuricemia: the case for conservative management. *Ann. Intern. Med.* 88, 666.

Lieberman, J. (1989). Enzymes in sarcoidosis: angiotensin-converting-enzyme (ACE). *Clin. Lab. Med.* 9, 745.

Lilijeqvist, J.A. and Edvardsson, N. (1989). *Torsade de pointes* tachycardias induced by overdosage of zimeldine. *J. Cardiovasc. Pharmacol.* 14, 666.

Lim, M., Linton, R.A.F., Wolff, C.B., and Band, D.M. (1981). Propranolol, exercise and arterial plasma potassium. *Lancet* ii, 591.

Lin, R.Y., Busher, J., Bogden, G.J., and Schwartz, R.A. (1985). Topical zinc sulfate augmentation of human delayed type skin test response. *Acta Derm. Venereol.* 65, 190.

Lin, H.Y., Rocher, L.L., McQuillan, M.A., Schmaltz, S., Palella, T.D., and Fox, I.H. (1989). Cyclosporine-induced hyperuricemia and gout. *N. Engl. J. Med.* 321, 287.

Linden, C.H. and Townsend, P.L. (1987). Metabolic acidosis after acute ibuprofen overdosage. *J. Pediatr.* 111, 922.

Linderman, R.D. (1976). Hypokalaemia: causes, consequences and correction. *Am. J. Med. Sci.* 272, 5.

Lindstedt, G., Lundberg, P-A., Hammond, G.L. and Vikko, R. (1985). Sex hormone binding globulin — still many questions. *Scand. J. Clin. Lab. Invest.* 45, 1.

Linford, S.M. and James, H.D. (1986). Sodium bicarbonate abuse: a case report. *Br. J. Psychiatry* 149, 502.

Linko, K. and Saxelin, I. (1986). Electrolyte and acid–base disturbances caused by blood transfusions. *Acta Anaesth. Scand.* 30, 139.

Linter, C.M. and Linter, S.P.K. (1986). Severe lactic acidosis following paraldehyde administration. *Br. J. Psychiatry* 149, 650.

Lipner, H.I., Ruzany, F., Dasgupta, M., Lief, P.D., and Bank, N. (1975). The behavior of carbenicillin as a nonreabsorbable anion. *J. Lab. Clin. Med.* 86, 183.

Lippmann, M., Yang, E., Au, E., and Lee, C. (1982). Neuromuscular blocking effects of tobramycin, gentamicin, and cefazolin. *Anesth. Anal.* 61, 767.

Lipsett, M.B., Combs, J.W., Catt, K., and Seigel, D.G. (1971). Problems in contraception. *Ann. Intern. Med.* 74, 251.

Lipsky, J.J., Lewis, J.C., and Novick W.J. Jr, (1984). Production of hypoprothrombinemia by moxalactam and 1-methyl-5-thiotetrazole in rats. *Antimicrob. Agents Chemother.* 25, 380.

Lipworth, B.J., McDevitt, D.G., and Struthers, A.D. (1989a). Systemic beta-adrenoceptor responses to salbutamol given by metered-dose inhaler alone and with pear shaped spacer attachment: comparison of electrocardiographic, hypokalaemic and haemodynamic effects. *Br. J. Clin. Pharmacol.* 27, 837.

Lipworth, B.J., McDevitt, D.G., and Struthers, A.D. (1989b). Prior treatment with diuretic augments the hypokalemic and electrocardiographic effects of inhaled albuterol. *Am. J. Med.* 86, 653.

Lisi, D.M. (1989). Muscle spasms and creatine kinase elevation following salbutamol administration. *Eur. Respir. J.* 2, 98.

Litwin, M., Smith, L., and Moore, F.D. (1959). Metabolic alkalosis following massive transfusion. *Surgery* 45, 805.

Liu, G.Z., Lyle, K.C., and Cao, J. (1987). Experiences with gossypol as a male pill. *Am. J. Obstet. Gynecol.* 157, 1079.

Liu, G.Z., Ch'iu-Hinton, K., Cao, J.A., Zhu, C.X., and Li, B.Y. (1988a). Effects of K salt or a potassium blocker on gossypol-related hypokalemia. *Contraception* 37, 111.

Liu, C.L., Mimouni, F., Ho, M., and Tsang, R. (1988b). In vitro effects of magnesium on ionized calcium concentration in serum. *Am. J. Dis. Child.* 142, 837.

Ljunghall, S., Akarstrom, G., Benson, L., Hetta, J., Rudberg, C., and Wide, L. (1984). Effects of epinephrine and norepinephrine on serum parathyroid hormone and calcium in normal subjects. *Exp. Clin. Endocrinol.* 84, 313.

LoCascio, V., Bonucci, E., Imbimbo, B., Ballanti, P., Tartarolti, D., Galvanini G., *et al.* (1984). Bone loss of glucocorticoid therapy. *Calcif. Tiss. Int.* 36, 435.

Lofaso, F., Baud, F.J., Halna du Frelay, X., Bismuth, C., Staikowsky, F., and Sidhom, M. (1987). Hypokalémie au cours d'intoxications massives par la chloroquine. Deux cas. *Presse Med.* 16, 22.

Longstretch, G.F. and Green, R. (1983). Folate status in patients receiving maintenance doses of sulfasalazine. *Arch. Intern. Med.* 143, 902.

Lonning, P.E., Bakke, P., Thorsen, T., Olsen, B., and Gulsvik, A. (1989). Plasma levels of estradiol, estrone, estrone sulfate and sex hormone binding globulin in patients receiving rifampicin. *J. Steroid Biochem.* 33, 631.

Lorch, V., Murphy, M.D, Hoersten, R., Harris, E., Fitzgerald, J., and Sinha, S.N. (1985). Unusual syndrome among premature infants: association with a new intravenous vitamin E product. *Pediatrics* 75, 598.

Lott, J.A. and Landesman, P.W. (1984). The enzymology of skeletal muscle disorders. *CRC Crit. Rev. Clin. Lab. Sci.* 20, 153.

Lott, J.A. and Stang, J.M. (1989). Differential diagnosis of patient with abnormal serum creatine kinase isoenzymes. *Clin. Lab. Med.* 9, 627.

Lott, J.A. and Wolf P.L. (1986a). Creatine kinase. In *Clinical enzymology. A case orientated approach* (ed. J.A. Lott and P.L. Wolf), p. 149. Field, Rich, New York.

Lott, J.A. and Wolf, P.L. (1986b). Amylase. In *Clinical enzymology. A case orientated approach.* (ed. J.A. Lott and P.L. Wolf), p. 75. Field, Rich, New York.

Lown, B., Black, H., and Moore, F.D. (1960). Digitalis, electrolytes and the surgical patient. *Am. J. Cardiol.* 6, 309.

Luft, D., Schmulling, R.M., and Eggstein, M. (1978). Lactic acidosis in biguanide treated diabetics: a review of 330 cases. *Diabetologia* 14, 75.

Lui, W.Y. (1979). Phenothiazine-induced dystonia associated with an increase in serum creatine phosphokinase. *Arch. Dis. Child.* 54, 150.

Luscher, T.F., Siegenthaler-Zaber, G., and Kuhlmann, U. (1983). Severe hyponatremic coma due to diphenylhydantoin intoxication. *Clin. Nephrol.* 20, 268.

Maatman, T.J., Gupta, M.K., and Montie, J.E. (1984). The role of serum prostatic acid phosphatase as a tumor marker in men with advanced adenocarcinoma of the prostate. *J. Urol.* 132, 58.

McBurney, E.I. and Rosen, D.A. (1984). Elevated creatine phosphokinase with isotretinoin. *J. Am. Acad. Dermatol.* 10, 528.

McClain, C.J., Soutor, C., Steele, N., Levina, A.S., and Silvis, S.E. (1980). Severe zinc deficiency presenting with acrodermatitis during hyperalimentation: Diagnosis, pathogenesis and treatment. *J. Clin. Gastronterol.* 2, 125.

McColl, K.E.L. and Goldberg, A. (1980). Abnormal porphyrin metabolism in diseases other than porphyria. *Clin. Haematol.* 9, 427.

McConkey, B., Crockson, R.A., Crockson, A.P. and Wilkinson, A.R. (1973). The effects of some antiinflammatory drugs on the acute phase proteins in rheumatoid arthritis. *Q. J. Med.* 42, 785.

McConnel, T.H. (1971). Fatal hypocalcaemia from phosphate absorption from laxative preparation. *JAMA* 216, 147.

McCormick, D.B. (1986). Vitamins. In *Textbook of clinical chemistry* (ed. N.W. Tietz), p. 927. W.B. Saunders, Philadephia.

McDonagh, A.J. and Harrington C.I. (1989). Pseudoporphyria complicating etretinate therapy. *Clin. Exp. Dermatol.* 14, 437.

Macfarlane, D.G. and Dieppe, P.A. (1985). Diuretic-induced gout in elderly women. *Br. J. Rheumatol.* 24, 155.

McIndoe, G.A., Menzies, K.W., and Reddy, J. (1981). Sulindac (Clinoril) and cholestatic jaundice. *N.Z. Med. J.* 94, 430.

MacIntyre, D., McLay, A.L.C., East, B.W., Williams, E.D., and Boddy, K. (1978). Silver poisoning associated with an anti-smoking lozenge. *Br. Med. J.* ii, 1749.

McIntyre, J.W.R., Russell, J.C., and Chambers, M. (1973). Oxalemia following methoxyfluorane anesthesia in man. *Anesth. Analg.* 52, 946.

McIvor, M.E. (1987). Delayed fatal hyperkalemia in a patient with acute fluoride intoxication. *Ann. Emerg. Med.* 16, 1165.

MacRury, S., Neilson, R., and Goodwin, K. (1987). Benylin dependence, metabolic acidosis and hyperglycaemia. *Postgrad. Med. J.* 63, 587.

Mactier, R.A. and Khanna, R. (1988). Hyperkalemia induced by indomethacin and naproxen and reversed by fluorocortisone. *South. Med. J.* 71, 799.

Magner, P.O., Robinson, L.H., Halperin, R.M., Zettle, R., and Halperin, M.L. (1988). The plasma potassium concentration in metabolic acidosis: a re-evaluation. *Am. J. Kidney Dis.* 11, 220.

Magnus, I.A. (1984). Drugs and porphyria. *Br. Med. J.* 288, 1474.

Maguire, J.F., Geha, R.S., and Umetsu, D.T. (1986). Myocardial specific creatine phosphokinase isoenzyme elevation in children with asthma treated with intravenous isoproterenol. *J. Allergy Clin. Immunol.* 78, 631.

Maislos, M., Sobel, R., and Shany, S. (1985). Leiomyoblastoma associated with intractable hypercalcemia and elevated 1,25-dihydroxycholecalciferol levels. Treatment by hepatic enzyme induction. *Arch. Intern. Med.* 145, 565.

Majumdar, S.K. (1981). Pyridoxine deficiency due to anticonvulsants. *J. Ind. Med. Assoc.* 76, 187.

Malas, K.L. and van Kammen, D.P. (1982). Markedly elevated creatine phosphokinase levels after neuroleptic withdrawal. *Am. J. Psychiatry* 139, 231.

Mall-Haefeli, M., Darragh, A., and Werner-Zodrow, I. (1983). Effects of various combined oral contraceptives on sex steroids, gonadotropins and SHBG. *Ir. Med. J.* 76, 266.

Mallette, L.E. and Eichhorn, E. (1986). Effects of lithium carbonate on human calcium metabolism. *Arch. Intern. Med.* 146, 770.

Mallette, L.E., Khouri, K., Zengotita, H., Hollis, B.W., and Malini, S. (1989). Lithium treatment increases intact and midregion parathyroid hormone and parathyroid volume. *J. Clin. Endocrinol. Metab.* 68, 654.

Malone, P.R., Davies, J.H., Standfield, N.J., Bush, R.A., Gosling, J.V. and Sheaver, R.J. (1986). Metabolic consequences of forced diuresis following prostatectomy. *Br. J. Urol.* 58, 406.

Mandel, H. and Berant, M. (1985). Oral contraceptives and breastfeeding: haematological effects on the infant. *Arch. Dis. Child.* 60, 971.

Manzione, N.C., Wolkoff, A.W., and Sassa, S. (1988). Development of porphyria cutanea tarda after treatment with cyclophosphamide. *Gastroenterology* 95, 1119.

Marasco, W.A., Gikas, P.W., Azziz-Baumgartner, R., Hyzy, R., Eldredge, C.J., and Stross, J. (1987). Ibuprofen-associated renal dysfunction. Pathophysiologic mechanisms of acute renal failure, hyperkalemia, tubular necrosis, and proteinuria. *Arch. Intern. Med.* 147, 2107.

Marel, G., Frame, B., and Parfitt, A.M. (1982). Lithium and calcium metabolism. *Am. J. Psychiatry* 139, 255.

Marin, F., Gonzalez Quintela, A., Moya, M., Suarez, E., and de Zarraga, M. (1989). Pseudohyperaldosteronism due to application of an antihemorrhoid cream. *Nephron* 52, 281.

Markman, M., Cleary, S., and Howell, S.B. (1986). Hypomagnesemia following high-dose intracavitary cisplatin with systemically administered sodium thiosulfate. *Am. J. Clin. Oncol.* 9, 440.

Marks, V. and Chapple, P.A. (1967). Hepatic dysfunction in heroin and cocaine users. *Br. J. Addict.* 62, 189.

Maronde, R.F., Milgrom, M., Vlachakis, N.D., and Chan, L. (1983). Response of thiazide-induced hypokalemia to amiloride. *JAMA* 249, 237.

Marsden, P. and Halperin, M.L. (1985). Pathophysiological approach to patients presenting with hypernatraemia. *Am. J. Nephrol.* 5, 229.

Marshall, A.W., Jakobovits, A.W., and Morgan, M.Y. (1982). Bromocriptine-associated hyponatraemia in cirrhosis. *Br. Med. J.* 285, 1534.

Marshall, J.C., Anderson, D.C., Burke, C.W., Galvao-Teles, A., and Russell-Fraser, T. (1972). Clomiphene citrate in man: increase in cortisol, luteinizing hormone, testosterone and steroid-binding globulin. *J. Endocrinol.* 53, 261.

Marshall, R.W., Selby, P.L., Chilvers, D.C., and Hodgkinson, A. (1984). The effect of ethinyl oestradiol on calcium and bone metabolism in peri- and postmenopausal women. *Horm. Metab. Res.* 16, 97.

Martin, B.J., McAlpine, J.K., and Devine, B.L. (1988). Hypomagnesaemia in elderly digitalised patients. *Scott. Med. J.* 33, 273.

Martin, R.R., Lisehora, G.R., Braxton, M., and Barcia, P.J. (1987). Fatal poisoning from sodium phosphate enema. Case report and experimental study. *JAMA* 257, 2190.

Martinez, R., Smith, D.W., and Frankel, L.R. (1989). Severe metabolic acidosis after acute naproxen sodium ingestion. *Ann. Emerg. Med.* 18, 1102.

Marwick, T.H. and Woodhouse, S.P. (1988). Severe hypophosphataemia induced by glucose-insulin-potassium therapy. A case report and proposal for altered protocol. *Int. J. Cardiol.* 18, 327.

Massara, F. and Cammani, F. (1970). Propranolol block of adrenaline-induced hypophosphataemia in man. *Clin. Sci.* 38, 245.

Massara, F., Martelli, S., Ghigo, E., Camanni, F., and Molinalti, G.M. (1979). Arginine induced hypophosphataemia and hyperkalemia in man. *Diabete Metab.* 5, 297.

Matsuoka, L.Y., Wortsman, J., Hanifan, N., and Holick, M.F. (1988). Chronic sunscreen use decreases circulating concentrations of 25-hydroxyvitamin D. A preliminary study. *Arch. Dermatol.* 124, 1802.

Mattar, J.A., Weil, M.H., Shubin, H., and Stein, L. (1974). Cardiac arrest in the critically ill. II Hyperosmolal states following cardiac arrest. *Am. J. Med.* 56, 162.

Matzen, T.A. and Martin, R.L. (1985). Magnesium deficiency psychosis induced by cancer chemotherapy. *Biol. Psychiatry* 20, 788.

Mavichak, V., Coppin, C.M., Wong, N.L., Dirks, J.H., Walker, V., and Sutton, R.A. (1988). Renal magnesium wasting and hypocalciuria in chronic cis-platinum nephropathy in man. *Clin. Sci.* 75, 203.

Maxwell, J.D., Hunter, J., Stewart, D.A., Ardeman, S., and William, R. (1972). Folate deficiency after anticonvulsant drugs: an effect of hepatic enzyme induction? *Br. Med. J.* i, 297.

Mazze, R.I. (1984). Fluorinated anaesthetic nephrotoxicity: an update. *Can. Anaesth. Soc. J.* 31, 16.

Meani, A. and Cartei, G. (1970). Contronto tra le variazioni del metabolismo triptofano acido nicotinico e quelle dei livelli ematici di ceruloplasmina e di transferrina nella gravidanza e nel tratlamento con contracettivi o con estrogeni. *Acta Vitaminol. Enzymol.* 24, 231.

Melby, J.C. (1986). The renin–angiotensin–aldosterone complex. *Am. J. Med.* 81 (suppl. 4C), 8.

Menard, D.B., Gisselbrecht, C., Marty, M., Reyes, F., and Dhumeaux, D. (1980). Anti-neoplastic agents and the liver. *Gastroenterology* 78, 142.

Mendis, S. (1988). Serum aluminium concentration in subjects cooking in aluminium cookware using water containing fluoride. *Med. Sci. Res.* 16, 739.

Mennen, M. and Slovis, C.M. (1988). Severe metabolic alkalosis in the emergency department. *Ann. Emerg. Med.* 17, 354.

Menon, P.A., Thach, B.T., Smith, C.H., Landt, M., Roberts, J.L., Hillman, R.E., *et al.* (1984). Benzyl alcohol toxicity in a neonatal intensive care unit. Incidence, symptomatology, and mortality. *Am. J. Perinatol.* 1, 288.

Menon, R.K., Mikhailidis, D.P., Bell, J.L., Kernoff, P.B.A., and Dandona, P. (1986). Warfarin administration increases uric acid concentrations in plasma. *Clin. Chem.* 32, 1557.

Menon, R.K., Gill, D.S., Thomas, M., Kernoff, P.B.A., and Dandona, P. (1987). Impaired carboxylation of osteocalcin in Warfarin-treated patients. *J. Clin. Endocrinol. Metab.* 64, 59.

Menzies, D.G., Conn, A.G., Williamson, I.J., and Prescott, L.F. (1989). Fulminant hyperkalaemia and multiple complications following ibuprofen overdose. *Med. Toxicol. Adverse Drug Exp.* 4, 468.

Mercer, C.W. and Logic, J.R. (1973). Cardiac arrest due to hyperkalemia following intravenous penicillin administration. *Chest* 64, 358.

Metcalfe, M.J. and Entrican, J.H. (1987). Carbenoxolone and hypokalaemia. *Lancet* ii, 1525.

Meyrick T.R.H., Payne, R.C.M., and Black, M.M. (1981). Isoniazid-induced pellagra. *Br. Med. J.* ii, 287.

Michos, N., Zulliger, H.W., and Fenzl, E. (1985). Pharmacokinetics and tolerability of suprofen. Experience with intramuscular application in healthy volunteers. *Arzneimittelforschung* 35, 738.

Mihas, A.A., Holley, P., Koff, R.S., and Hirschowitz, B.I. (1976). Fulminant hepatitis and lymphocyte sensitization due to propylthiouracil. *Gastroenterology* 70, 770.

Millar, J.W. (1980). Rifampicin-induced porphyria cutanea tarda. *Br. J. Dis. Chest* 74, 405.

Miller, A.R., Addis, B.J., and Clarke, P.D. (1982). Nitrofurantoin and chronic active hepatitis. *Ann. Intern. Med.* 97, 452.

Miller, L.K., Sanchez, P.L., Berg, S.W., Kerbs, S.B., and Harrison, W.O. (1983). Effectiveness of aztreonam, a new monobactam antibiotic, against penicillin-resistant gonococci. *J. Infect. Dis.* 148, 612.

Miller, N.L. and Finberg, L. (1960). Peritoneal dialysis for salt poisoning. *N. Engl. J. Med.* 263, 1347.

Milligan, A., Graham-Brown, R.A., Sarkany, I., and Baker, H. (1988). Erythropoietic protoporphyria exacerbated by oral iron therapy. *Br. J. Dermatol.* 119, 63.

Milne, D.B., Canfield, W.K., Mahalko, J.R., and Sandstead, H.H. (1984). Effect of oral folic acid supplements on zinc, copper, and iron absorption and excretion. *Am. J. Clin. Nutr.* 39, 535.

Mino, M., Nakagawa, S., Tamai, H., and Miki, M. (1983). Clinical evaluation of red blood cell tocopherol. *Ann. N.Y. Acad. Sci.* 393, 175.

Mino, M., Miki, M., Miyake, M., and Ogihara, T. (1989). Nutritional assessment of vitamin E in oxidative stress. *Ann. N.Y. Acad. Sci.*, 570, 296.

Misra, U.K., Nag, D., Khan, W.A., and Ray, P.K. (1988). A study of nerve conduction velocity, late responses and neuromuscular synapse functions in organophosphate workers in India. *Arch. Toxicol.* 61, 496.

MMWR (1983). Lead poisoning from Mexican folk remedies — California. *MMWR* 32, 554.

MMWR (1984). Lead poisoning-associated death from Asian Indian folk remedies — Florida. *MMWR* 33, 638, 643.

MMWR (1989). Lead poisoning associated with intravenous-methamphetamine use — Oregon, 1988. *MMWR* 38, 830.

Modi, K.B., Horn, E.H., and Bryson, S.M. (1985). Theophylline poisoning and rhabdomyolysis. *Lancet* ii, 160.

Mohamadi, M., Bivins, L., and Becker, K.L. (1979). Effect of thiazides on serum calcium. *Clin. Pharmacol. Ther.* 26, 390.

Mohar, J.A., Clark, R.M., Whang, R., and Waack, T.C. (1979). Nafcillin-associated hypokalaemia. *JAMA* 242, 544.

Molony, D.A. and Jacobson, H.R. (1986). Respiratory acid-base disorders. In *Fluids and electrolytes* (ed. J.P. Kokko and R.L. Tannen), p. 305. W.B. Saunders, Philadelphia.

Momblano, P., Pradere, B., Jarrige, N., Concina, D., and Bloom E. (1984). Metabolic acidosis induced by cetrimonium bromide. *Lancet* ii, 1045.

Monreal, M., Lafoz, E., Salvador, R., Roncales, J., and Navarro, A. (1989). Adverse effects of three different forms of heparin therapy: thrombocytopenia, increased transaminases, and hyperkalaemia. *Eur. J. Clin. Pharmacol.* 37, 415.

Montgomery, R.D. (1960). Magnesium metabolism in infantile protein malnutrition. *Lancet* ii, 74.

Montorsi, M., Negri, G., Radrizzani, D., Ferro, A., Zannini, P., Rebuffat, C., *et al.* (1984). Acid load after intravenous amino acid infusion: comparison of clorurated vs acetated solutions. *Ital. J. Surg. Sci.*, 14, 162.

Moore, C.M. (1988). Hypernatremia after the use of an activated charcoal-sorbitol suspension. *J. Pediatr.* 112, 333.

Moore, M.R. and Disler, P.B. (1988). Drug sensitive diseases — 1. Acute porphyrias. *Adverse Drug React. Bull.* 129, 484.

Moore, M.R. and McColl, K.E. (1989). Therapy of the acute porphyrias. *Clin. Biochem.* 22, 181.

Morgan, D.B. and Davidson, C. (1980). Hypokalaemia and diuretics: an analysis of publications. *Br. Med. J.* 280, 905.

Morgan, D.B., Cumberbatch, M., and Swaminathan, R. (1981). The relation between plasma, erythrocyte and total body potassium in patients with hypokalaemia. *Miner. Electrolyte Metab.* 5, 233.

Moriarty, A.T., Moorehead, W.R., Ryder, K.W. and Oei To. (1983). Sulfasalazine interference in total protein measurements with the Du Pont ACA, *Clin. Chem.* 29, 592.

Morita, Y., Nishida, Y., Kamatani, N., and Miyamoto, T. (1984). Theophylline increases serum uric acid levels. *J. Allergy Clin. Immunol.* 74, 707.

Morley, J.E., Sawin, C.T., Carlson, H.E., Longcope, C., and Hershman, J.M. (1981). The relationship of androgen to the thyrotropin and prolactin response to thyrotropin-releasing hormone in hypogonadal and normal men. *J. Clin. Endocrinol. Metab.* 52, 173.

Morris, R.C., Sebastian, A. and McSherry, E. (1972). Renal acidosis. *Kidney Int.* 1, 322.

Moses, A.M., Howanitz, J., van Gemert, M., and Miller, M. (1973). Clofibrate-induced antidiuresis. *J. Clin. Invest.* 52, 535.

Moses, A.M., Blumenthal, S.A., and Streeten, D.H.P. (1985). Drugs and water metabolism. In *Fluid, electrolyte and acid-base disorders* (ed. A.I. Arieff and R.A. DeFronzo), p. 1145. Churchill Livingstone, Edinburgh.

Moss, A.H., Gabow, P.A., Kaehny, W.D., Goodman, S.I., and Hant, L.L. (1980). Fanconi's syndrome and distal renal tubular acidosis after glue sniffing. *Ann. Intern. Med.* 92, 69.

Moss, M.H. and Rasen, A.R. (1962). Potassium toxicity due to intravenous penicillin therapy. *Pediatrics* 29, 1032.

Mostellar, M.E. and Tuttle, E.P. (1964). Effects of alkalosis on plasma concentration and urinary excretion of inorganic phosphate in man. *J. Clin. Invest.* 43, 138.

Motohara, K., Endo, F., and Matsuda, I. (1985). Effect of vitamin K administration on acarboxy prothrombin (PIVKA-II) levels in newborns. *Lancet* ii, 242.

Moynot, A., Zins, B., Naret C., Canaud, B., Polito, C., Judith D., *et al.* (1990). Traitement pendant un an de 43 malades hémodialysés chroniques par l'erythropoiétine récombinante humaine. *Presse Med.*, 19, 111.

MRC Working Party Report (1981). Adverse reactions to bendrofluazide and propranolol for the treatment of mild hypertension. *Lancet* ii, 538.

Mukherjee, A.B., Ghazanfari, A., Svoronos, S., Staton, R.C., Nakada, T., and Kwee, I.L. (1986). Transketolase abnormality in tolazamide-induced Wernicke's encephalopathy. *Neurology* 36, 1508.

Murchison, L.E., How, J., Bewsher, P.D. (1979). Comparison of propranolol and metoprolol in the management of hyperthyroidism. *Br. J. Clin. Pharmacol.* 8, 581.

Murphy, A., Cropp, C.S., Smith, B.S., Burkman, R.T., and Zacur, H.A. (1990). Effect of low-dose oral contraceptive on gonadotropins, androgens, and sex hormone binding globulin in nonhirsute women. *Fertil. Steril.* 53, 35.

Nanji, A.A. and Denegri, J.F. (1984). Hypomagnesemia associated with gentamicin therapy. *Drug Intell. Clin. Pharm.* 18, 596.

Nanji, A.A. and Lauener, R.W. (1984). Lactulose-induced hypernatremia. *Drug Intell. Clin. Pharm.* 18, 70.

Narins, R.G. and Gardner, L.B. (1981). Simple acid-base disturbances. *Med. Clin. N. Am.* 65, 321.

Narins, R.G., Jones, E.R., Townsend, R., Goodkin, D.A., and Shay, R.J. (1985). Metabolic acid-base disorders: pathophysiology, classification, and treatment. In *Fluid, electrolyte and acid-base disorders* (ed. A.I. Arieff and R.A. DeFronzo), p. 269. Churchill Livingstone, Edinburgh.

Neil-Dwyer, G. and Marus, A. (1989). ACE inhibitors in hypertension: assessment of taste and smell function in clinical trials. *J. Hum. Hypertens.* 3, 169.

Nemesanszky, E. (1986). Alkaline phosphatase. In *Clinical enzymology. A case orientated approach* (ed. J.A. Lott and P.L. Wolf), p. 47. Field, Rich, New York.

Nesher, G., Zimran, A., and Hershko, C. (1988). Reduced incidence of hyperkalemia and azotemia in patients receiving sulindac compared with indomethacin. *Nephron* 48, 291.

Newbury-Ecob, R.A. and Barbor, P.R.H. (1989). Hypophosphataemic rickets after ifosfamide treatment. *Br. Med. J.* 299, 258.

Newmann, J.H, Neff, T.A., and Ziporin, P. (1977). Acute respiratory failure associated with hypophosphatemia. *N. Engl. J. Med.* 296, 1101.

Newton, H.M.V., Morgan, D.B., Schorah, C.J., and Hullin, R.P. (1983). Relation between intake and plasma concentration of vitamin C in elderly women. *Br. Med. J.* 287, 1429.

Ng, R.H., Roe, C., Funt, D., and Statland, B.E. (1985). Increased activity of creatine kinase isoenzyme MB in a theophylline-intoxicated patient. *Clin. Chem.* 31, 1741.

Nicholls, M.G. (1987). Overview: angiotensin, angiotensin converting enzyme inhibition, and the kidney — congestive heart failure. *Kidney Int.* 31 (suppl. 20), S200.

Nicholls, M.G., Espiner, E.A., Ikram, H., and Maslowski, A.H. (1980). Hyponatraemia in congestive heart failure during treatment with captopril. *Br. Med. J.* 281, 909.

Nicholson, G.A., McLeod, J.G., Morgan, G., Meekin, M., Cowan, J., Bretag, A., *et al.* (1985). Variable distribution of serum creatine kinase reference values. Relationship to exercise activity. *J. Neurol. Sci.* 71, 233.

Nicolis, G.L., Kahn, T., Sanchez, A., and Gabrilove, J.L. (1981). Glucose-induced hyperkalemia in diabetic subjects. *Arch. Intern. Med.* 141, 49.

Nielsen, O.A., Johannessen, C.J., and Bardrum, B. (1988). Oxycarbazepine-induced hyponatremia, a cross sectional study. *Epilepsy Res.* 2, 269.

Nilsson, B., Holst, J., and von Schoultz, B. (1984). Serum levels of unbound 17 beta-oestradiol during oral and percutaneous postmenopausal replacement therapy. *Br. J. Obstet. Gynaecol.* 91, 1031.

Nilsson, O.S., Lindholm, T.S., Elmstedt, E., Lindback, A., and Lindholm, T.C. (1986). Fracture incidence and bone disease in epileptics receiving long-term anticonvulsant drug treatment. *Arch. Orthop. Trauma Surg.* 105, 146.

Nilsson, T.K., Tomic, R., and Ljungberg, B. (1989). Effects of high dose medroxyprogesterone acetate treatment on antithrombin III and other plasma proteins in males with renal cell or prostatic carcinoma. *Scand. J. Urol. Nephrol.* 23, 11.

Nisbeth, S.B., Parker, J.A., and Habal, F. (1985). Methyltestosterone-induced night blindness. *Can. J. Ophthalmol.* 20, 254.

Nishiyama, S., Kuwahara, T., and Matsuda, I. (1986). Decreased bone density in severely handicapped children and adults, with reference to the influence of limited mobility and anticonvulsant medication. *Eur. J. Pediatr.* 144, 457.

Norby, L.H., Ramwell, P., Weidig, J., Slotkoff, L., and Flamenbaum, W. (1978). Possible role for impaired renal prostaglandin production in pathognesis of hyporeninaemic hypoaldosteronism. *Lancet* ii, 1118.

Nordberg, G.F., Goyer, R.A., and Clarkson, T.W. (1985). Impact of effects of acid precipitation on toxicity of metals. *Environ. Health Perspect.* 63, 169.

Nordenvall, B., Backman, L., Larsson, L., and Tiselius, H.G. (1983). Effects of calcium, aluminum, magnesium and cholestyramine on hyperoxaluria in patients with jejunoileal bypass. *Acta Chir. Scand.* 149, 93.

Nordin, B.E.C. (1990). Calcium homeostasis. *Clin. Biochem.* 23, 3.

Nordin, B.E.C., Crilly, R.G., and Smith D.A. (1984). Osteoporosis. In *Metabolic bone and stone disease* (ed. B.E.C. Nordin), p. 1. Churchill Livingstone, Edinburgh.

Notrica, S., Miyada, D.S., Baysinger, V., and Nakamura, R.M. (1972). Effects of various medications on values from the HABA and BCG methods for determining albumin. *Clin. Chem.* 18, 1537.

Novak, M.A., Roth, A.S., and Levine, M.R. (1988). Calcium oxalate retinopathy associated with methoxyflurane abuse. *Retina* 8, 230.

Nugent, D.J., Bray, G.L., Counts, R.B., Clements, M.J., and Thompson, A.R. (1986). Danazol fails to increase factor VIII or IX levels in a double blind crossover study of patients with haemophilia A and B. *Br. J. Haematol.* 64, 493.

Nuti, R., Vattimo, A., Turchetti, V., and Righi, G. (1984). 25-Hydroxycholecalciferol as an antagonist of adverse corticosteroid effects on phosphate and calcium metabolism in man. *J. Endocrinol. Invest.* 7, 445.

Nylander, M., Friberg, L., and Lind, B. (1987). Mercury concentrations in the human brain and kidneys in relation to exposure from dental amalgam fillings. *Swed. Dent. J.* 11, 179.

O'Connell, T.X. (1981). Hypercalcemia induced by tamoxifen. *Am. J. Surg.* 141, 277.

O'Connor, D.T., Strause, L., Saltman, P., Parmer, R.J., and Cervenka, J. (1987). Serum zinc is unaffected by effective captopril treatment of hypertension. *J. Clin. Hypertens.* 3, 405.

O'Kelly, R., Magee, F., and McKenna, T.J. (1983). Routine heparin therapy inhibits adrenal aldosterone production. *J. Clin. Endocrinol. Metab.* 56, 108.

O'Reilly, R.A. and Aggeler, P.M. (1976). Covert anticoagulant ingestion: study of 25 patients and review of world literature. *Medicine* (Baltimore) 55, 389.

O'Sullivan, D. and Oyebode, F. (1987). Hyponatraemia and lofepramine. *Br. J. Psychiatry* 150, 720.

Odigwe, C.O., McCulloch, A.J., Williams, D.O., and Tunbridge, W.M. (1986). A trial of the calcium antagonist nisoldipine in hypertensive non-insulin-dependent diabetic patients. *Diabetic Med.* 3, 463.

Oettgen, H.F., Stephenson, P.A., Schwartz, M.K., Leeper, R.D., Tallal, L., Tan, C.C., *et al.* (1970). Toxicity of *E coli* L-asparaginase in man. *Cancer* 25, 253.

Ogawa, K., Hatano, T., Yamamoto, M., and Matsui, N. (1984). Influence of acute diuresis on calcium balance — a comparative study of furosemide and azosemide. *Int. J. Clin. Pharmacol. Ther. Toxicol.* 22, 401.

Ogunmekan, A.O. (1979). Predicting serum vitamin E concentrations from the age of normal and anticonvulsant drug-treated epileptic children using regression equations. *Epilepsia* 20, 295.

Oikkonen, M. (1984). Isoflurane and enflurane in long anaesthesias for plastic microsurgery. *Acta Anaesthesiol. Scand.* 28, 412.

Oikkonen, M. and Meretoja, O. (1989). Serum fluoride in children anaesthetized with enflurane. *Eur. J. Anaesthesiol.* 6, 401.

Okada, K., Takahashi, S., Nagura, Y., and Hatano, M. (1989*a*). Treatment of secondary hyperparathyroidism in patients on maintenance hemodialysis. *Nippon Jinzo Gakkai Shi* 31, 1085.

Okada, K., Nagura, Y., Takahashi, S., and Hatano, M. (1989*b*). Influence of 1-alpha-hydroxy vitamin D_3 (0.25 micrograms/day) and calcium carbonate on patients with chronic renal failure at the predialytic stage. *Nippon Jinzo Gakkai Shi* 31, 657.

Olson, R.E. (1984). The function and metabolism of vitamin K. *Annu. Rev. Nutr.* 4, 281.

Olson, R.E. (1987). Vitamin K. In *Hemostasis and thrombosis* (ed. R.W. Colman, J. Hirsh, V.J. Marder, and E.W. Salzman), p. 846. J.B. Lippincott, Philadelphia.

Olsson, R., Hellner, L., Lindstedt, G., Lundberg, P.A., and Teger-Nilsson, A.C. (1983). Plasma proteins in patients on long-term antiepileptic treatment. *Clin. Chem.* 29, 728.

Omaye, S.T., Schaus, E.E., Kutnink, M.A., and Hawkes, W.C. (1987). Measurement of vitamin C in blood components by high-performance liquid chromatography. *Ann. N.Y. Acad. Sci.* 498, 389.

Ong, E.L., Ellis, M.E., McDowell, D., Gebril, M., Weinkove, C., and Ead, R. (1988). Porphyria cutanea tarda in association with the human immunodeficiency virus infection. *Postgrad. Med. J.* 64, 956.

Oppe, T.E. and Redstone, D. (1968). Calcium and phosphorus level in healthy newborn infants given various types of milk. *Lancet* i, 1045.

Oppenheimer, S.J. and Snodgrass, G.J. (1980). Neonatal rickets. Histopathology and quantitative bone changes. *Arch. Dis. Child.* 55, 945.

Osborn, D.E., Rao, P.N., Greene, M.J., and Barnard, R.J. (1980). Fluid absorption during transurethral resection. *Br. Med. J.* 281, 1549.

Ott, S.M., Maloney, N.A., Klein, G.L., Alfrey, A.C., Ament, M.E., Coburn, J.W. *et al.* (1983). Aluminum is associated with low bone formation in patients receiving chronic parenteral nutrition. *Ann. Intern. Med.* 98, 910.

Ottosson, U.B., Carlstrom, K., Johansson, B.G., and von Schoultz, B. (1986). Estrogen induction of liver proteins and high-density lipoprotein cholesterol: comparison between estradiol valerate and ethinyl estradiol. *Gynecol. Obstet. Invest.* 22, 198.

Paasuke, R.T. and Brownell, A.K. (1986). Serum creatine kinase level as a screening test for susceptibility to malignant hyperthermia. *JAMA* 255, 769.

Packer, L. and Landvik, S. (1989). Vitamin E: Introduction to biochemistry and health benefits. *Ann. N.Y. Acad. Sci.* 570, 1.

Pahl, M.V., Vaziri, N.D., Ness, R., Nathan, R., and Maksy, M. (1984). Association of beta hydroxybutyrate acidosis with isoniazid intoxication. *J. Toxicol. Clin. Toxicol.* 22, 167.

Pak, C.Y.C. (1986). Calcium disorders: Hypercalcemia and hypocalcemia. In *Fluids and electrolytes* (ed. I.P. Kokko and R.C. Tanner), p. 472. W.B. Saunders, Philadelphia.

Palella, T.D. and Fox, I.H. (1989). In *The metabolic basis of inherited disease* (6th edn) (ed. C.R. Scriver, A.L. Beaudet, W.S. Sly, and D. Valle), p. 965. McGraw-Hill, New York.

Palestine, A.G., Austin, H.A., and Nussenblatt, R.B. (1986). Renal tubular function in cyclosporine-treated patients. *Am. J. Med.* 81, 419.

Paliard, P., Vitrey, D., Fournier, G., Belhadjali, J., Patricot, L., and Berger, F. (1978). Perhexiline maleate-induced hepatitis. *Digestion* 17, 419.

Pannall, P.R. and Maas, D.A. (1977). Danazol and thyroid function tests. *Lancet* i, 102.

Pantuck, E.J., Pantuck, C.B., Ryan, D.E., and Conney, A.H. (1985). Inhibition and stimulation of enflurane metabolism in the rat following a single dose or chronic administration of ethanol. *Anesthesiology* 62, 255.

Pappas N.J.J. (1989). Theoretical aspects of enzymes in diagnosis. Why do serum enzymes changes in hepatic, myocardial and other diseases? *Clin. Lab. Med.* 9, 595.

Parker, W.A. and Shearer, C.A. (1979). Phenytoin hepatotoxicity: A case report and review. *Neurology* 29, 175.

Parodi, A., Guarrera, M., and Rebora, A. (1988). Amiodarone-induced pseudoporphyria. *Photodermatology* 5, 146.

Parras, F., Patier, J.L., and Ezpeleta, C. (1987). Lead-contaminated heroin as a source of inorganic-lead intoxication. *N. Engl. J. Med.* 316, 755.

Parry, M.F. and Neu, H.C. (1978). A comparative study of ticarcillin plus tobramycin versus carbenicillin plus gentamicin for the treatment of serious infections due to gram-negative bacilli. *Am. J. Med.* 64, 961.

Paterson, C.R. (1980). Vitamin-D poisoning: Survey of causes in 21 patients with hypercalcaemia. *Lancet* i, 1164.

Paterson, K.R., Paice, B.J., and Lawson, D.H. (1984). Undesired effects of biguanide therapy. *Adverse Drug React. Acute Poisoning Rev.* 3, 173.

Paterson, Y. and Lawrence, E.F. (1972). Factors affecting creatine phosphokinase levels in normal adult females. *Clin. Chim. Acta* 42, 131.

Patrono, C. and Dunn, M.J. (1987). The clinical significance of inhibition of renal prostaglandin synthesis. *Kidney Int.* 32, 1.

Payne, R.B., Little, A.J., Williams, R.B., and Milner, J.R. (1973). Interpretation of serum calcium in patients with abnormal serum proteins. *Br. Med. J.* iv, 643.

Pearlman, C., Wheadon, D., and Epstein, S. (1988). Creatine kinase elevation after neuroleptic treatment. *Am. J. Psychiatry* 145, 1018.

Pearson, J.C., Dombrovskis, S., Dreyer, J., and Williams, R.D. (1983). Radio-immunoassay of serum prostatic acid phosphatase after prostatic massage. *Urology* 21, 37.

Pellock, J.M., Howell, J., Kendig, E.L. Jr, and Baker, H. (1985). Pyridoxine deficiency in children treated with isoniazid. *Chest* 87, 658.

Peltz, S. and Hashmi, S. (1989). Pentamidine-induced severe hyperkalemia. *Am. J. Med.* 87, 698.

Pendlebury, S.C., Moses, D.K., and Eadie, M.J. (1989). Hyponatraemia during oxcarbazepine therapy. *Hum. Toxicol.* 8, 337.

Pereira, A., Cervantes, F., and Rozman, C. (1985). Anemia macrocitica por deficit de acido folico y linfema no hodgkiniamo associados a la ingesta prolongade de difenilhidantoina. *Med. Clin.* 85, 503.

Peretz, A., Praet, J-P., Bosson, D., Rozenberg, S., and Bourdoux, P. (1989*a*). Serum osteocalcin in the assessment of corticosteroid induced osteoporosis. Effect of long and short term corticosteroid treatment. *J. Rheumatol.* 16, 363.

Peretz, A., Nere, T., and Famaey I.P. (1989*b*). Effects of chronic and acute corticosteroid therapy on zinc and copper status in rheumatoid arthritis patients. *J. Trace Elem. Electrolytes Health Dis.* 3, 103.

Pessayre, D., Feldmann, G., Degott, C., Ulmann, A., Roger, W., Erlinger, S., and Benhamou, J.P. (1979). Gold salt-induced cholestasis. *Digestion* 19, 56.

Petersen, L.R., Denis, D., Brown, D., Hadler, J.L., and Helgerson, S.D. (1988). Community health effects of a municipal water supply hyperfluoridation accident. *Am. J. Public Health* 78, 711.

Petren, S. and Vesterberg, O. (1987). Studies of transferrin in serum of workers exposed to organic solvents. *Br. J. Ind. Med.* 44, 566.

Pfeiffer, F.E., Homburger, H.A., Houser, O.W., Baker, H.L. Jr, and Yanagihara, T. (1987). Elevation of serum creatine kinase B-subunit levels by radiographic contrast agents in patients with neurologic disorders. *Mayo Clin. Proc.* 62, 351.

Phillips, P.J., Need, A.G., Thomas, D.W., Conyers, R.A.J., Edwards, J.B., and Lehmann, D. (1979). Nalidixic acid and lactic acidosis. *Aust. N.Z. J. Med.* 9, 694.

Pierides, A.M. and Alvasez-Ude, F. (1975). Clofibrate-induced muscle damage in patients with chronic renal failure. *Lancet* ii, 1279.

Pietila, K. and Koivula, T. (1984). Increase of serum angiotensin-converting enzyme activity after freezing. *Scand. J. Clin. Lab. Invest.* 44, 453.

Pietsch, J. and Meakins, J.L. (1976). Complications of povidone–iodine absorption in topically treated burns patients. *Lancet* i, 280.

Pietschmann, P., Woloszczuk, W., Panzer, R.S., Kyrle, P., and Smolen, J. (1988). Decreased serum osteocalcin levels in phenprocoumon-treated patients. *J. Clin. Endocrinol. Metab.* 66, 1071.

Pillans, P.I., Cowan, P., and Whitelaw, D. (1985). Hyponatraemia and confusion in a patient taking ketoconazole. *Lancet* i, 821.

Pinto, J., Huang, Y.P., and Rivlin, R.S. (1981). Inhibition of riboflavin metabolism in rat tissues by chlorpromazine, imipramine, and amitriptyline. *J. Clin. Invest.* 67, 1500.

Pironi, L., Cornia, G.L., Ursitti, M.A., Dallasta, M.A., Miniero, R., Fasano, F., *et al.* (1988). Evaluation of oral administration of folic acid and folinic acid to prevent folate deficiency in patients with inflammatory bowel disease treated with salicylazosulfapyridine. *Int. J. Clin. Pharmacol. Res.* 8, 143.

Pittman, J.G. (1963). Water intoxication due to oxytocin. *N. Engl. J. Med.* 268, 481.

Platts, M.M., Goode, G.C., and Hislop, J.S. (1977). Composition of the domestic water supply and the incidence of fractures and encephalopathy in patients on home dialysis. *Br. Med. J.* ii, 657.

Pollock, A.S. and Arieff, A.I. (1980). Abnormalities of cell volume regulation and their functional consequences. *Am. J. Physiol.* 239, F195.

Pontifex, A.H. and Garg, A.K. (1985). Lead poisoning from an Asian Indian folk remedy. *Can. Med. Assoc. J.* 133, 1227.

Poole-Wilson, P.A. (1987). Diuretics, hypokalaemia and arrhythmias in hypertensive patients: still an unresolved problem. *J. Hypertens.* (suppl. 5), S51.

Poor, G. and Mituszova, M. (1989). Saturnine gout. *Baillière's Clin. Rheumatol.* 3, 51.

Pople, I.K. and Phillips, H. (1988). Bone cement and the liver. A dose-related effect? *J. Bone Joint Surg.* 70, 364.

Porteous, C.E., Coldwell, R.D., Trafford, D.J., and Makin, H.L. (1987). Recent developments in the measurement of vitamin D and its metabolites in human body fluids. *J. Steroid. Biochem.* 28, 785.

Porter, K.G., McMaster, D., Elmes, M.E., and Love, A.H.G. (1977). Anaemia and low serum-copper during zinc therapy. *Lancet* ii, 774.

Porter, R.H., Cox, B.G., Heaney, D., Hostetter, T.H., Stinebaugh, B.J., and Suki, W.N. (1978). Treatment of hypoparathyroid patients with chlorthalidone. *N. Engl. J. Med.* 298. 577.

Postlethwaite, A.E. and Kelley, W.N. (1971). Uricosuric effect of radiocontrast agents. A study in man of four commonly used preparations. *Ann. Intern. Med.* 74, 845.

Prasad, A.S. (1985). Clinical, endocrinological and biochemical effects of zinc deficiency. *Clin. Endocrinol. Metab.* 14, 567.

Prasad, A.S., Lai, K.Y., Oberleas, D., Moghissi, K.S., and Stryker, J.C. (1975). Effect of oral contraceptive agents on nutrients: II. Vitamins. *Am. J. Clin. Nutr.* 28, 385.

Prasad, A.S., Brewer, G.J., Schoomaker, E.B., and Rabbani, P. (1978). Hypocupremia induced by zinc therapy in adults. *JAMA* 240, 2166.

Prescott, L.F. (1986*a*). Liver damage with non-narcotic analgesics. *Med. Toxicol.* 1 (suppl. 1), 44.

Prescott, L.F. (1986*b*). Effects of non-narcotic analgesics on the liver. *Drugs* 32 (suppl. 4), 129.

Primos, W., Bhatnager, A., Bishop, P., and Evans, O.B. (1987). Acute metabolic acidosis due to ibuprofen overdose. *J. Miss. State Med. Assoc.* 28, 233.

Probstfield, J.L., Statland, B.E., Gorman, L., and Hunning Lake, D.B. (1983). Alterations in human serum alkaline phosphatase and its isoenzymes by hypolipidemic agents: colestipol and clofibrate. *Metabolism* 32, 818.

Prouse, P., Shawe, D., and Gumpel, J.M. (1987). Macrocytic anaemia in patients treated with sulfasalazine for rheumatoid arthritis. *Br. Med. J.* 294, 90.

Purdie, D.W., Hay, A., and Abbas, S.K. (1987). Effects of danazol on mineral homeostasis in normal postmenopausal women: preliminary communication. *J. R. Soc. Med.* 80, 681.

Rado, J.P. (1988). Successful treatment of hyperkalemic quadriplegia associated with spironolactone. *Int. J. Clin. Pharmacol. Ther. Toxicol.* 26, 339.

Rado, J.P., Juhos, E., and Sawinsky, I. (1975). Dose-response relations in drug-induced inappropriate secretion of ADH: effects of clofibrate and carbamazepine. *Int. J. Clin. Pharmacol. Ther. Toxicol.* 12, 315.

Rahilly, G.T. and Berl, T. (1979). Severe metabolic alkalosis caused by administration of plasma protein fraction in end-stage renal failure. *N. Engl. J. Med.* 301, 824.

Rahman, H., Al Khayat, A., and Menon, N. (1986). Lead poisoning in infancy — unusual causes in the U.A.E. *Ann. Trop. Paediatr.* 6, 213.

Raisz, L.G. (1980). New diphosphonates to block bone resorption. *N. Engl. J. Med.* 302, 347.

Rajantie, J., Lamberg-Allardt, C., and Wilska, M. (1984). Does carbamazepine treatment lead to a need of extra vitamin D in some mentally retarded children. *Acta Paediatr. Scand.* 73, 325.

Ramanathan, J., Sibai, B.M., Pillai, R., and Angel, J.J. (1988). Neuromuscular transmission studies in preeclamptic women receiving magnesium sulfate. *Am. J. Obstet. Gynecol.* 158, 40.

Ranft, K. and Eibl-Eibesfeldt, B. (1990). Enterale Hyperoxalose bei Therapie mit Somatostatin-Analog. *Dtsch. Med. Wochenschr.* 115, 179.

Rao, P.N. (1987). Fluid absorption during urological endoscopy. *Br. J. Urol.* 60, 93.

Ratcliffe, W.A., Hazelton, R.A., Thomson, J.A., and Ratcliffe, J.G. (1980). The effect of fenclofenac on thyroid function test in vivo and in vitro. *Clin. Endocrinol.* 13, 569.

Ratzmann, G.W. (1985). On the insulin effect on the magnesium homeostasis. *Exp. Clin. Endocrinol.* 86, 141.

Ratzmann, G.W. and Zollner, H. (1985). Hypomagesiamie und Hypokaliamie wahrend des Insulin-Hypoglykamietestes. *Z. Gesamte. Inn. Med.* 40, 567.

Reedy, J.C. and Zwiren, G.T. (1983). Enema-induced hypocalcemia and hyperphosphatemia leading to cardiac arrest during induction of anesthesia in an outpatient surgery center. *Anesthesiology* 59, 578.

Refsum, H., Helland, S., and Ueland, P.M. (1989). Fasting plasma homocysteine as a sensitive parameter of antifolate effect: a study of psoriasis patients receiving low-dose methotrexate treatment. *Clin. Pharmacol. Ther.* 46, 510.

Reid, I.R., Chapman, G.E., Fraser, T.R., Davies, A.D., Surus, A.S., Meyer, J., *et al.* (1986). Low serum osteocalcin levels in glucocorticoid-treated asthmatics. *J. Clin. Endocrinol. Metab.* 62, 379.

Reid, J.L., Curzio, J., and Vincent, J. (1985). Bucindolol in essential hypertension. *Int. J. Clin. Pharmacol. Res.* 5, 293.

Reid, J.L., White, K.F., and Struthers, A.D. (1986). Epinephrine-induced hypokalemia: The role of beta adrenoceptors. *Am. J. Cardiol.* 57, 23F.

Rej, R. (1989). Aminotransferase in disease. *Clin. Lab. Med.* 9, 667.

Relman, A.S. (1978). Lactic acidosis. In *Acid-base and potassium homeostasis* (ed. B.M. Brenner and J.H. Stein), p.65. Churchill Livingstone, New York.

Resnick, L.M., Nicholson, J.P., and Laragh, J.H. (1987). Calcium, the renin-aldosterone system, and the hypotensive response to nifedipine. *Hypertension* 10, 254.

Resnick, L.M., Nicholson, J.P., and Laragh, J.H. (1989). The effects of calcium channel blockade on blood pressure and calcium metabolism. *Am. J. Hypertens.* 2, 927.

Reusz, G.S., Latta, K., Hoyer, P.F., Byrd, D.J., Ehrich, J.H.H., and Brodehl, J. (1990). Evidence suggesting hyperoxaluria as a cause of nephrocalcinosis in phosphate-treated hypophosphataemic rickets. *Lancet* 335, 1240.

Rey, E., Luquel, L., Richard, M.O., Mory, B., Offenstadt, G., and Olive, G. (1989). Pharmacokinetics of intravenous salbutamol in renal insufficiency and its biological effects. *Eur. J. Clin. Pharmacol.* 37, 387.

Reynolds, E.H. (1967). Effects of folic acid on the mental state and fit frequency of drug treated epileptic patients. *Lancet* i, 1086.

Reynolds, E.H. (1974). Iatrogenic nutritional effects of anticonvulsants. *Proc. Nutr. Soc.* 33, 225.

Reynolds, E.H. (1983). Mental effects of antiepileptic medications. A review. *Epilepsia* 24 (suppl. 2), S85.

Reynolds, E.H. and Trimble M.R. (1985). Adverse neuropsychiatric effects of anticonvulsant drugs. *Drugs* 29, 570.

Reynolds, J.E.F. (ed.) (1989). *Martindale: the extra pharmacopoeia,* (29th edn). The Pharmaceutical Press, London.

Reynolds, R.D. and Natta, C.L. (1985). Depressed plasma pyridoxal phosphate concentrations in adult asthmatics. *Am. J. Clin. Nutr.* 41, 684.

Richards, S.R. and Klingelberger, C.E. (1987). Intravenous ritodrine as a possibly provocative predictive test in gestational diabetes. A case report. *J. Reprod. Med.* 32, 798.

Richards, S.R., Chang, F.E., and Stempel, L.E. (1983). Hyperlactacidemia associated with acute ritodrine infusion. *Am. J. Obstet. Gynecol.* 146, 1.

Richens, A. and Rowe, D.J.F. (1970). Disturbance of calcium metabolism by anticonvulsant drugs. *Br. Med. J.* iv, 73.

Riikonen, R., Simell, O., Jaaskelainen, J., Rapola, J., and Perheentupa, J. (1986). Disturbed calcium and phosphate homeostasis during treatment with ACTH of infantile spasms. *Arch. Dis. Child.* 61, 671.

Riley, L.J. Jr, Cooper, M., and Narins, R.G. (1989). Alkali therapy of diabetic ketoacidosis: biochemical, physiological, and clinical perspectives. *Diabetes Metab. Rev.* 5, 627.

Ritch, P.S. (1988). Cis-dichlorodiammineplatinum II-induced syndrome of inappropriate secretion of antidiuretic hormone. *Cancer* 61, 448.

Ritter, M.A., Gioe, T.J., and Sieber, J.M. (1984). Systemic effects of polymethylmethacrylate. Increased serum levels of gamma-glutamyltranspeptidase following arthroplasty. *Acta Orthop. Scand* 55, 411.

Ritz, E. (1982). Acute hypophosphataemia. *Kidney Int.* 22, 84.

Rivers, J.M. (1987). Safety of high-level vitamin C ingestion. *Ann. N.Y. Acad. Sci.* 498, 445.

Rivers, J.K. and Barnetson, R.S. (1989). Naproxen-induced bullous photodermatitis. *Med. J. Aust.* 151, 167.

Rivey, M.P., Schottelius, D.D., and Berg., M.J. (1984). Phenytoin–folic acid: a review. *Drug Intell. Clin. Pharm.* 18, 292.

Robertson, G.L. (1988). Differential diagnosis of polyuria. *Annu. Rev. Med.* 39, 425.

Robertson, G.L., Bhoopalam, N., and Zelkowitz, L.J. (1973). Vincristine neurotoxicity and abnormal secretion of antidiuretic hormone. *Arch. Intern. Med.* 132, 717.

Robertson, N.J. (1985). Fatal overdose from a sustained-release theophylline preparation. *Ann. Emerg. Med.* 14, 154.

Rodriguez, M., Solanki, D.L., and Whang, R. (1989). Refractory potassium repletion due to cisplatin-induced magnesium depletion. *Arch. Intern. Med.* 149, 2592.

Roels, H., Lauwerys, R., Buchet, J.P., Genet, P., Sarhan, M.J., Hanotiau, I., et al. (1987). Epidemiological survey among workers exposed to manganese: effects on lung, central nervous system, and some biological indices. *Am. J. Ind. Med.* 11, 307.

Rofe, A.M., Conyers, R.A.J., Bais, R., and Edwards, J.B. (1979). Oxalate excretion in rats injected with xylitol or glycollate: stimulation by phenobarbitone pretreatment. *Aust. J. Exp. Biol. Med. Sci.* 57, 171.

Rogiers, P., Vermeier, W., Kesteloot, H., and Stroobandt, R. (1989). Effect of the infusion of magnesium sulfate during atrial pacing on ECG intervals, serum electrolytes, and blood pressure. *Am. Heart J.* 117, 1278.

Rolla, G. and Bucca, C. (1988). Magnesium, beta-agonists, and asthma. *Lancet* i, 989.

Romer, F.K. and Jacobsen, F. (1982). The influence of prednisone on serum angiotensin-converting enzyme activity in patients with and without sarcoidosis. *Scand. J. Clin. Lab. Invest.* 42, 377.

Rooney, P.J. and Housley, E. (1972). Trimethoprim–sulphamethoxazole in folic acid deficiency. *Br. Med. J.* ii, 656.

Rosa, R.M., Silva, P., Young, J.B., Landsberg, L., Brown, R.S., Rowe, J.W., et al. (1980). Adrenergic modulation of extrarenal potassium disposal. *N. Engl. J. Med.* 302, 431.

Rosalki, S.B. (ed.) (1984). In *Clinical biochemistry of alcoholism*, p. 65. Churchill Livingstone, New York.

Rosalki, S.B., Foo, A.Y., and Armtsen, K.W. (1989). Alkaline phosphatase of possible renal origin identified in plasma after colchicine overdose. *Clin. Chem.* 35, 702.

Rose, B.D. (1986). New approach to disturbances in the plasma sodium concentration. *Am. J. Med.* 81, 1033.

Rose, B.D. (1989). In *Clinical physiology of acid-base and electrolyte disorders* (3rd edn). McGraw-Hill, New York.

Rosen, R.A., Julian, B.A., Dubovsky, E.V., Galla, J.H., and Luke, R.G. (1988). On the mechanism by which chloride corrects metabolic alkalosis in man. *Am. J. Med.* 84, 449.

Rosenberg, H. and Fletcher, J.E. (1986). Masseter muscle rigidity and malignant hyperthermia susceptibility. *Anesth. Analg.* 65, 161. (E142)

Rosenblatt, J.E. and Edson, R.S. (1987). Metronidazole. *Mayo Clin. Proc.* 62, 1013.

Rosenblatt, S., Chanley, J.D., and Segal, R.L. (1989). The effect of lithium on vitamin D metabolism. *Biol. Psych.* 26, 206.

Rosenblum, M., Simpson, D.P., and Evenson, M. (1977). Fictitious Bartter's syndrome. *Arch. Intern. Med.* 137, 1244.

Rosenmund, A., Camponovo, F., and Kochli, H.P. (1986). Der Einfluss hormoneller Kontrazeptiva und der Schwangerschaft auf Eisenstoffwechsel, Plasmalactoferrinkonzentration und Granulozytenzahl der Frau. *Schweiz. Med. Wochenschr.* 116, 1411.

Rossner, S. and Wallgren, A. (1984). Serum lipoproteins and proteins after breast cancer surgery and effects of tamoxifen. *Atherosclerosis* 52, 339.

Roth, A., Miller, H.I., Belhassen, B., and Laniado, S. (1989). Slow-release verapamil and hyperglycemic metabolic acidosis. *Ann. Intern. Med.* 110, 171.

Rovelli, E., Luciani, L., Pagani, C., Albonico, C., Colleoni, N., and D'Amico, G. (1988). Correlation between serum aluminum concentration and signs of encephalopathy in a large population of patients dialyzed with aluminum-free fluids. *Clin. Nephrol.* 29, 294.

Roxe, D.M., Mistovich, M., and Barch, D.H. (1989). Phosphate-binding effects of sucralfate in patients with chronic renal failure. *Am. J. Kidney Dis.* 13, 194.

Rozkovec, A. and Marshall, A.J. (1983). New drugs: modern diuretic treatment. *Br. Med. J.* 286, 1971.

Ruder, H., Corvol, P., Mahoudeau, J.A., Ross, G.T. and Lipsett, M.B. (1971). Effects of induced hyperthyroidism on steroid metabolism in man. *J. Clin. Endocrinol. Metab.* 33, 382.

Ruokonen, A. and Kaar, K. (1985). Effects of desogestrel, levonorgestrel and lynestrenol on serum sex hormone binding globulin, cortisol binding globulin, ceruloplasmin and HDL-cholesterol. *Eur. J. Obstet. Gynecol. Reprod. Biol.* 20, 13.

Russell, R.G.G., Smith, R., Preston, C., Walton, R.J., and Woods, C.G. (1974). Diphosphonates in Paget's disease. *Lancet* i, 894.

Russell, R.M. (1980). Vitamin A and zinc metabolism in alcoholism. *Am. J. Clin. Nutr.* 33, 2741.

Rutten, J.M.J., Booij, L.H.D.J., Rulten, C.C.J., and Crul, J.F. (1980). The comparative neuromuscular blocking effects of some aminoglycoside antibiotics. *Acta Anesthesiol. Belg.* 4, 293.

Ryan, J.A.J. (1976). Complication of total parenteral nutrition. In *Total parenteral nutrition* (ed. E. Fischer), p. 55. Little Brown, Boston.

Ryan, M.P. (1986). Magnesium and potassium-sparing diuretics. *Magnesium* 5, 282.

Ryan, M.P. (1987). Diuretics and potassium/magnesium depletion. Directions for treatment. *Am. J. Med.* 82 (suppl. 3A), 38.

Ryan, T., Coughlan, G., McGing, P., and Phelan, D. (1989). Ketosis, a complication of theophylline toxicity. *J. Intern. Med.* 226, 227.

Ryder, R.E. (1987). The danger of high dose sodium bicarbonate in biguanide-induced lactic acidosis: the theory, the practice and alternative therapies. *Br. J. Clin. Pract.* 41, 730.

Ryle, P.R. and Thomson, A.D. (1984). Nutrition and vitamins in alcoholism. In *Clinical biochemistry of alcoholism* (ed. S.B. Rosalki), p. 188. Churchill Livingstone, Edinburgh.

Sabatini, S. and Kurtzman, N.A. (1984). The maintenance of metabolic alkalosis: factors which decrease bicarbonate excretion. *Kidney Int.* 25, 357.

Sabiniewicz, M. and Szajewski, J.M. (1979). Creatine phosphokinase and barbiturate overdosage. *Lancet* i, 152.

Sadik, W., Kovacs, L., Pretnar-Darovec, A., Mateo de Acosta, O., Toddywalla, V.S., Dhall, G.I., *et al.* (1985). A randomized double-blind study of the effects of two low dose combined oral contraceptives on biochemical aspects. *Contraception* 32, 223.

Sakemi, T., Ohchi, N., Sanai, T., Rikitae, O., and Maeda, T. (1988). Captopril-induced metabolic acidosis with hyperkalemia. *Am. J. Nephrol.* 8, 245.

Salata, R. and Klein, I. (1987). Effects of lithium on the endocrine system: a review. *J. Lab. Clin. Med.* 110, 130.

Salem, P., Khalyl, M., Jabboury, K., and Hashimi, L. (1984). Cis-diamminedichloroplatinum (II) by 5-day continuous infusion. A new dose schedule with minimal toxicity. *Cancer* 53, 837.

Salih, E.S., Zein, A.A., and Bayoumi, R.A. (1986). The effect of oral contraceptives on the apparent vitamin B_6 status in some Sudanese women. *Br. J. Nutr.* 56, 363.

Sallen, M.K., Efrusy, M.E., Kniaz, J.L., and Wolfson, P.M. (1983). Streptokinase-induced hepatic dysfunction. *Am. J. Gastroenterol.* 78, 523.

Salter, A.J. (1973). The toxicity profile of trimethoprim/sulphamethoxazole after four years of widespread use. *Med. J. Aust.* i (suppl.), 70.

Salusky, I.B., Coburn, J.W., Paunier, L., Sherrard, D.J., and Fine, R.N. (1984). Role of aluminum hydroxide in raising serum aluminum levels in children undergoing continuous ambulatory peritoneal dialysis. *J. Pediatr.* 105, 717.

Salway, J.G. (1989). *Drug–test interactions Handbook.* Chapman and Hall Medical, London.

Sangster, G., Kayl, S.B., Calman, K.C., and Dalton, J.F. (1984). Failure of 2-mercaptoethane sulphonate sodium (mesna) to protect against ifosfamide nephrotoxicity. *Eur. J. Cancer. Clin. Oncol.* 20, 435.

Sanpitak, N. and Chayutimonkul, L. (1974). Oral contraceptives and riboflavine nutrition. *Lancet* i, 836.

Sanwikarja, S., Kauffmann, R.H., te Velde, J., and Serlie, J. (1989). Tubulointerstitial nephritis associated with pyrazinamide. *Neth. J. Med.* 34, 40.

Saruta, T., Suzuki, H., Kawamura, M., and Itoh, H. (1985). Serum creatine phosphokinase levels during treatment with beta-adrenoreceptor blocking agents. *J. Cardiovas. Pharmacol.* 7, 805.

Sawhney, A.K. and Lott, J.A. (1986). Acetylcholinesterase and cholinesterase. In *Clinical enzymology. A case orientation approach* (ed. J.A. Lott and P.L. Wolf), p. 1. Field, Rich, New York.

Sawyer, W.T., Caravati, E.M., Ellison, M.J., and Krueger, K.A. (1985). Hypokalemia, hyperglycemia, and acidosis after intentional theophylline overdose. *Am. J. Emerg. Med.* 3, 408.

Scanlon, J.W. and Krakaur, R. (1980). Hyperkalemia following exchange transfusion. *J. Pediatr.* 96, 108.

Schade, R.W.B., Denmacker, P.N.M., and Vant Laar, A. (1977). Clofibrate effect on alkaline phosphatase: bone or liver fraction. *N. Engl. J. Med.* 297, 669.

Schatz, D.L., Palter, H.C., and Russell, C.S. (1968). Effects of oral contraceptives and pregnancy on thyroid function. *Can. Med. Assoc. J.* 99, 882.

Scheppach, W., Kortmann, B., Burghardt, W., Keller, F., Kasper, H., and Bahner, U. (1988). Effects of acetate during regular hemodialysis. *Clin. Nephrol.* 29, 19.

Schiele, F., Henry, J., Hitz, J., Petitclerc, C., Gueguen, R., and Siest, G. (1983). Total bone and liver alkaline phosphatases in plasma: biological variations and reference limits. *Clin. Chem.* 29, 634.

Schilsky, R.L. and Anderson, T. (1979). Hypomagnesemia and renal magnesium wasting in patients receiving cisplatin. *Ann. Intern. Med.* 90, 929.

Schindler, A.M. (1984). Isolated neonatal hypomagnesaemia associated with maternal overuse of stool softener. *Lancet* ii, 822.

Schindler, A.M. and Hiner, L.B. (1988). Hypernatremic metabolic alkalosis in a two-month old infant. *Hosp. Pract.* 23, 31. (N55)

Schlaeffer, F. (1988). Oxacillin-associated hypokalemia. *Drug Intell. Clin. Pharm.* 22, 695.

Schlienger, J.L., Kapfer, M.T., Singer, L., and Stephan, F. (1980). The action of clomipramine on thyroid function. *Horm. Metab. Res.* 12, 481.

Schmid, R. (1960). Cutaneous porphyria in Turkey. *N. Engl. J. Med.* 263, 397.

Schmidt, E., Poliwoda, H., Buhl, V., Alexanda, K., and Schmidt, F.W. (1972). Observations of enzyme elevations in the serum during streptokinase treatment. *J. Clin. Pathol.* 25, 650.

Schmidt, K.H., Hagmaier, V., Hornig, D.H., Vuilleumier, J.P., and Rutishauser, G. (1981). Urinary oxalate excretion after large intakes of ascrobic acid in man. *Am. J. Clin. Nutr.* 34, 305.

Schmidt, R.E. and Sesin, G.P. (1987). Hetastarch-induced hyperkalemia. *Drug Intell. Clin. Pharm.* 12, 922.

Schmutz, J.L., Cuny, J.F., Trechot, P., Weber, M., and Beurey, J. (1987). Les erythèmes pellagroïdes médicamenteux. Une observation d'erythème pellagroïde secondaire à l'isoniazide. *Ann. Dermatol. Venereol.* 114, 569.

Schnabel, R., Rambeck, B., and Janssen, F. (1984). Fatal intoxication with sodium valproate. *Lancet* i, 221.

Schneider, J., Muhlefllner, G., and Kaffarnik, H. (1980). Creatine kinase in hyperlipoproteinemic patients treated with clofibrate. *Artery* 8, 164.

Schneider, R.E. and Beeley, L. (1977). Megaloblastic anaemia associated with sulphasalazine treatment. *Br. Med. J.* i, 1638.

Schroeder, E.T. (1968). Alkalosis resulting from combined administration of a 'nonsystemic' antacid and a cation exchange resin. *Gastroenterology* 56, 868.

Schultz, R.E., Hanno, P.M., Levin, R.M., Wein, A.J., Pollack, H.M., and van Arsdalen, K.N. (1983). Percutaneous ultrasonic lithotripsy: choice of irrigant. *J. Urol.* 130, 858.

Schumer, W. (1971). Adverse effects of xylitol in parenteral alimentation. *Metabolism* 20, 345.

Schwartz, M.K. (1973). Interferences in diagnostic biochemical procedures. *Adv. Clin. Chem.* 16, 1.

Schwartz, R.H. and Jones, R.W.A. (1978). Transplacental hyponatraemia due to oxytocin. *Br. Med. J.* i, 152.

Schwartz, S.M., Carroll, H.M., and Scharschmidt, L.A. (1986). Sublimed (inorganic) sulfur ingestion. A cause of life-threatening metabolic acidosis with a high anion gap. *Arch. Intern. Med.* 146, 1437.

Schwartz, W.B. and Relman, A.S. (1953). Metabolic and renal studies in chronic potassium depletion resulting from overuse of laxatives. *J. Clin. Invest.* 32, 258.

Schweisfurth, H. and Schioberg-Schiegnitz, S. (1984). Assay and biochemical characterization of angiotensin-I converting enzyme in cerebrospinal fluid. *Enzyme* 32, 12.

Scoggin, C., McClellan, J.R., and Cary, J.M. (1977). Hyponatraemia and acidosis in association with topical treatment of burns. *Lancet* i, 959.

Seager, J. (1984). IgA deficiency during treatment of infantile hypothyroidism with thyroxine. *Br. Med. J.* 288, 1562.

Sebastian, A., McSherry, E., and Morris, R.C. Jr (1971). Renal potassium wasting in renal tubular acidosis (RTA): Its occurrence in types 1 and 2 RTA despite sustained correction of systemic acidosis. *J. Clin. Invest.* 50, 667.

Sebastian, A., Hulter, H.N., Kurtz, I., Maher, T., and Schambelan, M. (1982). Disorders of distal nephron function. *Am. J. Med.* 72, 289.

Sedman, A.B., Klein, G.L., Merritt, R.J., Miller, N.L., Weber, K.O., Gill, W.L., *et al.* (1985). Evidence of aluminum loading in infants receiving intravenous therapy. *N. Engl. J. Med.* 312, 1337.

Seely, E.W., Moore, T.J., LeBroff, M.S. and Brown, E.M. (1989*a*). A single dose of lithium carbonate acutely elevates intact parathyroid hormone levels in humans. *Acta Endocrinol.* 121, 174.

Seely, E.W., LeBoff, M.S., Brown, E.M., Chen, C., Posillico, J.T., Hollenberg, N.K., *et al.* (1989*b*). The calcium channel blocker diltiazem lowers serum parathyroid hormone levels in vivo and in vitro. *J. Clin. Endocrinol. Metab.* 68, 1007.

Selby, P.L. and Peacock, M. (1986*a*). Ethinyl estradiol and norethindrone in the treatment of primary hyperparathyroidism in postmenopausal women. *N. Engl. J. Med.* 314, 1481.

Selby, P.L. and Peacock, M. (1986*b*). The effect of transdermal oestrogen on bone, calcium-regulating hormones and liver in postmenopausal women. *Clin. Endocrinol.* 25, 543.

Seller, R.H., Greco, J., Banach, S., and Seth, R. (1975). Increasing the inotropic effect and toxic dose of digitalis by the administration of antikaliuretic drugs — further evidence for a cardiac effect of diuretic agents. *Am. Heart J.* 90, 56.

Sequeira, S.J. and McKenna, T.J. (1986). Chlorbutol, a new inhibitor of aldosterone biosynthesis identified during examination of heparin effect on aldosterone production. *J. Clin. Endocrinol. Metab.* 63, 780.

Sestili, M.A. (1983). Possible adverse health effects of vitamin C and ascorbic acid. *Semin. Oncol.* 10, 299.

Sevitt, L.H. and Wrong, D.M. (1968). Hypercalcaemia from calcium resin in patients with chronic renal failure. *Lancet* ii, 950.

Shaaban, M.M., Elewan, S.I., el-Sharkawy, M.M., and Farghaly, A.S. (1984). Effect of subdermal levonorgestrel contraceptive implants, Norplant, on liver functions. *Contraception* 30, 407.

Shah, I.A. and Brandt, H. (1983). Halothane-associated granulomatous hepatitis. *Digestion* 28, 245.

Shalev, A., Hermesh, H., and Munitz, H. (1987*a*). The hypouricemic effect of chlorprothixene. *Clin. Pharmacol. Ther.* 42, 562.

Shalev, O., Gilon, D., and Nubain, N.H. (1987*b*). Masked phenytoin-induced megaloblastic anaemia in beta-thalassemia minor. *Acta Haematol.* 77, 186.

Shannon, M. and Graef, J.W. (1989). Lead intoxication from lead-contaminated water used to reconstitute infant formula. *Clin. Pediatr.* 28, 380.

Shannon, M. and Lovejoy, F.H. Jr (1989). Hypokalemia after theophylline intoxication. The effects of acute vs chronic poisoning. *Arch. Intern. Med.* 149, 2725.

Shannon, R.S. and Barclay, R.P.C. (1974). Sodium citrate and hypernatraemia in infancy. *Br. Med. J.* iii, 503.

Shapiro, W. and Taubert, K. (1975). Hypokalaemia and digoxin-induced arrhythmias. *Lancet* ii, 604.

Sheffer, A.L., Fearon, D.T., and Austen, K.F. (1981). Clinical and biochemical effects of stanozol therapy for hereditary angioedema. *J. Allergy Clin. Immunol.* 68, 181.

Shek, C.C., Natkunam, A., Tsang, V., Cockram, C.S. and Swaminathan, R. (1990). Incidence causes and mechanism of hypercalcaemia in a hospital population in Hong Kong. *Q. J. Med.* 77, 1277.

Shelley, E.D., Shelley, W.B., and Burmeister, V. (1987). Naproxen-induced pseudoporphyria presenting a diagnostic dilemma. *Cutis* 40, 314.

Shelton, D. and Goulding, R. (1979). Silver poisoning associated with an antismoking lozenge. *Br. Med. J.* i, 267.

Shepherd, L.L., Hutchinson, R.J., Worden E.K., Koopmann C.F., and Coran A. (1989). Hyponatremia and seizures after intravenous administration of desmopressin acetate for surgical hemostasis. *J. Pediatr.* 114, 470.

Shergy, W.J., Gilkeson, G.S., and German, D.C. (1988). Acute gouty arthritis and intravenous nitroglycerin. *Arch. Intern. Med.* 148, 2505.

Sherlock, S. (1971). Halothane hepatitis. *Gut* 12, 324.

Sherman, R.A. and Ruddy, M.C., (1986). Suppression of aldosterone production by low-dose heparin. *Am. J. Nephrol.* 6, 165.

Shields, H.M. (1978). Rapid fall of serum phosphorus secondary to antacid therapy. *Gastroenterology* 75, 1137.

Shils, M.E. (1969). Experimental human magnesium depletion. *Medicine* (Baltimore) 48, 61.

Shin, Y.K. and Kim, Y.D. (1988). Ventricular tachyarrhythmias during cesarean section after ritodrine therapy: interaction with anesthetics. *South. Med. J.* 81, 528.

Shneerson, J.M. and Gazzard, B.G. (1977). Reversible malabsorption caused by methyldopa. *Br. Med. J.* ii, 1456.

Shojania, A.M., Hornady, G.J., and Barnes, P.H. (1971). The effect of oral contraceptives on folate metabolism. *Am. J. Obstet. Gynecol.* 111, 782.

Shorey, J., Bhardwaj, N., and Loscalzo, J. (1984). Acute Wernicke's encephalopathy after intravenous infusion of high-dose nitroglycerin. *Ann. Intern. Med.* 101, 500.

Sibai, B.M., Graham, J.M., and McCubbin, J.H. (1984). A comparison of intravenous and intramuscular magnesium sulfate regimens in preeclampsia. *Am. J. Obstet. Gynecol.* 150, 728.

Siebers, R.W., Burgess, C.D., Flatt, A., Beasley, R., and Crane, J. (1989). Unsuitability of the human erythrocyte as a model for in vivo sodium transport activation by beta 2 adrenergic agonists. *Ann. Clin. Biochem.* 26, 444.

Silverman, L.M., Christenson, R.H., and Grant, G.H. (1986). Aminoacids and proteins. In *Textbook of clinical chemistry* (ed. N.W. Tietz), p. 519. W.B. Saunders, Philadephia.

Silvis, S.E. and Paragas, P.D.J. (1972). Paresthesias, weakness, seizures, and hypophosphatemia in patients receiving hyperalimentation. *Gastroenterology* 134, 513.

Simmer, K., Iles, C.A., James, C., and Thompson, R.P. (1987). Are iron-folate supplements harmful? *Am. J. Clin Nutr.* 45, 122.

Simmons, M.A., Adcock, E. III., Bard, H., and Battaglia, F. (1974). Hypernatraemia and intracranial hemorrhage and NaHCO₃ administration in neonates. *N. Engl. J. Med.* 291, 6.

Simons, M.L. and Goldman, E. (1988). Atypical malignant hyperthermia with persistent hyperkalaemia during renal transplantation. *Can. J. Anaesth.* 35, 409.

Simpson, W.M. Jr (1971). Oral contraceptives and untoward effects coincident with their use. Review. *South. Med. J.* 64, 1184.

Singer, J. and Rotenberg, D. (1973). Demeclocycline-induced nephrogenic diabetes insipidus. *In-vivo* and *in-vitro* studies. *Ann. Intern. Med.* 79, 679.

Singh, H.P., Hebert, M.A., and Gault, M.H. (1972). Effect of some drugs on clinical laboratory values as determined by the Technicon® SMA 12-60. *Clin. Chem.* 18, 137.

Sipila, R., Skrifvars, B., and Tornroth, T. (1986). Reversible non-oliguric impairment of renal function during azapropazone treatment. *Scand. J. Rheumatol.* 15, 23.

Sivasubramanian, K.N., Hoy, G., Davitt, M.K., and Henkin, R.I. (1978). Zinc and copper changes after neonatal parenteral alimentation. *Lancet* i, 508.

Sjoden, G., Rosenqvist, M., Kriegholm, E., and Haglund, K. (1987). Calcium absorption and excretion in patients treated with verapamil. *Br. J. Clin. Pharmacol.* 24, 367.

Skinner, R., Pearson, A.D.J., Price, L., Cunningham, K., and Craft, A.W. (1989). Hypophosphataemic rickets after ifosfamide treatment in children. *Br. Med. J.* 298, 1560.

Skrede, S., Ro, J.S., and Mjolnerod, O. (1973). Effects of dextrans on the plasma protein changes during the postoperative period. *Clin. Chim. Acta* 48, 143.

Skrha, J., Sramkova, J., Rehak, F., and Pacovsky, V. (1986). Serum isoamylase activities during infusions of glucose and amino acids. *Eur. J. Clin. Invest.* 16, 35.

Sluiter, H.E., Hytsmans, F.T., Thien, T.A., Van Lier, H.J., and Koene, R.A. (1984). Haemodynamic, hormonal and diuretic effects of felodipine in healthy normotensive volunteers. *Drugs* 29 (suppl. 2), 26.

Small, M., Beastall, G.H., Semple, C.G., Cowan, R.A., and Forbes C.D. (1984). Alteration of hormone levels in normal males given the anabolic steroid stanozolol. *Clin. Endocrinol.* 21, 49.

Smilkstein, M.J., Smolinske, S.C., Kulig, K.W., and Rumack, B.H. (1988). Severe hypermagnesemia due to multiple-dose cathartic therapy. *West. J. Med.* 148, 208.

Smith, D.A. and Nordin, B.E.C. (1964). The effect of a high phosphorus intake on total and ultrafiltrable plasma calcium and phosphate clearance. *Clin. Sci.* 26, 479.

Smith, J.L. and Hodges, R.E. (1987). Serum levels of vitamin C in relation to dietary and supplemental intake of vitamin C in smokers and non smokers. *Ann. N.Y. Acad. Sci.* 498, 144.

Smith, J.L., Goldsmith, G.A., and Lawrence, J.D. (1975). Effects of oral contraceptive steroids on vitamin and lipid levels in serum. *Am. J. Clin. Nutr.* 28, 371.

Smith, N.J. and Espir, M.L.E. (1977). Raised plasma arginine vasopressin concentration in carbamazepine-induced water intoxication. *Br. Med. J.* ii, 804.

Smith, S.R., Galloway, M.J., Reilly, J.T., and Davies, J.M. (1988). Amiloride prevents amphotericin B related hypokalaemia in neutropenic patients. *J. Clin. Pathol.* 41, 494.

Smith, T.J., Gill, J.C., Ambruso, D.R., and Hathaway, W.E. (1989). Hyponatremia and seizures in young children given DDAVP. *Am. J. Hematol.* 31, 199.

Smith, T.W. (1988). Digitalis: Mechanisms of action and clinical use. *N. Engl. J. Med.* 318, 358.

Smith, T.W. and Willerson, J.T. (1971). Suicidal and accidental digoxin ingestion. *Circulation* 44, 29.

Smithells, R.W., Sheppard, S., and Schorah, C.J. (1976). Vitamin deficiencies and neural tube defects. *Arch. Dis. Child* 51, 944.

Snapp, K.R., Boyer, D.B., Peterson, L.C., and Svare, C.W. (1989). The contribution of dental amalgam to mercury in blood. *J. Dent. Res.* 68, 780.

Snider, D.E. (1980). Pyridoxine supplementation during isoniazid therapy. *Tubercle.* 61, 191.

Sola, R., Puig, L.L., Ballarin, J.A., Donate, T., and del Rio, G. (1987). Pseudoporphyria cutanea tarda associated with cyclosporine therapy. *Transplantation* 43, 772.

Somani, P., Temesy-Armos, P.N., Leighton, R.F., Goodenday, L.S., and Fraker, T.D. Jr (1984). Hyponatremia in patients treated with lorcainide, a new antiarrhythmic drug. *Am. Heart J.* 108, 1443.

Song, S., Chen, J.K., He, M.L., and Fotherby, K. (1989). Effect of some oral contraceptives on serum concentrations of sex hormone binding globulin and ceruloplasmin. *Contraception* 39, 385.

Song, Z.Y., Lu, Y.P., and Gu, X.Q. (1985). Treatment of yellow phosphorus skin burns with silver nitrate instead of copper sulfate. *Scand. J. Work Environ. Health* 11, 33.

Sonino, N. (1987). The use of ketoconazole as an inhibitor of steroid production. *N. Engl. J. Med.* 317, 812.

Sorrell, T.C., Forbes, I.J., Burness, F.R., and Rischbieth, R.H.C. (1971). Depression of immunological function in patients treated with phenytoin sodium (sodium diphenylhydantoin). *Lancet* ii, 1233.

Spargo, E. (1984). The acute effects of alcohol on plasma creatine kinase (CK) activity in the rat. *J. Neurol. Sci.* 63, 307.

Spaulding, W.B. (1979). Myalgia and elevated creatine phosphokinase with danazol in hereditary angioedema. *Ann. Intern. Med.* 90, 854.

Speires, C.J., Dollery, C.T., Inman, W.H.W., Rawson, N.S.B., and Witton, L.V. (1988). Postmarketing surveillance of enalapril. II: Investigation of the potential role of enalapril in death with renal failure. *Br. Med. J.* 297, 830.

Spencer, H., Karamer, L., Osis, D., and Wiatrowski, E. (1985). Effects of aluminum hydroxide on fluoride and calcium metabolism. *J. Environ. Pathol. Toxicol. Oncol.* 6, 33.

Sprague, S.M., Corwin, H.L., Wilson, R.S., Mayor, G.H., and Tanner, C.M. (1986). Encephalopathy in chronic renal failure responsive to deferoxamine therapy. Another manifestation of aluminum neurotoxicity. *Arch. Intern. Med.* 146, 2063.

Sprince, H., Parker, C.M., Smith, G.G., and Gonzales, L.J. (1975). Protective action of ascorbic acid and sulphur compounds against acetaldehyde toxicity: implication in alcoholism and smoking. *Agent Actions* 5, 164.

Stacpoole, P.W., Harman, E.M., Curry, S.H., Baumgartner, T.G., and Misbin, R.I. (1983). Treatment of lactic acidosis with dichloroacetate. *N. Engl. J. Med.* 309, 390.

Stahl, R.A., Kanz, L., Maier, B., and Schollmeyer, P. (1986). Hyperchloremic metabolic acidosis with high serum potassium in renal transplant recipients: a cyclosporine A associated side effect. *Clin. Nephrol.* 25, 245.

Standal, B.R., Kao-Chen, S.M., Yang, G.Y., and Chan, D.F.B. (1974). Early changes in pyridoxine status of patients receiving isoniazid therapy. *Am. J. Clin. Nutr.* 27, 479.

Steedman, D.J. (1988). Poisoning with sustained release potassium. *Arch. Emerg. Med.* 5, 206.

Steele, T.H. and Oppenheimer, S. (1969). Factors affecting urate excretion following diuretic administration in man. *Am. J. Med.* 47, 564.

Steele, T.H. and Rieselbach, R.E. (1967). The renal mechanism for urate homeostasis in normal man. *Am. J. Med.* 43, 868.

Steidl, L., Tolde, I., and Svomova, V. (1987). Metabolism of magnesium and zinc in patients treated with antiepileptic drugs and with magnesium lactate. *Magnesium* 6, 284.

Steiniche, T., Mosekilde, L., Christensen, M.S., and Melsen, F. (1989). Histomorphometric analysis of bone in idiopathic hypercalciuria before and after treatment with thiazide. *APMIS* 97, 302.

Steinmetz, P.R. and Lawson, L.R. (1970). Defect in urinary acidification induced *in vitro* by amphotericin B. *J. Clin. Invest.* 49, 596.

Stephens, W.P., Espir, M.L.E., Tattersall, R.B., Quinn, N.P., Gladwell, S.R.F., Galbraith, A.W., *et al.* (1977). Water intoxication due to carbamazepine. *Br. Med. J.* i, 754.

Sterns, R.H., Cox, M., Feig, P.U., and Singer, I. (1981). Internal potassium balance and the control of the plasma potassium concentration. *Medicine* (Baltimore) 60, 339.

Stevens, A.R. Jr and Wolff, H.G. (1950). Magnesium intoxication; absorption from intact gastrointestinal tract. *Arch. Neurol.* 63, 749.

Stewart, A.F., Keating, T., and Schwartz, P.E. (1985). Magnesium homeostasis following chemotherapy with cisplatin: a prospective study. *Am. J. Obstet. Gynecol.* 153, 660.

Stewart, J.A., Ackerly, C.C., Myers, C.F., Newman, R.A., and Krakoff, I.H. (1986). Clinical and clinical pharmacologic studies of 2-amino-1,3,4-thiadiazole (A-TDA:NSC4728). *Cancer Chemother. Pharmacol.* 16, 287.

Stewart, J.W., Harrison, W., Quitkin, F., and Leibowitz, M.R. (1984). Phenelzine-induced pyridoxine deficiency. *J. Clin. Psychopharmacol.* 4, 225.

Stewart, M.J. and Simpson, E. (1973). Prognosis in paracetamol self-poisoning: the use of plasma paracetamol concentration in a region. *Ann. Clin. Biochem.* 10, 173.

Stewart, P.M., Wallace, A.M., Valentino, R., Burt, D., Shackleton, C.L., and Edwards, C.R.W. (1987). Mineralocorticoid activity of liquorice: 11-β-hydroxysteroid dehydrogenase deficiency comes of age. *Lancet* ii, 821.

Stewart, P.M., Wallace, A.M., Atherden, S.M., Shearing, C.H., and Edwards, C.R. (1990). Mineralocorticoid activity of carbenoxolone: contrasting effects of carbenoxolone and liquorice on 11 β-hydroxysteroid dehydrogenase activity in man. *Clin. Sci.* 78, 49.

Stinebaugh, B.J. and Schloeder, F. (1972). Glucose-induced alkalosis in fasting subjects: relationship to renal bicarbonate reabsorption during fasting and refeeding. *J. Clin. Invest.* 51, 1326.

Stock, J.L., Coderre, J.A., and Mallette, L.E. (1985). Effects of a short course of estrogen on mineral metabolism in postmenopausal women. *J. Clin. Endocrinol. Metab.* 61, 595.

Stoff, J.S. (1982). Phosphate homeostasis and hypophosphatemia. *Am. J. Med.* 72, 489.

Stovner, J., Theodorsen, L., and Bjelke, E. (1972) Sensitivity to dimethyltubocurarine and toxiferine with special reference to serum proteins. *Br. J. Anaesth.* 44, 374.

Strandjord, R.E., Aanderud, S., Myking, O.L., and Johannessen, S.I. (1981). Influence of carbamazepine on serum thyroxine and triiodothyronine in patients with epilepsy. *Acta Neurol. Scand.* 63, 111.

Streicher, H.Z., Gabow, P.A., Moss, A.H., Kono, D., and Kaehny, W.D. (1981). Syndromes of toluene sniffing in adults. *Ann. Intern. Med.* 94, 758.

Strom, B.L., West, S.L., Sim, E., and Carson, J.L. (1989). The epidemiology of the acute flank pain syndrome from suprofen. *Clin. Pharmacol. Ther.* 46, 693.

Studd, J.W.W., Savvas, M., and Johnson, M. (1989). Correction of corticosteroid-induced osteoporosis by percutaneous hormone implants. *Lancet* i, 339.

Sueblinvong, V. and Wilson, J.F. (1969). Myocardial damage due to imipramine intoxication. *J. Pediat.* 74, 475.

Sugino, H., Kagoshima, M., and Katagiri, S. (1984). Effects of some drugs on plasma uric acid in rats — action of catecholamines and beta-blocking agents. *Nippon Yakurigaku Zasshi* 84, 293.

Suki, W.N., Yium, J.J., Von Minden, M., Saller-Hebert, C., Eknoyan, G., and Martinez-Maldonada, M. (1970). Acute treatment of hypercalcemia with furosemide. *N. Engl. J. Med.* 283, 836.

Sunderam, M.B.M. and Swaminathan, R. (1981). Total body potassium depletion and severe myopathy due to liquorice ingestion. *Postgrad. Med. J.* 57, 48.

Sunderam, S.G. and Manikkar, G.D. (1983). Hyponatraemia in the elderly. *Age Ageing* 12, 77.

Sunderrajan, S., Bauer, J.H., Vopat, R.L., Wanner-Barjenbruch, P., and Hayes, A. (1984). Post transurethral prostatic resection hyponatremic syndrome : case report and review of the literature. *Am. J. Kidney Dis.* 4, 80.

Sunderrajan, S., Brooks, C.S., and Sunderrajan, E.V. (1985). Nortriptyline-induced severe hyperventilation. *Arch. Intern. Med.* 145, 746.

Sussman, N.M. and McLain, L.W. (1979). A direct hepatotoxic effect of valproic acid. *JAMA* 242, 1173.

Suttie, J.W., Mummah-Schendel, L.L., Shab, D.V., Lyle, B.J., and Greger, J.L. (1988). Vitamin K deficiency from dietary vitamin K restriction in humans. *Am. J. Clin. Nutr.* 47, 475.

Suzuki, H., Yamazaki, N., Suzuki, Y., Hiraiwa, M., Shimoda, S., Mori, K., *et al.* (1984). Lowering effect of diphenylhydantoin on serum free thyroxine and thyroxine binding globulin (TBG). *Acta Endocrinol.* 105, 477.

Suzuki, N., Nonaka, K., Kono, N., Ichihara, K., Fukumoto, Y., Inui, Y., *et al.* (1986). Effects of the intravenous administration of magnesium sulphate on corrected serum calcium level and nephrogenous cyclic AMP excretion in normal human subjects. *Calcif. Tiss. Int.* 39, 304.

Suzuki, Y., Ichikawa, Y., Saito, E., and Homma, M. (1983). Importance of increased urinary calcium excretion in the development of secondary hyperparathyroidism of patients under glucocorticoid therapy. *Metabolism* 32, 151.

Swainson, C.P., Colls, B.M., and Fitzharris, B.M. (1985). Cis-platinum and distal renal tubule toxicity. *N.Z. Med. J.* 98, 375.

Swainson, C.P., Walker, R.J., and Bailey, R.R. (1989). Effects of cilazapril on renal function and hormones in hypertensive patients with renal disease. *Am. J. Med.* 87, 83S.

Swales, J.D. (1982). Magnesium deficiency and diuretics. *Br. Med. J.* 285, 1377.

Swaminathan, R., Morgan, D.B., Ionescu, M., and Hill, G.L. (1978). Hypophosphataemia and its consequences in patients following open heart surgery. *Anaesthesia* 33, 601.

Swaminathan, R., Bradley, P., Morgan, D.B., and Hill, G.L. (1979). Hypophosphataemia in surgical patients. *Surgery* 148, 448.

Swaminathan, R., Chin, R.K., Lao, T.T.H., Mak, Y.T., Panesar, N.S., and Cockram, C.S. (1989). Thyroid function in hyperemesis gravidarum. *Acta Endocrinol.* 120, 155.

Swartz, R., Dombrouski, J., Burnatowska-Hledin, M., and Mayor, G. (1987). Microcytic anemia in dialysis patients: reversible marker of aluminum toxicity. *Am. J. Kidney Dis.* 9, 217.

Swartz, R.D., Wesley, J.R., Somermeyer, M.G., and Lau, K. (1984). Hyperoxaluria and renal insufficiency due to ascorbic acid administration during total parenteral nutrition. *Ann. Intern. Med.* 100, 530.

Sweeney, J.D., Ziegler, P., Pruet, C., and Spaulding, M.R. (1989). Hyperzincuria and hypozincemia in patients treated with cisplatin. *Cancer* 63, 2093.

Swenson, E.R. (1986). Severe hyperkalemia as a complication of timolol, a topically applied β-adrenergic antagonist. *Arch. Intern. Med.* 146, 1220.

Swenson, R.D., Golper, T.A., and Bennett, W.M. (1982). Acute renal failure and rhabdomyolysis after ingestion of phenylpropanolamine-containing diet pills. *JAMA* 48, 1216.

Sybrecht, G.W. (1983). Influence of brotizolam on the ventilatory and mouth-occlusion pressure response to hypercapnia in patients with chronic obstructive pulmonary disease. *Br. J. Clin. Pharmacol.* 16, 425S.

Szatalowicz, V.L., Miller, P.D., Lacher, J.W., Gordon, J.A., and Schrier, R.W. (1982). Comparative effect of diuretics on renal water excretion in hyponatremic oedematous disorders. *Clin. Sci.* 62, 235.

Takahashi, H., Fukuyama, M., Yoneda, S., Okabavyashi, H., and Yoshimura, M. (1989). Comparison of nisoldipine and atenolol in the treatment of essential hypertension. *Arzneimittelforschung* 39, 379.

Taliani, U., Rossetti, A., Bonati, P.L., and Prati, G. (1988). Iposodiemia durante terapia con basse dosi di carbamazepina. Relazione su un caso clinico. *Acta Biomed. Ateneo. Parmense.* 59, 35.

Tannen, R.L. (1986). Potassium disorders. In *Fluids and electrolytes* (ed. J.P. Kokko and R.L. Tannen), p. 150. W.B. Saunders, Philadelphia.

Taves, D.R., Fry, B.W., Freeman, R.B., and Gillies, A.J. (1970). Toxicity following methoxyflurane anaesthesia II. Fluoride concentrations in nephrotoxicity. *JAMA* 214, 96.

Taylor, B.J. and Duffill, M.B. (1987). Pseudoporphyria from nonsteroidal anti-inflammatory drugs. *N.Z. Med. J.* 100, 322.

Teicher, A., Rosenthal, T., Kissin, E., and Sarova, I. (1981). Labetalol-induced toxic myopathy. *Br. Med. J.* 282, 1824.

Tennant, G.B., Smith, R.C., Leinster, S.J., O'Donnell, J.E., and Wardrop, C.A.J. (1981*a*). Acute depression of serum folate in surgical patients during preoperative infusion of ethanol-free parenteral nutrition. *Scand. J. Haematol.* 27, 327.

Tennant, G.B., Smith, R.C., Leinster, S.J., O'Donnell, J.E., and Wardrop, C.A.J. (1981*b*). Aminoacid infusion induced depression of serum folate after cholecystectomy. *Scand. J. Haematol.* 27, 333.

Tephly, T.R., Wagner, G., Sedman, R.L., and Piper, W. (1977). Effect of metals on heme biosynthesis and metabolism. *Fed. Proc.* 37, 35.

ter Wee, P.M., van Hoek, B., and Donker, A.J. (1985). Indomethacin treatment in a patient with lithium-induced polyuria. *Intens. Care Med.* 11, 103.

Texier, D., Chevallier, P., Perrotin, D., and Guilmot, J.L. (1982). Hypercalcaemia associated with resorbable haemostatic compresses. *Lancet* i, 688.

Thiebaud, D., Jaeger, P., Jacquet, A.F., and Burckhardt, P. (1986). A single-day treatment of tumor-induced hypercalcemia by intravenous amino-hydroxypropylidene bisphosphonate. *J. Bone Miner. Res.* 1, 555.

Thomas, D.W., Edwards, J.B., Gilligan, J.E., Lawrence, J.R., and Edwards, R.G. (1972). Complication following intravenous administration of solutions containing xylitol. *Med. J. Aust.* i, 1238.

Thomas, T.H., Ball, S.G., Wales, J.K., and Lee, M.R. (1978). Effect of carbamazepine on plasma and urine arginine-vasopressin. *Clin. Sci. Mol. Med.* 54, 419.

Thompson, C.B., June, C.H., Sullivan, K.M., and Thomas, E.D. (1984). Association between cyclosporin neurotoxicity and hypomagnesaemia. *Lancet* ii, 1116.

Thompson, M. and Dempsey, W. (1983). Hyperuricemia, renal failure, and elevated creatine phosphokinase after amoxapine overdose. *Clin. Pharm.* 2, 579.

Thomson, A.D. and Majumdar, S.K. (1981). The influence of ethanol on intestinal absorption and utilization of nutrients. *Clin. Gastroenterol.* 10, 263.

Thorp, J.M., Mackenzie, I., and Simpson, E. (1987). Gross hypernatraemia associated with the use of antiseptic surgical packs. *Anaesthesia* 42, 750.

Tiitinen, S., Nissila, M., Ruutsalo, H.M., and Isomaki, H. (1983). Effect of non steroidal anti-inflammatory drugs on the renal excretion of uric acid. *Clin. Rheumatol.* 2, 233.

Toft, H. and Roin, J. (1971). Effect of frusemide administration on calcium excretion. *Br. Med. J.* i, 437.

Toghill, P.J. and Smith, P.G. (1971). Folate deficiency and the pill. *Br. Med. J.* i, 608.

Tomic, R., Ljungberg, B., and Damber, J.E. (1988). Hormonal effects of high dose medroxyprogesterone acetate treatment in males with renal or prostatic adenocarcinoma. *J. Urol. Nephrol.* 22, 15.

Tomkin, G.H. (1973). Malabsorption of vitamin B_{12} in diabetic patients treated with phenformin: a comparison with metformin. *Br. Med. J.* iii, 673.

Tomkins, A. and Hussey G. (1989). Vitamin A, immunity and infection. *Nutr. Res. Rev.* 2, 17.

Toogood, J.H., Crilly, R.G., Jones, G., Nadeau, J., and Wells, G.A. (1988). Effect of high-dose inhaled budesonide on calcium and phosphate metabolism and the risk of osteoporosis. *Am. Rev. Respir. Dis.* 138, 57.

Toone, B.K., Wheeler, M., and Fenwick, P.B. (1980). Sex hormone changes in male epileptics. *Clin. Endocrinol.* 12, 391.

Tormey, W.P., Jina, A.G., and Stone, C. (1989). Potassium-sparing diuretics and hyperkalaemia. Still a problem. *Ir. Med. J.* 82, 179.

Tovey, D.L.A. and Lathe, G.H. (1968). Caeruloplasmin and green plasma in women taking oral contraceptives, in pregnant women, and in patients with rheumatoid arthritis. *Lancet* ii, 596.

Trachtenberg, J. and Pont, A. (1984). Ketoconazole treatment for advanced prostate cancer. *Lancet* ii, 433.

Travis, S.F., Sugerman, H.J., Ruberg, R.L., Dudrick, S.J., Delivoria-Papado-poulos, M., Miller, L.D., *et al.* (1971). Alterations of red-cell glycolytic intermediates and oxygen transport as a consequence of hypoposphataemia in patients receiving intravenous hyperalimentation. *N. Engl. J. Med.* 285, 763.

Trump, D.L. and Hortvet, L. (1985). Etoposide and very high dose cisplatin: salvage therapy for patients with advanced germ cell neoplasms. *Cancer Treat. Rep.* 69, 259.

Tsega, E. (1987). Long-term effect of high-dose, short-course chloroquine therapy on porphyria cutanea tarda. *Q. J. Med.* 65, 953.

Turetta, F., de Stefani, R., Milanesi, A., Cannizzaro, A., Padoan, A.M., and de Giorgio, P. (1985). Variation du calcium ionisé plasmatique au cours de l'angiographie en fluorescence. *J. Fr. Ophtalmol.* 8, 785.

Tuzhilin, S.A., Gonda, M., Carbonell, G., and Dreiling, D.A. (1982). Serum amylases and their inhibitors: 2. clinical and experimental observations-diet and steroid effects. *Am. J. Gastroenterol.* 77, 26.

Tymms, D.J. and Leatherdale, B.A. (1988). Lactic acidosis due to metformin therapy in a low-risk patient. *Postgrad. Med. J.* 64, 230.

Tyrer, L.B. (1984). Nutrition and the pill. *J. Reprod. Med.* 29 (suppl.), 547.

Ubbink, J.B., Delport, R., Becker, P.J., and Bissbort, S. (1989). Evidence of a theophylline-induced vitamin B6 deficiency caused by noncompetitive inhibition of pyridoxal kinase. *J. Lab. Clin. Med.* 113, 15.

Ubbink, J.B., Vermaak, W.J., Delport, R., and Serfontein, W.J. (1990). The relationship between vitamin B_6 metabolism, asthma, and theophylline therapy. *Ann. N.Y. Acad. Sci.* 585, 285.

Umeki, S., Tsukiyama, K., Okimoto, N., and Soejima, R. (1989). Urinastatin (Kunitz-type proteinase inhibitor) reducing cisplatin nephrotoxicity. *Am. J. Med. Sci.* 298, 221.

Umino, M., Miura, M., Kondo, T., Ohi, K., Yoshino, A., and Kubota, Y. (1985). Effect of thiamylal and diazepam on release of myoglobin and creatine phosphokinase by succinylcholine chloride during halothane anesthesia. *Bull. Tokyo Med. Dent. Univ.* 32, 91.

Valberg, L.S., Flanagan, P.R., and Chamberlain, M.J. (1984). Effects of iron, tin, and copper on zinc absorption in humans. *Am. J. Clin. Nutr.* 40, 536.

van Riel, P.L., van de Putte, L.B., Gribnau, F.W., and de Waal, R.M. (1984). Serum IgA and gold-induced toxic effects in patients with rheumatoid arthritis. *Arch. Intern. Med.* 144, 1401.

Vandenburg, M., Parfrey, P., Wright, P., and Lazda, E. (1981). Hepatitis associated with captopril treatment. *Br. J. Clin. Pharmacol.* 11, 105.

Varanos, S., Ansell, B.M., and Reeve, J. (1987). Vertebral collapse in juvenile chronic arthritis: Its relationship with glucocorticoid therapy. *Calcif. Tissue Int.* 41, 75.

Varkel, Y., Braester, A., Nusem, D., and Shkolnik, T. (1988). Methyldopa-induced syndrome of inappropriate antidiuretic hormone secretion and bone marrow granulomatosis. *Drug Intell. Clin. Pharm.* 22, 700.

Vaziri, N.D., Stokes, J., and Treadwell, T.R. (1981). Lactic acidosis, a complication of papaverine overdose. *Clin. Toxicol.* 18, 417.

Veech, R.L. and Gitomer, W.L. (1988). The medical and metabolic consequences of administration of sodium acetate. *Adv. Enzyme Regul.* 27, 313.

Vermeulen, A. and Thiery, M. (1982). Metabolic effects of the triphasic oral contraceptive trigynon. *Contraception* 26, 505.

Veterans Administration Co-Operative Study Group on Antihypertensive Agents. (1984). Low dose captopril for the treatment of mild to moderate hypertension. I. Results of a 14-week trial. *Arch. Intern. Med.* 144, 1947.

Vincens, M., Mercier-Bodard, C., Mowszowicz, I., Kuttenn, F., and Mauvais-Jarvis, P. (1989). Testosterone-estradiol binding globulin (TeBG) in hirsute patients treated with cyproterone acetate (CPA) and percutaneous estradiol. *J. Steroid Biochem.* 33, 531.

Vithayasai, P., Rojanasthien, N., and Punglumpoo, S. (1989). A case of hypomagnesemia hypocalcemia as a complication of aminoglycoside and review of the literature. *J. Med. Assoc. Thai.* 72, 413.

Vladutiu, O. and Reitz, M. (1980). Creatine kinase isoenzymes in aspirin intoxication. *Lancet* ii, 864.

Vlasses, P.H., Rotmensch, H.H., Swanson, B.N., Irvin, J.D., Johnson, C.L., and Ferguson, R.K. (1984). Indacrinone: natriuretic and uricosuric effects of various ratios of its enantiomers in healthy men. *Pharmacotherapy* 4, 272.

Vogelzang, N.J., Torkelson, J.L., and Kennedy, BJ. (1985). Hypomagnesemia, renal dysfunction, and Raynaud's phenomenon in patients treated with cisplatin, vinblastine, and bleomycin. *Cancer* 56, 2765.

Wagnerova, M., Wagner, V., Madlo, Z., Zavazal, V., Wokounova, D., Kriz, J., *et al* (1986). Seasonal variations in the level of immunoglobulins and serum proteins of children differing by exposure to air-borne lead. *J. Hyg. Epidemiol. Microbiol. Immunol.* 30, 127.

Wagnerova, M., Wagner, V., Znojemska, S. and Hrebacka J. (1988). Factors of humoral resistance in workers exposed to vinyl chloride with a view to smoking habits. *J. Hyg. Epidemiol. Microbiol. Immunol.* 32, 265.

Waibel-Treber, S., Minne, H.W., Scharla, S.H., Bremen, Th., Ziegler, R., and Leyendecker, A. (1989). Reversible bone loss in women treated with GnRH agonists for endometriosis and uterine leiomyoma. *Hum. Reprod.* 4, 384.

Walden, C.E., Knopp, R.H., Johnson, J.L., Heiss, G., Wahl, P.W., and Hoover, J.J. (1986). Effect of estrogen/progestin potency on clinical chemistry measures. The Lipid Research Clinics Program Prevalence Study. *Am. J. Epidemiol.* 123, 517.

Walker, B.J., Evans, P.A., Forsling, M.L., and Nelstrop, G.A. (1985). Somatostatin and water excretion in man: an intrarenal action. *Clin. Endocrinol.* 23, 169.

Walker, F.B. IV, Becker, D.M., Kowal-Nelley, B., and Krongaard, L.S. (1988). Lack of effect of warfarin on uric acid concentration. *Clin. Chem.* 34, 952.

Walker, J.F. (1988). HMG CoA reductase inhibitors. Current clinical experience. *Drugs* 36 (suppl. 3), 83.

Waller, P.C. and Ramsay, L.E. (1989). Predicting acute gout in diuretic-treated hypertensive patients. *J. Hum. Hypertens.* 3, 457.

Walter, G.F. and Maresch, W. (1987). Iertümliche Kochsalzintoxikation bei Neugeborenen. Morphologische Befunde und pathogenetische Diskussion. *Klin. Padiatr.* 199, 269.

Walter, U., Forthofer, R., and Witte, P.U. (1987). Dose-response relation of the angiotensin converting enzyme inhibitor ramipril in mild to moderate essential hypertension. *Am. J. Cardiol.* 59, 125D.

Walters, E.G., Barnes, I.C., Price, S.A., and Abi-Akbar, F. (1987). Hyponatraemia associated with diuretics. *Br. J. Clin. Pract.* 41, 841.

Walton, R.J., Russell, R.G.G., and Smith, R. (1975). Changes in the renal and extra renal handling of phosphate induced by sodium etidronate (EHDP) in man. *Clin. Sci.* 49, 45.

Wan, H.H. and Lye, M.D.W. (1980). Moduretic-induced metabolic acidosis and hyperkalaemia. *Postgrad. Med. J.* 56, 348.

Wandrup, J. and Kancir, C. (1986). Complex biochemical syndrome of hypocalcemia and hypoparathyroidism during cytotoxic treatment of an infant with leukemia. *Clin. Chem.* 32, 706.

Ward, D.J. (1963). Fatal hypernatraemia after saline emetic. *Br. Med. J.* ii, 432.

Ward, M.J. and Routledge, P.A. (1988). Hypernatraemia and hyperchloraemic acidosis after bleach ingestion. *Hum. Toxicol.* 7, 37.

Wardrop, C.A.J., Lewis, M.H., Tennant, G.B., Williams, R.H.P., and Hughes, L.E. (1977). Acute folate deficiency associated with intravenous nutrition with aminoacid-sorbitol-ethanol: prophylaxis with intravenous folic acid. *Br. J. Haematol.* 37, 521.

Warrell, R.P. Jr, Skelos, A., Alcock, N.W., and Bockman, R.S. (1986). Gallium nitrate for acute treatment of cancer-related hypercalcemia: clinicopharmacological and dose response analysis. *Cancer Res.* 46, 4208.

Warrell, R.P. Jr, Issacs, M., Alcock, N.W., and Bockman, R.S. (1987). Gallium nitrate for treatment of refractory hypercalcemia from parathyroid carcinoma. *Ann. Intern. Med.* 107, 683.

Warrell, R.P. Jr, Israel, R., Frisone, M., Snyder, T., Gaynor, J.J., and Bockman, R.S. (1988). Gallium nitrate for acute treatment of cancer-related hypercalcemia. A randomized, double-blind comparison to calcitonin. *Ann. Intern. Med.* 108, 669.

Wason, S., Lacouture, P.G., and Lovejoy, F.H. (1981). Single high-dose pyridoxine treatment for isoniazid overdose. *JAMA* 246, 1102.

Watkinson, M., Aggett, P.J., and Cole, T.J. (1985). Zinc and acute tropical ulcers in Gambian children and adolescents. *Am. J. Clin. Nutr.* 41, 43.

Watson, A., Coffey, L., Keogh, B., and McCann, S.R. (1983). Severe hypomagnesaemia and hypocalcaemia following gentamicin therapy. *Ir. Med. J.* 76, 381.

Watson, A.J., Watson, M.M., and Keogh, J.A. (1984). Metabolic abnormalities associated with tobramycin therapy. *Ir. J. Med. Sci.* 153, 96.

Webb, D.I., Chodos, R.B., Mahar, C.Q., and Faloon, W.W. (1968). Mechanism of vitamin B_{12} malabsorption in patients receiving colchicine. *N. Engl. J. Med.* 279, 845.

Webberley, M.J. and Murray, J.A. (1989). Life-threatening acute hyponatraemia induced by low dose cyclophosphamide and indomethacin. *Postgrad. Med. J.* 650, 950.

Weber, J.A. and van Zanten, A.P. (1987). Elimination of heparin interference in the determination of gamma-GT. *Clin. Chim. Acta* 169, 345.

Weimar, V.M., Weimar, G.W., and Ceilley, R.J. (1978). Estrogen-induced porphyria cutanea tarda complicating treatment of prostatic carcinoma. *J. Urol.* 120, 643.

Weinman, E.J., Eknoyan, G., and Suki, W.N. (1975). The influence of the extra-cellular volume on the tubular reabsorption of uric acid. *J. Clin. Invest.* 55, 283.

Weinstein, R.E., Bona, R.D., Altman, A.J., Quinn, J.J., Weisman, S.J., Bartolomeo, A., et al. (1989). Severe hyponatremia after repeated intravenous administration of desmopressin. *Am. J. Hematol.* 32, 258.

Weinstein, R.S., Bryce, G.F., Sappington, L.J., King D.W., and Gallagher, B.B. (1984). Decreased serum ionized calcium and normal vitamin D metabolite levels with anticonvulsant drug treatment. *J. Clin. Endocrinol. Metab.* 58, 1003.

Weiss, M., Hassin, D., Eisenstein, Z., and Bank, H. (1979). Elevated skeletal-muscle enzymes during quinidine therapy. *N. Engl. J. Med.* 300, 1218.

Weitekamp, M.R. and Aber, R.C. (1983). Prolonged bleeding times and bleeding diathesis associated with moxalactam administration. *JAMA* 249, 69.

Welborn, J., Meyers, F.J., and O'Grady, L.F. (1988). Renal salt wasting and carboplatinum. *Ann. Intern. Med.* 108, 640.

Welch, W.J., Ott, C.E., Lorenz, J.N., and Kotchen, T.A. (1986). Effects of chlorpropamide on loop of Henle function and plasma renin. *Kidney Int.* 30, 712.

Werther, C.A., Cloud, H., Ohtake, M., and Tamura, T. (1986). Effect of long-term administration of anticonvulsants on copper, zinc, and ceruloplasmin levels. *Drug Nutr. Interact.* 4, 269.

West, C., Carpenter, B.J., and Hakala, T.R. (1987). The incidence of gout in renal transplant recipients. *Am. J. Kidney Dis.* 10, 369.

West, R.J. and Lloyd, J.K. (1975). The effect of cholestyramine on intestinal absorption. *Gut* 16, 93.

Wester, P.O. (1975). Zinc during diuretic treatment. *Lancet* i, 578.

Whang, R. (1976). Hyperkalemia: diagnosis and treatment. *Am. J. Med. Sci.* 272, 19.

Whang, R., Oei, T.O., Aikawa, J.K., Ryan, M.P., Watanabe, A., Chrysant, S.G., et al. (1981). Magnesium and potassium interrelationships. Experimental and clinical. *Acta Med. Scand.* 647 (suppl.), 139.

Whang, R., Flink, E.B., Dyckner, T., Wester, P.O., Aikawa, J.K., and Ryan, M.P. (1985). Magnesium depletion as a cause of refractory potassium depletion. *Arch. Intern. Med.* 145, 1686.

Wharton, J.M., Demopulos, P.A., and Goldschlager, N. (1987). *Torsade de pointes* during administration of pentamidine isethionate. *Am. J. Med.* 83, 571.

Whitaker, K.B., Costa, D., and Moss D.W. (1979). Selective effects of clofibrate on alkaline phosphatase isoenzymes in serum. *Clin. Chim. Acta* 94, 191.

White, S.T., Voter, K., and Perry, J. (1985). Surreptitious warfarin ingestion. *Child Abuse Negl.* 9, 349.

Whyte, K.F., Addis, G.J., Whitesmith, R., and Reid, J.L. (1987). Adrenergic control of plasma magnesium in man. *Clin. Sci.* 72, 135.

Whyte, K.F., Reid, C., Addis, G.J., Whitesmith, R., and Reid, J.L. (1988a). Salbutamol induced hypokalaemia: the effect of theophylline alone and in combination with adrenaline. *Br. J. Clin. Pharmacol.* 25, 571.

Whyte, K.F., Whitesmith, R., and Reid, J.L. (1988*b*). The effect of diuretic therapy on adrenaline-induced hypokalaemia and hypomagnesaemia. *Eur. J. Clin. Pharmacol.* 34, 333.

Widman, L., Dyckner, T., and Wester, P.O. (1982). Effect of moduretic and aldactone on electrolytes in skeletal muscle in patients on long-term diuretic therapy. *Acta Med. Scand.* 661, 33.

Wilkins, M.R., Franklyn, J.A., Woods, K.L., and Kendall, M.J. (1985). Effect of propranolol on thyroid homeostasis of healthy volunteers. *Postgrad. Med. J.* 61, 391.

Wilkinson, R., Kapadi, A.L., Aston, E.M., and Ramsden, D.B. (1983). The effect of β-blockade therapy on serum thyroxine binding globulin (TBG) concentration. *Acta Endocrinol.* 103, 352.

Wilkinson, R., Lucas, G.L., Heath, D.A., Franklin, I.M., Boughton, B.J. (1986). Hypomagnesaemic tetany associated with prolonged treatment with aminoglycosides. *Br. Med. J.* 292, 818.

Willett, W.C. and MacMahon, B. (1984). Diet and cancer — an overview. *N. Eng. J. Med.* 310, 633.

Williams, C., Netzloff, M., Folkerts, L., Vargas, A., Garnica, A., and Frias J. (1984). Vitamin D metabolism and anticonvulsant therapy: effect of sunshine on incidence of osteomalacia. *South. Med. J.* 77, 834.

Williams, H.E. and Wandzilak, T.R. (1989). Oxalate synthesis, transport and the hyperoxaluric syndromes. *J. Urol.* 141, 742.

Williams, J.W., Vera, S.R., Peters, T.G., Luther, R.W., Bhattacharya, S., Spears, H., *et al.* (1986). Biliary excretion of aluminum in aluminum osteodystrophy with liver disease. *Ann. Intern. Med.* 104, 782.

Wills, M.R. (1990). Effects of renal failure. *Clin. Biochem.* 23, 55.

Wills, M.R. and Savory J. (1989). Aluminium and chronic renal failure: sources, absorption, transport and toxicity. *CRC Crit. Rev. Clin. Lab. Sci.* 27, 59.

Wilson, C., Azmy, A.F., Beattie, T.J., and Murphy, A.V. (1986). Hypermagnesemia and progression of renal failure associated with renacidin therapy. *Clin. Nephrol.* 25, 266.

Wilson, R.F., Dulchavsky, S.A., Soullier, G., and Beckman, B. (1987). Problems with 20 or more blood transfusions in 24 hours. *Am. Surg.* 53, 410.

Windsor, A.C.M., Hobbs, C.B., Treby, D.A., and Cowper, R.A. (1972). Effect of tetracycline on leucocyte ascorbic acid levels. *Br. Med. J.* i, 214.

Wing, S.S. and Fantus, I.G. (1987). Adverse immunologic effects of anti-thyroid drugs. *Can. Med. Assoc. J.* 136, 121.

Wolf, P.L. (1989). Lactate dehydrogenase isoenzymes in myocardial disease. *Clin. Lab. Med.* 9, 655.

Wolf, P.L., Williams, D., Coplon, N., and Coulson, A.S. (1972). Low aspartate transaminase activity in serum of patients undergoing chronic hemodialysis. *Clin. Chem.* 18, 567.

Wong, T.C., Palar, A.B., Kin, B.J., and Tricomi, V. (1972). Changes in serum and urinary electrolytes following intra-amniotic injection of hypertonic saline. *N.Y. State J. Med.* 72, 564.

Woods, H.F. and Alberti, K.G.M.M. (1972). Dangers of intravenous fructose. *Lancet* ii, 1354.

Wordsworth, B.P. and Mowat, A.G. (1985). Rapid development of gouty tophi after diuretic therapy. *J. Rheumatol.* 12, 376.

Wu, S.C., Secchi, M.B., Mancarella, S., Oltrona, L., Bettazzi, L., and Sale, M., (1989). Severa ipopotassiemia e rabdomiolisi da uso di spray nasale contenente 9-alfa-fluorprednisolone in soggetto normoteso. *Recenti Prog. Med.* 80, 195.

Wynn, V. (1977). Metabolic effects of danazol. *J. Int. Med. Res.* 5 (suppl. 3), 25.

Yao, F.S., Seidman, S.F., and Artusio, J.G. (1980). Disturbance of consciousness and hypocalcemia after neomycin irrigation, and reversal by calcium and physostigmine. *Anaesthesiology* 53, 69.

Yassa, R., Iskandar, H., Nastase, C., and Camille, Y. (1988). Carbamazepine and hyponatremia in patients with affective disorder. *Am. J. Psychiatry* 145, 339.

Yendt, E.R. and Cohanim, M. (1978). Prevention of calcium stones with thiazides. *Kidney Int.* 13, 397.

Young, D.S. (1990). *Effects of drugs on clinical laboratory tests* (3rd edn). AACC Press, Washington.

Young, G.A., Collins, J.P., and Hill, G.L. (1979). Plasma proteins in patients receiving intravenous amino acids or intravenous hyperalimentation after surgery. *Am. J. Clin. Nutr.* 32, 1192.

Young, G.P., Sullivan, J., and Hurley, T. (1973). Hypokalaemia due to gentamicin/cephalexin in leukaemia. *Lancet* ii, 855.

Yuen, W.C., Whiteoak, R., and Thompson, R.P.H. (1988). Zinc concentrations in leucocytes of patients receiving antiepileptic drugs. *J. Clin. Pathol.* 41, 553.

Yurtkuran, M., Dilek, K., Gullulu, M., Yavuz, M., and Muftuglu, A. (1989). Effects of sublingual administration of nifedipine on arterial pressure, plasma renin activity, and glomerular filtration rate in essential hypertension. *Angiology* 40, 791.

Zabrodski, R.M. and Schnurr, L.P. (1984). Anion gap acidosis with hypoglycemia in acetaminophen toxicity. *Ann. Emerg. Med.* 13, 956.

Zalin, A.M., Hutchinson, C.E., Jong, M., and Matthews, K. (1984). Hyponatraemia during treatment with chlorpropamide and Moduretic (amiloride plus hydrochlorothiazide). *Br. Med. J.* 289, 659.

Zaloga, G.P., Chernow, B., Pock, A., Wood, B., Zaritsky, A., and Zucker, A (1984) Hypomagnesemia is a common complication of aminoglycoside therapy. *Surg. Gynecol. Obstet.* 158, 561.

Zanella, M.T., Maltei, J.E., Draibe, S.A., Kater, C.E., and Ajzan, H. (1985). Inadequate aldosterone response to hyperkalemia during angiotensin converting enzyme inhibition in chronic renal failure. *Clin. Pharmacol. Ther.* 38, 613.

Zantvoort, F.A., Derkx, F.H.M., Boomsma, F., Roos, P.J., and Schalekamp, M.A.D.H. (1986). Theophylline and serum electrolytes. *Ann. Intern. Med.* 104, 134.

Zarrabi, M.H., Zucker, S., Miller, F., Derman, R.M., Romano, G.S., Hartnett, J.A., *et al.* (1979). Immunologic and coagulation disorders in chlorpromazine-treated patients. *Ann. Intern. Med.* 91, 194.

Zavagli, G., Ricci, G., Tataranni, G., Mapelli, G., and Abbasciano, V. (1988). Life-threatening hyponatremia caused by vinblastine. *Med. Oncol. Tumor Pharmacother.* 5, 67.

Zazgornik, J., Shaheen, F.A., Kopsa, H., Biesenbach, G., Kaiser, W., and Waldhausal, W. (1988). Severe hyperkalaemia, hyperchloraemia, hyporeninaemia and hyperaldosteronism in a cyclosporin-treated renal-transplant patient. *Nephrol. Dial. Transplant* 3, 826.

Zeana, C.D., Cerchez, E., and Blidaru, P. (1982). Hepatitis and renal tubular acidosis after anesthesia with methoxyflurane. *Med. Interne* 20, 295.

Zeharia, A., Levy, Y., Rachmel, A., Nitzan, M., and Steinherz, R. (1987). Hyperkalemia as a late side effect of prolonged adrenocorticotropic hormone therapy for infantile spasms. *Helv. Paediatr. Acta* 42, 433.

Zimran, A., Kramer, M., Plaskin, M., and Hershko, C. (1985). Incidence of hyperkalaemia induced by indomethacin in a hospital population. *Br. Med. J.* 291, 107.

Zsigmond, E.K. and Robins, G. (1972). The effect of a series of anti-cancer drugs on plasma cholinesterase activity. *Can. Anaesth. Soc. J.* 19, 75.

16. Disorders of muscle, bone, and connective tissue

H. G. M. SHETTY, P. A. ROUTLEDGE, and D. M. DAVIES

Drugs may produce localized or diffuse disorders of muscle, bone, and connective tissue. These tissues may also be involved as a part of a more generalized drug-induced disease, and when this is the case they are more appropriately dealt with elsewhere in this book. Consequently, parts of this chapter serve mainly as signposts to other chapters, although they do also provide reminders that symptoms and signs involving bones, joints, tendons, and subcutaneous tissues may be the earliest or predominant indications of an adverse drug reaction.

Muscles

Myalgia and cramps

Myalgia, sometimes accompanied by muscle cramps, may be an early symptom of drug-induced polyneuropathy, myopathy, or disorders of the extrapyramidal system, but it is usually soon overshadowed by other features of these conditions (which are discussed in detail in Chapter 18). The same is true of aching in the legs and back, which may be an early feature of vascular compression resulting from retroperitoneal fibrosis induced by methysergide and, possibly, other drugs, for more obvious indications of peripheral vascular insufficiency are not long delayed in such cases.

The pain accompanying venous thrombosis caused by oral contraceptives may be mistaken for myalgia until swelling, and possibly discolouration appear. Conversely, myalgia affecting the calves only while walking, an uncommon complication of oral contraceptive therapy (Davies and Lund 1965), may arouse suspicion of a vascular disorder when none is present. A syndrome of myalgia, arthralgia, and swelling affecting only the hands has been attributed to oral contraceptive therapy (Spiera and Plotz 1969) and in a case of this kind seen by one of us coldness and discolouration of the hands accompanied the attacks of pain. Slight muscular aching in patients taking oral contraceptives may be due to fluid retention caused by these compounds, and several other drugs can cause mild myalgia in this way.

Muscle cramps have also been described in association with diuretic, calcium antagonist, and β_2-agonist therapy. Diuretics may produce hyponatraemia, hypokalaemia, and hypomagnesaemia, which, in turn, cause muscle cramps. These and other adverse effects produced by diuretics are discussed in Chapter 15. In two patients who were not epileptic but had a history of idiopathic cramps, muscle pains and cramps, collapse, and seizures in the absence of electrolyte abnormalities have been attributed to metolazone therapy. The mechanism underlying this syndrome is unclear (Fitzgerald and Brennan 1976).

Oral salbutamol in doses of 4 mg thrice daily has been reported to cause muscle cramps in up to 45 per cent of patients (Palmer 1978). Terbutaline has also been shown to cause painful muscle cramps with persistent muscle twitching and tremor, and these signs and symptoms did not recur when the drug was replaced by orciprenaline (Zelman 1978), though Lotzof (1968) has reported that muscle cramps occur in about 8 per cent of patients receiving orciprenaline and that they disappear when potassium is given concurrently.

Keidar and associates (1982) have described severe cramps with nifedipine in three patients, in two of whom rechallenge with the drug reproduced their symptoms; and in other cases described by MacDonald (1982) paraesthesiae accompanied the cramps.

Doxazosin has been reported to cause muscle cramps in 1 per cent of patients (Young and Brogden 1988).

In some cases of myalgia there is associated elevation of serum muscle enzymes, indicating muscle damage.

Myalgia, muscle weakness, or both, and elevation of CK has been reported with several of the lipid-lowering drugs. Lovastatin causes this 'myopathy' within a few weeks to 2 years of commencement of therapy in a small number of patients (Tobert 1988). The creatine kinase (CK) levels may range from 8000 to 223 000 units per litre (Tobert 1988). There appears to be very little relationship between the magnitude of the CK elevation and the intensity of symptoms (Tobert 1988). Concomitant treatment with cyclosporin, erythromycin, gemfibrozil, or nicotinic acid appears greatly to increase the risk and severity of myopathy due to lovastatin (Tobert 1988; Norman *et al.* 1988; Corpier *et al.* 1988; Marais and Larson 1990), resulting in rhabdomyolysis and acute renal failure in some of the patients in whom these drugs were used concomitantly. The exact mechanism underlying this interaction is unclear, but it is of interest to note that nicotinic acid causes myalgia, cramps, and elevated CK and aspartate aminotransferase when used on its own (Litin and Anderson 1989). Lovastatin should be withheld in patients who have unexplained muscle pain or weakness with elevated CK and also in those who have conditions predisposing to rhabdomyolysis or renal failure (Tobert 1988). Frank myopathy has not been reported with simvastatin, but asymptomatic and transient elevation of CK has been observed in 3–4 per cent of the patients, the causal relationship being uncertain in some cases (Walker 1989). Because of the experience with lovastatin, simvastatin should be used with caution in patients receiving cyclosporin, gemfibrozil, or niacin (Walker 1989). Myalgia, weakness, stiffness, malaise, and elevation of CK is an uncommon adverse effect of clofibrate (Langer and Levy 1968; Smith *et al.* 1970; Sekowski and Samuel 1972), but asymptomatic elevation of muscle enzymes is frequent (Watermeyer *et al.* 1975). The dose of clofibrate should be reduced in patients with renal disease, who tend to develop myopathy most frequently (Goldberg *et al.* 1977). Bezafibrate has also been reported to cause muscle cramps, paresis, elevation of muscle enzymes, myoglobinaemia, and myoglobinuria, particularly in patients with impaired renal function (Rumpf *et al.* 1984).

Suxamethonium has been reported to cause myalgia in about 50 per cent of patients on the day after surgery (Glauber 1966; McGloughlin *et al.* 1988; O'Sullivan *et al.* 1988). The pain occurs mainly in the neck, shoulders, back, and chest and in some cases has been likened to being 'driven over by a bus' (Glauber 1966). The aetiology of this adverse effect is unknown. It is commoner in women (Hegarty 1956; Leatherdale *et al.* 1959), and in non-pregnant than in pregnant women (Crawford 1971; Datta *et al.* 1977; Thind and Bryson 1983). Suxa-

methonium administration results in release of CK and myoglobin, but there is no obvious relationship between the pain and the extent of the biochemical changes (Laurence 1987). The intensity of pain is also unrelated to strength or even the presence of visible fasciculations (Newnam and Loudon 1966; O'Sullivan *et al.* 1988). Waters and Mapleson (1971) have observed that the pain appears to be worse in patients whose muscles do not appear to fasciculate or to fasciculate very little. Irreversible damage to muscle spindles (Rack and Westbury 1966), potassium flux (Mayrhofer 1959), lactic acid (Konig 1956), and serotonin (Kaniaris *et al.* 1973) have all been implicated in the causation of pain. Injection of small, non-paralysing doses of a non-depolarizing relaxant such as tubocurarine (Blitt *et al.* 1981) or gallamine, 2–3 minutes before suxamethonium, reduces the frequency of myalgia by about 20–30 per cent (White 1962; Glauber 1966; Erkola *et al.* 1983); but the disadvantages of non-depolarizing drugs are that they diminish or abolish the intensity of fasciculations, which are useful indicators of the drug effect for the anaesthetist, and impair the intensity of neuromuscular block, so that more suxamethonium is required to produce the desired effect (Cullen 1971; Masey *et al.* 1983). Soluble aspirin 600 mg given 1 hour preoperatively has been shown to reduce the frequency of myalgia to 21 per cent compared with 57 per cent in patients given suxamethonium alone and 36 per cent in a group who received tubocurarine 0.05 mg per kg 3 minutes before induction (McGloughlin *et al.* 1988). Aspirin does not impair the intensity of neuromuscular block or abolish the visible fasciculations, and its exact mechanism of action in relieving the myalgia is not known. Although it has been claimed that diazepam is effective in preventing myalgia (Fahmy *et al.* 1979), it has not been shown to be so in a study comparing its effect with that of tubocurarine (Manchikanti 1984).

Myalgia has been described with a variety of other drugs. Danazol has been reported to cause myalgia, muscle cramps, muscle spasm, and elevation of CK (Buttram *et al.* 1985; Watts *et al.* 1985).

Severe myalgia, predominantly affecting the shoulder girdle and upper limbs, associated with elevation of CK, has occurred in hyperthyroid women treated with carbimazole for between 3 weeks and 3 months. Stopping the drug resulted in rapid resolution of symptoms and return of CK to normal concentrations (Page and Nussey 1989); it has been suggested that in such cases the cause may be 'tissue hypothyroidism' rather than a direct adverse effect of the drug (O'Malley 1989). A 37-year-old woman with Graves' disease developed generalized severe muscle pain, cramps, and biochemical and histological evidence of rhabdomyolysis during treatment with cyclosporin (Noppen *et al.* 1987), the symptoms recurring when the drug was given again. Three other cases of 'myopathy' have been attributed to cyclosporin (Goy *et al.* 1989), although the aetiological role of the drug in these cases has been questioned (Chassagne *et al.* 1989).

Other drugs that have been described to cause myalgia include cimetidine (Burland 1978), enalapril (Cooper *et al.* 1987), guanethidine (Stocks and Robertson 1966), intramuscular iron injections (Ben-Ishay 1961), nalidixic acid (Gleckman *et al.* 1979), and zidovudine (Richman *et al.* 1987).

Topical minoxidil therapy has been associated with a reversible 'pseudopolymyalgia' syndrome of severe pain in the pelvic and shoulder girdles, fatigue, anorexia, weight loss, and a normal erythrocyte sedimentation rate. The symptoms cleared a few days after stopping the drug and recurred on rechallenge (Colamarino *et al.* 1990). A similar syndrome has complicated treatment with enalapril (Le Loët *et al.* 1989) and dipyridamole (Chassagne *et al.* 1990).

Severe and widespread myalgia and joint pains may occur in patients who have been taking daily doses of corticosteroids equivalent to 10 mg or more of prednisone for 30 days or longer when steroid therapy is withdrawn. In a few cases the illness progresses until it resembles systemic lupus erythematosus, and death may ensue (Kriegel and Müller 1972). Whether this type of case represents an unmasked spontaneous lupus erythematosus, previously controlled by the steroid therapy, is not clear. It would seem rational to treat these disorders by administering steroids again in the maximum dosage previously taken by the patient. The dose is then reduced by small amounts (1–2.5 mg of prednisone or its equivalent) at intervals of several days or longer, depending on the patient's condition. Complete rest, heavy sedation, and analgesic therapy should also be given (Kriegel and Müller 1972).

Muscle damage

Drugs may damage muscular tissue in several ways. The most obvious is by local action following intramuscular injection, and severe damage of this kind has been caused by chlorpromazine (O'Connor 1980) and diclofenac (Müller-Vahl 1984). This is rarely disabling, unless necrosis (rhabdomyolysis) is extensive or the site of injection becomes infected, and is usually of clinical importance only because it may cause a rise in the serum concentration of enzymes originating in muscle, which may be misleading if the possibility is overlooked (see

Creatine kinase — Chapter 15). Repeated intramuscular injections of some drugs may cause severe fibrosis and contracture. The drugs most often implicated in western countries are the opiates (Mastaglia *et al.* 1971; Adams *et al.* 1983), but in India and South America the culprit is often an antibiotic (Blain and Lane 1983). Sterile abscesses and pain on injection have been described in between 18 and 75 per cent of patients treated with intramuscular pentamidine isethionate (Goa and Campoli-Richards 1987). Muscle damage, functional or anatomical, or both, may also accompany severe drug-induced muscle spasm of the kind described under Fractures and dislocations below; may rarely follow the use of suxamethonium (Gibbs 1978); or may occur as a rare adverse effect of drug abuse (amphetamine [Kendrick *et al.* 1977]; heroin [Schwartzfarb *et al.* 1977]; or phencyclidine [Cogen *et al.* 1978]). It is a feature of drug-induced myasthenia and myopathy.

The injury may be primary, due to a direct action of the drug on muscle tissue, muscle metabolic enzymes, or neuromuscular transmitters; or secondary, when it follows hypokalaemia induced by the drug concerned. It is also a feature of polymyositis and dermatomyositis, disorders occasionally precipitated by drug allergy. Traditionally, myasthenia and myopathy come within the province of the neurologist and they are dealt with in Chapter 18.

Rhabdomyolysis and myoglobinuria are very serious adverse effects of drugs. Rhabdomyolysis may result from a direct myotoxic effect of the drug; muscle ischaemia in drug overdose; or drug-induced malignant hyperthermia, the neuroleptic malignant syndrome, the central cholinergic syndrome, and polymyositis.

Aminocaproic acid, amphetamine, barbiturates, chloroquine, cocaine, colchicine, diphenhydramine, diuretics, doxylamine, emetics, heroin, laxatives, lovastatin, methadone, pentazocine, phencyclidine, retinoids, theophylline, and vincristine have been reported to cause rhabdomyolysis. For a detailed discussion of this disorder the reader is referred to a review by Köppel (1989).

Polymyositis and dermatomyositis

Penicillamine causes polymyositis, which may be mild, with elevation of muscle enzymes alone; moderately severe, with moderate muscular weakness; or severe, with marked muscular weakness, myolysis, and myocarditis, resulting in death (Wouters *et al.* 1982; Doyle *et al.* 1983). It causes dermatomyositis less frequently (Wouters *et al.* 1982). Polymyositis has also been attributed to cimetidine (Matthiesen 1979), in which case it has sometimes been accompanied by interstitial nephritis (Watson *et al.* 1983).

Death due to respiratory and renal failure has been reported in a young woman suffering from Chagas' disease, who developed acute polymyositis, toxic erythema, and purpura while taking nifurtimox (Shaw *et al.* 1982).

Dermatomyositis has occurred in an 11-year-old boy a few days after injection of the local anaesthetic carticaine for tooth extraction, but a causal relationship has not been established (Rose *et al.* 1985).

Eosinophilia–myalgia syndrome

This is a disease characterized by severe, incapacitating myalgia and a total peripheral blood eosinophil count of more than 1×10^9 cells per litre (Centres for Disease Control 1990; Kilbourne *et al.* 1990). In almost all the cases so far described the patients had taken over-the-counter dietary supplements containing L-tryptophan. The median dose ingested was 1.5 g daily for periods of a few weeks to several years. In some patients the syndrome appeared only after they had stopped taking the supplements.

Most of the affected patients are women. In addition to myalgia, a number of other symptoms and signs may occur — fatigue, arthralgia, fever, cough, dyspnoea, oedema and induration of the extremities with a tendency to involve the lower limbs more than the upper limbs, alopecia, transient maculopapular or urticarial rashes in the early stages and morphoea-like lesions in the late stages, mouth ulcers, myocarditis, right ventricular strain, tricuspid insufficiency, muscle cramps, paraesthesiae, and ascending polyneuropathy resembling the Guillain–Barré syndrome (Kaufman *et al.* 1990; Medsger 1990). Eosinophilia is found in all cases. The erythrocyte sedimentation rate is normal or only slightly elevated and serum CK concentrations are rarely elevated. Histological examination of the muscles shows perivascular accumulation of lymphocytes and plasma cells, but no evidence of myofibrillar degeneration, indicating that the myalgia is likely to be due to damage to the peripheral sensory nerves. In fact, sensory and motor neurological symptoms and electrophysiological evidence of axonal degeneration have been described in some patients. Although dyspnoea and hypoxaemia are common, the chest X-ray is often clear and rarely shows inflammatory infiltration (Kaufman *et al.* 1990; Medsger 1990).

The course of the disease is variable. In some patients it resolves quickly after discontinuing L-tryptophan

preparations, but in the majority it is severe, disabling, and chronic and may progress even after the drug is withheld (Kaufman *et al.* 1990). Of over 1400 cases reported in the USA between October 1989 and April 1990, a third have required hospitalization and 19 have died (Medsger 1990; Diggle 1990). Once the diagnosis is established, L-tryptophan tablets or food supplements containing this amino acid should be discontinued. Corticosteroids have been used in high doses in severe cases but their efficacy remains to be established (*Drugs and Therapeutics Bulletin* 1990; Kaufman *et al.* 1990).

Since the initial reports from New Mexico, USA, the syndrome has appeared in other parts of the USA, and in the UK and elsewhere in Europe. Retrospective analysis of cases has revealed that diffuse fasciitis with eosinophilia was first reported in 1974 in the USA, shortly after the introduction of L-tryptophan to the market (Shulman 1975), and the lack of cases over the next 14 years, despite continued use of the amino acid, with a sudden increase in the number of reports in 1989, suggests that L-tryptophan itself may not be the aetiological agent. One hypothesis is that a contaminant, which somehow gets incorporated into L-tryptophan during manufacture, may be responsible. Most of the patients with the syndrome in Oregon, USA appear to have obtained L-tryptophan in the first 5 months of 1989 from a single company that used aniline and anthranilic acid as starting compounds for tryptophan synthesis (Slutsker *et al.* 1990). Aniline and anilide complexes contained in adulterated rape seed oil have been proposed as a possible cause of the epidemic 'toxic-oil syndrome' that was described in Spain in 1981 (Kilbourne *et al.* 1983). The eosinophilia–myalgia syndrome has many clinical similarities to the toxic-oil syndrome, and both these conditions are associated with eosinophilia though their pathophysiology may be diferent. The serum IgE levels have been shown to be elevated in 37–50 per cent of patients with the toxic-oil syndrome but normal in most cases of eosinophilia–myalgia syndrome (Toxic Epidemic Syndrome Study Group 1982; Centers for Disease Control 1990; Kaufman *et al.* 1990).

Belongia and others (1990) have found an association between the outbreak of eosinophilia–myalgia syndrome in 1989 in Minnesota, USA and the use of reduced quantities of powdered carbon in a purification step together with the use of a new strain of *Bacillus amyloliquefaciens* (Strain V) for the fermentation process in the manufacture of tryptophan by one company. They have also described an absorbance peak on high-performance liquid chromatography of the tryptophan manufactured by that company, which was present in 9 of the 12 lots (75 per cent) used by the patients but only 3 of

11 lots (27 per cent) used by the controls. It has been suggested that 'the chemical constituent representing the peak may contribute to the pathogenesis or it may be a surrogate for another chemical that induces the syndrome'. Eosinophilia and a scleroderma-like syndrome have been observed in an individual with abnormal tryptophan metabolism (Sternberg *et al.* 1980) and alteration of bioavailability of tryptophan by a contaminant is thought to be the cause of 'fog fever' seen in cattle, which develop interstitial pneumonia with eosinophilic infiltrates (Blood and Radostits 1989). Plasma tryptophan levels before and after an oral dose in patients with the eosinophilia–myalgia syndrome and in normal subjects are similar, but the plasma L-kynurenine and quinolinic acid, which are metabolites of tryptophan, are significantly higher in patients with active disease compared with those in whom eosinophilia has resolved and normal subjects. These findings suggest activation of the enzyme indoleamine-2,3-dioxygenase, which may have a pathogenetic role in the syndrome (Silver *et al.* 1990). Further research is needed to clarify the aetiology and pathogenesis of this serious condition.

Bones

Osteoporosis and osteomalacia

Pain caused by drug-induced osteoporosis is usually acute in onset and commonly affects the back because of vertebral compression and collapse, but it may arise elsewhere due to spontaneous fractures of the ribs, pelvis, or other bones. Osteomalacia, too, may cause pain arising in the spine, though aching in other parts of the skeleton is likely, and spontaneous fractures are not uncommon. Sudden, or gradual and progressive, deformity of the spine may occur in either osteoporosis or osteomalacia. These disorders and their pathogeneses are discussed in Chapter 15.

Slipped epiphysis

It has been suspected for many years that slipping of the upper femoral epiphysis might have an endocrine basis. Harris (1950) concluded from experiments in rats that growth hormone decreases (while sex hormones increase) the shearing strength of the epiphyseal plate, thus predisposing to slipping of the epiphysis by altering the thickness of the third layer of the epiphyseal plate. He suggested that these findings might provide an explanation for the human disorder, especially when associated with the adiposogenital syndrome or with rapid

adolescent growth. This hypothesis was supported by a case report (Rennie and Michell 1974) which described the development of a slipped femoral disc in a 15-year-old girl during treatment with growth hormone. Fidler and Brook (1974) reported similar occurrences in two younger children treated with the hormone.

Fractures and dislocations

Since patients with drug-induced osteomalacia may develop spontaneous fractures (see above), it is obvious that they are even more likely to sustain fractures from falls or other kinds of trauma. Ingestion of aluminium-containing antacids in large quantities for prolonged periods may result in phosphate depletion, osteomalacia, and pseudofractures in patients with normal renal function (Spencer and Kramer 1983). In patients with chronic renal failure who are on dialysis, exposure to excessive amounts of aluminium in the dialysate is believed to have a direct toxic effect on mineralization of bone and this may result in a high frequency of spontaneous fractures (Schneider *et al.* 1984; Malluche and Faugère 1985).

Fractures caused by falls are strongly associated with the use of barbiturates in the elderly (MacDonald and MacDonald 1977). Apart from causing impaired awareness and unsteadiness (a possible hazard of all hypnotics and sedatives in the elderly), barbiturates stimulate hepatic enzymes involved in the metabolism of vitamin D, and may thus induce or aggravate osteomalacia (Marshall 1977) (see also Chapter 15). The findings of MacDonald and MacDonald (1977) gained support from a case–control study involving 1021 elderly patients with hip fractures and 5606 elderly controls, which showed a significantly increased risk of hip fractures in association with hypnotics and anxiolytics that have long half-lives, tricyclic antidepressants, and antipsychotics. The risk increased with increasing doses of these drugs (Ray *et al.* 1987). Patients taking levodopa plus benserazide for parkinsonism are more prone to fractures than those taking other antiparkinsonian drugs. This may partly be due to the increased mobility of the patients produced by the drugs and therefore an increased likelihood of accidental falls, but it is interesting to note that benserazide has caused skeletal changes in rats used for toxicity investigations (Barbeau and Roy 1976).

Repeated intramuscular injections into the deltoid may produce abduction deformity of the arm (Levin and Engel 1975) due to fibrosis of the muscle and contraction of fibrous tissue, which in extreme cases may lead to dislocation of the shoulder (Cozen 1977).

Muscle spasm severe enough to cause fracture–s0dislocation of the hips complicated myelography with meglumine iocarmate (Eastwood *et al.* 1978).

Aseptic (avascular, ischaemic) necrosis

The ordinary spontaneous fracture of bone has already been discussed; a special type of spontaneous fracture remains to be described.

Aseptic necrosis of bone is associated with certain types of drug therapy, as well as with trauma, a variety of natural disorders (Sutton 1968) or, very rarely, arteriography or radiotherapy (Kriegel and Müller 1972). The drug-induced disorder is almost always a complication of treatment with adrenal corticosteroids (Cruess 1977) or ACTH and occurs too often to be coincidental, even in rheumatoid arthritis and systemic lupus erythematosus, which appear to predispose to aseptic necrosis. It may be, however, that only in certain conditions (of which rheumatoid arthritis and systemic lupus erythematosus may be examples) do steroids induce avascular necrosis, a possibility strengthened by the observation that while avascular necrosis may affect patients with renal disease under treatment with steroids and renal dialysis it is said not to occur in children with the nephrotic syndrome treated only with steroids (Gregg *et al*. 1980). The head of the femur is the commonest site of involvement (Solomon 1973) but the head of the humerus, the tibia, the condyle of the mandible, and the carpal bones may also be affected. In corticosteroid-induced cases, dose appears to be the major predictor of the risk of avascular necrosis (Felson and Anderson 1987). Large doses of prednisolone (60 mg) for 14 days every 6 weeks (Watkins and Williams 1982) have resulted in avascular necrosis of the head of the femur. In these cases prednisolone had been given with a number of cytotoxic drugs in the treatment of Hodgkin's disease. Even short courses of dexamethasone in large doses have caused the disease (McCluskey and Gutteridge 1982). The pathogenesis of steroid-induced aseptic necrosis is still unclear, but among the more plausible suggestions are a steroid-induced vasculitis of the small vessels supplying the affected portion of bone, or fat embolism, the fat emboli originating in a liver rendered excessively fatty by the action of adrenal corticosteroids or ACTH (Sutton 1968). The fat embolism theory was not supported, however, by the histological studies of Solomon (1973), who examined 42 femoral heads removed from patients with avascular necrosis and concluded that the amount and the location of fat in the specimens was much the same as in specimens from patients with normal hips or from those suffering from other disorders of the femoral head. He proposed an alternative explanation for the disease, namely, that the diminished joint sensibility produced by the anti-inflammatory effect (and consequent analgesic effect) of steroids predisposes to microtrauma in osteoporotic bone, resulting in subarticular collapse of the femoral head.

Avascular necrosis is said to have complicated treatment with drugs of the 'phenylbutazone group' (Murray and Jacobson 1972), and has been caused by combination cancer chemotherapy (Harper *et al*. 1984).

Osteosclerosis, ectopic calcification, bone thickening, and bone destruction

Osteosclerosis may result from excessive doses of vitamin A or D, or fluorine, and is a rare feature of the milk–alkali syndrome. The bone changes of Vitamin A excess are normally believed to be short-lasting, although a patient with hyperostosis induced by vitamin A has been found to have permanent deformity of long bones and scoliosis after 12 years of follow-up (Ruby and Mital 1974). Chronic vitamin D poisoning may result in ectopic calcification in the muscles, tendons, ligaments, subcutaneous tissue, and other parts of the body. Excessive intake of vitamin A or fluoride may result in calcification, usually confined to the tendons and periarticular tissues (Kriegel and Müller 1972). Calcification may rarely occur at the site of intramuscular or subcutaneous injections (Kriegel and Müller 1972).

Thickening of the skull, mainly the diploic space, with no abnormalities of other bones, has been observed in patients on long-term treatment with phenytoin, some of whom were also on other anticonvulsant drugs (Kattan 1970). Sodium valproate therapy has been reported to cause generalized skeletal pain and osteosclerosis affecting the distal metaphyses of femur, radius, and ulna (John 1981). The mechanism of these manifestations is unclear. Long-term isotretinoin therapy for ichthyosis has been shown to be associated with arthralgia or myalgia and an ossification disorder resembling diffuse idiopathic skeletal hyperostosis. Although lowering the dose or withdrawal of the drug resulted in clinical improvement, the radiological changes persisted over the observation period (Pittsley and Yoder 1983).

Asymptomatic skeletal fluorosis resulting in osteosclerosis, predominantly affecting the axial skeleton, has been observed in patients on long-term treatment with niflumic acid and flufenamic acid capsules containing fluoride (Del Favero 1984; Vrhovac 1988). The biochemical abnormalities included hypocalcemia, hypocalciuria, high urinary fluoride, and raised serum alkaline phosphatase. Bone biopsy showed an increase in trabecular bone volume suggestive of bone fluorosis. The mechanism underlying the fluoride-induced changes in bone structure and the uneven distribution of osteosclerosis is unclear.

Clubbing of fingers associated with the ingestion of excessive doses of purgatives was described by Silk and others (1975), and other cases of this kind were subsequently described (Prior and White 1978; Malmquist *et al.* 1980), and a combination of clubbing of digits and hypertrophic osteoarthopathy due to purgative abuse has been described by Armstrong and others (1981). In the latter case the clubbing disappeared within 6 months of withdrawal of the purgative (senna in the form of Senokot), though at the time of the report the radiological abnormalities were still present.

Newman and Ling (1985) have shown a significant association between the use of non-steroidal anti-inflammatory drugs (NSAID) in patients with primary osteoarthrosis of the hip and acetabular destruction. The mechanism of this process is unclear, but it has been suggested that NSAID may inhibit the repair of necrotic bone, resulting in femoral head necrosis and trabecular microfractures (Newman and Ling 1985).

Joints

Arthralgia and arthritis

Mild arthralgia and arthritis may accompany almost any type of generalized skin eruption caused by drugs (discussed in Chapter 17); and more severe joint pains, with associated swelling, are an essential component of 'serum sickness', which can be induced by any one of a number of drugs (discussed in Chapter 25). A particularly severe example of arthropathy associated with a reaction of this kind has been reported as an adverse reaction to carbimazole (Bethel 1979); and the crippling arthritis attributed to vaccination against swine influenza (Hasler *v* United States 1981) may have had a similar cause. Arthritis has been observed in 0.5 per cent of patients receiving BCG immunotherapy (Torisu *et al.* 1978; Lamm *et al.* 1986; Ochsenkühn *et al.* 1990). It has been suggested that cross reactivity between BCG and HLA-B27 may underlie the pathogenesis of this arthritis (Ochsenkühn *et al.* 1990).

Arthralgia and arthritis may be the early manifestation of systemic lupus erythematosus, and it is now recognized that some cases of this disorder can be attributed to drug treatment. The drugs implicated and the complex mechanisms involved are described later in this chapter. This disorder may also appear for the first time during the withdrawal of steroid therapy. (See the section on Myalgia, under Muscles).

Another collagen disease that may present with aches and pains is arteritis. This uncommon disease may arise spontaneously or may be induced by drugs (Moser 1964), notably sulphonamides. Whether or not treatment with adrenal corticosteroids is usually responsible for the arteritis that may complicate rheumatoid arthritis remains in doubt. In addition to arthralgia and myalgia, arteritis may produce a confusing multiplicity of adverse effects, including malaise, fever, anaemia, rashes, wasting, peripheral neuropathy, hypertension, hepatitis, purpura, and a variety of other symptoms and signs resulting from arterial narrowing, necrosis, thrombosis, or haemorrhage. In the absence of treatment most cases run a progressive course resulting in death from haemorrhage, pulmonary oedema, renal failure, or a cerebrovascular accident.

Septic arthritis may occur as a result of faulty aseptic technique during intra-articular injections, or may complicate treatment with drugs that lower the body's resistance to infection, a subject discussed in detail in Chapter 23.

Quinidine has been reported to cause symmetrical, reversible polyarthritis with no immunological abnormalities on three occasions in one patient (Kertes and Hunt 1982).

Quinolones have been shown to cause erosions of articular cartilage and permanent damage to weight-bearing joints in immature dogs when administered in very high doses for prolonged periods (Neu 1988). Joint disease has been described in association with quinolone therapy in human patients, involving norfloxacin (Jeandel *et al.* 1989), perfloxacin (Kesseler *et al.* 1989), and ciprofloxacin (Ball 1986; Alfaham *et al.* 1987). Nalidixic acid (the oldest of the quinolones) has also caused arthralgia and arthritis (Bailey *et al.* 1972; Gleckman *et al.* 1979).

Joint effusion, which recurred on rechallenge, has been attributed to practolol therapy (Fraser and Irvine 1976). Although it has been reported that arthralgia is a common adverse effect of β-blockers, particularly metoprolol (Savola 1983, 1984; Sills and Bosco 1986), a case–control study of 127 patients attending a hypertension clinic found no significant association (Walker and Ramsay 1985). An acute febrile polyarthritis has been reported with the antihypertensive drug prazosin (Cairns and Jordan 1976). Captopril has been reported to cause a migratory polyarthralgia with a false-positive test (VDRL) for syphilis, both of which resolved on discontinuation of the drug (Malnick and Schattner 1989).

The most severe joint pain of all is caused by the arthritis of acute gout, which can be precipitated by certain types of drug therapy; these and the mechanisms involved are discussed in Chapter 15.

An interesting and unusual complication of treatment for gout has been described: telescoping of the fingers and toes developed in a patient with chronic tophaceous gout during treatment with allopurinol, due to rapid resorption, without replacement by new bone, of large and extensive osseous tophi (Gottlieb and Gray 1977).

Arthralgia may be a feature of the steroid-withdrawal syndrome, but, paradoxically, steroids very rarely cause arthralgia and arthritis (Newmark *et al.* 1974; Bailey and Armour 1974; Bennett and Strong 1975).

An unusual effect of steroids was reported by Tannenbaum (1972), who described a patient whose dermatitis of the distal phalanx of a finger was treated for 4 months with local applications of fluorinated steroids. The treatment resulted in disappearance of part of the underlying bone, which developed a 'pencil-sharpener' appearance that persisted during the 2 years of observation.

There is nothing to suggest that the most common collagen disease, rheumatoid arthritis, is ever induced by drugs, but iron–dextran complex (Imferon) when given by the 'total dose' method may cause an acute exacerbation of some of the symptoms and signs of this disorder, and this drug may cause arthralgia in patients not known to be suffering from rheumatoid arthritis.

Sodium aurothiomalate has also been reported to cause exacerbation of rheumatoid arthritis at the start of treatment (Reynolds 1989). Levamisole has been reported to worsen rheumatoid arthritis (Dinai and Pras 1975) and to cause arthritis in two patients with Crohn's disease (Segal *et al.* 1977) and in a patient with Behçet's syndrome on two occasions when it was given (Siklos 1977). Meclofenamic acid has been shown to aggravate psoriatic arthropathy (Meyerhoff 1983).

A polyarthritis has been described in association with clindamycin-induced colitis (Rollins and Moeller 1975). Painless deforming arthropathy has been reported with purgative abuse (Frier and Scott 1977) and is believed to be related to chronic purgative-induced bowel disease.

Arthritis has been attributed to treatment with propylthiouracil (Oh *et al.* 1983), methimazole (Hietarinta and Merilanti-Palo 1989), phenytoin (Stalnikowicz *et al.* 1982), cimetidine (CSM 1981), and ranitidine (SADRAC 1989).

Haemarthrosis

In patients who are on anticoagulant therapy, haemarthrosis has been described in the absence of obvious trauma (McLaughlin *et al.* 1966).

Shoulder–hand syndrome

A syndrome resembling the naturally occurring shoulder–hand syndrome, characterized by arthralgia affecting the shoulder and other joints of the upper limbs and sometimes accompanied by contractures and other changes, was first described many years ago as a complication of treatment with phenobarbitone (Maillard and Renard 1925). Subsequently, the barbiturates were implicated in similar cases reported in France (Maillard and Thomazi 1931), Bériel and Barber 1934; Castin and Gardien 1934; Arlet *et al.* 1967; Lequesne 1967), Scandinavia (Lövgren 1948), Holland (van der Korst *et al.* 1960) and, most recently, Chile (Cuchacovich and Kappes 1987). In the cases attributed to phenobarbitone the drug had been given in daily doses of 100–300 mg for periods varying from a few weeks to more than 20 years, and the condition was usually, though not invariably, bilateral. The way in which phenobarbitone produced these changes was not apparent.

In many patients, particularly those with bilateral disease, acute symptoms of burning pain, oedematous swelling, and decreased sweating were followed after an interval of 3–9 months by dystrophic changes in the hand and contractures of the fingers (van der Korst *et al.* 1960).

In the 1960s a number of reports were published suggesting antituberculous therapy as a cause of the shoulder–hand syndrome, suspicion falling mainly on isoniazid (see Kriegel and Müller 1972). Typically, there was a sudden onset of pain, tenderness, and stiffness in the joints of the hand accompanied by severe pain in the shoulder. Most patients also experienced widespread myalgia and arthralgia, and some felt tired and depressed. Although paraesthesiae were felt by some patients, no convincing objective signs of neuropathy appeared. The disease was commonest in men aged 40–50 years. In some cases, restriction of movement of the shoulders and fingers became apparent within a few days of onset of symptoms, and after a few weeks the acute pain subsided to leave a 'frozen shoulder', flexion deformity of the elbow, and tendon contractures of the hand (Good *et al.* 1965). Similar deformities have occurred in the lower limbs (McKusick and Hsu 1961). In one series of cases (McKusick and Hsu 1961) isoniazid was the only antituberculous agent common to all the treatment regimens, and suspicion that this drug was to blame was strengthened by a fall in the incidence of the rheumatic syndrome in certain hospitals when the routine daily dosage of isoniazid was reduced from 600 mg to 300 mg (McKusick 1965).

The mechanism by which isoniazid produces rheumatic disorders is unclear, but it has been suggested

(Good *et al.* 1965) that as isoniazid interferes with the metabolism of serotonin (Zarafonetis and Kalas 1960) an excess of this substance may produce fibrosis, as it has been shown to do when injected into the joints of animals, particularly those given isoniazid concurrently (Gum *et al.* 1960). There is no firm evidence that pyridoxine metabolism is involved in the production of the shoulder–hand syndrome, and prophylactic treatment with pyridoxine does not prevent the disorder (Good *et al.* 1965).

Complete immobility and severe pain of shoulder joint has been reported with antimony sodium tartrate injections. It occurred equally in the arm used for injection or in the other arm and the movement in the shoulder joint was regained 3–5 days after discontinuation of the drug (Davies 1968).

Disorders of growth

Corticosteroids

Long-term corticosteroid therapy in children inhibits hypophyseal growth hormone secretion and reduces the sensitivity of the peripheral tissues to the hormone, resulting in retardation of linear growth (Bondy 1985). It has been shown that the vitamin D_3 metabolites are reduced in the plasma of children on daily or intermittent long-term corticosteroid therapy for various disorders, and this may be the cause of inhibition of metabolism in cartilage and bone tissue rather than a direct effect of corticosteroids (Chesney *et al.* 1978; O'Reagan *et al.* 1979). Although corticotrophin (ACTH) is thought to produce less inhibition of growth than corticosteroids (Bondy 1985), it is recognized that it does inhibit growth hormone secretion and should therefore be used with caution in children if long-term therapy is required. It is difficult to assess objectively the contribution of corticosteroids and corticotrophin to growth retardation in many children who are taking them for serious systemic diseases that themselves may have a growth-suppressant effect. Withdrawal of corticosteroids before the end of puberty may result in normal growth in some children, but this may not be the case in all (Bondy 1985). Avoiding corticosteroids if at all possible and using them in smallest possible doses and intermittently are the best options in children to reduce the likelihood of growth impairment.

Tetracyclines

Tetracyclines are deposited in the growing bone and teeth of the fetus if administered during pregnancy and

of the infant and young child if administered in infancy or early childhood. At doses of 7–25 mg (*The Lancet* 1963) they may produce an inhibition of linear growth by about 40 per cent (Cohlan *et al.* 1963). The effect of tetracyclines on teeth is described in Chapter 9. These drugs should be avoided in pregnancy and in children under the age of 12 years (*British National Formulary* 1990).

Central nervous system stimulants

Use of methylphenidate, amphetamine, and pemoline in prepubertal children with the hyperactive or attention-deficit syndrome has been shown to be associated with a retardation of growth in weight and stature that is related to the dose of the drugs and absence of 'drug holidays' (Safer and Allen 1973; Roche *et al.* 1979; Dickinson et al. 1979). It has been suggested that these drugs may interfere with the release of growth hormone that is normally produced by slow-wave sleep (Barter and Kammer 1978).

Cocaine

Cocaine abuse during pregnancy has been associated with significant growth retardation and a variety of other problems in infants, including congenital abnormalities, withdrawal symptoms, and an increased incidence of preterm delivery, perinatal mortality, and intrauterine fetal death (Neerhof *et al.* 1989; Fulroth *et al.* 1989).

Lead

Shukla and associates (1989) have reported that exposure to high concentrations of lead *in utero*, or relatively high concentrations in the neonatal period has a detrimental effect on growth in stature of infants, but Sachs and Moel (1989) found no correlation between growth and blood lead at any concentration.

Connective tissues

Tendons

Tendons may be affected in drug-induced gout, as in the natural disorder. They may also be involved in ectopic calcification, described earlier.

Tenosynovitis affecting both Achilles tendons has been reported with ciprofloxacin therapy (McEwan and Davey 1988).

Spontaneous rupture of tendons may complicate treatment with steroid given by mouth or by local injection. The Achilles tendon is most often involved, but the patellar tendon can also rupture (Lee 1957; Cowan and Alexander 1961; Lee 1961; Smaill 1961; Melmed 1965; Ismail *et al.* 1969; Bedi and Ellis 1970). Cooney and others (1980) have claimed that rupture of tendons in patients taking corticosteroids is mainly due to natural connective tissue disorders affecting the tendons rather than to the steroids alone, and stated that no cases of tendon rupture had occurred in patients on high-dose steroid therapy for such diseases as asthma, skin disease, or lymphoproliferative conditions. Haines (1983), however, has described three patients who suffered bilateral rupture of the Achilles tendon while on systemic steroid therapy for chest diseases. He suggested that steroid therapy probably suppresses the repair of degenerated or partially ruptured tendons to such an extent that complete rupture can occur after minor strain.

Adipose tissue

Atrophy and hypertrophy

Atrophy of subcutaneous fatty tissue may develop at the site of injection or topical application of corticosteroids (Johns and Bower 1970). There may be a genetic susceptibility to the corticosteroid-induced lipoatrophy. Three cases of severe lipoatrophy occurring within the same family after intramuscular injection of triamcinolone have been reported (von Eickstedt and Elsässer 1988). Hypertrophy of the adipose tissue may occur at the periphery of atrophic lesions, or may be the predominant reaction, when it leads to the formation of lipomata (Kriegel and Müller 1972). Lipomatosis affecting the mediastinal (Teates 1970), paraspinal (Streiter *et al.* 1982), and epidural (Bischoff 1988) regions has been attributed to corticosteroid therapy.

Atrophy and hypertrophy of subcutaneous fatty tissue may also develop with bovine and porcine insulins (McNally *et al.* 1988). Purified insulins appear to cause lipoatrophy less frequently than the conventional insulins. Injection of a purer animal insulin or human insulin into and around the atrophic tissue may result in the reversal of this adverse effect. Repeated injections of insulin to the same site may result in lipohypertrophy. This adverse effect can be averted by using different sites for injecting insulin, but the variability in insulin absorption from different anatomical sites should be kept in mind (Koivisto and Felig 1980; McNalley *et al.* 1988).

Nodular panniculitis

This disorder, characterized by subcutaneous nodules that may be tender and may later disappear leaving depressions at the affected sites, has occasionally followed the withdrawal of corticosteroid therapy (Taranta *et al.* 1958; Roenick *et al.* 1964; Jaffe *et al.* 1971; Saxena and Nigam 1988).

Fibrous tissue

A number of migrainous patients under treatment with vasoconstrictor drugs have developed a disorder characterized by proliferation of fibrous tissue. Retroperitoneal fibrous tissue is mainly affected, but fibrotic changes have also been detected in the mediastinum, pleura, lungs, and pericardium. In most instances methysergide is believed to have been responsible for this disorder (Graham *et al.* 1964 1968; Utz *et al.* 1965; Graham *et al.* 1966) but in a small number of cases ergotamine or dihydroergotamine are also suspected to have initiated fibrotic changes or to have reactivated fibrosis originally induced by methysergide (Graham *et al.* 1966). The symptoms and signs of retroperitoneal fibrosis include persistent pain in the loins and groins, oliguria, and pain on micturition, due to compression of one or both ureters by enveloping fibrous tissue, and myalgia, coldness, and oedema in the lower extremities, caused by involvement of the great vessels. The condition tends to regress when methysergide treatment is withdrawn (when it is as well also to withhold ergotamine compounds), but regression is not invariable (Schwartz and Dunea 1966).

In order to guard against this reaction it is wise to use the smallest effective dose of methysergide and the period of continuous treatment should never exceed 6 months. At the end of this time methysergide should be withheld for at least 1 month and whenever possible ergotamine compounds should also be withheld during the rest period (*The Lancet* 1966). Throughout treatment the patient should be seen regularly to ensure that any symptoms and signs suggestive of retroperitoneal fibrosis are detected as early as possible.

A number of β-adrenoceptor blocking drugs have been associated with retroperitoneal fibrosis, including atenolol (Doherty *et al.* 1978; Johnson and McFarland 1980); propranolol (Pierce *et al.* 1981; Henri and Groleau 1981); oxprenolol (McCluskey *et al.* 1980); metoprolol (Thompson and Julian 1982); sotalol (Laakso *et al.* 1982); and timolol (Rimmer *et al.* 1983); these multiple reports relating to a single pharmacological group have strengthened the belief that there may be a causal relationship. Pryor and colleagues (1983) disputed this, but Bullimore (1984), in turn, disputed their conclusions, and the question appears to remain unanswered at the present time.

There have also been isolated reports of retroperitoneal fibrosis developing in patients treated with a variety of other drugs, such as aspirin, phenacetin, and codeine (Lewis et al. 1975), bromocriptine (Herzog et al. 1989; Vermersch et al. 1989), haloperidol (Jeffries et al. 1982), lysergic acid diethylamide (Aptekar and Michinson 1970), methyldopa (Iversen et al. 1975; Ahmad 1983), and in patients abusing co-proxamol (Distalgesic — a mixture of propoxyphene and paracetamol) (Critchley et al. 1985), but the evidence is insufficient to incriminate any of these drugs at the present time. It is interesting to note that lysergic acid diethylamide has structural similarity to methysergide, and bromocriptine is an ergot derivative.

Formaldehyde (1–10% solutions) used intravesically for the treatment of intractable haematuria has been reported to cause bladder wall fibrosis, ureteric fibrosis, and retroperitoneal fibrosis (Ferrie et al. 1983).

A fibrosing peritonitis has been recognized as one of the serious adverse reactions produced by the β-adrenoceptor blocking drug practolol as a part of the 'practolol syndrome' (Windsor et al. 1975; Eltringham et al. 1977; Marshall et al. 1977). This condition and the pericardial, pleural, skin, and eye disorders that may accompany it are discussed elsewhere in this book. Sclerosing peritonitis has also been described in association with propranolol (Ahmad 1981) and atenolol (Nillson and Pederson 1985).

The formation of fibrous plaques in the shaft of the penis, causing deformity and discomfort during erection are features of Peyronie's disease. This distressing condition has also been reported in patients under treatment with β-adrenoceptor blocking drugs, including labetalol (Kristensen 1979), metoprolol (Yudkin 1977), and propranolol (Osborne 1977; Wallis et al. 1977; Coupland 1977). Pryor and Kahn (1979) have reported a retrospective case–control study of 146 cases of Peyronie's disease, and Pryor and Castle (1982) a prospective study of 100 cases. It is now thought that atherosclerosis may be the aetiological factor in Peyronie's disease, and that the association of the latter with β-blocker therapy is coincidental (Pryor and Castle 1982; Chilton et al. 1982).

A case of rapidly progressive bilateral Dupuytren's contracture has been observed in a patient who had been under treatment with propranolol for some years (Coupland 1977) but this occurrence may well have been coincidental.

Cases of the carpal tunnel syndrome appear to have been precipitated by treatment with oestrogen–progestogen combinations or progestogens alone in high doses (Di Saia and Morrow 1977), danazol (Gray 1978; Sikka et al. 1983), and disulfiram (Howard 1982).

Drug-related systemic lupus erythematosus (D-RSLE)

A drug-related lupus-like syndrome, involving sulphadiazine, was first described by Hoffman (1945). Subsequently several drugs have been suspected of having caused this syndrome although a true association is doubtful in some cases (Table 16.1). Although a large number of patients develop such serological abnormalities as antinuclear antibodies while taking certain drugs (22 per cent of patients treated with isoniazid; 26 per cent of patients treated with chlorpromazine), D-RSLE itself occurs rarely (Hughes 1987).

Incidence of D-RSLE

Estimates of the incidence of the disorder have varied widely: *hydralazine* 1–21 per cent (Müller et al. 1955; Shulman and Harvey 1960, Lee and Siegel 1968; Alarcón-Segovia 1969; Perry et al. 1970; Lee and Chase 1975), with positive serological tests in 54 per cent (Perry et al. 1970); *anticonvulsants* 8 per cent or less (Wilske et al. 1965; Lee and Siegel 1968), with positive serological tests in 50–78 per cent (Alarcón-Segovia et al. 1972); *antituberculous drugs* 0.1 per cent (Lee et al. 1966), with positive serological tests on 10–67 per cent (Seligmann et al. 1965; Lee et al. 1966; Cannat and Seligmann 1966; Siegel et al. 1967; Alarcón-Segovia 1969; Rothfield et al. 1971); *procainamide* 5–-10 per cent (Fakhro, et al. 1967; Hope and Bates 1972; Bluestein et al. 1979), with positive serological tests in 50–74 per cent (Dubois et al. 1968; Lee and Chase 1975; Bluestein et al. 1979).

Aetiology

It is believed that the drugs act as immunogens, or haptens, which result in D-RSLE in predisposed individuals. The pathogenetic mechanisms are probably different for different drugs (Hughes et al. 1981). Hydralazine-related SLE is more common in slow acetylators, females, and in individuals possessing the histocompatibility antigen HLA DR4 (Batchelor et al. 1980; Mansilla-Tinoco et al. 1982). Among the pathogenetic mechanisms that have been suggested for one or other of a number of drugs are inhibition of enzymes; enhancement of formation of disulphide bonds; interference with cross-linkage of collagen and elastin; influence on the polymerization of macromolecular complexes; antagonism of some 'physiological' protective mechanisms or

TABLE 16.1
Drugs involved in reported cases of drug-related SLE

Group	Many or several reports and/or particularly convincing supporting evidence	Few or single reports and/or less convincing supporting evidence
Antiarrhythmic	procainamide	quinidine
Anticonvulsant	ethosuximide methoin phenytoin primidone troxidone	carbamazepine pheneturide
Antihypertensive	hydralazine methyldopa	clonidine guanoxan minoxidil reserpine

Anti-infective	isoniazid
	sulphasalazine
		griseofulvin
		nalidixic acid
		nitrofurantoin
		penicillin
		sodium amino-
		  salicylate (PAS)
		streptomycin
		sulphonamides
		  (other than
		  sulphasalazine)
		tetracycline

Antithyroid	thiouracils	methimazole
β-Adrenoceptor blockers	practolol	acebutolol labetalol pindolol propranolol
Miscellaneous	chlorpromazine	allopurinol ambenonium chloride chlorprothixene gold salts lithium methysergide nomifensine oral contraceptives oxyphenbutazone perphenazine phenylbutazone propafenone spironolactone zinc sulphate

TABLE 16.2
Clinical features of D-RSLE and SLE

Clinical features	Frequency (per cent)		
	Hydralazine	Procainamide	SLE
Arthralgia	84–95	77–91	92
Arthritis	50	18	–
Fever	50	45	84
Skin rash	25	5–18	72
Adenopathy	14	0–9	59
Myalgia	2–34	20–50	48
Pleuropulmonary	25–30	–	–
pleurisy	–	52	45
effusion	–	33	33
infiltrate	–	30	8
Pericarditis	2	14–18	31
Hepatosplenomegaly	8–75	20–33	5–10
CNS/seizures	0	0–2	16–25
Raynaud's phenomenon	–	5	23
Joint deformities	0	0	26
Renal involvement	2–20	0–5	46

(Based on the cases from Alarcón-Segovia 1969; Hahn and associates 1972; Perry 1973; Dubois 1969; Blomgren and associates 1972; and Dubois and Tuffanelli 1964)

change in structure, antigenicity, or both, of DNA and soluble nucleic acid and cytoplasmic nucleoprotein (Harpey *et al.* 1972; Harpey 1973); and alteration of lymphocyte function (Raftery and Denman 1973; Bluestein *et al.* 1979; Hughes *et al.* 1981; Ochi *et al.* 1983). The influence of rate of drug acetylation on the risk of development of some types of D-RSLE is discussed elsewhere in Chapter 3.

Clinical features

The classical features of D-RSLE resemble those of naturally occurring systemic lupus erythematosus (SLE) although there are some distinguishing features (Table 16.2). D-RSLE characteristically develops after a delay of 1 month to 5 years of treatment (Hughes 1987). There is a less pronounced female preponderance; only 48–61 per cent of cases induced by procainamide or hydralazine are females as against 89 per cent in naturally occurring SLE (Harpey 1974). Members of black races account for 30 per cent of cases of spontaneous SLE, but few develop D-RSLE (Dubois 1969; Perry 1973). The mean age of onset of D-RSLE is 55.2 years for procainamide and 52.8 years for hydralazine, as opposed to 27.5 years in spontaneous SLE (Alarcón-Sergovia 1969).

Renal involvement has been reported in approximately 20 per cent of patients (Alarcón-Segovia 1969; Björck *et al.* 1983). Central nervous system involvement is rare (Harmon and Portanova 1982), but pulmonary involvement may be commoner (Blomgren *et al.* 1972). D-RSLE associated with procainamide is more often accompanied by pericarditis than is the case with other drugs, and this may, rarely, cause cardiac tamponade and restrictive pericarditis (Browning *et al.* 1984).

Laboratory investigations

Antinuclear antibodies are invariably positive in D-RSLE and have been shown to be largely directed against nuclear histone (Fritzler and Tan 1978), predominantly histones H2A and H2B (Harmon and Portonova 1982). The non-complement-fixing nature of the antihistone antibodies may explain the low incidence of renal disease in D-RSLE (Fritzler and Tan 1978). The LE-cell phenomenon is quite marked in D-RSLE (Harmon and Portanova 1982). Unlike the situation in spontaneous SLE, D-RSLE is not usually associated with anti-double-stranded deoxyribonucleic acid (Winfield and Davis 1974). Complement levels are usually normal but hypocomplementaemia has been reported (Weinstein 1978). Anaemia, leucopenia, and hypergammaglobulinaemia may be present (Harmon and Portanova 1982). A circulating anticoagulant producing spontaneous abortion and deep vein thrombosis has been described in a 29-year-old woman who had D-RSLE associated with perphenazine (Steen and Ramsey-Goldman 1988). Evidence of circulating anticoagulant and elevation of IgM and a positive Coombs test has also been reported with D-RSLE involving chlorpromazine (Zarrabi *et al.* 1979).

Treatment and outcome

Withholding the offending drug usually results in resolution of symptoms in days or weeks, but they may persist for months or years in some patients (Alarcón-Segovia *et al.* 1967). Corticosteroid treatment may be necessary if there is pleuropericardial involvement (Harmon and Portanova 1982). Rarely, fatalities have been reported in patients with hydralazine-related (Sturman *et al.* 1988) and isoniazid-related SLE (Hoigné *et al.* 1975).

Drugs involved in D-RSLE

Space precludes provision of a comprehensive list of references concerning drugs for which there is overwhelming evidence of culpability, and these references can be found in the papers of the authors mentioned earlier under the heading 'Incidence of D-RSLE'. Since, however, interpretation of reports of a single case or only a very small number of cases relating to a particular drug may be considered debatable, readers may wish to evaluate these cases and other relevant evidence for themselves, and the following references are provided for this purpose. *Acebutolol* (Cody *et al.* 1979); *allopurinol* (Lee and Chase 1975); *ambenonium chloride* (Fries and Holman 1975); *β-adrenoceptor blockers (in general)* (Wilson *et al.* 1978); *carbamazepine* (Alarcón-Segovia *et al.* 1972); *chlorpromazine* (Zarrabi *et al.* 1979); *chlorprothixene* (Haid 1964); *clonidine* (Witman and Davis 1981); *gold salts* (Castleman and Mandebaum 1950; Kapp *et al.* 1967; Goetz 1969); *griseofulvin* (Alexander 1962); *guanoxan* (Bordman *et al.* 1967; Cotton and Montuschi 1967; Alarcón-Segovia 1977); *labetalol* (Griffiths and Richardson 1979); *lithium* (Presley *et al.* 1976; Shukla and Borison 1982); *methimazole* (Librik *et al.* 1970); *methoin* (Lindqvist 1957); *methyldopa* (Breckenridge *et al.* 1967; Sherman *et al.* 1967; Feltkamp *et al.* 1970; Harrington and Davis 1981; Dupont and Six 1982); *methysergide* (Racouchot *et al.* 1968); *minoxidil* (Tunkel *et al.* 1987); *nalidixic acid* (Rubinstein 1979); *nitrofurantoin* (Selroos and Edgren 1975); *nomifensine* (Garcia-Morteo and Maldonado-Cocco 1983); *oral contraceptives* (Schleicher 1968; Bole *et al.* 1969; Kay *et al.* 1969; Elias 1973); *oxyphenbutazone* (Cameron 1975); *penicillin* (Walsh and Zimmerman 1953; Paull 1955; Finegold and Middleton 1971); *perphenazine* (Steen and Ramsey-Goldman 1988); *pheneturide* (Dorfmann *et al.* 1972); *phenylbutazone* (Ogryzlo 1956; Farid and Anderson 1971); *pindolol* (Bensaid *et al.* 1979); *practolol* (Raftery and Denman 1973; Jachuck *et al.* 1977); *propafenone* (Guindo *et al.* 1986); *propranolol* (Harrison *et al.* 1976); *quinidine* (Kendall and Hawkins 1970); *spironolactone* (Uddin *et al.* 1979); *streptomycin* (Popkhristov and Kapnilov 1960); *sulphasalazine* (Crisp and Hoffbrand 1980; Carr-Locke 1982); *sulphonamides* (Hoffman 1945; Honey 1956; Rallison *et al.* 1961; Alarcón-Segovia *et al.* 1965); *tetracycline* (Domz *et al.* 1959); *zinc salts* (aggravation of hydralazine-induced SLE) (Fjellner 1979).

Drug-related pseudolupus

Venocuran, a proprietary preparation used in some European countries (but not in the UK) for the treatment of venous disorders, contains phenopyrazone, an extract of horse-chestnut (*Aesculus hippocastanum*), and glycosides derived from several plants, and has caused a syndrome in some ways resembling systemic lupus erythematosus but differing from it in that anti-

nuclear antibodies are absent, though antimitochondrial antibodies are present in 90 per cent of cases (these antibodies are uncommon in SLE). About 30 per cent of affected patients experience such symptoms as myalgia and arthralgia, and more than 10 per cent develop the full pseudolupus syndrome. Symptoms regress on withdrawal of the drug, and cortiocosteroid therapy appears to be beneficial. It is not known which constituent of the drug is responsible for the disorder (Grob *et al.* 1975).

Types of reaction

Of the signs and symptoms described in this chapter, those due to venous thrombosis, fluid depletion, disturbances of electrolytes and of uric acid metabolism, osteomalacia, osteoporosis, and some cases of osteosclerosis can undoubtedly be classified as Type A (see Chapter 3), as also can the dental and bone disorders induced by ACTH and corticosteroids, and the haemarthrosis complicating anticoagulant therapy. A few of the remaining disorders that have been mentioned can be labelled Type B, but in most of them the underlying mechanisms are too poorly understood to make classification possible.

References

Adams, E.M., Horowitz, H.W., and Sundstrom, W.R. (1983). Fibrous myopathy in association with pentazocine. *Arch. Intern. Med.* 143, 2203.

Ahmad, S. (1981). Sclerosing peritonitis and propranolol. *Chest* 79, 361.

Ahmad, S. (1983). Methyldopa and retroperitoneal fibrosis. *Am. Heart J.* 105, 1037.

Alarcón-Segovia, D. (1969). Drug-induced lupus syndromes. *Proc. Staff Meetings Mayo Clin.* 44, 664.

Alarcón-Segovia, D. (1977). Drug-induced antinuclear antibodies and lupus syndromes. *Curr. Ther.* 18, 85.

Alarcón-Segovia, D., Herskovic, T., Dearing, W.H., Bartholomew, L.G., Cain, J.C., and Shorter, R.G. (1965). Lupus erythematosus cell phenomenon in patients with chronic ulcerative colitis. *Gut* 6, 39.

Alarcón-Segovia, D., Wakim, K.G., Worthington, J.W., and Ward, L.E. (1967). Clinical and experimental studies on the hydralazine syndrome and its relationship to systemic lupus erythematosus. *Medicine* (Baltimore) 46, 1.

Alarcón-Segovia, D., Fishbein, E., Reyes, P.A., Dies, H., and Shwadsky, S. (1972). Antinuclear antibodies in patients on anticonvulsant therapy. *Clin. Exp. Immunol.* 12, 39.

Alexander, S. (1962). Lupus erythematosus in two patients after griseofulvin treatment of *Trichophyton rubrum* infection. *Br. J. Dermatol.* 74, 72.

Alfaham, M, Holt, M.E., and Goodchild, M.C. (1987). Arthropathy in a patient with cystic fibrosis taking ciprofloxacin. *Br. Med. J.* 295, 699.

Aptekar, R.G. and Michinson, J. (1970). Retroperitoneal fibrosis in two patients previously exposed to LSD. *Calif. Med.* 113, 77.

Arlet, J., Rascoul, A., Mole, J., and Roger, J.M. (1967). Observations de rhumatisme gardénalique. *Revue Rhum. Mal. Osteo-artic.* 34, 193.

Armstrong, R.D., Crisp, A.J., Grahame, R., and Woolfe, D.L. (1981). Hypertrophic osteoarthropathy and purgative abuse. *Br. Med. J.* 282, 1836.

Bailey, R.R. and Armour, P. (1974). Acute arthralgia after high-dose intravenous methylprednisolone. *Lancet* ii, 1014.

Bailey, R.R., Natale, R., and Linton, A.L. (1972). Nalidixic acid arthralgia. *Can. Med. Assoc. J.* 107, 604.

Ball, A.P. (1986). Overview of clinical experience with ciprofloxacin. *Eur. J. Clin. Microbiol.* 5, 214.

Barbeau, A. and Roy, M. (1976). Six-year results of treatment with levodopa plus benserazide in Parkinson's disease. *Neurology* 26, 399.

Barter, M. and Kammer, H. (1978). Methylphenidate and growth retardation. *JAMA* 239, 1742.

Batchelor, J.R., Welsh, K.I., Mansilla-Tinoco, R., Dollery, C.T., Hughes, G.R.V., Berstein, R., *et al.* (1980). Hydralazine-induced lupus erythematosus: influence of HLA-DR and sex on susceptibility. *Lancet* i, 1107.

Bedi, S.S. and Ellis, W. (1970). Spontaneous rupture of the calcaneal tendon in rheumatoid arthritis after local steroid injection. *Ann. Rheum. Dis.* 29, 494.

Belongia, E.A., Hedberg, C.W., Gleich, G.J., White K.E., Mayeno, A.N., Loegering, D.A., *et al.* (1990). An investigation of the cause of the eosinophilia–myalgia syndrome associated with tryptophan use. *N. Engl. J. Med.* 323, 357.

Ben-Ishay, D. (1961). Toxic reactions to intramuscular administration of iron–dextran. *Lancet* i, 476.

Bennett, W.M. and Strong, D. (1975). Arthralgia after high-dose steroids. *Lancet* i, 332.

Bensaid, J., Aldigier, J.C., and Gulde, N. (1979). Systemic lupus erythematosus syndrome induced by pindolol. *Br. Med. J.* i, 1603.

Bériel, M.M. and Barbier, J. (1934). Le rhumatisme gardénalique. *Presse Med.* 42, 67.

Bethel, R.G.H. (1979). Carbimazole-induced arthropathy. *Br. J. Clin. Pract.* 33, 294.

Bischoff, C. (1988). Epidural lipomatosis as a complication of long term corticosteroid medication. *Dtsch. Med. Wochenschr.* 113 1964.

Björck, S., Westberg, G., Svalander, C., and Mulec, H. (1983). Rapidly progressive glomerulonephritis after hydralazine. *Lancet* ii, 42.

Blain, P.G. and Lane, R.J.M. (1983). Drugs and muscle. *Adverse Drug React. Acute Poisoning Rev.* 2, 1.

Blitt, C.D., Carlson, G.L., Rolling, G.D., Hameroff, S.R., and Otto, C.W. (1981). A comparative evaluation of pretreatment with non-depolarizing neuromuscular blockers prior to the administration of succinylcholine. *Anesthesiology* 55, 687.

Blomgren, S.E., Condemi, J.J., and Vaughan, J.H. (1972). Procainamide-induced lupus erythematosus. Clinical and laboratory observations. *Am. J. Med.* 52, 338.

Blood, D.C. and Radostits, O.M. (1989). Specific diseases of uncertain aetiology. In *Veterinary Medicine* (ed. D.C. Blood and O.M. Radostits), p. 1405. Baillière Tindall, London.

Bluestein, H.G., Zvaifler, N.J., Weisman, M.H., and Shapiro, R.F. (1979). Lymphocyte alteration by procainamide in relation to drug-induced lupus erythematosus. *Lancet* i, 816.

Bole, G.G., Friedlander, M.M., and Smith, C.K. (1969). Rheumatic symptoms and serological abnormalities induced by oral contraceptives. *Lancet* i, 323.

Bondy, P.K. (1985). Disorders of the adrenal cortex. In *Williams textbook of endocrinology*, (7th edn) (ed. J.D. Wilson and D.W. Foster), p. 816. W.B. Saunders, Philadelphia.

Bordman, P.L., Robinson, K.C., and Dudley Hart, F. (1967). Guanoxan and systemic lupus erythematosus. *Br. Med. J.* i, 111.

Breckenridge, A., Dollery, C.T., Worlledge, S.M., Holborow, E.J., and Johnson, G.D. (1967). Positive direct Coombs test and antinuclear factor in patients treated with methyldopa. *Lancet* ii, 1265.

British National Formulary Number 19 (1990). Tetracyclines. p. 218. British Medical Association and the Royal Pharmaceutical Society of Great Britain.

Browning, C.A., Bishop, R.L., Heilpern, R.J., Singh, J.B., and Spodick, D.H. (1984). Accelerated constrictive pericarditis in procainamide induced systemic lupus erythematosus. *Am. J. Cardiol.* 53, 376.

Bullimore, D.W. (1984). Do beta-adrenoceptor blocking drugs cause retroperitoneal fibrosis? *Br. Med. J.* 288, 719.

Burland, W.L. (1978). In *Proceedings of the third international symposium on histamine H_2-receptor antagonists.* (ed. W. Creutzfeldt), p. 238. Excerpta Medica, Amsterdam.

Buttram, V.C., Reiter, R.C., and Ward, S. (1985). Treatment of endometriosis with danazol: report of a 6 year prospective study. *Fertil. Steril.* 43, 353.

Cairns, S.A. and Jordan, S.C. (1976). Prazosin treatment complicated by acute febrile polyarthritis. *Br. Med. J.* ii, 1424.

Cameron, D.C. (1975). Diffuse pulmonary disorder caused by oxyphenbutazone. *Br. Med. J.* ii, 500.

Cannat, A. and Seligmann, M. (1966). Possible induction of antinuclear antibodies by isoniazid. *Lancet* i, 185.

Carr-Locke, D.L. (1982). Sulphasalazine-induced lupus syndrome in a patient with Crohn's disease. *Am. J. Gastroenterol.* 77, 614.

Castin, P. and Gardien, P. (1934). Arthralgies et myalgies barbituriques *Presse Med.* 42, 1536.

Castleman, L. and Mandebaum, R.A. (1950). Gold poisoning and disseminated lupus erythematosus. *Am. Practit. Dig. Treat.* i, 561.

Centres for Disease Control (1990). Clinical spectrum of eosinophilia–myalgia syndrome — California. *MMWR* 39, 89.

Chassagne, P., Mejjad, O., Moore, N., Le Loët, X., and Deshayes, P. (1989). Myopathy as possible side-effect of cyclosporin. *Lancet* ii, 1104.

Chassagne, P., Mejjad, O., Noblet C., Gourmelen O., Moore, N., and Le Loët, X. (1990). Pseudopolymyalgia rheumatica with dipyridamole. *Br. Med. J.* 301, 875.

Chesney, R.W., Mazess, R.B., Hamstra, A.J., DeLuca, H.F., and O'Reagan, S. (1978). Reduction of serum 1,25-dihydroxy vitamin-D₃ in children receiving glucocorticoids. *Lancet* ii, 1123.

Chilton, C.P., Castle, W.M., Westwood, C.A., and Pryor, J.P. (1982). Factors associated in the aetiology of Peyronie's disease. *Br. J. Urol.* 54, 748.

Cody, R.J. Jr, Calabrese, L.H., Clough, J.D., Tarazi, R.C., and Bravo, E.L. (1979). Development of anti-nuclear antibodies during acebutolol therapy. *Clin. Pharmacol. Ther.* 25, 800.

Cogen, F.C., Rigg, G., Simmons, J.L., and Domino, E.F. (1978). Phencyclidine-associated acute rhabdomyolysis. *Ann. Intern. Med.* 88, 210.

Cohlan, S.Q., Bevelander, G., and Tiamsie, T. (1963). Growth inhibition of prematures receiving tetracycline: clinical and laboratory investigation. *Am. J. Dis. Child.* 105, 453.

Colamarino, R., Dubost, J.J., and Sauvezie, B. (1990). Polymyalgia and minoxidil. *Ann. Intern. Med.*. 113, 256.

Cooney, L.M. Jr, Aversa, J.M., and Newman, J.H. (1980). Insidious bilateral intrapatellar tendon rupture in a patient with systemic lupus erythematosus. *Ann. Rheum. Dis.* 39, 592.

Cooper, W.D., Sheldon, D., Brown, D., Kimber, G.R., Isitt, V.L., and Currie, W.J.C. (1987). Post-marketing surveillance of enalapril: experience in 11 710 hypertensive patients in general practice. *J. R. Coll. Gen. Pract.* 37, 316.

Corpier, C.L., Jones, P.H., Suki, W.N., Lederer, E.D., Quinones, M.A., Schmidt, S.W., *et al.* (1988). Rhabdomyolysis and renal injury with lovastatin use. Report of two cases in cardiac transplant recipients. *JAMA* 260, 239.

Cotton, S.G. and Montuschi, E. (1967). Guanoxan. *Br. Med. J.* iii, 174.

Coupland, W.W. (1977). Fibrosing conditions and propranolol. *Med. J. Aust.* ii, 137.

Cowan, M.A. and Alexander, S. (1961). Simultaneous bilateral rupture of Achilles tendons due to triamcinolone. *Br. Med. J.* i, 1658.

Cozen, L.N. (1977). Pentazocine injections as causative factor in dislocation of the shoulder. *J. Bone Joint Surg.* 59. 979.

Crawford, J.S. (1971). Suxamethonium muscle pains and pregnancy. *Br. J. Anaesth.* 43, 677.

Crisp, A.J. and Hoffbrand, B.I. (1980). Sulphasalazine-induced systemic lupus erythematosus in a patient with Sjögren's syndrome. *J. R. Soc. Med.*. 73, 60.

Critchley, J.A.J.H., Smith, M.F., and Prescott, L.F. (1985). Distalgesic abuse and retroperitoneal fibrosis. *Br. J. Urol.* 57, 486.

Cruess, R.L. (1977). Cortisone-induced avascular necrosis of the femoral head. *J. Bone Joint Surg.* 59, 308.

CSM (Committee on Safety of Medicines) (1981). Cimetidine and arthropathy. *Current Problems No. 7.* HMSO, London.

Cuchacovich, M.T. and Kappes, J.B. (1987) Shoulder–hand syndrome induced by phenobarbitone. *Rev. Med. Chil.* 115, 865.

Cullen, D.J. (1971). The effect of pretreatment with non-depolarizing muscle relaxants on the neuromuscular blocking action of succinylcholine. *Anesthesiology* 35, 572.

Datta, S., Crocker, J.S., and Alper, M.H. (1977). Muscle pain following administration of suxamethonium to pregnant and non-pregnant patients undergoing laparoscopic tubal ligation. *Br. J. Anaesth.* 49, 625.

Davies, A. (1968). Comparative trials of antimonial drugs in urinary Schistosomiasis. *Bull. WHO* 38 197.

Davies, D.M. and Lund, J.F. (1965). Myalgia and an oral contraceptive. *Lancet* ii, 1187.

Del Favero A. (1984). Antiinflammatory analgesics and drugs used in rheumatoid arthritis and gout. In *Side effects of drugs* Annual 8. (ed. M.N.G. Dukes), p. 100. Elsevier Science Publishers, Amsterdam.

Dickinson, L.D., Lee, J., Ringdahl, C., Schedewie, H.K., Kilgore, B.S., and Elders, M.J. (1979). Impaired growth in hyperkinetic children receiving pemoline. *J. Pediatr.* 94, 538.

Diggle, G. (1990). The eosinophilia–myalgia syndrome and L-tryptophan. *Health Trends* 22, 2.

Dinai, Y. and Pras, M. (1975). Levamisole in rheumatoid arthritis. *Lancet* ii, 556.

Di Saia, P.J. and Morrow, C.P. (1977). Unusual side-effects of megestrol acetate. *Am. J. Obstet. Gynecol.* 129, 460.

Doherty, C.G., McGeown, M.G., and Donaldson, R.A. (1978). Retroperitoneal fibrosis after treatment with atenolol. *Br. Med. J.* ii, 1786.

Domz, C.A., McNamara, D.H., and Holzappfez, H.F. (1959). Tetracycline provocation in lupus erythematosus. *Ann. Intern. Med.* 50, 1217.

Dorfmann, H., Kahn, M.F., and Deseze, S. (1972). Possibilité de lupus iatrogène induit par le phénéturide à propos de 2 observations). *Ann. Intern. Med.* 123, 331.

Doyle, D.R., McCurley, T.L., and Sergent, J.S. (1983). Fatal polymyositis in D-penicillamine treated rheumatoid arthritis. *Ann. Intern. Med.* 98, 327.

Drug and Therapeutics Bulletin (1990). L-Tryptophan and the eosinophilia–myalgia syndrome. *Drug Ther. Bull.* 28, 37.

Dubois, E.L. (1969). Procainamide induction of a systemic lupus erythematosus-like syndrome. *Medicine* (Baltimore) 48, 217.

Dubois, E.L. and Tuffanelli, D.L. (1964). Clinical manifestations of systemic lupus erythematosus: computer analysis of 520 cases. *JAMA* 190, 104.

Dubois, E.L., Molina, J., Bilitch, M., and Friou, G.J. (1968). Procainamide-induced serological changes in asymptomatic patients. *Arthritis Rheum.* 11, 477.

Dupont, A. and Six, R. (1982). Lupus-like syndrome induced by methyldopa. *Br. Med. J.* 285, 696.

Eastwood, J.B., Parker, B., and Reid, B.R. (1978). Bilateral central fracture dislocation of hips after myelography with meglumine iocarmate (Dimer X). *Br. Med. J.* i, 692.

Elias, P.M. (1973). Erythema nodosum and serological lupus erythematosus. Simultaneous occurrence in a patient using oral contraceptives. *Arch. Dermatol.* 108, 716.

Eltringham, W.K., Espiner, H.J., Windsor, C.W.O., Griffiths, D.A., Davies, J.D., Baddeley, H., *et al.* (1977). Sclerosing peritonitis due to practolol: a report of 9 cases and their surgical management. *Br. J. Surg.* 64, 229.

Erkola, O., Salmenperä, A., and Kuoppamäki, R. (1983). Five non-depolarizing muscle relaxants in precurarization. *Acta Anaesthesiol. Scand.* 27, 427.

Fahmy, N.R., Malek, N.S., and Lappas, D.G. (1979). Diazepam prevents some adverse effects of succinylcholine. *Clin. Pharmacol. Ther.* 26, 395.

Fakhro, A.M., Ritchie, R.F., and Lown, B. (1967). Lupus-like syndrome induced by procainamide. *Am. J. Cardiol.* 20, 367.

Farid, N. and Anderson, J. (1971). SLE-like reaction to phenylbutazone therapy. *Lancet* i, 1022.

Felson, D.T. and Anderson, J.J. (1987). A cross-study evaluation of association between steroid dose and bolus steroids and avascular necrosis of bone. *Lancet* i, 902.

Feltkamp, T.E.W., Dorhout, E.J., and Nieuwenhuis, M.G. (1970). Autoantibodies related to treatment with chlorthalidone and α-methyldopa. *Acta Med. Scand.* 187, 219.

Ferrie, B.G., Smith, P.J.B., and Kirk, D. (1983). Retroperitoneal fibrosis complicating intravesical formalin therapy. *J. R. Soc. Med.* 76, 831.

Fidler, M.W. and Brook, C.G.D. (1974). Slipped upper femoral epiphysis following treatment with human growth hormone. *J. Bone Joint Surg.* 56, 1719.

Finegold, I. and Middleton, E. Jr (1971). Positive lupus erythematosus preparations and penicillin sensitivity. *J. Allergy Immunol.* 48, 115.

Fitzgerald, M.X. and Brennan, M.J. (1976). Muscle cramps, collapse and seizures in two patients taking metolazone. *Br. Med. J.* i, 1381.

Fjellner, B. (1979). Drug-induced lupus erythematosus aggravated by oral zinc therapy. *Acta Derm.Venereol.* (Stockh.) 59, 368.

Fraser, D.M. and Irvine, N.A. (1976). Joint effusions and practolol. *Lancet* i, 89.

Frier, B.M. and Scott, R.D.M. (1977). Osteomalacia and arthropathy associated with prolonged abuse of purgatives. *Br. J. Clin. Pract.* 31, 17.

Fries, J.F. and Holman, H.R. (1975). SLE-like syndrome produced by drugs. In *Major problems in internal medicine 6*, p. 134. W.B. Saunders, Philadelphia.

Fritzler, M.J. and Tan, E.M. (1978). Antibodies to histones in drug-induced and idiopathic erythematosus. *J. Clin. Invest.* 62, 560.

Fulroth, R., Phillips, B., and Durand, D.J. (1989). Perinatal outcome of infants exposed to cocaine and/or heroin in utero. *Am. J. Dis. Child.* 143, 905.

Garcia-Morteo, O. and Maldonado-Cocco, J. A. (1983). Lupus-like syndrome during treatment with nomifensine. *Arthritis Rheum.* 26, 936.

Gibbs, J.M. (1978). A case of rhabdomyolysis associated with suxamethonium. *Anaesth. Intens. Care* 6, 141.

Glauber, D. (1966). The incidence and severity of muscle pains after suxamethonium when preceded by gallamine. *Br. J. Anaesth.* 38, 541.

Gleckman, R., Alvarez, S., Joubert D.W., and Mathews, S.J. (1979). Drug Therapy Reviews: Nalidixic acid. *Am. J. Hosp. Pharm.* 36, 1071.

Goa, K.L. and Campoli-Richards, D.M. (1987). Pentamidine isethionate. A review of its antiprotozoal activity, pharmacokinetic properties and therapeutic use in pneumocystis carinii pneumonia. *Drugs* 33, 242.

Goetz, G. (1969). Erythematodes-provokation durch Goldtherapie wegen primär-chronischer Polyarthritis. *Dtsch. Med. Wochenschr.* 94, 2045.

Goldberg, A.P., Sherrard, D.J., Hass, L.B., and Brunzell, J.D. (1977). Control of clofibrate toxicity in uraemic hypertriglyceridaemia. *Clin. Pharmacol. Ther.* 21, 317.

Good, A.E., Green, R.A., and Zarafonetis, C.J.D. (1965). Rheumatic symptoms during tuberculous therapy. A manifestation of isoniazid therapy. *Ann. Intern. Med.* 63, 800.

Gottlieb, N.L. and Gray, R.G. (1977). Allopurinol-associated hand and foot deformities in chronic tophaceous gout. *JAMA* 238, 1663.

Goy, J., Stauffer, J., Deruaz, J., Gillard, D., Kaufmann, U., Kuntzer, T., et al. (1989). Myopathy as a possible side-effect of cyclosporin. *Lancet* i, 1446.

Graham, J.R. (1964). Methysergide for prevention of headache (experience in five hundred patients over three years). *N. Engl. J. Med.* 270, 67.

Graham, J.R. (1968). Fibrosis associated with methysergide therapy. In *Drug-induced diseases*, Vol. 3 (ed. L. Meyler and H.M. Peck). Associated Scientific Publishers, Amsterdam.

Graham, J.R., Suby, H.I., Le Compte, P.R., and Sadowsky, N.L. (1966). Fibrotic disorders associated with methysergide therapy for headache. *N. Engl. J. Med.* 274, 359.

Gray, R.G. (1978). Bilateral carpal tunnel syndrome and arthritis associated with danazol administration. *Arthritis Rheum.* 21, 493.

Gregg, PJ., Barsoum, M.K., Soppitt, D., amd Jackson, R.H. (1980). Avascular necrosis of bone in children receiving high-dose steroid treatment. *Br. Med. J.* 281, 116.

Griffiths, I.D. and Richardson, J. (1979). Lupus-type illness associated with labetalol. *Br. Med. J.* ii, 496.

Grob, P.J., Müller-Schoop, J.W., Häcki, M.A., and Joller-Jemelka, H.I. (1975). Drug-induced pseudolupus. *Lancet* ii, 144.

Guindo, J., Rodriguez de la Serna, A., Borja, J., Oter, R., Jane, R., De Luna, A.B., et al. (1986). Propafenone and a syndrome of the lupus erythematosus type. *Ann. Intern. Med.*. 104, 589.

Gum, O.B., Smythe, C.J., Hamilton, S,K, Jr, and Moens, C. (1960). Effect of intra-articular serotonin and other amines on connective tissue proliferation of rabbit joints. *Arthritis Rheum.* 3, 447.

Hahn, B.H., Sharp, G.C., Irvin, W.S., Kantor, O.S., Gardner, C.A., Bagby, M.K., et al. (1972). Immune responses to hydralazine and nuclear antigens in hydralazine-induced lupus erythematosus. *Ann. Intern. Med.* 76, 365.

Haid, A. (1964). Case of drug systemic lupus erythematosus from chlorprothixene ('Taractan'). *Ugeskr. Laeg.* 126, 1112.

Haines, J.F. (1983). Bilateral rupture of the Achilles tendon in patients on steroid therapy. *Ann. Rheum. Dis.* 42, 652.

Harmon, C.E. and Portanova, J.P. (1982). Drug-induced lupus: clinical and serological studies. *Clin. Rheum. Dis.* 8, 121.

Harper, P.G., Trask, C., and Souhami, R.L. (1984). Avascular necrosis caused by combination chemotherapy without corticosteroids. *Br. Med. J.* 288, 267.

Harpey, J.P. (1973). Drugs and disseminated lupus erythematosus. *Adverse Drug React. Bull.* 43, 140.

Harpey, J.P. (1974). Lupus-like syndromes induced by drugs. *Ann. Allergy* 33, 256.

Harpey, J.P., Caille, B., Moulias, R., and Goust, J.M. (1972). Drug allergy and lupus-like syndrome (with special reference to pencillamine). In *Mechanisms in drug allergy* (ed. C.H. Dash and H.E.H. Jones), p. 51. Churchill Livingstone, Edinburgh.

Harrington, T.M. and Davis, D.E. (1981). Systemic lupus-like syndrome induced by methyldopa therapy. *Chest* 79, 696.

Harris, W.R. (1950). The endocrine basis for slipping of the upper femoral epiphysis. *J. Bone Joint Surg.* 32, 5.

Harrison, T., Sisca, T.S., and Wood, W.H. (1976). Propranolol-induced lupus erythematosus syndrome? *Postgrad. Med.*. 59, 241.

Hasler v United States (517 F Supp. 1262-E. D. Mich. 1981). *Clin-Alert* 1981, item No. 251 B.

Hegarty, P. (1956). Postoperative muscle pains. *Br. J. Anaesth.* 28, 209.

Henri, L. and Groleau, M. (1981). Retroperitoneal fibrosis after treatment with propranolol. *Drug Intell. Clin. Pharm.* 15, 696.

Herzog, A., Minne, H., and Ziegler, R. (1989). Retroperitoneal fibrosis in a patient with macroprolactinoma treated with bromocriptine. *Br. Med. J.* 298, 1315.

Hietarinta, M. and Merilanti-Palo, R. (1989). Methimazole-induced arthritis. *Scand. J. Rheumatol.* 18, 61.

Hoffman, B.J. (1945). Sensitivity to sulfadiazine resembling acute disseminated lupus erythematosus. *Arch. Dermatol. Syph.* 51 190.

Hoigné, R., Biedermann, H.P., and Naegeli, H.R. (1975). INH-induzierter systemischer Lupus erythematodes: 2. Beobachtungen mit Reexposition. *Schweiz. Med. Wochenschr.* 105, 1726.

Honey, M. (1956). SLE presenting with sulphonamide hypersensitivity reaction. *Br. Med. J.* i, 1272.

Hope, R.R. and Bates, L.A. (1972). The frequency of procainamide-induced systemic lupus erythematosus. *Med. J. Aust.* ii, 298.

Howard, J.F. (1982). Arthritis and carpal tunnel syndrome associated with disulfiram (Antabuse) therapy. *Arthritis Rheum.* 25, 1484.

Hughes, G.R.V. (1987). Recent development in drug-related systemic lupus erythematosus. *Adverse Drug React. Bull.* 123, 40.

Hughes, G.R.V., Rynes, R.I., Charavi, A., Ryan, P.F.J., Sewell, J., and Mansilla, R. (1981). The heterogenicity of serological findings and predisposing host factors in drug-induced lupus erythematosus. *Arthritis Rheum.* 24, 1070.

Ismail, A.M., Balakrishnan, R., and Rajakumar, M.K. (1969). Rupture of patellar ligament after steroid infiltration. Report of a case. *J. Bone Joint Surg.* 51, 503.

Iversen, B.M., Johannese, J.W., Nordahl, E., Ofstad, J., Thunold, S., and Willassen, Y. (1975). Retroperitoneal fibrosis during treatment with methyldopa. *Lancet* ii, 302.

Jachuck, S.J., Stephenson, J., Bird, T., Jackson, F.S., and Clark, F. (1977). Practolol-induced autoantibodies and their relation to oculo-cutaneous complication. *Postgrad. Med. J.* 53, 75.

Jaffe, N., Hie Won, L.H., and Vawter, G.F. (1971). Post-steroid panniculitis in acute leukaemia. *N. Engl. J. Med.* 284, 366.

Jeandel, C., Manciaux, M.A., Bannwarth, B., Pere, P., Penin, F., Netter, P., *et al.* (1989). Arthritis induced by norfloxacin. *J. Rheumatol.* 16, 560.

Jeffries, J.J., Lyall, W.A., Bezchlibnyk, K., Papoff, P.M., and Newman, F. (1982). Retroperitoneal fibrosis and haloperidol. *Am. J. Psychiatry* 139, 1524.

John, G. (1981). Transient osteosclerosis associated with sodium valproate. *Dev. Med. Child Neurol.* 23, 234.

Johns, A.M. and Bower, B.D. (1970). Wasting of napkin area after repeated use of fluorinated steroid ointment. *Br. Med. J.* i, 347.

Johnson, J.N. and McFarland, J.B. (1980). Retroperitoneal fibrosis associated with atenolol. *Br. Med. J.* 280, 864.

Kaniaris, P., Galanopoulou, T., and Varnos, D. (1973). Effects of succinylcholine on plasma 5-HT levels. *Anaesth. Analg.* 52, 425.

Kapp, W., Klunker, W., and Fellman, N. (1967). Auslösung eines Lupus erythematodes durch Goldtherapie bei primärchronischer Polyarthritis? *Dtsch. Med. Wochenschr.* 56, 1594.

Kattan, K.R. (1970). Calvarial thickening after Dilantin medication. *AJR* 110, 102.

Kaufman, L.D., Seidman, R.J., and Gruber, B.L. (1990). L-Tryptophan-associated eosinophilic perimyositis, neuritis and fasciitis. A clinicopathologic and laboratory study of 25 patients. *Medicine* (Baltimore). 69, 187.

Kay, D.R., Bole, G.G., and Ledger, W.J. (1969). The use of oral contraceptives and the occurrence of antinuclear antibodies and LE cells in women with early rheumatic disease. *Arthritis Rheum.* 12, 306.

Keidar, S., Binenboim, C., and Palant, A. (1982). Muscle cramps during treatment with nifedipine. *Br. Med. J.* 285, 1241.

Kendall, M.J. and Hawkins, C.F. (1970). Quinidine-induced lupus erythematosus. *Postgrad. Med. J.* 46, 729.

Kendrick, W.C., Hull, A.R., and Knochel, J.P. (1977). Rhabdomyolysis and shock after intravenous amphetamine administration *Ann. Intern. Med.* 86, 381.

Kertes, P. and Hunt, D. (1982). Polyarthritis complicating quinidine treatment. *Br. Med. J.* 284, 1373.

Kesseler, A., Lacassie, A., Hugot, J.P., Talon, Ph., Thomas, D., and Astier L. (1989). Perfloxacin induced joint disease in an adolescent with cystic fibrosis. *Ann. Pediatr.* 36, 275.

Kilbourne, E.M., Rigau-Perez, J.G., Heath, C.W. Jr, Zack, M.M., Falk, H., Martin-Marcos, M., *et al.* (1983). Clinical epidemiology of toxic-oil syndrome: manifestations of a new illness. *N. Engl. J. Med.* 309, 1408.

Kilbourne, E.M., Swygert, L.A., and Philen, R.M. (1990). Interim guidance on the eosinophilia–myalgia syndrome. *Ann. Intern. Med.* 112, 85.

Koivisto, V.A. and Felig, P. (1980). Alterations in insulin absorption and in blood glucose control associated with varying insulin injection sites in diabetic patients. *Ann. Intern. Med.* 92, 59.

König, W. (1956). Uber Beschwerden nach Anwendung von Succinylcholin. *Anaesthetist* 5, 50.

Köppel, C. (1989). Clinical features, pathogenesis and management of drug-induced rhabdomyolysis. *Med. Toxicol. Adverse Drug Experience* 4, 108.

Kriegel, W. and Müller, W. (1972). Drug-induced disease of the bones, joints and connective tissue. In *Drug-induced diseases*, (Vol. 4) (ed. L. Meyler and H.M. Peck). Associated Scientific Publishers, Amsterdam.

Kristensen, B.O. (1979). Labetalol-induced Peyronie's disease. *Acta Med. Scand.* 206, 511.

Laakso, M., Arvala, I., Tervonen, S., and Sotaranta, M. (1982). Retroperitoneal fibrosis associated with sotalol. *Br. Med. J.* 285, 1085.

Lamm, D.L., Stodgill, V.D., Stodgill, B.J., and Crispen, R.G. (1986). Complications of BCG immunotherapy in 1278 patients with bladder cancer. *J. Urol.* 135, 272.

The Lancet (1963). Toxicity of tetracyclines. *Lancet* ii, 283.

The Lancet (1966). Drugs and retroperitoneal fibrosis. *Lancet* i, 969.

Lane, R.J.M. and Mastaglia, F.L. (1978). Drug-induced myopathies in man. *Lancet* ii, 562.

Langer, T. and Levy, R.I. (1968). Acute muscular syndrome associated with the administration of clofibrate. *N. Engl. J. Med.* 279, 856.

Laurence, A.S. (1987). Myalgia and biochemical changes following intermittent suxamethonium administration. *Anaesthesia* 42, 503.

Leatherdale, R.A.L., Mayhew, R.A.J., and Hayton-Williams, D.S. (1959). Incidence of 'muscle pain' after short-acting relaxants: a comparison between suxamethonium chloride and suxamethonium bromide. *Br. Med. J.* i, 904.

Lee, H.B. (1957). Avulsion and rupture of the tendo calcaneus after injection of hydrocortisone. *Br. Med. J.* ii, 395.

Lee, M.L.H. (1961). Bilateral rupture of Achilles tendon. *Br. Med. J.* i, 1829.

Lee, S.L. and Chase, P.H. (1975). Drug-induced lupus erythematosus: a critical review. *Sem. Arthritis Rheum.* 5, 83.

Lee, S.L. and Siegel, M. (1968). Drug induced lupus erythematosus. In *Drug-induced diseases*, (Vol. 3) (ed. L. Meyler and H.M. Peck), p. 239. Associated Scientific Publishers, Amsterdam.

Lee, S.L., Rivero, I., and Siegel, M. (1966). Activation of systemic lupus erythematosus by drugs. *Arch. Intern. Med.* 117, 620.

Le Loët, X., Moore, N., and Deshayes, P. (1989). Pseudo-polymyalgia rheumatica during treatment with enalapril. *Br. Med. J.* 298, 325.

Lequesne, M. (1967). L'algo-dystrophie d'origine chimio-thérapique. Pseudorhumatisme de l'isoniazide, de l'éthionamide du phénobarbital et de l'iode radioactive. *Sem. Hop. Paris* 43, 2581.

Levin, B.E. and Engel, W.K. (1975). Iatrogenic muscle fibrosis. Arm levitation as an initial sign. *JAMA* 234, 621.

Lewis, C.T., Molland, E.A., Marshall, V.R., Tresidder, G.C., and Blandy, J.P. (1975). Analgesic abuse, ureteric obstruction and retroperitoneal fibrosis. *Br. Med. J.* ii, 76.

Librick, L., Sussman, L., Bejar, R., and Clayton, G.W. (1970). Thyrotoxicosis and collagen-like disease in three sisters of American-Indian extraction. *J. Pediatr.* 76, 64.

Lindqvist, T. (1957). Lupus erythematosus disseminatus after administration of mesantoin. Report of two cases. *Acta Med. Scand.* 158, 131.

Litin, S.C. and Anderson, C.F. (1989). Nicotinic acid-associated myopathy: a report of three cases. *Am. J. Med.* 86, 481.

Lotzof, L. (1968). Orciprenaline in the treatment of asthma. *Med. J. Aust.* i, 1105.

Lövgren, O. (1948). Om s.k. barbitursyrereumatism. *Svenska Läkartidn.* 45, 234.

McCluskey, D.R., Donaldson, R.A., and McGeown, M.G. (1980). Oxprenolol and retroperitoneal fibrosis. *Br. Med. J.* 281, 1459.

McCluskey, J. and Gutteridge, D.H. (1982). Avascular necrosis of bone after high doses of dexamethasone during surgery. *Br. Med. J.* i, 333.

MacDonald, J.B. (1982). Muscle cramps during treatment with nifedipine. *Br. Med. J.* 285, 1744.

MacDonald, J.B. and MacDonald E.T. (1977) Nocturnal femoral fracture and continuing widespread use of barbiturate hypnotics. *Br. Med. J.* ii, 483.

McEwan, S.R. and Davey, P.G. (1988). Ciprofloxacin and tenosynovitis. *Lancet* ii, 900.

McGloughlin, C., Nesbitt, G.A., and Howe, J.P. (1988). Suxamethonium-induced myalgia and the effect of pre-operative administration of oral aspirin. *Anaesthesia* 43, 565.

McKusick, A.B. (1965). Personal communication to Good *et al.* (1965).

McKusick, A.B. and Hsu, J.M. (1961). Clinical and metabolic studies of the shoulder-hand syndrome in tuberculous patients. In *Xth Congress of the International League against Rheumatism*, Vol. 2. Turin.

McLaughlin, G.E., McCarthy, D.J., and Segal, B.L. (1966). Hemarthrosis complicating anticoagulant therapy. *JAMA* 196, 1020.

McNally, P.G., Jowett, N.I., Kurinczuk, J.J., Peck, R.W., and Hearnshaw, J.R. (1988). Lipohypertrophy and lipoatrophy complicating treatment with highly purified bovine and porcine insulins. *Postgrad. Med. J.* 64, 850.

Maillard, G. and Renard, G. (1925). Un nouveau traitement de l'épilepsie: la phénolyl-méthylmalonylurée (Rutonal). *Presse Med.* 33, 315.

Maillard, G. and Thomazi, P. (1931). Douleurs provoquées par certains dérivés barbituriques au cours du traitement de l'épilepsie. *Presse Med.* 39, 851.

Malluche, H.H. and Faugère, M.C. (1985). Aluminium: toxin or innocent bystander in renal osteodystrophy. *Am. J. Kidney Dis.* vi, 336.

Malmquist, J., Ericsson, B., Hulten-Nosslin, M.B., Jeppsson, J-Q., and Ljungberg, O. (1980). Finger clubbing and aspartylglucosamine excretion in a laxative-abusing patient. *Postgrad. Med. J.* 56, 862.

Malnick, S.D.H. and Schattner, A. (1989). Arthralgia associated with captopril. *Br. Med. J.* 299, 394.

Manchikanti, L. (1984). Diazepam does not prevent succinylcholine-induced fasciculations and myalgia: a comparative evaluation of the effect of diazepam and D-tubocurarine pretreatments. *Acta Anaesthesiol. Scand.* 28, 523.

Mansilla-Tinoco, R., Harland, S.J., Ryan, P.J., Bernstein, R.M., Dollery, C.T., Hughes, G.R.V., *et al.* (1982). Hydralazine, antinuclear antibodies, and the lupus syndrome. *Br. Med. J.* 284, 936.

Marais, G.E. and Larson, K.K. (1990). Rhabdomyolysis and acute renal failure induced by combination lovastatin and gemfibrozil therapy. *Ann. Intern. Med.*. 112, 228.

Marshall, A.J., Baddeley, H., Barrit, D.W., Davies, J.D., Lee, R.E.J., Low-beer, T.S., *et al.* (1977). Practolol peritonitis: a study of 16 cases and a survey of small bowel function in patients taking β-adrenergic blockers. *Q. J. Med.* 46, 135.

Marshall, W. (1977). Barbiturates and fractures. *Br. Med. J.* ii, 640.

Masey, S.A., Glazebrook, C.W., and Goat, V.A. (1983). Suxamethonium: a new look at pretreatment. *Br. J. Anaesth.* 55, 729.

Mastaglia, F.L., Gardner-Medwin, D., and Hudgson, P. (1971). Muscle fibrosis and contracture in a pethidine addict. *Br. Med. J.* iv, 532.

Matthiesen, J. (1979). Polymyositis som en mulig bivirkning af cimetidin behandling. *Ugeskr Laeger* 141, 2762.

Mayrhofer, O. (1959). Die Wirksamheit von D-Tubocurarin zur Verhütung der Muskelschmerzen nach Succinylcholin. *Anaesthetist* 8, 313.

Medsger, J.A. Jr (1990). Tryptophan-induced eosinophilia–myalgia syndrome. *N. Engl. J. Med.* 322, 926.

Melmed, E.P. (1965). Spontaneous bilateral rupture of the calcaneal tendon during steroid therapy. *J. Bone Joint Surg.* 47, 104.

Meyerhoff, J.O. (1983). Exacerbation of psoriasis with meclofenamate. *N. Engl. J. Med.* 309, 496.

Moser, R.H. (1964). Collagen and collagen-like diseases. In *Diseases of medical progress* (2nd edn) (ed. R.H. Moser). Thomas, Springfield, Ohio.

Muller, J.C., Rast, C.L. Jr, Pryor, W.W., and Orgain, E.S. (1955). Late systemic complications of hydralazine (Apresoline) therapy. *JAMA* 157, 894.

Müller-Vahl, H. (1984). Aseptische Gewebsnekrose: eine schwerwiegende Komplikation nach intramuskulärer Injektion. *Dtsch. Med. Wochenschr.* 109, 786.

Murray, R.O. and Jacobson, H.G. (1972). *The radiology of skeletal disorders*, Vol.1, pp. 553, 560. Churchill Livingstone, Edinburgh.

Neerhof, M.G., MacGregor, S.N., Retzky, S.S., and Sullivan, T.P. (1989). Cocaine abuse during pregnancy: peripartum prevalence and perinatal outcome. *Am. J. Obstet. Gynecol.* 161, 633.

Neu, H.C. (1988). Quinolones: a new class of antimicrobial agents with wide potential uses. *Med. Clin. N. Am.* 72, 623.

Newman, N.M. and Ling, R.S.M. (1985). Acetabular bone destruction related to non-steroidal anti-inflammatory drugs. *Lancet* ii, 11.

Newmark, K.J., Mitra, S., and Berman, L.B. (1974). Acute arthralgia following high-dose intravenous methylprednisolone therapy. *Lancet* ii, 229.

Newnam, P.T.F. and Loudon, J.M. (1966). Muscle pain following administration of suxamethonium: the aetiological role of muscular fitness. *Br. J. Anaesth.* 38, 533.

Nillson, B.V. and Pederson, K.G. (1985). Sclerosing peritonitis associated with atenolol. *Br. Med. J.* 290, 518.

Noppen, M., Velkeniers, B., Dierckx, R., Bruyland, M., and Vanhaelst, L. (1987). Cyclosporin and myopathy. *Ann. Intern. Med.* 107, 945.

Norman, D.J., Illingworth, D.R., Munson, J., and Hosenpud, J. (1988). Myolysis and acute renal failure in a heart-transplant patient receiving lovastatin. *N. Engl. J. Med.* 318, 46.

Ochi, T., Goldings, E.A., Lipsky, P.E., and Ziff, M. (1983). Immunomodulatory effect of procainamide in man: inhibition of human suppressor T-cell activity *in vitro. J. Clin. Invest.* 71, 36.

Ochsenkühn, T., Weber, M.M., and Caselmann, W.H. (1990). Arthritis after *Mycobacterium bovis* immunotherapy for bladder cancer. *Ann. Intern. Med.*. 112, 882.

O'Connor, M. (1980). Muscle necrosis induced by intramuscular chlorpromazine. *Med. J. Aust.* i, 36.

Ogryzlo, M.A. (1956). The LE (lupus erythematosus) cell reaction. *Can. Med. Assoc. J.* 75, 980.

Oh, B.K., Von Overveld, G.P., and Macfarlane, J.D. (1983). Polyarthritis induced by propyl thiouracil. Case report. *Br. J. Rheumatol.* 22, 106.

O'Malley, B. (1989). Carbimazole-induced cramps. *Lancet* i, 1456.

O'Reagan, S., Chesney, R.W., Hamstra, A., Eisman, J.A., O'Gorman, A.M., and Deluca, H.F. (1979). Reduced serum 1, 25(OH)$_2$-vitamin D$_3$ levels in prednisolone treated adolescents with systemic lupus erythematosus. *Acta Paediatr. Scand.* 68, 109.

O'Sullivan, E.P., Williams, N.E., and Calvey, T.N. (1988). Differential effects of neuromuscular blocking agents on suxamethonium-induced fasciculations and myalgia. *Br. J. Anaesth.* 60, 367.

Osborne, D.R. (1977). Propranolol and Peyronie's disease. *Lancet* i, 131.

Page, S.R. and Nussey, S.S. (1989). Myositis in association with carbimazole therapy. *Lancet* i, 964.

Palmer, K.N.V. (1978). Muscle cramp and oral salbutamol. *Br. Med. J.* ii, 833.

Paull, A.M. (1955). Occurrence of the 'LE' phenomenon in a patient with a severe penicillin reaction. *N. Engl. J. Med.* 252, 128.

Perry, H.M. (1973). Late toxicity to hydralazine resembling systemic lupus erythematosus or rheumatoid arthritis. *Am. J. Med.* 54, 58.

Perry, H.M. Jr, Tan, E.M., Carmody, S., and Sakamoto, A. (1970). Relationship of acetyl transferase activity to antinuclear antibodies and toxic symptoms in hypertensive patients treated with hydralazine. *J. Lab. Clin. Med.* 76, 114.

Pierce, J.R., Throstle, D.C., and Warner, J.J. (1981). Propranolol and retroperitoneal fibrosis. *Ann. Intern. Med.* 95, 244.

Pittsley, R.A. and Yoder, F.W. (1983). Retinoid hyperostosis: skeletal toxicity associated with long-term administration of 13-cis-retinoic acid for refractory ichthyosis. *N. Engl. J. Med.* 308, 1012.

Popkhristov, P. and Kapnilov, S. (1960). Streptomycin as a factor producing and aggravating lupus erythematosus. *Vestn. Dermatol. Venerol.* 34, 10.

Presley, A.P., Kahn, A., and Williamson, N. (1976). Antinuclear antibodies in patients on lithium carbonate. *Br. Med. J.* ii, 280.

Prior, J. and White, I. (1978). Tetany and clubbing in a patient who ingested large quantities of senna. *Lancet* ii, 947.

Pryor, J.P. and Castle, W.M. (1982). Peyronie's disease associated with chronic degenerative arterial disease and not with beta-adrenoceptor blocking agents. *Lancet* i, 917.

Pryor, J.P. and Kahn, O. (1979). Beta-blockers and Peyronie's disease. *Lancet* i, 331.

Pryor, J.P., Castle, W.M., Dukes, D.C., Smith, J.C., Watson, M.E., and Williams, J.L. (1983). Do beta-adrenoceptor blocking drugs cause retroperitoneal fibrosis? *Br. Med. J.* 287, 639.

Rack, P.M.H. and Westbury, D.R. (1966). The effects of suxamethonium and acetylcholine on the behaviour of cat muscle spindles during dynamic stretching, and during fusimotor stimulation. *J. Physiol.* (Lond.) 186, 698.

Racouchot, J., Gaillard, L., and Guilane, J. (1968). Lupus erythémateux subaigu et méthysergide. *Lyon Med.* 220, 1766.

Raftery, E.B. and Denman, A.M. (1973). Systemic lupus erythematosus syndrome induced by practolol. *Br. Med. J.* ii, 452.

Rallison, M.L., O'Brien, J., and Good, R.A. (1961). Severe reactions to long-acting sulfonamides: erythema multiforme exudativum and lupus erythematosus following administration of sulfamethoxypyridazone and sulfadimethodine. *Pediatrics* 28, 908.

Ray, W.A., Griffin, M.R., Schaffner, W., Baugh, D.K., and Melton, J.L. (1987). Psychotropic drug use and the risk of hip fracture. *N. Engl. J. Med.* 316, 363.

Rennie, W. and Mitchell, N. (1974). Slipped femoral capital epiphysis occurring during growth hormone therapy. *J. Bone Joint Surg.* 56, 703.

Reynolds, J.E.F. (ed.) (1989). Analgesics and anti-inflammatory agents. In *Martindale The extra pharmacopoeia* (29th edn), p. 1. The Pharmaceutical Press, London.

Richman, D.D., Fischl, M.A., and Gvieco, M.H. (1987). The toxicity of azidothymidine (AZT) in the treatment of

patients with AIDS and AIDS-related complex: double-blind, placebo-controlled trial. *N. Engl. J. Med.* 317 192.

Rimmer, E., Richens, A., Forster, M.E., and Rees, R.W.M. (1983). Retroperitoneal fibrosis associated with timolol. *Lancet* i, 300.

Roche, A.F., Lipman, R.S., Overall, J.E., and Wellington, H. (1979). The effects of stimulant medication on growth of hyperkinetic children. *Pediatrics* 63, 847.

Roenick, H.H., Haberic, J.R., and Arundell, F.D. (1964). Poststeroid panniculitis. *Arch. Dermatol.* 90, 387.

Rollins, D.E. and Moeller, D. (1975). Polyarthritis associated with clindamycin-induced colitis. *JAMA* 231, 1228.

Rose, T., Nothjunge, J., and Schlote, W. (1985). Familial occurrence of dermatomyositis and progressive scleroderma after injection of a local anaesthetic for dental treatment. *Eur. J. Pediatr.* 143, 225.

Rothfield, N.F., Bierir, W.F., and Gardield, J.W. (1971). The induction of antinuclear antibodies by isoniazid: a prospective study. *Arthritis Rheum.* 14, 182.

Rubinstein, A. (1979). LE-like disease caused by nalidixic acid. *N. Engl. J. Med.* 301, 1288.

Ruby, L.K. and Mital, M.A. (1974). Skeletal deformities following chronic hypervitaminosis A. *J. Bone Joint Surg.* 56, 1283.

Rumpf, K.W., Barth, M., Blech, M., Kaiser, H., Koop, I., Arnold R., *et al.* (1984). Bezafibrat-induzierte Myolyse und Myoglbinurie bei Patienten mit eingeschränkter Nierenfunktion. *Klin. Wochenschr.* 62, 346.

Sachs, H.K. and Moel, D.I. (1989). Height and weight following lead poisoning in childhood. *Am. J. Dis. Child.* 143, 820.

SADRAC (Swedish Adverse Drug Reactions Advisory Committee) (1989). Ranitidine and arthralgia. *SADRAC Bull.* 55, 2.

Safer, D.J. and Allen, R.P. (1973). Factors influencing the suppressant effect of two stimulant drugs on the growth of hyperactive children. *Pediatrics* 51, 660.

Savola, J. (1983). Arthropathy induced by beta blockade. *Br. Med. J.* 287, 1256.

Savola, J. (1984). Arthropathy induced by beta blockade. *Br. Med. J.* 288, 238.

Saxena, A.K. and Nigam, P.K. (1988). Panniculitis following steroid therapy. *Cutis* 42, 341.

Schleicher, E. (1968). LE cells after oral contraceptives. *Lancet* i, 821.

Schneider, H., Kulbe, K.D., Weber, H., and Streicher, E. (1984). Aluminium-free oral phosphate binder. *Trace Elem. Med.* 1, 76.

Schwartz, F.D. and Dunea, G. (1966). Progression of retroperitoneal fibrosis despite cessation of treatment with methysergide. *Lancet* i, 955.

Schwartzfarb, L., Singh, G., and Marcus, D. (1977). Heroin-associated rhabdomyolysis with cardiac involvement. *Arch. Intern. Med.* 137, 1255.

Sekowski, I. and Samuel, P. (1972). Clofibrate-induced acute muscular syndrome. *Am. J. Cardiol.* 30, 572.

Segal, A.W., Pugh, S.F., Levi, A.J., and Loewi, G. (1977). Levamisole-induced arthritis in Crohn's disease. *Br. Med. J.* ii, 555.

Seligmann, M., Cannat, A., and Hamard, M. (1965). Studies on antinuclear antibodies. *Ann. N.Y. Acad. Sci.* 124, 816.

Selroos, O. and Edgren, J. (1975). Lupus-like syndrome associated with pulmonary reaction to nitrofurantoin. *Acta Med. Scand.* 197, 125.

Shaw, M., Petrone, J., Iglesias, D., Costantini, S., and Formentini, Y.E. (1982). Polimiositis aguda por nifurtimox. *Arch. Argent. Dermatol.* 32, 191.

Sherman, J.D., Love, D.E., and Harrington, J.F. (1967). Anemia, positive lupus and rheumatoid factors with methyldopa. A report of 3 cases. *Arch. Intern. Med.* 120, 321.

Shukla, R., Bornschein, R.L., Dietrich, K.N., Buncher, C.R., and Berger, O.G. (1989). Fetal and infant lead exposure: effects on growth in stature. *Pediatrics* 84, 604.

Shukla, V.R. and Borison, R.L. (1982). Lithium and lupus-like syndrome. *JAMA* 248, 921.

Shulman, L.E. (1975). Diffuse fasciitis with eosinophilia: a new syndrome? *Trans. Assoc. Am. Physicians* 88, 70.

Shulman, L.E. and Harvey, A.M. (1960). The nature of drug-induced systemic lupus erythematosus. *Arthritis Rheum.* 3, 464.

Siegel, M., Lee, S.L., and Peress, N.S. (1967). The epidemiology of drug-induced systemic lupus erythematosus. *Arthritis Rheum.* 10, 407.

Sikka, A., Kemman, E., Vrabik, R.M., and Brossman, L. (1983). Carpal tunnel syndrome associated with danazol therapy. *Am. J. Obstet. Gynecol.* 147, 103.

Siklos, P. (1977). Levamisole-induced arthritis. *Br. Med. J.* ii, 773.

Silk, D.B.A., Gibson, J.A., and Murray, C.R.H. (1975). Reversible finger clubbing in the case of purgative abuse. *Gastroenterology* 68, 790.

Sills, J.M. and Bosco, L. (1986). Arthralgia associated with beta-adrenergic blockade. *JAMA* 255 198.

Silver, R.M., Heyes, M.P., Maize, J.C., Quearry, B., Vionett-Fuasset, M., and Sternberg, E.M. (1990). Scleroderma, fasciitis and eosinophilia associated with the ingestion of tryptophan. *N. Engl. J. Med.* 322, 874.

Slutsker, L., Hoesly, F.C., Miller, L., Williams, L.P., Watson, J.C., and Fleming, D.W. (1990). Eosinophilia–myalgia syndrome associated with exposure to tryptophan from a single manufacturer. *JAMA* 264, 213.

Smaill, G.B. (1961). Bilateral rupture of Achilles tendons. *Br. Med. J.* i, 1657.

Smith, A.F., Macfie, W.G., and Oliver, M.F. (1970). Clofibrate serum enzymes and muscle pain. *Br. Med. J.* ii, 86.

Solomon, L. (1973). Drug-induced arthropathy and necrosis of the femoral head. *J. Bone Joint Surg.* 55, 246.

Spencer, H. and Kramer, L. (1983). Antacid-induced calcium loss. *Arch. Intern. Med.* 143, 657.

Spiera, H. and Plotz, C.M. (1969). Rheumatic symptoms and oral contraceptives. *Lancet* i, 571.

Stalnikowicz, R., Mosseri, M., and Shalev, O. (1982). Phenytoin-induced arthritis. *Neurology* 32, 1317.

Steen, V.D. and Ramsey-Goldman, R. (1988). Phenothiazine-induced systemic lupus erythematosus with superior vena cava syndrome: case report and review of the literature. *Arthritis Rheum.* 31, 923.

Sternberg, E.M., van Woert, M.H., Young, S.M., Magnussen, I.B., Baker, H., Gauthier, S., *et al.* (1980). Development of a scleroderma-like illness during therapy with L-5-hydroxy tryptophan and carbidopa. *N. Engl. J. Med.* 303, 782.

Stocks, A.E. and Robertson, A. (1966). The long-term therapy of severe hypertension with guanethidine. *Med. J. Aust.* i, 893.

Streiter, M.L., Schneider, H.L., and Proto, A.V. (1982). Steroid-induced thoracic lipomatosis: paraspinal involvement. *AJR* 139, 679.

Sturman, S.G., Kumararatne, D., and Beevers, D.G. (1988). Fatal hydralazine-induced systemic lupus erythematosus. *Lancet* ii, 1304.

Sutton, R.D. (1968). Aseptic necrosis of bone, a complication of corticosteroid therapy. In *Drug-induced diseases*, Vol. 3 (ed. L. Meyler and H.M. Peck), p. 171. Associated Scientific Publishers, Amsterdam.

Tanenbaum, M.H. (1972). Topical steroid atrophy: a disappearing digit. *JAMA* 220, 126.

Taranta, A., Mack, H., Hass, R.G., Hudson, J., and Cooper, N.S. (1958). Nodular panniculitis after massive prednisone therapy. *Am. J. Med.* 25, 52.

Teates, C.D. (1970). Steroid-induced mediastinal lipomatosis. *Radiology* 96, 501.

Thind, G.S. and Bryson, T.H.L. (1983). Single-dose suxamethonium and muscle pain in pregnancy. *Br. J. Anaesth.* 55, 743.

Thompson, J. and Julian, D.G. (1982). Retroperitoneal fibrosis associated with metoprolol. *Br. Med. J.* 284, 83.

Tobert, J.A. (1988). Efficacy and long-term adverse effect pattern of lovastatin. *Am. J. Cardiol.* 62, 28J.

Torisu, M., Miyahara, T., Shinohara, O., Ohsato, K., and Sonozaki, H. (1978). A new side effect of BCG immunotherapy — BCG-induced arthritis in man. *Cancer Immunol. Immunother.* 5, 77.

Toxic Epidemic Syndrome Study Group (1982). Toxic epidemic syndrome, Spain 1981. *Lancet* ii, 697.

Tunkel, A.R., Shuman, M., Popkin, M., Seth, R., and Hoffman, B. (1987). Minoxidil-induced systemic lupus erythematosus. *Arch. Intern. Med.* 147, 599.

Uddin, M.S., Lynfield, Y.L., Grosberg, S.J., and Stiefler, R. (1979). Cutaneous reaction to spironolactone resembling lupus erythematosus. *Cutis* 24 198.

Utz, D.C., Rooke, E.D., Spittell, J.A., and Bartholomew, L.G. (1965). Retroperitoneal fibrosis in patients taking methysergide. *JAMA* 191, 983.

van der Korst, J.K., Colenbrauer, H., and Cats, A. (1960). Phenobarbital and the shoulder–hand syndrome. *Ann. Rheum. Dis.* 25, 553.

Vermersch, P., Foissac-Gegoux, Ph., Caron, J., and Petit, H. (1989). Retroperitoneal fibrosis after treatment with bromocriptine. *Presse Med.* 18, 841.

von Eickstedt, K.W. and Elsässer, W. (1988). Corticotrophins and corticosteroids. In *Meyler's side effects of drugs* (11th edn) (ed. M.N.G. Dukes), p. 812. Elsevier Science Publishers, Amsterdam.

Vrhovac, B. (1988). Anti-inflammatory analgesics and drugs used in gout. In *Meyler's side effects of drugs* (11th edn) (ed.

M.N.G. Dukes), p. 170. Elsevier Science Publishers, Amsterdam.

Walker, F.J. (1989). Simvastatin: the clinical profile. *Am. J. Med.* 87: (suppl. 4A), 44S.

Walker, P.C. and Ramsay, L.E. (1985). Do β-blockers cause arthropathy? A case controlled study. *Br. Med. J.* 291, 1684.

Wallis, A.A., Bell, R., and Sutherland, P.W. (1977). Propranolol and Peyronie's disease. *Lancet* ii, 980.

Walsh, J.R. and Zimmerman, J.H. (1953). The demonstration of the 'LE' phenomenon in patients with penicillin hypersensitivity. *Blood* 8, 65.

Watermeyer, G.S., Mann, J.I., Truswell, A.S., and Levy, I. (1975). Type IIa hyperlipoproteinaemia: an evaluation of four therapeutic regimens. *S. Afr. Med. J.* 49, 631.

Waters, D.J. and Mapleson, W.W. (1971). Suxamethonium pains: hypothesis and observation. *Anaesthesia* 26, 127.

Watkins, S.M. and Williams, J.R.B. (1982). Avascular necrosis of bone after high doses of dexamethasone during neurosurgery. *Br. Med. J.* 284, 742.

Watson, A.J.S., Dalbow, M.H., Stachura, I., Fragola, A.J., Rubin, M.F., Watson, R.M., *et al.* (1983). Immunological studies in cimetidine-induced nephropathy and polymyositis. *N. Engl. J. Med.* 308, 142.

Watts, J.F., Edwards, R.L., and Butt, W.R. (1985). Treatment of premenstrual syndrome using danazol: preliminary report of a placebo-controlled double-blind, dose-ranging study. *J. Int. Med. Res.* 13, 127.

Weinstein, J. (1978). Hypocomplementemia in hydralazine-induced systemic lupus erythematosus. *Am. J. Med.* 65, 553.

White, D.C. (1962). Observations on the prevention of muscle pain after suxamethonium. *Br. J. Anaesth.* 34, 332.

Wilske, K.R., Shalit, I.E., Willkens, R.F., and Decker, J.L. (1965). Findings suggestive of systemic lupus erythematosus in subjects on chronic anticonvulsant therapy. *Arthritis Rheum.* 8, 260.

Wilson, J.D., Bullock, J.Y., Sutherland, D.C., Main, C., and O'Brien, K.P. (1978). Antinuclear antibodies in patients receiving non-practolol beta-blockers. *Br. Med. J.* i, 14.

Windsor, W.O., Kurrein, F., and Dyer, N.H. (1975). Fibrous peritonitis a complication of practolol therapy. *Br. Med. J.* ii, 68.

Winfield, J.B. and Davis, J.S. (1974). Anti-DNA antibody in procaine-induced lupus erythematosus. Determinations using DNA fractionated by methylated albumin-kieselguhr chromatography. *Arthritis Rheum.* 17, 97.

Witman, G. and Davis, R. (1981). A lupus erythematosus syndrome induced by clonidine hydrochloride. *Rhode Island Med. J.* 64, 147.

Wouters, J.M.G.W., van de Putte, L.B.A., Renier, W.O., and Joosten, E.M.G. (1982). D-Penicillamine-induced polymyositis. *Neth. J. Med.* 25, 159.

Young, R.A. and Brogden, R.N. (1988). Doxazosin. A review of its pharmacodynamic and pharmacokinetic properties, and therapeutic efficacy in mild or moderate hypertension. *Drugs* 35, 525.

Yudkin, J.S. (1977). Peyronie's disease in association with metoprolol. *Lancet* ii, 1355.

Zarafonetis, C.J.D. and Kalas, J.P. (1960). Serotonin degradation by ceruloplasmin and its inhibition by isoniazid and iproniazid. *Am. J. Med. Sci.* 239, 203.

Zarrabi, M.H., Zucker, S., Miller, F., Derman, R.M., Romano, G.S., Hartnett, J.A., *et al.* (1979). Immunologic and coagulation disorders in chlorpromazine-treated patients. *Ann. Intern. Med.* 91, 194.

Zelman, S. (1978). Terbutaline and muscular symptoms. *JAMA* 239, 930.

17. Skin disorders

R. H. FELIX and A. G. SMITH

Incidence

Adverse drug reactions more commonly affect the skin than any other organ. Approximately 30 per cent of reported drug reactions involve the skin: of these about 46 per cent are maculopapular rashes, 23 per cent urticarial, 10 per cent fixed eruptions, and 5 per cent erythema multiforme (Kuokkanen 1972). A recent study of over 15 000 consecutive inpatients identified an overall reaction rate of 2.2 per cent (Bigby *et al.* 1986). The most commonly implicated drugs with reaction rates per 1000 were amoxycillin (51), co-trimoxazole (34), ampicillin (33), cephalosporins (13), and blood products. No reactions were observed to digoxin, promethazine, spironolactone, methyldopa, aminophylline, or propranolol. These reaction rates are of value in assessing which of a number of a patient's drugs may have caused his rash. It must be remembered, however, that even those drugs with a low reaction rate in this study may be implicated: for example, digoxin as the cause of a psoriasiform eruption (David *et al.* 1982).

Diagnosis

In practice it is often difficult to diagnose a drug eruption confidently. Frequently, they correspond closely in morphology with various naturally occurring eruptions; more than one of the drugs a patient is receiving may be recognized as a possible cause of his rash; finally it is rare for additional *in vivo* or *in vitro* tests to clarify the situation greatly.

Drug rashes, like other drug reactions, may be divided into Type A (augmented) and Type B (bizarre) (see Chapter 3). An example of a Type A reaction is the captopril eruption due to kinin potentiation (Wilkin *et al.* 1980); and of a Type B reaction, the practolol eruption (Felix *et al.* 1974). In so far as Type A reactions are predictable (especially with hindsight), occur in a high proportion of patients taking the drug, are dose-related, and subside readily on drug withdrawal, their diagnosis presents less of a problem than with the generally less common Type B reactions. In these, diagnosis is complicated by low incidence rates, absence of dose-dependency, and even failure of resolution of the eruption on drug withdrawal as in some cases of penicillamine-induced pemphigus (Santa Cruz *et al.* 1981).

In some instances the characteristics of the reaction make it difficult to maintain the Type A–Type B dichotomy. Examples of this are the hlgh incidence of hydralazine-induced systemic lupus erythematosus in patients (especially females) who are slow acetylators and HLA DR4-positive (Batchelor *et al.* 1980); the 95 per cent incidence of eruption in patients with infectious mononucleosis treated with ampicillin (Pullen *et al.* 1967); and the 10-fold increase in reaction rate to co-trimoxazole in AIDS patients (De Raeve *et al.* 1988). In other groups these reactions would be designated Type B: here they might be termed augmentedly bizarre (Type AB).

In an attempt to justify the diagnosis of a drug rash consideration should be given to the following points.

1. *History* The interval between the initiation of drug therapy and the onset of the rash may be of value in diagnosis. Most cutaneous reactions occur within one week of exposure to the drug (Arndt and Jick 1976). This early onset is especially probable in Type A reactions; for example, for the captopril eruption the mean ($\pm$SD) latent period was 9 ± 4.4 days, whereas in the Type B practolol eruption it was 312 ± 240 days.

2. *Signs* Few drug eruptions are pathognomonic of a particular drug. Historical exceptions are the scaly reticulated and lichenoid purpura produced by carbromal, and the embedded palmar–plantar warts combined with raindrop pigmentation caused by arsenic. The mor-

phological pattern of the eruption may be of value in identifying the causative drug. Thus a lichenoid eruption is commoner with thiazides than with penicillins, so although penicillins cause more rashes overall than do thiazides a lichenoid eruption in a patient taking both types of drug is more likely to be due to the thiazide.

It is important to consider alternative aetiological candidates for any putative drug eruption. For example, most varieties of eczema are unrelated to systemic therapy, and drugs can be eliminated as likely causes. Thus, in an ongoing study of rashes in rheumatological patients receiving systemic therapy, the authors have identified discoid and asteatotic eczemas as the cause in approximately 90 per cent of cases. Treatment of the eczema effects resolution, without the need to alter systemic therapy.

3. *Continuation and discontinuation (dechallenge) of therapy* Most drug rashes will persist for as long as the drug is continued. There are some exceptions to this, as in the case of the transient maculopapular rash that may be produced by phenytoin (Wilson *et al.* 1978). The morbilliform eruption that may complicate therapy with penicillins may also fade with continued therapy.

The diagnostic value of continuation and discontinuation may be vitiated by the drug not being a sufficient cause of the eruption: thus, screening of ultraviolet light may abolish drug-associated photosensitivity. In most instances the eruption will resolve when the drug is withdrawn. In some instances, however, the pathological changes are not readily reversible. In hyperpigmentation induced by oral contraceptives, antimalarials, or chlorpromazine much of the pigment is bound in dermal macrophages and may persist for years. In other instances, the drug initiates immunological changes that may maintain the rash long after drug withdrawal, as with penicillamine pemphigus, or drug-induced lupus erythematosus.

4. *Challenge* The recurrence of a rash when a drug is readministered provides the best evidence of a causal relationship. Patients are often not enthusiastic about this procedure, and its use is contraindicated where the rash is part of an acute systemic disturbance, as in the pulmonary oedema and eosinophilia which may accompany the rash caused by nitrofurantoin. Another absolute contraindication to challenge is in the more severe skin disorders such as toxic epidermal necrolysis, and in exanthematous eruptions which may progress to erythroderma, namely, those due to isoniazid and streptomycin.

5. *Special tests* Epicutaneous and intracutaneous tests which suggest Type 1 hypersensitivity (Coombs and Gell classification) may be positive in some urticarial and maculopapular eruptions. Generally, the tests are more reliable with high-molecular weight compounds such as globulins and insulin.

Patch testing, indicating Type IV hypersensitivity, has been of some value in supporting the diagnosis of generalized eruptions due to diazepam, meprobamate, and practolol (Felix and Comaish 1974); carbamazepine (Houwerzijl *et al.* 1974); the tartrazine dyes, which are widely added to drugs and foods (Roeleveld and van Ketel 1976); and chloramphenicol (Rudzki *et al.* 1976).

Positive patch tests have also been demonstrated in toxic epidermal necrolysis due to ampicillin (Tagami *et al.* 1983). Patch testing carries less risk of anaphylaxis than does prick testing but, rarely, systemic symptoms have occurred as in a case of dyspnoea with piperazine patch testing (Fregert 1976).

Of *in vitro* tests (see Chapter 25), the radioallergosorbent (RAST) test has shown a good correlation with prick testing in penicillin allergy (Kraft and Wide 1976), but its use has not been widely extended to other drugs. The results of other *in vitro* tests have been disappointing. Lymphocyte transformation studies in a variety of drug reactions showed variously 13 per cent (Sarkany and Gaylarde 1978) and 32 per cent (Dobozy *et al.* 1981) positive reactions. Macrophage migration inhibition tests (Halevy *et al.* 1990) have produced positive responses in 70 per cent of cases of drug eruption. Thus these tests neither verify nor falsify the diagnosis of a drug reaction. They do, however, when positive, increase the probability that the drug tested caused the eruption.

In practice, a number of tests in which it is not sought to infer causation, but to increase the negative analogy between drug eruptions and their idiopathic 'look-alikes', are often more helpful. In differentiating between idiopathic and drug-related systemic lupus erythematosus, the absence of antibodies to double-stranded DNA and presence of antibodies to single-stranded DNA will point to drug induction. Histology may be valuable. For example, lichenoid drug eruptions, in contrast to idiopathic lichen planus, tend to have a thinner and parakeratotic epidermis, with a more varied and deeply extending dermal infiltrate (Ackerman 1978).

Whereas most skin diseases are diseases of the skin alone, the situation is not so reassuring in the case of drug rashes. In the cases of practolol, benoxaprofen (Halsey and Cardoe 1982), and amiodarone (McGovern *et al.* 1983) a high incidence of skin reaction was matched by a high incidence of internal organ involvement. Idiopathic urticaria and angioedema are practically never associated with dyspnoea and laryngeal oedema, but these life-threatening events may occur with the urticaria and angioedema of angiotensin-converting enzyme inhibiting drugs such as captopril and enalapril (Slater *et al.* 1988). Idiopathic pemphigus vulgaris is not associated with renal disease, but that associated with penicillamine treatment may be associated with minimal-change nephropathy (Savill *et al.* 1988). The rash *per se* may also be more significant than its idiopathic counterpart. For example, idiopathic cutaneous lichen planus does not undergo malignant change, whereas the lichenoid eruption induced by quinacrine hydrochloride may do so (Bauer 1981). Thus the dismissive listing of rashes under a drug's adverse reactions may cover a multitude of adverse effects.

Acneiform eruptions

Drugs may either exacerbate acne or precipitate its development in subjects without pre-existing acne. In the latter group the acne tends to be a more monomorphic papulo-pustular eruption, without conspicuous comedones, and of sudden onset, and to involve the extremities in addition to the face and trunk. The factors recognized as important in the aetiology of acne are: the sebum excretion rate (SER) and possibly obstruction to sebum flow; the hormonal control of the sebaceous gland; and the bacteriology of the gland. Drugs influencing any of these may produce acne.

Androgens increase SER, and synthetic androgens such as danazol (Greenberg 1979) can cause acne in women, as may oral contraceptives which contain a progesterone component with significant androgenic activity, such as 19-norethisterone. Increasingly, severe acne is being seen in athletes who take anabolic steroids (Kiraly *et al.* 1987). High doses of corticosteroids may cause a monomorphic acne (Hurwitz 1989); the mechanism is uncertain but may be by obstruction due to hyperkeratinization of the upper pilosebaceous duct.

A similar mechanism has been proposed for isoniazid which, especially in slow inactivators, may either induce or exacerbate acne (Oliwiecki and Burton 1988). Other antituberculous agents, such as rifampicin, ethambutol, and ethionamide have also been implicated in acneiform eruptions.

Of psychotropic drugs it is believed that phenothiazines may exacerbate acne, and lithium (Yoder 1975) certainly can. Medicines containing bromides and iodides are now less frequently prescribed but were recognized to cause acne, which might progress to bromoderma or iododerma. The potential acneogenic effect of halogens is emphasized by the occasional case report of halothane-induced acne (Guldager 1987).

The anticonvulsants phenobarbitone, phenytoin, and troxidone (trimethadione) have been thought to cause acne. A study of 243 patients on a variety of anticonvulsants, however, failed to show any increased prevalence of acne or increased SER (Greenwood *et al.* 1983).

PUVA therapy (the combination of long-wave ultraviolet light with oral methoxsalen [8-methoxypsoralen]) (Jones and Bleehan 1977) may cause acne. It was suggested that this might be a direct effect of the heat and UVA, but the effects of PUVA on immune function and thus on bacterial growth may also be relevant, as they probably are in the 15 per cent of patients treated with cyclosporin who develop acne (Bencini *et al.* 1986).

Fixed drug eruptions

Sometimes a drug induces lesions that recur at the same site on drug readministration. These fixed drug eruptions (FDE) are common; they have become increasingly so, and now approximate exanthematous eruptions in frequency (Alanko *et al.* 1989). Clinically, the lesion is circular and may evolve through macular, raised, and blistered stages. Characteristically, it is bright or a dusky red early and usually resolves with pigmentation. The limbs are more frequently affected than the trunk and involvement of genital skin and oral or genital mucous membranes is not rare. The time elapsing between drug ingestion and the appearance of the rash varies from a few to 24 hours.

Recently, wandering (Guin *et al.* 1987) and non-pigmenting (Shelley and Shelley 1987) variants have been described. Multifocal FDE (Sowden and Smith 1990) may be difficult to distinguish from erythema multiforme. In these cases the histology of intraepidermal vesiculation, and a denser and more varied dermal inflammatory infiltrate, involving the deep as well as superficial vessels favours the diagnosis of FDE.

Of the great many drugs that may cause FDE the phenazone derivatives, sulphonamides and trimethoprim, barbiturates, tetracyclines, and carbamazepine are the most common (Alanko *et al.* 1989). FDE may be seen even after administration of drugs that are only minimally absorbed (e.g. phenolphthalein) or after insoluble sulphonamides (e.g. succinylsulphathiazole and phthalylsulphathiazole [Tan and Copeman 1974]) or nystatin (Pareek 1980).

Reappearance of the eruption within two to three hours of oral challenge with the suspected drug is a useful and safe means of confirming the diagnosis, as systemic involvement is absent. In addition, patch testing at the site of the eruption, but not elsewhere, is often positive (Alanko *et al.* 1987).

Vesiculo-bullous (blistering) eruptions

Blisters are circumscribed elevated lesions that contain fluid; they may be subdivided into vesicles, if their diameter is less than 0.5 cm, and bullae, if greater. While such lesions may occur as part of the picture of toxic epidermal necrolysis, fixed drug eruption, or cutaneous vasculitis, this section deals with those instances in which the blister is the dominant lesion.

Bullae may occur in drug-induced coma and are generally at the site of pressure and trauma. Histological examination in patients with coma caused by heroin, methadone, and barbiturates (Mandy and Ackerman 1970) showed subepidermal bullae with intraepidermal spongiosis, associated with sweat gland necrosis. These lesions have been described in coma induced by a variety of drugs, including barbiturates (Beveridge and Lawson 1965), azapropazone (Barker and Cotterill 1977), glibenclamide (Wongpaitoon et al. 1981), and chlormethiazole (Banerjee et al. 1988).

In other instances, drugs may induce eruptions that are closely similar to idiopathic bullous dermatoses. Of these, drug-induced pemphigus with intraepidermal blistering and deposition of immunoglobulins is best recognized. The majority of cases have been described with penicillamine (Santa Cruz et al. 1981), and may occur in the treatment of rheumatoid arthritis, scleroderma, or Wilson's disease with this drug. Mostly the pemphigus is of the superficial blistering foliaceous or erythematosus subtypes, with only 15 per cent the suprabasal pemphigus vulgaris. Other drugs cited as inducing pemphigus are captopril, which is structurally related to penicillamine (Katz et al. 1987); penicillin (Duhra and Foulds 1988); rifampicin (Honeybourne et al. 1987); and, possibly, piroxicam (Martin et al. 1983).

Drug-induced bullous pemphigoid with immunoglobulin deposition and splitting at the dermoepidermal junction has been described with a few drugs, which include mefenamic acid (Shepherd et al. 1986); penicillamine (Brown and Dubin 1987); penicillin (Alcalay et al. 1988); and ibuprofen (Laing et al. 1988).

In the dermatitis herpetiformis variant, linear IgA bullous dermatosis, lithium carbonate (McWhirter et al. 1987) and vancomycin (Baden et al. 1988) have been cited as causes.

In porphyria cutanea tarda, blistering on areas exposed to light is associated with skin fragility, hypertrichosis, and hyperpigmentation. In contrast with the erythropoietic porphyrias, acute cutaneous photosensitivity is rare. The blistering occurs at the dermoepidermal junction, where there may be deposition of immunoglobulins, which is, however, greater around dermal blood vessels. Porphyria cutanea tarda may be precipitated by ethanol, androgens, oestrogens, griseofulvin, sulphonylureas, and the 4-aminoquinoline antimalarials (hydroxychloroquine and chloroquine) (Bruinsma 1987a).

Pseudoporphyria is clinically and histologically similar to porphyria cutanea tarda, but is not associated with any abnormalities of porphyrin metabolism. There may be signs of acute phototoxicity with erythema and oedema as in the case of nalidixic acid (Ramsay and Obreshkova 1974) and amiodarone (Parodi et al. 1988); or these may be lacking, as in examples due to tetracyclines, frusemide, naproxen (Judd et al. 1986), chlorthalidone (Barker et al. 1989), etretinate (McDonagh and Harrington 1989) and cyclosporin (Sola et al. 1987).

Nail changes

Drug-induced psoriasiform eruptions, such as those due to practolol (Kirkham and Holt 1976), may induce nail changes similar to those of idiopathic psoriasis. In contrast, lichenoid drug eruptions rarely involve the nails, although those produced by mepacrine (Bauer 1981) are exceptions. Nail plate dystrophy, either alone or as part of a more widespread cutaneous involvement, may be caused by the retinoids (Garioch and Simpson 1989) or penicillamine (Bjellerup 1989), and may also accompany the yellow nail syndrome (Ilchyshyn and Vickers 1983).

Photo-onycholysis has been reported with many drugs, including oral contraceptives (via their induction of porphyria) (Byrne et al. 1976), psoralens, tetracyclines, and fluoroquinolones (Baran and Juhlin 1987), and benoxaprofen (Halsey and Cardoe 1982).

Various cytotoxic drugs, including bleomycin, melphalan, dacarbazine, and cyclophosphamide, have been cited as causing hyperpigmentation, especially in longitudinal bands (Daniel and Scher 1984). More rarely, transverse white lines similar to Mee's lines of arsenic ingestion may occur with combination chemotherapy (James and Odom 1983). A number of recent reports have described longitudinal bands of pigmentation in association with zidovudine therapy (Groark et al. 1989).

Both the 9-aminoacridine (e.g. mepacrine) and the 4-aminoquinoline (e.g. chloroquine, hydroxychloroquine, and amodiaquine) antimalarials may produce pigmentary changes of the nails: these may be either a diffuse blue-brown colouration or longitudinal banding. In addition, Daniel and Scher (1984) describe increased nail pigmentation with phenothiazine and psoralen therapy and the yellow discolouration of 'gold nails'.

Alopecia

While a cicatricial alopecia may occur in, for example, a severe drug-induced lichenoid eruption of the scalp (Bauer 1981), the great majority of drug-induced alopecias are non-scarring. They are usually confined to the scalp, which shows diffuse involvement, and reversible on stopping therapy.

In alopecia due to cytotoxic agents and colchicine, direct damage occurs to the follicle in the actively growing anagen phase, and dystrophic hairs with tapering roots are shed about 2 weeks after the beginning of therapy. This pattern of anagen effluvium is also a feature of thallium poisoning. In all other described drug alopecias a telogen effluvium occurs with shedding of club-shaped hairs about 3 months after starting therapy. A telogen effluvium may also complicate drug-induced anagen effluvium.

The alopecia of cytostatic drugs may be regarded as a Type A response. While the severity is dose-related, some agents produce more severe hair loss than others; doxorubicin and vincristine produce severe loss; methotrexate and cyclophosphamide less, and cisplatin none (Brodin 1987).

Anticoagulants produce hair loss in a high percentage of patients — heparin and heparinoids (including dextran) in up to 50 per cent, coumarins in about 40 per cent, and with combinations of the two about 80 per cent (Fischer *et al.* 1953). Antithyroid drugs may produce hair loss, even when the patient is euthyroid. This has been described with methylthiouracil and propylthiouracil and also carbimazole (Papadopoulos and Harden 1966).

Alopecia, which may be severe, is well recognized with retinoid therapy (Mahrle *et al.* 1979). It is more common with etretinate than isotretinoin and takes the form of a dose-dependent telogen effluvium, with hair root dystrophy at high dosage.

Lithium (Dawber and Mortimer 1982) may definitely cause hair loss. In many other cases, such as with oral contraceptives, the evidence is conflicting, while in others the causal association of the telogen effluvium is with the condition treated and not with the treatment (Barth and Dawber 1989).

Hirsutism and hypertrichosis

Hirsutism may be defined as excessive growth of coarse terminal body hair in a male pattern in a female. Drugs with androgenic activity may produce hirsutism, with possible concomitant androgenic alopecia. Examples are testosterone, danazol, corticotrophin (ACTH), and metyrapone (Bergfeld and Redmond 1987).

Hypertrichosis may be distinguished as an increase in non-androgen-modulated hair, and thus may occur on sites such as the eyebrows, forehead, and cheeks. It may be caused by minoxidil (Burton and Marshall 1979), diazoxide (Burton *et al.* 1975), cyclosporin (Wysocki and Daley 1987), penicillamine, phenytoin, and psoralens.

Abnormalities of pigmentation

Abnormal pigmentation is mainly produced either by the deposition of drugs themselves in the skin, or by their stimulation of melanogenesis, or by a combination of these two factors.

Drug deposition

Therapeutic use of compounds containing silver, bismuth, and mercury has declined and with it the incidence of the pigmentation they may produce (Granstein and Sober 1981). Wet dressings of silver nitrate solution, however, remain a popular treatment for leg ulcers. Argyria does not seem to follow its use in this instance, although it is described with silver-containing antismoking lozenges (Shelton and Goulding 1979). The therapeutic use of gold salts may rarely be accompanied by the development of chrysiasis, in which there is a grey-blue photodistributed pigmentation of the skin and sclera, commonest in Caucasian women. Gold particles are deposited in dermal macrophages and melanogenesis is increased (Leonard *et al.* 1986). After long-term administration of systemic iron, a generalized haemochromatosis-like discolouration may appear (Pletcher *et al.* 1963).

The tetracycline derivative minocycline may rarely cause either a diffuse pigmentation in areas exposed to the sun, pigmentation located in scars, or a patchy pigmentation of the shins. Electron microscopy of involved skin demonstrates electron-dense cytoplasmic granules in dermal macrophages, which are probably deposits of the drug itself (Okada *et al.* 1989). Similar granules are also found in the involved skin of the photosensitivity-associated amiodarone pigmentation (Zachary *et al.* 1984), in which instance lipofuscin deposition also occurs in dermal macrophages. Intracytoplasmic granules, which again probably consist largely of the drug itself, also occur in pigmentation due to chlorpromazine (Benning *et al.* 1988) and to mepacrine (Leigh *et al.* 1979). Similar skin pigmentation has been attributed to quinidine, which is structurally related to mepacrine (Mahler *et al.* 1986). Most patients taking mepacrine develop a yellowing of the skin, and in a minority a blue-black discolouration of the shins, nails, and hard palate occurs. As well as with the 9-amino-acridines (e.g. mepacrine), pigmentation may occur with the 4-aminoquinoline group (e.g. chloroquine, hydroxy-chloroquine, and amodiaquine). With the latter, but not with mepacrine, there is a correlation between skin pigmentation and retinal damage.

Yellow discolouration of the skin may also be pro-duced by β-carotene, which is used in the treatment of erythropoietic protoporphyria; as with mepacrine, in contrast to jaundice, the sclerae are not discoloured. Clofazimine may directly stain the skin red within a few weeks of starting therapy; after 2–3 months black-brown or violaceous-brown staining may develop, which may be due to complexes of the drug with fatty acids derived from the leprosy bacilli (Sakurai and Skinsnes 1977).

Increased melanogenesis

Both corticotrophin (ACTH) and tetracosactrin contain the seven-amino-acid sequence common to peptides with melanocyte-stimulating activity, and their long-term administration leads to the Addisonian pattern of hyperpigmentation.

Chloasma (or melasma) due to epidermal (reversible) and dermal (relatively irreversible) pigmentation of the face occurs in about 5 per cent of women taking oral contraceptives. This appears to be due to a direct effect of oestrogens and progestogens on melanogenesis and not to stimulation of peptides related to melanocyte-stimulating hormone (MSH) (Smith *et al.* 1977). Simi-larly, no elevation of MSH was found in patients on phenytoin, of whom about 10 per cent may develop a chloasma pattern of pigmentation. Direct stimulation of melanocytes, as occurs with amphibian melanophores (Kuske and Krebs 1964) seems to be the likely mechan-ism. Likewise, no elevation of MSH has been demon-strated in the pigmentation of cytotoxic drug therapy (Kew *et al.* 1977). Busulphan may produce an Addison-ian pattern of pigmentation in up to 20 per cent of those receiving it. Bleomycin produces a similar incidence of hyperpigmentation, but of a different pattern, with streaking on the trunk and maximization of pigment over the extensor surfaces of joints. Cyclophosphamide, melphalan, doxorubicin, fluorouracil, and mustine hy-drochloride (Granstein and Sober 1981) may also pro-duce hyperpigmentation. More recently, cyclosporin (Brady and Wing 1989) and zidovudine (Merenich *et al.* 1989) have been recognized as causes of Addisonian hyperpigmentation. PUVA therapy (combining psora-len [8-methoxypsoralen] and long-wave ultraviolet light) is now widely used in the treatment of psoriasis and other dermatoses; the concomitant tanning is better guaranteed than is disease responsiveness.

Cutaneous vasculitis

The lesions of cutaneous vasculitis mainly involve the lower legs and evolve rapidly through red macules to urticated papules which become purpuric (palpable pur-pura), and in severe cases haemorrhagic blisters and ulcers may develop.

Histologically, the lesions involve the postcapillary venules, which show fibrinoid necrosis of their walls and a perivascular infiltrate of mononuclear cells and neu-trophils, the destruction of which (leucocytoclasis) pro-duces the nuclear dust of a leucocytoclastic vasculitis. It has been claimed that, in drug-induced vasculitis, mono-nuclear cells and eosinophils predominate and that leucocytoclasis and fibrinoid vascular lesions are incon-spicuous (Mullick *et al.* 1979). Other reports do not, however, stress these discriminants, and it may be that there is a change from neutrophilic and leucocytoclastic to mononuclear infiltration, which is solely a function of time (Zax *et al.* 1990).

The drugs mainly implicated are sulphonamides, thia-zides, chlorpropamide, phenylbutazone, indomethacin, hydantoin derivatives, propylthiouracil (Gammeltoft and Kristensen 1982), and radiographic contrast media (Kerdel *et al.* 1984). More recent reports have implicated diltiazem (Carmichael and Paul 1988), terbutaline (Enat *et al.* 1988), and the retinoids (Dwyer *et al.* 1989).

The term polyarteritis nodosa is best reserved for cases in which necrosis and vessel wall inflammation with leucocytoclasis occur in small to medium-sized arteries, corresponding to the occurrence of tender nodules along the course of a superficial artery. This pattern of vas-culitis is generally not associated with drug therapy, but an association with drug abuse (especially of methyl-amphetamine) has been described (Citron *et al.* 1970).

Erythema nodosum is characterized clinically by tender cutaneous nodules and histologically by a septal panniculitis with sometimes a mild vasculitis. In the minority of cases associated with drug therapy, sul-phonamides, salicylates, oral contraceptives (Dombar-dieri *et al.* 1977), or gold salts (Stone *et al.* 1973) are implicated.

Photosensitivity

Photosensitivity denotes reactions to normally harmless doses of ultraviolet or visible radiation. Drugs may induce photosensitivity either by direct mechanisms in which the presence of the drug, in either altered or unaltered form, in the skin is necessary, or by indirect effects on other organs. Examples of indirect photosensitivity are drug-associated lupus erythematosus, hepatic porphyria, and pellagra.

Lupus erythematosus and porphyria are dealt with elsewhere. Pellagra may be induced by isoniazid acting as an antagonist of niacin, and also by fluorouracil, mercaptopurine, chloramphenicol, the hydantoins, phenobarbitone, and azathioprine (Stadler *et al.* 1982).

Direct photosensitivity may be divided into phototoxic (usually Type A) and photoallergic (Type B) mechanisms. Phototoxic reactions occur in a high proportion of those exposed, are dose-dependent, may occur on first exposure, and have a short latency of minutes to a few hours; the opposite obtains in photoallergic reactions. Clinically, phototoxic reactions resemble sunburn and show the appropriate histology, with epidermal necrosis, dermoepidermal separation, and a sparse superficial lymphohistiocytic dermal infiltrate. Photoallergic reactions show a more varied morphology, which may be eczematous or papular and is less well localized; the histological appearances are of epidermal spongiosis, oedema of the papillary dermis, and a deeper lymphohistiocytic dermal infiltrate.

The action-spectrum of most drug photosensitizers is in the UVA range (320–400 nm) with some extension into UVB (290–320 nm), which is filtered off by window glass).

Predominantly phototoxic reactions

Amiodarone is structurally related to the psoralens and causes photosensitivity in nearly half of patients taking it (Ferguson *et al.* 1985); these changes may continue for up to 4 months after stopping therapy. The drug's action-spectrum is 334–460 nm.

The tetracyclines, especially demeclocycline, are more likely to cause photosensitivity than any other group of antibiotics. Their action spectrum is 320420 nm. Sulphonamides, especially sulphamethoxazole; griseofulvin; and ciprofloxacin (Granowitz 1989) have also been implicated.

A number of the non-steroidal anti-inflammatory drugs are photosensitizers. Benoxaprofen produced a high incidence of phototoxicity (Ferguson *et al.* 1982). Of currently prescribed anti-inflammatory drugs, piroxicam (McKerrow and Greig 1986) has been most frequently cited; its reaction has both features of phototoxicity and photoallergy. The propionic acid derivatives

azapropazone and tiaprofenic acid are also recognized photosensitizers.

Other groups of drugs with phototoxic potential include the thiazides (Addo *et al.* 1987), tricyclic antidepressants (Bruinsma 1987*b*), and the retinoids (Ferguson and Johnson 1986) — etretinate being more frequently implicated than isotretinoin. It is suggested that a metabolite of etretinate is responsible for its phototoxicity. Variation in patient capacity for degradation of this and other drugs producing phototoxicity may account for the comparative rarity of adverse reaction, which thus may have more affinity with Type B than Type A reactions.

Predominantly photoallergic reactions

Of the phenothiazines, chlorpromazine is the best recognized photosensitizer. It may cause both phototoxic and photoallergic reactions, with an action spectrum in the UVA range (Epstein 1968). Promethazine and thioridazine (Rohrborn and Brauninger 1987) are also photoallergens.

Quinine may induce photosensitivity in the form of oedema and erythema or a lichenoid eruption. Monochromator studies show delayed erythema induced by UVB, UVA, and visible radiation. Ferguson and others (1987) suggest that the reaction has greater affinity with phototoxicity than photoallergy. Quinidine may induce either a lichenoid or eczematous UVA-induced photodermatosis, as well as a livedo reticularis type of eruption on light-exposed areas (Manzi *et al.* 1989).

Flushing and erythema

Ethanol-induced flushing in patients taking chlorpropamide or tolbutamide is well recognized, and may be important in having a negative correlation with diabetic retinopathy and proteinuria. Similar reactions are described when ethanol is taken after griseofulvin, metronidazole, or a cephalosporin. These reactions are blocked both by the opiate antagonist naloxone and prostaglandin-synthetase inhibitors such as indomethacin; the latter group also inhibit the flushing caused by nicotinic acid (Wilkin 1983). Flushing may occasionally be seen after administration of bromocriptine, calcitonin, dacarbazine (DTIC), isoniazid, nitrofurantoin, or pentazocine and, rather more frequently, with calcium-channel blockers such as nifedipine and verapamil (Bork 1988).

Livedo reticularis is a red-blue network pattern of skin discolouration which develops in 50–90 per cent of patients receiving amantadine hydrochloride for Parkinson's disease (Vollum *et al.* 1971); more rarely it complicates bromocriptine therapy. Bromocriptine and pergolide

(Monk *et al.* 1984) may cause erythromelalgia (redness, swelling, and a sensation of heat, usually in the hands and feet) (see also Chapter 7). The induction of painful and swollen red hands and feet by cytotoxic drug therapy has also been described; the drug most frequently implicated has been cytosine arabinoside, usually in combination with other cytotoxic drugs in the treatment of leukaemia (Shall *et al.* 1988), but other cases have occurred in the treatment of Hodgkin's disease and various cancers. Exacerbation of these signs and symptoms by cyclosporin infusion is recorded by Kampmann and others (1989), who also cite instances due to hydroxyurea, fluorouracil, methotrexate, or mercaptopurine. The erythema does not appear to be due to any pathological vascular change.

Histologically, the skin shows individual epidermal cell necrosis, associated with spongiosis and a mild perivascular inflammatory infiltrate in the superficial dermis. The condition remits even if therapy is continued.

Skin necrosis

Skin necrosis may arise during therapy with either oral or parenteral anticoagulants. In oral therapy it has more often been recorded with warfarin than phenindione. Warfarin necrosis is said to occur in approximately 1 in every 1000 patients treated, obese women being most at risk. It mainly occurs between days 3 and 5 of therapy, especially after administration of a loading dose. Erythema is followed by painful oedema and then infarction and blistering. Histological examination of the affected skin shows epidermal necrosis with thrombi in dermal vessels and extravasation of red blood cells. It may be associated with the development of a deficiency of clotting factor VII (Russell-Jones and Cunningham 1979), but the role of this deficiency in the pathogenesis is obscure. Resolution occurs with continuing therapy.

Heparin necrosis is similar clinically and histologically. It usually occurs at the sites of injection, but may be distant (Levine *et al.* 1983). The onset of necrosis (at 6–13 days) is later than with warfarin. The pathogenesis seems to involve the immunological production of a platelet-aggregating factor. Because of this hypersensitivity to heparin, discontinuation of therapy is essential. Subsequent administration of warfarin has not been associated with recurrence (Kelly *et al.* 1981).

Cytotoxic drugs may produce skin necrosis in a number of ways. Most are vesicants and may irritate the vein through which they are being infused. If extravasation occurs, pain and erythema may be followed by necrosis and persistent ulceration (Bronner and Hood

1983). Lawrence and Dahl (1984) describe two patterns of skin necrosis in the treatment of psoriasis with methotrexate. One occurs in the psoriatic plaques soon after starting therapy, and the other in skin uninvolved by psoriasis but the site of another disorder, such as venous stasis, which may occur at any time during therapy. The histological changes are of epidermal necrosis without significant vascular abnormality. Methotrexate may also produce the radiation-recall phenomenon (an inflammatory response during chemotherapy at the site of previous irradiation). This may be so severe as to produce cutaneous necrosis (Logan *et al.* 1988). The radiation-recall phenomenon is also described with cyclophosphamide, vincristine, bleomycin, and doxorubicin.

Cutaneous necrosis may be produced by vasoconstriction. This may be caused by noradrenaline added to local anaesthetics, so such preparations should not be used at acral sites. β-Adrenoceptor blocking drugs may so impair cutaneous circulation as to cause necrosis (Gokal *et al.* 1979; Hoffbrand 1979). Pitressin, used in the treatment of bleeding oesophageal varices, may, rarely, cause skin necrosis (Greenwald *et al.* 1978; Wormser *et al.* 1982).

A number of drugs, but especially penicillamine, may alter dermal connective tissue. The changes are usually degenerative, but lesions like those of systemic sclerosis have been described (Miyagawa *et al.* 1987). Similar changes may occur with bleomycin (Cohen *et al.* 1973), when diffuse sclerosis of the hand and feet, resembling scleroderma, may progress to gangrene of the finger tips.

Pruritus

As with idiopathic rashes, pruritus is a common concomitant of drug rashes. The lone drug-induced pruritus, here considered, is rare.

Morphine and cocaine provoke pruritus; and the perception of opiate-induced itch is diminished by the selective antagonist naloxone (Greaves 1987).

In patients with pruritus, the possibility of drug hepatotoxicity must be considered. Drugs that may produce cholestasis, such as the contraceptive pill (Drill 1974) are far more likely to present with pruritus than those, such as ketoconazole, that may produce a hepatitis-like picture (Lewis *et al.* 1984).

When used in malaria (but not, for example, in rheumatoid arthritis), chloroquine produces pruritus in 8–20 per cent of African patients. The itch often occurs within a few hours of starting therapy and remits within 3 days, even with continuing treatment (Sowunmi *et al.* 1989).

Pruritus may complicate PUVA therapy; it appears to be related to the dose of UVA. It is usually not so severe as to prevent further treatment and is generally controlled by antihistamines (Wolff and Honigsmann 1981).

Urticaria

Drugs are commonly suspected of causing urticaria but proven cases of drug-induced urticaria are comparatively few, and only cases of acute urticaria are likely to be drug-induced. Chronic urticaria is rarely caused by a drug unless the patient is reacting to aspirin and continuing to take it.

Penicillin, salicylates, codeine, and imipramine (Rook *et al.* 1972) may cause acute urticaria, which can also occur after the administration of serum or toxoid, during a course of injections with pollen vaccines, or in 1–2 per cent of patients having blood transfusions (Dukes 1975).

Urticaria may be a feature of anaphylactic shock caused by drugs, including Dextran 70 and Dextran 40 (Ring and Messmer 1977; Furhoff 1977), and is particularly prone to occur in asthmatic subjects, usually at the beginning of the infusion.

Urticaria can be due to X-ray contrast media, when the chronic as well as the acute form can result. It has been caused by insulin (Lamkin et al 1976), including porcine insulin (Reisner *et al.* 1978); thyroid hormones; corticotrophin (ACTH); and synthetic corticosteroids given systematically or by intralesional injection. Generalized urticaria has been attributed to doxorubicin (Fallah-Sohy and Figueredo 1979). Acute urticaria caused specifically by alcohol (ethanol) was described by Ormerod and Holt (1983).

Erythema multiforme

Erythema multiforme is characterized by erythematous maculopapules that are most profuse peripherally. These emerge in crops over a period of a few days and then fade within 1–2 weeks. Each lesion increases in size centrifugally, attaining a diameter of 1–2 cm within 48 hours. The centre of the lesion becomes cyanotic or even purpuric, giving rise to the characteristic iris or target-shaped lesion. In more severe cases, vesicles and bullae appear, with haemorrhage into the skin lesions indicating that there has been a split at the dermoepidermal junction. Healing occurs without scarring, though hyperpigmentation may persist for a long time. The sites most commonly involved are the backs of the hands, palms, wrists, forearms, feet, elbows, and knees.

Bullous or vesicular lesions may be accompanied by mucosal lesions and constitutional disturbance (Stevens–Johnson syndrome).

In a 5-year study (Fellner 1971), it was found that erythema multiforme accounted for 5 per cent of drug reactions involving the skin.

Drugs most likely to cause erythema multiforme are sulphonamides and chemically related compounds, such as chlorpropamide, thiazide diuretics, and sulphones. Anticonvulsants of the hydantoin group (e.g. phenytoin) and succinimide group (e.g. ethosuximide) can cause a severe bullous erythema multiforme (Levantine and Almeyda 1972). In children and adolescents, hydantoins may give rise to severe oral lesions and palmar erythema multiforme but relatively little systemic illness (Rudner 1970). Other drugs that have been implicated are atropine, aspirin and other salicylates, benzodiazepines, carbamazepine, clindamycin, codeine, frusemide, gold salts, isoniazid, meprobamate, mercurial diuretics, penicillins, phenolphthalein, phenothiazines, propranolol, quinidine, sulindac (Husain *et al.* 1981), and tetracyclines. Eruptions resembling those of erythema multiforme have been reported in patients undergoing treatment with cyclophosphamide (Falkson and Schultz 1962), busulphan therapy (Dosik *et al.* 1970), and diltiazem (Berbis *et al.* 1989). The Stevens–Johnson syndrome is thought to have been provoked by cimetidine (Ahmed *et al.* 1978), diflunisal (Hunter *et al.* 1978), and topical sulphonamide applications (Gottschaek and Stone 1976).

Chan and others (1990) determined the incidence of erythema multiforme and Stevens–Johnson syndrome (and toxic epidermal necrolysis) requiring admission to hospital from 1972–1986. Drug therapies with reaction rates in excess of 1 per 100 000 treated patients included phenobarbitone, nitrofurantoin, sulphamethoxazole and trimethoprim, ampicillin, and amoxycillin.

Toxic erythema

This term embraces erythematous rashes resembling exanthemata and includes morbilliform rashes. The difficulty of ascribing such a rash to a drug is obvious, since such 'toxic' rashes are common from other causes. Sometimes 'toxic' rashes occur during drug administration and disappear even though the drug is continued, but if itching is marked it is less likely that the drug rash will clear. When the rash progresses, it may assume eczematous features leading to exfoliative dermatitis or to the scald-like lesions of toxic epidermolysis (see below). A severe morbilliform rash may be caused by amoxycillin and the esters bacampicillin, pivampicillin, and talampicillin. Toxic erythematous rashes may be accompanied by a drug-induced fever. A high incidence of toxic erythematous rashes may be expected during treatment with penicillin or chemically related antibiotics or with gold salts. Diltiazem can produce severe toxic erythema (Wakeel *et al.* 1988) as well as a distinctive exanthematous pustular eczematous eruption (Lambert *et al.* 1988).

Exfoliative dermatitis

This condition may be defined as redness of the entire skin (erythroderma) with widespread scaling due to exfoliation, which may have severe systemic effects including hypovolaemia, heart failure, intestinal malabsorption, hypoproteinaemia, and hypothermia. Withdrawal of the offending drug is mandatory, and treatment with systemic corticosteroid drugs may be required.

Drugs that can induce this serious disorder are gold; phenylbutazone (Mauer 1955) and oxyphenbutazone (Anderson *et al.* 1962); streptomycin (Harris 1950); the anticonvulsants phenytoin, methoin, and troxidone; and cimetidine (Yantis *et al.* 1980). Carbamazepine (Roberts and Marks 1981; Reed *et al.* 1982) and captopril (Solinger 1982) have also been incriminated. The eczematous reaction to chlorpromazine, at first resembling seborrhoeic eczema or photodermatitis, may progress to generalized exfoliative dermatitis; sulphonamides may also be a cause of exfoliative dermatitis (Payne and Giesecke 1987) and quinidine may cause either this disorder or a severe erythrodermic exacerbation of psoriasis.

Occasionally, patients who have been sensitized to a drug given topically (e.g. chloramphenicol, diphenhydramine) subsequently develop exfoliative dermatitis when the drug is given orally. In the investigation of suspected cases of drug-induced exfoliative dermatitis, it is therefore important to check that any drug that the patient is taking is not an analogue of any other drug that he might have applied topically in the past.

Toxic epidermal necrolysis (TEN)

This term was first applied by Lyell in 1956, and later reviewed by him in 1979, to a condition in which the skin changes are identical to scalded skin. TEN is characterized by large areas of erythema followed by a bullous phase in which there is separation of the epidermis — 'scalded skin syndrome'; mucous membrane involvement may precede the skin eruption by 10–14 days, so that the skin changes look identical to those of a severe form of erythema multiforme (Stevens–Johnson syndrome). With the apparent clinical overlap between TEN, the Stevens–Johnson syndrome, and erythema multiforme, Lyell (1990) now wonders if the term TEN is still appropriate or should be abandoned. Two of his original four cases presented with the more appropriate descriptions of a generalized bullous fixed drug eruption (GBDFE), because of their uniform eruptions and recurrences.

Drugs that have been implicated are barbiturates, pentamidine (Wang *et al.* 1970), oxyphenbutazone, phenolphthalein, hydantoin derivatives (e.g. phenytoin), penicillin, sulphonamides (commonly prescribed today as co-trimoxazole), dapsone (Schuppli 1960), chloramphenicol, plicamycin (mithramycin) (Eyster *et al.* 1971), gold salts, neomycin, nitrofurantoin, opium alkaloids, pentazocine, quinine, tetracyclines, and thiabendazole (Robinson and Samorodin 1976). Allopurinol has been held responsible in three cases (Kantor 1970; Stratigos *et al.* 1972; Bennett *et al.* 1977). Allopurinol can cause both Stevens–Johnson syndrome and TEN. Fatal Stevens–Johnson syndrome was reported in a patient taking captopril and allopurinol (Pennell *et al.* 1984) and it is inferred that potentiation of skin eruptions due to allopurinol can be induced by captopril. One case of pancytopenia and TEN was described by Fenton and English (1982).

Roujeau and others (1990) undertook a 5-year retrospective survey in France of all cases of TEN; the two drugs most commonly involved were sulphonamides and non-steroidal anti-inflammatory drugs; the survey emphasized the severity and rarity of this type of reaction.

Drug-related systemic lupus erythematosus

The common manifestations of drug-related lupus-like syndromes are an erythematous rash on the face, neck, and backs of hands associated with fever, weight loss, polyarthritis, myalgia, hepatosplenomegaly, and serositis (pleural and pericardial). The antinuclear factor is usually positive; lupus erythematosus cells are often seen; and in some cases antibodies to DNA may be found.

The anticonvulsant drug ethosuximide has been shown to produce the lupus syndrome combined with scleroderma of the extremities. These features cleared after the drug was stopped but readministration of ethosuximide for control of epilepsy resulted in prominent sclerodermatous changes which again resolved once the drug was withdrawn (Teoh and Chan 1975).

Drug-related systemic lupus erythematosus is discussed in detail in Chapter 16.

Psoriasiform eruptions

The β-adrenoceptor blocking drugs can produce a distinctive psoriasiform eruption involving the knees and other bony prominences, associated with hyperkeratosis of palms and soles. The rash may appear several months to years after starting the drug. The first β-blocking drug producing this type of rash was practolol (Felix *et al.* 1974, 1975). Other sites involved are the conjunctiva, lungs, and gastrointestinal tract — the oculomucocutaneous syndrome. Since then other β-blockers have been incriminated: oxprenolol (Holt and Waddington 1975), propranolol (Jensen *et al.* 1976), and atenolol (Gawkrodger and Beveridge 1985; Richards 1985).

The evidence for cross-reactivity between practolol and other β-blocking drugs with respect to adverse effects is conflicting; in two series (Felix *et al.* 1974; Zacharias 1976) a lack of cross-reactivity was observed, whereas cross-reactivity between practolol and atenolol was described by Jensen and others (1976). In a group of patients with glaucoma who were treated with topical β-blocking drugs and developed ocular or periocular dermatitis, or both (van Joost *et al.* 1979), positive patch tests examined were compatible with a delayed hypersensitivity reaction (a Type B reaction).

Acute exacerbation of psoriasis can occur in patients on β-blocking drugs. (Sondergaard *et al.* 1976); cyclic-AMP is low in psoriatic epidermis, and a reduction of cyclic-AMP by β-blockade could explain the production of the psoriasiform eruption. Indomethacin has a tendency to exacerbate psoriasis (Katayama and Kawada 1981); phenylbutazone and oxyphenbutazone (Reshed *et al.* 1983) can cause a severe form of the disease, generalized pustular psoriasis. These drugs inhibit prostaglandin synthetase, leading to a reduction of prostaglandins and cyclic-AMP; or, alternatively, reduced prostaglandin synthetase leads to the production of potent neutrophil chemotactic agents such as leukotriene B_4 (in pustular psoriasis there is an invasion of the epidermis by neutrophils).

Chloroquine and related drugs (Baker 1966) and lithium (Skott *et al.* 1977; Lowe and Ridgway 1978) can cause an exacerbation of psoriasis or even induce the disease in previously unaffected subjects (Thormann 1978). Psoriasiform rashes can be induced by glibenclamide (Goh 1987).

Lichenoid eruptions

In eruptions resembling lichen planus a drug may be suspected of being the cause when the rash is diffuse and severe and when improvement occurs following withdrawal of the drug. Mouth lesions can occur. Scaling, loss of hair, and anhidrosis are more likely to develop than with true lichen planus.

The term lichenoid drug eruptions can be used in two senses. First, drug eruptions similar to or identical with lichen planus; and, secondly, drug eruptions that do not necessarily resemble lichen planus clinically, but have histological features very like those of lichen planus or of drug eruptions resembling lichen planus. In this category special mention must be made of the eruptions associated with the β-adrenoceptor blocking drugs, in which, histologically, the features are those of a lichenoid drug eruption but morphologically the rash may be very similar to lichen planus. The rash due to labetalol, for example, is of this type (Gange and Wilson-Jones 1978), whereas other β-blocker drugs, for example, practolol and oxprenolol, produce a rash that is more psoriasiform in character, but with a lichenoid histology (see also section on Psoriasiform eruptions).

Gold salts, organic arsenicals, quinine, quinidine (Wolf *et al.* 1987), mepacrine, and chloroquine have long been recognized causes. Streptomycin rarely causes lichenoid rashes, but sodium aminosalicylate (PAS) (Shatin *et al.* 1953) is a well-recognized culprit. Amiphenazone (Baker *et al.* 1964), dapsone, frusemide, methyldopa (Stevenson 1971), penicillamine, phenothiazines (Groth 1961), spironolactone (Downham 1978), tetracycline, thiazide diuretics (Harber *et al.* 1959), and triprolidine can also cause lichenoid drug eruptions. Oral lichenoid reactions caused by non-steroidal anti-inflammatory drugs have been reported (Hamburger and Potts 1983). In a review of cutaneous adverse effects of β-adrenoceptor blocking drugs, lichenoid (see also section on Psoriasiform eruptions) and psoriasiform changes have been associated with many of the drugs, and they may may occur several years after the start of treatment (Richards 1985).

Purpura

The term 'purpura' describes the discolouration caused by extravasation of erythrocytes into the skin or the mucous membranes. The primary defect may be either in the platelets in clotting mechanisms, or in the blood vessels, but the majority of cases seen in dermatological practice are due to vascular lesions. There is no reliable physical sign that helps to distinguish thrombocytopenic from non-thrombocytopenic purpura.

Drugs may cause purpura by producing thrombocytopenia by a toxic or allergic mechanism, by damaging the blood vessel, or by affecting blood coagulation. Drug interaction can play an important role in drug-induced purpura either by enzyme induction or displacement of drugs from their protein-binding sites (but see Chapter 30).

A large number of drugs can cause purpura; allopurinol, antimetabolites, bismuth, carbimazole, chlorothiazide, digitoxin, dinitrophenol, ergot, frusemide, gold, indomethacin, mercurials, methyldopa, nitrofurantoin, oestrogens, organic arsenicals, oxytetracycline, phenobarbitone, potassium iodide, quinidine, salicylates, streptomycin, sulphonamides, tolbutamide, and troxidone.

Aspirin can produce purpura by an effect on the blood clotting mechanism, and in aspirin poisoning purpura may occur if the patient performs Valsalva's manoeuvre.

Adverse reactions to topical medicaments

As with reactions to ingested drugs, reactions to topical preparations may be divided into Types A and B. Of these Type B reactions, allergic contact dermatitis is the most important. Sensitization is more readily induced percutaneously than by any other route; which fact relates to the epidermal Langerhans cell's role as the afferent limb of the immune system (Wolff and Stingl 1983). Thus, nearly all subjects are capable of sensitization to topical dinitrochlorobenzene (Friedmann *et al.* 1983); and locally applied penicillin and streptomycin, in contrast to their administration systemically, produced so much contact dermatitis that their topical use was discontinued early on in their history.

Type A reactions

These may be divided into topical and systemic adverse effects. Drugs may be absorbed through the skin in sufficient amount to cause Type A systemic toxicity. This is most likely to occur with widespread diseased skin, in infants (with a high ratio of surface area to volume), in the thinned skin of old age, and when absorption is enhanced by the use of polythene dressings.

Toxicity from resorcinol (impaired thyroid function and methaemoglobinaemia) and boric acid (nephrotoxicity) is now rarely reported. Boric acid is a constituent of the widely used Eusol. While experimental work in animals suggests that such preparations may impair wound healing, the clinical impression of Eusol as a debriding agent remains favourable (Cunliffe 1990). Adverse systemic reactions to phenol in magenta paint, which also contains resorcinol (Rogers *et al.* 1978), and percutaneous salicylate poisoning (Anderson and Ead 1979) occur occasionally.

Corticosteroids are the most widely prescribed topical preparations, and the commonest cause of Type A reactions. As a rule these reactions occur only with the more potent (usually fluorinated) preparations. The fluorine atom is not essential for these effects, as they also occur with the non-fluorinated endogenous steroids of Cushing's syndrome; and mild expression of these effects has been described with 1% hydrocortisone (Guin 1981).

When the most potent steroids are used in large amounts (e.g. 300 g of clobetasol propionate per week) for long periods over large areas of diseased skin, hypothalamic–pituitary suppression with Cushingoid features may occur (Carruthers *et al.* 1975). Far more commonly troublesome are steroid-induced changes in the skin, of which the most prominent is thinning of both epidermis and dermis (Winter and Burton 1976). Dermal atrophy causes striae, telangiectasia, easy bruising, and fragile skin with poor wound healing.

Inappropriate steroid treatment may result in the potentiation of infection, with masking of its expression. This may occur with bacteria (widespread folliculitis), viruses (e.g. disseminated molluscum contagiosum), arthropods (widespread and atypical scabies), and with fungal infections — the so-called 'tinea incognito' of Ive and Marks (1968).

The more potent steroids will regularly induce rosacea and perioral dermatitis on the face (Cotterill 1979), and their withdrawal may be associated with the conversion of plaque to pustular psoriasis (Boxley *et al.* 1975).

Primary irritant contact dermatitis

Primary irritant contact dermatitis provides an instance of a Type A reaction occurring with topical drugs. It is common with both tar and dithranol used in the treatment of psoriasis, and may be avoided by initial use of low drug concentrations, followed by cautious increase. Allergic contact dermatitis may occur with both tar and, more rarely, dithranol (Lawlor and Hindson 1982).

Phototoxic reactions may complicate therapy with tar (Diette *et al.* 1983) and more commonly with topical psoralens (Weber 1974). Photoallergy occurring with topical preparations may be caused by their containing hexachlorophane (Wennersten *et al.* 1984) and *p*-aminobenzoic acid esters (Mathias *et al.* 1978), which are used in sunscreens.

Type B reactions

Allergic contact dermatitis

Allergic contact dermatitis is the major complication of topical therapy. It may be caused not only by the active ingredient of a cream or ointment but also by the base (e.g. lanolin), preservatives (e.g. parabens), emulsifiers (e.g. the Span group), and various fragrances.

Incidence

Fourteen per cent of 4000 consecutive patients with eczema from five European skin clinics who were tested by the International Contact Dermatitis Research Group (ICDRG) were considered to have allergic contact dermatitis to medicaments. Neomycin and benzocaine were the most frequent sensitizers (4 per cent each) (Cronin *et al.* 1970).

Predisposing factors

Patients with atopic eczema are no more likely to develop contact dermatitis than those with other forms of endogenous eczema (Bandmann *et al.* 1972). Certainly, sensitization is less readily induced experimentally in atopics (Forsbeck *et al.* 1976). Any patient with long-standing eczema of any sort, however, is likely to have had prolonged treatment with medicaments and thus the opportunity to become sensitized.

The prevalence of allergic contact dermatitis falls with advancing age (Hjorth and Fregert 1979); but it is wise to assume that the sensitized patient will remain so for life.

It is probable that drugs delivered in an occlusive ointment base are more likely to sensitize than when a cream base is used (Hjorth and Thomsen 1968). Creams, however, contain a greater number of potential sensitizers, such as humectants and preservatives, which are not required in ointments.

Not surprisingly, the prevalence of medicament sensitivity relates to the prevalence of medicament usage. Thus, neomycin allergy occurred in 1.7 per cent of tested patients in Warsaw and 19 per cent in Finland (Macdonald and Beck 1983).

Medicament dermatitis has a well-recognized association with stasis eczema and ulcers of the lower leg (Paramsothy *et al.* 1988). This may relate to local factors and an increased predisposition to acquire new sensitivities (amplicative medicament allergy), but it is also a function of chronicity of application. A similarly high prevalence of medicament sensitization obtains in chronic otitis externa and anogenital pruritus (Wilkinson *et al.* 1980).

Patch tests

Patch testing represents both a limited and comparatively safe form of challenge with the suspected allergen, and also the oldest (Jadasohn 1896) test of Type IV sensitivity.

The substances to be tested are applied to discs of filter paper stuck by heat to aluminium foil covered with polythene (the Al-test unit). The strips of foil are applied to the patient's back and left in place for 2 days, when they are removed and readings taken. Positive patch tests are indicated by an eczematous reaction at the test site, but as 20 per cent of reactions finally judged positive may develop over the next 5 days (Mitchell 1978), late readings are important, especially with neomycin.

The International Contact Dermatitis Research Group has developed a standard battery of patch test substances, which can be obtained commercially (from Cand. pharm. K. Trolle-Lassen, Hoyrups Alle 1, 2900 Hellerup, Denmark). This includes neomycin 20%, benzocaine 5%, wool alcohols (lanolin) 30%, parabens 3%, balsam of peru 25%, chinoform 5%, and ethylene diamine 1%. All are found in many topical preparations, and are common sensitizers. A battery of test substances is especially useful when the history is obscure. When the result of a test on a proprietary product is positive, it is desirable to retest with individual components of the preparation so that the allergen can be identified and the patient warned to avoid other products containing the allergen and other drugs that may cross-react with it.

The distinction between an irritant and allergic contact dermatitis may be difficult — both clinically and at patch testing. In the latter the following will favour allergic contact dermatitis: positivity at low concentration, itching rather than soreness, eczematous morphology rather than an erosion, spread beyond the site of application, and continued evolution of response following removal of the patches (Cronin 1980*a*).

As an awareness of cross-reaction between topical sensitizers and systemically administered drugs is relevant to safe prescription of both, medicament dermatitis will be discussed, with special emphasis on these cross-reactions. Most characteristically, when a patient has previously been sensitized to a topical drug and then receives the same or a related drug systemically he develops a symmetrical eczematous eruption, which may be maximal at the site of previous sensitization — the so-called systemic eczematous contact type eczema. For example, a patient with a history of a leg ulcer and treatment with creams containing parabens reacted severely to an intramuscular injection of ampicillin, which also contained the parabens as a preservative (Carradori *et al.* 1990).

Important sensitizers

Topical antibiotics and antibacterials Topical antibiotics are indicated in the treatment of primary bacterial infections of the skin like impetigo, and in combination with steroids in the treatment of impetiginized eczema (Leyden and Kligman 1977*a*). They should be avoided in the treatment of potentially chronic conditions like leg ulcers, where the risk of sensitization is great; this is especially true of sodium fusidate (Verbov 1970) and gentamicin (Cronin 1980b), which may later need to be given systemically.

Chlortetracycline is the least sensitizing antibiotic (Vickers 1961). Its topical formulation Aureomycin, however, contains lanolin and parabens, so it is possible for sensitization to occur to these ingredients.

Neomycin remains the commonest topical sensitizer amongst the antibiotics, and cross-reactions may occur with other aminoglycosides, such as framycetin, kanamycin, netilmicin, streptomycin, and tobramycin. Many patients sensitive to neomycin are also sensitive to bacitracin, but it is thought that the sensitization is simultaneous and independent. Systemic eczematization has been reported following the use of oral neomycin and the use of a bacitracin–neomycin dental preparation (Macdonald and Beck 1983).

Topical antibiotics are widely prescribed for acne. Clindamycin has been described as causing facial contact dermatitis (Coskey 1978) and also as producing allergy presenting as rosacea (de Kort and de Groot 1989). Actinac (containing chloramphenicol) is widely used in the UK, as are chloramphenicol eye drops and ointment. Although chloramphenicol sensitivity is rare (Cronin 1980c), it would seem prudent to avoid applying it topically long-term. While sensitivity to benzoyl peroxide (Leyden and Kligman 1977b) may occur, this and tretinoin are generally the most suitable topical treatments for acne.

Preparations containing clioquinol (iodochlorhydroxyquinoline, chinoform, Vioform) and chlorquinaldol are much used in combination with topical steroids and in medicated bandages (e.g. Quinaband). They are a not uncommon cause of contact dermatitis, and cross-reactions between clioquinol and chlorquinaldol and also the quinoline antimalarials may occur (Kernekamp and van Ketel 1980).

The imidazole topical antifungal preparations are weak sensitizers, but cases of contact dermatitis caused by them have been described (Samsoen and Jelen 1977). Such sensitization carries the risk of cross-reaction with orally administered ketoconazole (van Dijke et al. 1983) and itraconazole.

Anti-inflammatory drugs When a patient reacts adversely to a topical steroid preparation, it is usually to a constituent of the base. However, many reactions to the corticosteroid itself have now been described. These include cortisone, hydrocortisone butyrate, and pred-

nisolone, and a variety of fluorinated steroids such as clobetasol propionate and clobetasol butyrate (Guin 1984).

In general, there is little tendency for cross-reaction to occur between steroids, in spite of their close chemical relationship. Systemic eczematization to either endogenous or exogenous steroids has not yet been described. In addition to these instances of adverse cutaneous reaction to topical steroids, contact dermatitis to budesonide in a nasal aerosol has been described (Jerez et al. 1990)

Topical non-steroidal anti-inflammatory drugs have been used in the treatment of both eczema and as rubefacients. When bufexamac was in use for the treatment of eczema, cases of contact allergy to it were described (Lachapelle 1975). Sensitization to oxyphenbutazone cream was associated with cross-sensitization to phenylbutazone (Krook 1975). Contact allergy to ketoprofen was reported by Angelini and Vena (1983).

Antihistamine creams are readily available 'over the counter', and provide the risk of sensitization without there being any good evidence of their efficacy. Diphenhydramine hydrochloride (contained, for example, in Caladryl cream) is well recognized as a cause of medicament dermatitis (Coskey 1983). Subsequent oral administration may cause a generalized eruption maximal at the site of previous sensitization (Shelley and Bennett 1972).

Local anaesthetics Although creams containing local anaesthetics are widely used, especially for pruritus ani, low-potency topical corticosteroids are more effective and safer. In many countries, topical benzocaine is much used and is a common cause of contact dermatitis. Like amethocaine and procaine, benzocaine is an ester of *p*-aminobenzoic acid, and this relationship to the sulphonamides and the dye paraphenylenediamine entails the risk of cross-sensitization.

Cinchocaine (contained in Proctosedyl) is a quinoline derivative and does not cross-react with benzocaine, but may cross-react with clioquinol. It is well recognized as a sensitizer (Wilson 1966).

Lignocaine is an aminoacyl amide not chemically related to benzocaine or cinchocaine. It is widely used as a local anaesthetic and for cardiac arrythmias and in some topical preparations (e.g. Betnovate rectal ointment). Contact allergy from lignocaine is very rare, but has been described (Nurse and Rosner 1983).

Preservatives and stabilizers Preservatives and stabilizers are perhaps the commonest cause of medicament sensitization. Two per cent of patients patch-tested to ethylene diamine (a stabilizer present in TriAdcortyl cream and also used as a solvent, corrosion inhibitor, and lubricant in industry) produced positive reactions (Eriksen 1975). Such patients are at risk of developing systemic eczematous-type dermatitis if they later receive aminophylline (85% theophylline and 15% ethylenediamine) (Fisher 1976).

A number of antihistamines (antazoline, chloropyrilene, methapyrilene, pyrilamine, promethazine, and tripelennamine) are derivatives of ethylenediamine and should be avoided in patients sensitive to it. The risk of reaction, however, does not appear to be great (King and Beck 1983). Parabens are effective preservatives for cosmetics, drugs, and food. While they are not strong sensitizers, allergy to them is an especial problem in patients with leg ulcers, in contrast to their use in cosmetics. Systemic eczematization in patients sensitive to parabens has occurred as a consequence of the presence of parabens in Xylocaine (Aeling and Nuss 1974) and ampicillin (Carradori *et al.* 1990). Sensitized patients have the potential to cross-react with the so-called para-substances, such as *p*-phenylenediamine, para-substituted azo dyes, *p*-aminosalicylic acid, and benzocaine. Reports of such cross-reactions are, however, rare (Malten *et al.* 1976).

There has been a tendency to replace parabens in creams, with a concomitant increase in sensitivity to the substituted preservatives, such as sorbic acid (Coyle *et al.* 1981).

Contact urticaria

Contact urticaria refers to a wheal-and-flare response elicited within a few minutes to an hour after the skin is exposed to certain rapidly absorbable agents (Odom and Maibach 1976). It may be divided into non-immunological (Type A) and immunological (Type B) categories: of these the non-immunological is the more common.

Type A contact urticaria may be due to by Trafuril (a nicotinic acid ester), dimethyl sulphoxide (used to promote percutaneous penetration), sorbic acid (a preservative), benzoic acid (an antifungal agent and preservative), and cinnamic acid (sometimes present in sunscreens) (Fisher 1990).

Immunological contact urticaria (Type B) is the more significant, as later systemic administration of the drug or its relatives may induce anaphylaxis. It has been described as being caused by the following drugs: bacitracin, cephalosporins, chloramphenicol, gentamicin, neomycin, penicillin, streptomycin, benzocaine, and mustine hydrochloride (Fisher 1990). It should be noted that intradermal testing with bacitracin and streptomycin and closed patch testing with chloramphenicol, neomycin, and penicillin have all produced anaphylaxis.

References

Ackerman, A.B. (1978). *Histological diagnosis of inflammatory skin disease*, p. 210. Lea and Febiger, Philadelphia.

Addo, H.A., Ferguson, J., and Frain-Bell, W. (1987). Thiazide-induced photo-sensitivity: a study of 33 subjects. *Br. J. Dermatol.* 116, 749.

Aeling, J.L. and Nuss, D.D. (1974). Systemic eczematous 'contact-type' dermatitis medicamentosa caused by parabens. *Arch. Dermatol.* 110, 640.

Ahmed, A.H., McLarty, D.G., Sharma, S.K., and Masawe, A.E.J. (1978). Stevens–Johnson syndrome during treatment with cimetidine. *Lancet* ii, 433,

Alanko, K., Stubbs, S., and Reitamo, S. (1987). Topical provocation of fixed drug eruption. *Br. J. Dermatol.* 116, 561.

Alanko, K., Stubbs, S., and Kauppinen, K. (1989). Cutaneous drug reactions: clinical types and causative agents. *Acta Derm. Venereol.* (Stockh.) 69, 223.

Alcalay, J., David, M., Ingber, A., Hazaz, B., and Sandbank, M. (1988). Bullous pemphigoid mimicking bullous erythema multiforme: an untoward effect of penicillins. *J. Am. Acad. Dermatol.* 18, 345.

Anderson, J., Ashby, D.W., and Peaston, M.J.T. (1962). Exfoliative dermatitis due to hyroxyphenylbutazone ('Tanderil'). *Br. Med. J.* ii, 1064.

Anderson, J.A.R. and Ead, R.D. (1979). Percutaneous salicylate poisoning. *Clin. Exper. Dermatol.* 4, 349.

Angelini, G. and Vena, G.A. (1983). Contact allergy to ketoprofen. *Contact Dermatitis* 9, 234.

Arndt, K.A. and Jick, H. (1976). Rates of cutaneous reactions to drugs. A report from the Boston Collaborative Drug Surveillance Program. *JAMA* 235, 918.

Baden, L.A., Apovian, C., Imber, M.J., and Dover, J.S. (1988). Vancomycin-induced linear IgA bullous dermatosis. *Arch. Dermatol.* 124, 1186.

Baker, H. (1966). The influence of chloroquine and related drugs on psoriasis and keratoderma blenorrhagicum. *Br. J. Dermatol.* 78, 161.

Baker, H., Hughes, D.T.D., and Pegum, J.S. (1964). Lichenoid eruption due to amiphenazole. *Br. J. Dermatol.* 76, 186.

Bandmann, H.J., Calnan, C.D., Cronin, E., Frefert, S., Hiorth, N., Magnusson, B., *et al.* (1972). Dermatitis from applied medicaments. *Arch. Dermatol.* 106, 335.

Banerjee, A.K., Bendall, K., and Liddell, K. (1988). Bullous eruptions following chlormethiazole overdose. *Clin. Exp. Dermatol.* 13, 357.

Baran, R. and Juhlin, L. (1987). Drug-induced photoonycholysis. Three subtypes identified in a study of 15 cases. *J. Am. Acad. Dermatol.* 17, 1012.

Barker, D.J. and Cotterill, J.A. (1977). Skin eruptions due to azapropazone. *Lancet* i, 90.

Barker, E.J., Reed, K D., and Dixon, S.L. (1989). Chlorthalidone-induced pseudo-porphyria: clinical and microscopic findings of a case. *J. Am. Acad. Dermatol.* 21, 1026.

Barth, J H. and Dawber, R.P.R. (1989). Drug induced hair loss. *Br. Med. J.* 298, 675.

Batchelor, J.R., Welsh, K.I., Tinoco, R.M., Dollery, C.T., Hughes, G.R.V., and Bernstein, R., *et al.* (1980). Hydralazine-induced systemic lupus erythematosus: influence of HLA-DR and sex on susceptibility. *Lancet* i, 1107.

Bauer, F. (1981). Quinacrine hydrochloride drug eruption (topical lichenoid dermatitis): its early and late sequelae and its malignant potential. *J. Am. Acad. Dermatol.* 4, 239.

Bencini, P.L., Montagnino, G., Sala, F., De Vecchi, A., Crosti, C., and Tarantino, A. (1986). Cutaneous lesions in 67 cyclosporin-treated renal transplant recipients. *Dermatologica* 172, 24.

Bennett, T.O., Sugar, J., and Sahgal, S. (1977). Ocular manifestations of toxic epidermal necrolysis associated with allopurinol use. *Arch. Ophthalmol.* 95, 1362.

Benning, T.L., McCormack, K.M., Ingram, P., Kaplan, D.L., and Shelburne, J.D. (1988). Microprobe analysis of chlorpromazine pigmentation. *Arch. Dermatol.* 124, 1541.

Berbis, P., Alfonso, M.J., Levy, J.L., and Privat, Y (1989). Diltiazem associated erythema multiforme. *Dermatologica* 179, 90.

Bergfeld, W.F. and Redmond, G.P. (1987). Hirsutism. *Dermatol. Clin.* 5, 501.

Beveridge, G.W. and Lawson, A.A.H. (1965). Occurrence of bullous lesions in acute barbiturate intoxication. *Br. Med. J.* i, 835.

Bigby, M., Jick, S., Jick, H., and Arndt, K. (1986). Drug-induced cutaneous reactions: a report from the Boston Colloborative Drug Surveillance Program on 15,438 consecutive inpatients, 1975 to 1982. *JAMA* 256, 3358.

Bjellerup, M. (1989). Nail changes induced by penicillamine. *Acta Derm. Venereol.* (Stockh.) 69, 339.

Bombardierie, S., DiMunno, O., Dipunzio, C., and Pasero, G. (1977). Erythema nodosum associated with pregnancy and oral contraceptives. *Br. Med. J.* i, 1509.

Bork, K. (1988). *Cutaneous side effects of drugs*, p. 318. W.B. Saunders, Philadelphia.

Boxley, J.D., Dawber, R.P.R., and Summerly, R. (1975). Generalised pustular psoriasis on withdrawal of clobetasol propionate ointment. *Br. Med. J.* ii, 255.

Brady, A.J. and Wing, A.J. (1989). Hyperpigmentation due to cyclosporin therapy. *Nephrol. Dial. Transplant.* 4, 309.

Brodin, M.B. (1987). Drug-related alopecia. *Dermatol. Clin.* 5, 571.

Bronner, A.K. and Hood, A.F. (1983). Cutaneous complications of chemotherapeutic agents. *J. Am. Acad. Dermatol.* 9, 645.

Brown, M.D. and Dubin, H.V. (1987). Penicillamine-induced bullous pemphigoid-like eruption. *Arch. Dermatol.* 123, 1119.

Bruinsma, W. (1987a). *A guide to drug eruptions* (4th edn), p. 43. De Zwalu, Oosthuizen.

Bruinsma, W. (1987b). *A guide to drug eruptions* (4th edn), p. 32. De Zwalu, Oosthuizen.

Burton, J.L. and Marshall, A. (1979). Hypertrichosis due to minoxidil. *Br. J. Dermatol.* 101, 593.

Burton, J.L., Schutt, W.H., and Caldwell, J.W. (1975). Hypertrichosis due to diazoxide. *Br. J. Dermatol.* 93, 707.

Byrne, J.P.H., Boss, J.M., and Dawber, R.P.R. (1976). Contraceptive pill-induced porphyria cutanea tarda presenting with onycholysis of the finger nails. *Postgrad. Med. J.* 52, 535.

Carmichael, A.J. and Paul, C.J. (1988). Vasculitic leg ulcers associated with diltiazem. *Br. Med. J.* 297, 562.

Carradori, S., Peluso, A.M., and Faccioli, M. (1990). Systemic contact dermatitis due to parabens. *Contact Dermatitis* 22, 238.

Carruthers, R.J.G., August, P.J., and Staughton, R.C.D. (1975). Observations on the systemic effect of topical clobetasol propionate (Dermovate). *Br. Med. J.* iv, 203.

Chan, H.L., Stern, R.S., Arndt, K.A., Langlois, J., Jick, S.S., Jick, H., *et al.* (1990). The incidence of erythema multiforme, Stevens–Johnson syndrome and toxic epidermal necrolysis. A population-based study with particular reference to reactions caused by drugs among outpatients. *Arch. Dermatol.* 126, 43.

Citron, A.P., Halpern, M., McCarron, M., Lindbert, G.D., McCormick, R., Pincus, I.J., *et al.* (1970). Necrotizing angiitis associated with drug abuse. *N. Engl. J. Med.* 283, 1003.

Cohen, I.S., Mosher, M.B., O'Keefe, E.J., Klaus, S.N., and DeConti, R.C. (1973). Cutaneous toxicity of bleomycin therapy. *Arch. Dermatol.* 107, 553.

Coskey, R. J. (1978). Contact dermatitis due to clindamycin. *Arch. Dermatol.* 114, 446.

Coskey, R.J. (1983). Contact dermatitis caused by diphenhydramine hydrochloride. *J. Am. Acad. Dermatol.* 8, 204.

Cotterill, J.A. (1979). Perioral dermatitis. *Br. J. Dermatol.* 101, 259.

Coyle, H.E., Miller, E., and Chapman, R.S. (1981). Sorbic acid sensitivity from unguentum Merck. *Contact Dermatitis* 7, 56.

Cronin, E. (1980a). *Contact dermatitis*, p. 10. Churchill Livingstone, Edinburgh.

Cronin, E. (1980b). *Contact dermatitis*, p. 209. Churchill Livingstone, Edinburgh.

Cronin, E. (1980c). *Contact dermatitis*, p. 204. Churchill Livingstone,. Edinburgh.

Cronin, E., Bandmann, H.J., Calnan, C.D., Fregert, 5., Hjorth, N., Magnusson, B., *et al.* (1970). Contact dermatitis in the atopic. *Acta Derm. Venereol.* (Stockh.) 50, 183.

Cunliffe, W.J. (1990). Eusol — to use or not to use. *Dermatology in Practice* 8, 5.

Daniel, C.R. and Scher, R.K. (1984). Nail changes secondary to systemic drugs or unguentants. *J. Am. Acad. Dermatol.* 10, 250.

David, M., Livini, E., Stern, E., Feuerman, E.J., and Grinblatt, J. (1982). Psoriasiform eruption induced by digoxin: confirmation by re-exposure. *J. Am. Acad. Dermatol.* 5, 702.

Dawber, R. and Mortimer, P. (1982). Hair loss during lithium treatment. *Br. J. Dermatol.* 107, 124.

De Kort, W.J.A. and De Groot, A.C. (1989). Clindamycin allergy presenting as rosacea. *Contact Dermatitis* 20, 72.

DeRaeve, L., Song, M., and van Maldergem (1988). Adverse cutaneous drug reactions in AIDS. *Br. J. Dermatol.* 119, 521.

Diette, K. M., Gange, R.W., Stern, R.S., Arntd, K.A., and Parrish, J.A. (1983). Coal tar phototoxicity: kinetics and exposure parameters. *J. Invest. Dermatol.* 81, 347.

Dobozya, A., Hundyadi, J., Kenderessy, A.S., and Simon, J. (1981). Lymphocyte transformation test in detection of drug hypersensitivity. *Clin. Exper. Dermatol.* 6, 367.

Dosik, H., Hurewitz, D.J., Rosner, F., and Schwartz, J.M. (1970). Bullous eruptions and elevated leukocyte alkaline phosphatase in the course of busulphan-treated chronic granulocytic leukaemia. *Blood* 35, 543.

Downham, T.F. III (1978). Spironolactone-induced lichen planus. *JAMA* 240, 1138.

Drill, V.A. (1977). Benign cholestatic jaundice of pregnancy and benign cholestatic jaundice from oral contraceptives. *Am. J. Obstet. Gynecol.* 119 165.

Duhra, P. and Foulds, I.S. (1988). Penicillin-induced pemphigus vulgaris. *Br. J. Dermatol.* 118, 307.

Dukes, M.N.G. (ed.) (1975). Blood and blood products. In *Meyler's side effects of drugs*, Vol. 8, p. 725. Associated Scientific Publishers, Amsterdam.

Dwyer, J.M., Kenicer, K., Thompson, B.T., Chen, D., La Braico, J., Schiefferdecker, R., *et al.* (1989). Vasculitis and retinoids. *Lancet* ii, 494.

Enat, R., Katz, R., Munichor, M., and Pollack, S. (1988). Hypersensitivity vasculitis induced by terbutaline sulfate. *Ann. Allergy* 61, 275.

Epstein, S. (1968). Chlorpromazine photosensitivity: phototoxic and photoallergic reactions. *Arch. Dermatol.* 98, 354.

Eriksen, K.E. (1975). Allergy to ethylenediamine. *Arch. Dermatol.* 111, 791.

Eyster, F.E., Wilson, C.B., and Maibach, H.1. (1971). Mithramycin as a possible cause of toxic epidermal necrolysis (Lyell's syndrome). *Calif. Med.* 114, 42.

Falkson, G. and Schultz, E.J. (1962). Skin changes in patients treated with 5-fluorouracil. *Br. J. Dermatol.* 74, 224.

Fallah-Sohy, E. and Figueredo, A.T. (1979). Allergic reaction to doxorubicin. *JAMA* 74, 224.

Felix, R.H. and Comaish, J.S. (1974). The value of patch and other skin tests in drug eruptions. *Lancet* i, 1017.

Felix, R.H., Ive, F.A., and Dahl, M.G.C. (1974). Cutaneous and ocular reactions to practolol. *Br. Med. J.* iv, 321.

Felix, R.H., Ive, F.A., and Dahl, M.G.C. (1975). Skin reactions to beta-blockers. *Br. Med. J.* i, 626.

Fellner, M.J. (1971). Adverse effects of drugs on the skin. In *International Academy of Pathology Monograph The Skin* (ed. E. B. Helwig and F. K. Mostofi), p. 226. Williams and Wilkins, Baltimore.

Fenton, D.A. and English, J.B. (1982). Toxic epidermal necrolysis, leucopenia and thrombocytopenic purpura — a further complication of benoxaprofen therapy. *Clin. Exp. Dermatol.* 7, 277.

Ferguson, J. and Johnson, B.E. (1986). Photosensitivity due to retinoids: clinical and laboratory studies. *Br. J. Dermatol.* 115, 275

Ferguson, J., Addo, H.A., McGill, P.E., Woodcock, K.R., Johnson, B.E., and Frain-Bell, W. A. (1982). A study of benoxaprofen-induced photosensitivity. *Br. J. Dermatol.* 107, 429.

Ferguson, J., Addo, H.A., Jones, S., Johnson, B.E., and Frain-Bell, W.A. (1985). A study of cutaneous photosensitivity induced by amiodarone. *Br. J. Dermatol.* 113, 537.

Ferguson, J., Addo, H.A., Johnson, B.E., and Frain-Bell, W.A. (1987). Quinine-induced photosensitivity: clinical and experimental studies. *Br. J. Dermatol.* 117, 631.

Fischer, R., Bircher, J., and Reich, T. (1953). Der Haarausfall nach antekoagulierender Therapie. *Schweiz. Med. Wochenschr.* 83, 509.

Fisher, A.A. (1976). Allergic dermatitis medicamentosa: the systemic contact type variety. *Cutis* 18, 637.

Fisher, A.A. (1990). Contact urticaria due to occupational exposures. In *Occupational skin disease* (ed. R.M. Adams), p. 113. W.B. Saunders, Philadelphia.

Forsbeck, M., Hovmark, A., and Skog, E. (1976). Patch testing, tuberculin testing and sensitization with dinitrochlorobenzene and nitrosodimethylamine of patients with atopic dermatitis. *Acta Derm. Venereol.* (Stockh.) 56, 135.

Fregert, S. (1976). Respiratory symptoms with piperazine patch testing. *Contact Dermatitis* 2, 61.

Friedmann, P.S., Moss, C., Shuster, S., and Simpson, J.M. (1983). Quantitation of sensitization and responsiveness to dinitrochlorobenzene in normal subjects. *Br. J. Dermatol.* (suppl.), 25, 86.

Furhoff, A. K. (1977). Anaphylactoid reaction to dextran — a report of 133 cases. *Acta Anaesth. Scand.* 21, 161.

Gammeltoft, M. and Kristensen, J.K. (1982). Propylthiouracil induced cutaneous vasculitis. *Acta Derm. Venereol.* (Stockh.) 62, 171.

Gange, R.W. and Wilson-Jones, E. (1978). Bullous lichen planus caused by labetalol. *Br. Med. J.* i, 816.

Garioch, J. and Simpson, N.B. (1989). Etretinate and severe nail plate dystrophies. *Clin. Exp. Dermatol.* 14, 261.

Gawkrodger, D.J. and Beveridge, G.W. (1985). Psoriasiform reaction to atenolol. *Clin. Exp. Dermatol.* 9, 92.

Goh, C.L. (1987). Psoriasiform drug eruption due to glibenclamide. *Aust. J. Dermatol.* 28, 30.

Gokal, R., Dornan, T.L., and Ledingham, J.G.G. (1979). Peripheral skin necrosis complicating beta-blockade. *Br. Med. J.* i, 721.

Gottschaek, H.R. and Stone, 0.J. (1976). Stevens–Johnson syndrome from ophthalmic sulphonamide. *Arch. Dermatol.* 112, 513.

Granowitz, E.V. (1989). Photosensitivity rash in a patient being treated with ciprofloxacin. *J. Infect. Dis.* 160, 910.

Granstein, R.D. and Sober, A.J. (1981). Drug and heavy metal induced hyperpigmentation. *J. Am. Acad. Dermatol.* 5, 1.

Greaves, M.W. (1987). Pathophysiology of pruritus. In *Dermatology in general medicine* (3rd edn) (ed. T.B. Fitzpatrick, A.Z. Eisen, K. Uolff, I.M. Freedberg, and K.F. Austen). McGraw-Hill, New York.

Greenberg, R.D. (1979). Acne vulgaris associated with antigonadotrophic (Danazol therapy). *Cutis* 24, 431.

Greenwald, R.A., Rheingold, O.J., and Chiprut, R.0. (1978). Local gangrene: a complication of peripheral pitressin therapy for bleeding esophageal varices. *Gastroenterology* 74, 744.

Greenwood, R., Fcnwick, P.B.C., and Cunliffe, W.J. (1983). Acne and anticonvulsants. *Br. Med. J.* 287, 1669.

Groark, S.P., Hood, A.F., and Nelson, K. (1989). Nail pigmentation associated with zidovudine. *J. Am. Acad. Dermatol.* 21, 1032.

Groth, O. (1961). Lichenoid dermatitis resulting from treatment with the phenothiazine derivatives metopromazine and laevopromazine. *Acta Derm. Venereol.* (Stockh.) 41, 168.

Guin, J.D. (1981). Complications of topical hydrocortisone. *J. Am. Acad. Dermatol.* 4, 417.

Guin, J.D. (1984). Contact sensitivity to topical corticosteroids. *J. Am. Acad. Dermatol.* 10, 773.

Guin, J.D., Haynie, L.S., Jaekson, D., and Baker, G.F. (1987). Wandering fixed drug eruption: a mucocutaneous reaction to acetaminophen. *J. Am. Acad. Dermatol.* 17, 399.

Guldager, H. (1987). Halothane allergy as a cause of acne. *Lancet* i, 1211.

Halevy, S., Grunwald, M.H., Sandbank, M., Buimovice, B., Joshua, H., and Livini, E. (1990). Macrophage migration inhibition factor. (MIF) in drug eruption. *Arch. Dermatol.* 126, 48.

Halsey, J. P. and Cardoe, N. (1982). Benoxaprofen: side effect profile in 300 patients. *Br. Med. J.* 284, 1365.

Hamburger, J. and Potts, A.J.C. (1983). Non-steroidal anti-inflammatory drugs and oral lichenoid reactions. *Br. Med. J.* 287, 1258.

Harber, L.C., Lashinsky, A.M., and Bacy, R.L. (1959). Skin manifestations of photosensitivity due to chlorothiazide and hydrochlorothiazide. *J. Invest. Dermatol.* 33, 83.

Harris, W.C. (1950). Exfoliative dermatitis complicating streptomycin therapy. *Lancet* i, 325.

Hjorth, N. and Fregerts, S. (1979). In *Textbook of dermatology* (ed. A. Rook, D.S. WIlkinson, and F.J.G. Eblang), p. 371. Blackwell Scientific, Oxford.

Hjorth, N. and Thomsen, K. (1968). Differences in the sensitizing capacity of neomycin in creams and in ointments. *Br. J. Dermatol.* 80, 163.

Hoffbrand, B.I. (1979). Peripheral skin necrosis complicating beta-blockade. *Br. Med. J.* i, 1082.

Holt, P.J.A. and Waddington, E. Oculocutaneous reaction to oxprenolol (1975).*Br. Med J.* ii, 539.

Honeybourne, D., Longworth, S., and Shaffer, J. (1987). Rifampicin causing an exacerbation of pemphigus. *Br. J. Clin. Pract.* 41, 937.

Houwerzijl, J., DeGast, G.C., and Nater, J.P. (1974). Tests for drug allergy, *Lancet* ii, 655.

Hunter, J.A., Dorward, A.J., Knill-Jones, R., Gunn, R.T.S., and Mackie, R. (1978). Diflunisal and Stevens–Johnson syndrome. *Br. Med. J.* ii, 1088.

Hurwitz, R.M. (1989). Steroid acne. *J. Am. Acad. Dermatol.* 21, 1179.

Husain, Z., Runge, L.A., Jabbs, J.M., and Hyla, J.A. (1981). Sulindac-induced Stevens–Johnson syndrome. *J. Rheumatol.* 8, 176.

Ilchyshyn, A. and Vickers, C.F.H. (1983). Yellow nail syndrome associated with penicillamine therapy. *Acta Derm. Venereol.* (Stockh.) 63, 534.

Ive, F.A. and Marks, R. (1968). Tinea incognito. *Br. Med. J.* iii, 149.

Jadasohn, J. (1896). Zur Kenntnis der Arzneiexantheme. *Arch. Dermatol. Syphilol.* 34, 103.

James, W.D. and Odom, R.B. (1983). Chemotherapy-induced transverse white lines of the fingernails. *Arch. Dermatol.* 119, 334.

Jensen, H.A., Mikkelsen, H.I., Wadskov, S., and Sondergaard, J. (1976). Cutaneous reactions to propranolol (Inderal). *Acta Med. Scand.* 199, 363.

Jerez, J., Rodriguez, F., Garces, M., Martin-Gil, D., Jimenez, I., Anton, E., *et al.* (1990). Allergic contact dermatitis from budesonide. *Contact Dermatitis* 22, 231.

Jones, C. and Bleehan, S.S. (1977). Acne induced by PUVA treatment. *Br. Med. J.* ii, 866.

Judd, L.E., Henderson, D.W., and Hill, D.C. (1986). Naproxen-induced pseudo-porphyria: a clinical and ultrastructural study. *Arch. Dermatol.* 122, 451.

Kampmann, K.K., Graves, T., and Rogers, S.D. (1989). Acral erythema secondary to high-dose cytosine arabinoside with pain worsened by cyclosporin infusions. *Cancer* 63, 2482.

Kantor, G.L. (1970). Toxic epidermal necrolysis, azotaemia and death after allopurinol therapy. *JAMA* 212, 478.

Katayama, H. and Kawada, A. (1981). Exacerbation of psoriasis induced by indomethacin. *J. Dermatol.* (Tokyo) 8, 323.

Katz, R.A., Hood, A.F., and Anhalt, G.J. (1987). Pemphigus like eruption from captopril. *Arch. Dermatol.* 123, 20.

Kelly, R.A., Gelfand, J.A., and Pincus, S.H. (1981). Cutaneous necrosis caused by systemically administered heparin. *JAMA* 246, 1582.

Kerdel, F.A., Fraker, D.L., and Haynes, A. (1984). Necrotizing vasculitis from radiographic contrast media. *J. Am. Acad. Dermatol.* 10, 25.

Kernekamp, A.S. van W., and van Ketel, W.G. (1980). Persistence of patch test reactions to clioquinol (Vioform) and cross-sensitization. *Contact Dermatitis* 6, 455.

Kew, M.C., Mzamane, D., Smith, A.G., and Shuster, S. (1977). MSH levels in doxorubicin-induced hyperpigmentation. *Lancet* i, 811.

King, C.M. and Beck, M. (1983). Oral promethazine hydrochloride in ethylenediamine sensitive patients. *Contact Dermatitis* 9, 444.

Kiraly, C.L., Collan, Y., and Alen, M. (1987). Effect of testosterone and anabolic steroids on the size of sebaceous glands in power athletes. *Am. J. Dermatopathol.* 9, 515.

Kirkham, N. and Holt, S. (1976). Nail dystrophy after practolol. *Lancet* ii, 1137.

Kraft, D. and Wide, L. (1976). Clinical patterns and results in radioallergosorbent test (RAST) and skin tests in penicillin allergy. *Br. J. Dermatol.* 94, 593.

Krook, G. (1975). Contact sensitivity to oxyphenbutazone (Tanderil) and cross sensitivity to phenylbutazone (Butazolidin). *Contact Dermatitis* 1, 262.

Kuokkanen, K. (1972). Drug eruptions: a series of 464 cases in the Department of Dermatology, University of Turku, Finland during 1966–70. *Acta Allergolica* 27, 407.

Kuske, H. and Krebs, A. (1964). Hyperpigmentierungen vom Typus des Chloasmus nach Behandlung mit Hydantoin Preparaten. *Dermatologica* 129, 121.

Lachapelle, J.M. (1975). Contact sensitivity to bufexamac. *Contact Dermatitis* 1, 261.

Laing, V.B., Sheretz, E.F., and Flowers, F.P. (1988). Pemphigoid-like bullous eruption related to ibuprofen. *J. Am. Acad. Hematol.* 19, 91.

Lambert, D.G., Dalac, S., Beer, F., Chavannet, P., and Portier, H. (1988). Acute generalized exanthematous pustular dermatitis induced by diltiazem. *Br. J. Dermatol.* 118, 308.

Lamkin, N., Lieberman, P., Hashimoto, K., Morotiasti, M., and Sullivan, P. (1976). Allergic reactions to insulin — clinical conference. *J. Allergy Clin. Immunol.* 58, 213.

Lawlor, F. and Hindson, C. (1982). Allergy to dithranol. *Contact Dermatitis* 8, 137.

Lawrence, C.M. and Dahl, M.G.C. (1984). Two patterns of skin ulceration induced by methotrexate in patients with psoriasis. *J. Am. Acad. Dermatol.* 11, 1059.

Leigh, I M., Kennedy, C.T.C., Ramsey, J.D., and Henderson, W.J. (1979). Mepacrine pigmentation in systemic lupus erythematosus. *Br. J. Dermatol.* 101, 147.

Leonard, P.A., Moatamed, F., and Ward, J.R. (1986). Chrysiasis: the role of sun exposure in dermal hyperpigmentation secondary to gold therapy. *J. Rheumatol.* 13, 58.

Levantine, A. and Almeyda, J. (1972). Drug reactions: 20 cutaneous reactions to anticonvulsants. *Br. J. Dermatol.* 87, 246.

Levine, L.E., Bernstein, J.E., Soltani, K., Medenica, M.M., and Yung C.W. (1983). Heparin-induced cutaneous necrosis unrelated to injection sites. *Arch. Dermatol.* 119, 400.

Lewis, J.H., Zimmerman, H.J., Benson, G.D., and Ishak, K.G. (1984). Hepatic injury associated with ketoconazole therapy. *Gastroenterology* 86, 503.

Leyden, J.J. and Kligman, A.M. (1977a). The case for steroid–antibiotic combinations. *Br. J. Dermatol.* 96, 179.

Leyden, J.J. and Kligman, A.M. (1977b). Contact sensitivity to benzoyl peroxide. *Contact Dermatitis* 3, 273.

Logan, R.A., McFadden, J.P., and Eady, R.A.J. (1988). Reaction of cutaneous radionecrosis associated with methotrexate therapy for psoriasis. *Clin. Exp. Dermatol.* 13, 350.

Lowe, N.J. and Ridgway, H.B. (1978). Generalised pustular psoriasis precipitated by lithium carbonate. *Arch. Dermatol.* 114, 1788.

Lyell, A. (1956). Toxic epidermal necrolysis: an eruption resembling scalding of the skin. *Br. J. Dermatol.* 68, 355.

Lyell, A. (1979). Toxic epidermal necrolysis (the scalded skin syndrome): a reappraisal. *Br. J. Dermatol.* 100, 69.

Lyell, A. (1990). Requiem for toxic epidermal necrolysis. *Br. J. Dermatol.* 122, 837.

McDonagh, A.J. and Harrington, C.I. (1989). Pseudoporphyria complicating etretinate therapy. *Clin. Exp. Dermatol.* 14, 437.

MacDonald, R.H. and Beck, M. (1983). Neomycin: a review with particular reference to dermatological usage. *Clin. Exp. Dermatol.* 8, 249.

McGovern, B., Garan, H., Kelly, E., and Ruskin, J.N. (1983). Adverse reactions during treatment with amiodarone hydrochloride. *Br. Med. J.* 287, 175.

McKerrow, K.J. and Greig, D.E. (1986). Piroxicam induced photosensitive dermatitis. *J. Am. Acad. Dermatol.* 15. 1237.

McWhirter, J.D., Hashimoto, K., Fayne, S., and Ito, R. (1987). Linear IgA bullous dermatosis related to lithium carbonate. *Arch. Dermatol.* 123, 1120.

Mahler, R., Sissons, W., and Watters, K. (1986). Pigmentation induced by quinidine therapy. *Arch. Dermatol.* 122, 1062.

Mahrle, G., Orfanos, L.E., Ippen, H., and Hofbauer, M. (1979). Haarwachstum Leberwerke und Lichtempfindlichkeit unter oraler Retinoid Therapie bei Psoriasis. *Deutsch. Med. Wochenschr.* 104, 473.

Malten, K.E., Nater, J.P., and Van Ketel, W.G. (1976). *Patch testing guidelines*, p. 84. Dekker and van de Vegt, Nijmegen.

Mandy, S. and Ackerman, A.B. (1970). Characteristic traumatic skin lesions in drug-induced coma. *JAMA* 213, 253.

Manzi, S., Kraus, V.B., and St Clair, E.W. (1989). An unusual photoactivated skin eruption. Quinidine-induced livedo reticularis. *Arch. Dermatol.* 125, 417.

Martin, R.L., McSweeney, G.W., and Schneider, J. (1983). Fatal pemphigus vulgaris in a patient taking piroxicam. *N. Engl. J. Med.* 309, 795.

Mathias, C.G.T., Maiback, H.I., and Epstein, J. (1978). Allergic contact dermatitis due to para-aminobenzoic acid. *Arch. Dermatol.* 114, 1665.

Mauer, E.F. (1955). The toxic effects of phenylbutazone (Butazolidin). *N. Engl. J. Med.* 253, 404.

Merenich, J.A., Hannon, R.N., Gentry, R.H., and Harrison, S.M. (1989). Azidothymidine-induced hyperpigmentation mimicking primary adrenal insufficiency. *Am. J. Med.* 86, 469.

Mitchell, J.C. (1978). Day 7 (D 7) patch testing reading — valuable or not? *Contact Dermatitis* 4, 139.

Miyagawa, S., Yoshiolca, A., Hatoko, M., Okuchi, T., and Sakamoto, K. (1987). Systemic sclerosis-like lesions during long-term penicillamine therapy for Wilson's disease. *Br. J. Dermatol.* 116, 95.

Monk, B.E., Parkes, J.D., Du Vivier, A. (1984). Erythromelalgia following pergolide administration. *Br. J. Dermatol.* 111, 97.

Mullick, F.G., McAllister, H.A., Wagner, B.M., and Fenoglio, J.J. (1979). Drug related vasculitis. *Hum. Pathol.* 10, 313.

Nurse, D.S. and Rosner, S.A. (1983). Contact dermatitis due to lignocaine. *Contact Dermatitis* 9, 513.

Odom, R.B. and Maibach, H.I. (1976). Contact urticaria: a different contact dermatitis. *Cutis* 188, 672.

Okada, N., Moriya, K., Nishida, K., Kitano, Y., Kobayashi, T., Nishimura, H., *et al.* (1989). Skin pigmentation associated with minocycline therapy. *Br. J. Dermatol.* 121, 247.

Oliwiecki, S. and Burton, J.L. (1988). Severe acne due to isoniazid. *Clin. Exp. Dermatol.* 13, 276.

Ormerod, A.D. and Holt, P.J. (1983). Acute urticaria due to alcohol. *Br. J. Dermatol.* 108, 723.

Papadopoulos, S. and Harden, R.M. (1966). Hair loss in patients treated with carbimazole. *Br. Med. J.* ii, 150.

Paramsothy, Y., Collins, M., and Smith, A.G. (1988). Contact dermatitis in patients with leg ulcers. The prevalence of late positive reactions evidence against systemic amplicative allergy. *Contact Dermatitis* 18, 30.

Pareek, S.S. (1980). Nystatin-induced fixed eruption. *Br. J. Dermatol.* 103, 679.

Parodi, A., Guarrera, M., and Rebora, A. (1988). Amiodarone-induced pseudoporphyria. *Photodermatology* 5, 146.

Payne, F.E. and Giesecke, T.F. (1987). Multiple system reaction to trimethoprimsulfamethoxazole. *South. Med. J.* 80, 275.

Pennell, T.O., Nunan, M.J., O'Doherty, M.J., and Croft, D.N. (1984). Fatal Stevens–Johnson syndrome in a patient on captopril and allopurinol. *Lancet* i, 463.

Pletcher, W.D., Brody, G.C., and Myers, M.C. (1963). Haemochromatosis following prolonged iron therapy in a patient with hereditary nonspherocytic haemolytic anaemia. *Am. J. Med. Sci.* 246, 27.

Pullen, H., Wright, N., and Murdoch, J.McC. (1967). Hypersensitivity reactions to antibacterial drugs in infectious mononucleosis. *Lancet* ii, 1176.

Ramsay, C.A. and Obreshkova, E. (1974). Photosensitivity from nalidixic acid. *Br. J. Dermatol.* 91, 523.

Reed, M.D., Bertino, J.A., and Blumer, J.L. (1982). Carbamazepine-associated exfoliative dermatitis. *Clin. Pharmacol.* 1, 78.

Reisner, C., Moll, D.J., and Çudworth, A.G. (1978). Generalised urticaria precipitated by change to highly purified porcine insulin. *Br. Med. J.* ii, 56.

Reshad, H., Margreaves, G.K., and Vickers, C.F. (1983). Generalised pustular psoriasis precipitated by phenylbutazone and oxyphenbutazone. *Br. J. Dermatol.* 117, 273.

Richards, S. (1985). Cutaneous side effects of beta-adrenergic blockers. *Aust. J. Dermatol.* 26, 25.

Ring, J. and Messmer, K. (1977). Incidence and severity of anaphylactoid reactions to colloid volume substitutes. *Lancet* i, 466.

Roberts, D.L. and Marks, R. (1981). Skin reactions to carbamazepine. *Arch. Dermatol.* 117, 273.

Robinson, H.M. and Samorodin, C.S. (1976). Thiabendazole-induced toxic epidermal necrolysis. *Arch. Dermatol.* 112, 1757,

Roeleveld, D.G. and van Ketel, W.G. (1976). Positive patch tests to azo dye tartrazine. *Contact Dermatitis* 2, 180.

Rogers, S.C.F., Burrow, D., and Neill, D. (1978). Percutaneous absorption of phenol and methyl alcohol in magenta paint B.P.C. *Br. J. Dermatol.* 98, 559.

Rohrborn, W. and Brauninger, W. (1987). Thioridazine photoallergy. *Contact Dermatitis* 17, 241.

Roujeau, J.C., Guillaume, J.C., Fabre, J.P., Penso D., Flechet, M.L., and Givve, J. (1990). Toxic epidermal necrolysis (Lyell syndrome). Incidence and drug aetiology in France. 1981–85. *Arch. Dermatol.* 126, 37.

Rudner, E.J. (1970). Diphenylhydantoin therapy. *Arch. Dermatol.* 102, 561.

Rudzki, E., Grzywa, Z., and Maciejowska, E. (1976). Drug reaction with positive patch tests to chloramphenicol. *Contact Dermatitis* 2, 181.

Russel Jones, R. and Cunningham, J. (1979). Warfarin skin necrosis: role of Factor VII. *Br. J. Dermatol.* 101, 561.

Sakurai, I. and Skinsnes, 0.K. (1977). Histochemistry of B633 pigmentation: ceroid-like pigmentation in macrophages. *Int. J. Leprosy* 45, 343.

Samsoen, M. and Jelen, G. (1977). Allergy to Daktarin gel. *Contact Dermatitis* 3, 351.

Santa Cruz, D.J., Marcus, M.D., Prioleau, P.G., and Uitto, J. (1981). Pemphigus-like lesions induced by D-penicillamine. *Am. J. Dermatopathol.* 3, 85.

Sarkany, I. and Gaylarde, P.M. (1978). Role of lymphocyte transformation in drug allergy. *Australas. J. Dermatol.* 19, 45.

Savill, J.S., Chia, Y., and Pusey, C.D. (1988). Minimal change nephropathy and pemphigus vulgaris associated with penicillamine treatment of rheumatoid arthritis. *Clin. Nephrol.* 29, 267.

Schuppli, R. (1960). On severe toxic effects in the prophylactic use of drugs. *Dermatologica* 121, 15.

Shall, L., Lucas, G.S., Whittaker, J.A., and Holt, P.J.A. (1988). Painful red hands: a side-effect of leukaemia therapy. *Br. J. Dermatol.* 119, 249.

Shatin, M., Canizares, M.D., and Worthington, E.L. (1953). Lichen planus-like eruption due to para-amino salicylic acid. *J. Invest. Dermatol.* 21, 135.

Shelley, W.B. and Bennett, R.G. (1972). Primary contact sensitization site: a determinant for the localisation of a diphenydramine eruption. *Acta Derm. Venereol.* (Stockh.) 52, 376.

Shelley, W.B. and Shelley, E. (1987). Nonpigmenting fixed drug eruption as a distinctive reaction pattern: examples caused by sensitivity to pseudoephedrine hydrochloride and tetrahydrozoline. *J. Am. Acad. Dermatol.* 17, 403.

Shelton, D. and Goulding, R. (1979). Silver poisoning associated with an anti-smoking lozenge. *Br. Med. J.* i, 267.

Shepherd, A.N., Ferguson, J., Bewick, M., and Bouchier, I.A.D. (1986). Mefenamic acid-induced bullous pemphigoid. *Postgrad. Med. J.* 62, 67.

Skott, A., Mobacken, H., and Starmark, J.E. (1977). Exacerbation of psoriasis during lithium treatment. *Br. J. Dermatol.* 96, 445.

Slater, E.E., Merrill, D.D., Guess, H.A., Roylance, P.J., Cooper, W.D., Inman, W.D.H., *et al.* (1988). Clinical profile of angioedema associated with angiotensin-converting enzyme inhibition. *JAMA* 260, 967.

Smith, A.G., Shuster, S., Thody, A.J., and Peberdy, M. (1977). Chloasma, oral contraceptives and plasma immunoreactive beta-MSH. *J. Invest. Dermatol.* 68, 169.

Sola, R., Puig, L.L., Ballarin, J.A., Donate, T., and Del Rio, G. (1987). Pseudoporphyria cutanea tarda associated with cyclosporin therapy. *Transplantation* 43, 772.

Solinger, A.M. (1982). Exfoliative dermatitis from captopril. *Cutis* 29, 473.

Søndergaard, J., Wadskov, S., Jensen, H.A., and Mikkelsen, H.I. (1976). Aggravation of psoriasis and occurrence of psoriasiform cutaneous eruptions induced by practolol (Eraldin). *Acta Derm. Venereol.* (Stockh.) 56, 239.

Sowden, J.M. and Smith, A.G. (1990). Fixed drug eruption to mefenamic acid mimicking cyclical erythema multiforme. *Clin. Exp. Dermatol.* 15, 387.

Sowunmi, A., Walker, 0., and Salako, L.A. (1989). Pruritus and antimalarial drugs in Africans. *Lancet* ii, 213.

Stadler, R., Orfanos, C.E., and Immel, C. (1982). Medikamentos induzierte Pellagra. *Hautarzt* 33, 276.

Stevenson, C.J. (1971). Lichenoid eruptions due to methyldopa. *Br. J. Dermatol.* 85, 600.

Stone, R.L., Claflin, A., and Penneys, N.S. (1973). Erythema nodosum following gold sodium thiomalate therapy. *Arch. Dermatol.* 107, 602.

Stratigos, J.D., Bartsokas, St K., and Capetanakis, J. (1972). Further experiences of toxic epidermal necrolysis incriminating allopurinol, pyrazolone and derivates. *Br. J. Dermatol.* 86, 564.

Tagami, H., Tatsuta, K., Iwatski, K., and Yamada, M. (1983). Delayed hypersensitivity in ampiclllin-induced toxic epidermal necrolysis. *Arch. Dermatol.* 119, 910.

Tan, R.S. and Copeman, P.W.M. (1974). Fixed drug eruption due to 'nonabsorbable' sulphonamides. *Proc. R. Soc. Med.* 67, 198.

Teoh, P.C. and Chan, H.L. (1975). Lupus–scleroderma syndrome induced by by ethosuximide. *Arch. Dis. Child.* 50, 658.

Thormann, J. (1978). I.ithium og psoriasis. *Ugeskr. Laeger.* 140, 721.

van Dijke, C.P.H., Veerman, F.R., and Haverkamp, H.C.H. (1983). Anaphylactic reactions to ketoconazole. *Br. Med. J.* 287, 1673.

van Joost, T., Middlekamp Hup, J., and Ros, F.E. (1979). Dermatitis as a side effect of long term topical treatment with certain beta-blocking agents. *Br. J. Dermatol.* 101, 171.

Verbov, J.L. (1970). Sensitivity to sodium fusidate. *Contact Dermatitis Newsletter* 7, 153.

Vickers, C.F.H. (1961). Dermatitis medicamentosa. *Br. Med. J.* i, 1366.

Vollum, D.I., Parkes, J.D., and Doyle, D. (1971). Livedo reticularis during amantidine treatment. *Br. Med. J.* ii, 627.

Wakeel, R.A., Gavin, M.P., and Reefe, M. (1988). Severe toxic erythema caused by diltiazem. *Br. Med. J.* 296, 1071.

Wang, J.J., Freeman, A.I., Gaeta, J.F., and Sinks, L.F. (1970). Unusual complication of pentamidine in treatment of *Pneumocystis carinii* pneumonia. *J. Pediatr.* 77, 311.

Weber, G. (1974). Combined 8-methoxypsoralen and black light therapy for psoriasis. *Br. J. Dermatol.* 90, 317.

Wennersten, G., Thume, P., Brodthagen, H., Jansen, C., and Rystedt, I. (1984). The Scandinavian multicentre photopatch study: preliminary results. *Contact Dermatitis* 10, 305.

Wilkin, J.K. (1983). Flushing reaction. In *Recent advances in dermatology*, Vol. 6 (ed. A.J. Rook and H.I. Maibach), p. 157. Churchill Livingstone, Edinburgh.

Wilkin, J.M., Hammond, J.J., and Kirkendall, W.M. (1980). The captopril-induced eruption: a possible mechanism — cutaneous kinin potentiation. *Arch. Dermatol.* 116, 902.

Wilkinson, J.D., Hambly, E.M., and Wilkinson, D.S. (1980). Comparison of patch test results in two adjacent areas of England. II. Medicaments. *Acta Derm. Venereol.* (Stockh.) 60, 245.

Wilson, H.T.H. (1966). Dermatitis from anaesthetic ointments. *Practitioner* 197, 673.

Wilson, J.T., Hojer, B., Tomson, G., Raine, A., and Sjöquist, F. (1978). High incidence of concentration-dependent skin reaction in children treated with phenytoin. *Br. Med. J.* i, 1583.

Winter, G.D. and Burton, J.L. (1976). Experimentally induced steroid atrophy in the domestic pig and man. *Br. J. Dermatol.* 94, 107.

Wolf R., Dorfman, B., and Krakowski, A. (1987). Quinidineinduced lichenoid and eczematous photodermatitis. *Dermatologica* 174, 285.

Wolff, K. and Honigsmann, H. (1981). Clinical aspects of photochemotherapy. *Pharmacol. Ther.* 12, 381.

Wolff, K. and Stingl, G. (1983). The Langerhans cell. *J. Invest. Dermatol.* 80, 17.

Wongpaitoon, V., Mills, P.R., Russell, R.I., and Patrick, R.S. (1981). Intrahepatic cholestasis and cutaneous bullae associated with glibenclamide therapy. *Postgrad. Med. J.* 57, 244.

Wormser, G.P., Kornblee L.V., and Gottfried, E.B. (1982). Cutaneous necrosis following peripheral intravenous vasopressin therapy. *Cutis* 29, 249.

Wysocki, G.P. and Daly, T.D. (1987). Hypertrichosis in patients receiving cyclosporin therapy. *Clin. Exp. Dermatol.* 12, 191.

Yantis, P. L., Bridges, M. E., and Pitman, F. E. (1980). Cimetidine-induced exfoliative dermatitis. *Dig. Dis. Sci.* 25, 73.

Yoder, F. W. (1975). Acneiform eruption due to lithium carbonate. *Arch. Dermatol.* 111, 396.

Zacharias, F. J. (1976). Cross sensitivity between practolol and other beta-blockers? *Br. Med. J.* i, 1213.

Zachary, C.B., Slater, D.N., Holt, D.W., Storey, G.C.A., and McDonald, D.M. (1984). The pathogenesis of amiodaroneinduced pigmentation and photosensitivity. *Br. J. Dermatol.* 110, 451.

Zax, R.H., Hodge, S.J., and Callen, J.P. (1990). Cutaneous leucocytoclastic vasculitis: serial histopathologic evaluation demonstrates the dynamic nature of the infiltrate. *Arch. Dermatol.* 126, 69.

18. Neurological disorders

P. G. BLAIN and R. J. M. LANE

Introduction

In studying the neurotoxicity of drugs and other compounds it is sometimes useful to consider the nervous system as a federation of organs, each with different functional roles, biochemical processes, and, consequently, susceptibility to a specific toxic insult. Drugs may interfere with the functioning of neurones, neuroglia, and muscles at several levels so that neurological adverse effects have a broad spectrum of expression, from mild and possibly subtle changes in mental activity and behaviour to obvious muscle weakness. Many of these adverse reactions can be classified as Type A (see Chapter 3) from a knowledge of the pharmacokinetics and pharmacodynamics of the drug. Such a classification applies to adverse effects such as coma, syncope, seizures, some involuntary movement disorders, and many of the neuromuscular disorders. Many neurological reactions are not so classifiable, however, because of our ignorance of the underlying mechanisms. As we increase our understanding of the interaction between a drug's required and unwanted effects and an individual's genetic and environmental background, so many of the reactions previously classified as Type B may be seen to be Type A effects.

Genetic polymorphisms in drug metabolism may play a significant role in an individual's susceptibility to neurotoxicity. Clinical consequences of the slow acetylator phenotype include increased susceptibility to peripheral neuropathies induced by isoniazid, hydralazine, and dapsone. Following the administration of methoin, poor metabolisers of this drug have increased somnolence and intellectual impairment (Relling 1989). Some of the possible mechanisms underlying other neurological adverse reactions will be discussed, although for many our knowledge of the pathogenesis is minimal.

It is convenient to classify drug-induced neurological disorders in terms of the presenting clinical syndromes and neuroanatomical hierarchy, from cerebral cortex to muscle fibre (Lane and Routledge 1983).

Brain and meninges

Coma and encephalopathy

Coma implies bilateral cortical dysfunction or involvement of the brainstem reticular formation. Most drugs causing coma do so by interfering with synaptic transmission or cellular oxidative metabolism. The clinical features of drug-induced coma are similar regardless of the drug involved. Typically, the pupillary and corneal reflexes are preserved while other brainstem reflexes (e.g. the oculocephalic and · oculovestibular [caloric]responses) are lost early (Cartlidge 1981). In very deep coma, however, the pupillary and corneal reflexes may also be lost; indeed, drug overdosage must be excluded before a patient is diagnosed as 'brain-dead' (*The Lancet* 1976). Generalized flaccidity with depressed or absent tendon reflexes, and flexor or equivocal plantar responses is typical, although some patients, particularly following tricyclic antidepressant poisoning, may have hyperreflexia and extensor plantar responses. Myoclonus and convulsions may also be seen, either as a direct neurotoxic effect or secondary to anoxia: for example, a 74-year-old woman with multiple medical problems, including chronic renal failure, was admitted for treatment of a diabetic foot infection. On day 12 of therapy with ciprofloxacin and metronidazole, the patient experienced generalized myoclonus and muscle twitching. The dose of ciprofloxacin administered was too high in view of her renal failure (Schwartz and Calvert 1990).

The physical signs present in drug-induced stupor and coma, and their pharmacological basis have been reviewed in detail by Ashton and others (1989).

Drug-induced coma can arise in one of three ways: by a primary neurotoxic effect on the central nervous system;

by indirect effects on cerebral metabolism; and through alterations in cerebral blood flow. Drugs that produce sudden vasodilatation can cause syncope, due to the collapse of peripheral resistance, systemic and cerebral hypotension, and a diminished cerebral blood flow. Drug-induced hypotension is discussed in detail in Chapter 7.

Primary neurotoxic effects

Most cases of drug-induced coma are caused by overdose with drugs that are used therapeutically for their action on the central nervous system (Cartlidge 1981). They are principally psychoactive compounds, such as the benzo-diazepines, phenothiazines, antidepressants, and narco-tics. Coma of this kind can be regarded as a Type A reaction. Rarely, coma may also arise in cases of self-poisoning with other groups of drugs, such as pro-pranolol (Helson and Duque 1978) or chlorothiazide (Rongraff 1959), the mechanisms involved being as yet unknown.

In opiate poisoning the pupils are markedly con-stricted, and a hand lens may be required to detect a preserved light reflex. It should be noted that opiates form the basis of many 'over-the-counter' cough sup-pressants (codeine, pholcodine, and dextromethor-phan) and of some antidiarrhoeal agents. Naloxone is a very effective and specific opiate receptor antagonist, and should be administered to all cases of known or suspected opiate overdose. Since its half-life is only 1–2 hours, however, frequently repeated doses or an intra-venous infusion may be required to reverse an opiate-induced coma (Blain and Lane 1983a).

Primary neurotoxic effects are generally dose-related, and are more likely to occur under circumstances in which drug elimination or metabolism is reduced. For example, cimetidine is excreted largely unchanged in the urine and its accumulation in renal failure may cause coma (McMillan et al. 1978). Lignocaine is predomi-nantly metabolised by the liver, and coma has followed administration of a standard dose of this drug to a patient with liver failure (Selden and Sasahara 1967).

Considerable attention has been paid to the various neurotoxic effects of cyclosporin. Early reports linking this drug to the development of seizures, coma, encepha-lopathy, paresis, involuntary movements, and visual im-pairment were frequently obscured by additional drug-related and metabolic factors in bone marrow and organ transplant recipients, but the development of encepha-lopathy in cardiac transplant recipients, in whom such factors were not pertinent, has clearly demonstrated the drug's neurotoxic effects (Lane et al. 1988). The mechan-ism is controversial. Neurotoxicity is not clearly related to plasma concentrations of the whole drug, and cyclo-

sporin metabolites (Kunzendorf et al. 1988) and even the drug's solvent (Hoefnagels et al. 1988) have been impli-cated. It is likely that damage to the blood-brain barrier, possibly through effects on endothelial cells, is import-ant in pathogenesis (Lane et al. 1988; Zaal et al. 1988).

Heavy-metal poisoning from industrial or environ-mental exposure to lead or mercury may also cause encephalopathy and coma. Bismuth-containing com-pounds such as the peptic ulcer-healing drug bismuth chelate (tripotassium dicitratobismuthate, De-Nol) may be neurotoxic in the face of reduced renal function (Playford et al. 1990). Elimination of the drug shows complex kinetics due to storage and variable release rates from different tissues. Bismuth encephalopathy has occurred in epidemics in France. The clinical picture included a prodromal phase with changes in memory and behaviour, unsteadiness, cramps, and myalgia fol-lowed by the abrupt development of altered conscious-ness, myoclonus, and ataxia (Slikkerveer and de Wolff 1989). A 68-year-old man with a low creatinine clearance who took twice the recommended dose of bismuth che-late daily for 2 months (equivalent to 864 mg bismuth per day), developed global cerebral dysfunction with halluci-nations, ataxia, and an abnormal EEG. Whole blood bismuth concentration was 864 μg per litre but fell to 46 μg per litre 50 days after stopping the drug and giving treatment with dimercaprol. His mental function also recovered (Playford et al. 1990). Organic arsenicals, such as melarsoprol, can also cause severe encephalopathy with seizures and coma (Pialoux et al. 1988).

The encephalopathic effects of certain cytotoxic drugs have been increasingly appreciated. Cisplatin can, rarely, cause encephalopathy, seizures, and visual disturbances (Hitchins and Thomson 1988), while ifosfamide may cause a dose-related syndrome of mental dysfunction, ataxia, and seizures with encephalographic evidence of cortical abnormality, probably through its principal metabolite, chloroacetaldehyde (Goren et al. 1986). A 22-year-old man developed a severe encephalopathy, grand mal seizures, and visual disturbance after combi-nation therapy with cisplatin, vinblastine, and bleo-mycin for metastatic testicular carcinoma. This resolved over several months and was ascribed to the cisplatin combination therapy (Hitchins and Thomson 1988). Coma, unassociated with convulsions, may also occur following vincristine therapy (Whittaker et al. 1973). Antiviral agents may also rarely be encephalopathic: a 24-year-old man with disseminated herpes zoster devel-oped an encephalopathy and an 'immobilizing' myo-clonus after 7 days of vidarabine treatment (Vilter 1986).

Anticonvulsants also have encephalopathic potential and this, again, is generally dose-related. The incidence of such complications has declined significantly with the development of plasma concentration monitoring (Chadwick 1981). Phenytoin toxicity may develop as a result of interaction with drugs that impair its metabolism, such as oral contraceptives, chloramphenicol, and dicoumarol; or that compete for plasma protein binding sites, such as valproate (Bruni *et al.* 1980). Coma associated with valproate poisoning may be associated with gross cerebral oedema (Hintze *et al.* 1987), and the GABA agonist vigabatrin (Reynolds 1990) appears to have a propensity for causing disturbances in mood and behaviour in certain patients (Sander and Hart 1990), especially those with long-standing unstable epilepsy and pre-existing neuropsychiatric abnormalities (Ring and Reynolds 1990; Dam 1990; Robinson *et al.* 1990).

Metabolic disturbances

Coma secondary to metabolic disturbances can be caused by drugs, such as insulin and the oral hypoglycaemic drugs in therapeutic doses. Coma may be preceded by seizures in such cases, and hypoglycaemic coma due to sulphonylureas and biguanides is notoriously difficult to reverse, even with glucagon. The incidence of permanent cerebral damage in such cases is high. Coma related to drug-induced hepatic or renal damage is clinically similar to that occurring in hepatic or renal failure from other causes. Hyperreflexia and extensor plantar responses are common, as are rolling eye movements, in contrast to the paralysis of eye movements in coma directly due to drugs.

Finally, it is important to bear in mind that drugs affecting neurotransmitters can have potent effects when an underlying neurodegenerative disease is present. For example, anticholinergic drugs used in Parkinson's disease can exacerbate cholinergic deficit, producing a clinical picture of dementia (Kurlan and Como 1988).

Stroke

Cerebral venous thrombosis (Atkinson *et al.* 1970) and thrombotic strokes (Vessey 1973) have been described in patients taking oral contraceptives (Bickerstaff 1975). Retrospective studies by Vessey and Doll (1969) have shown that the absolute risk to the individual woman is small. Inman and Vessey (1968) provided data suggesting that of every million women using oral contraceptives, about 100 would be admitted to hospital and about 5 will die each year from thrombotic stroke attributable to these agents. Inman and others (1970) have suggested that the risk of thrombotic stroke is related to the oestrogen content of the oral contraceptive preparation and that low-dose preparations should be used when possible, but there is also evidence to suggest that the progestogen component of the contraceptive pill may play a part in some types of thromboembolic disease (Meade *et al.* 1980). Irey and others (1978) described the pathological findings in three young women who developed strokes while taking oral contraceptives and died. All three had thrombosis of major intracranial arteries with areas of focal intimal thickening, the latter presumably produced by the exogenous steroids. Evidence has also accumulated to implicate oral contraceptives in subarachnoid haemorrhage, particularly in women who smoke (RCGP 1977; Petitti and Wingerd 1978). Oral contraceptives are a cause of hypertension (Weir *et al.* 1971), which may predispose to strokes in some women. It is important to ensure that women who are at risk because of a history of thromboembolic disorders, hypertension, or migraine do not use oral contraceptives (Bickerstaff 1975).

The use of other drugs has also been associated with thrombosis of cerebral vessels. Six hours after intranasal use of cocaine, a man developed an acute infarction of the left putamen and caudate nucleus (Meza *et al.* 1989). After smoking 'crack' a 27-year-old man had a thrombosis of the right middle cerebral artery, which was felt to be due to vasospasm from the sympathomimetic action of cocaine (Golbe and Merkin 1986). A 34-year-old bodybuilder who had been taking various anabolic steroids for over 4 years developed an acute right hemiparesis and speech difficulties. He also had a simple partial seizure, and an EEG showed abnormal slow activity consistent with a left hemisphere lesion. He made a slow recovery with residual weakness of the right upper limb. The authors suggest that there is an increased risk of stroke with the illicit use of anabolic steroids (Frankle *et al.* 1988).

A 27-year-old man developed an intracerebral haemorrhage with cerebral vasculitis after a suicidal ingestion of decongestant tablets containing phenylpropanolamine (Maertens *et al.* 1987) and two young patients who developed strokes whilst taking phenylpropanolamine have been reported (Johnson *et al.* 1983).

Other drugs that may induce hypertension and so predispose to cerebral vascular accidents are discussed in Chapter 7.

Seizures

Drugs may precipitate seizures in epileptics, those with a low seizure threshold due to cerebral or systemic disease, or in apparently healthy people (although they often have a family history of epilepsy). Many drugs have been implicated (Chadwick 1981), but for most the association is probably circumstantial. It is not surprising that those drugs that easily cross the blood–brain barrier and enter the central nervous system are most commonly associated with convulsions; given intrathecally, they can also produce seizures (Wray *et al.* 1978; Chadwick 1981). The actual incidence of drug-induced seizures, however, is low. In a series of 12 617 medical inpatients, seizures attributed to drugs occurred in 17 (0.13 per cent) (BCDSP 1972). In this study, the occurrence of seizures was greatest in patients receiving intravenous penicillin (4 of 1245 patients), insulin (3 of 763 patients, all of whom were hypoglycaemic), and infusions of lignocaine for cardiac arrhythmias (2 of 349 patients).

Antibiotics, notably the synthetic penicillins and including oxacillin and carbenicillin (Whelton *et al.* 1971) have been associated with seizures: invariably the doses were high, or the patients had evidence of renal failure, or the drugs had been given intrathecally. Stupor and generalized myoclonus occurred following administration of ticarcillin (Kallay *et al.* 1979), a semi-synthetic penicillin, and the quinolone ciprofloxacin (*Drug Intelligence and Clinical Pharmacy* 1990) to patients with chronic renal failure. Ampicillin has also been reported to facilitate seizure activity (Serdaru *et al.* 1982).

Phenothiazines, most particularly chlorpromazine, prochlorperazine, and promazine, have been reported to cause seizures in non-epileptics (Jarvik 1970). Phenothiazines with a piperazine side chain (e.g. fluphenazine and trifluoperazine) may be less likely to induce seizures than those with an aliphatic side-chain (e.g. chlorpromazine). Tricyclic antidepressants, particularly imipramine and amitriptyline (Betts *et al.* 1968; Houghton 1971), may cause or precipitate seizures and should be used cautiously in epileptics. The subject of seizures in patients taking antidepressants (excluding monoamine oxidase inhibitors) was reviewed by Trimble (1978), who regarded maprotiline, together with flupenthixol and nomifensine, as least likely to increase fit frequency in known epileptic patients. This opinion was, however, based largely on experimental data, and an epidemiological study of reports to the Committee on Safety of Medicines of convulsions in patients taking antidepressants suggested that maprotiline is strongly epileptogenic and should be avoided in known epileptics (Edwards 1979). A recent study has suggested that the serotoninergic antidepressants, such as zimeldine and fluoxetine may be less epileptogenic than tricyclic compounds, and the highly selective serotonin re-uptake blocker fluvoxamine appears almost devoid of this property, a useful consideration in the management of chronic epilepsy when there is a significant prevalence of depression (Harmant *et al.* 1990)

Reports of anaesthetic agents causing seizures are infrequent, but ether, halothane (Smith *et al.* 1966), methohexitone, propanidid (Barron 1974), ketamine (Thompson 1972), and the steroid anaesthetic agent Althesin (alphaxolone and alphadolone) (Evans and Keogh 1977) have been implicated (though the latter is sometimes used in the management of status epilepticus). High plasma concentrations of local anaesthetics, such as mepivacaine or lignocaine, can cause signs of cerebral irritation and convulsions (Arthur *et al.* 1988), and toxic plasma concentrations of lignocaine, given as an antiarrhythmic drug, can be inadvertently achieved with therapeutic infusions in patients with cardiac failure, since there is often a decreased apparent volume of distribution of the drug in such patients. Rapid intravenous injection of lignocaine or theophylline may produce convulsions, most commonly in patients with liver disease.

Induction of hepatic drug-metabolizing enzymes increases the risk of convulsions caused by pethidine, because of the increased plasma concentrations of norpethidine. The mechanism by which the interaction of pethidine and monoamine oxidase inhibitors produces convulsions and hyperthermia is, however, not known. Disopyramide has been reported to cause seizures occasionally, and the β-adrenoceptor antagonist atenolol has been reported to precipitate seizures (Russell *et al.* 1979). Major seizures and coma have occurred in children with leukaemia treated with vincristine (Martin and Mainwaring 1973) and with pyrimethamine (Ragab 1973). Antituberculous treatment with cycloserine and isoniazid (Weinstein 1970) can be associated with seizures. Slow acetylators of isoniazid may be at a greater risk. The mechanism is possibly related to cerebral pyridoxine deficiency (Evans *et al.* 1960). Fraser and Harrower (1977) described one healthy patient who developed seizures and hyperglycaemia on therapeutic doses of nalidixic acid. Generalized seizures occurred in a breast-fed infant after its mother had taken indomethacin (Eeg-Olofsson *et al.* 1978) and mefenamic acid also appears to have epileptogenic potential (Prescott *et al.* 1981).

Seizures have been reported after the use of intravenous contrast media. Patients who are well hydrated and nursed with the head raised after the investigation are less likely to develop cerebral irritation from metrizamide (Chadwick 1981). Inhibition of cerebral hexokinase activity has been suggested as the mechanism by which seizures are induced by this agent (Bertoni *et al.* 1981). The probability of seizures being induced by contrast media appears to be greater in the presence of structural brain lesions, such as a glioma or metastases

(Onda *et al.* 1987). A non-convulsive state, presenting as lethargy and aphasia, has recently been reported following cerebral angiography with iothalamate (Vickrey and Bahls 1989). Diazepam withdrawal as a cause of seizures was stressed by Vyas and Carney (1975) because of the ubiquitous use of the drug. Withdrawal of other benzodiazepines carries the same risk (Ashton 1986). Other drugs of habituation, such as alcohol or the barbiturates, are associated with an increased risk of seizures following sudden withdrawal.

Abrupt cessation of baclofen therapy has been associated with various forms of seizure activity (Terrance and Fromm 1981; Barker and Grant 1982). Lithium therapy may be complicated by seizures (Demers *et al.* 1970), usually in patients with poor renal function. Accumulation in renal failure may also cause convulsions during treatment with nalidixic acid, cimetidine, or a cephalosporin. Overhydration from intravenous fluid therapy or water intoxication induced by oxytocin or carbamazepine may result in seizures. Rapid intravenous injection of Factor VIII has induced seizures (Small *et al.* 1983). Chloroquine preparations used for malarial prophylaxis have been reported to precipitate seizures. Both chloroquine and pyrimethamine are known to cause convulsions in high doses. Chloroquine inhibits glutamate dehydrogenase activity, reducing the production of the inhibitory neurotransmitter γ-aminobutyric acid. Women with low seizure thresholds appear particularly vulnerable to this adverse reaction (Fish and Espir 1988). Finally, excessive doses of known cerebral irritants, such as the respiratory stimulant doxapram, may also produce seizures, and high doses of terbutaline may cause cerebral irritation and seizure activity (Friedman *et al.* 1982).

Headache

Intracranial vascular causes

Drug-induced headaches most commonly result from the stretching of pain-sensitive cerebral blood vessel walls by vasodilatation or vasoconstriction, or by chemical irritation of the meninges. Vasodilator drugs that are most frequently implicated include amyl nitrite, glyceryl trinitrate, hydralazine, nifedipine, perhexilene, theophylline, and terbutaline. Headaches following administration of intravenous oestrogens and carmustine are associated with flushing, suggesting that they too may result from vasodilatation.

Prolonged drug use

Headache is sometimes a paradoxical complication of prolonged use of analgesics and antimigraine drugs;

ergotamine and other ergoline derivatives are particularly troublesome. Headache is an early neurological manifestation of ergotism, although the incidence of the more dramatic manifestations this condition in the migraine population appears to be very low (Hudgson and Hart 1964).

Drug withdrawal

Acute withdrawal of vasodilator drugs such as the ergots, methysergide, amphetamines, caffeine, alcohol (Lancer 1973), or the administration of vasoconstrictors such as bromocriptine and dopamine, may also cause headache.

Hypertension

Headache rarely results from hypertension but is a feature of the hypertensive crises induced by monoamine oxidase inhibitors taken in combination with sympathetic agonists such as amphetamines, ephedrine, tricyclic antidepressants, or foods containing tyramine (see Chapter 7). The combination of amitriptyline, metoclopramide, and levodopa plus carbidopa (Sinemet) produced hypertension and headache in a patient with Parkinson's disease (Rampton 1977). Administration or sudden withdrawal of clonidine or propranolol may precipitate headache, as may that of labetalol, although the incidence of headache with this drug decreases with continuing use, suggesting the development of tolerance (Bayne *et al.* 1980).

Intracranial fluid changes

Headache may result from changes in intravascular or extravascular fluid volume in the intracranial compartment, and develop after the administration of osmotic agents such as glycerol. This explanation has also been given for the development of headaches at the start of treatment with a variety of the non-steroidal anti-inflammatory analgesics (NSAID), notably indomethacin, which cause salt and water retention.

Aseptic meningitis

Apart from their ability to cause headache by intracranial volume changes, NSAID can do so by inducing a typical aseptic meningitis, with polymorphonuclear pleocytosis, raised protein, and low sugar in the CSF. Early reports of this complication with sulindac (Ballas and Donta 1982), tolmetin (Ruppert and Barth 1981), and ibuprofen (Giansiracusa *et al.* 1980) occurred in patients with lupus erythematosus, and were also reported following treatment with co-trimoxazole in such a patient (Kremer *et al.* 1983). More recently, an aseptic meningitis has been reported in otherwise healthy patients following the use of naproxen (Sylvia *et al.* 1988), and recurrent cases have been induced by ibuprofen therapy (Mifsud 1988; Chez *et al.* 1989). The latter authors reported increased intrathecal IgG synthesis in such cases, consistent with an antigen-specific immune response to the agent in the CNS.

Benign intracranial hypertension (BIH, pseudotumour cerebri)

BIH comprises headache associated with papilloedema and sometimes complicated by diplopia due to sixth nerve paresis, visual blurring, and visual field defects, due to cerebral oedema. Drugs that give rise to the syndrome include tetracyclines (*British Medical Journal* 1970; Pearson *et al.* 1981), nalidixic acid (Gedroyc and Shorvon 1982; Kilpatrick and Ebeling 1982), corticosteroids, both oral and topical (Neville and Wilson 1970; Hosking and Elliston 1978), nitrofurantoin (Sharma and James 1974), and the anaesthetic agents ketamine and nitrous oxide. Excess as well as a deficiency of vitamin A, and the use of etretinate (Bonnetblanc *et al.* 1983), may also be associated with the development of benign intracranial hypertension. Severe headache and papilloedema occurred in three patients treated with perhexilene maleate (Stephens *et al.* 1978). Cerebrospinal fluid pressures were not measured, but the results of other investigations suggested the diagnosis. BIH was recently reported to follow therapy with the gonadotrophin analogue lucoprotein acetate (Arber *et al.* 1990).

Davidson (1971), reviewing the ocular complications of oral contraceptives, described six patients with papilloedema, two of whom were diagnosed as cases of benign intracranial hypertension. Whether this can be attributed to the oral contraceptives is not certain, for benign intracranial hypertension may occur spontaneously in young, often obese, women. Bickerstaff (1975) pointed out, however, that Davidson's affected patients were all slim. Again, the mechanism by which the drugs produce intracranial hypertension may involve salt and water retention and intracranial fluid redistribution. It is of interest that many cases occur at the beginning or end of drug therapy.

Extrapyramidal system

Although disorders of this system are usually referred to as drug-induced extrapyramidal syndromes, other neuronal systems in the brain stem and spinal cord are probably involved. Patients may have symptoms and signs similar to those of idiopathic Parkinson's disease or may show involuntary movements now recognized to be

TABLE 18.1
Some of the drugs associated with extrapyramidal syndromes

Antimalarials	*Thioxanthines*
e.g. Amodiaquine	e.g. Chlorprothixene
Chloroquine	Thiothixene
Butyrophenones	*Tricyclic antidepressants*
e.g. Droperidol	e.g. Amitriptyline
Haloperidol	Desipramine
Trifluoperidol	Imipramine
	Miscellaneous
	e.g. Diazoxide
Phenothiazines	Diphenhydramine
e.g. Chlorpromazine	Levodopa
Fluphenazine	Lithium
Perphenazine	Methyldopa
Prochlorperazine	Metoclopramide
Promazine	Reserpine
Thioridazine	Tetrabenazine
Trifluoperazine	

characteristic effects of neuroleptic agents and some other drugs (Table 18.1). Several attempts have been made to classify the motor disorders (Duvoisin 1968) and a division into reversible and irreversible groups has been suggested (Lader 1970).

Drug-induced parkinsonism

This is probably the most common drug-induced disorder of involuntary movement. Clinically it resembles classical paralysis agitans except that resting tremor is less prominent. Many drugs have been implicated, most frequently those antipsychotic groups that antagonize dopaminergic neurotransmission. The clinical severity is variable and, paradoxically, patients suffering from naturally occurring Parkinson's disease do not appear to have increased sensitivity to these drugs (Dukes 1980). A 74-year-old man with parkinsonism developed progressive cognitive and behavioural dysfunction suggestive of Alzheimer's disease but which resolved on withdrawal of his anticholinergic antiparkinsonian drugs (Kurlan and Como 1988).

Almost all the phenothiazines have been associated with the production of parkinsonism, which has also been induced by the butyrophenones (e.g. haloperidol), reserpine, methyldopa (Rosenblum and Montgomery 1980), lithium, metoclopramide (Indo and Ando 1982), the tricyclic antidepressants, and tetrabenazine. A reversible parkinsonism has been reported in an elderly woman taking perhexilene maleate (Gordon and Gordon 1981).

Reduction of the dose of the drug usually produces a remission of symptoms and signs, although the administration of an anticholinergic drug can produce a rapid reversal of signs in acute severe drug-induced parkinsonism. There is no indication for concomitant prophylactic anticholinergic therapy in the treatment of affective psychosis, since there is strong evidence that this predisposes the patient to the development of an irreversible tardive dyskinesia; neither should levodopa be given, since it frequently aggravates the underlying psychotic condition. Parkinsonism, associated with an irreversible orofacial dyskinesia, has been reported in a patient taking amoxapine (Lapierre and Anderson 1983). Sulpiride, a selective D_2-receptor antagonist with antipsychotic and antidepressant properties, has been reported to induce parkinsonism and a persistent segmental dystonia 2 months after starting the drug (Miller and Jankovic 1990), but in general this drug seems to be less prone than others to produce this adverse effect.

The development of parkinsonism following exposure to a variety of neurotoxins has provided valuable insights into the pathogenesis of the idiopathic disorder. A severe parkinsonian syndrome developed in a 46-year-old man poisoned by cyanide. Magnetic resonance imaging (MRI) showed multiple areas of low signal intensity in the globus palidus and posterior putamen confirming the functional impairment of dopaminergic nigrostriatal neurones (Rosenberg et al. 1989). Chronic manganese poisoning may cause a complex of symptoms and signs similar to those found in idiopathic Parkinson's disease and accompanied by similar neuropathological findings (Yamada et al. 1986).

The illicit synthesis and use of 'designer' drugs containing the contaminant 1-methyl-4-phenyl-1,2,5,6-tetrahydro-pyridine (MPTP) has been associated with the rapid development of extrapyramidal dysfunction. The administration of MPTP to man and animals results in the appearance of a parkinsonian syndrome, closely related to idiopathic Parkinson's disease. MPTP interacts with the A and B forms of MAO but its main inhibitory effect results in an irreversible inhibition of MAO-B. The neurotoxicity of MPTP has been attributed to the formation of MPP+ from MPTP by MAO-B and the subsequent effects of MPP+ on mitochondrial respiration (Dostert and Strolin-Benedetti 1988). Parkinsonism induced by MPTP has been described as 'time-telescoped' Parkinson's disease and it is currently used as an animal model of the disease. MPP+ has been shown to be concentrated in neurones with a catecholamine uptake mechanism and this may explain the vulnerability of nigrostriatal dopaminergic neurones (Kopin and Markey 1988). The induction of an extrapyramidal syndrome by an exogenous chemical has given rise to speculation about the role of other environmental agents, such as pesticides, in the aetiology of chronic degenerative neurological diseases.

Akathisia

Akathisia is defined as involuntary continuous motor restlessness. The patient has a subjective desire to move about, pace the floor, alternately sit and stand, and stamp his feet. When the restlessness is confined to the feet it is termed tasikinesia. Although most commonly associated with levodopa therapy, it has apparently followed oxazepam withdrawal (Mendelsohn 1978) and can occur with the phenothiazines, butyrophenones (Weiner and Luby 1983), and amoxapine (Ross et al. 1983).

Acute dystonias

These dramatic and often alarming movement disorders are relatively common, particularly in children and young adults. The onset can be abrupt and may be mistaken for hysteria or even tetany. The muscles of the head and neck are mainly affected, with involuntary movement and spasm of the tongue, trismus, and facial grimacing and other orofacial dyskinesias. Oculogyric crises, torticollis and retrocollis, opisthotonus, axial dystonias, and a bizarre gait can occur, often accompanied by writhing movements of the limbs. The attacks are episodic and, although frightening to witness or experience, are usually painless. Between each episode muscle tone is normal, and during a subsequent attack different muscle groups may be affected.

Many of the antipsychotic drugs, such as the phenothiazines and butyrophenones, have been associated with acute dystonic reactions in the young. Other drugs include metoclopramide, tricyclic antidepressants, phenytoin (Chadwick et al. 1976), and carbamazepine (Joyce and Gunderson 1980), and propranolol in high dosage (Crawford 1977). Spasmodic torticollis occurred in a patient treated with chlorzoxazone for back pain (Rosin 1981).

The mechanism of action in dystonias may relate to an increased release of dopamine and subsequent receptor hypersensitivity as the plasma concentration of the drug declines. Usually the dystonia remits once the drug is withdrawn. Intravenous benztropine or diazepam are useful in severe cases. Administration of another antipsychotic drug can sometimes be used to treat a severe dystonia.

The incidence of these reactions depends upon the patient population studied. The Boston Collaborative Drug Surveillance Program (BCDSP 1973) reported drug-induced extrapyramidal symptoms in 18 (0.9 per cent) of 2049 patients. These were all inpatients, mainly on short-term treatment, only one of them having been under treatment with one of the offending drugs at the time of admission. The drugs involved were phenothiazines (in 15 out of 18 patients, trifluoperazine in 14 cases), butyrophenones, and tricyclic antidepressants. In all cases the symptoms disappeared when the drug was withdrawn. On the other hand, Ayd (1961) reported an overall incidence of approximately 39 per cent (with about 15 per cent drug-induced pseudoparkinsonism, 21 per cent akathisia, and 2.3 per cent acute dystonic reactions) in 3775 patients with major psychoses under treatment with phenothiazines. Obviously the epidemiology of this disorder warrants further study. About 2.5 per cent of a group patients treated with neuroleptic drugs develop acute dystonia within 48 hours of starting treatment (Rupniak *et al.* 1986).

Forty-seven railroad workers who were exposed to polychlorinated phenols, including the dioxin TCDD, while cleaning up a chemical spillage, were followed for over 6 years. There was a suggestion of an increase in action dystonias and postural intention tremor in a significant number of patients (Klawans 1987) although such an association has not been subsequently confirmed.

Chorea

Chorea usually presents as irregular, jerking, involuntary movements of the limbs. Often the slow writhing movements of athetosis or a dystonia are superimposed. The patient frequently attempts to disguise the movement by converting it into some reasonable action. There have been several reports of chorea occurring in patients taking the oral contraceptive pill (Riddoch *et al.* 1971; Bickerstaff 1975). This resolves within a couple of months of stopping the drug. Anabolic steroids (oxymethalone) have also been implicated (Tilzey *et al.* 1981). The most frequent association has been with the antipsychotic drugs and the anticonvulsants (especially phenytoin [Chadwick *et al.* 1976]). Choreoathetosis has been described in two patients intoxicated with phenytoin, with improvement after reduction of the dose (McLellan and Swash 1974). Long-term therapy with benzhexol caused choreiform movements that ceased on withdrawal and returned on direct challenge with the drug (Warne and Gubbay 1979). Amphetamines (Lundh and Tunving 1981), methadone (Wasserman and Yahr 1980), methylphenidate, amoxapine (Patterson 1983),

and cimetidine (Kushner 1982) are also reputed to produce chorea.

Nine days after acute poisoning with carbon monoxide a 24-year-old man developed choreoathetosis in the upper limbs and face. There were also memory disturbances that cleared within 6 months. A computed tomographic (CT) scan and nuclear magnetic resonance (NMR) showed symmetrical bilateral lesions in the globus pallidus (Meucci *et al.* 1989). Pemoline, an indirectly acting sympathomimetic drug with actions similar to amphetamine, has been reported to cause a choreoathetosis. A 49-year-old man developed a severe choreoathetosis with rhabdomyolysis and myoglobinuria after an increase in his dose of pemoline. This resolved after 48 hours (Briscoe *et al.* 1988).

Tremor

The problem of drug-induced tremor has been reviewed by Lane (1984). A large number of drugs can exacerbate physiological (postural) tremor, increasing both its frequency and amplitude. These include the tricyclic antidepressants, anticonvulsants (including sodium valproate), lithium, amiodarone, cimetidine (Bateman et al. 1981), and caffeine. Withdrawal of alcohol or benzodiazepines will also produce an increase in postural tremor. Paradoxically, both alcohol and primidone are effective in the treatment of benign (familial) essential tremor (Chakrabati and Pearace 1981).

Resting tremor is rarely drug-induced, and is not a notable feature of parkinsonism, but it has been reported with amiodarone (Lustman and Moncou 1974). Action tremors may be seen as part of drug-induced postural tremor and are particularly a feature of lithium and valproate toxicity. Frank cerebellar signs, including tremor, may occur in phenytoin toxicity.

Anticonvulsants at toxic plasma concentrations may produce asterixis and myoclonus (Chadwick *et al.* 1976). Myoclonus has also been reported in a patient with renal disease taking metoclopramide (Hyser and Drake 1983).

Gilles de la Tourette syndrome

This rare, enigmatic syndrome has occurred after haloperidol withdrawal in a child with a congenital encephalopathy (Singer 1981). Paradoxically, it has also occurred in four children treated with the central nervous system stimulants dextroamphetamine, methylphenidate, or pemoline for hyperactivity (Lowe *et al.* 1982).

Tardive dyskinesia

This condition is most frequently seen in psychiatric

hospitals in chronically ill patients treated with neuroleptic drugs. The extrapyramidal adverse effects of the neuroleptics include parkinsonism, dystonia, and akathisia (Stephen and Williamson 1984; Shaleve *et al.* 1987; Hardie and Lees 1988), but these develop early in treatment and are mitigated by the concurrent administration of anticholinergic antiparkinsonian drugs. The condition of tardive dyskinesia develops much later in treatment, particularly after high doses of the drugs; it is estimated to occur in 10–20 per cent of those patients treated with neuroleptic drugs for more than one year.

A tardive dyskinesia is characterized by abnormal involuntary movements that most frequently start in the face with repetitive blinking and abnormal movements of the lips and tongue, but often extend to include a torticollis and choreoathetoid movements of the limbs and trunk. The only effective treatment is withdrawal of the neuroleptic drug, when an initial exacerbation is usually followed by gradual improvement over several months (Task Force 1980). Lesser measures, such as dose reduction or a change of drug, may be all that are possible in chronically psychotic patients. Antiparkinsonian drugs are believed to aggravate the condition and should therefore also be discontinued (Barnes 1988). Tardive dyskinesia is best prevented from developing by using the minimum effective doses of neuroleptics for the shortest possible time in the treatment of those conditions for which there are no alternative treatments.

The condition has long been regarded as due to a dopamine-receptor hypersensitivity. There is recent evidence that reduced γ-aminobutyric acid (GABA) activity in striatal neurones may contribute to its development (Gerlach and Casey 1988). Tardive dyskinesia has been more extensively reviewed in articles by Barnes (1988) and the American Psychiatric Association (Task Force 1980).

Neuroleptic malignant syndrome (NMS)

This important and possibly under-diagnosed condition has been extensively reviewed (*The Lancet* 1984; Gibb and Lees 1985; Kellam 1987). The essential clinical features of the syndrome are extrapyramidal rigidity, altered consciousness, and autonomic dysfunction with pyrexia, profuse sweating, tachycardia, and labile blood pressure. The serum creatine kinase (CK) is typically raised and a leucocytosis and abnormal liver function tests are often found. Patients rapidly become dehydrated with associated abnormalities in plasma electrolytes and, if untreated, progress to coma, often with seizures, and death in 20–30 per cent of cases, usually from hypoventilation or aspiration pneumonia. Myo-

necrosis and myoglobinaemic renal failure, hepatic necrosis, and cardiovascular failure may also develop.

The condition appears to result from a sudden reduction in central dopaminergic function in the striatum and hypothalamus (Henderson and Wooton 1981; Burke *et al.* 1981) usually related to treatment with dopamine-receptor blocking drugs such as haloperidol, fluphenazine, chlorpromazine, thiothixene, thioridazine, trimeprazine, trifluoroperazine, and prochlorperazine, and most commonly occurs in patients with presumed pre-existing central neurotransmitter dysfunction, including schizophrenia and other psychotic states, for which the neuroleptic medication is being prescribed. The condition has also, however, been described in many other non-psychotic conditions in relation to neuroleptic medication, including preoperative sedation (Moyes 1973; Konikoff *et al.* 1984). The condition is also well described following abrupt reduction or withdrawal of the dopamine agonists levodopa and bromocriptine in Parkinson's disease, particularly in association with 'drug holidays', and with tetrabenazine and α-methyl-*p*-tyrosine, which deplete dopamine stores, in Huntington's chorea (Burke *et al.* 1981). It may occur with drug combinations that reduce dopamine receptor activity, such as dothiepin and phenelzine (Ritchie 1983) and amitriptyline and thioridazine (Eiser *et al.* 1982); and antipsychotic–anticholinergic combinations, the latter impairing the peripheral heat loss mechanisms (Gibb and Lees 1985).

Lithium has been reported to provoke NMS in patients taking neuroleptic drugs, such as haloperidol (Loudon and Waring 1976; Goekoop and Carbaat 1982), and following its use in the management of off-period dystonia in Parkinson's disease (Pfeiffer and Sucha 1985; Koehler and Mirandolle 1988). NMS has rarely been reported in relation to isolated therapy with a tricyclic antidepressant (Grant 1984). It is also clear that relatively mild forms of NMS can occur under similar clinical circumstances and that the diagnosis may be missed (Clarke *et al.* 1988; Mezaki *et al.* 1989; Domingo *et al.* 1989). Neuroleptics can produce a 'forme fruste' of NMS through their ability to interfere with central hypothalamic dopamine pathways and peripheral cholinergic and α-adrenergic thermoregulatory mechanisms. They also cause the release of calcium (Ca^{2+}) from the sarcoplasmic reticulum, and raise serum creatine kinase levels (Meltzer and Moline 1970; Anderson 1972).

There is a considerable degree of overlap between the clinical characteristics of NMS and the syndromes of acute lethal catatonia and malignant hyperthermia (MH).

Lethal catatonia is characterized by catatonia or stupor with waxy flexibility, occurring spontaneously in schizophrenia and other psychoses following a period of intensive agitation and hyperactivity. The typical extra-pyramidal rigidity of NMS is not generally seen and the pyrexia tends to be a late phenomenon. It has been suggested that NMS is an iatrogenic form of lethal catatonia with the addition of the extrapyramidal effects of neuroleptic medication or underlying basal ganglia disease (Kellam 1987). Acute lethal catatonia has become rare since the introduction of electroconvulsive therapy (ECT) and the various neuroleptic drugs.

Malignant hyperthermia (MH) shares with NMS the features of hyperpyrexia, its metabolic consequences, and muscular rigidity with release of CK and myoglobin, but is precipitated by anaesthetic agents (see below), and so the onset is generally more abrupt and the fever and increase in serum CK concentration more dramatic. The pathogenesis of MH appears to be distinct, in that the muscular rigidity of NMS is relieved by centrally acting drugs such as diazepam and lorazepam, and by pre-synaptic blockade with pancuronium and curare, all of which are ineffective in MH. Both, however, may be relieved by dantrolene, which prevents calcium release at the sarcoplasmic reticulum, indicating a common final pathway for the muscular signs and symptoms, including myonecrosis. Furthermore, MH is known to have a dominant pattern of inheritance and to recur following re-exposure to anaesthetics while NMS occurs sporadically and rarely, if ever, recurs. It is interesting to note that muscle taken from an NMS survivor showed abnormal contracture on exposure to halothane (but not to caffeine as would be expected in MH [Caroff et al. 1983]), and that pigs with the porcine stress syndrome (clinically similar to human MH) had low striatal dopamine levels (Hallberg et al. 1983). A recent study also found increased intracellular Ca^{2+} concentrations in NMS muscle fibres, as noted in patients with MH (Lopez et al. 1989).

Treatment of mild cases of NMS may require only supportive measures, removal of the neuroleptics, cooling, oxygen, intravenous hydration, and management of acidosis; but in most instances dantrolene sodium intravenously or orally, combined with bromocriptine orally, will be required and is generally rapidly effective (Gibb and Lees 1985). In refractory cases, intravenous benzodiazepines or even ECT may be required (Kellam 1987). This subject is also discussed in Chapter 28.

Levodopa-induced movement disorders

These are typically Type A reactions that remit when the dose is reduced or the drug withdrawn. Orthostatic hypotension and syncope are also Type A reactions to levodopa. Two particular adverse effects deserve further discussion.

The 'on–off' phenomenon

This is usually a result of long-term levodopa therapy. Several times a day the patient goes through a cycle of benefit from levodopa, but accompanied by involuntary movements ('on'), which suddenly changes to a state of akinesia and severe rigidity ('off') (Marsden et al. 1973). Although this phenomenon is dose-related it does not correspond to changes in blood concentrations of levodopa (Rosin et al. 1979). Smaller and more frequent doses of levodopa are often advocated to alleviate the condition and a change to bromocriptine is suggested (Fahn et al. 1979). Bromocriptine, however, may produce marked mental changes and, indeed, can cause alteration in dopamine receptor sensitivity. Price and colleagues (1978) suggested that the dopamine antagonist tiapride can alleviate levodopa-induced dyskinesias without the necessity of a reduction in levodopa dosage.

Akinesia paradoxica

This adverse effect can be very difficult to distinguish from parkinsonian bradykinesia (Ambani and van Woert 1973). In akinesia paradoxica the patient experiences a sudden sensation of extreme heaviness of both feet, trembling, and a tendency to fall forwards but an inability to start walking. There is no rigidity and, once walking starts, the gait is fairly normal. The phenomenon is dose-related and responds to a reduction in the dose of levodopa, unlike bradykinesia.

Other dyskinesias caused by levodopa

Oro-bucco-lingual-facial dyskinesias, which may progress to involve the trunk and limbs, can develop early in treatment with levodopa; fortunately they respond to a reduction in dose.

Neuropathies

Cranial neuropathies

The drugs that affect the functioning of the cranial nerves involved with vision and eye movements and with smell, taste, hearing, and balance, are discussed in greater detail in the relevant chapters on eye disorders (Chapter 19), and on ear, nose, and throat disorders (Chapter 20).

Visual evoked potentials (VEP) were studied in a patient who developed visual impairment during ethambutol treatment. The electroretinogram (ERG) and flash VEP were normal at the time of maximal visual loss, whereas pattern reversal VEP 2 and 5 months after the onset revealed evidence of severe bilateral optic nerve involvement, especially affecting macular fibres. Seven months after the onset, paramacular positive–negative–positive (PNP) complexes with a late positivity (scotomatous response) were recorded after pattern reversal and half-field stimulation, suggesting involvement of fibres subserving central vision. At a time when visual acuity was normal there was still electrophysiological evidence of a mild involvement of the anterior visual pathway. The papillomacular bundle seems to be especially involved in ethambutol eye toxicity (Petrera *et al.* 1988). Ethambutol-induced optic neuropathy may not always be reversible and two cases have been reported in which the toxic optic neuropathy was severe and irreversible despite prompt discontinuation of the drug (DeVita *et al.* 1987).

Visual and auditory neurotoxicity is reported in 42 out of 89 patients with transfusion-dependent anaemia receiving subcutaneous desferrioxamine. Seventy-one patients had abnormal visual evoked responses and 22 had abnormal audiograms with a high-frequency sensorineural deficit. The affected patients were younger, had lower serum ferritin levels, and were on higher doses of desferrioxamine (Freedman *et al.* 1988) than those unaffected.

Amiodarone has been implicated in the pathogenesis of optic neuropathy but the association has not been proven, although the incidence was significantly higher in patients treated with amiodarone than in an age-matched control group (Feiner *et al.* 1987). Lamellar inclusions were found in the large axons of the optic nerve from an asymptomatic subject and were interpreted as a drug-induced lipidosis (Mansour *et al.* 1988). Other reported neurotoxic effects of amiodarone include tremor, peripheral neuropathy, and ataxia. Some rarer effects include brainstem dysfunction with downbeat nystagmus, hemisensory loss and ataxia, dyskinesia, jaw tremor, and proximal myopathy. Electrophysiological examination showed a predominantly demyelinating peripheral neuropathy. These findings suggest that amiodarone neurotoxicity is not confined to the peripheral nervous system but also affects the central nervous system, including the basal ganglia and brain stem and their connections (Palakurthy *et al.* 1987). Amiodarone has been associated with mild visual loss secondary to a papilloedema and papillopathy. A patient developed bilateral toxic optic neuropathy 4 weeks after initiation of amiodarone therapy; 9 months later his vision was 20/50 in the right eye and 20/200 in the left (Nazarian and Jay 1988).

A 77-year-old man complained of 4 weeks of hearing loss and a progressive inability to walk. Previous treatment with a course of low-dose cytarabine was felt to be the cause of his acute cerebellar syndrome (Cersosimo *et al.* 1987).

Peripheral neuropathies

The pathological changes in a drug-induced peripheral neuropathy usually consist of axonal degeneration with secondary breakdown of the myelin sheath. Hypertrophy of Schwann cells occurs; the myelin debris undergoes phagocytosis; and eventually the axon regenerates along the existing basal laminal tubes of the Schwann cell. Neither the site of the damage nor its mechanism are known in most cases.

A rarer pathological process in drug-induced neuropathy is segmental demyelination. This is more variable, affecting some Schwann cells but not others, the axons remaining intact. The internodal myelin degenerates and undergoes phagocytosis, with baring of the axon. Remyelination follows from Schwann cell replication.

Most neuropathies may be of a mixed nature with one of the pathological processes dominating (Bradley and Thomas 1974). Patients with underlying systemic diseases such as diabetes mellitus, alcoholism, and various deficiency states have a lower threshold for the development of a drug-induced neuropathy. Drug accumulation can occur in patients with impaired renal or hepatic function and when drug-metabolising enzymes are inhibited by other drugs (e.g. cimetidine). About half the population of the United Kingdom (in other parts of the world the proportion may be different) have an increased risk of developing a neuropathy if given isoniazid because they are slow to metabolise the drug by acetylation. Genetically determined slow inactivation of the drug may result in prolonged high serum drug concentrations that potentiate neurotoxic effects. Isoniazid interferes with pyridoxine metabolism and this may also be the mechanism of action in ethionamide and, possibly, pencillamine neuropathies.

Vincristine and colchicine are specific in their action on axonal neurotubular transport mechanisms. In a case with a very high dose of cisplatin, serious derangement of central and peripheral neurones with muscle atrophy and effects on other organs was seen (Maeda *et al.* 1987). Chloramphenicol can produce a vitamin B_{12} deficiency; while nitrofurantoin, especially in renal or hepatic failure, inhibits oxidative decarboxylation of pyruvate. Perhexiline maleate (Heathfield and Carabott 1982) and amiodarone (Martinez-Arizala *et al.* 1983) are unique in producing a pure segmental demyelination. Possibly

TABLE 18.2
Clinical syndromes of drug-induced neuropathy

Paraesthesiae only	Sensorimotor neuropathy	Predominantly motor
Colistin	Amiodarone	Amitriptyline
Cyatarabine	Amitriptyline	Amphotericin
Methysergide	Carbutamide	Cimetidine
Nalidixic acid	Chlorambucil	Dapsone
Phenelzine	Chlorpropamide	Imipramine
Propranolol	Chloroquine	Sulphonamides
Streptomycin	Clioquinol	
Sulthiame	Clofibrate	*Localized*
	Colchicine	*neuropathy*
Sensory	Disopyramide	Amphetamines
neuropathy	Disulfiram	Amphotericin
Calcium carbimide	Ethambutol	Anticoagulants
Chloramphenicol	Glutethimide	Ethoglucid
Diamines	Gold	Mustine
Ergotamine	Hydralazine	Penicillin
Nitrofurazone	Indomethacin	
Procarbazine	Isoniazid	
Propylthiouracil	Methaqualone	
Sulfoxone	Methimazole	
Thiamphenicol	Metronidazole	
	Nitrofurantoin	
	Penicillamine	
	Perhexiline	
	Phenylbutazone	
	Phenytoin	
	Podophyllin	
	Streptomycin	
	Thalidomide	
	Tolbutamide	
	Vinblastine	
	Vincristine	

(Adapted from Argov and Mastaglia 1979)

their mechanism of action is through interference with glycolipid metabolism.

A summary of the drugs most commonly associated with a peripheral neuropathy and the predominant type of neuropathy produced is given in Table 18.2. It is probably more useful to consider the types of peripheral neuropathy produced and the drugs associated than simply to list the many drugs and their neurotoxic properties.

Mixed sensory and motor neuropathy

Sensory or sensorimotor distal polyneuropathy is probably the most commonly encountered drug-induced neuropathy. Patients present with the classical symptoms and signs of a mixed peripheral neuropathy. They complain of a symmetrical distal sensory loss, often more severe in the lower limbs and characterized by the classical 'glove and stocking' distribution. There may be painful dysaesthesiae and depressed tendon reflexes. This is the classical type of neuropathy associated with isoniazid and ethionamide. These drugs are structurally related and, as previously stated, isoniazid interferes with pyridoxine metabolism, causing an axonal neuropathy that resembles Wallerian degeneration (Ochoa 1970). If the drug is withdrawn at the early stage of the neuropathy, then symptoms and signs remit. The neuropathy is associated with doses of isoniazid in excess of 300 mg daily, and it is recommended that pyridoxine should be given concurrently with isoniazid when large doses are used or when the patient is malnourished and likely to be suffering from a vitamin deficiency (Biehl and Vilter 1954). Nitrofurantoin, commonly used in the treatment of urinary tract infections, has caused peripheral neuropathy, particularly in patients with chronic renal failure (Toole and Parrish 1973). Lindholm (1967) reported an incidence of peripheral neuropathy of 62 per cent in patients with normal renal function and, indeed, a subclinical neuropathy was induced in normal volunteers given 400 mg of nitrofurantoin daily for 2 weeks (Toole *et al.* 1968). Ethambutol can also cause a sensorimotor neuropathy in addition to an optic neuropathy. Thalidomide was an important cause of a predominantly sensory neuropathy, the patients complaining of a painful burning sensation in the extremities with cramping pains in the calves. The symptoms persisted in up to half the patients after drug withdrawal (*The Lancet* 1969). Follow-up of nine patients did not identify any reliable neurophysiological indicators of thalidomide-induced neuropathy, although a possible relationship with a slow acetylation polymorphism was suggested (Hess *et al.* 1986). A 67-year-old man developed a peripheral neuropathy with glove-and-stocking sensory disturbances after the administration of metronidazole for hepatic amoebiasis. The clinical picture appeared to be that of myeloneuropathy and a sural nerve biopsy showed severe loss of myelinated fibres, a low density of unmyelinated fibres, and axonal degeneration (Takeuchi *et al.* 1988).

The cytotoxic drugs mustine hydrochloride, procarbazine, vincristine, and vinblastine, cause a predominantly sensory polyneuropathy (Weiss *et al.* 1974*a,b*). Vincristine neuropathy commonly develops after 2 months of treatment and may be more likely to occur in patients with lymphoma. Loss of tendon reflexes is accompanied by severe pain in proximal muscles. Paraesthesiae, sometimes with a definite sensory loss, can develop. The neuropathy is axonal in type and usually improves spontaneously on withdrawal of the drug (*The*

Lancet 1973*a*). Some degree of sensorimotor neuropathy may occur in all patients on long-term treatment with this drug. When present, the motor weakness may be severe (Casey *et al*. 1973). A few patients also develop features of a painful proximal myopathy. Other neurological effects of cytotoxic drugs have been reviewed by Woodhouse and Blain (1983).

Over half of patients taking perhexiline maleate are found to have electrophysiological evidence of a neuropathy. A severe clinical neuropathy only develops after several months of treatment on daily doses of around 300 mg (Sebille 1978). In addition to dysaesthesiae and weakness, there may be evidence of cranial neuropathies, and a small number of patients develop intracranial hypertension. The neuropathy is slow to resolve following withdrawal of the drug and some degree of dysaesthesia may persist.

Patients on long-term phenytoin therapy (often 10 years or more) may develop a sensorimotor peripheral neuropathy (Lovelace and Horwitz 1968). These patients may have reduced vibration sense and depressed tendon reflexes, particularly if they have been on large doses of the drug (Dobkin 1977). A sural nerve biopsy from a 47-year-old man on chronic phenytoin therapy and with peripheral neuropathy showed loss of large myelinated nerve fibres and a non-random clustered distribution of segmental demyelination and remyelination and axonal shrinkage. Sixteen months after stopping the phenytoin, the patient had improved on clinical and electrophysiological examination (Ramirez *et al*. 1986). Irreversible cerebellar damage or an encephalopathy can also result from chronic phenytoin toxicity.

Chloroquine has been reported to cause a neuromyopathy, usually in patients taking 500 mg or more daily (Whisnant et al. 1963). A single case report has appeared of a neuropathy in a patient taking standard antimalarial therapy (Karstorp *et al*. 1973). A toxic myopathy and polyneuropathy may occur together with a cardiomyopathy (Estes *et al*. 1987). Rarely, a similar syndrome is caused by dapsone (Saqueton *et al*. 1969), disulfiram (Gardner-Thorpe and Benjamin 1971), and glutethimide (Haas and Marasigan 1968), the last drug being structurally related to thalidomide and also causing a cerebellar ataxia. Neuropathy is one of the most severe adverse effects of disulfiram. Frisoni and Di-Monda (1989) reviewed 37 cases of disulfiram neuropathy reported since 1971. There was no numerical sex prevalence, although the incidence was higher in women. Symptom onset latency was longer and the neurological deficits were milder below a dose threshold of 250 mg daily or less, suggesting that the disulfiram neuropathy was dose-dependent. In addition, chloral hydrate appeared to potentiate the neuropathy, but the mechanism is unknown. Digitalis toxicity may be associated with paraesthesiae or shooting pains in the arms, back, and legs (Batterman and Gutner 1948). Lely and Van Enter (1970) described adverse effects from digitoxin intoxication occurring accidentally in 179 patients of whom 2 per cent complained of vague pains in the calves and arms. No paraesthesiae or neuralgic pains were noted.

A 62-year-old woman positive for hepatitis B surface antigen and with cirrhosis of the liver presented with distal weakness and paraesthesiae during treatment with adenine arabinoside 5′-monophosphate. She recovered several weeks after the drug's withdrawal. Electrophysiological and histological investigations demonstrated axonal neuropathy. The dose was relatively low (120 mg per kg), and age and advanced liver disease may have contributed to the neurotoxicity (Kanterewicz *et al*. 1990). Twenty patients with AIDS or AIDS-related complex (ARC) received 2′,3′,dideoxycytidine in doses ranging from 0.03–0.25 mg per kg every 8 hours. Nine of the patients developed a mixed axonal neuropathy at between 9 and 12 weeks of treatment. The neuropathy was different from the slowly progressive painful neuropathy of AIDS since there was a sudden onset, motor involvement, and a temporal relationship to the drug (Dubinsky *et al*. 1989).

Almitrine dimesylate can induce a stereotypic sensory neuropathy associated with high plasma concentrations of the drug, but there is no evidence that these are due to slow oxidation of the parent compound (Belec *et al*. 1989). Almitrine is thought to cause a sensory neuropathy with sensory symptoms and signs confined to the distal parts of the lower limbs and involving large and small fibres with an axonal degeneration. Recovery is slow, taking 3 to 6 months after withdrawal of the drug (Bouche *et al*. 1989). A double-blind prospective study of the effects of almitrine dimesylate on peripheral nerve function in patients with chronic bronchitis confirmed that the drug may be associated with the development of a peripheral neuropathy with slow resolution (Allen and Prowse 1989). A longer follow-up of patients with clinical evidence of sensory peripheral neuropathy of the feet and lower legs found electrophysiological evidence of a distal axonopathy without denervation. The amplitudes of sensory potentials were reduced and conduction velocities were slightly decreased. On biopsy, mild neurogenic atrophy of muscles and a distal axonopathy were found, and light and electron microscopy confirmed axonal damage affecting myelinated fibres and to a lesser extent the unmyelinated fibres, and some degree of segmental demyelination (Gherardi *et al*. 1987). Clinical improvement was very slow and at 6–12 months many patients still had decreased vibration sensation and ankle reflexes and decreased motor nerve conduction velocities. In addition, there was evidence of subclinical disturbance of motor function in the upper limbs (Petit *et al.* 1987). Optic neuropathy has also been reported in a patient with sensorimotor neuropathy associated with almitrine that resolved completely 7 months after stopping the drug (Blondel *et al.* 1986).

Two cases of peripheral neuropathy were reported with cyclosporin (Blin *et al.* 1989). Colchicine may produce a mixed picture of neuropathy and myopathy. Electrophysiological investigation was reported to show myopathic motor unit potentials, early recruitment in proximal and truncal muscles, fibrillation, and positive sharp waves or complex repetitive discharges that correlated with the course of the weakness, all of which resolved rapidly after discontinuation of the drug. The accompanying signs of axonal neuropathy persisted for longer but with little functional consequence (Kuncl *et al.* 1989). The myopathy presents with proximal weakness and elevation of serum creatine kinase and an accompanying axonal polyneuropathy which slowly recovers. Electromyographic examination shows abnormal spontaneous activity. These features often result in a diagnosis of polymyositis or uraemic neuropathy, especially when there is decreased renal function and elevated serum colchicine. The myopathy is vacuolar, with marked accumulation of lysosomes and autophagic vacuoles. The pathogenesis probably involves disruption of the microtubular-dependent cytoskeletal network which interacts with lysosomes (Kuncl *et al.* 1987). (See also below under Vacuolar myopathy.)

The development of a polyneuropathy with the radio-sensitizing drug misonidazole was found to be associated with a high peak plasma concentration and a large area under the clearance curve (Melgaard *et al.* 1988).

Low doses of cisplatin (20 mg per m^2 weekly) have been reported to cause a primarily sensory neuropathy in patients with carcinomata and metastases and symptoms of painful paraesthesiae and numbness in a glove-and-stocking distribution. The neuropathy developed at a cumulative dose of between 100–640 mg per m^2 and recovery was incomplete despite withdrawal of the drug (Greenspan and Treat 1988). Cisplatin can also cause ototoxicity and has been reported to be associated with the clinical sign of Lhermitte, which is an indication of posterior column pathology and was considered to suggest spinal cord demyelination. The doses involved were high, and the sign resolved on cessation of the drug (Walther *et al.* 1987). The symptoms are those of a symmetrical, distal, predominantly sensory neuropathy of an axonal type with major involvement of propriocep-

tion. A postmortem examination in one case showed a degeneration of the posterior column ganglia. Early clinical findings included distal paraesthesiae and decreased tendon reflexes before the more serious findings of ataxia, pain, and Lhermitte's sign (Amiel *et al.* 1987).

Nerve biopsies from patients taking chloroquine for either connective tissue diseases or as antimalarial prophylaxis, who were suspected of having chloroquine-induced neuromyopathy, showed segmental demyelination and remyelination. Cytoplasmic inclusions were seen in Schwann cells, perineural and endothelial cells, and some interstitial cells, but never within axons themselves. Occasional curvilinear profiles were seen in perineural and Schwann cells with perineural calcification. These findings suggest that chloroquine neuropathy is due to primary involvment of Schwann cells (Tegner *et al.* 1988). A peripheral neuropathy in a patient with a psoriatic neuropathy was initially ascribed to hydroxychloroquine rather than naproxen but was shown to be related to therapeutic doses of naproxen on subsequent rechallenge (Rothenberg and Sufit 1987).

A case of painful legs and moving toes was reported as due to a neuropathy caused by a combination of vincristine and metronidazole; the symptoms resolved within 6 weeks of withdrawal of the drugs (Gastaut 1986). A predominantly sensory peripheral neuropathy is caused by vincristine. Ocular palsies, hoarseness, autonomic neuropathy with postural hypotension, reduced intestinal motility, and atony of the urinary bladder can also occur. The neurotoxicity is dose-related and cumulative with repeated doses up to 30–50 mg but recovery is slow (Legha 1986).

A 54-year-old man was reported to have developed lower limb paraesthesiae, mild distal global hypoaesthesia, and reduced ankle reflexes after taking 150 mg amitriptyline daily for 2 years. An electromyogram (EMG) showed a sensorimotor pattern in all limbs compatible with an axonal neuropathy. The clinical picture and electrophysiological changes resolved following withdrawal of the drug (Zampollo *et al.* 1988).

Motor neuropathies

A predominantly motor neuropathy can be associated with the use of sulphonamides, dapsone, nitrofurantoin, or amphotericin. A combined motor and sensory peripheral neuropathy occurring in a man treated with dapsone for dermatitis herpetiformis resolved when sulphapyridine was substituted for the dapsone (Ahrens *et al.* 1986). A motor neuropathy has also been reported with several tricyclic antidepressants, including amitriptyline and imipramine. An association between cimetidine and a motor neuropathy has been described (Walls and

Pearce 1980). Eade and others (1975) described a predominantly motor peripheral neuropathy associated with indomethacin, which regressed when the drug was stopped. A principally motor but, occasionally, ascending sensorimotor neuropathy, similar clinically to the Guillain–Barré syndrome, can occur in patients treated with gold (Dick and Raman 1982). Painful paraesthesiae and fasciculations may be prominent and there may be an accompanying encephalopathy. Resolution is accelerated by chelating agents such as dimercaprol (Perry and Jacobsen 1984). The cerebrospinal fluid protein may be elevated in these patients. A patient was described who developed an acute peripheral neuropathy of Guillain–Barré type shortly after starting captopril for moderate hypertension; this resolved after stopping the drug (Chakraborty and Ruddell 1987). A similar syndrome was seen in two cases of amitriptyline overdose (Leys*et al*. 1987) and occurred so commonly with zimeldine that the drug was withdrawn (Fagius *et al*. 1985).

Subacute myelo-opticoneuropathy (SMON)

In 1973, Nakae and others reported the appearance in Japan of a new syndrome, subacute myelo-opticoneur-opathy (SMON). Patients with this syndrome developed paraesthesiae in the limbs and an optic neuropathy. These symptoms were usually preceded by abdominal pain. The syndrome appeared to be associated with taking of large doses of between 1.1–1.3 g per day of clioquinol (Entero-Vioform). The number of cases reported has declined dramatically following a ban on the sale of clioquinol. The Japanese had taken particularly high doses of the drug, and although a case of dysaesthesiae following treatment with a preparation containing clioquinol has been reported in the United Kingdom (Terry 1971), the Japanese may have a genetic susceptibility to the development of this adverse effect.

Other neuropathies and radiculopathies

Facial numbness may occur with sulthiame treatment and has also been caused, together with a trigeminal neuropathy, by hydroxystilbamidine (Goldstein *et al*. 1963), trichloroethylene (Mitchell and Parsons-Smith 1969), and labetalol (Gabriel 1978). The mechanism of the cranial neuropathy associated with heavy trichloroethylene exposure is unknown. In severe cases there is destructive spread of the neuropathic process from the

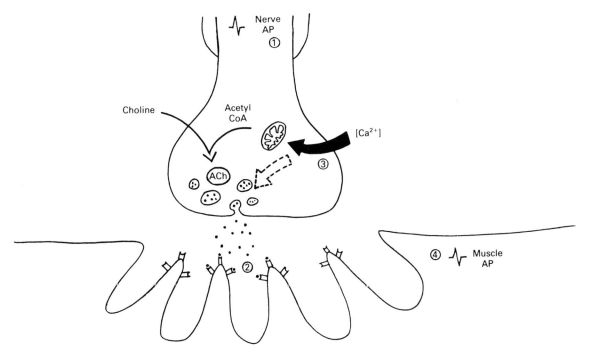

Fig. 18.1
Diagram of neuromuscular junction showing possible sites of action of drugs. 1. Presynaptic effect on nerve action potential (AP). 2. Postsynaptic acetylcholine (ACh) receptor blockade. 3. Effect on calcium (Ca²⁺) influx and neurotransmitter release. 4. Effect on muscle membrane and generation of muscle AP.

fifth cranial nerve nuclei up and down the brain stem. There is a suggestion that the chemical reactivates latent orofacial herpes simplex (Cavanagh and Buxton 1989) (see also Chapter 23).

Batterman and Gutner (1948) reported several patients under treatment with digitalis who developed aching in the lower third of the face, sometimes bilateral, together with a sharp stabbing pain reminiscent of trigeminal neuralgia.

An unusual sensory disturbance, in which patients developed discomfort, pain, and paraesthesiae in the perineal region following intravenous injections of hydrocortisone sodium phosphate, was described by Bartrop and Diba (1969). A similar syndrome is produced by intravenous injections of stilboestrol diphosphate (Honvan). Unilateral or bilateral sciatica and weakness of the legs (rarely progressing to paraplegia, as a result of chronic spinal arachnoiditis) may follow myelography (Shaw et al. 1978). This complication, although uncommon, is seen particularly after the use of iophendylate and less commonly with water-soluble contrast media such as methylglucamine iothalamate (meglumine iothalamate) (see also Chapter 27).

Danazol has been reported to cause carpal tunnel syndrome, probably as a result of fluid retention (Sikka et al. 1983). Finally, following injection with antitetanus serum, or vaccination against diphtheria, pertussis, rabies, or typhoid or paratyphoid fevers, a polyradiculitis similar to neuralgic amyotrophy may occur (Holliday and Bauer 1983). The patient usually experiences severe pain and then develops weakness and wasting of muscles, most often those innervated by the fifth and sixth cervical roots (Foster 1974). Less commonly a polyneuritis may be seen, sometimes taking the form of an acute ascending polyneuritis of the Guillain–Barré type (Miller and Stanton 1954). Ribera and Dutka (1983) report a case of the Guillain–Barré syndrome associated with the administration of hepatitis B vaccine.

A delayed distal axonopathy may occur with certain organophosphate compounds (Blain 1990). The original description of this syndrome involved triorthocresyl phosphate. The toxic effects were seen several weeks after acute exposure, and consisted of an ataxia and a mixed sensorimotor neuropathy principally affecting the lower limbs. Severe cases have shown marked motor effects resulting in a flaccid paralysis. The mechanism of this delayed neurotoxic effect is believed to be associated with the inhibition of a neuropathy target esterase (formerly called neurotoxic esterase). The neuropathological findings in this delayed neuropathy include a Wallerian degeneration rather than demyelination. Initially there is a focal lesion in large myelinated fibres that leads to axonal death distal to the lesion. Chronic effects following an acute single non-toxic exposure to organophosphates are less well defined and may be principally neuropsychological or behavioural. Neither delayed nor chronic toxic effects have been reported following exposure to carbamates, and both the plasma and red cell cholinesterases return rapidly to normal levels after acute poisoning with carbamates.

Neuromuscular junction

Drugs can block neuromuscular transmission by any one of four mechanisms (Argov and Mastaglia 1979) (Fig. 18.1):
1. presynaptic inhibition of propagation of the nerve action potential (local-anaesthetic-like effect);
2. postsynaptic curareform blockade of acetylcholine receptors;
3. combined presynaptic and postsynaptic effects, the presynaptic effect probably being due to impaired release of acetylcholine (membrane-stabilizing action) by inhibition of calcium movement through the nerve terminal membrane, and the postsynaptic effect due to a curareform blockade of acetylcholine receptors;
4. inhibition of ionic conductances across the muscle membrane, preventing generation of an end-plate potential.

Neuromuscular transmission is also compromised by compounds (such as the organophosphates) that inhibit acetylcholinesterase and increase the local concentration of acetylcholine at the neuromuscular junction (Blain 1990).

The drugs producing clinical neuromuscular blockade can be classified in terms of the mechanisms involved, and although many exert both presynaptic and postsynaptic effects one action usually predominates at therapeutic doses. It is more useful, therefore, to consider the clinical syndromes that may occur and the classes of drugs most likely to be implicated.

Postoperative respiratory depression

This is probably the most common clinical manifestation of a drug-induced neuromuscular blockade. Drugs given before or during the operation or in the immediate postoperative period prevent re-establishment of spontaneous respiration. Occasionally, postoperative respiratory depression can follow an apparently normal recovery, due to an interaction between a drug and the muscle relaxants used during anaesthesia with potentiation of their effects and duration of action, a phenomenon termed 'recurarization'.

Postoperative respiratory depression is produced most commonly by the aminoglycoside antibiotics (streptomycin, neomycin, gentamicin, and kanamycin), the polymyxins (polymyxin B, colistin), tetracyclines, and lincomycin and its derivative clindamycin. It has also been encountered following instillation of chloroquine into the peritoneum to prevent the formation of adhesions (Jin-Yen 1971). Paralysis of respiratory muscles usually predominates, occasionally accompanied by generalized weakness. Treatment usually involves assisted respiration, although in the case of direct suppression of neuromuscular transmission by drugs an infusion of calcium gluconate to overcome the presynaptic component of the block and the use of parenteral neostigmine to antagonize a postsynaptic curare-like effect may be useful (Argov and Mastaglia 1979).

Postoperative respiratory depression must be distinguished from suxamethonium apnoea (*The Lancet* 1973b). Patients with an atypical serum pseudocholinesterase are unable to inactivate the muscle relaxant suxamethonium. Although the abnormality is usually genetically determined, an acquired cholinesterase deficiency can also occur in hepatic failure. Drugs such as phenelzine and the potent anticholinesterase ecothiopate (used in ophthalmological preparations) may reduce serum pseudocholinesterase activity. Cimetidine and ranitidine are both reported to inhibit cholinesterases (Hansen and Bertl 1983). A number of other drugs are known to potentiate the neuromuscular-blocking effect of suxamethonium and they may also precipitate postoperative apnoea.

The chemical agents used in 'nerve gases' are potent and irreversible inactivators of plasma cholinesterases. The organophosphate and carbamate insecticides can also inactivate cholinesterases but, in the case of the organophosphates, poisoning with these agents is reversible with pralidoxime if this drug is given rapidly after exposure. Both organophosphate insecticides and nerve gases are extensively absorbed through intact skin.

Activation or unmasking of myasthenia gravis

The safety factor for neuromuscular transmission is already reduced in myasthenia gravis, and drugs known to affect neuromuscular transmission, clinically or experimentally, should be used with extreme caution. Large doses of thyroxine or corticosteroids can produce a sudden deterioration in myasthenia gravis, although by what mechanism is unknown.

Many of the drugs involved have a curare-like action on postsynaptic acetylcholine receptors. Withdrawal of the drug usually produces a remission of symptoms, although there are several reports of true myasthenia gravis being precipitated in predisposed patients. The drugs involved include the aminoglycoside antibiotics, chloroquine, procainamide, quinidine, β-adrenoceptor blocking drugs, phenytoin, and lithium. A reversible drug-induced myasthenic syndrome is distinguishable from naturally occurring myasthenia gravis by the presence of acetylcholine receptor antibodies in the latter.

Ampicillin and erythromycin are commonly regarded as the antibiotics of choice in myasthenia gravis. There is, however, a single report of the electrophysiological characteristics of the Eaton–Lambert syndrome occurring in patients taking these two drugs (Herishanu and Taustein 1971).

Drug-induced myasthenic syndrome

This is a relatively uncommon disorder, since drugs known to inhibit neuromuscular transmission rarely do so at therapeutic doses in normal individuals because of the high safety factor inherent in the system. Adverse effects are usually only seen when this safety factor is compromised, as in electrolyte disturbances such as hyperkalaemia or hypocalcaemia. High plasma drug concentrations occurring with diminished renal function may also predispose a patient to these effects.

The clinical picture is that of myasthenia gravis with a rapid onset but prompt remission on withdrawal of the drug. A drug-induced myasthenic syndrome has been reported in association with many of the drugs already mentioned, particularly the aminoglycoside antibiotics and polymyxins (e.g. polymyxin B), β-adrenoceptor blocking drugs, and the anticonvulsants phenytoin and troxidone. Carnitine has been reported to produce a myasthenic syndrome when given experimentally to reduce serum triglycerides in patients undergoing long-term haemodialysis (De Grandis *et al.* 1980). The metabolites of carnitine are structurally similar to acetylcholine and may compete at the receptor site. A myopathy with myasthenic features has been attributed to high doses of codeine linctus (Kilpatrick *et al.* 1982); the authors felt that the squill oxymel present in the linctus was responsible for the muscle weakness.

A 55-year-old man with idiopathic Parkinson's disease developed myasthenia gravis shortly after taking trihexyphenidyl. The myasthenic symptoms varied directly with the plasma trihexyphenidyl level but without any change in antiacetylcholine receptor antibody titre (Ueno *et al.* 1987).

Mechanism of action of specific drugs at the neuromuscular junction

Penicillamine

Penicillamine causes a myasthenic syndrome that is clinically and electrophysiologically identical to myasthenia gravis and is similarly characterized by the presence of acetylcholine receptor antibodies in nearly all affected patients (Alberb et al. 1980). Most reported cases have been in patients with rheumatoid arthritis, Wilson's disease, or primary biliary cirrhosis. The onset of myasthenia varies from 2 days to 8 years from the start of therapy although symptoms usually present after about 8 months. The doses involved have varied from 250–1500 mg per day, with no clear association between cumulative dose and severity of symptoms. Why only a small number of patients develop the condition is not clear. The first symptoms are usually diplopia and ptosis. Although bulbar symptoms and signs may occur, when involvement is generalized it is usually mild and respiratory difficulty is unusual. The patients respond to edrophonium and in over 70 per cent of cases withdrawal of the drug results in a gradual remission of symptoms and signs. There is also a progressive fall of acetylcholine receptor antibody titres and electrophysiological improvement. In patients who fail to remit an anticholinesterase drug (e.g. neostigmine) is useful.

It has been suggested that the drug unmasks latent myasthenia gravis in individuals possessing the HLA A1 B8 phenotype commonly found in the naturally occurring disease. The drug-induced condition differs in several respects, however, from the natural condition. The modal age of onset, mid-40s, is much later than in females with classical myasthenia gravis. The rate of fall of acetylcholine receptor antibody titres and subsequent clinical and electrophysiological improvement is far more rapid following withdrawal of the drug than in the spontaneous disease. No association with thymoma has been reported, athough thymic hyperplasia and the presence of striated muscle antibodies are documented. Penicillamine therapy can result in generation of antibodies to platelets (causing thrombocytopenia), skin basement membrane (precipitating pemphigus), kidney (causing a nephritis and Goodpasture's syndrome), and nuclear constituents (causing systemic lupus erythematosus). The presence of striated muscle antibodies may be related to the development of thymic hyperplasia, and the increased frequency in patients with rheumatoid arthritis may reflect a non-specific effect of the drug on the immune system. Experimental work has shown that penicillamine binds covalently to a subunit of the acetylcholine receptor molecule and affects the affinity of the acetylcholine binding site (Bever et al. 1982). Such antigenic modulation could also act as a stimulus and result in acetylcholine receptor antibody production. An identical clinical syndrome, including the production of acetylcholine-receptor antibodies, has been described in a patient with rheumatoid arthritis treated with chloroquine (Schumm et al. 1981).

β-Adrenoceptor blocking drugs

β-Adrenoceptor blocking drugs are associated with a number of subjective adverse effects, including muscle fatigue and peripheral coldness as well as neurological symptoms. In therapeutic doses, propranolol has a postsynaptic curare-like effect in vivo, competitively inhibiting the acetylcholine receptor and producing a rapid fall in the amplitude of miniature endplate potentials. Prolonged curarization due to propranolol has been reported in postoperative patients (Rozen and Whan 1977). Practolol, pindolol, sotalol, and oxprenolol can also produce postsynaptic blockade. In doses far in excess of those commonly used, propranolol has a presynaptic effect (local anaesthetic action) on the propagation of the nerve action potential and inhibits neurotransmitter release. Chloroquine, lincomycin, and lithium have similar actions. The symptoms of fatigability and weakness, commonly found in hypertensive patients taking propranolol, may be a result of its curare-like action. The drug has central effects and an action on peripheral blood flow and these may contribute to this tiredness. Lipophilicity may be associated with an increased incidence of neurological symptoms (Lewis and McDevitt 1986). Skeletal muscle tremor, the most frequent dose-limiting adverse effect, may be reduced by changing the drug or starting at a low dose (Lulich et al. 1986).

Phenytoin

Phenytoin has both presynaptic and postsynaptic effects. The presynaptic action is predominant at therapeutic doses and is believed to be due to a change in calcium flux across the nerve terminal membrane. Aggravation of myasthenia gravis and a myasthenic syndrome have been described in patients with phenytoin intoxication, and this may be due to a combination of decreased transmitter release and a postsynaptic curareform blockade.

Skeletal muscle

Complaints of weakness, cramps, and muscle aching are more commonly attributed to an underlying medical disorder than to the drugs prescribed for a patient. Although serious drug-induced myopathies are rare, it is likely that mild subclinical effects are quite common. The subject has been extensively reviewed by Lane and Routledge (1983), Blain and Lane (1983b), Blain (1984), and Lane (1988). Consequently, only the more recent observations in this area will be considered. It is probably most convenient to consider the main clinical syndromes as classified by Lane and Mastaglia (1978).

Focal myopathy

The intramuscular injection of any drug can produce focal inflammation from traumatic necrosis, haematoma formation, or low-grade infection ('needle myopathy'). Over several months or years, repeated intramuscular injections may produce severe fibrosis and contractures. In the West, the drugs of abuse such as opiates and tranquillizers are most commonly implicated, while on the Indian subcontinent repeated intramuscular injections of antibiotics into the deltoid muscles of children have been reported to produce severe contractures (Shanmagasundaram 1980). It must always be remembered that phenytoin can crystallize at the site of an intramuscular injection, causing haemorrhagic necrosis of the muscle and also producing an erratic and unpredictable absorption of the anticonvulsant. Ideally, phenytoin should never be given by intramuscular injection.

Acute and subacute painful proximal myopathy

Muscle pain and cramps are such common symptoms that they are often not investigated. They may indicate an underlying myopathy, however, and raised serum concentrations of muscle enzymes or electromyographic changes suggesting a mild myopathy have been reported in patients treated with the diuretics bumetanide and metolazone, danazol (Spauding 1979), salbutamol (Palmer 1978), cytotoxic agents, cimetidine, and lithium (Tyrer and Shopsin 1980). When symptoms and signs have been more dramatic and investigations, including muscle biopsy, have been pursued, three underlying mechanisms have been definable on histological grounds.

Necrotizing myopathy

A necrotizing myopathy can be produced by a number of drugs, including aminocaproic acid (ε-aminocaproic acid, EACA) (Lane et al. 1979), ethanol (acute intoxication), opiates (Blain and Lane 1984), colchicine,

quinine, chloroquine (MacDonald and Engel 1970), clofibrate, emetine (which is also cardiotoxic) (Fewings et al. 1973; Bradley et al. 1976), dimethylsulphoxide (DMSO), and vincristine (which more commonly produces a peripheral neuropathy).

The myopathy induced by EACA is sudden in onset and usually occurs many weeks after starting the drug. Although doses in excess of 32 g per day have been taken by many patients without evidence of muscle damage, the myopathy usually occurs when the dose is greater than 18 g a day. The mechanism of action may possibly be related to intravascular coagulation and ischaemic damage to the muscle. Biopsies from these patients often show capillary occlusion and fibrin deposits. Myoglobinuria may be found (Brodkin 1980). Withdrawal of the drug usually results in a rapid recovery.

Clofibrate, although no longer widely prescribed in the United Kingdom, was reported to produce a necrotizing myopathy, especially in patients with renal failure, the nephrotic syndrome, or hypothyroidism (Bridgman et al. 1972; Pierides et al. 1975; Rumf et al. 1976). Once the drug was withdrawn the patient rapidly recovered. It has been demonstrated that patients developing this myopathy frequently have a raised plasma free fraction of chlorophenoxyisobutyric acid, the active metabolite of clofibrate. There has also been a report of reversible electrocardiographic changes of a cardiomyopathy in a young boy given clofibrate during the treatment of diabetes insipidus (Smals et al. 1977). The pathogenesis of clofibrate myopathy is not clear but it may be due to an interference in cholesterol synthesis that affects muscle membrane structure and function, impairment of lipid metabolism by inhibition of mitochondrial carnitine palmityl transferase leading to an increase in lipoprotein lipase activity resulting in muscle necrosis, or the local production of a toxic metabolite. A number of new hypolipidaemic agents have been introduced recently and some can, like clofibrate, cause raised CK levels and features of a painful proximal myopathy (Shetty and Routledge 1990). These include lovastatin, simvastatin, gemfibrozil, and bezafibrate, when used alone or, particularly, when given in combination (Tolbert 1988). Heavy physical activity may exacerbate the mild underlying myopathy. Nicotinic acid has been reported to cause a similar syndrome in this context (Litin and Anderson 1989). It has been suggested that lovastatin might inhibit production of mevalonic acid and thus ubiquinone formation, which is vital to mitochondrial oxidative phosphorylation (Maher et al. 1989).

Steroids commonly produce a chronic painless proximal myopathy, although an acute painful myopathy has been observed in patients treated for severe asthma with large doses of intravenous hydrocortisone (MacFarlane and Rosenthal 1977; van Marle and Woods 1980) and in patients taking a 17-hydroxycorticosteroid (Perkoff *et al.* 1959). A painful proximal myopathy has also occurred in patients treated with propranolol (Forfar *et al.* 1979) and labetalol (Teicher *et al.* 1981), and with the vitamin A analogue isotretinoin (Hodak *et al.* 1986). This drug can also cause apparently symptomless elevation of serum CK levels in occasional patients (Dicken 1984; Lane and Cream, personal observations).

Cyclosporin has been implicated as a cause of this syndrome (Noppen *et al.* 1987; Goy *et al.* 1989; Grezard *et al.* 1990), and biopsy findings such as accumulations of subsarcolemmal mitochondria and increased amounts of glycogen and lipid in atrophic fibres have been reported (Goy *et al.* 1989). Concurrent administration of other drugs and somewhat inadequate documentation of these cases raised doubts regarding the association but a further carefully studied case has clearly established a relationship (Fernandez-Sola *et al.* 1990).

Confusion has also surrounded the role of zidovudine in the production of myalgia and proximal myopathy in patients with AIDS and AIDS-related complex (ARC). It was known that, prior to the introduction of zidovudine, HIV-infected patients could develop a necrotizing myopathy with little inflammatory infiltration ('HIV myopathy') in addition to a more commonly encountered inflammatory myopathy, but the incidence of this complication was greatly increased when use of the drug became widespread. Indeed, up to one-third of AIDS and ARC patients develop a myopathy after treatment for about one year, using 1–1.2 g of the drug daily, though this largely resolves on drug withdrawal. Evidence suggested, however, that zidovudine itself had only a very mild intrinsic myotoxic action. It now seems that the drug exacerbates an underlying low-grade HIV-related inflammatory myopathy (Dalakas *et al.* 1990; Lane *et al.* 1991). The drug appears to act primarily by inhibiting mitochondrial function and causing structural mitochondrial abnormalities, resulting in a characteristic microvacuolation and myofibrillary aggregation at light-microscopic level, with the development of 'ragged red fibres' of mitochondrial myopathy in more severe cases (Dalakas *et al.* 1990).

A patient who developed an acute painful proximal myopathy associated with the use of amiodarone has been reported. This was accompanied by hypothyroidism and a neuropathy, and the patient improved on drug withdrawal. Muscle biopsy demonstrated an acute necrotizing myopathy but the mechanism was unclear (Clouston and Donnelly 1989).

Vacuolar myopathy

Severe hypokalaemia can cause a myopathy that is often associated with prolonged use of diuretics, purgatives, and licorice and glycyrrhizinic acid derivatives such as carbenoxolone (Lane and Mastaglia 1978). Amphotericin has also caused this type of myopathy (Drutz *et al.* 1970). A hypokalaemic myopathy generally occurs when the serum potassium concentration is between 1–2 mmol per litre, especially if there is an accompanying hypochloraemic alkalosis. The weakness is generalized and often severe, with depressed tendon reflexes. Psychiatric symptoms such as dysphoria and hallucinations may occur. Electromyography shows evidence of muscle membrane damage, and the histological picture on biopsy is similar to that found in hypokalaemic periodic paralysis. Return of the serum potassium concentration to normal usually results in a remission of clinical symptoms and signs, although serial muscle biopsies may show more persistent changes. A less acute fall in serum potassium concentration can produce a chronic painless proximal or generalized myopathy. Colchicine taken in excess or in therapeutic doses in patients with renal or hepatic impairment may also produce myalgia, with proximal weakness and depressed or absent tendon reflexes and markedly raised serum CK levels. Muscle biopsy in such cases may also show a vacuolar myopathy, but this is due to an accumulation of lysosomes and autophagic vacuoles without fibre necrosis (Kuncl *et al.* 1987). The drug appears, however, to produce a complex neuromyopathy rather than a myopathy in isolation, and in such cases there is usually evidence of additional axonal neuropathy (*The Lancet* 1987) and defective neuromuscular transmission (Besana *et al.* 1987).

Myositis

Drugs such as hydralazine, procainamide (Fontiveros *et al.* 1980), and sulphacetamide (Mackie and Mackie 1979) can precipitate a syndrome similar to systemic lupus erythematosus. This may be accompanied by a myositis and is more common in patients who are slow acetylators so that, ideally, patients given these drugs should have their acetylator status determined. A painful inflammatory myopathy has also been reported in patients treated with penicillamine (Fernandes *et al.* 1977).

Eosinophilia–myalgia syndrome

An eosinophilic myositis, with eosinophilic perivasculitis and fasciitis, is a feature of the eosinophilia–myalgia syndrome (EMS). This syndrome, which comprises fatigue and intense myalgia, and often multisystem involvement with arthralgia, fever, cough, dyspnoea, skin rash, and oedema, and evidence of myocarditis, pancreatitis, pneumonitis, and ascending polyneuritis, is characterized by an eosinophil count exceeding 2×10^9 cells per litre (*Drug and Therapeutics Bulletin* 1990; Belongia *et al.* 1990). EMS was first reported in 1989 in New Mexico (Eidson *et al.* 1990) and there have now been more than 1400 cases with 19 deaths reported from the United States, mostly in women. These cases appear to have been associated with the ingestion of over-the-counter powders and capsules containing L-tryptophan produced by a single Japanese manufacturer. The epidemic in 1989–90 followed a change in the manufacturing process which resulted in the appearance of a contaminant comprising less than 0.5% of the product (Belongia *et al.* 1990). Independent studies have suggested that the contaminant may be a bacitracin-like peptide; injected bacitracin can induce eosinophilia in monkeys and might be produced in the fermentation process used to produce L-tryptophan (Barnhart *et al.* 1990). Similar cases reported from Europe have involved the prescription of drugs containing L-tryptophan containing drugs (van Garsse and Boeykens 1990; Douglas *et al.* 1990; Walker *et al.* 1990) but it would seem likely that a similar explanation pertains. This has led to the withdrawal of all products for the treatment of depression containing this amino acid.

Rhabdomyolysis

A more severe form of necrotizing myopathy, usually accompanied by myoglobinuria, may be caused by any of the drugs that produce an acute or subacute painful myopathy. The disorder is most often seen, however, with drugs of abuse such as opiates (Richter *et al.* 1971; Blain *et al.* 1985), amphetamines (Grossman *et al.* 1974), phencyclidine, and alcohol. It has also been reported following accidental ingestion of paraphenylenediamine (Baud *et al.* 1983). The onset is acute with severe muscle pain, tenderness, and swelling. Generalized weakness is often found, the proximal muscles being more severely affected than the distal, and patients may be areflexic. Seizures and coma or depression of the level of consciousness may occur and about half the patients develop acute renal failure secondary to acute tubular necrosis. Serum muscle enzymes and myoglobin levels are grossly elevated and electromyographic testing in the acute phase shows myopathic changes, frequently associated with increased spontaneous insertional activity due to surface membrane damage. Biopsy at this stage may show severe necrosis, with nearly every muscle fibre in the section destroyed. In milder cases, however, the changes may be slight, with scattered focal necrosis, phagocytosis, and degeneration. Inflammatory infiltrates may also be seen.

Narcotics or alcohol are directly toxic to muscle, and the damage may accumulate through repeated use. Experimentally, narcotics alter membrane transport mechanisms and cellular energy production, and both narcotics and alcohol cause morphological changes in muscle cells when they are exposed to sublethal concentrations. The rhabdomyolysis associated with phencyclidine overdose may be secondary to extreme motor excitation rather than direct muscle toxicity.

The major complications of acute non-traumatic rhabdomyolysis are hyperkalaemia and acute renal failure. The acute tubular necrosis may be secondary to plugging of the renal tubules by an interaction between myoglobin and tubular proteins, or may result from a direct toxic action of myoglobin on the kidney (Grossman *et al.* 1974). Hyperkalaemia is common and it may cause dangerous cardiac arrhythmias. There may also be characteristic changes in serum calcium and phosphate concentrations following release of phosphate from damaged muscle cells. Initially there is a paradoxical hypocalcaemia in the oliguric phase of the renal failure, followed by a rebound hypercalcaemia in the diuretic phase. The presence of pigment casts in the urine, a raised plasma creatine kinase, and myoglobinuria are diagnostic of rhabdomyolysis in a patient with acute renal failure (Grossman *et al.* 1974). The myoglobinuria may be transient but a raised serum myoglobin concentration as measured by radioimmunoassay is always found. Hypophosphataemia has been found to precipitate rhabdomyolysis in alcoholics and in patients undergoing treatment for diabetic ketoacidosis. It has also been caused by the administration of calcium supplements following parathyroidectomy (Lane 1988).

Chronic painless proximal myopathy

This is probably the most common type of drug-induced muscle disease. Severe cases are uncommon but milder forms may be overlooked, particularly if the drug involved is a steroid and is used to treat a condition, such as polymyositis, in which muscle weakness and wasting may be interpreted as part of the clinical presentation of the disease. Quantitative electromyography in patients treated with steroids for prolonged periods suggests that there is a high incidence of a subclinical myopathy (Yates 1970). The syndrome may also be caused by chloroquine, drug-induced hypokalaemia, rifampicin (Jenkins and Emerson 1981), by alcohol and opiate abuse, and by perhexiline maleate (Tomlinson and Rosenthal 1977).

Steroid myopathy can be caused by any steroid, but fluorinated steroids such as triamcinolone, dexamethasone, and betamethasone are most often implicated. The myopathy is not clearly related to the dose or duration of treatment. Clinically, the muscle weakness is symmetrical and initially affects the proximal leg muscles. Proximal arm muscles are also affected, and in severe cases distal and axial muscles may be involved. Wasting can be severe, particularly of the quadriceps and glutei. Reflexes are frequently preserved but may be diminished if the wasting is profound. Usually serum enzyme levels (CK, aldolase, and AST) and serum myoglobin concentration are normal in steroid myopathy but raised during an exacerbation of inflammatory muscle disease. The histological picture in steroid myopathy shows a remarkably selective Type 2b fibre atrophy. Experimentally, steroids affect cell surface membranes and alter the resting membrane potential. There is experimental evidence that the effects on enzyme systems are secondary to an initial binding with a specific glucocorticoid receptor in the muscle cytosol. This complex binds to DNA in the cell nucleus and presumably affects RNA production. Glucocorticoids appear to initiate several important changes including a decrease in protein synthesis. The Type 2 fast-twitch, glycolytic muscle fibres are much more severely affected than the Type 1 slow-twitch, oxidative fibres. The highly selective involvement of Type 2b fibres in steroid myopathy may be related to inhibition of myophosphorylase activity in fibres that have a limited ability to utilize other energy sources in oxidative phosphorylation. Such biochemical changes may also explain the ultrastructural alterations in Cushing's disease and steroid myopathy, such as the development of intermyofibrillary vacuoles, excessive accumulation of cytoplasmic glycogen, and subsarcolemmal mitochondrial aggregation.

Myotonia

In myotonia the muscle fibres undergo prolonged contraction due to repetitive firing of action potentials by the muscle membrane. The muscle cannot relax properly after a voluntary contraction. Several agents are known to induce myotonia in animals but not necessarily in man. These include the antilipidaemic drugs triparanol and clofibrate (Kwiencinski 1978), propranolol, veratrum alkaloids, aconitine, 20,25-diazocholesterol, 2,4-dichlorphenoxyacetate, and several other monocarboxylic aromatic acids. Myotonia can also occur when there is a low extracellular chloride concentration. Some drugs can unmask or aggravate myotonia, particularly in patients with myotonia congenita or dystrophia myo-

tonica. A reversible myotonia has been observed in a patient taking propranolol who was subsequently found to have dystrophia myotonica (Blessing and Walsh 1977). Depolarizing muscle relaxants (e.g. suxamethonium) can cause difficulties with intubation and ventilation during general anaesthesia in myotonic patients (Mitchell et al. 1978) but non-depolarizing agents (e.g. tubocurarine) do not have this effect. Propranolol, pindolol, barbiturates, and fenoterol can also aggravate myotonia. Frusemide, ethacrynic acid, and acetazolamide can induce myotonia in vitro and may produce clinical exacerbations. The muscle pains, cramps, and weakness, of which many patients complain when taking these diuretics, may result from the induction of a subclinical myotonia. Muscle cramps have also been reported in a patient taking nifedipine (MacDonald 1982).

Malignant hyperthermia

This is a serious and sometimes fatal response to various anaesthetic agents. Predisposition to the condition is inherited as an autosomal dominant trait and it is not strictly a drug-induced myopathy. Some affected individuals have a clinical myopathy, particularly central-core disease, often with a raised plasma CK concentration, although this is not a reliable indicator. Many patients who develop hyperthermia with a particular anaesthetic may have undergone anaesthesia previously without complications. There is an in vitro test for the identification of susceptible individuals but it requires considerable expertise in interpretation (Ellis et al. 1978). A platelet bioassay for screening patients also exists. Many anaesthetic agents are believed to induce malignant hyperthermia (the most frequently implicated being halothane and suxamethonium), including methoxyflurane, enflurane, isoflurane, trichloroethylene, ethylene, diethyl ether, cyclopropane, chloroform, and possibly ketamine (Page et al. 1972). It is also suspected that nitrous oxide and some local anaesthetics may induce the disorder.

A reaction usually occurs during anaesthesia but may begin immediately after operation. There is a severe pyrexia, metabolic acidosis, often general muscle rigidity, and myoglobinuria. The temperature may exceed 40°C (104°F). Apart from supportive measures, the specific emergency drug treatment consists of intravenous dantrolene.

A similar disorder affects the pig, which has been used as an animal model. There appears to be an abnormality in the control of the release of calcium and its reuptake by the sarcoplasmic reticulum. Excessive amounts of calcium within the muscle cytoplasm produce a sustained contraction that leads to hyperthermia, subsequent acidosis, hyperkalaemia, and muscle damage. Recent studies have demonstrated linkage between the hyperthermia gene and the ryanodine receptor (calcium release channel of the sarisplasmic reticulum) gene in the 19q12–13.2 locus of chromosome 19, and genetic screening for susceptibility to MH is now possible (MacLennan *et al.* 1990). (This condition is also discussed in Chapter 28).

Suxamethonium myalgia

Although unrelated to MH, a much more common phenomenon is suxamethonium myalgia with muscle pain, which occurs in about half the patients receiving this drug, on the day following surgery. The drug is known to cause release of CK and myoglobin (Laurence 1987) but there is no clear relationship between biochemical changes or the extent of fasciculation induced by the drug and subsequent symptoms. It has been suggested that the drug induces Ca^{2+}-stimulated phospholipid hydrolysis, leading on the one hand to myalgia mediated by prostanoids (*The Lancet* 1988) and to enzyme efflux due to membrane damage by free radical mediated peroxidation (Jackson *et al.* 1987) on the other. Treatment with soluble aspirin 600 mg per hour preoperatively appears to halve the incidence of this complication (McGloughlin *et al.* 1988).

Disorders of bladder function

The bladder has a somatic nerve supply by the pudendal nerves, an autonomic nerve supply from sympathetic fibres carried in the hypogastric nerve, and parasympathetic fibres carried in the pelvic splanchnic nerves. The bladder base and neck and the proximal urethra are rich in α-adrenergic receptors while the bladder vault has β-adrenergic receptors. The act of micturition is a spinal reflex that can be inhibited by higher cortical centres. Micturition is initiated by contraction of the detrusor muscle following parasympathetic stimulation. There is distension of the posterior part of the urethra, reflex relaxation of the external urethral sphincter, and voiding of urine.

Urinary retention

Inhibition of parasympathetic postganglionic cholinergic neurones decreases bladder tone and can produce retention of urine. especially if there is already some degree of outflow obstruction from prostatic hypertro-

phy. This may be an adverse effect of drugs that are used therapeutically for their anticholinergic activity. This group includes benzhexol, benztropine, atropine, dicyclomine, hyoscine, methixene, orphenadrine, propantheline, and other derivatives of the belladonna alkaloids. Many compounds have an unwanted anticholinergic activity in addition to their intended therapeutic action, and can produce urinary retention. The major groups of drugs that have such an unwanted effect are the tricyclic antidepressants and the phenothiazines. Tricyclic antidepressants also stimulate α-adrenoceptors following blockade of neuronal reuptake of noradrenaline and produce constriction of the bladder neck. Monoamine oxidase inhibitors and disopyramide have also caused urinary retention. Oral and parenteral forms (but not preparations for inhalation) of β-adrenoceptor agonists, such as ephedrine, salbutamol, and terbutaline, have been associated with urinary retention. Theophylline preparations given intravenously (but not those given orally) have produced episodes of urinary retention associated with high plasma theophylline concentrations (Hassan 1983).

Urinary incontinence

Difficulty in the control of micturition, resulting in urinary incontinence, has been reported as a complication of treatment with prazosin (Thien *et al.* 1978), benoxaprofen, metoprolol, and the depot phenothiazines (Shaikh 1978). Kiruluta and others (1981) found that prazosin depressed the urethral pressure profile in urodynamic studies. The mechanism was thought to be by selective blockade of postsynaptic α-adrenoceptors in the proximal urethra. Total urinary incontinence occurred within 24 hours of the concurrent administration of phenoxybenzamine and methyldopa but not with either drug on its own. A subsequent challenge confirmed this interaction (Fernandez *et al.* 1981). Urinary incontinence was reported in two patients taking clonazepam. On discontinuing treatment normal bladder control was regained (Sandyk 1933).

Ureteric function

Ureteric activity is not affected by drugs acting on the autonomic nervous system since the ureteric muscle has no nerve supply. The initiation and propagation of peristaltic waves is an inherent property of ureteric muscle, controlled by a pacemaker focus in the calyces.

References

Ahrens, E.M., Meckler, R.J., and Callen, J.P. (1986). Dapsone-induced peripheral neuropathy. *Int. J. Dermatol.* 25, 314.

Alberb, J.W., Hodach, R.J., Kimmel, D.W., and Treacy, W.L. (1980). Penicillamine associated myasthenia gravis. *Neurology* 30, 1246.

Allen, M.B. and Prowse, K. (1989). Peripheral nerve function in patients with chronic bronchitis receiving almitrine or placebo. *Thorax* 44, 292.

Ambani, L.M. and van Woert, M.H. (1973). Start hesitation — a side effect of long-term levodopa therapy. *N. Engl. J. Med.* 288, 1113.

Amiel, H., Gherardi, R., Giroux, C., Salama, J., Breau, J.L., and Delaporte, P. (1987). Neuropathy caused by cisplatin. 7 cases including one with an autopsy study. *Ann. Med. Intern.* (Paris) 138, 96.

Anderson, K.E. (1972). Effects of chlorpromazine, imipramine and quinidine on the mechanical activity of single skinned muscle fibres in the frog. *Acta Psychol. Scand.* 85, 532.

Arber, N., Fadila, R., Pinkhas, J., Shirin, H., Melamed, E., and Sidi, Y. (1990). Pseudotumour cerebri associated with leuprorelin acetate. *Lancet* i, 668.

Argov, Z. and Mastaglia, F.L. (1979). Disorders of neuromuscular transmission caused by drugs. *N. Engl. J. Med.* 301, 409.

Arthur, G.R., Feldman, H.S., and Covino, B.G. (1988). Alterations in the pharmacokinetic properties of amide local anaesthetics following local anaesthetic-induced convulsions. *Acta Anaesthesiol. Scand.* 32, 522.

Ashton, C.H. (1986). Adverse effects of prolonged benzodiazepine use. *Adverse Drug React. Bull.* No. 118, 440.

Ashton, C.H., Teoh, R., and Davies, D.M. (1989). Drug-induced stupor and coma: some physical signs and their pharmacological basis. *Adverse Drug React. Acute Poisoning Rev.* 8, 1.

Atkinson, E.A., Fairburn, B., and Heathfield, K.W.G. (1970). Intracranial venous thrombosis as a complication of oral contraception. *Lancet* i, 914.

Ayd, F.J. (1961). A survey of drug induced extrapyramidal reactions. *JAMA* 175, 1054.

Ballas, Z.K. and Donta, S.T. (1982). Sulindac-induced aseptic meningitis. *Arch. Intern. Med.* 142, 165.

Barker, I. and Grant, I.S. (1982). Convulsions after abrupt withdrawal of baclofen. *Lancet* ii, 556.

Barnes, T.R.E. (1988). Tardive dyskinesia. *Br. Med. J.* 296, 150.

Barnhart, E.R., Maggio, V.L., Alexander, L.R., Turner, W.E., Patterson D.G. Jr, Needham L.L., *et al.* (1990). Bacitracin-associated peptides and contaminated L-tryptophan, *Lancet* 336, 742.

Barron, D.W. (1974). Propanidid in epilepsy. *Anaesthesia* 9, 445.

Bartrop, D. and Diba, Y.T. (1969). Paraesthesiae after intravenous efcortesol. *Lancet* i, 529.

Bateman, D.N., Bevan, P., Langley, B.P., Mastaglia. F., and Wandless, 1. (1981). Cimetidine induced postural and action tremor. *J. Neurol. Neurosurg. Psychiatry* 44, 9.

Batterman, R.C. and Gutner, L.B. (1948). Hitherto undescribed neurological manifestations of digitalis toxicity. *Am. Heart J.* 36, 582.

Baud, F., Bismuth, C., Galliot, M., Garnier, R., and Peralma. A. (1983). Rhabdomyolysis in para-phenylene diamine intoxication. *Lancet* ii, 514.

Bayne, L., McLeod, P.J., and Ogilvie, R.I. (1980). Antihypertensive drugs. In *Meyler's side effects of drugs* (9th edn) (ed. M.N.G. Dukes), p. 317. Excerpta Medica, Amsterdam.

BCDSP (Boston Collaborative Drug Surveillance Program) (1972). Drug-induced convulsions. *Lancet* ii, 677.

BCDSP (Boston Collaborative Drug Surveillance Program) (1973). Drug-induced extrapyramidal syndromes. *JAMA* 224, 889.

Belec, L., Larrey, D., De-Cremoux, H., Tinel, M., Louarn, F., Pessayre, D., *et al.* (1989). Extensive oxidative metabolism of dextromethorphan in patients with almitrine neuropathy. *Br. J. Clin. Pharmacol.* 27, 387.

Belongia, E.A., Hedberg, C.W., Gleich, G.J., White K.E., Mayeno, A.N., Loegering, D.A., *et al.* (1990). An investigation of the cause of the eosinophilia–myalgia syndrome associated with tryptophan use. *N. Engl. J. Med.* 323, 357.

Bertoni, J.M., Schwartzman. R.J., van Horn, G., and Partin, J. (1981). Asterixis and encephalopathy following metrizamide myelography: investigations into possible mechanisms and review of the literature. *Ann. Neurol.* 9, 366.

Besana, C., Comi, G., Baldini, V., Ciboddo, G., and Bianchi, R. (1987). Colchicine myoneuropathy. *Lancet* ii, 1271.

Betts, T.A., Kalra. P.L., Cooper, R., and Jeavons, P.M. (1968). Epileptic fits as a probable side-effect of amitriptyline. *Lancet* i, 390.

Bever, C.T., Chang. H.W., Penn, A.S., Jaffe, I.A., and Bock, E. (1982). Penicillamine-induced myasthenia gravis: effects of penicillamine on acetylcholine receptor. *Neurology* (N.Y.) 32, 1077.

Bickerstaff, E. R. (1975). *Neurological complications of oral contraceptives.* Clarendon Press, Oxford.

Biehl, U.P. and Vilter, R.W. (1954). Effects of isoniazid on pyridoxine metabolism. *JAMA* 156, 1549.

Blain, P.G. (1984). Adverse effects of drugs on skeletal muscle. *Adverse Drug React. Bull.* 104, 384.

Blain, P.G. (1990). Aspects of pesticide toxicology. *Adverse Drug React. Acute Poisoning Rev.* 9, 37.

Blain, P.G. and Lane., R.J.M. (1983a). Drugs and muscle. *Adverse Drug React. Acute Poisoning Rev.* 2, 1.

Blain, P.G. and Lane, R.J.M. (1983b). Dihydrocodeine overdose treated with naloxone infusion *Br. Med. J.* 287, 1547.

Blain, P.G., and Lane, R.J.M. (1984). Opiate induced rhabdomyolysis. *Br. Med. J.* 289, 228

Blain, P.G., Lane, R.J.M., Bateman, D.N., and Rawlins, M.D. (1985). Opiate induced rhabdomyolysis. *Hum. Toxicol.* 4, 71.

Blessing, W. and Walsh. J.C. (1977). Myotonia precipitated by propranolol therapy. *Lancet* i, 73.

Blin, O., Desnuelle, C., Pellissier, J.F., Pouget, J., Serratrice, G., Vialettes, B., *et al.* (1989). Peripheral neuropathy and cyclosporin (apropos of 2 cases). *Therapie* 44, 55.

Blondel, M., Arnott, G., Defoort, S., Bouchez, B., Persuy, P., Masingue, M., *et al.* (1986). Eleven cases of neuropathy induced by almitrine, of which one had optic neuropathy. *Rev. Neurol.* 142, 683.

Bonnetblanc, J.M., Hugon, J., Dumas, M., and Rupin, D. (1983). Intracranial hypertension with etretinate. *Lancet* ii. 974.

Bouche, P., Lacomblez, L., Leger, J.M., Chaunu, M.O.P., Ratinahirana, H., Brunet, P., *et al.* (1989). Peripheral neuropathies during treatment with almitrine: report of 46 cases. *J. Neurol.* 236, 29.

Bradley, W.G. and Thomas, P.K. (1974). The pathology of peripheral nerve disease. In *Diseases of voluntary muscle* (3rd edn) (ed. J.N. Walton), p. 234. Churchill Livingstone, Edinburgh.

Bradley, W.G., Fewings, J.D., Harris, J.B., and Johnson, M.A. (1976). Emetine myopathy in the rat. *Br. J. Pharmacol.* 57, 29.

Bridgman, J.F., Rosen, S.M., and Thorp, J.M. (.1972). Complications during clofibrate treatment of nephrotic syndrome hyperlipoproteinaemia. *Lancet* ii, 506.

Briscoe, J.G., Curry, S.C., Gerkin, R.D., and Ruiz, R.R. (1988). Pemoline-induced choreoathetosis and rhabdomyolysis. *Med. Toxicol. Adverse Drug Exp.* 3, 72.

British Medical Journal (1970). Benign intracranial hypertension. *Br. Med. J.* iii, 536.

Brodkin, H. M. (1980). Myoglobinuria following epsilon aminocaproic acid (EACA) therapy. Case report. *J. Neurosurg.* 53, 690.

Bruni, J., Gallo, J.M., Lee, C.S., Pethalski, R.J., and Wilder, B.J. (1980). Interaction of valproic acid with phenytoin. *Neurology* (N.Y.) 30, 1233.

Burke, R.E., Fahn, S., Mayeux, R., Weinberg, H., Louis, K., and Willner, J.H. (1981). Neuroleptic malignant syndrome caused by dopamine-depleting drugs in the patient with Huntington's disease. *Neurology* (N.Y.) 31, 1022.

Caroff, S., Rosenberg, H., and Gerber, J.C. (1983). Neuroleptic malignant syndrome and malignant hyperthermia. *Lancet* i, 244.

Cartlidge, N.E.F. (1981). Drug-induced coma. *Adverse Drug React. Bull.* No. 88.

Casey, E.G., Jelife, A.M., LeQuesne, P.M., and Millett, Y.L. (1973). Vincristine neuropathy: Clinical and electrophysiological observations. *Brain* 96, 69.

Cavanagh, J.B. and Buxton, P.H. (1989). Trichloroethylene cranial neuropathy: is it really a toxic neuropathy or does it activate latent herpes virus? *J. Neurol. Neurosurg. Psychiatry* 52, 297.

Cersosimo, R.J., Carter, R.T., Matthews, S.J., Coderre, M., and Karp, D.D. (1987). Acute cerebellar syndrome, conjunctivitis, and hearing loss associated with low-dose cytarabine administration. *Drug Intell. Clin. Pharmacol.* 21, 798.

Chadwick, D., Reynolds, E.H., and Marsden. C.D. (1976). Anticonvulsant-induced dyskinesias: A comparison with dyskinesias induced by neuroleptics. *J. Neurol. Neurosurg. Psychiatry* 39, 1210.

Chadwick, D.W. (1981). Convulsions associated with drug therapy. *Adverse Drug React. Bull.* 87, 316.

Chakrabati, A. and Pearace, J.M.S. (1981). Essential tremor: Response to primidone. *J. Neurol. Neurosurg. Psychiatry* 44, 650.

Chakraborty, T.K. and Ruddell, W.S. (1987). Guillain–Barré neuropathy during treatment with captopril. *Postgrad. Med. J.* 63, 221.

Chez, M., Gila, C.A., Ransohoff, R.M., Longworth, D.L., and Weida, C. (1989). Ibuprofen-induced meningitis: detection of intrathecal IgG synthesis and immune complexes. *Neurology* 39, 1578.

Clarke, C.E., Shand, D., Yuill, G.M., and Green, M.H.P. (1988). Clinical spectrum of neuroleptic malignant syndrome. *Lancet* ii, 969.

Clouston, P.D. and Donnelly, P.E. (1989). Acute necrotising myopathy associated with amiodarone therapy. *Aust. N.Z. J. Med.* 19, 483.

Crawford, J.P. (1977). Dystonic reaction to high dose propranolol. *Br. Med. J.* iii, 1156.

Dalakas, M.C., Illa, I., Pezeshkpour, G.H., Laukatis, J.P., Cohen, B., and Griffin, J.L. (1990). Mitochondrial myopathy caused by long-term zidovudine therapy. *N. Engl. J. Med.* 322, 1098.

Dam, M. (1990). Vigabatrin and behaviour disturbances. *Lancet* 335, 605.

Davidson, S.I. (1971). Reported adverse effects of oral contraceptives on the eye. *Trans. Ophthalmol. Soc. U.K.* 91, 561.

De Grandis, D., Mezzina, C., Fiaschi, A., Pinelli, P., Bazato, G., and Morachiello. M . (1980). Myasthenia due to carnitine treatment. *J. Neurol. Sci.* 46, 365.

Demers, R., Lukesh, R., and Prichard, J. (1970). Convulsion during lithium therapy. *Lancet* ii, 315.

DeVita, E.G., Miao, M., and Sadun, A.A. (1987). Optic neuropathy in ethambutol-treated renal tuberculosis. *J. Clin. Euro. Ophthalmol.* 7, 77.

Dick, D.J. and Raman. D. (1982). The Guillain–Barré syndrome following gold therapy. *Scand. J. Rheumatol.* 1, 119.

Dicken, C.H. (1984). Retinoids: a review. *J. Am. Acad. Dermatol.* 11, 541.

Dobkin, B.H. (1977). Reversible subacute peripheral neuropathy induced by phenytoin. *Arch. Neurol.* 34. 189.

Domingo, P., Munoz, J., Bonastre, M., Lloret, J., and Ris, J. (1989). Benign type of malignant syndrome. *Lancet* i, 50.

Dostert, P and Strolin-Benedetti, M. (1988). The bases of MPTP neurotoxicity. *Encephale* 14, 399.

Douglas, A.S., Eagles, J.M., and Mowat, N.A.G. (1990). Eosinophilia–myalgia syndrome associated with tryptophan. *Br. Med. J.* 301, 387.

Douglas, C.R. and Harms, R.H. (1990). An evaluation of a stepdown amino-acid feeding program for commercial pullets to 20 weeks of age. *Poult. Sci.* 69, 763.

Drug and Therapeutics Bulletin 1990). L-tryptophan and the eosinophilia–myalgia syndrome. *Drug Ther. Bull.* 28, 37.

Drug Intelligence and Clinical Pharmacy (1990). Potential neurologic toxicity related to ciprofloxacin. *Drug Intell. Clin. Pharm.* 24, 138.

Drutz, D.J., Fan. J.H., Tai, T.Y., Cheng, J.T., and Hsieh, W.C. (1970). Hypokalemic rhabdomyolysis and myoglobinuria following amphotericin B therapy. *JAMA* 211, 824.

Dubinsky, R.M., Yarchoan, R., Dalakas, M., and Broder, S. (1989). Reversible axonal neuropathy from the treatment of AIDS and related disorders with 2′,3′-dideoxycytidine (ddC). *Muscle–Nerve* 12, 856.

Dukes, M.N.G. (ed.) (1980). *Meyler's side effects of drugs* (9th edn). Excerpta Medica, Amsterdam.

Duvoisin, R.C. (1968). Neurological reactions to psychotropic drugs. In *Psychopharmacology: a review of progress 1957–1967*, p. 111. U.S. Government Printing Office, Washington.

Eade, O.E., Acheson, E.D., Cuthbert, M.F., and Hawkes, C.H. (1975). Peripheral neuropathy and indomethacin. *Br. Med. J.* ii, 66.

Edwards, J.G. (1979). Antidepressants and convulsions. *Lancet* ii, 1368.

Eeg-Olofsson, O., Malmros, I., Carl-Eric, E., and Steen, B. (1978). Convulsions in a breast-fed infant after maternal indomethacin. *Lancet* ii, 215.

Eidson, M., Philen, R.M., Sewell, C.M., Voorhees, R., and Kilbourne, E.M. (1990). L-tryptophan and eosinophilia–myalgia syndrome in New Mexico. *Lancet* 335, 645.

Eiser, R., Neff, M.S., and Slifkin, R.F. (1982). Acute myoglobinuric renal failure, a consequence of the neuroleptic malignant syndrome. *Arch. Intern. Med.* 142, 601.

Ellis. F.R., Harriman, D.G.F., and Currie, S. (1978). Screening for malignant hyperthermia in susceptible patients. In *Second international symposium on malignant hyperthermia* (ed. J.A. Aldreta and B.A. Britt), p. 273. Grune and Stratton, New York.

Estes, M.L., Ewing-Wilson, D., Chou, S.M., Mitsumoto, H., Hanson, M., Shirey, E., *et al.* (1987). Chloroquine neuromyotoxicity. Clinical and pathologic perspective. *Am. J. Med.* 82, 447.

Evans, D.A.P., Manley, K.A., and McKusick, V.A. (1960). Genetic control of isoniazid metabolism in man. *Br. Med. J.* ii, 485.

Evans, J.M. and Keogh, J.A.M. (1977). Adverse reactions to intravenous anaesthetic induction agents. *Br. Med. J.* ii, 735.

Fahn, S., Cote, L.J., Snider, S.R., Barrett. R.E., and Isgreen, W.P. (1979). The role of bromocriptine in the treatment of parkinsonism. *Neurology* (N.Y.) 29, 1077.

Feiner, L.A., Younge, B.R., Kazmier, F.J., Stricker, B.H., and Fraunfelder, F.T. (1987). Optic neuropathy and amiodarone therapy. *Mayo Clin. Proc.* 62, 702.

Fernandes, L., Swinson, D.R., and Hamilton. E.B.D. (1977). Dermatomyositis complicating penicillamine treatment. *Ann. Rheum. Dis.* 36, 94.

Fernandez-Sola, J., Campistol, J., Casademont, J., Grau, J.M., and Urbano-Marquez, A. (1990). Reversible cyclosporin myopathy. *Lancet* 335, 362.

Fernandez, P.G., Sahni. S., Galway. B.A., Granter, S., and McDonald, J. (1981). Urinary incontinence due to interaction of phenoxybenzamine and alpha-methyldopa. *Can. Med. Assoc. J.* 124. 174.

Fewings, J.D., Burns, R.J., and Kakulas, B.A. (1973). A case of acute emetine myopathy. In *Clinical studies in myology* (ed. B.A. Kakulas), p. 594. Excerpta Medica, Amsterdam.

Fish, D.R. and Espir, M.L.E. (1988). Convulsions associated with anti-malarial drugs: implications for people with epilepsy. *Br. Med. J.* 297, 526.

Fontiveros, E.S., Cumming, W.J.K., and Hudgson, P. (1980). Procainamide-induced myositis. *J. Neurol. Sci.* 45, 143.

Forfar, J.C., Brown. G.J., and Cull, R.E. (1979). Proximal myopathy after beta-blockade. *Br. Med. J.* ii. 1331.

Foster, J.B. (1974). Clinical features of some miscellaneous neuromuscular disorders. In *Diseases of voluntary muscle* (3rd edn) (ed. J.N. Walton), p. 890. Churchill Livingstone, Edinburgh .

Frankle, M.A., Eichbert, R., and Zachariah, S.B. (1988). Anabolic androgenic steroids and a stroke in an athlete: case report. *Arch. Phys. Med. Rehabil.* 69, 623.

Fraser, A.G. and Harrower, A.D.B. (1977). Convulsions and hyperglycaemia associated with nalidixic acid. *Br. Med. J.* ii. 1518.

Freedman, M.H., Boyden, M., Taylor, M., and Skarf, B. (1988). Neurotoxicity associated with deferoxamine therapy. *Toxicology* 49, 283.

Friedman, R., Zitelli, B., Jardine, B., and Fireman, P. (1982). Seizures in a patient receiving terbutaline. *AJDC* 136, 1091.

Frisoni, G.B. and Di-Monda, V. (1989). Disulfiram neuropathy: a review and report of a case. *Alcohol Alcohol.* 24, 429.

Gabriel, R. (1978). Circumoral paraesthesiae and labetalol. *Br. Med. J.* i, 580.

Gardner-Thorpe, C. and Benjamin, S. (1971). Peripheral neuropathy after disulfiram administration. *J. Neurol. Neurosurg. Psychiatry* 34, 253.

Gastaut, J.L. (1986). Painful legs and moving toes. A drug-induced case. *Rev. Neurol.* 142, 641.

Gedroyc, W. and Shorvon, S.D. (1982). Acute intracranial hypertension and nalidixic acid therapy. *Neurology* (N.Y.) 32, 212.

Gerlach, J. and Casey, D.E. (1988). Tardive dyskinesia. *Acta Psychiatr. Scand.* 77, 369.

Gherardi, R., Baudrimont, M., Gray, F., and Louarn, F. (1987). Almitrine neuropathy. A nerve biopsy study of 8 cases. *Acta Neuropathol.* 73, 202.

Giansiracusa, D.F., Blumberg, S., and Kantrowitz, F.G. (1980). Aseptic meningitis associated with ibuprofen. *Arch. Intern. Med.* 140, 1553.

Gibb, W.R.G. and Lees, A.J. (1985). The neuroleptic malignant syndrome — a review. *Q. J. Med.* 56, 421.

Glazer, W.M., Bower, M.B., Charney, D.S., and Heninger, G.R. (1989). The effect of neuroleptic discontinuation on psychopathology, involuntary movements, and biochemical measures in patients with persistent tardive dyskinesia. *Biol. Psychiatry* 26, 224.

Goekoop, J.G. and Carbaat, P.A.T.H. (1982). Treatment of neuroleptic malignant syndrome with dantrolene. *Lancet* ii, 49.

Golbe, L.I. and Merkin, M.D. (1986). Cerebral infarction in a user of free-base cocaine ('crack'). *Neurology* (N.Y.) 36, 1602.

Goldstein, N.P., Gibilisco, J.A., and Rushton, J.G. (1963). Trigeminal neuropathy and neuritis. *JAMA* 184, 458.

Gordon, M. and Gordon, A.S. (1981). Perhexiline maleate as a cause of reversible parkinsonism and peripheral neuropathy. *J. Am. Geriatr. Soc.* 29, 259.

Goren, M.P., Wright, R.K., Pratt, C.B., and Pell, F.E. (1986). Dechlorethylation of ifosfamide and neurotoxicity. *Lancet* ii, 1219.

Goy, J.J., Stauffer, J.C., Deruaz, J.P., Gillard, D., Kaufmann, U., Kuntzer, T., *et al.* (1989). Myopathy as possible side-effect of cyclosporine. *Lancet* i, 1446.

Grant, R. (1984). Neuroleptic malignant syndrome. *Br. Med. J.* 288, 1690.

Greensplan, A. and Treat, J. (1988). Peripheral neuropathy and low dose cisplatin. *Am. J. Clin. Oncol.* 11, 660.

Grezard, O., Lebranchuy, Y., Birmele, B., Sharobeem, R. Nivet, H., and Bagros, P.H. (1990). Cyclosporin-induced muscular toxicity. *Lancet* 335, 177.

Grossman, R.A., Hamilton, R.W., Morse, B.M., Penn, A.S., and Goldberg, M. (1974). Nontraumatic rhabdomyolysis and acute renal failure. *N. Engl. J. Med.* 291, 807.

Haas, D.C. and Marasigan, A. (1968). Neurological effects of glutethimide. *J. Neurol. Neurosurg. Psychiatry* 31, 561.

Hallberg, J.W., Draper, D.D., Topel, D.G., and Altrogge, D.M. (1983). Neural catecholamine deficiencies in the porcine stress syndrome. *Am. J. Vet. Res.* 44, 368.

Hansen, W.E. and Bertl, S. (1983). Inhibition of cholinesterases by ranitidine. *Lancet* i 235.

Hardie, R.J. and Lees, A.J. (1988). Neuroleptic-induced Parkinson's syndrome: clinical features and results of treatment with levodopa. *J. Neurol. Neurosurg. Psychiatry* 51, 850.

Harmant J., van Ryckevorsel-Harmant, K., de Barsy, Th., and Hendrickx, B. (1990). Fluvoxamine: an antidepressant with low (or no) epileptogenic effect. *Lancet* 336, 386.

Hassan, S.N. (1983). Urinary retention with theophylline. *South. Med. J.* 76, 408.

Heathfield, K.W.G. and Carabott. F. (1982). Adverse effects of perhexiline. *Lancet* i, 507.

Helson, L. and Duque, L. (1978). Acute brain syndrome after propranolol. *Lancet* i, 98.

Henderson, V.W. and Wooton, G.F. (1981). Neuroleptic malignant syndrome: a pathogenetic role for dopamine receptor blockade? *Neurology* (N.Y.) 31, 132.

Herishanu, Y. and Taustein, I. (1971). The electromyographic changes induced by antibiotics: a preliminary study. *Confin. Neurol.* 33. 41.

Hess, C.W., Hunziker, T., Kupfer, A., and Ludin, H.P. (1986). Thalidomide-induced peripheral neuropathy. A prospective clinical, neurophysiological and pharmacogenetic evaluation. *J. Neurol.* 233, 83.

Hintze, G., Klein, H.H., Prange, H., and Kreuzer, H.IL. (1987). A case of valproate intoxication with extensive brain oedema. *Klin. Wochenschr.* 65, 424.

Hitchins, R.N. and Thomson, D.B. (1988). Encephalopathy following cisplatin, bleomycin and vinblastine therapy for non-seminomatous germ cell tumour of testis. *Aust. N.Z. J. Med.* 18, 67.

Hodak, E., Gadoth, N., David, M., and Sandbank, M. (1986). Muscle damage induced by isotretinoin. *Br. Med. J.* 293, 435.

Hoefnagels, W.A.J., Gerritsen, E.J.A., Brouver, O.F., and Souverijn, J.H.N. (1988). Cyclosporin encephalopathy associated with fat embolism induced by the drug's solvent. *Lancet* ii, 901.

Holliday, P.L. and Bauer, R.B. (1983). Polyradiculoneuritis secondary to immunization with tetanus and diphtheria toxoids. *Arch. Neurol.* 40, 56.

Hosking, G.P. and Elliston. H. (1978). Benign intracranial hypertension in a child with eczema treated with topical steroids. *Br. Med. J.* i, 550.

Houghton, A.W.S. (1971). Convulsions precipitated by amitriptyline. *Lancet* i, 138.

Hudgson, P. and Hart, J.A.L. (1964). Acute ergotism: report of a case and a review of the literature. *Med. J. Aust.* ii, 589.

Hyser, C.L. and Drake. M.E. (1983). Myoclonus induced by metoclopramide therapy. *Arch. Intern. Med.* 143, 2201.

Indo, T. and Ando, K. (1982). Metoclopramide-induced parkinsonism. Clinical characteristics of ten cases. *Arch. Neurol.* 39, 494.

Inman, W.H.W. and Vessey, M.P. (1968). Investigation of deaths from pulmonary, coronary and cerebral thrombosis and embolism in women of childbearing age. *Br. Med. J.* ii, 193.

Inman, W.H.W., Westerholm, B., and Engelund, A. (1970). Thromboembolic disease and the steroidal content of oral contraceptives: a report to the Committee on Safety of Drugs. *Br. Med. J.* ii, 203.

Irey, N.S., McAllister, H.A., and Henry. J.M. (1978). Oral contraceptives and stroke in young women: a clinico-pathologic correlation. *Neurology* 28. 1216.

Jackson, M.J., Wagenmakers, A.J.M., and Edwards, R.H.T. (1987). The effects of inhibitors of arachidonic acid metabolism on efflux of intracellular enzymes from skeletal muscle following experimental damage. *Biochem. J.* 241, 403.

Jarvik, M.E. (1970). Drugs used in the treatment of psychiatric disorders. In *The pharmacological basis of therapeutics* (4th edn) (ed. L.S. Goodman and A. Gilman), p. 189. Macmillan, London.

Jenkins, P. and Emerson, P.A. (1981). Myopathy induced by rifampicin. *Br. Med. J.* 283, 105.

Jin-Yen, T. (1971). Clinical and experimental studies on mechanism of neuromuscular blockade by chloroquine diorotate. *Jpn J. Anesth.* 20, 491.

Johnson, D.A., Etter, H.S., and Reeves, D.M. (1983). Stroke and phenylpropanolamine use. *Lancet* ii, 970.

Joyce, R.P. and Gunderson, C.H. (1980). Carbamazepine-induced orofacial dyskinesia. *Neurology* (N.Y.) 30, 1333.

Kallay. M.C., Tabechian, H., Riley, G.R., and Chessin, L.N. (1979). Neurotoxicity due to ticarcillin in patient with renal failure. *Lancet* i, 608.

Kane, J.M. and Smith J.M. (1982). Tardive dyskinesia. *Arch. Gen. Psychiatry* 39, 473.

Kanterewicz, E., Bruguera, M., Viola, C., Lamarca, J., and Rodes, J. (1990). Toxic neuropathy after adenine arabinoside treatment in chronic HBsAg-positive liver disease. *J. Clin. Gastroenterol.* 12, 90.

Karstorp, A., Ferngren, H., Lundbergh, P., and Lving Tunell, U. (1973). Neuromyopathy during malaria suppression with chloroquine. *Br. Med. J.* iv, 736.

Kellam, A.M.P. (1987). The neuroleptic malignant syndrome, so called. *Br. J. Psychiatry* 150, 752.

Kilpatrick, C. and Ebeling, P. (1982). Intracranial hypertension in nalidixic acid therapy. *Med. J. Aust.* i, 252.

Kilpatrick, C., Braund, W., and Burns, R. (1982). Myopathy with myasthenic features possibly induced by codeine linctus. *Med. J. Aust.* ii, 410.

Kiruluta, G.H., Mercer, A.R., and Winsor, G.M. (1981). Prazosin as cause of urinary incontinence. *Urology* 18, 618.

Klawans, H.L.K. (1987). Dystonia and tremor following exposure to 2,3,7,8-tetrachlorodibenzo-p-dioxin. *Mov. Disord.* 2, 255.

Koehler, P.J. and Mirandolle, J.F.M. (1988). Neuroleptic malignant-like syndrome and lithium. *Lancet* ii, 1499.

Konikoff, F., Kuritzky A., Jerushahmi, Y., and Theodo, E. (1984). Neuroleptic malignant syndrome induced by a single injection of haloperidol. *Br. Med. J.* 289, 1228.

Kopin, I.J. and Markey, S.P. (1988). MPTP toxicity: implications for research in Parkinson's disease. *Annu. Rev. Neurosci.* 11, 81.

Kremer, I., Ritz. R., and Brummer, F. (1983). Aseptic meningitis as an adverse effect of co-trimoxazole. *N. Engl. J. Med.* 308, 1481.

Kushner. M.J. (1982). Chorea and cimetidine. *Ann. Intern. Med.* 96, 126.

Kuncl, R.W., Cronblath, D.R., Avila, O., and Duncan, G. (1989). Electrodiagnosis of human colchicine myoneuropathy. *Muscle Nerve* 12, 360.

Kuncl, R.W., Duncan, G., Watson, D., Alderson, K., Rogawski, M.A., and Peper, M. (1987). Colchicine myopathy and neuropathy. *N. Engl. J. Med.* 316, 1562.

Kunzendorf, V., Brockmoller, J., Jochinsen, F. Keller, F. Watz, G., and Offermann, G. (1988). Cyclosporin metabolites and central nervous system toxicity. *Lancet* i, 1223.

Kurlan, R. and Como, P. (1988). Drug-induced alzheimerism. *Arch. Neurol.* 45, 356.

Kwiencinski, H. (1978). Myotonia induced with clofibrate in rats. *J. Neurol.* 219, 107.

Lader, M.H. (1970). Drug-induced extrapyramidal syndromes. *J. R. Coll. Physicians Lond.* 5, 87.

Lancer, J.W. (l973). *The mechanism and management of headache* (2nd edn), p. 49. Butterworth, London.

The Lancet (1969). Thalidomide neuropathy. *Lancet* ii, 713.

The Lancet (1973a). Neurotoxicity of vincristine. *Lancet* i, 980.

The Lancet (1973b). Suxamethonium apnoea. *Lancet* i, 246.

The Lancet (1976). Diagnosis of brain death. A paper endorsed by the Conference of the Royal Colleges and Faculties of the U.K. *Lancet* ii, 1069.

The Lancet (1984). Neuroleptic malignant syndrome. *Lancet* i, 545.

The Lancet (1987). Colchicine myoneuropathy. *Lancet* ii, 668.

The Lancet (1988). Suxamethonium myalgia. *Lancet* ii, 944.

Lane, R.J.M. (1984). Drugs and tremor. *Adverse Drug React. Bull.* 106, 392.

Lane, R.J.M. (1988). Muscle involvement in systemic and iatrogenic disease. In *Recent advances in clinical neurology*, Vol. 5 (ed. C. Kennard), p 201. Churchill Livingstone, Edinburgh.

Lane, R.J.M. and Mastaglia, F.L. (1978). Drug-induced myopathies in man. *Lancet* ii, 562.

Lane, R.J.M. and Routledge, P.G. (1983). Drug-induced neurological disorders. *Drugs* 26, 124.

Lane, R.J.M., McLelland, N.J., Martin, A.M., and Mastaglia, F.L. (1979). Epsilon-aminocaproic acid (EACA) myopathy. *Postgrad. Med. J.* 55, 282.

Lane, R.J.M., Roche, S.W., Leung, A.A.W., Greco, A., and Lange, L.S. (1988). Cyclosporin neurotoxicity in cardiac transplant recipients. *J. Neurol. Neurosurg. Psychiatry* 51, 1434.

Lane, R.J.M., Davies, P.T.G., McLean, K.A., McCormack, S., Moss, J., and Woodrow, D.A. (1991). Muscle pathology in HIV infection: the role of zidovudine and significance of tubuloreticular inclusions. *Brain* (in press).

Lapierre, Y.D. and Anderson, K. (1983). Dyskinesia associated with amoxapine antidepressant therapy: A case report. *Am. J. Psychiatry* 140, 493.

Laurence, A.S. (1987). Myalgia and biochemical changes following intermittent suxamethonium administration. *Anaesthesia* 42, 503.

Legha, S.S. (1986). Vincristine neurotoxicity. Pathophysiology and management. *Med. Toxicol.* 1, 421.

Lely, A.H. and van Enter, C.H.J. (1970). Large-scale digitoxin intoxication. *Br. Med. J.* iii, 737.

Lewis, R.V. and McDevitt, D.G. (1986). Adverse reactions and interactions with beta-adrenoceptor blocking drugs. *Med. Toxicol.* 1, 343.

Lindholm, T. (1967). Electromyographic changes after nitrofurantoin (Furadantin) therapy in non-uraemic patients. *Neurology (N.Y.)* 17, 1017.

Litin, S.C. and Anderson, C.F. (1989). Nicotinic acid-associated myopathy: a report of three cases. *Am. J. Med.* 86, 481.

Lopez, J.R., Sanchez, V., and Lopez, M.J. (1989). Sarcoplasmic ionic calcium concentration in neuroleptic malignant syndrome. *Cell Calcium* 10, 223.

Loudon, J.B. and Waring, H. (1976). Toxic reactions to lithium and haloperidol. *Lancet* ii, 1088.

Lovelace, R.E. and Horwitz, S.J. (1968). Peripheral neuropathy in long-term diphenylhydantoin therapy. *Arch. Neurol.* 18, 69.

Lowe, T.L., Cohen, D.J., Detlor, J., Kramonitzer, M.W., and Straywitz, B.A. (1982). Stimulant medications precipitate Tourette's syndrome. *JAMA* 247, 1168.

Lulich, K.M., Goldie, R.G., Ryan, G., and Paterson, J.W. (1986). Adverse reactions to beta-2 agonist bronchodilators. *Med. Toxicol.* 1, 286.

Lundh, H. and Tunving, K. (1981). An extrapyramidal choreiform syndrome caused by amphetamine addiction. *J. Neurol. Neurosurg. Psychiatry* 44, 728.

Lustman, F., Moncu, G. (1974). Amiodarone and neurological side-effects. *Lancet* i, 568.

Macdonald, J.B. (1982). Muscle cramps during treatment with nifedipine. *Br. Med. J.* 285, 1744.

MacDonald. R.D. and Engel, A.G. (1970). Experimental chloroquine myopathy. *J. Neuropathol. Exp. Neurol.* 29, 479.

MacFarlane, I.A. and Rosenthal, F.D. (1977). Severe myopathy after status asthmaticus. *Lancet* ii, 615.

McGloughlin, C., Nesbitt, G.A., and Howe, J.P. (1988). Suxamethonium induced myalgia and the effect of preoperative administration of oral aspirin. *Anaesthesia* 43, 565.

Mackie, B.S. and Mackie, L.E. (1979). Systemic lupus erythematosus–dermatomyositis induced by sulphacetamide eye drops. *Australas. J. Dermatol.* 29, 49.

McLellan, D.L. and Swash, M. (1974). Choreoathetosis and encephalopathy induced by phenytoin. *Br. Med. J.* ii, 204.

MacLennan *et al.* 1990. Ryanodine receptor gene is a candidate for predisposition to malignant hyperthermia. *Nature* 343, 559.

Nature 343, 559.

McMillan, M.A., Ambis, D., and Siegel, J.H. (1978). Cimetidine and mental confusion. *N. Engl. J. Med.* 298, 284.

Maeda, K., Ueda, M., Ohtaka, H., Koyama, Y., Ohgami, M., and Miyazaki, H. (1987). A massive dose of vincristine. *Jpn J. Clin. Oncol.* 17, 247.

Maertens, P., Lum, G., Williams, J.P., and White, J. (1987). Intracranial haemorrhage and cerebral angiopathic changes in a suicidal phenylpropanolamine poisoning. *South. Med. J.* 80, 1584.

Maher, V.M.G., Pappu, A., Illingworth, D.R., and Thompson, G.R. (1989). Plasma mevalonate response in lovastatin-related myopathy. *Lancet* ii, 1098.

Mansour, A.M., Puklin, J.E., and O'Grady, R. (1988). Optic nerve ultrastructure following amiodarone therapy. *J. Clin. Neurol. Ophthalmol.* 8, 231.

Marsden, C.D., Parkes, J.D., and Rees. J.E. (1973). A year's comparison of treatment of patients with Parkinson's disease with levodopa combined with carbidopa versus treatment with levodopa alone. *Lancet* ii, 1459.

Martin, J. and Mainwaring, D. (1973). Coma and convulsions associated with vincristine therapy. *Br. Med. J.* iv, 282.

Martinez-Arizala, A., Sobol, S.M., McCarty, G.E., Nichols, B.R., and Rakita, L. (1983). Amiodarone neuropathy. *Neurology* 33, 643.

Meade, T.W., Greenberg, G., and Thompson, S.G. (1980). Progestogens and cardiovascular reactions associated with oral contraceptives and a comparison of the safety of 50- and 30 μg oestrogen preparations. *Br. Med. J.* 280, 1157.

Melgaard, B., Kohler, O., Sand-Hansen, H., Overgaard, J., Munck-Hansen, J., and Paulson, O.B. (1988). Misonidazole neuropathy. A prospective study. *J. Neurooncol.* 6, 227.

Meltzer, H.Y. and Moline, R. (1970). Plasma enzymatic activity after exercise. Study of psychiatric patients and their relatives. *Arch. Gen. Psychiatry* 22, 390.

Mendelsohn, G. (1978). Withdrawal reactions after oxazepam. *Lancet* i 565.

Meucci, G., Rossi, G., and Mazzoni, M. (1989). A case of transient choreoathetosis with amnesic syndrome after acute monoxide poisoning. *Ital. J. Neurol. Sci.* 10, 513.

Meza, I., Estrada, C.A., Mopntalvo, J.A., Hidalgo, W.N., and Andresen, J. (1989). Cerebral infarction associated with cocaine use. *Henry Ford Hosp. Med. J.* 37, 50.

Mezaki, T., Ohtani, S.I., Abe, K., Hirono, N., Udaka, F., and Kameyama, M. (1989). Benign type of malignant syndrome. *Lancet* i, 49,

Mifsud, A.J. (1988). Drug-related recurrent meningitis. *J. Infect.* 17, 151.

Miller. H.G. and Stanton, J.B. (1954). Neurological sequelae of prophylactic inoculation. *Q. J. Med.* 23, 1.

Miller, L.G. and Jankovic, J. (1990). Sulpiride-induced tardive dystonia. *Mov. Disord.* 5, 83.

Mitchell, A.B.S. and Parsons-Smith. B.G. (1969). Trichloroethylene neuropathy. *Br. Med. J.* i, 422.

Mitchell, M.M., Ali, H.H., and Savarese, J.J. (1978). Myotonia and neuromuscular blocking agents. *Anesthesiology* 49, 44.

Moyes, D.G. (1973). Malignant hyperpyrexia caused by trimeprazine. *Br. J. Anaesth.* 45, 1163.

Nakae, K., Yamamoto, S., and Shigematsu, I. (1973). Relation between subacute myelo-optic neuropathy (SMON) and clioquinol: nation-wide survey. *Lancet* i, 171.

Nazarian, S.M. and Jay, W.M. (1988). Bilateral optic neuropathy associated with amiodarone therapy. *J. Clin. Neurol. Ophthalmol.* 8, 25.

Neville, B.G.R. and Wilson, J. (1970). Benign intracranial hypertension following corticosteroid withdrawal in childhood. *Br. Med. J.* iii, 554.

Noppen, M., Velkeniers, B., Dierckx, R., Bruyland, M., and Vanhadst, L. (1987). Cyclosporin and myopathy. *Ann. Intern. Med.* 107, 945.

Ochoa, J. (1970). Isoniazid neuropathy in man. Quantitative electron microscopy study. *Brain* 93, 831.

Onda, K., Tekada, N., and Tanaka, R. (1987). Clinical course and CT findings in patients with contrast media associated figures. *No-To-Shinkei* 39, 331.

Page, P., Morgan, M., and Loh, L. (1972). Ketamine anaesthesia in paediatric procedures. *Acta Anaesthesiol. Scand.* 16, 155.

Palakurthy, P.R., Iyer, V., and Mecker, R.J. (1987). Unusual neurotoxicity associated with amiodarone therapy. *Arch. Intern. Med.* 147, 881.

Palmer, K.N.V. (1978). Muscle cramp and oral salbutamol. *Br. Med. J.* ii, 833.

Patterson, J.F. (1983). Amoxapine-induced chorea. *South. Med. J.* 76, 1077,

Pearson, M.G., Littlewood, S.M., and Bowden, A.N. (1981). Tetracycline and benign intracranial hypertension. *Br. Med. J.* 282, 568.

Perkoff, G.T., Silber, T., and Tyler, F.H. (1959). Studies in disorders of muscle. Xll. Myopathy due to the administration of therapeutic amounts of 17-hydroxycorticosteroids. *Am. J. Med.* 26, 1891.

Perry, R. and Jacobsen, E.S. 91984). Gold-induced encephalopathy. Case report. *J. Rheumatol.* 11, 233.

Petit, H., Leys, D., Hurtevent, J.F., Parent, M., Caron, J., Salomez, J.L., *et al.* (1987). Neuropathies and almitrine. 14 cases. *Rev. Neurol.* 143, 510.

Petitti. D.B. and Wingerd, J. (1978). Use of oral contraceptives, cigarette smoking and risk of subarachnoid haemorrhage. *Lancet* ii, 234.

Petrera, J.E., Fledelius, H.C., and Trojaborg, W. (1988). Serial pattern evoked potential recording in a case of toxic optic neuropathy due to ethambutol. *Electroencephalogr. Clin. Neurophysiol.* 71, 146.

Pfeiffer, R.F. and Sucha, E.L. (1985). On–off induced malignant hyperthermia. *Ann. Neurol.* 18, 138.

Pialoux, G., Kernbaum, S., and Vachon, F. (1988). Arsenical-induced encephalopathy during the treatment of African trypanosomiasis. *Bull. Soc. Pathol. Exot. Filiales* 81, 555.

Pierides, A.M., Alvarex-Ude, F., Kerr. D.N.S., and Skillen, A.W. (1975). Clofibrate-induced muscle damage in patients with chronic renal failure. *Lancet* ii, 1279.

Playford, R.J., Matthews, C.H., Campbell, M.J., Delves, H.T., Hla, K.K., Hodgson, H.J., *et al.* (1990). Bismuth induced encephalopathy caused by tripotassium dicitrato bismuthate in a patient with chronic renal failure. *Gut* 31, 359.

Prescott, L.F., Balali-Mood, M., Critchley, J.A.J.H., and Proudfoot, A.T. (1981). Avoidance of mefenamic acid in epilepsy. *Lancet* ii, 418.

Price. P., Parkes, J.D., and Marsden. C.D. (1978). Tiapride in Parkinson's disease. *Lancet* ii, 1106.

Ragab, A.H. (1973). Pyrimethamine in central nervous system leukaemia. *Lancet* i, 1061.

Ramirez, J.A., Mendell, J.R., Warmoltgs, J.R., and Griggs, R.C. (1986) Phenytoin neuropathy: structural changes in the sural nerve. *Ann. Neurol.* 19, 162.

Rampton, D.S. (1977). Hypertensive crisis in a patient given Sinemet, metoclopramide, and amitriptyline. *Br. Med. J.* ii, 607.

RCGP (1977). (Royal College of General Practitioners Oral Contraceptive Study). *Lancet* ii, 727.

Relling, M.V. (1989). Polymorphic drug metabolism. *Clin. Pharm.* 8, 852.

Reynolds, E.H. (1990). Vigabatrin: rational treatment for chronic epilepsy. *Br. Med. J.* 300, 277.

Ribera, E.F. and Dutka, A.J. (1983). Polyneuropathy associated with administration of hepatitis B vaccine. *N. Engl. J. Med.* 309, 614.

Richter, R.W., Challener. Y.B., Pearson, J., Kagen, L.J., Hamilton, L.L., and Ramsey, W.H. (1971). Acute myoglobinuria associated with heroin addiction. *JAMA* 216, 1172.

Riddoch, D., Jefferson, M., and Bickerstaff. E.R. (1971). Chorea and the oral contraceptives. *Br. Med. J.* iv, 217.

Ring, H.A. and Reynolds, E.H. (1990). Vigabatrin and behaviour disturbance. *Lancet* i, 970.

Ritchie, P. (1983). *Br. Med. J.* 287, 561.

Roberts, W.C. (1989). Safety of fenofibrate. US and worldwide experience. *Cardiology* 76, 169.

Robinson, M.K., Richens, A., and Oxley, R. (1990). Vigabatrin and behaviour disturbances. *Lancet* 336, 504.

Rongraff, M.E. (1959). Chlorothiazide overdosage effects in a two-year-old child. *Pa Med.* 62, 694.

Rosenberg, N.L., Myers, J.A., and Martin, W.R. (1989). Cyanide-induced Parkinsonism: clinical, MRI and 6-fluoro-dopa PET studies. *Neurology* (N.Y.) 39, 142.

Rosenblum, A.M. and Montgomery, E.B. (1980). Exacerbation of parkinsonism by methyldopa. *JAMA* 244, 2727.

Rosin, A.J., DeVereux, D., Eng, N., and Calne, D.B. (1979). Parkinsonism with 'on–off' phenomena. *Arch. Neurol.* 36, 32.

Rosin, M.A. (1981). Chlorzoxazone-induced spasmodic torticollis. *JAMA* 246, 2575.

Ross, D.R., Walker, J.I., and Peterson, J. (1983). Akathisia induced by amoxapine. *Am. J. Psychiatry* 140, 115.

Rothenberg, R.J. and Sufit, R.L. (1987). Drug-induced peripheral neuropathy in a patient with psoriatic arthritis. *Arthritis Rheum.* 30, 221.

Rozen, M.S. and Whan, R.McK. (1977). Prolonged curarisation associated with propranolol therapy. *Lancet* i, 73.

Rumpf, K., Albers, R., and Scheler, F. (1976). Clofibrate induced myopathy syndrome. *Lancet* i, 249.

Rupniak, N.M., Jenner, P., and Marsden, C.D. (1986). Acute dystonia induced by neuroleptic drugs. *Psychopharmacology* 88, 403.

Ruppert, G.B. and Barth, W.F. (1981). Tolmetin-induced aseptic meningitis. *JAMA* 245, 67.

Russell, D., Veger, J., Bunae, U. B., and Efskind, P.S. (1979). Epileptic seizures precipitated by atenolol. *J. Neurol. Neurosurg. Psychiatry* 42, 484.

Sander, J.W. and Hart, Y.M. (1990). Vigabatrin and behaviour disturbances. *Lancet* 335, 57.

Sandyk, R. (1983). Urinary incontinence associated with clonazepam therapy. *S. Afr. Med. J.* 64, 230.

Saqueton, A.C., Lonncz, A.L., Vick, N.A., and Hamer, R.D. (1969). Dapsone and peripheral motor neuropathy. *Arch. Dermatol.* 100, 214.

Schumm, F., Wietholter, H., and Fateh-Moghadam, A. (1981). Myasthenie-syndrom unter Chloroquin-therapie. *Dtsch. Med. Wochenschr.* 52, 1715.

Schwartz, M.T. and Calvert, J.F. (1990). Potential neurologic toxicity related to ciprofloxacin. *Drug Intell. Clin. Pharm.* 24, 188.

Sebille, A. (1978). Prevalence of latent perhexilene neuropathy. *Br. Med. J.* i, 1321.

Selden, R., and Sasahara, A.A. (1967). Central nervous system toxicity induced by lidocaine. Reports of a case in a patient with liver disease. *JAMA* 202, 908.

Serdaru, M., Diquet, B., and Lhermitte, F. (1982). Generalised seizures and ampicillin. *Lancet* ii, 617.

Shaikh, A. (1978). Urinary incontinence during treatment with depot phenothiazines. *Br. Med. J.* i, 1698.

Shalev, A., Hermesh, H., and Munitz, H. (1987). Severe akathisia causing neuroleptic failure. *Acta Psychiatr. Scand.* 76, 715.

Shanmagasundaram, T.K. (1980). Post-injection fibrosis of skeletal muscle: a clinical problem. *Int. Orthop.* 4, 31.

Sharma, D.B. and James, A. (1974). Benign intracranial hypertension associated with nitrofurantoin therapy. *Br. Med. J.* ii, 771.

Shaw. M.D.M., Russell, J.A., and Grossart. K.W. (1978). The changing pattern of spinal arachnoiditis. *J. Neurol. Neurosurg. Psychiatry* 41, 97.

Shetty, H.G.M. and Routledge, P.A. (1990). Adverse effects of hypolipidaemic drugs. *Adverse Drug React. Bull.* 142, 532.

Sikka, A., Keramann, E., Vrablek. R.M., and Grossman, L. (1983). Carpal tunnel syndrome associated with danazol therapy. *Am. J. Obstet. Gynecol.* 147, 102.

Singer, W.D. (1981). Transient Gilles de la Tourette syndrome after chronic neuroleptic withdrawal. *Dev. Med. Child Neurol.* 23, 518.

Slikkerveer, A. and de Wolff, F.A. (1989). Pharmacokinetics and toxicity of bismuth compounds. *Med. Toxicol. Adverse Drug Exp.* 4, 303.

Small, M., Durward, W.F., and Forbes, C.D. (1983). Seizures after infusion of factor Vlll. *Br. Med. J.* 286, 1106.

Smals, A.G.H., Beex, L.V.A., and Kloppenborg, P.W.C. (1977). Clofibrate-induced muscle damage with myoglobinuria and cardiomyopathy. *N. Engl. J. Med.* 296, 942.

Smith, P.A., Macdonald, T.R., and Jones, C.S. (1966). Convulsions associated with halothane anaesthesia. *Anesthesia* 21, 229.

Spaulding, W.B. (1979). Myalgia and elevated creatine phosphokinase with danazol in hereditary angioedema. *Ann. Intern. Med.* 90, 854.

Stephen, P.J. and Williamson, J. (1984). Drug-induced Parkinsonism in the elderly. *Lancet* ii, 1082.

Stephens, W.P., Eddy, J.D., Parsons, L.M., and Singh, S.P. (1978). Raised intracranial pressure due to per hexiline maleate. *Br. Med. J.* i, 21.

Sylvia, L.M., Forlenza, S.W., and Brocavich, J.M. (1988). Aseptic meningitis associated with naproxen. *Drug Intell. Clin. Pharm.* 22, 399.

Takeuchi, H., Yamada, A., Touge, T., Miki, H., Nishioka, M., and Hashimoto, S. (1988). Metronidazole neuropathy: a case report. *Jpn J. Psychiatry Neurol.* 42, 291.

Task Force (1980). Task Force on late neurological effects of antipsychotic drugs. Tardive dyskinesia: summary of a task force report of the American Psychiatric Association. *Am. J. Psychiatry* 137, 1163.

Tegner, R., Tome, F.M., Godeau, P., Lhermitte, F., and Fardeau, M. (1988). Morphological study of peripheral nerve changes induced by chloroquine treament. *Acta Neuropathol.* 75, 253.

Teicher, A., Rosenthal, T., Kissin, E., and Sarova, I. (1981). Labetalol induced toxic myopathy. *Br. Med. J.* 282, 1824.

Terrance, C.G. and Fromm, G.H. (1981). Complications of baclofen withdrawal. *Arch. Neurol.* 38, 588.

Terry, S.I. (1971). Transient dysaesthesiae and persistent leucocytosis after clioquinol therapy. *Br. Med. J.* iii, 745.

Thien, T.H., Delaere, K.R.J., Debruyne, F.M.J., and Keone, R.A.P. (1978). Urinary incontinence caused by prazosin. *Br. Med. J.* i, 622.

Thompson, G.E. (1972). Ketamine-induced convulsions. *Anesthesiology* 37, 662.

Tilzey, A., Heptonstall, J., and Hamblin, T. (1981). Toxic confusional state and choreiform movements after treatment with anabolic steroids. *Br. Med. J.* 283, 349.

Tolbert, J.A. (1988). Efficacy and long-term adverse effect pattern of lovastatin. *Am. J. Cardiol.* 62, 28J.

Tomlinson, I.W.K. and Rosenthal, F.D. (1977). Proximal myopathy after perhexiline maleate treatment. *Br. Med. J.* ii, 1319.

Toole, J.F. and Parrish, M.L. (1973). Nitrofurantoin polyneuropathy. *Neurology* (N.Y.) 23, 554.

Toole, J.F., Gergen, J.A., Hayes, D.M., and Felts, J.H. (1968). Neural effects of nitrofurantoin. *Arch. Neurol.* 18, 680.

Trimble, M. (1978). Non-monoamine oxidase inhibitor antidepressants and epilepsy: A review. *Epilepsia* 19, 241.

Tyrer, S. and Shopsin, B. (1980). Neural and neuromuscular side-effects of lithium. In *Handbook of lithium therapy* (ed. F.N. Johnson), p. 289. MTP Press, Lancaster.

Ueno, S., Takahashi, M., Kajiyama, K., Okahisa, N., Hazama, T., Yorifuji, S., and Tarui, S. (1987). Parkinson's disease and myasthenia gravis: adverse effect of trihexyphenidyl on neuromusclar transmission. *Neurology* (N.Y.) 37, 832.

van Garsse L.G.M.M., and Boeykens, P.P.H. (1990). Two patients with eosinophilia myalgia syndrome associated with tryptophan. *Br. Med. J.* 301, 21.

van Marle, W. and Woods, K. L. (1980). Acute hydrocortisone myopathy. *Br. Med. J.* 281, 271.

Vessey, M.P. (1973). Oral contraceptives and stroke. *N. Engl. J. Med.* 288, 906.

Vessey, M.P. and Doll, R. (1969). Investigation of relation between use of oral contraceptives and thromboembolic disease: a further report. *Br. Med. J.* ii, 651.

Vickrey, B.G. and Bahls, F.H. (1989). Non-convulsive status epilepticus following cerebral angiography. *Ann. Neurol.* 25, 199.

Vilter, R.W. (1986). Vidarabine-associated encephalopathy and myoclonus. *Antimicrob. Agents Chemother.* 29, 933.

Vyas, I. and Carney. M.W.P. (1975). Diazepam and withdrawal fits. *Br. Med. J.* ii, 44.

Walker, K.G., Eastmond, C.J., Best, P.V., and Matthews, K. (1990). Eosinophilia–myalgia syndrome associated with prescribed L-tryptophan. *Lancet* 336, 695.

Walls, T.J. and Pearce, S.J. (1980). Motor neuropathy associated with cimetidine. *Br. Med. J.* 281, 974.

Walther, P.J., Rossitch, E. Jr, and Bullard, D.E. (1987). The development of Lhermitte's sign during cisplatin chemotherapy. Possible drug-induced toxicity causing spinal cord demyelination. *Cancer* 60, 2170.

Warne, R.W. and Gubbay, S.S. (1979). Choreiform movements induced by anticholinergic therapy. *Med. J. Aust.* i, 465.

Wasserman, S. and Yahr, M.D. (1980). Choreic movements induced by the use of methadone. *Arch. Neurol.* 37, 727.

Weiner, W.J. and Luby. E.D. (1983). Persistent akathisia following neuroleptic withdrawal. *Ann. Neurol.* 13, 466.

Weinstein, L. (1970). Drugs used in the chemotherapy of leprosy and tuberculosis. In *The pharmacological basis of therapeutics* (4th edn) (ed. L.S. Goodman and A. Gilman), p. 1311. Macmillan, London.

Weir, R.J., Briggs. E., Browning, J., Mack. A., Naismith, L., Taylor, L., *et al.* (1971). Blood pressure in women after one year of oral contraception. *Lancet* i, 467.

Weiss, H.D., Walker, M.D., and Wiernik. P.H. (1974*a*). Neurotoxicity of commonly used antineoplastic agents. *N. Engl. J. Med.* 291, 75.

Weiss, H.D., Walker, M.D., and Wiernik. P.H. (1974*b*). Neurotoxicity of commonly used antineoplastic agents. *N. Engl. J. Med.* 291, 127.

Whelton, A., Carter, G.G., Garth, M.A., Darwish, M.O., and Walker, W.G. (1971). Carbenicillin-induced acidosis and seizures. *JAMA* 218, 1942.

Whisnant, J.P., Espinosa, R.E., Kierland. R.R., and Lambert, E.H. (1963). Chloroquine neuromyopathy. *Proc. Staff Meet. Mayo Clin.* 38, 501.

Whittaker, J.A., Parry, D.H., Bunch, C., and Weatherall, D.J. (1973). Coma associated with vincristine therapy. *Br. Med. J.* iii, 335.

Woodhouse, K.W. and Blain, P.G. (1983). Some organ-specific adverse reactions to cytotoxic drugs. *Adverse Drug React. Acute Poisoning Rev.* 2, 123.

Wray, A.R., Templeton, J., and Laird. J.D. (1978). Seizure following lumbar myelography with metrizamide. *Br. Med. J.* ii, 1787.

Yamada, M., Ohno, S., Okayasu, I., Okeda, R., Hatakeyama S., Watanabe, H., *et al.* (1986). Chronic manganese poisoning: a neuropathological study with determination of manganese distribution in the brain. *Acta Neuropathol.* 70, 273.

Yates, D.A.H. (1970). Steroid myopathy. In *Muscle diseases* (ed. J.N. Walton, N. Canal, and G. Scarlato), p. 482. Excerpta Medica, Amsterdam.

Zaal, M.J.W., de Vries, J., and Boen-Tan, Y.T.N. (1988). Is cyclosporin toxic to endothelial cells? *Lancet* ii, 956.

Zampollo, A., Sozzi, G., and Basso, F. (1988). Amitriptyline related peripheral neuropathy. Case report. *Ital. J. Neurol. Sci.* 9, 89.

19. Eye disorders

S. I. DAVIDSON and M. HICKEY-DWYER

Introduction

Almost all categories of drugs have been known to have toxic effects on the visual apparatus. Such toxicity may also be teratogenic, resulting in congenital ocular abnormalities.

All ocular structures are potentially vulnerable to drug-induced damage and unfortunately such effects may be irreversible and, indeed, may progress after withdrawal of the precipitating drugs. The majority of reports of ocular toxicity involve corticosteroids, the anti-inflammatory, and the antimalarial drugs, together with the phenothiazines and other tranquillizers (Davidson 1973).

In addition to the information provided here, readers will find it helpful to refer to the encyclopaedic contributions of Grant (1986) and Fraunfelder (1989).

Eyelids and periorbital tissues

Allergic drug reactions involving the eyelids and periorbital tissues are characterized by lid oedema and erythema. The initial treatment of hyperthyroidism with antithyroid drugs or radioactive iodine may cause acute periorbital oedema and induce or exacerbate exophthalmos (Slansky *et al.* 1967). A rapid onset of exophthalmos may occur with the use of lithium carbonate but this will resolve on discontinuing the drug (Rabin and Evans 1981), and long-term high-dosage corticosteroid therapy may also give rise to this problem (Cohen *et al.* 1981), as may vitamin A.

Whitening of the eyelashes and eyebrows (poliosis) may occur with amodiaquine, chloroquine, and hydroxychloroquine. Discolouration of the skin of the head and neck, involving the eyelids, often follows long-term treatment with chlorpromazine in large doses, the skin assuming a bronze or purplish-grey hue — the so-called purple-people syndrome (Feldman and Frierson 1964). Grey-brown pigmentation occurs in ochronosis induced by long-continued application of phenolic solutions to the skin. A more localized pigmentation, usually confined to the fornices, may result from the local application of solutions or ointments containing silver salts or adrenaline. Photosensitivity involving the eyelids may be caused by many drugs, but particularly the phenothiazines, sulphonamides, sulphonylurea derivatives, tetracyclines, and thiazide diuretics (Kirshbaum and Beerman 1964), but when the offending drug is withdrawn resolution of the skin lesions is usual. Alopecia of the eyelids and eyebrows has been attributed to actinomycin D, thallium, and vitamin A.

Striated muscle in the eyelids contracts in response to systemic administration of choline, acetylcholine, and nicotine. Adrenergic-neurone blocking drugs or ganglion-blocking drugs inhibit the normal sympathetic tone of Müller's muscle, which is responsible for adjustment of the height of the upper lid, causing a ptosis, an effect used therapeutically to counteract the lid retraction of dysthyroid eye disease, while sympathomimetic drugs produce lid retraction. Overdose of antimyasthenic drugs can result in the redevelopment of the initial myasthenic ptosis.

Conjunctiva

Application to the eye of any type of solution or ointment may result in inflammation of the conjunctiva in sensitive subjects. Conjunctival involvement in systemic drug toxicity is rare. The practolol-induced oculomucocutaneous syndrome resulted in subconjunctival fibrosis with occlusion of lacrimal ductules and destruction of the lacrimal glands, resulting in a severe and progressive dry-eye syndrome. In some cases this progressed to corneal ulceration, perforation, and endophthalmitis with loss of the eye (Wright 1975; Wright and Fraunfelder 1976). Fortunately this syndrome occurred only in about 0.2 per cent of patients taking the drug and has not been found to occur with other β-blocking agents.

Isotretinoin, used in the treatment of dermatological disorders, such as acne vulgaris, causes blepharoconjunctivitis in 40 per cent of patients (Blackman *et al.* 1979; Windhorst and Nigra 1982).

An important conjunctival reaction to systemic drug administration is the Stevens–Johnson syndrome. This is an idiosyncratic reaction with sight-threatening complications. There is an acute onset of an exudative conjunctivitis of variable degree which, if severe, may lead to symblepharon formation and corneal scarring with resultant diminished vision and even blindness. The acute exudative conjunctivitis is associated with fever and an erythematous bullous eruption of the skin. Drugs particularly implicated in this syndrome are the barbiturates, carbamazepine, chloramphenicol, chlorpropamide, phenytoin, and the sulphonamides.

It is worth noting that rifampicin may cause orange staining of hydrophilic (soft) contact lenses, due to excretion of the drug in the tears (Lyons 1979).

The cornea

The cornea is an avascular transparent structure. Its transparency is maintained by a normally functioning sodium-potassium pump in the endothelium, regular orientation of collagen fibres that compose the stroma, and a superficial intact epithelium, which in turn is dependent upon a normal tear film. Disturbance of any of these structures results in loss of transparency which may impair vision.

Corneal epithelial deposits may occur with the chronic systemic administration of several drugs, the most important of which are amiodarone, amodiaquine, chloroquine, hydroxychloroquine (Bernstein 1967), chlorpromazine, and clofazimine (Font *et al.* 1989). It is likely that the corneal epithelial deposits associated with amiodarone, chloroquine, or hydroxychloroquine are due to drug-induced corneal phospholipidosis. The deposits appear as fine granules in the epithelium, coloured grey or yellowish-brown, assuming a whorl-like pattern — the so-called cornea verticillata (vortex dystrophy). While vision is not seriously affected, the deposits may give rise to an appearance of haloes round lights or complaints of photophobia. Although most patients taking amiodarone develop a keratopathy after a few months (D'Amico *et al.* 1981), it is less common with chloroquine, appearing in 30–70 per cent of patients. The corneal deposits gradually disappear on withdrawal

of the culprit drug. Corneal opacities, which may be reversible, may occur with the use of oral isotretinoin (Weiss and Degnan 1981; Fraunfelder 1983).

Corneal stromal deposits have long been recognized to occur with metals such as copper, gold, mercury, and silver, and have also been attributed to chlorpromazine (Rashussen *et al.* 1976), clofazimine, and indomethacin (Burns 1968).

Chronic parenteral administration of gold compounds may give rise to deposition of gold in the cornea — ocular chrysiasis — which is dose-related, requiring administration of, usually, 0.5–1.5 g over several months before the corneal changes are noted (Kameyama *et al.* 1977). With the slit-lamp microscope, glittering opacities are visible deep in the epithelium (Bron *et al.* 1979); these will disappear if the drug is discontinued. In a more advanced stage, fine dust-like granules are seen throughout the corneal stroma with greatest density in the deeper layers. Vision is not affected.

Corneal calcification has complicated treatment with topical tretinoin (Avisar *et al.* 1988).

Reference has been made previously to the practolol oculomucocutaneous syndrome, in which the conjunctiva became involved. The cornea was affected slightly in most patients with superficial punctate lesions or small erosions, but severely in other patients, with central stromal opacification, ulceration, and (more rarely) perforation.

Although it has been suggested that contraceptive hormones may have an effect on tear production, may alter the corneal curvature, result in corneal oedema, or induce contact lens intolerance, controlled evaluation has not substantiated these observations (Reilingh *et al.* 1978).

Fluorouracil (5-fluorouracil) may cause circumcorneal oedema and corneal erosions (Caravella *et al.* 1981). Steroid drops or ointments should never be applied to the eye if there is any possibility that the lesion to be treated may be due to herpes simplex or to a fungal infection, because severe keratitis, ulceration, and even perforation of the globe may occur in these circumstances. Some authorities consider that steroid preparations should never be applied topically to the eye unless recommended by an ophthalmologist.

The pupil

Iritis is rarely caused by drugs, but it has been reported as part of an adverse reaction to chloroquine, and to eye drops or ointments containing ecothiopate iodide, demecarium bromide, or dyflos. Cysts of the iris may also result from treatment with the last three drugs.

Paresis (rather than paralysis) of accommodation and dilatation of the pupil often occurs with drugs administered systemically in the management of hypertension, parkinsonism, disturbances of the gastrointestinal tract, and allergies. Indeed, this is most probably the commonest ocular adverse reaction to systemic drug therapy. The anticholinergic action of such parasympatholytic agents results in symptoms of blurring of vision, which are more marked in younger patients than in presbyopes.

Pupillary dilatation may precipitate acute angle-closure glaucoma in patients with a predisposition to this disorder because of shallow anterior chambers — indeed, it is semidilatation of the pupil that is most dangerous. In patients who are under treatment for glaucoma, however, either open-angle or narrow-angle, parasympatholytic drugs are *not* contraindicated (Davidson 1975; *Drug and Therapeutics Bulletin* 1975).

Certain proprietary preparations for the common cold may induce mydriasis, for example, Contact 400 and Quinasp (Davidson 1973). Pupillary dilatation occurs in drug abuse with amphetamines and lysergic acid derivatives (Verin *et al.* 1977).

It must also be borne in mind that corticosteroids, especially when applied locally, cause a rise in intraocular pressure and may occasionally precipitate glaucoma in a patient predisposed to this condition.

Miosis resulting from systemic use of drugs is not common, the most familiar drugs being morphine and other opiate-like drugs that have a central action.

The lens

The normal lens is clear and avascular. Without doubt the commonest, and most important, drug-induced lens change is that due to corticosteroids. The lens opacities that occur are typically bilateral and posterior subcapsular in situation and can result from the use of a variety of glucocorticoids, when applied to the cornea (Crews 1965), to the skin (Costagliola *et al.* 1989), or when given by inhalation (Allen *et al.* 1989). The lens opacities develop slowly, and are irreversible and, because of their position relative to the nodal point of the eye, they cause a significant impairment of visual acuity even if the opacities are slight. In general 7.5 10 mg of prednisolone (or an equivalent dose of another steroid) per day for 12–18 months is unlikely to result in cataract formation, but individual susceptibility varies (Skalka and Prahal 1980).

Long-term administration and administration of the phenothiazines in high doses often results in the deposition of fine yellowish-brown granules beneath the anterior lens capsule. Vision is not significantly impaired, but the lesions are irreversible (Delong *et al.* 1965).

Although posterior subcapsular lens opacities have been suspected to occur in patients taking allopurinol (Fraunfelder *et al.* 1982a), particularly on exposure to ultraviolet light (Lerman *et al.* 1982, 1984), this has not been supported by further investigation (Jick and Brandt 1984).

Lens opacities have also been reported as adverse reactions to locally applied antibacterial drugs, ecothiopate iodide, demecarium bromide, and dyflos.

Drug-induced myopia is a rare and idiosyncratic reaction which is *not* attributable to parasympathomimetic contraction of the ciliary muscle resulting in spasm of accommodation for near vision; nor is there constriction of the pupil. Although the mechanism of acute idiosyncratic transient myopia is not fully understood, it appears that some alteration in the lens (degree of hydration?) is responsible for the change in refraction, possibly associated with shallowing of the anterior chamber. When the offending drug is withdrawn, the myopia disappears spontaneously within a few days (Dralands and Garvin 1972; Schroeder and Schwarzer 1978). Drugs noted to have produced acute transient myopia include acetazolamide (Maddalena 1968), sulphonamides (Maddalena 1968; Bovino and Marcus 1982), tetracyclines, and the thiazide diuretics (D'Alena and Robinson 1969). In the early stages of the treatment of diabetes mellitus with insulin or oral hypoglycaemic agents, there may be a fluctuating myopia.

The retina

Whilst retinal toxicity apparently results in abnormalities of the retinal pigment epithelium, the retinal photoreceptors often show associated changes.

The most frequently used drugs liable to cause retinal toxicity are the 4-aminoquinolines — chloroquine, hydroxychloroquine, and amodiaquine. Chloroquine is slowly eliminated and probably about 80 per cent of the drug is retained, the highest concentrations being found in melanin-containing tissues, particularly the retinal pigment epithelium. It is likely that toxicity involving the retinal pigment epithelium results in drug-induced lysosomal abnormalities, the photoreceptor lesions appearing to be secondary to retinal pigment epithelium dysfunction during 4-aminoquinoline therapy (Mackenzie 1983a). Although retinal toxicity is infrequent (probably about 1–2 per cent), avoidance is imperative, as permanent visual loss, even blindness, may occur. Initial symptoms are often non-specific (blurred vision, photophobia) but later impaired colour vision, reduction in visual acuity, loss of the foveal reflex, disturbances in macular pigmentation, and scotomata to red targets may be clinically apparent.

It appears that retinal toxicity is not idiosyncratic but dose-related; hydroxychloroquine is safer. The daily dose, rather than the total drug accumulation, seems to determine the development of retinopathy (Mackenzie 1983a). Although toxicity is low with 250 mg chloroquine (or 400 mg hydroxychloroquine) per day, to prevent overdose the dose should be calculated from the patient's *lean* body-weight and should not exceed 4 mg per kg per day of chloroquine or 6.5 mg per kg per day of hydroxy-chloroquine (Mackenzie 1983b).

Prolonged administration of a phenothiazine eventually results in a brown discolouration of the macula due to lipofuscin deposition in retinal ganglion cells. This is a harmless effect (Meier-Ruge 1977) and is not related to the retinal toxicity that may occur with thioridazine in patients receiving more than 600–800 mg per day within a 1–2 month period (Meredith *et al.* 1978). Although stopping thioridazine usually results in resolution of symptoms and fundal changes, as with chloroquine, retinal changes may progress, even after withdrawal of the drug (Brinkley *et al.* 1979).

Cardiac glycosides, principally digoxin, have long been recognized to give rise to visual disturbances when dosage has been excessive. Dazzling or glare phenomena and disturbances of colour vision predominate in the symptomatology but are reversible (Leopold 1968). Central scotomata with reduction of visual acuity have, however, been reported, suggesting that it is the retinal receptor cells that are principally involved (see Visual hallucinations).

Retinal vascular abnormalities, such as central retinal vein or artery occlusion and retinal perivasculitis, as well as macular oedema, have been observed in patients taking sex hormones for contraceptive (Davidson 1971) or other purposes (Rock *et al.* 1989), but whether these observations are significant remains unproven.

Overdosage with quinine has long been recognized as a cause of sudden loss of vision with variable recovery. Both eyes are always affected, the ophthalmoscopic findings being variable — retinal (macular) oedema, hyperaemia of the disc, occasionally a macular red spot, or even normal fundi. Recovery of central vision occurs but this is usually associated with persistent attenuation of the retinal arterioles and pallor of the optic nerve head. The mechanism of the retinal toxicity remains obscure. Electrodiagnostic tests would seem to indicate involvement of the photoreceptors and pigment epithelium in the early stages, but there also appears to be a direct toxic effect on the retinal ganglion cells. No treatment has proved of value (Bateman *et al.* 1985).

High dosage of the antioestrogen agent tamoxifen has resulted in deposition in the maculae of fine yellow-white refractile opacities and is also associated with cystoid macular oedema. Corneal deposits may also present as a vortex dystrophy (Mckeown *et al.* 1981; Kaiser-Kupfer *et al.* 1981).

Retinal detachment may complicate treatment with eye drops containing ecothiopate iodide, demecarium bromide, or dyflos.

The optic nerve

Toxic optic neuropathy always involves both eyes and generally has a rapid onset with a reduction in vision associated with hyperaemia and oedema of the optic discs or, in more chronic cases, optic atrophy.

Ethambutol may give rise to toxic optic neuropathy if the dosage exceeds 15 mg per kg daily (Barron *et al.* 1974); below this dosage level the risk is slight. An early symptom of toxicity is impaired colour vision (dys-chromatopsia), and patients should be warned of this possibility. Unilateral visual loss soon becomes bilateral, field loss being central. The early onset of toxicity may be identified by testing colour vision with Ishihara plates or the Farnsworth–Munsell '100 hue' test. The vitamin B_{12} analogue cobamamide (dibencozide), has been useful in some cases of ethambutol toxicity (Quere *et al.* 1976). Another antituberculous drug, isoniazid, may cause toxic optic neuropathy which may be associated with a peripheral neuropathy (Kass *et al.* 1957).

Optic neuropathy induced by chloramphenicol generally arises in prolonged treatment of children with cystic fibrosis (Harley *et al.* 1970). Visual loss is always bilateral, of varying severity, and usually accompanied by central scotomata. On examination, the discs appear hyperaemic and swollen but sometimes atrophic. If the symptoms are recognized early and the drug withdrawn, there may be some return of visual function. There is evidence to indicate that vitamin B_{12} given to such children in conjunction with chloramphenicol may prevent development of optic neuropathy.

Disulfiram, used in the management of alcoholism, can also cause a toxic optic neuropathy (Humblet 1953; Norton and Walsh 1972), but on cessation of treatment there is a rapid recovery of vision, usually within a month (Walsh and Hoyt 1982).

Clioquinol is a halogenated hydroxyquinoline used to treat gastrointestinal disturbances that has been associated with an epidemic of subacute myelo-optic neuropathy (SMON) (Kono *et al.* 1971; see also Chapter 18).

Severe visual loss may occur (Oakley 1973) and withdrawal of the drug may result in some recovery of visual function.

Swelling of the optic nerve head (papilloedema) as a result of drug therapy is invariably associated with an increase in cerebrospinal fluid pressure without any evidence of brain tumour or other brain disease — so-called benign intracranial hypertension or pseudotumour cerebri. Systemic corticosteroids, commonly prednisolone or triamcinolone, have given rise to this syndrome, most often in children when the corticosteroids are withdrawn or reduced. This may be due to adrenocortical insufficiency (*The Lancet* 1964) and management consists of temporarily increasing the corticosteroid and then reducing it more slowly. Tetracyclines (including minocycline — Le Bris *et al.* 1988) can also produce benign intracranial hypertension, particularly in infants but it is reversible on cessation of the drug (van Dyk and Swan 1969). The antibacterial nalidixic acid may also induce intracranial hypertension with papilloedema, principally in infants and children; this disappears on drug withdrawal, being probably due to a metabolic acidosis (Boreus and Sundstrom 1967). More commonly, however, nalidixic acid gives rise to reversible visual disturbances such as photopsia, photophobia, or temporary loss of vision as well as disturbances of colour vision. Excessive amounts of vitamin A cause elevated intracranial pressure with papilloedema, and in children this may occur within 12 hours of the administration of 100 000 units (Crews 1974). Finally, as oral contraceptives may cause benign intracranial hypertension, papilloedema may also accompany the use of these preparations (Davidson 1971). This subject is also discussed in Chapter 18.

Although colour vision disturbances are rare, they are important as they may be the presenting symptom of drug toxicity. Any drug that is toxic to the optic nerve may cause a disturbance in colour vision which may be assessed with Ishihara colour plates or the Farnsworth–Munsell '100 hue' test. Xanthopsia has been described in patients taking barbiturates, methaqualone, oral contraceptives, streptomycin, sulphonamides, or thiazide diuretics, and a recent case implicated desferrioxamine (Benc *et al.* 1989), but the most frequently prescribed drug causing this problem is digitalis and, indeed, xanthopsia is a useful pointer to the presence of digoxin toxicity (Arronson and Ford 1980). This visual problem is dose-related and occurs when the serum digoxin is above $2 \mu g$ per litre. As electroretinographic studies have shown a reduced sensitivity to red, there is probably a direct toxic effect on the cones. The red–green defect is reversible.

Disturbances of ocular movements

Extraocular muscle palsies secondary to drugs are caused by a toxic effect on either nerve or muscle. Drugs that may cause such palsies are cardiac glycosides; chloroquine; heavy metals (e.g. gold, lead, and thallium); quinine; the rauwolfia alkaloids such as reserpine (rarely used nowadays); and the sulphonamides.

Barbiturates may cause abnormal pursuit movements and total ophthalmoplegia (Tedeschi *et al.* 1983). External ophthalmoplegia and oculogyric crises can occur when toxic serum levels are reached. Gaze palsies may also be produced (Edis and Mastaglia 1977).

Involuntary eye movements can occur due to levodopa treatment (Shimizu *et al.* 1977). Overdosage of thioridazine may produce ocular motility disturbances and has been reported to cause internuclear ophthalmoplegia (Cook *et al.* 1981).

Many drugs give rise to nystagmus, usually reversible on withdrawal of the precipitating agent, and examples of such drugs include chlordiazepoxide, diazepam, fenfluramine, mephenesin, phenytoin, and salicylates, usually with high dosage (Siddal 1966; Davidson 1973). Downbeat nystagmus can be caused by carbamazepine (Wheeler *et al.* 1982), and lithium (Engelhardt and Neundörfer 1988; Williams *et al.* 1988; Halmagyi *et al.* 1989), and vertical nystagmus may occur with barbiturates, particularly in children. Vestibular nystagmus can follow from the toxic effects of streptomycin on the vestibular apparatus (*Adverse Drug Reaction Bulletin* 1969).

Oculogyric crises (sudden uncontrollable elevation of both eyes accompanied by neck retraction and twitching of the shoulder girdle muscles) can be produced by the piperazine series of the phenothiazines (Apt 1967). These are due to extrapyramidal change and are dose-related. So-called tardive oculogyric crises have been observed in elderly women treated with antipsychotic drugs for 3–16 years, as part of tardive dyskinesia (Fitzgerald and Jankovic 1989).

Higher visual centres

Visual hallucinations

Higher visual centre dysfunction may be clinically manifest by complaints either of perception of unformed visual images (e.g. flashes of light) or of formed visual images (hallucinations). Overdosage of drugs acting on the central nervous system may cause such symptoms; they usually disappear on withdrawal of the offending drug.

Visual hallucinations may be caused by bromides, chlorpromazine and frusemide (Willetts 1969), pentazocine, primidone, and salicylates (Davidson 1973). Atropine, either orally or topically, may produce visual hallucinations, and ketamine may cause visual hallucinations and nightmares which may recur for months (Hawks et al. 1971). Again, digitalis may cause visual hallucinations (Volpe and Soave 1979), as can oral contraceptives, the latter possibly altering the circulation of the occipital cortex. Cannabis and lysergic acid derivatives cause vivid visual hallucinations.

Transient amaurosis

As has been mentioned previously, nalidixic acid may produce this effect, possibly related to its action of raising intracranial pressure.

Cortical blindness

Transient cortical blindness has been reported in children given vincristine (Byrd et al. 1981), and in adults following the use of the immunosuppressant cyclosporin (Hughes 1990), the cytotoxic drug cisplatin (Lindeman et al. 1990), and arteriography of various types (Lantos 1989). Excessive doses of salicylates or barbiturates can produce cortical blindness, and it should be noted that undue reduction of high blood pressure in hypertensives and arteriopaths can also cause blindness.

Fetal abnormalities

Drugs taken by mothers in the first trimester of pregnancy can cause malformations of the developing eye and adnexa. Phenytoin has been reported to cause optic nerve hypoplasia (Hoyt and Billson 1978). Busulfan has given rise to microphthalmos and pigmentary degeneration of the retina (Saraux and Lefrancois 1977). Troxidone (trimethadione), another anticonvulsant, has given rise to the fetal trimethadione syndrome, affecting children of epileptic mothers taking this drug and characterized by V-shaped eyebrows, epicanthus and, more rarely, myopia and strabismus, associated with a number of non-ocular congenital anomalies (Zackai et al. 1975). Clomiphene has been reported to cause congenital retinal aplasia (Laing et al. 1981). Teratogenesis affecting the eyes of children of mothers who have taken warfarin during early pregnancy has been well documented; anomalies reported include optic atrophy, microphthalmos, lens opacity, and large eyes (Shaul and Hall 1977).

Isotretinoin is a potent teratogen in man. In addition to many non-ocular malformations, it causes microph-7thalmos and maldevelopment of the visual pathways (Benke 1984; Hill 1984). This subject is also discussed in Chapter 5.

Systemic effects of topical ophthalmic therapy

Although most of these effects are discussed in other chapters, they are also mentioned here to emphasize their importance.

Absorption of instilled drops may be reduced by advising patients to occlude the nasolacrimal duct immediately after instillation of drops by pressing over the lacrimal punctum to minimize nasal mucosal absorption. The systemic effects that may arise from topical ocular therapy may be considered in three main groups: cardiovascular and respiratory effects, autonomic effects, and central nervous system effects.

Cardiovascular system

Systemic absorption of topical β-blocker agents used in the management of glaucoma, such as carteolol, levobunolol, metipranolol, and timolol, may result in bradycardia, hypotension, or cardiac failure. Caution must therefore be taken when prescribing for patients with poor cardiac function, as the negative inotropic effect of such drops can precipitate cardiac failure. Such β-blockers are contraindicated in patients with bradycardia and heart block, and must not be prescribed for patients who are already taking verapamil (Pringle and MacEwen 1987). These non-selective β-blocking agents may also precipitate bronchospasm in patients who suffer from asthma or chronic obstructive airway disease. While betaxolol is more cardioselective, it too may cause bronchospasm in patients with asthma and chronic airway disease, and thus should also be avoided.

The topical use of adrenaline in the eye may induce extrasystoles, and may also cause faintness, pallor, sweating, tachycardia, and occipital headache with a marked rise in blood pressure (Lansche 1966). Dipivefrine, a prodrug of adrenaline, may have similar effects. It is therefore advisable to avoid these drugs in patients with cardiac disease or hyperthyroidism (Davidson 1974). Systemic absorption of phenylephrine drops produces elevation of both systolic and diastolic blood pressure, usually associated with a reflex bradycardia (Wilensky and Woodward 1973) which is particularly likely to occur in premature infants (Borromeo-McGrail *et al.* 1973). Accordingly, it is advisable to avoid 10% solutions of the drug and use a lower strength (2.5%) for pupillary dilatation. Phenylephrine drops are contra-indicated in patients who are already taking monoamine oxidase inhibitors, and should be used with caution in patients on tricyclic antidepressants or atropine, as well as patients with hypertension, advanced arteriosclerotic changes, aneurysms, orthostatic hypotension, or long-standing insulin-dependent diabetes mellitus (Fraunfelder and Meyer 1987).

Anticholinesterase miotic drops (ecothiopate iodide), which are occasionally used in the management of glaucoma, depress serum pseudocholinesterase and erythrocyte cholinesterase levels asymptomatically. Such patients are at risk of prolonged apnoea if given suxamethonium in conjunction with a general anaesthetic because of the persistence of suxamethonium, which is not broken down at the normal rate because of the lack of the specific active enzyme (Pantuck 1966).

Autonomic nervous system

The autonomic nervous system may be affected by the systemic absorption of cholinergic drugs, such as pilocarpine, anticholinesterase agents (e.g. eserine and ecothiopate iodide), or sympathomimetic drugs (e.g. phenylephrine).

Pilocarpine, which may be used in frequent doses when treating acute angle-closure glaucoma, may cause the symptoms and signs of acute systemic cholinergic toxicity: nausea, vomiting, sweating, abdominal cramps, diarrhoea, and salivation. There may be respiratory distress due to bronchiolar spasm, tachycardia, or bradycardia, and hypotension. Muscular weakness, tremor, and confusion may occur in severe cases. The drug may cause symptomatic atrioventricular block (Littmann *et al.* 1987) in as low a dose as 2.5 ml of a 4% solution of pilocarpine (Davidson 1974).

Treatment with anticholinesterases results in decreased amounts of cholinesterase, with accumulation of acetylcholine in neural tissues or effector organs, which produces abdominal cramps, diarrhoea, increased sweating, and weakness. Occasionally, rhinorrhoea, peripheral muscle cramps, and salivation occur, as well as neurological symptoms of paraesthesiae, hyperaesthesia, and pyramidal tract signs; but usually symptoms and signs are mild and disappear soon after discontinuation of the drug. For severe toxic symptoms treatment with atropine may be necessary.

Central nervous system effects

The anticholinergic group of drugs used to dilate the pupil — tropicamide, cyclopentolate, homatropine, and atropine — may produce manifestations of central nervous system toxicity, the very young and the elderly being particularly susceptible. Toxicity may be manifest by a confusional psychosis, cortical disturbances, or cerebellar dysfunction. These ill effects occur most frequently with cyclopentolate and are dose-dependent (Fraunfelder and Meyer 1987).

Miscellaneous

Hypoplasia of the bone marrow and even aplastic anaemia (Davidson 1974; Abrams *et al.* 1980; Fraunfelder *et al.* 1982*b*; Flach 1982) have occurred during the chronic use of chloramphenicol drops. Iodide drops have been reported to induce thyrotoxicosis (Andre *et al.* 1988).

Finally it is worth pointing out that vitamin A, in the form of 'antiwrinkle' cream applied to the skin of the lids, can be absorbed systemically.

References

Abrams,S.M., Degnan, T.J., and Vinciguerra, V. (1980). Marrow aplasia following topical application of chloramphenicol ointment. *Arch. Intern. Med.* 140, 567.

Adverse Drug Reaction Bulletin (1969). Drugs and the eye. *Adverse Drug React. Bull.* 17. 45.

Allen, M.B., Ray, S.G., Leitch, A.G., Dhillon, B., and Collen, B. (1989).Steroid aerosols and cataract formation. *Br. Med. J.* 299, 432.

Andre, F., Bielefeld, P., Besancenot, J.F., Belleville, I., Sgro, C., and Martin, F. (1988). False innocuousness of eye drops apropos of one case of thyrotoxicosis induced by iodide. *Therapie* 43, 431.

Apt, L. (1967). In *Symposium on ocular therapy No. 4*, Vol. 2 (ed. I.H.Leopold), p. 102. C.V. Mosby, St Louis.

Arronson, J.K. and Ford, A.R. (1980). The use of colour vision measurement in the diagnosis of digoxin toxicity. *Q. J. Med.* 195, 273.

Avisar, R., Deutsch, D., and Savir, H. (1988). Corneal calcification in dry eye disorders associated with retinoic acid treatment. *Am. J. Ophthalmol.* 106, 753.

Ballin, N., Becker, B., and Goldman, M.L. (1966). Systemic effects of epinephrine applied topically to the eye. *Invest. Ophthalmol.* 5, 125.

Barron, G.J., Tepper, L., and Iovine, G. (1974) Ocular toxicity from ethambutol. *Am. J. Ophthalmol.* 77, 256.

Bateman, D.N., Blain, P.G., Woodhouse, K.W., Rawlins, M.D., Dyson, H., Heyworth, R., *et al.* (1985). Overdosage: lack of efficacy of techniques intended to enhance elimination. *Q. J. Med.* 1, 54 and 125.

Bene, C., Manzier, A., Bene, D., and Kranias, G. (1989). Irreversible ocular toxicity from single 'challenge' dose of deferoxamine. *Clin. Nephrol.* 31, 45.

Benke, P.J. (1984). Isoretinoin teratogen syndrome. *JAMA* 251, 3267.

Bernstein, H.M. (1967). Chloroquine ocular toxicity. *Surv. Ophthalmol.* 12, 415 .

Blackman, H.J., Peck, F.L., Olsen,T.G., and Bergsma, D.R. (1979). Blepharoconjunctivitis: a side effect of 13-cis-retinoic acid therapy for dermatologic diseases. *Ophthalmology* (Rochester) 86, 753.

Boreus, L.O. and Sundstrom, B. (1967). Intracranial hypertension in a child during treatment with nalidixic acid. *Br. Med. J.* ii, 744.

Borromeo-McGrail, V., Bordiuk, J.M., and Keitel, H. (1973). Systemic hypertension following ocular administration of 10% phenylephrine in the neonate. *Pediatrics* 51, 1032.

Bovino, J.A. and Marcus, D.F. (1982). The mechanism of transient myopia induced by sulfonamide therapy. *Am. J. Ophthalmol.* 94, 99.

Brinkley, J.R., Dubois, E.L., and Ryan, S.J. (1979). Longterm course of chloroquine retinopathy after cessation of medication. *Am. J. Ophthalmol.* 88, 1.

Bron, A. J., McLendon, B.F., and Lamp, A.V. (1979). Epithelial deposition of gold in the cornea in patients receiving systemic therapy. *Am. J. Ophthalmol.* 88, 354.

Burns, C.A. (1968). Indomethacin induced retinal sensitivity and corneal deposits. *Am. J. Ophthalmol..* 66, 825.

Byrd, R.L., Rohrbaugh, T.M., Raney, R.B. Jr, and Norris, D.G. (1981). Transient cortical blindness secondary to vincristine therapy in childhood malignancies. *Cancer* 47, 37.

Caravella, L.P., Burns, J.A., and Zangmeister, M. (1981). Punctal canalicular stenosis related to systemic fluorouracil therapy. *Arch. Ophthalmol.* 99, 284.

Cohen, B.A., Som, P.M., Haffner, P.H., and Friedman, A. H. (1981). Case report — steroid exophthalmos. *J. Comp. Assist. Tomogr.* 5, 907.

Cook, F.F., Davis, G., and Russo, L.S. (1981). Internuclear ophthalmoplegia caused by phenothiazine intoxication. *Arch. Neurol.* 38, 465.

Costagliola, C., Cati-Giovanelli, B., Piccirillo, A., and Delfino, M. (1989). Cataracts associated with long-term topical steroids. *Br. J. Dermatol.* 120, 472.

Crews, S.J. (1965). Adverse reactions to corticosteroid therapy in the eye. *Proc. R. Soc. Med.* 58, 533.

Crews, S.J. (1974). Adverse drug reactions in neuro-ophthalmology. In *Aspects of neuro-ophthalmology* (ed. S.I. Davidson), p. 155. Butterworth, London.

Cronin, T.P. (1964). Cataract with topical use of corticosteroid and idoxuridine. *Arch. Ophthalmol.* 72, 198.

D'Alena, P. and Robinson, M. (1969). Hygroton-induced myopia. *Calif. Med.* 110, 134.

D'Amico, D.J., Kenyon, K.R., and Ruskin J.N. (1981). Amiodarone keratopathy: drug induced lipid storage disease. *Arch. Ophthalmol.* 99, 257.

Davidson, S.I. (1971). Reported adverse effects of oral contraceptives on the eye. *Trans. Ophthalmol. Soc. U.K.* 91, 561.

Davidson, S.I. (1973). Reports of ocular adverse reactions. *Trans. Ophthalmol. Soc. U.K.* 93, 495.

Davidson, S.I. (1974). Systemic effects of eye drops. *Trans. Ophthalmol. Soc. U.K.* 94, 487.

Davidson, S.I. (1975). In *Recent advances in ophthalmology* (ed. P.D. Trevor-Roper), p. 284. Churchill Livingstone, Edinburgh.

De Juan, E. Jr and Maumenee, A.E. (1982). Steroid glaucoma. *Invest. Ophthalmol. Vis. Sci.* 22 (suppl.) Abstract 23.

DeLong, S.L.,. Poley, B.J., and McFarlane, J.R. (1965). Ocular changes associated with long term chlorpromazine therapy. *Arch. Ophthalmol.* 73, 611.

Donshik, P.C., Cavanaugh, H.D., Boruchoss, S.A., and Dohlman, C.H. (1981). Posterior subcapsular cataracts induced by topical corticosteroids following keratoplasty for keratoconus. *Ann. Ophthalmol.* 13, 29.

Dralands, L. and Garvin, P. (1972). The injurious effect of systemic medications on the visual apparatus. *Bull. Soc. Belge Ophthalmol.* 160, 447.

Drug and Therapeutics Bulletin (1975). Tricyclic antidepressives and glaucoma: what is the risk? *Drug Ther. Bull.* 13, 7.

Edis, R.H. and Mastaglia, F.L. (1977). Vertical gaze palsy in barbiturate intoxication. *Br. Med. J.* i, 144.

Engelhardt, A. and Neundörfer, B. (1988). Downbeat nystagmus in lithium medication. *Nervenarzt* 59, 624.

Espildora, C.J., Vicuna, C.P., and Diaz, B.E. (1981). Cortisone glaucoma; concerning 44 eyes. *J. Fr. Ophtalmol.* 4, 503.

Feldman, P.E. and Frierson, B.D. (1964). Dermatological and ophthalmological changes associated with prolonged chlorpromazine therapy. *Am. J. Psychiatry* 121, 187.

Fitzgerald, P.M. and Jankovic, J. (1989). Tardive oculogyric crises. *Neurology* (N.Y.) 39, 1434.

Flach, A.J. (1982). Fatal aplastic anaemia following topical administration of ophthalmic chloramphenicol. *Am. J. Ophthalmol.* 94, 420.

Font, R.L., Sobul, W., and Matoba, A. (1989). Polychromatic corneal and conjunctival crystals secondary to clofazimine. *Ophthalmology* 96, 311.

Fraunfelder, F.T. (1983). Ocular side effects of isotretinoin therapy. *JAMA* 250, 2545.

Fraunfelder, F.T. (1989). *Drug induced ocular side effects and drug interactions* (3rd edn). Lea and Febiger, Philadelphia.

Fraunfelder, F.T. and Meyer, S.M. (1987). Systemic reactions to ophthalmic drug preparations. *Medical Toxicology and Adverse Drug Experience* (Auckland) 2, 287.

Fraunfelder, F.T., Hanna, C., Dreis, M.W., and Cosgrove, K.W. Jr (1982a). Cataracts associated with allopurinol therapy. *Am. J. Ophthalmol.* 94, 137.

Fraunfelder, F.T., Bagby, G.C., and Kelly, D.J. (1982b). Fatal aplastic anemia following topical administration of ophthalmic chloramphenicol. *Am. J. Ophthalmol.* 93, 356.

Grant, W.M. (1986). *Toxicology of the eye.* Charles C. Thomas, Illinois.

Halmagyi, G.M., Lessell, I., Curthoys, I.S., Lessell, S., and Hoyt, W.F. (1989). Lithium-induced downbeat nystagmus. *Am. J. Ophthalmol.* 107, 664.

Harley, R.D., Huang, N.N., Macri, C.M., and Green, W.R. (1970). Optic neuritis and optic atrophy following chloramphenicol in cystic fibrosis patients. *Trans. Am. Acad. Ophthalmol. Otolaryngol.* 74, 1011.

Hawks, W.M. Jr, Levin, K.J., and Lowe, E. (1971). Some side effects of ketamine hydrochloride during ophthalmoscopic examination. *J. Pediatr. Ophthalmol. Strabismus* 8, 171.

Hill, R.M. (1984). Isoretinoin teratogenicity. *Lancet* i, 1465.

Hoyt, C.S. and Billson, F.A. (1978). Maternal anticonvulsants and optic nerve hypoplasia. *Br. J. Ophthalmol.* 62, 3.

Hughes, R.L. (1990). Cyclosporine-related central nervous system toxicity in cardiac transplantation. *N. Engl. J. Med.* 323, 420.

Humblet, M. (1953). Neurite rétrobulbaire chronique par Antabuse. *Bull. Soc. Belge Ophtalmol.* 104, 297.

Jick, H. and Brandt, D.E. (1984). Allopurinol and cataracts. *Am. J. Ophthalmol.* 98, 355.

Kaiser-Kupfer, M.I., Kupfer, C., and Rodrigues, M.M. (1981). Tamoxifen retinopathy. *Ophthalmology* 88, 89.

Kameyama, M.K., Uchida, Y., Namiki, O., and Morisaki, N. (1977). A study of corneal chrysiasis in rheumatoid arthritis patients. *Jpn J. Clin. Ophthalmol.* 31, 1053.

Kass, K., Mandel, W., Cohen, M., and Dressler, S.H. (1957). Isoniazid as a cause of optic neuritis and atrophy. *JAMA* 164, 1740.

Kirshbaum, B.A. and Beerman, H. (1964). Photosensitisation due to drugs: a review of some of the recent literature. *Am. J. Med.* 248, 445.

Kono, R., Inoue, Y., and Hinuma, Y. (1971). Joint discussion on SMON. *Nippon Rinsho* 29, 775.

Laing, I.A., Steer, C.R., Dudgeon, J., and Brown, J.K. (1981). Clomiphene and congenital retinopathy. *Lancet* ii, 1107.

The Lancet (1964). Intracranial hypertension and steroids. *Lancet* ii, 1052.

Lansche, R.K. (1966). Systemic reactions to topical epinephrine and phenylephrine. *Am. J. Ophthalmol.* 61, 95.

Lantos, G. (1989). Cortical blindness due to osmotic disruption of the blood–brain barrier by angiographic contrast media — CT and MRI studies. *Neurology* (N.Y.) 39, 567.

Le Bris, P., Glacet-Bernard, A., and Meyrignac, C.L. (1988). Papilloedema and minocycline. *J. Fr. Ophtalmol.* 11, 681.

Leopold, I.H. (1968). Ocular complications of drugs. *JAMA* 205, 631.

Lerman, S., Megaw, J.M., and Gardner, K. (1982). Allopurinol therapy and cataractogenesis in humans. *Am. J. Ophthalmol.* 94, 141.

Lerman, S., Megaw, J., and Fraunfelder, F.T. (1984). Further studies on allopurinol therapy and human cataracts. *Am. J. Ophthalmol.* 97, 205.

Lindeman, G., Kefford, R., and Stuart-Harris, R. (1990). Cyclosporine-related central nervous system toxicity. *N. Engl. J. Med.* 323, 420.

Littmann, L., Kempler, P., Rohla, M., and Penyvesi, I. (1987). Severe symptomatic atrioventricular block induced by pilocarpine eye drops. *Arch. Intern. Med.* 174, 586.

Lyons, R.W. (1979). Orange contact lenses from rifampicin. *N. Engl. J. Med.* 300, 372.

Mackenzie, A.H. (1983a). Pharmacologic actions of 4-aminoquinoline compounds. Plaquenil symposium. *Am. J. Med.* 75, 5.

Mackenzie, A.H. (1983b). Dose refinements in long-term therapy of rheumatoid arthritis with antimalarials. Plaquenil symposium. *Am. J. Med.* 75, 40.

McKeown, C.A., Schwartz, M., Blom, J., and Maggiano, J.M. (1981). Tamoxifen retinopathy. *Br. J. Ophthalmol.* 65, 177.

Maddalena, M.A. (1968). Transient myopia associated with acute glaucoma and retinal oedema following vaginal administration of sulfanilamide. *Arch. Ophthalmol.* 80, 186.

Meier-Ruge, W. (1977). Toxicological testing on the retina. In *Arzneimittel-nebenwirkunqen an Auge* (ed. O. Hockwin and H.R. Koch), p. 300. Fischer, Stuttgart.

Meredith, T.A., Aaberg, T.M., and Willerson, W.D. (1978). Progressive chorioretinopthy after receiving thioridazine. *Arch. Ophthalmol.* 96, 1172.

Norton, A. and Walsh, F.B. (1972). Disulfiram-induced optic neuritis. *Trans. Am. Acad. Ophthalmol. Otorhinolaryngol.* 76, 1263.

Oakley, G.P. Jr (1973). The neurotoxicity of the halogenated hydroxyquinolines. *JAMA* 225, 395.

Pantuck, E.J. (1966). Ecothiopate iodide drops and prolonged response to suxamethonium. *Br. J. Anaesthesia* 38, 406.

Pringle, S.D. and MacEwen, C.J. (1987). Severe bradycardia due to interaction of timolol eye drops and verapamil. *Br. Med. J. Clin. Res.* 294, 155-6.

Quere, M.A., Ballerau, L., and Baikoff, G. (1976). Le traitement des neurites optiques graves à l'éthambutol. *Bull. Soc. Ophtalmol. Fr.* 76, 935.

Rabin, P.L. and Evans, D.C. (1981). Exophthalmos and elevated thyroxine levels in association with lithium therapy. *J. Clin. Psychiatry* 42, 398.

Rashussen, K., Kirk, L., and Faurbye, P. (1976). Deposits in the lens and cornea of the eye during long-term chlorpromazine medication. *Acta Psychiatr. Scand.* 53, 1.

Reilingh, A.D.V., Vi Reinera, M.D., and van Bijsterveld, 0.P. (1978). Contact lens tolerance and oral contraceptives. *Ann. Ophthalmol.* 10, 947.

Rock, T., Dinary, Y., and Romen, M. (1989). Retinal periphlebitis after hormone treatment. *Ann. Ophthalmol.* 21, 75.

Saraux, H. and Lefrancois, A. (1977). Retinal degeneration seen in a child after busulphan treatment of the mother during pregnanqy. *Klin. Monatsbl. Augenheilkd.* 170 818.

Schroeder, W. and Schwarzer, J. (1978). Transient myopia with angle closure glaucoma. *Klin. Monatsbl. Auqenheilkd.* 172, 762.

Shaul, W.L. and Hall, J.G. (1977). Multiple congenital anomalies associated with oral anticoagulants. *Am. J. Obstet. Gynecol.* 127, 191.

Shimizu, N., Cohen, B., Bala, S.P., Mendoza, M., and Yahr, M.D. (1977). Ocular dyskinesias in patients with Parkinson's disease treated with levodopa. *Ann. Neurol.* 1, 167.

Siddall, J.R. (1966). Ocular toxic changes associated with chlorpromazine and thioridazine. *Can. J. Ophthalmol.* 1, 190.

Skalka, H.W. and Prahal, J.T. (1980). Effect of corticosteroids on cataract formation. *Arch. Ophthalmol.* 98, 1773.

Slansky, H.H., Kolbert, G., and Gartner, S. (1967). Exophthalmos induced by steroids. *Arch. Ophthalmol.* 77, 579.

Smith, M.S. (1979). Amitriptyline ophthalmoplegia. *Ann. Intern. Med.* 91, 793.

Tedeschi, G., Bittencourt, P.R., Smith, A.I., and Richens, A. (1983). Specific oculomotor deficits after amylobarbitone. *Psychopharmacology* (Berlin) 79, 187.

Valerio, M., Carones, A.V., and DePoli, A. (1965). Monolateral cataract from local corticosteroid therapy. *Boll. Oculist* 44, 127.

van Dyk, H.J.L. and Swan, K.C. (1969). In *Symposium on ocular therapy*, Vol. 2 (ed. I.H. Leopold), p. 71. C.V. Mosby, St Louis.

Verin, P., Vilby, A., Maurin, J.F., and Hubert, G. (1977). Dilated pupil and amphetamines and lysergic acid. *Ann. Oculist* 210, 453.

Vie, R. (1980). Glaucoma and amaurosis associated with long-term application of topical corticosteroids to the eyelids. *Acta Derm. Venereol.* (Stockh.) 60, 541.

Volpe, B.T. and Soave, R. (1979). Formed visual hallucinations as digitalis toxicity. *Ann. Intern. Med.* 91, 865.

Walsh, F.B. and Hoyt, W.F. (1982). In *Clinical neuro-ophthalmology* (4th edn) (ed. N.R. Miller), p. 298. Williams and Wilkins, Baltimore.

Weiss, J. and Degnan, M. (1981). Bilateral corneal opacities: occurrence in a patient treated with oral isotretinoin. *Arch. Dermatol.* 117, 182.

Wheeler, S.D., Ramsey, R.l., and Weiss, J. (1982). Drug induced down-beat nystagmus. *Ann. Neurol.* 12, 227.

Wilensky, J.T. and Woodward, H.J. (1973). Acute systemic hypertension after conjunctival instillation of phenylephrine hydrochloride. *Am. J. Ophthalmol.* 76, 156.

Willetts, G.S. (1969). Ocular side effects of drugs. *Br. J. Ophthalmol.* 53, 252.

Williams, D.P., Troost, B.T., and Rodgers, J. (1988). Lithium-induced downbeat nystagmus. *Arch. Neurol.* 45, 1022.

Windhorst, D.B. and Nigra, T. (1982). General clinical toxicology of oral retinoids. *J. Am. Acad. Dermatol.* 6, 675.

Wright, P. (1975). Untoward effects associated with practolol administration: oculomucocutaneous syndrome. *Br. Med. J.* i, 595.

Wright, P. and Fraunfelder, F.T. (1976). In *Symposium on ocular therapy No. 9*, Vol. 2 (ed. I.H. Leopold), p. 97. Wiley, New York.

Zackai, E.H., Mellman, W.J., and Neiderer, B. (1975). The fetal trimethadione syndrome. *J. Pediatr.* 87, 280.

20. Ear, nose, and throat disorders

C. DIAMOND

The ear

The study of adverse drug reactions affecting the ear, nose, and throat system has had both an expected and an unexpected benefit. As expected, awareness of possible adverse effects has enabled the medical profession to prevent harm coming to patients and thereby to fulfil its first commandment: *primum non nocere*. The unexpected benefit has been the new knowledge gained concerning the normal physiological mechanisms of hearing and, to a lesser extent, of taste and smell. Search for the mechanism of the adverse reaction has often illuminated the mechanism of the normal physiological process. This may be illustrated by a single example at this stage. Streptomycin was first introduced into clinical medicine in 1945 by Hinshaw and Feldman. They treated 34 tubercular patients with this new drug and noted a striking response to therapy in some of them. The preliminary report (Hinshaw and Feldman 1945) is a model of good practice. They made modest claims for the benefits of the drug. They recorded that one of their patients had transient deafness and three of their patients had apparent disturbance of vestibular function when large doses were administered for prolonged periods. Having recorded the adverse effect, they pondered about the mechanism of the adverse reaction and tentatively suggested it might be caused by a selective neurotoxic effect on the eighth cranial nerve. The quest for the ototoxic mechanism has led to a great deal of animal and clinical research, as a result of which it is now known that streptomycin damages the hair cells of the cochlea and the hair cells of the vestibular apparatus and does not damage the eighth nerve itself. The knowledge gained by this research has resolved a problem of cochlear physiology, namely, the source of the cochlear microphonic electrical potential. There are two main cochlear electrical potentials evoked by auditory stimuli: the cochlear microphonic (CM) and the eighth nerve compound action potential (AP). When the eighth nerve is severed AP disappears, as one would expect, but CM persists. The source of CM was initially a mystery. Animal and human studies have shown that when the cochlear hair cells are destroyed by aminoglycoside antibiotics CM disappears while AP persists. It has thus been demonstrated that CM is generated by the cochlear hair cells.

Ototoxic adverse reactions were known for a long time before streptomycin was introduced. Hawkins (1967) has suggested that the Shamans, priest doctors of the Incas in ancient Peru, were aware of the ototoxic effects of wormseed, source of the anthelmintic chenopodium oil, and of Peruvian bark, source of the antimalarial cinchona alkaloids. Peruvian bark was introduced into Spain in 1632 by Jesuit missionaries returning from South America. In England in 1692 Richard Morton, Physician in Ordinary to King William III, wrote in his *Pyretologia* — a book of fevers — of his experience of the bark and of its temporary ototoxic effect, '. . . I have never known anyone suffer a misfortune as a result of using the Bark, other than to experience a distressing type of hearing loss at the time of use. . . .' (quoted by Stephens 1982); thus the fact that certain drugs can have an ototoxic effect has been known for centuries.

Deafness has been reported in association with a number of medications that are no longer in use, for example, arsenic (Salvarsan), strychnine, and valerian (Mawson 1967). In this chapter, however, consideration will only be given to drugs and therapeutic substances that are in current use. Ototoxic industrial compounds will not be considered, although some of these compounds can harm people who do not encounter them as industrial hazards. For example, some individuals have suffered deafness and vertigo after using hair dyes containing paraphenylenediamine, which is a recognized labyrinthine poison (Lumsden and McDowell 1968); also the organophosphorus insecticide malathion is reported to have produced profound permanent sensorineural deafness in a young man who used a spray

Table 20.1
Major ototoxic drugs in order of decreasing incidence of toxicity (Friedlander, 1979)

Drug	Cochlear toxicity	Vestibular toxicity
Minocycline		+ + + +
Kanamycin	+ + +	+
Amikacin	+ + + +	
Neomycin	+ + +	+
Streptomycin	+	+ + +
Viomycin	+ +	+ +
Gentamicin	+	+ + +
Tobramycin	+	+ + +
Ethacrynic acid	+ + +	+
Frusemide	+ + + +	
Vancomycin	+ + + +	
Quinine	+ + + +	
Salicylates	+ + + +	
Polymyxin B†		+ + + +
Colistin†		+ + + +

* ototoxicity is indicated on a scale of 0 to + + + +
† applied topically
After I.R. Friedlander (1979). Reprinted by permission of the *New England Journal of Medicine* 301, 213.

containing this chemical in his father's orchard (Harell *et al.* 1978*a*). In the latter example the reaction appears to have been a Type B reaction.

Friedlander (1979) has compiled a table of the major ototoxic drugs showing their relative incidence and listing their cochlear and vestibular toxicity under separate columns (Table 20.1).

Ototoxic antibiotics

Aminoglycoside antibiotics

The number of aminoglycoside antibiotics with ototoxic properties has grown steadily since streptomycin was first used in patients in 1945. The list includes capreomycin, dihydrostreptomycin, framycetin, gentamicin, kanamycin, neomycin, paromomycin, tobramycin, and viomycin. Although they do not belong to the group, it is convenient to consider polymyxin B and polymyxin E (colistin), vancomycin, and ristocetin with the aminoglycoside antibiotics. All these drugs can damage both the auditory and vestibular parts of the inner ear but they do tend to cause preferential damage to one or the other. This is illustrated by Table 20.1. In addition, all the aminoglycosides are nephrotoxic. The search for less toxic aminoglycosides has led to the production of the semisynthetic aminoglycosides amikacin and netilmicin. In equipotent dosages amikacin and gentamicin have an equivalent degree of auditory toxicity (Smith *et al.* 1977).

The potential margin of safety of netilmicin appears to be much greater than that of gentamicin and amikacin. Netilmicin and gentamicin are equipotent in their antibacterial action, yet 150 mg per kg of netilmicin produces less cochlear damage than 50 mg per kg of gentamicin in guinea pigs (Brummet *et al.* 1978). If a new drug appears to be less ototoxic than others in animals, it does not necessarily follow that it will be less ototoxic in humans. Tjernstrom (1980) carried out a prospective evaluation of both auditory and vestibular function in 76 patients receiving treatment with netilmicin. Audiometry and electronystagmography were performed before, during, and after treatment. Only one patient showed any ototoxic effect and the adverse reaction in this patient was a subclinical reversible disturbance of vestibular function. There have been several other trials that suggest that netilmicin is significantly less ototoxic in humans than gentamicin and amikacin and is also less ototoxic than tobramycin (Lerner *et al.* 1983).

Nature and mechanism of aminoglycoside antibiotic ototoxicity

It has been repeatedly demonstrated in animal and human studies that the principal structural lesion produced by these drugs is a degeneration of the sensory (hair) cells. The hair cells of the cochlea are confined to the organ of Corti. The vestibular hair cells are found in the macula of the saccule, the macula of the utricle, and the ampullae of the three semicircular canals. Kohonen (1965) and many other investigators have shown that, although these drugs differ in the degree of cochlear damage they cause, the pattern of cochlear hair cell injury is common to all members of the group. Damage is greatest in the outer hair cells at the base of the cochlea (which respond to high-frequency sound) and diminishes progressively towards the apex and helicotrema. This is reflected in the audiogram, which reveals a high tone sensorineural deafness with lesser impairment of the hearing for the middle and lower sound frequencies (Fig. 20.1). Severe damage results in total deafness in all frequencies. Hair cell degeneration is irreversible and the deafness produced by it is therefore permanent. The vestibular disturbance produced by the aminoglycosides does not cause acute vertigo such as is seen in patients with Ménière's disease. Instead, an unusual and highly characteristic type of disequilibrium is produced, in which the patient experiences a vertical oscillation of his surroundings every time he moves. The patient seldom has symptoms while he is confined to bed but when he is able to walk he does so with the feet wide apart and has great difficulty walking in a straight line. Objects in his visual field appear to bounce up and down in time with

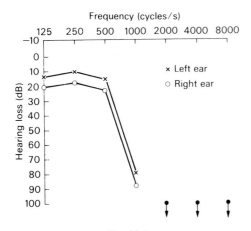

Frequency (cycles/s)

× Left ear
○ Right ear

FIG. 20.1

Bilateral high-tone deafness following daily neomycin irrigation of the pleural cavity after removal of a mesothelioma in a 47-year-old man.

each footfall. As soon as the patient stops moving the bouncing of his surroundings ceases. The term 'bobbing oscillopsia' has been applied to this symptom. This pattern of disequilibrium was described shortly after the introduction of streptomycin (Brown and Hinshaw 1946; Wallner 1949), and has also been described in patients receiving gentamicin (Ramsden and Ackrill 1982). True rotational vertigo is rare in aminoglycoside vestibulo-toxicity. Caloric tests and rotational tests show a loss of labyrinthine function. Frequently nystagmus is not detectable clinically. It can often be demonstrated by electronystagmography, however. Although the hair cell damage in the vestibule is permanent, as it is in the cochlea, the patient's balance steadily improves after a few months and improvement can sometimes continue for up to 2 years. This is the result of adaptive changes in the central mechanisms of balance control and these adaptive changes develop more readily in younger than in older patients.

The mechanism of aminoglycoside ototoxicity has not yet been fully explained. It has been well established that, following intramuscular injection, the concentration of these drugs in the perilymph is much higher than their concentration in the serum, or in the brain, or in the cerebrospinal fluid and the half-life of some of these antibiotics in the perilymph is 10 times longer than their half-life in the blood stream (Meyer zum Gut-tesberge and Stupp 1969). Stupp and others (1973) have also shown that the degree of damage to the cochlear hair cells is directly proportional to the concentration achieved by the aminoglycoside in the inner ear fluids. It was previously considered that the ototoxic mechanism

might be explained on a pharmacokinetic basis by the prolonged high concentration of these drugs in the inner ear fluids. Doubt has been cast on this explanation because, although the perilymph concentration may be high, the concentration in the inner ear tissue (as opposed to the perilymph) does not appear to be significantly higher than the concentration in the liver (Toyoda and Tachibana 1978) or in the heart, lung, and spleen (Desrochers and Schacht 1982). It has been pointed out that the concentration of aminoglycosides in perilymph associated with complete hair cell loss following chronic drug administration was only 0.5 per cent of the cytotoxic drug concentration *in vitro* (Brummet and Fox 1982). It has therefore been suggested that the hair cells of the inner ear may be intrinsically more sensitive or more susceptible to damage by aminoglycosides than are the cells of the liver, lung, heart, and spleen. Spoendlin (1966) has suggested that the aminoglycosides may produce their ototoxic effect on the hair cells in the same way that they exert their antibacterial activity, namely, by inhibition of protein synthesis. It has been suggested more recently that there is a specific interaction between aminoglycosides and cell membrane lipids with disturbance of calcium ion binding and phosphorylation processes (Fee 1980; Schacht 1986). It is generally agreed that the mechanism of ototoxicity cannot be fully explained on such a biochemical basis or on a pharmacokinetic basis at present.

One of the most puzzling features of aminoglycoside ototoxicity is the latency of onset of the damage in some cases. Deafness has often been noticed within a few days of starting an aminoglycoside in low dosage and such an occurrence suggests a direct assault on the cochlear hair cells by the antibiotic, leading to hair cell degeneration. It has frequently been reported, however, that deafness or vertigo began some time after administration of the drug had ceased and thereafter progressed remorselessly. This appears to be incompatible with a mechanism of direct injury to the hair cells. Wilson and Ramsden (1977) have thrown considerable light on this problem by demonstrating the changes produced by intravenous tobramycin on the electrocochleogram of three patients. When peak serum levels exceeded the accepted maximum safe level of 8–10 mg per litre, an immediate dramatic reduction in the electrical output of the cochlea was observed. This recovered fully as the serum tobramycin level fell. Although electrocochleography revealed objective measurable reduction of hearing acuity, none of the three patients noticed any subjective auditory or vestibular symptoms. Yung and Dorman (1986) also showed diminished electrical output of the cochlea by electrocochleography in three patients receiving tobramycin. Interestingly enough they found no alteration in the electrocochleograms of 10 patients receiving 8-hour intravenous infusions of cisplatin. The speed of onset and recovery of the electrical changes produced by the aminoglycoside is so rapid that the changes cannot be explained by a process of structural damage followed by tissue repair. It is suggested that the electrical changes are due to alterations in the ionic composition of the endolymph that are initially reversible, and that when hair cell damage occurs it is secondary to these changes in the endolymph. If this is correct, the primary site of ototoxic injury is more likely to be in the tissues responsible for maintaining the homoeostasis of the endolymph. Hawkins (1973) postulated that the primary ototoxic effect is on the secretory tissues (stria vascularis and spiral ligament) and on the reabsorptive tissues (outer sulcus and spiral prominence). If the primary site of ototoxic injury is in the secretory and reabsorptive tissues, then after a latent interval these damaged tissues would be unable to maintain endolymph homoeostasis and would thereby cause hair cell damage of delayed onset.

Topical administration (non-aural) of aminoglycoside antibiotics

The risk of ototoxic damage from the topical use of neomycin was the subject of a leading article in the *British Medical Journal* (1969) and is now widely recognized. It has been repeatedly shown that absorption, and therefore ototoxicity, can occur after oral, peritoneal, or intrabronchial administration, as well as after wound irrigation (Fig. 20.1). There still appears, however, to be a tendency to regard the aminoglycosides as 'the non-absorbable' antibiotics. Weinstein and others (1977) illustrated their absorption very clearly. They studied 10 patients undergoing total hip-replacement surgery who received intraoperative wound irrigation with a 1% neomycin solution. The serum concentration of neomycin was estimated during the first 4 hours of the postoperative period. All 10 patients showed striking systemic absorption of neomycin. Ototoxicity following the use of 0.1% gentamicin cream to a fairly small area of skin was reported by Drake (1974). The patient applied the cream four times daily to a paronychial infection of her great toes. After 2 days of treatment she developed bilateral tinnitus. The medication was stopped for 2 days and the tinnitus subsided, but recurred when she resumed topical application of the drug.

Little and Lynn (1975) reported a case of deafness in a 20-year-old man suffering from burns covering 10 per cent of the body surface. His burned area of skin was repeatedly sprayed with an antibiotic aerosol containing neomycin, bacitracin, and polymyxin. On the fifteenth day of treatment he complained of mild hearing loss and within the following 48 hours he developed severe permanent bilateral sensorineural deafness. The ototoxicity of topical antibiotics can be overlooked in young children who have not developed speech. Bamford and Jones (1978) studied six young boys who received burns covering 10–22 per cent of their body surfaces. Their ages at the time of the burns were between 8 and 16 months. The burns were treated with sprays containing neomycin, bacitracin, and polymyxin. All six suffered a retardation of speech and language development, and audiometry (when they were old enough for this test) showed quite severe hearing losses.

The occurrence of such case reports prompted the Committee on Safety of Medicines (1977) to send a notice to all doctors in the UK warning them of the ototoxic potential of aerosols containing neomycin.

Other ototoxic antibiotics

Apart from minocycline, few of the other antibiotics commonly cause ototoxic damage when they are administered systemically.

Minocycline

This antibiotic inflicts its ototoxic damage almost exclusively upon the vestibule and causes severe vertigo and a powerful suppression of the normal caloric responses of the ear. Early reports gave conflicting accounts of the incidence of adverse reactions. Gould and Brockler (1972) recorded a 30 per cent incidence of vertigo in a small series of patients and Yeadon and Garratt (1975) recorded a 7 per cent incidence of vestibular upset in a large-scale trial in general practice. In a series of 19 patients, Williams and others (1975) reported that treatment with minocycline had to be abandoned in 17 patients (89 per cent) because of severe vertigo. In an important review article, Allen (1976) concluded that the average reported incidence of vestibular adverse effects was in the region of 76 per cent and felt, therefore, that minocycline should not be recommended for general use. There have been no convincing reports of hearing loss due to minocycline, and guinea-pig studies have shown no histological damage to the ear by this drug. It has been suggested that minocycline may act centrally on the pontomedullary region of the brain and that it may not have a direct peripheral action on the ear.

Erythromycin

Ototoxic adverse reactions occur rarely with this drug

but they are particularly interesting because they develop with dramatic suddenness, and swift recovery usually takes place when the drug is stopped. Erythromycin has been in clinical use since the 1950s but there are probably only about 36 reported cases of ototoxic damage in the English-language literature. The typical symptoms exhibited by the patients are tinnitus, subjective hearing loss, and sometimes an impairment of balance. The hearing loss is sensorineural and usually affects the low, middle, and high frequencies, producing a flat audiometric pattern unlike the principally high-tone hearing loss seen with aminoglycoside toxicity. Seven patients developed reversible deafness while receiving intravenous erythromycin (Mintz et al. 1973; Karmody and Weinstein 1977; Quinnan and McCabe 1978). Three patients suffered transient deafness following oral erythromycin in dosages ranging between 2 and 4 g daily. One of these patients had severe diabetic nephropathy (Eckman et al. 1975) and the other two suffered from both hepatic disease and azotaemia (van Marion et al. 1978). Only 2–5 per cent of orally administered erythromycin is excreted in the urine, while the rest is concentrated in the liver and excreted in the bile. Advanced renal failure, however, causes a twofold prolongation of the half-life of erythromycin in the body (Lee et al. 1955). It seems reasonable to conclude that, in all 10 cases, ototoxicity was the result of very high peak blood concentrations of erythromycin. Mery and Kanfer (1979) reported three elderly patients with severe renal insufficiency who received total doses of 7–12 g of erythromycin over 4–6 days. They developed bilateral symmetrical sensorineural deafness which recovered within 2 weeks of stopping the drug. The authors concluded that the daily dosage of erythromycin should not exceed 1.5 g in patients with a raised serum creatinine. In two patients on continuous ambulatory peritoneal dialysis, erythromycin caused an approximately 60 decibel sensorineural hearing loss which recovered shortly after the drug was discontinued (Taylor et al. 1981). The authors pointed out that, although liver function tests were normal in both patients, excretion of erythromycin is delayed in patients with end-stage renal failure. This has been emphasized by a report from Kroboth and others (1983) of a 52-year-old woman on home dialysis for polycystic disease of the kidneys. She was given 1 g of erythromycin lactobionate intravenously every 6 hours and developed deafness on the second day. The drug was stopped and her hearing improved. Miller (1982) reported the case of a 71-year-old lady without renal or hepatic disease who was given 1 g of erythromycin lactobionate 6-hourly intravenously. After three doses she noticed deafness and her audiogram showed a 60 decibel

hearing loss across the frequency range in both ears. Her hearing recovered quickly after the drug was discontinued. It is important to emphasize that the ototoxic reaction is seen with any salt or ester of the drug. It is an event to be expected at very high serum concentrations. The mechanism of ototoxicity of erythromycin is not known and animal studies have not proved helpful. From a clinical standpoint the ototoxic reaction bears a close resemblance to salicylate ototoxicity and is quite different from aminoglycoside ototoxicity.

Chloramphenicol

This drug is reputed to be ototoxic when given systemically. For many years this reputation was based on a single case report by Gargye and Dutta (1959), who attributed bilateral sensorineural deafness in a child to treatment with an excessive dosage of chloramphenicol (estimated as 125 mg per kg body weight daily for 26 days). The child received the medication from an unqualified practitioner, however, and was not seen by the authors until 10 months after receiving the drug. The child was 20 months old at the time of this treatment and, understandably enough, no formal assessment of his hearing ability before the chloramphenicol therapy is recorded, and the possibility of congenital deafness cannot be ruled out. Iqbal and Srivatsav (1984) added a second case to the literature when they reported an 18-year-old Indian girl who was given a 17-day course of chloramphenicol for typhoid fever. About one month after completion of treatment she developed tinnitus and deafness in one ear. Investigation revealed a high-tone hearing loss and a reduced caloric response in the affected ear. A few months later she developed fever again and was given a 7-day course of chloramphenicol. About a month after her second course of chloramphenicol she developed bilateral tinnitus and deafness and over the following 5 months she progressed to a complete bilateral deafness with bilateral loss of caloric responses. There have been other reports of partial hearing loss in patients receiving chloramphenicol and ampicillin for treatment of meningitis but little weight can be given to them because meningitis itself frequently causes partial or complete deafness. The paucity of reports of ototoxicity after systemic administration of a drug that has been in widespread use since 1948 casts doubt upon the ototoxic reputation of systemic chloramphenicol.

Cephalexin

The cephalosporins have not been regarded as potentially ototoxic drugs. Sennesael and others (1982), however, reported two patients with renal disease who developed dizziness and vertigo while taking cephalexin. The drug was stopped and the dizziness disappeared within 4 weeks in both patients. Audiometry was normal in both patients but electronystagmography demonstrated a temporary unilateral labyrinthine dysfunction.

Ampicillin

There is no convincing evidence that this drug is ototoxic although, on several occasions, it has been reported to cause deafness when used in the treatment of patients with meningitis. As has been already mentioned, deafness is a well-recognized complication of meningitis. Nadol (1978) has reported that partial or complete hearing loss as a sequel of bacterial meningitis occurred in 21 per cent of patients over the age of 2½ years who survived the illness. A search of the literature has failed to find any reports of deafness following treatment with ampicillin for extracranial infections.

Teicoplanin

This glycopeptide antibiotic is structurally and antigenically similar to vancomycin and may have similar adverse effects. Maher and others (1986) record the case of a 39-year-old man with Down's syndrome who received teicoplanin for infective endocarditis. An audiogram on the eighth day of treatment was normal. An audiogram on the thirty-first day of treatment showed a 60 decibel sensorineural hearing loss at the 8 kHz frequency in both ears. The hearing for the other frequencies was normal. The drug was stopped and serial audiograms over the following 5 months showed that the high-tone hearing loss persisted. A study of the comparative ototoxicity of teicoplanin and tobramycin in guinea pigs demonstrated that both drugs were equally ototoxic to the vestibule but that teicoplanin was somewhat less toxic to the cochlea than tobramycin (Cazals *et al.* 1987).

Antibiotic ear drops and antiseptics

The use of ototoxic antibiotics in ear drops and powders is the subject of considerable controversy and further work needs to be done to establish the degree of risk involved. It has been demonstrated that gentamicin, neomycin, polymyxin, streptomycin, chloramphenicol, and erythromycin can cause inner ear damage in guinea-pigs after instillation into the middle-ear cleft (Stupp *et al.* 1973). Many other workers have shown this effect after placing various antibiotic solutions and powders into the middle ears of different experimental animals. In addition, propylene glycol, the vehicle used in chlor-

amphenicol ear drops and other aural preparations, has been suspected of ototoxicity. Morizono and Johnstone (1975) studied the effects of placing solutions of propylene glycol into the middle ears of guinea-pigs. They reported that propylene glycol in concentrations of 10% or more always caused irreversible inner-ear deafness. Their experiments were repeated by Vernon and others (1978) with certain modifications, and diametrically opposite results were obtained. Vernon's group found no adverse effects on the middle ear or inner ear with 10% propylene glycol solutions placed in the middle ear. In addition, when they instilled 90% propylene glycol into the middle ear they found no inner-ear damage, though some middle-ear dysfunction was produced by this high concentration. The use of topical chloramphenicol in ears has largely been abandoned by otologists in Great Britain, but ear drops containing aminoglycoside antibiotics and polymyxin are used frequently in otitis media. Chronic forms of tubotympanic otitis media often fail to respond to treatment when antibiotic therapy is given solely by the systemic route. Chronic suppurative otitis media is, of course, an ototoxic disease and is associated with an insidious inner-ear deafness. Most otologists believe that pus in the middle ear is more dangerous than antibiotic solution in the middle ear. Although antibiotic solutions diffuse easily into the inner ear from the healthy middle ears of experimental animals, similar diffusion does not appear to take place in infected human middle ears with the dilute antibiotic solutions used in clinical practice. Nevertheless, there are a few scattered reports in the literature of sudden deterioration in hearing immediately after the instillation of topical drops containing a solution of a single antibiotic or a mixture of antibiotics and steroids. In the majority of these reports there was some recovery of hearing provided the ear drops were discontinued. Editorials in the *Medical Journal of Australia* (1975) and in *The Lancet* (1976) expressed concern about the possible toxicity of antibiotic ear drops. Kohonen and Tarkkanen (1969), writing on the use of antibiotic ear drops in otitis media, stated: 'Widespread clinical use with very few known complications suggests that the risk cannot be very large, but it is, on the other hand, possible that moderate hearing losses in chronically infected ears have been unduly attributed to infection only'. Ward and Rounthwaite (1978) summed up the general view when they stated: '. . . the topical application of neomycin to the external ear canal or to the middle ear is considered by most to be innocuous with only occasional hypersensitivity skin reactions'.

There is a need, however, for prospective, double-blind, controlled trials to assess the validity of these clinical impressions or assumptions. One such trial has been reported by McKelvie and others (1975). They carried out repeated audiometric testing on patients with chronic middle ear infections over a 4-year period. Half of the ears were treated with gentamicin ear drops and the other half with placebo drops. The placebo used was the vehicle for the gentamicin ear drops. They found no adverse effect of gentamicin ear drops on the cochlea. In a more recent series of 124 patients with otitis media treated with antibiotic ear drops over a 12–24 month period, it was concluded that a small degree of sensorineural hearing loss (approximately 2–11 decibels) may be attributable to the ear drops (Podoshin *et al.* 1989). The authors felt that the possibility of hearing loss due to the use of antibiotic ear drops could not be ignored. Although many otologists feel that clinical expediency justifies the use of antibiotic ear drops in chronic otitis media, the slight potential risk of ototoxicity should be remembered and the drops should be stopped immediately if the patient notices any loss of hearing Some patients have suffered unexplained inner-ear deafness following myringoplasty procedures to repair tympanic membrane perforations. Suspicion has fallen on chlorhexidine antiseptic solution used to cleanse the skin of the pinna and external auditory canal preoperatively. Many surgeons now pack the external canal to prevent any possible diffusion of antiseptic solution through the middle ear to the inner ear. Bismuth– iodoform–paraffin paste (BIPP) is a standard postoperative dressing in ENT surgery. Iodoform intoxication has been reported when large amounts of this substance are used to pack the sizeable cavities created by maxillary sinus surgery. Fortunately, iodoform intoxication is not a problem when BIPP packs are used in the relatively small cavities associated with middle-ear and mastoid operations (O'Connor *et al.* 1977).

Ototoxic diuretics

There have been several reports of both transient and permanent deafness following treatment with ethacrynic acid and frusemide (Pillay *et al.* 1969; Schwartz *et al.* 1970; Lloyd-Mostyn and Lord 1971), and it is clear from the reports that impaired renal function enhances the ototoxic effect of these diuretics. The speed of onset of deafness can be quite startling, especially when the diuretics are administered by rapid intravenous injection. Hanzelik and Peppercorn (1969) record one patient with previously normal hearing who complained of tinnitus and hearing loss within 5 minutes of receiving 10 mg of ethacrynic acid intravenously. Examination 10 minutes later confirmed her deafness. The hearing returned to normal after 8 hours.

Vestibular damage with disturbance of balance appears to be rare. Gomolin and Garshick (1980) reported the unusual case of a 40-year-old man who developed deafness and dizziness accompanied by fine nystagmus in all directions during an intravenous infusion of ethacrynic acid. The hearing returned to normal and the nystagmus disappeared within an hour of stopping the drug.

Two other loop diuretics, bumetanide and piretanide, are ototoxic. In animal studies, they have a similar degree of ototoxicity (Rybak and Whitworth 1986). Ethacrynic acid is more ototoxic than frusemide in humans. The ototoxic potential of bumetanide is similar to that of ethacrynic acid but its diuretic potential is 40 times greater. Thus, a lower dose of bumetanide may be expected to have the same diuretic effect but a lower ototoxic effect (Oliveira 1989*a*).

Nature and mechanism of diuretic ototoxicity

Although there are many reports of permanent deafness from diuretics, the majority of patients suffering from diuretic-induced ototoxicity experience immediate and short-lived deafness. Vestibular damage with disturbance of balance occurs rarely. This contrasts markedly with aminoglycoside-induced ototoxicity, in which deafness is more often delayed and permanent deafness and vestibular disturbance is a common finding. Despite the marked difference in their clinical features, there are striking similarities between the two types of ototoxicity.

Mathog and others (1970) have shown that both ethacrynic acid and frusemide produce a primary depression of the electrical output of the cochlea with almost complete recovery in one hour in experimental animals. This bears a strong resemblance to the changes in the electrocochleograms following intravenous tobraycin reported by Wilson and Ramsden (1977) (see above). Mathog and others (1970) also showed that ethacrynic acid in doses above 10 mg per kg produced a delayed severe secondary depression of cochlear electrical output with evidence of outer hair cell degeneration in the basal and middle turns of the cochlea. Matz and others (1969), reporting on the temporal bone of a patient with permanent deafness due to ethacrynic acid, showed that the structural lesion produced was outer hair-cell damage, most marked in the basal turn of the cochlea. It seems possible, therefore, that the reversible deafness may be due to short-term alterations in the composition of the endolymph and that long-term changes in the endolymph cause hair-cell damage and permanent deafness. Cohn and his co-workers (1971) reported complete reversal of the K^+/Na^+ ratio in the endolymph 10 minutes after the intravenous administration of ethacrynic acid in dogs. Frusemide and ethacrynic acid are chemically dissimilar, but they have a similar diuretic action and a similar ototoxic action. It has therefore been suggested that their ototoxic action is due to their diuretic properties, which alter the ionic composition of the inner ear fluids. It would seem unwise, however, to extrapolate the results from experiments in the dog to the human cochlea because this reversal of relative endolymph concentrations of sodium and potassium appears to be species-dependent. Bosher (1980) has shown that ethacrynic acid administered intravenously to guinea-pigs and rats caused only small changes in the concentrations of sodium and potassium in the endolymph. The mechanism of ototoxicity caused by diuretics in humans is unknown and remains the subject of interesting speculation.

Salicylate ototoxicity

In general, ototoxicity caused by salicylates is not serious, provided that the drug is withdrawn as soon as symptoms appear, because the damage is usually reversible. Large amounts of salicylates are consumed and therefore ototoxic effects are commonly encountered. Ototoxic symptoms can occur with all salicylates and with salicylate compounds, for example, Benorylate (salicylate and paracetamol) and sulphasalazine (salicylate and sulphonamide). Tinnitus and deafness are prominent symptoms and vertigo is also experienced sometimes when the serum salicylate concentration reaches toxic levels. The therapeutic serum level of salicylate is 200–300 mg per litre and symptoms of salicylism occur as the concentration approaches 300 mg per litre. Effective dosage, therefore, must be close to toxic dosage. Since symptoms appear promptly with peak serum salicylate levels, one would expect aspirin deafness to be strongly dependent on the unit dosage used. This is confirmed in a report by the Boston Collaborative Drug Study Program, which records an overall incidence of salicylate-induced deafness of 11 per 1000 patients exposed. With unit dosage of 600–899 mg, however, the rate was only 1 per 1000 and, with 900–1199 mg, 45 per 1000, rising to 150 per 1000 when unit doses larger than 1200 mg were used (Porter and Jick 1977). Pearlman (1966) records that two women suffered from deafness as a result of the application of an ointment containing 5% salicylic acid to the skin. Both women had psoriasis involving more than 90 per cent of the skin surface. Serum salicylate levels of 350 mg per litre and 240 mg per litre were achieved.

In humans, the hearing loss from salicylate toxicity is a reversible sensorineural hearing loss affecting all frequencies fairly evenly. There may perhaps be a tendency for the upper frequencies to be slightly more susceptible to damage than are the lower frequencies in some patients (Waltner 1955; Myers *et al.* 1965; McCabe and Day 1965; Ramsden *et al.* 1985). Tinnitus frequently precedes the onset of deafness. Imbalance is much less commonly reported. There is considerable evidence from animal experiments to show that salicylate ototoxicity is not associated with hair cell damage. Electrophysiological studies in guinea-pigs (Mitchell *et al.* 1973) and in adult cats (Stypulkowski 1990) have shown that the cochlear microphonic potential (CM) is not decreased by salicylate administration but the compound nerve action potential (AP) is temporarily diminished by the drug. Similar preservation of the CM and reversible diminution of the AP has been recorded in two patients suffering from salicylate overdosage (Ramsden *et al.* 1985). de Moura and Hayden (1968), in a temporal bone examination of a woman affected by salicylate ototoxicity, found no evidence of hair cell damage or other structural abnormality attributable to salicylates. It has been suggested that the ototoxic effects of salicylates are due to a temporary metabolic blockade at the hair cell/neural interface, the chemical transmitter at which is as yet unidentified (Ramsden *et al.* 1985). This biochemical mechanism is consistent with the classification of salicylate ototoxicity as a Type A reaction.

Ototoxicity of quinine and chloroquine

Both these drugs are used in the treatment of malaria, and both have been responsible for inner-ear damage.

Quinine has been given in large doses to a multitude of patients without causing any deafness. Individual susceptibility or idiosyncrasy seems to be an important factor. The hearing loss is predominantly in the low tones. Tinnitus is an early symptom. The deafness is not usually severe and is reversible in the majority of patients if the drug is withdrawn early.

Chloroquine has been observed to cause tinnitus and perceptive deafness. The deafness tends to occur after prolonged high dosage and is usually irreversible. Its onset may take place after the drug has been discontinued (Toone *et al.* 1965), exhibiting the same peculiar latency so frequently noted with the aminoglycoside antibiotics. Chloroquine has a strong affinity for melanin and therefore tends to accumulate in melanin-containing cells. If labelled chloroquine is injected into pigmented rats it accumulates in the melanin-rich cells of the stria vascularis and is retained there for a prolonged period. It is not found in the endolymph or perilymph. In albino rats, no accumulation of chloroquine takes place in any part of the inner ear (Dencker and Lindquist 1975). This again suggests that the primary ototoxic injury is likely to be to the stria vascularis and that damage to this tissue causes a gradual change in the composition of the endolymph, which damages the hair cells. Melanin-rich cells are present in retina and in the inner ear. Patients with deafness and vertigo following chloroquine therapy may also suffer from visual disturbances (Dwivedi and Mehra 1978). Chloroquine deafness is unconmon in Western Europe and the USA, but Obiako (1979) reported a series of 50 patients seen in the University of Nigeria teaching hospital during a period of less than 2 years who had suffered deafness after treatment with chloroquine phosphate injections. Chloroquine is very frequently prescribed in the west, and other, malarious regions of Africa because practically every complaint is provisionally blamed on malaria; and, because of a widespread faith in and willingness to pay extra for injections, it is often quite unnecessarily given parenterally — with obvious dangers when the re-use of needles is common.

Ototoxicity of cytotoxic drugs

Mustine hydrochloride (nitrogen mustard) is now acknowledged to be an ototoxic drug. Deafness is most common in patients who have had a regional perfusion that included the circulation to the ear. This produces a correspondingly higher blood level in the area of the cochlear blood supply. Deafness seldom follows intravenous administration, but Schuknecht (1964) described a 30-year-old woman who received mustine hydrochloride for Hodgkin's disease in a dose of 0.8 mg per kg body-weight by injection while fully alert. Immediately afterwards she noticed tinnitus, a bilateral decrease in hearing, and vertigo. An audiogram showed a bilateral symmetrical perceptive deafness. Cummings (1968) demonstrated in cats that mustine hydrochloride produced structural damage in the hair cells of the organ of Corti. Bleomycin may produce ototoxic damage when given in high dosage, whether administered systemically or topically to the middle ear (Ballantyne 1973).

Cisplatin (cis-platinum) is an inorganic heavy metal with antineoplastic properties which has been used in the chemotherapy of testicular tumours. Although its more prominent adverse effects involve the gastrointestinal and renal systems, auditory symptoms have also been produced. Temporary tinnitus and high-tone deafness were noted in 20 per cent of a series of patients by Higby and his colleagues (1974). Since then, numerous other papers showing that ototoxic damage by this drug is not just an occasional occurrence have been published. Rybak (1981) reviewed the literature and noted that the published incidence of ototoxicity varied from 9 to 90 per cent in the series he surveyed. Schaefer and others (1981) recorded a case of a man with vestibular damage as well as cochlear hearing loss attributed to the use of this drug. In their series of 24 patients treated with cisplatin, Strauss and colleagues (1983) reported that 25 per cent of their patients suffered ototoxic injury. They stated that the treatment factors that appear to increase the ototoxic effect are: high dose per treatment, prolonged therapy, total cumulative dosage, and bolus administration. In common with most other authors, they reported that the effect was a high-tone sensorineural deafness and that the maximal loss at any single frequency did not exceed 25 decibels. Van der Hulst and colleagues (1988) used special high-frequency audiometers to measure the hearing loss in between 8 kHz and 20 kHz. The hearing thresholds routinely tested in clinical practice are those in the 0.125 kHz–8 kHz range. These authors demonstrated that in the majority of patients with cisplatin deafness, the hearing loss began between 10 kHz and 18 kHz. Hearing loss at these high frequencies would not be noticed by the patient and would not be recordable with standard clinical audiometers. Laurell and Jungnelius (1990) carefully assessed the ototoxic effect of high-dose (100–120 mg per m² body-surface) cisplatin on 54 patients. In this series 81 per cent showed significant high-frequency hearing loss while 41 per cent also showed significant loss of hearing for the middle frequencies used in human speech. They found the ototoxic effect was determined more by the amount of the single dose than by the accumulated dose. No ototoxic effects were seen below a peak plasma concentration of 1 μg per litre. The ototoxic effect was not increased by pre-existing hearing loss per se but was slightly increased by age. They calculated a risk factor that could be applied for second and subsequent courses of cisplatin therapy. They estimated that after each course of high-dosage cisplatin 25 per cent of patients would sustain a 25 per cent deterioration of their remaining high-frequency (3 kHz–8 kHz) hearing threshold. In the majority of patients the hearing loss is permanent, but some cases of partial and even of complete recovery have been reported. Human and animal histopathological studies have demonstrated severe destruction of the outer hair cells in the basal turn of the cochlea similar to that seen in aminoglycoside ototoxicity (Kopelman et al. 1988).

Vincristine is a cytotoxic drug known to have neurotoxic properties. Mahajan and others (1981) reported the first recorded case of sensorineural deafness after treatment with this drug. Their patient was a 73-year-old woman who had two acute episodes of deafness following vincristine therapy. After the first episode of deafness her hearing recovered completely within 2 months. Later she had a recurrence of her tumour and was given a second course of treatment. Once again she became deaf and recovered her hearing over a period of 2 months.

Misonidazole is a potent antitumour agent that selectively increases the effect of ionizing radiations on poorly oxygenated tumour cells. It was used as a radiosensitizer in a series of 21 patients by Waltzman and Cooper (1981). Hearing loss secondary to the drug developed in 11 (52 per cent) of the patients. The hearing loss was sensorineural and all the affected patients experienced complete or partial recovery of hearing within a few weeks. The authors found no relationship between the degree of hearing loss and the age, sex, and previous hearing status of the patient, with the dose of the drug used, or with the anatomical site of the tumour.

Ototoxicity of β-adrenoceptor blockers

Initially these drugs were considered to be relatively free from adverse effects in the ear, though propranolol was known to cause mild reversible inner ear disturbance occasionally (Lloyd Mostyn 1969). Practolol, however, had some totally unexpected adverse effects, including deafness, following long-term use (Wright 1975). The type of deafness caused by practolol differs from any other known type of drug-induced deafness. In addition to inducing a sensorineural deafness, it can cause conductive deafness. The conductive deafness is due to a sterile effusion into the middle-ear cleft (serous otitis media) and responds to myringotomy and the insertion of a tympanostomy tube. The sensorineural deafness either improves or remains static when the drug is withdrawn (Jones et al. 1977). The ototoxic mechanism is unknown. Practolol was withdrawn from general use and is now reserved for short-term use in hospitals only. Up to the end of 1977 a total of 1878 cases of adverse reactions to practolol had been reported to the Committee on Safety of Medicines. In 150 of these, deafness was noted to have occurred but in only 36 was it the main complaint (Committee on Safety of Medicines 1978, personal communication).

Miscellaneous ototoxic drugs and vaccines

Desferrioxamine

Desferrioxamine is a chelating agent introduced in 1963 for treatment of iron overload resulting from long-term blood transfusion therapy. Deafness was recorded in patients with thalassaemia receiving treatment with desferrioxamine but initially the deafness was attributed to the thalassaemia (De Virgiliis et al. 1979). Serious auditory and visual disturbances attributable to the use of desferrioxamine were, however, reported by Olivieri and colleagues (1986) and have been confirmed by others (Cases et al. 1988; Wonke et al. 1989). The drug causes a sensorineural hearing loss maximal in the higher sound frequencies. In severe cases, the deafness extends into the middle and lower sound frequencies. Partial and sometimes complete recovery of hearing may occur when the drug is stopped. Some patients show no recovery and have required hearing aids to ameliorate the permanent deafness. The incidence of damage to the hearing was almost 25 per cent in the 89 patients treated by Olivieri and colleagues (1986). They stopped treatment and approximately one-third of affected patients regained normal or next to normal hearing within 3 weeks. Desferrioxamine treatment was restarted after a rest period of some months with a lower dosage of the drug without causing any further hearing loss. There was a 26 per cent incidence of damage to the hearing in the 50 patients reported by Wonke and others (1989). Five of these patients (10 per cent) had severe hearing loss. Treatment with desferrioxamine was stopped in these five patients and was replaced by chelation with Ca-DTPA (calcium diethylene triamine pentacetic acid) with zinc supplements. Hearing recovered completely within 19 months in one patient and improved substantially in the other four patients while chelation with Ca-DTPA was being administered.

Propoxyphene hydrochloride

This mild analgesic, which is used fairly widely in North America, is reported to have caused a moderate degree of sensorineural deafness and vestibular disturbance in a young man who mistakenly took approximately four times the recommended dosage for a period of 6 days (Lupin and Harley 1976). A case of total permanent deafness following chronic propoxyphene abuse has been recorded by Harell and his colleagues (1978b). These authors believe that ototoxicity is often overlooked because severe propoxyphene intoxication is frequently fatal.

Naproxen

Chapman (1982) reported the case of a patient who developed permanent bilateral sensorineural deafness and acute renal failure from treatment with the non-steroidal anti-inflammatory drug naproxen. His report draws attention to the possibility of other prostaglandin-synthetase-inhibiting drugs being ototoxic. Since then there have been occasional reports of auditory complications caused by mefenamic acid (Morris and Fletcher 1986).

Nortriptyline

This may produce deafness not detectable by routine pure-tone audiometry. Smith and others (1972) described an 8-year-old enuretic who received the drug for 9 months. Although his pure-tone thresholds were normal, his tone-decay and speech-discrimination tests were depressed. These recovered after the drug was stopped, suggesting that the drug had produced a more subtle type of ototoxic damage.

Imipramine

Racy and Ward-Racy (1980) reported four patients who received imipramine for depression and developed tinnitus as an adverse reaction. The tinnitus was reduced or abolished by reducing the dosage of imipramine. This is a helpful report, because many tinnitus sufferers are treated with imipramine for depression caused by tinnitus.

Propylthiouracil

Both unilateral sensorineural deafness and systemic lupus erythematosus were produced by this drug in a patient described by Smith and Spalding (1972). Fortunately, termination of the drug led to recovery both from the lupus erythematosus and from the hearing impairment.

Bromocriptine

This drug has been implicated as the cause of deafness in three patients suffering from hepatic encephalopathy (Lanthier et al. 1984). A high-tone hearing loss was produced, which improved when the dosage was reduced, suggesting that the ototoxicity is reversible.

Indomethacin

Vertigo and tinnitus have been recorded in patients given this drug, together with vomiting, confusion, and ataxia (Hart and Boardman 1965; Rothermich 1966). It is uncertain whether all of these symptoms are of central origin.

Quinidine

The adverse effects of quinidine therapy (cinchonism) include tinnitus and deafness. Rosketh and Storstein (1963) quote the occurrence of vertigo and tinnitus in 24 of a series of 274 patients treated with quinidine.

Dantrolene

The possibility that this skeletal muscle relaxant may have ototoxic potential has been raised by Pace-Balsan and Ramsden (1988). They reported the case of a 19-year-old girl with athetoid cerebral palsy. She was known to have normal hearing in the left ear and a longstanding, non-progressive, sensorineural deafness of 70 decibels in the right ear, the cause of which had never been positively identified. On the fifth day of dantrolene treatment she suddenly developed a 70 decibel hearing loss in the previously normal left ear and lost all her remaining hearing in the previously partially deaf right ear. There was no associated tinnitus or vertigo and no recovery of hearing took place. The authors stated that it is only by reporting such possible cases of ototoxic damage that suspicion may be aroused.

Vaccines

Sudden hearing loss following vaccination or the therapeutic use of antisera is, fortunately, a rare event. The majority of reported cases have occurred following the administration of tetanus antitoxin, and a few have occurred after vaccinations against whooping cough and rabies. Mair and Elverland (1977) recorded the case of a young girl who developed a local hypersensitivity reaction on her arm at the site of a routine revaccination against tetanus and diphtheria. She also developed a unilateral, irreversible, total hearing loss at the same time. The authors reviewed the literature and suggested that a hypersensitivity reaction accounts for the deafness in these patients. Healy (1972) postulated that mumps vaccine was responsible for a unilateral perceptive deafness found on routine audiological screening in a boy whose hearing had been normal on screening one year earlier. In the intervening year he had been given the mumps virus vaccine, but had suffered no illness.

Relative frequency of ototoxic damage

It is difficult to give more than a rough estimate of the incidence of ototoxic damage. The Boston Collaborative Drug Surveillance Program monitors adverse reactions in a continuing series of patients admitted to medical wards, and therefore reports on a highly selected sample. In 1973, it reported that 32 out of 11 526 medical in-patients (3 per 1000) developed deafness attributed to

TABLE 20.2
Incidence of ototoxic damage

Drug	Incidence per 1000 patients exposed	
	In 1973 report	In 1977 report
Aspirin (plain, buffered, and enteric coated)	11	11
Aminoglycoside antibiotics	13	7
Ethacrynic acid	7	10
Quinidine	3	1

drugs. In 1977, the numbers monitored had risen to 32 812 and the number of patients with deafness attributed to drugs was 53 (1.6 per 1000) (Porter and Jick 1977). The principal drugs implicated are indicated in Table 20.2.

Arcieri and others (1970) studied the records of 1327 patients treated with gentamicin and found significant ototoxicity in 31 cases (2.3 per cent). Gailiunas and others (1978) estimated that the incidence of gentamicin ototoxicity was 1.8 per cent in the general population of patients receiving the drug, but 30 per cent among patients on long-term haemodialysis.

Brummet and Morrison (1990) have suggested that the reported incidence of hearing loss due to aminoglycoside drugs may be exaggerated. They point out that the definition of ototoxicity in most clinical studies of aminoglycosides is an increase in pure-tone threshold, from a base-line audiogram, of either 15 decibels or more at two frequencies, or 20 decibels or more at a single frequency. In their study of 20 volunteers who were not taking any known ototoxic drugs, they found test–retest differences of 15 decibels or more at two frequencies in 33 per cent, and of 20 decibels or more at a single frequency, in 20 per cent of the volunteers. They concluded that many of the audiometric threshold changes reported to represent aminoglycoside ototoxicity may actually represent the normal variation in audiometric threshold movements found in normal individuals.

Factors influencing ototoxicity

Drug concentration in the inner ear

This is probably the most important single factor in the production of ototoxic damage. It will be affected by the dose of the drug given, by the route of administration, and by the rate of excretion.

Intolerance

There is no doubt that some individuals show a markedly heightened sensitivity to ototoxic drugs. In an interesting clinical experiment, Meyer zum Guttesberge and Stupp (1969) gave 26 otosclerotic patients a standard dose of streptomycin preoperatively and took perilymph samples at stapedectomy. Five hours after injection, the average level of streptomycin in the perilymph was $260 \mu g$ per litre. Very large variations in the level, however, were found among the 26 patients, and in some cases the level in the perilymph was many times higher than that in the serum. It is tempting to speculate that intolerance may be due to abnormally high ability of an individual to accumulate the drug in the inner ear.

Renal and hepatic disease

Many ototoxic drugs (for example, the aminoglycoside antibiotics) are excreted by the kidney. If renal function is impaired, the serum level and inner ear concentration of the drug can increase alarmingly. Since many ototoxic drugs are also nephrotoxic, it is unwise to assume that if renal function is normal at the beginning of treatment it will remain so throughout. Berk and Chalmers (1970) reported five cases of ototoxic damage by oral neomycin in patients with hepatic cirrhosis. Two of these patients had normal renal function throughout treatment, while two others had relatively low serum antibiotic levels despite the presence of renal failure. All five received large total doses of neomycin (750–2500 g) over periods ranging from 8 to 24 months before ototoxic damage became apparent. The authors emphasize that, despite minimal absorption of the drug from the gut and correspondingly low serum levels, and even in the presence of normal renal function, oral neomycin can be harmful.

Ballantyne (1970) also reported sensorineural hearing loss in 6 of 13 patients treated with oral neomycin for hepatic failure; 4 had no ascites and were treated with neomycin alone, while 2 had ascites and received diuretics as well.

Placental transport

The develolping otocyst is most vulnerable to damage by drugs and viral infections during the first 3 months of fetal life. Mature development is achieved by the sixth fetal month.

Thalidomide

Livingstone (1965) reported 14 children with congenital bilateral meatal atresia due to their mothers being given thalidomide; 3 had perceptive deafness in addition to outer and middle ear damage.

Isotretinoin

This vitamin A derivative is a well known teratogen. John and Ganti (1987) reported two infants with microtia and anotia and associated nervous systems malformations, born to mothers who had used isotretinoin during pregnancy for severe acne.

Chloroquine and quinine

Matz and Naunton (1968) reported on the temporal bone of a child whose mother had taken 250 mg chloroquine twice daily during the first trimester. The specimen showed complete cochlear damage. In this family, two siblings also developed profound sensorineural hearing loss following their mother's taking chloroquine during pregnancy. In three other pregnancies she did not take chloroquine and these had resulted in three children with normal hearing.

McKinna (1966) reported two cases of congenital deafness in infants whose mothers had taken a high dose of quinine during pregnancy in an effort to induce abortion. Histological examination of the temporal bone revealed degenerative changes in the spiral ganglion cells of the inner ear.

Streptomycin

Conway and Birt (1965) reported on 17 children whose mothers had received streptomycin during pregnancy. Four of the children showed a mild unilateral high-tone hearing loss. These authors concluded that the risk of fetal ear damage with streptomycin therefore appears to be small.

Ototoxic synergism

Mutual potentiation of ototoxicity seems to be possible when, for example, an ototoxic antibiotic and diuretic are used simultaneously. Meriwether and others (1971) recorded two patients who were receiving non-toxic doses of an aminoglycoside antibiotic and who developed deafness following a standard intravenous dose of ethacrynic acid. Both had normal renal function. West and others (1973) showed particularly severe cochlear damage in guinea-pigs exposed to kanamycin and ethacrynic acid. Ototoxic synergism between gentamicin and frusemide was suspected in a group of patients reported by Thomsen and colleagues (1976). A possible explanation of the ototoxic synergism experienced with

aminoglycoside antibiotics and loop diuretics has been suggested by Ohtani and others (1978a,b). They found that the kanamycin concentration in rabbit serum, cerebrospinal fluid, and perilymph was much higher after a single injection of kanamycin with frusemide than after a single injection of kanamycin alone. They obtained a similar result when they substituted the newer loop diuretic bumetanide for frusemide. They concluded that the ototoxic interaction is caused by the inhibiting effect of the diuretic on the excretion of the aminoglycoside. Thus, the enhancement of the ototoxicity is related to the diuretic potency of the diuretic used. (This subject is also discussed in Chapter 30.)

There is also some evidence to suggest increased sensitivity to drug-induced deafness in patients with diminished cochlear function from any cause such as, for example, presbyacusis, previous otitis media, or acoustic trauma. Dayal and others (1971) showed that guinea-pigs exposed to a combination of kanamycin and the noise generated by children's incubators sustained hair cell damage. Neither agent produced hair cell damage when acting alone. Since premature children are often given aminoglycoside antibiotics while being nursed in incubators, the work of these authors may be of practical importance. It appears that, in guinea-pigs, kanamycin in small dosages increases the susceptibility of hair cells to noise and that this increased susceptibility lingers for 20 days after the drug has been stopped (Gannon et al. 1979).

Prevention of ototoxicity

Jolicoeur (1972) makes a number of recommendations, which may be summarized as follows:

1. the dose of ototoxic drug used should be determined by the weight of the patient and should be the smallest dose compatible with efficient treatment;
2. treatment should not be unduly prolonged, and patients should be questioned daily regarding tinnitus, vertigo, and diminution of hearing;
3. hearing should be measured before, during, and some weeks after treatment;
4. in a patient with renal disease, the dose of the ototoxic compound should be reduced;
5. renal function should be checked throughout treatment, and it should be borne in mind that in elderly patients there is an increased likelihood of impaired renal function.
6. it should be remembered that patients who already have some sensorineural damage will be more vulnerable to the effects of ototoxic drugs;
7. patients should be kept in a proper state of hydration.

Ramsden and Ackrill (1982) emphasized the value of daily estimation of serum peak and trough levels of drugs when aminoglycosides are being administered. In day-to-day control of the dosage levels they found trough levels more helpful than peak levels.

As in so many other fields, awareness of the danger is the most important single factor in prevention. A great variety of ingenious attempts have been made to reduce the ototoxicity of aminoglycosides and cisplatin by biochemical methods. It was hoped that giving vitamin A, or vitamin B complex, or vitamin C with aminoglycosides would reduce ototoxicity but these have been found to be ineffective. Some experimental evidence suggests that administering an aminoglycoside in the form of its pantothenic or glucuronate salt might decrease ototoxicity but this has not been substantiated in practice. It has been proposed that calcium ions might reduce the ototoxic effect of streptomycin by competing for receptor sites in the inner ear. It has also been suggested that glycosaminoglycan acids might exert a protective role against ototoxicity. Similarly, substances that inhibit the production of free radicals by aminoglycosides have also been considered to be helpful in reducing ototoxicity. For reasons not fully understood, hyperglycaemia appears to reduce the toxic effects of kanamycin on the guinea-pig cochlea. The possibility of combining glucose administration with aminoglycoside therapy has therefore been considered. There is evidence giving more reason for hope that fosfomycin, a phosphonic acid antibiotic may ameliorate the toxic effects of aminoglycosides and cisplatin. A number of trials have shown that fosfomycin reduced the ototoxicity of aminoglycosides both in experimental animals and humans. Fosfomycin has also been shown to exert a protective effect against the ototoxic and nephrotoxic effects of cisplatin in a number of experimental animals (Oliveira 1989*b*). If further studies confirm that it is an effective antidote in clinical practice, its use would help to prevent or reduce the ototoxicity of aminoglycosides and cisplatin.

The nose

It is well recognized that drugs can produce nasal obstruction, nasal bleeding, and anosmia.

Nasal obstruction

Rhinitis medicamentosa caused by the prolonged use of vasoconstrictor drops and sprays in the nose is probably still the commonest form of iatrogenic nasal obstruction.

Hypersensitivity reactions

Topical antibiotics used in the nose may cause hypersensitivity reactions and are not recommended. Nasal allergy caused by drugs and foods is well recognized, and aspirin, for example, can produce nasal obstruction and profuse rhinorrhoea in allergic individuals. Asthma, nasal polyps, and aspirin allergy form a familiar triad in ENT practice. Presley (1988) reported an interesting case of severe rhinitis with profuse rhinorrhoea and grossly oedematous swelling of the nasal mucosa in a 76-year-old man receiving penicillamine. He also had cutaneous lesions and a skin biopsy was compatible with penicillamine-induced pemphigus foliaceus. Penicillamine was stopped and all symptoms cleared rapidly.

Nasal drops and sprays

Ephedrine, amphetamine, and privine all lose vasoconstrictor efficacy if used over a long period, and produce an increasing amount of after-congestion (Wilson and Schild 1968). The chronic and often severe mucosal swelling thus produced can cause extreme narrowing of the nasal passages. It is fortunate that so many patients obtain relief from their obstruction within a short time of stopping the drug. Neonates are particularly at risk from the excessive use of these drops because they are obligate nasal breathers and do not develop oral breathing until some time between the ages of 2–6 months. Nasal obstruction in neonates can cause severe respiratory distress. Osguthorpe and Shirley (1987) record the case of a child started on phenylephrine nasal drops at birth. The parents instilled the drops before each feed (every 3–4 hours). At the age of 3 weeks the infant was having multiple daily episodes of apnoea and cyanosis. Clinical examination, blood tests, and radiological investigations revealed oedematous obstructing turbinates, polycythaemia, cardiomegaly, and prominence of the pulmonary vasculature. Most paediatricians advocate limiting the therapy to 5–7 days in order to avoid rhinitis medicamentosa.

Nasal preparations of sodium cromoglycate and beclomethasone dipropionate are now available for the treatment of allergic rhinitis. These drugs were first introduced for intrabronchial administration in patients with asthma, and a few complications from their use in this way have been reported. There have been no reports so far of serious adverse effects with the intranasal use of these drugs in standard dosage. Minor symptoms of sneezing, stinging, and some blood-stained nasal discharge are sometimes encountered but are not serious.

Block (1975) reported some degree of nasal congestion in three patients using intranasal sodium cromoglycate. Mygind and others (1978) followed up a group of 33 patients who had prolonged treatment lasting from 9–36 months with beclomethasone dipropionate. They found no adverse effects with a daily dose of 200–400 µg. Heroman and co-workers (1980), however, recorded the disturbing case of a 4-year-old girl who developed adrenal suppression and cushingoid changes following treatment with 0.1% dexamethasone nasal drops. She suffered from chronic serous otitis media and was given 3 drops in each nostril 4 times daily for 8 weeks. The short corticotrophin stimulation test confirmed the adrenal suppression. The drops were stopped and eventually her appearance returned to normal and her adrenal function was adequate on retesting. It is clear that topical nasal steroids must be used with great caution in children until a safe dosage has been established.

A case of Cushing's syndrome due to the abuse of betamethasone nasal drops is reported by Stevens (1988) in a young man who took them in excessive dosage (approximately 130 ml in 10 weeks). Stevens calculated that this dose was equivalent to 20 mg of prednisolone daily.

The anticholinergic drug ipratropium bromide has been used intrabronchially for its bronchodilator effect for many years. It has recently become available in the form of an intranasal aerosol for the treatment of watery rhinorrhoea and perennial rhinitis and has proved very effective. No significant systemic effects were noted in a trial of 40 patients on long-term treatment. Mild nasal adverse effects occurred but usually resolved during the trial as patients adjusted the dosage (Milford *et al.* 1990).

Antihypertensives

Drugs such as methyldopa, reserpine, and guanethidine, which inhibit adrenergic function, give rise to nasal congestion and obstruction due to their unopposed parasympathetic activity. This is usually a fairly minor symptom that patients tolerate quite well once the cause is explained to them. This is clearly a Type A reaction. The angiotensin-converting-enzyme (ACE) inhibitor enalapril was reported as the cause of severe nasal obstruction in a 45-year-old woman with a history suggestive of mild allergic rhinitis (Finnerty *et al.* 1986). After 4 weeks' treatment she developed severe nasal obstruction that was not relieved by intranasal sodium cromoglycate, nasal steroids, or oral antihistamines. Enalapril was stopped and the nasal blockage cleared within 2 days. Enalapril was restarted a fortnight later and nasal obstruction recurred within 2 days. This seems likely to have been a Type B reaction typical of drug allergy.

Oral contraceptives

These drugs have been blamed for the occurrence of nasal congestion, together with a plugged feeling in the ear and a distortion of sound (presumably due to obstruction of the Eustachian tube), in a number of patients (Banovetz 1972). In some cases, changing from a sequential to a concomitant contraceptive or vice versa relieves the problem. In the *Interim report on oral contraceptives and health* by the Royal College of General Practitioners (1974), which covered 46 000 women in 1400 practices observed over 4 years, there was a well-marked increase in the incidence of nasal catarrh and allergic rhinitis in women taking these drugs.

Epistaxis

Nasal bleeding in patients receiving long-term anticoagulant therapy is a frequent cause of referral to an ENT clinic and warfarin is probably the drug most commonly implicated. Dipyridamole, which inhibits platelet aggregation and adhesion, is another well-documented cause of epistaxis.

More recently attention has been drawn to the effect of aspirin and other non-steroidal anti-inflammatory drugs, which also alter platelet function. In a study of 53 patients admitted to an ENT ward for epistaxis, Watson and Shenoi (1990) found that four times as many of the patients were taking non-steroidal anti-inflammatory drugs as in a matched control group admitted to the same ward with other diagnoses. The authors recommended that doctors and their patients should be warned of the possible risk of epistaxis as well as of gastrointestinal haemorrhage before beginning treatment with non-steroidal anti-inflammatory drugs.

Anosmia

Although chemically induced anosmia is an occupational hazard in workers exposed to carbon dioxide, carbon disulphide, and phosphorus oxychloride (MacIntyre 1971), it is rarely caused by drugs. The application of cocaine, the repeated use of vasoconstrictor drops, and the use of topical neomycin have been held responsible for anosmia (Rebattu *et al.* 1972). Kerekovic and Curkovic (1971) have pointed out that the aminoglycoside antibiotics can be olfactotoxic as well as ototoxic. In a series of 300 patients treated with streptomycin they found 8 cases of complete anosmia and 13 cases of hyposmia attributable to the antibiotic.

592   **Textbook of adverse drug reactions**

Buccal cavity and salivary glands
(see also Chapter 9)

A very large number of drugs are known to cause stomatitis, and the list grows yearly. Mercurial diuretics, now seldom used, remain a well-remembered cause. Oral antibiotics, particularly the tetracyclines and chloramphenicol, can induce a vitamin B deficiency and also a monilial infection of the oral cavity, both well-recognized factors in the development of glossitis, stomatitis, and pharyngitis. Fortunately the monilial infection will respond quickly to treatment with nystatin.

It is less well known that a wide variety of modern cytotoxic drugs can produce stomatitis. Mention may be made of the oral ulceration caused by cyclophosphamide, chlorambucil, and bleomycin. Although oral or intramuscular methotrexate fairly often causes stomatitis, it is strikingly rare after intravenous administration. Mercaptopurine, colaspase (asparaginase), actinomycin D, azotomycin, plicamycin (mithramycin), mitomycin, fluorouracil, and bendamustine (Imet 3393) are all recognized causes of stomatitis, while the antileukaemic drug daunorubicin is reported to have caused oropharyngeal ulceration in 12 of 38 children treated by Holton and others (1968).

Dentists are familiar with the oral lesions caused by the local application of salicylates, but the unsuspecting physician may be confused by this kind of ulceration. Even the aspirin-fortified chewing gum used for relief of throat discomfort after tonsillectomy has been known to produce these ulcers. It is interesting that sublingual isoprenaline not uncommonly causes buccal ulceration, and pancreatic extract can cause severe oral ulceration, presumably by enzymic digestion of the mucous membrane because of the patient's failure to swallow quickly enough.

There have been a small number of reports of buccal ulceration caused by chloroquine, griseofulvin, barbiturates, the indanedione group of anticoagulants, and more recently by gold therapy (Glenert 1984) and by proguanil (Daniels 1986).

Xerostomia and sialorrhoea

Dryness of the mouth and throat is a very well known adverse effect of drugs with anticholinergic or atropine-like activity. The list of such drugs is extensive and includes:
1. antihistamines, e.g. diphenhydramine and deptropine;
2. antihypertensives, e.g. methyldopa, guanethidine, clonidine, and the rauwolfia alkaloids;
3. anorectic agents, e.g. fenfluramine and diethylpropion;
4. antiarrhythmic drugs, e.g. disopyramide;
5. benzodiazepine hypnotics, e.g. flurazepam;
6. butyrophenones, e.g. haloperidol.

The major tranquillizer loxapine, the vasodilator guancidine, and the pituitary inhibitor bromocriptine also produce xerostomia as an unwanted effect.

By way of contrast, drugs that have cholinergic effects will produce an excessive flow of saliva. In addition, their cholinergic action on the nasal and bronchial mucosa will cause excessive nasal and bronchial secretion. Deanol (2-dimethylaminoethanol) is used in the management of several neurological disorders and is thought to be effective through its conversion in the body to choline and acetylcholine. Nesse and Carroll (1976) report the case of a woman who received deanol therapy for 3 weeks and developed sialorrhoea, rhinorrhoea, and dyspnoea due to increased bronchial secretion. When the drug was discontinued, symptomatic improvement was apparent within 16 hours, and by the second day the lungs were clear and the rhinorrhoea and sialorrhoea had ceased. The cholinergic and anticholinergic adverse effects are clearly Type A reactions.

In 1988 the WHO record file contained five cases of hypersalivation and also 10 cases of gynaecomastia attributed to the ACE inhibitor captopril (Adverse Drug Reactions Advisory Committee 1988). The mechanism of captopril-induced sialorrhoea is unknown at present.

Hyperplasia and hypertrophy of the gums

This seems a somewhat bizarre complication of drug treatment, but its occurrence after the use of phenytoin was well documented by Bergmann (1967) and also by Livingston and Livingston (1969), who estimated the incidence to be as high as 40 per cent in the 15 000 patients they surveyed. Neither the occurrence nor the degree of hyperplasia is related to the dosage, and it may be due to a hypersensitivity reaction. In most cases the gums return to normal within a year of stopping the drug. It is suggested that phenytoin should not be used as the drug of first choice in epileptic children receiving orthodontic treatment, or for female epileptics, especially during adolescence.

A great deal has been written about the possible adverse effects of oral contraceptives. Hypertrophic gingivitis has been recorded (Lynn 1967; Lindhe and Bjorn 1968; El-Ashiry *et al.* 1970) as a complication of these drugs, but the incidence appears to be low. Giustiniani and co-workers (1987) reported a case of gingival hyperplasia in a patient receiving verapamil. The drug was stopped and the hyperplasia settled. Treatment with diltiazem was started after an interval and the gingival hyperplasia recurred. In a series of 107 patients who had had renal transplants, Slavin and Taylor (1987) recorded that 51 per cent of the patients treated with nifedipine and cyclosporin, but only 8 per cent of those receiving cyclosporin alone developed hyperplasia. Bowman and others (1988) recorded gingival hyperplasia in a 72-year-old man who received diltiazem. They pointed out that calcium is known to be involved in the control of tissue growth and suggested that the calcium-blocking effect of these agents may be part of the common pathogenesis of drug-induced gingival hyperplasia.

Disturbances of taste

Many medicaments induce abnormalities of taste by processes not yet properly understood, for example, gold salts, levodopa, the biguanides, oxyfedrine, lincomycin, ethambutol, and aspirin (Rollin 1978; Guerrier and Uziel 1979). Minor taste disturbances have been reported in patients receiving griseofulvin (Fogan 1971), metronidazole (Powell 1968), and lithium carbonate (Duffield 1973). Transitory disturbance of taste has also been reported during the intravenous injection of the hypotensive diazoxide and the cytotoxic drug carmustine. The antibiotic carbenicillin, the antihistamine azelastine, and the antiarrhythmic drug propafenone have been reported to cause a transient bitter or altered taste sensation.

Interest in the drug-induced disorders of taste was sparked by the classic paper by Henkin and others (1967), who studied the effect of the chelating agent penicillamine on taste sensation. They found that the drug caused a loss of taste sensation in only 4 per cent of patients with Wilson's disease, in which the body stores an excessive amount of copper. In diseases, however, in which the body stores copper normally, for example, rheumatoid arthritis, scleroderma, cysteinuria, and idiopathic pulmonary fibrosis, they found that penicillamine caused a loss of taste sensation in 32 per cent of patients. Further studies led Henkin and Bradley (1969) to the conclusion that a deficiency of copper and zinc ions and an excess of the thiol group brought about a decrease in taste sensitivity. This prompted the authors to recommend oral administration of copper and zinc in the treatment of abnormalities of taste (Henkin and Bradley 1970). It has also been postulated, however, that penicillamine-induced taste disturbance is due to a direct effect of the drug on the receptor cells (Lyle 1974). Day and Golding (1974) found that taste disturbance was dose-related. If the dosage of penicillamine is below 900 mg

daily, there is a 25 per cent incidence of taste disturbance in patients with Wilson's disease. The incidence climbs to 50 per cent when the daily dosage exceeds 900 mg. It would appear that taste disturbance is reversible within a period of 8–10 weeks, whether or not penicillamine is discontinued (Jaffe 1968). Topronin and pyritinol, which have therapeutic actions similar to penicillamine, have also been reported to cause a similar taste disturbance.

The ACE inhibitor captopril is known to cause temporary loss of taste and the incidence of this effect increases with increasing dosage. Both penicillamine and captopril contain a sulphydryl group and it has been suggested that this component of the drugs is responsible for the taste loss. Dysgeusia has also been reported with the non-sulphydryl ACE inhibitor enalapril. Transient disturbances of taste (and of smell) have been encountered with the calcium antagonists nifedipine and diltiazem (Berman 1985; Levenson and Kennedy 1985). Transient taste loss has also recently been reported with the use of etidronate, one of the diphosphonate group of drugs used in the treatment of hypercalcaemia found in various disease states (Jones et al. 1987) and also as a remedy for senile osteoporosis and Paget's disease. The role of sulphydryl groups and of calcium in the mechanism of taste disturbance remains to be elucidated.

Some drugs have a selective action on the sense of taste in that they depress the taste sensation of salty substances without diminishing the taste of sweet, sour, or bitter items. Acetazolamide, a carbonic anhydrase inhibitor, has been shown to alter the taste sensation of carbonated drinks and to eliminate the tingle associated with carbonation. Graber and Kelleher (1988) reported that when acetazolamide was taken as a prophylactic against mountain sickness it abolished the carbonated tingle of beer and soda water and gave these drinks an unpleasant taste. They included in their report a translation of a Scandinavian study by Hansson (1961) demonstrating that both the systemic use of acetazolamide and the use of mouth rinses containing carbonic anhydrase inhibitors reduced the taste of salt and enhanced the taste of sweetness. It would seem likely that the drug exerts its effect by causing a local change in the normal working environment of taste receptor buds and is the consequence of inhibition of carbonic anhydrase. This would represent a Type A reaction. Support is given to the theory of a peripheral rather than a central selective action on taste sensation in a study by Lang and others (1988). They reported on the effect of chlorhexidine 0.2% mouth rinses taken by a group of 24 volunteers, who noted a significant and selective impairment in taste perception for salt but not for sucrose (sweet), citric acid (sour), or quinine (bitter). The altered taste sensation began on the first day of using chlorhexidine rinses and continued until the last day of use of the rinse, returning to normal when the mouth rinses were discontinued. (This subject is also discussed in Chapter 9.)

Salivary gland disorders

Salivary gland swelling has been reported as an adverse effect of insulin, phenylbutazone, oxyphenbutazone, iodides, and also occasionally of some hypertensive drugs. Shaper (1966) reported that 3–5 per cent of his diabetic patients in Uganda developed parotid gland enlargement when started on insulin therapy or after an increase in dosage, while Lawrence (1965) mentioned that this had occurred in 20 of his patients. The swelling can be painful, and a number of these patients were referred to an ENT specialist on account of 'earache'. Salivary gland swelling caused by phenylbutazone and oxyphenbutazone has been mistaken for mumps (Gross 1969; Mirsky 1970). In the patient described by Chen and colleagues (1977), the oxyphenbutazone-induced swelling of parotid and submandibular salivary glands was accompanied by pyrexia and transient eosinophilia. They suggested that the reaction was an allergic response (Type B reaction) producing oedema and spasm of the smooth muscle in the salivary ducts.

Harden (1968) proved beyond doubt that the salivary gland swelling caused by iodides was dose-dependent. He described a patient who developed bilateral submandibular salivary gland tenderness and swelling after taking the equivalent of 6 g of iodine per day for 36 hours in the form of a cough medicine. The medicine was discontinued, and 48 hours later the swelling had disappeared. The medicine was restarted 14 days later and once more the swelling occurred, but again it disappeared 3 days after stopping the drug. Harden demonstrated that whenever the plasma iodine concentration rose above 11 mg per 100 ml, the glandular swelling reappeared. He stated that the true incidence of salivary gland enlargement resulting from iodine administration was uncertain, and reports in the literature are few. It is important none the less to consider iodide administration in the differential diagnosis of painful salivary gland enlargement, as extensive investigation may be avoided and rapid cure achieved by withdrawal of the drug. Either the submandibular or the parotid glands may be affected. The pathogenesis is uncertain. It is well known that iodide is concentrated in saliva to many times the plasma level. The drug is also concentrated in the thyroid, stomach, and breasts. (This subject is also discussed in Chapter 9.)

The throat

The oesophagus

Drugs pass from the mouth to the stomach through the oesophagus so rapidly that adverse drug reactions in this organ are seldom seen. If the passage of drugs through the oesophagus is delayed, however, the risk of local damage appears to be increased.

McCall (1975) attributed a case of oesophageal ulceration with fatal haemorrhage to the use of slow-release potassium chloride (Slow-K) tablets. The patient had an aneurysmal dilatation of the left atrium sufficient to impede the passage of oesophageal contents.

Howie and Strachan (1975) first drew attention to the hold-up of Slow-K in the oesophagus after cardiac surgery in patients with enlarged hearts, and observed that this delayed passage of the drug produced oesophageal ulceration and stricture formation. Their barium studies showed a Slow-K tablet lodged in a compressed segment of the oesophagus, and they pointed out that the risk of taking this drug would be increased in those patients who required a prolonged period of recumbency.

There have been a number of reports of oesophageal ulceration due to emepronium bromide, a drug used for urinary incontinence and nocturia. The drug is frequently taken without water before going to bed. It is a parasympatholytic agent with peripheral actions similar to those of atropine. Although oral ulceration has been described in confused elderly patients who may have had difficulty in swallowing, oesophageal ulceration by this drug has also been reported in fit, young people who have no known oesophageal problems (Strouthidis et al. 1972; Puhakka 1978). An alternative formulation, emepronium carrageenate, is claimed to have less of an irritant effect in the oesophagus. Similar oesophageal ulcers have been found in people without oesophageal obstruction after swallowing tetracycline (Crowson et al. 1976), doxycycline (Schneider 1977), clindamycin (Sutton and Gosnold 1977), co-trimoxazole (Bjarnason and Bjornsson 1981), theophylline (Enzenauer et al. 1984), and also bacampicillin and clorazepate.

Carlborg and others (1983) have documented a series of 40 patients with endoscopically proven oesophageal ulcers following ingestion of tablets or capsules containing oxytetracycline, doxycycline, or limecycline. In their series, doxycycline in capsule form caused most of the ulcers. This suggests that capsules are more prone to lodge and dissolve in the oesophagus than tablets. After recommendations from the Swedish Adverse Reaction Committee in 1979, doxycycline capsule preparations were withdrawn from the Swedish market. The number of doxycycline-induced ulcers in Sweden appears to have diminished as a result of this decision.

Evans and Roberts (1976) studied the passage through the oesophagus of barium sulphate tablets (made to the size and shape of aspirin tablets) in 98 consecutive patients during routine radiological screening. In 57 patients, the tablets remained in the oesophagus for longer than 5 minutes. One patient, with no radiological abnormality of the oesophagus, retained a tablet for 45 minutes. The incidence of retention of the tablets in the oesophagus was found to be increased more than twofold in those patients with radiologically demonstrated oesophageal abnormalities. Oesophageal irritation with stenosis or ulceration has been reported with fluorouracil, large doses of chloral hydrate, or very large doses of aspirin. A single tablet of ferrous sulphate that lodged in the hypopharynx caused severe swelling and ulceration of the hypopharynx and cervical oesophagus (Abbarah *et al*. 1976). The lesson of these reports is that tablets or capsules should always be washed down with a glass of water, especially if they are taken after meals, preferably in the erect position. Special precautions must be taken with patients who are recumbent or who have any degree of oesophageal obstruction. A very detailed review of the adverse effects of certain tablets and capsules on the upper gastrointestinal tract has been published by Al-Dujaili and others (1983).

The larynx

Glottic oedema is the most dangerous element of angioedema (angioneurotic oedema), and is seen more commonly in the hereditary form of this disease than in the sporadic form due to food and drug allergies. The dangers of X-ray contrast media in iodine-sensitive individuals have been known for a long time. Seymour (1969) reported a case of glottic oedema during angiography which required an emergency laryngostomy. This occurred despite the fact that the patient was given an antihistamine and hydrocortisone before the injection of the contrast medium. When the reaction began, adrenaline was administered but failed to influence significantly the development of tissue oedema. Glottic oedema has also been reported following treatment with colaspase (L-asparaginase) (Storti and Quaglino 1970) and with penicillin (Dunn 1967).

Laryngospasm resulting from the use of barbiturates is well known to anaesthetists, and intravenous thiopentone is notorious in this respect. Doxapram and ethamivan are central nervous stimulants and non-specific analeptics. They can cause muscle twitching, and both have been known to cause laryngospasm.

Although the laryngeal changes in myxoedema are very well recognized by ENT specialists, it is surprising to find that no cases of hoarseness following treatment with antithyroid drugs are described in recent literature. Virilization of the larynx after treatment with testosterone or anabolic steroids was, however, very well documented by Kambic and Lenart (1969) and by Johanson and others (1969). They point out that many anabolic agents are included in low dosage in various combination preparations under names that do not indicate the presence of an androgen. Whenever a woman complains of a change in her voice, one should carefully enquire about any drugs she may be taking. The use of drostanolone propionate in hormone-dependent breast cancer is a fairly common cause of virilization of the larynx in Great Britain today.

The introduction of inhaled steroids has been a major advance in the treatment of patients with asthma. Adverse effects have been few, consisting mainly of mild sore throats, oropharyngeal candidiasis, and hoarseness. Williams and others (1983) studied a group of 14 patients with hoarseness who were receiving inhaled steroids. Incomplete adduction of the vocal cords on phonation was found in 9 of these 14 patients, and the authors postulated that this was the cause of the hoarseness and was due to steroid-induced myopathy of the adductor muscles. They found that the muscle weakness was related to the dose and potency of the inhaled steroid and that the weakness and dysphonia were reversed when the inhaled steroid was stopped. Resolution sometimes took a few weeks to be complete. This is an unexpected adverse reaction and the theory of causation is ingenious. *The Lancet* (1984) expressed the opinion that the steroid myopathy explanation was plausible but unproven. It certainly cannot account for all the cases of hoarseness in patients taking inhaled steroids. In 5 of the 14 patients in the series mentioned, no vocal cord abnormality was present. Candidiasis was thought to be the sole cause of hoarseness in three of these five patients, and in the remaining two there was neither candidiasis nor vocal cord abnormality, and no organic cause for the hoarseness was found. Although steroid inhalers are commonly prescribed, the incidence of hoarseness associated with their use is small. The hoarseness is generally mild and reversible. The reason for the hoarseness in some cases remains obscure and the steroid myopathy theory has still to be proven.

References

Abbarah, T.R., Fredell, J.E., and Ellenz, G.B. (1976). Ulceration by oral ferrous sulphate. *JAMA* 236, 2320.

Adverse Drug Reactions Advisory Committee (1988). Hyper-salivation and gynaecomastia associated with captopril. *Adverse Reactions Newsletter, No. 1.* WHO Collaborating Centre for International Drug Monitoring, Uppsala.

Al-Dujaili, H., Salole, E.G., and Florence, A.T. (1983). Drug formulation and oesophageal injury. *Adverse Drug React. Acute Poisoning Rev.* 2, 235.

Allen, T.C. (1976). Minocycline. *Ann. Intern. Med.* 84, 482.

Arcieri, G.M., Falco, F.G., Smith, H.M., and Hobson, L.B. (1970). Clinical research experience with gentamicin: incidence of adverse reactions. *Med. J. Aust.* i (suppl.), 30.

Ballantyne, J. (1970). Iatrogenic deafness. *J. Laryngol. Otol.* 84, 967.

Ballantyne J. (1973). Ototoxicity: a clinical review. *Audiology* 12, 325.

Bamford, M.F.M. and Jones, L.F. (1978). Deafness and biochemical imbalance after burns treatment with topical antibiotics in young children. Report of 6 cases. *Arch. Dis. Child.* 53 326.

Banovetz, J.D. (1972). In *Drugs of choice* (ed. W. Modell), p. 645. C.V. Mosby, St Louis.

Bergmann, C.L. (1967). Dilantin (diphenylhydantoin): its effect on the gingival tissues. *Dent. Dig.* 73, 63.

Berk, D.P. and Chalmers, T. (1970). Deafness complicating antibiotic therapy of hepatic encephalopathy. *Ann. Intern. Med.* 73, 393.

Berman, J.L. (1985). Dysomnia, dysgeusia and diltiazem. *Ann. Intern. Med.* 102, 717.

Bjarnason, I. and Bjornsson, S. (1981). Oesophageal ulcers. An adverse reaction to co-trimoxazole. *Acta Med. Scand.* 209, 431.

Block. S.H. (1975). Side effects of cromolyn sodium therapy. *J. Pediatr.* 87, 502.

Bosher, S.K. (1980). The nature of the ototoxic actions of ethacrynic acid upon the mammalian endolymph system. 1. Functional aspects. *Acta Otolaryngol.* 89, 407.

Boston Collaborative Drug Surveillance Program (1973). Drug-induced deafness. *JAMA* 224, 515.

Bowman, J.M., Levy, B.A., and Grubb, R.V. (1988). Gingival overgrowth induced by diltiazem. *Oral Surg. Oral Med. Oral Pathol.* 65, 183.

British Medical Journal (1969). Deafness after topical neomycin. *Br. Med. J.* iv, 181.

Brown, H.A. and Hinshaw, H.C. (1946). Toxic reaction of streptomycin on the eighth nerve apparatus. *Proc. Staff Meet. Mayo Clin.* 21, 347.

Brummett, R. E. and Fox, K.E. (1982). Studies of aminoglycoside ototoxicity in animal models. In *The aminoglycosides. Microbiology, clinical use and toxicology* (ed. A. Whelton and H.C. Neu), p. 419. Marcel Dekker, New York.

Brummett, R.E., Fox, K.E., Brown R.T., and Himes, D.L. (1978). Comparative ototoxic liability of netilmicin and gentamicin. *Arch. Otolaryngol.* 104, 579.

Brummett, R. E. and Morrison, M. S. (1990). The incidence of aminoglycoside antibiotic induced hearing loss. *Arch. Otolaryngol. Head Neck Surg.* 116, 406.

Carlborg, B., Densert, O., and Lindquist, C. (1983). Tetracycline induced oesophageal ulcers. A clinical and experimental study. *Laryngoscope* 93, 184.

Cases, A., Kelly, J., Sabater, J., Campistol, J.M., Torras, A. Montoliu, J., *et al.* (1988). Acute visual and auditory neurotoxicity in patients with end-stage renal disease receiving desferrioxamine. *Clin. Nephrol.* 29, 176.

Cazals, Y., Erre, J.P., Aurousseau, C., and Aran, J.M. (1987). Ototoxicity of teicoplanin in the guinea pig. *Br. J. Audiol.* 21, 27.

Chapman, P. (1982) . Naproxen and sudden hearing loss. *J. Laryngol. Otol.* 96, 163.

Chen, J.H., Ottolenghi, P., and Distenfeld, H. (1977). Oxyphenbutazone-induced sialadenitis. *JAMA* 238, 1399.

Cohn, E.S., Gordes, E.H., and Brusilow, S.W. (1971). Ethacrynic acid effect on the composition of cochlear fluids. *Science* 171, 910.

Committee on Safety of Medicines (1977). *Adverse Reactions Series No. 14*, London.

Conway, N. and Birt, B.D. (1965). Streptomycin in pregnancy; effect on the foetal ear. *Br. Med. J.* ii, 260.

Crowson, T.D., Head, L.H., and Ferrante, W.A. (1976). Esophageal ulcers associated with tetracycline therapy. *JAMA* 235, 2747.

Cummings, C.W. (1968). Experimental observations on the ototoxicity of nitrogen mustard. *Laryngoscope* 78, 530.

Daniels, A.M. (1986). Mouth ulceration: incidence study. *Lancet* i, 269.

Day, A. T. and Golding, J. (1974). Hazards of penicillamine therapy in the treatment of rheumatoid arthritis. *Postgrad. Med. J.* 50 (suppl.), 71.

Dayal, V.S., Kokshanian, A., and Mitchell, D.P. (1971). Combined effects of noise and kanamycin. *Ann. Otol. Rhinol. Laryngol.* 80, 897.

de Moura, L.E.P. and Hayden, R.C. (1968). Salicylate ototoxicity: a human temporal bone report. *Arch. Otolaryngol.* 87, 368.

Dencker, L. and Lindquist, N.G. (1975). Distribution of labelled chloroquine in the inner ear. *Arch. Otolaryngol.* 101, 185.

Desrochers, C.S. and Schacht, J. (1982). Neomycin concentrations in inner ear tissues and other organs of the guinea pig after chronic drug administration. *Acta Otolaryngol.* 93, 233.

De Virgiliis, S., Argiolu, F., Sanna, G., Cornacchia, G., Cossu, P., Cao, A., *et al.* (1979). Auditory involvement in thalassemia major. *Acta Haematol.* 61, 209.

Drake, T.E. (1974). Reaction to gentamicin sulfate cream. *Arch. Dermatol.* 110, 638.

Duffield, J.E. (1973). Side effects of lithium carbonate. *Br. Med. J.* i, 491.

Dunn, J.H. (1967). Oral penicillin and anaphylactoid reactions. *JAMA* 202, 552.

Dwivedi, G. S. and Mehra, Y.N. (1978). Ototoxicity of chloroquine phosphate. *J. Laryngol. Otol.* 92, 701.

Eckman, M.R., Johnson, T., and Riess, R. (1975). Partial deafness after erythromycin. *N. Engl. J. Med.* 292, 649.

El-Ashiry, G.M., El-Karfawy, A.H., Nasr, M.F., and Younis, N. (1970). Comparative study of the influence of pregnancy and oral contraceptives on the gingivae. *Oral Surg.* 30, 472.

Enzenauer, R.W., Bass, J.W., and McDonnell, J.T. (1984). Oesophageal ulceration associated with oral theophylline. *N. Engl. J. Med.* 310, 261.

Evans, K.T. and Roberts, G.M. (1976). Where do all the tablets go? *Lancet* ii, 1237.

Fee, W.E. (1980). Aminoglycoside ototoxicity in the human. *Laryngoscope* 90 (suppl.), 24.

Finnerty, A., Littley, M., and Reid, P. (1986). Enalapril-induced nasal blockage. *Lancet* ii, 1395.

Fogan, L. (1971). Griseofulvin and dysgeusia: implications? *Ann. Intern. Med.* 74, 795.

Friedlander, I.R. (1979). Ototoxic drugs and the detection of ototoxicity. *N. Engl. J. Med.* 301, 213.

Gailiunas, J. Jr, Dominguez-Moreno, M., Lazarus, J.M., Lowrie, E.G., Gottlieb, M.N., and Merrill, J.P. (1978). Vestibular toxicity of gentamicin. *Arch. Intern. Med.* 138, 1621.

Gannon, R.P., Tso, S.S., and Chung, D.Y. (1979). Interaction of kanamycin and noise exposure. *J. Laryngol. Otol.* 93, 341.

Gargye, A.K. and Dutta, D.V. (1959). Nerve deafness following chloromycetin therapy. *Indian J. Pediatr.* 26, 265.

Giustiniani, S., Robustelli della Cuna, F., and Marieni, M. (1987). Hyperplastic gingivitis during diltiazem therapy. *Int. J. Cardiol.* 15, 247.

Glenert, U. (1984). Drug stomatitis due to gold therapy. *Oral Surg. Oral Med. Oral Pathol.* 58, 52.

Gomolin, I.H. and Garshick, E. (1980). Ethacrynic acid-induced deafness accompanied by nystagmus. *N. Engl. J. Med.* 303, 702.

Gould, W.J. and Brockler, K.H. (1972). Minocycline therapy. *Arch. Otolaryngol.* 96, 291.

Graber, M. and Kelleher, S. (1988). Side effects of acetazolamide: the champagne blues. *Am. J. Med.* 84, 979.

Gross, L. (1969). Oxyphenbutazone-induced parotitis. *Ann. Intern. Med.* 70, 1229.

Guerrier, Y. and Uziel, A. (1979). Clinical aspects of taste disorders. *Acta Otolaryngol.* 87, 232.

Hansson, H.P.J. (1961). On the effect of carbonic anhydrase inhibition on the sense of taste: an unusual side effect of a medication (trans. D. Vigertz). *Nord. Med.* 65, 566.

Hanzelik, E. and Peppercorn, M. (1969). Deafness after ethacrynic acid. *Lancet* i, 416.

Harden, R.McG. (1968). Submandibular adenitis due to iodide administration. *Br. Med. J.* i, 160.

Harell, M., Shea, J.J., and Emmett, J.R. (1978a). Bilateral sudden deafness following combined insecticide poisoning. *Laryngoscope* 88, 1348.

Harell M., Shea, J.J., and Emmett, J.R. (1978b1). Total deafness with propoxyphene abuse. *Laryngoscope* 88, 1518.

Hart, F.D. and Boardman, P.L. (1965). Indomethacin and phenylbutazone: a comparison. *Br. Med. J.* ii, 1281.

Hawkins, E. Jr (1967). In *Deafness in childhood* (ed. F. McConnell and P.H. Ward). Vanderbilt University Press, Nashville.

Hawkins, E. (1973). Ototoxic mechanisms. *Audiology* 12, 383.

Healy, C.E. (1972). Mumps vaccine and nerve deafness. *Am. J. Dis. Child.* 123, 612.

Henkin, R.I. and Bradley, D.F. (1969). Regulation of taste acuity by thiols and metal ions. *Proc. Nat. Acad. Sci. USA.* 62, 30.

Henkin R.I. and Bradley D.F. (1970). Hypogeusia corrected by Ni^{++} and Zn^{++}. *Life Sci.* 9, 701.

Henkin R.I., Keiser, H.R., Jaffe, I.A., Sternlieb, I, and Scheinberg, I.H. (1967). Decreased taste sensitivity after D-penicillamine reversed by copper administration. *Lancet* ii, 1268.

Heroman, W.M., Bybee, D.E., Cardin, J., Bass, J.W., and Johnsonbaugh, R.E. (1980). Adrenal suppression and cushingoid changes secondary to dexamethasone nose drops. *J. Pediatr.* 96, 500.

Higby, D.J., Wallace, H.J., Albert, D., and Holland, J.F. (1974). Diamminodichloroplatinum in the chemotherapy of testicular tumours. *J. Urol.* 112, 100.

Hinshaw, H.C. and Feldman, W.H. (1945). Streptomycin in the treatment of clinical tuberculosis: a preliminary report. *Proc. Staff Meet. Mayo Clin.* 20, 313.

Holton, C.P., Lonsdale, D., Nora, A.H., Thurman, W.G., and Vietti, T.J. (1968). Clinical study of daunomycin (NSC-82151) in children with acute leukemia. *Cancer* 22, 1014.

Howie, A.D. and Strachan, R.W. (1975). Slow release potassium chloride treatment. *Br. Med. J.* ii, 176.

Iqbal, S. and Srivatsav, C.B.P. (1984). Chloramphenicol toxicity: a case report. *J. Laryngol. Otol.* 98, 523.

Jaffe, I.A. (1968). Effects of penicillamine on the kidney and taste. *Postgrad. Med. J.* 44 (suppl.), 15.

Jahn, A. F. and Ganti, K. (1987). Major auricular malformations due to accutane (isotretinoin). *Laryngoscope* 97, 832.

Johanson, A.J., Brasel, J.A., and Blizzard, R.M. (1969). Growth in patients with gonadal dysgenesis receiving fluoxymesterone. *J. Pediatr.* 75, 1015.

Jolicoeur, G. (1972). Ototoxic changes due to drugs. In *Drug-induced diseases*, Vol. 4 (ed. L. Meyler and H.M. Peck), p. 540. Associated Scientific Publishers, Amsterdam.

Jones, P.B.B., McCloskey, E.V., and Kanis, J.A. (1987). Transient taste loss during treatment with etidronate. *Lancet* ii, 637.

Jones, R.F.McN., Wright, H.D., and Ballantyne, J.C. (1977). Practolol and deafness. *J. Laryngol. Otol.* 91, 963.

Kambic, V. and Lenart, I. (1969). Modifications cliniques et histologiques de la muqueuse laryngienne des femmes après le traitement par la testostérone. *J. Fr. Otorhinolaryngol.* 18, 97.

Karmody, C. S. and Weinstein, L. (1977). Reversible sensorineural hearing loss with intravenous erythromycin lactobionate. *Ann. Otol. Rhinol. Laryngol.* 86, 9.

Kerekovic, M. and Curkovic, M. (1971). Olfactotoxicity of streptomycin. *Int. Rhinol.* 9, 97.

Kohonen, A. (1965). Effect of some ototoxic drugs upon the pattern and innervation of cochlear sensory cells in the guinea pig. *Acta Otolaryngol.* (suppl.) 208, 1.

Kohonen, A. and Tarkkanen, J. (1969). Cochlear damage from ototoxic antibiotics by intratympanic application. *Acta Otolaryngol.* 68, 90.

Kopelman, J., Budnick, A.S., Sessions, R.B., Kramer, M.B., and Wong, G.Y, (1988). Ototoxicity of high dose cisplatin by bolus administration in patients with advanced cancers and normal hearing. *Laryngoscope* 98, 858.

Kroboth, P.D., McNeil, M.A., Kreeger, A., Dominguez, J., and Rault, R. (1983). Hearing loss and erythromycin pharmacokinetics in a patient receiving haemodialysis. *Arch. Intern. Med.* 143, 1263.

The Lancet (1976). Ear-drops. *Lancet* i, 896.

The Lancet (1984). Inhaled steroids and dysphonia. *Lancet* i, 375.

Lang, N.P., Catalanotto, F.A., Knöpfli, R.U., and Antczak, A.A.A. (1988). Quality-specific taste impairment following the application of chlorhexidine digluconate mouth rinses. *J. Clin. Periodontol.* 15, 43.

Lanthier, P.L., Morgan, M.Y., and Ballantyne, J. (1984). Bromocriptine associated ototoxicity. *J. Laryngol. Otol.* 98, 399.

Laurell, G. and Jungnelius, U. (1990). High dose cisplatin treatment: hearing loss and plasma concentrations. *Laryngoscope* 100, 724.

Lawrence, R.D. (1965). Evanescent parotitis in diabetes. *Br. Med. J.* ii, 1432.

Lee, C.C., Anderson, R.C., and Chen, K.K. (1955). Renal clearance of erythromycin. *Proc. Soc. Exp. Biol. Med.* 88, 584.

Lerner, A.M., Cone, L.A., Jansen, W., Reyes, M.P., Blair, D.C., Wright, G.E., *et al.* (1983). Randomised controlled trial of the comparative efficiency, auditory toxicity, and nephrotoxicity of tobramycin and netilmicin. *Lancet* i, 1123.

Levenson, J.L. and Kennedy, K. (1985). Dysomnia, dysgeusia and nifedipine. *Ann. Intern. Med.* 102, 135.

Lindhe, J. and Bjorn, A.L. (1968). Influence of hormonal contraceptives on gingiva of women. *Dent. Dig.* 74, 389.

Little, P.J. and Lynn, K.L. (1975). Neomycin toxicity. *N.Z. Med. J.* 81, 445.

Livingston, S. and Livingston, H.L. (1969). Diphenylhydantoin gingival hyperplasia. *Am. J. Dis. Child.* 117, 265.

Livingstone, G. (1965). Congenital ear abnormalities due to thalidomide. *Proc. R. Soc. Med.* 58, 493.

Lloyd-Mostyn, R.H. (1969). Tinnitus and propranolol. *Br. Med. J.* ii, 766.

Lloyd-Mostyn, R.H. and Lord, I.J. (1971). Ototoxicity of intravenous frusemide. *Lancet* ii, 1156.

Lumsden, R.B. and McDowell, G.D. (1968). In *Logan Turner's diseases of the nose, throat, and ear* (7th edn) (ed. J.P. Stewart and J.F. Birrell), p. 533. Wright, Bristol.

Lupin, A.J. and Harley, C.H. (1976). Inner ear damage related to propxyphene ingestion. *Can. Med. Assoc. J.* 114, 596.

Lyle, W.H. (1974). Penicillamine and zinc. *Lancet* ii, 1140.

Lynn, B.D. (1967). The 'pill' as an etiologic agent in hypertrophic gingivitis. *Oral Surg.* 24, 333.

McCabe, P.A. and Day, F.L. (1965). The effect of aspirin on auditory sensitivity. *Ann. Otol. Rhinol. Laryngol.* 74, 312.

McCall, A.J. (1975). Slow-K ulceration of oesophagus with aneurysmal left atriuim. *Br. Med. J.* iii, 230.

MacIntyre, I. (1971). Prolonged anosmia. *Br. Med. J.* ii, 709.

McKelvie, P., Johnstone, I. Jamieson, I., and Brooks, C. (1975). The effect of gentamicin ear drops on the cochlea. *Br. J. Audiol.* 9, 45.

McKinna, A.J. (1966). Quinine-induced hypoplasia of the optic nerve. *Can. J. Ophthalmol.* 1, 261.

Mahajan, S.L., Ikeda, Y., Myers, T.J., and Baldini, M.G. (1981). Acute acoustic nerve palsy associated with vincristine therapy. *Cancer* 47, 2404.

Maher, E.R., Hollman, A., and Gruneberg, R.N. (1986). Teicoplanin induced ototoxicity in Down's syndrome. *Lancet* i, 613.

Mair, I.W.S. and Elverland, H.H. (1977). Sudden deafness and vaccination. *J. Laryngol. Otol.* 91, 323.

Mathog, R.H., Thomas, W.G., and Hudson, W.R. (1970). Ototoxicity of new and potent diuretics. *Arch. Otolaryngol.* 92, 7.

Matz, G.J. and Naunton, R.F. (1968). Ototoxicity of chloroquine. *Arch. Otolaryngol.* 88, 370.

Matz, G.J., Beal, D.D., and Krames, L. (1969). Ototoxicity of ethacrynic acid demonstrated in a human temporal bone. *Arch. Otolaryngol.* 90, 152.

Mawson, S.R. (1967). *Diseases of the ear*, p. 441. Edward Arnold, London.

Medical Journal of Australia (1975). Ear drops and iatrogenic deafness. *Med. J. Aust.* ii, 626.

Meriwether, W.D., Mangi, R.J., and Serpick, A.A. (1971). Deafness following standard intravenous dose of ethacrynic acid. *JAMA* 216, 795.

Mery, J.P. and Kanfer, A. (1979), Ototoxicity of erythromycin in patients with renal insufficiency. *N. Engl. J. Med.* 301, 944.

Meyer zum Guttesberge, A. and Stupp, H.F. (1969). Streptomycin spregelin der Perelymphe des Menschen. *Acta Otolaryngol.* 67, 171.

Milford, C.A., Mugliston, T.A., Lund, V.J., and Mackay, I.S. (1990). Long-term safety and efficacy study of intranasal ipratropium bromide. *J. Laryngol. Otol.* 104, 123.

Miller, S.M. (1982). Erythromycin ototoxicity. *Med. J. Aust.* ii, 242.

Mintz, U., Amir, J., Pinkhas, J., and De Vries, A. (1973). Transient perceptive deafness due to erythromycin lactobionate. *JAMA* 255, 1122.

Mirsky, S. (1970). Salivary gland reaction to phenylbutazone. *Can. Med. Assoc. J.* 102, 91.

Mitchell, C., Brummet, R.E., Himes, D., and Vernon. J. (1973). Electrophysiological study of the effect of sodium salicylate upon the cochlea. *Arch. Otolaryngol.* 98, 297.

Morizono, T. and Johnstone, B.M. (1975). Ototoxicity of chloramphenicol ear drops with propylene glycol as solvent. *Med. J. Aust.* ii, 634.

Morris, D.L. and Fletcher, A. (1986). Hyperacusis after treatment with mefenamic acid. *Br. Med. J.* 293, 823.

Morton, R. (1692). *Pyretologia: seu exercitationes de morbus universalis acutis.* Samuel Smith, London (quoted by Stephens, S.D.G. 1982).

Myers, E.N., Bernstein, J.M., and Fosriporolous, G. (1965). Salicylate ototoxicity, a clinical study. *N. Engl. J. Med.* 273, 587.

Mygind, N., Sørensen, H., and Pedersen, C.B. (1978). The nasal mucosa during long-term treatment with beclomethasone dipropionate aerosol. *Acta Otolaryngol.* 85, 437.

Nadol, J.B. (1978). Hearing loss as a sequela of meningitis. *Laryngoscope* 88, 739.

Nesse, R. and Carroll, B.J. (1976). Cholinergic side-effects associated with deanol. *Lancet* ii, 50.

Obiako, M.N. (1979). Chloroquine ototoxicity: an iatrogenic tragedy. *Ghana Med. J.* 18, 179. Quoted in *Side effects of drugs annual 7 — 1983* (ed. M.N.G. Dukes), p. 295. Associated Scientific Publishers, Amsterdam.

O'Connor, A.F.F., Freeland, A.P., Heal, D.J., and Rossouw, D.S. (1977). Iodoform toxicity following the use of BIPP: a potential hazard. *J. Laryngol. Otol.* 91, 903.

Ohtani, I., Ohtsuki, K., Omata, T., Ouchi, J., and Saito, T. (1978*a*). Potentiation and its mechanisms of cochlear damage resulting from furosemide and aminoglycoside antibiotics. *Otorhinolaryngol.* (Fukuoka) 40, 53.

Ohtani, I.,, Ohtsuki, K., Omata, T., Ouchi, J., and Saito, T. (1978*b*). Interaction of bumetanide and kanamycin. *Otorhinolaryngol.* (Fukuoka) 40, 216.

Oliveira, J.A.A. (1989*a*). *Audiovestibular toxicity of drugs*, Vol. 2, p. 140. CRC Press Inc., Boca Raton, Florida.

Oliveira, J.A.A. (1989*b*). *Audiovestibular toxicity of drugs*, Vol. 1, p. 138. CRC Press Inc., Boca Raton, Florida.

Olivieri, N.F., Buncic, J. R., Chew, E., Gallant, T. Harrison, R.V., Keenan, N., *et al.* (1986). Visual and auditory neurotoxicity in patients receiving subcutaneous deferoxamine infusions. *N. Engl. J. Med.* 314, 869.

Osguthorpe, J.D. and Shirley, R. (1987). Neonatal respiratory distress from rhinitis medicamentosa. *Laryngoscope* 97, 829.

Pace-Balzan, A. and Ramsden, R.T. (1988). Sudden bilateral sensorineural hearing loss during treatment with dantrolene sodium (dantrium). *J. Laryngol. Otol* 102, 57.

Pearlman, L.V. (1966). Salicylate intoxication from skin application. *N. Engl. J. Med.* 274, 164.

Pillay, V.K.G., Schwartz, F.D., Aimi, K., and Kark, R.M. (1969). Transient and permanent deafness following treatment with ethacrynic acid in renal failure. *Lancet* i, 77.

Podoshin, L., Fradis, M., and Ben-David, J. (1989). Ototoxicity of ear drops in patients suffering from chronic otitis media. *J. Laryngol. Otol.* 103, 46.

Porter, J. and Jick, H. (1977). Drug-induced anaphylaxis, convulsions, deafness, and extrapyramidal symptoms. *Lancet* i, 587.

Powell, S.J. (1968). Metronidazole. An anti-infective agent of growing importance. *Medicine Today* 2, 44.

Presley, A.P. (1988). Penicillamine-induced rhinitis. *Br. Med. J.* 296, 1332.

Puhakka, H.J. (1978), Drug-induced corrosive injury of the oesophagus. *J. Laryngol. Otol.* 42, 927.

Quinnan, G.U. and McCabe, W.R. (1978). Ototoxicity of erythromycin. *Lancet* i, 1160.

Racy, J. and Ward-Racy, A. (1980). Tinnitus in imipramine therapy. *Am. J. Psychiatry* 137, 854.

Ramsden, R.T. and Ackrill, P. (1982). Bobbing oscillopsia from gentamicin toxicity. *Br. J. Audiology* 16, 147.

Ramsden, R.T., Latif, A., and O'Malley, S. (1985). Electrocochleographic changes in acute salicylate overdosage. *J. Laryngol. Otol.* 99, 1269.

Rebattu, J.P., Lafon, H., and Cajgfinger, H. (1972). La pathologie iatrogène en oto-rhino-laryngologie. *Lyon Med.* 118, 787.

Rollin, H. (1978). Drug related gustatory disorders. *Ann. Otol. Rhinol. Laryngol.* 87, 1.

Rosketh, R. and Storstein, O. (1963). Quinidine therapy of chronic auricular fibrillation. *Arch. Intern. Med.* 111, 184.

Rothermich, N.O. (1966). An extended study of indomethacin. *JAMA* 195, 531.

Royal College of General Practitioners (1974). *Interim report on oral contraceptives and health.* London.

Rybak, L.P. (1981). Cis-platinum associated hearing loss. *J. Laryngol. Otol.* 95, 745.

Rybak, L.P and Whitworth, C. (1986). Comparative ototoxicity of furosemide and piretamide. *Acta Otolaryngol.* 101, 59.

Schacht, J. (1986). Molecular mechanisms of drug-induced hearing loss. *Hear. Res.* 22, 297.

Schaefer, S.D., Wright, C.G., Post, J.D., and Frenkel, E.P. (1981). Cis-platinum vestibular toxicity. *Cancer* 47, 857.

Schneider, R. (1977). Doxycycline esophageal ulcers. *Am. J. Digest. Dis.* 22, 805.

Schuknecht, H.F. (1964). The pathology of several disorders of the inner ear which cause vertigo. *South. Med. J.* 57, 1161.

Schwartz, G.H., David, D.S., Riggio, R.R., Stenzel, K.H., and Rubin, A.L. (1970). Ototoxicity induced by furosemide. *N. Engl. J. Med.* 282, 1413.

Sennasael, J. Verbeelen, D., and Lauwers, S. (1982). Ototoxicity associated with cephalexin in 2 patients with renal failure. *Lancet* ii, 1154.

Seymour, J. (1969). Severe laryngeal oedema during injection with sodium metrizoate (Triosil). *Br. Heart J.* 31, 529.

Shaper, A.G. (1966). Parotid gland enlargement and the insulin–oedema syndrome. *Br. Med. J.* i, 803.

Slavin, J. and Taylor. J. (1987). Cyclosporin, nifedipine and gingival hyperplasia. *Lancet* ii, 739.

Smith, C.R., Baughman, K.L., Edwards, C.Q., Rogers, J.F., and Leitman, P.S. (1977). Controlled comparison of amikacin and gentamicin. *N. Engl. J. Med.* 296, 349.

Smith, K.E. and Spaulding, J.S. (1972). Ototoxic reaction to propylthiouracil. *Arch. Otolaryngol.* 96, 368.

Smith, K.E. Reece, C.A., and Kauffman, R. (1972). Ototoxic reaction associated with the use of nortriptyline hydrochloride. *J. Pediatr.* 80, 1046.

Spoendlin, H. (1966). Zur Ototoxizität des Streptomyzins. *Practica Otorhinolaryngol.* 28, 305.

Stephens, S.D.G. (1982). Some historical aspects of ototoxicity. *Br. J. Audiol.* 16, 76.

Stevens, D.J. (1988). Cushing's syndrome due to abuse of betamethasone nasal drops. *J. Laryngol. Otol.* 102, 219.

Storti, E. and Quaglino, D. (1970). Dysmetabolic and neurological complications in leukaemic patients treated with L-asparaginase. *Recent Results Cancer Res.* 33, 344.

Strauss, M., Towfighi, J., Lord, S., Lipton, A., Harvery, H.A., and Brown, B. (1983). Cis-platinum ototoxicity: clinical experience and temporal bone histopathology. *Laryngoscope* 93, 1554.

Strouthidis, T.M., Mankikar, G.D., and Irvine, R.E. (1972). Ulceration of the mouth due to emepronium bromide. *Lancet* i, 72.

Stupp, H.F., Kupper, F., Lagler, H., and Sousand Quante, M. (1973). Inner ear concentrations and ototoxicity of different antibiotics in local and systemic application. *Audiology* 12, 350.

Stypulkowski, P.H. (1990). Mechanisms of salicylate ototoxicity. *Hear. Res.* 46, 113.

Sutton, D.R. and Gosnold, J.K. (1977). Oesophageal ulceration due to clindamycin. *Br. Med. J.* i, 1598.

Taylor, R., Schofield, I.S., Ramos, J.M., Blint, A.J., and Ward, M.K. (1981). Ototoxicity of erythromycin in peritoneal dialysis patients. *Lancet* ii, 935.

Thomsen, J. Bech, P., and Szpirt, W. (1976). Otologic symptoms in chronic renal failure. The possible role of aminoglycoside–furosemide interaction. *Arch. Otorhinolaryngol.* 214, 71.

Tjernstrom, O. (1980). Prospective evaluation of vestibular and auditory function in 76 patients treated with netilmicin. *Scand. J. Infect. Dis.* (suppl. 23), 122.

Toone, E.C., Hayden, G.D., and Ellman, H.M. (1965). Ototoxicity of chloroquine. *Arthr. Rheum.* 8, 475.

Toyoda, Y. and Tachibana, M. (1978). Tissue levels of kanamycin in correlation with oto and nephrotoxicity. *Acta Otolaryngol.* 86, 9.

van der Hulst, R.J.A.M., Dreschler, W.A., and Uranus, N.A.M. (1988). High frequency audiometry in prospective clinical research of ototoxicity due to platinum derivatives. *Ann. Otol. Rhinol. Laryngol.* 97, 133.

van Marion, W.F., van der Meer, J.W.M., Kalff, M.W., and Scnicht, S.M. (1978). Ototoxicity of erythromycin. *Lancet* ii, 214.

Vernon, J., Brummett, R., and Walsh, T. (1978). The ototoxic potential of propylene glycol in guinea pigs. *Arch. Otolaryngol.* 104, 726.

Wallner, L.J. (1949). The otologic effects of streptomycin therapy. *Ann. Otol. Rhinol. Laryngol.* 58, 111.

Waltner, J.G. (1955). The effect of salicylates on the inner ear. *Ann. Otol.* 64, 617.

Waltzman, S.B.G. and Cooper, J.S. (1981). Nature and incidence of misonidazole-produced ototoxicity. *Arch. Otolaryngol.* 107, 52.

Ward, K.M. and Rounthwaite, F.J. (1978). Neomycin ototoxicity. *Ann. Otol. Rhinol. Laryngol.* 87, 211.

Watson, M.G. and Shenoi, P.M. (1990). Drug-induced epistaxis. *J. R. Soc. Med.* 83, 162.

Weinstein, A.J., McHenry, M.C., and Gavan, T.L. (1977). Systemic absorption of neomycin irrigation solution. *JAMA* 238, 152.

West, B.A., Brummett, R.E., and Himes, D.L. (1973). Interaction of kanamycin and ethacrynic acid. *Arch. Otolaryngol.* 98, 32.

Williams, A.J., Baghat, M.S., Stableforth, D.E., Cayton, R.M., Shenoi, P.M., and Skinner, C. (1983). Dysphonia caused by inhaled steroids: recognition of a characteristic laryngeal abnormality. *Thorax* 38, 813.

Williams, D.N., Laughlin, L.W., and Yhu-Hsiung Lee (1975). Minocycline: possible vestibular side effects. *Lancet* ii, 744.

Wilson, A. and Schild, H.O. (1968). *Applied pharmacology*, p. 150. Churchill, London.

Wilson, P. and Ramsden, R.T. (1977). Immediate effects of tobramycin on human cochlea and correlation with serum tobramycin levels. *Br. Med. J.* i, 259.

Wonke, B., Hoffbrand, A.V., Aldouri, M., Wickens, D., Flynn, D., Stearns, M., *et al.* (1989). Reversal of desferrioxamine induced auditory neurotoxicity during treatment with Ca-DTPA. *Arch. Dis. Child.* 64, 77.

Wright, P. (1975). Untoward effects associated with practolol administration: oculomucocutaneous syndrome. *Br. Med. J.* i, 595.

Yeadon, A. and Garratt, P.R. (1975). Minocycline (Minocin): a large-scale assessment in general practice. *Clin. Trials J.* 12, 3.

Yung, M.W. and Dorman, E.B. (1986). Electrocochleography during intravenous infusion of cisplatin. *Arch. Otolaryngol. Head Neck Surg.* 112, 823.

21. Psychiatric disorders

K. DAVISON and F. HASSANYEH

Introduction

Adverse drug reactions account for a substantial amount of psychiatric morbidity which is increasing as new and ever more potent drugs are introduced. A survey of adverse drug reactions in general practice revealed that neuropsychiatric reactions accounted for 30 per cent of cases, second only to gastrointestinal reactions (Martys 1979). The Boston Collaborative Drug Surveillance Program (BCDSP 1971) recorded adverse psychiatric reactions in 2.7 per cent of 9000 hospital patients receiving non-psychiatric drugs.

Problems of ascertainment

The difficulties attaching to establishing the validity of any alleged drug reaction are greatly magnified for psychiatric reactions. The latter may be delayed in onset, and some reactions may persist for weeks or months after drug withdrawal. Confounding placebo effects, intercurrent illness, and psychiatric effects of the condition being treated are especially significant. As it is rarely possible to control these variables, most of the time only drug associations are reported, the strength of which must then be assessed on the basis of frequency and consistency, temporal association, relation to drug plasma levels, and the response to rechallenge. Correct identification of the psychiatric syndromes encountered is another problematic area. Many reports emanate from non-psychiatrists, who tend to equate hallucinations and delusions with 'psychosis' or even 'schizophrenia', and apathy with 'depression' when the correct diagnosis is 'delirium' (see below). Application of a recognized diagnostic system, such as the International Classification of Diseases (ICD-9) (WHO 1977) or that of the American Psychiatric Association (DSM-III-R) (APA 1987) would help to obviate this difficulty. These problems emphasize importance of national systems of reporting adverse drug reactions, such as that of the Committee on Safety of Medicines in the United Kingdom.

Predisposing factors

An important variable in the production of adverse psychiatric reactions is personal predisposition. The risk is increased in those with pre-existing impairment of brain function, such as the elderly or brain-damaged, or with past or present psychiatric illness, or a history of alcohol or drug abuse, but those with unblemished psychiatric records are by no means immune. Although a family history of affective disorder (depression or mania) predisposes to the drug precipitation of the same conditions (Whitlock and Evans 1978), the relationship is less clear-cut for paranoid or schizophreniform psychoses (Davison 1976). These disorders can also appear in those without such predisposition.

Other predisposing factors include extreme youth (Prescott 1979), concurrent physical disease (James 1975), and stressful environments, such as intensive treatment units (Tomlin 1977; Davison 1989a).

In addition to drug-related factors, such as dose, duration, and drug interaction, adverse reactions are correlated with the number of drugs being taken concomitantly. In a survey of 1000 patients the incidence of adverse reactions reached 81.4 per cent in those receiving six or more drugs (Hurwitz 1969).

Types of reaction

The vast majority of adverse psychiatric drug reactions are of Type A in that they are dose-dependent or recognizably related to the known pharmacological properties of the drug. Even when a reaction occurs at therapeutic plasma drug levels there is often an interaction of an identifiable drug effect with individual predisposition.

Reactions may appear to be idiosyncratic merely because the full range of a drug's pharmacological effects is not completely identified.

Classification

Adverse psychiatric reactions to drugs, formerly given the generic label 'toxic psychosis', are now more precisely classified (McClelland 1985) into several distinct syndromes, as follows:

1. behavioural toxicity (minimal or borderline reactions);
2. delirium (DSM-III-R) (confusional state, acute brain syndrome);
3. affective reactions (DSM-III-R organic mood disorder);
   a) depression
   b) mania and hypomania;
4. paranoid and schizophreniform psychoses (DSM-III-R organic delusional disorder);
5. hallucinatory states (DSM-III-R organic hallucinosis);
6. dementia (DSM-III-R) and pseudodementia
7. neuropsychiatric states (encephalopathies).

DSM-III-R also lists a number of specific 'psycho-active substance-induced organic mental disorders', including reactions to amphetamine; caffeine; cannabis; cocaine; hallucinogens; inhalants; opioids; phencyclidine; sedative, hypnotic, and anxiolytic drugs; and 'unspecified psycho-active substances', each with its own criteria-based syndromes (APA 1987).

Behavioural toxicity

This term includes a number of symptoms and behavioural changes which can occur singly or in combination, for example, drowsiness, insomnia, vivid dreams and nightmares, mild depression or excitement, anxiety, irritability, sensitivity to noise, listlessness, and restlessness (McClelland 1985). Such symptoms may be the precursors of a more florid psychiatric disorder, such as delirium. The drugs commonly associated with these symptoms are listed in Table 21.1.

Delirium

Delirium is characterized by a reduction in the level of conscious awareness (clouding), manifested clinically as disorientation in time or space, or both, usually worse at night. Fluctuation between lucidity and clouding is com-

TABLE 21.1
Drugs liable to induce behavioural toxicity

Drowsiness	Antihistamines
	Antihypertensive drugs
	Benzodiazepines
	Phenothiazines
	Tricyclic antidepressants
Vivid dreams and nightmares	Antihypertensive drugs
	Baclofen
	β-Adrenoceptor blockers
	Fenfluramine
	Hypnotic withdrawal
Behavioural changes	Benzodiazepines
	Levodopa
	Lithium with neuroleptic drugs
	Methyldopa with haloperidol

mon, however, hence other evidence, such as patchy amnesia and noisy nocturnal restlessness, must be taken into account. The patient's mood is characteristically labile, fluctuating between apathy, excitement, anxiety, depression, perplexity, and hostility. Paranoid misinterpretation of the environment is common. Conversations are misheard as referring to the patient, and nearby voices are misinterpreted as those of relatives who are being refused access. Occasionally actual auditory hallucinations occur, for example, other patients or staff are heard to be threatening harm or conspiring together to kill the patient. Hallucinations are more often visual and may take the form of grotesque faces, recognizable figures, or animals. Behaviour disturbances, often based on paranoid ideation, include wandering, attempts to abscond from the hospital ward, and aggressive outbursts (Davison 1989b). The drugs principally associated with the induction of delirium are listed in Table 21.2.

Depression

Depressive reactions to drugs vary from mild mood changes with weepiness, loss of interest, and impaired concentration, to severe psychoses with psychomotor retardation, suicidal thinking, insomnia, anorexia, and delusions of sin, disease, poverty, or bodily disintegration. Drowsiness and lethargy alone should not be construed as depressive symptoms. The drugs mainly involved are listed in Table 21.3.

Mania and hypomania

A degree of euphoria is common in behavioural toxicity but specific manic or hypomanic reactions are infrequent.

TABLE 21.2
Drugs liable to cause delirium

Antibacterial drugs	Cycloserine
	Isoniazid
	Penicillin
	Rifampicin
	Streptomycin
	Sulphonamides
Anticholinergic drugs	Antiparkinsonian drugs
	Atropine
	Homatropine
	Hyoscine
	Tricyclic antidepressants
Anticonvulsants	Phenytoin
	Sodium valproate
Cardiovascular drugs	β-Adrenoceptor blockers
	Digitalis
	Diuretics
Dopamine agonists	Amantadine
	Bromocriptine
	Levodopa
Tranquillizers and hypnotics	Barbiturates
	Benzodiazepines
	Phenothiazines
Miscellaneous	Chloroquine
	Cimetidine
	Disulfiram
	Oral hypoglycaemic drugs
Drug withdrawal	Barbiturates
	Benzodiazepines

TABLE 21.3
Drugs liable to induce depression

Analgesics	Indomethacin
	Pentazocine
Antihypertensive drugs	Clonidine
	Methyldopa
	Reserpine
Major tranquillizers	Chlorpromazine
	Fluphenazine
	Thioridazine
Miscellaneous	Anticancer agents
	Levodopa
	Steroids
Stimulant withdrawal	Amphetamines
	Anorectic drugs

The concept of 'secondary mania' as a response to physical disease or toxins has become established in the last decade; a familial tendency to affective disorder is not a necessary precondition (Krauthammer and Klerman 1978).

Hypomania is characterized by elevated mood, often accompanied by excitement, arrogant hostility, overactivity, insomnia, pressure of speech, and boastful overconfidence. Mania is a more extreme form, often with grandiose or paranoid delusions.

Paranoid and schizophreniform psychoses

Paranoid psychoses are characterized by delusions of persecution, with or without auditory hallucinations, in the absence of clouding of consciousness. The additional association of bizarre delusions, incoherent thought and emotional withdrawal, blunting or incongruity warrants the description 'schizophreniform'. The clinical resemblance to natural schizophrenia can be close, but a family history of schizophrenia is rarely found (Davison 1976). The drugs commonly associated are listed in Table 21.4.

TABLE 21.4
Drugs liable to induce paranoid and schizophreniform psychoses

Anti-infective drugs	Antibacterial drugs
	Antimalarials
Antiparkinsonian drugs	Anticholinergic drugs
	Bromocriptine
	Levodopa
Cardiovascular drugs	Antihypertensive drugs
	β-Adrenoceptor blockers
	Digitalis
	Stramonium
CNS depressants	Anticonvulsants
	Antihistamines
	Barbiturates
	Bromides
CNS stimulants	Amphetamines
	Anorectic drugs
	Cocaine
	Nasal decongestants
Hallucinogens	Cannabis
	LSD
	MDMA
	Phencyclidine
Miscellaneous	Disulfiram
	Indomethacin
	Steroids

Hallucinatory states

The hallucinations involved are usually visual but occur without other features of delirium or psychosis. They can be extremely vivid and are often in colour and of animals. Sometimes they take a microptic or 'Lilliputian'

TABLE 21.5
Drugs liable to induce isolated visual hallucinations

Analgesics	Indomethacin
Antiparkinsonian drugs	Anticholinergic drugs Bromocriptine Levodopa
Cardiovascular drugs	β-Adrenoceptor blockers Digitalis
Psychotropic drugs	Benzodiazepines Bromides Tricyclic antidepressants

form (Harper and Knothe 1973). The drugs principally concerned are listed in Table 21.5.

Dementia and pseudodementia

Dementia is a deterioration, usually irreversible, of intellect, memory, and personality and normally secondary to organic cerebral disease. Although it is described in association with certain drugs, for example, the combination of levodopa, benzhexol, and amantadine (Wolf and Davis 1973), most examples turn out to be chronic delirious states which are reversible and therefore should more properly be labelled as pseudodementia (Davison 1981).

Neuropsychiatric states

These are combinations of any of the psychiatric syndromes listed above with neurological features such as involuntary movements, ataxia, dysarthria, and epileptiform fits. An example is the paranoid–hallucinatory psychosis, accompanied by cerebellar signs and symptoms, that may be induced by phenytoin (Logan and Freeman 1969).

Drugs and their adverse psychiatric effects

The various drug-induced psychiatric disorders and the drugs that may cause them will now be considered in greater detail.

Drugs acting mainly on the nervous system

Antimuscarinic drugs

Antimuscarinic, often less accurately termed 'anticholinergic', drugs include:

1. atropine and related alkaloids, used as cycloplegics or for premedication (e.g. hyoscine, homatropine);
2. synthetic tertiary amines, used as gut antispasmodics (e.g. dicyclomine and piperidolate hydrochloride);
3. synthetic quaternary ammonium compounds, also used as gut antispasmodics (e.g. propantheline bromide);
4. antiparkinsonian agents (e.g. benzhexol, orphenadrine, procyclidine, and benztropine hydrochlorides);
5. antihistamines;
6. tricyclic antidepressants (see section on Psychotropic drugs);
7. phenothiazines (see section on Neuroleptics);
8. ipratropium, a bronchodilator;
9. terodiline, used to treat urinary frequency;

The profound behavioural disturbances engendered by antimuscarinic drugs have been known since the recognition of poisoning by belladonna, so-called because of its use as a pupil dilator for beauty enhancement, derived from the wild plant deadly nightshade (*Atropa belladonna*). The syndrome induced is reasonably consistent and has become known as the 'central anticholinergic syndrome'. Its features include (Longo 1966):

1. impaired concentration and memory;
2. drowsiness and withdrawal;
3. excitement;
4. ataxia and asynergia;
5. hallucinations, usually visual;

These features are accompanied by the characteristic dry mouth, hot, dry skin, dilated pupils, and tachycardia. The central anticholinergic syndrome usually clears rapidly after withdrawal of the offending drug but it can also be terminated by intravenous physostigmine (Ullman *et al.* 1970).

Atropine and hyoscine

These drugs, used for preoperative medication, can induce both preanaesthetic (Smiler *et al.* 1973) and postanaesthetic excitement (Eckenhoff *et al.* 1961). The administration of atropine to control cardiac arrhythmia after infarction induced delirium accompanied by slow cerebration, somnolence, and inattention in 5 of 30 patients (Erikssen 1969). Hyoscine has induced memory impairment in normal subjects, reversed by physostigmine (Drachman 1977), which confirms the importance of cerebral cholinergic activity for normal memory function. Reduced activity of cerebral choline acetyltransferase (CAT), an enzyme involved in the production of acetycholine, is a notable feature of senile dementia of the Alzheimer type (Perry *et al.* 1977).

The use of mydriatic eye drops containing atropine and homatropine (Hoefnagel 1961), hyoscine (Freund and Merin 1970), or cyclopentolate (Shihab 1980; Khurana *et al.* 1988) is associated with the precipitation of behavioural toxicity and delirium, often accompanied by auditory and visual hallucinations and subsequent amnesia. Contamination of drinks with these eye drops is sometimes undertaken for criminal purposes, the delirious victim being more easily robbed (Brizer and Manning 1982).

The use of stramonium, which contains varying proportions of atropine and hyoscine, for hallucinogenic purposes, either alone (Dean 1963) or in a belladonna–stramonium mixture (Goldsmith *et al.* 1968; DiGiacomo 1968), or from the flowers of the plant *Datura stramonium* (Jimson weed, angel's trumpet, devil's trumpet) (Hall *et al.* 1977), is a potent precipitant of the central anticholinergic syndrome. A review of 212 cases of abuse leading to toxicity revealed visual hallucinations in 44.8 per cent, disorientation in 21.2 per cent, hyperactivity and combativeness in 13.7 per cent, amnesia in 10 per cent, dilated pupils in 17 per cent, dry mouth in 15 per cent, ataxia in 14.6 per cent, fever in 10 per cent, tachycardia in 8.5 per cent, skin flush in 6.1 per cent, and hypertension in 1 per cent. Five patients died after responding inappropriately to visual hallucinations (Gowdy 1972).

Antiparkinsonian drugs

Although these drugs can induce excited delirium with visual hallucinations in therapeutic doses (Porteous and Ross 1956), many reports refer to the effects of their abuse for euphoriant (Kaminer *et al.* 1982) or hallucinogenic purposes (Stephens 1967). Thus, toxic psychoses due to the abuse of benztropine (Woody and O'Brien 1974), benzhexol (Marriott 1976; Crawshaw and Mullen 1984), and procyclidine (Coid and Strang 1982) have been reported. The last report described a manic reaction, with overactivity, pressure of speech, and disinhibition.

A dementia-like state occurring in a 74-year-old man with Parkinson's disease recovered after the discontinuation of biperiden hydrochloride 2 mg twice daily (Kurlan 1988).

Histamine H₁-receptor blocking agents

These drugs are the antihistamines used in the treatment of allergic and vestibular disorders. Some are constituents of antitussive preparations for example, diphenhydramine in Benylin. Many have significant antimuscarinic properties and are therefore liable to induce the usual range of associated psychiatric disorders. Additionally, brompheniramine inhibits central dopamine uptake (Farnebo *et al.* 1970) and chlorpheniramine inhibits both central serotonin and noradrenaline uptake (Carlsson and Lingqvist 1969). Drowsiness is the commonest problem encountered with the use of antihistamines (Young 1964), although tolerance to this effect develops rapidly (Nicholson 1983). It is attributed to inhibition of central H₁-receptor excitatory effects. Astemizole and terfenadine cause less sedation and psychomotor impairment because they only penetrate the blood–brain barrier to a slight extent (Wood 1986).

Toxic psychoses of central anticholinergic type have occurred with diphenhydramine (Sachs 1948; Nigro 1968; Lambert 1987; Schreiber *et al.* 1988), cyclizine (Gott 1968), and pheniramine (Waldman and Pelner 1950). A schizophreniform psychosis, without delirium, has been reported with the last-named drug (Yapalater and Rockwell 1950) and isolated auditory, visual, or tactile hallucinations have been caused by it (Jones *et al.* 1973) and by dimenhydrinate (Malcolm and Miller 1972). These drugs are sometimes abused for their hallucinogenic properties (Malcolm and Miller 1972; Jones *et al.* 1973).

Parkinsonism, akathisia, tardive dyskinesia, and depression are described in association with both cinnarizine (Capellà *et al.* 1988) and flunarizine (Chouza *et al.* 1986). Twenty-two cases of depression in association with flunarizine were reported to the Netherlands Centre for Monitoring of Adverse Reactions to Drugs (Meyboom *et al.* 1986).

CNS stimulants

Amphetamine is the generic name for the racemic mixture of β-phenylisopropylamine. It was first synthesized as long ago as 1887 but independently resynthesized in 1927 by Alles and found to have peripheral sympathomimetic and CNS-stimulant properties (Angrist 1983). The D-isomer (dextroamphetamine) was soon isolated and the methyl derivative (methylamphetamine) synthesized. These substances induce euphoria, relieve fatigue, and enhance verbal and motor activity. Effects of a single dose last several hours; tolerance and psychological dependence develop; hence, both oral (Sadusk 1966) and intravenous (Hawks *et al.* 1969) abuse are common. Formerly employed in the treatment of depression and obesity, amphetamine is now used mainly in the treatment of narcolepsy and occasionally for attention-deficit disorder in children. The psychiatric effects of amphetamines are thought to be mediated via an increase in available dopamine at central receptor sites (Moore 1977; Angrist 1983).

Acute amphetamine intoxication is characterized by hyperalertness, hyperactivity, loquacity, euphoria, grandiosity, irritability, distractibility, hostility, aggressiveness, and impaired judgement. These effects develop within 20–60 minutes after oral ingestion or immediately after intravenous injection and are sometimes accompanied by chest or abdominal pain. Hypertension or hyperpyrexia are potentially fatal complications (Lake and Quirk 1984).

More familiar is the amphetamine psychosis. First reported in narcoleptics treated with amphetamine (Young and Scoville 1938), it subsequently occurred mainly in amphetamine-abusers (Connell 1958). In a classical monograph, Connell (1958) reviewed 34 case reports from the 1938–57 literature and reported 42 new cases. He described the clinical picture of amphetamine psychosis as 'primarily a paranoid psychosis with ideas of reference, delusions of persecution, and auditory and visual hallucinations in a setting of clear consciousness.' He pointed out that the mental picture may be indistinguishable from acute or chronic paranoid schizophrenia and has often been misdiagnosed as such, an observation that has since been repeatedly confirmed (Angrist 1983). The psychosis usually clears within a week of withdrawing the drug but if it persists in the absence of amphetamine derivatives in the urine a diagnosis of schizophrenia is possible (Connell 1958). Connell's patients displayed no family history of schizophrenia. The evocation of a psychosis so closely resembling schizophrenia by amphetamine, an indirect dopamine agonist, is one of the pillars of the central dopamine excess hypothesis of the pathogenesis of schizophrenia (Crow et al. 1976).

Amphetamine psychoses usually develop in a setting of prolonged consumption of high doses (Lake and Quirk 1984) but a single oral dose of 55 mg has precipitated a psychosis (Beamish and Kiloh 1960). Typical amphetamine psychoses have been evoked in experimental subjects in 1–5 days by giving oral dexamphetamine in doses of 20–190 mg per day (Griffiths et al. 1972) and 5–50 mg per hour (Angrist and Gershon 1970), or in 1 hour by methylamphetamine intravenously in doses from 55 to 640 mg (Bell 1973).

Amphetamine withdrawal, especially after prolonged consumption, induces lethargy, anxiety, somnolence, nightmares, and depression, sometimes of suicidal intensity, within 3 days and often persisting for weeks (Lake and Quirk 1984). Withdrawal delirium has also been recorded (Young et al. 1961; Deveaugh-Geiss and Pandurangi 1982).

Ephedrine is closely allied, chemically and pharmacologically, to amphetamine but has a much longer pedigree, having been used in the form of a herbal extract by the ancient Chinese over 5000 years ago (Chen and Schmidt 1925). It is now used clinically as a bronchodilator and nasal decongestant, is marketed in the USA as a legal cocaine substitute under the title of Ma Huang incense (Siegel 1980), and is often a constituent of stimulant 'look-alike' street drugs (Lake and Quirk 1984). It possesses sympathomimetic and dopaminergic agonist properties (Angrist et al. 1977) so that its adverse psychiatric effects are similar to those of amphetamine.

Whitehouse and Duncan (1987) reported a case of ephedrine psychosis and reviewed 20 case reports from the literature. They described the typical clinical picture as a paranoid psychosis with delusions and auditory hallucinations, in a setting of clear consciousness, with 45 per cent of patients experiencing visual hallucinations. Sixty per cent of their patients were taking ephedrine for asthma, the remainder largely for its euphoriant effect. The duration of ephedrine consumption varied from 3 days to 25 years, and in 80 per cent of cases was at least a year. The daily dose of ephedrine immediately before the psychotic episode ranged from 125 mg to 2500 mg (mean 510 mg). A schizophreniform picture, with 'first rank' symptoms is also seen (Roxanas and Spalding 1977).

Delirium is also occasionally precipitated (Kane and Florenzano 1971), usually when ephedrine is combined with other drugs as it is in the proprietary cough mixture Phensedyl, which is liable to abuse (Abed and Clark 1987).

Mephentermine is a sympathomimetic amine with a chemical structure resembling methylamphetamine that is used as a pressor agent and as a nasal decongestant inhalant (Weiner 1985). It possesses both α-adrenergic and β-adrenergic activity but its neurostimulatory effects are relatively slight (Reynolds 1982). Brief paranoid psychoses have been described after abuse of the contents of inhalers (Greenberg and Lustig 1966; Angrist et al. 1970), and a persistent schizophreniform psychosis has been reported in a physician who regularly injected himself with this drug (Joshi and Bhat 1988).

Phenylpropanolamine (PPA) is a sympathomimetic amine with a chemical structure similar to amphetamine but a much weaker stimulant effect on the CNS. It stimulates sympathetic activity indirectly by displacing noradrenaline and other endogenous monoamine neurotransmitters from their storage sites, and may have direct effects on α and β receptors (Lake and Quirk 1984). PPA exists in four isomeric forms. The usual preparation used as an ephedrine substitute, for nasal decongestion, and bronchial relaxation, is D-L-norephedrine. Another isomer, D-norpseudoephedrine (cathine) is also a constituent of the khat plant whose leaves are chewed by natives of East Africa and the Arabian peninsula. PPA is also abused as a street-drug 'look-alike' amphetamine substitute (Lake and Quirk 1984) in preparations with names such as 'pink ladies', 'black beauties', and 'speckled pups' (Mueller 1983).

In 1979 the Swedish Adverse Drug Reaction Committee received 61 reports of psychiatric disturbance associated with the ingestion of preparations containing PPA (Norvenius *et al.* 1979). These included restlessness, irritability, aggressiveness, and insomnia. Psychotic episodes, including delirium, visual hallucinations, paranoid delusions, and acute mania occurred in five subjects, three of them young children. A review of 34 reports of psychiatric emergencies after PPA ingestion found 30 psychotic episodes, 5 of which were acute mania (Lake and Quirk 1984). Amphetamine-like paranoid psychoses also develop (Kane and Green 1966; Dietz 1981; Rieger 1981) during which homicidal (Cornelius *et al.* 1984) or sexually disinhibited behaviour (Mueller 1983) may become apparent. Major depression is also reported (Twerski 1987). Similar reactions occur with the use of nasal sprays containing PPA (Wharton 1970). In several of the cases reported fits or hypertension also developed (Mueller 1983; Cornelius *et al.* 1984).

In the United Kingdom in 1984, the Committee on Safety of Medicines (CSM 1985) received 16 reports of visual hallucinations in children receiving the decongestant Actifed, which contains PPA and the antihistamine triprolidine, and several reports were published (Sankey *et al.* 1984; Bain 1984; Drennan 1984; Miller 1984). Actifed is sometimes abused and can then induce a paranoid psychosis (Leighton 1982; Lambert 1987). Subjects with pre-existing psychiatric disorders are particularly vulnerable (Scavullo and Dementi 1986).

On the other hand, Puder and Morgan (1987) conclude, from an analysis of 53 published reports, that the attribution of toxicity to PPA has been exaggerated, due to observer bias.

Khat (*Catha edulis*) is a plant whose leaves are chewed for their stimulating effect. It is grown mainly in the Yemen, Somalia, and Ethiopia but is also found in Turkestan, Afghanistan, Kenya, Uganda, Tanzania, Zaire, and Zimbabwe (McKee 1987). For many years the sole active ingredient was thought to be norpseudoephedrine (see above), but a labile active compound with sympathomimetic properties, present only in fresh leaves less than 5 days old, has been identified and named cathinone. Other compounds of similar structure, the cathedulins, have also been isolated (Kalix 1984; McKee 1987).

The acute effects in man are those of sympathetic stimulation, including tachycardia, tachypnoea, hypertension, facial and conjunctival congestion, and headache. Psychiatric effects include excitement, increased alertness, insomnia, anorexia, anxiety, and aggressive behaviour. Paranoid (Critchlow and Seifert 1987), schizophreniform (Gough and Cookson 1984), and manic (Giannini and Castellani 1982) psychoses induced by chewing khat have been reported in both indigenous and expatriate East Africans and Arabs (Dhadphale and Arap Mengech 1987). Psychological dependence is also recognized (Eddy *et al.* 1965). British clinicians should be aware of the effects of khat as it is imported into Britain (Mayberry *et al.* 1984; McLaren 1987) or grown locally (Giannini and Castellani 1982) by users. Further details are provided by Kalix (1984) and McKee (1987).

Pemoline is a weak CNS stimulant used in the treatment of attention-deficit disorder in children. Although its pharmacological effects resemble those of amphetamine it is structurally unrelated. It possesses dopamine-agonist properties and, like methylphenidate, it has provoked chorea and Gilles de la Tourette's syndrome (multiple tics accompanied by involuntary coprolalic utterances) (Mitchell and Matthews 1980; Bonthala and West 1983).

Abuse and dependence occur and manic (Sternbach 1981) and paranoid–hallucinatory psychoses (Polchert and Morse 1985) have been reported.

Phenylephrine is a vasoconstrictive sympathomimetic, used in eye drops and nasal sprays and as a hypertensive agent. Abuse of the nasal spray has induced paranoid (Snow *et al.* 1980) and manic (Waters and Lapierre 1981) psychoses.

Propylhexedrine is a constituent of nasal decongestant inhalers, abuse of which has provoked a paranoid psychosis (Anderson 1970).

Caffeine is a methylated xanthine with central stimulant properties used in many proprietary analgesic compounds. It is also available as a look-alike street drug and is the active constituent of coffee and Coca-Cola. Excessive caffeine intake can induce a picture resembling an anxiety state (Greden 1974) or psychotic reactions resembling mania, depression, or schizophrenia (Lake and Quirk 1984).

Anorectic drugs, centrally acting appetite suppressants, are sympathomimetics with amphetamine-like properties and corresponding psychiatric adverse effects and liability to abuse (Willis 1976). The descending order of stimulant potency is dexamphetamine, phentermine, chlorphentermine, mazindol, diethylpropion, and fenfluramine (Nir 1980).

Phentermine increases brain noradrenaline and dopamine but has no effect on serotonin (Garattini *et al.* 1978). Paranoid psychoses of the amphetamine type have been reported (Rubin 1964; Brooke *et al.* 1988; Devan 1990), usually after the taking of doses above the recommended level or in previously psychotic patients (Rubin 1964).

Mazindol was reported to the Australian Adverse Reaction Committee, in 1981, as a cause of paranoid–hallucinatory psychoses of the amphetamine type.

Over 20 reports of paranoid psychoses with auditory, and sometimes visual, hallucinations in association with either therapeutic (Brooke *et al.* 1988; Carney 1988) or excessive doses of diethylpropion (Petursson 1979) have appeared. A similar psychosis occurred one week after withdrawal of diethylpropion 75 mg daily taken for a month (Fookes 1976). Its abuse potential is stated to be restricted by its anxiety-provoking effect (Angrist 1983).

Fenfluramine is an indirect serotonin agonist (Garattini 1989) and this may be responsible for the depression which may occur in association with its consumption (Imlah 1970; Mullen *et al.* 1977) or withdrawal (Harding 1972). The dextroisomer, which is the more specifically serotonergic and more anorectic (Garattini 1989), has recently become available as well as the commoner racemic mixture. Psychoses (Innes *et al.* 1977) and delirium (Brandon 1969) have also been reported. The UK Committee on Safety of Medicines received only two reports of fenfluramine-related psychosis between 1963 and 1986 (Watters and Le Ridant 1986), whereas the Swedish equivalent (SADRAC 1987) received 19 reports of adverse reactions to fenfluramine in 1985–87, of which 10 described serious psychiatric disorders during or shortly after fenfluramine ingestion. These included depression in four, mania in three, paranoid psychosis in two, and delirium in one. Seven of the patients, however, had a previous history of psychiatric disorder so that the causal relationship with use of fenfluramine was not fully established in these cases. Certainly, known schizophrenic patients are liable to relapse after taking fenfluramine (Murphy and Watters 1986).

Phenmetrazine has been widely abused for its euphoriant effects (Glatt 1957), particularly in Scandinavia, where intravenous use was popular (Angrist 1983). Paranoid psychoses have been reported (Bethell 1957; Evans 1959; Simma 1960; Mendels 1964; Wittstock 1967), as well as withdrawal depression (Clein 1957; Glatt 1957).

Methylphenidate, introduced as an anorectic and also used in the treatment of narcolepsy, has been abused with the production of auditory hallucinations (Lucas and Weiss 1971) and paranoid psychoses (McCormick and McNeil 1963; Spensley 1972; Spensley and Rockwell 1972). Like pemoline, methylphenidate has induced Gilles de la Tourette's syndrome (see above) (Golden 1974).

Cocaine is a potent CNS stimulant, used clinically as a topical local anaesthetic but also widely abused by smoking, sniffing, or injection. It is present in the leaves of the coca plant, grown and extensively chewed in Central and South America. The free-base preparation, 'crack', extracted from the commoner hydrochloride, readily evokes dependence and increases the risk of psychosis (Honer *et al.* 1987), as smoking it leads to rapidly peaking plasma levels in contrast to the more gradual effects of sniffed cocaine hydrochloride (Strang and Edwards 1989). Cocaine possesses adrenergic, dopaminergic, and serotoninergic agonist properties (Post 1975). From a review of the literature, Manschreck *et al.* (1987) list the psychiatric complications of cocaine consumption as follows:

intoxication elevated mood, anxiety, and panic, misperceptions and hallucinations, disturbed attention and judgement, loss of impulse control, loquacity, stereotypic behaviour, enhanced sexuality, agitation, maladaptive behaviour, psychosis, and death;
withdrawal craving, depression, anhedonia, increased dreaming, suicidal behaviour, and insomnia;
psychoses schizophreniform, manic, and paranoid pyschoses, delirium, hallucinosis, and dementia.
possible long-term effects paranoid features, impairment of memory, attention or perception, dementia, and other residual patterns.

Siegel (1978) recorded the experience of visual, auditory, tactile, olfactory and gustatory hallucinations in 15 (17.7 per cent) of 85 recreational cocaine users. The characteristic formication experience ('cocaine bugs', Magnan's sign) occurred in 11 (13 per cent), but only after several days of intensified ingestion. A high prevalence of depression has been noted in cocaine abusers, presumably as a withdrawal effect (Siegel 1982; Gawin and Kleber 1986).

Dopamine agonists

Drugs such as levodopa that increase the level of brain dopamine are associated with a high incidence of psychiatric disorder. In animals levodopa also reduces brain serotonin (Everett and Borcherding 1970) and increases noradrenaline levels (Randrup and Munkvad 1966) in animals; if this effect occurs in man, it may be a contributory factor in the genesis of psychiatric complications. For example, a review of 908 patients receiving levodopa for Parkinson's disease revealed psychiatric complications in 20 per cent (Goodwin 1971), including delirium in 4.4 per cent, depression in 4.2 per cent, overactivity, restlessness, and agitation in 3.6 per cent, paranoid delusional psychosis in 3.6 per cent, and hypomania in 1.5 per cent. Similar observations have been made on several other large series (Goodwin et al. 1971; Murphy 1973), but a higher prevalence of up to 55.5 per cent has been reported in postencephalitic parkinsonism (Calne et al. 1969). Apart from mood changes (Mindham et al. 1976), psychiatric reactions to levodopa appear to be dose-dependent, and a critical dose of the drug is often identifiable (Celesia and Barr 1970).

Claims have been made that depression occurs in half of all patients receiving levodopa (Pearce 1984), but mood disorder is independently correlated with Parkinson's disease (Mindham 1970), so that the effect of the drug is not easily disentangled. Depression is often associated with the 'off' phase of the 'on–off' phenomenon associated with levodopa treatment of Parkinson's disease (Nissenbaum et al. 1987). Claims of relief of depression, not attributable solely to motor improvement, in parkinsonian patients receiving levodopa are also made by some (O'Brien et al. 1971), although denied by others (Marsh and Markham 1973).

Analysis of the psychopathology in eight patients who developed psychoses while taking levodopa found delusions, visual and auditory hallucinations, distortion of reality, and behavioural disturbance, preceded by a prodromal phase of increasing anxiety and nightmares. In six there was evidence of associated clouding of consciousness but in two the sensorium was clear and these psychoses were schizophreniform in character (Celesia and Barr 1970). These authors comment on the mean latent interval of 4 months before the onset of psychosis and the association of dyskinetic, dystonic, or myoclonic movements in six of the eight cases. Predictably on theoretical grounds, the use of levodopa in the treatment of parkinsonism induced in schizophrenic patients by neuroleptic drugs leads to deterioration in their mental state (Yaryura-Tobias et al. 1970, 1972).

Levodopa, in combination with carbidopa, bromocriptine, or selegiline, has released abnormal sexual behaviour, including masochism (Quinn et al. 1983) and hypersexuality (Lin and Ziegler 1976).

Many experienced clinicians are convinced that levodopa accelerates the development of dementia in Parkinson's disease (Pearce 1984), although occasional reports of improvement in cognitive function in demented patients receiving levodopa have appeared (O'Brien et al. 1971). Memory impairment has been found to correlate with the degree of fluctuation rather than the absolute level of plasma dopamine (Huber et al. 1989).

Bromocriptine is a dopamine agonist used in the treatment of parkinsonism, to reduce the elevated serum prolactin levels associated with some pituitary adenomata, and to suppress lactation in nursing mothers. It is a monoamide of lysergic acid but lacks the hallucinogenic properties of the diethyl amide (LSD) (Goodkin 1980). Its psychotogenic properties are likely to be connected with its elevation of brain dopamine (Turner et al. 1984). Psychiatric complications were observed in 8 of 92 patients (8.7 per cent) treated for parkinsonism for up to 30 months (Calne et al. 1978) and in 35 of 445 (7.9 per cent) similar patients (Pearce and Pearce 1978). These reactions are similar to those induced by levodopa but the psychotic features are more florid and may persist for up to 6 weeks after the discontinuation of of the bromocriptine.

Puerperal psychoses of manic or schizomanic type have been reported after suppression of lactation by bromocriptine in doses of 7.5-30 mg daily (Brook and Cookson 1978; Vlissides et al. 1978). Recovery occurred 1–7 days after stopping treatment. Of 600 patients receiving doses of 7.5–100 mg daily for pituitary tumours, 8 (1.3 per cent) developed psychoses with auditory and tactile hallucinations, paranoid delusions, and mood changes without delirium (Turner et al. 1984). Of the 8 cases, 5 were diagnosed as having schizophreniform psychoses, 2 hypomania, and one a paranoid psychosis. None gave any previous personal or family history of psychiatric problems. Recovery invariably followed withdrawal of the drug. Several reports of similar cases have appeared (Steinbeck and Turtle 1979; Le Feuvre et al. 1982; Proctor et al. 1983).

Similar psychotic reactions also occur in association with the related drugs piribedil (Gerner et al. 1976) and lisuride (Turner et al. 1984). Psychoses also sometimes develop when bromocriptine is withdrawn (Lipper 1976; Shukla et al. 1985).

General anaesthetics

Postanaesthetic excitement is particularly common after the use of cyclopropane and ether (Eckenhoff et al. 1961), and delirium and hallucinosis after ketamine (Coppel et al. 1973; Garfield 1974). Halothane and isoflurane can induce fatigue, depression, delirium, anger, and tension, all of which may persist for up to 4 weeks (Davison *et al.* 1975). A dentist who inhaled nitrous oxide daily for 3 months developed a paranoid psychosis with some persisting memory impairment (Brodsky and Zuniga 1975).

Opioid analgesics

Opioid receptors and naturally occurring opioid peptides, the endorphins and enkephalins, are present in the brain (Snyder 1978). The latter act as neuromodulators and neurotransmitters in the regulation of pain, perception, response to stress, and mood. Opioid administration suppresses endorphin production and withdrawal induces a temporary relative deficiency of endogenous opioids (Gold *et al.* 1980). These effects are relevant to the psychotoxic properties of the opioid analgesics (Pickar *et al.* 1982).

Considering the extensive use of morphine in critically ill patients, it shows surprisingly little psychotoxicity. Occasional examples of over-sedation, progressing to stupor and accompanied by paranoid thinking, have been reported (D'Souza 1987; Leipzig *et al.* 1987), and visual hallucinations also occur (Jellema 1987; Kalso and Vainio 1988). Opioids, particularly morphine and diamorphine, have euphoriant effects and are liable to abuse and the induction of physical and psychological dependence. The physical withdrawal syndrome includes nausea and vomiting, muscle aches, lacrimation and rhinorrhoea, pupillary dilatation, piloerection, sweating, diarrhoea, yawning, fever, and insomnia (APA 1987). These symptoms are, not unnaturally, often accompanied by depression and agitation (Dackis and Gold 1984) but a schizophreniform psychosis can also develop (Uhde *et al.* 1982).

Pentazocine, a synthetic opioid analgesic, is associated with a variety of psychiatric effects, including coloured visual hallucinations in 7 per cent of recipients (Wood *et al.* 1974), depression (Kane and Pokorny 1975), insomnia and nightmares (Alexander and Spence 1974), and paranoid–hallucinatory psychoses (Blazer and Haller 1975; Goldstein 1985).

Of other opioid analgesics, butorphanol provokes vivid dreams, depersonalization, and visual hallucinations (Koch-Weser and Vandam 1980); and buprenorphine has caused hallucinations when administered epidurally (MacEvilly and O'Carroll 1989); methadone can induce visual hallucinations (Jellema 1987); and pethidine can induce delirium (Eisendrath *et al.* 1987) and hallucinatory psychoses (Fogarty and Murray 1987). Dihydrocodeine (Taylor *et al.* 1978) produces similar effects to pentazocine but at about half the frequency. A paranoid–hallucinatory psychosis after withdrawal of dextropropoxyphene has been described (Harris and Harper 1979).

Other analgesics

Salicylate intoxication can induce visual hallucinations (Greer *et al.* 1965) or progress to delirium (Beringer 1984; Blum 1987).

Non-steroidal anti-inflammatory drugs

These drugs have analgesic and anti-inflammatory properties. Indomethacin, a methoxylated indole derivative, may be associated with the development of severe headache and depression (Prescott 1975) and the production of paranoid–hallucinatory psychoses (Carney 1977), mania (Bishop *et al.* 1987), and visual hallucinations (Braddock and Heard 1986). The related drug sulindac has induced delirium (Thornton 1980) and paranoid psychoses (Kruis and Barger 1980). Visual hallucinations have been reported in a 75-year-old female after two doses of 300 mg fenbufen (Morris and Hardway 1985) but this occurred in only one of 5201 patients in a postmarketing survey (Brook and Jackson 1982). Ibuprofen, a prostaglandin synthesis inhibitor, has also been reported to have provoked a paranoid psychosis (Griffith *et al.* 1982).

Anticonvulsants

Epileptic patients have an increased risk of developing a psychiatric disorder, even without the effects of medication, so that psychotoxic effects of anticonvulsant drugs may be unsuspected or difficult to isolate. Combinations of drugs are often employed, which further enhances their synergistic toxic propensities. Plasma drug levels are helpful in diagnosis, but psychiatric reactions can develop at subtherapeutic levels (e.g. McDanal and Bolman 1975) and without physical signs such as ataxia and nystagmus (Reynolds 1982). A therapeutic test by withdrawing or replacing the suspect drug may be the only way to apportion responsibility for the patient's condition correctly. The role of folate deficiency induced by anticonvulsants in provoking psychiatric disorder is controversial (Reynolds 1968; Snaith *et al.* 1970).

Phenobarbitone is still widely used as an anticonvulsant. In addition to drowsiness, depression, and delirium (Tollefson 1980) its long-term use may induce a subacute impairment of intellectual function (Trimble and Reynolds 1976), especially in children (Trimble *et al.* 1980). Excitement, irritability, aggression, and a hyperkinetic syndrome can also occur in children (Ounsted 1955).

Primidone is metabolised to phenobarbitone and thus shares the same adverse effects, including excess sedation, delirium, mood swings, paranoid psychoses, and personality changes (Booker 1972).

Phenytoin has been noted for its psychotoxicity since its introduction (Blair *et al.* 1939). The spectrum of reactions reported includes delirium accompanied by visual and tactile hallucinations (Glaser 1972), somatic delusions, and paranoid (McDanal and Bolman 1975) or schizophreniform psychoses (Franks and Richter 1979). The non-delirious psychoses may develop at therapeutic blood levels (Logan and Freeman 1969; McDanal and Bolman 1975). Acute intoxication induces nystagmus at a blood level of $20\,\mu$g per ml, cerebellar ataxia at $30\,\mu$g per ml, and drowsiness at $40\,\mu$g per ml. Associated neuropsychiatric symptoms include slurred speech, delirium, restlessness, and visual hallucinations (Glaser 1972). Chronic intoxication can induce a reversible cerebral degenerative picture (pseudodementia) (Logan and Freeman 1969). Phenytoin is also implicated in the subacute cognitive impairment referred to above (Reynolds 1982).

Sodium valproate increases the level of brain γ-aminobutyric acid (GABA). It is able to provoke dose-related delirium, visual hallucinations, and hyperactivity, particularly in children (Trimble and Reynolds 1976; Reynolds 1982; Chadwick 1985). A 'valproate encephalopathy', with semi-stupor and dystonic posturing is a rare complication (Reynolds 1982). Exacerbation of both acute and chronic schizophrenia has been reported (Lautin *et al.* 1980; Meldrum 1982).

Carbamazepine, in addition to being used as an anticonvulsant, is also employed in the control of trigeminal neuralgia and manic–depressive psychosis. Its mood-controlling effect may be related to limbic receptor stabilization, a property it shares with lithium (Dorus *et al.* 1983). The drug can induce drowsiness, anxiety, and restlessness (Tollefson 1980), delirium (Reynolds 1982), major depression (Gardner and Cowdry 1986), and schizophreniform psychoses (Franks and Richter 1979; Matthew 1988).

Ethosuximide is used in the treatment of petit mal epilepsy, mostly in children and young adults. A wide spectrum of psychiatric reactions to it is reported, including anxiety, depression, paranoid–hallucinatory psychoses (Roger *et al.* 1968; Buchanan 1972), lethargy and euphoria (Stores 1975), night terrors, aggression, and paranoia (Tollefson 1980).

Clonazepam, like the other benzodiazepines, possesses anticonvulsant properties. Its use is associated with the development of personality changes in the form of irritability and aggression (Trimble and Reynolds 1976), and occasionally with paranoid psychoses (White *et al.* 1982; Jaffe and Gibson 1986).

Muscle relaxants

Baclofen is a muscle relaxant, structurally similar to GABA, that acts by inhibiting GABA-mediated spinal reflexes. Centrally, baclofen is variously postulated to inhibit dopaminergic activity (Olpe *et al.* 1977) or to enhance it by amphetamine-like effect (Wolf *et al.* 1982). Psychiatric symptoms that have been reported include visual and auditory hallucinations, paranoia, euphoria, depression, anxiety, suicidal attempts, and aphrodisiac effects (Jones and Lance 1976); they usually clear within 24 hours of withdrawal of the drug. Catatonia and mutism (Pauker and Brown 1986) and paranoid–hallucinatory psychoses have also been described (Yassa and Iskandar 1988). Swigar and Bowers (1986) have reviewed from the literature eight examples of psychiatric disorder due to withdrawal of baclofen, and added one of their own. Symptoms observed included severe anxiety, insomnia, agitation, disorientation, paranoid delusions, and auditory, visual and formicatory hallucinations. One case developed mania (Arnold *et al.* 1980). The association of dystonic features in several cases suggests a dopamine supersensitivity effect. Others developed tonic and clonic movements or grand mal seizures. These patients had taken baclofen for at least 6 months and the withdrawal effects developed within 12–72 hours and usually subsided with restoration of the drug.

Tizanidine has caused depression that remitted within 2 days of the drug being withdrawn and reappeared on rechallenge, following its use for the relief of spasticity in a patient with multiple sclerosis (Nab and Hommes 1987).

Psychotropic drugs

Hypnotics and anxiolytics

Benzodiazepines are safe and effective drugs for short-term administration as hypnotics, anxiolytics, anticonvulsants, muscle relaxants, and amnesic agents for minor surgery. Their effects are mediated through enhancement of the actions of brain γ-aminobutyric acid (GABA) by interaction with specific benzodiazepine receptors (Braestrup *et al.* 1983). These drugs are now consumed rather less extensively, but in 1980 it was estimated that 40 billion tablets daily were being ingested worldwide (Tyrer 1980). Studies in the Northern Region of the National Health Service in England show a 40 per cent fall in the number of prescriptions for benzodiazepine anxiolytics but an 8 per cent rise in those for benzodiazepine hypnotics between 1980 and 1986 (Chaplin 1988).

Benzodiazepines are usefully classified according to the duration of their elimination half-lives and those of their metabolites. Those with a half-life over 24 hours may be termed long-acting and include diazepam, chlordiazepoxide, flurazepam, and clorazepate. Desmethyldiazepam, the major active metabolite of diazepam, chlordiazepoxide, and clorazepate have half-lives of 30–200 hours. Intermediate to short-acting drugs have half-lives of 5–24 hours and include oxazepam, lorazepam, temazepam, lormetazepam, and loprazolam. Nitrazepam, the half-life of which is 18–34 hours, is on the borderline between long-acting and intermediate-acting drugs. Triazolam and midazolam, with half-lives of 2–4 hours are ultra-short-acting. Hangover effects and the risk of drug accumulation are commoner with long-acting drugs. Rebound insomnia (Kales *et al.* 1983) or nocturnal delirium (Patterson 1987) are liable to appear with ultra-short-acting drugs.

The adverse mental effects of short-term benzodiazepine use are those of sedation, depressing effects on psychomotor function (Hindmarch 1980), and impairment of ability to drive or operate machinery (Betts and Birtle 1982). With longer-term consumption these effects increase and more obvious psychomotor impairment may appear, with ataxia, dysarthria, inco-ordination, diplopia, muscle weakness, vertigo, defective memory, and mental confusion. A possible contribution to traffic accidents is claimed (Skegg *et al.* 1979). A chronic schizophreniform psychosis associated with the consumption of a high dose of lorazepam (30 mg daily) has been reported (Fraser and Ingram 1985). These effects are more easily elicited in the elderly, in whom benzodiazepines are a common cause of delirium, falls, and fractures (Jarvis 1981).

The amnesic effect is useful in anaesthesia (Dundee and Pandit 1972), but triazolam can induce transient global amnesia ('traveller's amnesia') (Morris and Estes 1987). Other unusual reactions include mania with alprazolam (Burke 1987; Goodman and Charney 1987), the similar drug, adinazolam (Papart *et al.* 1986), and clorazepate (Bourgeois *et al.* 1987). Visual hallucinations are reported in children (Pfefferbaum *et al.* 1987). Chronic use can induce depression or emotional dulling (Lader and Petursson 1981) or provoke suicide (Priest and Montgomery 1987), and it is blamed, especially when combined with alcohol (Terrell 1988), for the appearance of antisocial actions, such as shoplifting or sexual misbehaviour, and for outbursts of rage and violence (Lader and Petursson 1981). Impairment of

cognitive function (Lader 1987) and increase in the ventricular–brain ratio on CAT-scans (Lader *et al.* 1984) in chronic benzodiazepine consumers are described but contradictory observations are reported by other workers (Poser *et al.* 1983).

The major hazard of long-term benzodiazepine consumption is, however, the development of both psychological and physical dependence. Physical dependence is manifested primarily by an abstinence syndrome on reducing or withdrawing the drug, rather than through increasing tolerance and escalation of dosage or drug-seeking behaviour (Tyrer 1987). The risk of dependence is correlated with high and continuous dosage, previous drug dependence, dependent personality traits, high levels of psychological dependence, and the use of short-acting benzodiazepines (Tyrer 1987). The majority of benzodiazepine-dependent patients can withdraw the drug gradually without problems (Tyrer *et al.* 1981) and only about 30 per cent of patients receiving a benzodiazepine for 6 months develop a withdrawal syndrome (Owen and Tyrer 1983).

The withdrawal syndrome appears within 2–3 days of withdrawing a short-acting benzodiazepine and within 7 days of a long-acting one. The more severe symptoms usually subside after about 2 weeks but symptoms in diminishing intensity may persist for several months (Ashton 1984). This syndrome consists of somatic and psychological symptoms of anxiety together with dysphoria; abnormal perceptual experiences, including visual and auditory hallucinations; a sensation of continuous movement; and feelings of depersonalization and unreality. In some 5 per cent of cases obsessive–compulsive disorder (Matthews and Drummond 1987), delirium (Foy *et al.* 1986; Heritch *et al.* 1987), paranoid (Bleich *et al.* 1987), or schizophreniform psychoses with first-rank symptoms (Roberts and Vass 1986) develop. Neurological symptoms include paraesthesiae and numbness; tremor; muscle pain, stiffness, weakness and fasciculation; ataxia; and blurred or double vision. Hypersensitivity to sound, light, taste, and smell are common, as are headache and tinnitus; and formication and itching can occur. Major or temporal lobe fits may also appear. Gastrointestinal symptoms of the irritable-bowel syndrome type are common (Ashton 1986).

Withdrawal symptoms can be minimized by gradual reduction of dosage. The detailed symptomatology of the withdrawal syndrome and problems encountered in its management are well described by Ashton (1984).

Benzodiazepine withdrawal is thought to decrease GABA activity, resulting in a surge of excitatory neurotransmitters normally controlled by GABA (Ashton 1984), or possibly a decrease in endogenous opioid activity (Millan and Duka 1981). Dependence can be prevented by only using benzodiazepines intermittently and for periods of no longer than 4–6 weeks (CSM 1988).

A provocative apologia for benzodiazepines has been delivered by Kraupl-Taylor (1989) and a balanced account of their benefits and risks was provided by Tyrer (1987). McClelland (1990) has comprehensively reviewed forensic aspects of their use.

Buspirone, a new anxiolytic drug, is an azaspirodecanedione that enhances brain dopaminergic and adrenergic activity and inhibits serotonin and acetylcholine activity. Its addition to the medication of a controlled manic–depressive patient is thought to have precipitated a recurrence of mania (Liegghio and Yeragani 1988).

Barbiturates, although highly effective, have been largely superseded as hypnotics and anxiolytics because of their propensity to induce physical dependence and their danger in overdose. Intoxication leads to drowsiness and delirium, often accompanied by ataxia, dysarthria, and nystagmus (Gibson 1966). More rarely, a paranoid–hallucinatory psychosis develops (Isbell *et al.* 1950). Withdrawal after long-term ingestion induces agitation and tremor, leading to delirium, often followed by epileptiform seizures (Barry and Weintraub 1978).

Bromides were widely used as sedatives and anticonvulsants in the 19th and early 20th centuries. In 1927 bromide intoxication accounted for 8 per cent (Wuth 1927) and in 1965 1 per cent (Ewing and Grant 1965) of admissions to American psychiatric hospitals. Bromides are now rarely prescribed but they do occasionally appear in unexpected guise, for example, in antacid mixtures (Deleu *et al.* 1985). Bromides are thought to act on the CNS by displacing the chloride ion, and their serum half-life of 12 days facilitates cumulative toxicity.

Mild bromide intoxication induces fatigue, drowsiness, weakness, emotional lability, depression, memory impairment, self-neglect, insomnia, and disorientation. More severe intoxication provokes delirium, stupor, coma, excitement, delusions, hallucinations, paranoia, slurred speech, ataxia, and seizures (Trump and Hochberg 1976; Raskind *et al.* 1978). Skin rashes occur in 20–30 per cent of cases. Misdiagnosis as schizophrenia or dementia is common (Levin 1946, 1948, Carney 1971; Raskind *et al.* 1978).

A serum bromide concentration of 150 mg per 100 ml (19 mEq per litre) or over is invariably associated with clinical toxicity. Levels of 72 mg per 100 ml (9 mEq per litre) or over are strongly suggestive of toxicity but even lower levels may be toxic in the elderly (Raskind *et al.* 1978). Treatment with sodium or ammonium chloride and a diuretic is usually effective but recovery from the psychiatric disorder may take up to 10 days (Perkins 1950).

Chlormethiazole possesses sedative, hypnotic, and anticonvulsant properties, probably mediated via catecholaminergic and GABA-ergic systems. Its adverse effects are those of sedation and ataxia but, more importantly, it can induce physical dependence after as little as 10 days' treatment. Sudden withdrawal then provokes delirium and epileptiform seizures, similar to barbiturate withdrawal effects (Hession *et al.* 1979).

Neuroleptics (major tranquillizers)

This group of drugs, used in the control of disturbed behaviour of whatever cause and in the long-term treatment of schizophrenia, includes the phenothiazines, which can be classified into three groups (British National Formulary 1990 p. 155) as follows:

1. chlorpromazine, methotrimeprazine, and promazine, characterized by pronounced sedative effects but moderate antimuscarinic and extrapyramidal adverse effects;

2. pericyazine, pipothiazine, and thioridazine, which have moderate sedative effects, marked antimuscarinic effects, but fewer extrapyramidal adverse effects;

3. fluphenazine, perphenazine, prochlorperazine, and trifluoperazine, which have fewer sedative and antimuscarinic effects but more pronounced extrapyramidal adverse effects.

Other neuroleptics resemble group 3 in their effects and include the butyrophenones (ben-, dro-, halo-, and triflu-peridol), diphenylbutylpiperidines (fluspirilene and pimozide), thiothanxenes (flu- and zuclo-penthixol) and oxypertine. Their antipsychotic effect is thought to derive from postsynaptic dopamine-receptor blockade, resulting in increased dopamine synthesis and turnover (Cooper *et al.* 1986), but they also block adrenergic receptors to varying degrees. Metoclopramide, also a neuroleptic, lacks antipsychotic effect but displays pronounced antiemetic properties.

Withdrawal syndromes with headache, insomnia, restlessness, sweating, nausea, and vomiting occur (Gardos *et al.* 1978), sometimes accompanied by dyskinesias (Perenyi *et al.* 1985). Neuroleptic withdrawal can also precipitate a schizophreniform psychosis, even in manic–depressive patients (Witschy *et al.* 1984), which is attributed to dopamine-receptor supersensitivity. Dose-related lethargy and sedation are common with Group 1 drugs (Hollister 1975) and exacerbation of depression and the negative symptoms of schizophrenia, such as apathy, affective flattening, and impaired volition, are described, although it is often difficult to isolate drug effects from the features of the illness (Prosser *et al.* 1987). Metoclopramide can also precipitate a depressive syndrome (Feder 1987; Weddington and Banner 1986).

Paradoxically, these drugs can have antidepressant effects in some patients (Robertson and Trimble 1981). Another type of paradoxical reaction is the precipitation of delirium of the central anticholinergic type, often preceded by restlessness and agitation, by phenothiazines of Groups 1 and 2, particularly after parenteral administration (Mariani 1988), but also by oral metoclopramide (Fishbain and Rogers 1987).

The extrapyramidal adverse effects of the neuroleptics include parkinsonism, dystonia, and akathisia (Stephen and Williamson 1984; Shalev *et al.* 1987; Hardie and Lees 1988). These develop early and are mitigated by the concurrent administration of anticholinergic antiparkinsonian agents. The condition of tardive dyskinesia develops later, particularly after high doses, and is estimated to afflict 10–20 per cent of those exposed to neuroleptic treatment for more than one year. This disorder is described in Chapter 18.

The neuroleptic malignant syndrome, an extrapyramidal syndrome induced by neuroleptic drugs, is occasionally accompanied by catatonic symptoms, including negativism, mutism, stupor, posturing, and muscle-tone anomalies such as waxy flexibility (Gelenberg and Mandel 1977; Cremona-Barbaro 1983). The other features of this condition are described in Chapters 18 and 28.

Antidepressant drugs

Tricyclic antidepressants These drugs, which include amitriptyline, amoxapine, butriptyline, clomipramine, desipramine, dothiepin, doxepin, imipramine, lofepramine, nortriptyline, protriptyline, and trimipramine, inhibit the central presynaptic uptake of noradrenaline and serotonin in varying proportions, thus increasing the availability of these neurotransmitters at the postsynaptic receptor (Hauger and Paul 1983). The relationship of these actions to their antidepressant effects remains unclear, as there are many contradictory observations (Oswald *et al.* 1972). Many of their adverse effects are, however, related to their antimuscarinic properties.

The Boston Collaborative Drug Surveillance Program (BCDSP 1972) reported adverse reactions of all kinds in 15.4 per cent of patients receiving tricyclic antidepressants, classified as major in 4.6 per cent. Analysis of data from a drug surveillance system in Berlin and Munich psychiatric hospitals revealed that in 1979–1982 tricyclic drugs caused 7.4 adverse drug reactions necessitating drug withdrawal per 100 drug exposures compared with only 3.1 by newer antidepressants such as mianserin,

nomifensine, and zimeldine (Schmidt *et al.* 1986). These reactions were of toxic delirium, delusions, visual hallucinations, urinary retention, and sweating, which are recognizable as features of the central anticholinergic syndrome (see above). Additive antimuscarinic effects of concomitant neuroleptic treatment enhance toxicity, although neuroleptic drugs also increase tricyclic blood levels (Linnoila *et al.* 1982; Siris *et al.* 1982). Delirium occurred in 13 per cent of 150 patients but in patients over age 40 the incidence was 35 per cent (Davies *et al.* 1971). Undue sedation is another common unwanted reaction. Children (Preskorn *et al.* 1988) and the elderly (Jarvis 1981) are the most susceptible to all these effects.

The induction of mania is not uncommonly attributed to tricyclic therapy (van Scheyen and van Kammen 1979), although some argue that switches from depression to mania are independent of concurrent medication (Angst 1987; Soloman *et al.* 1990). In those with pre-existing personal or family history of bipolar disorder it is reasonable to attribute this effect to an interaction with the subject's constitutional predisposition, possibly reflected in neurotransmitter levels. Without such a background, unless every depressed patient is assumed to be potentially liable to become manic, a postulated latent bipolar predisposition is only a circular assumption; the predisposition must have been present because the mania developed! A simpler concept is to regard mania in these circumstances as an exaggerated Type A drug effect.

Rapid cycling of mood in manic–depressive patients has been attributed to tricyclic antidepressants (Wehr and Goodwin 1979) and mania is sometimes provoked by tricyclic withdrawal (Mirin *et al.* 1981; Gupta and Narang 1986). More typical withdrawal symptoms are recognized, usually after the ingestion of high doses over a long period, including insomnia, nightmares, nausea and vomiting, and agitation and anxiety in both adults (Kramer *et al.* 1961) and children (Law *et al.* 1981). The combination of amitriptyline with alcohol is occasionally abused for its euphoriant effect (Hyatt and Bird 1987).

Heterocyclic antidepressant drugs This heterogeneous group of drugs, which includes iprindole, maprotiline, mianserin, trazodone, and viloxazine has various physical adverse effects, but relatively few adverse psychiatric reactions. Trazodone, which inhibits serotonin uptake, amongst other effects (Riblet *et al.* 1979), can induce mania (Knobler *et al.* 1986; Lennhof 1987; Zmitek 1987), and its withdrawal is associated with the production of anxiety, depersonalization, nightmares, and insomnia (Menza 1986). Reduction in the dose of trazodone has been reported to have provoked a sensation of bugs crawling on the skin, relieved by restoration of the original dose of 300 mg daily (Peabody 1987).

The unicyclic aminoketone antidepressant, bupropion, not yet available in Britain, is associated with the development of paranoid–hallucinatory psychoses, visual hallucinations, and delirium (Golden *et al.* 1985), although double-blind studies found the overall incidence of these symptoms to be no greater with bupropion than with a placebo or with amitriptyline (Johnston *et al.* 1986). Bupropion has a chemical structure similar to amphetamine and diethylpropion, and this is regarded as significant for its psychotogenic potential, which is possibly mediated via its dopaminergic effect (Golden *et al.* 1988).

Selective serotonin (5-HT)-uptake inhibitors These newly introduced antidepressant drugs include fluoxetine, fluvoxamine, femoxetine, sertraline, and citalopram. Zimeldine was withdrawn by the manufacturer after the appearance of an influenza-like reaction and Guillain–Barré syndrome. They do not bind to any of the neurotransmitter receptors, except that of serotonin, and thus have limited toxicity potential (Doogan and Caillard 1988) and are much safer than tricyclic drugs in overdose (Cassidy and Henry 1987). They can induce anxiety, insomnia, and headache (Cooper 1988). Fluoxetine (Lebegue 1987) and sertraline (Laporta *et al.* 1987) have been reported to precipitate mania. Interaction with tricyclic drugs enhances the toxic effects of the latter (Vaughan 1988).

Monoamine oxidase inhibitors (MAOI) Combined treatment with MAOI and tricyclic antidepressants is sometimes undertaken for resistant depression (White and Simpson 1984) but the risk of inducing delirium, seizures, hyperthermia, or a hypertensive crisis is considerable (White and Simpson 1981; Graham *et al.* 1982). Trimipramine and amitriptyline are relatively safe in combination with a MAOI, but it is recommended that the tricyclic be started first. The greatest risk attaches to the combination of a MAOI with a serotonin uptake inhibitor drug, such as clomipramine or the newer drugs of this class (see above), which should never be used (Lader 1990), as there is a risk of provoking the life-threatening 'serotonin syndrome' of hyperthermia, tremor, and convulsions. The persistence of plasma levels of the long-acting metabolite of fluoxetine, norfluoxetine, means that at least 5 weeks must elapse after cessation of fluoxetine before it is safe to commence a MAOI (CSM 1989). The possibility of interaction persists for at least 2 weeks after MAOI withdrawal.

MAOI are occasionally associated with the development of delirium and auditory and visual hallucinations,

either alone (White 1987) or in combination with other drugs such as cyproheptadine (Kahn 1987). Schizophreniform psychoses are also reported (Sheehy and Maxmen 1978).

Tranylcypromine possesses amphetamine-like properties, and examples of dependence, with tolerance, escalation of dosage and withdrawal symptoms are reported (Le Gassicke 1963; Ben-Arie and George 1979). The others do not induce such dependence, but withdrawal symptoms, including headache, shivering, paraesthesiae, and nightmares can occur after prolonged treatment (Pitt 1974). In one large series, abrupt withdrawal of phenelzine provoked panic, headache, shaking, sweating, nausea, and perceptual disturbances in 25 per cent of patients (Tyrer 1984).

L-Tryptophan This amino acid and serotonin (5-HT) precursor, formerly used as an antidepressant, often in conjunction with others, has recently been withdrawn from general use on account of an epidemic of the potentially dangerous tryptophan-related eosinophilia–myalgia syndrome (Medsger 1990), possibly due to a contaminant (*The Lancet* 1990; Belongia *et al.* 1990).

L-Tryptophan was liable to induce nausea, drowsiness, and headache and, combined with a MAOI, mania (Goff 1985) or excited delirium (Baldessarini 1984).

Lithium salts Lithium carbonate and citrate are used in the prophylaxis and treatment of mania and recurrent depression and of certain forms of aggressive and self-mutilating behaviour. Lithium enhances serotonin (Bunney and Garland-Bunney 1987) and decreases catecholamine activity (Linnoila *et al.* 1983). Because of its narrow therapeutic/toxic ratio, plasma levels of lithium must be monitored regularly and kept within the range of 0.6–1.2 mmol per litre 12 hours after the last dose.

Adverse effects at therapeutic levels are common but they usually respond to a decrease in dose. They include tremor, nausea, diarrhoea, thirst and polyuria, oedema, and weight gain. Occasionally, delirium with psychotic features is provoked (Kamlana 1989). Lithium toxicity develops at plasma levels above 1.5 mmol per litre and becomes a medical emergency at 2 mmol per litre. Psychiatric features include delirium and stupor.

Wernicke's encephalopathy has resulted from persistent diarrhoea and vomiting secondary to a high lithium intake (Epstein 1989). Apart from overdose, such toxicity is more likely with impaired renal function, excessive sodium loss due to profuse sweating, vomiting, or diarrhoea, or the ingestion of a diuretic. Interaction with NSAID and ACE-inhibitors may increase lithium plasma levels and toxicity may develop without raised plasma levels with concurrent ingestion of calcium-channel blocking agents, methyldopa, carbamazepine, and phenytoin.

There is evidence that long-term lithium therapy can induce mild impairment of cognitive function (Lund *et al.* 1982) in as many as 10 per cent of cases (Vestergaard *et al.* 1988). Certainly, overdose has produced permanent memory impairment (Saxena and Mallikarjuna 1988).

In addition to the relapse of the underlying disorder that may follow lithium withdrawal (Mander 1986), other withdrawal symptoms, including anxiety, insomnia, and irritability (Klein *et al.* 1981) or delirium (Wilkinson 1979) can occur.

Attention has been drawn to the neurotoxic effects of the combination of lithium and haloperidol, which include irreversible cerebellar and extrapyramidal damage and cognitive impairment (Cohen and Cohen 1974; Donaldson and Cunningham 1983). Similar reactions are described in combination with thioridazine (Spring 1979), thiothixene (Fetzer *et al.* 1981), and fluphenazine (Singh 1982). Lithium alone, however, can evoke neurological symptoms. Episodes of sleep-walking have been reported after the addition of various neuroleptics to patients established on lithium (Charney *et al.* 1979).

Other psychoactive drugs and substances

Hallucinogens

These substances include lysergic acid diethylamide (LSD,'acid'), mescaline, dimethoxymethylamphetamine (DOM, 'STP') (Davison 1976), methylenedioxy-amphetamine (MDMA, 'ecstasy') (Edwards 1989), psilocybin (in certain mushrooms) (Young *et al.* 1982), phencyclidine ('angel dust') (Pearlson 1981), cannabis (Ashton 1987), and volatile hydrocarbons contained in various solvents, glues, and petrol (Ron 1986; Ashton 1990). These drugs are unusual because they produce changes in thought, perception, and mood without necessarily altering consciousness. This has resulted in the application of various names to the category, for example, phantastica, psychedelic (mind-expanding), and psychotomimetic. They are all subject to abuse and liable to precipitate a range of psychiatric syndromes that differ little between the drugs.

LSD can be taken as the paradigm and its psychiatric reactions can be classified as follows (Davison 1976).

Acute reaction   The acute reaction to LSD occurs after oral doses of as little as 100 μg and lasts 2–10 hours. The usual sequence is:

1. somatic symptoms — dizziness, weakness, tremors, nausea, drowsiness, paraesthesiae, and blurred vision;

2. perceptual symptoms — altered shapes and colours, difficulty in focusing, sharpened sense of hearing, and 'synaesthesia';
3. psychological symptoms — alterations in mood, tension, distorted time sense, difficulty in expressing thoughts, depersonalization, dream-like feelings, and visual hallucinations.

These effects are often elaborated into a complex visual and emotional experience with mystical and ecstatic qualities — the 'trip', which may be enjoyable (good trip) or frightening (bad trip). This condition is distinguished from schizophrenia by the preponderance of visual hallucinations and retention of insight (Davison 1976). Dilated pupils, increased tendon reflexes, incoordination, and ataxia are common physical signs. Tolerance develops quickly and is lost quickly.

Prolonged psychotic reaction   The prolonged psychotic reaction, which by definition lasts for more than 48 hours, accounts for 63 per cent of the reported adverse reactions to LSD (Smart and Bateman 1967). Cohen (1960) reviewed the adverse reactions to 25 000 LSD administrations in about 5000 subjects in America and found that psychotic reactions lasting longer than 48 hours occurred at a rate of 0.8 per 1000 in experimental subjects and 1.8 per 1000 in patients receiving LSD as therapy. In a similar review of British experience, Malleson (1971) found a psychosis rate of 9 per 1000. In the latter series 9 patients recovered in less than 2 weeks, and 3 in 2–12 weeks; in 7 the psychosis lasted more than 12 weeks and in 10 it persisted indefinitely. The onset of the psychosis could be delayed for up to 8 weeks after a single dose of LSD. Typical symptoms included paranoid delusions, schizophreniform auditory hallucinations, and overwhelming panic. This type of reaction closely resembles naturally occurring schizophrenia (Davison 1976).

Chronic psychosis (amotivational syndrome)   The repeated consumption of LSD over a period of years produces, in some individuals, the insidious development of a mental state characterized by withdrawal, shallow affect, paranoid ideas, and bizarre thinking centred on religious mysticism. Orientation and recent memory are usually unaffected but there may be some effect on remote memory (Glass and Bowers 1970), and some display a schizophrenic type of thought disorder (Tucker and Quinlan 1972).

Spontaneous recurrences (flashbacks)   These occur after use of any of the major hallucinogens and consist of spontaneous recurrences of the acute hallucinatory reaction weeks, months, or even up to 5 years after the last ingestion of the drug, after a intervening normal interval

(Abraham 1983). Although these experiences are often frightening and bizarre (for example, one subject had recurring visual hallucinations of decomposing people), insight is usually retained. Their occurrence is related to the frequency of prior drug ingestion, but in view of the short half-life of about 3 hours for LSD the phenomenon is unlikely to be due to persistence of the drug in the brain (Alarcon *et al.* 1982).

The molecular resemblance of LSD (and psilocybin) to serotonin (5-HT) is likely to be more than coincidence, as LSD is a serotonin antagonist at central synapses. It also stimulates dopamine-sensitive adenyl cyclase, however, and its effects are blocked by dopamine antagonist drugs, so that its psychotogenic properties may be due to its dopamine agonist action (Hamon 1984).

The psychiatric effects of the other hallucinogens listed above are similar, except for a greater tendency to provoke delirium or induce withdrawal symptoms. Detailed reviews are available for LSD (Strassman 1984), MDMA (Climko *et al.* 1986), psilocybin (Peden *et al.* 1981), phencyclidine (Pearlson 1981), cannabis (Negrete 1983; Thornicroft 1990) and organic solvents (King *et al.* 1981; Ron 1986).

Herbal and other unorthodox medicines

Khat and datura intoxication and the psychiatric effects of rauwolfia derivatives are discussed above. Euphoriant and hallucinogenic effects can develop in association with the smoking of several varieties of herbal cigarette containing yohimbe, broom, Californian poppy, catnip, cinnamon, damiana, hops, hydrangea, juniper, kava-kava, kola, lobelia, passion flower, periwinkle, prickly poppy, snakeroot, wild lettuce, and wormwood. Other vegetable hallucinogens include mandrake (*Mandragora officinarum*) and nutmeg (*Myristica fragrans*) (Penn 1986).

Ginseng, the powdered root of *Panax ginseng*, has long been used in the Far East as a general tonic and promoter of virility but is now a cult in Western countries. The 'ginseng abuse syndrome' is said to induce excitation, arousal, nervousness, tremor, and hypertension (Siegel 1979) and, combined with phenelzine, ginseng has provoked mania (Jones and Runikis 1987).

Sassafras is the dried inner bark of the root *Sassafras albidum* which contains about 3 per cent of volatile oil and is used as an antirheumatic and a soft-drink flavouring. The volatile oil contains 80–95% safrole (isosafrole, 1-allyl-3,4,-methylenedioxybenzene), which is hepatotoxic and carcinogenic in rats. It is a minor component of other essential oils, including star anise, camphor, mace, nutmeg, bay laurel, and cinnamon (Penn 1986). A 19-

year-old male developed a schizophreniform psychosis after taking 500–750 mg isosafrole daily for 2 weeks; this resolved 3 weeks after the isosafrole was withdrawn (Keitner *et al.* 1984).

The ink cap fungus (*Coprinus atramentarius*), a constituent of some health foods, contains disulfiram (Penn 1986) and is thus liable to interact with alcohol to produce an unpleasant systemic reaction.

X-ray contrast media

Metrizamide, a contrast medium used in myelography and ventriculography, has been implicated in the production of a wide range of psychiatric effects, usually transient. A review of 2500 cervical myelograms revealed 1 per cent with such reactions, including delirium, depression, visual hallucinations, paranoid psychosis, nightmares, anxiety, and somnolence (Nyegaard and Company 1977). Mania (Kuventus *et al.* 1984) and organic personality change and memory impairment lasting for six months are also reported (Wade *et al.* 1986).

Specific antidotes

Naloxone, a specific opiate antagonist, is known to produce a variety of psychiatric effects, including dysphoria, visual hallucinations, racing thoughts, and daydreams (Woods 1956). Naltrexone, also an opiate antagonist, has induced depression (Hollister 1986). Flumazenil, a specific benzodiazepine antagonist of potential value in the treatment of benzodiazepine poisoning, has provoked psychomotor agitation and benzodiazepine-withdrawal symptoms (Bateman 1988).

Disulfiram (Antabuse)

Disulfiram is used to prevent relapses in abstinent alcoholics. From its first introduction in 1948, reports of serious adverse psychiatric reactions, in the absence of alcohol ingestion, appeared in as many as 10–20 per cent of recipients (Gottesfeld *et al.* 1951; Macklin *et al.* 1953), but the frequency declined after reduction in the recommended daily dose to 200 mg (Liddon and Satran 1967). Concurrent ingestion of metronidazole, which has a disulfiram-like effect with alcohol and was formerly thought to suppress the craving for alcohol, increases the risk of a psychotic reaction (Rothstein and Clancy 1969). The majority of reactions are delirious in nature (Liddon and Satran 1967), often with reversible neurological signs (Hotson and Langston 1976), but schizophreniform (Knee and Razani 1974) and manic (Usdin and Robinson 1951) psychoses are described. Of 52 published cases, 21 were regarded as clinically schizophrenic and a further 9 as having suffered acute schizophrenic episodes (Knee and Razani 1974). An example of the Capgras syndrome (delusion that relatives and friends have been replaced by identical doubles) has been reported after the ingestion of 500 mg disulfiram daily for 2 weeks (Daniel *et al*. 1987). Established schizophrenia is also aggravated by disulfiram (Heath *et al*. 1965). A connection with schizophrenia is provided by the inhibition of the enzyme dopamine β-hydroxylase by disulfiram, leading to an excess of available dopamine at the synaptic cleft, one of the postulated mechanisms underlying schizophrenia. Minor tranquillizers are, however, reported to be more effective than dopamine-antagonist neuroleptic drugs in the treatment of disulfiram psychoses (Knee and Razani 1974).

Antibacterial drugs

Acute non-anaphylactic reactions with psychiatric features, occurring after intramuscular aqueous procaine penicillin, were first described in 1951 (Batchelor *et al*. 1951) but subsequently designated Hoigné's syndrome (Hoigné and Schoch 1959; Hoigné 1962). Over 100 case reports have since been published. The psychiatric profile commonly described is summarized by Ilechukwu (1990) as follows:
(a) reaction within one minute of injection;
(b) characteristic symptoms of:
  (i) extreme apprehension or fear of death;
  (ii) auditory/vestibular, visual, gustatory (penicillin taste), olfactory, and kinaesthetic disturbances, including illusions and hallucinations;
  (iii) depersonalization, perceptual changes in body image;
(c) absence of anaphylactic features; patients often able to continue procaine penicillin treatment, and the condition subsiding rapidly with reassurance or sedation.
There are also physical symptoms, including tachycardia, hypertension, and cyanosis.

The experience can occasionally develop, in susceptible people, into a chronic neurosis of the post-traumatic stress syndrome type (Ilechukwu 1990).

This reaction is attributed to the effects of the procaine moiety being inadvertently injected intravascularly and affecting the limbic region of the brain (Ilechukwu 1990). However, similar reactions are reported with other depot penicillins (Hoigné *et al*. 1984).

A 30-year-old female developed weight loss, anorexia, insomnia, confusion, thought disorder, and auditory hallucinations after 10 days' treatment with amoxycillin, 14 years after a similar episode while taking ampicillin

(Beal *et al*. 1986). Four children aged 18 months to 10 years became irritable and aggressive when their sinusitis was treated with the combination of amoxycillin and clavulanic acid (Augmentin), although amoxycillin alone was without adverse effect (Macknin 1987).

Delirium and paranoid–hallucinatory psychoses have been reported in association with streptomycin (Porot and Destaing 1950) and chloramphenicol therapy (Perreau and Maurice 1950). Nightmares have been reported with oral erythromycin (Black and Dawson 1988; Williams 1988) and delirium, accompanied by paranoid delusions and visual hallucinations, with the intravenous form (Umstead and Neumann 1986). Gentamicin has provoked acute delirium (Kane and Byrd 1975). Co-trimoxazole (a mixture of 80% sulphamethoxazole and 20% trimethoprim) induced catatonic stupor in a 72-year-old female on two separate occasions (Saxe 1988), and has also provoked bizarre mannerisms followed by a generalized convulsion (Mermel *et al*. 1986).

Ofloxacin, a quinolone derivative and gyrase inhibitor, one of a class of antimicrobial agents structurally related to nalidixic acid, has provoked mania followed by depression and induced a schizophrenia-like psychosis with catatonic features (Zaudig and von Bose 1987). These authors report receiving information about an increasing number of psychoses due to ofloxacin.

The parenteral cephalosporin ceftazidime has been associated with the occurrence of headaches, dizziness, convulsions, and visual hallucinations and, in one case, visual and auditory hallucinations in the absence of delirium (Al-Zahawi and Sprott 1988).

Isoniazid has a structural formula similar to niacin (nicotinamide, vitamin B$_3$) and also to iproniazid, a monoamine oxidase inhibitor. It interferes with the conversion of tryptophan to niacin by inducing a deficiency of pyridoxine co-enzymes so that it can evoke various manifestations of niacin deficiency, such as pellagra, especially in malnourished patients. Pellagra classically presents with dermatitis, diarrhoea, and dementia, although the psychiatric disorder can assume other forms (Shah *et al*. 1972).

Pellagra has been found in association with isoniazid therapy, both clinically (McConnell and Cheetham 1952) and pathologically (Ishii and Nishihara 1985). The latter authors described eight cases diagnosed at post-mortem, of whom six were thought to have manifested schizophrenia or a schizophrenic reaction in life, and McConnell and Cheetham's case also displayed schizophrenic and catatonic features. Treatment with niacin is invariably effective (Wallach and Gershon 1972).

Isoniazid is also associated with the production of delirium (Hall *et al*. 1980) and paranoid–hallucinatory psychoses without delirium (Wallach and Gershon 1972; Ball and Rosser 1989). These psychiatric disorders usually clear rapidly after withdrawal of the drug but there are at least eight reports of psychoses persisting for weeks or months (Wallach and Gershon 1972). Recrudescence of schizophrenia after 10 years' remission has been reported with isoniazid in a dose of 8 mg per kg body-weight per day (Ferrara and Peterson 1952).

A long list of psychiatric symptoms has been attributed to cycloserine treatment, including anxiety, irritability, drowsiness or insomnia, poor concentration, memory lapses, confusion, disorientation, hallucinations, paranoid delusions, and delirium. Cases are variously classified as schizophrenic reactions, depression, mania, or toxic delirium (Wallach and Gershon 1972). Cycloserine tends to activate schizophrenic patients, increasing agitation and hallucinations and inducing disorientation (Simeon et al. 1970).

The combination of isoniazid and cycloserine is also associated with the development of a similar range of psychoses (Wallach and Gershon 1972). Both drugs can induce epileptiform convulsions and peripheral neuropathy which, unlike the psychiatric complications, are prevented by giving pyridoxine (Cohen 1969).

Dapsone in a daily dose of 200 mg induced a psychotic reaction of violence, delusions, and visual and auditory hallucinations (Garrett 1971). This is claimed to be rare since the recommended dose was reduced to 100 mg daily (Browne 1971).

Antimalarial drugs

Chloroquine is used not only in malaria but also in the treatment of skin disorders and arthritis, and mepacrine is now more commonly used for giardiasis and tapeworm infestation than for malaria. Mepacrine (Greiber 1947; Perk 1947; Engel 1966; James et al. 1987) and chloroquine (Kabir 1969) have both been associated with the development of paranoid–hallucinatory psychoses, sometimes with manic features (Torrey 1968). Chloroquine also induces behavioural toxicity (Good and Shader 1977) and was suspected of causing a mini-epidemic of psychosis amongst young overseas volunteers (Ragan et al. 1985).

Antiviral drugs

Amantadine, an antiviral also used in the treatment of Parkinson's disease, has induced mania, depression, delirium, lethargy, nightmares, night terrors (Flaherty and Bellur 1981), and aggressive behaviour (Stewart 1987), and has precipitated an acute psychotic exacerbation in controlled schizophrenic patients (Hausner 1980; Nestelbaum et al. 1986). Coloured Lilliputian hallucinations occurred in a patient receiving 200 mg daily (Harper and Knothe 1973).

Acyclovir is active against the herpes virus. In 1988, the Australian Adverse Drug Reaction Advisory Committee intimated that 6 of 32 adverse reports received about acyclovir involved hallucinations or paranoid ideas after intravenous treatment, and one report was of delirium with visual hallucinations after taking the drug by mouth. Patients with renal impairment are the most vulnerable (Jones and Beier-Hanratty 1986). Depression with paranoid delusions and suicidal ideas (Sirota et al. 1988) or with fatigue and lethargy (Krigel 1986) has also been reported.

Ganciclovir has provoked delirium in 3 per cent of the subjects of clinical trials (Davey 1990).

Antifungal drugs

Intrathecal amphotericin has provoked acute delirium, resolving when the dose was reduced (Winn et al. 1979). Griseofulvin is associated with fatigue, depression, irritability, and insomnia, all these symptoms being aggravated by alcohol (Tester-Dalderup 1984).

Anticancer drugs

The difficulty of distinguishing drug effects from those of the underlying disorder is an obvious problem in this group. The temporal relationship between starting the suspected drug and the onset of psychiatric effects, and the effects of drug withdrawal or dose reduction on the psychiatric symptoms are particularly important in assessing the role of the drug.

Interferons, naturally occurring proteins with complex effects on immunity and cell function, are used in the treatment of advanced malignant disease (Priestman 1980) and severe viral infections (Ho 1987). Dose-related psychiatric effects, described in up to 17 per cent of patients (Renault et al. 1987), are reminiscent of the postviral fatigue syndrome. They include fatigue, impaired concentration, anxiety, and depression, which clear after cessation of treatment (Adams et al. 1984; Renault et al. 1987). Anorexia is common and often severe (Priestman 1980; Davey 1990). Delirium (Honisberger et al. 1983; Smedley et al. 1983; Renault et al. 1987), and visual hallucinations (Rohatiner et al. 1983) have also been reported.

The alkylating agents dacarbazine and hexamethylmelamine are both associated with adverse psychiatric reactions. Delirium and depression were reported in 5 per cent of patients receiving dacarbazine, and similar syndromes, with the addition of hallucinations and suicidal attempts, in 20 per cent of patients receiving hexamethylmelamine (Peterson and Popkin 1980).

Antimetabolites have been incriminated in psychiatric syndromes. A multifocal leukoencephalopathy with delirium, tremor, ataxia, irritability, and somnolence, mitigated by folic acid administration, is associated with treatment with methotrexate, which inhibits the enzyme dihydrofolate reductase, necessary for the synthesis of purines and pyrimidines (Kay *et al.* 1972). Intravenous fluorouracil is associated with decreased concentration, mood lability, and a parkinsonian syndrome (Peterson and Popkin 1980); and when used topically for actinic keratosis, it has been reported to induce mild to moderate depression in 25 per cent of cases (Milstein 1980). The combination of cyclophosphamide, methotrexate, and fluorouracil (CMF) is especially psychotoxic (Maguire *et al.* 1980), although this effect can be mitigated by restricting the duration of its use to 6 months (Hughson *et al.* 1986).

Other anticancer agents implicated in psychiatric adverse reactions include plicamycin (mithramycin), which has caused agitation; vincristine and vinblastine, which have induced depression; colaspase (asparaginase), which has produced delirium or depression (Weiss *et al.* 1974*a,b*; Peterson and Popkin 1980); and procarbazine, a mild monoamine oxidase inhibitor, which has been associated with mania (Mann and Hutchinson 1967). Interleukin-2 provokes psychiatric disturbance in a high proportion of recipients: of 44 patients with metastatic cancer receiving it, 43 per cent developed behavioural disturbance, severe in 27 per cent; 13.6 per cent developed hallucinations; 16 per cent developed paranoid delusions; and 50 per cent became delirious. Nearly all patients complained of fatigue, anorexia, and somnolence (Denicoff *et al.* 1987).

Visual hallucinations have developed in association with cyclosporin immunosuppression (Katirji 1987).

Dermatological drugs

Oral etretinate, used in the treatment of psoriasis and erythrokeratoderma (Borbujo *et al.* 1987; Henderson and Highet 1989), and isotretinoin (Hazen *et al.* 1983), used for severe acne, have been associated with severe depression. Topical application of the insect repellent, diethyltoluamide (DEET), has induced a manic reaction which responded to a single dose of haloperidol and the withdrawal of DEET (Poe *et al.* 1987).

Hormones

Corticosteroids and corticotrophin (ACTH) are used in a wide variety of medical disorders. Animal observations show that cortisone enhances cerebral catecholamine synthesis (Iuvone *et al.* 1977) and hippocampal serotonin levels (De Kloet *et al.* 1982). Psychotoxic effects are therefore to be expected.

Fairly soon after the introduction of corticotrophin and cortisone therapy, psychoses with a mixture of schizophrenic and affective symptoms were reported (Clark *et al.* 1952). The Boston Collaborative Drug Surveillance Program (BCDSP 1971) noted that steroids were the commonest cause of serious psychiatric reactions in medical wards and depression was the most frequent response. Analysis of 718 consecutive admissions receiving prednisone (BCDSP 1972) found 21 patients (3 per cent) with acute psychiatric reactions, including 13 with psychoses and 8 with inappropriate euphoria. Psychotic symptoms included auditory hallucinations, paranoid delusions, and violent behaviour; 6 patients were manic and 2 severely depressed. A definite dose-related effect was identified, the incidence of psychiatric disorder rising from 1.3 per cent on doses of prednisone below 40 mg daily to 18.4 per cent on doses over 80 mg daily. Psychoses can, however, appear at low doses (Greeves 1984). Similar observations have been made with prednisolone (Greeves 1984; Glynne-Jones *et al.* 1986) and corticotrophin (Cass *et al.* 1966). From a review of 14 cases, Hall and colleagues (1979) described steroid psychoses as 'spectrum' disorders, with symptoms ranging from affective, through schizophreniform, to those of an organic brain syndrome (delirium), these syndromes alternating in individual patients. Although a high incidence of steroid-related psychiatric reactions is found in patients with underlying conditions that predispose to mental disturbance, for example, multiple sclerosis (Minden *et al.* 1988), the majority of cases show no identifiable pre-existing psychiatric vulnerability (Hall *et al.* 1979; Ling *et al.* 1981). Children are particularly susceptible (Rutgers *et al.* 1988), even to inhaled budesonide (Lewis and Cochrane 1983). Steroid psychoses have been relieved by spacing out the daily dose or switching to an enteric-coated formulation (Glynne-Jones *et al.* 1986), both of which reduce peak blood levels. Successful treatment or prophylaxis of steroid psychoses with lithium (Falk *et al.* 1979; Goggans *et al.* 1983) or clonazepam (Viswanathan and Glickman 1989), in patients whose steroid therapy must be maintained, has been reported.

As might be expected with drugs with euphoriant effects, steroids can induce psychological dependence, and withdrawal is then resisted (Kimball 1971; Morgan *et al.* 1973). There appears to be also a degree of physical dependence, as rapid withdrawal of high doses provokes a withdrawal syndrome of anorexia, nausea, lethargy, joint and muscle pain, weakness, and skin desquamation (Hargreave *et al.* 1969), not attributable to pituitary–adrenal suppression (Bacon *et al.* 1966). Withdrawal psychoses of manic (Venkatarangam *et al.* 1988) or schizophreniform (Judd *et al.* 1983) type also occur.

The pituitary–adrenal suppression induced by long-term steroid therapy may be associated with psychiatric symptoms, including anxiety, depression, depersonalization, irritability, emotional lability, fatigue, and memory difficulties (Wolkowitz and Rapaport 1989).

Anabolic steroids are used by some athletes and body-builders to increase muscle size and strength (Wilson and Griffin 1980). Interviews with 31 users of 17-alkylated steroids (methandrostrenolone, oxandrolone, and oxymetholone) yielded 3 who had experienced paranoid–hallucinatory episodes and a further 4 with transient psychotic symptoms; 4 met diagnostic criteria for mania and 5 developed major depression during or immediately after a course of these substances (Pope and Katz 1987). Other reported reactions include an acute schizophrenic episode in a young athlete who was taking anabolic steroids surreptitiously (Annitto and Leyman 1980), aggressive behaviour (Barker 1987), and hypomania (Freinhar and Alvarez 1985). Eight weightlifters developed dependence on anabolic steroids, continuing their use despite adverse effects and then suffering withdrawal effects (Brower *et al.* 1990). Withdrawal depression occurred in 5 of 41 recipients and a further 2 experienced depression when not taking steroids (Pope and Katz 1988).

Depression accompanied by paranoid delusions and visual and auditory hallucinations has been reported in a 40-year-old man who received methyltestosterone 10 mg twice daily for 2 weeks for impotence (Pope and Katz 1987).

The association of psychiatric disorder, especially depression, with the use of oral contraceptives has long been a subject of controversy. Oestrogens influence presynaptic serotonin neurotransmission, and progestogens enhance MAO activity (Grant and Pryse-Davies 1968), both of which mechanisms might affect mood (Weizman *et al.* 1988). A literature review in 1970 (*British Medical Journal* 1970) concluded that depression occurred in 6–7 per cent of recipients compared with 1–2 per cent of controls. Subsequent controlled studies on large groups of women, however, failed to demonstrate any increase in depression in users compared with controls (e.g. Fleming and Seager 1978).

Isolated cases of paranoid–hallucinatory and schizo-affective psychoses have been reported (Daly *et al.* 1967; Kane 1968), including one example after hormone withdrawal in a woman with a past history of puerperal psychosis (Keeler *et al.* 1964). The incidence of serious psychiatric illness, as measured by first referral to hospital for specialist treatment, was studied in 9504 women taking oral contraceptives, 4144 using a diaphragm, and 3098 using an intrauterine device (Vessey *et al.* 1985). Referral rates for non-psychotic conditions in the oral contraceptive, diaphragm, and intrauterine device groups were 3.0, 2.6, and 2.8 per 1000 woman-years of observation, respectively. For psychotic disorders the rates were 0.46, 0.43, and 0.53. No relationship to duration of use or type of pill was identified. This technique would, however, have missed minor mood changes not requiring hospital referral. The change in formulation of contraceptive pills in recent years is likely to render this controversy obsolete.

The abrupt withdrawal of oestrogens in two male-to-female transsexuals precipitated paranoid schizophreniform psychoses which were regarded as analogous to a puerperal psychosis (Mallet *et al.* 1989; Faulk 1989).

A 36-year-old woman developed an acute paranoid psychosis 2 days after completing a 5-day course of 150 mg clomiphene daily, which settled after 2 days (Altmark *et al.* 1987).

Cardiovascular drugs

Digitalis preparations have long been known to precipitate delirium ('délire digitalique' was described by Duroziez in 1874), even after allowing for the contributory effect of associated cardiac disorder (Carr 1926). Associated symptoms include restlessness, excitement, ideas of reference, paranoid delusions, and coloured visual hallucinations (King 1950; Church and Marriott 1959). A paranoid psychosis with delusions and auditory hallucinations, without delirium, also occurs (Gorelick *et al.* 1978). Non-specific symptoms are also common in digitalis intoxication, including anorexia, fatigue, generalized weakness, dizziness, nightmares, listlessness, and somnolence (Lely and Van Enter 1970). Depression (Eisentrath and Sweeney 1987) and pseudodepression (depression-associated symptoms without mood change) are also reported (Wamboldt *et al.* 1986).

Although psychiatric symptoms due to digitalis are usually associated with elevated serum levels, and therefore often associated with cardiotoxic effects (De Graff and Lyon 1963), they can occur at normal therapeutic levels (Eisentrath and Sweeney 1987). Predisposition to develop digitalis toxicity is enhanced by increasing age, myocardial ischaemia or infarction, hypoxaemia, hypothyroidism, potassium or magnesium deficiency, renal insufficiency, and interaction with concurrent drug therapy (Wamboldt *et al.* 1986). The development of chorea associated with fatigue, disorientation, and fear as a complication of digoxin therapy suggests the possible implication of elevated brain dopamine in the production of psychic effects (Wedzicha *et al.* 1984). Peripheral and central catecholamine release is associated with the arrhythmogenic action of digitalis (Roberts *et al.* 1963; Saxena and Bhargava 1975) and could also play a part in inducing psychic effects.

β-Adrenoreceptor blocking drugs are used in the treatment of angina, hypertension, cardiac arrhythmias, anxiety and, topically, glaucoma. Some are lipid-soluble and others are water-soluble. The latter (e.g. atenolol, nadolol, and sotalol) enter the brain less readily, and psychiatric effects are correspondingly less common. β-Adrenergic receptors exist both peripherally and in the brain (Nahorski 1976) and propranolol also possesses serotonin-antagonist properties (Middlemiss *et al.* 1977).

Propranolol was the first of the group to appear, in the 1960s, and has therefore most often been linked with adverse effects. In 4708 patients receiving propranolol, drowsiness and fatigue were reported in 3.1 per cent, sleep disorders in 0.4 per cent, increased dreams and nightmares in 1 per cent, hypnagogic and hypnopompic hallucinations in 0.5 per cent, and depression in 0.7 per cent (Paykel *et al.* 1982). Although the overall prevalence of depression associated with propranolol is reported to be only around 1 per cent (Paykel *et al.* 1982) individual well-documented cases have been reported (Waal 1967; Prichard and Gillam 1969; Hansson *et al.* 1972; Petrie *et al.* 1982). Observations on depression and β-blocking drugs generally are contradictory. Thus, Carney and others (1987) found that 77 patients with coronary artery disease showed less depression with β-blocking agents than with alternative drugs, whereas Avorn and colleagues (1986) found that the likelihood of receiving tricyclic antidepressant treatment was 50–100 per cent greater with β-blocker therapy than with other antihypertensive therapy.

Dose-related visual hallucinations, usually nocturnal, occur in about 10 per cent of patients receiving propranolol (Fleminger 1978; Paykel *et al.* 1982). Delirium, often associated with visual and tactile hallucinations, has occurred both during propranolol therapy (Topliss and Bond 1977; Helson and Duque 1978) and after its abrupt withdrawal (Patterson 1985; Golden *et al.* 1989). Schizophrenia-like psychoses are reported to occur at

therapeutic doses (Koehler and Guth 1977; Steinert and Pugh 1979; Gershon *et al.* 1979; Thompson 1979) and, paradoxically, propranolol has been employed in large doses in the management of resistant schizophrenia (Yorkston *et al.* 1974).

Drowsiness and fatigue (6.8 per cent), insomnia (2.6 per cent), and depression (0.3 per cent) were reported in 367 patients receiving oxprenolol (Paykel *et al.* 1982). Vivid dreams (Freeman and Knight 1975) and schizophreniform psychoses (Steinert and Pugh 1979) also occur. Isolated cases of depression with metoprolol (Assayheen and Michell 1982) and nadolol therapy (Russell and Schuckit 1982) have also been described. Pindolol is associated with vivid dreams and nightmares, visual hallucinations, sedation, and depression (Paykel *et al.* 1982) and practolol, now restricted to intravenous injection for cardiac arrhythmias, with vivid dreams and depression (Wiseman 1971). Atenolol provoked delirium, with visual hallucinations and paranoid ideation, in an 85-year-old man when the dose was increased from 100 to 200 mg daily (Arber 1988).

Of the 1721 patients with adverse reactions to topical ocular timolol reported to the National Registry of Drug-Induced Ocular Side-Effects between 1978 and 1985 (Shore *et al.* 1987), 369 (21 per cent) experienced neurological or psychiatric effects, including depression (16.8 per cent of the 369), confusion (13.3 per cent), headache (12.2 per cent), fatigue (10.8 per cent), hallucinations (10.5 per cent), dizziness (9.7 per cent), sensory disorder (9.5 per cent), impotence (4.6 per cent), psychosis (3.5 per cent), somnolence (1.9 per cent), or myasthenia, myalgia, peripheral neuropathy, insomnia, and malaise (7 per cent). Psychiatric effects accounted for 163 (44 per cent) cases, with a median age of 65 years, but they remitted within a week of drug withdrawal. Both ocular timolol (Nolan 1982) and betaxolol (Orlando 1986) have provoked acute suicidal depression with recovery within 10 days of withdrawal of the drug.

Diuretics are the commonest cause of adverse drug reactions in the elderly (Williamson and Chopin 1980; Jarvis 1981). There is little evidence of intrinsic toxicity and their psychiatric effects are mediated indirectly through disturbance of water and electrolyte metabolism. Thus, hyponatraemia causes a range of effects, including weakness, confusion, postural giddiness, and hypotension, and transient hemiparesis (Sundaram and Mankikar 1983). Weakness, apathy, agitation, insomnia, confusion, disorientation, bizarre hallucinations, and delusions, accompanied by hypokalaemia and hyponatraemia, in patients receiving diuretics for hypertension were diagnosed as psychotic depression by Lewis (1971) but were thought by Paykel and colleagues

(1982) to be suffering from hypokalaemic apathy with delirium.

Although reserpine is an effective treatment for mild hypertension, with few adverse effects, it has now largely been superseded. It is of historical interest, however, as one of the first drugs recognized as a precipitant of a depressive syndrome (Schroeder and Perry 1955). Estimates of the incidence varied from 6–20 per cent (Goodwin *et al.* 1972). The onset was often delayed and insidious, and commoner at high doses (Freis 1954) and in patients with a previous depressive history (Muller *et al.* 1955). The depression is attributed to the central noradrenaline-depleting effect of reserpine (Mendels and Fraser 1974). It also produces central dopamine depletion (Cooper *et al.* 1986) and this may account for its former effective use as an antipsychotic.

Methyldopa is a centrally acting drug of which the mode of action is not fully determined. It is known to deplete both serotonin and dopamine and to be metabolised to α-methylnoradrenaline, which may act as a false transmitter or stimulate medullary α-2-adrenoceptors that inhibit noradrenaline release (Cooper *et al.* 1986; Ryall 1989).

Paykel and colleagues (1982) reviewed the extensive literature on the psychiatric effects of methyldopa, including reports of 2320 patients, and discovered a high incidence of drowsiness (32.5 per cent) but comparatively low frequencies of sleep disorder (0.8 per cent), vivid dreams, and nightmares (1.9 per cent) and depression (3.6 per cent). Nevertheless, the incidence of early waking (15 per cent) (a symptom of biological depression) and depression (13 per cent) was commonest in association with methyldopa therapy in 7954 patients interviewed annually for 5 years while receiving treatment for hypertension with various drugs (Curb *et al.* 1986). As with other drugs, the occurrence of depression is greater in those with a previous depressive history (Bant 1978). Isolated cases of delirium have been reported (Dubach 1963), one after the addition of haloperidol (Thornton 1976), and loss of concentration and forgetfulness have been described (Adler 1974).

Adrenergic-neurone blockers, which include guanethidine, debrisoquine, and bethanidine, act peripherally by blocking the release of noradrenaline. Guanethidine has also been shown to deplete serotonin and noradrenaline centrally in animals (Paykel *et al.* 1982).

Complaints of fatigue and lack of energy are common, 40 per cent being reported in one series (Ruedy and Davies 1967). In a literature review, Paykel and colleagues (1982) found low incidences of depression with all three drugs: guanethidine 1.9 per cent of 725, debrisoquine 0.4 per cent of 466, and bethanidine 1.3 per cent of 149 patients; but they accepted that isolated examples of genuine depressive reactions occur, especially to guanethidine.

Clonidine, also employed as a prophylactic against migraine and in the relief of opiate withdrawal symptoms, is a presynaptic α-adrenoceptor agonist which inhibits the release of central noradrenaline. It also has indirect central serotonin-inhibiting effects (Svensson *et al.* 1975).

Drowsiness, lethargy, and fatigue were reported in 47.6 per cent of 791 cases, but sleep disturbance occurred in only 4.7 per cent and depression in 1.5 per cent of the same series (Paykel *et al.* 1982). Isolated examples of paranoid psychosis (Raftos *et al.* 1973), anxiety, reversible delirium (Kellett and Hamilton 1970; Hoffman and Lodogama 1981), and visual and auditory hallucinations (Brown *et al.* 1980) have been reported. A withdrawal syndrome may develop after abrupt cessation of long-term clonidine therapy, with symptoms of sympathetic overactivity including insomnia, anxiety, tremor, sweating, restlessness, vivid dreams, headache, nausea, vomiting, diarrhoea, abdominal pain, salivation, and hiccup (Paykel *et al.* 1982). Other withdrawal effects include delirium and the exacerbation of pre-existing manic and schizophrenic psychoses (Adler *et al.* 1982). Clonidine has also been proposed as a treatment for mania (Jimerson *et al.* 1980) and schizophrenia (Freedman *et al.* 1982).

Prazosin has postsynaptic α-adrenoceptor-blocking and vasodilator properties. It has provoked delirium in patients with renal failure (Chin *et al.* 1986), and the development of auditory hallucinations has been reported (Patterson 1988).

Hydralazine acts by direct relaxation of vascular smooth muscle but may have central hypotensive effects (Ingenito *et al.* 1970). Paykel and colleagues (1982) have reviewed the literature on adverse psychiatric effects and cite examples of mania, anxiety, and 'nervousness' associated with hydralazine therapy. Although long-term administration is known to precipitate a systemic lupus erythematosus syndrome, the psychoses that often occur with that condition have not been observed (Alarcon-Segovia *et al.* 1967).

Calcium channel blockers (CCB) are classified into four groups, according to chemical structure. These are:
1. *piperazines* cinnarizine and flunarizine;
2. *phenylalkylamines* verapamil;
3. *dihydropyridines* nifedipine, felodipine, and nicardipine;
4. *benzothiazepines* diltiazem.

Cinnarizine and flunarizine are used mainly as antihistamines and peripheral vasodilators, the others are employed mainly in the treatment of cardiac arrhythmias, angina, and hypertension but occasionally for neurological disorders such as migraine, Gilles de la Tourette's syndrome, tardive dyskinesia and dystonia, and some psychiatric disorders (Biriell *et al.* 1989).

CCB produce a number of pharmacological effects that can influence neuropsychiatric function. Thus by blocking calcium influx through slow calcium channels they influence intracellular calcium homoeostasis, which is important for neuronal metabolism and signal processing (Abdel-Latif 1986). Also, there are specific binding sites for CCB in the brain reminiscent of benzodiazepine receptors (Snyder and Reynolds 1985). In addition, CCB affect the synthesis and release of neurotransmitters (Turner and Goldin 1985; Hullett *et al.* 1988) and can act as competitive antagonists at α-adrenergic receptors (Triggle 1982).

There is some evidence that intracellular calcium concentrations are elevated in mania and some cases of depression (Dubovsky and Franks 1986), so that calcium blockade might be expected to influence the development and course of affective disorders. CCB, and particularly verapamil, are claimed to have similar pharmacological and clinical effects to lithium (Höschl and Kozený 1989).

Verapamil is an effective treatment for mania (Giannini *et al.* 1984; Höschl and Kozený 1989). Although there is a single report of its apparent efficacy in depression (Höschl 1983), a double-blind trial failed to find any greater antidepressant effect than with placebo (Höschl and Kozeny 1989). A syndrome of peripheral paraesthesiae and suicidal thoughts remitted within a week of discontinuation of verapamil (Kumana and Mahon 1981). Delirium has also been reported with a dose of 320 mg daily (Jacobsen *et al.* 1987).

Nifedipine is associated with the induction of depression (Ahmad 1984; Hullett *et al.* 1988), mania (Tacke 1987), and paranoid–hallucinatory psychoses (Kahn 1986). Treatment-resistance in established cases of severe depression has been related to concurrent nifedipine therapy (Eccleston and Cole 1990).

The WHO Collaborating Centre for International Drug Monitoring has published details of eight cases of depression associated with diltiazem therapy reported from Canada, the USA, and the UK (Biriell *et al.* 1989). In some the depression was extremely severe. The latency of onset ranged from less than a day to 2 months. There was a positive rechallenge in two cases and recovery followed within 2 weeks of cessation of the drug in all but one instance. In five cases the daily dose was 180 mg or more and a dose-related effect was observed. Manic (Palat *et al.* 1984) and paranoid–hallucinatory psychoses

have also been reported (Bushe 1988) and an example of the Capgras syndrome (delusions that close relatives and friends have been replaced by doubles) occurred in a 79-year-old woman after one week on diltiazem 20 mg daily, remitting within 3 days of its withdrawal (Franklin *et al.* 1982).

Observations of akathisia (Jacobs 1983) and short-term improvement in tardive dyskinesia with diltiazem (Falk *et al.* 1988) suggest a dopaminergic effect.

The use of intravenous lignocaine, itself chemically related to cocaine, is associated with the production of delirium, accompanied by visual hallucinations, paranoid delusions, and disturbed behaviour (Graham *et al.* 1981; Turner 1982; Saravay *et al.* 1987). Reports of 'doom anxiety' and depression (Saravay *et al.* 1987) are difficult to disentangle aetiologically from the underlying physical condition.

Procainamide, also related to cocaine, has provoked manic episodes (Rice *et al.* 1988), in one case repeatedly (McCrum and Guidry 1978).

Tocainide, a primary amine analogue of lignocaine, is also associated with the development of delirium and paranoid psychoses, in two cases at serum levels of 6.7 and 10.2 mg per litre (Currie and Ramsdale 1984). The UK Committee on Safety of Medicines had received four reports of confusional states, four of hallucinatory episodes, and six of paranoid psychoses associated with tocainide up to July 1985 (CSM 1986). Depression has also been reported (Bikadaroff 1987).

The CSM also recorded one case of delirium, seven of hallucinations, and nine of paranoid psychoses associated with mexiletine during the same period (CSM 1986). Holt (1988) reported the appearance of visual hallucinations in two elderly patients receiving the drug.

Flecainide, related to lignocaine, is associated with the production of a severe depressive psychosis (Drerup 1988) and the development of visual hallucinations (Ramhamadany *et al.* 1986).

Disopyramide is associated with the production of paranoid–hallucinatory psychoses (Padfield *et al.* 1977; Ahmad *et al.* 1979), which have been attributed to its anticholinergic effects (Padfield *et al.* 1977), although the psychoses described are not typical of anticholinergic reactions (see above).

Nightmares, hallucinations, and behavioural disturbances occurred in 4 of 135 children (3 per cent) being treated with amiodarone for cardiac arrhythmias (Coumel and Fidelle 1980).

Quinidine is the optical isomer of quinine and both drugs induce the syndrome of nausea, tinnitus, and blurred vision known as cinchonism. Quinidine has been inculpated in the genesis of a dementia picture at therapeutic blood levels in three patients (Billig and Buongiorno 1985) and has induced an acute paranoid–hallucinatory psychosis in two patients at subtherapeutic blood levels (Deleu and Schmedding 1987). Quinine has provoked a similar psychosis at homoeopathic doses (Jerram and Greenhalgh 1988) and a manic psychosis in an elderly lady taking 300 mg at night for a year to relieve nocturnal cramp (Verghese 1988).

Angiotensin-converting-enzyme (ACE) inhibitors, which include captopril, enalapril, and lisinopril, inhibit the conversion of angiotensin I to angiotensin II and are used in the treatment of hypertension and cardiac failure. Captopril crosses the blood–brain barrier (Evered *et al.* 1980), and intracerebral angiotensin II is known to influence plasma levels of catecholamines and steroids in dogs (Scholkens *et al.* 1980).

Captopril is associated with mood elevation and the precipitation of outright mania in patients with a personal or family history of depression (Zubenko and Nixon 1984; McMahon 1985). 'Neurological' adverse effects, including lethargy, headache, and confusion, were recorded in only 0.2 per cent of cases surveyed by the New Zealand Drug Monitoring Programme (Edwards *et al.* 1987). Delirium due to hyponatraemia secondary to polydipsia induced by captopril has also been reported (Al-Mufti and Arieff 1985).

The vasodilator isosorbide dinitrate has induced visual hallucinations in an elderly female patient (Rosenthal 1987). Intravenous epoprostenol (prostacylin), given for Raynaud's phenomenon, provoked depression in three women (Ansell *et al.* 1986).

Bronchodilators

Salbutamol is a β-adrenoceptor agonist, so it is no surprise that it possesses antidepressant activity (Widlocher *et al.* 1977; Lecrubier *et al.* 1980) and can provoke manic reactions (Jacquot and Bottari 1981) and induce psychological dependence (Edwards and Holgate 1979), and is liable to abuse (Brennan 1983; Thompson *et al.* 1983). Paranoid psychoses without clouding of consciousness, accompanied by visual, auditory, and tactile hallucinations occur with salbutamol taken either orally (Ray and Evans 1978), by inhalation (Khanna and Davies 1986), or by both routes (Gluckman 1974; Whitehouse and Novosel 1989). The lowest oral dose to have induced a psychosis is 8 mg daily (Ray and Evans 1978). The minimum toxic dose of inhaled salbutamol is difficult to estimate, as most of the reported cases had exceeded the prescribed frequency of use. A 73-year-old male reported by Khanna and Davies (1986) became acutely depressed and experienced vivid visual and auditory persecutory hallucinations lasting an hour after each inhalation of 2.5 mg of nebulized salbutamol.

Both theophylline and aminophylline (a mixture of theophylline with ethylenediamine) can induce an excited state bordering on mania (McClelland 1985) and aminophylline has precipitated delirium in dose of 900 mg daily of a sustained-release preparation (Ramsay *et al.* 1980). A 58-year-old female receiving 1.2 g theophylline daily for asthma developed episodic bizarre behaviour with alternating stupor and wild flailing of limbs, catatonic posturing, and emotional lability when the dose was increased to 2 g daily. Blood levels, at 65.8 mg per litre were well above the therapeutic range of 10–20 mg per litre and the behaviour settled when the blood level fell to 13.4 mg per litre after 24 hours (Wasser *et al.* 1981).

Gastrointestinal drugs

Cimetidine is an histamine H₂-receptor blocker, used to control gastric acid secretion in the treatment of peptic ulcer, which has long been known to precipitate delirium (Kinnell and Webb 1979) and paranoid psychoses (Graham 1979; Adler *et al.* 1980), and to induce visual hallucinations (Agarwal 1978). Depressive syndromes have also been reported (Jefferson 1979). Early reports involved only elderly patients, often with renal (Bories *et al.* 1980) or hepatic (Nouel *et al.* 1980) impairment and elevated serum levels (Kimelblatt *et al.* 1980), but it is now clear that psychiatric reactions can occur at any age and at therapeutic blood levels (Papp and Curtis 1984). Intravenous administration in the elderly (Niv *et al.* 1986) or critically ill is particularly psychotoxic (Peura and Johnson 1985). An interaction with imipramine, allegedly provoking depression and paranoid psychosis, has been reported (Miller *et al.* 1987). Delirium usually develops within 2 days of starting cimetidine therapy and remits within 2–3 days of its discontinuation (Sonnenblick *et al.* 1982).

Ranitidine, with neurochemical and clinical effects similar to those of cimetidine but formerly thought to be free from adverse psychiatric effects, is now known to induce delirium (Hughes *et al.* 1983; Mandal 1986; MacDermott *et al.* 1987), depression (Billings and Stein 1986), mania (Patterson 1987; Delerue *et al.* 1988), and visual hallucinations (Price *et al.* 1985). A psychosis with delusions of creatures crawling over the body and penetrating the skin, without delirium, cleared within a week of withdrawing ranitidine 300 mg daily (Lesser *et al.* 1987).

There appears to be no cross-toxicity between cimetidine and ranitidine, as examples of ranitidine being used with impunity after cimetidine toxicity (Pedrazolli *et al.* 1983) and vice versa (Hughes *et al.* 1983) have been reported.

An encephalopathy secondary to use of bismuth salts for dyspepsia was formerly prevalent in France, Belgium, and Australia, presumably reflecting the popularity of bismuth in those countries. Collignon and colleagues (1979) analysed 99 case reports and added a further 7. Typically, a prodromal stage of headache, insomnia, asthenia, and mental sluggishness is followed by delirium with visual, auditory, and gustatory hallucinations, hostility, and excitement, often progressing to coma. At the same time myoclonic jerks, ataxia, dysarthria, and convulsions appear. Although several deaths have occurred, a gradual recovery on stopping taking bismuth is usual. The condition disappeared from France after bismuth was banned by the French Department of Health in 1978. Intestinal infection was postulated as the mechanism whereby sufficient relatively insoluble bismuth salts were absorbed to induce toxicity (*The Lancet* 1980).

Diagnosis

Some of the difficulties have been described previously. The sudden development of an unexpected psychiatric disorder shortly after the exhibition of a drug should certainly arouse suspicion. Insidiously developing disorders in patients with a constant drug intake over a long period are more difficult to recognize. Any drug, no matter how blameless its reputation, can be implicated. If in doubt, a therapeutic test by reducing or withdrawing the suspect drug may clarify the position.

Management

Whenever possible a drug identified as psychotoxic should be discontinued. If continued medication is essential, a different drug with similar pharmacological effects should be used but, if this is not practicable, the offending drug may have to be continued in reduced dosage.

Behavioural toxicity, hallucinosis, and delirium as a rule subside quickly after drug withdrawal. Specific psychiatric syndromes may persist and then require treatment in their own right with antidepressant medication or electroplexy (ECT) for depression, or with neuroleptic drugs for paranoid or schizophreniform psychoses, bearing in mind that psychotropic drugs are themselves a substantial source of psychiatric morbidity (see above).

The ultimate prognosis is usually good and specific treatment can usually be withdrawn within 2 weeks of the resolution of the syndrome.

Prevention

George and Kingscombe (1980) propose the following guidelines for minimizing the risk of adverse drug reactions, both somatic and psychiatric:

1. question whether drug therapy is really needed;
2. use appropriately reduced doses for children and the elderly;
3. avoid polypharmacy as far as possible;
4. introduce and withdraw drugs gradually;
5. avoid using known toxic drugs if at all possible.

The wider use of plasma drug level estimation may assist both diagnosis and prevention (Mucklow 1978).

Conclusion

Adverse drug reactions account for an appreciable amount of psychiatric morbidity. Doctors and pharmacists should be alert to this possibility, as it is a category of psychiatric disorder that often responds with gratifying rapidity to relatively simple measures.

References

Abdel-Latif, A.A. (1986). Calcium-mobilising receptors, polyphosphoinositides, and the generation of second messengers. *Pharmacol. Rev.* 38, 227.

Abed, R.T. and Clark, P.J. (1987). Acute psychotic episode caused by the abuse of phensedyl. *Br. J. Psychiatry* 151, 868.

Abraham, H.D. (1983). Visual phenomenology of the LSD flashback. *Arch. Gen. Psychiatry* 40, 884.

Adams, F., Quesada, J.R., and Gutterman, J.U. (1984). Neuropsychiatric manifestations of human leukocyte interferon therapy in patients with cancer. *JAMA* 252, 938.

Adler, L.E., Sadja, L., and Wilets, G. (1980). Cimetidine toxicity manifested as paranoia and hallucinations. *Am. J. Psychiatry* 137, 1112.

Adler, L.E., Bell, J., Kirch, D., Friedrich, E., and Freedman, R. (1982). Psychosis associated with clonidine withdrawal. *Am. J. Psychiatry* 139, 110.

Adler, S. (1974). Methyldopa-induced decrease in mental activity. *JAMA* 230, 1428.

Agarwal, S.K. (1978). Cimetidine and visual hallucinations. *JAMA* 240, 214.

References

Ahmad, S. (1984). Nifedipine-associated acute psychosis. *J. Am. Geriatr. Soc.* 32, 408.

Ahmad, S., Sheikh, A.I., and Meeran, M.K. (1979). Disopyramide-induced acute psychosis. *Chest* 76, 712.

Alarcón, R.D., Dickinson, W.A., and Dohn, H.H. (1982). Flashback phenomena. Clinical and diagnostic dilemmas. *J. Nerv. Ment. Dis.* 170, 217.

Alarcón-Segovia, D., Wakim, K.G., Worthington, J.W., and Ward, L.E. (1967). Clinical and experimental studies on the hydralazine syndrome and its relation to systemic lupus erythematosus. *Medicine* (Baltimore) 46, 1.

Alexander, J.I. and Spence, A. (1974). CNS effects of pentazocine. *Br. Med. J.* ii, 224.

Al-Mufti, H.I. and Arieff, A.I. (1985). Captopril-induced hyponatraemia with irreversible neurologic damage. *Am. J. Med.* 79, 769.

Altmark, D.,Tomer, R., and Segal, M. (1987). Psychotic episode induced by ovulation-initiating treatment. *Israel J. Med. Sci.* 23, 1156.

Al-Zahawi, M.F. and Sprott, M.S. (1988). Hallucinations in association with ceftazidime. *Br. Med. J.* 297, 858.

Anderson, E.D. (1970). Propylhexedrine (Benzedrex) psychosis. *N.Z. Med. J.* 71, 302.

Angrist, B. (1983). Psychoses induced by CNS stimulants and related drugs. In *Stimulants: neurochemical, behavioral and clinical perspectives* (ed. I. Creese), p. 1. Raven Press, New York.

Angrist, B. and Gershon, S. (1970). The phenomenology of experimentally induced amphetamine psychosis — preliminary observations. *Biol. Psychiatry* 2, 95.

Angrist, B.M., Schweitzer, J.W., Gershon, S., and Friedhoff, A.J. (1970). Mephentermine psychosis: misuse of the Wyamine inhaler. *Am. J. Psychiatry.* 126, 1315.

Angrist, B., Rotrosen, J., Kleinberg, D., Merriam, V., and Gershon, G. (1977). Dopaminergic agonist properties of ephedrine — theoretical implications. *Psychopharmacology* 55, 115.

Angst, J. (1987). Switch from depression to mania. *J. Psychopharmacol* 1, 13.

Annitto, W.J. and Leyman, W.A. (1980). Anabolic steroids and acute schizophrenic episode. *J. Clin. Psychiatry* 41, 143.

Ansell, D., Belch, J.J.S., and Forbes, C.D. (1986). Depression and prostacyclin infusion. *Lancet* ii, 509.

APA (American Psychiatric Association) (1987). *Diagnostic and statistical manual of mental disorders* (3rd edn revised). APA, Washington DC.

Arber, N. (1988). Delirium induced by atenolol. *Br. Med. J.* 297, 1048.

Arnold, E.S., Rudd, S.M., and Kirshner, H. (1980). Manic psychosis following rapid withdrawal from baclofen. *Am. J. Psychiatry* 137, 1466.

Ashton, C.H. (1984). Benzodiazepine withdrawal: an unfinished story. *Br. Med. J.* 288, 1135.

Ashton, C.H. (1986). Adverse effects of prolonged benzodiazepine use. *Adverse Drug React. Bull.* 118, 440.

Ashton, C.H. (1987). Cannabis: dangers and possible uses. *Br. Med. J.* 294, 141.

Ashton, C.H. (1990). Solvent abuse. Little progress after 20 years. *Br. Med. J.* 300, 135.

Assayheen, T.A. and Michell, G. (1982). Metoprolol in hypertension. *Med. J. Aust.* i, 73.

Avorn, J., Everitt, D.E., and Weiss, S. (1986). Increased antidepressant use in patients prescribed beta-blockers. *JAMA* 255, 357.

Bacon, P.A., Myles, A.B., Beardwell, C.G., Daly, J.R., and Savage, O. (1966). Corticosteroid withdrawal in rheumatoid arthritis. *Lancet* ii, 935.

Bain, J. (1984). Visual hallucinations in children receiving decongestants. *Br. Med. J.* 288, 1688.

Baldessarini, R.J. (1984). Treatment of depression by altering monoamine metabolism. Precursors and metabolic inhibitors. *Psychopharm. Bull.* 34, 259.

Ball, R. and Rosser, R. (1989). Psychosis and anti-tuberculosis therapy. *Lancet* ii, 205.

Bant, W.P. (1978). Anti-hypertensive drugs and depression: a re-appraisal. *Psychol. Med.* 8, 275.

Barker, S. (1987). Oxymethalone and aggression. *Br. J. Psychiatry* 151, 564.

Barry, D. and Weintraub, M. (1978). Barbiturate management of withdrawal syndromes. *Drug Therapy* 8, 83.

Batchelor, R.C.L., Horne, C.O., and Rogerson, H.L. (1951). An unusual reaction to procaine penicillin in aqueous suspension. *Lancet* ii, 195.

Bateman, D.N. (1988). Adverse reactions to antidotes. *Adverse Drug React. Bull.* 133, 496.

BCDSP (Boston Collaborative Drug Surveillance Program) (1971). Psychiatric side-effects of non-psychiatric drugs. *Semin. Psychiatry* 3, 435.

BCDSP (Boston Collaborative Drug Surveillance Program) (1972). Acute adverse reactions to prednisone in relation to dosage. *Clin. Pharmacol. Ther.* 13, 694.

Beal, D.M., Hudson, B., and Zaiaic, M. (1986). Amoxicillin-induced psychosis. *Am. J. Psychiatry* 143, 255.

Beamish, P. and Kiloh, L.G. (1960). Psychosis due to amphetamine consumption. *J. Ment. Sci.* 106, 337.

Bell, D.S. (1973). The experimental reproduction of amphetamine psychosis. *Arch. Gen. Psychiatry* 29, 35.

Belongia, E.A., Hedberg, C.W., Gleich, G.J., White K.E., Mayeno, A.N., Loegering, D.A., *et al.* (1990). An investigation of the cause of the eosinophilia–myalgia syndrome associated with tryptophan use. *N. Engl. J. Med.* 323, 357.

Ben-Arie, O. and George, G.C.W. (1979). A case of tranylcypromine (Parnate) addiction. *Br. J. Psychiatry* 135, 273.

Beringer, T.R.O. (1984). Salicylate intoxication in the elderly due to benorylate. *Br. Med. J.* 288, 1344.

Bethell, M.F. (1957). Toxic psychosis caused by 'Preludin'. *Br. Med. J.* i, 30.

Betts, T.A. and Birtle, J. (1982). Effect of two hypnotic drugs on actual driving performance next morning. *Br. Med. J.* 285, 852.

Bikadoroff, S. (1987). Depression provoked by tocainide. *Can. J. Psychiatry* 32, 219.

Billig, N. and Buongiorno, P. (1985). Quinidine-induced organic mental disorders. *J. Am. Geriatr. Soc.* 33, 504.

Billings, R.F. and Stein, M.B. (1986). Depression associated with ranitidine. *Br. J. Psychiatry* 143, 915.

Biriell, C., McEwen, J., and Sanz, E. (1989). Depression associated with diltiazem. *Br. Med. J.* 299, 796.

Bishop, L.C., Bisset, A.D., and Benson, J.I. (1987). Mania and indomethacin. *J. Clin. Psychopharmacology* 7, 203.

Black, R.J. and Dawson, T.A.J. (1988). Erythromycin and nightmares. *Br. Med. J.* 296, 1070.

Blair, D., Bailey, K.C., and McGregor, J.S. (1939). Treatment of epilepsy with epanutin. *Lancet* ii, 363.

Blazer, D.G. and Haller, L. (1975). Pentazocine psychosis. A case of persistent delusions. *Dis. Nerv. Syst.* 36, 404.

Bleich, A., Grinspoon, A., and Garb, R. (1987). Paranoid reaction following alprazolam withdrawal. *Psychosomatics* 28, 599.

Blum, A. (1987). Salicylate-induced delirium. *Psychosomatics* 28, 344.

Bonthala, M.C. and West, A. (1983). Pemoline-induced chorea and Gilles de la Tourette's syndrome. *Br. J. Psychiatry* 143, 300.

Booker, H.E. (1972). Primidone toxicity. In *Anti-epileptic drugs* (ed. D.M. Woodbury, J.K.Penry, and R.P. Schmidt). Raven Press, New York.

Borbujo, M.J.M., Casado, J.Z.M., Garijo, L.M.B., and Soto, M.J. (1987). Etretinate. Depression and behavioral changes: case report. *Med. Clin.* 89, 577.

Bories, P., Michel, H., Duclos, B., Berand, J-J., and Mironze, J. (1980). Use of ranitidine, without mental confusion, in patients with renal failure. *Lancet* ii, 755.

Bourgeois, M., Goumilloux, R., Peyre, F., Assens, F., and Degeilh, B. (1987). Virage maniaque sous clorazépate. *Ann. Med-Psychol.* (Paris) 145, 855.

Braddock, L.E. and Heard, R.N.S. (1986). Visual hallucinations due to indomethacin: a case report. *Int. Clin. Psychopharmacol.* 1, 263.

Braestrup, C., Nielsen, M., Honore, T., Jensen, L.H., and Petersen, E.N. (1983). Benzodiazepine receptor ligands with positive and negative efficacy. *Neuropharmacology* 22, 1451.

Brandon, S. (1969). Unusual effect of fenfluramine. *Br. Med. J.* iv, 557.

Brennan, P. (1983). Inhaled salbutamol: a new form of drug abuse. *Lancet* ii, 1030.

British Medical Journal (1970). Depression and oral contraception. *Br. Med. J.* iv, 127.

Brizer, D.A. and Manning, D.W. (1982). Delirium induced by poisoning with anti-cholinergic agents. *Am. J. Psychiatry* 139, 1343.

Brodsky, L. and Zuniga, J. (1975). Nitrous oxide: a psychotogenic agent. *Compr. Psychiatry* 16, 185.

Brook, N.M. and Cookson, I.B. (1978). Bromocriptine-induced mania? *Br. Med. J.* i, 790.

Brook, P.G. and Jackson, D. (1982). UK general practice experience of fenbufen in elderly patients. *Eur. J. Rheumatol. Inflamm.* 2, 326.

Brooke, D., Kerwin, R., and Lloyd, K. (1988). Di-ethylpropion hydrochloride-induced psychosis. *Br. J. Psychiatry* 152, 572.

Brower, K.J., Eliopulos, G.A., Blow, F.C., Catlin, D.H., and Beresford, T.P. (1990). Evidence for physical and psychological dependence on anabolic androgenic steroids in eight weight lifters. *Am. J. Psychiatry* 147, 510.

Brown, M.J., Salmon, D., and Rendell, M. (1980). Clonidine hallucinations. *Ann. Intern. Med.* 93, 456.

Browne, S.G. (1971). Anti-leprosy drugs. *Br. Med. J.* iv, 558.

Buchanan, R.A. (1972). Ethosuximide toxicity. In *Anti-epileptic drugs* (ed. D.M. Woodbury, J.K.Penry, and R.P. Schmidt). Raven Press, New York.

Bunney, W.E. Jr, and Garland-Bunney, B.L. (1987). Mechanisms of action of lithium in affective illness: basic and clinical implications. In *Psychopharmacology: third generation of progress* (ed. H.Y. Meltzer), p. 553. Raven Press, New York.

Burke, W.J. (1987). Benzodiazepine-induced hypomania. *J. Clin. Psychopharmacol.* 7, 356.

Bushe, C.J. (1988). Organic psychosis caused by diltiazem. *J. R. Soc. Med.* 81, 296.

Calne D.B., Stern, G.M., Spiers, H.S.D., and Laurence, D.R. (1969). L-dopa in post-encephalitic Parkinsonism. *Lancet* i, 744.

Calne, D.B., Plotkin, C., Williams, A.C., Nutt, J.G., Neophytides, A., and Teychenne, P.F. (1978). Long-term treatment of Parkinsonism with bromocriptine. *Lancet* i, 735.

Capellà, D., Laporte, J-R., Castel, J-M., Tristán, C., Cos, A., and Morales-Olivas, F.J. (1988). Parkinsonism, tremor and depression induced by cinnarizine and flunarizine. *Br. Med. J.* 297, 722.

Carlsson, A. and Lindqvist, M. (1969). Central and peripheral monoaminergic membrane pump blockade by some additive analgesics and antihistamines. *J. Pharm. Pharmacol.* 21, 460.

Carney, M.W.P. (1971). Five cases of bromism. *Lancet* ii, 523.

Carney, M.W.P. (1977). Paranoid psychosis with indomethacin. *Br. Med. J.* ii, 994.

Carney, M.W.P. (1988). Diethylpropion and psychosis. *Br. J. Psychiatry* 152, 146.

Carney, R.M., Rich, M.W., te Velde, A., Saini, J., Clark, K., and Freedland, K.E. (1987). Prevalence of major depressive disorder in patients receiving beta-blocker therapy versus other medication. *Am. J. Med.* 83, 223.

Carr, J.G. (1926). Digitalis delirium. *Med. Clin. N. Am.* 9, 1391.

Cass, L.J., Alexander, L., and Enders, M. (1966). Complications of corticotrophin therapy in multiple sclerosis. *JAMA* 197, 173.

Cassidy, S. and Henry, J. (1987). Fatal toxicity of antidepressant drugs in overdose. *Br. Med. J.* 295, 1021.

Celesia, G.C. and Barr, A.N. (1970). Psychosis and other psychiatric manifestations of levodopa therapy. *Arch. Neurol.* 23, 193.

Chadwick, D.W. (1985). Concentration–effect relationships of valproic acid. *Clin. Pharmacokinet.* 10, 155.

Chaplin, S. (1988). Benzodiazepine prescribing. *Lancet* i, 120.

Charney, D.S., Kales, A., Soldatos, C.R., and Nelson, J.C. (1979). Somnambulistic episodes secondary to combined lithium-neuroleptic treatment. *Br. J. Psychiatry* 135, 418.

Chen, K.K. and Schmidt, C.F. (1925). The action of ephedrine, the active constituent of the Chinese drug Ma Huang. *J. Pharmacol. Exp. Ther.* 24, 339.

Chin, D.K.F., Ho, A.K.C., and Tse, C.Y. (1986). Neuropsychiatric complications related to use of prazosin in patients with renal failure. *Br. Med. J.* 293, 1347.

Chouza, C., Scaramelli, A., Caamano, J.L., De Medina, O., Aljanati, R., and Romero, S. (1986). Parkinsonism, tardive dyskinesia, akathisia, and depression induced by flunarizine. *Lancet* i, 1303.

Church, G. and Marriott, J.H.L. (1959). Digitalis delirium: a report on three cases. *Circulation* 20, 549.

Clark, L.D., Bauer, W., and Cobb, S. (1952). Preliminary observations on mental disturbances occurring in patients under therapy with cortisone and ACTH. *N. Engl. J. Med.* 246, 205.

Clein, L. (1957). Toxic psychosis caused by Preludin. *Br. Med. J.* i, 282.

Climko, R.P., Roehrich, H., and Sweeney, D.R. (1986). 'Ecstasy': a review of MDMA and MDA. *Int. J. Psychiatry Med.* 16, 359.

Cohen, A.C. (1969). Pyridoxine in the prevention and treatment of convulsions and neurotoxicity due to cycloserine. *Ann. N.Y. Acad. Sci.* 166, 346.

Cohen, S. (1960). Lysergic acid diethylamide: side effects and complications. *J. Nerv. Ment. Dis.* 139, 30.

Cohen, W. and Cohen, N. (1974). Lithium carbonate, haloperidol and irreversible brain damage. *JAMA* 230, 1283.

Coid, J. and Strang, J. (1982). Mania secondary to procyclidine ('Kemadrin') abuse. *Br. J. Psychiatry* 141, 81.

Collignon, R., Bruyer, R., Rectem, D., Indekeu, P., and Laterre, E.C. (1979). Analyse sémiologique de l'encéphalopathie bismuthique. Confrontation avec sept cas personnels. *Acta Neurol. Belg.* 79, 73.

Connell, P.H. (1958). Amphetamine psychosis. *Maudsley Monograph No 5.* London.

Cooper, G.L. (1988). The safety of fluoxetine — an update. *Br. J. Psychiatry* 153 (suppl. 3), 77.

Cooper, J.R., Bloom, F.E., and Roth, R.H. (1986). *The biochemical basis of neuropharmacology.* Oxford University Press.

Coppel, D.L., Bovill, J.G., and Dundee, J.W. (1973). The taming of ketamine. *Anaesthesia* 28, 293.

Cornelius, J.R., Soloff, P.H., and Reynolds, C.F. (1984). Paranoid homicidal behavior and seizures associated with phenylpropanolamine. *Am. J. Psychiatry* 141, 120.

Coumel, P. and Fidelle, J. (1980). Amiodarone in the treatment of cardiac arrhythmias in children: 135 cases. *Am. Heart J.* 100, 1063.

Crawshaw, J.A. and Mullen, P.E. (1984). A study of benzhexol abuse. *Br. J. Psychiatry* 145, 300.

Cremona-Barbaro, A. (1983). Neuroleptic-induced catatonic symptoms. *Br. J. Psychiatry* 142, 98.

Critchlow, S. and Seifert, R. (1987). Khat-induced psychosis. *Br. J. Psychiatry* 150, 247.

Crow, T.J., Johnstone, E.C., Deakin, J.F.W., and Longden, A. (1976). Dopamine and schizophrenia. *Lancet* ii, 563.

CSM (Committee on Safety of Medicines) (1985). Actifed syrup and hallucinations in children. *Current Problems* 14, 2. HMSO, London.

CSM (Committee on Safety of Medicines) (1986). Update: recurrent ventricular tachycardia: adverse drug reactions. *Br. Med. J.* 292, 50.

CSM (Committee on Safety of Medicines) (1988). Benzodiazepines: dependence and withdrawal symptoms. *Current Problems* 21, 1. HMSO, London.

CSM (Committee on Safety of Medicines) (1989). Fluvoxamine and fluoxetine — interaction with monoamine oxidase inhibitors. *Current Problems* 26, 1. HMSO, London.

Curb, J.D., Maxwell, M.H., Schneider, K.A., Taylor, J.O., and Schulman, N.B. (1986). Adverse effects of anti-hypertensive medication in the Hypertension Detection and Follow-up Program. *Prog. Cardiovasc. Dis.* 29 (suppl. 1), 73.

Currie, P. and Ramsdale, D.R. (1984). Paranoid psychosis induced by tocainamide. *Br. Med. J.* 288, 606.

Dackis, C.A. and Gold, M.S. (1984). Depression in opiate addicts. In *Substance abuse and psychopathology* (ed. S.M. Mirin). American Psychiatric Press, Washington DC.

Daly, R.J., Kane, F.J., and Ewing, J.A. (1967). Psychosis associated with the use of a sequential oral contraceptive. *Lancet* ii, 444.

Daniel, D.G., Swallows, A., and Wolff, F. (1987). Capgras delusions and seizures in association with therapeutic doses of disulfiram. *South. Med. J.*, 80, 1577.

Davey, P.G. (1990). New anti-viral and anti-fungal drugs. *Br. Med. J.* 300, 793.

Davies, R.K., Tucker, G.J., Harrow, M., and Detre, T.P. (1971). Confusional episodes and anti-depressant medication. *Am. J. Psychiatry* 128, 95.

Davison, K. (1976). Drug-induced psychoses and their relationship to schizophrenia. In *Schizophrenia today* (ed. D. Kemali, G. Bartholini, and D. Richter), p. 105. Pergamon Press, Oxford.

Davison, K. (1981). Toxic psychosis. *Br. J. Hosp. Med.* 26, 530.

Davison, K. (1989a). Adverse psychiatric reactions to drugs used in the ITU. *Care of the Critically Ill* 5, 9.

Davison, K. (1989b). Acute organic brain syndromes. *Br. J. Hosp. Med.* 41, 89.

Davison, L.A., Steinhelber, J.C., and Eger, E.I. (1975). Psychological effects of halothane and isoflurane anaesthesia. *Anesthesiology* 43, 313.

Dean, E.S. (1963). Self-induced stramonium intoxication. *JAMA* 185, 882.

De Graff, A.C. and Lyon, A.F. (1963). The neurotoxic effects of digitalis. *Am. Heart J.* 65, 839.

De Kloet, E.R., Kovacs, G.L., Szabo, G., Telegdy, G., Bohar, B., and Versteeg, D.H.G. (1982). Decreased serotonin turnover in the dorsal hippocampus of rat brain shortly after adrenalectomy: selective normalisation after cortisone substitution. *Brain Res.* 239, 659.

Delerue, O., Muller, J-P., Destee, A., and Warot, P. (1988). Mania-like episodes associated with ranitidine. *Am. J. Psychiatry* 145, 271.

Deleu, D. and Schmedding, E. (1987). Acute psychosis as idiosyncratic reaction to quinidine: report of two cases. *Br. Med. J.* 294, 1001.

Deleu, D., De Keyser, J., and Ebinger, G. (1985). Bromide intoxication due to chronic intake of a bromide containing antacid. *Acta Gastro-Enterol. Belg.* 48, 509.

Denicoff, K.D., Rubinon, D.R., and Papa, M.Z. (1987). The neuropsychiatric effects of treatment with interleukin-2 and lymphokine-activated killer cells. *Ann. Intern. Med.* 107, 293.

Devan, G.S. (1990). Phentermine and psychosis. *Br. J. Psychiatry* 156, 442.

Deveaugh-Geiss, J. and Pandurangi, A. (1982). Confusional paranoid psychosis after withdrawal from sympathomimetic amines: two case reports. *Am. J. Psychiatry* 139, 1190.

Dhadpale, M. and Arap Mengech, H.N.K. (1987). Khat-induced paranoid psychosis. *Br. J. Psychiatry* 150, 876.

Dietz, A.J. (1981). Amphetamine-like reactions to phenyl-propanolamine. *JAMA* 245, 601.

DiGiacomo, J.N. (1968). Toxic effect of stramonium simulating LSD trip. *JAMA* 204, 265.

Donaldson, I.M.G. and Cunningham, J. (1983). Persisting neurologic sequelae of lithium carbonate therapy. *Arch. Neurol.* 40, 747.

Doogan, D.P. and Caillard, V. (1988). Sertraline: a new anti-depressant. *J. Clin. Psychiatry* 49 (suppl.), 46.

Dorus, E., Cox, N.J., Gibbons, R.D., Shaughnessy, R., Pandey, G.N., and Cloninger, R. (1983). Lithium ion transport and affective disorders within families of bipolar patients. *Arch. Gen. Psychiatry* 40, 545.

Drachman, D.A. (1977). Memory and cognitive function in man: does the cholinergic system have a specific role. *Neurology* 27, 783.

Drennan, P.C. (1984). Visual hallucinations in children receiving decongestants. *Br. Med. J.* 288, 1688.

Drerup, U. (1988). Zentral nervose Nebenwirkungen unter antiarrhythmika-Therapie. Psychotische Depression unter Flecainid. *Dtsch. Med. Wochenschr.* 113, 386.

D'Souza, M. (1987). Unusual reaction to morphine. *Lancet* ii, 98.

Dubach, U.C. (1963). Methyldopa and depression. *Br. Med. J.* i, 261.

Dubovsky, S.L. and Franks, R.D. (1983). Intracellular calcium ions in affective disorders: a review and an hypothesis. *Biol. Psychiatry* 18, 781.

Dundee, J.W. and Pandit, S.K. (1972). Anterograde amnesic effects of pethidine, hyoscine and diazepam in adults. *Br. J. Clin. Pharmacol.* 44, 140.

Duroziez, P. (1874). De délire et du coma digitaliques. *Gaz. Hebdom. Med. Chir.* 11, 780.

Eccleston, D. and Cole, A.J. (1990). Calcium channel blockade and depressive illness. *Br. J. Psychiatry* 156, 889.

Eckenhoff, J.E., Kneale, D.H., and Dripps, R.D. (1961). The incidence and etiology of post-anesthetic excitement. *Anesthesiology* 22, 667.

Edwards, G. (1989). Blasted with ennui. Dangers in another drug fashion. *Br. Med. J.* 298, 136.

Edwards, I.R., Coulter, D.M., Beasley, D.M.G., and Macintosh, D. (1987). Captopril: 4 years of post-marketing surveillance of all patients in New Zealand. *Br. J. Clin. Pharmacol.* 23, 529.

Edwards, J.G. and Holgate, S.T. (1979). Dependency upon salbutamol inhalers. *Br. J. Psychiatry* 134, 624.

Eddy, N., Halbach, H., Isbell, H., and Seevers, M. (1965). Drug dependence: its significance and characteristics. *Bull. WHO* 32, 721.

Eisendrath, S.J. and Sweeney, M.A. (1987). Toxic neuro-psychiatric effects of digoxin at therapeutic serum concentrations. *Am. J. Psychiatry* 144, 506.

Eisendrath, S.J., Goldman, B., Douglas, J., Dimatteo, L., and van Dyke, L. (1987). Meperidine-induced delirium. *Am. J. Psychiatry* 144, 1062.

Engel, G.L. (1966). Quinacrine effects on the central nervous system. *JAMA* 197, 235.

Epstein, R.S. (1989). Wernicke's encephalopathy following lithium-induced diarrhoea. *Am. J. Psychiatry* 144, 806.

Erikssen, J. (1969). Atropine psychosis. *Lancet* i, 53.

Evans, J. (1959). Psychosis and addiction to phenmetrazine (Preludin). *Lancet* ii, 152.

Evered, M.D., Robinson, M.M., and Richardson, M.A. (1980). Captopril given intracerebroventricularly, subcutaneously or by gavage inhibits angiotensin-converting enzyme activity in the rat brain. *Eur. J. Pharmacol.* 68, 443.

Everett, G.M. and Borcherding, J.W. (1970). L-dopa: effects on concentrations of dopamine, norepinephrine and serotonin in brains of mice. *Science* 168, 849.

Ewing, J.A. and Grant, W.J. (1965). The bromide hazard. *South. Med. J.* 58, 148.

Falk, W.E., Mahnke, M.W., and Poskanzer, D.C. (1979). Lithium prophylaxis of corticotrophin-induced psychosis. *JAMA* 241, 1011.

Falk, W.E., Wojick, J.D., and Greenberg, A.J. (1988). Diltiazem for tardive dyskinesia and tardive dystonia. *Lancet* i, 824.

Farnebo, L-O., Fuxe, K., Hanberger, B., and Ljungdahl, H. (1970). Effect of some anti-parkinsonian drugs on catecholamine neurons. *J. Pharm. Pharmacol.* 22, 733.

Faulk, M. (1989). Psychosis in a transsexual. *Br. J. Psychiatry* 155, 285.

Feder, R. (1987). Metoclopramide and depression. *J. Clin. Psychiatry* 48, 38.

Ferrara, M.A. and Peterson, E.B. (1952). Isoniazid in tuberculous psychotic patients. *N. Engl. J. Med.* 249, 1070.

Fetzer, J., Kader, G., and Danahy, S. (1981). Lithium encephalopathy: a clinical, psychiatric and EEG evaluation. *Am. J. Psychiatry* 138, 1622.

Fishbain, D.A. and Rogers, A. (1987). Delirium secondary to metoclopramide. *J. Clin. Psychopharmacol.* 7, 281.

Flaherty, J. and Bellur, S. (1981). Mental side effects of amantadine therapy. *J. Clin. Psychiatry* 42, 344.

Fleming, O. and Seager, C.P. (1978). Incidence of depressive symptoms in users of the oral contraceptive. *Br. J. Psychiatry* 132, 431.

Fleminger, R. (1978). Visual hallucinations and illusions with propranolol. *Br. Med. J.* i, 1182.

Fogarty, T. and Murray, G.B. (1987). Psychiatric presentation of meperidine toxicity. *J. Clin. Psychopharmacol.* 7, 116.

Fookes, B.H. (1976). Schizophrenia-like reaction to diethylpropion. *Lancet* ii, 1206.

Foy, A., Drinkwater, V., March, S., and Mearrick, P. (1986). Confusion after admission to hospital in elderly patients using benzodiazepines. *Br. Med. J.* 293, 1986.

Franklin, G.S., Brown, J.W., and Freedman, M.L. (1982). Shared Capgras syndrome and nifedipine. *Lancet* ii, 222.

Franks, R.D. and Richter, A.J. (1979). Schizophrenia-like psychosis associated with anticonvulsant toxicity. *Am. J. Psychiatry* 136, 973.

Fraser, A.A. and Ingram, I.M. (1985). Lorazepam dependence and chronic psychosis. *Br. J. Psychiatry* 147, 211.

Freedman, R., Kirch, D., Bell, J., Adler, L.E., Pecevich, M., Pachtman, E., and Denver, P. (1982). Clonidine treatment of schizophrenia. *Acta Psychiatr. Scand.* 65, 35.

Freeman, J.W. and Knight, L.W. (1975). Oxprenolol and hydralazine in the treatment of hypertension. *Med. J. Aust.* i (suppl.), 12.

Freinhar, J.P. and Alvarez, W. (1985). Androgen-induced hypomania. *J. Clin. Psychiatry* 46, 354.

Freis, E.D. (1954). Mental depression in hypertensive patients treated for long periods with large doses of reserpine. *N. Engl. J. Med.* 251, 1006.

Freund, M. and Merin, S. (1970). Toxic effects of scopolamine eye drops. *Am. J. Ophthalmol.* 70, 637.

Garattini, S. (1989). Reduction of food intake by manipulation of central serotonin. In *Serotonin in behavioural disorders* (ed. D. Eccleston and D.P. Doogan). *Br. J. Psychiatry* 155 (suppl. 8), 41.

Garattini, S., Borroni, E., and Mennini, T. (1978). Differences and similarities among anorectic agents. In *Central mechanisms of anorectic drugs* (ed. S. Garratini and R Samanin), p.127. Raven Press, New York.

Gardner, D.L. and Cowdry, R.W. (1986). Development of melancholia during carbamazepine treatment in borderline personality disorder. *J. Clin. Psychopharmacol.* 6, 236.

Gardos, G., Cole, J.O., and Tarsy, D. (1978). Withdrawal syndromes associated with anti-psychotic drugs. *Am. J. Psychiatry* 135, 1321.

Garfield, J.M. (1974). Psychologic problems in anesthesia. *Am. Fam. Physician* 10, 60.

Garrett, A.S. (1971). Anti-leprosy drugs. *Br. Med. J.* iv, 300.

Gawin, F.H. and Kleber, H.D. (1986). Abstinence symptomatology and psychiatric diagnosis in cocaine abusers. Clinical observations. *Arch. Gen. Psychiatry* 43, 107.

Gelenberg, A.J. and Mandel, M.R. (1977). Catatonic reaction to high-potency neuroleptic drugs. *Arch. Gen. Psychiatry* 34, 947.

George, C.F. and Kingscombe, P.M. (1980). Can adverse drug reactions be prevented? *Adverse Drug React. Bull.* 80, 288.

Gerner, R.H., Post, R.M., and Bunney, W.E. (1976). A dopaminergic mechanism in mania. *Am. J. Psychiatry* 133, 1177.

Gershon, E.S., Goldstein, R.E., Moss, A.J., and van Kammen, D.P. (1979). Psychosis with ordinary doses of propranolol. *Ann. Intern. Med.* 90, 938.

Giannini, A. and Castellani, S. (1982). A manic-like psychosis due to Khat. *J. Toxicol. Clin. Toxicol.* 19, 455.

Giannini, A.J., Houser, W.L., Loiselle, R.H., Giannini, M.C., and Price, W.A. (1984). Anti-manic effects of verapamil. *Am. J. Psychiatry* 141, 1602.

Gibson, I.I.J.M. (1966). Barbiturate delirium. *Practitioner* 197, 345.

Glaser, G.H. (1972). Diphenylhydantoin toxicity. In *Anti-epileptic drugs* (ed. D.M. Woodbury, J.K. Penry, and R.P. Schmidt), p. 219. Raven Press, New York.

Glass, G.S. and Bowers, M.B. (1970). Chronic psychosis associated with long-term psychotomimetic drug abuse. *Arch. Gen. Psychiatry* 23, 97.

Glatt, M.M. (1957). Toxic psychosis caused by Preludin. *Br. Med. J.* i, 460.

Gluckman, L. (1974). Ventolin psychosis. *N.Z. Med. J.* 80, 411.

Glynne-Jones, R., Vernon, C.C., and Bell, G. (1986). Is steroid psychosis preventable by divided doses? *Lancet* ii, 1404.

Goff, D.C. (1985). Two cases of hypomania following the addition of L-tryptophan to a monoamine oxidase inhibitor. *Am. J. Psychiatry* 142, 1487.

Goggans, F.C., Weisberg, L.J., and Koran, L.M. (1983). Lithium prophylaxis of prednisone psychosis: a case report. *J. Clin. Psychiatry* 44, 111.

Gold, M.S., Pottash, A.L.C., and Extein, I. (1980). Anti-endorphin effects of methadone. *Lancet* ii, 972.

Golden, G.S (1974). Gilles de la Tourette's syndrome following methyl-phenidate administration. *Dev. Med. Child Neurol.* 16, 76.

Golden, R.N., James, S.P., Sherer, M.A., Rudorfer, M.V., Sack, D.A., and Potter, W.Z. (1985). Psychoses associated with bupropion treatment. *Am. J. Psychiatry* 142, 1459.

Golden, R.N., Rudorfer, M.V., Sherer, M.A., Linnoila, M., and Potter, W.Z. (1988). Bupropion in depression: biochemical effects and clinical response. *Arch. Gen. Psychiatry* 45, 139.

Golden, R.N., Hoffman, J., Falk, D., Provenzale. D., and Curtis, T.E. (1989). Psychoses associated with propranolol withdrawal. *Biol. Psychiatry* 25, 351.

Goldsmith, S.R., Frank, I., and Ungerlieder, J.T. (1968). Poisoning from ingestion of a stramonium-belladonna mixture: Asthmador. *JAMA* 204, 169.

Goldstein, G. (1985). Pentazocine. *Drug Alcohol Depend.* 14, 313.

Good, M.I. and Shader, R.I. (1977). Behavioral toxicity and equivocal suicide associated with chloroquine and its derivatives. *Am. J. Psychiatry* 134, 798.

Goodkin, D.A. (1980). Mechanism of bromocriptine-induced hallucinations. *N. Engl. J. Med.* 302, 1479.

Goodman, W.K. and Charney, D.S. (1987). A case of alprazolam, but not lorazepam, inducing manic symptoms. *J. Clin. Psychiatry* 48, 117.

Goodwin, F.K. (1971). Psychiatric side-effects of levodopa in man. *JAMA* 218, 1915.

Goodwin, F.K., Murphy, D.L., Brodie, H.K.H., and Bunney, E.W. (1971). Levodopa: alterations of behaviour. *Clin. Pharmacol. Ther.* 12, 383.

Goodwin, F.K., Ebert, M.H., and Bunney, W.E. (1972). Mental effects of reserpine in man: a review. In *Psychiatric complications of medical drugs* (ed. R.I. Shader), p. 73. Raven Press, New York.

Gorelick, D.A., Kussin, S.Z., and Kahn, I. (1978). Paranoid delusions and auditory hallucinations associated with digoxin intoxication. *J. Nerv. Ment. Dis.* 166, 817.

Gott, P.H. (1968). Cyclizine toxicity. Intentional abuse of a proprietary anti-histamine. *N. Engl. J. Med.* 279, 596.

Gottesfeld, B.H., Lasser, L.M., Conway, E.J., and Mann, N.M. (1951). Psychiatric implications of the treatment of alcoholism with tetraethylthiuram disulfide. *Q. J. Stud. Alcohol* 12, 184.

Gough, S.P. and Cookson, I.B. (1984). Khat-induced schizophreniform psychosis in the UK. *Lancet* i, 455.

Gowdy, J.M. (1972). Stramonium intoxication. Review of symptomatology in 212 cases. *JAMA* 221, 585.

Graham, C.F., Turner, W.M., and Jones, J.K. (1981). Lidocaine–propranolol interactions. *N. Engl. J. Med.* 304, 1301.

Graham, J.R. (1979). Psychotic reactions to cimetidine; presumably an idiosyncrasy. *Med. J. Aust.* ii, 491.

Graham, P.M., Potter, J.M., and Paterson, J.W. (1982). Combination of monoamine oxidase inhibitor/tricyclic antidepressant interaction. *Lancet* ii, 440.

Grant, R.H.E. and Pryse-Davies, J. (1968). Effect of oral contraceptives on depressive mood changes and on endometrial monoamine oxidase and phosphatases. *Br. Med. J.* iii, 777.

Greden, J.F. (1974). Anxiety or caffeinism: a diagnostic dilemma. *Am. J. Psychiatry* 131, 1089.

Greenberg. J.R. and Lustig, N. (1966). Misuse of Dristan inhaler. *N.Y. J. Med.*, 66, 613.

Greer, H.D., Ward, H.P., and Corbrin, K.B. (1965). Chronic salicylate intoxication in adults. *JAMA* 193, 555.

Greeves, J.A. (1984). Rapid-onset steroid psychosis with very low dose of prednisolone. *Lancet* i, 1119.

Greiber. M.F. (1947). Psychoses associated with the administration of atabrine. *Am. J. Psychiatry* 104, 306.

Griffith, J.D., Cavanaugh, J., Held, J., and Oates, J.A. (1972). Dextroamphetamine: evaluation of psychotomimetic properties in man. *Arch. Gen. Psychiatry* 26, 97.

Griffith, J.D., Smith, C.H., and Smith, R.C. (1982). Paranoid psychosis in a patient receiving Ibuprofen, a prostaglandin synthesis inhibitor: case report. *J. Clin. Psychiatry* 43, 499.

Gupta, R. and Narang, R.L. (1986). Mania induced by gradual withdrawal from long-term treatment with imipramine. *Am. J. Psychiatry* 143, 260.

Hall, R.C.W., Popkin, M.K., and McHenry, L.E. (1977). Angel's trumpet psychosis: a CNS anti-cholinergic syndrome. *Am. J. Psychiatry* 134, 312.

Hall, R.C.W., Popkin, M.K., Stickney, S.K., and Gardner, E.R. (1979). Presentation of the steroid psychoses. *J. Nerv. Ment. Dis.* 167, 229.

Hall, R.C.W., Stickney, S.K., and Gardner, E.R. (1980). Behavioral toxicity of non-psychiatric drugs. In *Psychiatric presentations of medical illness: somatopsychic disorders* (ed. R.C.W. Hall), p. 137. Spectrum Publications, New York.

Hamon, M. (1984). Common neurochemical correlates to the action of hallucinogens. In *Hallucinogens: neurochemical, behavioral and clinical perspectives* (ed. B.L. Jacobs), p. 143. Raven Press, New York.

Hansson, L., Malmcrona, R., Olander, R., Rosenhall, L., Westerlund, A., Aberg, H., et al. (1972). Propranolol in hypertension. *Klin. Wochenschr.* 50, 365.

Hardie, R.J. and Lees, A.J. (1988). Neuroleptic-induced Parkinson's syndrome: clinical features and results of treatment with levodopa. *J. Neurol. Neurosurg. Psychiatry* 51, 850.

Harding, T. (1972). Depression following fenfluramine withdrawal. *Br. J. Psychiatry* 121, 338.

Hargreave, F.E., McCarthy, D.S., and Pepys, J. (1969). Steroid 'pseudorheumatism' in asthma. *Br. Med. J.* i, 443.

Harper, R.W. and Knothe, B.U.C. (1973). Coloured hallucinations with amantadine. *Med. J. Aust.* i, 444.

Harris, B. and Harper, M. (1979). Psychosis after dextropropoxyphene. *Lancet* ii, 743.

Hauger, R.L. and Paul, S.M. (1983). Neurotransmitter receptor plasticity: alterations by antidepressants and antipsychotics. *Psychiatr. Ann.* 13, 399.

Hausner, R.S. (1980). Amantadine-associated recurrence of psychosis. *Am. J. Psychiatry* 137, 240.

Hawks, D., Mitcheson, M., Ogborne, A., and Edwards, G. (1969). Abuse of methylamphetamine. *Br. Med. J.* ii, 715.

Hazen, P.G., Carney, J.F., Walker, A.E., and Stewart, J.J. (1983). Depression: a side-effect of 13-cis-retinoic acid therapy. *J. Am. Acad. Dermatol.* 9, 278.

Heath, R.G., Nesselhof, W., Bishop, M.P., and Byers, L.W. (1965). Behavioral and metabolic changes associated with administration of tetraethylthiuram disulfide (Antabuse). *Dis. Nerv. Syst.* 26, 99.

Helson, L. and Duque, L. (1978). Acute brain syndrome after propranolol. *Lancet* i, 98.

Henderson, C.A. and Highet, A.S. (1989). Depression induced by etretinate. *Br. Med. J.* 298, 964.

Heritch, A.J., Capwell, R., and Roy-Byrne, P.P. (1987). A case of psychosis and delirium following withdrawal from triazolam. *J. Clin. Psychiatry* 48, 168.

Hession, M.A., Verma, S., and Bhakta, K.G.M. (1979). Dependence on chlormethiazole and effects of its withdrawal. *Lancet* i, 953.

Hindmarch, I. (1980). Psychomotor function and psychoactive drugs. *Br. J. Clin. Pharmacol.* 10, 189.

Ho, M. (1987). Interferon for the treatment of infections. *Annu. Rev. Med.* 38, 51.

Hoefnagel, D. (1961). Toxic effects of atropine and homatropine eyedrops in children. *N. Engl. J. Med.* 264, 168.

Hoffman, W.F. and Lodogama, L. (1981). Delirium secondary to clonidine therapy. *N.Y. State J. Med.* 81, 382.

Hoigné, R. (1962). Acute side-reactions to penicillin. *Acta Med. Scand.* 171, 201.

Hoigné, R. and Schoch, K. (1959). Anaphylaktischer Schock und akute nichtallergische Reaktionen nach Procaine-Penicillin. *Schweiz. Med. Wochenschr.* 89, 1350.

Hoigné, R., Keller, H., and Sonntag, R. (1984). Penicillins, cephalosporins and tetracyclines. In *Meyler's side effects of drugs* (10th edn) (ed. M.N.G. Dukes), p. 146. Elsevier, Amsterdam.

Hollister, L.E. (1975). Complications from the use of tranquillising drugs. *N. Engl. J. Med.* 257, 170.

Hollister, L.E. (1986). Drug-induced psychiatric disorders and their treatment. *Med. Toxicol.* 1, 428.

Holt, P. (1988). Visual hallucinations. *N.Z. Med. J.* 101, 29.

Honer, W.G., Gewirtz, G., and Turey, M. (1987). Psychosis and violence in cocaine smokers. *Lancet* ii, 451.

Honisberger, L., Fielding, J.W., and Priestman, T.J. (1983). Neurological effects of recombinant human interferon. *Br. Med. J.* 286, 719.

Höschl, C. (1983). Verapamil for depression? *Am. J. Psychiatry* 140, 1100.

Höschl, C. and Kožený, J. (1989). Verapamil in affective disorders: a controlled, double-blind study. *Biol. Psychiatry* 25, 128.

Hotson, J.R. and Langston, W. (1976). Disulfiram-induced encephalopathy. *Arch. Neurol.* 33, 141.

Huber, S.J., Schulman, H.G., and Paulson, G.W. (1989). Dose-dependent memory impairment in Parkinson's disease. *Neurology* 39, 438.

Hughes, J.D., Reed, W.D., and Serjeant, C.S. (1983). Mental confusion associated with ranitidine. *Med. J. Aust.* ii, 12.

Hughson, A.V.M., Cooper, A.F., McArdle, C.S., and Smith, D.C. (1986). Psychological impact of adjuvant chemotherapy in the first two years after mastectomy. *Br. Med. J.* 293, 1268.

Hullett, F.J., Potkin, S.G., Levy, A.B., and Ciasca, R. (1988). Depression associated with nifedipine-induced calcium channel blockade. *Am. J. Psychiatry* 145, 1277.

Hurwitz, N. (1969). Predisposing factors in adverse reactions to drugs. *Br. Med. J.* i, 536.

Hyatt, M.C. and Bird, M.A. (1987). Amitriptyline augments and prolongs ethanol-induced euphoria. *J. Clin. Psychopharmacol.* 7, 277.

Ilechukwu, S.T.C. (1990). Acute psychotic reactions and stress response syndromes following intramuscular aqueous procaine penicillin. *Br. J. Psychiatry* 156, 554.

Imlah, N.W. (1970). Unusual effect of fenfluramine. *Br. Med. J.* ii, 178.

Ingenito, A.J., Barrett, J.P., and Procita, L. (1970). Centrally-mediated peripheral hypotensive effects of reserpine and hydralazine when perfused through the isolated in situ cat brain. *J. Pharmacol. Exp. Ther.* 170, 210.

Innes, J.A., Watson, M.L., Ford, M.J., Munro, J.F., Stoddart, M.E., and Campbell, D.B. (1977). Plasma fenfluramine levels, weight loss and side effects. *Br. Med. J.* ii, 1322.

Isbell, H., Altschule, S., Kornetsky, C.H., Eisenman, A.J., Flanary, H.G., and Fraser, H.F. (1950). Chronic barbiturate intoxication. *Arch. Neurol. Psychiatry* 64, 1.

Ishii, N. and Nishihara, Y. (1985). Pellagra encephalopathy among tuberculous patients: its relationship to isoniazid therapy. *J. Neurol. Neurosurg. Psychiatry* 48, 628.

Iuvone, M.P., Morasco, J., and Dunn, A.J. (1977). Effect of cortisone on the synthesis of [3H] catecholamines in the brains of CD-1 mice. *Brain Res.* 120, 571.

Jacobs, M.B. (1983). Diltiazem and akathisia. *Ann. Intern. Med.* 99, 794.

Jacobsen, F.M., Sack, D.A., and James, S.P. (1987). Delirium induced by verapamil. *Am. J. Psychiatry* 144, 248.

Jacquot, M. and Bottari, R. (1981). Etat maniaque ayant été déclenché par la prise orale de salbutamol. *Encephale* 7, 45.

Jaffe, R. and Gibson, E. (1986). Clonazepam withdrawal psychosis. *J. Clin. Psychopharmacol.* 6, 193.

James, I.M. (1975). Disease and adverse drug reactions. *Adverse Drug React. Bull.* 51, 172.

James, J.J., James, N.S., Morgenstern, M., and Gwinn, J. (1987). Quinacrine-induced toxic psychosis in a child. *Pediatr. Infect. Dis.* 6, 427.

Jarvis, E.H. (1981). Drugs and the elderly patient. *Adverse Drug React. Bull.* 86, 312.

Jefferson, J.W. (1979). Central nervous system toxicity of cimetidine: a case of depression. *Am. J. Psychiatry* 136, 346.

Jellema, J.G. (1987). Hallucinations during sustained-release morphine and methadone administration. *Lancet* ii, 392.

Jerram, T. and Greenhalgh, N. (1988). Quinine psychosis. *Br. J. Psychiatry* 152, 864.

Jimerson, D.C., Post, R.M., Stoddard, F.J., Gillin, J.C., and Bunney, W.E. Jr (1980). Preliminary trial of the noradrenergic agonist clonidine in psychiatric patients. *Biol. Psychiatry* 15, 45.

Johnston, J.A., Lineberry, C.G., and Frieden, C.S. (1986). Prevalence of psychosis, delusions and hallucinations in clinical trials with bupropion. *Am. J. Psychiatry* 143, 1192.

Jones, B.D. and Runikis, A.M. (1987). Interaction of ginseng with phenelzine. *J. Clin. Psychopharmacol.* 7, 201.

Jones, I.H., Stevenson, J., Jordan, A., Connell, H.M., Hetherington, H.D.G., and Gibney, G.N. (1973). Pheniramine as an hallucinogen. *Med. J. Aust.* i, 382.

Jones, P.G. and Beier-Hanratty, S.A. (1986). Acyclovir: neurologic and renal toxicity. *Ann. Intern. Med.* 104, 892.

Jones, R.F. and Lance, J.W. (1976). Baclofen (Lioresal) in the long-term management of spasticity. *Med. J. Aust.* i, 654.

Joshi, U.G. and Bhat, S.M. (1988). Mephentermine dependence with psychosis. A case report. *Br. J. Psychiatry* 152, 129.

Judd, F.K., Burrows, G.D., and Norman, T.R. (1983). Psychosis after withdrawal of steroid therapy. *Med. J. Aust.* ii, 350.

Kabir, S.M.A. (1969). Chloroquine psychosis. *Trans. R. Soc. Trop. Med. Hyg.* 63, 549.

Kahn, D.A. (1987). Possible toxic interaction between cyproheptadine and phenelzine. *Am. J. Psychiatry* 144, 1242.

Kahn, J.K. (1986). Nifedipine-associated acute psychosis. *Am. J. Med.* 81, 705.

Kales, A., Soldatos, S.R., Bixler, E.O., and Kales, J.D. (1983). Rebound insomnia and rebound anxiety: a review. *Pharmacology* 26, 121.

Kalix, P. (1984). The pharmacology of Khat. *Gen. Pharmacol.* 15, 179.

Kalso, E. and Vainio, A. (1988). Hallucinations during morphine but not during oxycodone treatment. *Lancet* ii, 912.

Kaminer, Y., Munitz, H., and Wijsenbeek, H. (1982). Trihexyphenidyl ('Artane') abuse — euphoriant and anxiolytic. *Br. J. Psychiatry* 140, 473.

Kamlana, S.H. (1989). Lithium-induced paranoid hallucinatory state. *Br. J. Psychiatry* 154, 273.

Kane, F.J. (1968). Psychiatric reactions to oral contraceptives. *Am. J. Obstet. Gynecol.* 102, 1053.

Kane, F.J. and Byrd, G. (1975). Acute toxic psychosis associated with gentamicin therapy. *South. Med. J.* 68, 1283.

Kane, F.J. and Florenzano, R. (1971). Psychosis accompanying use of bronchodilator compound. *JAMA* 215, 2116.

Kane, F.J. and Green, B.Q. (1966). Psychotic episodes associated with the use of common proprietary decongestants. *Am. J. Psychiatry* 123, 484.

Kane, F.J. and Pokorny, A. (1975). Mental and emotional disturbance with pentazocine. *South. Med. J.* 68, 808.

Katirji, M.B. (1987). Visual hallucinations and cyclosporine. *Transplantation* 43, 768.

Kay, H.E.M., Knapton, P.J., and O'Sullivan, J.P. (1972). Encephalopathy in acute leukemia associated with methotrexate therapy. *Arch. Dis. Child.* 47, 344.

Keeler, M.H., Kane, F., and Daly, R. (1964). An acute schizophrenic episode following abrupt withdrawal of Enovid in a patient with previous post-partum psychiatric disorder. *Am. J. Psychiatry* 120, 1123.

Keitner, G.I., Sabaawi, M., and Haier, R.J. (1984). Isosafrole and schizophrenia-like psychosis. *Am. J. Psychiatry* 141, 997.

Kellett, R.J. and Hamilton, M. (1970). The treatment of benign hypertension with clonidine. *Scott. Med. J.* 15, 137.

Khanna, P.B. and Davies, R. (1986). Hallucinations associated with the administration of salbutamol via a nebuliser. *Br. Med. J.* 292, 1430.

Khurana, A.K., Ahluwalia, B.K., Rajan, C., and Vohra, A.K. (1988). Acute psychosis associated with topical cyclopentolate hydrochloride. *Am. J. Ophthalmol.* 105, 91.

Kimball, C.P. (1971). Psychological dependence on steroids? *Ann. Intern. Med.* 75, 111.

Kimelblatt, B.J., Cerra, F.B., and Callieri, G. (1980). Dose and serum concentration relationships in cimetidine associated mental confusion. *Gastroenterology* 78, 791.

King, J.T. (1950). Digitalis delirium. *Ann. Intern. Med.* 33, 1360.

King, M.D., Day, R.E., Oliver, J.S., Lush, M., and Watson, J.M. (1981). Solvent encephalopathy. *Br. Med. J.* 283, 663.

Kinnell, H.G. and Webb. A. (1979). Confusion associated with cimetidine. *Br. Med. J.* ii, 1438.

Klein, H., Broucek, B., and Griel, W. (1981). Lithium withdrawal triggers psychotic states. *Br. J. Psychiatry* 139, 255.

Knee, S.T. and Razani, J. (1974). Acute organic brain syndrome: a complication of disulfiram therapy. *Am. J. Psychiatry* 123, 1284.

Knobler, H.Y., Itzchaky, S., Emanuel, P., Mester, R., and Maizel, S. (1986). Trazodone-induced mania. *Br. J. Psychiatry* 149, 787.

Koch-Weser, J. and Vandam, L.D. (1980). Butorphanol. *N. Engl. J. Med.* 302, 381.

Koehler, K. and Guth, W. (1977). Schizophrenie-ähnlicke Psychose nach Einnahme von Propranolol. *Munch. Med. Wochenschr.* 119, 443.

Kramer, J.C., Klein, D.F., and Fink, M. (1961). Withdrawal symptoms following discontinuation of imipramine therapy. *Am. J. Psychiatry* 118, 549.

Kräupl-Taylor, F. (1989). The damnation of benzodiazepines. *Br. J. Psychiatry* 154, 697.

Krauthammer, C. and Klerman, G.L. (1978). Secondary mania. Manic symptoms associated with physical illness or drugs. *Arch. Gen. Psychiatry* 35, 1333.

Krigel, R.L. (1986). Reversible neurotoxicity due to oral acyclovir in a patient with chronic lymphocytic leukaemia. *J. Infect. Dis.* 154, 189.

Kruis, R and Barger, R. (1980). Paranoid psychosis with sulindac. *JAMA* 243, 1420.

Kumana, C.R. and Mahon, W.A. (1981). Bizarre perceptual disorder of extremities in patients taking verapamil. *Lancet* i, 1324.

Kurlan, R. (1988). Drug-induced Alzheimerism. *Arch. Neurol.* 45, 356.

Kuventus, J.A., Silverman, J.J., and Sprague, M. (1984). Manic syndrome after metrizamide myelography. *Am. J. Psychiatry* 141, 700.

Lader, M. (1987). Long-term benzodiazepine use and psychological functioning. In *The benzodiazepines in current clinical practice* (ed. H. Freeman and Y. Rue), p. 55. Royal Society of Medicine, London.

Lader, M. (1990). Interactions that matter: Monoamine oxidase inhibitors. *Prescribers'.* 30, 48.

Lader, M. and Petursson, H. (1981). Benzodiazepine derivatives — side effects and dangers. *Biol. Psychiatry* 16, 1195.

Lader, M., Ron, M., and Petursson, H. (1984). Computed axial brain tomography in long term benzodiazepine users. *Psychol. Med.* 14, 203.

Lake, C.R. and Quirk, R.S. (1984). CNS stimulants and the look-alike drugs. *Psychiatr. Clin. N. Am.* 7, 689.

Lambert, M.T. (1987). Paranoid psychoses after abuse of proprietary cold remedies. *Br. J. Psychiatry* 151, 548.

The Lancet (1980). Idiosyncratic neurotoxicity: clioquinol and bismuth. *Lancet* i, 857.

The Lancet (1990). Contaminated L-tryptophan. *Lancet* i, 1152.

Laporta, M., Chouinard, G., Goldbloom, D., and Beauclair, L. (1987). Hypomania induced by sertraline, a new serotonin re-uptake inhibitor. *Am. J. Psychiatry* 144, 1513.

Lautin A, Angrist, B., Stanley, M., Gershon, S., Heckl, K., and Karobath, M. (1980). Sodium valproate in schizophrenia. Some biochemical correlates. *Br. J. Psychiatry* 137, 240.

Law, W., Petti, T.A., and Kazdin, A.E. (1981). Withdrawal symptoms after graduated cessation of imipramine in children. *Am. J. Psychiatry* 138, 647.

Lebegue, B. (1987). Mania precipitated by fluoxetine. *Am. J. Psychiatry* 144, 1620.

Lecrubier, Y., Puech, A.J., Jouvent, R., Simon, P., and Widlocher, D. (1980). A beta-adrenergic stimulant (salbutamol) versus clomipramine in depression: a controlled study. *Br. J. Psychiatry* 136, 354.

Le Feuvre, C.M., Isaacs, A.J., and Franks, O.S. (1982). Bromocriptine-induced psychosis in acromegaly. *Br. Med. J.* 285, 1315.

Le Gassicke, J. (1963). Tranylcypromine. *Lancet* i, 270.

Leighton, K.M. (1982). Paranoid psychosis after abuse of Actifed. *Br. Med. J.* 285, 1315.

Leipzig, R.M., Goodman, H., Gray, G., Erle, B., and Reidenberg, M.M. (1987). Reversible narcotic-induced mental status impairment in patients with metastatic cancer. *Pharmacology* 35, 47.

Lely, A.H. and van Enter, C.H.J. (1970). Large scale digoxin intoxication. *Br. Med. J.* iii, 737.

Lennhof, M. (1987). Trazodone-induced mania. *J. Clin. Psychiatry* 48, 423.

Lesser, I.M., Miller, B.L., Boone, K., and Lowe, C. (1987). Delusions in a patient treated with histamine H2 receptor antagonists. *Psychosomatics* 28, 501.

Levin, M. (1946). Transitory schizophrenias produced by bromide intoxication. *Am. J. Psychiatry* 103, 229.

Levin, M. (1948). Bromide psychosis: four varieties. *Am. J. Psychiatry* 104, 798.

Lewis, L.D. and Cochrane, G.M. (1983). Psychosis in a child inhaling budesonide. *Lancet* ii, 634.

Lewis, W.H. (1971). Iatrogenic psychotic depressive reaction in hypertensive patients. *Am. J. Psychiatry* 127, 1416.

Liddon, S.C and Satran, R. (1967). Disulfiram (Antabuse) psychosis. *Am. J. Psychiatry* 123, 1284.

Liegghio, N.E. and Yeragani, V.K. (1988). Buspirone-induced hypomania: a case report. *J. Clin. Psychopharmacol.* 8, 226.

Lin, J.T.Y. and Ziegler, D.K. (1976). Psychiatric symptoms with initiation of carbidopa-levodopa treatment. *Neurology* 26, 699.

Ling, M.H.M., Perry, P.J., and Tsuang, M.T. (1981). Side effects of corticosteroid therapy. Psychiatric aspects. *Arch. Gen. Psychiatry* 38, 471.

Linnoila, M., George, L, and Guthrie, S. (1982). Interaction between antidepressants and perphenazine in psychiatric patients. *Am. J. Psychiatry* 139, 1329.

Linnoila, M., Karoum, F., Rosenthal, N., and Potter, W.Z. (1983). ECT and lithium carbonate. Their effects on norepinephrine metabolism in patients with primary major depression. *Arch. Gen. Psychiatry* 40, 677.

Lipper, S. (1976). Psychosis in patient on bromocriptine and levodopa with carbidopa. *Lancet* ii, 571.

Logan, W. and Freeman, J. (1969). Pseudo-degenerative disease due to diphenylhydantoin intoxication. *Neurology* 21, 631.

Longo, V.G. (1966). Behavioural and EEG effects of atropine and related compounds. *Pharmacol. Rev.* 18, 965.

Lucas, A.R. and Weiss, M. (1971). Methylphenidate hallucinosis. *JAMA* 217, 1079.

Lund, Y., Nissen, M, and Rafaelson, O.J. (1982). Long-term lithium treatment and psychological function. *Acta Psychiatr. Scand.* 65, 233.

McClelland, H.A. (1985). Psychiatric disorders. In *Textbook of adverse drug reactions* (3rd edn) (ed. D.M. Davies), p. 549. Oxford University Press.

McClelland, H.A. (1990). The forensic implications of benzodiazepine usage. In *Benzodiazepines: current concepts* (ed. I. Hindmarch, G. Beaumont, S. Brandon, and R.E. Leonard), p. 227. John Wiley, New York.

McConnell, R.B. and Cheetham, H.D. (1952). Acute pellagra during isoniazid therapy. *Lancet* ii, 959.

McCormick, T.C. Jr and McNeil, T.W. (1963). Acute psychosis and Ritalin abuse. *Am. J. Med.* 59, 99.

McCrum, I.D. and Guidry, J.R. (1978). Procainamide-induced psychosis. *JAMA* 240, 1265.

McDanal, C.E. and Bolman, W.M. (1975). Delayed idiosyncratic psychosis with diphenylhydantoin. *JAMA* 231, 1063.

MacDermott, A.J., Insole, J., and Kaufman, B. (1987). Acute confusional episodes during treatment with ranitidine. *Br. Med. J.* 294, 1616.

MacEvilly, M. and O'Carroll, C. (1989). Hallucinations after epidural buprenorphine. *Br. Med. J.* 298, 928.

McKee, C.M. (1987). Medical and social aspects of qat in Yemen: a review. *J. R. Soc. Med.* 80, 762.

Macklin, E.A., Simon, A., and Crook, G.H. (1953). Psychotic reactions in problem drinkers treated with disulfiram (Antabuse). *Arch. Neurol. Psychiatry* 69, 415.

Macknin, M.L. (1987). Behavioral changes after amoxicillin-clavulanate. *Pediatr. Infect. Dis.* 6, 873.

McLaren, P. (1987). Khat psychosis. *Br. J. Psychiatry* 150, 712.

McMahon, T (1985). Bipolar affective symptoms associated with use of captopril and abrupt withdrawal of pargyline and propranolol. *Am. J. Psychiatry* 142, 759.

Maguire, G.P., Tait, A., Brooke, M., Thomas, C., Howat, J.M.T., Sellwood, R.A., *et al.* (1980). Psychiatric morbidity and physical toxicity associated with adjuvant chemotherapy after mastectomy. *Br. Med. J.* 281, 1179.

Malcolm, R. and Miller, W.C. (1972). Dimenhydrinate (Dramamine) abuse: hallucinogenic experiences with a proprietary anti-histamine. *Am. J. Psychiatry* 128, 1012.

Malleson, N. (1971). Acute adverse reactions to LSD in clinical and experimental use in the UK. *Br. J. Psychiatry* 118, 229.

Mallet, P., Marshall, E.J., and Blacker, C.V.R. (1989). 'Puerperal psychosis' following male to female sex reassignment. *Br. J. Psychiatry* 155, 257.

Mandal, S.K. (1986). Psychiatric side-effects of ranitidine. *Br. J. Clin. Pract.* 40, 260.

Mander, A.J. (1986). Is there a lithium withdrawal syndrome. *Br. J. Psychiatry* 149, 498.

Mann, A.M. and Hutchinson, J.R. (1967). Manic reaction associated with procarbazine hydrochloride therapy of Hodgkin's disease. *Can. Med. Assoc. J.* 97, 1350.

Manschreck, T.C., Allen, D.F., and Neville, M. (1987). Freebase psychosis: cases from a Bahamian epidemic of cocaine abuse. *Compr. Psychiatry* 28, 555.

Mariani, P.J. (1988). Adverse reactions to chlorpromazine in the treatment of migraine. *Ann. Emerg. Med.* 17, 380.

Marriot, P. (1976). Dependence on antiparkinsonian drugs. *Br. Med. J.* i, 152.

Marsh, G.G. and Markham, C.H. (1973). Does levodopa alter depression and psychopathology in Parkinsonism patients. *J. Neurol. Neurosurg. Psychiatry* 36, 925.

Martys, C.R. (1979). Adverse reactions to drugs. *Br. Med. J.* ii, 1194.

Matthew, G. (1988). Psychiatric symptoms associated with carbamazepine. *Br. Med. J.* 296, 1071.

Matthews, H.P. and Drummond, L.M. (1987). Obsessive-compulsive disorder on diazepam withdrawal. *Br. J. Psychiatry* 150, 272.

Mayberry, J., Morgan, G., and Perkin, E. (1984). Khat-induced schizophreniform psychosis in UK. *Lancet* i, 455.

Medsger, T.A. (1990). Tryptophan-induced eosinophilia–myalgia syndrome. *N. Engl. J. Med.* 322, 926.

Meldrum, B. (1982). GABA and acute psychoses. *Psychol. Med.* 12, 1.

Mendels, J. (1964). Paranoid psychosis associated with phenmetrazine addiction. *Br. J. Psychiatry* 110, 865.

Mendels, J. and Fraser, A. (1974). Brain biogenic amine depletion and mood. *Arch. Gen. Psychiatry* 30, 447.

Menza, M.A. (1986). Withdrawal syndrome in a depressed patient treated with trazodone. *Am. J. Psychiatry* 143, 1195.

Mermel, L.A., Doro, J.M., and Kabad, U.M. (1986). Acute psychosis in a patient receiving trimethoprim–sulfamethoxazole intravenously. *J. Clin. Psychiatry* 47, 269.

Meyboom, R.H.B., Ferrari, M.N., and Dieleman, B.P. (1986). Parkinsonism, tardive dyskinesia, akathisia and depression induced by flunarizine. *Lancet* ii, 292.

Middlemiss, D.N., Blakeborough, L., and Leather, S.R. (1977). Direct evidence for an interaction of beta-adrenergic blockers with the 5-HT receptor. *Nature* 267, 289.

Millan, M.J. and Duka, T.H. (1981). Anxiolytic properties of opiates and endogenous opioid peptides and their relationship to the actions of benzodiazepines. *Mod. Probl. Pharmacopsychiatry* 17, 123.

Miller, M.G. (1984). Visual hallucinations in children receiving decongestants. *Br. Med. J.* 288, 1688.

Miller, M.E., Perry, C.J., and Siris, S.G. (1987). Psychosis in association with combined cimetidine and imipramine treatment. *Psychosomatics* 28, 217.

Milstein, H.G. (1980). Mental depression secondary to fluorouracil therapy for actinic keratoses. *Arch. Dermatol.* 116, 1100.

Minden, S.L., Orau, J., and Schildkraut, J.J. (1988). Hypomanic reactions to ACTH and prednisone treatment for multiple sclerosis. *Neurology* 38, 1631.

Mindham, R.H.S. (1970). Psychiatric symptoms in Parkinsonism. *J. Neurol. Neurosurg. Psychiatry* 33, 188.

Mindham, R.H.S., Marsden, C.D., and Parkes, J.D. (1976). Psychiatric symptoms during l-dopa therapy for Parkinson's disease and their relationship to physical disability. *Psychol. Med.* 6, 23.

Mirin, S.M., Schatzberg, A.F., and Creasey, D.E. (1981). Hypomania and mania after withdrawal of tricyclic antidepressants. *Am. J. Psychiatry* 138, 87.

Mitchell, E. and Matthews, K.L. (1980). Gilles de la Tourette's syndrome associated with pemoline. *Am. J. Psychiatry* 137, 1618.

Moore, K.E. (1977). The actions of amphetamine on neurotransmitters: a brief review. *Biol. Psychiatry* 12, 451.

Morgan, H.G., Boulnois, J., and Burns-Cox, C. (1973). Addiction to prednisone. *Br. Med. J.* ii, 93.

Morris, D.E. and Hardway, R.L. (1985). Visual hallucinations induced by fenbufen. *Br. Med. J.* 290, 822.

Morris, H.H. and Estes, M.L. (1987). Traveller's amnesia. Transient global amnesia secondary to triazolam. *JAMA* 258, 945.

Mucklow, J.C. (1978). Value of plasma drug level estimation. *Adverse Drug React. Bull.* 73, 260.

Mueller, S.M. (1983). Neurologic complications of phenylpropanolamine use. *Neurology* 33, 650.

Mullen, A., Wilson, C.W.M., and Wilson, B.P.M. (1977). Dreaming, fenfluramine and vitamin C. *Br. Med. J.* i, 70.

Muller, J.C., Pryor, W.W., and Gibbons, J.E. (1955). Depression and anxiety occurring during rauwolfia therapy. *JAMA* 159, 836.

Murphy, D.D. (1973). Mental effects of l-dopa. *Annu. Rev. Med.* 24, 209.

Murphy, D. and Watters, J. (1986). Psychosis induced by fenfluramine. *Br. Med. J.* 292, 992.

Nab, H.W. and Hommes, O.R. (1987). Depression associated with tizanidine. *Br. Med. J.* 295, 612.

Nahorski, S.R. (1976). Association of high affinity stereospecific binding of 3H-propranolol to cerebral membranes with beta-adrenoreceptors. *Nature* 259, 488.

Negrete, J.C. (1983). Psychiatric effects of cannabis abuse. In *Cannabis and health hazards* (ed. K.O. Fehr and H. Kalant), p. 577. Addiction Research Foundation, Toronto.

Nestelbaum, Z., Siris, S.G., Rifkin, A., Klar, H., and Reardon, G.T. (1986). Exacerbation of schizophrenia associated with amantadine. *Am. J. Psychiatry* 1443, 1170.

Nicholson, A.N. (1983). Antihistamines and sedation. *Lancet* ii, 211.

Nigro, S.A. (1968). Toxic psychosis due to diphenhydramine hydrochloride (benadryl). *JAMA* 203, 301.

Nir, I. (1980). CNS stimulants and anorectic drugs. In *Meyler's side effects of drugs* (9th edn) (ed. M.N.G. Dukes), p. 11. Excerpta Medica, Amsterdam.

Nissenbaum, H., Quinn, N.P., Brown, R.G., Toone, B., Gotham, A-M., and Marsden, A.M. (1987). Mood swings with the 'on-off' phenomenon in Parkinson's disease. *Psychol. Med.* 17, 899.

Niv, Y., Zlatkis, L., and Kosakov, K. (1986). Cimetidine encephalopathy. *Ann. Intern. Med.* 105, 977.

Nolan, B.Y. (1982). Acute suicidal depression associated with the use of timolol. *JAMA* 247, 1567.

Norvenius, G., Widerlov, E., and Lonnerholm, G. (1979). Phenylpropanolamine and mental disturbances. *Lancet* ii, 1367.

Nouel, O., Bernuau, J., and Lebar, M. (1980). Cimetidine-induced mental confusion in patients with cirrhosis. *Gastroenterology* 79, 780.

Nyegaard & Company. (1977). Summarising notes from the Amipaque symposium. Quoted by Dukes, M.N.G. and Ansell, G. (1980). Radiological contrast media and radiopharmaceuticals. In *Meyler's side effects of drugs*

(9th edn) (ed. M.N.G. Dukes), p. 749. Excerpta Medica, Amsterdam.

O'Brien, C.P., DiGiacomo, J.N., Fahn, S., and Schwartz, G.A. (1971). Mental effects of high-dose levodopa. *Arch. Gen. Psychiatry* 24, 61.

Olpe, H.R., Koella, W.P., and Wolf, P. (1977). The action of baclofen on neurons of the substantia nigra and of the ventral tegmental area. *Brain Res.* 134, 577.

Orlando, R.G. (1986). Clinical depression associated with betaxolol. *Am. J. Ophthalmol.* 102, 275.

Ounsted, C. (1955). The hyperkinetic syndrome in epileptic children. *Lancet* ii, 303.

Oswald, I., Brezinova, V., and Dunleavy, D.L.F. (1972). On the slowness of action of tricyclic anti-depressant drugs. *Br. J. Psychiatry* 120, 673.

Owen, R.T. and Tyrer, P. (1983). Benzodiazepine dependence: a review of the evidence. *Drugs* 25, 385.

Padfield, P.L., Smith, D.A., Fitzsimons, E.J., and McCruden, D.C. (1977). Disopyramide and acute psychosis. *Lancet* i, 1152.

Palat, G.K., Hooker, E.A., and Movahed, A. (1984). Secondary mania associated with diltiazem. *Clin. Cardiol.* 7, 611.

Papart, P., Ansseau, M., Cerfontaine, J-L., and Frank, G. (1986). Adinozalam-induced mania. *Am. J. Psychiatry* 143, 684.

Papp, K.A. and Curtis, R.M. (1984). Cimetidine-induced psychosis in a 14-year old girl. *Can. Med. Assoc. J.* 131, 1081.

Patterson, J.F. (1985). Psychosis following discontinuation of a long-acting propranolol preparation. *J. Clin. Psychopharmacol.* 5, 125.

Patterson, J.F. (1987). Triazolam syndrome in the elderly. *South. Med. J.* 80, 1425.

Patterson, J.F. (1988). Auditory hallucinations induced by prazosin. *J. Clin. Psychopharmacol.* 8, 228.

Pauker, S.L. and Brown, R. (1986). Baclofen-induced catatonia. *J. Clin. Psychopharmacol.* 6, 387.

Paykel, E.S., Fleminger, R., and Watson, J.P. (1982). Psychiatric side-effects of anti-hypertensive drugs other than reserpine. *J. Clin. Psychopharmacol.* 2, 14.

Peabody, C.A. (1987). Trazodone withdrawal and formication. *J. Clin. Psychiatry* 48, 385.

Pearce, I. and Pearce, J.M.S. (1978). Bromocriptine in Parkinsonism. *Br. Med. J.* i, 1402.

Pearce, J.M.S. (1984). Drug treatment in Parkinson's disease. *Br. Med. J.* 288, 1777.

Pearlson, G.D. (1981). Psychiatric and medical syndromes associated with phencyclidine (PCP) abuse. *Johns Hopkins Med. J.* 148, 25.

Peden, N.R., Macaulay, K.E.C., Bissett, A.E., Crooks, J., and Pelosi, A.J. (1981). Clinical toxicology of 'magic mushroom' ingestion. *Postgrad. Med. J.* 57, 543.

Pedrazolli, S., Petrin, P., Pasquali, C., Millitello, C., Sperti, C., Fregonese, V., *et al.* (1983). Cimetidine-induced mental confusion in a patient with Zollinger–Ellison syndrome. *Arch. Surg.* 118, 256.

Penn, R.G. (1986). Adverse reactions to herbal and other unorthodox remedies. In *Iatrogenic diseases* (3rd edn) (ed.

P.F. D'Arcy and J.P. Griffin), p. 898. Oxford University Press.

Perenyi, A., Frecska, E., Bagdy, G., and Revai, K. (1985). Changes in mental condition, hyperkinesias and biochemical parameters after withdrawal of chronic neuroleptic treatment. *Acta Psychiatr. Scand.* 72, 430.

Perk, D. (1947). Mepacrine psychosis. *J. Ment. Sci.* 93, 756.

Perkins, H.A. (1950). Bromide intoxication. *Arch. Intern. Med.* 85, 783.

Perreau, O. and Maurice, H. (1950). Les troubles psychiques au cours de la fièvre typhoïde traitée par la chloromycétine. *Sem. Hop. Paris* 26, 1060.

Perry, E.K., Gibson, P.H., Blessed, G., Perry, R.H., and Tomlinson, B.E. (1977). Neurotransmitter enzyme abnormalities in senile dementia. *J. Neurol. Sci.* 34, 247.

Peterson, L.G. and Popkin, M.K. (1980). Neuropsychiatric effects of chemotherapeutic agents for cancer. *Psychosomatics* 21, 141.

Petrie, W.M., Maffucci, J., and Woosley, R.L. (1982). Propranolol and depression. *Am. J. Psychiatry* 139, 92.

Petursson, H. (1979). Diethylpropion and paranoid psychoses. *Aust. N.Z. J. Psychiatry* 13, 67.

Peura, D.A. and Johnson, L.F. (1985). Cimetidine for prevention and treatment of gastro-duodenal mucosal lesions in an intensive care unit. *Ann. Intern. Med.* 103, 173.

Pfefferbaum, B., Butler, P.M., Mullins, D., and Copeland, D.R. (1987). Two cases of benzodiazepine toxicity in children. *J. Clin. Psychiatry* 48, 450.

Pickar, D., Extein, I., and Gold, P.W. (1982). Endorphins and affective illness. In *Endorphins and opiate agonists in psychiatric research* (ed. N.S. Shah and A.S. Donald). Plenum Press, New York.

Pitt, B. (1974). Withdrawal symptoms after stopping phenelzine. *Br. Med. J.* ii, 332.

Poe, R.O., Snyder, J.W., Stubbins, J.F., and Garrettson, L.K. (1987). Acute manic psychosis following the dermal application of *N,N*-diethyl-*m*-toluamide (DEET) in an adult. *Am. J. Psychiatry* 144, 1103.

Polchert, S.E. and Morse, R.M. (1985). Pemoline abuse. *JAMA* 254, 946.

Pope. H.G. and Katz, D.L. (1987). Bodybuilder's psychosis. *Lancet* i, 863.

Pope, H.G. and Katz, D.L. (1988). Affective and psychotic symptoms associated with anabolic steroid use. *Am. J. Psychiatry* 145, 487.

Porot, M. and Destaing, F. (1950). Stréptomycine et troubles mentaux. *Ann. Med. Psychol.* 108, 47.

Porteous, H.B. and Ross, D.N. (1956). Mental symptoms in Parkinsonism following benzhexol therapy. *Br. Med. J.* ii, 138.

Poser, W., Poser, S., Roscher, D., and Argyrakis, A. (1983). Do benzodiazepines cause cerebral atrophy? *Lancet* i, 715.

Post, R.M. (1975). Cocaine psychosis: a continuum model. *Am. J. Psychiatry* 132, 225.

Prescott, L.F. (1975). Anti-inflammatory analgesics and drugs used in the treatment of rheumatoid arthritis and gout. In *Meyler's side effects of drugs*, Vol. 8 (ed. M.N.G. Dukes), p. 207. Excerpta Medica, Amsterdam.

Prescott, L.F. (1979). Factors predisposing to adverse drug reactions. *Adverse Drug React. Bull.* 78, 280.

Preskorn, S.H., Weller, E., Jerkovich, G., Hughes, C.W., and Weller, R. (1988). Depression in children: concentration-dependent CNS toxicity of tricyclic anti-depressants. *Psychopharmacol. Bull.* 24, 140.

Price, W., Coli, L., Brandstetter, R.D.M., and Gotz, V.P. (1985). Ranitidine-associated hallucinations. *Eur. J. Clin. Pharmacol.* 29, 375.

Prichard, B.N.C and Gillam, P.M.S. (1969). Treatment of hypertension with propranolol. *Br. Med. J.* i, 7.

Priest, R.G. and Montgomery, S.A. (1987). Benzodiazepines and dependence: a College statement. *Bull. R. Coll. Psychiatrists* 12, 107.

Priestman, T.J. (1980). Initial evaluation of human lympho-blastoid interferon in patients with advanced malignant disease. *Lancet* ii, 113.

Proctor, A.W., Littlewood, R., and Fry, A.H. (1983). Bromo-criptine-induced psychosis in acromegaly. *Br. Med. J.* 286, 50.

Prosser, E.S., Csernansky, J.G., Kaplan, J., Thiemann, S., Becker, T.J., and Hollister. (1987). Depression, parkinsonian symptoms, and negative symptoms in schizophrenics treated with neuroleptics. *J. Nerv. Ment. Dis.* 175, 100.

Puder, K.S. and Morgan, J.P. (1987). Persuading by citation: an analysis of 53 published reports of phenylpropanolamine's clinical toxicity. *Clin. Pharmacol. Ther.* 42, 1.

Quinn, N.P., Toone, B., Lang., A.E., Marsden,C.D., and Parkes, J.D. (1983). Unmasking of latent sexual deviation (masochism) in 2 cases by dopaminergic drugs. *Br. J. Psychiatry* 142, 296.

Raftos, J., Bauer, G.E., Lewis, R.G., Stokes, G.S., and Mitchell, A.S. (1973). Clonidine in the treatment of severe hypertension. *Med. J. Aust.* i, 786.

Ragan, E., Wilson, R., Li, F., Spasoff, R., Bigelow, G., and Spinner, N. (1985). Psychotic symptoms in volunteers serving overseas. *Lancet* ii, 37.

Ramhamadany, E., Mackenzie, S., and Ramsdale, D.R. (1986). Dysarthria and visual hallucinations due to fle-cainide toxicity. *Postgrad. Med. J.* 62, 61.

Ramsay, L.E., Mackay, A., Eppel, M.L., and Oliver, J.S. (1980). Oral sustained-release aminophylline in medical out-patients. *J. Clin. Pharmacol.* 10, 101.

Randrup, A. and Munkvad, I. (1966). DOPA and other naturally occurring substances as causes of stereotypy and rage in rats. *Acta Psychiatr. Scand.* 42 (suppl. 191), 193.

Raskind, M.A., Kitchell, M., and Alvarez, C. (1978). Bromide intoxication in the elderly. *J. Am. Geriatr. Soc.* 26, 222.

Ray, I. and Evans, C.J. (1978). Paranoid psychosis with Ven-tolin (salbutamol tablets BP). *Can. Psychiatr. Assoc. J.* 23, 427.

Renault, P.F., Hoofnagle, J.H., Park, Y., Mullen, K.D., Peters, M., Jones, B., *et al.* (1987). Psychiatric complications of long-term interferon alfa therapy. *Arch. Intern. Med.* 147, 1577.

Reynolds, E.H. (1968). Mental effects of anticonvulsants and folate metabolism. *Brain* 91, 197.

Reynolds, E.H. (1982). The pharmacological management of epilepsy associated with psychiatric disorders. *Br. J. Psychiatry* 141, 549.

Riblet, L.A., Gatewood, C.F., and Mayol, R.F. (1979). Comparative effects of trazodone and tricyclic antidepressants on uptake of selected neurotransmitters by isolated rat brain synaptosomes. *Psychopharmacology* (Berlin) 63, 99.

Rice, H., Haltzman, S., and Tucek, C. (1988). Mania associated with procainamide. *Am. J. Psychiatry* 145, 129.

Rieger, G. (1981). Paranoid-halluzinorische Psychosen nach Einnahme von D-Nor-pseudoephedrin-haltigen Appetit-zuglern. *Nervenarzt* 52, 423.

Roberts, J., Rynta, J., Reilly, J., and Cairoli, V.J. (1963). Influence of reserpine and BTM10 on digitalis-induced ventricular arrhythmia. *Circ. Res.* 13, 149.

Roberts, K. and Vass, N. (1986). Schneiderian first-rank symptoms caused by benzodiazepine withdrawal. *Br. J. Psychiatry* 148, 593.

Robertson, M.M. and Trimble, M.R. (1981). Neuroleptics as antidepressants. *Neuropharmacology* 20, 1335.

Roger, J., Grangeon, H., Guey, J., and Lob, H. (1968). Psychological and psychiatric symptoms in treatment of epileptics with ethosuccimide. *Encephale* 57, 407.

Rohatiner, A.Z.S., Prior, P.F., Burton, A.C., Smith, A.T., and Balkwill, F.R. (1983). CNS toxicity of interferon. *Br. J. Cancer* 47, 419.

Ron, M.A. (1986). Volatile substance abuse: a review of possible long-term neurological, intellectual and psychiatric sequelae. *Br. J. Psychiatry* 148, 235.

Rosenthal, R. (1987). Visual hallucinations and suicidal ideation attributed to isosorbide dinitrate. *Psychosomatics* 28, 555.

Rothstein, E. and Clancy, D.D. (1969). Toxicity of disulfiram combined with metronidazole. *N. Engl. J. Med.* 280, 1006.

Roxanas, M.G. and Spalding, J. (1977). Ephedrine abuse psychosis. *Med. J. Aust.* ii, 639.

Rubin, R.T. (1964). Acute psychotic reaction following ingestion of phentermine. *Am. J. Psychiatry* 120, 1124.

Ruedy, J. and Davies, R.O. (1967). A comparative clinical trial of guanoxan and guanethidine in essential hypertension. *Clin. Pharmacol. Ther.* 8, 38.

Russell, J.W. and Schuckit, M.A. (1982). Anxiety and depression in patients on nadolol. *Lancet* ii, 1286.

Rutgers, A.W.F., Links, T.P., Coultre, R.L., and Begeer, J.H. (1988). Behavioural disturbances after effective ACTH treatment of the dancing-eyes syndrome. *Dev. Med. Child Neurol.* 30, 408.

Ryall, R.W. (1989). *Mechanisms of drug action on the central nervous system.* Cambridge University Press.

Sachs, B.A. (1948). The toxicity of benadryl. *Ann. Intern. Med.* 29, 135.

SADRAC (Swedish Adverse Drug Reactions Advisory Committee) (1987). Fenfluramine — psychiatric reactions. *SADRAC Bull. No 49.*

Sadusk, J.R. (1966). Non-narcotic addiction: size and extent of the problem. *JAMA* 196, 707.

Sankey, R.J., Nunn, A.J., and Sills, J.A. (1984). Visual hallucinations in children receiving decongestants. *Br. Med. J.* 288, 1369.

Saravay, S.M., Marke, J., Steinberg, M.D., and Rabiner, C.J. (1987). Doom anxiety and delirium in lidocaine toxicity. *Am. J. Psychiatry* 144, 159.

Saxe, T.G. (1988). Severe depression from TMP–SMX. *Drug Intell. Clin. Pharm.*, 22, 267.

Saxena, P.R. and Bhargara, K.P. (1975). The importance of a central adrenergic mechanism in the cardiovascular responses to ouabain. *Eur. J. Pharmacol.* 31, 332.

Saxena, S. and Mallikarjuna, P. (1988). Severe memory impairment with acute overdose lithium toxicity. A case report. *Br. J. Psychiatry* 152, 853.

Scavullo, B.C. and Dementi, B. (1986). Psychotic reactions following the naive ingestion of phenylpropanolamine in psychiatric patients. *J. Am. Coll. Toxicol.* 5, 577.

Schmidt, L.G., Grohmann, R., Muller-Oerlinghausen, B., Ochsenfahrt, H., and Schonhofer, P.S. (1986). Adverse drug reactions to first and second-generation antidepressants. A critical evaluation of drug surveillance data. *Br. J. Psychiatry* 148, 38.

Scholkens, B.A., Jung, W., Rascher, W., Schonig, A., and Ganten, D. (1980). Brain angiotensin II stimulates release of pituitary hormones, plasma catecholamines and increases blood pressure in dogs. *Clin. Sci.* 59, 53s.

Schreiber, W., Pauls, A.M., and Kreig, J.C. (1988). Toxische Psychose als Akutmanifestation der Diphenhydramin-vergiftung. *Dtsch. Med. Wochenschr.* 113, 180.

Schroeder, H.A. and Perry, H.M. (1955). Psychosis apparently produced by reserpine. *JAMA* 159, 839.

Shah, D.R., Pandey, S.K., and Rathi, R. (1972). Psychiatric manifestations of pellagra. *J. Assoc. Physicians India* 20, 575.

Shalev, A., Hermesh, H., and Munitz, H. (1987). Severe akathisia causing neuroleptic failure. *Acta Psychiatr. Scand.* 76, 715.

Sheehy, L.M. and Maxmen, J.S. (1978). Phenelzine-induced psychosis. *Am. J. Psychiatry* 135, 1422.

Shihab, Z.M. (1980). Psychotic reaction in an adult after topical cyclopentolate. *Ophthalmologica* 181, 228.

Shore, J.H., Fraunfelder, F.T., and Meyer, S.M. (1987). Psychiatric side-effects from topical ocular timolol, a beta-adrenergic blocker. *J. Clin. Psychopharmacol.* 7, 264.

Shukla, S., Turner, W.J., and Newman, G. (1985). Bromocriptine-related psychosis and treatment. *Biol. Psychiatry* 20, 326.

Siegel, R.K. (1978). Cocaine hallucinations. *Am. J. Psychiatry* 135, 309.

Siegel, R.K. (1979). Ginseng abuse syndrome. *JAMA* 241, 1614.

Siegel, R.K. (1980). Cocaine substitutes. *N. Engl. J. Med.* 302, 817.

Siegel, R.K. (1982). Cocaine smoking. *J. Psychoactive Drugs* 14, 321.

Simeon, J., Fink, M., Itil, T.M., and Ponce, D. (1970). D-cycloserine therapy of psychosis by symptom provocation. *Compr. Psychiatry* 11, 80.

Simma, K. (1960). Uber Preludin-Halluzinose. *Wien. Klin. Wochenschr.* 24, 441.

Singh, S.V. (1982). Lithium carbonate and fluphenazine decanoate producing irreversible brain damage. *Lancet* ii, 278.

Siris, S.G., Cooper, T.B., Rifkin, A.E., Bremer, R., and Lieberman, J.A. (1982). Plasma imipramine concentrations in patients receiving concomitant fluphenazine decanoate. *Am. J. Psychiatry* 139, 104.

Sirota, P., Stoler, M., and Meshulam, B., (1988). Major depression with psychotic features associated with acyclovir therapy. *Drug Intell. Clin. Pharm.* 22, 306.

Skegg, D.C.G., Richards, S.M., and Doll, R. (1979). Minor tranquillizers and road accidents. *Br. Med. J.* i, 917.

Smart, R.G. and Bateman, K. (1967). Unfavourable reactions to LSD: a review and analysis of the available case reports. *Can. Med. Assoc. J.* 97, 1214.

Smedley, H., Katrak, M., Sikora, K., and Wheeler, T. (1983). Neurological effects of recombinant human interferon. *Br. Med. J.* 286, 262.

Smiler, B.G., Bartholomew, E.G., Sivak, B.J., Alexander, G.D., and Brown, E.M. (1973). Physostigmine reversal of scopolamine delirium in obstetric patients. *Am. J. Obstet. Gynecol.* 116, 326.

Snaith, R.P., Mehta, S., and Raby, A.H. (1970). Serum folate and vitamin B12 in epileptics with and without mental illness. *Br. J. Psychiatry* 116, 179.

Snow, S.S., Logan, T.P., and Hollander, M.H. (1980). Nasal spray addiction and psychosis: a case report. *Br. J. Psychiatry* 136, 297.

Snyder, S.H. (1978). The opiate receptor and morphine-like peptides in the brain. *Am. J. Psychiatry* 135, 645.

Snyder, S.H. and Reynolds, I.J. (1985). Calcium antagonist drugs: receptor interactions that clarify therapeutic effects. *N. Engl. J. Med.* 313, 995.

Soloman, R.L., Rich, C.L., and Darko, D.F. (1990). Antidepressant treatment and the occurrence of mania in bipolar patients admitted for depression. *J. Affect. Dis.* 18, 253.

Sonnenblick, M., Rosin, A.J., and Weissberg, N. (1982). Neurological and psychiatric side-effects of cimetidine — report of 3 cases with review of the literature. *Postgrad. Med. J.* 58, 415.

Spensley, J. (1972). Folie à deux with méthylphénidate psychosis. *J. Nerv. Ment. Dis.* 155, 288.

Spensley, J. and Rockwell, D.A. (1972). Psychosis during methylphenidate abuse. *N. Engl. J. Med.* 286, 880.

Spring, G.K. (1979). Neurotoxicity with combined use of lithium and thioridazine. *J. Clin. Psychiatry* 40, 135.

Steinbeck, K. and Turtle, J.R. (1979). Treatment of acromegaly with bromocriptine. *Aust. N.Z. J. Med.* 9, 217.

Steinert, J. and Pugh, C.R. (1979). Two patients with schizophrenic-like psychoses after treatment with beta-adrenergic blockers. *Br. Med. J.* i, 790.

Stephen, P.J. and Williamson, J. (1984). Drug-induced Parkinsonism in the elderly. *Lancet* ii, 1082.

Stephens, D.A. (1967). Psychotoxic effects of benzhexol hydrochloride. *Br. J. Psychiatry* 113, 213.

Sternbach, (1981). Pemoline-induced mania. *Biol. Psychiatry* 16, 987.

Stewart, J.T. (1987). Adverse behavioral effects of amantadine therapy in Huntington's disease. *South. Med. J.* 80, 1324.

Stores, G. (1975). Behavioural effects of anti-epileptic drugs. *Dev. Med. Child Neurol.* 17, 647.

Strang, J. and Edwards, G. (1989). Cocaine and crack. *Br. Med. J.* 299, 337.

Strassman, R.J. (1984). Adverse reactions to psychedelic drugs. A review of the literature. *J. Nerv. Ment. Dis.* 172, 577.

Sunderam, S.G. and Mankikar, G.D. (1983). Hyponatraemia in the elderly. *Age Ageing* 12, 77.

Svensson, T.H., Bunney, B.S., and Aghajanian, G.K. (1975). Inhibition of both noradrenergic and serotonergic neurons in brain by the alpha-adrenergic agonist clonidine. *Brain Res.* 92, 291.

Swigar, M.E. and Bowers, M.B. (1986). Baclofen withdrawal and neuropsychiatric symptoms: a case report and review of other case literature. *Compr. Psychiatry* 27, 396.

Tacke, U. (1987). Mania induced by biochemical imbalance. *Br. Med. J.* 295, 1485.

Task Force on late neurological effects of antipsychotic drugs. (1980). Tardive dyskinesia: summary of a task force report of the American Psychiatric Association. *Am. J. Psychiatry* 137, 1163.

Taylor, M., Galloway, D.B., Petrie, J.C., Davidson, J.F., Gallon, S.C., and Moir, D.C. (1978). Psychotomimetic effects of pentazocine and dihydrocodeine tartrate. *Br. Med. J.* ii, 1198.

Terrell, H.B. (1988). Behavioral dyscontrol associated with combined use of alprazolam and alcohol. *Am. J. Psychiatry* 145, 1313.

Tester-Dalderup, C.B.M. (1984). Anti-fungal drugs. In *Meyler's side effects of drugs* (10th edn) (ed. M.N.G. Dukes), p. 516. Elsevier, Amsterdam.

Thompson, M.K. (1979). Schizophrenia-like psychosis after treatment with beta-blockers. *Br. Med. J.* i, 1084.

Thompson, P.J., Dhillon, P., and Cole, P. (1983). Addiction to aerosol treatment. The asthmatic alternative to glue sniffing. *Br. Med. J.* 287, 1515.

Thornicroft, G. (1990). Cannabis and psychosis. Is there epidemiological evidence for an association? *Br. J. Psychiatry* 157, 25.

Thornton, T.L. (1980). Delirium associated with sulindac. *JAMA* 243, 1630.

Thornton, W.E. (1976). Dementia induced by methyldopa with haloperidol. *N. Engl. J. Med.* 294, 1222.

Tollefson, G. (1980). Psychiatric implications of anti-convulsant drugs. *J. Clin. Psychiatry* 41, 295.

Tomlin, P.J. (1977). Psychological problems in intensive care. *Br. Med. J.* ii, 441.

Topliss, D. and Bond, R. (1977). Acute organic brain syndrome after propranolol treatment. *Lancet* ii, 1133.

Torrey, E.F. (1968). Chloroquine seizures: report of four cases. *JAMA* 204, 115.

Triggle, D.J. (1982). Biochemical pharmacology of calcium blockers. In *Calcium blockers* (ed. S.F. Flaim and R. Zelis), p. 37. Urban and Schwarzenberg, Baltimore.

Trimble, M. and Reynolds, E.H. (1976). Anti-convulsant drugs and mental symptoms. A review. *Psychol. Med.* 6, 169.

Trimble, M.R., Corbett, J.A., and Donaldson, D. (1980). Folic acid and mental symptoms in children with epilepsy. *J. Neurol. Neurosurg. Psychiatry* 43, 1030.

Trump, D.L. and Hochberg, M.C. (1976). Bromide intoxication. *Johns Hopkins Med. J.* 138, 119.

Tucker, G.J. and Quinlan, D. (1972). Chronic hallucinogenic drug use and thought disturbance. *Arch. Gen. Psychiatry* 27, 443.

Turner, T.H., Cookson, J.C., Wass, J.A.H., Drury, P.L., Price, P.A., and Besser, G.M. (1984). Psychotic reactions during treatment of pituitary tumours with dopamine agonists. *Br. Med. J.* 289, 1101.

Turner, T.J. and Goldin, S.M. (1985). Calcium channels in rat brain synaptosomes: identification and pharmacological characterization: high affinity blockade by organic Ca¢ channel blockers. *J. Neurosci.* 5, 841.

Turner, W.M. (1982). Lidocaine and psychotic reactions. *Ann. Intern. Med.* 97, 149.

Twerski, B. (1987). Sympathomimetic-induced depression. *Am. J. Psychiatry* 144, 252.

Tyrer, P.J. (1980). Dependence on benzodiazepines. *Br. J. Psychiatry* 137, 576.

Tyrer, P. (1984). Clinical effects of abrupt withdrawal from tricyclic antidepressants and monoamine oxidase inhibitors after long term treatment. *J. Affect. Dis.* 6, 1.

Tyrer, P. (1987). Benefits and risks of benzodiazepines. In *The benzodiazepines in current clinical practice* (ed. H. Freeman and Y. Rue), p. 3. Royal Society of Medicine, London.

Tyrer, P., Rutherford, D., and Huggett, T. (1981). Benzodiazepine withdrawal symptoms and propranolol. *Lancet* i, 520.

Uhde, T.W., Redmond, D.E.Jr, and Kleber, H.D. (1982). Psychosis in the opioid addicted patient. *J. Clin. Psychiatry* 43, 240.

Ullman, K.C., Groh, R.H., and Wolff, F.W. (1970). Treatment of scopolamine-induced delirium. *Lancet* i, 252.

Umstead, G.S. and Neumann, K.H. (1986). Erythromycin ototoxicity and acute psychotic reaction in cancer patients with hepatic dysfunction. *Arch. Intern. Med.* 146, 897.

Usdin, G.L. and Robinson, K.E. (1951). Psychosis during Antabuse administration. *Arch. Neurol. Psychiatry* 66, 38.

van Scheyen, J.D. and Van Kammen, D.P. (1979). Clomipramine-induced mania in unipolar depression. *Arch. Gen. Psychiatry* 36, 560.

Vaughan, D.A. (1988). Interaction of fluoxetine with tricyclic antidepressants. *Am. J. Psychiatry* 145, 1478.

Verghese, C. (1988). Quinine psychosis. *Br. J. Psychiatry* 153, 575.

Venkatarangam, S.H.M., Kutcher, S.P., and Notkin, R.M. (1988). Secondary mania with steroid withdrawal. *Can. J. Psychiatry* 33, 631.

Vessey, M.P., McPherson, M., Lawless, M., and Yeates, D. (1985). Oral contraception and serious psychiatric illness: absence of an association. *Br. J. Psychiatry* 146, 45.

Vestergaard, P., Paulstrup, I., and Schou, M. (1988). Prospective studies on a lithium cohort. *Acta Psychiatr. Scand.* 78, 434.

Vlissides, D.N., Gill, D., and Castelow, J. (1978). Bromo-criptine-induced mania? *Br. Med. J.* i, 510.

Viswanathan, R. and Glickman, L. (1989). Clonazepam in the treatment of steroid-induced mania in a patient after renal transplant. *N. Engl. J. Med.* 320, 319.

Waal, H.J. (1967). Propranolol-induced depression. *Br. Med. J.* ii, 50.

Wade, J.D., Hart, R.P., and Suter, C. (1986). Neuropsychological implications of metrizimide myelography. *Lancet* ii, 102.

Waldman, S. and Pelner, L. (1950). Toxic psychosis due to overdosage with prophenpyridamine (trimeton): report of 2 cases with recovery. *JAMA* 143, 1334.

Wallach, M.B. and Gershon, S. (1972). Psychiatric sequelae to tuberculosis chemotherapy. In *Psychiatric complications of medical drugs* (ed. R.I. Shader), p. 201. Raven Press, New York.

Wamboldt, F.S., Jefferson, J.W., and Wamboldt, M.Z. (1986). Digitalis intoxication misdiagnosed as depression by primary care physicians. *Am. J. Psychiatry* 143, 219.

Wasser, W.G., Bronheim, H.E., and Richardson, B.K. (1981). Theophylline madness. *Ann. Intern. Med.* 95, 91.

Waters, B.G.H. and Lapierre, Y.D. (1981). Secondary mania associated with sympathomimetic drug use. *Am. J. Psychiatry* 138, 837.

Watters, K and Le Ridant, A. (1986). Psychosis induced by fenfluramine. *Br. Med. J.* 292, 1465.

Weddington, W.W. Jr and Banner, A. (1986). Organic affective syndrome associated with metoclopramide: case report. *J. Clin. Psychiatry* 47, 208.

Wedzicha, J.A., Gibb, W.R., Lees, A.J., and Hoffbrand, B.I. (1984). Chorea in digoxin toxicity. *J. Neurol. Neurosurg. Psychiatry* 47, 419.

Wehr, T.A. and Goodwin, F.K. (1979). Rapid cycling in manic-depressives induced by tricyclic anti-depressants. *Arch. Gen. Psychiatry* 36, 555.

Weiner, N. (1985). Norepinephrine, epinephrine, and the sympathomimetic amines. In *The pharmacological basis of therapeutics* (7th edn) (ed. A.G. Gilman, L.S. Goodman, T.W. Rall, and F. Murad). Macmillan, New York.

Weiss, H.D., Walker, M.D., and Wiernik, P.H. (1974a). Neurotoxicity of commonly used anti-neoplastic agents. *N. Engl. J. Med.* 291, 75.

Weiss, H.D., Walker, M.D., and Wiernik, P.H. (1974b). Neurotoxicity of commonly used anti-neoplastic agents. *N. Engl. J. Med.* 291, 128.

Weizman, A., Morgenstern, H., Kaplan, B., Amiri, Z., Tyano, S., Ouadia, Y., et al. (1988). Up-regulatory effect of triphasic oral contraceptive on platelet ^{3}H-imipramine binding sites. *Psychiatr. Res.* 23, 23.

Wharton, B.K. (1970). Nasal decongestants and paranoid psychosis. *Br. J. Psychiatry* 117, 439.

White, K. and Simpson, G. (1981). Combined MAOI-tricyclic anti-depressant treatment: a re-evaluation. *J. Clin. Psychopharmacol.* 1, 264.

White, K. and Simpson, G. (1984). The combined use of MAOIs and tricyclics. *J. Clin. Psychiatry* 45, 67.

White, M.C., Silverman, J.J., and Harrison, J.W. (1982). Psychosis associated with clonazepam therapy for blepharospasm. *J. Nerv. Ment. Dis.* 170, 117.

White, P.D. (1987). Myoclonus and episodic delirium associated with phenelzine: a case report. *J. Clin. Psychiatry* 48, 340.

Whitehouse, A.M. and Duncan, J.M. (1987). Ephedrine psychosis rediscovered. *Br. J. Psychiatry* 150, 258.

Whitehouse, A.M. and Novosel, S. (1989). Salbutamol psychosis. *Biol. Psychiatry* 26, 631.

Whitlock, F.A. and Evans, L.E.J. (1978). Drugs and depression. *Drugs* 15, 53.

Widlocher, D., Lecrubier, Y., Jouvent, R., Puech, A.J., and Simon, P. (1977). Antidepressant effect of salbutamol. *Lancet* ii, 767.

Wilkinson, D.G. (1979). Difficulty in stopping lithium prophylaxis? *Br. Med. J.* i, 235.

Williams. N.R. (1988). Erythromycin: a case of nightmares. *Br. Med. J.* 296, 214.

Williamson, J. and Chopin, J.M. (1980). Adverse reactions to prescribed drugs in the elderly: a multicentre investigation. *Age Ageing* 9, 73.

Willis, J.H. (1976). Abuse of non-amphetamine appetite suppressants. *Lancet* i, 37.

Wilson, J.D. and Griffin, J.E. (1980). The use and misuse of androgens. *Metabolism* 29, 1278.

Winn, R.E., Bower, M.J., and Richards, M.J. (1979). Acute toxic delirium: neurotoxicity of intrathecal amphotericin B. *Arch. Intern. Med.* 139, 706.

Wiseman, R.A. (1971). Practolol: accumulated data on unwanted effects. *Postgrad. Med. J.* (suppl.), 47, 68.

Witschy, J.K., Malone, G.L., and Holden, L.D. (1984). Psychosis after neuroleptic withdrawal in a manic-depressive patient. *Am. J. Psychiatry* 141, 105.

Wittstock, P. (1967). Schizophrenie-ähnliche exogene Psychose bei Preludin-Sucht. *Nervenarzt* 38, 39.

Wolf, M.E., Almy, G., Toll, M., and Mosnaim, A.D. (1982). Mania associated with the use of baclofen. *Biol. Psychiatry* 17, 757.

Wolf, S.M. and Davis, R.L. (1973) Permanent dementia in idiopathic Parkinsonism treated with levodopa. *Arch. Neurol.* 29, 276.

Wolkowitz, O.M. and Rapaport, M. (1989). Longstanding behavioral changes following prednisone withdrawal. *JAMA* 261, 1731.

Wood, A.J.J., Moir, D.C., Campbell, C., Davidson, J.F., Gallon, S.C., Henney, E., et al. (1974). CNS effects of pentazocine. *Br. Med. J.* i, 305.

Wood, S.F. (1986). Oral antihistamine or nasal steroid in hay fever. *Clin. Allergy* 16, 195.

Woods, L.A. (1956). The pharmacology of nalorphine. *Pharmacol. Rev.* 8, 175.

Woody, G.E. and O'Brien, C.P. (1974). Anticholinergic toxic psychosis in drug abusers treated with benztropine. *Compr. Psychiatry* 15, 439.

World Health Organisation. (1977). *Manual of the international statistical classification of diseases, injuries, and causes of death* (9th rev.). WHO, Geneva.

Wuth, O. (1927). Rational bromide treatment. *JAMA* 88, 2013.

Yapalater, A.R. and Rockwell, F.V. (1950). Toxic psychosis due to prophenpyridamine (Trimeton). Report of a case. *JAMA* 143, 428.

Yaryura-Tobias, J., Wolpert, A., Dana, L., and Merlis, S. (1970). Action of L-dopa in drug-induced extra-pyramidalism. *Dis. Nerv. Syst.* 31, 60.

Yaryura-Tobias, J.A., Diamond, B., and Merlis, S. (1972). Psychiatric manifestations of levodopa. *Can. Psychiatr. Assoc. J.* 17 (suppl. II), 123.

Yassa, R.Y. and Iskandar, H.L. (1988). Baclofen-induced psychosis: two cases. *J. Clin. Psychiatry* 49, 318.

Yorkston, N.J., Zaki, S.A., Malik, M.K.U., Morrison, R.C., and Havard, C.W.H. (1974). Propranolol in the control of schizophrenic symptoms. *Br. Med. J.* iv, 633.

Young, D. and Scoville, W.B. (1938). Paranoid psychosis in narcolepsy and possible danger of benzedrine treatment. *Med. Clin. N. Am.* 22, 637.

Young, G.G., Simson, C.B., and Frohman, C.E. (1961). Clinical and biochemical studies of an amphetamine withdrawal psychosis. *J. Nerv. Ment. Dis.* 132, 234.

Young, G.O. (1964). A sustained-release antihistamine. *Practitioner* 193, 664.

Young, R.E., Hutchison, S., Milroy, R., and Kesson, C.M. (1982). The rising price of mushrooms. *Lancet* i, 213.

Zaudig, M and von Bose, M. (1987). Oxoflavin-induced psychosis. *Br. J. Psychiatry* 151, 563.

Zmitek, A. (1987). Trazodone-induced mania. *Br. J. Psychiatry* 151, 274.

Zubenko, G.S., and Nixon, R.A. (1984). Mood-elevating effect of captopril in depressed patients. *Am. J. Psychiatry* 141, 110.

22. Disorders of blood cells and haemostasis

Part 1 Disorders of blood cells

G. H. JACKSON and S. J. PROCTOR

Introduction

As the number of pharmacological agents in use increases, and the understanding of the biology of the haematopoietic system improves, the nature of the effects of drugs on the haematopoietic system becomes a more fertile area for research. It is the intention in this chapter to attempt to relate the such effects to possible mechanisms. For many interactions this is not possible and only speculative unproven mechanisms can be considered. For drug reactions which are well known in the literature, the simple expedient of tabulating them has been used and the reader is referred to the original paper or reviews on the subject.

In order to understand fully the effects of drugs on the developing blood elements, a short resumé of the biology of blood cell development and the growth factors involved in normal marrow activity has been given. As many of these growth factors have been cloned and produced in recombinant form for clinical use, a brief resumé of the potential clinical use of such factors will also be included, as such agents, like other drugs, also have some deleterious effects on haematopoiesis.

Biology of blood cell development

The human bone marrow is a large vascular organ comprising some 4 per cent of lean body-weight in the mature adult. The relative size of the haematopoietic marrow in infancy and childhood is greater, and in the ageing adult the relative amount of haematopoietic marrow declines. Thus the effects of drugs on paediatric and geriatric populations can be different. Throughout life the marrow is the site of normal haematopoiesis, a finely controlled process that allows the production of all circulating blood cells at a rate determined by the body's variable demand, in which a small undifferentiated self-renewing population of pluripotent stem cells gives rise to large numbers of fully mature cells including erythrocytes, granulocytes, platelets, macrophages, and T and B lymphocytes. The production of mature cells is complex and strictly regulated, so that stable blood cell levels are maintained in health and yet these can alter swiftly in response to trauma or infection. Normally $4\mu10^8$ white cells and $1\mu10^{10}$ red cells are replaced per hour (Metcalf 1987). The neutrophil count can increase 10-fold, however, in response to severe infection within a matter of 24 hours. Clearly, to allow such an amplification of cell numbers during differentiation there must be a number of stages between the stem cell and the fully differentiated end cell. Each stage is associated with a gradual loss of potential and a decline in proliferative capacity such that the mature granulocyte has only a life span of some 48 hours and mature platelets of some 5 days.

In the mid-60s, cell culture systems that allowed investigation of proliferation and differentiation of cells from the bone marrow were developed. Such biological systems have been further refined and, in addition, it is now possible to grow bone marrow in long-term culture and analyse not only haematopoietic progeny but also bone marrow stromal cells. The control of the haematopoietic system to allow the production of large numbers of cells at a rate depending on variable demand is extremely complex, and it is only recently that the regulation of the system has begun to be unravelled. Interest has centred on a group of glycoproteins which have been shown to stimulate the growth of intermediate cells in the haematopoietic system (Fig. 22.1) (Balkwill 1989). These include erythropoietin, granulocyte–macrophage colony-stimulating factor (GM-CSF), granulocyte colony-stimulating factor (G-CSF), macrophage colony-stimulating factor (M-CSF) and multi-CSF, often referred to as interleukin-3 (IL-3). The haematopoietic

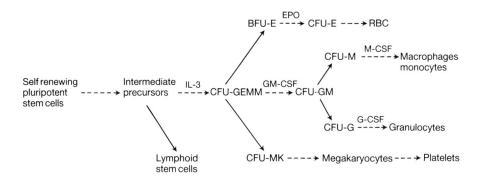

FIG. 22.1.

Model of haematopoiesis, from pluripotent self-renewing stem cell to non-dividing end cell, showing some sites of action of some of the haematopoietic growth factors.

CFU–GEMM	colony-forming unit, granulocyte–erythroid–macrophage–megakaryocyte		CFU–MK	colony-forming unit, megakaryocyte
			IL–3	interleukin 3
CFU–GM	colony-forming unit, granulocyte–macrophage		GM–CFS	granulocyte–macrophage colony-stimulating factor
BFU–E	burst-forming unit, erythroid			
CFU–E	colony-forming unit, erythroid		G–CSF	granulocyte colony-stimulating factor
CFU–G	colony-forming unit, granulocyte		M–CFS	macrophage colony-stimulating factor
CFU–M	colony-forming unit, macrophage		EPO	erythropoietin

lineages affected by these agents are diagrammatically demonstrated in Figure 22.1. Chromosomal localization of the above biological response modifiers is now known and most have been cloned, and recombinant DNA technology has allowed their development for clinical use. The bone marrow micro-environment and the inter-actions of the above growth factors with all elements and/or production by elements of the bone marrow stroma is, at the present time, being dissected, but there is little doubt that the bone marrow, stroma, and matrix are critically involved in the regulation of haematopoiesis (Dexter 1987). It is thus evident that drugs that induce bone marrow failure may affect haematopoiesis through effects on the stem cell, the bone marrow micro-environment, or any of the intermediate stages between stem cell and the mature end cell.

Bone marrow failure

Peripheral blood cytopenia arising primarily as a result of a specific failure of bone marrow precursor cells, rather than the production of abnormal cells or the production of normal cells that are subjected to an abnormal environment, is termed bone marrow failure. The remaining cells within the bone marrow appear normal and the marrow stroma does not seem to be altered.

Bone marrow failure can take two forms: aplastic anaemia, in which the pluripotent stem cell is damaged

leading to pancytopenia, and single-cell cytopenias where the failure lies in one or other of the committed cell lines, the other cell lines being unaffected.

Aplastic anaemia

Aplastic anaemia is usually defined as peripheral blood pancytopenia associated with a hypocellular marrow. The remaining cells within the marrow and the marrow architecture are normal, and the finding of abnormal cells or excess fibrosis within the marrow excludes a diagnosis of aplastic anaemia (Gordon-Smith 1989; Adamson and Erslev 1990).

The presenting features are those of bone marrow failure, including anaemia, neutropenia, and thrombo-cytopenia; the onset of symptoms may be insidious. The reader is directed to haematological texts (Gordon-Smith and Lewis 1989; Adamson and Erslev 1990) for a review of diagnosis and treatment options.

Drug-induced aplastic anaemia can be divided into two forms: (a) inevitable, and (b) idiosyncratic. These two categories may be regarded as Type A and Type B reactions respectively (see Chapter 3).

Inevitable (dose-dependent, Type A) drug-induced aplastic anaemia

Many cytotoxic chemotherapeutic agents have a low therapeutic index and are toxic to normal dividing cells as well as malignant cells. As the haematopoietic system is constantly 'turning over' it is, therefore, not surprising

TABLE 22.1
*Cytotoxic agents that regularly induce
bone marrow aplasia*

Actinomycin D	Etoposide
Amsacrine	Fluorouracil
Azathioprine	Hydroxyurea
Busulphan	Lomustine (CCNU)
Carboplatin	Melphalan
Carmustine (BCNU)	Mercaptopurine
Chlorambucil	Methotrexate
Cisplatin	Mitomycin
Cyclophosphamide/ifosfamide	Mitozantrone
Cytarabine	Plicamycin (mithramycin)
(cytosine arabinoside)	Procarbazine
Doxorubicin (adriamycin)	Thioguanine
Epirubicin	Thiotepa

TABLE 22.2
Drugs strongly linked with aplastic anaemia

Antibacterials	Chloramphenicol
	Co-trimoxazole
	Sulphonamides
Anti-inflammatory agents	Benoxaprofen
	Gold
	Indomethacin
	Oxyphenbutazone
	Penicillamine
	Phenylbutazone
	Piroxicam
Antithyroid drugs	Carbimazole
	Thiouracils
Antimalarials	Amodiaquine
	Mepacrine
	Pyrimethamine
Anticonvulsants	Phenytoin
Antidepressants	Chlorpromazine
	Prothiaden

that temporary aplasia is frequently encountered with many forms of cytotoxic chemotherapy. Indeed, bone marrow aplasia is the dose-limiting toxicity of a large number of these agents (Table 22.1). This is largely predictable and, with careful attention to dosage, is usually reversible. Autologous bone marrow transplantation has been developed to avoid the aplasia induced by these agents in the therapy of haematological malignancy. This allows doses of drugs to be increased when marrow toxicity would otherwise have limited them. Occasionally, repeated or prolonged courses of therapy, particularly with alkylating agents (e.g. busulphan), can produce prolonged and unpredictable aplasia. Aplasia can also develop as part of the evolution of many haematological disorders, thus complicating the relevance of a particular therapeutic agent in this context.

Idiosyncratic (dose-independent, Type B) aplastic anaemia

The association between aplastic anaemia and drug therapy has long been recognized. The relative rarity of aplastic anaemia and the absence of appropriate tests mean that a causal association between aplastic anaemia and drug therapy is not easy to prove. Investigation of the aetiology of aplastic anaemia is complicated by the observation that there can be a delay of 1–6 months between exposure to the supposed causative drug or agent and the development of the anaemia. This situation is further complicated, as the slow onset of symptoms often leads to symptomatic treatment that may further complicate retrospective analysis of the drug history. The literature is littered with case reports of aplastic anaemia developing in patients taking any one of a number of drugs, but clearly this does not prove cause and effect and only careful case–control studies will yield valuable data.

There are only a few therapeutic compounds for which the link between a drug and aplastic anaemia is strong (Table 22.2). The idiosyncratic induction of aplastic anaemia by these compounds has made it difficult to study mechanisms, and it is still not known if these drugs are toxic to the pluripotential stem cell population, either directly or via the immune system, or whether their toxicity is exerted via another mechanism such as the induction of damage to the bone marrow stroma.

Chloramphenicol

Chloramphenicol, an early antibiotic which is still widely used, particularly in the third world, was one of the first agents to be associated with the development of aplastic anaemia.

Its antimicrobial action depends upon the binding to the rRNA of bacterial ribosomes and the inhibition of bacterial protein synthesis. It does not inhibit eukaryotic ribosomes, although it may bind to the ribosomal RNA found within mitochondria. This may prove to be the basis for chloramphenicol-induced aplasia, but clearly another factor, possibly genetic, must be involved.

Aplasia can be dose-related with serum levels $>25\ \mu$g per ml (Yunis 1973), and with extended therapy (Oski 1979). Inhibition of mitochondrial ferrochelatase results in diminished iron uptake by erythroid precursors causing anaemia. Thrombocytopenia and agranulocytosis may follow, but are reversible within 2–3 weeks of stopping the drug (Oski 1979).

The idiosyncratic aplasia is irreversible and often fatal, but very rare, occurring in only one case per 25–$40\mu 10^3$

courses of treatment (Wallerstein *et al.* 1969). Often slight delay in presentation occurs, and prognosis is poor in those developing aplasia up to 2 months after stopping the drug (Polak *et al.* 1972). There is a suspicion that the risk of aplasia is greater with the oral use of the drug, but this is uncertain (Ristuccia 1985). Cases have been ascribed to ocular use of chloramphenicol (Carpenter 1975; Stevens and Mission 1987). Liver dysfunction and aplasia have also been linked (Casale *et al.* 1982). Monitoring blood levels will not predict the risk of aplasia and must be put into perspective, as the risk is less than that from anaphylaxis due to penicillin (Rudolph and Price 1973). Chloramphenicol is a very cheap and useful drug and the presently accepted uses have been reviewed by Smyth and Pallet (1988).

Non-steroidal anti-inflammatory drugs

Non-steroidal anti-inflammatory agents (NSAID) have been associated with the development of agranulocytosis and aplastic anaemia. Phenylbutazone and oxyphenbutazone, both pyrazole derivatives, either had their indications restricted or, in some countries, were withdrawn from the market because of their association with the development of aplastic anaemia or agranulocytosis (Inman 1977). Other NSAID associated with aplastic anaemia or agranulocytosis include benoxaprofen, indomethacin, piroxicam, and sulindac. A number of other NSAID, including aspirin, have been linked with aplastic anaemia, but purely anecdotally.

Gold and penicillamine

Gold and penicillamine, both second-line agents in the treatment of patients with rheumatoid arthritis, have been linked with the development of aplastic anaemia. Again the exact mechanisms are not understood. Both gold and penicillamine therapy usually induce thrombocytopenia and/or neutropenia before aplastic anaemia, so regular blood count monitoring is valuable in patients taking these second-line agents. Cessation of therapy is advised if a patient's platelet or white cell count falls. Gold may be removed from the body in patients with gold-induced aplastic anaemia using the agent dimercaprol, although there is no evidence that this therapy will hasten recovery. Confirmatory reports on aplasia and gold therapy (Williams *et al.* 1987) continue to appear.

Other drugs

Further reports of antithyroid drugs in this context have been published (Retsagi *et al.* 1988). Additional agents implicated in the development of pancytopenia include zidovudine (Mir and Costello 1988), which is used in the treatment of HIV-positive patients, and this effect may

TABLE 22.3
Drugs reported to induce pure red blood cell aplasia

Azathioprine	Old *et al.* 1978
Carbamazepine	Medberry *et al.* 1987
Chloramphenicol	Alter *et al.* 1978
Chlorpropamide	Planas *et al.* 1980; Gill *et al.* 1980
Co-trimoxazole	Ammus and Yunis 1987
Dapsone—*see* Maloprim	
Fenoprofen	Ammus and Yunis 1987
Gold (sodium aurothiomalate)	Reid and Patterson 1977
Halothane	Ammus and Yunis 1987
Isoniazid	Ammus and Yunis 1987
Maloprim (dapsone/pyrimethamine)	Ammus and Yunis 1987
Penicillin	Ammus and Yunis 1987
Pentachlorophenol	Ammus and Yunis 1987
Phenobarbitone	Ammus and Yunis 1987
Phenylbutazone	Alter *et al.* 1978
Phenytoin	Alter *et al.* 1978
Pyrimethamine—*see* Maloprim	Ammus and Yunis 1987
Sulphasalazine	Ammus and Yunis 1987
Sulphathiazide	Ammus and Yunis 1987
Sulphonamides	Alter *et al.* 1978
Sulphonylureas	Alter *et al.* 1978
Thiamphenicol	Ammus and Yunis 1987
Tolbutamide	Ammus and Yunis 1987

be potentiated by the addition of gancyclovir (Jacobson *et al.* 1988). Additional anecdotal cases have involved lorazepam (El Sayed and Symonds 1988), and methazolamide, a carbonic anhydrase inhibitor (Mogk and Cyrlin 1988).

Red cell aplasia

Pure red cell aplasia (PRCA) is a haematological disorder characterized by anaemia, reticulocytopenia, and erythroid hypoplasia or aplasia. The marrow is usually cellular and the myeloid and megakaryocytic lines are normal. PRCA has been reported in association with a number of drugs (see Table 22.3). In most cases the mechanism of drug-induced PRCA is unknown. Phenytoin-induced PRCA is possibly mediated via a humoral immune mechanism, but in most cases no antibody or cytotoxic factor has been discovered in the serum. There is no specific indication that the drugs act by modifying erythropoietin release or activity.

TABLE 22.4
Drugs reported to induce agranulocytosis

Acetazolamide	Meprobamate
Allopurinol	Methimazole
Amitriptyline	Methyldopa
Amodiaquine	Oxyphenbutazone
Benzodiazepines	Paracetamol
Captopril	Penicillamine
Carbamazepine	Penicillins and
Carbimazole	semi-synthetic
Cephalosporins	penicillins
Chloramphenicol	Pentazocine
Chloroquine	Phenacetin
Chlorothiazide	Phenothiazines
Chlorpromazine	Phenylbutazone
Chlorpropamide	Phenytoin
Chlorthalidone	Procainamide
Cimetidine	Propranolol
Co-trimoxazole	Propylthiouracil
Clindamycin	Pyrimethamine
Dapsone	Quinidine
Desipramine	Quinine
Disopyramide	Ranitidine
Ethacrynic acid	Rifampicin
Fansidar	Sodium aminosalicylate
(pyrimethamine/sulfadoxine)	(*p*-aminosalicylic acid)
Gentamicin	Streptomycin
Gold	Sulphadoxine
Hydralazine	Sulphonamides
Hydrochlorothiazide	Tetracyclines
Imipramine	Tocainide
Indomethacin	Tolbutamide
Isoniazid	Vancomycin
Levamisole	

The acquired variety of this disorder is usually immunogenic and may be associated with a tumour of the thymus (Krantz 1976). This form of the disorder is rare but can be treated effectively by removal of the thymus. Transitory erythroblastopenia of childhood, which may mimic red cell aplasia, is now causally associated with parvovirus infection (Kurtzman *et al.* 1987).

Little has been added to the literature on red cell aplasia and drug involvement in the last few years, though a report from Itoh and others (1988) suggests that methyldopa might cause red cell aplasia by suppression of erythroid colony-forming units.

Drug-induced granulocytopenia

Agranulocytosis or neutropenia, although rare, can be severe and even life-threatening. Adverse drug reactions are thought to be a common cause of neutropenia, although study of drug-induced neutropenia is difficult because it is not predictable, numerous agents have been implicated (Table 22.4), and there is not an ideal animal

model for study. Clearly there are a number of drugs, particularly cytotoxic agents, that produce predictable and usually reversible bone marrow aplasia which can particularly affect the granulocyte count, and these agents have been discussed earlier in the section on aplastic anaemia.

Idiosyncratic drug-induced agranulocytoses usually fall into two main categories. First, allergic or immune-mediated destruction of both immature myeloid precursors and mature granulocytes. This type of reaction is more common in the older female patient and it generally occurs early in a course of treatment to which the patient has previously been exposed. The second type of reaction usually involves dose-related toxicity from the effects of the drug on protein synthesis or cell replication. This interaction is often non-selective, and other haematopoietic and non-haematopoietic tissues may be involved. Antithyroid drugs and phenothiazines are particular examples of drugs that act in this way.

Platelet–drug interactions

Thrombocytopenia due to reduced platelet production

Platelets are derived from megakaryocytes, which are predominantly non-proliferative cells. Study of megakaryocytes is complicated by the fact that the precursors are capable of cell division and endomitosis (nuclear reduplication so that diploid and polydiploid forms exist). In spite of the problems, clonogenic assays of megakaryocyte progenitors do exist (Nakeff and Bryan 1978). Unfortunately, the exact mechanisms of drug actions on the megakaryocyte progenitors remain unknown. This phenomenon is rare, though alcohol (Levine *et al.* 1986), α-interferon (Talpaz *et al.* 1987), oestrogens (Cooper and Bigelow 1960), and thiazide diuretics (Bottiger and Westerholm 1972) have all been implicated.

Drug-induced autoimmune thrombocytopenia

Large numbers of compounds (Table 22.5) have been reported to induce autoimmune thrombocytopenia, although only a few have been consistently linked with this disorder. These include gold (Walker *et al.* 1986), heparin (Warkentin *et al.* 1990), methyldopa (Manohitharajah *et al.* 1971) quinidine and quinine (Shulman 1972), rifampicin (Blajchman *et al.* 1970), and sulphonamides (Hamilton and Sheets 1978).

Heparin is of particular interest in that it commonly produces a mild thrombocytopenia, possibly by inducing platelet aggregation, and it can also, rarely, induce

TABLE 22.5
*Drugs reported to induce autoimmune
thrombocytopenia*

Acetazolamide	Bertino *et al.* 1957
Actinomycin	Hodder *et al.* 1985
Allopurinol	Rosenbloom and Gilbert 1981
Alpha-interferon	Abdi *et al.* 1986
Amiodarone	Weinberger *et al.* 1987
Ampicillin	Brooks 1974
Aspirin	Garg and Sarker 1974
Carbamazepine	Ponte 1983
Carbenicillin	Conti *et al.* 1984
Cephalosporins	Lown and Barr 1987
Chenodeoxycholic acid	Conti *et al.* 1984
Chloroquine	Nieweg *et al.* 1963
Chlorothiazide	Bottiger and Westerholm 1972
Chlorpheniramine	Eisner *et al.* 1975
Chlorpropamide	Bottiger and Westerholm 1972
Chlorthalidone	Bottiger and Westerholm 1972
Cimetidine	Glotzback 1982
Co-trimoxazole	Claas *et al.* 1979
Cyclophosphamide	Mueller-Eckhardt *et al.* 1983
Danazol	Arrowsmith and Dreis 1986
Desferrioxamine	Walker *et al.* 1985
Diazepam	Conti and Gandolfo 1983
Diazoxide	Wales and Wolff 1967
Diclofenac	Kramer *et al.* 1986
Digoxin	Pirovino *et al.* 1981
Diltiazem	Baggott 1987
Frusemide	Bottiger and Westerholm 1972
Gentamicin	Chen *et al.* 1980
Glymidine	Von dem Borne *et al.* 1986
Gold	Bottiger and Westerholm 1972
Hydrochlorothiazide	Okafor *et al.* 1986
Imipramine	Karpatkin *et al.* 1977
Isoniazid	Zorab 1960
Levamisole	El-Ghobari and Capella 1977
Meprobamate	Karpatkin *et al.* 1977
Methyldopa	Pai and Pai 1988
Mianserin	Stricker *et al.* 1985
Minoxidil	Peitzman and Martin 1980
Morphine	Cimo *et al.* 1982
Nitrofurantoin	Bottiger and Westerholm 1972
Oxprenolol	Hare and Hicks 1979
Oxyphenbutazone	Handley 1971
Penicillamine	Harrison and Hickman 1975
Penicillin	Conti *et al.* 1984
Phenylbutazone	Tolot *et al.* 1976
Phenytoin	Cimo *et al.* 1977
Piroxicam	Meisner *et al.* 1985
Procainamide	Giordano *et al.* 1987
Quinidine	Christie *et al.* 1985
Quinine	Christie *et al.* 1985
Ranitidine	Gafter *et al.* 1987
Rifampicin	Pau and Fisher 1987
Sodium aminosalicylate (*p*-aminosalicylic acid)	Eisner and Kasper 1972
Sodium valproate	Barr *et al.* 1982
Sulphasalazine	Pena *et al.* 1985
Sulphonamides	Hamilton and Sheets 1978
Thioguanine	Karpatkin *et al.* 1977

Table 22.5 continued

Valproate—*see* Sodium valproate	
Vancomycin	Walker and Heaton 1985
Vitamin A (isotretinoin)	Johnson and Rapini 1987

a severe thrombocytopenia that is immunologically mediated. Heparin-associated immune thrombocytopenia usually begins within 3 to 15 days of commencing therapy although it may occur more rapidly if the patient has been previously exposed to heparin. The incidence appears to be higher in patients treated with bovine heparin and seems to be dose-related. Heparin-induced thrombocytopenia is strongly associated with thrombosis, particularly arterial thrombosis, and has a high mortality (see also Chapter 7). Paradoxically, bleeding problems are rare despite anticoagulation and thrombocytopenia. Clearly, a rapid switch to oral anticoagulation will avoid this complication, but if heparin is to be continued for some time then the platelet count should be regularly monitored and if it falls significantly an alternative antithrombotic therapy should be used (Warkentin *et al.* 1990).

In any patient with acute thrombocytopenia of unknown aetiology, all medications should be stopped or, if this is not possible, the drugs should be changed. Usually the platelet count rises within 7 days, although it is occasionally delayed, and the patient should be managed in the standard way. Once a patient has demonstrated drug sensitivity in this way then the drug should be carefully avoided in the future.

Red cell–drug interactions

Immune-mediated red cell destruction

Drug-induced haemolytic anaemia has been recognized for some time; it is usually a relatively benign process although severe and even fatal cases may occur. It must be distinguished from spontaneous forms of autoimmune haemolytic anaemia and other types of drug-induced non-immune red cell destruction, which usually occur upon exposure of inherently defective red cells to a drug or its metabolites. The incidence of immune haemolytic anaemia appears to be increasing, possibly due to the introduction of numerous new drugs and escalation in numbers of drug prescriptions.

There are four major mechanisms of drug-induced immune haemolysis, although it is not always easy in individual cases to be certain that the haemolysis is drug-induced or sure of the mechanisms involved.

Hapten-induced haemolysis

Most drugs are substances of low molecular weight that are unable to stimulate an immune response on their own. In hapten-induced immune haemolysis the drug binds to the red cell membrane and the drug–red cell complex stimulates an immune response. Penicillin (White *et al.* 1968), cephalosporin (Gralnick *et al.* 1971), and tetracycline (Wenz *et al.* 1974) can induce this type of immune response when given in high doses for long periods. Usually an IgG antibody is responsible for this type of haemolysis, which will be detected in a direct antiglobulin test. If the antibody is eluted from the patient's red blood cells then it will not react with other red cells unless they have been preincubated with the drug or are drug-coated. Interestingly, while a number of patients on high doses of penicillin develop a positive direct antiglobulin reaction very few develop haemolytic anaemia.

Cephalosporins and semi-synthetic penicillins also cross-react with penicillin and can bind to the red cell membrane and in some instances induce immune haemolytic anaemia.

Tetracycline and tolbutamide may also bind to red cell membranes and thus act as haptens for an immune response.

Drug-induced autoantibody production

Certain drugs, particularly methyldopa, levodopa, and mefenamic acid (Breckenridge *et al.* 1967; Scott *et al.* 1968; Bernstein 1979; Beutler 1985), are capable of inducing autoantibodies against red blood cells. In this situation the drug does not act as a hapten but may act to suppress the normal controls on the immune system, allowing the expression of autoantibodies against normally occurring red cell antigens. Alternatively, the drug may alter the red cell membrane so that one or more of the membrane proteins appear foreign, hence inducing an autoantibody against the red cell. Usually this type of haemolysis is slow in onset and generally mild, and the IgG-coated red cells are sequestered in the spleen. The IgG will be detectable on both the red cell and also in the serum, and will react with a number of different red cells without preincubation with the offending drug. A number of patients receiving methyldopa will develop a positive direct antiglobulin test, but few will develop clinically significant haemolysis.

Immune complex mechanisms

In this type of reaction there is formation of a complex between the drug, an immunoglobulin, and a drug-membrane binding site. Usually, red blood cell destruction is intravascular following completion of the complement cascade, although there may be some destruction in the liver and spleen. This type of haemolysis can be fairly brisk. The direct antiglobulin reaction is usually only positive to components of the complement cascade. Drugs implicated are shown in Table 22.6.

TABLE 22.6
Drugs reported to induce haemolysis following formation of an immune complex

Antimony (Stibophen)	Harris 1956
Chlorpropamide	Logue *et al.* 1970
Methotrexate	Woolley *et al.* 1983
Quinidine	Croft *et al.* 1968
Quinine	Muirhead *et al.* 1958
Rifampicin	Lakshminarayan *et al.* 1973

Non-immunological protein absorption

Cephalosporin antibiotics can induce the non-specific absorption of plasma proteins to the red blood cell membrane, which may produce a positive direct antiglobulin reaction; but haemolysis has not been seen. This type of interaction may, however, interfere with blood cross-matching in patients receiving cephalosporin therapy.

Non-immune red cell damage

Oxidation damage to red cells

As oxygen is transferred from the haemoglobin molecule during oxygen transfer in the tissues, highly reactive oxygen species such as the superoxide anion can be generated (Carrell *et al.* 1975), which are capable of denaturing haemoglobin and inactivating vital red blood cell enzymes. The red cell has a number of antioxidant defence mechanisms, which include catalase and reduced glutathione working through the enzymes glutathione peroxidase and glutathione transferase. The most important red cell enzyme that protects against oxidant stress is glucose-6-phosphate dehydrogenase (G6PD) (Beutler 1978).

Drugs that act as oxidants *in vivo* or which increase the generation of activated oxygen species may produce high levels of oxidative stress in the red cell. Red cells that have a lowered reducing capacity due to enzyme deficiency, such as G6PD deficiency, cannot operate effective reduction pathways to prevent haemolysis.

Extensive lists of drugs that can be given safely to G6PD-deficient individuals are available and readers are

Table 22.7

Drugs that have been clearly shown to cause clinically significant haemolytic anaemia in G6PD deficiency

Acetanilide	Phenylhydrazine
Methylene blue	Primaquine
Nalidixic acid	Sulphacetamide
Naphthalene	Sulphamethoxazole
Niridazole	Sulphanilamide
Nitrofurantoin	Sulphapyridine
Pamaquine	Thiazolesulphone
Phenazopyridine	Toluidine blue

referred to the excellent text produced by Beutler (1978) for details.

In Table 22.7 are listed the drugs that have clearly been associated with significant haemolysis in G6PD-deficient patients (Beutler 1985). Interestingly, deficiency of the enzymes glutathione reductase and glutathione peroxidase is not associated with haemolytic anaemia (Beutler 1985). Ballin and colleagues (1988) reported a case of oxidative haemolysis in an infant caused by ascorbic acid.

Haemolysis due to non-oxidative drugs

A large number of chemicals have been associated with non-immune, non-oxidative red cell destruction (Table 22.8). Beutler (1985) has discussed the varying mechanisms. Lead, for example, shortens the life-span of red cells probably by inhibiting the enzyme pyrimidine 5′-nucleotidase producing basophilic stippling of red cells. Lead also inhibits several enzymes involved in the synthesis of haem. Copper can cause haemolysis, which can be seen in Wilson's syndrome, but the mechanism is unclear. Among commonly used drugs, cisplatin (Getaz *et al.* 1980; Levi *et al.* 1981) and penicillamine (Harrison and Hickman 1976) are most frequently associated with non-oxidative red cell destruction. The exact mechanisms of destruction are not known.

Table 22.8

Agents that may cause haemolysis by non-oxidative mechanism

Aniline	Nitrobenzene
Arsine	*p*-Aminosalicylic
Chlorate	acid
Cisplatin	Penicillamine
Copper	Phenazopyridine
Formaldehyde	Resorcin
Lead	Sulphasalazine
Mephenesin	Zinc ethylene *bis*
	(dithiocarbamate)

Drug-induced megaloblastic anaemia

Megaloblastic anaemia is a disorder with characteristic abnormalities of the blood and bone marrow induced by impaired DNA synthesis. RNA and protein synthesis continue normally giving rise to the well-recognized morphological changes of megaloblastic anaemia.

Drugs can impair DNA synthesis in a number of ways (listed in Table 22.9) and will eventually produce a

Table 22.9

Drugs that may induce megaloblastic anaemia

Drugs that interfere with vitamin B$_{12}$ metabolism
Alcohol
Colchicine
Metformin
Neomycin
Nitrous oxide
Phenformin
Sodium aminosalicylate (*p*-aminosalicylic acid)
Vitamin C (in large doses)

Drugs that interfere with folate metabolism
(a) Dihydrofolate reductase inhibitors
Aminopterin
Methotrexate
Pentamidine
Proguanil
Pyrimethamine
Triamterene
Trimethoprim

(b) Impaired folate absorption/utilization
Alcohol
Cycloserine
Metformin
Nitrofurantoin
Oral contraceptive agents
Phenobarbitone
Phenytoin
Primidone
Sulphasalazine

Drugs that interfere with DNA synthesis directly
Acyclovir
Azathioprine
Cytarabine
Floxuridine
Fluorouracil
Hydroxyurea
Mercaptopurine
Thioguanine
Zidovudine

Mechanism unknown
Benzene
Tetracycline
Vinblastine
Vitamin A

megaloblastic anaemia (Ammus and Yunis 1989; Scott and Weir 1980; Stibbins and Bertino 1976).

Zidovudine (AZT), a thymidine analogue, inhibits the retroviral enzyme reverse transcriptase and has been shown to be a potent inhibitor of the HIV virus. It is, however, a toxic drug inducing macrocytosis in most patients, and in some cases produces a severe megaloblastic anaemia often associated with neutropenia. B_{12} and folate levels are usually normal (Mir and Costello 1988; Youle and Gazzard 1990). These adverse effects can limit or even preclude the drug's use. In a double-blind, randomized, placebo-controlled trial, a 25 per cent or greater fall in haemoglobin was observed in 40 per cent of patients given AZT.

The correct approach to patients who develop severe red cell aplasia on AZT is not known although these patients seem to have a poor prognosis.

Drug-induced sideroblastic anaemia

Sideroblastic anaemia results from disordered haem synthesis and is associated with the accumulation of iron in mitochondria, forming typical ring sideroblasts. Usually the red blood cells are hypochromic, although a dimorphic picture is commonly seen. The reticulocyte count is low or normal and bone marrow aspiration usually reveals erythroid hyperplasia with numerous basophilic normoblasts and plentiful ring sideroblasts. These changes have been described in association with a number of drugs (see Table 22.10). The anaemia may be quite severe, necessitating transfusion. Removal of the drug in question and/or pyridoxine therapy usually results in reversal of the changes and resolution of the associated anaemia.

TABLE 22.10
Drugs that may induce sideroblastic anaemia

Alcohol	Hines 1960
Chloramphenicol	Beck *et al.* 1967
Cycloserine	Haden 1967, Tomlin 1973
Isoniazid	Verwilghen *et al.* 1965
Penicillamine	Ramselaar *et al.* 1987
Phenacetin	Popovic *et al.* 1973
Pyrazinamide	McCurdy *et al.* 1966

Antituberculous drugs, including isoniazid and pyrazinamide, are associated with the development of sideroblastic anaemia. Isoniazid probably interferes with the synthesis of δ-aminolaevulinic acid, an important precursor in haem synthesis. Pyrazinamide may interfere with vitamin B_6 metabolism.

Chloramphenicol also interferes with haem synthesis, producing anaemia which is distinct from the rarer aplastic anaemia.

Methaemoglobinaemia

The iron of haem in red cells normally stays in the divalent form. The loss of an additional electron can create a trivalent form of iron known as methaemoglobin. Normally the cell copes with this stress through the NADH reducing system via the enzyme NADH diaphorase. Certain drugs and chemicals have the capacity to increase greatly the rate at which this occurs, and it is a more common occurrence in children than in adults. Details of the agents involved are discussed by Beutler (1985). Recent additions to the list of agents that cause methaemoglobinaemia are metoclopramide (Kearns and Fisher 1988) and prilocaine, a local anaesthetic (Menahem 1988). Both reactions were seen in children. The observation has been confirmed recently when prilocaine–lignocaine cream used as local skin anaesthetic in children aged 1–6 years caused an increase in levels of methaemoglobin (Frayling *et al.* 1990). This caused no clinical symptoms, but users are warned against frequent use in paediatric patients.

Drug-induced haematological tumours

Drug-induced myelodysplasia and leukaemia

Cytotoxic drugs

A number of studies have demonstrated that long-term survivors of certain malignancies, such as Hodgkin's disease (Tucker *et al.* 1988), ovarian carcinoma (Einhorn *et al.* 1982), and childhood malignancies (Tucker *et al.* 1987) treated with cytotoxic chemotherapy and radiotherapy are at risk of developing myelodysplasia and acute non-lymphocytic leukaemia. Alkylating agents, in particular, have been implicated in most studies as being leukaemogenic. The additional toxicity of radiotherapy when used in conjunction with chemotherapy is disputed, and the incidence varies in different series. In the United Kingdom, for example, secondary leukaemia after therapy for Hodgkin's disease therapy occurs in less than one per cent of cases (Proctor and Evans 1985), whereas in series from North America the incidence has been as high as 7 per cent. Carcinogenic mechanisms of cytotoxic chemotherapy have been difficult to study. Direct DNA damage or prolonged immunosuppression have been suggested as possible mechanisms. The risk of secondary leukaemia remains small and clearly should not restrict the use of chemotherapy essential for cure or prolonged survival in those with otherwise incurable disease. As improvements in treatment regimens continue, however, and cure rates increase, careful consideration of the long-term adverse effects of cytotoxic chemotherapy will be important (see also Chapter 24).

Growth hormone therapy

Reports have been published suggesting that there is possibly an increased incidence of leukaemia in children who are receiving treatment with recombinant growth hormone (Watanabe *et al.* 1988; Delemarre-van de Waal *et al.* 1988). Watanabe and others (1988), reviewing the incidence in Japan, found a fivefold increase. Fisher and colleagues (1988), reviewing the use of growth hormone replacement therapy, indicated that the association is restricted to Japanese data and the overall incidence in Europe and North America is 11 cases in 22 000 patients, representing a twofold increase. Fisher (1988) suggests that the risk is very small and insufficient to indicate the withholding of growth hormone treatment. It is also pertinent to suggest that certain disorders, such as Fanconi's anaemia, may present with the problem of small stature, and subsequent leukaemia in such cases would in no way be related to growth factor therapy but be part of the progression of the underlying syndrome.

Drug-induced non-Hodgkin's lymphoma (NHL) and solid tumours

Cytotoxic drugs

Following the successful therapy of Hodgkin's disease the problems of secondary non-Hodgkin's lymphoma or other solid tumours have emerged. The cumulative risk of developing a secondary NHL at 10 years is approximately 1.8 per cent and of secondary cancer 8.8 per cent (Cosset *et al.* 1990). Alkylating agents used in primary chemotherapy are regarded as being involved in this process (see also Chapter 24).

References

Abdi, E.A., Brien, W., and Venner, P.M. (1986). Autoimmune thrombocytopenia related to interferon therapy. *Scand. J. Haematol.* 36, 515.

Adamson, J.W. and Erslev, A.J. (1990). Aplastic anaemia. In *Hematology* (4th edn.) (ed. W.J. Williams, E. Beutler, A.J. Erslev and M.A. Lichtman), p. 158. McGraw-Hill, New York.

Alter, B.P., Potter, N.U., and Li, F.P. (1978). Classification and aetiology of the aplastic anaemias. *Clin. Haematol.* 7, 431.

Ammus, S.S. and Yunis, A.A. (1987). Acquired pure red cell aplasia. *Am. J. Haematol.* 24, 311.

Ammus, S.S. and Yunis, A.A. (1989). Drug-induced red cell dyscrasias. *Blood Reviews* 3, 71.

Arrowsmith, J.B. and Dreis, M. (1986). Thrombocytopenia after treatment with danazol. *N. Engl. J. Med.* 315, 585.

Baggott, L.A. (1987). Diltiazem-associated immune thrombocytopenia. *Mt Sinai J. Med.* 54, 500.

Balkwill, F.R. (1989). The colony-stimulating factors. In *Cytokines in cancer therapy* (ed. F.R. Balkwill), p. 114. Oxford University Press.

Ballin, A., Brown, E.J., Koren, G., and Zipursky, A. (1988). Vitamin C-induced erythrocyte damage in premature infants. *J. Pediatr.* 113, 114.

Barr, R.D., Copeland, S.A., Stockwell, M.L., Morris, N., and Kelton, J.C. (1982). Valproic acid and immune thrombocytopenia. *Arch. Dis. Child.* 57, 681.

Beck, E.A., Ziegler, G., Schmid, R., and Lüdin, H. (1967). Reversible sideroblastic anaemia caused by chloramphenicol. *Acta Haematol.* (Basel) 38, 1.

Bernstein, R.M. (1979). Reversible haemolytic anaemia after levodopa–carbidopa. *Br. Med. J.* i, 1461.

Bertino, J.E., Rodman, T., and Myerson, R.M. (1957). Thrombocytopenia and renal lesions associated with acetazolamide (Diamox) therapy. *Arch. Intern. Med.* 99, 1006.

Beutler, E. (1978). *Hemolytic anaemia in disorders of red cell metabolism.* Plenum Press, New York.

Beutler, E. (1985). Chemical toxicity of the erythrocyte. In *Toxicology of the blood and bone marrow* (ed. R.D. Irons), p. 39. Raven Press, New York.

Blajchman, M.A., Lowry, R.C., Pettit, J.E., and Stradling, P. (1970). Rifampicin-induced immune thrombocytopenia. *Br. Med. J.* iii, 24.

Bottiger, L.E. and Westerholm, B. (1972). Drug-induced thrombocytopenia. *Acta Med. Scand.* 191, 541.

Breckenridge, A., Dollery, C.T., Worlledge, S.M., Holborrow, E.J., and Johnson, G.D. (1967). Positive direct Coombs tests and antinuclear factor in patients treated with methyldopa. *Lancet* ii, 1265.

Brooks, A.P. (1974). Thrombocytopenia during treatment with ampicillin. *Lancet* ii, 723.

Carpenter, G. (1975). Chloramphenicol eye drops and marrow aplasia. *Lancet* ii, 326.

Carrell, R.W., Winterbourn, C.C., and Rachmilewitz, E.A. (1975). Activated oxygen and haemolysis. *Br. J. Haematol.* 30, 259.

Casale, T.B., Macher, A.M., and Fauci, A.S. (1982). Complete haematologic and hepatic recovery in a patient with chloramphenicol hepatitis–pancytopenia syndrome. *J. Pediatr.* 101, 1025.

Chen, J-H., Wiener, L., and Distenfeld, A. (1980). Immunologic thrombocytopenia induced by gentamicin. *N.Y. State J. Med.* 80, 1134.

Christie, D.J., Mullen, P.C., and Aster, R.H. (1985). Fab-mediated binding of drug-dependent antibodies to platelets in quinidine- and quinine-induced thrombocytopenia. *J. Clin. Invest.* 75, 310.

Cimo, P.L., Pisciotta, A.V., Desai, R.G., Pino G.L., and Aster, R.H. (1977). Detection of drug-dependent antibodies by the ⁵¹Cr platelet lysis test: documentation of immune thrombocytopenia induced by diphenylhydantoin, diazepam, and sulfisoxazole. *Am. J. Haematol.* 2, 65.

Cimo, P.L., Hammond, J.J., and Moake, J.L. (1982). Morphine-induced immune thrombocytopenia. *Arch. Intern. Med.* 142, 832.

Claas, F.H., van der Meer, J.W.M., and Langerak, J. (1979). Immunological effect of co-trimoxazole on platelets. *Br. Med. J.* ii, 898.

Conti, L. and Gandolfo, G.M. (1983). Benzodiazepine-induced thrombocytopenia. Demonstration of drug-dependent platelet antibodies in two cases. *Acta Haematol.* 70, 386.

Conti, L., Fidani, P., Christolini, A., Francesconi, M., Gandolfo, G.M., and Mazzucconi, M.G. (1984). Detection of drug-dependent IgG antibodies with anti-platelet activity by the antiglobulin consumption assay. *Haemostasis* 14, 480.

Cooper, B.A. and Bigelow, F.S. (1960). Thrombocytopenia associated with the administration of diethylstilbestrol in man. *Ann. Intern. Med.* 52, 907.

Cosset, J.M., Henry-Amar, M., and Meerwaldt, J.H. (1990). Long term toxicity of Hodgkin's disease treatment. *4th International Conference on Malignant Lymphoma, Lugano* 12, (Abstract).

Croft, J.D., Swisher, S.N. Jr, Gilliland, B.C., Bakemeier, R.F., Leddy, J.P., and Weed, R.I. (1968). Coombs test positivity induced by drugs: mechanisms of immunologic reactions and red cell destruction. *Ann. Intern. Med.* 68, 176.

Delemarre-Van De Waal, H.A., Odink, R.J.H., De Grauw, T.J., and De Waal, F.C. (1988). Leukaemia in patients treated with growth hormone. *Lancet* i, 1159.

Dexter, T.M. (1987). Stem cells in normal growth and disease. *Br. Med. J.* 295, 1192.

Einhorn, N., Eklund, G., Frazen, S., Lambert, B., Lindsten, J., and Soderhall, S. (1982). Late side effects of chemotherapy in ovarian carcinoma: a cytogenetic, hematologic and statistical study. *Cancer* 49, 2234.

Eisner, E.V. and Kasper, K. (1972). Immune thrombocytopenia due to a metabolite of para-aminosalicylic acid. *Am. J. Med.* 53, 790.

Eisner, E.V., LaBocki, N.L., and Pinkney, L. (1975). Chlorpheniramine dependent thrombocytopenia. *JAMA* 231, 735.

El Sayed, S. and Symonds, R.P. (1988). Lorazepam induced pancytopenia. *Br. Med. J.* 296, 1332.

El Ghobari, A.F. and Capella, H.A. (1977). Levamisole-induced thrombocytopenia. *Br. Med. J.* ii, 555.

Fisher, D.A., Job, J.C., Preece, M., and Underwood, L.E. (1988). Leukaemia in patients treated with growth hormone. *Lancet* i, 1159.

Frayling, I.M., Addison, G.M., Chattergee, K., and Meakin, G. (1990). Methaemoglobinaemia in children treated with prilocaine–lignocaine cream. *Br. Med. J.* 301, 153.

Gafter, U., Komlos, L., Weinstein, T., Zevin, D., and Levi, J. (1987). Thrombocytopenia, eosinophilia, and ranitidine. *Ann. Intern. Med.* 106, 477.

Garg, S.K. and Sarker, C.R. (1974). Aspirin-induced thrombocytopenia on an immune basis. *Am. J. Med. Sci.* 267, 129.

Getaz, E.P., Beckley, S., Fitzpatrick, J., and Dozier, A. (1980). Cisplatin-induced hemolysis. *N. Engl. J. Med.* 302, 334.

Gill, M.J., Ratliff, D.A., and Harding, L.K. (1980). Hypoglycaemic coma, jaundice and pure red blood cell aplasia following chlorpropamide therapy. *Arch. Intern. Med.* 140, 714.

Giordano, N., Sancasciani, S., Cantore, M., Fioravanti, A., Gandolfo, G., Conti, L., *et al.* (1987). Thrombocytopenic purpura associated with piroxicam. *Clin. Exp. Rheumatol.* 5, 298.

Glotzback, R.E. (1982). Cimetidine-induced thrombocytopenia. *South. Med. J.* 75, 232.

Gordon-Smith, E.C. (1989). Aplastic anaemia — aetiology and clinical features. In *Clinical haematology*, Vol. 2 (ed. E.C. Gordon-Smith), p. 1. Baillière, London.

Gordon-Smith, E.C. and Lewis, S.M. (1989). Aplastic anaemia and other types of bone marrow failure. In *Postgraduate haematology* (3rd edn) (ed. A.V. Hoffbrand and S.M. Lewis), p. 83. Heinemann, London.

Gralnick, H.R., McGinniss, M., Elton, W., and McCurdy, P. (1971). Hemolytic anemia associated with cephalothin. *JAMA* 217, 1193.

Haden, H.T. (1967). Pyridoxine-responsive sideroblastic anemia due to antituberculous drugs. *Arch. Intern. Med.* 20, 602.

Hamilton, H.E. and Sheets, R.F. (1978). Sulfisoxazole-induced thrombocytopenic purpura. *JAMA* 239, 2586.

Handley, A.J. (1971). Thrombocytopenia and LE cells after oxyphenbutazone. *Lancet* i, 245.

Hare, D.L. and Hicks, B.H. (1979). Thrombocytopenia due to oxprenolol. *Med. J. Aust.* ii, 259.

Harris, J.W. (1956). Studies on the mechanism of drug induced hemolytic anaemia. *J. Lab. Clin. Med.* 47, 760.

Harrison, E.E. and Hickman, J.W. (1975). Hemolytic anemia and thrombocytopenia associated with penicillamine ingestion. *South. Med. J.* 68, 113.

Harrison, E.E. and Hickman, J.W. (1976). D-pencillamine and haemolytic anaemia. *Lancet* i, 38.

Hines, J. (1960). Reversible megaloblastic and sideroblastic abnormalities in alcoholic patients. *Br. J. Haematol.* 16, 87.

Hodder, F.S., Kempert, P., McCormack, S., Bennets, G.A., Katz, J., and Cairo, M.S. (1985). Immune thrombocytopenia following actinomycin-D therapy. *J. Pediatr.* 107, 611.

Inman, W.H.W. (1977). Study of fatal bone marrow depression with special reference to phenylbutazone and oxyphenbutazone. *Br. Med. J.* i, 1500.

Itoh, K., Wong, P., Asai, T., Yoshida, S., and Fukuda, T. (1988). Pure red cell aplasia induced by α-methyldopa. *Am. J. Med.* 84, 1088.

Jacobson, M.A., Miranda, P.D., Gordon, S.M., Blum, R., Volberding, P., and Mills, J. (1988). Prolonged pancytopenia due to combined gancyclovir and zidovudine therapy. *J. Infect. Dis.* 158, 489.

Johnson, T.M. and Rapini, R.P. (1987). Isotretinoin-induced thrombocytopenia. *J. Am. Acad. Dermatol.* 17, 838.

Karpatkin, M., Siskind, G.W., and Karpatkin, S. (1977). The platelet factor 3 immuno injury technique re-evaluated: development of a rapid test for antiplatelet antibody: detection in various clinical disorders, including immunologic drug-induced and neonatal thrombocytopenias. *J. Lab. Clin. Med.* 82, 400.

Kearns, G.L. and Fisher, D.H. (1988). Metoclopramide induced methemoglobinaemia. *Pediatrics* 82, 364.

Kramer, M.R., Levene, C., and Hershko, C. (1986). Severe reversible autoimmune haemolytic anaemia and thrombocytopenia associated with diclofenac therapy. Case report. *Scand. J. Haematol.* 36, 118.

Krantz, S.B. (1976). Diagnosis and treatment of pure red cell aplasia. *Med. Clin. North Am.* 60, 945.

Kurtzman, G.J., Ozawa, K., Cohen, B., Hanson, G., Oseas, R., and Young, N.S. (1987). Chronic bone marrow failure due to persistent B19 parvovirus infection. *N. Engl. J. Med.* 317, 287.

Lakshminarayan, S., Sahn, S.A., and Hudson, L.D. (1973). Massive haemolysis caused by rifampicin. *Br. Med. J.* 282, 2003.

Levi, J.A., Aroney, R.S., and Dalley, D.N. (1981). Haemolytic anaemia after cisplatin treatment. *Br. Med. J.* 282, 2003.

Levine, R.F., Spivak, J.L., and Meagher, R.C. (1986). Effect of ethanol on thrombopoiesis. *Br. J. Haematol.* 62, 345.

Logue, G.L., Boyd, A.E., and Rosse, W.F. (1970). Chlorpropamide induced immune hemolytic anaemia. *N. Engl. J. Med.* 283, 900.

Lown, J.A. and Barr, A. (1987). Immune thrombocytopenia induced by cephalosporins specific for thiomethyltetrazole side chain. *J. Clin. Pathol.* 40, 700.

Manohitharajah, S.M., Jenkins, W.J., Roberts, P.D., and Clark, R.C. (1971). Methyldopa and associated thrombocytopenia. *Br. Med. J.* i, 494.

McCurdy, P.R., Donohoe, R.F., and Magovern, M. (1966). Reversible anemia caused by pyrazinoic acid (pyrazinamide). *Ann. Intern. Med.* 64, 1280.

Medberry, C.A., Pappas, A., and Ackerman, B.H. (1987). Carbamazepine and erythroid arrest. *Drug Intell. Clin. Pharm.* 21, 439.

Meisner, D.J., Carlson, R.J., and Gottlieb, A.J. (1985). Thrombocytopenia following sustained-release procainamide. *Arch. Intern. Med.* 145, 700.

Menahem, S. (1988). Prilocaine hydrochloride and neonatal methaemoglobinaemia. *Aust. N.Z. J. Obstet. Gynaecol.* 28, 76.

Metcalf, D. (1987). The molecular control of normal and leukaemic granulocytes and macrophages. *Proc. R. Soc. Lond. (Biol.)* 230, 389.

Mir, N. and Costello, C. (1988). Zidovudine and bone marrow. *Lancet* ii, 1195.

Mogk, L.G. and Cyrlin, M.M. (1988). Blood dyscrasias and carbonic anhydrase inhibitors. *Ophthalmology* (Rochester) 95, 768.

Mueller-Eckhardt, C., Küenzlen, E., Kiefel, V., Vahrson, H., and Graubner, M. (1983). Cyclophosphamide-induced immune thrombocytopenia in a patient with ovarian carcinoma successfully treated with intravenous gamma globulin. *Blut* 46, 165.

Muirhead, E.E., Halden, E.R., and Groves, M. (1958). Drug dependent Coombs (antiglobulin) test and anemia. Observations on quinine and acetophenetidine. *Arch. Intern. Med.* 101, 87.

Nakeff, A. and Bryan, J. E. (1978). Megakaryocyte proliferation and its regulation as revealed by CFU-M analysis. In *Hemopoetic cell differentiation* (ed. D.W. Golde, M.J. Cline, D. Metcalf, and C.F. Fox), p. 241. Academic Press, New York.

Nieweg, H.O., Bouma, H.G., DeVries, K., and Jansz, A. (1963). Haematological side effects of some antirheumatic drugs. *Ann. Rheum. Dis.* 22, 440.

Okafor, K.C., Griffin, C., and Ngole, P.M. (1986). Hydrochlorothiazide-induced thrombocytopenic purpura. *Drug Intell. Clin. Pharm.* 20, 60.

Old, C.W., Flannery, E.P., Grogan, T.M., Stone, W.H., and San Antonio, R.P. (1978). Azathioprine-induced pure red cell aplasia. *JAMA* 240, 552.

Oski, F.A. (1979). Hematological consequences of chloramphenicol therapy. *J. Pediatr.* 94, 515.

Pai, R.G. and Pai, S.M. (1988). Methyldopa-induced reversible immune thrombocytopenia. *Am. J. Med.* 85, 123.

Pau, A.K. and Fisher, M.A. (1987). Severe thrombocytopenia associated with once-daily rifampin therapy. *Drug Intell. Clin. Pharm.* 21, 882.

Peitzman, S.J. and Martin, C. (1980). Thrombocytopenia and minoxidil. *Ann. Intern. Med.* 92, 874.

Pena, J.M., Gonzalez, J.J., Garciaal, J., Barbado, F.J., and Vazquez, J.J. (1985). Thrombocytopenia and sulfasalazine. *Ann. Intern. Med.* 102, 277.

Pirovino, M., Ohnhaus, E.E., and Vonfelte, A. (1981). Digoxin-associated thrombocytopenia. *Eur. J. Clin. Pharmacol.* 19, 205.

Planas, A.T., Kranwinkel, R.N., Solitsky, H.B., and Pezzimenti, J.F. (1980). Chlorpropamide induced pure red blood cell aplasia. *Arch. Intern. Med.* 140, 707.

Polak, B.C.P., Wesseling, H., Schut, D., Herxheimer, A., and Meyler, L. (1972). Blood dyscrasias attributed to chloramphenicol. *Acta Med. Scand.* 192, 409.

Ponte, C.D. (1983). Carbamazepine-induced thrombocytopenia, rash and hepatic dysfunction. *Drug Intell. Clin. Pharm.* 17, 642.

Popovic, K., Sknulovic, D., and Sknulovic, M. (1973). Sideroblastic anemia in chronic phenacetin misuse. *Clin. Toxicol.* 6, 585.

Proctor, S.J. and Evans, R.G.B. (1985). Recognition of a chronic relapsing form of Hodgkin's disease in a population of patients demonstrating no second tumours. *Clin. Radiol.* 36, 461.

Ramselaar, A.C., Pekker, A.W., Huber-Bruning, O., and Bijlsma, J.W. (1987). Acquired sideroblastic anaemia after aplastic anaemia caused by D-pencillamine therapy for rheumatoid arthritis. *Ann. Rheum. Dis.* 46, 156.

Reid, G. and Patterson, A.C. (1977). Pure red cell aplasia after gold treatment. *Br. Med. J.* ii, 1457.

Retsagi, G., Kelly, J.P., and Kaufman, D.W. (1988). Risk of agranulocytosis and aplastic anaemia in relation to use of antithyroid drugs. *Br. Med. J.* 297, 262.

Ristuccia, A.M. (1985). Chloramphenicol: clinical pharmacology in pediatrics. *Ther. Drug Monit.* 7, 159.

Rosenbloom, D. and Gilbert, R. (1981). Reversible flu-like syndrome, leukopenia, and thrombocytopenia induced by allopurinol. *Drug Intell. Clin. Pharm.* 15, 286.

Rudolph, A.E. and Price, E.V. (1973). Penicillin reactions among patients in venereal disease clinics: a national survey. *JAMA* 223, 499.

Scott, G.L., Myles, A.B., and Bacon, P.A. (1968). Auto-immune haemolytic anaemia and mefenamic acid therapy. *Br. Med. J.* iii, 534.

Scott, J.M. and Weir, D.G. (1980). Drug induced megaloblastic change. *Clin. Haematol.* 9, 587.

Shulman, N.R. (1972). Immunologic reactions to drugs. *N. Engl. J. Med.* 287, 408.

Smyth, E.G. and Pallett, A.P. (1988). Clinicians's guide to antibiotics. Chloramphenicol. *Br. J. Hosp. Med.* 39, 424.

Stevens, J.D. and Mission, G.P. (1987). Ophthalmic use of chloramphenicol. *Lancet* ii, 1456.

Stibbins, R. and Bertino, J.R. (1976). Megaloblastic anaemia produced by drugs. *Clin. Haematol.* 5, 619.

Stricker, B.H., Barendregt, J.N., and Claas, F.H. (1985). Thrombocytopenia and leucopenia with mianserin-dependent antibodies. *Br. J. Clin. Pharmacol.* 19, 102.

Talpaz, M., Kantarijan, H.M., McCredie, K.B., Keating M.J., Trujillo J., and Gutterman J. (1987). Clinical investigation of human alpha-interferon in chronic myelogenous leukaemia. *Blood* 69, 1280.

Tolot, F., Prost, G., Guignot, B., and Pelletier, M. (1976). Manifestations multiples d'intolérance à une association d'anti-inflammatoires. Rôle de la phénylbutazone. *Semin. Hop. Paris* 52, 185.

Tomlin, G.H. (1973). Isoniazid as a cause of neuropathy and sideroblastic anaemia. *Practitioner* 211, 773.

Tucker, M.A., Meadows, A.T., Boice, J.D. Jr, Stovall, M., Oberlin, O., Stone, B.J., *et al.* (1987). Leukemia after therapy with alkylating agents for childhood cancer. *J. Natl Cancer Inst.* 78, 459.

Tucker, M.A., Coleman, C.A., Cox, R.S., Varghese, A., and Rosenberg, S.A. (1988). Risk of second cancers after treatment for Hodgkin's disease. *N. Engl. J. Med.* 318, 76.

Verwilghen, R., Reybrouk, G., Callens, L., and Cusemans, J. (1965). Antituberculous drugs and sideroblastic anaemia. *Br. J. Haematol.* 11, 92.

von dem Borne, A.E.G.Kr., Pegels, J.G., van der Stadt, R.J., van der Plas-van Dalen, C.M., and Helmerhorst, F.M. (1986). Thrombocytopenia associated with gold therapy: a drug induced autoimmune disease?. *Br. J. Haematol.* 63, 509.

Wales, J. and Wolff, F. (1967). Haematological side effects of diazoxide. *Lancet* i, 53.

Walker, D.J., Saunders, P., and Griffiths, I.D. (1986). Gold induced thrombocytopenia. *J. Rheumatol.* 13, 225.

Walker, J.A., Sherman, R.A., and Eisinger, R.P. (1985). Thrombocytopenia associated with intravenous deferoxamine. *Am. J. Kidney Dis.* 6, 254.

Walker, R.W. and Heaton, A. (1985). Thrombocytopenia due to vancomycin. *Lancet* i, 932.

Wallerstein, R.O., Condit, P.K., Kasper, C.K., Brown, J.W., and Morrison, F.R. (1969). State-wide study of chloramphenicol therapy and fatal aplastic anemia. *JAMA* 208, 2045.

Warkentin, T.E. and Kelton, J.G. (1990). Heparin and platelets. *Hematol. Oncol. Clin. North Am.* 4, 243.

Watanabe, S., Tsunematsu, Y., Fujimoto, J., and Komiyama, A. (1988). Leukaemia patients treated with growth hormone. *Lancet* i, 1159.

Weinberger, I., Rotenberg, Z., Fuchs, J., Ben Sasson, E., and Agmon, J. (1987). Amiodarone-induced thrombocytopenia. *Arch. Intern. Med.* 147, 735.

Wenz, B., Klein, R.L., and Lacezari, P. (1974). Tetracycline-induced immune hemolytic anemia. *Transfusion* 14, 265.

White, J.M., Brown, D.L., Hepner, G.W., and Worledge, S.M. (1968). Pencillin induced haemolytic anaemia. *Br. Med. J.* iii, 26.

Williams, L.M.E., Joos, R., Proot, F., and Immesoete, C. (1987). Gold induced aplastic anaemia. *Clin. Rheumatol.* 6600.

Woolley, P.V.III, Sacher, R.A., Priego, V.M., Schanfield, M.S., and Bonnem, E.M. (1983). Methotrexate-induced immune haemolytic anaemia. *Br. J. Haematol.* 54, 543.

Youle, M. and Gazzard, B. (1990). The treatment of HIV disease. In *Clin. Haematology*, Vol. 3 (ed. C. Costello), p. 153. Baillière, London.

Yunis, A.A. (1973). Chloramphenicol induced bone marrow suppression. *Sem. Hematol.* 10, 225.

Zorab, P.A. (1960). Fulminating purpura during antituberculosis drug treatment. *Tubercle* 41, 219.

22. Part 2 Disorders of haemostasis

P. CAREY and S. J. PROCTOR

Introduction

In the normal state, haemostasis is maintained by a complex series of dynamically interacting mechanisms involving vascular endothelium, platelets, plasma coagulation proteins and enzymes and their inhibitors, and the components of the fibrinolytic system. Drugs may affect this delicate balance in a wide variety of ways. Groups of drugs, such as oral and parenteral anticoagulants, and thrombolytic, antiplatelet, and antifibrinolytic agents are used deliberately to manipulate haemostatic mechanisms. Adverse haemostatic reactions to these agents may result from overdosage, abnormal sensitivity in individuals to usual dosage, interactions with other drugs or agents, or idiosyncratic reactions. These drugs may also cause non-haemostatic adverse effects, which are discussed elsewhere in this book. Adverse haemostatic effects of other drugs usually occur because of a predominant effect on one particular component of the coagulation system.

This section will briefly review the physiological mechanisms of haemostasis, and then consider adverse reactions to those agents that are used deliberately to manipulate those mechanisms, dealing mainly with haemostatic and adverse effects. Lastly, adverse haemostatic effects of other drugs will be reviewed according to which component of the coagulation system is predominantly affected. The adverse reaction of thrombocytopenia has been dealt with in the previous chapter and is not further considered.

Normal haemostasis

The maintenance of the integrity of the vascular compartment while preserving the fluidity of the blood requires continuous interaction between various mechanisms, which exist in a dynamic equilibrium. The major components will be described here separately and briefly, to clarify the causes of the adverse drug reactions discussed later.

Platelets

These are non-nucleated discoid structures that circulate in the blood at a level of $150-200\mu 10^9$ per litre. Their outer membrane is extensively invaginated to form an interconnecting canalicular system of tubules that provides a large phospholipid surface that facilitates many plasma coagulation reactions. Several different types of glycoprotein molecule project from the membrane surface, acting as receptors for other coagulation proteins including thrombin, fibrinogen, and von Willebrand factor (VWF). These variously facilitate calcium release within the platelet, aggregation to other platelets, and attachment to damaged endothelium. Calcium release causes contractile proteins inside the outer membrane, to effect shape changes in the activated platelet encouraging irreversibilty of the aggregation phenomenon and forming a stable platelet plug at the site of injury. Activation is associated with release of inclusion body contents. Dense bodies within the platelet contain vasoactive substances, such as 5-hydroxytryptamine, and aggregation stimulators including ADP, ATP, and adrenaline; α-granules contain coagulation proteins such as fibrinogen, factor V, factor VIII, β-thromboglobulin and thrombospondin. Calcium ions also stimulate the production of the potent vasoconstrictor thromboxane A_2 (TXA$_2$) from arachidonic acid available from the platelet membrane via the pathway shown in Fig. 22.2.

The amount of free calcium ion available is heavily influenced by cyclic adenosine monophosphate (c-AMP).

In general, high levels of c-AMP are associated with low levels of Ca^{++}, and vice versa.

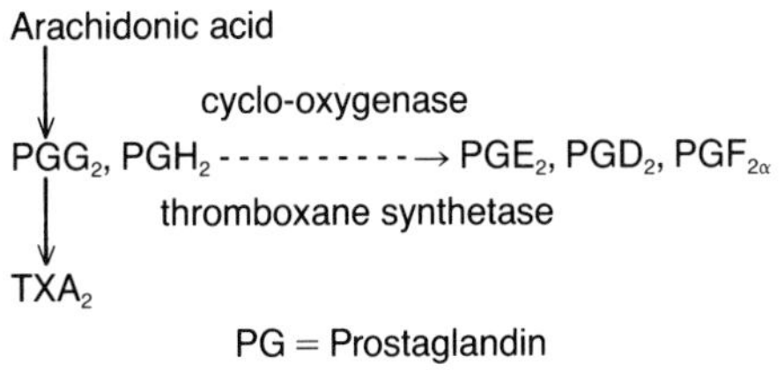

Arachidonic acid

cyclo-oxygenase

PGG_2, PGH_2 - - - - - - - - - → PGE_2, PGD_2, $PGF_{2\alpha}$

thromboxane synthetase

TXA_2

PG = Prostaglandin

FIG. 22.2.

Drugs may thus affect platelet function by several mechanisms, including interference with surface receptors, calcium availability, and prostaglandin metabolism.

Plasma coagulation

The formation of a stable fibrin clot from circulating soluble fibrinogen is mediated by a sequence of enzymatic reactions, depicted in simplified form in Fig. 22.3. The intrinsic pathway is activated by damaged endothelium, and the extrinsic pathway by exposure to extravascular tissue thromboplastins. After pathway activation, circulating inactive polypeptide factors are sequentially converted to active serine proteases, which in turn activate the next in sequence, providing an amplifying cascade of molecular activation. The reactions occur on a phospholipid surface and require Ca^{++} at various points.

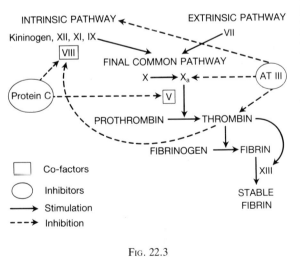

FIG. 22.3

These reactions are controlled by a number of feedback mechanisms. Two inhibitors are shown which are relevant to drugs used for anticoagulant therapy. The cofactors factor V and factor VIII catalyse, respectively, the activation of factor X by factor IX_a and the activation of prothrombin by factor X_a, enabling these reactions to occur many times faster. These co-factors are inhibited by protein C and its co-factor protein S, which are vitamin K-dependent and thus affected by oral anticoagulation in addition to factors II, VII, IX, and X. The inhibitor antithrombin III (ATIII) inhibits factor X_a and also IX_a, XI_a, and XII_a. Heparin acts as a co-factor for this inhibitor.

Fibrinolysis

Once a haemostatic plug has formed and maintained the integrity of the vessel, the prevention of its propagation and its eventual removal occurs by fibrinolysis. This is not a separate process but is continuously interacting with coagulation. Fibrin is digested by the enzyme plasmin. Plasminogen is the inert precursor of plasmin and circulates in the blood. Activation of plasminogen to form plasmin is brought about by tissue plaminogen activator (tPA), produced by vascular endothelium. tPA also has a binding site for fibrin, thus localizing the activation of plasminogen to the site of clot.

Plasminogen activator inhibitor, also produced by vascular endothelium, is a rapid inactivator of non-fibrin-bound tPA, preventing unwanted plasminogen activation in the circulation. In addition to fibrinolysis, plasminogen activation causes the cleavage of platelet and endothelial glycoprotein receptors for VWF and fibrinogen, thus impairing aggregation, a decrease in factors V and VIII, and an increase in fibrin degradation products (FDP), which inhibit plasma coagulation. Drugs that cause plasminogen activation are used in thrombolytic therapy.

Vascular endothelium

The balance between coagulation and fibrinolysis is regulated to a large extent by the endothelial cell lining of the circulation. Against clot formation it provides a barrier protecting the blood from extravascular procoagulant stimuli, inhibits platelet aggregation, and encourages vasodilatation by producing prostacyclin, inhibits plasma coagulation by producing ATIII and thrombomodulin (which binds thrombin and causes activation of protein C), and encourages fibrinolysis by producing tPA.

On the other hand, the endothelium expresses VWF, encouraging platelet adhesion, producing plasminogen activator inhibitor and, when damaged, initiating the intrinsic coagulation cascade.

Drugs used to manipulate haemostatic mechanisms

Oral anticoagulants

These agents are widely used for the prophylaxis and treatment of venous thrombosis and the prevention of arterial thromboembolism in cardiac disease, especially following prosthetic valvular replacement.

They are classified according to their structure into the coumarins, which include warfarin, the single most widely used agent; and the indanediones, of which phenindione is the most commonly prescribed example. They work by antagonizing the action of vitamin K, thus inhibiting production by the liver of functional forms of factors II, VII, IX, and X. They also inhibit the production of the co-factor inhibitor protein C.

Dosage requirements vary between individuals. Maintenance of an adequate therapeutic anticoagulant effect while minimizing the risk of haemorrhagic complications requires regular laboratory monitoring and appropriate dose adjustment. The most widely accepted control method uses the prothrombin time test performed with a thromboplastin reagent that has been standardized directly or indirectly against an international standard reference material. Test result times are expressed as a ratio of 'normal', standardized for the particular thromboplastin reagent used, and expressed as an international normalized ratio (INR). Therapeutic ranges for the INR lie within the limits of 2.0–4.5 and vary according to the indication for anticoagulation (British Society for Haematology 1984).

The dose required to maintain an individual within the therapeutic range may vary with time. Interaction with other concomitantly administered drugs is a major cause of difficulty with control.

Haemorrhage

Spontaneous bleeding, including bruising, subconjunctival haemorrhage, epistaxis, haemoptysis, haematemesis, melaena, haematuria, menorrhagia, and intracranial bleeding, are more common in patients taking oral anticoagulants, especially when control is poor.

It is difficult to assess the true incidence of haemorrhage. Two British studies of large series of patients on long-term anticoagulation indicated an incidence for bleeding episodes of 1 in 23–25 treatment-years (Forfar 1979; Sixty-plus Reinfarction Group 1980). Risk is increased with age (Gurwitz *et al.* 1988). Higher incidences have been reported for short-term treatment (Marple and Wright 1950). In a study of 565 patients (Landefeld and Goldman 1989) the monthly risk of major bleeding

dropped from 3 per cent per month for the first month to 0.3 per cent per month following the first year of therapy. There is a clear relationship in these studies between the occurrence of haemorrhage and laboratory evidence of over-anticoagulation. Apart from drug interaction, poor control may result from lack of compliance, intercurrent illness, alcohol ingestion, or dietary factors.

Drug interactions affecting control of oral anticoagulant therapy

Drugs may affect oral anticoagulation in several ways. Those that reduce the intestinal absorption of vitamin K will potentiate the anticoagulant effect. Potentiation may also occur as a result of displacement of the anticoagulant from plasma albumin binding increasing the level of active free drug. Agents may affect the metabolism of anticoagulants by the microsomal enzymes in the liver either by inducing these enzymes, enhancing drug elimination, and reducing anticoagulant effect, or by inhibiting enzymes and potentiating anticoagulation. Warfarin exists as a mixture of the R and S optical isomers, the latter being some five times more active than the former in terms of anticoagulant effect. There are differences in the microsomal metabolism of the two isomers, and in the presence of some drugs effects may occur because of preferential metabolism of one isomer. Table 22.11 lists some drugs that may have an important interaction with oral anticoagulant treatment.

TABLE 22.11
Drugs that may affect oral anticoagulation

1. Drugs that may potentiate oral anticoagulants

Anabolic steroids	Chloramphenicol	Erythromycin
Amiodarone	Cimetidine	Metronidazole
Amitriptyline	Clofibrate	Norfloxacin
Aspirin	Co-trimoxazole	Oxyphenbutazone
Azapropazone	Danazol	Phenylbutazone
Chloral hydrate	Dextrothyroxine	Sulphonamides

2. Drugs that may reduce the effect of oral anticoagulants

Alcohol (chronic)	Dichloralphenazone	Primidone
Carbamazepine	Griseofulvin	Rifampicin
Cholestyramine	Phenytoin	Vit K preparations

Changes in, or short-term intermittent courses of, concomitant therapy are much more likely to cause difficulty with anticoagulant control than stable long-term therapy with a constant dose of another agent.

Skin necrosis and protein C deficiency

The occasional occurrence of a necrotic skin rash during

the induction phase of warfarin therapy has been recognized to be due to diffuse thrombosis in small vessels in patients with heterozygous protein C deficiency (McGehee *et al.* 1983; Samama *et al.* 1984; Broekmans and Bertina 1990). This coagulation inhibitor is also vitamin K-dependent and has a half-life of 6 hours, similar to that of factor VII, but shorter than those of the other vitamin K-dependent factors (Weiss *et al.* 1987). Thus, during the early stages of oral anticoagulation there is a state of increased tendency to thrombosis, especially when protein C levels are already low.

Warfarin resistance

The commonest reason for failure to achieve anticoagulation with oral agents is poor patient compliance. Occasionally, however, a patient may be genuinely resistant to anticoagulation with warfarin (see Chapter 3). Satisfactory control can then usually be achieved with an indanedione.

Non-haemostatic adverse reactions

Effects on the fetus

Warfarin is a small molecule that crosses the placenta producing a risk of fetal haemorrhage, particularly in the later stages of pregnancy (Bonnar 1977). Additionally, there appears to be a risk of non-haemorrhagic teratogenic effects in the first trimester (Shaul *et al.* 1975; Hall *et al.* 1980). Accordingly, the British Society for Haematology guidelines (1984) for patients requiring anticoagulation during pregnancy recommend the use of heparin in monitored dosage, though oral anticoagulants may be used between the 12th and 36th weeks. This subject is also considered in Chapter 5.

Hypersensitivity (allergic) reactions

Skin rashes and alopecia have been reported with coumarin drugs but are excessively rare. Rashes and other reactions, such as neutropenia, thrombocytopenia, diarrhoea, and hepatitis are more common with the indanediones, and it is for this reason that the coumarin warfarin is the most widely used agent. These subjects are considered further in other parts of this book.

Heparin

This parenteral anticoagulant is widely used for the initial treatment and for the prevention of venous and arterial thrombosis and for maintaining blood fluidity in vascular catheters and extracorporeal circulations.

Standard heparin is a naturally occurring sulphated glycosaminoglycan usually derived from bovine or porcine lung and intestinal mucosa. It has a heterogeneous molecular weight varying from 5000 to 30 000. A specific tetrasaccharide sequence binds to antithrombin III (AT III), enhancing this molecule's inhibition of thrombin and activated factors X, XI, and XII. Heparin also binds directly to thrombin, exerting an important anticoagulant effect. This is greater for the higher-molecular-weight forms, which bind to both AT III and thrombin in a ternary complex. Lower-molecular weight forms more specifically inhibit X_a activity.

Heparin has a short half-life in the circulation of about 90 minutes. It may be given by intermittent bolus or continuous intravenous infusion, of which the latter method avoids wide fluctuations and is associated with fewer haemorrhagic complications (Salzman *et al.* 1975; Glazier and Crowell 1976). Subcutaneous administration is usually used for low-dose prophylaxis but can also be used to deliver full-dose anticoagulation (Walker *et al.* 1987).

Maintenance of adequate anticoagulation, while minimizing the risk of haemorrhage, requires dosage adjustment according to results of laboratory control tests. Conventionally, the partial thromboplastin time (PTT) test is used. This has a more useful response curve over the therapeutic range than the thrombin time, though the latter is more sensitive to small amounts of heparin. Alternatively, an indirect assay of heparin may be performed, usually by assessing X_a inactivation with a chromogenic substrate.

Haemorrhage

Spontaneous haemorrhage, particularly soft-tissue bleeding such as wound haemorrhage following surgery, cannula insertions, and intramuscular injections, and including the potentially dangerous complication of retroperitoneal bleeding, may occur. Risk increases with heparin dose; patient age, particularly in women (Holm *et al.* 1985); severity of concomitant illness; administration of other agents interfering with coagulation, such as aspirin (Walker and Jick 1980); and uraemia or previous bleeding tendency (Salzman *et al.* 1975).

The relatively reduced antithrombin effect compared with anti-factor X activity of low-molecular-weight (LMW) heparin fractions suggested the theoretical possibility of a more favourable ratio of antithrombotic effect to haemorrhagic risk for these agents. Clinical study has indicated good results as regards efficacy and safety for LMW heparin in prophylaxis after hip surgery (Turpie *et al.* 1986), but clear safety advantages over standard heparin have not been demonstrated (Samama *et al.* 1989).

Thrombocytopenia

Heparin may cause thrombocytopenia by an immune mechanism and this is discussed in Part 1 of this chapter.

Osteoporosis

Long-term heparin therapy (lasting over 6 months) has been reported to be associated with bone demineralization (Avioli 1975; de Swiet et al. 1983) (see also Chapter 16).

Thrombolytic therapy

Thrombolytic agents are used in the management of proximal deep-vein thrombosis; serious pulmonary embolism; acute arterial thromboembolic disease, including myocardial infarction; and for the unblocking of vascular catheters.

The agents available all act directly or indirectly as activators of plasminogen, reacting more or less selectively with fibrin-bound plasminogen. Streptokinase (SK) is a protein derived from β-haemolytic streptococcal culture. Urokinase (UK) is a trypsin-like protease derived from human urine, with similar thrombolytic properties but avoiding the problem of inactivation by antistreptococcal antibodies. These agents have been in regular clinical use for over a decade. Subsequent studies and the development of recombinant DNA technology have yielded further agents such as acylated plasminogen–streptokinase complex (APSAC), recombinant single-chain and double-chain tissue plasminogen activator (r-tPA), and recombinant single-chain urokinase plasminogen activator (r-scuPA) (Marder and Sherry 1988). Thrombolytic agents produce maximal activation of fibrin-bound plasminogen, but the various agents differ in their propensity to activate plasma plasminogen, resulting in fibrinogen proteolysis and a so-called lytic state. This effect is minimal with r-tPA and r-scuPA, which are more fibrin-selective, moderate with UK, and greatest with SK and APSAC (Marder and Sherry 1988).

Haemorrhage

Despite the relatively hypocoagulable state that may result from thrombolytic therapy, the incidence of major bleeding complications is about 5 per cent (Goldhaber et al. 1984), and is mainly related to sites of invasive procedures, provided that therapy is not used inappropriately in patients with recent trauma or surgery, peptic ulceration, hypertension, or pre-existing coagulation impairment. Impressive results in terms of reduction of mortality and limitation of ventricular damage have been obtained with thrombolytic therapy used early in myocardial infarction, especially when sequential aspirin treatment follows the initial thrombolysis (GISSI 1987; ISIS 1988; AIMS Trial Study Group 1988; van der Werf and Arnold 1988). The question is whether the more fibrin-selective agents are associated with fewer adverse haemorrhagic effects. The fact that most bleeding episodes are in any case associated with sites of tissue injury makes this less likely. The most extensive studies available to answer this question have compared SK with r-tPA. SK was associated with a greater degree of hypofibrinogenaemia than r-tPA in the 1988 TIMI study (Rao et al. 1988), but no greater incidence of haemorrhagic complications. The recent GISSI-2 study (1990), comparing r-tPA and SK in a randomized study of 12 490 patients, found a slightly but significantly higher incidence for major bleeds in the SK group (1 per cent) compared with the r-tPA group (0.5 per cent), although this was more marked in patients receiving sequential heparin (half the patients in each group) and the heparin at their dosage did not improve the therapeutic endpoints (mortality and severe LV damage). Also the incidence of stroke was higher in the r-tPA group (1.1 per cent vs. 0.9 per cent in the SK group), although this was not statistically significant. On this evidence the differences in incidence of haemorrhagic adverse effects of these types of thrombolytic agent appear relatively marginal.

Antifibrinolytic agents

These drugs inhibit plasminogen activation. Aminocaproic acid and tranexamic acid bind to plasminogen by its lysine binding site and prevent association with fibrin so that activation cannot occur. They are useful systemically for troublesome mucosal bleeding such as epistaxis and menorrhagia especially in haemophilia and von Willebrand's disease. They may also be used to treat systemic fibrinolysis and, if necessary, to attempt to reverse the effect of thrombolytic therapy. Tranexamic acid is also used as a topical agent.

These agents may precipitate ureteric obstruction by clot, if there is haematuria, which is therefore a contraindication to their use. They should not be given to patients with recent thromboembolic disease.

Antiplatelet agents

A number of drugs with antiplatelet effects, such as aspirin, dipyridamole, prostacyclin, ticlopidine, and dextran are used in the treatment or secondary prevention of such arterial thromboembolic diseases as myocardial infarction, transient ischaemic attacks, and peripheral vascular disease.

Many other drugs may have incidental unwanted effects on platelet function mediated via similar mechanisms and these are discussed in the next section.

Antiplatelet effects of drugs may only become apparent as abnormalities on *in vitro* testing, or may cause prolongation of the bleeding time, purpura or mucocutaneous bleeding, or haemorrhagic problems following trauma or surgery. Difficulties are more frequently encountered if there is an underlying haemorrhagic disorder or concomitant anticoagulant therapy.

Aspirin acts as an inhibitor of cyclo-oxygenase (Roth and Majerus 1975) thereby inhibiting platelet production of TXA_2. Prostacyclin production by endothelial cells is also inhibited, but because endothelial cells are able to synthesize cyclo-oxygenase the antiplatelet effect is greater, and a low dose of aspirin is probably optimal (Kallmann *et al.* 1987).

Dipyridamole inhibits platelet phosphodiesterase, causing a rise in platelet c-AMP and hence reduced Ca^{++} availability.

Prostacyclin, in addition to being a potent vasodilator, is an inhibitor of platelet aggregation as it also causes an increase in c-AMP.

Ticlopidine inhibits the binding of VWF and fibrinogen to platelet receptors and thereby inhibits platelet aggregation and adhesion.

Dextran is a neutral polysaccharide with a large molecular mass (40–70 kDaltons). Molecules are absorbed onto the platelet surface impairing aggregation and adhesion.

Adverse reactions to drugs not primarily used to manipulate haemostatic mechanisms

Drugs interfering with platelet function

Cyclo-oxygenase inhibitors

Aspirin has been discussed above. Many non-steroidal anti-inflammatory drugs, such as ibuprofen, indomethacin, naproxen, phenylbutazone, and sulphinpyrazone, have a similar effect (Simon and Mills 1980). In some cases this effect is reversible, whereas in the case of aspirin the effect on the bleeding time lasts for 5–7 days (i.e. for the life of the affected platelets, rather than the half-life in the circulation of the drug).

Drugs increasing platelet c-AMP levels

In addition to dipyridamole and prostacyclin (see above), theophylline and caffeine have this effect, and may prolong the bleeding time.

Drugs interfering with the platelet surface

Dextran (see above) is used therapeutically for this purpose, but if it or hydroxyethyl starch are used as plasma expanders the antiplatelet effect may be an unwanted adverse reaction.

High doses of the penicillin antibiotic family can cause prolongation of the bleeding time in normal volunteers and may cause bleeding problems in patients (Sattler *et al.* 1986). The proposed mechanism of action is via binding to the platelet membrane and interference with adhesion (Cazenave *et al.* 1973). Similar effects have been reported with moxalactam, some cephalosporins, and nitrofurantoin.

Non-thrombocytopenic purpura

The clinical manifestation of purpura is most often due to thrombocytopenia or to defective platelet function. A similar picture can, however, be caused by damage to small blood vessels either by immunological mechanisms or by changes in vascular permeability. A list of drugs that have been associated with this phenomenon is given in Table 22.12 (Bloom and Thomas 1987).

TABLE 22.12
Drugs associated with non-thrombocytopenic purpura

Aspirin	Digoxin	Oestrogens
Allopurinol	Frusemide	Penicillins
Arsenicals	Gold salts	Phenacetin
Atropine	Iodides	Piperazine
Barbiturates	Indomethacin	Procaine
Belladonna	Isoniazid	Quinine
Chloral hydrate	Mercury	Quinidine
Chloramphenicol	Meprobamate	Reserpine
Chlorothiazide	Methyldopa	Sulphonamides
Chlorpropamide	Nifedipine	Tolbutamide
Coumarins		

Drugs affecting plasma coagulation

Hypoprothrombinaemia

Reduction in the vitamin K-dependent clotting factors has been mentioned above in connection with oral anticoagulation. Depletion of these factors with prolongation of the prothrombin time is a recognized adverse effect of cephalosporin antibiotic therapy (Betchold 1984 *et al.* 1984; Conjera *et al.* 1988).

Factor X deficiency

Acquired factor X deficiency with an associated clinical bleeding disorder has been reported as a complication of treatment with the cytotoxic drug amsacrine (Carter and Winfield 1988).

Disseminated intravascular coagulation

This widespread inappropriate deposition of fibrin in the circulation occurs secondarily to a wide variety of causes involving extensive tissue damage. The cytotoxic drug colaspase (asparaginase), commonly used in the treatment of acute lymphoblastic leukaemia, is recognized occasionally to cause this phenomenon (Legnani *et al.* 1988).

Thrombotic thrombocytopenic purpura (TTP)

This rare disorder is characterized by the inappropriate deposition of platelet plugs in the microcirculation; it manifests as thrombocytopenia and a microangiopathic haemolytic anaemia associated with fever, renal failure, and neurological abnormalities. The aetiology is thought to be due to endothelial damage. The immunosuppressive drug cyclosporin A, frequently used in organ and bone marrow transplantation, has been implicated as one potential cause (Dzik *et al.* 1987).

Thrombosis
(See also Chapter 7)

Many interacting factors have been recognized to be associated with an increased risk of arterial or venous thromboembolic disease. The following drug associations are important:

Oral contraceptive pill

Epidemiological studies have shown that oestrogen-containing oral contraceptive preparations constitute a risk factor for thrombosis and that a decreased oestrogen content lowers the excess risk for venous but not arterial thrombotic disease (Vessey and Mann 1978; Böttiger *et al.* 1980). This risk must be balanced against that of pregnancy or of other contraceptive methods (Sachs *et al.* 1984).

Lupus anticoagulant

This acquired anticardiolipin antibody, first detected in systemic lupus erythematosus, interferes with *in vitro* plasma coagulation, causing prolongation of the partial thromboplastin time, but associated clinically with a predisposition to thrombosis rather than a bleeding diathesis. It has also been found in patients under treatment with procainamide (Heyman *et al.* 1988).

Factor IX concentrates

These preparations, used for the treatment of bleeding episodes in congenital factor IX deficiency, often contain other prothrombin complex factors and are sometimes used to supplement replacement therapy in other haemorrhagic states, such as liver disease, emergency reversal of oral anticoagulant overdosage, and DIC. There is an incidence of thromboembolic complications with their use (Kasper 1975).

Type of reaction

Most of the adverse reactions described above are of Type A, the exceptions being immune thrombocytopenia and, possibly, osteoporosis, diessseminated intravascular coagulation, thrombotic thrombocytopenic purpura, and thrombosis due to lupus anticoagulant, which are of Type B (see Chapter 3).

References

AIMS Trial Study Group (1988). Effect of intravenous APSAC on toxicity after acute myocardial infarction: Preliminary report of a placebo-controlled clinical trial. *Lancet* i, 545.

Avioli, L.V. (1975). Heparin induced osteopenia: an appraisal. *Adv. Exp. Med. Biol.* 52, 375.

Betchold, H., Andrassy, K., and Jahnchen, E. (1984). Evidence for impaired hepatic vitamin K metabolism in patients treated with *N*-methyl thiotetrazole cephalosporins. *Thromb. and Haemost.* 51, 358.

Bloom, A. L. and Thomas, D. P. (1987). *Haemostasis and thrombosis* (2nd edn). Churchill Livingstone, Edinburgh.

Bonnar, J. (1977). Acute and chronic coagulation disorders in pregnancy. In *Recent advances in blood coagulation 2.* (ed. L. Poller), p. 363. Churchill Livingstone, Edinburgh.

Böttiger, L.E., Boman, G., Ekland, G., and Westerholm, B. (1980). Oral contraceptives and thromboembolic disease: effects of lowering oestrogen content. *Lancet* i, 1097.

British Society for Haematology (1984). Guidelines on oral anticoagulant control.

Broekmans, A. W. and Bertina, R. M. (1990). Protein C. In *Recent advances in blood coagulation 4* (ed. L. Poller), p. 117. Churchill Livingstone, Edinburgh.

Carter, C. and Winfield, D.A. (1988). Factor X deficiency during treatment of relapsed acute myeloid leukaemia with amsacrine. *Clin. Lab Haematol.* 10, 225.

Cazenave, J.P., Packman, M.A., Guccione, M.A., and Mustard, J.F. (1973). Effects of penicillin G on platelet aggregation release and adherence to collagen. *Proc. Soc. Exp. Biol. Med.* 142, 159.

Conjera, A., Bell, W., and Lipsky, J.J. (1988). Cefotetan and hypoprothrombinemia. *Ann. Intern. Med.* 108, 643.

de Swiet, M., Dorrington-Ward, P., Fidler, J., Horsman, A., Katz, D., Letsky, E., *et al.* (1983). Prolonged heparin therapy in pregnancy causes bone dimineralization. *Br. J. Obstet. Gynaecol.* 90, 1129.

Dzik, W.H., Georgi, B.A., Khettry, V., and Jenkins, R.L. (1987). Cyclosporin associated thrombotic thrombocytopenic purpura following liver transplantation: successful treatment with plasma exchange. *Transplantation* 44, 570.

Forfar, J.C. (1979). A seven year analysis of haemorrhage in patients on long term anticoagulant treatment. *Br. Heart J.* 42, 128.

GISSI (Gruppo Italiano per lo studio della streptochinasi nell 'infarto miocardico') (1987). Long-term effects of intravenous thrombolysis in acute myocardial infarction: final report of the GISSI study. *Lancet* ii, 871.

GISSI-2 (Gruppo Italiano per lo studio della soppravivenza nell 'infarto miocardico') (1990). A factorial randomized trial of alteplase versus streptokinase and heparin versus no heparin among 12 490 patients with acute myocardial infarction. *Lancet* ii, 65.

Glazier, R.L. and Crowell, E.B. (1976). Randomised prospective trial of continuous vs intermittent heparin therapy. *JAMA* 236, 1365.

Goldhaber, S.Z., Buring, J.E., Lipnick, R.J., and Hennekens, C.H. (1984). Pooled analyses of randomized trials of streptokinase and heparin in phlebographically documented acute deep vein thrombosis. *Am. J. Med.* 76, 393.

Gurwitz, J.H., Goldberg, R.J., Holden, A., Knapic, N., and Ansell, J. (1988). Age related risks of long term oral anticoagulant therapy. *Arch. Intern. Med.* 148, 1733.

Hall, J.D., Pavli, R.M., and Wilson, K.M. (1980). Maternal and fetal sequelae of anticoagulation during pregnancy. *Am. J. Med.* 68, 122.

Heyman, M.R., Flores, R.M., Edelman, B.B., and Corlier, N.H. (1988). Procainamide induced lupus anticoagulant. *South. Med. J.* 81, 934.

Holm, H.A., Abildgaard, U., and Kalvenes, S. (1985). Heparin assays and bleeding complications in treatment of deep vein thrombosis with particular reference to retroperitoneal bleeding. *Thromb. Haemost.* 53, 278.

ISIS-2 (Second International Study of Infarct Survival) and Collaborative Group) (1988). Randomized trial of intravenous streptokinase, oral aspirin, both or neither among 17 187 cases of suspected acute myocardial infarction. *Lancet* ii, 349.

Kallmann, R., Niewenhuis, H.K., de Groot, P.G., van Gijn, J, and Sixma, J.J., *et al.* (1987). Effects of low doses of aspirin, 10 mg and 30 mg daily, on bleeding time, thromboxane production and 6-keto-PGF$_{1\alpha}$ excretion in healthy subjects. *Thromb. Res.* 45, 355.

Kasper, C.K. (1975). Factor IX concentrates: thromboembolic complications. *Thromb. Haemost.* 33, 640.

Landefeld, C.S. and Goldman, L. (1989). Major bleeding in outpatients treated with warfarin: incidence and prediction by factors known at the start of outpatient therapy. *Am. J. Med.* 87, 144.

Legnani, C., Paleredi, G., Pession, A., Poggi, M., and Vecchi, V. (1988). Intravascular coagulation phenomenon associated with prevalent fall in fibrinogen and plasminogen during L-asparaginase treatment in leukaemic children. *Haemostasis* 18, 179.

Marder, V. and Sherry, S. (1988). Thrombolytic therapy: current status. *N. Engl. J. Med.* 23, 1512.

Marple, C. D. and Wright, I. S. (1950). *Thromboembolic conditions and their treatment with anticoagulants.* Charles C. Thomas, Springfield, Illinois.

McGehee, W.G., Klotz, T.A., Epstein, D.J., and Rappaport, S.I. (1983). Coumarin induced necrosis in a patient with familial protein C deficiency. *Blood* 62 (suppl.), 304(a).

Rao, A.K., Pratt, C., and Berke, A. (1988). Thrombolysis in myocardial infarction (TIMI) trial phase 1: hemorrhagic complications and changes in plasma fibrinogen and fibrinolytic system in patients treated with recombinant tissue plasminogen activator and streptokinase. *J. Am. Coll. Cardiol.* 11, 1.

Roth, D.J. and Majerus, P.W. (1975). The mechanism of the effect of aspirin on human platelets: acetylation of a particulate fraction protein. *J. Clin. Invest.* 56, 624.

Sachs, B.P., Masterton, T., Jewett, J.F., and Guyer, B. (1984). Reproductive mortality in Massachusetts in 1981. *N. Engl. J. Med.* 311, 1667.

Salzman, E.W., Deykin, D., Shapiro, R.M., and Rosenberg, R.D. (1975). The management of heparin therapy. Controlled prospective trial. *N. Engl. J. Med.* 191, 1046.

Samama, M., Horrelou, M.H., Soria, J., Conard, J., and Nicholas, G. (1984). Successful programme of anticoagulation in severe protein C deficiency and skin necrosis at the initiation of oral anticoagulant treatment. *Thromb. Haemost.* 51, 132.

Samama, M., Boissel, J.P., Combe-Tamzali, S., and Leizorovicz, A. (1989). Clinical studies with low molecular weight heparin in the prevention and treatment of venous thromboembolism. *Ann. N.Y. Acad. Sci.* 556, 386.

Sattler, F.R., Weittekamp, M.R., and Ballard, J.O. (1986). Potential for bleeding with the new beta lactam antibiotics. *Ann. Intern. Med.* 105, 924.

Shaul, W.L., Emery, H., and Hall, J.G. (1975). Chondroplasia punctata and maternal warfarin use during pregnancy. *Am. J. Dis. Child.* 129, 360.

Simon, L.S. and Mills, J.A. (1980). Non-steroidal anti-inflammatory drugs. *N. Engl. J. Med.* 302, 1179.

Sixty-plus Reinfarction Group (1980). A double-blind trial to assess long term oral anticoagulant therapy in elderly patients with myocardial infarction. *Lancet* ii, 989.

Turpie, A.G.G., Levine, M.N., Hirsch, J., Carter, C.J., Jay, R.M., Powers, P.J., *et al.* (1986). A randomized controlled trial of a low molecular weight heparin (enoxaparin) to prevent deep vein thrombosis in patients undergoing elective hip surgery. *N. Engl. J. Med.* 315, 925.

van der Werf, F. and Arnold, A.E.R. (1988). The European Cooperative Study Group for recombinant tissue type plasminogen activator: Intravenous tissue plasminogen activator and size of infarct, left ventricular function and survival in acute myocardial infarction. *Br. Med. J.* 297, 1374.

Vessey, M.P. and Mann, J.I. (1978). Female sex hormones and thrombosis – epidemiological aspects. *Br. Med. Bull.* 34, 157.

Walker, A.M. and Jick, H. (1980). Predictors of bleeding during heparin therapy. *JAMA* 244, 1209.

Walker, M.G., Shaw, J.W., Thomson, G.J.L., Cumming, J.G.R., and Lea Thomas, M. (1987). Subcutaneous calcium heparin versus intravenous sodium heparin in treatment of established acute deep vein thrombosis of the legs: a multicentre prospective randomised trial. *Br. Med. J.* 294, 1189.

Weiss, P., Soff, G.A., Halkin, M., and Seligsohn, U. (1987). Decline of proteins C and S and factor II, VII, IX and X during initiation of warfarin therapy. *Thromb. Res.* 45, 783.

23. Effect of drugs on infections

D. M. DAVIES

Introduction

Some drugs can aggravate existing infections, reactivate quiescent infections, or predispose to new infections. They do this by weakening host defences against the micro-organisms; changing the environment of the organisms, so facilitating their multiplication; encouraging the emergence of more virulent organisms; or by making treatment with antimicrobial drugs less effective.

The host is protected against infection by the barriers presented to micro-organisms by properly functioning organs, and by intact skin and mucosal surfaces and the antimicrobial properties of the secretions produced by these. Other defences include active white blood cells and tissue macrophages; a lymphatic system of adequate mass and function; and effective inflammatory and immune responses. Drugs can undermine these defences in several ways. Some diminish the mass of lymphoid tissue, change the number and behaviour of white blood cells, reduce the intensity of the inflammatory reaction, and alter the immune response. A variety of drugs may damage blood-forming tissues, so reducing the number of circulating polymorphonuclear cells, while other agents induce changes in the function or response of these cells or of macrophages. Preparations of sex hormones may cause alterations in bodily structure and biochemistry that appear to predispose to infection. Antibacterial therapy alters the pattern of the body's bacterial flora, and this may lead to multiplication of drug-resistant organisms normally kept in check by force of numbers of their drug-susceptible fellows. Treatment with antibacterial drugs may also be responsible for changes within bacterial species, whereby resistant organisms flourish while drug-sensitive strains die out; and the survivors may possibly be more invasive than were the dead; and some resistant organisms are capable of transferring their powers of resistance to previously vulnerable neighbours.

Some of these actions deserve further consideration. Corticotrophin and adrenal glucocorticoids (but not deoxycorticosterone) damage lymphocytes and reduce the mass of lymphoid tissue (Sayers and Travis 1970). Under the influence of steroid therapy the number of circulating eosinophils diminishes and the migration and activity of phagocytes are impeded. The inflammatory process, characterized by oedema and capillary dilatation followed by capillary and fibroblast proliferation, collagen deposition and, finally, scar formation, is inhibited (Spain 1961). In man, antibody production is not inhibited as it is in some animal species, and other elements of the immune response also remain unimpaired; but delayed hypersensitivity is suppressed (Sayers and Travis 1970).

Most antineoplastic agents act, by various mechanisms, on cell growth; and some that are used for immunosuppression are particularly active in preventing lymphocyte proliferation and function. Such actions explain why these drugs suppress bone marrow activity, damage immunologically competent cells, and impair the immune response, so making patients more susceptible to infections of all kinds. These infections are not necessarily prevented by nursing such patients in a sterile environment, since the infecting organisms often come from the patient's own respiratory tract or gut (Lessof 1972). Some of these drugs also change certain elements of the inflammatory response in tissues. As examples: povidone–iodine, applied locally, may inhibit leucocyte migration and fibroblast aggregation in wounds (Vilijanto 1980); nitrogen mustard interferes with the release of lactic acid by phagocytes (Walter and Israel 1974), so diminishing their effectiveness against some micro-organisms; indomethacin impairs the mobility of polymorphonuclear leucocytes, while diclofenac aggravates the impairment of bactericidal activity present in rheumatoid arthritis (Youinou and Le Goff 1987); cimetidine reduces the number of suppressor/cytotoxic lymphocytes in mice (Osband et al. 1981), an observation that may have implications in human disease; Intralipid, a lipid emulsion used for parenteral nutrition, has been shown to impair the clearance of bacteria from the circulation and to enhance the virulence of bacteria in animals, and to inhibit the chemotaxis of human neutrophil leucocytes *in vitro*, and these findings suggest that the emulsion may increase the risk of bacterial infection in some patients (Fischer *et al.* 1980), as well as fungal infections (see below); iron–dextran appears to have an effect on macrophage activity, possibly because of the large dextran complexes present in the plasma (Becroft *et al.* 1977).

The relationship between infection and iron and desferrioxamine is a complex and fascinating one (*Lancet* 1974; Sussman 1974; Bullen *et al.* 1978). Some workers have claimed that iron-deficient human infants have an increased susceptibility to infection (Arbeter *et al.* 1971), possibly because of impaired cellular immunity (Joynson *et al.* 1972; MacDougall *et al.* 1975) and disturbances in granulocyte function (Chandra 1944; Likhite *et al.* 1976; Yetgin *et al.* 1979; Swarup-Mitra and Sinha 1982). Lymphocyte function and the immune response may also be impaired in iron deficiency; but, paradoxically, Masawe and others (1974) have pointed out that iron deficiency appears to protect against some infections. To complicate matters further, Masawe and colleagues (1974) drew attention to experiments *in vitro* and in laboratory animals (e.g. Fletcher and Goldstein 1970) demonstrating that elemental iron promotes the growth, multiplication, and virulence of many micro-organisms; and it is well recognized that patients with iron overload are more susceptible than normal subjects to a variety of infections. The implications of these relationships as regards medical treatment are considered further under some of the specific infections discussed below.

It has long been known that tears, saliva, and nasal secretions have antibacterial properties (Wilson and Miles 1955). It has also been observed that nasal secretions carry antibodies to certain viruses (Allison 1972). It would not therefore be surprising if impaired secretion of tears predisposed to infection of the eyes, and reduced production of saliva to infection of the buccal mucosa and salivary glands, and clinical experience suggests that this is so. Elderly patients under treatment with drugs with anticholinergic properties (for example, tricyclic antidepressants) are prone to develop oral and lingual ulcers (Hall 1972), and it may be that these are infective in origin; but as yet there is no evidence that treatment with drugs that reduce nasal secretion predisposes to viral infections.

Antimicrobial properties have also long been attributed to another bodily secretion, gastric juice. In 1933 Kemps presented evidence to show that certain infections occur more commonly in people with hypochlorhydria than in those with normal gastric acid secretion, and in the following year Hurst, physician to Guy's Hospital, suggested that British servicemen due to be posted to the tropics should have gastric test meals and not be sent abroad if they had achlorhydria, which would make them vulnerable to certain tropical infections. The question of whether or not the reduction of gastric acidity produced by drugs used for this purpose may predispose to infection by ingested organisms normally destroyed by gastric acid has been the subject of much discussion (Steffen 1977; *British Medical Journal* 1978). Some workers (Ruddell *et al.* 1980; Deane *et al.* 1982; Stockbrugger *et al.* 1981) have found significant alteration in the pattern of gastric microflora during cimetidine treatment, while others (Milton-Thompson *et al.* 1982) have detected no such change. Clinical observations relating to this vexed question are discussed below under specific infections.

Almost all the adverse effects described in this chapter are the result of either the normal pharmacological action or the known chemical properties of the drugs concerned and can therefore be regarded as Type A reactions (see Chapter 3).

Bacterial infections

Some years after the introduction of the antibiotics, the emergence and spread of organisms (particularly staphylococci) resistant to many or all of the antibiotics available at the time became a serious problem. It has been observed that a high incidence of antibiotic-resistant organisms is often related to usage of a particular antibiotic (Knight and Holzer 1954; Alder and Gillespie 1967), and that a reduction in the use of an antibiotic is often followed by a reduction in the frequency with which resistant strains are isolated (Kirby and Ahern 1953). If the use of antibiotics brings about an increase in population of resistant organisms, then this effect can be regarded as a drug reaction, though not an *adverse* reaction unless it can be shown that resistant organisms are more invasive (that is, more likely to cause new cases of infection) than non-resistant strains. Some studies (Williams *et al.* 1959, 1960; Barber *et al.* 1960; Jessen *et al.* 1959; McDonald *et al.* 1960) suggest that this may be the case.

An interesting change in bacterial metabolism following prolonged antibacterial therapy has been reported (Maskell *et al.* 1976). Patients given long-term, low-dose treatment with co-trimoxazole (sulphamethoxazole–trimethoprim) have occasionally been found to have become infected with bacteria dependent on thymine or thymidine for growth, and resistant to co-trimoxazole. The organisms may survive *in vivo* because of the availability of thymine in the infected tissues; but they may not grow on culture media deficient in thymine, and this fact may be misinterpreted as meaning that the organisms are fully sensitive to the antibacterial agents against which they are being tested.

The factors that determine the emergence of strains of micro-organisms resistant to one or more antibacterial drugs are very complex, and for further information the reader is referred to comprehensive reviews (Brumfitt and Hamilton-Miller 1987), but there seems little doubt that excessive and inappropriate use of these drugs, particularly those with a very broad spectrum of activity, aggravates the situation and has led to the emergence of resistant organisms not only of familiar species but also those rarely encountered as pathogens in earlier times (e.g. *Acinetobacter* spp., *Corynebacterium jeikeium*, *Pseudomonas maltophila*, *Serratia* spp., and *Staphylococcus epidermidis*) which are now responsible for serious infections at a variety of sites (Midtvedt 1989). Restricted and circumspect administration tends to reduce the development of resistant organisms.

It has been known for some time that there is an increased incidence of complications during and after surgical operations in patients undergoing long-term steroid therapy (Winstone and Brooke 1961; Hill *et al.* 1967; Russell 1968; Ehrlich and Hunt 1969; Ginn 1969); and Engquist and others (1974) have shown that operations performed under 'steroid cover' are more likely to be followed by wound infection than operations on patients not so treated. Steroids, and also non-steroidal anti-inflammatory drugs, have also been shown to increase the risk of serious complications of operative treatment for diverticular disease of the colon, so that caution should be exercised when prescribing such drugs for patients with a history of diverticulosis (Corder 1987), and it is suggested that these drugs impair the ability of the colon to limit or terminate inflammatory processes occurring within diverticula or, alternatively or in addition, may mask symptoms, so that patients present with more advanced disease.

Staphylococcal infections

Broad-spectrum antibiotics, notably the tetracyclines, so alter the normal flora of the gut that pathogenic organisms resistant to the drugs may multiply inordinately for want of competition from their absent friends.

Staphylococcal diarrhoea and enterocolitis are well-recognized complications of treatment with broad-spectrum antibacterial drugs such as the tetracyclines, the combination of penicillin and streptomycin (Cook *et al.* 1957), neomycin (Tisdale *et al.* 1960), and kanamycin (Finegold and Gaylor 1960), not only when these drugs are given orally but also when they are given parenterally (Lundsgaard-Hansen *et al.* 1960) if some of the drug is excreted into the gut (as is the case with the tetracyclines). Staphylococcal enterocolitis is a very serious complication, with a mortality rate as high as 60 per cent (Spaulding 1962). Fortunately, in recent times the disease is said to have virtually disappeared, and it has been suggested that some of the cases attributed to *Staphylococcus aureus* may have been caused by *Clostridium difficile* (Phillips and Eykyn 1987). It should still, however, be included in the differential diagnosis (though less likely than infection with *Cl. difficile* — see below) when the condition of a patient who was previously making good progress deteriorates abruptly and anorexia, and abdominal pain or distension develop or worsen. Other infections due to resistant staphylococci that may follow antibacterial therapy include acute arthritis, osteomyelitis, parotitis, pneumonia, endocarditis, and septicaemia (Smith 1964).

Staphylococcal infections may also complicate treatment with corticosteroids (Clifton and Stuart-Harris 1962; Berntsen and Freyberg 1961), and immunosuppressive drugs (Andrews and Bagshawe 1966; Smith and Cleve 1957), and have followed the use of indomethacin for closure of patent ductus arteriosus in premature infants (Hersen *et al.* 1988).

During treatment of acne vulgaris with isotretinoin, marked changes occur in the skin, including almost total suppression of sebum production which, in turn, leads to dryness, inflammatory changes, and alteration in the bacterial population. The organism present in acne, *Propionibacterium acnes*, falls significantly in number, together with Gram-negative commensals. Colonization of the skin and anterior nares with *Staphylococcus aureus* follows in most patients, of whom a relatively small proportion develop folliculitis, furuncles, or even cellulitis, usually during or shortly after a course of treatment (Leyden and James 1987). Paronychia and pyogenic granuloma-like lesions may also arise (Blumenthal 1984).

Streptococcal infections

In animal experiments it has been shown that streptococcal infection of blood and tissues is markedly enhanced following cortisone injections (Mogabgab and Thomas

1950). Streptococcal infection commonly arises in patients suffering from drug-induced agranulocytosis, and may complicate treatment with steroids or cytotoxic drugs. Unlike staphylococcal infection, it can rarely, if ever, be attributed to antibacterial therapy.

Infection with *E. coli* and other Gram-negative organisms

These bacteria have always been less susceptible to antibacterial drugs than Gram-positive organisms, but whether there has been any great increase in resistant strains is uncertain, and there is little evidence to suggest that resistant Gram-negative organisms are essentially more virulent than the drug-sensitive strains. It does seem, however, that with the increasing use of broad-spectrum antibiotics there has been an increase in the prevalence of serious infections that are caused by Gram-negative organisms (Finland *et al.* 1959). Treatment with an antibacterial drug may occasionally be complicated by infection with coliform organisms resistant to this and other drugs. Septicaemia may occur and has a high mortality rate (Smith 1964). Coliform infections may also complicate long-term treatment with corticosteroid drugs and immunosuppressive agents (Altemeier *et al.* 1967).

Ureteric dilatation analogous to that occurring in pregnancy is seen in some patients taking oral contraceptives (Marshall *et al.* 1966; Guyer and Delany 1970), and in some cases this appears to predispose to infection with coliform organisms.

Other Gram-negative organisms causing septicaemia in association with treatment with antibacterial agents or immunosuppressants, or (in premature infants given this drug for closure of a patent ductus arteriosus) indomethacin (Hersen *et al.* 1988), are *Klebsiella* spp., *Pseudomonas* spp., *Paracolon* bacteria, and *Proteus* spp. (Smith 1964).

It has been observed (Evans *et al.* 1967) that when corticosteroid creams, ointments, or sprays are used to treat varicose ulcers, these often increase rapidly in size and depth and commonly become severely infected with *Ps. aeruginosa (Ps. pyocyanea)*. Antibiotics or antibacterial substances contained in some preparations of this kind fail to prevent these secondary infections. While topical corticosteroids can be valuable in the treatment of stasis eczema, it is most important to prevent the medicament from entering any abrasion or ulcer within the treated area.

Barry and Reeve (1974) have observed a high incidence of Gram-negative sepsis in Polynesian babies given injections of iron-dextran soon after birth as pro-

phylactic or curative treatment for iron-deficiency anaemia. When this treatment was abandoned there was a dramatic fall in the incidence of infection. These workers suggest that iron given in this way may overcome immune mechanisms and promote infection (see earlier), and they advise against this method of treatment.

Salmonellosis

The suggestion that treatment with cimetidine (or, presumably, other H_2-receptor blocking agents, omeprazole, and the mineral antacids) might predispose to infection with salmonellae and to certain other infections is discussed below under the heading Brucellosis.

Cholera

The possibility that patients taking drugs that reduce gastric acidity might be more susceptible to infection with *Vibrio cholerae* or certain other infections is discussed below under the heading Brucellosis.

Helicobacter pylori (formerly *Campylobacter pyloridis*) infection

The question of whether or not duodenal ulcer is an infective disease caused by this curved or spiral Gram-negative bacterium remains unanswered, but it has been shown that some effects of tripotassium dicitratobismuthate, the most effective agent in eliminating the organism from the stomach and duodenum, are abolished by aspirin. The clinical relevance of this observation, however, is not apparent. For a helpful review and discussion of the whole problem the reader is referred to an editorial in the *Proceedings of the Royal College of Physicians of Edinburgh* (1990).

Clostridial infections

Pseudomembranous colitis is an uncommon infection of the colon caused by *Clostridium difficile*. As a natural disease it may, rarely, occur in otherwise healthy people or, more often, in patients already suffering from some predisposing condition such as chronic colonic obstruction or carcinoma, leukaemia, or uraemia (Larson 1987). Most frequently, however, it complicates treatment with antimicrobial drugs: clindamycin and lincomycin are the commonest culprits, followed by ampicillin and amoxicillin; but almost all commonly used antimicrobial agents have been implicated at times, including, paradoxically, vancomycin (Miller and Ringler 1987; Hecht and Olinger 1989) and metronidazole (Daly and Chowdary 1983), which are the drugs of first and second choice, respectively, for the treatment of the condition.

Drugs other than antimicrobials that have been suspected of having induced *Cl. difficile* colitis are cytarabine (Roda 1987) and a combination of cytotoxic agents used to treat ovarian carcinoma (Satin *et al.* 1989); and a case without evidence of *Cl. difficile* infection but firmly diagnosed by colonoscopy and biopsy has been attributed to the antidiabetic drug chlorpropamide (Gupta and Sachar 1985). This subject is also discussed in Chapter 10.

Yersinia enterocolitica infections

It is known that patients with iron overload are prone to systemic yersiniosis (Robins-Browne *et al.* 1978; Hoen *et al.* 1988), a condition that rarely, if ever, occurs in patients with normal iron stores, and long-term iron therapy has been associated with liver abscess caused by this organism (Leighton and MacSween 1987). But, paradoxically, the treatment of iron overload with desferrioxamine also appears to predispose to this disorder, the suggested explanation being that the supply of exogenous siderophores, such as desferrioxamine, enables the organism to overcome the handicap of being unable to synthesize iron-binding components (Robins-Browne and Prpic 1983).

Legionella infections

The case of a patient under treatment with cyclosporin for rheumatoid arthritis who developed legionnaires' disease attributed to the drug therapy has been reported (Pillemer *et al.* 1989).

Brucellosis

It was suggested some time ago that the risk of contracting brucellosis might be increased during treatment with the older antacids (Steffen 1977; *British Medical Journal* 1978) and, more recently, a case has been described in which a young man taking cimetidine contracted brucellosis (*Br. melitensis*) by eating infected cheese that proved harmless to other members of his family (Cristiano and Paradisi 1982). Presumably, treatment with other drugs that reduce gastric acidity might also predispose to this disorder, as well as to such serious intestinal infections as cholera and salmonellosis; and omeprazole has certainly been implicated in recurrent enteric infection (Littman 1990). It should, however, be noted that as far as brucellosis and cimetidine are concerned an expla-

nation not involving reduction of gastric acidity has been put forward by Thorne (1982), namely that cimetidine lowers the number of suppressor/cytotoxic T lymphocytes with consequent acute exacerbation of latent or chronic brucellosis.

Listeriosis

Meningitis caused by *Listeria monocytogenes* has occurred as a complication of therapy with steroids (Sobrevilla *et al.* 1962) and with antilymphocyte globulin (Girmenia *et al.* 1988).

Nocardiosis

This disorder, a systemic infection caused by a Grampositive filamentous bacterium, has been associated with a variety of malignant and autoimmune diseases, chronic lung conditions, diabetes, plasma protein abnormalities, and certain rare diseases of other types (Mitchell 1987). In some cases, treatment with cytotoxic drugs, corticosteroids, or immunosuppressive agents appears to have increased the risk of infection, and a case in which low-dose methotrexate for rheumatoid arthritis was suggested as a cause has been reported (Keegan and Byrd 1988).

Tuberculosis

Experiments in animals demonstrated that tuberculosis infection worsened when the infected animal was given adrenal corticosteroids in large doses (D'Arcy Hart and Rees 1950; Spain and Molamut 1950), and subsequent studies suggested that the disease in man could be induced, reactivated, or aggravated by corticosteroid therapy (Fred *et al.* 1951; Harris-Jones and Pein 1952; Mackinnon 1959; King *et al.* 1951; Popp *et al.* 1951). This risk came to be regarded as a considerable one, but after analysing data supplied by 50 chest physicians in England, Scotland, and Wales for the years 1959 and 1960, Mayfield (1962) concluded that in this country during the years under review corticosteroid therapy had not made any significant contribution either to the incidence of new cases of tuberculosis or to the relapse rate of old cases, and he failed to find any striking evidence of especially acute or insidious disease. Nevertheless, he agreed that British experience might not reflect exactly the situation elsewhere, and he suggested that a careful search (including a chest X-ray) should be made for past or present tuberculosis before corticosteroid treatment is started; that chest X-rays should be repeated periodically throughout treatment and for a year thereafter; and that in some cases, notably when old tuberculosis lesions are present, cover of corticosteroid treatment by antituberculous drugs should be considered.

Following a more recent study, in a population with a high prevalence of tuberculosis (Cowie and King 1987), it was concluded that the risk of tuberculosis in asthmatics, attributable to corticosteroid therapy, is not great enough to justify the routine use of antituberculosis prophylaxis.

Mixed bacterial infections

Respiratory infections

The risk of non-specific respiratory tract infections among previously healthy recruits to the Singapore armed services increased during prophylactic antimalarial therapy with a combination of dapsone and pyrimethamine (Maloprim), particularly while they were engaged in strenuous physical activity, and it was suggested that the antimalarial combination caused some degree of immunosuppression (Lee and Lau 1988).

Hidradenitis suppurativa

Some cases of hidradenitis suppurativa, the term applied to recurrent boils affecting the axillary apocrine sweat glands, anogenital area, and breasts, and caused by a variety of anaerobic bacteria, have been attributed, fairly convincingly, to the use of combined oral contraceptives (Stellon and Wakeling 1989).

Muscle abscesses

Abscesses, some sterile and some containing mixed organisms, have long been known to follow the intramuscular injection of such irritant drugs as paraldehyde and quinine, and a more recent example involved chloroquine (Ahmed and Fahal 1989).

Pyoderma

Atypical pyoderma of the nose, caused by a mixture of staphylococci and streptococci has occurred in a patient under treatment with isotretinoin (Helpern 1985).

Viral infections

The defences against viral infection include the natural resistance of cells at the primary site of infection, the activity of macrophages, and the effects of circulating antibody and cell-mediated immunity (Allison 1972). Drugs may interfere with one or more of these protective mechanisms.

In monkeys infected with smallpox, viraemia persisted longer in those concurrently treated with steroids than in those not so treated, and deaths from the infection were confined to the steroid-treated animals, three-quarters of which died (Rao et al. 1968). In mice, the severity of viral hepatitis is increased by treatment with corticosteroids (Datta and Isselbacher 1969). In other experiments it was shown that the multiplication of Coxsackie virus and the viruses of poliomyelitis, Rift Valley fever, and encephalomyelitis was enhanced by corticosteroids or ACTH (Findley and Howard 1952).

In man, corticosteroid therapy appears to increase the severity of established herpes zoster (Irons 1964; Eckhardt and Hebard 1961; Merselis et al. 1964), herpes simplex (Montgomerie et al. 1969; Diderholm et al. 1969; Wiest et al. 1989), ocular herpes simplex (Crompton 1965), chickenpox (Domart et al. 1964; Roschlau 1967; Finkel 1961; Hennemann 1960; Lust et al. 1960; Weinstein 1962), and vaccinia (MacKenzie et al. 1969). Corticosteroid therapy may also predispose to poliomyeltis and cytomegalovirus infection (Wiest et al. 1989). Vaccination against smallpox may result in severe gangrenous vaccinia in patients taking corticosteroids (Levy 1969).

In animals, immunosuppression by cyclophosphamide potentiates the infectivity and ill-effects of some members of the arborvirus, enterovirus, and herpesvirus groups (Allison 1972). In man, infection with herpes zoster, herpes simplex, varicella, cytomegalovirus, measles, or the Epstein–Barr virus has complicated treatment with immunosuppressive drugs such as azathioprine, cyclosporin, methotrexate, and the murine monoclonal antibody muromonab-CD3 (OKT3), often combined with corticosteroids (Meadow et al. 1969; Montgomerie et al. 1969; Lessof 1972; D'Arcy and Griffin 1972; British Medical Journal 1976; Pullan et al. 1976; Lewis et al. 1978; Mayer et al. 1988; Franson et al. 1987; Ren and Chan 1988; Junker et al. 1989).

It has been known for years that exposure to trichloroethylene, in industry or during general anaesthesia, is occasionally followed by neuropathy of the trigeminal nerve. It has been generally accepted that the cause is a direct toxic effect of the chemical on some part of the nerve tract, though as far back as 1944 Humphrey and McClelland suspected that the lesion might be due to an indirect effect of the chemical in reactivating latent herpes simplex infection of the nerve; but they were not able to prove their hypothesis because of the inadequacy of investigative methods available at that time. Much more recently the problem has been readdressed by Cavanagh and Buxton (1989), who present detailed and very convincing evidence of the involvement of the virus in the induction of trigeminal palsies following trichloroethylene exposure.

Fungal infections

Candida infections of mouth, oesophagus, gut, and anus may occur during treatment with antibiotics (Dunlop and Murdoch 1960), usually, but not invariably (Hachiya *et al*. 1982), those with a broad antibacterial spectrum, and some observers believe that such infections remain confined to the mucosal surfaces unless the patient is also being treated with corticosteroids (Torack 1957). Other workers (Braude and Rock 1959) have observed, however, that systemic candidiasis can be precipitated by antibiotics alone in debilitated patients (Harrell and Thompson 1958; Braude and Rock 1959). According to Symmers (1966), broad-spectrum antibiotics have little effect on susceptibility to fungal infections other than candidiasis or, more rarely, geotrichosis.

Oral and oesphageal or laryngeal candidiasis may complicate treatment with corticotrophin or corticosteroids when they are given systemically, or may occur when aerosol sprays containing such steroids as dexamethasone and beclomethasone are used for the treatment of asthma (Dennis and Itkin 1964; Hayes 1965; McAllen *et al*. 1974; Milne and Crompton 1974; Kesten *et al*. 1988; Salzman and Pyszczynski 1988), but it is claimed that children are relatively immune to this complication (Godfrey *et al*. 1974). Acute disseminated candidiasis has complicated long-term corticosteroid therapy (Boyd and Chappell 1961) and combined treatment with corticosteroids and antibiotics (Bendel and Rade 1961).

Other fungal infections attributed to ACTH or corticosteroid therapy include pulmonary aspergillosis (Nabarro 1960; Sidransky and Pearl 1961; Wiest *et al*. 1989), coccidioidomycosis (Aguardo *et al*. 1988), cryptococcosis (Goldstein and Rambo 1962; Bennington *et al*. 1964; Jacobs 1963; Meyler 1966; Wiest *et al*. 1989), histoplasmosis (Dismukes *et al*. 1978), mucormycosis (phycomycosis, zygomycosis) (Hutter 1959; Rex *et al*. 1988; Sane *et al*. 1989), and sporotrichosis (Kaufman 1962).

Immunosuppressive therapy in organ transplantation has been held responsible for aspergillosis and candidiasis (Lessof 1972); and low-dose methotrexate therapy has been associated with cryptococcosis (Altz-Smith *et al*. 1987).

Cases of mucormycosis (phycomycosis, zygomycosis), some fatal, have occurred in patients treated with desferrioxamine during long-term haemodialysis (Veis *et al*. 1987; Sombolos *et al*. 1988; Daly *et al*. 1989).

There has been controversy over the role of oral contraceptives in genital candidiasis. Yaffee and Grots (1965) suggested that these drugs predisposed to vulval and vaginal candidiasis, often resistant to treatment, but this has been disputed by Morris and Morris (1969) and

Lazan (1971), and by Davidson and Oates (1985) who studied patients from three different centres over a period of 8 years and found no correlation between oral contraceptive use and genital candidal infection.

Stark and others (1978) have suggested that previous treatment with cimetidine predisposes to *Candida* peritonitis in patients with perforated ulcer, but Hassan and Browne (1978) disputed this. Triger and colleagues (1981) comment that suppression of gastric acid production may permit overgrowth of *Candida* within the gastrointestinal tract, and they describe three cases of systemic candidiasis complicating acute hepatic failure in patients treated with cimetidine.

Kochar and others (1988) described a patient whose duodenal ulcer, which had failed to heal after treatment with cimetidine for 3 months, was found to have been infiltrated with *Candida albicans*. The lesion began to heal satisfactorily when ranitidine was substituted for cimetidine and the antifungal drug nystatin was added to the treatment regimen. The authors postulated that in this case the reduction of gastric acidity together with the effects of cimetidine on the immune system and on leucocyte function were responsible for invasive candidiasis. Earlier, Minoli and colleagues (1987) had claimed that short-term cimetidine therapy is not complicated by invasive candidiasis.

A number of cases have been reported in which patients receiving prolonged intravenous infusions of nutrients such as amino acids and lipids ('intravenous hyperalimentation') developed *Candida* septicaemia (Curry and Quie 1971; Vogel *et al*. 1972). This type of treatment probably predisposes to infection because of the long duration of intravenous cannulation, but why in these circumstances the risk of fungal infection is much greater than that of bacterial infection is uncertain.

Application of steroids to the skin, particularly under occlusive dressings, may predispose to local fungal infections (Gill *et al*. 1963), sometimes atypical in appearance and size (Peterkin and Khan 1969; Ive and Marks 1968).

Protozoal infections

Experiments in animals have demonstrated that the effects of protozoal infections are aggravated by corticosteroid therapy (Kass and Finland 1953). In man, amoebiasis has been attributed to steroid therapy (Eisert *et al*. 1959) and activation of latent amoebic infections has also been described (Mody 1959; Stuiver and Goud 1978; Amin 1978). Indeed, in countries in which amoebiasis is endemic, it is now considered prudent to endeavour to exclude occult intestinal amoebiasis before using steroids more than briefly (de Glanville, personal communication). Infection with *Pneumocystis carinii* has followed treatment with ACTH (Aguardo *et al.* 1988; Goetting 1986); corticosteroids (Woodward and Sheldon 1961; Kozeny *et al.* 1987); immunosuppressive agents (Lessof 1972), including methotrexate used in low doses for rheumatoid arthritis (Perruquet *et al.* 1983); antilymphoma therapy (Browne *et al.* 1986); and desferrioxamine (Kouides *et al.* 1988). As far as some of the immunosuppressant agents are concerned, findings in patients infected with the human immunodeficiency virus may be relevant: it has been shown that the risk of these patients developing *Pneumocystis carinii* pneumonia is closely linked to the absolute count of CD4 cells in the blood, a count of less than 200 cells per mm^3 making infection very likely (Phair *et al.* 1990). The use of antilymphocyte globulin, antithymocyte globulin and, particularly, OKT3 will produce a similar effect and may explain differing incidences of this infection in different populations of transplant recipients.

Reactivation of latent cryptosporidial infection has been attributed to diarrhoea induced by the laxative docusate calcium and the antibiotic erythromycin in a diabetic patient (Holley and Thiers 1986). The erythromycin was replaced by cephalexin, and the patient was also given prednisone and azathioprine, so it is difficult to decide which of these drugs was the culprit.

Toxoplasmosis may complicate treatment with immunosuppressive drugs and may be due to reactivation of organisms lying dormant in the patient's own tissues. It should be suspected when unexplained fever or focal neurological signs appear in patients under treatment with these drugs (Cohen 1970).

Szanto (1971) reported a case in which *Trichomonas vaginalis* infection appeared to follow systemic administration of oxytetracycline, and responded to treatment with metronidazole only after the oxytetracycline was withheld. He suggested that oxytetracycline might have interfered in some way with the action of metronidazole.

It now seems firmly established that there is a relationship between iron and amoebiasis. It has been shown experimentally (Latour and Reeves 1965; Diamond *et al.* 1978) that *Entamoeba histolytica* needs iron for growth, has a high requirement for the element, and obtains it from the host. It might therefore be expected that an excess of body iron would increase susceptibility to amoebiasis, while iron deficiency would protect against infection (unless outweighed by the impairment of certain bodily defences against infection, thought to occur in iron deficiency — see earlier); and these expectations appear to have been fulfilled. Iron overload was found to be commoner in black Africans who had died of amoe-

biasis than in the general population (Bothwell *et al.* 1984). Iron deficiency, on the other hand, appeared to protect against amoebiasis in milk-drinking African nomads, and when some of these subjects were treated with oral iron the infection rate rose sharply, but this did not happen when the iron was given by injection (Murray *et al.* 1980), and it was concluded that it is the intestinal content of iron rather than the iron state of the body as a whole that is important in controlling the growth of *Entamoeba histolytica*.

It has also been observed that there is a tendency for malarial infections to occur or flare up when iron deficiency anaemia is treated (Masawe *et al.* 1974; Murray *et al.* 1975; Murray *et al.* 1978), and injections of iron-dextran (Imferon) in infants appeared to increase their chances of contracting malaria (Oppenheimer *et al.* 1984). (See also above under Infection with *E. coli* and other Gram-negative organisms.)

Nematode infections

In some parts of the world infection with *Strongyloides stercoralis* is encouraged by treatment with corticosteroids and immunosuppressive drugs (Cruz *et al.* 1966; Purtilo *et al.* 1974) or corticosteroids alone (Higenbottam and Heard 1976); and a case has also been described in which an existing infection was thought to have been aggravated by treatment with cimetidine in a patient undergoing chemotherapy for lymphoma (Ainley *et al.* 1986). The disease may manifest itself by gastrointestinal discomfort, diarrhoea, pruritus, urticaria, pneumonia, and pulmonary infarction with haemoptysis, and widespread dissemination of larvae may prove fatal.

Arthropod infestation

Of several members of a family suffering from Norwegian scabies, only one proved refractory to benzyl benzoate therapy. This patient was also under treatment with etretinate, and it was postulated that reduction of skin sebum, a recognized effect of etretinate, enhanced susceptibility to the infestation, since it is known that *S scabiei* favours areas of skin in which sebum secretion is minimal (Zlotogorski and Leibovici 1987).

Interference with the efficacy of antimicrobial therapy

Some drugs may harm patients suffering from infections by reducing the effectiveness of other drugs being used in treatment. (See also Chapter 3.)

Antibiotic combinations

Chloramphenicol, a bacteriostatic drug, weakens the bactericidal action of penicillin in pneumococcal meningitis in animals (Wallace *et al*. 1965), and tetracycline has the same effect on the disease in man (Lepper and Dowling 1951). Staphylococci sensitive to lincomycin but resistant to erythromycin become less susceptible to the first of these drugs when the second is administered concurrently (Griffith *et al*. 1965). In streptococcal infections, penicillin has been found to be more effective than erythromycin, while a combination of these drugs was the least successful form of treatment (Strom 1955). Neomycin and kanamycin reduce the absorption of orally administered penicillin (Cheng and White 1962). The antibacterial effect of gentamicin is reduced by benzylpenicillin and by carbenicillin (McLaughlin and Reeves 1971), which has the same effect on kanamycin (Stockley 1974) and ticarcillin (Bint and Burtt 1980), but it has been suggested that this interaction is not likely to be clinically significant except in patients with severe renal impairment in whom prolonged high concentrations of the penicillin would be expected and doses would be given infrequently (Bint and Burtt 1980). In laboratory experiments nitrofurantoin reduces the antibacterial effect of nalidixic acid on a variety of Gram-negative bacteria (Stille and Ostner 1966; Piguet 1969).

Other drug combinations

When phenobarbitone is given at the same time as griseofulvin, the serum concentrations of the antifungal drug may be lower than when it is given alone (Busfield *et al*. 1963; Riegelman *et al*. 1970), and its therapeutic effect may be impaired (Lorenc 1967). It has been postulated that an increased rate of metabolism of griseofulvin by hepatic microsomal enzymes stimulated (induced) by phenobarbitone is to blame, but an alternative explanation is that phenobarbitone decreases absorption of griseofulvin by stimulating bile secretion, which in turn stimulates peristalsis (Stockley 1974).

The absorption of tetracyclines is reduced by antacids containing bismuth, calcium, magnesium, or aluminium salts, and by calcium-containing foods. This effect is probably due to tight chemical binding of the antibiotic to the antacid (chelation), but it is possible that alteration in gastrointestinal pH plays a part (Stockley 1974), since sodium bicarbonate also markedly reduces absorption of tetracyclines (Barr *et al*. 1971). Aluminium compounds also impair the absorption of isoniazid when they are given concurrently, so an interval should be left between the administration of the two medicines; and both aluminium and magnesium antacids impair absorp-

tion of 4-quinolone antibacterial drugs (especially ciprofloxacin), so that these groups of drugs should not be given within 2–4 hours of each other. Ferrous sulphate has a similar effect on tetracycline absorption (Neuvonen *et al*. 1970), due to chelation, but the clinical importance of this interaction has been questioned (Bateman 1970), and further doubt about its clinical relevance has been raised by retrospective studies of the efficacy of tetracyclines in patients who were taking iron tablets (Crooks *et al*. 1977). Some of these interactions can be avoided if the drugs are given separately at an interval of 3 hours or more (Gothoni *et al*. 1972).

It has been shown experimentally that cyclamates, present as sweetening agents in a variety of food and drink, reduce the absorption of lincomycin (Wagner 1969), but whether or not this is clinically relevant is uncertain (Stockley 1974). The absorption of lincomycin is also impaired by kaolin (Wagner 1961), which might well be prescribed for symptomatic treatment at the same time as the antibiotic is being used as a specific remedy. An interval of 2 hours, however, between the administration of the drugs prevented the interaction (Wagner 1968) (see also Bint and Burtt 1980, and Chapter 30).

Sulphonamides inhibit bacterial growth by interference with the uptake by the bacteria of *p*-aminobenzoic acid, but enough of this substance is provided by the metabolic products of the local anaesthetics procaine and benzocaine, and of the 'antifibrotic' drug potassium *p*-aminobenzoate, to overcome this inhibitory effect. Fortunately, the occasions on which this situation is likely to arise are few and far between; nevertheless, the potential interaction should be kept in mind.

Interactions of antimicrobial drugs in infusion solutions

A number of antibacterial agents may be inactivated when dissolved in infusion fluids, either by the fluids themselves or by other drugs added to them. Information on the stability of antibacterial drugs in infusion solutions and possible adverse interactions between drugs added to these fluids is provided by the current *British National Formulary*.

Masking of infection by drugs

The 'masking' of infection by some drugs has been described by Lundsgaard-Hansen (1972) in these terms: 'The temporary, more or less complete suppression of clinical and laboratory signs and symptoms without actual eradication of the basic disease. Following cessation of therapy, the clinical manifestations usually reappear, being often atypical and sometimes deceivingly innocent.'

The problems presented by masking of infection by antibacterial drugs have been outlined by Davies (1979): 'The arrival of the sulphonamides and antibiotics brought new masking hazards. When treated with antibacterial drugs, some abdominal disorders lost their classical diagnostic symptoms and signs. Because of rapid and impressive cures in a few cases, too much was expected of the new drugs; and lulled into an unjustified sense of security, some doctors became *blasé* when dealing with abdominal emergencies, taking less care in their observation of the case and with their diagnosis. Worse, they supposed that conditions for which surgical intervention had hitherto been regarded as mandatory could now be cured by drugs. In consequence, appendices, gall-bladders, and obstructed portions of the gut perforated and intra-abdominal abscesses and peritonitis followed, often with quite atypical symptoms and signs. In other cases the treatment of comparatively trivial infections at one site suppressed their signs and symptoms, and delayed the diagnosis of more severe infections elsewhere in the body, often with very serious results. Thus, the treatment of pharyngitis, sinusitis, or otitis media with antibacterial drugs masked the symptoms and signs of meningitis or of a developing brain abscess, in some cases even rendering angiographic studies unhelpful. Empyema was missed when pneumonia seemed to have responded satisfactorily to treatment. The aetiology of pleural effusion became more difficult to diagnose if the patient had received antibacterial drugs at the onset of the illness, for no longer was an apparently sterile pleural fluid, containing a preponderance of lymphocytes, virtually diagnostic of postprimary tuberculosis in a young patient. Other types of tuberculosis were also masked by short-term treatment of seemingly mild respiratory infections with a popular combination of penicillin and streptomycin. Again, in the early days of antibiotic therapy reports were published of cases in which the treatment of gonorrhoea with penicillin temporarily suppressed, but did not cure, concurrent syphilitic infection.'

Adrenal corticosteroids may not only encourage infections but also disguise them by suppressing the 'calor, rubor, and dolor' of the inflammatory response; and examples of such a happening continue to occur, including the masking of symptoms and signs of diverticulitis (Corder 1987). The same may possibly be true, though to a lesser degree, of the anti-inflammatory drugs phenylbutazone, oxyphenbutazone, and indomethacin,

and the last-named drug is known to have masked the signs of osteomyelitis developing in a patient with rheumatoid arthritis (Block 1972).

Acknowledgement

I am grateful to Dr R. Freeman, Reader in Bacteriology, University of Newcastle upon Tyne, for helpful advice.

References

Aguardo, J.L., Greaves, T., Hutchinson, H.T., and McCarthy, J.M. (1988). Pneumonia in infants given adrenocorticotropic hormone for infantile spasms. *J. Pediatr.* 112, 508.

Ahmed, M.E. and Fahal, A.H. (1989). Acute gluteal abscesses: injectable chloroquine as a cause. *J. Trop. Med. Hyg.* 92, 317.

Ainley, C.C., Clarke, D.G., Timothy, A.R., and Thompson, R.P.H. (1986). *Strongyloides stercoralis* hyperinfection associated with cimetidine in an immunosuppressed patient: diagnosis by endoscopic biopsy. *Gut* 27, 337.

Alder, V.G. and Gillespie, W.A. (1967). Influence of neomycin sprays on the spread of resistant staphylococci. *Lancet* ii, 1062.

Allison, A.C. (1972). Immunity against viruses. In *The scientific basis of medicine, annual reviews* (ed. I. Gilliland and J. Francis), p. 51. Athlone, London.

Altemeier, W.A., Todd, J.C., and Inge, W.W. (1967). Gram-negative septicaemia: a growing threat. *Ann. Surg.* 166, 530.

Altz-Smith, M., Kendall, L.G., and Stamm, A.M. (1987). Cryptococcosis associated with low-dose methotrexate for arthritis. *Am. J. Med.* 83, 179.

Amin, N. (1978). Amoebiasis and corticosteroids. *Br. Med. J.* ii, 1084.

Andrews, H.J. and Bagshawe, K.D. (1966). Acquisition of *Staphylococcus aureus* by patients undergoing cytotoxic therapy in an ultra-clean isolation unit. *J. Hyg. (Camb.)* 64, 501.

Arbeter, A., Echeverri, L., Fraco, D., Munson, D., Velez, H., and Vitale, J.J. (1971). Nutrition and infection. *Fed. Proc.* 30, 1421.

Barber, M., Dutton, A.A.C., Beard, M.A., Elmes, P.C., and Williams, R. (1960). Reversal of antibiotic resistance in hospital staphylococcal infection. *Br. Med. J.* i, 11.

Barr, W.H., Adir, J., and Garrettson, L. (1971). Decrease of tetracycline absorption in man by sodium bicarbonate. *Clin. Pharmacol. Ther.* 12, 779.

Barry, D.M.J. and Reeve, A.W. (1974). Iron and infection in the newborn. *Lancet* ii, 1385.

Bateman, F.J.A. (1970). Effects of tetracyclines. *Br. Med. J.* iv, 802.

Becroft, D.M.O., Dix, M.R., and Farmer, K. (1977). Intramuscular iron-dextran and susceptibility of neonates to bacterial infections. *In vitro* studies. *Arch. Dis. Child.* 52, 778.

Bendel, W.L. and Rade, G.J. (1961). Acute disseminated candidiasis in aplastic anaemia. Potentiation by antibiotics and steroids. *Arch. Intern. Med.* 108, 916.

Bennington, J.L., Haber, S.L., and Morgenstern, N.L. (1964) Increased susceptibility to cryptococcosis following steroid therapy. *Dis. Chest* 45, 262.

Berntsen, C.A. and Freyberg, R.H. (1961). Rheumatoid patients after five or more years of corticosteroid treatment. A comparative analysis of 183 cases. *Ann. Intern. Med.* 54, 938.

Bint, A.J. and Burtt, I. (1980). Adverse antibiotic drug interactions. *Drugs* 20, 57.

Blackman, H.J., Peck, G.L., Olsen, G., and Bergsma, D.R. (1979). Blepharoconjunctivitis: a side effect of 13-*cis*-retinoic acid therapy for dermatologic disease. *Ophthalmology* 86, 753.

Block, S.H. (1972). Indomethacin. *JAMA* 222, 1062.

Blumenthal, G. (1984). Paronychia and pyogenic granuloma-like lesions with isotretinoin. *J. Am. Acad. Derm.* 10, 677.

Bothwell, T.H., Adams, E.B., Simon, M., Isaacson, C., Simjee, A.E., Killichurum, S., *et al.* (1984) The iron status of black subjects with amoebiasis. *S. Afr. Med. J.* 65, 601.

Boyd, J.F. and Chappell, A.G. (1961). Fatal mycetosis due to *Candida albicans* after combined steroid and antibiotic therapy. *Lancet* ii, 19.

Braude, A.L. and Rock, J.A. (1959). The syndrome of acute disseminated moniliasis in adults. *Arch. Intern. Med.* 104, 91.

British Medical Journal (1976). Measles encephalitis during immunosuppressive therapy. *Br. Med. J.* i, 1552.

British Medical Journal (1978). Antacids and brucellosis. *Br. Med. J.* i, 739.

Browne, M.J., Hubbard, S.M., Longo, D.L., Fisher, R., Wesley, R., Ihde, D.C., *et al.* (1986). Excess prevalence of *Pneumocystis carinii* pneumonia in patients treated for lymphoma with combination chemotherapy. *Ann. Intern. Med.* 104, 338.

Brumfitt, W. and Hamilton-Miller, J.M.T. (1987). Principles and practice of antimicrobial chemotherapy. In *Avery's Drug treatment* (3rd edn), (ed. T.M. Speight), p. 1216. Churchill Livingstone, Edinburgh.

Bullen, J.J., Rogers, H.J., and Griffiths, E. (1978). Role of iron in bacterial infection. *Immunology* 80, 1.

Busfield, D., Child, K.J., Atkinson, R.M., and Tomich, E.G. (1963). An effect of phenobarbitone on blood levels of griseofulvin in man. *Lancet* ii, 1042.

Cavanagh, J.B. and Buxton, P.H. (1989). Trichloroethylene cranial neuropathy: is it really a toxic neuropathy or does it activate latent herpes virus? *J. Neurol. Neurosurg. Psychiatry* 52, 297.

Chandra, R.K. (1944). Reduced bactericidal capacity of polymorphs in iron deficiency. *Arch. Dis. Child.* 48, 864.

Cheng, S.H. and White, A. (1962). Effect of orally administered neomycin on the absorption of penicillin V. *N. Engl. J. Med.* 267, 1296.

Clifton, M. and Stuart-Harris, C.H. (1962). Steroid therapy in chronic bronchitis. *Lancet* i, 1311.

Cohen, S.N. (1970). Toxoplasmosis in patients receiving immunosuppressive therapy. *JAMA* 211, 657.

Cook, J., Elliott, C., Elliott-Smith, A., Frisby, B.R., and Gardner, A.M.M. (1957). Staphylococcal diarrhoea; with an account of two outbreaks in the same hospital. *Br. Med. J.* i, 542.

Corder, A. (1987). Steroids, non-steroidal anti-inflammatory drugs, and serious septic complications of diverticular disease. *Br. Med. J.* 295, 1238.

Cowie, R.L. and King, R.M. (1987). Pulmonary tuberculosis in corticosteroid-treated asthmatics. *S. Afr. Med. J.* 72, 849.

Cristiano, P. and Paradisi, F. (1982). Can cimetidine facilitate infections by oral route? *Lancet* ii, 45.

Crompton, D.O. (1965). Corticosteroids exacerbate ocular herpes simplex. *Med. J. Aust.* i, 487.

Crooks, J., Stevenson, I.H., Shepherd, A.M.M., and Muir, D.C. (1977). In *Drug interactions* (ed. D. Grahame-Smith), p. 3. Macmillan, London.

Cruz, T., Reboucas, G., and Rochas, H. (1966). Fatal strongyloidiasis in patients receiving corticosteroids. *N. Engl. J. Med.* 275, 1093.

Curry, C.R. and Quie, P.G. (1971). Fungal septicaemia in patients receiving parenteral hyperalimentation. *N. Engl. J. Med.* 285, 1221.

Daly, A.L., Velaquez, L.A., Bradley, S.F., and Kaufman, C.A. (1989). Mucormycosis: association with deferroxamine therapy. *Am. J. Med.* 87, 768.

Daly, J.J. and Chowdary, K.V.S. (1983). Pseudomembranous colitis secondary to metronidazole. *Dig. Dis. Sci.* 28, 573.

D'Arcy Hart, P. and Rees, R.J.W. (1950). Enhancing effect of cortisone on tuberculosis in the mouse. *Lancet* ii, 391.

D'Arcy, P.F. and Griffin, J.P. (1972). *Iatrogenic diseases.* Oxford University Press.

Datta, D.V. and Isselbacher, K.J. (1969). Effects of corticosteroids on mouse hepatitis virus infection. *Gut* 10, 522.

Davidson, F. and Oates, J.K. (1985). The pill does not cause 'thrush'. *Br. J. Obstet. Gynaecol.* 92, 1265.

Davies, D.M. (1979). In *Topics in therapeutics, No. 5* (ed. D.M. Davies and M.D. Rawlins), p. 120. Pitman Medical, Tunbridge Wells.

Deane, S., Youngs, D., Poxon, V., Keighley, M.R.B., Alexander-Williams, J., and Burdon, D.W. (1982). Cimetidine and gastric microflora. *Br. J. Surg.* 67, 371 (abstr. 51).

Dennis, M. and Itkin, I.H. (1964). Effectiveness and complications of aerosol dexamethasone phosphate in severe asthma. *J. Allergy* 35, 70.

Diamond, L.S., Harlow, D.R., Phillips, B.P., and Keister, D.B. (1978). *Entamoeba histolytica*: iron and nutritional immunity. *Arch. Invest. Med. (Mex.)* Suppl.1, 9, 329.

Diderholm, H., Stenram, U., Tegner, K.B., and Willen, R. (1969). Herpes simplex hepatitis in an adult. *Acta Med. Scand.* 186, 151.

Dismukes, W.E., Royal, S.A., and Tynes, B.S. (1978). Disseminated histoplasmosis in corticosteroid-treated patients. Report of five cases. *JAMA* 240, 1495.

Domart, A., Hazard, J., Labram, C., Husson, R., and Portos, J.L. (1964). Varicelle hémorrhagique avec pneumopathie chez un adult traité par la delta-cortisone pour leucose aiguë. *Presse Med.* 72, 235.

Dunlop, D.M. and Murdoch, J. McC. (1960). Dangers of antibiotic treatment. *Br. Med. Bull.* 16, 67.

Eckhardt, W.F. and Hebard, G.W. (1961). Severe herpes zoster during corticosteroid therapy. *Arch. Intern. Med.* 108, 594.

Ehrlich, H.P. and Hunt, T.K. (1969). The effects of cortisone and anabolic steroids on the tensile strength of healing wounds. *Ann. Surg.* 170, 203.

Eisert, J., Hannibal, J.E. Jr, and Sanders, S.L. (1959). Fatal amebiasis complicating corticosteroid management of pemphigus vulgaris. *N. Engl. J. Med.* 261, 843.

Engquist, A., Backer, O.G., and Jarnum, S. (1974). Incidence of postoperative complications in patients subjected to surgery under steroid cover. *Acta Chir. Scand.* 140, 343.

Evans, C.D., Harman, R.R.M., and Warin, R.P. (1967). Varicose ulcers and the use of topical corticosteroids. *Br. Med. J.* iv, 482.

Findley, G.M. and Howard, E.M. (1952). The effects of cortisone and adrenocorticotrophic hormone on poliomyelitis and other virus infections. *J. Pharm. Pharmacol.* 4, 37.

Finegold, S.M. and Gaylor, D.W. (1960). Enterocolitis due to phage type 54 staphylococci resistant to kanamycin, neomycin, paromycin, and chloramphenicol. *N. Engl. J. Med.* 263, 1110.

Finkel, K.C. (1961). Mortality from varicella in children receiving adrenocorticosteroids and adrenocorticotrophin. *Pediatrics* 28, 436.

Finland, M., Jones, W.F., and Barnes, M.W. (1959). Occurrence of serious bacterial infections since introduction of antibacterial agents. *JAMA* 170, 2188.

Fischer, G.W., Hunter, K.W., Wilson, S.R., and Mease, A.D. (1980). Diminished bacterial defences with Intralipid. *Lancet* ii, 819.

Fletcher, J. and Goldstein, E. (1970). The effect of parenteral iron preparations on experimental pyelonephritis. *Br. J. Exp. Pathol.* 51, 280.

Franson, T.R., Kauffman, H.M. Jnr, Adams, M.B., Leman, J. Jnr, Cabrera, E., and Hanacik, L. (1987) Cyclosporine therapy and refractory *Pneumocystis carinii* pneumonia: a potential association. *Arch. Surg.* 122, 1034.

Fred, L., Rivo, J.B., and Barrett, T.F. (1951). Development of active pulmonary tuberculosis during ACTH and cortisone therapy. *JAMA* 147, 242.

Gill, K.A. Jr, Katz, H.I., and Baxter. D.L. (1963). Fungus infections occurring under occlusive dressings. *Arch. Dermatol.* 88, 348.

Ginn, H.E. (1969). Late medical complications of renal transplantation. *Arch. Intern. Med.* 123, 537.

Girmenia, C., Iori, A.P., Arcese, W., Martino, P., Antonini, G., and Bozzao, L. (1988). Fatal listeria meningitis in immunosuppressed patients. *Lancet* i, 794.

Godfrey, S., Hambleton, G., and König, P. (1974). Steroid aerosols and candidiasis. *Br. Med. J.* ii, 387.

Goetting, M.G. (1986). Fatal *Pneumocystis carinii* pneumonia from ACTH therapy for infantile spasms. *Ann. Neurol.* 19, 307.

Goldstein, E. and Rambo, O.N. (1962). Cryptococcal infection following steroid therapy. *Ann. Intern. Med.* 56, 114.

Gothoni, G., Neuvonen, P.J., Mattila, M., and Hackman, R. (1972). Iron–tetracycline interaction: effect of time interval between the drugs. *Acta Med. Scand.* 191, 409.

Griffith, L.J., Ostrander, W.E., Mullins, C.G., and Beswick, D.E. (1965). Drug antagonism between lincomycin and erythromycin. *Science* 147, 746.

Gupta, R. and Sachar, D.B. (1985). Chlorpropamide-induced cholestatic jaundice and pseudomembranous colitis. *Am. J. Gastroenterol.* 78, 811.

Guyer, P.B. and Delany, D. (1970). Urinary tract dilatation and oral contraceptives. *Br. Med. J.* iv, 588.

Hachiya, K.A., Kobayashi, R.H., and Antonson, D.L. (1982). Candida esophagitis following antibiotic usage. *Pediatr. Infect. Dis.* 1, 168.

Hall, M.R.P. (1972). Drugs and the elderly. *Adverse Drug React. Bull.* 35, 108.

Harrell, E.R. and Thompson, S.R. (1958). Systemic candidiasis (moniliasis) complicating treatment of bacterial endocarditis, with review of literature and report of apparent cure of one case with parenteral mycostatin. *Ann. Intern. Med.* 49, 207.

Harris-Jones, J.N. and Pein, N.K. (1952). Disseminated lupus erythematosus complicated by miliary tuberculosis during cortisone therapy. *Lancet* ii, 115.

Hassan, K.E. and Browne, M.K. (1978). Candida peritonitis and cimetidine. *Lancet* ii, 1054.

Hayes, M. (1965). Esophageal moniliasis. *Am. J. Gastroenterol.* 43, 143.

Hecht, J.R. and Olinger, E.J. (1989). *Clostridium difficile* colitis secondary to intravenous vancomycin. *Dig. Dis. Sci.* 34, 148.

Helpern, D.J. (1985). Atypical pyoderma as a side effect of isotretinoin. *J. Am. Acad. Derm.* 13, 1045.

Hennemann, G. (1960). Varicella and cortisone: what should be our therapeutic attitude? *Arch. Fr. Pediatr.* 17, 38.

Hersen, V.C., Krause, P.J., Eisenfeld, L.I., Pontious, L., and Maderazo, E.G. (1988). Indomethacin-associated sepsis in very-low-birthweight infants. *AJDC* 142, 555.

Higenbottam, T.W. and Heard, B.E. (1976). Opportunistic pulmonary strongyloidiasis complicating asthma treated with steroids. *Thorax* 31, 226.

Hill, R.B., Dahrling, B.E. II, Starzi, T.E., and Rifkind, D. (1967). Death after transplantation. An analysis of 60 cases. *Am. J. Med.* 42, 327.

Hoen, B., Renoult, E., Jonon, B., and Kessler, M. (1988). Septicaemia due to *Yersinia enterocolitica* in a long-term haemodialysis patient after a single desferrioxamine administration. *Nephron* 50, 378.

Holley, H.P. and Thiers, B.H. (1986). Cryptosporidiosis in a patient receiving immunosuppressive therapy: possible reactivation of latent infection. *Dig. Dis. Sci.* 31, 1004.

Humphrey, J.H.C. and McClelland, M. (1944). Cranial nerve palsies with herpes following general anaesthesia. *Br. Med. J.* i, 315.

Hutter, R.V.P. (1959). Phycomycetous infection (mucormycosis) in cancer patients: a complication of therapy. *Cancer* 12, 330.

Irons, G.V. (1964). Steroids and herpes zoster. *JAMA* 189, 649.

Ive, F.A. and Marks, R. (1968). Tinea incognita. *Br. Med. J.* iii, 149.

Jacobs, H.W. (1963). Unusual fatal infectious complications of steroid-treated liver disease. *Gastroenterology* 44, 519.

Jessen, O., Faber, V., Rosendel, K., and Eriksen, K.R. (1959). Some properties of *Staphylococcus aureus* possibly related to pathogenicity. *Acta Pathol. Microbiol. Scand.* 47, 316, 327.

Joynson, D.H.M., Jacobs, A., Walker, D.M., and Dolby, A.E. (1972). Defect of cell-mediated immunity in patients with iron-deficiency anaemia. *Lancet* ii, 1058.

Junker, A.K., Chan, K.W., and Lirenman, D.S. (1989). Epstein–Barr virus infections following OKT3 treatment. *Transplantation* 47, 574.

Kass, E.H. and Finland, M. (1953). Adrenocortical hormones in infection and immunity. *Annu. Rev. Microbiol.* 7, 361.

Kaufman, J.H. (1962). Cutaneous sporotrichosis and candidiasis occurring in a patient on prolonged steroid therapy. *J. Mich. State Med. Assoc.* 61, 190.

Keegan, J. and Byrd, J.W. (1988). Nocardiosis associated with low-dose methotrexate for rheumatoid arthritis. *J. Rheumatol.* 15, 1585.

Kesten, S., Hyland, R.H., Pruzanski, W.R., and Kortan, P.P. (1988). Esophageal candidiasis associated with beclomethasone diproprionate aerosol therapy. *Drug Intell. Clin. Pharm.* 22, 568.

King, E.Q., Johnson, J.B., Batten, G.S., and Henry, W.L. (1951). Report of a case of rapidly progressive pulmonary tuberculosis following cortisone therapy for rheumatoid arthritis. *JAMA* 147, 238.

Kirby, W.M.M. and Ahern, J.J. (1953). Changing patterns of resistance of staphylococci to antibiotics. *Antibiotics Chemother.* 3, 831.

Knight, V. and Holzer, A.R. (1954). Studies on staphylococci from hospital patients; predominance of strains of group III phage patterns which are resistant to multiple antibiotics. *J. Clin. Invest.* 33, 1190.

Kochar, R., Talwar, P., Singh, S., and Mehta, S.K. (1988). Invasive candidiasis following cimetidine therapy. *Am. J. Gastroenterol.* 83, 102.

Kouides, P.A., Slapak, C.A., Rosenwasser, L.J., and Miller, K.B. (1988). *Pneumocystis carinii* pneumonia as a complication of desferrioxamine therapy. *Br. J. Haematol.* 70, 383.

Kozeny, G.A., Quinn, J.P., Bansal, V.K., Vertuno, L.L., and Hano, E. (1987). *Pneumocystis carinii* pneumonia: a lethal complication of 'pulse' methylprednisone therapy. *Int. J. Artif. Organs* 10, 304.

The Lancet (1974). Iron and resistance to infection. *Lancet* ii, 325.

Larson, H.E. (1987). Clostridial infection of gastrointestinal tract — pseudomembranous colitis. In *Oxford textbook of medicine* (2nd edn) (ed. D.J. Weatherall, J.G.G. Ledingham, and D.A. Warrell), p. 5.274. Oxford University Press.

Latour, N.G. and Reeves, R.E. (1965). An iron requirement for growth of *Entamoeba histolytica* in culture; and the antiamoebal activity of 7-iodo-8-hydroxy-quinoloine-5-sulfonic acid. *Exp. Parasitol.* 17, 203.

Lazan, A. (1971). Gynecologic moniliasis: incidence with various contraceptive methods. *J. Med. Soc. N.J.* 68, 37.

Lee, P.S. and Lau, E.Y.L. (1988). Risk of acute non-specific respiratory tract infection in healthy men taking dapsone–pyrimethamine for prophylaxis against malaria, *Br. Med. J.* 296, 893.

Leighton, P.M. and MacSween, H.M. (1987). *Yersinia* hepatic abscesses subsequent to long-term iron therapy. *JAMA* 257, 964.

Leyden, J.J. and James, W.D. (1987). *Staphylococcus aureus* infection as a complication of isotretinoin. *Arch. Dermatol.* 123, 606.

Lepper, M.H. and Dowling. H.F. (1951). Treatment of pneumococcic meningitis with penicillin compared with penicillin plus aureomycin. *Arch. Intern. Med.* 88, 489.

Lessof, M.H. (1972). The current status of transplantation immunology. In *The scientific basis of medicine: annual reviews, 1972* (ed. I. Gilliland and J. Francis), p. 122. Athlone, London.

Levy, J.S. (1969). Vaccinia gangrenosum; rare complication of smallpox vaccination. *South. Med. J.* 62. 1408.

Lewis, M.J., Cameron, A.H., Shah. K.J.. Purdham. D.R., and Mann. J.R. (1978). Giant-cell pneumonia caused by measles and methotrexate in childhood leukaemia in remission. *Br. Med. J.* i, 330.

Likhite, V., Rodvein, R., and Crosby, W.H. (1976). Depressed phagocytic function exhibited by polymorphonuclear leucocytes from chronically iron-deficient rabbits. *Br. J. Haematol.* 34, 251.

Lorenc, E. (1967). A new factor in griseofulvin treatment failures: case report. *Mo. Med.* 64, 32.

Lundsgaard-Hansen, P. (1972). Masking effects of drugs. In *Drug-induced disease*, Vol. 4 (ed. L. Meyler and H.M. Peck), p. 208. Associated Scientific Publishers, Amsterdam.

Lundsgaard-Hansen, P., Sen, A., Roos, B., and Waller, U. (1960). Staphylococcic enterocolitis: Report of six cases with two fatalities after intravenous administration of *N*-(pyrrolidinomethyl) tetracycline. *JAMA* 173, 1008.

Lust, M., Ghins, P., and Hennemanne. G. (1960). Varicella and cortisone. *Scalpel* 113, 575.

McAllen, M.K., Kochanowski, S.J.. and Shaw, K.M. (1974). Steroid aerosols in asthma: an assessment of betamethasone valerate and a 12-month study of patients on maintenance treatment. *Br. Med. J.* i, 171.

McDonald, J.C.. Miller, D.L.. Williams, R.E.O., and Jevons, M.P. (1960). Nasal carriers of penicillin-resistant staphylococci in recruits to the Royal Air Force. *Proc. R. Soc. Med.* 53, 255.

MacDougall, L.G., Anderson, R., MacNab, G.M., and Katz, J. (1975). The immune response in iron-deficient children: impaired cellular defense mechanisms with altered humoral components. *J. Pediatr.* 86, 833.

MacKenzie, N.G., Chapman, O.W., and Middleton, P.J. (1969). Progressive vaccinia with chronic lymphatic leukaemia. *N.Z. Med. J.* 70. 324.

Mackinnon, J. (1959). Tuberculosis occurring during steroid therapy. *Br. Med. J.* ii, 1375.

McLaughlin, J.E. and Reeves, D.S. (1971). Clinical and laboratory evidence for inactivation of gentamicin by carbenicillin. *Lancet* i. 261.

Marshall. S., Lyon, R.P., and Minkler, D. (1966). Ureteral dilatation following use of oral contraceptives. *JAMA* 198, 782.

Masawe, A.E.J.. Muindi, J.M.. and Swai. G.B.R. (1974). Infections in iron deficiency and other types of anaemia in the tropics. *Lancet* ii. 314.

Maskell, R., Okubadejo, O.A., and Payne. R.H. (1976). Thymine-requiring bacteria associated with co-trimoxazole therapy. *Lancet* i. 834.

Mayer, G., Watschinger, B., Pohanka, E., Graf, H., and Popow, T. (1988). Cytomegalovirus infection after kidney transplantation using cyclosporin A and low-dose prednisolone immunosuppression. *Nephrol. Dial. Transplant.* 3, 464.

Mayfield, R.B. (1962). Tuberculosis occurring in association with corticosteroid treatment. *Tubercle* 43, 55.

Meadow, S.R., Weller. R.O., and Archibald, R.W.R. (1969). Fatal systemic measles in a child receiving cyclophosphamide for nephrotic syndrome. *Lancet* ii. 876.

Merselis J.G., Kaye, D., and Hook, E.W. (1964). Disseminated herpes zoster. A report of 17 cases. *Arch. Intern. Med.* 113, 679.

Meyler, L. (ed.) (1966). Hormones and synthetic substitutes. In *Side effects of drugs*, Vol. V, p. 415. Associated Scientific Publishers, Amsterdam.

Midtvedt, T. (1989). Penicillins, cephalosporins, and tetracyclines. in *Side effects of drugs — Annual 13* (ed. M.N.G. Dukes and L. Beeley), p. 210. Elsevier, Amsterdam.

Miller, S.N. and Ringler, R.P. (1987). Vancomycin-induced pseudomembranous colitis. *J. Clin. Gastroenterol.* 9, 114.

Milne, L.J.R. and Crompton, G.K. (1974). Beclomethasone dipropionate and oropharyngeal candidiasis. *Br. Med. J.* iii, 797.

Milton-Thompson, G.J., Lightfoot, N.F., Ahmet, Z., Hunt, R.H., Barnard. J., Bavin, P.M.G., *et al.* (1982). Intragastric acidity. bacteria. nitrite, and *N*-nitroso compounds before, during, and after cimetidine treatment. *Lancet* i, 1091.

Minoli, G., Teruzzi, V., Butti, G.C., Plada, A., Porro, A., Mandelli, P., *et al.* (1987). Invasive candidiasis does not complicate short-term treatment of duodenal ulcer. *Gastrointest. Endosc.* 33, 227.

Mitchell, R.G. (1987). Nocardiosis. In *Oxford textbook of medicine*, (2nd edn), (ed. D.J. Weatherall, J.G.G. Ledingham, and D.A. Warrell), p. 5.317. Oxford University Press.

Mogabgab, W.J. and Thomas, L. (1950). Quoted by Fred *et al.* (1951) (see above).

Mody, V.R. (1959). Corticosteroids in latent amoebiasis. *Br. Med. J.* ii, 1399.

Montgomerie. J.Z.. Becroft, D.M.O., Croxson, M.C., Doak, P.B., and North. J.D.K. (1969). Herpes simplex virus infection after renal transplantation. *Lancet* ii, 867.

Morris, C.A. and Morris, D.F. (1969). 'Normal' vaginal microbiology of women of childbearing age in relation to use of oral contraceptives and vaginal tampons. *J. Clin. Pathol.* 20, 636.

Murray, M.J., Murray, A.B., and Murray, C.J. (1980). The salutary effect of milk on amoebiasis and its reversal by iron. *Br. Med. J.* i, 1351.

Murray, M.J., Murray, A.B., Murray N.J., and Murray, M.B. (1975). Refeeding-malaria and hyperferraemia. *Lancet* i, 636.

Murray, M.J., Murray, A.B., Murray, M.B., and Murray, C.J. (1978). The adverse effects of iron repletion on the course of certain infections. *Br. Med. J.* ii, 1113.

Nabarro, J.D.N. (1960). The pituitary and adrenal cortex in general medicine. *Br. Med. J.* ii, 625.

Neuvonen, P.J., Gothoni, G., Hackman, R., and Bjorksten, K. af. (1970). Interference of iron with the absorption of tetracyclines in man. *Br. Med. J.* iv, 532.

Oppenheimer, S.J., Gibson, F.D., Macfarlane, S.B., Moody, J.B., and Hendrickse, R.G. (1984). Iron supplementation and malaria. *Lancet* i, 389.

Osband, M.E., Shen, T.J., Shlesinger, M., Brown, A., Hamilton, D., Cohen, E., *et al.* (1981). Successful tumour immunotherapy with cimetidine in mice. *Lancet* i, 636.

Perruquet, J.L., Harrington, T.M., and Davis, D.E. (1983). *Pneumocystis carinii* pneumonia following methotrexate therapy for rheumatoid arthritis. *Arthritis Rheum.* 26, 1291.

Peterkin, G.A.G. and Khan, S.A. (1969). Iatrogenic skin disease. *Practitioner* 202, 117.

Phair, J., Munoz, A., Detels, R., Kaslow, R., Rinaldo, C., Saah, A., and the Multicenter AIDS Cohort Study Group (1990). The risk of *Pneumocystis carinii* pneumonia among men infected with human immunodeficiency virus type I. *N. Engl. J. Med.* 322, 161.

Phillips, I. and Eykyn, S.J. (1987). Staphylococci. In *Oxford textbook of medicine* (2nd edn), (ed. D.J. Weatherall, J.G.G. Ledingham, and D.A. Warrell), p. 5.191. Oxford University Press.

Piguet, D. (1969). *In vitro* inhibitive action of nitrofurantoin on the bacteriostatic activity of nalidixic acid. *Ann. Inst. Pasteur*, Paris 116, 43.

Pillemer, S.R., Webb, D., and Yocum, D.E. (1989). Legionnaires' disease in a patient with rheumatoid arthritis treated with cyclosporine. *J. Rheumatol.* 16, 117.

Popp, C.G., Ottosen, P., and Brasher, C.A. (1951). Cortisone and pulmonary tuberculosis. *JAMA* 147, 241.

Proceedings of the Royal College of Physicians of Edinburgh (1990). Duodenal ulcer: an infectious disease? *Proc. R. Coll. Phys. Edinb.* 20, 3.

Pullan, C.R., Noble, T.C., Scott, D.J., Wizniewski, K., and Gardner, P.S. (1976). Atypical measles infections in leukaemic children on immunosuppressive treatment. *Br. Med. J.* i, 1562.

Purtilo, D.T., Meyers, D.M., and Connor, D.H. (1974). Fatal strongyloidiasis in immunosuppressed patients. *Am. J. Med.* 56, 488.

Rao, A.R., Sukumar, M.S., Kamalakshi, S., Paramasivan, T.V., Parasuraman, A.B., and Shantha, M. (1968). Experimental variola in monkeys. *Indian J. Med. Res.* 56, 1855.

Ren, E.C. and Chan, S.H. (1988). Possible enhancement of Epstein–Barr infections by the use of OKT3 in transplant recipients. *Transplantation* 45, 988.

Rex, J.H., Ginsberg, A.M., Fries, L.F., Pass, H.I., and Kwon-Chung, K.J. (1988). *Cunninghamella bertholletiae* infection associated with deferrioxamine therapy. *Rev. Infect. Dis.* 10, 1187.

Riegelman, S., Rowland, M., and Epstein, W.L. (1970). Griseofulvin-phenobarbital interaction in man. *JAMA* 213, 426.

Robins-Browne, R.M. and Prpic, J.K. (1983). Desferrioxamine and systemic yersiniosis. *Lancet* ii, 1372.

Robins-Browne, R.M., Rabson, A.R., and Koorrnhof, H. (1978). Generalized infection with *Yersinia enterocolitica* and the role of iron. *Contrib. Microbiol. Immunol.* 5, 277.

Roda, P. (1987). *Clostridium difficile* colitis induced by cytarabine. *Am. J. Clin. Oncol.* 10, 451.

Roschlau, G. (1967). Two cases of generalized fatal varicella during treatment with large doses of corticosteroids. *Münch. Med. Wochenschr.* 109, 1889.

Ruddell, W.S.J., Axon, A.T.R., Findlay, J.M., Bartholomew, B.A., and Hill, M.J. (1980). Effect of cimetidine on gastric bacterial flora. *Lancet* i, 672.

Russell, P.S. (1968). Kidney transplantation. *Am. J. Med.* 44, 776.

Salzman, G.A. and Pyszczynski, D.R. (1988). Oropharyngeal candidiasis in patients treated with beclomethasone dipropionate delivered by metered-dose inhaler alone and with Aerochamber. *J. Allergy Clin. Immunol.* 81, 424.

Sane, A., Manzi, S., Perfect, J., Herzberg, A.J., and Moore, J.O. (1989). Deferoxamine treatment as a risk factor for zygomycete infection. *J. Infect. Dis.* 159, 151.

Satin, A.J., Harrison, C.R., Hancock, K.C., and Zahn, C.M. (1989). Relapsing *Clostridium difficile* toxin-associated colitis in ovarian cancer patients treated with chemotherapy. *Obstet. Gynecol.* 74, 487.

Sayers, G. and Travis, R.H. (1970). Adrenocorticotropic hormone, adrenocortical steroids and their synthetic analogs. In *The pharmacological basis of therapeutics* (4th edn) (ed. L.S. Goodman and A. Gilman), pp. 1622, 1624. Macmillan, New York.

Sidransky, H. and Pearl, M.A. (1961). Pulmonary fungus infections associated with steroid and antibiotic therapy. *Dis. Chest* 39, 630.

Smith, F.P. and Cleve, E.A. (1957). Infections complicating cortisone therapy. *N. Engl. J. Med.* 256, 104.

Smith, T.J. (1964). Antibiotic-induced diseases. In *Diseases of medical progress* (ed. R.H. Moser), p. 9. Thomas, Springfield, Ill.

Sobrevilla, L.A., Tedeschi, L.G., Cronin, J.F., and Kantrowitz, W. (1962). *Listeria monocytogenes* meningitis as a complication of steroid therapy. *Boston Med. Q.* 13, 62.

Sombolos, K., Kalekou, H., Barboutis, K., and Tzarou, V. (1988). Fatal phycomycosis in a haemodialysed patient receiving deferroxamine. *Nephron* 49, 169.

Spain, D.M. (1961). Steroid alterations in the histopathology of chemically induced inflammation. In *Inflammation and diseases of connective tissue* (ed. L.C. Mills and J.W. Mayer). Saunders, Philadelphia.

Spain, D.M. and Molamut, N. (1950). Effects of cortisone on development of tuberculous lesions in guinea pigs and on their modification by streptomycin therapy. *Am. Rev. Tuberc. Pulm. Dis.* 62, 373.

Spaulding, W.B. (1962). Dangers in the use of some potent drugs. *Can. Med. Assoc. J.* 87, 1275.

Stark, F.R., Ninos, N., Hutton, J., Katz, R., and Butler, M. (1978). *Candida* peritonitis and cimetidine. *Lancet* ii, 744.

Steffen, R. (1977). Antacids: a risk factor in travellers' brucellosis? *Scand. J. Infect. Dis.* 9, 311.

Stellon, A.J. and Wakeling, M. (1989). Hidradenitis suppurativa associated with oral contraceptives. *Br. Med. J.* 298, 28.

Stille, W. and Ostner, K.H. (1966). Antagonismus Nitrofurantoin–Nalidixinsäure. *Klin. Wochenschr.* 44, 155.

Stockbrugger, R.W., Eugenidis, N., Bartholomew, B.A., Walter, C.L., Thompson, R.E.M., Hill, M.J., *et al.* (1981). Cimetidine treatment, intragastric bacterial overgrowth and its consequences. *Gastroenterology* 80, 1295.

Stockley, I. (1974). *Drug interactions and their mechanisms*, p. 35. Pharmaceutical Press, London.

Strom, J. (1955). The question of antagonism between penicillin and chlortetracycline, illustrated by therapeutical experiments in scarlatina. *Antibiotic Med.* 1, 6.

Stuiver, P.C. and Goud, Th.J.L.M. (1978). Corticosteroids and liver amoebiasis. *Br. Med. J.* ii, 394.

Sussman, M. (1974). Iron and infection. In *Iron in biochemistry and medicine* (ed. A. Jacobs and M. Worwood), p. 649. Academic Press, New York.

Swarup-Mitra, S. and Sinha, A.K. (1982). PMN function in nutritional anaemias: phagocytosis and bacterial killing. *Indian J. Med. Res.* 75, 259.

Symmers, W.St.C. (1966). Septicaemia candidosis. In *Symposium on candida infections* (ed. H.I. Winner and R. Hurley), p. 208. Churchill Livingstone, Edinburgh.

Szanto, S. (1971). Trichomonas and oxytetracycline. *Br. Med. J.* ii, 467.

Thorne, R.D. (1982). Cimetidine and brucellosis. *Lancet* ii, 217.

Tisdale, W., Fenster, L.F., and Klatskin, G. (1960). Acute staphylococcal enterocolitis complicating oral neomycin therapy in cirrhosis. *N. Engl. J. Med.* 263, 1014.

Torack, R.M. (1957). Fungus infections associated with antibiotics and steroid therapy. *Am. J. Med.* 22, 872.

Triger, D.R., Goepel, J.R., Slater, D.N., and Underwood, J.C.E. (1981). Systemic candidiasis complicating acute hepatic failure in patients treated with cimetidine. *Lancet* ii, 837.

Veis, J.H., Contiguglia, R., Klein, M., Mishell, J., Alfrey, A.C., and Shapiro, J.I. (1987). Mucormycosis in deferoxamine-treated patients on dialysis. *Ann. Intern. Med.* 107, 258.

Viljanto, J. (1980). Disinfection of surgical wounds without inhibition of normal wound healing. *Arch. Surg.* 115, 253.

Vogel, C.M., Kingsburg, R.J., and Baue, A.E. (1972). Intravenous hyperalimentation: a review of two and one-half years' experience. *Arch. Surg.* 105, 414.

Wagner, J.G. (1961). Biopharmaceutics: absorption aspects. *J. Pharm. Sci.* 50, 359.

Wagner, J.G. (1968). Aspects of pharmacokinetics and biopharmaceutics in relation to drug activity. *Am. J. Pharmacol.* 141, 5.

Wagner, J.G. (1969). Cyclamates antagonistic to antibiotics. *J. Am. Diet. Assoc.* 54, 121.

Wallace, J.F., Smith, R.H., Garcia, M., and Petersdorf, R.G. (1965). Antagonism between penicillin and chloramphenicol in experimental pneumococcal meningitis. *Antimicrob. Ag. Chemother.* 5, 439.

Walter, J.B. and Israel, M.S. (eds) (1974). *General pathology*, p. 96. Churchill Livingstone, Edinburgh.

Weinstein, L. (1962). Corticotrophin and corticosteroids in human viral infections. *Med. Clin. North Am.* 46, 1141.

Wiest, P.M., Flanigan, T., Salata, R.A, Shales, D.M., and Katzman, M. (1989). Serious infectious complications of corticosteroid therapy for COPD. *Chest* 95, 1180.

Williams, R.E.O., Blowers, R., Garrod, L.P., and Shooter, R.A. (1960). *Hospital infections: causes and prevention*, p. 29. Lloyd-Luke, London.

Williams, R.E.O., Jevons, M.P., Shooter, R.A., Hunter, C.J.W., Girling, J.A., Griffiths, J.D., *et al.* (1959). Nasal staphylococci and sepsis in hospital patients. *Br. Med. J.* ii, 658.

Wilson, G.S. and Miles, A.A. (1955). *Topley and Wilson's Principles of bacteriology and immunity* (4th edn), pp. 1163, 1167. Arnold, London.

Winstone, N.E. and Brooke, B.N. (1961). Effects of steroid treatment on patients undergoing operation. *Lancet* i, 973.

Woodward, S.C. and Sheldon, W.H. (1961). Subclinical *Pneumocystis carinii* pneumonitis in adults. *Bull. Johns Hopkins Hosp.* 109, 148.

Yaffee, H.S. and Grots, I. (1965). Moniliasis due to norethynodrel with mestranol. *N. Engl. J. Med.* 272, 647.

Yetgin, S., Altay, C., Ciliv, G., and Lalely, Y. (1979). Myeloperoxide activity and bactericidal function of PMN in iron deficiency. *Acta Haematol.* 61, 10.

Youinou, P. and Le Goff, P. (1987). Drug-induced impairment of polymorphonuclear bactericidal ability in rheumatoid arthritis. *Ann. Rheum. Dis.* 46, 50.

Zlotogorski, A. and Liebovici, V. (1987). Does etretinate exacerbate scabies? *Br. J. Dermatol.* 116, 882.

24. Neoplastic disorders

J. S. MALPAS

The role of hormones, immunosuppressants, and cyto-toxic agents in the causation of neoplasia is now well established. As a result, some agents, such as phenyl-butazone, have been withdrawn, and others such as stilboestrol have ceased to be used for indications such as bleeding in the first trimester of pregnancy. The degree of risk associated with the use of oestrogen replacement therapy in causing breast cancer, the relationship of the contraceptive pill to the causation of cancer of the breast, or its possible protective effect in reducing the incidence of cancer of the ovary, are now major concerns in the field of public health. One of the most striking recent advances has been the publication of studies of large numbers of adults and children followed up over a considerable period of time following cancer therapy, in whom second malignant neoplasms (SMN) have been identified (Draper *et al.* 1986; Meadows *et al.* 1989; van Leeuwen *et al.* 1989; Falkson *et al.* 1989). In addition, some large series have now been the subject of case controls (Kaldor *et al.* 1990*a*, *b*), which have enabled the relative risks for individual chemotherapeutic agents to be calculated. An account of these findings and an examination of the factors influencing the occurrence of drug-associated neoplasia is the subject of this chapter.

In 1979, the International Agency for Research on Cancer (IARC) published a list of chemical substances including drugs in the order of certainty that they might be carcinogenic to man. An abbreviated list referring to the drugs presently in use is given in Table 24.1. Group 1 comprised drugs for which there was strong evidence of a causal association between exposure and cancer in man. Group 2 included drugs that were probably carcinogens, with those most likely to be so included in the A category. Groups 2B and 3 contained drugs of undecided or unlikely potential. Since then many more agents, particularly those used for treating cancer, could be added to the list, and agents such as chlorambucil would probably now feature in Group 1.

TABLE 24.1
Drugs that are carcinogenic to man

Group 1
Diethylstilboestrol
Melphalan
Mustine hydrochloride (mechlorethamine, nitrogen mustard)
Group 2A
Cyclophosphamide
Chlorambucil
Groups 2B and 3
Isoniazid
Phenytoin

(Modified from IARC.)

Hormones as carcinogens

Herbst and Scully (1970) reported seven cases of adeno-carcinoma of the vagina in adolescent girls in the Eastern United States. This clustering of cases alerted Herbst to the finding in the eighth case that the mother had been treated with diethylstilboestrol during the first trimester of pregnancy. A retrospective analysis showed some of the other seven mothers had also been treated in this way. Greenwald and others (1971) confirmed this association, and eventually 333 cases of clear-cell carcinoma were found to be associated with stilboestrol therapy. This unequivocal demonstration of the carcinogenicity of stilboestrol not only alerted doctors to the possible hazards of short-term intensive administration, but also to the possibility that long-term low-dose hormonal therapy, such as that used in oral contraception or in hormonal replacement therapy after the menopause, might be hazardous.

Oral contraceptives

The role of oral contraceptives in the induction of breast cancer is still the subject of debate. It should be remembered that combination oral contraceptives which contain a synthetic oestrogen (usually ethinyl oestradiol) and a synthetic progestogen effectively stop ovarian function. This should therefore mimic the effect of the menopause and theoretically reduce the risk of breast cancer (Pike 1986). Epidemiological studies have found little evidence that this occurs, and the present position is still unclear. It may be that some women are at increased risk (Brinton *et al.* 1986; Pike 1986). The likelihood is that the dose of oestrogen in the preparation provides a higher level of oestrogen than would be circulating naturally. With the newer formulation of contraceptive combinations, with a lower quantity of oestrogen, it is hoped that the risk will decrease.

The role of oral contraception in other gynaecological cancer is less clear. There has been a suggestion (Vessey *et al.* 1983) that invasive carcinoma of the cervix was increased in patients on oral contraceptives. In the Oxford Family Planning Association study 13 cases were found in users of 'the pill', and none in users of intra-uterine devices. Since the association with virus infection has become established, it may be possible that this is not an independent factor but related to sexual behaviour.

There is now good evidence of a reduction in the risk of endometrial carcinoma when oestrogen and progestogens are given together (CASH study 1983*a*,*b*), and a reduced risk of ovarian cancer in the case–control studies of Rosenberg and colleagues (1982), Cramer and others (1982), and Pike (1986), when long-term contraceptive agents were used. The risk of developing endometrial cancer was approximately halved in those women taking the pill, and it appeared that the protection lasted for at least 10 years after stopping the treatment.

Oestrogen replacement

The increasing use of oestrogen replacement therapy in women in an attempt to prevent menopausal symptoms and osteoporosis has produced concern that this might be provoking an increase in the incidence of carcinoma of the breast. Kendall and Horton (1990) concluded that there was no evidence that hormone replacement therapy caused an increase in breast cancer, but concern has arisen from the results of a Swedish study by Bergkvist and co-workers (1989). This was a prospective study of over 23 000 Swedish women on hormone replacement therapy, comparing them with a group in the same geographical area. The study found no increased risk of breast cancer in the population as a whole, but subgroup analysis revealed major differences. In those treated

with oestradiol for 9 years, there was an increased risk of 1.8 times that of the control population with regard to the development of breast cancer. The risk rose to fourfold in those treated with oestradiol and progestogen for 4 years. This study conflicts with the finding of Gambrell and colleagues (1983), who found that the incidence of carcinoma was less in those women taking a combined oestrogen and progestogen preparation.

Endometrial carcinoma was found to be increased by Smith and others (1975) and Ziel and Finkel (1975), in studies in which they determined the incidence in menopausal and postmenopausal women who were given oestrogen alone. The risk of 'unopposed' oestrogen therapy was 4.5 times greater in those on therapy than in controls. The risk increased the longer the duration of therapy, rising to nearly 14-fold after 7 years. Other studies (McDonald *et al.* 1977; Gray *et al.* 1977) confirmed this.

Elwood (1981) found that patients presenting with endometrial carcinoma had a far better survival when they had had oestrogen, the non-users having a death rate some five times that of those women who had used oestrogens.

In conclusion, hormones may be shown to play an aetiological role in the production of cancer. Paradoxically, while promoting it in one organ, they can protect against it in another, and the administration of mixtures of hormones, as in the use of low-dose oral contraceptives, may negate any carcinogenic activity. Furthermore, the aggressiveness of the cancer produced seems to be modified by the nature of the hormonal stimulus.

Immunosuppressive drugs as carcinogens

This section will deal with those drugs that are specifically used to depress immune reactions and have been employed, for example, to prevent rejection of marrow or kidney grafts. Many drugs have an immunosuppressive effect, but are not used for that purpose therapeutically, and will not therefore be considered.

The first reports of a greater than expected incidence of malignant disease following renal or bone marrow transplantation started to appear in the late 1970s (Kinlen *et al.* 1979; Calne *et al.* 1979). At that time, immunosuppression was usually achieved with a combination of drugs, such as steroids and azathioprine or steroids and cyclophosphamide. Another agent that was commonly added was methotrexate. A major feature was the incidence of lymphoid malignancy (Kinlen *et al.* 1979). It was unusual for other malignancies to occur, and if this happened they were usually rare mesenchymal sarcomas. There was also a definite time relationship to the onset of the lymphoma. Another notable feature was the predilection for the central nervous system.

At that time the hypothesis was that in some way 'immune surveillance' of the body, which inhibited the growth of clones of malignant cells, was disturbed, possibly by reducing specific cells in the lymphoid system called 'natural killer cells'. This hypothesis is less favoured now, for it would be expected (if it were the case) that a wide variety of the more common malignancies could be seen, and this does not prove to be so. One of the most commonly used immunosuppressive agents, which is given over a long period of time, is azathioprine, which is related to mercaptopurine. Although carcinogenic, azathioprine is, like cyclophosphamide, not thought to be very active in this respect. It would be surprising if these agents were limited in carcinogenic action to the lymphoid system only, and the mechanism therefore remains unclear.

Azathioprine

This drug has been shown to induce an increased number of malignancies of the lymphoid and mesenchymal tissues in the course of renal transplantation (Kinlen et al. 1979) or in the control of autoimmune diseases such as rheumatoid arthritis (Isomaki et al. 1982). The increased incidence over that observed in a control population is related to the dose and length of treatment.

Cyclosporin

Calne and colleagues (1979) first reported the occurrence of lymphoma in three transplant patients receiving cyclosporin. This association has been confirmed and, of 5550 transplant patients receiving cyclosporin by 1984, lymphoproliferative disorders had been diagnosed in 40, an incidence of 0.7 per cent (*Martindale* 1989). Reduction of the dose or avoidance of combinations with other carcinogenic immunosuppressants reduces the incidence of cancer.

Cyclophosphamide

Cyclophosphamide has been found to increase the incidence of bladder, lymphoproliferative, and myeloproliferative tumours. Elliot et al. (1982) reported the development of bladder cancer in two women treated with cyclophosphamide for lupus nephritis, and Baltus and others (1983) showed that the risk of malignancy in 81 patients with rheumatoid arthritis treated with cyclophosphamide was 4.1 times as great as in 81 control subjects.

Cytotoxic agents and second malignant tumours
(See also Chapter 22)

By far the greatest number of second malignant tumours (SMN) occur in patients who are treated for cancer with cytotoxic agents. The exponential rise of SMN in patients who are surviving for 5, 10, or more years is a major cause for concern, especially in those tumours like Hodgkin's disease or Wilms' tumour, where cure is probable. It is true that the phenomenon is being seen only as the price of success, and it must be kept in perspective as a relatively rare occurrence, but given that there might be a propensity to form malignant tumours in a particular person, there is no doubt that it is important to study these patients and to try and identify which are the cytotoxic drugs responsible, and what host factors put a patient particularly at risk.

Several methods have been used to study SMN. Individual case reports have been important to establish risk, but have been little use in quantifying it. The two most useful methods have been cohort and case–control studies. In cohort studies, specific groups of patients are observed for a number of years to identify specific malignancies. The person–years of observation are calculated from the start of observation to last follow-up, death, or diagnosis of SMN, whichever is the first. Tumour incidence rates from the general population specific for age, sex, race, and calendar year are multiplied by the accumulated person–years to decide the number of expected tumours. The observed number is then divided by the expected number to get the relative risk. The 95 per cent confidence interval is then calculated, and the degree of significance of the finding can be stated. Although there are a number of criticisms of this method, this type of study has been informative.

Another type of analysis is the case–control study, in which the exposure to chemotherapy of individuals who develop SMN (cases) and those who do not (controls) is compared. The controls are matched as closely as possible, and ideally the largest number possible is obtained, although it is important that they be collected without bias.

These two methods have been used in most of the studies described below, and have enabled not only the time scale of production of SMN to be studied, but more recently have identified the causative agents.

Evidence from studies on Hodgkin's disease

A number of reports have demonstrated that survivors of Hodgkin's disease treated with chemotherapy develop SMN (Arsenau *et al.* 1972; Coltman and Dixon 1982; Boivin *et al.* 1984; Valagussa *et al.* 1986; Tucker *et al.* 1988). Among the first reports of a greater than expected number of SMN in Hodgkin's disease was that of Arsenau and others (1972), who noted an increase in non-lymphomatous malignant tumours, and related this to the non-intensive chemotherapy being given at that time.

Subsequent studies showed that this increase particularly took the form of myeloblastic leukaemia (Valagussa *et al.* 1986; Tucker *et al.* 1988). The evidence has come from either single institution or collaborative trial groups. Although most groups have reported a dozen or more leukaemias, these numbers have been insufficient in themselves to allow for an examination of risk factors. In adult Hodgkin's disease, Kaldor and colleagues (1990*b*) have combined the data for 12 population-based cancer registries in Europe and Canada, and six large hospitals in Europe. They have carried out a case–control study on 163 cases of leukaemia following treatment. They show that there was a relative risk of leukaemia of 9 (95 per cent confidence intervals 4.1–20), as compared with patients treated with radiotherapy alone. Table 24.2 shows the distribution of acute non-lymphocytic leukaemia according to type of chemotherapy in the series given.

Table 24.3 gives estimates of the relative risk of acute non-lymphocytic leukaemia for patients with selected chemotherapy regardless of radiotherapy received. With these data it is only possible to calculate the relative rates for combinations of drugs used frequently, that is, mustine hydrochloride (mechlorethamine, nitrogen mustard), and procarbazine, cyclophosphamide and procarbazine, and doxorubicin and dacarbazine. Relatively few patients received single agents. In 55 patients who received mustine hydrochloride and procarbazine, the relative risk was 6.4; for cyclophosphamide and procarbazine, 11; and for chlorambucil, over 27, although in this case the number of patients receiving the agent was small.

In children with Hodgkin's disease, Meadows and colleagues (1989) have recorded second neoplasms in

TABLE 24.2
Distribution of cases of acute non-lymphocytic leukaemia according to chemotherapy

Chemotherapy	Cases (n)	Controls (n)
Combinations		
Mustine hydrochloride (mechlorethamine, nitrogen mustard) + prednisolone	115	187
Cyclophosphamide + procarbazine	17	21
Chlorambucil + procarbazine	7	9
Doxorubicin + dacarbazine	19	19
Other combinations containing an alkylating agent	45	59
Combinations with no alkylating agent	9	12
Single agents		
Carmustine	3	3
Bleomycin	5	3
Lomustine	9	5
Chlorambucil	16	10
Cyclophosphamide	8	19
Cytarabine	1	6
Mustine hydrochloride	9	5
Procarbazine	7	9
Thiotepa	3	3
Vinblastine	26	41
Vincristine	3	6

(After Kaldor *et al.* 1990 *a,b*)

TABLE 24.3
Relative risk of acute non-lymphocytic leukaemia for patients with selected chemotherapy histories, irrespective of radiotherapy received

Chemotherapy history	Cases (n)	Controls (n)	Relative risk
MP only			
<6 cycles	30	89	4.7 (2.2–10)
>6 cycles	20	28	14.0 (5.1–37)
Any	50	117	6.4 (3.0–13)
CP only			
<6 cycles	1	4	3.3 (0.33–33)
>6 cycles	3	1	38.0 (3.6–410)
Any	4	5	11.0 (2.6–48)
ChP only	1	5	2.8 (0.29–27)
Chlorambucil only	3	1	27 (2.5–300)
MP + CP only	1	2	7.3 (0.59–90)
MP + DD only	2	8	4.1 (0.65–26)
MP + lomustine only	3	2	12.0 (1.5–91)
MP + vinblastine only	4	11	4.7 (1.2–19)

MP = mustine hydrochloride (mechlorethamine, nitrogen mustard) + procarbazine and no other alkylating agent
CP = cyclophosphamide + procarbazine and no other alkylating agent
ChP = combinations including chlorambucil + procarbazine and no other alkylating agent
DD includes doxorubicin and dacarbazine and no other alkylating agent
Figures in brackets are 95 per cent confidence intervals
(After Kaldor *et al.* 1990 *a,b*)

TABLE 24.4
*Alkylating agent dose and risk of leukaemia or
non-Hodgkin lymphoma*

AAD score	Leukaemia/NHL risk
1	0.02
2	0.02
4	0.03
6	0.06
8	0.10
8810	0.10

(After Meadows *et al.* 1989)

series from 11 major hospitals. Solid tumours, non-lymphocytic leukaemia, and non-Hodgkin lymphoma developed in 18, 17, and 3 patients respectively in the 979 children at risk. The study proposed an alkylating agent dose (AAD) risk for each patient. The score was calculated as follows: a single alkylating agent of at least 6 months' duration was assigned a score of 1; for double alkylating agents given for 6 months, a score of 2 was given. Thus, 6 months' MOPP or COPP were given a score of 2 because these contain two alkylating agents. The AAD scores were calculated for each individual patient. The study shows a close correlation between total alkylating agent received, the AAD score, and the risk for leukaemia and non-Hodgkin lymphoma (Table 24.4).

These adult and paediatric studies go a long way to indicate that alkylating agents (in particular mustine hydrochloride, cyclophosphamide, chlorambucil, and procarbazine) can be placed in the IARC's Group 1. Does Hodgkin's disease reveal anything more about the drugs used in its treatment? The vinca alkaloids vinblastine and vincristine have formed part of treatment programmes over many years, and have been used rela-

tively infrequently as single agents. van Leeuwen and others (1989) reviewed the relative risk for various combinations of cytotoxic agents used in treating 744 patients with Hodgkin's disease admitted to the Netherlands Cancer Institute from 1966 to 1983. No excess risk was observed in Hodgkin's patients treated with vinblastine alone, so that this suggests that vinblastine does not play an important role in increasing leukaemia risk.

Evidence from studies on ovarian cancer

Corroboration of these findings in alkylating agents can be found in the study of other cancers, and in particular ovarian cancer. Green and co-workers (1986) estimated the cumulative 10-year risk of contracting leukaemia for 333 women treated with cyclophosphamide as 5.4 per cent. The incidence peaked at 5–6 years, and subsequently declined. Kaldor and colleagues (1990*a*), again using a case–control method, studied the incidence of acute leukaemia in patients following chemotherapy for ovarian cancer. The data were taken from 11 population-based registries in Europe and Canada, and two large hospitals in Europe. One hundred and fourteen cases of leukaemia were identified, and matched in the manner previously described. Because single agents are given more frequently in ovarian cancer than in other conditions such as Hodgkin's disease, the patient-years of observation were considerably greater for single agents, and allowed the order of risk to be ranked (Table 24.5).

Carcinogenicity of cytotoxic agents

It can be seen from the above studies that chlorambucil, melphalan, and thiotepa present a high relative risk

TABLE 24.5
Distribution of cases and controls with acute non-lymphocytic leukaemia according to type of chemotherapy, with relative risks according to type and dose, among patients who received only one form of chemotherapy

Drug	Low dose				High dose			
	Cases	Controls	Median dose (mg) (controls)	Relative risk	Cases	Controls	Median dose (mg) (controls)	Relative risk
Chlorambucil	2	2	170	14.0	5	2	3200	23.0
Cyclophosphamide	4	14	1200	2.2	8	15	22 500	4.1
Melphalan	9	18	170	12.0	17	18	400	23.0
Thiotepa	4	5	30	8.3	5	6	600	9.7
Treosulfan	1	3	64 000	3.6	7	2	260 000	33.0

Low and high doses were defined with respect to median dose in the controls.
(After Kaldor *et al.* 1990*a,b*)

while treosulfan and cyclophosphamide rank rather lower. Cyclophosphamide was also found to be less leukaemogenic in children than other agents (de Vathaire *et al.* 1989) in a study of 634 children treated between 1942 and 1969, which showed that in 280 children treated with non-alkylating agents or cyclophosphamide the relative risk was 2.9, whereas with all other alkylating agents the relative risk was 7.4. Further evidence of the relative safety of cyclophosphamide has come in a study from Curtis and others (1990), who found 24 cases of acute myeloid leukaemia in 13 734 women treated for breast cancer with chemotherapy. When compared with another group of 7974 women who had received no chemotherapy, the relative risk was 11.5 per cent (95 per cent confidence interval 7.4–17.1). In a case–control study the relative risk for melphalan in the women with breast cancer was 44.6 (95 per cent confidence interval 4.9–409), and for cyclophosphamide 1.3 (95 per cent confidence interval 0.3–6.6), once again emphasizing the different potential of different alkylating agents for producing SMN. A study by Falkson and others (1989) showed that 23 of 1460 patients receiving mitolactol (dibromodulcitol, DBD) for adjuvant treatment of breast cancer developed leukaemia or myelodysplasia. The authors concluded that DBD is one of the most potent leukaemogenic agents in use, and recommended that it should no longer be employed as an adjuvant. This study did not, however, calculate a relative risk for the drug, so that its exact place in the order of carcinogenicity is difficult to determine.

TABLE 24.6
Leukaemogenicity of cytotoxic agents in order of potential, based on reported relative risks

1. Chlorambucil
2. Melphalan
3. Procarbazine
4. Thiotepa
5. Mustine hydrochloride (mechlorethamine, nitrogen mustard)
6. Cyclophosphamide
7. Vinblastine

It ought to be possible now to assign an order of leukaemogenicity to commonly used chemotherapeutic agents; this would be of importance in the planning of treatment programmes. As an approximation, on evidence so far, it is suggested that the order is that shown in Table 24.6.

Anticonvulsant hydantoins and malignant lymphoma

Members of the hydantoin group of drugs, particularly phenytoin, are known to produce changes in lymphoid tissue (Rosenfeld *et al.* 1961; Anthony 1970; *The Lancet* 1971; Tashima and de los Santos 1974; Li *et al.* 1975; Wilden and Scott 1978). Sometimes the disorder presents as a syndrome comprising fever, rash, lymphadenopathy and, occasionally, enlargement of the liver and spleen. In some instances histological changes have been interpreted as indicative of malignant lymphoma, but have resolved after withdrawal of the drug suspected of causing the reaction. Classical Hodgkin's disease and non-Hodgkin's lymphoma have also been attributed to these drugs, but the current opinion is that the causal association suggested is probably not valid.

Phenacetin abuse and carcinoma

Long-continued abuse of analgesic drug combination containing phenacetin is likely to have been responsible for some cases of transitional cell carcinoma of the renal pelvis (*The Lancet* 1969; *British Medical Journal* 1969; Bengtsson and Angervall 1970). Fortunately, in most countries phenacetin is no longer used.

Host-related factors

It is increasingly important to recognize the role of chemotherapy and host interaction, especially when assessing the safety of chemotherapeutic drug regimens. The role of immunological status has been referred to above. More recently the importance of genetic abnormalities or tumour cell phenotype has become apparent. Draper and colleagues (1986), in a follow-up study of 882 retinoblastoma patients treated with surgery, radiotherapy, or chemotherapy, compared the outcome of these treatments in 384 children known to have the genetic form of the disease with that in 498 others who had the non-genetic form. Comparing the incidence of SMN in children with genetic disease treated by radiotherapy and chemotherapy, or chemotherapy alone, a total of 10 patients had a second malignancy, while none were noted in the non-genetic group, showing that there was an increased susceptibility of SMN when there was already an underlying genetic defect.

Pui and others (1989) studied the risk of development of acute myeloid leukaemia during initial remission of

733 consecutive children treated with intensive chemotherapy for acute lymphoblastic leukaemia. In the study, 13 patients developed myelogenous leukaemia. While there was a wide variation in the karyotype at diagnosis of the acute lymphoblastic patients who eventually developed AML, an unusual finding was the frequency with which a T cell phenotype was found. Of 98 patients with T cell phenotypes, 5 developed AML, while in 635 without the phenotype 8 developed AML. This is significant (p=0.004), and in a multivariate analysis of risk factors remains highly significant (p=0.001). Thus genetic and phenotype changes may produce susceptibility to the action of cytotoxic drugs.

Conclusion

Since the review by Ross (1985) in the third edition of this book, it has become apparent that hormones, immunosuppressants, and chemotherapeutic agents can induce malignancy, and that it is now possible to arrange these last in an order of the risk that malignancy may occur. This must be increasingly important to the medical oncologist designing curative therapies. It is also necessary to remember that underlying genetic abnormalities or surface phenotypes of the tumour being treated will influence susceptibility, and this is likely to be of increasing importance.

References

Anthony, J.J. (1970). Malignant lymphoma associated with hydantoin drugs. *Arch. Neurol.* 22, 450.

Arsenau, J.C., Sponzo, R.W., Levin, D.L., Schnipper, L.E., Bonner, H., Young, R.C., *et al.* (1972). Nonlymphomatous malignant tumours complicating Hodgkin's disease. Possible association with intensive therapy. *N. Engl. J. Med.* 287, 1119.

Baltus, J.A., Boersma, J.W., Hartman, A.P., and Vandenbroucke, J.P. (1983). The occurrence of malignancies in patients with rheumatoid arthritis treated with cyclophosphamide: a controlled retrospective follow-up. *Ann. Rheum. Dis.* 42, 368.

Bengtsson, U. and Angervall, L. (1970). Analgesic abuse and tumours of the renal pelvis. *Lancet* i, 305.

Bergkvist, L., Adami, H.O., Persson, I., Hoover, R., and Schairer, C. (1989). The risk of breast cancer after oestrogen and oestrogen–progestogen replacement. *N. Engl. J. Med.* 321, 293.

Boivin, J.F., Hutchison, G.B., Lyden, M., Godbold, J., Chorosh, J., and Schottenfeld, D. (1984). Second primary cancers following treatment of Hodgkin's disease. *J. Natl Cancer Inst.* 72, 233.

Brinton, L.A., Hoover, R., and Fraumeni, J.F. (1986). Menopausal oestrogens and breast cancer risk: an expanded case–control study. *Br. J. Cancer* 54, 825.

British Medical Journal (1969). Phenacetin and bladder cancer. *Br. Med. J.* iv, 701.

Calne, R.Y., Rolles, K., White, D.J., Thiru, S., Evans, D.B., McMaster, P., *et al.* (1979). Cyclosporin A initially as the only immunosuppressant in 34 recipients of cadaveric organs — 33 kidneys, 2 pancreases and 2 livers. *Lancet* ii, 1033.

CASH (Centers for Disease Control: Cancer and steroid hormone study) (1983*a*). *JAMA* 249, 1596.

CASH (Centers for Disease Control: Cancer and steroid hormone study) (1983*b*). *JAMA* 249, 1600.

Coltman, C.A., and Dixon, D.O. (1982). Second malignancies complicating Hodgkin's disease — the National Cancer Institute experience. *Cancer Treat. Rep.* 66, 1023.

Cramer, D.W., Hutchison, G.B., Welch, W.R., Scully, R.E., and Knapp, R.C. (1982). Factors affecting the association of oral contraceptives and ovarian cancer. *N. Engl. J. Med.* 307, 1047.

Curtis, R.E., Boice, J.D., Moloney, W.C., Ries, L.G., and Flannery, J.T. (1990). Leukaemia following chemotherapy for breast cancer. *Cancer Res.* 50, 2741.

De Vathaire, F., Schweisguth, O., Rodary, C., Francois, P., Sarrazin, D., Oberlin, O., *et al.* (1989). Long term risk of second malignant neoplasm after a cancer in childhood. *Br. J. Cancer* 59, 448.

Draper, G.J., Sanders, B.M., and Kingston, J.E. (1986). Second primary neoplasms in patients with retinoblastoma. *Br. J. Cancer* 53, 661.

Elliott, R.W., Essenhigh, D.M., and Morvey, A.R. (1982). Cyclophosphamide treatment of systemic lupus erythematosus: risk of bladder cancer exceeds benefit. *Br. Med. J.* 284, 1160.

Elwood, J.M. (1981). Estrogens and endometrial cancer: some answers and further questions. *Can. Med. Assoc. J.* 124, 1129.

Falkson, G., Gelman, R.S., Dreicer, R., Turmey, D.C., Alberts, A.S., Coccia-Portugal, M.A., *et al.* (1989). Myelodysplastic syndrome and acute nonlymphocytic leukaemia secondary to mitolactol treatment in patients with cancer. *J. Clin. Oncol.* 9, 1252.

Gambrell, R.D., Maier, R.C., and Sanders, B.I. (1983). Decreased incidence of breast cancer in postmenopausal estrogen–progestogen users. *Obstet. Gynecol.* 62, 435.

Gray, L.A., Christopherson W.M., and Hoover, R.N. (1977). Estrogen and endometrial cancer. *Obstet. Gynecol.* 49, 385.

Greene, M.H., Harris, E.L., and Gershenson, D.M. (1986). Melphalan may be a more potent leukaemogen than is cyclophosphamide. *Ann. Intern. Med.* 105, 360.

Greenwald, P., Barlow, J.J., Nasca, P.C., and Burnett, W.S. (1971). Vaginal cancer after maternal treatment with synthetic oestrogens. *N. Engl. J. Med.* 285, 390.

Herbst, A.L. and Scully, R.E. (1970). Adenocarcinoma of the vagina in adolescence; a report of 7 cases including 6 clear cell carcinomas (so-called mesonephromas). *Cancer* 25, 745.

International Agency for Research on Cancer (1979). *Evaluation of the carcinogenic risk of chemicals to humans*. IARC Monographs, Supplement 1. IARC, Lyon, France.

Isomaki, H.I.A., Hakulinen, T., and Joutsenlahti U. (1982). Excess risk of lymphomas, leukaemia and myeloma in patients with rheumatoid arthritis. *Ann. Rheum. Dis.* 41, (suppl. i), 34.

Kaldor, J.M., Day, N.E., Pettersson, F., Clarke, E.A., Pedersen, D., Mehnert, W., *et al.* (1990a). Leukaemia following chemotherapy for ovarian cancer. *N. Engl. J. Med.* 322, 1.

Kaldor, J.M., Day, N.E., Clarke, A., van Leeuwen, F.E., Henry-Amar, M., Fiorentino, M.V., *et al.* (1990b). Leukaemia following Hodgkin's disease. *N. Engl. J. Med.* 322, 7.

Kendall, M.J. and Horton, R.C. (1990). Clinical pharmacology and therapeutics: reviews in medicine. *Postgrad. Med. J.* 66, 166.

Kinlen, L.J., Sheil, A.G.R., Peto, J., and Doll, R. (1979). Collaborative United Kingdom–Australasian study of cancer in patients treated with immunosuppressive drugs. *Br. Med. J.* ii, 1461.

The Lancet (1969). Analgesic abuse and tumours of the renal pelvis. *Lancet* i, 1233.

The Lancet (1971). Is phenytoin carcinogenic? *Lancet* ii, 1071

Li, F.P., Willard, D.R., Goodman, R., and Vawter, G. (1975). Malignant lymphoma after diphenylhydantoin (Dilantin) therapy. *Cancer* 36, 1359.

McDonald, T.W., Annegers, J.F., O'Fallow, W.M., Dockerty, M.B., Malkasian, G.D., and Kurlord, L.T. (1977). Exogenous estrogen and endometrial carcinoma — a case controlled study. *Am. J. Obstet. Gynecol.* 127, 572.

Martindale. The extra pharmacopoeia, Vol. 29 (1989) (ed. J.E.F. Reynolds), p. 614. Pharmaceutical Press, London.

Meadows, A.T., Obringer, A.C., Marrero, O., Oberlin, O., Robison, L., Fossati-Bellani, F., *et al.* (1989). Second malignant neoplasms following childhood Hodgkin's disease; treatment and splenectomy as risk factors. *Med. Pediatr. Oncol.* 17, 477.

Pike, M.C. (1986). Epidemiology of cancer. In *Introduction to the cellular and molecular biology of cancer* (ed. S.L.M.

Franks and W. Teich), p. 63. Oxford University Press.

Pui, C-H., Behm, F.G., Raimondi, S.C., Dodge, R.K., George, S.L., Rivera, G.K., *et al.* (1989). Secondary acute myeloid leukaemia in children treated for acute lymphoid leukaemia. *N. Engl. J. Med.* 321, 136.

Rosenberg, L., Shapiro, S., Slone, D., Kaufman, D.W., Idelmrich, S.P., Miethinen, O.S., *et al.* (1982). Epithelial ovarian cancer and combination oral contraceptives. *JAMA* 247, 2310.

Rosenfeld, S., Swiller, A.I., Shenoy, Y.M.V., and Morrison, A.N. (1961). Syndrome simulating lymphosarcoma induced by diphenylhydantoin. *JAMA* 176, 491.

Ross, W.M. (1985). Neoplastic disorders. In *Textbook of adverse drug reactions* (3rd edn) (ed. D.M. Davies), p. 607. Oxford University Press.

Smith, D.C., Ross, P., Thompson, D.J., and Herrmann, W.l. (1975). Association of exogenous estrogen and endometrial carcinoma. *N. Engl. J. Med.* 293, 1164.

Tashima, C.K. and de los Santos, R. (1974). Lymphoma and anticonvulsive therapy. *JAMA* 228, 286.

Tucker, M.A., Coleman, C.N., Cox, R.S., Varghese, A., and Rosenberg, S.A. (1988). Risk of second cancers after treatment for Hodgkin's disease. *N. Engl. J. Med.* 318, 76.

Valagussa, P., Santoro, A., Fossati-Bellani, F., Banfi, A., and Bonadonna, G. (1986). Second acute leukaemia and other malignancies following treatment for Hodgkin's disease. *J. Clin. Oncol.* 4, 830.

Van Leeuwen, F.E., Somers, R., Taal, B.G., Van Heerde, P., Coster, B., Doseman, T., *et al.* (1989). Increased risk of lung cancer, non-Hodgkin's lymphoma, and leukaemia following Hodgkin's disease. *J. Clin. Oncol.* 7, 1046.

Vessey, M.P., Lawless, M., McPherson, K., and Yeates, D. (1983). Neoplasm of the cervix uteri and contraception: a possible adverse effect of the Pill. *Lancet* ii, 392.

Wilden, J.N. and Scott, C.A. (1978). A pseudolymphomatous reaction in soft tissue associated with phenytoin sodium. *J. Clin. Pathol.* 31, 761.

Ziel, H.K. and Finkel, W.D. (1975). Increased risk of endometrial carcinoma among users of conjugated estrogens. *N. Engl. J. Med.* 293, 1167.

25. Drug allergy and tests for its detection

E-S. K. ASSEM

Part 1 Drug allergy

Introduction

Drug allergy continues to present an immense challenge both as a special type of adverse drug reaction (ADR) and as a special discipline of allergy. By definition 'drug allergy' is mediated by immunological mechanisms. The term 'hypersensitivity', used as an alternative to 'allergy' in other parts of this book and elsewhere, lacks precision and will not be used in this chapter. Allergic drug reactions are of Type B (see Chapter 3).

Epidemiology

Though well appreciated, allergic and other ADR may be grossly under-reported, and a high proportion may be unrecognized or misdiagnosed, for instance anaesthetic reactions (Youngman *et al.* 1983; Dundee 1986; Nimmo 1988). Allergy constitutes a small proportion of all ADR, approximately 20 per cent (Lakshmanan *et al.* 1986; Laurence and Bennett 1987). One of the reasons of misdiagnosis is the occurrence of an unrecognized or unusual manifestation.

Although drug allergy is a rare cause of death, it may contribute significantly to patient morbidity. To support this statement, the author wishes to refer to a relatively well-defined (and not so subtle as other types) reaction, anaphylaxis. Anaesthetics are among the many causes of anaphylactic reaction (AR). Around 3.5 million general anaesthetics (GA) are given in the UK every year and according to conservative estimates between 175 and 800 AR occur (Assem 1990*b*). A 4 per cent mortality suggests 7–32 deaths per annum. Frequencies of reactions are available for other groups of drugs, for example, β-lactam antibiotics, non-steroidal anti-inflammatory drugs, and iodinated radiocontrast media (Assem 1984*b*), and extension of these calculations would certainly point to the magnitude of the problem.

Distinctive features of allergic drug reactions

1. They have no correlation with known pharmacological properties of the drug (unlike toxic reactions).
2. There is no linear relationship with drug dosage (unlike toxic reactions).
3. They often include a rash, angioedema (angioneurotic oedema), the serum sickness syndrome, anaphylaxis, and asthma, which are reactions similar to those of classical protein allergy.
4. They require an induction period on primary exposure but not on readministration.
5. They disappear on cessation of therapy and reappear after readministration of a small dose.
6. They usually occur in a minority of persons receiving the drug.
7. Desensitization may be possible.

Some, if not all, of these criteria are not specific; for example, the reaction to a small dose may be due to idiosyncrasy. There are also instances of drug allergy that do not fulfil the above criteria. The lack of history of a sensitizing dose of penicillin is not uncommon, and in this case previous exposure may have been to penicillin-like compounds that may be present in many natural substances. Another example is the occasional persistence of symptoms and signs or even the appearance of fresh ones after the cessation of therapy. Hyposensitization may not be possible, because of the development of reactions during this process.

Factors affecting the incidence of allergic reactions

There are several factors predisposing to allergy during drug therapy: (1) the drug and (2) the patient (the so-called constitutional factors); (3) the disease for which the drug is given.

The drug as an allergen

An antigen is an agent capable of inducing antibody formation. Antigens may or may not produce allergy.

Effect of molecular size

Drugs that are themselves macromolecules, such as protein or peptide hormones, and dextrans, which are polysaccharides, act as complete antigens, while simple chemicals cannot do so. Simple chemicals may be arbitrarily defined as those having a molecular weight less than 500–1000. Macromolecular contaminants, which may result from the production processes or storage of simple chemicals, may be a cause of allergic reactions to these preparations.

It has been suggested that standard preparations of benzylpenicillin contain high-molecular-weight contaminants (macromolecular fractions [MMF], separable by dextran gel 'Sephadex' chromatography) that evoke reactions in allergic subjects (Batchelor *et al.* 1967; Knudsen *et al.* 1967; Stewart 1967). This fact has not turned out, however, to be as important as was thought. On the other hand, macromolecular contaminants are important in the allergenicity of semi-synthetic penicillins such as ampicillin (Knudsen *et al.* 1970).

Formation of antigens from simple chemicals

Simple chemicals that are incomplete antigens are called 'haptens'. The fact that simple chemicals may induce antibody formation and hypersensitivity of immediate or delayed type, or both, was established many years ago (Landsteiner 1945; Gell *et al.* 1948).

Hapten–protein conjugates of many chemicals, which can now be prepared *in vitro*, can be shown to be antigenic. Irreversible conjugation of the simple chemical with proteins by covalent bonds seems to be essential for the formation of a complete antigen. There is evidence suggesting that a similar mechanism occurs *in vivo*. Reversible binding, which frequently occurs between drugs and plasma proteins, is generally inadequate for the sensitization process.

Having stated the prerequisites for formation of proper antigens from simple chemicals, and having assumed that conjugation of metabolites of chemically simple drugs takes place *in vivo* prior to the immune response, it still remains to be seen if exceptions to these rules can emerge. One such possible exception is the group of neuromuscular blockers with a bis-quaternary ammonium structure. These compounds are certainly allergenic, and seem to behave like 'proper' antigens in eliciting histamine release from basophil leucocytes of allergic individuals (Assem 1977*b*, 1983*b*, 1984*a*; Didier *et al.* 1987).

Simple chemicals vary greatly in their ability to induce allergy. Some rarely, if ever, do so; others can cause an immunological response in virtually every subject, and allergy in many of those receiving them. It is important to stress the fact that the presence of an immunological response does not necessarily mean allergy. A drug may induce an immunological response, as evidenced by the formation of hapten-specific antibodies, without the production of clinical manifestations of allergy. Probably everyone who receives penicillin develops antibodies against the penicilloyl group, which is the 'major' haptenic determinant derived from penicillin. It has also been reported that penicillin antibodies were found in almost all subjects who denied ever having received penicillin therapy during their lifetime (Levine *et al.* 1966), and it was suggested that these antibodies represented an immunological response to penicillins in foods such as milk and dairy products. A naturally occurring immunoglobulin-G (IgG) antibody-like substance capable of binding to the quaternary ammonium group and to neuromuscular blockers (NMB) was also detected in human and animal sera (Assem 1990*a*). If confirmed, this preliminary finding could have some important bearings, both as an 'immunological' phenomenon and as a clue as to how 'spontaneous' sensitization to NMB could occur.

The importance of drug metabolites

The ability of simple chemicals to react covalently with proteins *in vitro* can be correlated with their immunogenicity *in vivo* in experimental animals, as shown by the frequency of induction of contact sensitivity and anaphylactic reactions (Eisen 1959). There are many simple chemicals, however, that do not react with protein *in vitro* but which are capable of inducing antibody formation *in vivo*. Most of the drugs that are currently used for therapeutic purposes cannot react *in vitro* with proteins. The ability of some of these compounds to produce allergic reactions and induce antibody formation may be explained by the formation *in vivo* of metabolites that react with proteins. Since our knowledge about the various metabolites of most drugs is limited, little is known about the various haptenic determinant groups that are derived from the drugs that are capable of inducing an immunological response.

In theory, any of the various degradation products of any compound, whether arising from metabolic processes in the body or by non-metabolic processes that may even take place before the drug is administered, may be capable of becoming an antigen and inducing allergy.

In inst⁻ nces where a drug gives rise to more than one allergen, the relative importance of each allergen may vary in different patients; but, on the whole, one of these is likely to be the main allergen in most allergic patients. The best-known example (and perhaps the only clear one) is penicillin allergy, which will be discussed at length later in this chapter.

The various ways in which a drug (a simple chemical) can become antigenic are shown in Fig. 25.1.

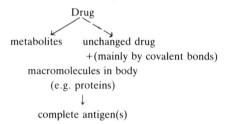

FIG. 25.1 Formation of antigens from simple chemicals.

Allergy to 'inactive' ingredients of drug preparations

Ingredients (such as vehicles and excipients) other than the active drug(s) in any preparation may themselves be responsible for an allergic reaction to a medicinal preparation.

Allergenicity of different preparations of the same drug or closely related derivatives

It has been found in the case of penicillin that, in general, allergic reactions to semi-synthetic compounds are much more frequent than reactions to natural penicillins (benzylpenicillin and phenoxymethylpenicillin; Idsøe et al. 1968). This is probably due in part to the previously mentioned 'contamination' with antigenic macromolecules. Such contaminants could be (1) polymers of the drug; (2) enzymes (i.e. bacterial amidase) used to cleave side chains of natural penicillins prior to their replacement with new side chains; (3) contaminants of the enzyme; or (4) penicilloylated enzyme or contaminants.

It seems likely that additives or formulations that are used to prolong the action of penicillin (e.g. procaine) may themselves be allergens; or may increase the antigenicity and allergenicity of penicillin; that is, they may act as 'adjuvants'. The effect of adding a β-lactamase inhibitor (e.g. clavulanic acid) to certain penicillin preparations (there is one with amoxycillin) on the occurrence of allergic reactions has not been properly evaluated. We have only examined the effect of β-lactamase inhibitors in *in vitro* tests for penicillin allergy (see Part 2 — Tests for drug allergy).

Route of administration

The severity and manifestations of allergy depend to some extent on the route of administration; thus, for example, anaphylactic reactions are usually more dramatic when the drug is given by injection than when it is given orally. Oral administration of drugs, for example, oral penicillin preparations, however, can occasionally cause as rapid and severe a reaction as that produced by injection (Simmonds *et al.* 1978).

Coincidental drug therapy

It has been reported (BCDSP 1972) that patients suffering from gout and treated with allopurinol have a significantly higher incidence of 'reaction' (skin rash) to ampicillin, which is probably allergic in nature. It is tempting to speculate that drug interactions, apart from producing changes in the pharmacological or toxic effects, might also enhance or reduce the allergic reaction to a drug.

The patient

The permissive role played by the host in producing an allergic reaction is the subject of much speculation but only a few known facts. In view of the several steps involved in the production of an allergic response to a simple chemical, many variables may be considered as contributory host factors.

Genetic predisposition

Association with other allergies

Patients with a history of allergic disease such as 'atopic' disease (eczema, hay fever, or asthma) or drug reactions, whether definitely allergic or due to an unidentified mechanism, have a significantly higher incidence of allergic drug reactions. This fact, although previously disputed, is becoming more generally accepted, and surveys or proper epidemiological studies support it (e.g. the survey by Hurwitz 1969). Penicillin allergy occurs more often in atopic than in non-atopic patients (Levine *et al.* 1966).

In my experience, this is true of allergy to many other drugs (Assem 1977*a,b*, 1983*a,b*), and not only of allergic drug reactions, but also of reactions simulating allergy but apparently not mediated by immunological mechanisms, for example asthma induced by aspirin and other non-steroidal anti-inflammatory drugs (non-immunological anaphylactic-like ['anaphylactoid'] reactions, described later). Another example is the anaphylactic-like reaction produced by narcotic analgesics (Assem 1976). Caution should, however, be exercised since we do not

clearly understand the mechanism of anaphylactoid reactions and some of them may eventually turn out to be
immunological in nature, as has already happened in the
case of anaphylactoid reactions to neuromuscular blockers, as explained below.

Definitive genetic studies

Correlation with HLA serotypes One of the recent
approaches to the question of genetic aspects of allergy is
to study its possible association with the major histocompatibility (HLA) antigens. This has been carried out in
patients with reagin (mainly IgE)-mediated allergy to
ragweed pollen, using highly purified preparations of
various pollen allergens (Marsh *et al.* 1973). Quantitative
prick-in skin tests were used to classify patients according to the intensity of skin response to each allergen. The
results suggested a significant correlation between a
particular HLA serotype and the ability to develop
reagin-mediated allergy to a particular allergen (as detected by skin testing). This correlation was highly significant, firstly in the case of allergens that were of
relatively simple chemical structure, and secondly where
the individual differences in response, particularly when
judged by the concentration of allergen required to elicit
a response, were clearly distinguishable. Thus, these two
conditions may be necessary in order to show a marked
association in a population as genetically polymorphic
as man.

It should be pointed out that the skin response to an
allergen may be influenced by several factors other than
the amount of reagin (or IgE) present in the skin; it is the
net result of all these factors, which may be regulated by
different genes.

The influence of HLA type on drug-induced immune
responses is complex, and it is interesting that HLA
typing may help in the assessment of whether or not
particular drug reactions are likely, especially if carried
out in conjunction with genetic determinants of drug
metabolism. The best example is hydralazine-related
systemic lupus erythematosus (SLE) which is 10 times
more frequent in DR4 patients than in the population at
large (Welsh and Batchelor 1981).

*Individual differences in the immune response to specific
chemicals* Genetically controlled individual differences in immunological responses to specific chemicals
or groups of chemicals were found in experimental animals such as the guinea-pig (Chase 1958). They have also
been shown in the immune response of mice of different
strains to various antigens ranging from simple polypeptides containing as little as two or three amino acids, to
large molecules, such as ovomucoid (McDevitt and
Benacerraf 1969; Levine and Vaz 1970; Benacerraf and

McDevitt 1972; McDevitt and Bodmer 1972). It has
been shown that certain strains of mice respond to the
injection of minute amounts of some of these antigens by
producing high titres of reaginic antibodies (Levine and
Vaz 1970).

Studies in drug allergy in man Genetically determined
immune responses to simple chemicals or chemical
groups of similar nature to those previously mentioned
have not as yet been demonstrated in man. At present,
the only drug allergy for which it may be possible to
study these aspects in man is penicillin allergy. Although
several of our penicillin-allergic patients have a family
history of penicillin allergy, it could not be concluded
that this was due to genetically determined specific
immune response to penicillin. The main reason for this
situation is the frequent occurrence in penicillin-allergic
patients and their relations of allergy to a wide variety of
unrelated chemicals. Among over 200 patients allergic to
penicillin, however, we have seen no more than 5 with
personal and family histories of allergy to penicillin
alone.

We believed that family studies in subjects who are
allergic to penicillin and in non-allergic subjects who
also produce penicillin antibodies, but who do not manifest allergy (which requires a special class of antibodies
of which these subjects produce little, if any), might
throw some light on another interesting aspect, namely
the pattern of immune response to various degradation
products of the penicillin nucleus. Extensive investigations were carried out with conjugates of three metabolites that act as antigenic determinants: the 'major'
determinant (the penicilloyl group); and two 'minor'
determinants (the penicillenate and penicillamine groups).
Using various techniques to measure the antibodies
specific to these three determinants, we have not yet
detected any family-specific patterns (Assem and
Vickers, unpublished).

Possible influence of genetic factors in drug metabolism
Genetically determined variations in the metabolism of
some drugs in turn influence the occurrence of adverse
drug reactions other than allergy. Examples are prolonged apnoea after suxamethonium administration in
patients with pseudocholinesterase deficiency, the polyneuritis due to isoniazid in patients who are slow inactivators of this drug, and the higher incidence of
hydralazine-related SLE in slow acetylators. At present
there is merely speculation that elements of this sort
may to some extent determine the incidence, type, or
manifestations of allergic drug reactions. Perhaps differences in specific and non-specific hydroxylating enzymes

may be of importance in this respect (Remmer and Schuppel 1972).

Other factors that influence the patient's response

A large number of other non-specific factors may influence the response to antigenic stimuli. These include genetic factors which operate through alterations in enzyme systems, age, sex (e.g. the higher incidence of hydralazine-related SLE in females), and perhaps nutritional factors. Epidemiological studies have shown that adverse reactions of all kinds are commoner in patients who are aged 60 years and over, and in women (Hurwitz 1969).

The occurrence of disease in organs that take part in drug metabolism may play some role in the immunological response. Epidemiological surveys did not show, however, that patients with liver or kidney disease or diabetes mellitus have a greater incidence of adverse drug reactions (Hurwitz 1969), which suggests the possible limitations of surveys of this type.

The disease

Glandular fever and ampicillin rash

When patients with glandular fever (Pullen *et al.* 1967), certain viral infections, or leukaemia are given ampicillin, many develop a skin rash which several investigators claim to be of non-allergic nature, since the allergy tests they have carried out have been negative (Knudsen 1969). There are two important points to be made here. First, ampicillin is not the only penicillin to cause a rash, though it may do so more frequently than the others. We have investigated patients with a similar rash following other penicillins including the two natural penicillins, benzylpenicillin and phenoxymethylpenicillin. Secondly, it seems more likely that the rash is due to allergy caused by an immunological abnormality induced by the disease, for other abnormalities of this kind are well known to occur in glandular fever: namely, the presence of heterophile antibodies (detected by the Paul–Bunnell test) and cold agglutinins; and the occurrence of false-positive serological tests for syphilis.

As in other infections, the virus that is thought to cause glandular fever may act as an 'adjuvant' (see below).

Adjuvant effect

In experimental work designed to induce sensitization (allergy) or potentiation of the response to an antigen in the way of increasing the amount of antibody produced, certain micro-organisms are used, such as tubercle ba-

cilli (in complete Freund's adjuvant) and *Bordetella pertussis*. It is therefore reasonable to speculate that patients with infections due to these organisms might have a higher incidence of drug allergy.

It has been suggested that the incidence of drug allergy is higher during infection, and that, when given prophylactically, antibiotics and other chemotherapeutic agents produce allergic reactions less frequently than when they are administered during infections. This was thought to be caused by an adjuvant effect produced by bacterial infections, partly due to bacterial endotoxin (Munoz 1964). It is also possible that the tissue injury produced by infection may create more possible binding sites for haptens. The final stage of allergic reactions may also be potentiated by bacterial products. This is suggested by the finding that the injection of *B. pertussis* vaccine potentiates the toxic effects of histamine in mice (Kind 1958).

Immunological mechanisms

The four main immunological mechanisms involved in drug allergy (and in allergy in general) are shown in Table 25.1.

TABLE 25.1
Immunological mechanisms of allergic reactions
(according to Coombs and Gell classification, 1968)

Type I	Immediate-type (or anaphylactic) which is mediated by anaphylactic (reaginic) antibodies of the IgE, or possibly the IgG, class of immunoglobulins.
Type II	Autoallergy (autoimmunity), autosensitization being mediated by lymphocytes or antibodies.
Type III	Arthus-type, mediated by IgG, IgM, and complement 1. Typical Arthus reaction. 2. Conditions reproduced by special types of late responses to antigen challenge. 3. Immune-complex disease, serum sickness, or apparently similar syndromes.
Type IV	Delayed-type hypersensitivity (also described as cell-mediated immunity due to mediation by sensitized lymphocytes).

It is important to stress that, apart from allergy and its underlying mechanisms, some immune responses to drugs appear to be quite harmless, for example, the symptomless formation of hapten-specific antibodies. There is evidence suggesting that this is the most common type of response to at least some, if not all, of the drugs that are capable of inducing an immunological stimulus. In certain instances these antibodies seem to inhibit the damaging influence that may be produced by the simultaneous occurrence of the other varieties of immunological responses. In these cases, the antibodies may be described as 'blocking' antibodies. This functional class of antibodies may also be induced by hyposensitization (desensitization) procedures. The best known example is the almost invariable production of non-sensitizing IgG and IgM anti-penicilloyl antibodies in patients who have received penicillin therapy. In fact, these antibodies are also found in the majority of human subjects who have not been exposed to penicillin in this way but who, presumably, have encountered penicillins present in the air or in food, particularly milk and dairy products (though this should not happen if farmers adhere to the regulations prohibiting the sale of milk from cattle treated with penicillin).

Type I (the anaphylactic reaction)

This reaction deserves detailed consideration because of its acute nature, its potentially fatal outcome, and its usefulness in illustrating how the knowledge of mechanism helps both in diagnosis and treatment.

Fatal anaphylactic reactions to drugs are very rare (e.g. 10 cases were reported by the Registrar General of England and Wales in 1963; 7 of these were due to penicillin). These figures may be an underestimate, for doctors are understandably reluctant to attribute a patient's death to therapy and may attribute it to disease if it is at all reasonable to do so. In the USA, penicillin was again the most common cause of fatal anaphylactic reactions: it was implicated in 32 out of 43 anaphylactic deaths in the American Armed Forces (Delage and Irey 1972), and it was suggested 100–500 patients die annually from anaphylactic reactions to penicillin (Parker 1965, 1980, 1982). The incidence of minor (non-fatal) anaphylactic reactions to drugs is not known, but they are presumably much more frequent than fatal reactions. Estimates of the overall frequency of Type I reactions to the β-lactam antibiotics range from 0.7 to 8 per cent, and many investigators have reported an incidence higher than 2 per cent (Smith et al. 1966; Idsøe et al. 1968; Sullivan et al. 1981). The incidence may have declined in recent years, however, as compared with the early 1960s (Parker 1980). Other drugs have also come to prominence as causes of anaphylactic and anaphylactoid reactions (see below).

Anaphylactic antibodies

The anaphylactic reaction (immediate-type allergy) is the reaction mediated by certain classes of antibodies known collectively as anaphylactic (tissue-sensitizing) antibodies. Various species produce their own characteristic anaphylactic antibodies.

Various classifications are applied to these antibodies. The term 'homocytotropic' antibody was introduced by Becker and Austen (1968) to describe a specialized class of anaphylactic antibodies capable of attaching to certain target cells of the same species. Homocytotropic antibodies may further be classified into reaginic and non-reaginic. Antibodies mediating the anaphylactic reaction in man are of the reaginic type. They belong mainly to the most recently discovered γE (IgE) class of immunoglobulins.

Two points must be stressed with regard to anaphylactic antibodies. First, non-IgE antibodies may be involved in anaphylactic reactions. Suggestive evidence has been reported by various authors (e.g. Assem and Schild 1968; Assem and McAllen 1970; Parish 1973; Assem and Turner-Warwick 1976; Scott 1987). This possibility seems to be more likely with certain allergens, for example, penicillin (Assem and Schild 1968; Assem 1972a — see also Part 2 dealing with the detection of drug allergy). Secondly, there is controversy about whether IgE can cross the 'species barrier'; for example, whether or not human IgE antibodies can sensitize rat mast cells (Perelmutter and Khera 1969; Plautt et al. 1973). This procedure was initially introduced as a practical solution to the problem of obtaining human or other primate tissues for the in vitro detection of immediate-type allergy.

Mechanism of the anaphylactic reaction

The anaphylactic reaction results from the interaction between the specific allergen and the cell-fixed anaphylactic antibodies. The cells that are particularly involved in this reaction include tissue mast cells and basophil leucocytes, and anaphylactic antibodies seem to have special affinity for these cells. The interaction between the allergen and anaphylactic antibodies fixed to these cells triggers a process which seems to involve several steps inside these cells, ultimately leading to the release of pharmacological mediators. The released mediators in turn act on certain target organs or tissues, such as vascular and bronchial smooth muscle. Thus, the reaction affects two types of cell populations; the first are 'sensitized' cells, which recognize the allergen and react to it by elaborating the pharmacological mediators, and the second are the 'effector' cells, responding to these mediators. The released mediators seem to produce their effect through 'specific' receptors on the surface of 'effector' cells, such as the bronchial smooth muscle in asthma.

In order that the antigen–antibody interaction may initiate the anaphylactic mechanism, two criteria should be fulfilled:

1. for any particular cell, sensitization requires that there should be more than one antibody molecule per cell (they indeed exist in hundreds of thousands) (Ishizaka et al. 1973);
2. two or more identical groups (antigenic determinants or sites) should be present in the antigen, since the main mechanism of allergen-initiated reaction is a 'bridging' process of two adjacent antibody molecules (Stanworth 1973).

Immunological concepts in Type I allergy to drugs

The aforementioned concepts have the following important consequences:

Eliciting of allergic reactions by skin and other tests

The manifestations of immediate allergic reactions cannot be produced unless both the antigen and antibodies have multiple combining groups. This explains the very frequent failure of drugs to elicit a positive skin test. This occurs in the case where the unconjugated drug is not protein-reactive, and in the case of a univalent conjugate (one haptenic residue per molecule of conjugate). On the occasions when the simple chemical itself or its derivatives react rapidly with protein, as in the case of penicillin, an immediate-type reaction may be produced.

Although a molecule bearing a single determinant (monovalent hapten) which is still capable of binding to a single antibody molecule is generally incapable of triggering an allergic reaction, it may, however, elicit a reaction under a special condition: if it has an additional chemical group that provides the possibility of a second though non-identical binding site (Raffel 1973). In contrast, contact hypersensitivity, which is an example of delayed hypersensitivity, unlike the immediate type, can be elicited frequently by the chemical itself.

Inhibition of allergic reactions by monovalent haptens

While a non-reactive chemical, or a monovalent conjugate thereof, is incapable of eliciting an allergic reaction, it can produce the opposite effect, namely, inhibition of reaction to a complete antigen, when applied simultaneously. This can be shown by inhibition of a 'direct' skin test, passive cutaneous anaphylaxis, or even of the reaction to a drug administered systemically to a patient who is allergic to this particular drug (de Weck et al. 1973).

The clinical applications and mechanisms of inhibition of allergic reactions by monovalent haptens, and the immunological changes observed after hyposensitization therapy will be discussed.

Hyposensitization procedures

A patient allergic to a drug may be hyposensitized by gradually increasing the drug dosage up to the desired level, followed by repeated administration of the dose that is considered adequate. Hyposensitization can be maintained only by repeated administration of the drug, or the whole procedure should be repeated when another course of drug therapy is required (Holgate 1988).

Biochemical mechanisms and metabolic requirements of the anaphylactic reaction

It is thought that the bridging effect of antigen between adjacent antibody molecules induces configurational changes in the Fc region of the cell-fixed antibody molecule (the part of antibody attached to cell membrane), which in turn initiates a series of biochemical events inside sensitized cells (e.g. mast cells). These biochemical events lead to the release or synthesis and release of various pharmacological mediators of this reaction. This process is considered to be secretory in nature. It requires calcium and energy (it can be inhibited by metabolic inhibitors which are, on the whole, toxic), but does not require oxygen. Sodium cromoglycate, the 'prophylactic' antiasthma and antiallergy drug, may be considered as the prototype of non-toxic inhibitors of the mediator-secretion process. Its action is not, however, fully understood (Foreman and Pearce 1989) and is limited because of lack of absorption after oral administration. It is only effective if applied directly: by inhalation in asthma, as an aerosol or drops in rhinitis, or as eye drops in allergic conjunctivitis.

Pharmacological mediators of anaphylaxis

The mediators released, or formed and released, in this reaction depend on the species and tissues involved; for example, the two main mediators released from sensitized human lung tissue are histamine and slow-reacting substance of anaphylaxis (SRSA), derived from arachidonic acid, like prostaglandins (Jakschik et al. 1977; Bach et al. 1977). Slow-reacting substance of anaphylaxis has now been identified as mainly consisting of leukotrienes C_4 and D_4 and E_4 (Samuelson 1981; Piper 1983). The list of mediators is expanding all the time. Other candidates identified in various species are 5-hydroxytryptamine; kinins (e.g. bradykinin) (Brocklehurst and Lahiri 1962); thromboxanes (TX), for example, TXA_2, the main component of the so-called rabbit-aorta-contracting substance (Piper and Vane 1969; Hamberg *et al.* 1975; Dawson *et al.* 1976; Samuelson *et al.* 1978); platelet-activating factor (PAF: acetylglyceryl ether phosphorylcholine), formed in a wide range of cell types from precursor cell-membrane phospholipids through the concerted action of phospholipase A_2 and acetyl-CoA (Henson and Benveniste 1971; Henson and Pinckard 1977; Snyder 1985; Morley 1989); eosinophil chemotactic factor (Kay and Austen, 1971); and dopamine (in ruminants — [Eyre and Deline 1971]). At present the list of mediators or possible contenders is huge, and it exceeded 50 different substances several years ago (*The Lancet* 1983).

Non-immunological mechanisms

Anaphylactic-like reactions

Anaphylactic-like (anaphylactoid) reactions that are not immunologically mediated may be produced by the various mechanisms listed in Table 25.2. At the cellular level (mast cell or basophil leucocyte) histamine release may be due to an idiosyncratic susceptibility to a certain chemical grouping. Physical processes may also trigger the release of histamine and other mediators; one example is the release of histamine by hyperosmolar solutions of iodinated radiocontrast media (Assem *et al.* 1983). When anaphylactoid reactions occur with drugs that are known to interact with (stimulate or block) certain receptors, for example, neuromuscular blockers, it is tempting to speculate that the underlying mechanism may be a receptor abnormality. Caution is needed, however, since the mechanism may still turn out to be immunological (as in the case of neuromuscular blockers, see below).

Several groups of drugs are capable of inducing reactions of this type, though they may also induce immunologically mediated reactions. These drugs include preanaesthetic medications, intravenous anaesthetic induction agents, iodinated radiographic contrast media, aspirin-like drugs, and plasma substitutes (Assem 1977*b*; Watkins and Ward 1978; Watkins 1979; Assem 1983*a,b*; Assem *et al.* 1983; Szczeklik 1983).

In the past, a proportion of patients with the so-called 'anaphylactoid' reaction to neuromuscular blockers was considered under this category for a variety of reasons, including: (1) this proportion of patients reacted on their first clinical exposure to NMB (Assem 1977*b*, 1983*b*); (2) NMB were included among direct, 'non-immune' histamine-releasers (Paton 1957). It turned out, however, that IgE antibodies (which mediate anaphylaxis) to

NMB could be detected in the serum of those patients (Baldo and Fisher 1983; Harle *et al.* 1984; see Charpin *et al.* 1983; Vervloet *et al.* 1983; Didier *et al.* 1987; see Moneret-Vautrin *et al.* 1988*a,b*; Assem and Ling 1988; Assem and Symons 1989; Assem 1989, 1990*b*). This example (see Part 2 of this Chapter for further discussion of NMB) illustrates how wrong assumptions can arise.

TABLE 25.2
Mechanisms of production of drug reactions simulating manifestations of anaphylaxis

1. *Direct release of pharmacological mediators* such as histamine and 5-hydroxytryptamine:
   (a) as a process that does not normally occur: a qualitative abnormality: idiosyncrasy;
   (b) as a process that normally occurs to a much smaller extent: a quantitative abnormality: intolerance;
   (c) as a qualitative abnormality that normally occurs in other species, e.g. dextran reaction in rats, cremophor or miscellophor reaction in dogs.

2. *Direct (non-immune) activation of the complement system*

3. *Direct agonist or antagonist effects of the drug on 'target' or 'shock' organs*:
   (a) as a qualitative abnormality, e.g. aspirin-induced bronchospasm (also other non-steroidal anti-inflammatory drugs, NSAID);*
   (b) as a quantitative abnormality: intolerance.

4. *Indirect effect on 'shock' organs* by interfering with the response to drugs or normal homoeostatic mechanisms, e.g. the autonomic regulatory mechanisms, balance between pathways of mediator synthesis or metabolism (lipoxygenase and cyclo-oxygenase pathways of arachidonic acid metabolism),* balance between mediators with opposite effects (broncho-constrictor and bronchodilator prostaglandins).*

* Among the possible explanations of asthma induced by NSAID

The formation of circulating antibodies that produce reactions not of the classical immediate type

Examples of this in penicillin allergy are the accelerated reaction which appears 2–48 hours after the start of penicillin therapy, and the retarded reaction that occurs 3 days or more after such treatment. Another example is the drug-induced illness resembling serum sickness, which may be caused by such drugs as penicillin and aspirin. Antibodies producing the Arthus reaction are also included in this category. In all these examples, the formation of immune complexes and the activation of complement takes place, thus initiating the inflammatory response or tissue damage.

Delayed-type hypersensitivity

The relation of circulating antibodies to this type of reaction is obscure, and the condition can be transferred by lymphocytes but not by serum. It has now been established that the reaction is mediated by sensitized T lymphocytes, which respond to the specific allergen (and non-specifically to certain mitogens) by producing lymphokines, which consist of a large number of protein or polypeptide substances and which are considered to be the putative soluble mediators of delayed-type hypersensitivity reactions (Dumonde et al. 1969). Among the activities of lymphokines are release of histamine and SRS (mainly leukotrienes C_4 and D_4) (Thueson et al. 1979; Sedgwick et al. 1981; Ezeamuzie and Assem 1982, 1983a, 1984, 1985a–d, 1986, 1987; Kaplan et al. 1985).

Contact sensitivity is an example of delayed hypersensitivity. The induction of contact cutaneous sensitivity occurs as a result of the conjugation of hapten to epidermal proteins. There is evidence that the ability of chemical compounds to elicit allergic contact dermatitis can be correlated with the affinity for sulphydryl-containing proteins of the skin. On subsequent exposure to the same haptens this process is repeated and the resulting conjugate elicits an allergic reaction by reacting with sensitized cells (Schild 1962; Calnan 1968).

Autoallergy and related phenomena

The formation of hapten–protein conjugates in the body may induce marked changes in the carrier protein molecule, depending on the degree of substitution with haptenic groups. In this way body proteins may no longer be recognized as 'self'. This may lead to the formation of a wide variety of antibodies; some of them are organ-specific (for example, antibodies against the formed elements of the blood) while others are not. This process (autoimmunization) may be associated with, or cause, illness (autoallergy).

The development of autoantibodies, for example red blood cell antibodies (detected by a positive Coombs test) or antinuclear antibodies, may not necessarily be associated with illness. In fact, in general, autoimmune disease (autoallergy) occurs in a minority of these patients, particularly if they have no strong disposition to such illnesses.

Drug-related systemic lupus erythematosus-like syndrome

One of the best examples used to illustrate the mechanisms involved in drug-induced autoallergy is the drug-related systemic lupus erythematosus syndrome (D-RSLE) (Harpey et al. 1972). The list of drugs capable of inducing this syndrome is shown in Table 16.1, Chapter 16.

Factors contributing to lupus induction or activation by drugs

Genetic predisposition

(a) Lupus diathesis: strong predisposition requires a weak stimulus, and *vice versa*; (b) the rate of drug metabolism, for example slow acetylation of isoniazid and hydralazine (Perry et al. 1970), and of procainamide (Woosley et al. 1978) appears to be a predisposing factor.

Pharmacological action of the drug involved

(a) Inhibition of certain enzymes, for example, DNAase (hydralazine); (b) enhancement of formation of disulphide bonds (hydralazine) (some other factors activate rheumatoid arthritis in a similar way); (c) interference with cross-linkage of collagen and elastin (penicillamine); (d) influence on polymerization of macromolecular complexes (penicillamine); (e) antagonism of some 'physiological' protective mechanisms (e.g. antiallergy).

Possibility (e) may explain the mechanism in the case of β-blockers, particularly in view of findings indicating that catecholamines have some anti-inflammatory and antiallergy effects (predominantly due to stimulation of β-adrenoceptors). Since the antiallergy effects were not $β_1$ or $β_2$ 'selective' (Assem and Schild 1971), we were not surprised to find that autoimmune phenomena such as the development of antinuclear antibodies in patients receiving β-receptor blocking drugs were not related to the 'selectivity' of these agents in regard to the subclasses of β-receptors ($β_1$ and $β_2$) (Assem 1975, 1977a). The significance of the various autoantibodies that were found in patients with practolol 'reactions' other than SLE is still unclear.

Changes in structure or antigenicity, or both, of DNA and soluble nuclear and cytoplasmic nucleoprotein

(a) Antigenicity of photochemical products of DNA and procainamide > photo-oxidized DNA > native DNA; (b) enhancement of the antigenicity of soluble nucleoprotein by hydralazine; (c) agents that may interact with viruses: for example, penicillamine interacting with polio virus and producing the lupus syndrome in certain strains of mice and the possible interaction of some drugs with oncorna virus nucleic acid; (d) enhanced production of drug metabolites that react with autoantigen through enzyme induction.

Modulation by the autonomic nervous system of immune responses and allergic reactions

A brief summary of these concepts will be given here; for further information the reader is referred to some key reviews (Sutherland and Robison 1966; Szentivanyi 1969; Assem 1971, 1973; Barnes 1989). Most of these concepts appear to stem from work on asthma and atopy, in which the neural (autonomic) mechanisms intermingle with immune and inflammatory reactions. There is evidence to suggest that the autonomic nervous system has an influence on various immunological mechanisms, and that it may possibly modulate allergic reactions by interfering with the different steps of these reactions. Adrenergic mechanisms seem to play an important role in immediate-type and delayed-type (cell-mediated) immune reactions, as suggested by the modulatory effect of adrenergic drugs. Cholinergic mechanisms may also play some role in the regulation of immediate-type allergy, as suggested by the potentiation of antigen-induced mediator release by cholinergic drugs. Cholinergic agents also enhance the cytotoxic action of sensitized lymphocytes. Both adrenergic and cholinergic agents trigger the proliferation of, and DNA synthesis in, spleen colony-forming cells.

More recently, the inflammatory aspect of asthma was associated with additional neural mechanisms: non-adrenergic non-cholinergic mechanisms, with possible involvement of many neuropeptides. A great deal of work is required in order to assess the importance of these mechanisms.

Clinical manifestations of drug allergy

Allergic reactions to drugs produce widely variable clinical manifestations. I do not intend to give more than a brief outline of these reactions and an incomplete list of drugs causing them. Chemical compounds that constitute an industrial hazard will not be mentioned. It is important to stress that minor reactions are fairly frequent, but serious ones are rare.

Clinical manifestations of allergy to a single drug may be single or multiple, and they vary from person to person as a result of involvement of different 'target' organs. The reasons for this variability are not very clear. Of special importance is the extent of dissemination of the causative antigens, which may be influenced by the dosage and route of administration. The site at which the simple chemical undergoes metabolic processes that lead to the formation of haptenic determinants is also of importance. The localization of the reaction may also depend on the formation of organ-specific antibodies, as mentioned previously.

Anaphylaxis

Immediate reactions may be manifested by urticaria, rhinitis, bronchial asthma, angioedema (angioneurotic oedema), and anaphylaxis. These manifestations are the counterpart of the classical allergy to foreign protein.

Anaphylactic reactions develop within a few minutes of the administration of the offending drug, and perhaps in less than a minute in some cases. The principal manifestations are those of peripheral circulatory collapse (shock), which may be associated with one or more of the other immediate reactions. It is important to differentiate anaphylaxis from vasovagal syncope, which may be produced by psychogenic causes, such as fear, the sight of blood, or painful stimuli. Recovery from vasovagal attacks takes place soon after lying down. The drugs and diagnostic agents that may cause anaphylactic reactions include β-lactam antibiotics (penicillins and cephalosporins), streptomycin, neuromuscular-blocking drugs, intravenous anaesthetics, local anaesthetic agents, organic mercurials, radio-opaque iodides, plasma expanders (dextrans, polygelatin, and starch derivatives), non-steroidal anti-inflammatory drugs (NSAID), narcotic analgesics, preanaesthetic medications, streptokinase, heparin, vitamin K_1 oxide (reactions to injections of other vitamins such as vitamins B_1 and B_{12} have also been reported), bromsulphthalein, sodium dehydrocholate (Decholin), and demeclocycline.

It should be added that some of the above-mentioned drugs, such as radio-opaque organic iodides, NSAID, anaesthetic agents, narcotic analgesics, and plasma expanders may possibly produce a reaction resembling anaphylaxis by mechanisms other than allergy. Radio-opaque organic iodides may cause angiotoxic damage and the direct release of histamine without the apparent mediation of an antigen–antibody interaction (Mann 1961; Assem *et al.* 1983). Histamine release by these agents may be caused by hyperosmolarity or activation of the alternative pathway of the complement system (causing the generation of anaphylatoxins). Further discussion will be included in Part 2 of this chapter.

Skin manifestations

Allergic reactions to drugs are most frequently manifested by skin eruptions; these have also been reported after placebo administration (Samter and Berryman 1964). The different varieties of reactions are: urticarial, morbilliform, maculopapular, vesicular, bullous, exfoliative, and eczematous eruptions; purpura; contact dermatitis; fixed eruptions; erythema nodosum; erythema multiforme; photosensitivity; and pruritus.

Urticaria is a typical example of immediate cutaneous sensitivity (Type I, or anaphylactic; but it may be mediated by other mechanisms, e.g. Type III) while contact dermatitis is a typical manifestation of delayed-type hypersensitivity. Skin manifestations of what were previously called 'connective tissue' diseases, which are associated with (and probably caused by) autoallergy, such as lupus erythematosus, which may be induced by drugs, may be included in this list.

As with many other manifestations of drug-induced disease, photosensitivity may be due to toxic or allergic reactions (Harber and Baer 1969; Ring and Przbilla 1989). Recent interest has focused on the photosensitizing effect of non-steroidal anti-inflammatory drugs, especially propionic acid derivatives (Ring et al. 1987).

Certain varieties of these reactions are produced more frequently by certain drugs. Erythema multiforme and nodosum are seen particularly in allergy to sulphonamides, barbiturates, pyrazolone derivatives, phenytoin, bromides, iodides, and troxidone. Fixed drug eruptions are most commonly due to phenolphthalein, amidopyrine, barbiturates, sulphonamides, and mepacrine. Photosensitivity occurs characteristically with sulphonamide derivatives (including those with no antibacterial activity, such as the thiazide diuretics and sulphonylurea compounds), phenothiazines, and tetracyclines. The sulphonamide derivatives seem to produce true photoallergic reactions. Drug-induced Stevens–Johnson syndrome is caused most frequently by barbiturates and sulphonamides. Carbamazepine may also induce this syndrome. The author has seen two severe cases due to the latter drug.

A few reports on allergy to β-adrenoceptor blocking drugs such as propranolol, practolol, and oxprenolol have been published. The skin rashes were psoriasiform, exfoliative, or urticarial eruptions, and were frequently associated with autoimmune phenomena, particularly the development of antinuclear antibodies and lupus erythematosus cells (Assem and Banks 1973; Raftery and Denman 1973; Assem 1975, 1977a) (see also Chapter 17).

Of all the cases of skin eruptions associated with the administration of β-adrenoceptor blocking drugs, and reported by various authors, only eight of ours (representing 40 per cent of our series) showed direct evidence of allergy to these agents. Such evidence was obtained in vitro by the lymphocyte stimulation (transformation) test. This and the delayed skin response in some patients suggested a delayed-type hypersensitivity.

It is not known whether the other syndromes that have been associated with practolol administration are due to immunologically mediated reactions, but autoallergy has been suspected at least in some (see the review by Amos 1979). Various organs may be involved, particularly the skin and, more seriously, the eyes (keratoconjunctivitis sicca and its sequelae [Wright 1975; Behan et al. 1976]) and serous membranes, particularly the peritoneum (sclerosing peritonitis [Brown et al. 1974]) and the pleura (MacKay and Axford 1976). The ears (Wright 1975), the kidneys (Farr et al. 1975), liver (Brown et al. 1978), lung (Marshall et al. 1977), pericardium (Assem 1977a), and the laryngotracheal region (Assem 1977a) may also be affected.

An alternative (non-immune) mechanism of skin eruptions induced by long-term therapy with β-adrenoceptor blocking drugs has been postulated by Jensen and others (1976). These authors suggested that such eruptions could be explained by a reduction in the concentration of cyclic adenosine $3',5'$-monophosphate inside epidermal cells, a mechanism that is related to the pharmacological action of these drugs.

Fever

This is one of the commonest manifestations of drug allergy in man, and many drugs, including most antibiotics and other chemotherapeutic agents, can cause fever with and without other manifestations. Pyrexia is, however, rare with some drugs, tetracycline, for instance. The underlying mechanisms have not been fully elucidated. In experimental animals drug fever may be caused by the interaction of antigen with circulating antibody (in the rabbit) or by delayed hypersensitivity (in the guinea-pig). (See the review by Cluff and Johnson [1964] for further discussion.) In the former case (circulating antibody–antigen interaction) endogenous pyrogens are produced by phagocytic leucocytes which are stimulated by the engulfment of immune complexes (Dinarello and Wolff 1978, 1982). In delayed hypersensitivity, lymphokines produced by antigen-stimulated lymphocytes seem to play some role (Chao et al. 1977), probably due to activation of phagocytic leucocytes.

It has now been established that the endogenous pyrogen produced by phagocytic leucocytes is 'interleukin 1' (Dinarello 1984, 1989) and that the pyrogens act by increasing arachidonate metabolites, particularly prostaglandin E_1, in the anterior hypothalamus (in the vicinity of the thermoregulatory centre) (Foreman 1989). This subject is also discussed in Chapter 28.

Serum sickness syndrome

This syndrome may be produced by penicillin, aspirin, streptomycin, sulphonamides, and thiouracils. Like serum sickness produced by foreign serum or proteins, the disease occurs in different forms depending on the time of onset in relation to the therapeutic course. The onset of the primary form typically occurs 7–12 days after the start of therapy. The accelerated form occurs in 2 hours to 3 days. A retarded form occurs within a few weeks of drug therapy, or even after the discontinuation of therapy. The main features of this syndrome are fever, arthralgia, urticaria, and maculopapular eruptions. Lymphadenopathy, dyspnoea, wheezing, angioedema, and eosinophilia occur less frequently. The symptoms may be mild and transitory, lasting from a few hours to 4 days, or may be very serious and continue for several weeks. A variety of other complications may develop, for example, brachial plexus neuritis or other types of mononeuritis multiplex, the Guillain–Barré syndrome, optic neuritis, nephritis, carditis, and polyarteritis nodosa.

Laboratory studies may disclose albumin and hyaline casts in the urine, eosinophilia, several types of circulating antibodies and, rarely, plasmacytosis (Arbesman and Reisman 1971).

Neuropathy

This mainly occurs in the serum sickness syndrome. Mononeuritis and polyneuritis are thought to be due to perineural oedema. Peripheral neuritis is a fairly common manifestation of polyarteritis nodosa, in which ischaemia of the peripheral nerves seems to be the underlying mechanism. (See also Chapter 18.)

Lymphadenopathy

The enlargement of lymph nodes occurs in serum sickness. Cellular proliferation in lymph nodes and spleen may be explained by a marked antigenic stimulation. Rarely, patients receiving long-term phenytoin therapy have clinical and pathological changes highly suggestive of lymphoma (Saltzstein and Ackerman 1959; see also Chapter 24). Lymph node enlargement subsides rapidly after cessation of therapy. We reported one patient with allergy to phenylbutazone and a condition resembling Hodgkin's disease (Littlejohns *et al.* 1973) which disappeared after stopping this drug. A few more patients with somewhat similar clinical manifestations have been investigated in our laboratory, but lymph node biopsy which was obtained in one of them did not show the characteristics of Hodgkin's disease (Assem 1976).

Haematological manifestations

Haematological disorders induced by drugs may be due to inherited biochemical abnormalities, drug toxicity, or allergy. Some of the drugs that have been proved or suggested to be capable of producing immunological responses, and changes affecting the blood, are included in the lists given in Chapter 22. In some of these the evidence is only circumstantial and it may be hard to exclude the possibility that the reactions produced by them are manifestations of cytotoxicity or some unrevealed biochemical abnormality.

Thrombocytopenia

It has been suggested that platelet antibodies that were found in patients with thrombocytopenia due to some drugs (for example, Sedormid) were formed in response to a loose hapten–platelet complex (Ackroyd 1964). It is doubtful whether such a complex would form an adequate antigen, and it seems more likely that these haptens can react irreversibly with platelet, tissue, or plasma proteins (i.e. the antigen may not be located on platelets) by an as yet unidentified pathway. Platelet antibodies are capable of agglutinating normal platelets *in vitro*, in the presence of the specific hapten, and when complement is added lysis of platelets occurs. At present the mechanisms of platelet agglutination and lysis *in vivo* and *in vitro* are not well understood (Ackroyd 1964; Shulman 1963, 1964).

Haemolytic anaemia

Drug-induced allergic haemolytic anaemia is produced by mechanisms similar to those of thrombocytopenia. Red cell antibodies seem to occur much more frequently than haemolytic reactions. It is important to remember that some of the above-mentioned drugs, such as sulphonamides and phenacetin, are also capable of causing haemolysis of cells deficient in glucose 6-phosphate dehydrogenase (Prankerd 1963; Dacie 1962). Also, some of the reported instances of allergic haemolytic reactions that were apparently induced by antibiotics or other chemotherapeutic agents have been due to virus disease, particularly the myxovirus group, producing 'autosensitization' (Isacson 1967).

Leucopenia and agranulocytosis

Leucocyte agglutinins have been found in cases of agranulocytosis produced by certain drugs. These agglutinins, however, could be demonstrated in most cases only when the offending drug was given a few hours before the collection of blood for testing or, as is the case of some drugs such as sulphapyridine, by the addition of a small amount of the drug to the serum to be tested. This strongly suggests that the antigen(s) corresponding to these agglutinins is not located on the white cells.

In addition to the presence of leucocyte agglutinins in the blood of subjects with amidopyrine-induced agranulocytosis, recipients of sensitized donor blood also developed agranulocytosis (Moeschlin and Wagner 1952; Moeschlin 1958).

The relationship between antinuclear factor and leucopenia in systemic lupus erythematosus is not understood. It seems that agranulocytosis may be produced either by the removal and destruction of agglutinated white cells, or the interaction of drug, antibody, and granulocyte precursors in the bone marrow, producing maturation arrest. The onset of clinical features is usually more or less sudden, and this limits the value of routine white cell counts as a precaution.

Leucopenia or agranulocytosis due to drugs containing a thiourea group is thought to be due to 'toxicity' (an expression of idiosyncrasy in many instances) rather than to allergy. A good example of the usefulness of studies on structure–activity relationship with respect to adverse effects is the replacement of the thiourea group in metiamide (a histamine H_2-receptor antagonist that caused leucopenia) by a cyanoguanidine moiety, thus forming cimetidine, which is less likely to have that effect (Brimblecombe et al. 1975; but see Chapter 22).

Hypoplastic anaemia and pancytopenia

At present evidence that the hypoplastic conditions of the bone marrow that are produced by drugs are due to an immunological response is not conclusive. The induction of this condition by relatively small amounts of some drugs in some people can be explained by mechanisms other than allergy. It has been suggested that bone marrow failure may be due to unsuspected biochemical abnormality.

Thrombocytopenic purpura

Symmers (1962) reported several cases of thrombocytopenic purpura that were probably due to drug allergy. (Blood disorders induced by drugs are also discussed in Chapter 22.)

Liver disease

Drug-induced hepatocellular disorders are probably not allergic: on the other hand, some cases of cholestatic jaundice probably are. This may be the case with drugs of the phenothiazine group, where jaundice may be produced after a small dose, and other phenomena that are suggestive of allergy may occur, for example, rashes, fever, blood and tissue eosinophilia, and blood dyscrasias. The inability to detect circulating antibodies in this type of reaction does not make the diagnosis of drug allergy untenable since the antigen may react with antibodies fixed to liver cells, thereby producing liver injury.

It may be that the low recurrence rate (below 40 per cent) of cholestatic jaundice when the drug is given again is evidence against the hypothesis of an allergic mechanism unless one postulates that desensitization occurs in 60 per cent of those who develop this reaction.

Latent cholestatic jaundice and, less frequently, overt jaundice may occur in association with systemic manifestations of drug allergy due to penicillin, sulphonamides, sodium aminosalicylate (PAS), and esters of the macrolide antibiotics (erythromycin and oleandomycin). For further information the reader is referred to Chapter 11 and to the reviews by Sherlock (Sherlock 1965; Sherlock and Ajdukiewicz 1972). The absence of proper material for skin tests and the inadvisability of carrying out passive sensitization by the Prausnitz–Kustner reaction are obvious limitations to these diagnostic methods. Antituberculous drugs other than PAS, and methyldopa, may cause either a hepatitis-like condition, or cholestatic jaundice (Assem et al. 1969; Assem 1972b; Toghill et al. 1974; Hoffbrand et al. 1974). The hepatitis-like picture, which may rarely be caused by isoniazid allergy (Assem et al. 1969), may suggest that allergy may also account for the hepatitis caused by iproniazid, another hydrazine derivative with monoamine-oxidase-inhibiting activity.

Vasculitis and connective tissue disease

This group of reactions has far less clearly defined manifestations than the previously mentioned categories. This is due to the lack of specific organ localization. Little is understood about the underlying mechanisms, and the evidence for the involvement of immunological processes is indirect and based more on speculative assumptions than on valid criteria. Studies of this group may perhaps, however, cast some light on the pathogenesis of connective tissue diseases in general.

Lupus erythematosus-like syndrome

A clinical syndrome resembling systemic lupus erythematosus (SLE) with or without the LE-cell phenomenon, associated with treatment with various drugs, notably hydralazine (Morrow et al. 1953), has been mentioned earlier. It is not established that this disease is due to drug allergy. Although it is reversible in the majority of cases, it may persist for years or become irreversible in some cases. It has been suggested that the drug merely unveils latent disease. In favour of this idea is the fact that some patients with so-called hydralazine-related LE have had an antecedent history suggestive of

SLE (Holley 1964). The finding that some patients may have further attacks of SLE following the discontinuation of the drug is not necessarily in favour of this theory. Apart from the LE-cell phenomenon and the antinuclear factors, a positive Coombs test, and occasionally, haemolytic anaemia may be associated with the SLE syndrome. This subject is also discussed in Chapter 16.

Acute vasculitis

Acute vasculitis, predominantly affecting small vessels, and ranging from mild cellular infiltration to acute necrosis, may be caused by drugs. The drugs most commonly implicated are penicillin, sulphonamides, and thiouracils (Symmers 1962). The clinical manifestations are petechial skin lesions, proteinuria, haematuria, and renal failure. Clinical features often include fever, dermatitis, arthralgia, oedema and, less frequently, myositis, coronary arteritis, and gastrointestinal bleeding.

Chronic vasculitis

The prolonged administration of some drugs, such as hydrazines, thiouracils, phenytoin, sulphonamides, penicillin, and iodides, may produce polyarteritis or some other variants of chronic inflammatory vascular disease (McCormick 1950). Rose and Spencer (1957) doubted the aetiological relationship of drugs to polyarteritis nodosa. It is also doubtful whether the administration of drugs for short periods can produce vasculitis in which fresh lesions appear months or years after the drug has been withdrawn. It is possible, however, that acute vasculitis may become a chronic condition through some self-perpetuating mechanisms.

Polymyositis

Allergy to penicillin, and perhaps other drugs also, may be manifested by polymyositis (Parker 1965). We have encountered a patient allergic to penicillin who developed an exacerbation of the symptoms of polymyositis following a skin test with penicilloyl-polylysine.

Pulmonary manifestations

Bronchial asthma is the most common pulmonary manifestation of drug allergy. It may occur as a manifestation of systemic or local anaphylaxis (affecting respiratory airways without involvement of other systems). Non-steroidal anti-inflammatory drugs may induce asthma attacks, particularly in those who already had suffered from asthma. Such asthma is frequently associated with angioedema. Its mechanism is complex; some of the possible explanations are shown in Table 25.2.

Hilar lymphadenopathy and pulmonary eosinophilia occur much less frequently, and pneumonitis with pulmonary oedema is very rare. Pneumonitis may be caused by cytotoxic anticancer drugs, but may also be produced by a wide range of other drugs (Cooper *et al.* 1986). (See also Chapter 8.)

Nephropathy

Glomerulonephritis is often associated with the serum sickness syndrome or acute vasculitis due to drug allergy. Acute interstitial nephritis may probably be produced by drug allergy (Baker and Williams 1963) to, for example, sulphonamides, phenindione, phenazone, and penicillins (benzylpenicillin, ampicillin, and methicillin [Baldwin *et al.* 1968]). With cephalosporins the mechanism is different, since certain derivatives (e.g. cephaloridine) are nephrotoxic. Allergy to cephalosporins may, however, cause kidney disease such as interstitial nephritis (Wiles *et al.* 1979). A few cases of interstitial nephritis due to phenylbutazone have also been reported (McMenamin *et al.* 1976; Russell *et al.* 1978). Among the other features found in those cases were skin rashes, eosinophilia, and hepatitis. A somewhat similar syndrome due to allopurinol has also been reported (McKendrick and Geddes 1979).

Focal or diffuse glomerulonephritis, often with classic 'wire-loop' changes, is present in the kidneys in the majority of patients who die with SLE. The deposition of γ-globulin and complement on the basement membrane has been demonstrated by immunofluorescent techniques. Clinically the disease may manifest itself by acute nephritis, typical nephrotic syndrome, or varying degrees of chronic renal failure. A large number of drugs may produce the nephrotic syndrome, but allergy has not been proved in these cases. The 'nephropathy' that may be produced by phenacetin and perhaps other analgesic drugs is probably not due to allergy.

Recently, it has been shown that the kidney may be involved in anaphylactic reactions (Assem *et al.* 1986; Assem and Abdullah 1987*a,b*; Assem *et al.* 1987; Abdullah *et al.* 1988; Abdullah and Assem 1989; Ghanem *et al.* 1989; see also Wiles *et al.* 1979). Mast cells have been shown in kidney tissue, in the interstitium of the cortex and outer medulla. Sensitization of kidney mast cells with IgE antibody has been demonstrated. *In vitro* experiments on sensitized human, guinea-pig and rat kidney have shown that the most likely consequence of an anaphylactic reaction affecting the kidney is increased glomerular capillary permeability (evidence of which may be sought from urine testing for protein) and renal vasoconstriction, a phenomenon difficult to demonstrate clinically. (See also Chapter 12.)

Cardiac manifestations

Myocarditis

Myocarditis may be associated with the serum sickness syndrome. It has also been reported after sulphonamides, neoarsphenamine, iodides, penicillin, and other sensitizing drugs (Rich 1958).

Cardiac involvement in anaphylaxis

There is strong evidence from work on isolated (*in vitro*), perfused hearts of experimental animals (Langendorff preparation [LP], usually perfused with buffer and not blood) that the heart, apart from being secondarily affected in systemic anaphylaxis (as a result of haemodynamic changes, hypoxia, effects of mediators released from other tissues, etc.), may be directly involved in systemic anaphylaxis. This phenomenon is described as 'cardiac anaphylaxis' (CA) (Hadji and Benveniste 1980; Levi *et al.* 1981; Burke *et al.* 1982; Levi *et al.* 1982; Ezeamuzie and Assem 1983b; Levi *et al.* 1984; Machado *et al.* 1985 a,b; Assem and Ghanem 1988; Ghanem 1988; Ghanem *et al.* 1988a,b, 1989; Assem and Ezeamuzie 1989). In the LP, gross CA is manifested by gross cardiac dysfunction occurring rapidly (1–2 min) after addition of the specific allergen to the perfusion fluid. This challenge causes concomitant release of various pharmacological mediators (the same mediators of anaphylaxis as mentioned before, histamine, etc.), which can readily explain the dysfunction. The development of cardiac arrhythmias (and A–V conduction block) has been associated with the effect of histamine (mainly through H_2-receptors, a small part through H_1-receptors, which are involved in A–V conduction block) (Levi *et al.* 1982; Machado *et al.* 1985a), which is released from tissue mast cells (also from basophil leucocytes, in the presence of blood) during the reaction, but which may also occur as a consequence of coronary vasoconstriction. Other manifestations of CA include coronary vasoconstriction and weakened myocardial contractility, which are due to thromboxane A_2, leukotrienes C_4, D_4, and E_4 (slow-reacting substance of anaphylaxis), prostaglandin D_2 and $F_{2\alpha}$, and platelet activating factor (PAF-acether; acetyl-glyceryl ether phosphorylcholine, AGEPC) (Burke *et al.* 1982; Levi *et al.* 1984; Machado *et al.* 1985b). The cell origin of the latter group of mediators is far more varied than histamine, including tissue mast cells, and endothelial cells (which release PAF, Camussi *et al.* 1983); also leucocytes and mononuclear cells (including phagocytes). Platelets (*in vivo*) are also a source of PAF and

thromboxane A_2. Thus, the *in vivo* reaction would be expected to involve a wider variety of mediators than the *in vitro* preparation, perfused with buffer.

The consensus of opinion is that human heart and guinea-pig heart are similar in their response to allergen challenge and histamine (Levi *et al.* 1981, 1982), and it is reasonable to assume that the cardiac arrhythmias and changes in ECG associated with anaphylactic shock in man are partly due to a primary cardiac anaphylaxis, and not solely to the hypoxia caused by the bronchospasm or respiratory arrest common in severe anaphylaxis.

Mechanism

Mast cells have been found in heart tissues of man and experimental animals. They are located in the connective tissue surrounding coronary vasculature, and in the innermost and outermost layers of cardiac tissue (subepicardial and subendocardial) (Ghanem 1988; Ghanem *et al.* 1988a,b). The sensitization of cardiac mast cells with IgE molecules, thus paving the way for a local reaction in the heart, has also been demonstrated both by mediator release (histamine and arachidonic acid metabolites, Marone *et al.* 1986) and immuno-histochemical studies (Assem and Ghanem 1988).

Prevention of allergic drug reactions

Pretreament allergy testing

The indications and limitations for 'prophylactic'/ 'predictive' testing are discussed in Part 2 of this chapter, dealing with the detection of drug allergy.

Skin testing

The predictive value of skin tests and their limitations in penicillin allergy are discussed in Part 2 of this chapter. There is no doubt that they provide some help in preventing allergic reactions to penicillin.

RAST tests for IgE antibodies to anaesthetics (see Part 2)

A variety of radioallergosorbent tests (RAST) for IgE antibodies to anaesthetics, using a variety of solid-phase components, have been developed recently. Sepharose beads were used by some workers (Baldo and Fisher 1983; Harle *et al.* 1984; Didier *et al.* 1987; Moneret-Vautrin *et al.* 1988a,b). Paper RAST for anaesthetics (NMB and thiopentone) were subsequently developed by the author, in conjunction with Pharmacia Ltd; these are simple and reliable, and their value was shown in patients who have had anaphylactic reactions under general anaesthesia (Assem and Ling 1988; Assem 1990*a,b*). Their value 'after the event' has paved the way for prospective 'screening' trials (before general anaesthesia), with the hope of reducing anaesthetic morbidity and mortality.

Elimination of antigenic material

Sources of antigenic material in drug preparations have been discussed earlier. It is possible to eliminate some of them.

Allergen-specific inhibition procedures

Allergic drug reactions may be inhibited prophylactically in different ways, as illustrated in Fig. 25.2.

Hapten inhibition

One of the practical outcomes of the failure of monovalent haptens to produce an allergic reaction is that if an excess of a hapten and a modest amount of an antigen are used together in challenging the sensitized cells (e.g.

mast cells), the ineffective hapten, competing with the antigen, will inhibit the reaction to the antigen. The ineffectiveness of a monovalent hapten may be predicted from its chemical structure, and is indicated by the lack of a reactive group other than the single haptenic determinant. Further confirmation of this property can be obtained by work in experimental animals (Raffel 1973).

This concept of hapten inhibition has been used in the treatment of penicillin allergy, using non-reactive monovalent penicilloyl haptens, such as benzylpenicilloyl-formyl-L-lysine (BPO-Flys) (de Weck *et al.* 1973; Fig. 25.3). Such monovalent hapten conjugates (BPO-Flys) may not, however, be entirely risk-free, and their success depends on the relative importance of the penicilloyl determinant (compared with other determinants) in the individual patient. This may explain the unsuccessful cases reported by other authors (Basomba *et al.* 1978).

A more recent and successful application of the principle of hapten inhibition of anaphylactic drug reactions is the use of 'dextran 1' (very low molecular weight, only 1 kD) to prevent anaphylactic reactions to the clinical dextrans, which have a much higher molecular weight (>40 kD). The intravenous injection of 20 ml of a 15% solution of dextran 1, before the infusion of the clinical dextrans is thought to have practically eliminated the risk of severe anaphylactic reactions and fatalities related to these clinical dextrans (Lingstrom *et al.* 1988).

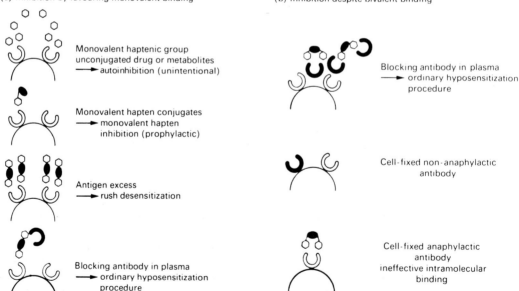

FIG. 25.2
Illustration of the various immunological mechanisms of inducing inhibition of the anaphylactic reaction to drugs, with particular reference to the nature of binding, whether monovalent or bivalent, by cell-fixed anaphylactic antibodies to the allergen.

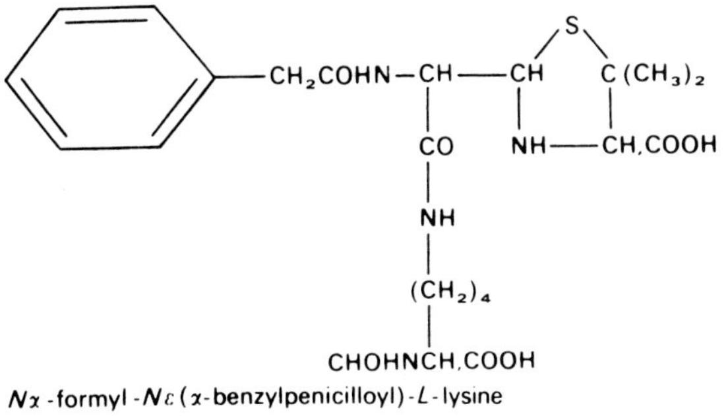

$N\alpha$ -formyl -$N\varepsilon$ (α-benzylpenicilloyl) -L-lysine

FIG. 25.3

Example of a monovalent penicilloyl conjugate capable of inhibiting allergic reactions to the penicilloyl determinant, the 'major' haptenic determinant in penicillin allergy (De Weck *et al.* 1973).

Inhibition by antigen excess

This may occur in what is described as 'rush desensitization', in which increasing amounts of an allergen are given, eventually reaching an excess.

Spontaneous autoinhibition and hyposensitization

Since most drugs are simple chemicals, and can thus act as haptens, the bulk of a free drug, given in the usual dose, or its metabolites, may inhibit the allergic response to the small chemically conjugated fraction of the drug forming an antigen. In fact, this seems to be the way by which many allergic patients inadvertently escape reactions. Although this process may occur spontaneously, one cannot predict its occurrence.

Induction of immunological tolerance by use of a tolerogen

These methods are potentially useful in the induction of prolonged desensitization to drugs, unlike those above. Chemical modification of allergens may produce a general reduction in the immune response to these agents, or may render them simple immunogens capable of inducing the formation of harmless antibodies, akin to those occurring frequently with certain substances, for example penicillin, as mentioned previously. Three different methods are described here as examples of a multitude of approaches that may be of potential value:

1. modification of protein allergens by conjugation with certain chemicals, for example, polyethylene glycol may render them less allergenic, that is, reaginic antibody production may be suppressed (Lee and Sehon 1978);
2. presentation of the hapten (in the case of drugs) as a conjugate with a carrier that is recognized by T

lymphocytes as 'self'. The mechanism of tolerance here is probably the reduction in the co-operation between B and T lymphocytes in the production of hapten-specific antibodies, including those capable of inducing disease. An example of such a tolerogen is penicilloyl-isologous IgG conjugate (Borel *et al.* 1976). This is still in the experimental stage, and the induction of auto-allergy might be a potential risk;

3. suppression of response to allergen by presentation of the hapten in a special way, for example, as hapten-coated liposomes (Schwenk *et al.* 1978).

All of these procedures involve taking a risk that is not justifiable, except when the underlying disease is serious and no adequate replacement for the drug in question is available. In this situation every possible measure to reduce the risk of reaction should be undertaken, by giving an appropriate cover of antiallergy drugs, by careful supervision of the patient, and by having adequate resuscitation facilities for combating acute allergic reactions.

Tests with immunologically cross-reactive agents

The best illustration of the practical value of this preventive measure can be shown in the case of cross-allergenicity between penicillin and cephalosporin derivatives (Assem and Vickers 1974), and between different neuro-muscular blockers (Assem 1984*a*,*b*).

Prophylactic antiallergy drugs

A 'strict' example of these drugs is disodium cromoglycate, which is used mainly for allergic (atopic) asthma (for mode of action see Kay 1987; Foreman and Pearce 1989). Cromoglycate has no effect when given orally and its injection into humans is not recommended. In theory, it should prevent drug-induced asthma, particularly when immediate-type allergy is the underlying mechanism. The author had no success with it, however, when it was given to patients by inhalation prior to challenge with a test-dose of the causative drug. It is hoped that more effective drugs with this action (with no limitations on route of administration), mainly preventing the release of pharmacological mediators of immediate type allergy, will be developed in due course. They would be invaluable in prevention of potentially fatal reactions.

Catecholamines, particularly those with predominant β-receptor agonist effects, have been shown to inhibit mediator release in anaphylaxis, and to inhibit the synthesis of some mediators like histamine and SRSA (leukotrienes C_4, D_4, and E_4, see review by Assem 1973).

These drugs, or other suitable preparations, may be

given as a prophylactic measure in patients with suspected or established allergy undergoing hyposensitization therapy, starting the day before, or at least a few hours before drug therapy is begun, and continuing until the danger of reaction is over.

Prevention of allergic reactions to penicillin

Before treatment is initiated, the doctor should ask about previous penicillin therapy and previous penicillin reactions. He should also enquire about any history of other allergic disorders, such as asthma and hay fever. The incidence of penicillin allergy in patients with such disorders, which are cited as examples of an atopic constitution, is greater than in non-atopic people. This history of such allergies should be considered as restricting indications for penicillin treatment to cases not manageable by other antibiotics (Levine *et al.* 1966; Idsøe *et al.* 1968; Levine and Zolov 1969). Certain other diseases seem to be associated with a higher incidence of penicillin allergy, such as glandular fever in which the incidence of skin reactions to ampicillin is said to be of the order of 90 per cent. Thus it seems logical to suggest that penicillin therapy, particularly ampicillin, should be avoided if glandular fever is suspected, even if one accepts the possibility that the rash is caused by a temporary abnormality in immune response.

The report of the potential value of a 'purified' benzylpenicillin preparation (Knudsen *et al.* 1967), Purapen G (Beecham), in reducing the incidence of penicillin allergy does not seem to have achieved general acceptance. Purified preparations of semi-synthetic penicillins, such as ampicillin (Knudsen *et al.* 1970), however, particularly in preparations given by injection, have achieved approval of many investigators.

Treatment of drug allergy

Acute allergic reactions/anaphylactic shock

The emergency kit should include parenteral preparations of adrenaline, an antihistamine, aminophylline, and hydrocortisone hemisuccinate or methylprednisolone, and a steroid aerosol. Immediate reactions are best treated with adrenaline and a parenterally administered antihistamine (but see below). Many aspects of the treatment of severe reactions are outside the scope of this review. The following is a brief account of some of the main lines of treatment.

Adrenaline

In anaphylactic reactions adrenaline BP, 0.3–1 ml of 1:1000 solution, should be given. The route of administration is decided according to whether shock (hypotension) is present or not; intramuscular or subcutaneous injection is adequate if blood pressure shows a small change (useful in laryngeal oedema and bronchospasm). A patient in shock requires immediate treatment to restore perfusion of the brain and heart, and absorption of subcutaneous or intramuscular adrenaline is unreliable in shock. Thus, if the reaction is severe (for example, an anaphylactic reaction during general anaesthesia; the severity of reaction is partly due to intravenous injection of the causative agent) adrenaline at a lower concentration, 1:10 000 (100 μg per ml) or less should be given intravenously. Hypotension is treated with a bolus injection of 4–8 μg initially; repeated if necessary, with monitoring of the ECG if possible. In cardiovascular collapse 2–4 μg per min is given, and a total of 100–500 μg may be necessary. Careful titration is necessary in order to prevent ventricular dysrhythmia (which could further add to histamine-induced dysrhythmia) and myocardial ischaemia (Sullivan 1982; Horak *et al.* 1983). Adrenaline is useful in counteracting bradydysrhythmia (atropine is an alternative; including bradydysrhythmia induced by histamine due to atrioventricular conduction block).

Intravenous volume expansion

The intravascular volume should be expanded with crystalloids (Ringer–lactate solution) or colloids (5% albumin, dextran, polygelatin, or cellulose derivatives), as 20–37% of the intravascular volume may be lost suddenly in anaphylactic reactions. Bicarbonate 0.5–1 mEq per kg is given if hypotension is prolonged or acidosis (to be monitored) is present or likely.

Aminophylline

This drug is used mainly to treat bronchospasm; giving an initial dose of 5–6 mg per kg over 20 minutes, and following with a maintenance dose of 0.9 mg per kg per hour. Isoprenaline infusion may be needed in severe, sustained bronchospasm (disadvantages: hypotension, tachyarrhythmias, and ventricular ectopics; possible advantages: reduction of pulmonary vascular resistance [if raised], positive inotropic and chronotropic effects and dromotropic [increasing conduction velocity] effects, useful in severe bradydysrhythmia).

Antihistamines

In theory, antihistamines should be of some value, though one of their limitations is that histamine is only one of the multitude of mediators of anaphylaxis. Their practical value has not, however, been well established, except in acute urticarial reactions. Nevertheless, it is reasonable to give 10 mg chlorpheniramine intramuscularly. Intravenous injection of antihistamines is probably best avoided because of the risk of hypotension. Chlorpheniramine is an example of a histamine H_1-antagonist; H_2-antagonists, such as cimetidine, are of no value unless combined with H_1-antagonists. In severe anaphylaxis, combined treatment with both types of antagonist is probably better than an H_1-antagonist alone, in view of the possibility of cardiac involvement in the anaphylactic reaction (see above). Persistent hypotension, not associated with bronchospasm may also be treated with the two types of antagonist combined.

Corticosteroids

Hydrocortisone hemisuccinate 0.1–1 g, or methyl prednisolone (up to 2 g) may be given intravenously in severe cases.

Rationale

The effect of corticosteroids on immediate-type allergy is surrounded by much confusion. It is true that, in order to prevent a reaction, corticosteroids have to be administered in repeated doses, starting at least 12 hours before the exposure to the causative agent. It has been shown by Church and others (1972) that this treatment in sensitized rats would prevent histamine release in local anaphylaxis induced by the intraperitoneal injection of antigen. They also have a prophylactic effect in man, causing inhibition of histamine release from mast cells, for example, in skin (Greaves and Plummer 1974), and from basophil leucocytes (Assem 1985). Despite the ineffectiveness of corticosteroids 'after the event', they possess the following properties, which apart from giving them the benefit of the doubt, provide a reasonable argument in favour of their use in patients with systemic reactions:

1. corticosteroids potentiate the α-effects of catecholamines, thus, to some extent, antagonizing the effect of various substances that contribute to vasodilatation, increased vascular permeability, and oedema, which is particularly dangerous when it affects the mucous membranes of the glottis and larynx;
2. they help to restore the response to catecholamines, for example, restoration of β-receptor-mediated relaxation of bronchial smooth muscle, which is believed to contribute to their usefulness in status asthmaticus;
3. their anti-inflammatory effect may help in counteracting some manifestations of allergic reactions;
4. one expects them to suppress delayed reactions;

5. they inhibit the synthesis of some mediators of immediate-type allergy, for example, histamine and prostaglandin $F_{2\alpha}$, which plays a role in immediate-type allergy and possibly in other mechanisms or types of allergy.

It should be added that, since airways obstruction produced by oedema in the larynx and glottis seems to be a source of fatalities due to drug reactions, steroid aerosols may be of value.

Supportive measures

Measures for counteracting cardiovascular collapse have to be maintained until the patient is out of danger. Specific therapeutic action should be taken and, for instance, antibiotics (preferably bactericidal) be given for prevention and treatment of infection in the case of agranulocytosis. Among the specific measures, penicillinase may be mentioned as a possible therapeutic approach in immediate reactions to penicillin (Becker 1956, 1960; Minno and Davis 1957) particularly in the case of long-acting preparations. Its value in immediate reactions, however, has been disputed (Levine 1966).

Desensitization

If no satisfactory alternative to the offending drug is found, and if there are indications that its use is essential (for example, penicillin in bacterial endocarditis), hyposensitization should be attempted. The procedure should be carried out in hospital, in an intensive care unit so that facilities for monitoring and resuscitation are at hand. Various hyposensitization regimens, including rush desensitization (which is a practical proposition), may be used in, for example, penicillin allergy (Holgate 1988). It should be stressed that maintenance of hyposensitization requires maintenance of exposure to the drug; return to the sensitized state occurring rapidly after interruption, and the whole procedure has to be repeated if further drug therapy is required. There is no agreed regimen of prophylactic medication and anti-allergy cover. Treatment may include:

1. inhibitors of mediator release or synthesis;
2. the continued use of available competitive or noncompetitive antagonists to the various pharmacological mediators;
3. physiological antagonists, for example bronchodilators, if asthma is likely to occur.

References

Abdullah, N.A. and Assem E-S.K. (1989). Role of thromboxane A_2 and leukotriene C_4 in the antigen-induced vasoconstriction in perfused, sensitized guinea-pig kidney. *Agents Actions* 27, 150.

Abdullah N.A., Assem E-S.K., and Damerau B. (1988). Anaphylatoxin-induced release of histamine from *in vitro* perfused guinea-pig kidney. *Agents Actions* 23, 181.

Ackroyd, J.F. (1964). The diagnosis of disorders of the blood due to drug hypersensitivity caused by an immune mechanism. In *Immunological methods*, p. 453. Blackwell, Oxford.

Amos, H.E. (1979). Immunological aspects of practolol toxicity. *Int. J. Immunopharmacol.* 1, 9.

Arbesman, C.E. and Reisman, R.E. (1971). Serum sickness and anaphylaxis. In *Immunological disease*, Vol. II (ed. M. Samter), p. 405. Little Brown, Boston.

Assem, E-S.K. (1971). Cyclic 3′,5′-adenosine monophosphate and the anaphylactic response. In *Effects of drugs on cellular control mechanisms* (ed. B.R. Rabin and R.B. Freedman), p. 259. Macmillan, London.

Assem, E-S.K. (1972a). The passive sensitization of human lung as a test for drug allergy. In *Mechanisms in drug allergy* (ed. C.H. Dash and H.E.H. Jones), p. 112. Churchill Livingstone, Edinburgh.

Assem, E-S.K. (1972b). IgE and other *in vitro* tests in the diagnosis and follow-up of drug allergy. In *Mechanisms in drug allergy* (ed. C.H. Dash and H.E.H. Jones), p. 179. Churchill Livingstone, Edinburgh.

Assem, E-S.K. (1973). Modulation by the autonomic nervous system of immune responses and allergic reactions. *Allergol. Immunopathol.* (suppl. 1), 117.

Assem, E-S.K. (1975). Specific immunological responses to propranolol and practolol in man. *Br. J. Clin. Pharmacol.* 2, 184.

Assem, E-S.K. (1976). Immunological and non-immunological mechanisms of some of the desirable and undesirable effects of anti-inflammatory and analgesic drugs. *Agents Actions* 6, 212.

Assem, E-S.K. (1977a). Autoimmune phenomena and autoallergy in patients treated with β-adrenoceptor blocking drugs. In *Cardiovascular drugs,* Vol. 2 *β-Adrenoceptor blocking drugs* (ed. G. Avery), p. 209. Adis, Sydney.

Assem, E-S.K. (1977b). Examples of the correlation between the structure of certain groups and adverse effects mediated by immune and non-immune mechanisms (with particular reference to muscle relaxants and steroid anaesthetics). In *Drug design and adverse effects* (ed. H. Bundgaard, P. Juul, and H. Kofod), p. 209. Munksgaard, Copenhagen.

Assem, E-S.K. (1983a). Reactions to general and local anaesthetics. In *Allergic reactions to drugs* (ed. A.L. de Weck and H. Bundgaard) *Handbook of experimental pharmacology* Vol. 63, p. 259. Springer-Verlag, Berlin.

Assem, E-S.K. (1983b). Reactions to neuromuscular blocking drugs. In *Allergic reactions to drugs* (ed. A.L. de Weck and H. Bundgaard) *Handbook of experimental pharmacology* Vol. 63, p. 299. Springer-Verlag, Berlin.

Assem, E-S.K. (1984a). Characteristics of basophil histamine release by neuromuscular blocking drugs in patients with anaphylactoid reactions. *Agents Actions* 14, 435.

Assem, E-S.K (1984b). Diagnostic and predictive test procedures in patients with life-threatening anaphylactic and anaphylactoid drug reactions. *Allergol. Immunopathol.* (Madrid) 12, 61.

Assem, E-S.K. (1985). Inhibition of histamine release from basophil leucocytes of asthmatic patients treated with corticosteroids. *Agents Actions* 16, 256.

Assem, E-S.K. (1989). Drug allergy. *Curr. Opin. Immunol.* 1, 660.

Assem, E-S.K. (1990a). Naturally occurring IgG-antibody-like substance reacting with quaternary ammonium group and neuromuscular blockers: a common finding in humans and other species. *Int. Arch. Allergy Appl. Immunol.* 91, 426.

Assem, E-S.K. (1990b). Anaphylactic anaesthetic reactions: the value of paper radioallergosorbent tests for IgE antibodies to muscle relaxants and thiopentone. *Anaesthesia* 45, 1032.

Assem, E-S.K. and Abdullah, N.A.(1987a). Experimental renal anaphylaxis: release of histamine and study of its effect on renal perfusion. *Agents Actions* 20, 141.

Assem, E-S.K. and Abdullah, N.A. (1987b). Release of thromboxane B_2 and leukotriene C_4 and reduction in renal perfusion in experimental anaphylactic reaction of isolated guinea-pig kidney. *Int. Arch. Allergy Appl. Immunol.* 82, 212.

Assem, E-S.K. and Banks, R. (1973). Practolol-induced drug eruption. *Proc. R. Soc. Med.* 66, 179.

Assem, E.-S.K. and Ezeamuzie, I.C. (1989). Suxamethonium-induced histamine release from the heart of naive animals and suxamethonium-sensitized guinea-pig: evidence suggesting spontaneous sensitization in naive animals, and relevance to anaphylactoid reaction in man. *Agents Actions* 27, 146.

Assem, E.-S.K. and Ghanem, N.S. (1988). Demonstration of IgE-sensitized mast cells in human heart and kidney. *Int. Arch. Allergy Appl. Immunol.* 87, 101.

Assem, E.-S.K. and Ling, B.Y. (1988). Fatal anaphylactic reaction to suxamethonium: new screening test suggests possible prevention. *Anaesthesia* 43, 958.

Assem, E-S.K. and McAllen, M.K. (1970). Serum reagins and leucocyte response in patients with house-dust mite allergy. *Br. Med. J.* ii, 504.

Assem, E-S.K. and Schild, H.O. (1968). Detection of allergy to penicillin and other antigens by *in vitro* passive sensitization and histamine release from human and monkey lung. *Br. Med. J.* iii, 272.

Assem, E-S.K. and Schild, H.O. (1971). Antagonism by beta-adrenoceptor blockers of the antianaphylactic effect of isoprenaline. *Br. J. Pharmacol.* 42, 620.

Assem, E-S.K. and Symons, I.E. (1989). Anaphylaxis due to suxamethonium in a seven year old child: a 14 year follow-up with allergy testing. *Anaesthesia* 44, 121.

Assem, E-S.K. and Turner-Warwick, M. (1976). Cytophilic antibodies in bronchopulmonary aspergillosis, aspergilloma and cryptogenic pulmonary eosinophilia. *Clin. Exp. Immunol.* 26, 67.

Assem, E-S.K. and Vickers, M.R. (1974). Tests for penicillin allergy in man. II. The immunological cross-reaction between penicillins and cephalosporins. *Immunology* 27, 255.

Assem, E-S.K., Ndoping, N., Nicholson, H., and Wade, J.R. (1969). Liver damage and isoniazid allergy. *Clin. Exp. Immunol.* 5, 439.

Assem, E-S.K., Bray, K., and Dawson, P. (1983). The release of histamine from human basophils by radiological contrast agents. *Br. J. Radiol.* 56, 647.

Assem, E-S.K., Abdullah, N.A., and Ghanem, N.S. (1986). Renal histamine: release by immune stimuli. *Agents Actions* 19, 141.

Assem, E-S.K., Abdullah, N.A., and Cowie, A.G.A. (1987). Kidney mast cells, IgE and release of inflammatory mediators capable of altering renal haemodynamics. *Int. Arch. Allergy Appl. Immunol.* 84, 212.

Bach, M.K., Brashler, J.R., and Gorman, R.R. (1977). On the structure of slow reacting substance of anaphylaxis: evidence of biosynthesis from arachidonic acid. *Prostaglandins* 14, 21.

Baker, S.B. and Williams, R.T. (1963). Acute interstitial nephritis due to drug sensitivity. *Br. Med. J.* ii, 1655.

Baldo, B.A. and Fisher, M.M. (1983). Substituted ammonium ions as allergenic determinants in allergy to muscle relaxants. *Nature* (Lond.) 306, 262.

Baldwin, D.S., Levine, B.B., McCluskey, R.T., and Gallo, G.R. (1968). Renal failure and interstitial nephritis due to penicillin and methicillin. *N. Engl. J. Med.* 279, 1245.

Barnes, P.J. (1989). Neural mechanisms in airway inflammation. In *Textbook of immunopharmacology* (ed. M.M. Dale and J.C. Foreman), p. 242. Blackwell, Oxford.

Basomba, A., Pelaez, A., VillaManzo, I.G., and Campos, A. (1978). Allergy to penicillin unsuccessfully treated with a haptenic inhibitor (benzylpenicilloyl-N_2-formyl-lysine, BPO-Flys). A case report. *Clin. Allergy* 8, 341.

Batchelor, F.R., Dewdney, J.M., Feinberg, J.G., and Weston, R.D. (1967). A penicilloylated protein impurity as a source of allergy to benzyl-penicillin and 6-amino-penicillanic acid. *Lancet* i, 1175.

BCDSP (Boston Collaborative Drug Surveillance Program) (1972). Excess of ampicillin rashes associated with allopurinol or hyperuricaemia. *N. Engl. J. Med.* 286, 505.

Becker, E.L. and Austen, K.F. (1968). Anaphylaxis. In *Textbook of immunopathology*, Vol. I (ed. P.A. Meischer and H.J. Muller-Eberhard), p. 76. Grune and Stratton, London.

Becker, R.M. (1956). Effect of penicillinase on circulating penicillin. *N. Engl. J. Med.* 254, 952.

Becker, R.M. (1960). Penicillinase treatment of penicillin reactions. *Practitioner* 184, 447.

Behan, P.O., Behan, W.H.M., Zacharias, F.J., and Nicholls, J.T. (1976). Immunological abnormalities in patients who had the oculomucocutaneous syndrome associated with practolol therapy. *Lancet* ii, 984.

Benacerraf, B. and McDevitt, H.O. (1972). Histocompatibility-linked immune response genes. *Science* 175, 273.

Borel, Y., Kilham, L., Hyslop, N., and Borel, H. (1976). Isologous IgG-induced tolerance to benzyl penicilloyl. *Nature* 261, 49.

Brimblecombe, R.W., Duncan, W.A.M., Durant, G.J., Emmett, J.C., Ganellin, C.R., and Parsons, M.E. (1975). Cimetidine — a non-thiourea H_2-receptor antagonist. *J. Int. Med. Res.* 3, 86.

Brocklehurst, W.E. and Lahiri, S.C. (1962). The production of bradykinin in anaphylaxis. *J. Physiol.* Lond. 160, 15P.

Brown, P., Baddeley, H., Read, A.E., Davies, J.D., and McGarry, J. (1974). Sclerosing peritonitis, an unusual reaction to a β-adrenergic blocking drug (practolol). *Lancet* ii, 1477.

Brown, P.J.E., Lesna, M., Hamlyn, A.N., and Record, C.O. (1978). Primary biliary cirrhosis after long-term practolol administration. *Br. Med. J.* i, 1591.

Burke, J.A., Levi, R., Guo, Z.-G., and Corey, E.J. (1982). Leukotrienes C_4, D_4 and E_4: effects on human and guinea-pig cardiac preparation *in vitro*. *J. Pharmac. Exp. Ther.* 221, 235.

Calnan, C.D. (1968). Allergic contact dermatitis. In *Clinical aspects of immunology* (2nd edn) (ed. P.G.H. Gell and R.R.A. Coombs), p. 756. Blackwell, Oxford.

Camussi, G., Aglietta, M., Malavasi, F., Tetta, C., Piacibello, W., Sanavio, F., et al. (1983). The release of platelet-activating factor from human endothelial cells in culture. *J. Immunol.* 131, 2397.

Chao, P., Francis, L., and Atkins, E. (1977). The release of an endogenous pyrogen from guinea pig leukocytes *in vitro*: a new model for investigating the role of lymphocytes in fevers induced by antigens in hosts with delayed hypersensitivity. *J. Exp. Med.* 145, 1288.

Charpin, J., Vervloet, D., and Nizankovska, E. (1983). Detection of serum IgE antibodies that react with alcuronium and tubocurarine after life-treatening reactions to muscle relaxant drugs. In *Proceedings of XIth International Congress of Allergology and Clinical Immunology* (ed. J.E. Kent and M.A. Ganderton), p. 67. Macmillan, London.

Chase, M.W. (1958). Antibodies to drugs. In *Sensitivity reactions to drugs* (ed. M.L. Rosenheim and R. Moulton), p. 125. Blackwell, Oxford.

Church, M.K., Collier, H.O., and James, G.W. (1972). The inhibition by dexamethasone and disodium cromoglycate of anaphylactic bronchoconstriction in the rat. *Br. J. Pharmacol.* 46, 56.

Cluff, L.E. and Johnson, J.E. (1964). Drug fever. *Prog. Allergy* 8, 149.

Coombs, R.R.A and Gell, P.G.H. (1968). Classification of allergic reactions responsible for clinical hypersensitivity and disease. In *Clinical aspects of immunology* (ed. P.G.H. Gell and R.R.A. Coombs), p. 575. Blackwell, Oxford.

Cooper, J.A.D., White D.A., and Matthay R.A. (1986). Drug-induced pulmonary disease. Part 2: Noncytotoxic drugs. *Am. Rev. Respir. Dis.* 133, 488.

Dacie, J.V. (1962). Haemolytic reactions to drugs. *Proc. R. Soc. Med.* 55, 28.

Dawson, D., Boot, J.R., Cockerill, A.F., Mallen, D.N.B., and Osborne, D.J. (1976). Release of novel prostaglandins and thromboxanes after immunological challenge of guinea-pig lung. *Nature* 62, 699.

Delage, C. and Irey, M.S. (1972). Anaphylactic deaths: a clinico-pathologic study of 43 cases. *J. Forensic Sci.* 17, 525.

de Weck, A.L., Schneider, C.H., Spengler, H., Toffler, O., and Lazary, S. (1973). Inhibition of allergic reactions by monovalent haptens. In *Mechanisms in allergy: reagin-mediated hypersensitivity* (ed. L. Goodfriend, A.H. Sehon and R.P. Orange), p. 323. Dekker, New York.

Didier, A., Cador, D., Bongrand, P., Furtoss, R., Fourneron, P., Senft, M., *et al.* (1987). Role of the quaternary ammonium ion determinant in allergy to muscle relaxants. *J. Allergy Clin. Immunol.* 79, 578.

Dinarello, C.A. (1984). Interleukin-1. *Rev. Infect. Dis.* 6, 51.

Dinarello, C.A. (1989). Interleukin-1. In *Textbook of immunopharmacology* (2nd edn) (ed. M.M. Dale and J.C. Foreman). Blackwell, Oxford.

Dinarello, C.A. and Wolff, S.M. (1978). Pathogenesis of fever in man. *N. Engl. J. Med.* 298, 607.

Dinarello, C.A. and Wolff, S.M. (1982). Molecular basis of fever in humans. *Am. J. Med.* 72, 800.

Dumonde, D.C., Wolstencroft, R.A., Panayi, G.S., Mathew, M., Morley, J., and Howson, W.T. (1969). Lymphokines: non-antibody mediators of cellular immunity generated by lymphocyte activation. *Nature* 224, 38.

Dundee, J.W. (1986). Adverse reactions to drugs and anaesthetists. *Anaesthesia*, 41, 351.

Eisen, H.N. (1959). Hypersensitivity to simple chemicals. In *Cellular and humoral aspects of the hypersensitivity states* (ed. H.S. Lawrence), p. 89. Holber-Harper, New York.

Eyre, P. and Deline, T.R. (1971). Release of dopamine from bovine lung by specific antigen and by compound 48/80. *Br. J. Pharmacol.* 42, 423.

Ezeamuzie, I.C. and Assem, E-S.K. (1982). Histamine and SRS release from human leucocytes by lymphokines. *Int. J. Immunopharmacol.* 4, 378P.

Ezeamuzie, I.C. and Assem, E-S.K. (1983a). A study of histamine release from human basophils and lung mast cells by products of lymphocyte stimulation. *Agents Actions* 13, 222.

Ezeamuzie, I.C. and Assem, E.-S.K. (1983b). Effects of leukotrienes C_4 and D_4 on guinea-pig heart and the participation of SRS-A in the manifestations of guinea-pig cardiac anaphylaxis. *Agents Actions* 13, 182.

Ezeamuzie, I.C. and Assem, E-S.K. (1984). Modulation of the effect of histamine-releasing lymphokine on human basophils. *Agents Actions* 14, 501.

Ezeamuzie, I.C. and Assem, E-S.K. (1985a). Histamine-releasing lymphokine: characteristics of its production. *Agents Actions* 14, 21.

Ezeamuzie, I.C. and Assem, E-S.K. (1985b). Basophil receptors for histamine-releasing lymphokine. *Int. J. Immunopharmacol.* 7, 339P.

Ezeamuzie, I.C. and Assem, E-S.K. (1985c). Release of slow reacting substance (SRS) from human leucocytes by lymphokine. *Int. J. Immunopharmacol.* 7, 533.

Ezeamuzie, I.C. and Assem, E-S.K. (1985d). Histamine-releasing lymphokine: preliminary evidence of membrane receptors on basophils. *Agents Actions* 17, 131.

Ezeamuzie, I.C. and Assem, E-S.K. (1986). Histamine releasing factor is not an interferon. *Agents Actions* 18, 159.

Ezeamuzie, I.C. and Assem, E-S.K. (1987). Antigen-induced formation of a lymphokine with possible role as a mediator of the late component of dual hypersensitivity reaction: a case report. *Int. Arch. Allergy Appl. Immunol.* 82, 221.

Farr, M.J., Wingate, J.P., and Shaw, J.N. (1975). Practolol and the nephrotic syndrome. *Br. Med. J.* ii, 68.

Foreman, J.C. (1989). Pyrogenesis. In *Textbook of immunopharmacology* (ed. M.M. Dale and J.C. Foreman), p. 223. Blackwell, Oxford.

Foreman, J.C. and Pearce, F.L. (1989). Cromoglycate. In *Textbook of imunopharmacology* (ed. M.M. Dale and J.C. Foreman), p. 262. Blackwell, Oxford.

Gell, P.G.H., Harington, C.R., and Michel, R. (1948). Antigenic function of simple chemical compounds: correlation of antigenicity with chemical reactivity. *Br. J. Exp. Pathol.* 29, 578.

Ghanem, N.S. (1988). *A comparative study of functional and morphological properties of cardiac mast cells.* Ph.D. Thesis, London University.

Ghanem, N.S., Assem, E-S.K., Leung, K.B.P., and Pearce, F.L. (1988a). Guinea pig mast cells: comparative study of morphology, fixation and staining properties. *Int. Arch. Allergy Appl. Immunol.* 85, 351.

Ghanem, N.S., Assem, E-S.K., Leung, K.B.P., and Pearce, F.L. (1988b). Cardiac and renal mast cells: morphology, distribution, fixation and staining properties in the guinea pig and preliminary comparison with human. *Agents Actions* 23, 123.

Ghanem, N.S., Abdullah, N.A., and Assem, E-S.K. (1989). The cardiac and renal effects of complement fragment $C5_a$ des Arg are partly mediated by the release of histamine and archidonic acid metabolites. *Agents Actions* 27, 138.

Greaves, M.W. and Plummer, V.M. (1974). Glucocorticoid inhibition of antigen-evoked histamine release from human skin. *Immunology* 27, 359.

Hadji, L. and Benveniste, J. (1980). Experimental cardiac anaphylaxis to an anaesthetic adjuvant as a model for drug allergy. *Allergol. Immunopathol.* 8, Abstr. 486.

Hamberg, M., Svensson, J., and Samuelson, B. (1975). Thromboxanes: a novel group of biologically active compounds derived from prostaglandin endoperoxides. *Proc. Natl Acad. Sci. USA*, 72, 2994.

Harber, L.C. and Baer, R.L. (1969). Classification and characteristics of photoallergy. In *The biologic effects of ultraviolet radiation* (ed. F. Urbach), p. 519. Pergamon, New York.

Harle, D.G., Baldo, B.A., and Fisher, M.M. (1984). Detection of IgE antibodies to suxamethonium after anaphylactoid reactions during anaesthesia. *Lancet* i, 121.

Harpey, J.P., Caille, B., Moulias, R., and Goust, J.M. (1972). Drug allergy, and lupus-like syndrome (with special reference to penicillamine). In *Mechanisms in drug allergy* (ed. C.H. Dash and H.E.H. Jones), p. 51. Churchill Livingstone, Edinburgh.

Henson, P.M. and Benveniste, J. (1971). Antibody–leucocyte–platelet interactions. In *Biochemistry of acute allergic reactions* (ed. F.K. Austin and E.L. Becker), p. 111. Blackwell, Oxford.

Henson, P.M. and Pinckard, R.N. (1977). Basophil-derived activating factor (PAF) as an *in vivo* mediator of allergic reactions: Demonstration of specific desensitization of platelets to PAF during IgE-induced anaphylaxis in the rabbit. *J. Immunol.* 119, 2179.

Hoffbrand, B.I., Fry, W., and Bunton, G.L. (1974). Cholestatic jaundice due to methyldopa. *Br. Med. J.* iii, 559.

Holgate, S.T. (1988). Penicillin allergy: how to diagnose and when to treat. *Br. Med. J.* 296, 1213.

Holley, H.L. (1964). Drugs and the lupus diathesis. *J. Chron. Dis.* 1, 17.

Horak, A., Raine, R., Opie, L.H., and Lloyd, E.A. (1983). Severe myocardial ischaemia induced by intravenous adrenaline. *Br. Med. J.* 286, 519.

Hurwitz, N. (1969). Predisposing factors in adverse reactions to drugs. *Br. Med. J.* i, 536.

Idsøe, O., Guthe, T., Wilcox, R.R., and de Weck, A.L. (1968). Nature and extent of penicillin side effects with particular reference to fatalities from anaphylactic shock. *Bull. WHO*, 38, 159.

Isacson, E.P. (1967). Myxoviruses and autoimmunity. *Prog. Allergy* 10, 256.

Ishizaka, T., Soto, C.S., and Ishizaka, K. (1973). Mechanisms of passive sensitization. III. Number of IgE molecules and their receptor sites on human basophil granulocytes. *J. Immunol.* 3, 500.

Jakschik, B.A., Falkenheim, S., and Parker, C.W. (1977). Precursor role of arachidonic acid in release of slow reacting substance from rat basophilic leukemia cells. *Proc. Natl Acad. Sci. USA*, 74, 4577.

Jensen, H.A., Mikkelsen, H.I., Wadskov, S., and Sondergaard, J. (1976). Cutaneous reactions to propranolol (Inderal). *Acta Med. Scand.* 199, 363.

Kaplan, A.P., Haak-Frendscho, M., Fauci, A., Dinarello, C., and Halbert, E. (1985). A histamine releasing factor from activated mononuclear cells. *J. Immunol.* 135, 2027.

Kay, A.B. (1987). The mode of action of anti-allergic drugs. *Clinical Allergy* 17, 153.

Kay, A.B. and Austen, K.F. (1971). The IgE-mediated release of an eosinophil leucocyte chemotactic factor from human lung. *J. Immunol.* 107, 899.

Kind, L.S. (1958). The altered reactivity of mice after inoculation with *Bordetella pertussis* vaccine. *Bacteriol. Rev.* 22, 173.

Knudsen, E.T. (1969). Ampicillin and urticaria. *Br. Med. J.* i, 846.

Knudsen, E.T., Robinson, O.P.W., Croydon, E.A.P., and Tees, E.C. (1967). Cutaneous sensitivity to purified benzylpenicillin. *Lancet* i, 1184.

Knudsen, E.T., Dewdney, J.M., and Trafford, J.A.P. (1970). Reduction in incidence of ampicillin rash by purified ampicillin. *Br. Med. J.* i, 469.

Lakshmanan, M.C., Hershey, C.O., and Breslau, D. (1986). Hospital admissions caused by iatrogenic disease. *Arch. Intern. Med*, 146, 1931.

The Lancet (1983). Inflammatory mediators of asthma. *Lancet* ii, 829.

Landsteiner, K. (1945). *The specificity of serological reactions* (revised edn). Harvard University Press.

Laurence, D.R. and Bennett, P.N. (1987). Adverse drug reactions. In *Clinical pharmacology*, p. 153. Churchill Livingstone, Edinburgh.

Lee, W.Y. and Sehon, A.H. (1978). Suppression of reaginic antibodies with modified allergens. I. Reduction in allergenicity of protein allergen by conjugation to polyethylene glycol. *Int. Arch. Allergy Appl. Immunol.* 56, 159.

Levi, R., Malm, J., Bowman, F.A., and Rosen, M.R. (1981). The arrhythmogenic actions of histamine on human atrial fibres. *Circ. Res.* 49, 625.

Levi, R., Chenouda, A.A., Trzeciakowski, J.P., Guo, Z.-G., Aaronson, L.M., Luskind, R.D., *et al.* (1982). Dysrhythmia caused by histamine release in guinea-pig and human hearts. *Klin. Wochenschr.,* 60, 965.

Levi, R., Burke, J.A., Guo Z.-G., Hattori, Y., Hoppens, C.M., McManus, L.M., *et al.* (1984). Acetylglyceryl ether phosphorylcholine (AGEPC). A putative mediator of cardiac anaphylaxis in the guinea-pig. *Circ. Res.* 54, 117.

Levine, B.B. (1966). Immunochemical mechanisms of penicillin allergy. A haptenic model system for the study of allergic diseases of man. *N. Engl. J. Med.* 275, 1115.

Levine, B.B. and Vaz, N.M. (1970). Effect of combinations of inbred strain, antigen, and antigen dose on immune responsiveness and reagin production in the mouse. A potential mouse model for immune aspects of human atopic allergy. *Int. Arch. Allergy Appl. Immunol.* 39, 156.

Levine, B.B. and Zolov, D.M. (1969). Prediction of penicillin allergy by immunological tests. *J. Allergy* 43, 231.

Levine, B.B., Redmond, A.P., Fellner, M.J., Voss, H.E., and Levytska, V. (1966). Penicillin allergy and the heterogeneous immune responses of many to benzylpenicillin. *J. Clin. Invest.* 45, 1895.

Lingstrom, K-G., Renck, H., Hedin, H., Richter, W., and Wiholm, B-E. (1988). Hapten inhibition and dextran anaphylaxis. *Anaesthesia* 43, 729.

Littlejohns, D.W., Assem, E-S.K., and Kennedy, C.T.C. (1973). Immunological evidence for two forms of allergy to pyrazolone drugs. *Rheumatol. Phys. Med.* 12, 57.

Machado, F.R.DaS., Assem, E.S.K., and Ezeamuzie, I.C. (1985a). Cardiac anaphylaxis: the role of different mediators, Part 1: histamine. *Allergol. Immunopathol.* 13, 259.

Machado, F.R.DaS., Assem, E.S.K., and Ezeamuzie, I.C. (1985b). Cardiac anaphylaxis, Part II: the role of prostaglandins, thromboxanes and leukotrienes. *Allergol. Immunopathol.* 13, 335.

McCormick, R.V. (1950). Periarteritis occurring during propylthiouracil therapy. *JAMA* 144, 1453.

McDevitt, H.O. and Benacerraf, B. (1969). Genetic control of specific immune responsiveness. *Adv. Immunol.* 11, 31.

McDevitt, H.O. and Bodmer, W.F. (1972). Histocompatibility antigens, immune responsiveness and susceptibility to disease. *Am. J. Med.* 52, 1.

MacKay, A.D. and Axford, A.T. (1976). Pleural effusions after practolol. *Lancet* i, 89.

McKendrick, M.W. and Geddes, A.M. (1979). Allopurinol hypersensitivity. *Br. Med. J.* i, 988.

McMenamin, R.A., Davies, L.M., and Craswell, P.W. (1976). Drug-induced interstitial nephritis, hepatitis, and exfoliative dermatitis: a case report. *Aust. N.Z. J. Med.* 6, 583.

Mann, M.R. (1961). The pharmacology of contrast media. *Proc. R. Soc. Med.* 54, 473.

Marone, G., Triggiani, M., Cirillo, R., Giacummo, A., Hammerstrom, S., and Condorelli, M. (1986). IgE-mediated activation of human heart *in vitro*. *Agents Actions* 18, 194.

Marsh, D.G., Bias, W.B., Hsu, S.H., and Goodfriend, L. (1973). Association between major histocompatibility (HLA) antigens and specific reaginic antibody responses in allergic man. In *Mechanisms in allergy: reagin-mediated hypersensitivity* (ed. L. Goodfriend, A.H. Sehon, and R.P. Orange), p. 113. Dekker, New York.

Marshall, A.J., Barrit, D.W., Griffiths, D.A., Laszlo, G., Eltringham, W.K., Davies, J.D., *et al.* (1977). Respiratory disease associated with practolol therapy. *Lancet* ii, 1254.

Minno, A.M. and Davis, G.M. (1957). Penicillinase in the treatment of penicillin reactions. *JAMA* 165, 222.

Moeschlin, S. (1958). Agranulocytosis due to sensitivity to drugs. In *Sensitivity reactions to drugs* (ed. M.L. Rosenheim and R. Moulton), p. 77. Blackwell, Oxford.

Moeschlin, S. and Wagner, K. (1952). Agranulocytosis due to occurrence of leucocyte agglutinins. *Acta Haematol.* 8, 29.

Moneret-Vautrin, D.A., Gueant, J.L., Kamel, L., Laxenaire, M.C., El Kholty, S., and Nicholas, J.P. (1988a). Anaphylaxis to myorelaxants: cross-sensitivity studied by radioimmunoassays compared to intradermal tests in 34 cases. *J. Allergy Clin. Immunol.* 82, 745.

Moneret-Vautrin, D.A., Laxenaire, M.C., Gueant, J.L., and Widmer, S. (1988b). Predictive tests of the re-use of a myorelaxant, in case of anaphylaxis to myorelaxants. *N. Engl. Reg. Allergy Proc.* 9, 254.

Morley, J. (1989). Platelet activating factor. In *Textbook of immunopharmacology* (ed. M.M. Dale and J.C. Foreman), p. 186. Blackwell, Oxford.

Morrow, J.D., Schroeder, H.A., and Perry, H.M. Jr (1953). Studies on the control of hypertension by hyphex; toxic reactions and side effects. *Circulation* 8, 829.

Munoz, J. (1964). Effect of bacteria and bacterial products on antibody response. *Adv. Immunol.* 4, 397.

Nimmo, W.S. (1988). Reporting adverse reactions to anaesthetic drugs: a new way forward. *Anaesthesia* 43, 627.

Parish, W.E. (1973). Reaginic and non-reaginic antibody reactions on anaphylactic participating cells. In *Mechanisms in allergy: reagin-mediated hypersensitivity* (ed. L. Goodfriend, A.H. Sehon and R.P. Orange), p. 197. Dekker, New York.

Parker, C.W. (1965). Drug reactions. In *Immunological diseases* (ed. M. Samter and H.L. Alexander), p. 663. Little Brown, Boston.

Parker, C.W. (1980). Drug allergy. In *Clinical immunology* (ed. C.W. Parker), p. 1372. Saunders, Philadelphia.

Parker, C.W. (1982). Allergic reactions in man. *Pharmacol. Rev.* 34, 85.

Paton, W.D.M. (1957). Histamine release by compounds of simple chemical structure. *Pharmacol. Rev.* 9, 269.

Perelmutter, L. and Khera, K. (1969). Rat mast cells in human reagin detection. *Lancet* i, 1269.

Perry, H.M., Tan, E.M., Carmody, S., and Sakamoto, A. (1970). Relationship of acetyl transference activity to antinuclear antibodies and toxic symptoms in hypertensive patients treated with hydralazine. *J. Lab. Clin. Med.* 76, 114.

Piper, P. (1983). Leukotrienes. *Trends Pharmacol. Sci.* 3, 75.

Piper, P.J. and Vane, J.R. (1969). Release of additional factors in anaphylaxis and its antagonism by anti-inflammatory drugs. *Nature* 223, 29.

Plautt, M., Lichtenstein, L.M., and Bloch, K.J. (1973). Failure to obtain histamine release from rat mast cells exposed to human allergic serum and specific antigen or IgE myeloma protein and anti-IgE. *J. Immunol.* 3, 1022.

Prankerd, T.A.J. (1963). Haemolytic effects of drugs and chemical agents. *Clin. Pharmacol. Ther.* 4, 334.

Pullen, H., Wright, N., and Murdoch, J.McC. (1967). Hypersensitivity reactions to antibacterial drugs in infectious mononucleosis. *Lancet* ii, 1176.

Raffel, S. (1973). Hapten-induced anaphylactic reactions. In *Mechanisms in allergy: reagin-mediated hypersensitivity* (ed. L. Goodfriend, A.H. Sehon and R.P. Orange), p. 313. Dekker, New York.

Raftery, E.B. and Denman, A.M. (1973). Systemic lupus erythematosus induced by practolol. *Br. Med. J.* ii, 452.

Remmer, H. and Schuppel, R. (1972). The formation of antigenic determinants. In *Hypersensitivity to drugs*, Vol. 1 (ed. M. Samter and C.W. Parker), p. 67. Pergamon, Oxford.

Rich, A.R. (1958). Tissue reactions produced by sensitivity to drugs. In *Sensitivity reactions to drugs* (ed. M.L. Rosenheim and R. Moulton), p. 196. Blackwell, Oxford.

Ring, J. and Przbilla, B. (1989). UV radiation and allergy. *Allergologie, XIVth Congress of the European Academy of Allergology and Clinical Immunology, Proceedings* (suppl.) S75.

Ring, J., Przbilla, B., and Ruzicka, Th. (1987). Nonsteroidal anti-inflammatory drugs induce UV-dependent histamine and leukotriene release from peripheral human leukocytes. *Int. Arch. Allergy Appl. Immunol.* 82, 344.

Rose, G.A. and Spencer, H. (1957). Polyarteritis nodosa. *Q. J. Med.* 26, 43.

Russell, G.L., Bing, R.F., Walls, J., and Pettigrew, N.M. (1978). Interstitial nephritis in a case of phenylbutazone hypersensitivity. *Br. Med. J.* i, 1322.

Saltzstein, S.L. and Ackerman, L.V. (1959). Lymphadenopathy induced by anticonvulsant drugs and mimicking clinically and pathologically malignant lymphomas. *Cancer* 12, 164.

Samter, M. and Berryman, G.H. (1964). Drug allergy. *Ann. Rev. Pharmacol.* 4, 265.

Samuelson, B. (1981). Oxidative products of arachidonate, a new group of compounds, including slow-reacting substance (SRS-A). In *Biochemistry of acute allergic reactions* (ed. E.L. Becker, A.S. Simon, and K.F. Austen), p. 1. Alan R. Liss, New York.

Samuelson, B., Hamberg, M., Roberts, L.J., Oates, J.A., and Nelson, N.A. (1978). Nomenclature for thromboxanes. *Prostaglandins* 16, 857.

Schild, H.O. (1962). The mechanism of contact sensitization. *J. Pharm. Pharmacol.* 14, 1.

Schwenk, R., Lee, W.Y., and Sehon, A.H. (1978). Specific suppression of anti-hapten reaginic antibody titers with hapten-coated liposomes. *J. Immunol.* 120, 1612.

Scott, J.R. (1987). A review of in vitro assays for IgG and IgG₄ antibodies: concept and potential applications. *N. Engl. Reg. Allergy Proc.* 8, 385.

Sedgwick, J.D., Holt, P.G., and Turner, K. (1981). Production of a histamine-releasing lymphokine by antigen- or mitogen-stimulated human peripheral T-cells. *Clin. Exp. Immunol.* 45, 409.

Sherlock, S. (1965). Hepatic reactions to therapeutic agents. *Ann. Rev. Pharmacol.* 5, 429.

Sherlock, S. and Ajdukiewicz, A. (1972). Hepatic reactions to drugs. In *Mechanisms in drug allergy* (ed. C.H. Dash and H.E.H. Jones), p. 103. Churchill Livingstone, Edinburgh.

Shulman, N.R. (1963). Mechanisms of blood-cell destruction in individuals sensitized to foreign antigens and its implications in autoimmunity. *Trans. Am. Assoc. Physicians* 76, 72.

Shulman, N.R. (1964). A mechanism of cell destruction in individuals sensitized to foreign antigens and its implications in autoimmunity. *Ann. Int. Med.* 60, 506.

Simmonds, J., Hodges, S., Nicol, F., and Barnett, D. (1978). Anaphylaxis after oral penicillin. *Br. Med. J.* ii, 1404.

Smith, J.W., Johnson, J.E., and Leighton, E.C. (1966). Studies on the epidemiology of adverse drug reactions. II. An evaluation of penicillin allergy. *N. Engl. J. Med.* 274, 998.

Snyder, F. (1985). Chemical and biochemical aspects of platelet activating factor: a novel class of acetylated ether-linked choline-phospholipids. *Med. Res. Rev.* 5, 107.

Stanworth, D.R. (ed.) (1973). Structural basis of reagin activity. In *Immediate hypersensitivity*, p. 212. North-Holland, Amsterdam.

Stewart, G.T. (1967). Allergenic residues in penicillin. *Lancet* i, 1177.

Sullivan, T.J. (1982). Cardiac disorders in penicillin induced anaphylaxis: association with intravenous therapy. *JAMA*, 248, 2161.

Sullivan, T.J., Wedner, H.J., Shatz, G.S., Yecies, L.D., and Parker, C.W. (1981). Skin testing to detect penicillin allergy. *J. Allergy Clin. Immunol.* 68, 171.

Sutherland, E.W. and Robison, G.A. (1966). The role of cyclic 3′,5′-AMP in responses to catecholamines and other hormones. *Pharmacol. Rev.* 18, 145.

Symmers, W.St.C. (1962). The occurrence of angiitis and other generalized diseases of connective tissues as a consequence of the administration of drugs. Symposium on drug sensitization. *Proc. R. Soc. Med.* 55, 20.

Szczeklik, A. (1983). Analgesics and non-steroidal anti-inflammatory drugs. In *Allergic reactions to drugs* (ed. A De Weck and H. Bundgaard), p. 277. Springer-Verlag, Berlin.

Szentivanyi, A. (1969). The beta adrenergic theory of the atopic abnormality in bronchial asthma. *J. Allergy* 42, 203.

Thueson, D.O., Speck, L.S., Lett-Brown, M.A., and Grant, J.A. (1979). Histamine-releasing activity (HRA). I. Production by mitogen or antigen-stimulated human mononuclear cells. *J. Immunol.* 123, 626.

Toghill, P.J., Smith, P.G., Benton, P., Brown, R.C., and Mathews, H.L. (1974). Methyldopa liver damage. *Br. Med. J.* iii, 545.

Vervloet, D., Nizankoweska, E., Arnaud, A., Senft, M., Alazia, M., and Charkin, J. (1983). Adverse reactions to suxamethonium and other muscle relaxants under general anaesthesia. *J. Allergy Clin. Immunol.* 71, 552.

Watkins, J. (1979). Anaphylactoid reactions to intravenous substances. *Br. J. Anaesth.* 51, 51.

Watkins, J. and Ward, A.M. (eds) (1978). *Adverse response to intravenous drugs.* Academic Press, London.

Welsh, K.I. and Batchelor, J.R. (1981). HLA and drug reactions. In *Drug reactions and the liver* (ed. M. Davis, J.M. Tredger and R. Williams), p. 111. Pitman Medical, London.

Wiles, C.M., Assem, E-S.K., Cohen, S.L., and Fisher, C. (1979). Cephradine-induced interstitial nephritis. *Clin. Exp. Immunol.* 36, 342.

Woosley, R.L., Drayer, D.E., Reidenberg, M.M., Nies, A.S., Carr, K., and Oates, J.A. (1978). Effect of acetylator phenotype on the rate at which procainamide induces antinuclear antibodies and the lupus syndrome. *N. Engl. J. Med.* 298, 1157.

Wright, P. (1975). Untoward effects associated with practolol administration: oculomucocutaneous syndrome. *Br. Med. J.* i, 595.

Youngman. P.R., Taylor, K.M., and Wilson, J.D. (1983). Anaphylactoid reactions to neuromuscular agents: a commonly undiagnosed condition? *Lancet* ii, 597.

25. Part 2 Tests for detecting drug allergy

Introduction

Before the diagnosis of an allergic drug reaction can be made, several problems have to be solved. First, one has to seek evidence of a drug reaction and to distinguish it from coincidental disease (the disease for which treatment is being given or a complication thereof, or other diseases that may be present or develop). Secondly, the culprit(s) in the case of multiple therapy has to be identified; this is the most frequent and difficult problem. Thirdly, allergy has to be distinguished from other unwanted drug effects. Proper medical history taking, clinical findings, and investigations (proper tests) all help to achieve these goals. Identification of the drug responsible for the reaction is important for obvious reasons. Testing for drug allergy is complicated. The second and third of these difficulties, which will be discussed in detail, are largely related to: (a) the diversity of immune reactions and the problem of finding an appropriate *in vivo* test or, more importantly, an *in vitro* correlate; (b) an allergic drug reaction may be due to the drug, to any of a wide variety of degradation products (often arising *in vivo* and occasionally *in vitro*), or to impurities introduced during the preparation and storage. The possibility of immunological cross-reactions with other drugs should also be kept in mind; (c) the lack of proper testing material, which represents one of the major limitations to the reliability of the testing procedures, for example, giving false-negative results. Alternatively, even when positive (e.g. when a wheal and flare response results in a direct skin test or *in vitro* leucocyte histamine release), these tests may not necessarily indicate an allergy, since such changes may be induced in other ways, as will be explained later.

Possible investigations in patients with suspected drug allergy are listed in Table 25.3. (Patch tests for investigating contact dermatitis are described in Chapter 17.)

Penicillin as a model study: skin tests

Despite modern technology and the availability of alternative test procedures, including the *in vitro* tests to be described, skin testing is still widely used for the diagnosis of allergy (e.g. immediate-type allergy in asthma and hay fever). In the latter examples the matter is relatively straightforward, and the risk of testing, particularly by the prick-in method, is minimal. In our own experience prick-in tests in drug allergy are totally unreliable, and intradermal tests are used, despite a definite risk. Unlike intradermal tests for inhalant allergies, intradermal tests for drug allergy are not very reliable, even when an apparently appropriate antigen is used. This was clearly shown by our studies in penicillin allergy (Assem and Vickers 1974a, 1975), in which skin-test false-negatives were frequently encountered.

False-positives (to intradermal testing) are of particular importance with certain drugs, for example, neuro-muscular blockers (NMB) and narcotic analgesics, particularly when high concentrations of these drugs are used (Assem 1984a, 1991; also see discussion of routine skin testing). They are more common in this type of skin test than they are in the prick/scratch test. Prick tests with NMB may give false-negatives, however, particularly with low drug concentrations (Farrell *et al.* 1988; Assem and Symons 1989; Assem 1990b, 1991).

Patch tests may be used in testing for reactions other than immediate-type allergy, particularly in delayed-type hypersensitivity and with agents that are capable of inducing contact dermatitis (such as local anaesthetics, Assem and Moorthy 1988).

Our model study for the evaluation of skin tests in drug allergy was carried out in a series of patients with penicillin allergy. This will be described at length here in order to illustrate several important points which are encountered in any drug allergy. The special importance of penicillin allergy and its medicolegal aspects are also discussed later in this chapter.

The importance of the testing material

The possible structural features of allergens capable of eliciting an anaphylactic reaction are shown in Figure 25.4. There have been several reports confirming the importance of skin test material in establishing the diag-

TABLE 25.3
Possible investigations in patients with drug allergy

In vivo

1. Skin tests:
   (a) direct skin test;
   (b) Prausnitz–Kustner reaction.
2. Other challenge tests.

In vitro

Specific allergy tests

1. Serological studies:
   (a) detection of antibodies against different haptenic determinants;
   (b) identification of antibody classes (IgG, IgM, IgA, IgD, IgE), and subclasses (particularly of IgG); Radioallergosorbent test for IgE antibodies*
2. Detection of tissue-sensitizing antibodies (and allergen-induced mediator release, e.g. histamine, from sensitized tissue/cells):
   (a) in serum, by passive sensitization;
   (b) cell-bound, by direct allergen challenge, e.g. leucocyte (basophil) histamine release
3. Detection of delayed-type hypersensitivity (cell-mediated immunity):
   (a) the lymphocyte transformation tests;
   (b) the macrophage migration inhibition test.
4. Other tests for antibody- or cell-mediated immunity, e.g. rosette formation by antigen-coated red cells around sensitized basophil leucocytes or lymphocytes.
5. Detection of immune complexes containing the specific hapten.

Non-specific tests for allergy

1. Total serum IgE, total leucocyte-bound IgE.
2. Indirect methods for detecting drug-specific antibodies by co-precipitation procedures, using radioisotope-labelled or unlabelled drugs:
   (a) measurement of binding to the globulin fraction of serum, using ammonium sulphate for precipitation of that fraction;
   (b) measurement of binding to serum immunoglobulins, using anti-human immunoglobulin serum for their precipitation.
3. Tests for autoantibodies, lupus erythematous cells, eosinophil count, etc.

Confirmation of anaphylactic or anaphylactoid reaction in plasma/serum:
   (a) histamine/methylhistamine;
   (b) eosinophil cationic protein;
   (c) tryptase

---

* most important

nosis of pencillin allergy and predicting cases that are likely to develop anaphylactic reaction (Finke *et al.* 1965; Siegel and Levine 1965; Levine and Zolov 1969; Bierman and van Arsdel 1969). Levine and colleagues

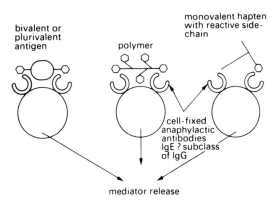

FIG. 25.4
Diagrammatic representation of the structure of test antigens capable of eliciting an anaphylactic reaction in drug allergy.

(1967) carried out a long-term prospective study of the predictive value of immediate skin tests in 218 patients with a history of penicillin allergy. Skin tests were carried out with both benzylpenicilloyl-polylysine and the 'minor determinants' mixture (which includes benzyl-penicillin and sodium benzylpenicilloate) to determine the benzylpenicilloyl specificity and the minor haptenic determinant specificity, respectively. Positive results were obtained in only 15 per cent when the two preparations of test material were used. Penicillin alone gave a positive result in less than 5 per cent. These results were obtained in patients with a past history of penicillin allergy, and the incidence of positive skin tests in patients without such a history was much smaller. These results have an important bearing on the practicability of routine skin testing, which will be discussed later.

Apart from the major and minor haptenic determinants mentioned previously, it has been suggested that standard preparations of benzylpenicillin contain high-molecular-weight contaminants that evoke reactions in allergic subjects (Batchelor *et al.* 1967; Knudsen *et al.* 1967; Stewart 1967). These contaminants may be of some use as eliciting antigens in skin tests (Stewart 1967; Assem and Schild 1968), although they may be of minor importance as a cause of allergy (de Weck *et al.* 1968).

The carrier effect

It is generally believed that in order to induce an allergic response to any simple chemical such as penicillin, the drug itself or, more commonly, its metabolites must first combine, irreversibly with some large carrier molecule, such as a protein (Assem 1967). It is therefore important to know whether the antibodies formed are specific also towards the carrier protein molecule. Levine (1962,

1963) has shown that when rabbits and guinea-pigs are immunized with a benzylpenicilloyl-protein conjugate then the antibodies formed are adapted to the entire benzylpenicilloyl group, the lysine side chain, and to some adjoining structures of the immunizing carrier protein. The identification of the protein with which penicillin or its metabolites combines *in vivo* would be extremely useful since it could lead to the preparation of the correct complete antigen for use in *in vitro* diagnostic tests.

Levine and Price (1964) have compared penicilloyl-polylysine (BPO:PL), penicilloyl human serum albumin (BPO:HSA), and penicilloyl human γ-globulin (BPO:HGG) as elicitors of the wheal and flare reaction in patients with a past history of penicillin allergy. They found that BPO:PL was more effective than BPO:HSA and BPO:HGG. This is probably due to the open structure of polylysine, which allows more contact between benzylpenicilloyl groups and the large antibenzylpenicilloyl combining sites than would be allowed by the more rigid structural configuration of the benzylpenicilloyl-protein conjugates.

Vickers and Assem (1974) have used benzylpenicilloyl conjugates with PL, HSA, HGG, bovine serum albumin (BSA), and bovine γ-globulin (BGG), the first three being evaluated in skin tests. BPO:HSA gave positive skin tests in a slightly higher proportion of patients (7 out of 14) than with either benzylpenicillin (5 out of 14) or BPO:PL (5 out of 14).

Skin tests with conjugates of some minor determinants and comparison with the penicilloyl conjugate

Assem and Vickers (1975) carried out a study to assess the value of skin tests with antigens prepared from the major haptenic determinant, the benzylpenicilloyl group, and two minor determinants, the benzylpenicillenate and penicillamine groups, using human serum albumin as a carrier in all conjugates, and comparing the results with those obtained with benzylpenicillin. This study included 22 patients with established penicillin allergy; among them were the 14 patients used for the study of the previously mentioned 'carrier' effect.

No positive skin responses were obtained for any determinant in 10 control subjects. Of the 22 patients allergic to penicillin tested, 10 responded to the benzylpenicilloyl group, 8 to benzylpenicillenate, and 10 to penicillamine. The BPO responses were generally greater than the benzylpenicillenate responses, and four of the patients responded to the benzylpenicilloyl group in the absence of a response to penicillenate and penicillamine.

This study and the study on carrier effect clearly show the limitations of skin testing with benzylpenicillin alone.

Limitations

Availability of proper testing material to the non-specialist

The unmodified penicillin is the only testing material that is readily available to the doctor who is not a specialist in allergy, and even the latter may not have the proper facilities and material to detect penicillin allergy. Although a penicilloyl-polylysine preparation is commercially available (Sigma Chemical Co.), it is used only by specialists and its wide use is inadvisable and impracticable. This imposes a great limitation on the value of skin tests as carried out in general practice. The risk involved in skin tests will be discussed later.

Other limitations of skin tests

Though the antibodies that mediate immediate-type hypersensitivity are skin-sensitizing antibodies, that is, they become 'fixed' to skin, and therefore can be detected by applying the test antigen to skin, it is still possible that other types of antibodies which are not skin-sensitizing may play a part in the allergic reaction (Levine *et al.* 1966). It is therefore not certain that potential anaphylaxis will always be detected by cutaneous testing, even when the appropriate antigen and proper techniques are employed.

It has also been shown (Vickers and Assem 1974; Assem and Vickers 1975) that skin tests compare unfavourably with some of the *in vitro* tests (such as the lymphocyte transformation test), which will be discussed later.

The overall predictive value of skin tests

In over 150 cases, including the previously mentioned small group of patients who have undergone extensive and quantitative studies, an immediate response to benzylpenicillin was obtained in only 22 per cent of allergic patients, and 36 per cent with the best carrier. Our results contradict those of other workers in the field of penicillin allergy. Levine and Zolov (1969) state that 'skin tests were found to be valuable predictive tests for immediate (including anaphylactic) and urticarial allergic reactions to penicillin'. This comment was based on a prospective study of 218 patients with past histories of penicillin allergy on whom such tests were performed.

The skin tests performed in this study used benzylpenicilloyl-polylysine and a minor determinant mixture. A further report by the Penicillin Study Group of the American Academy of Allergy (Green and Rosenblum 1971) found that whereas these reagents have a predictive accuracy of about 84 per cent in immediate reactions, test doses employing benzylpenicillin itself have an accuracy of 55 per cent. In other words, more than half of all individuals who are actually sensitive (immediate reactors) could be recognized by penicillin skin testing. The skin reaction rate was particularly high in patients who experienced penicillin reactions of the immediate type within 30 minutes.

In a more recent series of 740 patients reported by Sullivan and others (1981), skin tests were carried out with benzylpenicillin, penicilloic acid, and penicilloyl-polylysine. Sixty-three per cent of the patients gave a positive result, but the incidence of skin-test positives was inversely related to the length of time that had elapsed between clinical reactions and skin testing. The maximum incidence (93 per cent) was obtained in patients who were tested 7–12 months after reactions, while the incidence in those tested after 10 years was only 22 per cent.

Despite the marked discrepancies in the proportions of positive skin tests in patients allergic to penicillin, in the experience of different investigators, there is an overall agreement on its value, particularly in the hands of specialists, even when the results are negative (Bierman and van Arsdel 1969).

Investigation of the cross-allergenicity between penicillins and cephalosporins

In patients with suspected or proven allergy to penicillin a skin test with a cephalosporin derivative (e.g. cephaloridine) should be carried out. Not only will this help in deciding whether a cephalosporin derivative may be given as a replacement for penicillin in patients with penicillin allergy, but it may also help in the confirmation of suspected penicillin allergy, since cephalosporins may give a stronger response and a higher incidence of positive reactions than penicillin in patients allergic to penicillin (Assem and Vickers 1974b).

Medicolegal aspects

The medicolegal aspects of penicillin allergy, particularly in relation to the question of whether skin tests for penicillin allergy should be carried out as a routine, have been borne out by several cases of fatal penicillin reactions that have occurred in Malaysia and Singapore (Horne 1973; Eravelly 1974).

Fatal anaphylactic reactions to penicillin are very rare. They seem to occur in about 1–2 per 100 000 patients treated with penicillin (Idsøe et al. 1968), compared with an overall incidence of penicillin allergy of 0.7–10 per cent reported in different studies in different countries. The incidence of minor (non-fatal) anaphylactic reactions is estimated to be about 1–5 per 10 000 patient-courses of penicillin (Levine and Zolov 1969).

In a study of 151 fatal anaphylactic reactions by Idsøe and others (1968), 14 per cent of the patients had evidence of previous allergies of some kind; 70 per cent had received penicillin previously; and one-third of these had already experienced sudden allergic reactions to penicillin. In 30 per cent there was no history of previous penicillin therapy, and one should assume that these patients had been exposed to penicillin previously. This may be explained by forgetfulness by the patient, lack of records, the patient not having been told that he had had penicillin, or by 'hidden contacts' such as milk, which may contain penicillin when obtained from cattle treated with this drug.

The point at law in all these cases was, apparently, to what extent was there negligence because of failure to give a test injection? It is known from the previously mentioned work, including our own (Assem and Vickers 1972, 1974a,b; Vickers and Assem 1974), that the test is of limited value — but how limited?

Views on routine testing before penicillin therapy

With regard to the question of routine tests before starting penicillin therapy, the following quotations from two leading groups of workers in the field of penicillin allergy may provide an answer.

'At the present time, it is not recommended that prior skin testing of patients about to be treated with penicillin be instituted as a routine clinical procedure' (Levine 1964).

'When dealing with the problem of prospective skin tests, it seems illogical to advise against it on the ground that they are potentially dangerous. If prospective testing is not performed, the patient may receive a much larger dose of the allergen, the only safeguard being the prior history-taking by the physician, but this is potentially a more dangerous procedure than a skin test. Mostly for practical reasons, however, routine skin tests with penicillin or penicilloyl-polylysine, or both, prior to penicillin administration, cannot be generally advocated, although they might be justified in special situations' (Idsøe et al. 1968).

Several leading articles discussing the unreliability and potential risk of skin tests have been published (e.g. in the *British Medical Journal* 1964, 1968). Another article (*Canadian Medical Association Journal* 1967) suggests that skin testing in general practice is undesirable: 'Such tests should be undertaken, if possible, by specialists trained and experienced in allergy skin test-ing, in co-operation with a competent laboratory'.

These quotations are representative of the generally held view that routine prospective testing for penicillin allergy cannot be advocated at present. The authors of many reviews on the subject prefer, however, to leave the doctor to come to a similar conclusion by himself.

Skin tests have been recommended before starting penicillin therapy, especially for patients who have a history of sensitivity and for patients who have had any allergic disorder, but even skin tests made with diluted penicillin solution, especially intradermal tests, may present danger. A prick/scratch test is preferred. A positive test is undoubtedly significant, but a negative test does not ensure safety when the full therapeutic dose is subsequently administered (Allan 1966).

Hazards of penicillin test injections

There is a definite risk involved in these test injections. Even minute concentrations may provoke anaphylactic reactions, such as have sometimes been experienced in connection with a skin test (Ettinger and Kaye 1964; Resnik and Shelley 1966) and after the intradermal injection of as little as 0.02 ml of a concentration of 1000 units of penicillin per ml (Berger and Eisen 1955). Rose (1953) and Driagin (1966) reported fatal anaphylactic reactions as a result of intradermal testing with penicil-lin. Fatal anaphylaxis may rarely follow the relatively safe scratch test (Dogliotti 1968). In fact, an accidental scratch with a needle contaminated with traces of peni-cillin has been reported as provoking anaphylactic shock (Wirth 1963). These reports perhaps represent rare inci-dents, however, and other investigators (e.g. Levine and Zolov 1969; Sullivan *et al.* 1981; and the author) have not encountered any serious systemic reactions to skin testing.

A relatively minor risk in skin testing is antigenicity of the test material used, which may occur in non-allergic patients who may be tested either because of suspicion of allergy, or because of routine procedures. This risk is more likely when hapten-macromolecule conjugates are used. It seems logical to use conjugates with homolo-gous proteins in order to avoid risk, and to obtain better results as pointed out previously in connection with the carrier effect. In Parker's view (1972), however, the use of hapten conjugates with homologous or autologous proteins, which would be expected to simulate those involved in drug allergy in man, appears to be of little real advantage, and their use in skin testing may produce undesirable effects, such as autosensitization. He rightly suggests the use of non-antigenic macromolecules (such as small polypeptides) as carriers for haptens in test conjugates. Even small polypeptides, however, may be antigenic, but less so than large macromolecules.

Conclusions

1. Skin tests as carried out by a specialist are not very reliable, particularly if they are performed a long time (years) after a clinical reaction. They are even less reliable in the hands of the non-specialist with no access to proper test material. The desirable range of testing material may not be available even to the specialist. It is also important to mention that potential anaphylaxis may not be detected by cutaneous testing, even when appropriate antigens and proper techniques are employed.

2. Skin and other test injections are risky, and in the allergic subject a fatal anaphylactic reaction may follow these procedures.

3. In view of 1 and 2 (which is a weak argument) and, above all, for practical reasons, routine prospective skin testing and other *in vivo* test procedures cannot gener-ally be advocated. They are probably not of much use in patients who have received penicillin on two or more occasions without developing adverse effects. It should be added, however, that allergy may develop in some patients who have previously received several courses of penicillin without adverse effects. As a compromise solution, these tests are indicated in selected patients:

(a) patients with a personal or family history of estab-lished or suspected allergy of any sort;

(b) where parenteral administration is planned, since any reaction may then be more serious than when the drug is given orally;

(c) if the patient has been treated with semi-synthetic penicillins, particularly by injection, or such a treat-ment, which carries a greater risk of allergy (Idsøe *et al.* 1968) is contemplated;

(d) patients with a suspected disease associated with a higher incidence of allergic drug reactions or immu-nological abnormalities, such as glandular fever, where the incidence of 'reactions' to ampicillin is said to be particularly high (Pullen *et al.* 1967). Although it is not known whether the skin test would be of value in this condition, it would perhaps help in reducing the anxiety about a possible reaction to penicillin therapy.

Indication for repeating a false-negative skin test

Negative skin tests may be obtained after a definitely allergic drug reaction. In fact this state may persist for days, weeks, or even a few months, and seems to occur particularly after severe reactions. Assem and Schild (1968) have reported an example after a severe anaphyl-actic reaction to penicillin. This was not surprising since temporary desensitization may follow exposure to a massive dose of allergen (see Fig. 25.2 in Part 1). It is also comparable in some respects to the occasionally dramatic improvement in some asthmatic patients following a severe reaction (unintentional) to an injection of allergen given during the course of hyposensitization therapy (McAllen *et al.* 1967). Sullivan and others (1981) have also reported a lower incidence of skin-test positives in the first 6 months after clinical reactions to penicillin, than between the seventh and twelfth months, when the incidence of positives was at its height (93 per cent).

Routine skin testing in other important allergies: anaesthesia

According to Fisher (1989) the prick test with anaesthetics (including in particular neuromuscular blockers [NMB], such as suxamethonium) is the simplest and cheapest and could be performed in an emergency, out of hours or prior to office anaesthesia. According to the author, these points are valid, but as stated earlier there are limitations to the value of prick testing with NMB and opioids (also see Assem 1989*b*). Though useful with suxamethonium, the test is not as reliable with other NMB, where false-positives occur frequently in normal subjects. Furthermore, false-negatives also occur with low concentration (Farrell *et al.* 1988; Assem and Symons 1989; Assem 1990*b*, 1991). Intradermal injection of high concentration, though less likely to give false negatives, carries the risk of anaphylactic reaction (Farrell *et al.* 1988; Assem 1990*b*). The author saw a case of systemic anaphylaxis (hypotension, bronchospasm, tachycardia, skin flushing) following a negative prick test and miscalculation of the dilution of a neuromuscular blocker before its use in an intradermal test. These limitations point to the importance of *in vitro* testing (see below).

Alternative procedures to direct skin testing

The Prausnitz–Kustner reaction

If it is felt that a serious reaction may result from test injections, the latter should be preceded by skin scratch tests. A passive transfer by injection of serum from a sensitized donor intradermally in a normal recipient, which constitutes the Prausnitz–Kustner reaction, may prove useful when great risk is likely from a direct skin test in the patient. Nowadays, if the test is ever to be carried out, the donor serum should be tested for hepatitis B and human immunodeficiency virus (HIV).

In vivo tests

Indications for *in vivo* challenge tests other than in the skin

Although the skin test is the most widely used of the tests for drug allergy, other challenge tests may be necessary. Thus, one may cite the following examples:

1. if the 'target organ' is likely to be of particular importance in connection with the route of exposure of the allergen. Thus, bronchial or nasal challenge is indicated when the allergen is inhaled, owing to contamination of the air; this may occur, and seemingly cause respiratory allergy in the form of airways obstruction (asthma) or rhinitis, in occupations such as, for example, drug manufacturing.

We have come across other examples where nurses or pharmacists developed asthmatic attacks while, or at some time after, reconstituting penicillin preparations or breaking their containers, or cleaning a drug cupboard;

2. if the manifestations of drug reactions are more or less localized in certain organs, though the drugs are given systemically either orally or by injection; for example, asthma induced by aspirin, or by intravenous anaesthetics or preanaesthetic medications;

3. if the skin test is obviously unreliable or gives nonspecific reactions, as in the case of narcotic analgesics, and competitive neuromuscular blocking agents such as tubocurarine. In these instances, if *in vivo* challenge tests are at all desirable, a small test dose may be given intravenously (Assem 1977*a*);

4. a test dose may be given by the conventional route, for example, intravenously, if the skin test is negative.

The risks of *in vivo* testing cannot be overemphasized. A remarkable example was a case of fatal anaphylactic reaction that resulted from the instillation of one drop of a local anaesthetic (as a test) in the conjunctival sac of an allergic patient (Adriani 1972).

Nowadays, all such procedures should be carried out in an intensive care unit.

In vitro tests

'There is an urgent need for *in vitro* tests for drug allergy, because skin testing is known to be unreliable and sometimes dangerous' (*British Medical Journal* 1968). Several laboratories in the world are now engaged on this problem. The techniques now available, though still of limited value in the prediction of drug allergy, particularly in urgent situations (Assem and Schild 1968; Assem 1972*a,b*; Assem and Vickers 1972; Assem 1983*a,b*; 1984*a,b*; Assem and Moorthy 1988; Assem 1989*b*; Assem and Symons 1989; Fisher 1989; Assem 1990*b*), may be of great help in the management of 'cold' cases. Some of them are also restricted in the range of allergies they can detect. So until more reliable and quick methods are developed to cope with urgent situations and to cover the desired range of drugs, preventive measures will be far from satisfactory. Recent expansion has been greatest in the range of allergies that can be detected by solid-phase assays of IgE antibodies. The detection of these antibodies is valuable in the diagnosis of anaphylaxis (see radioallergosorbent test, RAST, below). There is little room for optimism, however, because there is a far greater limitation than all those mentioned above: the enormous cost (see routine testing in anaesthetic practice, below).

Serological studies

The detection of drug-specific circulating antibodies proves only the occurrence of an immunological response to that particular drug, not evidence of allergy. This is best illustrated in connection with penicillin.

The usefulness of serological investigations will certainly improve when we know more about all the haptenic determinants of every allergenic drug. When this is combined with the study of the different classes of antibodies, the predictive and diagnostic value of these tests will perhaps reach a satisfactory level. Work along these lines is going on at several centres. The study by Levine and others (1966) on the correlation between the serological and the clinical findings in human penicillin allergy provides a useful approach to this problem.

'When the metabolites of a drug acting as haptenic determinants have not been identified, or their synthesis and conjugation to carrier molecules is not possible, it may be possible to devise a method of circumventing this problem. An example is the generation of practolol metabolites using the rat liver mixed-function-oxidase complex *in vitro* (Amos *et al.* 1977).'

Methods of detection of the various classes of hapten-specific antibodies

It is desirable at this stage to describe the basic details of some techniques. In order to establish the various immunoglobulin classes of antibodies directly against any particular haptenic determinant, the following reagents should be available: (1) conjugate of the haptenic determinant; (2) serum containing antibodies against the hapten; (3) antiserum against the various human immunoglobulin classes (IgG, IgM, IgA, IgD, and IgE). There are simpler methods, however, for detecting certain classes of antibodies, for example, the use of SH-reducing agents (e.g. mercaptoethanol) for distinguishing agglutinating IgM antibodies, which lose this prop-

erty after reduction. Leaving aside these simpler techniques, which are of limited value, the three reagents are used in what are called 'double-antibody techniques' (e.g. human antibodies against a drug metabolite and, say, rabbit antihuman immunoglobulins), and the ensuing positive reaction can be illustrated by double-agglutination techniques with their variants, or double-precipitation techniques, again with their variants. A variant of the latter is shown in Fig. 25.5. Though this procedure, as such, is not used in routine allergy diagnosis, it illustrates the basic principles of a radioimmunoassay, be it for the detection of allergen-specific antibodies and their immunoglobulin class or the antigens (or even haptens and other simple molecules, for example, histamine; see assay of 'markers' of allergic reactions).

The haptenic conjugate used in this experiment was prepared by the conjugation of the penicilloyl determinant to ^{125}I-labelled human serum albumin. The first step was to separate the proteins in the human serum (placed in the wells on either side of the middle trough) including the various immunoglobulins, by electrophoresis in agar gel covering a glass slide. The antiserum specific to any particular immunoglobulin class in man or in experimental animals was then placed in the central trough (if the antibodies against the hapten were not precipitating) together with the labelled hapten-protein conjugate (antigen). The antigen diffused towards the separated immunoglobulins, producing precipitin arcs which contained: (1) the labelled penicilloyl antigen; (2) its antibody of the particular class; Fig. 25.5 shows: (a) IgG precipitating hapten-specific antibodies in rabbit antiserum; (b) IgG non-precipitating antibodies in human serum; (c) IgM non-precipitating antibodies in human serum); and (3) the second antibody used in precipitating hapten-specific antibodies (goat antiserum) against human IgG and IgM (Fig. 25.5 (a) and (b) respectively). The precipitin arcs seen by the naked eye are only markers, but the essential step is to establish by autoradiography where the labelled antigen has precipitated in relation to these markers.

In place of the latter procedure, and for quantitative assay, one could carry out the co-precipitation or double-antibody procedures (labelled antigen + specific antibody of a particular immunoglobulin class, the first antibody, and the second antibody raised in another species, against any particular immunoglobulin class of the first antibody) in a test tube and count the radioactivity in the precipitate, which correlates with the amount of hapten-specific antibody of the particular immunoglobulin class in the tested serum. Labelling antibodies or antigens may employ radioisotopes, most commonly ^{125}I, or enzymes such as alkaline phosphatase (enzyme-linked immunoassay). In the latter procedure the enzyme activity in the precipitate is determined and the amount of antibody is worked out from a calibration curve.

The introduction of solid-phase techniques, where either the antigen or antibody is conjugated to dextran, agarose, or paper, and of radioimmunoassays of many drugs (Butler 1978) will no doubt have its impact on methods of detecting, identifying, and quantifying antibodies to drugs and their metabolites. Commercial kits

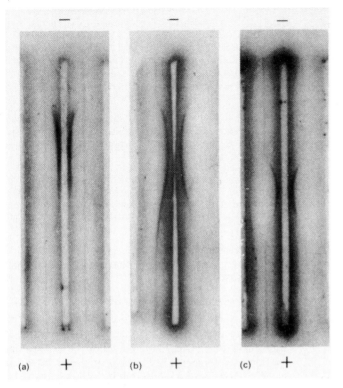

(a)   +   (b)   +   (c)   +

Fig. 25.5
Illustration of the identification of the immunoglobulin classes of penicilloyl-specific antibodies by radio-immunoelectrophoresis and autoradiography (see text). (a) Precipitating IgG antibodies in antiserum raised in a rabbit; (b) and (c)
IgG and IgM antibodies (non-precipitating and
requiring a second, precipitating antibody, goat
anti-human IgG and anti-human IgM antisera to
show them) in the sera of a normal subject and a
subject allergic to penicillin, respectively.

for the detection of certain drug allergies by antibody
measurement, using solid-phase techniques, either radioallergosorbent (RAST) or enzyme-linked immunosorbent assays (ELISA), are now available (discussed under
RAST, below).

When autoimmunization is suspected, for example, in
haemolytic anaemia or thrombocytopenia, tests for
specific antibodies are indicated, both with regard to the
drug, and the 'autoantigen'. An example of such an
exercise was initiated in relation to practolol (Assem and
Banks 1973; also see Part 1 on Mechanisms).

The possible assignment of different functions to different antibody classes, for example, the reaginic (skin-
sensitizing) antibody producing immediate-type allergic
reactions, forms the basis of a number of *in vitro* tests,
which will be mentioned briefly.

In vitro tests for immediate-type drug allergy

Detection of reaginic antibodies in vitro

Almost all the initial work on these antibodies in man
has been done in connection with atopy, particularly in
asthma and hay fever. Application of these tests to
certain drug allergies has been successful and it is reasonable to assume that in due course they will have a wider
use. The most prominent feature of reaginic antibodies is

their capacity to sensitize either autologous or homologous cells, which on subsequent challenge with the
specific antigen will release pharmacologically active
mediators, such as histamine, slow-reacting substance
(leukotrienes C_4, D_4, and E_4), bradykinin, 5-hydroxy-
tryptamine, and platelet-activating factor. These mediators of immediate allergic reactions may be estimated
either by bioassays, biochemical methods with or without the use of radioisotopes, or by radioimmunological
techniques, as in the case of bradykinin. The following
methods are now available:

1. Sensitization of tissue, for example by passive
sensitization of chopped lung. Since reaginic antibodies
are, in general, species-specific, human allergy may be
detected by use of homologous tissue or tissue from a
closely related species, such as the monkey. The use of
human and monkey lung for this purpose has been
reported by Assem and Schild (1968) and Assem
(1972a). Other tissues or cells, for example, basophil
leucocytes, may also be sensitized *in vitro*, and if these
tissues are contractile (e.g. intestine or appendix), contraction of their smooth muscle may be elicited on
subsequent challenge with the antigen (Schultz–Dale
reaction). There is some controversy concerning the
possibility of passively sensitizing rat peritoneal mast
cells with human reagins (Perelmutter *et al.* 1970; Plautt
et al. 1973).

2. Measurement of antigen-induced histamine release from the patient's leucocytes (Lichtenstein and Osler 1964). The leucocyte histamine-release test has been found to be very valuable, not only in the diagnosis of truly anaphylactic reactions to a wide variety of drugs but also in equally life-threatening anaphylactoid reactions (Assem and Vickers 1974a,b, 1975; Assem 1977b, 1983a,b, 1984a,b; Hirshman et al. 1982, Assem et al. 1983) which appear not to be immunologically mediated. These two 'types' of immediate reaction are clinically indistinguishable, the anaphylactoid type being identified by exclusion (lack of evidence of an immune mechanism and occurrence at first exposure). The test would not only show the release with the drug causing the clinical reaction, but generally not with others that are not structurally or pharmacologically related, but also would indicate if the patient is likely to react to related drugs that might be considered as potential alternatives. In addition, the test should also predict anaphylactoid reactions, should the need for a 'screening test' arise. It also provides a valuable tool to study the underlying abnormality and the mechanism (e.g. hyperosmolarity in the case of iodinated radiocontrast media) and characteristics of the mediator release process in the anaphylactoid reaction, for example, if the process is cytotoxic or 'secretory' in nature (Assem 1984c).

Caution against the term 'anaphylactoid'   Although mediator release, for example, from basophils as in the leucocyte histamine-release test, can be triggered independently from IgE antibodies as a result of a physicochemical process (e.g. hyperosmolarity, high or low temperature, polybasic compounds, i.e. effect of positive charges, or by anaphylatoxins: complement fragments C5a and C3a), it is difficult to explain most of the so-called anaphylactoid reactions and the mediator release involved. In the days before the development of tests for IgE antibodies to NMB (described below), reactions to these drugs were divided into truly anaphylactic and anaphylactoid, partly based on the history of prior exposure or its absence, and partly on whether there was evidence of an immune response to these drugs or not (Assem 1977a,b).

Anaphylactoid reactions to NMB, defined according to these criteria, were investigated by the leucocyte histamine-release test and were found to give a positive result (like truly anaphylactic reactions). We wanted to know what was the mechanism of histamine release in that case (loosely described as 'idiosyncratic'), and we went on to study the characteristics of histamine release (Assem 1977b, 1983b, 1984c). It was interesting to find that the characteristics of drug-induced histamine release from patients' leucocytes were identical to those of 'true' anaphylactic reactions (Assem 1984c). Histamine release could, however, be induced by the drug on its own (without any 'artificial' conjugation), which would be unusual with a simple chemical acting as hapten and not as a complete antigen. Despite this finding and the absence of any history of previous clinical exposure, we could not rule out the possibility that the reaction was truly anaphylactic (IgE-mediated). The reason for this was the demonstration that histamine release could not be elicited with compounds possessing a single quaternary ammonium

group (QAG); only those with two or three QAG could release histamine; that is, those that share this requirement (bivalency or polyvalency) in order to be able to elicit an anaphylactic reaction (Fig. 25.4). Therefore, it seemed possible that NMB behaved like very small antigens. Evidence to support this possibility was obtained from other *in vitro* tests. *In vitro* passive sensitization of human skin slices showed some response, drug-induced histamine release from slices that had been preincubated with patients' sera. Furthermore, patients' lymphocytes responded to the drug by increased mitosis and DNA synthesis, as shown by the increased incorporation of ^{3}H-thymidine (Assem 1983b).

Subsequent work has shown that patients who have had anaphylactoid reactions to NMB (defined as above) had high levels of IgE antibodies to these agents (Baldo and Fisher 1983; Harle et al. 1984; Didier et al. 1987; Assem and Ling 1988; Moneret-Vautrin et al. 1988; Assem and Symons 1989; Assem 1990a,b).

3. Measurement of the release of isotopically labelled 5-hydroxytryptamine from platelets (Caspary and Comaish 1967).

The detection of immediate-type allergy by IgE tests

The discovery of IgE (see Part 1 of this chapter) and the consequent introduction of IgE tests for the detection of immediate-type allergy have been two of the most important developments in the field of allergy in recent years. The importance of the latter development can be seen in the light of other test procedures.

For over 50 years the passive cutaneous transfer in man (known as the Prausnitz–Kustner reaction) has been the principal indirect test for immediate-type allergy (anaphylaxis). This carries the risk of transmitting viral hepatitis and human immunodeficiency viral (HIV) infection. An alternative procedure is passive cutaneous anaphylaxis in monkeys (Stanworth 1973). This test is feasible only for some research workers. Before the introduction of IgE tests, all *in vivo* tests for anaphylactic antibodies in serum relied on the biological assay of these antibodies or, rather, the 'tissue-sensitizing' or 'reaginic activity' of serum, which is mediated at least in part by IgE antibodies. These tests, apart from being laborious, are available only in some research centres, and require the use of tissues from man or other primates for passive sensitization. They are qualitative, but only semi-quantitative, even when more than one dilution of the serum to be tested is used. The number of sera that can be tested in a single experiment is limited, and there are no agreed standards for assessing the 'reaginic activity' of serum. Each group of research workers may use its own reference sera, but these cannot be kept for long periods of time because of the eventual loss of activity and have to be replaced at intervals.

The measurement of allergen-specific IgE antibodies in serum by the radio-allergosorbent test (RAST) (Wide *et al.* 1967) is free from some of these problems, but it has its own limitations (see below). An alternative non-isotopic method is the enzyme-linked immunoassay (ELISA) procedure (Voller *et al.* 1976).

Detection and measurement of allergen-specific IgE

So far, it seems that the RAST analysis, which can be carried out as originally described by Wide and others (1967) or by a variety of modifications, is the best method for this type of non-biological assay of tissue-sensitizing antibodies. It is based on the direct measurement of allergen-specific IgE, with two assumptions: (a) that tissue-sensitizing antibodies belong at least in part to the IgE class of immunoglobulins; and (b) all allergen-specific IgE antibodies are tissue-sensitizing. In the RAST analysis the allergen is conjugated to an insoluble carrier and this conjugate is used for the detection of allergen-specific IgE. The place of RAST in allergy diagnosis is difficult to assess, partly owing to technical problems. In respiratory allergy caused by inhalant allergens the results are more reliable than in food allergies (Thompson and Bird 1983).

In allergy to drugs that are simple chemicals (molecular weight less than 1000) the RAST analysis is at present of limited value, one of the main reasons being that the drug itself, or its various metabolites, which may be more important in the production of allergy, act only as haptens. The preparation of hapten conjugates in an insoluble form, which is essential for the RAST procedure, is a big problem that has been partly solved by direct conjugation of the drug to an insoluble matrix. To our knowledge the RAST analysis has so far been applied mainly (with only a very few exceptions, where it was used mainly for research purposes — see Assem 1977 [in the 1st, and repeated in this, edition of this book]; Wiles *et al.* 1979; Jarisch 1981; Baldo and Fisher 1983; Smal *et al.* 1988; Harle *et al.* 1984, 1986, 1988; Assem and Ling 1988; Assem and Symons 1989; Assem 1990*a,b*, 1991) in penicillin and anaesthetic allergies (commercial kits are available). Experience with these two RAST will be discussed in detail at the end of this chapter.

Non-specific correlates of immediate-type allergy

As in the case of intrinsic asthma, where there is a possibility of an allergy to unidentifiable allergens, the use of the RAST procedure is at present out of the question for allergy to many drugs. The reason for this in these drug allergies is somewhat different: the haptenic determinants are either unknown, or methods of preparing antigens from them are not available.

The practical value of total serum IgE estimation

Many patients with suspected drug allergy present an immediate diagnostic problem requiring quick action. In these patients, skin tests, despite their potential risk and their limited value, may provide the best possible diagnostic aid. Naturally, skin tests should be avoided if the risk of a reaction is potentially high, and in patients with a widespread skin rash. Since the skin test often gives a false-negative result, due to the reasons previously explained, and a false-positive with some drugs (e.g. narcotic analgesics), the estimation of total serum IgE by the radio-immunosorbent technique (RIST), or alternative procedures, may provide additional diagnostic help. Kits for the RIST tests are commercially available, and results may be obtained within one day, which is not possible with other *in vitro* tests. It is of particular value where a RAST analysis is not feasible, and biological *in vitro* tests are not available. It is also of value when other *in vitro* tests are negative, or their results are either of doubtful significance, or cannot distinguish between true allergic reactions and conditions simulating allergic reactions. Examples of these situations are the direct histamine-releasing effect of some drugs (Paton 1957) and the possible effect of some drugs on other *in vitro* correlates of allergy (not necessarily those which are strict correlates of immediate-type allergy), such as the lymphocyte transformation test (LTT). Thus in the histamine release test carried out on the patients' own leucocytes, a positive result may be either due to immediate-type allergy, or to direct histamine-releasing effect, that is, where such a reaction is not mediated by anaphylactic antibodies. In the LTT several drugs may possibly inhibit the response of sensitized cells to antigen.

In all these cases, and when other allergies can be excluded (because this test is a non-specific correlate of immediate-type allergy), a positive result will confirm the diagnosis of allergy, but a negative result will not exclude it.

Despite the shortcomings of the RIST analysis, it is potentially useful in a number of respects other than the confirmation of the diagnosis of drug allergy. Thus it is a useful aid in sorting out further diagnostic problems in patients with established allergy. Further, an immediate-type allergy may be confirmed in retrospect by a decreasing serum IgE level (Assem 1972*b*); it is also useful in the follow-up of effects of hypersensitization (Assem and McAllen 1973).

Reversed leucocyte anaphylaxis test

We have observed, in patients with allergic asthma and rhinitis, that total serum IgE may be normal in over two-thirds and that, in nearly a half, leucocyte (basophil)-bound IgE was apparently higher than normal (Assem and McAllen 1970; Assem and Vickers 1972). These conclusions were based on the indirect measurement of leucocyte-bound IgE by challenging these cells with antihuman IgE serum and measuring the amount of histamine released by this treatment. The mechanism of this response is comparable to that of the antigen-induced histamine release from leucocytes sensitized with anaphylactic antibodies. The response, however, of leucocytes to anti-IgE (called 'reversed' anaphylaxis because anti-IgE takes the role of the antigen), like the total serum IgE estimation, appears to be related to the total amount of cell-bound IgE and not to the cell-bound IgE antibodies against the allergen in question. Thus, both are non-specific correlates of immediate-type allergy, but 'reversed' anaphylaxis is the more sensitive of the two tests. This is partly owing to the increased 'releasability' of histamine from the basophils of allergic patients. Immunoglobulin E (IgE) in allergic patients may also differ from that in normal subjects (Assem and Attallah, 1981).

Other in vitro *correlates of immediate-type allergy*

The basophil-degranulation test The degranulation of actively sensitized mast cells and basophil leucocytes on exposure to antigen is a correlate of immediate-type allergy. Tests for it are comparable with the previously mentioned methods in which the response of these cells is detected by measuring released pharmacological mediators. One of the drawbacks of these tests is, however, the lack of good quantitative correlation between the observed degranulation and the amount of mediator released. Apart from the relative inaccuracy of assessing the degree of degranulation, there is the inability of this technique to detect the synthesis of some mediators, for example, SRSA and possibly histamine, which is activated by antigen challenge.

Shelley and Juhlin (1962), in an attempt to develop a useful test for reaginic antibodies, used an indirect test in the presence of non-sensitized basophils, allergic sera, and antigen. An indirect test using rabbit basophils, which are more plentiful, was described by Shelley (1961) and was used by other investigators (Katz *et al.* 1964) to study drug allergy. The reproducibility of this test has been questioned, and in view of the established species specificity of the reagins, doubt as to the relationship between the results obtained and reaginic antibodies has been expressed (Hubscher and Goodfriend 1969).

The red-cell-linked antigen–antiglobulin reaction This test, in which antiserum specific to IgE is utilized, has been used to investigate allergy to aspirin, penicillin, penicillamine, insulin, and proteolytic enzymes. Other antihuman immunoglobulin sera may also be used in

order to establish the profile of antibodies belonging to various other immunoglobulin classes (IgG, IgM, IgA, and IgD) (Steele and Coombs 1964; Devey *et al.* 1970; Newhouse *et al.* 1970; Amos *et al.* 1971; Wheeler 1971; Assem and Vickers 1975). There is a vague notion that the relative proportion of these antibodies to IgE antibodies may influence the outcome of an allergic reaction by inhibiting the antigen-induced response in anaphylactic sensitization, that is, by behaving as 'blocking' antibodies and interfering with the latter reaction in a number of different ways. This is thought to have some bearing on the mechanism of action of hyposensitization therapy (Assem and McAllen 1973).

The leucocyte double-layer agglutination method This test is based on rosette formation, due to immunocytoadherence between sensitized leucocytes, particularly basophils and red blood cells coated with antigen (Fitzpatrick *et al.* 1967). The value of the leucocyte aggregation test, which is based on a somewhat similar principle, in penicillin allergy in man has been reported by Levacher *et al.* (1983).

Methods for detecting delayed-type hypersensitivity

This type of allergic reaction (Type IV in the Coombs and Gell classification [1968]), also described as cell-mediated immune response, may be detected by two main tests.

The lymphocyte transformation test

When first introduced, the lymphocyte transformation test was considered to be an *in vitro* correlate of delayed-type hypersensitivity (Coulson and Chalmers 1967). Since a positive lymphocyte transformation test may be obtained in conditions which are considered as classical examples of immediate-type allergy (Girard *et al.* 1967), this test may be made more specific for cell-mediated immunity by introducing modifications that would make it possible to assess the response of 'thymus-derived' or 'thymus-processed' lymphocytes (T lymphocytes).

This test has been applied to drug allergy by several authors (Holland and Mauer 1964; Vischer 1966; Kunz *et al.* 1967; Fellner *et al.* 1967; Denman and Denman 1968; Halpern *et al.* 1969; Assem *et al.* 1969; Assem and Vickers 1972, 1974*a,b*; Vickers and Assem 1974; Sarkany 1976).

Several important points in this technique, apart from the correlation of results with the type(s) of immunological mechanism, have been pointed out by some of the above authors.

The macrophage migration inhibition test

Again, when this test was first introduced, it was thought

to correlate with cell-mediated immunity (David *et al.* 1964*a*). It was also said to require both hapten and carrier for its expression, supporting the same notion (David *et al.* 1964*b*).

In this test, which is carried out by a variety of technical variations, a macrophage migration-inhibition factor (MIF) is generated by the incubation of sensitized lymphocytes with antigen (Dumonde *et al.* 1969). Two variations of this technique are (1) the use of isolated blood lymphocytes for incubation with antigen, followed by measurement of MIF (i.e. a two-stage procedure), and (2) the use of whole-blood leucocytes in a single-stage procedure.

It does seem at present that the initial assumptions may not be right. An example of the evidence in favour of the latter conclusion is the demonstration by Ortiz-Ortiz and others (1974) that inhibition of leucocyte migration in patients with penicillin allergy could be passively transferred by patients' sera.

Other *in vitro* tests suggested as correlates of cell-mediated immunity

Cytotoxic activity The cytotoxic activity of sensitized lymphocytes has been successfully utilized as an *in vitro* test in contact dermatitis (Deleschise and Turk 1970).

Immunocyto-adherence

When this test (a lymphocyte rosette formed between sensitized lymphocytes and antigen-coated red cells) was first introduced it was thought to correlate with cell-mediated immunity (Perrudet-Badoux and Frei 1969), but later work by Roberts and others (1971) has cast doubt on this.

Binding of labelled drugs to sensitized lymphocytes

This is another variation of the tests for demonstrating sensitized lymphocytes, which seems more likely to correlate with antibody-mediated allergy rather than cell-mediated immune reactions (Dwyer and Mackay 1970).

Methods of detecting cytotoxic antibodies

Target cells may be labelled with a suitable radioisotope, or an intracellular substance (such as an enzyme, potassium, histamine, etc) may be used as a marker to detect cell damage in the presence of specific antibody (auto-antibody) and complement. An example of the application of this technique is the detection of immunologically mediated leucopenia (Assem 1977*b*).

Detection of immune complexes

Immune complexes, representing an alternative mechanism of drug-induced immune tissue damage, may be

demonstrated by different techniques. An interesting example was reported by Williams and others (1977) who found immune complexes in the serum of one patient with serum-sickness-like syndrome and jaundice, apparently due to halothane (see Chapter 11). Metabolites of halothane were associated with these complexes.

Practical experience with important drug allergies

Penicillin allergy

Experience with penicillin RAST

In penicillin allergy, some workers (Wide and Juhlin 1970, 1971; Juhlin and Wide 1972) have used this technique to detect serum IgE antibodies against the penicilloyl groups (the main haptenic determinant formed during the degradation of penicillin), using phenoxy-methyl-penicilloyl-polylysine conjugated to an insoluble polysaccharide (Sephadex or cellulose) as an immunosorbent. More recently the range of penicillin RAST has been extended to include the penicilloyl determinant of phenoxymethylpenicillin (penicillin V), ampicillin, and amoxycillin (available from Pharmacia).

For a number of years (since 1970, see the first edition of this book), we have used the RAST procedure for the detection of penicillin allergy, after a prior study (unpublished) in allergic airways disease (allergic asthma and rhinitis, including hay fever). We used particulate conjugates of three antigenic determinants derived from benzylpenicillenate and penicillamine. This addition improved the value of RAST in penicillin allergy, as predicted from our biological test procedures, which have shown that some patients seemed to be predominantly allergic to one or both of these two minor determinants (Assem and Vickers 1975).

Despite the apparent simplicity of this test, we found that it was less reliable than some biological tests, such as antigen-induced histamine release from isolated leucocytes. Furthermore, it detects allergen-specific IgE antibodies without testing their biological activity, and does not detect other anaphylactic antibodies (e.g. particular examples are IgG_2 [Assem and Turner-Warwick 1976] and IgG_4 [Scott 1987]) that may possibly mediate immediate-type allergy, as mentioned in Part 1 of this Chapter. It should be added that antibody classes other than IgE, particularly if present in great excess, may interfere with the estimation of allergen-specific IgE antibodies in a way similar to their possible interference with the detection of IgE antibodies by passive sensitiz-ation procedures (Assem and McAllen 1973). There is another source of artefact, namely the presence of high levels of IgE in serum, which may be non-allergic-specific in general, or may be specific to an allergen other than the one in question.

Comparison of the relative value of some of the *in vitro* tests

Various authors have made limited comparisons be-tween different *in vitro* tests. Assem and Vickers (1972, 1974a,b, 1975) have reported wider comparisons.

The specific *in vitro* tests for immediate-type allergy used in our study (histamine release from leucocytes and detection of reagins by passive lung sensitization) have an established diagnostic value but are too elaborate for routine use. They are generally positive in allergy to pollen, house-dust, and other inhalant allergens. On the other hand, in penicillin allergy these tests are frequently (in about 50 per cent of cases) negative even when penicilloyl conjugates are used (see also Assem and Schild 1968) and diagnostically not superior to skin tests apart from the safety aspect. The reason for the relatively frequent negative results even in established cases of penicillin allergy is probably the choice of an inadequate antigen. When better test reagents are used (e.g. peni-cilloyl conjugates to other carrier proteins), the *in vitro* tests emerge as more sensitive and more reliable than skin tests (Vickers and Assem 1974). A more important improvement was obtained by using conjugates of hap-tenic determinants other than the penicilloyl determi-nant (Assem and Vickers 1975). Tests with β-lactamase inhibitors, such as clavulanic acid (in patients who have had reactions while receiving penicillin preparations containing these inhibitors) suggested that these sub-stances did not 'specifically' contribute to the reaction (histamine release was smaller than with the penicillin component). They also had no significant effect on histamine release by penicilloyl conjugates (excluding the possibility of using them for inhibition of reactions).

The test of histamine release from leucocytes, which detects active sensitization, has a higher incidence of positive results than the lung test, which is based on passive sensitization.

The lymphocyte stimulation test gives fewer negative results than the previously mentioned *in vitro* correlates of immediate-type allergy. This is not surprising since the allergic drug reaction of most patients is likely to be due to a combination of various immunological mechan-isms: immediate-type or Type I, delayed-type or Type IV, etc., Coombs and Gell classification 1968. Another

reason is the frequent ability of the drug itself to produce lymphocyte stimulation, while in strict correlates (tests) of immediate-type allergy the use of appropriate drug conjugates is of critical value. The ability of the drug itself to stimulate the incorporation of [³H]-thymidine by the lymphocytes of allergic patients is presumably due to the formation of conjugates in the lymphocyte culture; de Weck (1971) suggested that penicillin reacts with the membrane of cells in culture, and is presented in this way to antigen-sensitive cells.

In patients with penicillin allergy, negative results were frequently (over 60 per cent) obtained with the drug itself in tests for immediate-type allergy, but not in the lymphocyte stimulation test (less than 40 per cent). This may lead to misinterpretation (regarding type of immune mechanism) of the lymphocyte stimulation test in conditions where drug conjugates have not been used.

On the whole, the lymphocyte stimulation test offered little help in distinguishing the immunological mechan-ism involved in drug allergy in the majority of patients; it made little difference whether they had normal or raised IgE and whether they had a late reaction in the skin test or not.

Anaesthetic allergies

Anaesthetic RAST

Baldo and Fisher (1983) have used the RAST test (sepharose beads used as solid phase to which the hapten was directly conjugated) in the investigation of anaphyl-actoid reactions of patients to NMB, some of whom were shown to have 'drug-specific' IgE antibodies although there had been no previous exposure to those drugs. These findings were of particular interest, since they suggested that allergy even to such specific drugs might be induced by prior exposure to apparently remotely related chemicals or drugs.

Paper anaesthetic RAST

Paper RAST for IgE antibodies to NMB and thiopen-tone were developed by Assem (Assem and Ling 1988; Assem and Symons 1989; Assem 1989a, 1990a,b). They were evaluated by Assem (1990b), in a retrospective 18-year series of patients with 'anaphylactoid' reactions during general anaesthesia. RAST for NMB proved to be valuable and reliable, and confirmed NMB as the most common cause of the so-called anaphylactoid reac-tion during general anaesthesia. These reactions were, therefore, truly anaphylactic.

TABLE 25.4
Comparison of the results of various in vitro *tests with the response to skin testing in patients with drug allergy*

	Response to skin test				Incidence in all patients tested (per cent)
	Immediate only	Delayed only	Immediate + delayed	Negative	
No. of patients	18 (30%)	4 (7%)	11 (18%)	27 (45%)	55 (33 out of 60)
% with raised serum IgE	56	25	46	19	37 (23 out of 62)
% with positive leucocyte test	70	100	100	12	56 (20 out of 36)
% with passive lung sensitization test	50	100	93	12	46 (18 out of 39)
% with positive lymphocyte stimulation test	100	100	100	66	88 (23 out of 26)

Comparison between various tests

Paper RAST tests were valuable in the preliminary investigation of anaesthetic reactions. Both skin tests and the leucocyte histamine-release test with a wide range of drug concentrations (particularly with NMB) are required in further testing of patients with positive RAST.

The leucocyte histamine-release test, however, may give positive reactions to drugs causing release of histamine that is probably not immunologically mediated but is due to a direct action of the drug. Thus some drugs, such as morphine, may induce the release of pharmacologically active substances such as histamine without the mediation of an immunological mechanism (see review by Paton 1957).

Is there a place for 'screening' for specific IgE antibodies to anaesthetics?

The case for routine screening for anaesthetic allergies is stronger than that for penicillin allergy (penicillin skin test, see above). Certain anaesthetics are always given intravenously, and the incidence of reactions to these may be more frequent than to penicillin. Although anaphylactic anaesthetic reactions are rare according to most surveys (1/4500–1/20 000 general anaesthetics, Fisher 1975; Fisher and Baldo 1984; Vervloet 1985), they have attracted much controversy in recent years. The debate was highlighted by medicolegal arguments that followed fatal cases of anaphylaxis, of which the first was reported by Assem and Ling (1988). This patient, a 40-year-old woman, suffered cardiovascular collapse, cardiac ischaemia, and cardiac arrest during the induction of anaesthesia. A newly developed paper RAST showed a high level of IgE antibodies to the NMB given. The other two most relevant points were the absence of a history of previous anaesthesia, and manifestations that suggested the heart as the principal target of reaction. There was argument as to whether the paper RAST could be used for preoperative screening (Assem and Ling 1988; Fisher 1989; Assem 1989*b*).

The second case, which occurred in Scotland, raised more debate, because the sheriff suggested that, since a test (RAST for IgE antibodies to NMB and thiopentone) had then become available, anaesthetists 'should consider screening people coming onto their waiting lists for elective surgery at the initial consultation, particularly when the patient was female', had previously had suxamethonium as part of anaesthesia, and/or had shown signs of other allergy'. Although the debate that followed was overwhelmingly against routine screening, but not testing of patients considered at risk (Assem and Ling 1988; Brahams 1989; Noble and Yap 1989; Watkins 1989; Watkins and Milford Ward 1989; Noble 1989; Lunn 1989; Jones 1989; Fisher 1989; Assem 1989*b*), the general conclusion was that this question could not be addressed until there had been further evaluation of these tests, pilot prospective studies, full appraisal of the frequency of allergic reactions and their contribution to anaesthetic morbidity and mortality, consideration of cost and who will pay it and of 'cost-effectiveness', and careful consideration of medicolegal implications.

Comparison between skin tests and other tests in various drug allergies

A comparison was carried out between the *in vitro* tests listed in Table 25.4 and the skin (intradermal) test in 60 patients; 45 of these had penicillin allergy, and were tested both with benzylpenicillin and benzylpenicilloyl polylysine, and 15 had allergy to other drugs, which were tested with the unmodified drugs. A summary of this study (Assem and Vickers 1972) is shown in Table 25.4.

Newly developed tests to confirm an anaphylactic or anaphylactoid reaction

The aim of the tests mentioned so far is to detect drug allergy, mainly in 'cold cases'. There is another set of blood (and sometimes urine) tests that can be applied to samples collected shortly after the 'event' to confirm a reaction or to 'monitor' it, e.g. following a test dose. Sequential blood samples have to be collected, starting within minutes of the reaction, and up to 24 hours.

Plasma/serum levels of released mediators

Three mediators/markers of reaction have been developed in the past few years:

1. histamine/methylhistamine may be measured in plasma or urine (Lorenz *et al.* 1981; Keyzer *et al.* 1985; Assem and Osei 1990; Assem *et al.* 1990);
2. tryptase (Schwartz *et al.* 1989; Matsson *et al.* 1991);
3. eosinophil cationic protein (Venge *et al.* 1988; Assem *et al.* 1990).

These mediators reach peak levels in plasma/serum within one hour of an anaphylactic or anaphylactoid reaction. The first two are liberated from mast cells.

Measurement of complement components and activation products

See Watkins *et al.* (1978); Watkins (1987).

Further reading

de Weck, A.L. and Bundgaard, H. (eds) (1983). *Allergic reactions to drugs*. Springer, Heidelberg.

References

Adriani, J. (1972). Etiology and management of adverse reactions to anaesthetics. *Int. Anesthesiol. Clin.* 10, 127.

Allan, F.N. (1966). Allergic reactions to drugs. *Practitioner* 196, 788.

Amos, H.E., Lake, B.G., and Atkinson, H.A.C. (1977). Allergic drug reactions: an *in vitro* model using a mixed function oxidase complex to demonstrate antibodies with specificity for a practolol metabolite. *Clin. Allergy* 7, 423.

Amos, H.E., Wilson, D.V., Taussig, M.J., and Carlton, S.J. (1971). Hypersensitivity reactions to acetylsalicylic acid. Detection of antibodies in human sera using acetylsalicylic acid attached to proteins through the carboxyl group. *Clin.Exp. Immunol.* 8, 563.

Assem, E-S.K. (1967). Drug allergy. *Br. J. Hosp. Med.* 2, 199.

Assem, E-S.K. (1972*a*). The passive sensitization of human lung as a test for drug allergy. In *Mechanisms in drug allergy* (ed. C.H. Dash and H.E.H. Jones), p. 112. Churchill Livingstone, Edinburgh.

Assem, E-S.K. (1972*b*). IgE and other *in vitro* tests in the diagnosis and follow-up of drug allergy. In *Mechanisms in drug allergy* (ed. C.H. Dash and H.E.H. Jones), p. 179. Churchill Livingstone, Edinburgh.

Assem, E-S.K. (1977*a*). Examples of the correlation between the structure of certain groups of drugs and adverse effects mediated by immune and non-immune mechanism (with particular reference to muscle relaxants and steroid anaesthetics). In *Drug design and adverse effects* (ed. H. Bundgaard, P. Juul, and H. Kofod), p. 209. Munksgaard, Copenhagen.

Assem, E-S.K. (1977*b*). Leucocyte histamine release and lymphocyte transformation tests in drug reactions. *Bull. Soc. Catalana Pediatr.* 37, 183.

Assem, E-S.K. (1983*a*). Reactions to local and general anaesthetics. In *Allergic reactions to drugs, Handbook of experimental pharmacology*, Vol. 63 (ed. A.L. de Weck and H. Bundgaard), p 259. Springer, Heidelberg.

Assem, E-S.K. (1983*b*). Reactions to neuromuscular blockers. In *Allergic reactions to drugs, Handbook of experimental pharmacology*, Vol. 63 (ed. A.L. de Weck and H. Bundgaard), p. 299. Springer, Heidelberg.

Assem E-S.K. (1984*a*). Allergic reactions during anaesthesia: methods of detection. In *Anaesthesia Review 2* (ed. L. Kaufman), p. 49. Churchill Livingstone, Edinburgh.

Assem, E-S.K. (1984*b*). Diagnostic and predictive test procedures in patients with life-threatening anaphylactic and anaphylactoid drug reactions. *Allergol. Immunopathol.* (Madr.) 12, 61.

Assem, E-S.K. (1984*c*). Characteristics of basophil histamine release by neuromuscular blocking drugs in patients with anaphylactoid reactions. *Agents Actions* 14, 435.

Assem, E-S.K. (1989*a*). Drug allergy. *Curr. Opin. Immunol.* 1, 660.

Assem, E-S.K. (1989*b*). Anaphylaxis. *Anaesthesia* 44, 517.

Assem, E-S.K. (1990*a*). Naturally occurring IgG-antibody-like substance reacting with quaternary ammonium groups and neuromuscular blockers: a common finding in humans and other species. *Int. Arch. Allergy Appl. Immunol.* 91, 426.

Assem, E-S.K. (1990*b*). Anaphylactic anaesthetic reactions: value of paper radioallergosorbent tests for IgE antibodies to muscle relaxants and thiopentone. *Anaesthesia* 45, 1032.

Assem, E-S.K. (1991). *In vivo* and *in vitro* tests in anaphylactic reactions to anaesthetic agents. *Agents Actions* 33, 208.

Assem E-S.K. and Atallah, N.A. (1981). Increased release of histamine by anit-IgE from leucocytes of asthmatic patients and possibly heterogeneity of IgE. Clin. Allergy 11, 367.

Assem, E-S.K and Banks, R. (1973). Practolol-induced drug eruption. *Proc. R. Soc. Med.* 66, 179.

Assem, E-S.K. and Ling, B.Y. (1988). Fatal anaphylactic reaction to suxamethonium: new screening test suggests possible prevention. *Anaesthesia* 43, 958.

Assem, E-S.K. and McAllen, M.K. (1970). Serum reagins and leucocyte response in patients with house-dust mite allergy. *Br. Med. J.* ii, 504.

Assem, E-S.K. and McAllen, M.K. (1973). Changes in challenge tests following hyposensitization with mite extract. *Clin. Allergy* 3, 161.

Assem, E-S.K. and Moorthy, A.P. (1988). Allergy to local anaesthetics: an approach to definitive diagnosis. *Br. Dent. J.* 164, 44.

Assem, E-S.K. and Osei, D. (1990). A modified assay for the detection of histamine release *in vivo* and *in vitro* in man. *Agents Actions* 30, 287.

Assem, E-S.K. and Schild, H.O. (1968). Detection of allergy to penicillin and other antigens by *in vitro* passive sensitization and histamine release from human and monkey lung. *Br. Med. J.* iii, 272.

Assem, E-S.K. and Symons, I.E. (1989). Anaphylaxis due to suxamethonium in a 7-year old child: a 14-year follow-up with allergy testing. *Anaesthesia* 44, 121.

Assem, E-S.K. and Turner-Warwick, M. (1976). Cytophilic antibodies in bronchopulmonary aspergillosis, aspergilloma and cryptogenic pulmonary eosinophilia. *Clin. Exp. Immunol.* 26, 67.

Assem, E-S.K. and Vickers, M.R. (1972). Serum IgE and other *in vitro* tests in drug allergy. *Clin. Allergy* 2, 325.

Assem, E-S.K. and Vickers, M.R. (1974a). Immunological response to penicillamine in penicillin-allergic patients and normal subjects. *Postgrad. Med. J.* 50, 65.

Assem, E-S.K. and Vickers, M.R. (1974b). Tests for penicillin allergy in man. II. The immunological cross-reaction between penicillins and cephalosporins. *Immunology* 27, 255.

Assem, E-S.K. and Vickers, M.R. (1975). Investigation of the response to some haptenic determination in penicillin allergy in man. *Clin. Allergy* 5, 43.

Assem, E-S.K., Ndoping, N., Nicholson, H., and Wade, J.R. (1969). Case report. Liver damage and isoniazid allergy. *Clin. Exp. Immunol.* 5, 439.

Assem, E-S.K., Bray, J., and Dawson, P. (1983). The release of histamine from basophils by radiological contrast agents. *Br. J. Radiol.* 56, 647.

Assem, E-S.K., Gelder, C.M., Spiro, S.G., Baderman,H., and Armstrong, F.R. (1990). Anaphylaxis induced by peanuts. *Br. Med. J.* 300, 1377.

Baldo, B.A. and Fisher, M.McD. (1983). Detection of serum IgE antibodies that react with alcuronium and tubocurarine after life-threatening reactions to muscle relaxant drugs. *Anaesth. Intens. Care* 11, 194.

Batchelor, J.R., Dewdney, J.M., Feinberg, J.G., and Weston, R.D. (1967). A penicilloylated protein impurity as a source of allergy to benzylpenicillin and 6-amino-penicillanic acid. *Lancet* i, 1175.

Berger, A.J. and Eisen, B. (1955). Feasibility of skin testing for penicillin sensitivity. *JAMA* 159, 191.

Bierman, C.W. and van Arsdel, P.P. Jr (1969). Penicillin allergy in children: the role of immunological tests in its diagnosis. *J. Allergy* 43, 267.

Brahams, D. (1989). Fatal reaction to suxamethonium: case for screening by radioallergosorbent test? *Lancet* i, 1400.

British Medical Journal (1964). Testing sensitivity to penicillin. *Br. Med J.* i, 1329.

British Medical Journal (1968). Allergy testing. *Br. Med. J.* iii, 262.

Butler, V.P. (1978). The immunological assay of drugs. *Pharm. Rev.* 29, 103.

Canadian Medical Association Journal (1967). Prevention of penicillin anaphylaxis. *Can. Med. Assoc. J.* 97, 128.

Caspary, E.A. and Comaish, J.S. (1967). Release of serotonin from human platelets in hypersensitivity states. *Nature* 214, 286.

Coombs, R.R.A. and Gell, P.G.H. (1968). Classification of allergic reactions responsible for clinical hypersensitivity and disease. In *Clinical aspects of immunology* (2nd edn) (ed. P.G.H. Gell and R.R.A. Coombs), p. 575. Blackwell, Oxford.

Coulson, A.S. and Chalmers, D.G. (1967). Response of human blood lymphocytes to tuberculin PPD in tissue culture. *Immunology* 12, 417.

David, J.R., Al-Askari, S., Lawrence, H.S., and Thomas, L. (1964a). Delayed hypersensitivity *in vitro*. The specificity of inhibition of cell migration by antigens. *J. Immunol.* 93, 264.

David, J.R., Lawrence, H.S., and Thomas, L. (1964b). Delayed hypersensitivity *in vitro* III. The specificity of hapten-protein conjugates in the inhibition of cells migration. *J. Immunol.* 93, 279.

Deleschise, J. and Turk, J.L. (1970). Lymphocyte cytotoxicity: a possible *in vitro* test for contact dermatitis. *Lancet* ii, 75.

Denman, E.J. and Denman, A.M. (1968). The lymphocyte transformation test and gold hypersensitivity. *Ann. Rheum. Dis.* 27, 582.

Devey, M., Sanderson, C.J., Carter, D., and Coombs, R.R.A. (1970). IgD antibody to insulin. *Lancet* ii, 1280.

de Weck, A.L. (1971). Immunochemical mechanisms of hypersensitivity to antibiotics, solution to the penicillin allergy problem. In *New concepts in allergy and clinical immunology* (ed. U. Serafini, A.W. Frankland, C. Masala, and J.M. Jamar), p. 208. Excerpta Medica, Amsterdam.

de Weck, A.L., Schneider, C.G., and Guthersohn, J. (1968). The role of penicilloylated protein impurities, penicillin polymers and dimers in penicillin allergy. *Int. Arch. Allergy* 33, 535.

Didier, A., Cador, D., Bongrand, P., Furtoss, R., Fourneron, P., Senft, M. *et al.* (1987). Role of the quaternary ammonium ion determinant in allergy to muscle relaxants. *J. Allergy Clin. Immunol.* 79, 578.

Dogliotti, M. (1968). An instance of fatal reaction to the penicillin scratch test. *Dermatologica* 136, 489.

Driagin, G.B. (1966). Anaphylactic shock with fatal outcome following an intradermal test for sensitivity to penicillin. *Terarkh* 38, 118.

Dumonde, D.C., Wolstencroft, R.A., Panayi, G.A., Matthew, N., Morely, J., and Howson, W.T. (1969). Lymphokines:

non-antibody mediators of cellular immunity generated by lymphocyte activation. *Nature* 224, 38.

Dwyer, J.M. and MacKay, I.R. (1970). Antigen-binding lymphocytes in human blood. *Lancet* i, 164.

Eravelly, J. (1974). Skin tests for penicillin allergy. *Malay Med. Assoc. Newsletter* 6, 1.

Ettinger, E. and Kaye, D. (1964). Systemic manifestations after a skin test with penicilloyl-polylysine. *N. Engl. J. Med.* 271, 1105.

Farrell, A.M., Gowland, G., McDowell, J.M., Simpson, K.H., and Watkins, J. (1988). Anaphylactoid reaction to vecuronium followed by systemic reaction to skin testing. *Anaesthesia* 43, 207.

Fellner, M.J., Baer, F.L., Ripps, C.S., and Hirschhorn, K. (1967). Response lymphocytes to penicillin: comparison with skin tests and circulating antibodies in man. *Nature* 216, 803.

Finke, S.R., Grieco, M.H., Connell, J.T., Smith, E.C., and Sherman, W.B. (1965). Results of comparative skin test with penicilloyl-polylysine and penicillin in patients with penicillin allergy. *Am. J. Med.* 38, 71.

Fisher, M.McD. (1975). Severe histamine-mediated reactions to intravenous drugs used in anaesthesia. *Anaesth. Intens. Care* 3, 180.

Fisher, M.McD. (1989). Anaphylaxis. *Anaesthesia* 44, 516.

Fisher, M.M. and Baldo, B.A. (1984). Anaphylactoid reactions during anaesthesia. *Clin. Anaesthesiol.* 2, 677.

Fitzpatrick, M.E., Connolly, R.C., Lea, D.J., O'Sullivan, S.A., Augustin, R., and MacCaulay, M.B. (1967). *In vitro* detection of human reagins by double-layer leucocyte agglutination: method and controlled blind study. *Immunology* 12, 1.

Girard, J.P., Rose, N.R., Kunz, M.L., Kobayashi, S., and Arbesman, E.C. (1967). *In vitro* lymphocyte transformation in atopic patients: induced by antigens. *J. Allergy* 39, 65.

Green, G.R. and Rosenblum, A. (1971). Report of the penicillin study group American Academy of Allergy. *J. Allergy Clin. Immunol.* 48, 331.

Halpern, B., Ky, N.T., and Amache, N. (1969). *In vitro* lymphoblast transformation test (L.T.T.) as a tool for the study of drug hypersensitivity. In *Proceedings of the European Society for the Study of Drug Toxicity*, Vol.10, p. 27. Excerpta Medica, Amsterdam.

Harle, D.G., Baldo, B.A., and Fisher, M.M. (1984). Detection of IgE antibodies to suxamethonium after anaphylactoid reactions during anaesthesia. *Lancet* i, 930.

Harle, D.G., Baldo, B.A., Smal, M.A., Wajon, P., and Fisher, M.M. (1986). Detection of thiopentone-reactive IgE antibodies following anaphylactoid reactions during anaesthesia. *Clin. Allergy* 16, 493.

Harle, D.G., Baldo, B.A., and Wells, J.V. (1988). Drugs as allergens: detection and combining site specificities of IgE antibodies to sulphamethoxazole. *Molecular Immunol.* 25, 1347.

Hirshman, C.A., Peters, J., and Cartwright-Lee, I. (1982). Leukocyte histamine release to thiopental. *Anesthesiology* 56, 64.

Holland, P. and Mauer, A.M. (1964). Drug-induced *in vitro* stimulation of peripheral lymphocytes. *Lancet* i, 1368.

Horne, G.O. (1973). The implications of fatal penicillin anaphylactic reaction. *Singapore Med. J.* 14, 467.

Hubscher, T. and Goodfriend, L. (1969). Role of human reaginic and hemagglutinating antibodies in the indirect rabbit basophil degranulation reaction. *Int. Arch. Allergy* 35, 298.

Idsøe, O., Guthe, T., Willcox, R.P., and de Weck, A.L. (1968). Nature and extent of penicillin side reactions, with particular reference to fatalities from anaphylactic shock. *Bull. WHO* 38, 159.

Jarisch, R., Roth, A., Boltz, A., and Sandor, A. (1981). Diagnosis of penicillin allergy by means of Phadebas RAST penicilloyl G and V and skin tests. *Clin. Allergy* 11, 155.

Jones, C.S. (1989). RAST screening for antibodies to anaesthetics. *Lancet* ii, 381.

Juhlin, L. and Wide, L. (1972). IgE antibodies and penicillin allergy. In *Mechanisms in drug allergy* (ed. C.H. Dash and H.E.H. Jones), p. 139. Churchill Livingstone, Edinburgh.

Katz, H.I., Gill, K.A., Baxter, D.L., and Mischella, S.L. (1964). Indirect basophil degranulation test in penicillin allergy. *JAMA* 188, 351.

Keyzer, J.J., Breukelman, H., Wolthers, B.G., Richardson, F.J., and DeMonchy, J.G.R. (1985). Measurement of *N*-methylhistamine concentrations in plasma and urine during anaphylactoid reactions. *Agents Actions* 16, 76.

Knudsen, E.T., Robinson, O.P.W., Croydon, E.A., and Tees, E.C. (1967). Cutaneous sensitivity to purified benzylpenicillin. *Lancet* i, 1184.

Kunz, M.L., Reisman, R.E., and Arbesman, C.E. (1967). Evaluation of penicillin hypersensitivity by two newer immunological procedures. *J. Allergy* 40, 135.

Levacher, M., Rouveix, B., and Badenoch-Jones, P. (1983). Diagnosis of penicillin-allergy — an evaluation of the leucocyte aggregation test in man. *Clin. Allergy* 13, 21.

Levine, B.B. (1962). *N*(alpha-*D*-penicilloyl) amines as univalent hapten inhibitors of antibody dependent allergic reactions to penicillin. *J. Med. Pharm. Chem.* 5, 1025.

Levine, B.B. (1963). Studies on the dimensions of the rabbit antibenzyl-penicilloyl antibody combining sites. *J. Exp. Med.* 177, 161.

Levine, B.B. (1964). Studies on the immunological mechanisms of penicillin allergy. I. Antigenic specificities of guinea-pig skin sensitizing rabbit antibenzylpenicillin antibodies. *Immunology* 7, 527.

Levine, B.B. and Price, V.H. (1964). Studies on the immunological mechanisms of penicillin allergy. II. Antigenic specificities of allergic wheal-and-flare skin responses in patients with histories of penicillin allergy. *Immunology* 7, 542.

Levine, B.B. and Zolov, D.M. (1969). Prediction of penicillin allergy by immunological tests. *J. Allergy* 43, 231.

Levine, B.B., Redmond, A.P., Fellner, M., Voss, H.E., and Levytska, V. (1966). Penicillin allergy and the heterogenous immune responses of man to benzylpenicillin. *J. Clin. Invest.* 45, 1895.

Levine, B.B., Redmond, A.P., Voss, H.E., and Zolov, D.M. (1967). Prediction of penicillin allergy by immunological tests. *Ann. N.Y. Acad Sci.* 145, 298.

Lichtenstein, L.M. and Osler, A.G. (1964). Studies on the mechanism of hypersensitivity phenomena. IX. Histamine release from human leukocytes by ragweed pollen antigen. *J. Exp. Med.* 120, 507.

Lorenz, W., Doenicke, A., Schoning, B., and Neugebaur, E. (1981). The role of histamine in adverse reactions to intravenous agents. In *Adverse reactions of anaesthetic drugs* (ed. J. A. Thornton), p. 169. Elsevier, Amsterdam.

Lunn, J.N. (1989). RAST screening for antibodies to anaesthetics. *Lancet* ii, 381.

Matsson, P., Enander, I., Shaw, M., Andersson, A-S., Nystrand, J., Schwartz, L., *et al.* (1991). Mast cell activation analysis by an immunodiagnostic assay for tryptase. *Agents Actions.* (In press.)

McAllen, M., Heaf, P.J.D., and Mcinroy, P. (1967). Depot grass pollen injections in asthma: effect of repeated treatment on clinical response and measured bronchial sensitivity. *Br. Med. J.* i, 22.

Moneret-Vautrin, D.A., Gueant, J.L., Kamel, L., Laxenaire, M.C., El Kholty, S., and Nicholas, J.P. (1988). Anaphylaxis to myorelaxants: cross-sensitivity studied by radio-immunoassays compared to intradermal tests in 34 cases. *J. Allergy Clin. Immunol.* 82, 745.

Newhouse, M.L., Tagg, B., Pocock, S.J., and McEwan, A.C. (1970). An epidemiological study of workers producing enzyme washing powders. *Lancet* i, 689.

Noble, D.W. (1989). RAST screening for antibodies to anaesthetics. *Lancet* ii, 381.

Noble, D.W. and Yap, P.L. (1989). Screening for antibodies to anaesthetics. *Br. Med. J.* 299, 2.

Ortiz-Ortiz, L., Zamacona, G., Garmilla, C., and Arellano, M.T. (1974). Migration inhibition test on leucocytes from patients allergic to penicillin. *J. Immunol.* 113, 993.

Parker, C.W. (1972). Practical aspects of diagnosis and treatment of patients who are hypersensitive to drugs. In *Hypersensitivity to drugs*, Vol. 1 (ed. M. Samter and C.W. Parker), p. 367. Pergamon, Oxford.

Paton, W.D.M. (1957). Histamine release by compounds of simple chemical structure. *Pharmacol. Rev.* 9, 269.

Perelmutter, L., Liakopoulou, A., and Larose, C. (1970). Detection of human IgE-type reagins utilising rat mast cells. *J. Allergy* 45, 126.

Perrudet-Badoux, A. and Frei, P.C. (1969). On the mechanism of 'rosette' formation in human and experimental thyroiditis. *Clin. Exp. Immunol.* 5, 117.

Plautt, M., Lichtenstein, L.M., and Bloch, K.J. (1973). Failure to obtain histamine release from rat mast cells exposed to human allergic serum and specific antigen or IgE myeloma protein and anti-IgE. *J. Immunol.* 111, 1022.

Pullen, H., Wright, N., and Murdoch, J.McC. (1967). Hypersensitivity reactions to antibacterial drugs in infectious mononucleosis. *Lancet* ii, 1176.

Resnik, S.S. and Shelley, W.B. (1966). Penicilloyl-polylysine skin test: anaphylaxis in absence of penicillin sensitivity. *JAMA* 196, 740.

Roberts, C.I., Brandriss, M.W., and Vaughan, J.H. (1971). Failure of immunocytoadherence to demonstrate delayed hypersensitivity. *J. Immunol.* 106, 1056.

Rose, B. (1953). Allergic reactions to penicillin: a panel discussion *J. Allergy* 24, 383.

Sarkany, I. (1967). Lymphocyte transformation in drug hypersensitivity. *Lancet* i, 743.

Schwartz, L.B., Yunginger, J.W., Miller, J., Bokhari, R., and Dull, D. (1989). Time course of appearance and disappearance of human mast cell tryptase in the circulation after anaphylaxis. *J. Clin. Invest.* 83, 1551.

Scott, J.R. (1987). A review of *in-vitro* assays for IgG and IgG$_4$ antibodies: concept and potential applications. *N. Engl. Reg. Allergy Proc.* 385.

Shelley, W.B. (1961). New serological test for allergy in man. *Nature* 195, 1181.

Shelley, W.B. and Juhlin, L. (1962). A new test for detecting anaphylactic sensitivity. *Nature* 191, 1056.

Siegel, B.B. and Levine, B.B. (1965). Antigenic specificities of skin sensitizing antibodies in patients with immediate systemic allergic reactions to penicillin. *J. Allergy* 36, 488.

Smal, M.A., Baldo, B.A. and Harle, D.G. (1988). Drugs as allergens: the molecular basis of IgE binding to trimethoprim. *Allergy* 43,184.

Stanworth, D.R. (ed.) (1973). Molecular basis of the allergic response. In *Immediate hypersensitivity*, p. 212. North-Holland, Amsterdam.

Steele, A.V.S. and Coombs, R.R.A. (1964). The red cell linked antigen test for incomplete antibodies to soluble proteins. *Int. Arch. Allergy* 28, 11.

Stewart, G.T. (1967). Allergenic residues in penicillin. *Lancet* ii, 1177.

Sullivan, T.J., Wedner, H.J., Shatz, G.S., Yecies, L.D., and Parker, C.W. (1981). Skin testing to detect penicillin allergy. *J. Allergy Clin. Immunol.* 68, 171.

Thompson, R.A. and Bird, I.G. (1983). How necessary are specific IgE antibody tests in asthma? *Lancet* i, 169.

Venge, R., Dahl, R., and Peterson, C.G.B. (1988). Eosinophil granule proteins in serum after allergen challenge of asthmatic patients and the effects of anti-asthmatic medication. *Int. Arch. Allergy Appl. Immun.* 87, 306.

Vervloet, D. (1985). Allergy to muscle relaxants and related compounds. *Clin. Allergy* 15, 501.

Vickers, M.R. and Assem, E-S.K. (1974). Tests for penicillin allergy in man. I. Carrier effect on response to penicilloyl conjugates. *Immunology* 26, 425.

Vischer, T.L. (1966). Lymphocyte cultures in drug hypersensitivity. *Lancet* ii, 467.

Voller, A., Bidwell, D.E., Barlett, A., Fleck, D.G., Perkins, M., and Oladehin, B. (1976). A microplate enzyme immunoassay for toxoplasma antibody. *J. Clin. Pathol.* 29, 150.

Watkins, J. (1987). Investigation of allergic and hypersensitivity reactions to anaesthetic agents. *Br. J. Anaesth.* 59, 104.

Watkins, J. (1989). Suxamethonium anaphylaxis. *Lancet* ii, 171.

Watkins, J. and Milford Ward, A. (1989). Screening for antibodies to anaesthetics. *Br. Med. J.* 299, 326.

Watkins, J., Udnoon, S., and Tausig, P.E. (1978). Mechanisms of adverse response to intravenous agents in man. In *Adverse response to intravenous drugs* (ed. J. Watkins and A.M. Ward), p. 71. Academic Press, London.

Wheeler, A.W. (1971). A method for measuring different classes of immunoglobulins specific for the penicilloyl group. *Immunology* 21, 547.

Wide, L. and Juhlin, L. (1970). *In vitro* method for detecting penicillin allergy of immediate type. In *Abstracts: VII International Congress of Allergology, Florence*, p. 110. Excerpta Medica, Amsterdam.

Wide, L. and Juhlin, L. (1971). Detection of penicillin allergy of immediate type by radioimmunoassay of reagins (IgE) to penicilloyl conjugates. *Clin. Allergy* 1, 171.

Wide, L., Bennich, H., and Johansson, S.G.O. (1967). Diagnosis of allergy by an *in vitro* test for allergen antibodies. *Lancet* ii, 1105.

Wiles, C.M., Assem, E-S.K., Cohen, S.L., and Fisher, C. (1979). Cephradine-induced interstitial nephritis. *Clin. Exp. Immunol.* 36, 342.

Williams, B.D., White, N., Amlot, P.L., Slaney, J., and Toseland, P.A. (1977). Circulating immune complexes after repeated halothane anaesthesia. *Br Med. J.* ii, 159.

Wirth, L. (1963). On anaphylactic shock due to penicillin. *Milit Med.* 128, 245.

26. Systemic toxicity of topical antiseptics

J. F. DUNNE

Compounds in common use

Fifty years after the discovery of antibiotics the need for non-selective germicides capable of killing living cells on contact is as great as ever. Whereas less reliance is now placed upon them as antiseptics in the treatment of infective skin lesions they are still routinely needed for presurgical skin preparation, and they remain ubiquitous in the home not only in topical antiseptic preparations but also as preservatives in toiletries, cosmetics, household cleaning products and, in very small quantities, in orally administered pharmaceutical products and some processed foods. They are also vital as disinfectants whenever a risk of cross-infection with dangerous pathogens, including human immunodeficiency virus, hepatitis B virus, mycobacteria, cytomegalovirus, and human papillomavirus, creates a need for rigorous decontamination procedures.

A wide range of germicidal substances has been used for these purposes, preservatives being particularly numerous. Those most commonly used as antiseptics and disinfectants are alcohols, ampholytic and cationic surfactants, chlorhexidine salts, dyes, chlorinated compounds, formaldehyde and glutaraldehyde, hydrogen peroxide, iodine, mercurials, and phenols. Some of these substances, particularly the dyes, are bacteriostatic rather than bactericidal and are limited in their spectrum of activity. Others, including formaldehyde, glutaraldehyde and the less refined phenols, are highly effective germicides but too corrosive to be applied directly to skin or mucosal surfaces. Yet others are potent sensitizers and a few, although apparently innocuous to the skin, are significantly absorbed and have demonstrable systemic toxicity. Little attention was paid to the possibility of transdermal absorption of antiseptics until the early 1970s, when it was discovered that hexachlorophane, one of the most widely used of a new generation of locally non-irritant substances, was both extensively absorbed and potentially neurotoxic. This was a misjudgement that is unlikely to be repeated. Transdermal absorption has become accepted as a simple and relatively efficient means of sustaining plasma concentrations of glyceryl trinitrate and some other drugs with an evanescent action, and it may ultimately provide a practicable means for administering others that are largely metabolised during the first pass through the liver (Corbo et al. 1990).

Many of the antiseptics that are still widely used, including the simpler derivatives of phenol, such as cresols and resorcinol, precipitate proteins. More complex derivatives such as the halogenated biphenols, which include hexachlorophane, are less irritant and have more selective antibacterial activity. Highly ionized salts of mercury, silver, and zinc also precipitate proteins; in the case of mercury, this is presumably due to the affinity of the metallic ion for sulphydryl groups. The weakly ionized organic mercurials and colloidal silver salts are less irritant to the tissues and are bacteriostatic rather than bactericidal in nature.

Many of the traditional and still widely used antiseptics share a basic common mechanism of action. Chlorine-containing compounds, including hypochlorites and chloramines, probably act as result of oxidation of hypochlorous acid. All iodine-containing preparations, including the iodophores, seem to be dependent on the release of elemental iodine, but the mechanism of action remains unclear. Other acidic compounds such as boric acid and benzoic acid also presumably act in part through a hydrogen-ion effect, but the potent bacteriostatic activity of their salts, including sodium borate and aliphatic esters of parahydroxybenzoic acid, indicates that the anionic configuration is also important.

Other compounds exert a more specific, and consequently more selective, germicidal effect. Acridine and rosaniline dyes, which are most efficient in alkaline media and bactericidal only against Gram-positive organisms are presumed to act on the cellular functions that underlie the differential staining properties. Cationic surface-active agents are presumed to act by altering the permeability of the bacterial cell membrane but, unexpectedly, this effect does not correlate closely with their bactericidal action. The bactericidal action of some other types of compounds, such as the furans, is often attenuated by the emergence of resistant strains. This, together with their characteristic selectivity of action, suggests that they act by interfering with enzymatic processes regulating bacterial growth.

Efficacy

The ideal germicide should be effective against all microbial forms, including yeasts and fungi, as well as bacteria. In general Gram-positive forms are more vulnerable, while spores are more resistant than vegetative forms. Exceptions are common, however, and some organisms show striking resistance to specific compounds. Solutions of cetrimide can become contaminated with *Pseudomonas* spp. (Lee and Fialkow 1961), while soaps and handcreams containing hexachlorophane can become contaminated with Gram-negative organisms (Ayliffe *et al*. 1969). The halogens hold advantage in that they exert a wide-ranging bactericidal action even in high dilution. For this reason, the British Medical Association's code of practice for control of cross infection recommends the use of hypochlorite solution, 10 000 ppm, to disinfect spillages of body fluids (British Medical Association 1989).

In most instances, however, *in vitro* performance gives an unduly favourable impression of therapeutic potential. Pus, serum, and organic debris greatly reduce the efficacy of most germicides. This commonly results from poor penetration, as is the case with products containing either the highly polar cationic surfactants or substances with an evanescent action, such as the peroxides and chlorine-containing compounds. In other instances, more specific factors are of importance. The activity of cationic surfactants, for example, is reduced by soaps. In the last analysis, efficacy needs to be established by bacteriological evidence obtained within clinical trials. Using this criterion, the United States Food and Drug Administration concluded in 1974 that only 19 of several hundred germicidal compounds then available had demonstrable antiseptic activity and that, of these, only five — tincture of iodine, hexylresorcinol, and three cationic surfactants — were safe and effective in clinical use.

Local reactions

Tissue damage

Many of the long-established antiseptics, including cresols, resorcinol, and other simple derivatives of phenol, form complexes with protein and penetrate deeply into tissue. This is an advantage in cauterizing animal bites, for which a 5% solution of phenol is still recommended. These preparations can, however, cause extensive necrosis even on intact skin, and accidental spillage should be treated immediately by thorough swabbing, preferably with glycerine or alcohol, or with water. Several cases of laryngeal oedema, one of which was fatal, have recently been attributed to a throat spray containing 1.4% phenol (Committee on Safety of Medicines 1990).

Iodine, the rapidly degraded chlorine-containing compounds, and the cationic surfactants usually cause only superficial damage, although most can traumatize intact skin when occlusive dressings are applied. Weak solutions of cetrimide seem particularly safe in this respect, since they are widely used with apparent safety as a diaper soak.

Of particular concern are compounds that readily penetrate intact skin without causing local irritation. At first, the absorption of hexachlorophane into the dermis was regarded as advantageous when a sustained antiseptic effect was needed, for example, to prevent umbilical sepsis in neonates or to eliminate pyogenic staphylococci among the health workers who cared for them (Shemano and Nickerson 1954). Such use was immediately contraindicated when hexachlorophane was shown to have potent neurotoxic properties. Excessive use of otherwise safe antiseptics during surgery can also have serious effects. The use of chlorhexidine, which is highly neurotoxic, as a preoperative skin disinfectant in aural surgery has resulted in nerve deafness (Bicknell 1971), and a fatal case of fulminating allergic serositis has been described after use of povidone iodine to sterilize the peritoneal cavity during closure of a colostomy (WMCADRR 1988).

Sensitization

Virtually all topical antiseptics have been implicated as sensitizing agents, although some induce allergic reactions much more frequently than do others. Contact dermatoses, generalized erythematous rashes, and photosensitivity have each been associated with commonly used compounds, and a large proportion of these reactions result from the repeated application of germicides in toiletries and cosmetics. Previously bithionol and subsequently hydroxybenzoates were widely used in this context, but both were largely superseded when patch testing showed them to be frequently implicated in cases of allergic contact dermatitis (Schorr and Mohajerin 1966; Epstein 1966; Schorr 1968;). Ten years ago a new preservative system — methylchloroisothiazolinone plus methylisothiazolinone (or kathon) — gained wide acceptance as a preservative. Unfortunately, however, history has seemingly been repeated. The prevalence of sensitization has been estimated to be about 1 per cent in North America and Britain, but elsewhere in Europe rates in excess of 8 per cent have been recorded (de Groot and Herxheimer 1990). In Holland, kathon has been implicated as the causative agent in over one quarter of a series of 119 patients with proven cosmetic-related allergic contact dermatitis (de Groot *et al.* 1988). Compulsory labelling of all ingredients in cosmetics and toiletries, which was introduced in the USA 10 years ago, could do much to reduce the scale of the problem.

None of the products that is widely used in skin preparations is entirely free from sensitizing potential. Iodine frequently induces erythematous rashes, and a systemic reaction with fever occasionally occurs. Contact dermatitis is also occasionally seen following the application of chlorhexidine (Restell 1965) and cetrimide (Morgan 1968). Exceptionally, the reported reactions have been severe. Severe shock has been associated with the use of 1% cetrimide solution as a preoperative skin preparation (Sharvill 1965), while fatal exfoliative dermatitis has been attributed to topical application of iodine (Seymour 1937). Povidone–iodine — which is a complex of iodine with polyvinylpyrrolidone — has rarely, however, been associated with sensitization reactions in patients with a normal immune status (Feldtman *et al.* 1979).

Sensitizing potential is not related to irritant capacity. Noxythiolin and polynoxylin, which act by slowly releasing formaldehyde, have a relatively low sensitizing potential. Nitrofurazone, in contrast, once used in skin grafting because of its negligible irritant effect, was estimated to cause sensitization in up to 6 per cent of patients treated for more than a few days (Downing and Brecker 1948).

Photosensitivity can be a serious consequence of exposure to germicidal agents. In its most severe form it may be disabling for many months and, once sensitized, patients are at risk of developing generalized dermatitis on re-exposure. More frequently, however, it results only in transient contact dermatitis on areas of skin exposed to light. Soaps and cosmetics containing either bithionol (Kinmont 1969) or bromsalans (Ison and Tucker 1968) have been withdrawn from use in many countries on these grounds (US Department of Health 1974).

Systemic reactions

Results of ingestion

Some germicides with particularly low systemic toxicity are used as orally administered urinary antiseptics. These include methenamine, which gradually releases formaldehyde in acidic solution; mandelic acid; nalidixic acid; and the furan derivative nitrofurantoin. Because of their greater propensity to induce sensitivity reactions, the last two are normally reserved for treatment of refractory infections.

Several germicides have been administered orally to treat intestinal infections. Hexylresorcinol, in particular, was once considered to be of value in the treatment of hookworm and ascariasis. In general, however, germicides are irritant to the gastrointestinal tract and many of the longer established substances are dangerously corrosive. Simple derivatives of phenol cause intense pain and vomiting when they are swallowed. Shock, pulmonary oedema, and respiratory failure supervene in potentially fatal cases. Cautious gastric lavage and aspiration using olive oil is of value if undertaken shortly after ingestion. In severe cases narcotic analgesics, maintenance of respiration and fluid balance, parenteral steroids, and broad-spectrum antibiotics offer the only hope of survival. Peritoneal dialysis may be necessary to prevent a precipitate rise in serum potassium concentrations (Thomas 1969).

Formaldehyde, which is also highly corrosive, is metabolised to formic acid. Intense acidosis, which rapidly induces cardiac and renal failure, requires infusion of sodium bicarbonate. Haemodialysis is claimed to be of value.

Iodine is less corrosive, partly because it forms complexes with partially digested starch and proteins. Large doses of the tincture, however, cause vomiting and bloody diarrhoea, and death has occasionally resulted from circulatory collapse. Lavage with starch solution or milk is useful in the early stages. Otherwise, treatment is symptomatic.

Surface-active quaternary compounds cause paralysis by depolarizing cholinergic neuromuscular junctions. Supportive treatment with artificial respiration and anti convulsant therapy has been successful (Arena 1964).

Results of percutaneous absorption

Percutaneous absorption of corrosive antiseptics such as phenol and formaldehyde can produce dangerous acute systemic toxicity. Other substances, notably mercury salts, cause insidious poisoning as a consequence of systemic accumulation. This now commonly results from the sustained use of 'skin-lightening' preparations by women in sub-Saharan Africa and the Caribbean. These are illicitly traded preparations that contain either mercury salts or hydroquinone. Regular use of soaps containing aminomercuric chloride frequently results in contact dermatitis, and cases of nephrotic syndrome due to membranous nephropathy have been described (Barr *et al*. 1972; Kibukamusoke *et al*. 1974). Other signs of systemic poisoning ascribed to this abuse include chronic gingivitis, erythroderma, purpura, conjunctivitis, neuritis, aplastic anaemia, and personality changes (Kasilo and Yetunde 1990).

Susceptibility of neonates and infants

Neonates and infants are particularly vulnerable to poisoning from percutaneous absorption of toxic substances. Their surface area is relatively large in proportion to their mass, and their skin, particularly when occluded by diapers, is highly absorptive. Borax and boric acid preparations have long been recognized as dangerous in the treatment of diaper rash. Although not locally irritant, they have been implicated in several cases of fatal poisoning when used in this way (Goldbloom and Goldbloom 1953; Maxson 1954; Valdes-Dapena and Arey 1962; Skipworth *et al*. 1967). The initial clinical signs were of gastrointestinal irritation, followed by diffuse erythema and later by desquamation of the skin. Signs of meningeal irritation, oliguria, and circulatory collapse were usually followed by death within 5 days, and widespread haemorrhagic effusions were apparent at autopsy. Management was directed primarily to maintaining fluid and electrolyte balance, and successful use of exchange transfusion and peritoneal dialysis has been reported (Segar 1960; Wong *et al*. 1964; Baliah *et al*. 1969).

Among other illustrations of the susceptibility of infants to otherwise acceptably safe germicides are cases of extensive haemolysis induced by use of preparations containing picric acid to treat extensive burns, and an outbreak of methaemoglobinaemia in a premature baby unit that was attributed to the use of trichlorocarbanilide — a disinfectant contained in some soaps, shampoos, and proprietary skin cleaners — in a diaper rinse (Fisch *et al*. 1963).

Outstanding in this context, however, is the neurotoxic potential of the substituted phenolic compound, hexachlorophane. In 1971 this compound was more widely used in medicinal and cosmetic products than any other germicide. It acts selectively against Gram-positive organisms and, at recommended dosages, it seems to be virtually devoid of any toxic or sensitizing effect on the skin. Unlike other antiseptics, it only becomes fully effective when the epidermis becomes impregnated as a result of repeated daily application. Its long-sustained effect was considered to justify its use in skin preparations employed in hospitals, and particularly in premature baby units where effective protection against staphylococcal sepsis is vital.

The first suspicion that percutaneous absorption might be both extensive and detrimental was raised in a case report (Herter 1959) of an infant who developed generalized erythema and transient signs of cerebral damage — including convulsions, nystagmus, and unilateral facial paralysis — after being rubbed down with 3% hexachlorophane on 4 successive days. A decade later it was suggested that hexachlorophane baths might contribute to the encephalopathy seen among patients in burns units (Larson 1968). Concern intensified when it was reported that rats became paraplegic when dosed with amounts sufficient to generate the plasma concentrations attained in neonates bathed daily in hexachlorophane. On autopsy, these animals were found to have diffuse spongy degenerative changes in the white matter of the brain (Kimbrough and Gaines 1971; Curley *et al*. 1971).

Irrefutable evidence of danger was provided shortly afterwards when 20 infants died in France following exposure to a baby powder that, by error, contained 6% hexachlorophane (Federal Register 1972). An erythematous diaper rash was followed by a progressive neurological deficit culminating in a state of decerebrate rigidity, and the anticipated cerebral oedema and vacuolation of the white matter were found at autopsy. Doubt remains, however, as to whether hexachlorophane ever induced such changes when used as recommended. Similar changes were demonstrated in the reticular substance in 21 of 250 children aged under 5 years who were autopsied at hospitals affiliated to the University of Washington (WHO 1973). Although the incidence and extent of the changes correlated inversely with age and weight and directly with exposure to hexachlorophane, the interpretation of these findings was guarded: the children were certified to have died from other causes, and several factors, including extreme prematurity, may have contributed to the neuropathology; in a few instances lesions occurred in children who had had little or no exposure to hexachlorophane, and no such correlation could be established with respect to similar changes detected in the long spinal tracts in other children.

Absorption of hexachlorophane through adult human skin occurs far less readily (Ulsamer and Marzulli 1973). The highest plasma concentration that was measured following 3–6 weeks of daily whole-body washing with a

3% emulsion was about one-third of the threshold toxic dose in rats, and for hand washing the average value was some 30-fold less. None the less, hexachlorophane is reputed to have been detected in cord blood of neonates following its topical use by the mother (Curley *et al.* 1971), and a series of retrospective surveys undertaken in Sweden generated data that at first aroused, but later tended to allay, suspicion of a teratogenic potential (Halling 1977; Källén 1978; Swedish National Board of Health and Welfare 1978).

Hexachlorophane preparations are no longer recommended for use in infants or children and the concentrations allowed in surgical scrubs and other products are widely subject to regulation. No national drug regulatory authority has taken any formal restrictive action as a result of the concerns expressed in Sweden regarding teratogenicity, although the United States Food and Drug Administration has advised 'surgeons, nurses and other health care personnel who are or who may become pregnant to avoid hexachlorophane antibacterial scrubs' (Food and Drug Administration 1978).

Various formulations of other compounds, including chlorhexidine, iodophores, and triclosan, that have an activity, after repeated application, similar to that of hexachlorophane, are now promoted for hand washing. As yet, no suspicion has been raised that regular topical use of these compounds results in toxic systemic absorption in adults. Iodine, however, is concentrated in breast milk and derangements of thyroid function in neonates have been attributed to the use of iodine-containing vaginal preparations by nursing mothers (Postellon and Aronow 1982). More recently, it has been shown that premature infants exposed to topical iodinated antiseptics absorb quantities of iodine sufficient to inhibit thyroid-hormone synthesis transiently in a large proportion of cases (Smerdely *et al.* 1989). Since primary hypothyroidism causes severe neurological and intellectual impairment when treatment is delayed, and because premature infants are at greater risk of psychomotor retardation for other reasons, it is clearly prudent to avoid treating them with iodine-containing drugs.

Delayed systemic reactions

Corrosive antiseptics inevitably fall under suspicion as potential carcinogens. There is no clinical evidence to confirm or refute this possibility, but formaldehyde has been identified as a mutagen and carcinogen under experimental conditions (Auerbach *et al.* 1977; Swenberg *et al.* 1980). Although its safety for sterilizing dialysis equipment has been questioned (Goh and Cestero 1982), the quantities contained in — or generated by — topical antiseptics are unlikely to pose a tangible health risk.

References

Arena, J.M. (1964). Poisonings and other health hazards associated with the use of detergents. *JAMA* 190, 50.

Auerbach, C., Moutschen-Dahmen, J., and Moutschen, J. (1977). Genetic and cytogenetical effects of formaldehyde and related compounds. *Mutat. Res.* 39, 317.

Ayliffe, G.A.J., Barrowcliff, D.F., and Lowbury E.J. (1969). Contamination of disinfectants. *Br. Med. J.* i, 505.

Baliah, T.B., Macleish, H., and Drummond, K.N. (1969). Acute boric acid poisoning. *Can. Med. Assoc. J.* 101, 166.

Barr, R.D., Rees, P.H., Cordy, P.E., Kungu, A., Woodger, B.A., and Cameron, H.M. (1972). Nephrotic syndrome in adult Africans in Nairobi. *Br. Med. J.* ii, 131.

Bicknell, G. (1971). Sensorineural deafness following myringoplasty operations. *J. Laryngol. Otol.* 85, 957.

British Medical Association (1989). *A code of practice for sterilisation of instruments and control of cross infection.* BMA, London.

Committee on Safety of Medicines (1990). *Current Problems, No.2.* HMSO, London.

Corbo, M., Liu, J.C., and Chien, Y.W. (1990). Bioavailability of propranolol following oral and transdermal administration in rabbits. *J. Pharm. Sci.* 79, 584.

Curley, A., Hawk, R.E., Kimbrough, R.D., Nathenson, G., and Finberg, L. (1971). Dermal absorption of hexachlorophane in infants. *Lancet* ii, 296.

de Groot, A.C. and Herxheimer, A. (1990). Isothiazolinone preservative: cause of a continuing epidemic of cosmetic dermatitis. *Lancet* i, 314.

de Groot, A.C., Bruynzeel, D.P, Bos, J.D., van Joost, T., van der Meeren, H.L.M., Jagtman, B.A., *et al.* (1988). The allergens in cosmetics. *Arch. Dermatol.* 124, 1525.

Downing, J.G. and Brecker, S.W. (1948). Further studies in use of furacin in dermatology. *N. Engl. J. Med.* 239, 862.

Epstein, E. (1966). Allergy to dermatologic agents. *JAMA* 198, 517.

Federal Register (1972). *Fed. Reg.* 37, 20163.

Feldtman, R.W, Adrassy, R.J., and Page, C.R (1979). Povidone–iodine skin sensitivity observed with possibly altered immune status. *JAMA* 242, 239.

Fisch, R.O., Berglund, E.B., Bridge, A.G., Finley, R.R., Quie, P.G.., and Raile, R. (1963). Methaemoglobinaemia in a hospital nursery. *JAMA* 185, 760.

Food and Drug Administration (1978). Hexachlorophene — interim caution regarding use in pregnancy. *F.D.A. Drug Bull.* Aug/Sept 1978.

Goh, K-O. and Cestero, R.V.M. (1982). Health hazards of formaldehyde. *JAMA* 247, 2778.

Goldbloom, R.B. and Goldbloom, A. (1953). Boric acid poisoning. *J. Pediatr.* 43, 631.

Halling, H. (1977). Suspected link between exposure to hexachlorophene and birth of malformed infants. *Lakartidningen* 74, 542 (cited by W. Check [1978]. New study shows hexachlorophene is teratogenic in man. *JAMA* 240, 513).

Herter, W.B. (1959). Hexachlorophene poisoning. *Kaiser Fed. Med. Bull.* 7, 228.

Ison, A.E. and Tucker, J.B. (1968). Photosensitive dermatitis from soaps. *N. Engl. J. Med.* 278, 81.

Källén, B. (1978). Hexachlorophene teratogenicity in humans disputed. *JAMA* 240, 1585.

Kasilo, O.J. and Yetunde, O. (1990). Epidemiology and toxicology of the bleaching agents: hydroquinone, mercury and misuse of corticosteroids. Drug and toxicology information service. University of Zimbabwe, No.19.

Kibukamusoke, J.W., Davies, D.R., and Hutt, M.S.R. (1974). Membranous neuropathy due to skin lightening creams. *Br. Med. J.* ii, 646.

Kimbrough, R.D. and Gaines, T.B. (1971). Hexachlorophene effects on the rat brain. *Arch. Environ. Health* 23, 114.

Kinmont, P.D.C. (1969). Deodorants. *Practitioner* 202, 88.

Larson, D.L. (1968). Studies show that hexachlorophene causes burn syndrome. *J. Am. Hosp. Assoc.* 42, 63.

Lee, J.C. and Fialkow, P.J. (1961). Benzalkonium chloride source of hospital infection with Gram-positive bacteria. *JAMA* 177, 708.

Maxson, W.T. (1954). Case report of boric acid poisoning from topical application. *JAMA* 156, 286.

Morgan, J.K. (1968). Iatrogenic epidermal sensitivity. *Br. J. Clin. Pract.* 22, 261.

Postellon, D.C. and Aronow, R. (1982). Iodine in mother's milk. *JAMA* 247, 463.

Restell, M. (1965). Reactions to chlorhexidine and cetrimide. *Lancet* i, 918.

Schorr, W.F. (1968). Paraben allergy: a cause of intractable dermatitis. *JAMA* 204, 859.

Schorr, W.F. and Mohajerin, A.H. (1966). Paraben sensitivity. *Arch. Dermatol.* 93, 721.

Segar, W.B. (1960). Peritoneal dialysis in the treatment of boric acid poisoning. *N. Engl. J. Med.* 262, 798.

Seymour, W.B. (1937). Poisoning from cutaneous application of iodine. *Arch. Intern. Med.* 59, 952.

Sharvill, D. (1965). Reaction to chlorhexidine and cetrimide. *Lancet* i, 771.

Shemano, I. and Nickerson, M. (1954). Cutaneous accumulation and retention of hexachlorophene-C^{14}. (Abstract) *Fed. Proc. Fed. Am. Soc. Exp. Biol.* 13, 404.

Skipworth, G.B., Goldstein, N., and McBride, W.P. (1967). Boric acid intoxication from a 'medicated talcum powder'. *Arch. Dermatol.* 95,83.

Smerdely, R., Lim, A., Boyages, S.C., Waite, K., Wu, D., Roberts, V., *et al.* (1989). Topical iodine-containing antiseptics and neonatal hypothyroidism in very-low-birthweight infants. *Lancet* ii, 661.

Swedish National Board of Health and Welfare (1978). Reference Group for Malformations and Development Disturbances. *Report on a study of deliveries in women employed in medical occupations.*

Swenburg, J.A., Kerns, W.D., Mitchell, R.I., Gralla, E.J., and Pavkov, K.L. (1980). Induction of squamous cell carcinomas of the rat nasal cavity by inhalation exposure to formaldehyde vapor. *Cancer Res.* 40, 3398.

Thomas, B.B. (1969). Peritoneal dialysis and lysol poisoning. *Br. Med. J.* iii, 720.

Ulsamer, A.G. and Marzulli, F.N. (1973). Hexachlorophene concentrations in blood associated with the use of products containing hexachlorophene. *Food Cosmet. Toxicol.* 11, 625.

United States Department of Health (1974). *Health Educ. Welfare Newsletter* 44.

Valdes-Dalpena, M.A. and Arey, J.B. (1962). Boric acid poisoning. *J. Pediatr.* 61, 531.

WMCADRR (West Midlands Centre for Adverse Drug Reaction Reporting) (1988). Povidone iodine: sensitivity reactions. *Newsletter* June 1988.

WHO (World Health Organization) 1973. Neuropathy in newborn infants bathed with hexachlorophane. *Wkly Epidemiol. Rec.* 19, 207.

Wong, L.C., Heimbach, M.D., and Truscott, D.R. (1964). Boric acid poisoning: report of eleven cases. *Can. Med. Assoc. J.* 90, 1018.

27. Toxicity of opaque media used in X-ray diagnosis

G. ANSELL

Introduction

The opacity of radiological contrast media is dependent upon the fact that they contain substances of high atomic number that absorb X-rays. Soluble contrast media are based on formulations containing iodine, which has an atomic number of 53. The soluble salts of barium (atomic number 56), are highly poisonous, and the preparations used in radiological practice therefore consist of suspensions of insoluble barium sulphate. The pharmacological aspects of contrast media have been described by Knoefel (1971), Miller and Skukas (1977), Grainger (1982), Carr (1988), and Enge and Edgren (1989). Adverse effects of contrast media and other complications of radiological investigations have been comprehensively reviewed by Ansell and Wilkins (1987). In this chapter attention will be focused on the main clinical implications of adverse reactions.

Urography, computed tomography, and angiography

Conventional contrast media used for excretion urography, computed tomography, and angiography are water-soluble tri-iodinated derivatives of benzoic acid. The conventional ionic media in current use include diatrizoate (Hypaque, Urografin, Renografin), iothalamate (Conray), metrizoate (Triosil, Isopaque), and iodamide (Uromiro). In terms of toxicity, on an equiosmolar basis, there is little difference between these compounds. Modifications of the cations, using varying ratios of sodium, methylglucamine, and calcium can affect the toxicity in specific circumstances, and these are discussed in greater detail in the appropriate sections of the text.

If large doses of contrast media are administered to animals to determine the LD_{50}, a characteristic syndrome occurs (Hoppe 1959). As lethal dose levels are approached, the animals become apprehensive. Vomiting, urination, and defaecation occur, followed by muscle twitching and convulsions. At a later stage, capillary breakdown develops in the lungs, causing pulmonary haemorrhage and right heart failure.

Experimentally, the toxicity of large doses is increased by rapid injection. Whereas the LD_{50} of sodium diatrizoate (Hypaque) by slow intravenous drip in the dog is 13 200 mg per kg, with *rapid* injection of 90% Hypaque the LD_{50} drops to 2700 mg per kg (3 ml per kg) (Bernstein *et al.* 1961).

A major factor in the toxicity of these conventional ionic contrast media is their hypertonicity. To overcome this problem, ratio 3 lower osmolar media have been introduced containing three atoms of iodine per particle in solution. Sodium methylglucamine ioxaglate (Hexabrix), an ionic medium, is a mono-acid dimer. The first non-ionic medium was metrizamide (Amipaque). This has now been superseded by the newer non-ionic media, iopamidol (Niopam), iohexol (Amipaque), iopromide (Ultravist), and ioversol (Optiray). These lower osmolar media, particularly the non-ionic media, generally cause fewer acute adverse effects. Present evidence suggests that they have an appreciably increased margin of safety, but some severe reactions and deaths have occurred even with the non-ionic media. The low-osmolar media are considerably more expensive than conventional ionic media and, in the majority of institutions, this has tended to limit their use to higher-risk situations (Grainger 1987). Conventional ionic contrast media are still in widespread use and the literature on adverse reactions discussed in this chapter relates mainly to these.

In clinical use, adverse reactions to contrast media may be considered under three main categories:

1. reactions following the use of very large total doses of contrast media;
2. reactions occurring when a concentrated bolus of contrast medium has been delivered to a critical area such as the myocardium, brain, spinal cord, or kidney;
3. idiosyncratic reactions, in a susceptible patient, to a dose of contrast medium that would be harmless to most patients.

The reactions in the first two categories can be predicted to some extent from results of animal experiments, since they depend largely on the known chemotoxic effects of contrast media and on their hypertonicity. Idiosyncratic reactions, on the other hand, are still poorly understood. Severe reactions are uncommon and death is rare, so that accumulation of data for analysis requires large-scale surveys (Pendergrass et al. 1958; Ansell 1968, 1970a; Ansell et al. 1980; Witten et al. 1973; Shehadi and Toniolo 1980; Hobbs 1981). Katayama (1988) and Palmer (1989) reported surveys comparing the incidence of adverse reactions with ionic and non-ionic media.

Chemotoxic effects

Effects on the cardiovascular system

Routine electrocardiographic monitoring of patients undergoing excretion urography with conventional ionic contrast media has shown that significant ECG changes may occur after intravenous injection of large doses of contrast media, particularly in patients with a preexisting abnormal ECG, coronary artery disease, or congestive heart failure. These changes are more common after bolus injections (Stadalnik et al. 1977). In patients with a history of angina, ischaemic ECG changes with or without chest pain have occurred following bolus injections of contrast media into the superior vena cava for digital subtraction angiography (DSA), and one patient developed ventricular fibrillation (Hesselink et al. 1984).

Arrhythmias have also been noted following contrast cardiac computed tomography in patients with known coronary artery disease, particularly after recent myocardial infarction (Foster and Griffin 1987).

In patients with incipient cardiac failure, there is particular risk of precipitating pulmonary oedema when large doses of ionic contrast media are used in high-dose urography (Ansell 1968; Davies et al. 1975). Pulmonary oedema can also be shown to occur in experimental animals, the severity being related to the dose of contrast medium and speed of injection (Måre and Violante 1983). Pretreatment with methylprednisolone at 24 hours and 30 minutes before the injection causes a significant decrease in this experimental pulmonary oedema (Måre et al. 1985). Pulmonary oedema may be partly due to volume of fluid administered, but the main factor is the high osmotic load of the contrast medium. This causes withdrawal of fluid from the interstitial tissues into the intravascular compartments with resulting hypervolaemia. The cardiotoxic and chemotoxic actions of contrast medium may also be a factor in the causation of pulmonary oedema. With sodium-containing contrast media, the high sodium load may be an aggravating factor, and low-osmolar media are preferable. Pulmonary oedema has, however, occurred in a patient with renal failure after administering iohexol (Dawson 1983).

Malins (1978) has also reported the development of pulmonary oedema following aortography under general anaesthesia, in patients with myocardial disease, and he has stressed the importance of preangiographic cardiological assessment.

Occasionally, increased pulmonary capillary permeability, due to anaphylactic shock, may cause a noncardiogenic type of pulmonary oedema (Chamberlin et al. 1979; Soloman 1986).

In angiocardiography, large doses of concentrated contrast medium are injected very rapidly and any preexisting cardiovascular abnormality may increase the risk of adverse effects. Fischer (1968) reviewed the complex haemodynamic changes that can take place with ionic contrast media. There may be a brief initial hypertensive phase followed by more prolonged hypotension due in part to peripheral vasodilatation and, in some cases, to depression of cardiac contractility. Alterations also occur in cardiac output and pulse rate. At the same time there are frequently transitory electrocardiographic changes, and arrhythmias may occasionally develop. In addition to its direct effect on the cardiovascular system, the hypertonicity of the contrast medium causes an increase in the serum osmolality. Extracellular fluid is drawn into the vascular compartment and there are changes in the serum electrolytes with a tendency to acidosis (Levin et al. 1969; Lichtman et al. 1975). The hypervolaemia resulting from haemodilution produces a rise in the left ventricular end-diastolic and left atrial pressures which may induce pulmonary oedema (Foda et al. 1965).

With right heart injections there may be transient pulmonary hypertension, and occasionally this is severe.

Rapid injections may cause severe dyspnoea and uncontrollable bouts of coughing (Foda *et al*. 1965). The risks of pulmonary angiography are, moreover, increased in patients with pre-existing pulmonary hypertension (Mills *et al*. 1980). Blockage of the pulmonary capillaries by clumps of erythrocytes may be an important factor in causing pulmonary hypertension. It was formerly believed that this was due to aggregation of erythrocytes in the pulmonary capillaries, but Aspelin and Schmid-Schönbein (1978) suggest that the hypertonic contrast media increase the rigidity of the walls of the erythrocytes so that they are unable to pass through the pulmonary capillaries. By comparison, ioxaglate, iopamidol, and iohexol cause only minor changes in the red cell membrane (Staubli *et al*. 1982; Aspelin 1983). In patients with normal pulmonary artery pressure undergoing pulmonary angiography, Iohexol caused significantly less increase in pulmonary artery pressure than diatrizoate and therefore appears safer (Tajima *et al*. 1988).

The coronary circulation is one of the critical areas where contrast media may produce vital changes. Contrast medium entering the coronary arteries after injections into the ascending aorta is usually partially diluted unless the catheter is misplaced at the opening of a coronary artery. With selective coronary arteriography, the injections are made directly into the right and left coronary arteries. Ionic contrast medium in the coronary circulation may cause decreased myocardial contractility, transient electrocardiographic abnormalities, arrhythmias and, in extreme cases, ventricular fibrillation. The latter is more likely to occur following injections into the right coronary artery.

The experimental work on dogs by Gensini and Di Giorgi (1964) indicated that high concentrations of sodium were toxic to the myocardium and that methylglucamine exerted a protective effect. Pure methylglucamine contrast medium was, however, subsequently found to produce an increased incidence of ventricular fibrillation when used for coronary arteriography, and it was shown that physiological quantities of sodium were desirable in the medium (Simon *et al*. 1972).

Coronary arteriography, when required, is usually performed in association with left ventriculography. An increase in left ventricular end-diastolic pressure may occur after either coronary arteriography or left ventriculography. Since the coronary injections are the more dangerous part of the procedure, they should be performed first, before myocardial depression has occurred. If the left ventricular end-diastolic pressure then rises above 40 mmHg (5.3 kPa) left ventriculography should be delayed (Levin and Baltaxe 1972). The new low-osmolar contrast media cause few myocardial and

haemodynamic changes (Gerber *et al*. 1982; Benotti 1988), and are therefore preferred for coronary arteriography and cardioangiography. If non-ionic contrast media are used for coronary arteriography, adequate heparinization is important to prevent a possible higher risk of thromboembolic phenomena. A meticulous technique is imperative and blood should not be withdrawn into the injection syringe (Grollman *et al*. 1988; Hwang *et al*. 1989).

During ventriculography, manipulation of the cardiac catheter in the ventricle may cause arrhythmias. Accidental intramural injections of contrast medium into the myocardium usually produce only transitory evidence of myocardial damage. Perforation of the myocardium, with injection of contrast medium into the pericardium, may give rise to pericardial tamponade. The hypertonic contrast medium causes an accumulation of fluid in the pericardial sac; this can usually be treated by aspiration, but if there is considerable bleeding, thoracotomy may be required (Popper *et al*. 1967).

Delayed cardiac tamponade may also occur after accidental injection of non-ionic contrast medium into the pericardium (Gallant and Studley 1990).

Effects on renal function

For a number of years, high doses of contrast medium were commonly used for excretion urography, particularly when visualization of the renal tract was required in patients with impaired renal function. Large doses of contrast medium may also be used during contrast computed tomography, in cardioangiography, and in other vascular investigations, venography, and therapeutic techniques.

Bergman and others (1968) showed that dehydration before high-dose urography could result in transient renal failure. There appeared to be a particular risk of renal failure developing from high-dose urography in azotaemic and dehydrated diabetic patients (Pillay *et al*. 1970). Moreover, renal failure has occurred in diabetes with a dose as little as 36 ml (17 g iodine) despite adequate hydration (Kamdar *et al*. 1977).

Kleinknecht and colleagues (1972) point out that sodium restriction or the use of diuretics in the days preceding administration of contrast media result in dehydration of the patient. It is now generally accepted that contrast media have a nephrotoxic potential. The earlier literature on this subject has been comprehensively reviewed by Mudge (1980), while Dawson and Trewhella (1990) provide a recent overview.

Variations in methodology have led to some divergence of conclusions but in most studies dehydration, insulin-dependent diabetes, and pre-existing renal impairment with azotaemia have been indicated to be major risk factors for contrast nephropathy. Other important risk factors include cardiac failure, a contrast medium dose exceeding 125 ml, and multiple studies (van Zee *et al.* 1978; D'Elia *et al.* 1982; Martin-Paredero *et al.* 1983; Taliercio *et al.* 1986). In infants undergoing angiocardiography, Gruskin and others (1970) showed that doses of diatrizoate above 3 ml per kg could cause significant renal damage including medullary necrosis.

The proximity of contrast medium injections to the renal circulation is also relevant: whereas conventional renal angiography involving injections of diatrizoate into the renal arteries caused a significant increase in serum creatinine and transient proteinuria, these changes were not noted after digital vascular imaging of the renal arteries using a similar dose of diatrizoate injected intravenously (Khoury *et al.* 1983). In patients undergoing renal angiography, an analysis by Cochran and others (1983) showed that the probability of acute renal damage increased with the number of risk factors involved.

Other possible risk factors include: patients in the older age group (Martin-Paredero *et al.* 1983), hypertension, vascular disease, proteinuria (Cochran *et al.* 1983), antibiotic nephrotoxicity (Barshay *et al.* 1973), cholecystography (Ihle *et al.* 1982), and hyperuricaemia. Urography in hyperuricaemic children with Burkitt's lymphoma may lead to irreversible renal failure (Mandell *et al.* 1983). There are also variations in the reported incidence of deterioration of renal function following contrast media. van Zee and others (1978) reported a minimal overall incidence of 0.8 per cent following high-dose urography, and an incidence of 8.5 per cent in non-diabetic, but 58 per cent in diabetic, patients with renal impairment. For angiography with large doses of contrast medium, Martin-Paredero and colleagues (1983) reported an overall rate of 11.3 per cent, while for patients with pre-existing renal disease the incidence of acute renal dysfunction was 41.7 per cent. In a recent prospective study Parfree and co-workers (1989) suggest a rate of 9 per cent in diabetic patients with pre-existing renal insufficiency. This improved rate may be partly due to selection and careful attention to hydration. Patients who develop renal failure following contrast media seem prone to a recurrence if the examination is subsequently repeated (Feldman *et al.* 1974).

Renal biopsy following high-dose urography has shown that histological changes similar to osmotic nephrosis may occur, but the significance of these changes is still not certain (Moreau *et al.* 1975).

Berdon and others (1969) suggested that some cases of contrast media nephropathy might be due to precipi-

tation of Tamm–Horsfall protein in the urine but this now appears unlikely since Dawson and colleagues (1984) were unable to confirm that urographic contrast media do precipitate this protein. Arteriography with diatrizoate may cause transient proteinuria and enzymuria (Nicot *et al.* 1984). Trewhella and associates (1990) demonstrated the release of vasopressin following the injection of contrast media and this may reduce renal perfusion. In animal experiments, nephrotoxicity from contrast media has been induced by sodium depletion and administration of indomethacin (Vari *et al.* 1988).

Ionic contrast media cause an early transient rise in uric acid excretion and a marked rise in oxalate excretion at 24 hours (Gelman *et al.* 1979). This may be relevant in the causation of renal failure, particularly in urate nephropathy (Karasick and Karasick 1981). Acute renal failure due to contrast media may also occur as a result of haemolysis after angiocardiography (Catterall *et al.* 1981) or in association with myoglobinuria (Winearls *et al.* 1980).

Kovnat and others (1973) described an unusual case in which aortography with diatrizoate was followed by a syndrome of nephrogenic diabetes insipidus that gradually improved over a period of 3–4 months.

Kerdel and colleagues (1984) report two cases of acute nephritis and necrotizing vasculitis after contrast studies in patients with malignant disease.

For some years it had become accepted that in myelomatosis there was a small but definite risk of causing transient or fatal renal failure as a result of excretion or retrograde urography (Brown and Battle 1964). Subsequently, *in vitro* tests by Lasser and others (1966) and by Cwynarski and Saxton (1969) showed that the earlier urographic media, such as diodone and acetrizoate, and the cholangiographic medium iodipamide all caused precipitation of myeloma protein, but that diatrizoate and iothalamate did not. On this basis, it was suggested that myelomatosis should no longer be regarded as a contraindication to excretion urography provided that dehydration was avoided. Cases of renal failure in myelomatosis have now, however, been reported in which the urographic contrast medium was diatrizoate, although dehydration was a possible complicating factor (Gross *et al.* 1968; Myers and Witten 1971). Shulman (1977) has described a fatal case of renal failure following urography in myelomatosis, despite the fact that the patient was well hydrated and the urine alkalinized. Renal failure has also occurred following renal angiography (McEvoy *et al.* 1970) and cerebral angiography (Ansell 1976) in unsuspected cases of myelomatosis. Gassmann and others (1983) report 26 cases of myeloma in whom urography was performed with methylglucamine iothalamate without significant deterioration of renal function. They conclude that if there is a definite indication for urography, this may be performed but compression and dehydration should be avoided and the urine alkalinized. Nevertheless, it must be accepted that there is a moderately increased risk of renal failure in myelomatosis and that contrast media should be avoided unless there are compelling reasons for their use. A fatal reaction with massive intravascular thrombosis has been reported by Burchardt and others (1981) following urography with diatrizoate in a patient with Waldenström's IgM paraproteinaemia.

When excretion urography is undertaken in the presence of renal failure, large quantities of contrast medium may remain in the circulation for several days, and extrarenal excretion may occur both through the liver (resulting in a cholecystogram) and through the small intestine (van Waes 1972). The contrast medium can, however, be removed rapidly by dialysis, and this may be necessary if a sensitivity reaction occurs.

Examination of the urine after intravenous urography may give rise to misleading results. The contrast medium causes an increase in the specific gravity of the urine. There may be a false-positive test for protein when the sulphasalicylic acid or nitric acid ring test is used, but the bromophenyl dye test (Albutest) is not affected. There may also be a false-positive black copper reduction reaction when a Clinitest tablet is added to the urine, thereby simulating the finding in alcaptonuria (Lee and Schoen 1966). Diatrizoate crystalluria may occur in some patients after excretion urography if the urine is cooled to room temperature. This may be confused with other types of crystalluria in routine microscopy of the urine. It is uncertain whether diatrizoate crystalluria has any relevance to contrast medium-induced renal failure (Ramsay et al. 1982).

Methylglucamine contrast media may interfere with the urinary estimation of catecholamines in phaeochromocytoma (McPhaul et al. 1984).

In summary, there is now increasing evidence that contrast media may aggravate renal failure in some patients. Usually the deterioration of renal function is transitory but occasionally it is permanent and may be fatal. The clinical criteria for the examination therefore require careful individual assessment in every patient. In some cases, alternative examinations such as ultrasound or isotope renography may provide adequate information. Patients with diabetes or myelomatosis are at particular risk, but there is also an increased risk in those with incipient cardiac failure and possibly also in those with gout. Dehydration should be avoided prior to the examination. Such dehydration may be caused by restriction of fluids, vomiting, and diarrhoea, by diuretics,

or even by prolonged salt restriction. It is probably also unwise to repeat high-dose contrast examinations within 7 days. Careful attention to hydration is important before and after administration of contrast media but this may not always prevent contrast nephropathy. Golman and Almén (1985) reviewed animal and clinical studies of contrast media nephrotoxicity and concluded that iohexol appeared to be the least toxic of the various contrast media currently available but, at very high dose levels, it can be nephrotoxic in animals. A number of cases of renal failure have now been reported after nonionic contrast media particularly after cardiac angiography (Evans et al. 1987; Elliott and Roger 1988). Dose appeared to be an important factor (Taliercio et al. 1989). In a randomized controlled trial, Schwab and others (1989) were unable to demonstrate a significant difference in nephrotoxicity of the non-ionic contrast medium iopamidol in comparison with the conventional ionic medium diatrizoate. The earlier optimism that contrast media nephropathy could be avoided by using non-ionic media is therefore no longer justified. Nevertheless, where an examination involving contrast medium is considered essential in higher-risk patients, it is probably preferable to use a non-ionic medium: the dose of contrast medium used should be the minimum that is consistent with diagnostic requirements, and multiple examinations should be avoided whenever possible.

In contrast nephropathy, elevation of serum creatinine may or may not be accompanied by oliguria and, unless the patient is monitored, the early stages may be overlooked. Older and co-workers (1980) reported that a prolonged nephrogram at 30 minutes or 24 hours after administration of contrast medium could be a useful predictor of possible incipient renal failure. Likewise, Love and others (1989) suggest that a cortical attenuation level of 55–110 Hounsfield units (HU) in an unenhanced CT scan of the kidneys 24 hours after administration of a contrast medium may indicate subclinical renal impairment with a high risk of nephropathy on subsequent exposure to contrast medium; and that a cortical attenuation in excess of 140 HU appears to be an early indicator of contrast nephropathy. Golman and Almén (1985) suggest that clearance studies of contrast medium remaining in the plasma, after examination in susceptible patients, could give an early warning of potential nephrotoxicity in individual patients and allow appropriate remedial therapy to be started. Surgery and procedures that may be associated with renal ischaemia should be deferred to allow elimination of residual contrast medium, particularly if excretion has been slowed by impaired renal function.

Accidental overdosage in children

Doses of contrast medium used for urography in children often tended to be relatively larger than those used in adults. In addition, the tendency to increasing dosage of contrast media may cause confusion. During a 12-month period, three cases of accidental overdosage in infants occurred in the UK with fatal results in two (Ansell 1970*b*). Fatalities due to accidental overdosage during urography have also been reported from the USA by McClennan and colleagues (1972) and by Kassner and others (1973). The usual presenting features are haemorrhagic pulmonary oedema and cardiac arrest, but convulsions may also occur. A case of pulmonary oedema with reversible cardiac arrest has been recorded in an infant receiving only 3.3 ml per kg of 45% sodium diatrizoate (Ansell 1976). The toxic effect of high doses in infants appears to be due partly to the chemotoxicity of the contrast medium and partly to the hyperosmolar state which may cause pulmonary oedema or cerebral symptoms due to hypertonic dehydration (Giammona *et al*. 1963). The low glomerular filtration rate in neonates may also result in delayed excretion of the contrast medium (Nogrady and Dunbar 1968). The new non-ionic low-osmolar media are preferable for use in infants.

The need for continuing vigilance to avoid contrast overdose is illustrated in a report by Junck and Marshall (1986). Owing to problems with the film changer, a 7-year-old child with coarctation of the aorta received a massive overdose totalling 340 ml Renografin 76 during five injections into the aortic arch. This caused status epilepticus, supraventricular tachycardia, hypertension, hyperthermia, and coma followed by disseminated intravascular coagulation and renal failure with death at 33 hours. A high concentration of contrast medium persisted in the brain and it was suggested that in patients with severe neurological complications and renal failure, prompt dialysis should be undertaken to remove excess contrast medium.

Effects on the central nervous system

Contrast media entering the cerebral circulation may alter the blood–brain barrier. Leakage across this barrier may directly damage the neural tissues, which are particularly sensitive to water-soluble contrast media. Gonsette and Andre-Balisaux (1967) used autoradiographic techniques in animals to measure these effects. Hilal (1966) showed that intracarotid injections of large doses of ionic contrast medium in the dog produced convulsions, hypotension, and bradycardia, and that these effects were partly related to the osmolarity of the contrast medium. Fischer and others (1965, 1968) used the haemodynamic changes following intracarotid injection to assess the neurotoxicity of different contrast media. Sodium salts of contrast media were found to be more toxic than methylglucamine salts in the cerebral circulation, but there was little difference in toxicity between the diatrizoate, iothalamate, and metrizoate anions.

Lundervold and Engeset (1976), using polygraphic recordings during cerebral angiography, confirmed that hypotension, bradycardia, and even transient asystole may occur. These changes were more marked when the posterior cerebral arteries had been filled, suggesting that they were due to involvement of centres in the hypothalamus or brain stem. Bradycardial reactions are often followed by tachycardia and hypertension. These reflex cardiovascular changes may be more serious in patients with coronary artery disease. Focal electroencephalographic (EEG) changes may also occur on the side of the injection and, if prolonged, may be followed by evidence of neurological involvement. Premedication with atropine decreased the incidence of cardiovascular changes but did not affect the focal EEG changes. The severity of both electrocardiographic (ECG) and EEG changes was increased by repeated injections and by larger doses of contrast medium. These authors also advocate premedication with hypertonic mannitol in patients with cerebral tumours. EEG recordings taken within a few hours after cerebral angiography may give rise to misleading localizing signs of the lesion (Binnie *et al*. 1971).

Confusional states may occur following cerebral angiography (Haley 1984). Neurological complications may also occur following aortic arch angiography (McIvor *et al*. 1987).

Experimental studies suggest that the reduced neurotoxicity of the new low-osmolar contrast media should be advantageous in cerebral angiography (Gonsette and Liesenborgh 1980). They cause less pain and discomfort and fewer EEG changes, but clinical complications due to other factors such as thromboembolism are not prevented (Nakstad *et al*. 1982; Skalpe 1988). Whereas ionic contrast media have a moderate anticoagulant effect, this is minimal with non-ionic media, and this may be a potential cause of thromboembolism (Robertson 1987).

Intravenous administration of contrast media may also occasionally cause convulsions in patients who have a predisposition to epilepsy, or when very large doses are administered (Ansell 1970*a*). It has been suggested that the liability of contrast media to cause convulsions and tetany may be partially due to depression of the serum calcium (Kutt *et al*.1966).

Convulsions may occur during contrast computed tomographic examinations in patients with cerebral tumours: diazepam is valuable in prophylaxis (Pagani *et al.* 1984). Benear and associates (1985) suggest that patients with thrombotic thrombocytopenic purpura may have an increased liability to contrast media convulsions.

Paraplegia is a rare complication of aortic angiography. In earlier investigations using the more neurotoxic contrast media, such as diodone and acetrizoate, the incidence of neurological complications following abdominal aortography was 0.22 per cent (McAfee 1957). Occasional cases of paraplegia have also been reported following aortography with 65% diatrizoate and 60% metrizoate (Ansell 1968). Bronchial arteriography with 70% diatrizoate has similarly been followed by paresis (Feigelson and Ravin 1965). Mishkin and others (1973) believed that the relative rarity of published reports did not reflect the true incidence of these complications. They quoted five cases notified to them during a 3-month period in 1973. There were four cases of tetraplegia (three being due to parathyroid arteriography, and one following angiography of the posterior fossa). In the fifth case, paraplegia followed attempted renal angiography. When these neurological complications occur following angiography, the iodine content of the cerebrospinal fluid is raised. Treatment of similar cases by irrigation of the subarachnoid space with isotonic saline has given encouraging results. Systemic steroid therapy should also be started as soon as this mishap is suspected.

Accidental injection of ionic contrast medium into the subarachnoid space by misplacement of the needle during aortography or vertebral arteriography produces clonic spasms, which may be fatal. This mishap should also be treated by irrigation of the subarachnoid space (McCleery and Lewtas 1966).

Effects on blood vessels

The intra-arterial injection of conventional contrast media results in vasodilatation and pain. This is mainly due to the hypertonicity of the media, but Lindgren (1970) has shown that chemotoxicity is also an important factor, since acetrizoate has a more severe action than an equiosmolar solution of diatrizoate. The effect is also more marked with increasing concentrations of contrast medium. Contrast medium may also damage endothelium at the capillary level. Acetrizoate produced more marked changes than diatrizoate, and sodium salts appear to be more vasoactive than methylglucamine salts (Harrington and Wiedeman 1965). The local tolerance of irritant substances is, of course, much higher with intravenous injection than it is with intra-arterial injection. In a

series of patients undergoing high-dose urography with methylglucamine or sodium salts of diatrizoate, however, Penry and Livingstone (1972) found that the incidence of arm pain was highest in those receiving the pure sodium media. Electron microscopy studies of the veins of rabbits showed minor endothelial changes that were related to the proportion of sodium in the diatrizoate mixture. Severe arm pain may sometimes occur after intravenous injection of 70% sodium iothalamate, and occasional cases of venous thrombosis have occurred with this and with other media (Ansell 1976).

In peripheral arteriography, pain is a problem with conventional contrast media, even when they are used in low concentrations. The low-osmolar contrast media are less irritant and cause less pain. In a comparative trial by Murphy and others (1988), iohexol produced considerably less pain than methylglucamine diatrizoate, but ioxaglate (Hexabrix) caused the least pain.

Effects on blood

Stemerman and others (1971) described what they believed to be the first reported case of pancytopenia due to diatrizoate. Over a period of 15 days, the patient had three urographic examinations and a renal angiogram with diatrizoate for the investigation of hypertension. One hour after angiography, there was a severe anaphylactic reaction with dizziness, pruritus, dyspnoea, pyrexia, and hypotension. This was followed by a decrease in haematocrit, platelets, and leucocytes, and a hypoplastic bone marrow, but 4 months later the blood picture was normal. This patient had also received penicillin and cephalothin, but the timing of the reaction suggests that the diatrizoate was responsible. More recently, repeated acute thrombocytopenia has been described following diatrizoate (Shojania 1985; Lacey *et al.* 1986; Chang *et al.* 1989). Transient benign eosinophilia may occur 24–72 hours after excretion urography. This appears to have no significance (Vincent *et al.* 1977).

Richards and Nulsen (1971) described severe sickling following cerebral angiography in two patients who were homozygous for sickle cell haemoglobin (SS), and McNair (1972) reported a fatality due to acute thrombosis following selective coronary arteriography. Acute haemolysis occurred in a patient with sickle-cell disease following left ventricular angiography with diatrizoate (Rao *et al.* 1985). *In vitro* experiments showed that severe sickling occurred when blood samples from SS patients were mixed with concentrations of diatrizoate above 35 per cent. This appeared to be partly due to the acidic nature of the contrast medium, and the degree of sickling was reduced but not eliminated by buffering the medium to pH 7.4. Although few cases have been described up till now, the risk of sickling is probably greater during angiography when relatively high concentrations of contrast medium are produced as compared with slow intravenous injections where admixture of blood will tend to decrease the blood concentration of the contrast medium. *In vitro* studies indicate that the non-ionic medium iopamidol causes significantly less sickling than conventional contrast media (Rao *et al.* 1982).

Bernstein (1970) found that when blood is diluted with 90% sodium diatrizoate *in vitro*, there is initially a decrease in red cell diameter due to the hypertonic environment, but as more contrast medium is added the red cells show an increase in diameter due to damage to the cell wall. Contrast media may also cause alterations in the shape of the red cell (Schiantarelli *et al.* 1973) and increased rigidity of the cell wall (Aspelin and Schmid-Schönbein 1978). These changes in the red cells also increase the microviscosity of the contrast medium–blood mixture. The greatest increase of microviscosity occurs with diatrizoate. Despite its low osmolality, metrizamide also caused a marked increase of microviscosity. The new low-osmolar media ioxaglate, iopamidol, and iohexol caused a much lower increase in microviscosity and only minor change in red cell membrane and shape (Staubli *et al.* 1982; Aspelin 1983). This shows that although osmolality is an important factor in contrast-medium toxicity it is not the only factor and the structure of the contrast medium molecule is also relevant.

When blood is aspirated into a syringe during the administration of contrast medium the red cells are subjected to a very high concentration of the medium. This will render them liable to subsequent haemolysis with liberation of haemoglobin and possibly other toxic substances. It is therefore preferable to avoid reinjection of the blood with the contrast medium. If stasis occurs after aspiration of blood into a syringe containing non-ionic contrast medium, clot formation may occur with a risk of thromboembolism (Robertson 1987). Dawson and colleagues (1988) found that clot formation occurred on two occasions in styrene acrylonitrile syringes but not in polypropylene syringes. Haemoglobinuria has been reported following cardioangiography with diatrizoate (Cohen *et al.* 1969).

Administration of large doses of ionic contrast media during angiography may cause hypocoagulability of the blood with inhibition of clotting and increased fibrinolytic activity. These coagulation defects may persist up to 24 hours after angiography and are believed to be due to interference with the protein factors responsible for coagulation (Stein and Hilgartner 1968). It has also been suggested that depression of the serum calcium may play a part in the hypocoagulable state (Chandra and Abraham 1973). Ionic contrast media potentiate the anticoagulant action of heparin *in vitro* and this may cause problems in monitoring anticoagulant therapy (Parvez *et al.* 1982). Cardiac catheterization without injection of contrast media, on the other hand, may cause increased coagulability of the blood (Bjork 1968). Protamine sulphate causes precipitation of diatrizoate and may cause an embolus if administered through an arteriography catheter (Iannone 1975). Hexabrix is precipitated by papaverine (Pilla *et al.* 1986).

The possible significance of protein-binding by contrast media has been reviewed by Lasser (1971). There is evidence that contrast media can activate serum complement by the 'alternative pathway' and this may be one of the factors in systemic reactions (Lasser *et al.* 1980; Lasser 1989). Disseminated intravascular coagulation may, rarely, occur as a result of a severe adverse reaction to contrast medium (Zeman 1977).

Depression of ionized calcium by chelating agents present in contrast media may affect cardiac function (Caulfield *et al.* 1975; Mallette and Gomez 1983). The diatrizoate ion also binds calcium directly whereas iopamidol does not bind calcium (Morris *et al.* 1982). The hypocalcaemia induced by contrast media may cause a transient increase in parathormone secretion (Berger *et al.* 1982). Batches of contrast medium may become contaminated by nickel during their manufacture: Leach and Sunderman (1987) found hypernickelaemia in patients undergoing coronary arteriography with Revografin 76.

Idiosyncratic reactions

There is probably no single factor that can explain the spectrum of idiosyncratic reactions. These range from anaphylactoid-type reactions such as urticaria, sneezing, epiphora, salivary gland enlargement, angioneurotic oedema, and bronchospasm, to the cardiovascular group with fainting, hypotensive collapse, or cardiac arrest. Other types of reaction include flushing, arm pain, nausea, vomiting, abdominal pain, paraesthesia, chest pain, dyspnoea, rigors, headache, tetany, convulsions, and coma (Ansell 1970a).

The incidence of reactions to ionic contrast media reported in various surveys ranged from 1 in 13 to 1 in 30 for minor reactions that required no treatment. For intermediate reactions that required some treatment but did not cause undue alarm for the patient's safety the rates varied from 1 in 57 to 1 in 130. The reported incidence of severe reactions requiring intensive treatment ranged from 1 in 1000 to 1 in 4000, while the incidence of fatal reactions varied from 1 in 15 000 to 1 in 93 000 (Shehadi and Toniolo 1980; Ansell *et al.* 1980; Hobbs 1981; Hartman *et al.* 1982). Differences may be partly due to the criteria used for assessing reactions and variations in dosage. Under-reporting of reactions may also be a problem.

It is now generally agreed that the incidence of mild and moderate reactions is considerably reduced with non-ionic media. In a double-blind trial of 1000 patients, Jacobson and others (1988) found an incidence of mild to moderate reactions in 31.2 per cent after conventional ionic medium and 7.7 per cent after non-ionic medium. The low-osmolar medium ioxaglate (Hexabrix) appears to cause more vomiting and histaminoid reactions (Spataro *et al.* 1987). In a large non-randomized Japanese survey of 337 647 cases (Katayama 1988), the combined incidence of 'severe' and 'very severe' reactions was approximately 0.25 per cent with ionic media and 0.04 per cent with non-ionic media, a ratio of approximately 6. It was not possible to assess the mortality rate. Several unreported deaths have been associated with non-ionic media (Grainger and Dawson 1990). In an Australian survey of 106 211 patients, Palmer (1989) found a significantly lower incidence of 'moderate' and 'severe' reactions with ionic media. This effect was evident in both 'high risk' and 'low risk' patients.

Although some severe or even fatal reactions may occur with small doses of contrast medium, there is evidence to suggest that the incidence of severe reactions is increased with higher doses (Ansell *et al.* 1980; Lasser *et al.* 1987). Katayama (1988) also found an increased incidence of severe and very severe reactions to ionic media with bolus injections and to a lesser extent with drip infusions. This was less apparent with non-ionic media. Older patients and those with heart disease appear to be at greater risk of severe reactions. Electrocardiographic abnormalities may occur in such patients following intravenous urography, and the incidence of these ECG changes increased with higher doses of contrast medium and with rapid injection (Stadalnik *et al.* 1977; Pfister and Hutter 1980). As previously discussed, there is also a risk of precipitating pulmonary oedema in patients with incipient congestive heart failure.

Hypotensive collapse is usually the most important feature of severe reactions. Impairment of venous return due to abdominal compression may occasionally cause hypotension, but it is probably not a major factor in most cases. With profound hypotension, there may be loss of consciousness and even convulsions. Cardiac arrhythmias may develop, or there may be transient ECG changes that may be misinterpreted as evidence of cardiac infarction. Sudden cardiac arrest may occur, but

with immediate and vigorous treatment there is a reasonable prospect of recovery. Hypotensive collapse is sometimes due to vagal overactivity. These patients have bradycardia instead of the more usual tachycardia (Andrews 1976).

Patients with a history of allergy or reactions to other drugs have an increased risk of reactions to contrast media and this is particularly high in asthmatic patients, in whom the risk of a severe reaction is increased by a factor of 5 (Ansell *et al.* 1980). Bronchospasm may occur during the injection, and as little as 0.5 ml to 1 ml of contrast medium may produce a severe attack with cyanosis. Bronchospasm may develop with any of the contrast media but its incidence appears possibly to be higher when methylglucamine is present in the medium (Ansell 1970*a*). In 140 asthmatic patients undergoing urography with methylglucamine diatrizoate, Witten and others (1973) found the incidence of 'acute' reactions to be 6 per cent. Subclinical bronchospasm can be demonstrated following the bolus injection of ionic contrast media, and this is more common in asthmatic patients. The incidence of subclinical bronchospasm is much reduced with iopamidol or iohexol and it has been suggested that these media should be used when urography is required in patients with asthma or obstructive airways disease (Dawson *et al.* 1983). Severe bronchospasm has, however, occurred in a high-risk patient with iopamidol (unpublished). Katayama (1988) found that in patients with a history of asthma, the incidence of severe and very severe reactions was 1.88 per cent using ionic media and 0.23 per cent with non-ionic media. Iopamidol and iohexol cause less histamine release than diatrizoate or iothalamate (Assem *et al.* 1983).

In patients with a previous history of a reaction to an ionic contrast medium, there is an 11-fold increased risk of a severe reaction. Approximately 40 per cent of such patients may be expected to develop a further reaction on rechallenge, but many of these repeat reactions are, of course, only minor or intermediate in type. It appears possible that certain ethnic groups, for example, Indians, may have a higher risk of reactions, but the reason for this is uncertain (Ansell *et al.* 1980). According to Witten and others (1973), patients with a history of 'iodism' have an increased liability to contrast medium reactions of all types. There is probably an increased risk of reactions in toxic or dehydrated patients.

Parotid gland swelling was rarely recorded following excretion urography with smaller doses of contrast media (Sussman and Miller 1956), but with the introduction of high-dose urography, and with delayed excretion due to renal failure, the condition became more frequent (Talner *et al.* 1971). It still appears, however, that it is an idiosyncratic reaction occurring in only a small proportion of patients, and it may recur in the same patient with repeated examinations. The swelling usually occurs 2–4 days after the contrast medium has been administered and may last several days. In these delayed cases, there may be both organically bound iodine and free iodide in the saliva. Evanescent salivary gland enlargement may also occur within a few minutes of the contrast medium injection and subside over a period of a few hours (Navani *et al.* 1972). In one patient, parotid gland swelling was associated with paralysis of the facial nerve (Koch *et al.* 1969).

Armour and co-workers (1986) described a patient with transitory parotid swelling occurring shortly after contrast injection, accompanied by transitory enlargement of the pancreas noted on CT. This was associated with mild back pain.

Two recent studies (Panto and Davies 1986; McCullough *et al.* 1989) have shown that delayed reactions in the week following exretion urography are not uncommon. Approximately 12 per cent of patients reported a 'flu-like' illness resembling iodism and approximately 4.5 per cent had delayed skin rashes. These delayed skin rashes appeared to be more common with contrast media that contained methylglucamine and with non-ionic media. Symptoms suggestive of parotid enlargement were reported in between 1 and 2 per cent of patients and there was a trend to a higher incidence after non-ionic media.

Heydenreich and Olholm Larsen (1977) have described a case of true iododerma which occurred 4 days after high-dose urography in a patient with renal failure. A number of other delayed severe skin reactions with bullous changes and vasculitis have recently been reported (Reuter and Eugester 1985; Grunwald *et al.* 1985; Ansell and Wilkins 1987, p. 6; Kaftori *et al.* 1988). Some of these cases had features suggesting a possible immunological process. While some of these severe delayed skin reactions have been due to conventional ionic media, there appears to be a disproportionate trend to involvement of non-ionic media. With the small number of cases so far reported, this may be fortuitous but it merits further evaluation. Likewise, two fatal cases of Stevens–Johnson syndrome have occurred following the use of non-ionic media for intravenous urography in patients with lupus syndromes (Goodfellow *et al.*1986; Savill *et al.* 1988). Gelmers (1984) has also reported exacerbation of systemic lupus erythematosus following myelography with the non-ionic agent metrizamide. Transient hyperthyroidism may, rarely, occur following the administration of high doses of contrast medium (Shetty *et al.* 1974; Ansell and Wilkins 1987, p. 14).

Miscellaneous

Some reports (Chagnac *et al.* 1985; Anzola *et al.* 1986; van den Bergh *et al.* 1986) indicate that contrast media may precipitate a myasthenic crisis in patients with myasthenia gravis, particularly in those with a thymoma. This may occur with ionic or non-ionic media.

Stinchcombe and Davies (1989) reported an acute toxic myopathy starting 1 hour after intravenous urography with iopamidol. There was severe muscle pain and a raised serum creatine kinase. The condition resolved over the next 3 days.

Mozley (1981) reported a fatal case of malignant hyperthermia which followed the injection of 100 ml of diatrizoate.

Weinstein and others (1985) reported a patient with a malignant VIPoma in whom iodinated contrast media caused release of vasoactive intestinal polypeptide with a marked increase in watery diarrhoea.

Prevention and treatment of reactions

Although there has been considerable research on the subject, the causes of idiosyncratic reactions to contrast media are still uncertain. Siegle and Lieberman (1978) reviewed the evidence in favour of histamine release while Lasser and others (1980) favoured the theory of complement activation. Lasser (1988*a*) suggests that release of bradykinin may be an important factor in contrast media reactions. Bolz and colleagues (1986) reported a severe delayed reaction to iohexol, which was associated with evidence of monocyte stimulation. In a few patients there may be a true allergic hypersensitivity (Ansell and Wilkins 1987, p. 19). Lalli (1980) believes that fear is the major factor in the causation of reactions to contrast media. It seems probable, indeed, that a number of different mechanisms may be involved. Injection of methylglucamine diatrizoate into dehydrated dogs may produce a syndrome with many of the features that occur in severe contrast media reactions in patients (Katzberg *et al.* 1983).

There is no completely reliable method of preventing contrast media reactions. Whilst the incidence of reactions is reduced with non-ionic media, cost has so far tended to limit their use to higher-risk patients (Grainger and Dawson 1990). In a large randomized study of patients receiving conventional ionic media, Lasser and others (1987) showed that a dose of 32 mg methylprednisolone at 12 and 2 hours before the contrast injection produced a significant reduction in the overall incidence of all grades of reaction by approximately one-third as compared with administration of placebo tablets. A single dose of methylprednisolone at 2 hours before the injection was no better than placebo. For high-risk patients, when time permits, Lasser (1988b) advocates a 3-day course of 32 mg methylprednisolone daily with the last dose 2 hours before injection of the medium. Where prolonged pretreatment is not possible, a single injection of steroid 6 hours before injection of the contrast medium might be effective. For patients with a previous history of reactions, Greenberger (1984) suggests that steroid prophylaxis may be supplemented by 50 mg diphenhydramine orally. He also suggests 25 mg ephedrine orally, provided that there is no cardiac contraindication. Pretreatment with corticosteroid does not, however, completely eliminate the risk of reactions. Likewise, severe reactions and deaths have also occurred after non-ionic media. For particularly high-risk patients, such as those with a history of previous reactions to ionic contrast media or with a history of asthma, it would seem logical to use a combination of corticosteroid pretreatment and non-ionic media. Non-ionic media would also be preferable in cardiac patients. In patients with asthma, it would be rational to supplement steroid prophylaxis with disodium cromoglycate.

Other prophylactic regimens that may be considered in particular circumstances include combined administration of H_1 and H_2-antagonists (Ring et al. 1985), aminocaproic acid (Michel 1982; Pinet et al. 1982), and hyposensitization (Agardh et al. 1983). Greenberger and Patterson (1988), however, advise against the use of cimetidine in prophylaxis, and a severe reaction to contrast medium has been reported following prophylaxis with H_1 and H_2-antagonists and prednisolone (Böckmann et al. 1989).

In their survey among radiologists in the USA, Fischer and Doust (1972) showed that pretesting was unreliable in predicting the risk of a contrast medium reaction. A patient may have no reaction to a small dose of contrast medium and yet develop a fatal reaction to a larger dose (Ansell 1968). On the other hand, the test dose itself may even cause death. Shehadi (1975) concluded that pretesting was of no significant value, but the data in his paper actually showed that in patients with positive pretests, the risks of subsequent reactions were increased by a factor of 12 and there were two deaths (0.5 per cent mortality).

In a recent survey, Katayama and Tanaka (1988) found that a positive pretest to 1 mg contrast medium intravenously was associated with an adverse reaction in 48 per cent of cases as compared with 7.4 per cent in those with a negative pretest. A positive pretest therefore appears to be an indicator of increased risk, but it

must be emphasized that a negative pretest does not exclude the possiblity of a reaction. Yocum and others (1978) describe a more refined and safer testing procedure for use in patients with a previous history of reactions to contrast medium.

Reactions are unpredictable: they may even occur de novo in patients who have previously received contrast medium without incident. The major modes of death are cardiovascular, respiratory, and neurological. Over 90 per cent of severe and fatal reactions commence within the first 20 minutes after injection of contrast medium (Ansell and Wilkins 1987, p. 25). It is therefore important for the patient to be under close observation during this period so that effective treatment can be started immediately, to minimize mortality. A scheme for emergency treatment is essential (Ansell 1986; Ansell and Wilkins 1987, p. 25; Cohan et al. 1988), with facilities to treat cardiac arrest, pulmonary oedema, respiratory impairment, etc. Treatment will depend on the clinical manifestations but, in severe reactions, intravenous steroids are usually given on an empirical basis, with oxygen adminstration as required. van Sonnenberg and colleagues (1987) have shown that non-cardiogenic hypotensive shock usually responds best to fluid replacement, but vasopressors may occasionally be required. Subcutaneous adrenaline is primarily indicated for bronchospasm and other allergic type reactions, but caution is required to avoid cardiac arrhythmias. Intravenous aminophylline may be helpful in bronchospasm. Intravenous dilute adrenaline (1/10 000) may occasionally be indicated in the treatment of anaphylactic collapse, but extreme care is required. Vagal reactions may require intravenous atropine (0.6 mg). Intravenous antihistamines are useful in angioedema but they may aggravate hypotensive reactions. Chemotoxic convulsions require intravenous diazepam and oxygenation. Other manifestations may require appropriate treatment as clinically indicated.

Venography

Large doses of contrast medium may also be used for peripheral venography, and the systemic effects are similar to those occurring in the investigations considered above. Albrechtsson and Ollsson (1976) drew attention to the risk of venous thrombosis following venography with conventional contrast media. This is reduced with the low-osmolar media (Albrechtsson and Ollsson 1979; Lea Thomas et al. 1982, 1984). Venography also carries an increased risk when the circulation of the leg is severely compromised. If extravasation of contrast medium occurs, this may lead to skin necrosis and gangrene

(Lea Thomas 1987); this risk may be less with low osmolar media.

Intravenous cholangiography

With the introduction of the new imaging techniques there has been a considerable decline in the use of intravenous cholangiography, but some institutions still consider the technique of value (Thompson *et al.* 1984; Daly *et al.* 1987; Bar-Meir *et al.* 1989).

The range of reactions to the intravenous injection of iodipamide (Biligrafin) or ioglycamide (Biligram) for cholangiography is similar to that following the use of urographic media (see above), but reactions are frequently more severe. Other symptoms, such as liver pain or severe diarrhoea, may also occur (particularly after combined oral and intravenous media), and hepatotoxic reactions that appear to be dose-related (Scholtz *et al.* 1974; Sutherland *et al.* 1977). Finby and Blasberg (1964) suggested that there was an increased incidence of toxic reactions when intravenous cholangiography was performed immediately after an oral cholecystogram. It was also suggested that the oral cholecystogram might exert a blocking action on the excretion of iodipamide. Although there has subsequently been no absolute confirmation of their findings, it is now generally considered wiser for the examinations to be separated by an interval of several days. Other drugs found to interfere with the excretion of iodipamide or ioglycamide include phenobarbitone (Nelson *et al.* 1973), oral contraceptives (Lindgren *et al.* 1974), corticosteroids (Wangermez 1975), and tolbutamide (Klumair and Pflanzer 1977).

The hypotensive action of iodipamide is increased by rapid injection (Saltzman and Sundström 1960) and the injection should always be given slowly, taking a minimum of 5 to 10 minutes. A more prolonged infusion technique over 15 to 30 minutes is preferable. In the most recent UK survey (Ansell *et al.* 1980), the incidence of minor reactions was significantly reduced with infusions lasting longer than 20 minutes; somewhat surprisingly, no significant difference was demonstrated for intermediate and severe reactions, but the number of cases involved was small. The overall incidence of minor reactions was 1 in 13, intermediate reactions 1 in 25, and severe reactions 1 in 2300. There were no deaths in this series, but the mortality rate in the earlier survey was 1 in 5000 (Ansell 1970*a*). Shehadi (1975) quotes an incidence of 1 in 441 for severe reactions with 1 death in 3097 cases. Knutsen and Teisberg (1978) suggest that there may be an increased risk of severe reactions in patients with lymphoproliferative disorders.

Lalli (1984) analysed 28 deaths following intravenous cholangiography. The majority were attributed to cardiac arrest or pulmonary oedema. Although iodipamide and ioglycamide are used in smaller doses than urographic agents, they are significantly more toxic.

The dosage of contrast medium used in infusion cholangiography was the subject of debate. Cooperman and others (1968) did not find that there was any significant advantage in increasing the dose of 50% iodipamide used in the infusion from 20 ml to 40 ml. Nolan and Gibson (1970) claimed that a dose of 1 ml per kg of 50% iodipamide in an infusion provided improved visualization of the common bile duct and gall-bladder. This dose is unnecessarily high, however, and likely to increase the incidence of toxic reactions. Miller and colleagues (1969) showed that there is a transport maximum for the excretion of contrast medium through the liver and they have produced diagnostic cholangiograms using as little as 3–5 ml of ioglycamide in an infusion. Moreover, the use of slow infusion techniques allows the liver to excrete the cholangiographic medium more efficiently (Whitney and Bell 1972). The value of low-dose infusion cholangiography in patients with normal liver function was confirmed by Ansell and Faux (1973) using doses of 10 ml of 50% iodipamide. When jaundice is present, results are often disappointing even with higher dose levels of iodipamide, and it is unusual for the biliary tract to be visualized when the serum bilirubin exceeds 52 μmol per litre. Ultrasound examination, transhepatic cholangiography, and endoscopic retrograde cholangiopancreatography (ERCP) are now the investigations of choice in jaundiced patients.

Craft and Swales (1967) reported two cases of renal failure following iodipamide administration. The risks are probably higher in patients with liver damage, who may be unduly susceptible to hypotension. Incipient renal damage may be an aggravating factor. Mudge (1971) has shown that both iodipamide and oral cholecystographic media have a uricosuric action analogous to that of probenecid. He therefore advocated that all patients receiving these media should be adequately hydrated, to avoid the risk of uric acid crystalluria.

Blum and others (1984) reported a case of nonoliguric renal failure which occurred following oral cholecystography and intravenous cholangiography on the same day. Hyperuricaemia may have been an aggravating factor. Iodipamide also causes precipitation of Bence-Jones protein and is therefore a potential cause of renal failure in myelomatosis (Lasser *et al.* 1966).

Two newer intravenous cholangiographic media, iodoxamate (Cholovue, Endobil) and iotroxate (Biliscopin), have been introduced. They are excreted more efficiently than the older media and can be used in smaller doses. They are believed to be less toxic but the numbers of cases examined are insufficient for adequate assessment. These media may also cause slight or moderate alterations in liver function with intrahepatic cholestasis, iodoxamate being possibly more liable to do so than iotroxate (Dohmen *et al.* 1981).

Waldenström's monoclonal IgM paraproteinaemia is an absolute contraindication to intravenous cholangiography with ioglycamide or iodipamide, since Bauer and others (1974) have shown that these media react with the patient's plasma to cause a lethal gel-like intravascular precipitate. Other types of paraproteinaemia (IgG and mixed forms) do not appear to react with either ioglycamide or iodipamide in this fashion.

A more detailed discussion will be found in Ansell and Wilkins (1987, p. 209).

Media administered by other routes

Oral cholecystography

Of the current oral cholecystographic media, the most widely used are iopanoic acid (Telepaque), ipodate (Biloptin, Oragrafin) and iocetamic acid (Cholebrin). Diarrhoea or vomiting, or both, are not uncommon following their administration and may occasionally be severe enough to cause collapse or even to precipitate myocardial infarction in a predisposed individual. Other adverse effects include headache, dysuria, and skin rashes (Ansell 1976).

Tishler and Gold (1969) found that a slight transient increase in serum creatinine commonly followed oral cholecystography, and that there might also be a false-positive sulphosalicylic acid test for protein. Bunamyodil (Orabilix) has been incriminated as a cause of renal failure, and the use of large doses appeared to be a major factor (Setter *et al.* 1963). The majority of cases of renal failure following oral cholecystography have been due to this medium. Schiro and others (1971), however, have reported a case of transient renal failure after the administration of 6 g of iopanoic acid. Cholecystographic media have a uricosuric action, and it is therefore important to ensure that the patient is adequately hydrated in order to avoid the risk of uric acid crystalluria (Mudge 1971). In the cases of renal failure following oral cholecystography described by Teplick and others (1965), the risk appeared to be higher in patients with liver disease. Oral cholecystographic media should not be administered in the presence of jaundice. There is commonly a slight rise in serum bilirubin following oral cholecystography, and the bromsulphthalein (BSP) retention test is also increased (Bolt *et al* 1961; Monroe and Longmore 1966). Cholecystographic media are excreted in breast milk and the examination is probably best avoided during lactation (Nelson 1979).

The physiological factors influencing the absorption and excretion of oral cholecystographic media have been comprehensively reviewed by Berk and others (1974, 1983). It is probable that drugs that influence liver function will affect the excretion of cholecystographic media. Experimental work in dogs by Nelson and others (1973) has shown that pretreatment with phenobarbitone increases the excretion of iopanoate in the bile, presumably as a result of enzyme induction. The excretion of iodipamide, on the other hand, is decreased by this procedure.

Because of their relatively slow excretion, the oral cholecystographic media may cause elevation of serum protein-bound iodine levels for up to 3 or 4 months, but the serum butanol-extractable iodine usually returns to within normal limits in 1 month. Jacobsson and Saltzman (1971) have reviewed the effects of the various iodinated contrast media on serum iodine levels. Clinical and experimental studies suggest that the liberation of iodine from cholecystographic media may actually produce minor alterations of thyroid function for up to 3 months after administration, causing a slight degree of thyroid suppression in euthyroid individuals (Constantinescu *et al.* 1973) and increased hormonal synthesis in cases of thyroid adenoma (Mahlstedt and Joseph 1973). Fairhurst and Naqvi (1975) have reported two cases of frank thyrotoxicosis after oral cholecystography. Thrombocytopenic purpura may occur as a rare complication of oral cholecystography: at least five cases have been described (Hysell *et al.* 1977; Curradi *et al.* 1981; Insauti *et al.* 1983). There appears to be increased destruction of the platelets by an immunological factor in the serum that combines with the contrast medium to cause platelet lysis.

Alimentary tract

Barium sulphate

Barium sulphate is insoluble and is used in an aqueous suspension. It has hitherto been regarded as a relatively innocuous substance when administered in the form of a barium meal, but recently there have been reports of several deaths after accidental aspiration of large quantities of high-density barium used for double-contrast examinations in elderly debilitated patients with disordered swallowing, particularly when this is due to neurological causes (Ansell and Wilkins 1987, p. 218; Gray *et al.* 1989). Accidental inhalation of gas-forming granules of Carbex may give rise to laryngeal spasm (Mills 1990).

It has recently been recognized that barium examinations may rarely cause allergic reactions varying in severity from erythema or periorbital oedema to loss of consciousness with severe anaphylactic collapse and generalized urticaria. It has been suggested that this may be due to one or more of the additives used in the barium suspension, as, for example, the preservative methyl parabens (Schwartz *et al.* 1984). Gelfand and others (1985) suggested that glucagon may be responsible for some cases. In a survey of 106 reactions by Janower (1986), however, only 11 patients had received glucagon, but most reactions occurred with double-contrast techniques. Feczo and associates (1989) reported a fatal hypersensitivity reaction in an asthmatic patient during a barium enema.

Thick barium may precipitate obstruction in an oesophageal stricture (Ansell and Wilkins 1987, p. 219).

Constipation is common after barium meals or barium enemas (Smith *et al.* 1988); patients should be warned of this and should be advised to take a laxative if appropriate. Barium meals should not be performed if there is any possibility of large bowel obstruction, since absorption of water in the colon may cause inspissation of the barium and may thereby convert a subacute to an acute obstruction. In elderly patients without any organic obstruction, there is still sometimes prolonged stasis of barium in the colon for 4–6 weeks after a barium meal, and lactulose appears to be useful in clearing the colon of barium in these cases (Prout *et al.* 1972). Barium retained in the appendix may rarely form an obstructing faecolith and cause acute appendicitis (Young 1958). Prolonged retention of barium may occur in the distal loop as a result of barium enemas in colostomy patients (Ansell and Wilkins 1987, p. 227). In small bowel lesions there is little risk of an obstruction being aggravated by barium, since the large amount of fluid present usually prevents inspissation, but impaction of barium has been reported in the small bowel in an infant with cystic fibrosis (Fischer and Nice 1984). Toxic dilatation of the colon may be aggravated by a barium enema (Ansell and Wilkins 1987, p. 233).

Perforation is a rare but serious hazard of barium enema examinations. In the majority of cases reported in the literature, a self-retaining catheter had been used. Rectal biopsy preceding a barium enema may also contribute to perforation. Intraperitoneal perforation is associated with severe pain and collapse, but a large extraperitoneal perforation may initially cause few symptoms. After recovery from shock, the patient may appear deceptively well in the early stages, but unex-

pected deterioration and death frequently occur approximately 12 hours later (Ansell 1976). In a series of cases with perforation following barium enema, analysed by Zheutlin and others (1952), the mortality of cases treated surgically was 47 per cent, while in patients treated conservatively it was 58 per cent. Faecal contamination of the peritoneum is an important aggravating factor, but studies by Nahrwold and others (1971) in dogs have shown that even sterile barium sulphate causes severe peritoneal irritation, with outpouring of fluid into the peritoneal cavity causing hypovolaemia. The prognosis in these animals was markedly improved by early and continued administration of large volumes of intravenous fluids. Gardiner and Miller (1973) successfully used this approach in four patients with perforation following a barium enema. Residual barium in the peritoneum eventually causes fibrogranulomatous changes and may give rise to recurrent small bowel obstruction or ureteral occlusion (Zheutlin *et al.* 1952; Herrington 1966). Barium granuloma in the rectum, due to extraperitoneal leakage, may present as an indurated ulcer or stricture resembling carcinoma (Lull *et al.* 1971)

Retroperitoneal emphysema following double-contrast enema appears to have a less serious prognosis and may resolve with conservative therapy (Ansell and Wilkins 1987, p. 233).

Venous intravasation of barium may rarely occur during barium enema examinations and is usually associated with a high mortality due to pulmonary embolism of barium but occasional patients have survived (Ansell and Wilkins 1987, p. 237).

ECG abnormalities commonly occur during barium enema examinations, particularly in the elderly or in patients with heart disease (Eastwood 1972).

Le Frock and others (1975) showed that transient bacteraemia may occur after barium enemata. This may be important in patients with valvular disease or prostheses, or in those with immune deficiency (Hammer 1977).

Reports in the French literature suggest that a barium encephalopathy may, rarely, occur following prolonged stasis of barium in the bowel or after intraperitoneal rupture of a barium enema (Dupuy *et al.* 1980; Deixonne *et al.* 1983). Fukuda and co-workers (1989) reported a non-hepatic hyperammonaemic encephalopathy following a rectal rupture during a barium enema. They suggested that this might be due to bacterial production of ammonia.

Gastrografin

Gastrografin is a 76% aqueous solution of sodium and methylglucamine diatrizoate with 0.1% of the wetting agent Tween 80. Originally the main indication for its use was in the investigation of suspected perforation. Gastrografin has an osmolarity of 1900 milliosmols per litre, approximately six times that of normal plasma (Harris *et al.* 1964). This hypertonicity has a marked cathartic effect on the gastrointestinal tract. This can result in a severe hypovolaemia, which can be particularly serious in cases where the plasma volume is initially low — in, for example, dehydrated or malnourished children. Collapse may also occur in debilitated adults. Somewhat surprisingly in view of the cathartic action of Gastrografin, it appears possible that its administration postoperatively may occasionally be the cause of ileus (Davies and Williams 1971). Animal experiments suggest that administration of Gastrografin adversely affects the prognosis in intestinal ischaemia (Stordahl *et al.* 1989). Water-soluble contrast media may be absorbed if there has been a perforation or an area of intestinal ischaemia (Hay and Cant 1990). Hypersensitivity reactions may also occur (Ansell and Wilkins 1987, p. 227). Care should be taken to ensure that Gastrografin is not inhaled, since its hyperosmolar action may cause the onset of pulmonary oedema (Chiu and Gambach 1974; Ansell 1986).

Dilute solutions of Gastrografin are frequently used to opacify the bowel during abdominal CT. The low-osmolar media are now preferable to Gastrografin for oral examination of the gastrointestinal tract. There is still some risk if they are inhaled (Rust *et al.* 1982) but this is less than with Gastrografin. The adverse effects due to hypertonic media in the gastrointestinal tract are also reduced. There is less dilution of the low-osmolar media during the passage through the bowel, so that the small intestine and colon can be well visualized and they can even be used in suspected colonic obstruction in appropriate circumstances.

The hyperosmolar property of Gastrografin has been used with advantage in the non-operative treatment of uncomplicated meconium ileus: a high Gastrografin enema is administered under fluoroscopic control, and large volumes of fluid are drawn into the bowel, loosening the viscid meconium and allowing it to be passed per rectum. As with oral Gastrografin, this may cause hypovolaemia, with an increase in haemocrit and serum osmolality and a profound reduction in cardiac output. Acute hypomagnesaemia has also been reported (Godson *et al.* 1988). It is, therefore, important that the infant should be adequately hydrated before the procedure. Additional intravenous fluids should be administered during the examination, and the water balance should be monitored for several hours (Rowe *et al.* 1971). Gastrografin enemata have also been used in adults to treat

chronic constipation, but a case of caecal perforation has been reported due to overdistension resulting from the hyperosmolar action of retained medium (Seltzer and Jones 1978). Inflammatory changes have been reported in the colonic mucosa following prolonged retention of a diatrizoate enema (Creteur *et al.* 1983).

Ross (1972) has shown that acid gastric juice causes the precipitation of diatrizoate, so that Gastrografin may, rarely, form a dense precipitate in the stomach. Gallitano and others (1976) have also reported precipitation of diatrizoate following stasis in an achlorhydric stomach. It is therefore preferable to aspirate any retained Gastrografin after the examination, when it is possible to do so. Precipitation of diatrizoate has also occurred within the intragastric balloon of a Sengstaken–Blakemore tube, preventing the tube from being withdrawn (Hugh *et al.* 1970).

Endoscopic and percutaneous cholangiography

Acute pancreatitis is an occasional complication of ERCP. An analysis by Hamilton and others (1983) suggests that multiple injections of contrast medium with opacification of the pancreatic duct are relevant factors. Significant quantities of contrast medium may be absorbed after ERCP and facilities should be available to treat contrast media reactions (Sable *et al.* 1983). Kone and colleagues (1986) reported three cases of acute renal failure related to the use of contrast medium for the purpose of percutaneous transhepatic cholangiographic examination.

Bronchography

Iodized oil (Lipiodol) is now rarely used for bronchography. Propyliodone (Dionosil), a derivative of diodone, is available as either an aqueous or an oily preparation. It is generally held that aqueous Dionosil is more irritant than the oily suspension, but in a comparison of the two media (Walker and Ma 1971) this was not confirmed. The aqueous preparation provided better coating of the proximal bronchi, whereas with the oily preparation there was more peripheral filling. Mild pyrexial reactions were not uncommon and appeared to be related to the degree of peripheral filling and retention of contrast medium in the lungs. In more severe cases, a pneumonic reaction may occur. This is occasionally associated with an eosinophilia, suggesting an allergic type of reaction. Wardman and others (1983) reported three severe delayed pneumonic reactions to Dionosil after bronchograms performed under general anaesthesia. McAlister (1989) reported a death from respiratory failure where

Dionosil that had been heated in an autoclave was used for bilateral bronchography under general anaesthesia. Heating of the medium should be avoided. Dionosil remaining in the tissues is hydrolysed with the liberation of diodone. Although this is irritant, it is absorbed. Absorption of diodone from the lung may rarely cause allergic-type reactions such as skin rashes.

In a series of paediatric bronchograms, Robinson and colleagues (1971) noted segmental collapse as a complication in 45 per cent of cases. occurring more commonly when aqueous contrast media had been used. Collapse was also more common when halothane and oxygen had been used as the anaesthetic agent. This appeared to be due to the highly diffusible nature of the gas, which was apparently absorbed in the lungs faster than it could be replaced. The presence of a partial bronchial block by contrast medium would enhance this effect. Collapse was also more common in asthmatic children. Bronchial block due to bronchospasm may also occur when bronchography is being performed under local anaesthesia in adult asthmatics, and intravenous aminophylline should be available to treat it (Beales and Saxton 1968).

Transient changes in lung function may occur after bronchography, owing to retention of contrast medium in the bronchi. Lung function usually returns to normal within 24 hours, but after bilateral bronchograms the diffusing capacity may be impaired for up to 72 hours, so that chest operations are best deferred for at least 3 days after bronchography (Bhargava and Woolf 1967).

Bronchography may be performed following fibreoptic bronchoscopy by injecting Dionosil through the suction channel of the bronchoscope. Goldman and co-workers (1987) have shown that this can produce marked arterial oxygen desaturation, particularly after bilateral bronchograms. Morcos and others (1989) have used iotrolan, a new non-ionic dimer, for bronchography through the fibreoptic bronchoscope. This is more fluid than Dionosil and is less likely to block the suction channel. It also appears to cause less arterial oxygen desaturation. One patient receiving a large volume of iotrolan had moderately severe nausea and vomiting for several hours.

When the cricothyroid route is used for bronchography, Dionosil may be accidentally injected into the soft tissues of the neck. There are often no immediate symptoms, but after a period varying from a few hours to 2 days a chemical inflammatory response may develop, with severe dysphagia and pain on movement of the neck. If untreated, this may last for 2 weeks. A short course of steroids with antibiotic cover may, however, produce dramatic relief of symptoms (Zucherman and Jacobson 1962).

Death during bronchography is rare. The commonest single cause is probably overdosage of local anaesthetic.

Lymphography

The complications of lymphography have been reviewed by Macdonald (1987). Iodized oils are usually used as contrast media. They can cause iodism or allergic reactions. Allergic reactions to the patent blue violet dye injected prior to the lymphangiogram to enable the lymphatics to be visualized may also occur. This dye causes incidental blue discolouration of the skin and urine. Extravasation of contrast medium into the skin may rarely cause a delayed dermatitis. Swelling of the limb may occur after lymphatic obstruction.

There is inevitably some degree of pulmonary oil embolism after lymphography, causing some impairment of pulmonary function. This is usually symptomless but it may be a major hazard if the patient has pre-existing poor lung function. Operations and anaesthesia may be poorly tolerated in the immediate post-lymphography period. Oil embolism may also cause a chemical pneumonitis. The risk of cerebral oil embolism is increased if lymphography is performed shortly after radiotherapy to the lungs.

Mild hypothyroidism has occurred after lymphography (Heidemann et al. 1982).

Myelography, cisternography, and ventriculography

Myelography with iophendylate (Myodil, Pantopaque) may occasionally be followed by evidence of an aseptic meningeal reaction with pyrexia, headache, and photophobia (Curtin 1971). There may be a lymphocytosis in the cerebrospinal fluid, with elevated protein and a low sugar content. Symptoms may appear shortly after the examination, or may be delayed for 2 or 3 weeks or even longer. Systemic steroid therapy appears to be helpful in treating these cases. Mason and Raaf (1962) reported a rare case of progressive neurological disease leading to death due to an extensive adhesive arachnoiditis. Howland and Curry (1966) showed that a mixture of blood and iophendylate in the cerebrospinal fluid (CSF) may produce a severe arachnoiditis, and it is therefore probably inadvisable to inject this medium in the presence of a bloody CSF. Retained iophendylate by itself usually causes a milder arachnoid reaction which may or may not be associated with clinical signs (Bergeron et al. 1971). In a review of 111 cases of myelography with iophendylate, Keogh (1974) found that severe pain in the sacrum and buttocks occurred in 12.6 per cent of the patients. Severe headache has been reported due to iophendylate in the cisterna magna in the hypophyseal region (Avrahami and Cohn 1982). In the USA, it was customary to remove as much as possible of the iophendylate at the conclusion of the examination. In the UK, where smaller volumes were used, it was usual to rely on spontaneous absorption of the medium, which takes place slowly over a period of years. Elevation of the serum protein-bound iodine may persist for as long as 10 years after a myelogram (White 1972). Lieberman and others (1976) reported a case of chronic urticaria caused by retained iophendylate. The preparation has now fallen into disuse for myelography and is currently the subject of litigation in relation to arachnoiditis.

Ionic water-soluble media such as diatrizoate are extremely toxic in the subarachnoid space and are liable to cause convulsions that may be fatal. Accidental intrathecal injection of ionic media should be treated by lavage of the subarachnoid space with isotonic saline (McCleery and Lewtas 1966; Tartiere et al. 1989).

A dimer of iothalamate, methylglucamine iocarmate (Dimer-X), was briefly used for sacroradiculography but required special precautions to ensure that it did not come into contact with the spinal cord itself to avoid possible convulsive effects. Clonic muscle spasms following Dimer-X radiculography have, rarely, caused fractures (Eastwood et al. 1978). Neurological changes due to disc herniation may also be aggravated by radiculography, causing a cauda equina syndrome (Perrigot et al. 1976).

Metrizamide (Amipaque) was the first non-ionic contrast medium to be used for myelography. This had a much reduced epileptogenic activity and could therefore be used for lumbar myelography (Dugstad and Eldevik 1977), thoracic myelography (Skalpe and Sortland 1977), or cervical myelography (Amundsen 1977). It has also been used in low concentration for examining the basal cisterns (Robertson et al. 1977). The commonest adverse effects of intrathecal metrizamide are headaches, nausea, and vomiting. These usually occur several hours after the examination when the contrast medium is in contact with the cerebral hemispheres. These adverse effects are therefore more frequent after cervical myelography or cisternography, and the incidence is related to the amount of contrast medium entering the cranial cavity. Other less common adverse effects include dizziness, increased pain, hypotension, paraesthesiae, myoclonia, weakness of the arms or legs, disturbances of micturition, meningism, and allergic reactions.

An unusual psychiatric syndrome with transient confusion and disorientation occurs in a few patients following metrizamide myelography (Sortland et al. 1977; Gelmers 1979). In some cases, this has been associated with asterixis or dysphasia (Smith and Laguna 1980; Vincent 1980). Reversible visual defects and auditory syndromes have also been reported (Leavengood et al. 1981; Hauge and Falkenberg 1982). In rare instances, there have been persisting neurological syndromes following myelography with metrizamide (Bastow and Goodwin-Austin 1979; Kelly et al. 1980; Davis et al. 1982). A number of epileptiform attacks have occurred following metrizamide, particularly in patients with a history of epilepsy. Buchman and others (1987) have reviewed the neurological complications of metrizamide myelography. Non-convulsive absence status epilepticus with confusion and disorientation responds dramatically to intravenous diazepam (Obeid et al. 1988). Latack and colleagues (1984) reported a case of hyperthermia after metrizamide myelography.

Lundervold and Sortland (1977) have monitored the electroencephalogram in patients undergoing examination with metrizamide. In 13 per cent of cases there were minor non-specific changes, but in 4 per cent there were more marked abnormalities believed to be due to a direct toxic action of metrizamide on the cerebral cortex. Metrizamide may also be used for ventriculography; indeed, somewhat higher concentrations are tolerated within the ventricular cavity, providing escape into the subarachnoid space is avoided (Gonsett 1977). The incidence of cerebral complications due to metrizamide myelography is related to the amount of contrast medium that enters the cranium. Computed tomography shows that this is absorbed into the surface of the cerebral cortex. There may also be slight cerebral oedema (Cala 1981). Metrizamide causes inhibition of the enzyme hexokinase and it has been suggested that it may interfere with glucose metabolism in the brain (Bertoni et al. 1981).

Postmyelographic reactions are more common in women (Maley 1989). Steiner and associates (1986) found an increased incidence of complications after metrizamide myelography in diabetics while Gelmers (1984) reported a transitory exacerbation of systemic lupus erythematosus following metrizamide myelography.

Ahlgren (1973) showed that adhesive arachnoiditis was not uncommon after use of Dimer-X. Metrizamide, on the other hand, does not appear to cause arachnoiditis in clinical use, although Haughton and others (1977) have shown that, at higher concentrations, it may cause arachnoiditis in monkeys. The risk of this experimental metrizamide arachnoiditis is not increased by the presence of blood in the CSF. A bloody CSF need not therefore be a contraindication to myelography with metrizamide (Haughton and Ho 1982). Arachnoiditis was at one time regarded as an incidental finding of relatively little importance, but analysis by Ahlgren (1980) has shown that it can be a significant cause of late symptoms such as persistent backache.

Much of the literature on water-soluble myelography has been based on the use of metrizamide but this has now largely been replaced by the newer non-ionic media iopamidal and iohexol. These have produced fewer adverse effects than metrizamide and they do not so far appear to have given rise to the psychiatric syndromes, but slight EEG changes may occur even with the newer media (Drayer *et al.* 1984; Hindmarsh *et al.* 1984). Mood and cognitive changes are less frequent with iopamidol or iohexol than with metrizamide (Hammeke *et al.* 1984; Ratcliff *et al.* 1986). In a recent comparison of iopamidol and iohexol by Davies and colleagues (1989), there was a slightly higher incidence of headache and delayed adverse effects with iopamidol. Computed tomography of the brain following iopamidol myelography shows penetration of the contrast medium into the cortex similar to that occurring with metrizamide (Drayer *et al.* 1983). Seizures have been reported in a very few patients following myelography with iopamidol (Carella *et al.* 1982; Lipman *et al.* 1983).

A liberal fluid intake is believed to reduce postmyelographic complications but in a case of encephalopathy with confusion and disorientation reported by Donaghy and others (1985) there was evidence of dilutional hyponatraemia and it seems that water intoxication may have been a contributing factor.

Kendall (1989) in a review of 634 paediatric myelograms draws attention to the risk of mechanical factors causing an increase in focal neurological signs of spinal cord tumours. Where available, magnetic resonance imaging is preferable if an intraspinal mass is suspected.

Iotrolan is a new non-ionic dimer which is isotonic with cerebrospinal fluid (Hoffman *et al.* 1987). This new medium is currently being evaluated.

References

Agardh, C-D., Arner, B., Ekholm, S., and Boijsen, E. (1983). Desensitisation as a means of preventing untoward reactions to ionic contrast media. *Acta Radiol. [Diagn.]* (Stockh.) 24, 235.

Ahlgren, P. (1973). Long term side effects after myelography with water soluble contrast media: Conturax, Conray meglumin 282 and Dimer-X. *Neuroradiology* 6. 206.

Ahlgren, P. (1980). Early and late side effects of water soluble contrast media for myelography and cisternography: a short review. *Invest. Radiol.* 15 (suppl. 6), S264.

Albrechtsson, U. and Ollsson, C-G. (1976). Thrombotic side-effects of lower-limb phlebography. *Lancet* i, 723.

Albrechtsson, U. and Ollsson, C-G. (1979). Thrombosis following phlebography with ionic and non-ionic media. *Acta Radiol. [Diagn.]* (Stockh.) 20, 46.

Amundsen, P. (1977). Metrizamide in cervical myelography. Survey and present state. *Acta Radiol. [Diagn.]* (Stockh.) 355 (suppl.) 314.

Andrews, E.J. (1976). The vagus reaction as a possible cause of severe complications of radiological procedures. *Radiology* 121, 1.

Ansell, G. (1968). A national survey of radiological complications interim report. *Clin. Radiol.* 19, 175.

Ansell, G.(1970*a*). Adverse reactions to contrast agents: scope of problem. *Invest. Radiol.* 5, 374.

Ansell, G. (1970*b*). Fatal overdose of contrast medium in infants. *Br. J. Radiol.* 43, 395.

Ansell, G. (ed.) (1976). *Complications in diagnostic radiology.* Blackwell, Oxford.

Ansell, G. (1986). *Notes on radiological emergencies* (3rd edn). Blackwell, Oxford.

Ansell, G. (1988). Radiological contrast media and radiopharmaceuticals. In *Meyler's side effects of drugs* (11th edn) (ed. M.N.G. Dukes), p. 961. Elsevier, Amsterdam.

Ansell, G. and Faux, P.A. (1973). Low-dose infusion cholangiography. *Clin. Radiol.* 24, 95.

Ansell, G. and Wilkins, R.A. (1987). *Complications in diagnostic imaging* (2nd edn). Blackwell Scientific, Oxford.

Ansell, G., Tweedie, M.C., West, C.R., Evans. P., and Couch, L. (1980). The current status of reactions to intravenous contrast media. *Invest. Radiol.* 15 (suppl. 6). S32.

Anzola, G.P., Capra, R., Magoni, M., and Vignolo, L.A. (1986). Myasthenic crisis during intravenous iodinated contrast injection. *Ital. J. Neurol. Sci.* 7, 273.

Armour, T.E., McClennan, B.L., and Glazer, H.S. (1986). Pancreatic mumps: a transient reaction to IV contrast media (case report). *AJR* 147, 188.

Aspelin, P. (1983). Personal communication.

Aspelin, P. and Schmid-Schonbein, H. (1978). Effect of ionic and non-ionic contrast media on red cell aggregation in-vitro. *Acta Radiol. [Diagn.]* (Stockh.) 19, 766.

Assem, E-S.K., Bray, K., and Dawson, P. (1983). The release of histamine from human basophils by radiological contrast agents. *Br. J. Radiol.* 56, 647.

Avrahami, E. and Cohn, D.F. (1982). Zur Problem der post-myelographischen Kopfschmerzen. *Schweiz. Arch. Neurol. Neurochir. Psychiatr.* 130, 157.

Bar-Meir, S., Ramsby, G.R., and Conn, H.O. (1989). Meglumine iodoxamate (Cholovue) in the cholangiographic visualization of the biliary tree in cirrhosis. A double blind diagnostic trial. *Clin. Trials J.* 26, 238.

Barshay, M.E., Kaye, J.H., Goldman, R., and Coburn, J.W. (1973). Acute renal failure in diabetic patients after intravenous infusion pyelography. *Clin. Nephrol.* 1, 35.

Bastow, M. and Goodwin-Austin, R.B. *(1979).* Cervical myelopathy after metrizamide myelography. *Br. Med. J.* ii, 1262.

Bauer, K., Tragi, K.H., and Bauer, G. (1974). Intravasale Denaturierung von Plasmaproteinen bei einer IgM-Para-proteinamie, ausgelöst durch ein intravenös verabreichtes lebergängiges Röntgenkontrastmittel. *Wien. Klin. Wochenschr.* 86, 766.

Beales, J.S.M. and Saxton, H.M. (1968). The radiographic demonstration of bronchospasm and its relief by aminophylline. *Br. J. Radiol.* 41, 899.

Benear, J.B., Vannata, J.B., Hosty, T.A., and Hughes, W.L. (1985). Contrast-induced seizure associated with thrombotic thrombocytopenic purpura: case report. *Arch. Intern. Med.* 145, 363.

Benotti, J.R. (1988). The comparative effects of ionic versus nonionic agents in cardiac catheterization. *Invest. Radiol.* (suppl. 2), S366.

Berdon, W.E., Schwartz, R.H., Becker, J., and Baker, D. (1969). Tamm–Horsfall proteinuria. Its relationship to prolonged nephrogram in infants and children and to renal failure in adults with multiple myeloma. *Radiology* 92, 714.

Berger, R.E., Gomez, L.S., and Mallette, L.E. (1982). Acute hypocalcaemic effects of clinical contrast media injection. *AJR* 138, 283.

Bergeron, R.T., Rumbaugh, C.L., Fang, H., and Cravioto, H. (1971). Experimental Pantopaque arachnoiditis in the monkey. *Radiology* 99, 95.

Bergman, L.A., Ellison, M.R., and Dunea, G. (1968). Acute renal failure after drip-infusion pyelography. *N. Engl. J. Med.* 279, 177.

Berk, R.N., Leopold, G.R., and Fordren, J.S. (1983). Imaging of the gallbladder. In *Advances in internal medicine*, Vol. 28, p. 387. Year Book Medical Publishers, Chicago.

Berk, R.N., Loeb, P.M., Goldberger, L.E., and Sokoloff, J. (1974). Oral cholecystography with iopanoic acid. *N. Engl. J. Med.* 290, 204.

Bernstein, E.F. (1970). Discussion. In Symposium on Contrast media toxicity. *Invest. Radiol.* 5, 416.

Bernstein, E.F., Palmer, J.D., Aaberg, T.A., and Davis, R.L. (1961). Studies of the toxicity of Hypaque 90% following rapid intravenous injection. *Radiology* 76, 88.

Bertoni, J.M., Schwatzman, R.J., van Horn, G., and Partin, J. (1981). Asterixis and encephalopathy following metrizamide myelography: investigations into possible mechanisms and review of the literature. *Ann. Neurol.* 9, 366.

Bhargava, R.K. and Woolf, C.R. (1967). Changes in diffusing capacity after bronchography. *Am. Rev. Resp. Dis.* 96, 827.

Binnie, C.D., Bernstein, D.C., Booth, A.E., McCaul, I.R., Margerison, J.H., and Scott, J.F. (1971). Clinical and electroencephalographic sequelae of carotid angiography. *Acta Radiol. [Diagn.]* (Stockh.) 6, 626.

Bjork, L. (1968). The effect of cardiac catheterization and angiocardiography on the coagulation activity of the blood. *AJR* 102, 441.

Blum, M., Liron, M., and Aviram, A. (1984). Acute renal failure following cholecystography. *Am. J. Proctol. Gastroenterol. Colon. Rect. Surg.* 35, 11.

Böckman, S., Bodman, K.F., and Schuster, H.P. (1989). Anaphylaktischer Schock nach Röntgenkontrastmittel trotz Prämedikation mit Ausbildung eines akuten Myokardinfarktes. *Intensivmedizin Notfallmedizin* 26, 385.

Bolt, R.J., Dillon, R.J., and Pollard, H.M. (1961). Interference with bilirubin excretion by a gall bladder dye (Bunamiodyl). *N. Engl. J. Med.* 265, 1043.

Bolz, K-D., Bolle, R., Due, J., and Østerud, B. (1986). Severe contrast medium reaction after iohexol (Omnipaque) with in vivo proven monocyte stimulation. *Tidsskr. Nor. Laegeforen.* 106, 2493.

Brown, M. and Battle, J.D. (1964). The effect of urography in renal function in patients with multiple myeloma. *Can. Med. Assoc. J.* 91, 786.

Buchman, A.S., Klawans, H.L., and Russell, E.J. (1987). Review: metrizamide and its neurological complications *Clin. Neuropharmacol.* 10, 1.

Burchardt, C.P., Flenker, H., and Schoop, H.J. (1981). Todlicher Kontrastmittelzwischenfall bei unbehandeltem Morbus Waldenström. *Dtsch. Med. Wochenschr.* 106, 1223.

Cala, L.A. (1981). Cerebral absorption of metrizamide. *Lancet* ii, 922.

Carella, A., Federico, F., Di Cuonzo, P., Vinjau, E., and Lamberti, P. (1982). Adverse side effects of metrizamide and iopamidol in myelography. *Neuroradiology* 22, 247.

Carr, D.H. (1988). *Contrast media.* Churchill Livingstone, Edinburgh.

Catterall, J.R., Ferguson, R.J., and Miller, H.C. (1981). Intravascular haemolysis with acute renal failure after angiocardiography. *Br. Med. J.* 282, 779.

Caulfield, J.B., Zir, L., and Harthorne, J.W. (1975). Blood calcium levels in the presence of angiographic contrast material. *Circulation* 52, 119.

Chagnac, Y., Hadani, M., and Goldhammer, Y. (1985). Myasthenic crisis after intravenous administration of iodinated contrast agent. *Neurology* 35, 1219.

Chamberlin, W.H., Stockman, G.D., and Wray, N.P. (1979). Shock and non-cardiogenic pulmonary edema following meglumine diatrizoate for intravenous pyelography. *Am. J. Med.* 67, 684.

Chandra, R. and Abraham, J. (1973). Preliminary studies on in vitro and in vivo effects of 50% Hypaque on coagulation in man. *Angiology* 24,199.

Chang, J.C., Lee, D., and Gross, H.M. (1989). Acute thrombocytopenia after IV administration of a radiographic contrast medium. *AJR* 152, 947.

Chiu, C.L. and Gambach, R.R. (1974). Hypaque pulmonary edema. A case report. *Radiology* 111, 91.

Cochran, S.T., Wong, W.W., and Roe, D.J. (1983). Predicting angiography induced acute renal function impairment: clinical risk model. *AJR* 141, 1027.

Cohan, R.H., Dunnick, N.R., and Bashore, T.M. (1988). Review article. Treatment of reactions to radiographic contrast material. *AJR* 151, 263.

Cohen, L.S., Kokko, J.P., and Williams, W.H. (1969). Haemolysis and haemoglobinuria following angiography. *Radiology* 92, 329.

Constantinescu, A., Negoescu, I., Don, M., and Heltianu, C. (1973). Effects of administration of some indigenous radiologic contrast media upon the thyroid function. Clinical and experimental studies. *Rev. Roum. Endocrinol.* 10, 49.

Cooperman, L.R., Rossiter, S.B., Reimer, G.W., and Ng, E. (1968). Infusion cholangiography. Thirteen years experience with 1600 cases. *AJR* 104, 880.

Craft, I.L. and Swales, J.D. (1967). Renal failure after cholangiography. *Br. Med. J.* ii, 736.

Creteur, V., Douglas, D., Galante, M., and Margulis, A.R. (1983). Inflammatory colonic changes produced by contrast material. *Radiology* 147, 77.

Curradi, F., Abbritti, G., and Gray, J.M. (1981). Acute thrombocytopenia following oral cholecystography with iopanoic acid. *Clin. Toxicol.* 18, 221.

Curtin, J.A. (1971). Pantopaque hypersensitivity meningitis. *Ann. Intern. Med.* 74, 838.

Cwynarski, M.T. and Saxton, H.M. (1969). Urography in myelomatosis. *Br. Med. J.* i, 486.

Daly, J., Fitzgerald, T., and Simpson, C.J. (1987). Pre-operative intravenous cholangiography as an alternative to routine operative cholangiography in elective cholecystectomy. *Clin. Radiol.* 38, 161.

Davies, A.M., Evans, N., and Chandy, J. (1989). Outpatient lumbar radiculography — comparison of iopamidol and iohexol and a literature review. *Br. J. Radiol.* 62, 716.

Davies, N.P. and Williams, J.A. (1971). Tubeless vagotomy and pyloroplasty and the 'Gastrografin test'. *Am. J. Surg.* 122, 368.

Davies, P., Roberts, M.B., and Roylance, J. (1975). Acute reaction to urographic contrast media. *Br. Med. J.* ii, 434.

Davis, C.E., Smith, C., Harris, R. (1982). Persistent movement disorder following metrizamide myelography. *Arch. Neurol.* 39, 128.

Dawson, P. (1983). Personal communication.

Dawson, P. and Trewhella, M. (1990). Intravascular contrast agents and renal failure. *Clin. Radiol.* 41, 373.

Dawson, P., Freedman, D.B., Howell, M.J., and Hine, A.L. (1984).Contrast medium induced acute renal failure and Tamm–Horsfall protein. *Br. J. Radiol.* 57, 577.

Dawson, P., Pitfield, J., and Britton, J. (1983). Contrast media and bronchospasm: a study with iopamidol. *Clin. Radiol.* 34, 227.

Dawson, P., McCarthy, P., and Allison, D.J. (1988). Non-ionic contrast agents; red cell aggregation and coagulation. *Br. J. Radiol..* 61, 963.

D'Elia, J.A., Gleason, R.E., Alday, M., Malarick, C., Godley, K., Warram, *et al.* (1982). Nephrotoxicity from angiographic contrast media: a prospective study. *Am. J. Med.* 72, 719.

Deixonne, B., Baumel, H., and Mauras, Y. (1983). Un cas de barytopéritoine avec atteinte neurologique intérêt du dosage du barium dans les liquides biologiques. *J. Chir.* (Paris) 120, 611.

Dohmen, J.P.M., Lemmens, J.A.M., and Lamers, J.J.H. (1981). A double blind comparison of meglumine iotroxate (Biliscopin) and meglumine iodoxamate (Cholovue). *Diagn. Imaging* 50, 305.

Donaghy, M., Fletcher, N.A., and Schott, G.D. (1985). Encephalopathy after iohexol myelography. *Lancet.* ii, 887.

Drayer, B.P., Allen, S., and Vassalo, C. (1984). Comparative safety of intrathecal iopamidol vs metrizamide for myelography. *Invest. Radiol.* 9 (suppl.), S 259.

Drayer, B.P., Vassalo, C., Sudilovsky, A., Luther, J.S., Wilkins, R.H., Allen, S., *et al.* (1983). A double-blind trial of iopamidol versus metrizamide for lumbosacral myelography. *J. Neurosurg.* 58, 531.

Dugstad, G. and Eldevik, P. (1977). Lumbar myelography. *Acta Radiol. [Diagn.]* (Stockh.) 355 (suppl.), 17.

Dupuy, F., Bestagne, M.H., Rodor, F., Poyen, B., and Jouglard, J. (1980). Encéphalopathie convulsive et sulfate de barium. *Therapie* 35, 447.

Eastwood, G.L. (1972). E.C.G. abnormalities associated with the barium enema. *JAMA* 219, 719.

Eastwood, J.B., Parker, B., and Reid, B.R. (1978). Bilateral central fracture dislocation of hips after myelography with meglumine iocarmate (Dimer-X). *Br. Med. J.* i, 692.

Elliott, C. and Roger, M. (1988). Acute renal failure following low osmolality radiocontrast dye. *Clin. Cardiol.* 11, 420.

Enge, I. and Edgren, J. (1989). *Patient safety and adverse events in contrast medium examinations.* Excerpta Medica international congress series 816. Elsevier, Amsterdam.

Evans, J.R., Shankel, S.W., and Cutler, R.E. (1987). Low osmolar contrast agents and nephrotoxicity. *Ann. Intern. Med.* 107, 116.

Fairhurst, B.J. and Naqvi, N. (1975). Hyperthyroidism after cholecystography. *Br. Med. J.* iii, 630.

Feczo, P.J., Simms, S.S., and Bakiri, N. (1989). Fatal hypersensitivity during a barium enema. *AJR* 153, 275.

Feigelson, H.H. and Ravin, H.A. (1965). Transverse myelitis following selective bronchial arteriography. *Radiology* 85, 663.

Feldman, H.A., Goldfarb, S., and McCurdy, D.K. (1974). Recurrent radiographic dye induced renal failure. *JAMA* 229, 72.

Finby, N. and Blasberg, G. (1964). A note on the blocking of hepatic excretion during cholangiographic study. *Gastroenterology* 46, 276.

Fischer, H.W. (1968). Hemodynamic reactions to angiographic media. A survey and commentary. *Radiology* 91, 66.

Fischer, H.W. and Cornell, S.H. (1965). The toxicity of sodium and methylglucamine salts of diatrizoate, iothalamate and metrizoate. Experimental study following carotid injection. *Radiology* 85, 1013.

Fischer, H.W. and Doust, V.L. (1972). An evaluation of pretesting in the problem of serious and fatal reactions to excretory urography. *Radiology* 103, 497.

Fischer, H.W., Reuter, S.R., and Moscow, N.P. (1968). Further toxicity studies with methylglucamine contrast agents. *Invest. Radiol.* 5, 324.

Fischer, W.W. and Nice, C.M. (1984). Barium impaction as a cause of small bowel obstruction in an infant with cystic fibrosis. Pediatr. Radiol. 14, 230.

Foda, M.T., Castillo, C.A., Corliss, R.J., McKenna, D.H., Crumpton, C.W., and Rowe, G.G. (1965). The intravascular pressure response in man to contrast substance used for angiography. *Am. J. Med. Sci.* 250, 390.

Foster, C.J., Griffin, J.F. (1987). A comparison of the incidence of cardiac arrhythmias produced by two intravenous contrast media in coronary artery disease. *Clin. Radiol.* 38, 399.

Fukuda, M., Ono, I., Takemasa, T., Fukajawa, S., and Itoh, K. (1989). A fatal case with non-hepatic hyperammonemic encephalopathy following rupture of the rectum during barium enema examination. *Shashin Igaku* 44, 2217.

Gallant, M.J. and Studley, J.G.N. (1990). Case report: delayed cardiac tamponade following accidental injection of non-ionic contrast medium into the pericardium. *Clin. Radiol.* 41, 139

Gallitano, A.L., Kondi, E.S., Phillips, E., and Ferris, E. (1976). Near-fatal hemorrhage following gastrografin studies. *Radiology* 118, 35.

Gardiner, H. and Miller, R.E. (1973). Barium peritonitis. A new therapeutic approach. *Am. J. Surg.* 125, 350.

Gassmann, W., Haferlach, T., Schmitz, N., Kayzer, W., and Loffler, H. (1983). Zur Problematik der intravenosen Urographie bei Patienten mit Plasmozytom. *Schweiz. Med. Wochenschr.* 113, 301.

Gelfand, D.W., Sowers, J.C., De Ponte, K.A., Summer, T.E., and Ott, D.J. (1985). Anaphylactic and allergic reactions during double control studies: is glucagon or barium suspension the allergen? *AJR* 144, 405.

Gelman, M.L., Rowe, J.W., Coggins, C.H., and Athanasoulis, C. (1979). Effect of an angiographic contrast medium on renal function. *Cardiovasc. Med.* 4, 313.

Gelmers, H.J. (1979). Adverse side effects of metrizamide in myelography. *Neuroradiology* 18, 119.

Gelmers, H.J. (1984). Exacerbation of systemic lupus erythematosus, aseptic meningitis and acute mental symptoms following metrizamide lumbar myelography. *Neuroradiology* 26, 65.

Gensini, G.G. and Di Giorgi, S. (1964). Myocardial toxicity of contrast agents used in angiography. *Radiology* 82, 24.

Gerber, K.H., Higgins, C.B., Yuh, Y-S., and Koziol, J.A. (1982). Regional hemodynamic and metabolic effects of ionic and non-ionic contrast media in normal and ischaemic states. *Circulation* 65, 1307.

Giammona, S.T., Lurie, P.R., and Segar, W.E. (1963). Hypertonicity following selective angiocardiography *Circulation* 28, 1096.

Godson, C., Ryan, M.P., and Brady, H.R. (1988). Acute hypomagnesaemia complicating the treatment of meconium ileus equivalent in cystic fibrosis. *Scand. J. Gastroenterol.* 23 (suppl. 143) 148.

Goldman, J.M., Currie, D.C., Morgan, A.D., and Collins, J.V. (1987). Arterial oxygen saturation during bronchography via the fibreoptic bronchoscope. *Thorax* 42, 694.

Golman, K. (1980). Discussion. *Invest. Radiol.* 15, 588.

Golman, K. and Almén, T. (1985). Contrast media induced nephrotoxicity: survey and present state. *Invest. Radiol.* (suppl. 20), S 92.

Gonsette, R.E. (1977). Ventriculography with metrizamide. *Acta Radiol. [Diagn.]* (Stockh.) 355 (suppl.), 247.

Gonsette, R.E. and Andre-Balisaux, G. (1967). La perméabilité des vaisseaux cérébraux. L'étude systématique de la tolérance des capillaires cérébraux pour les produits de contraste utilisés en artériographie. *Acta Radiol.* (Stockh.) 270 (suppl.), 228.

Gonsette, R.E. and Liesenborgh, L. (1980). New contrast media in cerebral angiography: animal experiments and preliminary clinical studies. *Invest. Radiol.* 15 (suppl. 6), S270.

Goodfellow, T., Haldstock, G.E., Brunton, F.J., and Bamforth, J. (1986). Fatal acute vasculitis after high dose urography with iohexol. *Br. J. Radiol.* 59, 620.

Grainger, R.G. (1982). Intravascular contrast media — the past, the present and the future. *Br. J. Radiol.* 55, 1.

Grainger, R.G. (1987). Annotation: Radiological contrast media. *Clin. Radiol.* 38, 3.

Grainger, R.G. and Dawson, P. (1990). Low osmolar contrast media: an appraisal (editorial). *Clin. Radiol.* 42, 1.

Gray, C., Sivaloganathan, S., and Simkins, K.C. Aspiration of high-density barium contrast medium causing acute pulmonary inflammation — report of two fatal cases in elderly women with disordered swallowing. *Clin. Radiol.* 40, 397.

Greenberger, P.A. (1984). Contrast media reactions. *J. Allergy Clin. Immunol.* 74, 600.

Greenberger, P.A. and Patterson, R. (1988). Adverse reactions to radiocontrast media. *Progr. Cardiovasc. Dis.* 31, 239.

Grollman, J.H., Liu, C.R., Astone, R.A., and Lurie, M.D. (1988). Thromboembolic complications in coronary angiography associated with the use of non-ionic contrast medium. *Cathet. Cardiovasc. Diagn.* 14, 159.

Gross, M., McDonald, H., and Waterhouse, K. (1968). Anuria following urography with meglumine diatrizoate (Renografin) in multiple myeloma. *Radiology* 90, 780.

Grunwald, M.H., Halevi, S., and Livni, E. (1985). Bullous lichen planus after intravenous pyelography. *J. Am. Acad. Dermatol.* 13, 512.

Gruskin, A.B., Oetliker, O.H., Wolfish, N.L., Gootman, N.L., Bernstein, J., and Edelman, C.M. (1970). Effects of angiography on renal function and histology in infants and piglets. *J. Pediatr.* 76, 41.

Haley, E.C. (1984). Encephalopathy following arteriography: a possible toxic effect of contrast agents. *Ann. Neurol.* 15, 100

Hamilton, I., Lintott, D.J., Rothwell, J., and Axon, A.T.R. (1983). Acute pancreatitis following endoscopic retrograde cholangiopancreatography. *Clin. Radiol.* 34, 543.

Hammeke, T.A., Haughton, V.M., Grogan, J.P., and Pfeiffer, M.F. (1984). A preliminary study of cognitive and affective alterations following intrathecal administration of iopamidol or metrizamide. *Invest. Radiol.* 19 (suppl.), S 268.

Hammer, J.L. (1977). Septicaemia following barium enema. *South. Med. J.* 70, 1361.

Harrington, G.J. and Weideman, M.P. (1965). The effect of contrast media on endothelial permeability. *Radiology* 84, 1108.

Harris, P.D., Neuhauser, E.B.D., and Gerth, R. (1964). The osmotic effect of water soluble contrast media on circulating plasma volume. *AJR* 91, 694.

Hartman, G.W., Hattery, R.R., Witten, D.M., and Williamson, B. (1982). Mortality during excretory urography: Mayo Clinic experience. *AJR* 139, 919.

Hauge, O. and Falkenberg, H. (1982). Neuropsychologic reactions and other side effects after metrizamide myelography. *Am. J. Neuroradiol.* 3, 229.

Haughton, V.M. and Ho, K-G. (1982). Effect of blood on arachnoiditis from aqueous myelographic contrast media. *AJR* 139, S69.

Haughton, V.M., Ho, K-C., Larsen, S.J., Unger, G.F., and Correa-Paz, F. (1977). Experimental production of arachnoiditis with water-soluble myelographic media. *Radiology* 123, 681.

Hay, M. and Cant, P.J. (1990). Case report: renal excretion of enteral Gastrografin in the absence of free intestinal perforation. *Clin. Radiol.* 41, 137.

Heidemann, P.H., Stubbe, P., Schurrnbrand, P., and Prindull, G. (1982). Iodine-induced hypothyroidism and goitre following Lipiodol TH Iymphangiography. *Eur. J. Pediatr.* 138, 82.

Herrington, J.L. (1966). Barium granuloma within the peritoneal cavity: ureteral obstruction 7 years after barium enema and colonic perforation. *Ann. Surg.* 164, 162.

Hesselink, J.R., Hayman, L.A., Chung, J.G., McGinnis, B.D., Davis, K.R., and Taveras, J.M. (1984). Myocardial ischaemia during intravenous DSA in patients with cardiac disease. *Radiology* 153, 577.

Heydenreich, G. and Olholm Larsen, P. (1977). Iododerma after high-dose urography in an oliguric patient. *Br. J. Dermatol.* 97, 567.

Hilal, S.K. (1966). Haemodynamic changes associated with the intra-arterial injection of contrast media. New toxicity tests and a new experimental contrast medium. *Radiology* 86, 615.

Hindmarsh, T., Ekholm, S.E., Kido, D., Sahler, L., and Sands, M. (1984). Lumbar myelography with iohexol and metrizamide a double-blind clinical trial. *Acta Radiol. [Diagn.]* (Stockh.) 25, 365.

Hobbs, B.B. (1981). Adverse reactions to intravenous contrast agents in Ontario 1975–1979. *J. Can. Assoc. Radiol.* 32, 8.

Hoffman, B., Becker, H., and Wenzel-Hora, B.I. (1987). Influence of spread and retention of iotrolan in the subarachnoid space on the side effects in myelography. *Neuroradiology* 29, 380.

Hoppe, J.O. (1959). Some pharmacological aspects of radioopaque compounds. *Ann. N.Y. Acad. Sci.* 78, 727.

Howland, W.J. and Curry, J.L. (1966). Pantopaque arachnoiditis. Experimental study of blood as potentiating agent and corticosteroids as ameliorating agent. *Acta Radiol.* (Stockh.) 5, 1032.

Hugh, T.B., Hennessy, W.B., Gunner, W., Hanks, T.J., and Eckert, G.M. (1970). Precipitation of contrast medium causing impaction of Sengstaken–Blakemore oesophageal tube. *Med. J. Aust.* 1, 60.

Hwang, M.H., Piao, Z.E., Murdock, D.K., Giardina, J.J., Pacold, I., Loeb, H.S., et al. (1989). The potential risk of thrombosis during coronary angiography using non-ionic contrast media. *Cathet. Cardiovasc. Diagn.* 16, 209.

Hysell, L.K., Hysell, J.W., and Gray, J.M. (1977). Thrombocytopenic purpura following iopanoic acid ingestion. *JAMA* 237, 361.

Iannone, L.A. (1975). Protamine–renografin chemical embolus. *Am. Heart J.* 90, 678.

Ihle, B.U., Byrnes, C.A., and Simenhoff, M.L. (1982). Acute renal failure due to interstitial nephritis from radio contrast agents. *Aust. N.Z. Med.* 12, 630.

Insauti, C.L.G., Lechin, F., and van der Digs, B. (1983). Severe thrombocytopenia following oral cholecystography. *Am. J. Hematol.* 14, 285.

Jacobson, B.F., Jorulf, H., Kalantar, M.S., and Narasimhan, D.L. (1988). Nonionic versus ionic contrast media in intravenous urography. Clinical trial in 1000 consecutive patients. *Radiology* 167, 601.

Jacobsson, L. and Saltzman, G.F. (1971). Effect of iodinated roentgenographic contrast media on butanol-extractable protein-bound and total iodine in serum. *Acta Radiol. [Diagn.]* (Stockh.) 11, 310.

Janower, M.L. (1986). Hypersensitivity reactions after barium studies of the upper and lower gastrointestinal tract. *Radiology* 161, 139.

Junck, L. and Marshall, W.H. (1986). Fatal brain edema after contrast-agent overdose. *AJNR* 7, 522.

Kaftori, J.K., Abraham, Z., and Gilhar, A. (1988). Toxic epidermal necrolysis after excretory pyelography. *Int. J. Dermatol.* 27, 346.

Kamdar, S., Weidmann, P., Makoff, D.L., and Massry, S.G. (1977). Acute renal failure following use of radiographic contrast dyes in patients with diabetes mellitus. *Diabetes* 26, 643.

Karasick, S. and Karasick, D. (1981). Acute urate nephropathy induced by Ticrynafen and exacerbated by urographic contrast medium. *Urol. Radiol.* 3, 51.

Kassner, E.G., Elguezabal, A., and Pochaczezsky, R.C. (1973). Death during intravenous urography. Overdosage symptoms in young infants. *N.Y. State J. Med.* 73, 1958.

Katayama, H. (1988). Report of the Japanese committee on the safety of contrast media. A scientific poster session presented at the Radiological Society of North America Meeting November 1988.

Katayama, H. and Tanaka, T. (1988). Clinical survey of adverse reactions to contrast media. *Invest. Radiol.* 23 (suppl. 1), S 88.

Katzberg, R.W., Morris, T.W., Schulman, G., Faillace, R.T., Boylan, L.M., Foley, M.J., et al. (1983). Reactions to intravenous contrast media. Part 1: Severe and fatal cardiovascular reactions in a canine dehydration model. *Radiology* 147, 327.

Kelly, R.E., Daroff, R.B., Sheremata, W.A., and McCormick, J.R. (1980). Unusual effects of metrizamide lumbar myelography. Constellation of aseptic meningitis, communicating hydrocephalus and Guillain–Barré syndrome. *Arch. Neurol.* 37, 588.

Kendall, B. (1989). Safety aspects and tolerability of non-ionic contrast media — subarachnoid use. In *Patient safety and adverse events in contrast media examinations* (ed. I. Enge and J. Edgren). Excerpta Medica Medical International Congress Series 816, p. 47. Elsevier, Amsterdam.

Keogh, A.J. (1974). Meningeal reactions seen with myelography. *Clin. Radiol.* 25, 361.

Kerdel, F.A., Fraker, D.L., and Haynes, H.A. (1984). Necrotising vasculitis from radiographic contrast media. *J. Am. Acad. Dermatol.* 10, 25.

Khoury, G.A. Hopper, J.C., Varghese, Z., Farrington, K., Dick, R., Irving, J.D., et al. (1983). Nephrotoxicity of ionic and non-ionic contrast material in digital vascular imaging and selective renal arteriography. *Br. J. Radiol.* 56, 631.

Kleinknecht, D., Jungers, P., and Michel, J.R. (1972). Les accidents anuriques après urographie par perfusion chez l'insuffisant rénal, en dehors du myélome. *Sem. Hop. Paris* 48, 3383.

Klumair, J. and Pflanzer. K. (1977). Der Einfluss oraler anti-diabetica (Sulphonylharnstoffe) auf die Ausscheidung intravenöser Gallenkontrastmittel. *Fortschr. Röntgenstr.* 126, 66.

Knoefel, P.K. (ed.) (1971). Radiocontrast agents. In *International encyclopedia of pharmacology and therapeutics.* Section 76, Vols 1 and 2. Pergamon, Oxford.

Knutsen, K.M. and Teisberg, P. (1978). Serious adverse reactions in intravenous cholangiography (with Biligram) in lymphoproliferative disorders. *Tidskr. Nor. Laegeforen.* 98, 328.

Koch, R.L., Byl, F.M., and Firpo, J.J. (1969). Parotid swelling with facial paralysis: complication of intravenous urography. *Radiology* 92, 1043.

Kone, B.C., Watson, A.J., Gimenez, L.F., and Kadir, S., (1986). Acute renal failure following percutaneous transhepatic cholangiography: a retrospective study. *Arch. Intern. Med.* 146, 1405.

Kovnat, P.J., Lin, K.Y., and Popky, C. (1973). Azotaemia and nephrogenic diabetes insipidus after arteriography. *Radiology* 108, 541.

Kutt, H., Verebely, K., Bang. N., Streuli, F., and McDowell, F. (1966). Possible mechanisms of complications of angiography. *Acta Radiol.* (Stockh.) 5, 276.

Lacey, J., Bober-Sorcinelli, K.E., Farber, L.R. and Guckman, M.G. (1986). Acute thrombocytopenia induced by parenteral radiographic contrast medium. *AJR* 146, 1298.

Lalli, A.F. (1980). Contrast media reactions: data analysis and hypothesis. *Radiology* 131, 1.

Lalli, A.F. (1984). Contrast media deaths. *Australas. Radiol.* 28, 133.

Lasser, E.C. (1971). Metabolic basis of contrast material toxicity. Status 1971. *AJR* 113, 415.

Lasser, E.C. (1988*a*). A general and personal perspective on contrast material research. *Invest. Radiol.* 23 (suppl. 1), S 71.

Lasser, E.C. (1988*b*). Pretreatment with corticosteroids to prevent reactions to IV contrast material: overview and implications. *AJR* 150, 257.

Lasser, E.C. (1989). Allergy and allergic-like reactions in relation to contrast media. *Patient safety and adverse events in contrast medium examinations* (ed. I. Enge and J. Edgren), p. 57. Elsevier, Amsterdam.

Lasser, E.C., Lang, J.H., and Zawadzki, Z.A. (1966). Contrast media/myeloma protein precipitates in urography. *JAMA* 198, 945.

Lasser, E.C., Lang, J.H., Hamblin, A.E., Lyon, S.G., and Howard, M. (1980). Activation systems in contrast idiosyncrasy. *Invest. Radiol.* 15 (suppl. 6), S2.

Lasser, E.C., Lang, J.H., Sovak, M., Kolb, W., Lyon, S., and Hamlin. A.E. (1977). Steroids: theoretical and experimental basis for utilization in prevention of contrast media reactions. *Radiology* 125, 1.

Lasser, E.G., Berry, C.C., Talner, L.B., Santini, L.C., Lang, E.K., and Gerber, F.H. (1987). Pretreatment with corticosteroids to alleviate reactions to intravenous contrast material. *N. Engl. J. Med.* 317, 845.

Latack, J.T., Gabrielsen, T.O., and Knake, J.E. (1984). Hyperthermia after metrizamide myelography. *AJNR* 5, 649.

Lea Thomas, M. (1987). Phlebography. In *Complications in diagnostic imaging* (2nd edn) (ed. G. Ansell), p. 288. Blackwell Scientific, Oxford.

Lea Thomas, M., Walters, H.L., and Briggs, G.M. (1982). A double blind comparative study of the tolerance of sodium and meglumine ioxaglate (Hexabrix) with meglumine iothalamate (Conray) in ascending phlebography of the leg. *Australas. Radiol.* 26, 288.

Lea Thomas, M., Keeling, F.P., Piaggio, R.B., and Treweeke, P.S. (1984). Contrast agent induced thrombophlebitis following leg phlebography: iopamidol versus meglumine iothalamate. *Br. J. Radiol.* 57, 205.

Leach, C.A. and Sunderman, F.W. (1987). Hypernickelemia following coronary arteriography caused by nickel in the radiographic contrast medium. *Ann. Cli. Lab. Sci.* 17, 137.

Leavengood, J.M., Wilson, W.B., Stears, J., and Posner J.B. (1981). Reversible visual defects following metrizamide (Amipaque) myelography. *Neurology* 31 (No. 4 Pt 2), 69.

Lee, S. and Schoen, I. (1966). Black-copper reduction reaction simulating alcaptonuria — occurrence after intravenous urography. *N. Engl. J. Med.* 275, 266.

LeFrock, J., Ellis, C.A., Klainer, A.S., and Weinstein, L. (1975). Transient bacteraemia associated with barium enema. *Arch. Intern. Med.* 135, 835.

Levin, A.R., Grossman, H., Schubert, E.T., Winchester, P., and Gilladoga, A. (1969). Effect of angiocardiography on fluid and electrolyte balance. *AJR* 105, 777.

Levin, D.C. and Baltaxe, H.A. (1972). Effect of radioopaque contrast material on left ventricular end diastolic pressure. *N.Y. State J. Med.* 72, 2619.

Lichtman, M.A., Murphy, M.S., Whitbeck, A.A, Pogal, M., and Lipchik, E.O. (1975). Acidification of plasma by the red cell due to radiographic contrast materials. *Circulation* 52, 943.

Lieberman, P., Siegle, R.L., Caplan, R.J., and Hashimoto, K. (1976). Chronic urticaria and intermittent anaphylaxis. Reaction to iophendylate. *JAMA* 236, 1495.

Lindgren, P. (1970). Haemodynamic responses to contrast media. *Invest. Radiol.* 5, 424.

Lindgren, P., Saltzman, G.F., and Zeuchner, E. (1974). Intravenous cholecystography after peroral contraceptives. A preliminary report. *Acta Radiol. [Diagn.]* (Stockh.) 15, 217.

Lipman, J.C., Wang, A-M., Brooks, R.M., and Rumbaugh, C.L. (1983). Seizure after intrathecal administration of iopamidol. *AJNR* 9, 787.

Love, L., Lind, J.A., and Olson, M.C. (1989). Persistent CT nephrogram: significance in the diagnosis of contrast nephropathy. *Radiology* 172, 125.

Lull, G., Bryne, P., and Sanowski, A. (1971). Barium sulfate granuloma of the rectum. A rare entity. *JAMA* 217, 1102.

Lundervold, A. and Engeset, A. (1976). Cerebral angiography. In *Complications in diagnostic radiology* (ed. G. Ansell), p. 151. Blackwell Scientific, Oxford.

Lundervold, A. and Sortland, O. (1977). EEG disturbances following myelography, cisternography and ventriculography with metrizamide. *Acta Radiol. [Diagn.]* (Stockh.) 355 (suppl.), 379.

McAfee, J.G. (1957). A survey of complications of abdominal aortography. *Radiology* 68, 828.

McAlister, W.H. (1989). Death associated with bronchography. Question role of heating the contrast agent. *Pediatr. Radiol.* 19, 458.

McCleery, W.N.C. and Lewtas, N.A. (1966). Subarachnoid injection of contrast medium — a complication of vertebral angiography. *Br. J. Radiol.* 39, 122.

McClennan, B.L., Kassner, E.G., and Becker, J.A. (1972). Overdose at excretory urography: toxic cause of death. *Radiology* 105, 383.

McCullough, M., Davies, P., and Richardson, R. (1989). A large trial of intravenous Conray 325 and Niopam 300 to assess immediate and delayed reactions. *Br. J. Radiol.* 62, 260.

MacDonald, J.S. (1987). Lymphography. In *Complications in diagnostic imaging* (2nd edn) (ed. G. Ansell and R.A. Wilkins), p. 300. Blackwell Scientific, Oxford.

McEvoy, J., McGeown, M.G., and Kumar, R. (1970). Renal failure after radiological contrast media. *Br. Med. J.* iv, 717.

McIvor, J., Steiner, T.J., Perkin, G.D., Greenhalgh, R.M., and Rose, F.C. (1987). Neurological morbidity of arch and carotid arteriography: the influence of contrast medium and radiologist. *Br. J. Radiol.* 60, 117.

McNair, J.D. (1972). Selective coronary angiography. Report of a fatality in a patient with sickle cell hemoglobin. *Calif. Med.* 117, 71.

McPhaul, M., Punzi, H.A., Sandy, A., Borganelli, M., Rose, R., and Kaplan, N.M. (1984). Snuff-induced hypertension in pheochromocytoma. *JAMA* 252, 2860.

Mahlstedt, J. and Joseph, K. (1973). Decompensation of autonomous thyroid adenoma after long-term iodine intake. *Dtsch. Med. Wochenschr.* 98, 1748.

Maley, P. (1989). Sex and age related differences in postmyelographic adverse reactions. A prospective study of 1765 myelographies. *Neuroradiology* 31, 331.

Malins, A.F. (1978). Pulmonary oedema after radiological investigation of peripheral occlusive vascular disease. Adverse reaction to contrast media. *Lancet* i, 413.

Mallette, L.E. and Gomez, L.S. (1983). Systemic hypocalcaemia after clinical injections of radiographic contrast media: amelioration by omission of calcium chelating agents. *Radiology* 147, 677.

Mandell, G.A., Swacus, J.R., Rosenstock, J., and Buck, B.E. (1983). Danger of urography in hyperuricaemic children with Burkitt's lymphoma. *J. Can. Assoc. Radiol.* 34, 273.

Måre, K., Violante, M., and Zack, A. (1985). Pulmonary edema following high intravenous doses of diatrizoate in the rat: effect of corticosteroid pretreatment. *Acta Radiol. [Diagn.]* (Stockh.) 26, 477.

Martin-Paredero, V., Dixon, S.M., Baker, J.D., Takiff, H., Gomes, A.S., Busuttili, R.W., *et al.* (1983). Risk of renal failure after major angiography. *Arch. Surg.* 118, 1417.

Mason, M.S. and Kaaf, J. (1962). Complications of Pantopaque myelography. Case report and review. *J. Neurosurg.* 19, 1032.

Michel, J.R. (1982). Prevention of shocks induced by intravenous urography. In *Contrast media in radiology* (ed. M. Amiel), p. 11. Springer-Verlag, Berlin.

Miller, G., Fuchs, W.A., and Preisig, R. 1969). Die Infusioncholangiographie in physiologischer Sicht. *Schweiz. Med. Wochenschr.* 99, 577.

Miller, R.E. and Skukas, J. (eds) (1977). *Radiographic contrast agents.* University Park Press, Baltimore.

Mills, J.O.M. (1990). Inhalation of Carbex. *Clin. Radiol.* 41, 69.

Mills, S.R., Jackson, D.C., Older, R.A., Heaston, D.K., and Moore, A.V. (1980). The incidence, etiologies and avoidance of complications of pulmonary angiography in a large series. *Radiology* 136, 295.

Mishkin, M.M., Baum, S., and Di Chiro, G. (1973). Emergency treatment of angiography-induced paraplegia and tetraplegia. *N. Engl. J. Med.* 288, 1184.

Monroe, L.S. and Longmore, W.J. (1966). Inhibition of sulfobromophthalein (BSP) conjugation with glutathione by iopanoic acid (Telepaque). *Gastroenterology* 50, 396.

Moore, R.D., Steinberg, E.P., Powe, N.R., White, R.I., Vrinker, J.A., Fishman, E.K., *et al.* (1989). Frequency and determinants of adverse reactions induced by high-osmolality contrast media. *Radiology* 170, 727.

Morcos, S.K., Baudouin, S.V., Anderson, P.B., Beedie, R., and Bury, R.W. (1989). Iotrolan in selective bronchography via the fibreoptic bronchoscope. *Br. J. Radiol.* 62, 383.

Moreau, J.F., Droz, D., Sabto, J., Jungers, P., Kleinknecht, D., Hinglais, N., *et al.* (1975). Osmotic nephrosis induced by water-soluble tri-iodinated contrast media in man. A retrospective study of 47 cases. *Radiology* 115, 329.

Morris, S., Sahler, L.G., and Fischer, H.W. (1982). Calcium binding by radiopaque media. *Invest. Radiol.* 17, 501.

Mozley, P.D. (1981). Malignant hyperthermia following intravenous iodinated contrast media. Report of a fatal case. *Diagn. Gynecol. Obstet.* 3, 81.

Mudge, G.H. (1971). Uricosuric action of cholecystographic agents. A possible factor in nephrotoxicity. *N. Engl. J. Med.* 284, 929.

Mudge, G.H. (1980). Nephrotoxicity of urographic radiocontrast drugs. *Kidney Int.* 18, 540.

Murphy, G., Campbell, D.R., and Fraser, D.B. (1988). Pain in peripheral arteriography: an assessment of conventional versus ionic and non-ionic low osmolality contrast agents. *J. Canad. Assoc. Radiol.* 39: 103.

Myers, G.H. and Witten, D.M. (1971). Acute renal failure after excretion urography in multiple myeloma. *AJR* 113, 583.

Nahrwold, D.L., Isch, J.H., Benner, R.E., and Miller, R.E. (1971). Effect of fluid administration and operation on the mortality rate in barium peritonitis. *Surgery* 70, 778.

Nakstad, P., Sortland, O., Aaserud, O., Lundervold, A. (1982). Cerebral angiography with the non-ionic water-soluble contrast medium iohexol and meglumine-ca-metrizoate. *Neuroradiology* 23, 199.

Navani, S., Taylor, C.E., Kaufman, S.A., and Parlee, R.H. (1972). Evanescent enlargement of salivary glands following tri-iodinated contrast media. *Br. J. Radiol.* 45. 19.

Nelson, J.A. (1979). Personal communication.

Nelson, J.A., Pepper, H.W., Goldberg, H.I., Moss, A.A.. and Amberg, J.R. (1973). Effect of phenobarbital on iodipamide and iopanoate bile excretion. *Invest. Radiol.* 8, 126.

Nicot, G.S., Merle, L.J., Charmes, J.P., Valette, J.P., Nouaille, Y.D., Lachatre, G.F. *et al.* (1984). Transient glomerular proteinuria, enzymuria, and nephrototoxic reaction induced by radiocontrast media. *JAMA* 252, 2432.

Nogrady, M.B. and Dunbar, J.S. (1968). Delayed concentration and prolonged excretion of urographic contrast medium in the first month of life. *AJR* 104, 289.

Nolan, D.J. and Gibson, M.J. (1970). Improvements in intravenous cholangiography. *Br. J. Radiol.* 43, 652.

Obeid, T., Yaqub, B., Panayiotopoulas, C., Jasser, S., Shabaan A., and Hawass, N.E. (1988). Absence status epileptics with computed tomographic brain changes following metrizamide myelography. *Ann. Neurol.* 24, 582.

Older, R.A., Korobkin, M., Cleeve, D.M., Schaaf, R., and Thompson, W.M. (1980). Contrast-induced acute renal failure. Persistent nephrogram as clue to early detection. *AJR* 134, 339.

Pagani, J.G., Hayman, L.A., Bigelow, R.H., Libshitz, H.I., and Lepke, R.A. (1984). Prophylactic diazepam in prevention of contrast media-induced seizures in glioma patients undergoing cerebral computed tomography. *Cancer* 54, 2200.

Palmer, F.J. (1989). The Royal Australasian College of Radiologists' (RACR) survey of reactions of intravenous ionic and non-ionic contrast media. In *Patient safety and adverse events in contrast medium examination.* Excerpta Medica International Congress Series 816, p. 137. Elsevier, Amsterdam.

Panto, P.N. and Davies, P. (1986). Delayed reactions to urographic contrast media. *Br. J. Radiol.* 59, 41.

Parfree, P.S., Griffiths, S.M., Barrett, B.J., Paul, M.D., Genge, M., Withers, J. *et al.* (1989). Contrast material-induced renal failure in patients with diabetes mellitus, renal insufficiency, or both. A prospective controlled study. *N. Engl. J. Med.* 320, 143.

Parvez, R., Moncada, R.; Messmore, H.L., and Fareed. J. (1982). Ionic and non-ionic contrast media interaction with anticoagulant drugs. *Acta Radiol. [Diagn.]* (Stockh.) 23, 401.

Pendergrass, H.P., Tondreau, R.L., Pendergrass, E.P., Ritchie, D.J., Hildrith, E.A., and Askowitz, S.I. (1958). Reactions associated with intravenous urography — historical and statistical review. *Radiology* 71, 1.

Penry, J.B. and Livingstone, A. (1972). A comparison of diagnostie effectiveness and vascular side-effects of various diatrizoate salts used for intravenous pyelography. *Clin. Radiol.* 23, 362.

Perrigot, M., Pierot-Deseilligny, E., Bussec, B., and Held, J-P. (1976). Paralysies survenus dans les suites d'une radiculographie au Dimer X. *Nouv. Presse Med.* 5, 1120.

Pfister, R.C. and Hutter, A.M. Jr. (1980). Cardiac alterations during intravenous urography. *Invest. Radiol.* 15 (suppl. 6), S239.

Pillay, T.J., Beshany, S.E., and Shields, J.B. (1986). Incompatibility of Hexabrix and papaverine. *AJR* 146, 1300.

Pillay, K.G., Robbins, P.C., Schwartz. F.D., and Kark, R.M. (1970). Acute renal failure following intravenous urography in patients with long-standing diabetes mellitus and azotaemia. *Radiology* 95, 633.

Pinet, A., Lyonett, D., Maillet, P., and Groleau, J.M. (1982). Adverse reactions to intravenous urography. Results of a national survey. In *Contrast media in radiology* (ed. M. Amiel), p. 14. Springer-Verlag, Berlin.

Popper, R.W., Schumacher. D., and Quinn. C.H. (1967). Cardiac tamponade due to hypertonic contrast medium in the pericardial sac. Clinical observations and experimental study. *Circulation* 35, 933.

Prout, B.J., Datta, S.B., and Wilson, T.S. (1972). Colonic retention of barium in the elderly after barium-meal examination and its treatment with lactulose. *Br. Med. J.* iv, 530.

Ramsay, A.W., Spector, M., Rodgers, A.L., Miller, R.L., and Knapp, D.R. (1982). Crystalluria following excretory urography. *Br. J. Urol.* 54. 341.

Rao, A.K., Thompson, R., Durlacher, L., and James, F. (1985). Angiographic contrast agent-induced acute hemolysis in a patient with hemoglobin SC disease. *Arch. Intern. Med.* 145, 759.

Rao, V.M., Rao, A.K., Steiner, R.M., Burka, E.R., Grainger, R.G., and Ballas, S.K. (1982). The effect of ionic and non-ionic contrast media on the sickling phenomenon. *Radiology* 144, 291.

Ratcliff, G., Sandler, S., and Latchaw, R. (1986). Cognitive and affective changes after myelography: a comparison of metrizamide and iohexol. *AJNR* 7, 683.

Reuter, F.W. and Eugester, C. (1985). Akuter Iodismus mit Sialadenitis, allergischer Vasculitis and Konjunctivitis nach Verabreichung jodhaltiger Kontrastmittel. *Schweiz. Med. Wochenschr.* 115, 1646.

Richards, D. and Nulsen, F.E. (1971). Angiographic media and the sickling phenomenoh. *Surg. Forum* 22, 403.

Ring, J., Rothernberger, K-H., and Clauss, W. (1985). Prevention of anaphylactoid reactions after radiographic contrast media infusion by combined H_1- and H_2-receptor antagonists: results of a prospective clinical trial. *Int. Arch. Allergy Appl. Immunol.* 78, 9.

Robertson, G.H., Ellis, G., Brismar, J., and Taveras, J.M. (1977). Cisternography with metrizamide and hypocycloidal tomography. *Acta Radiol. [Diagn.]* (Stockh.) 355 (suppl.), 314.

Robertson, H.J.E. (1987). Blood clot formation in angiographic syringes containing non-ionic media. *Radiology* 162, 621.

Robinson, A.E., Hall, K.D., Yokoyama, K.N., and Capp, M.P. (1971). Pediatric bronchography: the problem of segmental pulmonary loss of volume. 1. A retrospective survey of 165 pediatric bronchograms. *Invest. Radiol.* 6, 89.

Ross, L.S. (1972). Precipitation of meglumine diatrizoate 76% (Gastrografin) in the stomach. Observations on the insolubility of diatrizoate in the normal range of gastric acidity. *Radiology* 105, 19.

Rowe, M.I., Furst, A.H., Altman, D.H., and Poole, C.A. (1971). The neonatal response to Gastrografin enema. *Pediatrics* 48, 29.

Rust, R.J., Cohen, M.D., and Ulbricht. T.M. (1982). Clinical radiographic and pathologic effects of Amipaque on rabbit lung. Comparison with barium and Gastrografin. *Acta Radiol. [Diagn.]* (Stockh.) 23, 553.

Sable, R.A., Rosenthal, W.S., and Seigle, J. (1983). Absorption of contrast medium during ERCP. *Dig. Dis. Sci.* 28, 801.

Saltzman, G.F. and Sundstrom, K-A. (1960). The influence of different contrast media for cholangiography on blood pressure and pulse rate. *Acta Radiol.* 54, 353.

Savill, J.S., Barrie, R., Ghosh, S., Muhlemann, M., Dawson, P., and Pusey, C.D. (1988). Fatal Stevens–Johnson syndrome following urography with iopamidol in systemic lupus erythematosus. *Postgrad. Med. J.* 64, 392.

Schiantarelli, P., Peroni, F., Tirone, P., and Rosati, G. (1973). Effects of iodinated contrast media on erythrocytes. 1. Effects of canine erythrocytes on morphology. *Invest. Radiol.* 8. 199.

Schiro, J.C., Ricci, J.A., Tristan, T.A., and Levin, D.M. (1971). Transient renal insufficiency secondary to iopanoic acid. *Pennsylvania Med. J.* 74, 53.

Scholtz, F.J., Johnson, D.O., and Wise, R.E. (1974). Hepatotoxicity in cholangiography. *JAMA* 229, 1724.

Schwab, S.J., Hlatky, M.A., Pieper, K.S., Davidson, C.J., Morris, K.G., Skelton, T.N., *et al.* (1989). Contrast nephrotoxicity, a randomised controlled trial of a non-ionic and an ionic radiographic contrast agent. *N. Engl. J. Med.* 320, 149.

Schwartz, E.E., Glick, S.N., Foggs, M.B., and Silverstein, G.S. (1984). Hypersensitivity reactions after barium enema examination. *AJR* 143, 937.

Seltzer, S.E. and Jones, B. (1978). Cecal perforation associated with gastrografin enema. *AJR* 130, 997.

Setter, J.G., Maher, J.F., and Schreiner, G.E. (1963). Acute renal failure following cholecystography. *Acta Radiol.* (Stockh.) 3, 353.

Shehadi, W.H. (1975). Adverse reactions to intravascularly administered contrast media: a comprehensive study based on a prospective study. *AJR* 124, 145.

Shehadi, W.H. and Toniolo. G. (1980). Adverse reactions to contrast media. A report from the Committee on safety of contrast media of the International Society of Radiology. *Radiology* 137, 299.

Shetty, S.P.. Murthy, G.G.. Shreeve. W.W., Nawaz, A.M., and Ryder, S.W. (1974). Hyperthyroidism after pyelography. *N. Engl. J. Med.* 291, 682.

Shojania, M. (1985). Immune-mediated thrombocytopenia due to an iodinated contrast medium. *Can. Med. Assoc. J.* 133, 123.

Shulman, G. (1977). Bence–Jones myelomatosis and intravenous pyelography. *S. Afr. Med. J.* 51, 574.

Siegle, R.L. and Lieberman, P. (1978). A review of untoward reactions to iodinated contrast material. *J. Urol.* 119, 581.

Simon, A.L., Shabetai, R.. Lang. J.H., and Lasser, E.C. (1972). The mechanism of production of ventricular fibrillation in coronary angiography. *AJR* 114, 810.

Skalpe, I.C. (1988). Complications in cerebral angiography with iohexol (Omnipaque) and meglumine metrizoate (Isopaque Cerebral). *Neuroradiology* 30, 69.

Skalpe, I.C. and Sortland. O. (1977). Thoracic myelography with metrizamide. *Acta Radiol. [Diagn.]* (Stockh.) 355 (suppl.), 57.

Slasky. B.S. (1981). Acute renal failure, contrast media, and computer tomography. *Urology* 28, 309.

Smith, H.J., Jones, K., and Hunter, T.B. (1988). What happens to patients after upper and lower gastrointestinal tract barium studies? *Invest. Radiol.* 23, 822.

Smith, M.S. and Laguna, J.F. (1980). Confusion, dysphasia, and asterixis following metrizamide myelography. *J. Can. Sci. Neurol.* 7, 309.

Soloman, D.R. (1986). Anaphylactoid reaction and noncardiac pulmonary edema following intravascular administration of contrast media. *Am. J. Emerg. Med.* 4, 146.

Sortland. O., Lundervold, A., and Nesbakken, K. (1977). Mental confusion and epileptic seizures following cervical myelography with metrizamide — report of a case. *Acta Radiol. [Diagn.]* (Stockh.) 355 (suppl.), 403.

Spataro, R.F., Katzberg, R.W., Fischer, H.W., and McMannis, M.J. (1987). High-dose clinical urography with the low-osmolality contrast agent Hexabrix: comparison with a conventional contrast agent. *Radiology* 162, 9.

Stadalnik, R.C., Vera, Z., DaSilva, O., Davies, R., Kraus, J.F., and Mason, D.T. (1977). Electrocardiographic response to intravenous urography: prospective evaluation of 275 patients. *AJR* 129, 825.

Staubli, M., Braunschweig, J., and Tillman, U. (1982). Changes in the rheological properties of blood as induced by sodium/meglumine ioxoglate as compared with sodium/meglumine diatrizoate and metrizamide. *Acta Radiol. [Diagn.]* (Stockh.) 23, 401.

Stein, H.L. and Hilgartner, M.W. (1968). Alteration of coagulation mechanism of blood by contrast media. *AJR* 104, 458.

Steiner, E., Simon, J.H., Ekholm, S.E., Erickson, J., Kido, D.K., and Okawara, S-H. (1986). Neurologic complications in diabetes after metrizamide lumbar myelography. *AJR* 146, 1057.

Stemerman, M., Goldstein, M.L., and Schulman, P.L. (1971). Pancytopenia associated with diatrizoate. *N. Y. State J. Med.* 11, 1220.

Stinchcombe, S.J. and Davies, P. (1989). Acute toxic myopathy: a delayed adverse effect of intravenous urography with iopamidol 370. *Br. J. Radiol.* 62, 949.

Stordahl, A., Haider, T., and Laerum, F. (1989). Acute lethality after enteral administration of contrast media in anaesthetised rats with intestinal ischaemia. *Acta Radiol. [Diagn.]* (Stockh.) 30, 213.

Sussman, R.M. and Miller, J. (1956). Iodide mumps after intravenous urography. *N. Engl. J. Med.* 255, 433.

Sutherland, L.R., Edwards, L.A., Medline, A., Wilkinson, R.W., and Connon, J.J. (1977). Meglumine iodipamide (Cholografin) hepatotoxicity. *Ann. Intern. Med.* 86, 437.

Tajima, H., Kumazaki, T., Tajima, N., and Ebata, K. (1988). Effect of iohexol and diatrizoate on pulmonary arterial pressure following pulmonary angiography. A clinical comparison in man. *Acta Radiol. [Diagn.]* (Stockh.) 29, 487.

Taliercio, C.P., Vliestra, R.E., Fisher, L.D., and Burnett, J.C. (1986). Risks of renal dysfunction with cardiac angiography. *Ann. Intern. Med.* 104, 501.

Taliercio, C.P., McCallister, S.H., Holmes, D.R., Ilstrup, D.M., and Vliestra, R.E. (1989). Nephrotoxicity of nonionic contrast media after cardiac angiography. *Am. J. Cardiol.* 64, 815.

Talner, L.B., Lang, J.H., Brasch, R.C., and Lasser, E.C. (1971). Elevated salivary iodine and salivary gland enlargement due to iodinated contrast media. *AJR* 112, 380.

Tartiere, J., Gerard, J-L., Peny, J., Hurpe, J-M., and Quesnel, J. (1989). Acute treatment after accidental intrathecal injection of hypertonic contrast medium. *Anesthesiology* 71, 169.

Tejler, L., Almen, T., and Holtas, S. (1977). Proteinuria following nephroangiography, 1. Clinical experiences. *Acta Radiol. [Diagn.]* (Stockh.) 18, 634.

Acta Radiol. [Diagn.]n, R.M., and Sanen, F.J. (1965). Acute renal failure following oral cholecystography. *Acta Radiol.* (Stockh.) 3, 353.

Thompson, G.J.L., Simpson, C.J., and Hansell, D.T. (1984). The early diagnosis of acute gallbladder disease: the accuracy of overnight eight-hour infusion cholangiography. *Br. J. Radiol.* 57, 685.

Thompson, W.M., Mills, S.R., Bates, M., Hedlung, L., and Rommel, J. (1983). Pulmonary angiography with iopamidol and renografin 76 in normal and pulmonary hypertensive dogs. *Acta Radiol. [Diagn.]* (Stockh.) 24, 425.

Tishler, J.M. and Gold, R. (1969). A clinical trial of oral cholecystographic agents: Telepaque, Sodium Oragrafin and Calcium Oragrafin. *J. Can. Assoc. Radiol.* 20, 102.

Trewhella, M., Dawson, P., Forsling, M., McCarthy, P., and O'Donnell, C. (1990). Vasopression release in response to intravenously injected contrast media. *Br. J. Radiol.* 63, 97.

van den Bergh, P., Kelly, J.J., Carter, B., and Munsat, T.I. (1986). Intravascular contrast media and neuromuscular junction disorders. *Ann. Neurol.* 19, 206.

van Sonnenberg, E., Neff, C.C., and Pfister, R.C. (1987). Life-threatening reactions to contrast media administration: comparison of pharmacologic and fluid therapy. *Radiology* 162, 15.

van Waes, P.F.G.M. (1972). *High-dose urography in oliguric and anuric patients.* Excerpta Medica, Amsterdam.

van Zee, B.E., Hoy, W.E., Talley, T.E., and Jaenike, J.R. (1978). Renal injury associated with intravenous pyelography in nondiabetic and diabetic patients. *Ann. Intern. Med.* 89, 51.

Vari, R.C., Laksmi, A., Natarajan, L.A., Whitescarver, S.A., Ott, C.E., and Jackson, B.A. (1988). Induction, prevention and mechanisms of contrast-media-induced acute renal failure. *Kidney Int.* 33, 699.

Vincent, F.M. (1980). Asterixis after metrizamide myelography. *JAMA* 244, 2727.

Vincent, M.E., Gerzof, S.G., and Robbins, A.H. (1977). Benign transient eosinophilia following intravenous urography. *JAMA* 237, 2629.

Walker, H.G. and Ma, H. (1971). Oily and aqueous propyliodone (Dionosil) as bronchographic contrast agents. *J. Can. Assoc. Radiol.* 22, 148.

Wangermez, J. (1975). La prévention des accidents par la cholangiographie-perfusion. Comparison entre les corticoïdes et l'acide tranéxamique. *J. Radiol. Electrol.* 56, 142.

Wardman, A.G., Willey, R.F., Cooke, N.J., Crompton, G.K., and Grant, I.W.B. (1983). Unusual pulmonary reaction to propyliodone (Dionosil) in bronchography. *Br. J. Dis. Chest* 77, 98.

Weinstein, G.S., O'Doriso, T.M., and Joehl, R.J. (1985). Exacerbation of diarrhoea after iodinated contrast agents in a patient with a VIPoma. *Digest. Dis. Sci.* 30, 588.

White, A.G. (1972). Prolonged elevation of serum protein-bound iodine following myelography with Myodil. *Br. J. Radiol.* 39, 112.

Whitney, B. and Bell, G.D. (1972). Simple bolus injection or slow infusion for intravenous cholangiography? Measurement of iodipamide (Biligrafin) excretion using a rhesus monkey model. *Br. J. Radiol.* 45, 891.

Winearls, C.G., Ledingham, J.G.G., and Dixon, A.J. (1980). Acute renal failure precipitated by radiographic contrast medium in a patient with rhabdomyolysis. *Br. Med. J.* 281, 1603.

Witten, D.M., Hirsch, F.D., and Hartman, G.W. (1973). Acute reactions to urographic contrast medium. Incidence, clinical characteristics and relationship to history of hypersensitivity states. *AJR* 119, 832.

Yocum, M.W., Heller, A.M., and Abels, R.I. (1978). Efficacy of intravenous pretesting and antihistamine prophylaxis in radio-contrast media-sensitive patients. *J. Allergy Clin. Immunol.* 62, 309.

Young, M.O. (1958). Acute appendicitis following retention of barium in the appendix. *Arch. Surg.* 77, 1011.

Zeman, R.K. (1977). Disseminated intravascular coagulation following intravenous pyelography. *Invest. Radiol.* 12, 203.

Zheutlin, N., Lasser, E.C., and Rigler, L.G. (1952). Clinical studies on the effect of barium in the peritoneal cavity following rupture of the colon. *Surgery* 32, 967.

Zucherman, S.D. and Jacobson, G. (1962). Transtracheal bronchography. Complications of injection outside the trachea. *AJR* 87, 840.

Zweiman, B., Mishkin, N.M., and Hildreth, E.A. (1975). An approach to the performance of contrast studies in contrast reactive persons. *Ann. Intern. Med.* 83, 159.

28. Disorders of temperature regulation

K. W. WOODHOUSE

Normal body temperature control

Human body temperature is controlled within a narrow range. Normally, a circadian rhythm occurs with a relative peak in the late afternoon and early evening and a trough in the early hours of the morning (Bernheim *et al.* 1979). A variety of physiological and behavioural mechanisms have evolved to maintain thermoregulation. For example, if we feel cold, the behavioural response is to put on an extra sweater or light the fire; the physiological responses include vasoconstriction to reduce heat loss and shivering to generate heat. By contrast, a perception of heat results in shedding of clothes, vasodilatation, and sweating (Bernheim *et al.* 1979).

Fever

Practically all drugs can cause fever under certain circumstances — certainly adverse drug reactions should always be considered in patients with obscure or unexplained pyrexia.

Production of fever

The usual mechanism by which fever is brought about in infective and inflammatory illnesses is probably by the generation of endogenous pyrogen (Atkins and Bodel 1979). A variety of cells, including polymorphs, monocytes, Kupffer cells, and alveolar macrophages are capable of producing these compounds after appropriate stimulation by, for example, antigen/antibody reaction (Atkins and Bodel 1971) or by exposure to bacterial endotoxin (Rawlins and Cranston 1972).

Endogenous pyrogen has been shown to affect cells in the preoptic region of the hypothalamus (Cooper *et al.* 1967); it causes fever by increasing the firing rates of temperature-sensitive neurones in this 'thermoregulatory centre', thus increasing the hypothalamic temperature 'set point'. It seems that several intermediaries are involved in this series of events, including prostaglandins and other arachidonic acid metabolites (Laburn *et al.* 1977) and brain monoamines such as noradrenaline and serotonin (Feldberg and Myers 1963; Atkins and Bodel 1979).

Classification of drug-induced fever

Drugs may induce fever by a variety of mechanisms including:
1. acting as a direct or indirect pyrogen or by causing inflammation or tissue damage;
2. causing pyrogen release as part of their pharmacological action;
3. altering thermoregulation by central, peripheral, or metabolic means;
4. inducing hypersensitivity reactions;
5. causing immunosuppression;
6. as a result of patient idiosyncrasy.

Fever as a result of inflammation, tissue damage, or pyrogenic activity

Many drugs cause a local inflammatory phlebitis following intravenous infusion, with resultant fever. These include hypertonic fluids, amphotericin (Seabury 1961), and a variety of antibiotics, such as erythromycin, vancomycin, and cephalosporins (Berger *et al.* 1976). A more serious local reaction is the development of a sterile abscess, again resulting in fever. This may occur following repeated intramuscular injections of drugs such as paraldehyde (Hayward and Boshell 1957) or pentazocine (Parks *et al.* 1971).

Local inflammatory responses and associated fever are also frequent following vaccine administration. Pneumococcal vaccine is a good example (Uhl *et al.* 1978). Regarding the more commonly used vaccines in children, it is quite difficult to obtain accurate figures for the incidence of febrile reactions. As early as 1945, Sako

(1945) observed systemic reactions with fever following pertussis vaccination in 7.1 per cent of subjects. More recently higher fever than 38°C has been reported in 44 per cent of children given diphtheria/pertussis/tetanus toxoid/poliomyelitis vaccine (Ipp *et al*. 1987). The use of paracetamol as a prophylactic antipyretic has been recommended (Ipp *et al*. 1987).

Some drugs appear to have a systemic pyrogenic action. In some instances, particularly with agents derived from micro-organisms, this is likely to be due to contamination with bacterial or other pyrogens; examples include colaspase (asparaginase) (Ekert *et al*. 1972) and amphotericin (Seabury and Dascomb 1958). Certainly, purification of amphotericin significantly reduces the occurrence of febrile reactions to it (Tynes *et al*. 1963; Groel 1963).

Other drugs may, however, be exogenous pyrogens themselves. Bleomycin administered systemically or into a body cavity is certainly pyrogenic (Dinarello *et al*. 1973), and it has been suggested that at least part of this action may be due to the drug rather than contaminants; similarly, interferon, administered either intramuscularly (Scott *et al*. 1981) or intrathecally (Ruutiainen *et al*. 1983), almost invariably causes a temperature rise. This drug is a biological product, and it has been suggested that the fever is due to contaminants; even highly purified preparations, however, cause fever and it is likely that interferon is inherently pyrogenic (Scott *et al*. 1981).

Fever due to pyrogen release as part of pharmacological action

The intended action of drugs can itself directly or indirectly induce fever. Perhaps the best example of this is the Jarisch–Herxheimer reaction, which may occur in some patients treated with penicillins for syphilis. Endotoxin is released from dead spirochaetes, resulting in fever 6–8 hours after starting therapy; this is often accompanied by rash, rigors, myalgia, and malaise (Gelfand *et al*. 1976).

In addition, several types of malignant cells, for example, those of acute leukaemia, histiocytic lymphoma, and Hodgkin's disease, can secrete endogenous pyrogen, resulting in fever as part of the disease process (Bernheim *et al*. 1979; Atkins and Bodel 1971). Treatment of the disease by chemotherapy may theoretically result in cell death, release of further pyrogen, and subsequent fever (Bodel *et al*. 1980), although it must be said that most fevers in patients with cancer who receive chemotherapy are due to intercurrent infections.

In the case of streptokinase, a drug which is frequently pyrogenic, at least some of the fever may be due to the release of unspecified metabolites during thrombolysis

(Kakkar *et al*. 1969). It is unlikely to be due to contamination with bacterial endotoxin or other agents, as the fever generally begins 14–20 hours into treatment, peaking at 24–36 hours. A febrile response to endotoxin would be expected to begin within 1–2 hours of starting therapy.

Fever due to altered thermoregulation

Drugs may theoretically modify thermoregulation in several ways: (a) centrally, (b) peripherally, and (c) by affecting metabolism and heat production. In practice, central effects are probably most important. Although drugs with anticholinergic properties such as atropine, antihistamines, and tricyclic antidepressants can decrease sweating, and sympathomimetics such as amphetamines can produce vasoconstriction, the fever they produce in overdose (Mikolich *et al*. 1975; Noble and Matthew 1969; Jordan and Hempson 1960; Judge and Dumard 1953) is due at least in part to central rather than these peripheral actions.

Experimental evidence for central thermomodulatory effects of some drugs is strong: catecholamines, serotonin, anticholinergics, and prostaglandins have all been shown to give temperature rises in various species of experimental animals when injected intraventricularly (Cranston 1979; Hellon 1975).

Tricyclic antidepressant overdose is frequently associated with fever (Noble and Matthews 1969), and this may well be due to increased concentrations of catecholamines in the synaptic cleft. Intraventricular administration of the tricyclic desmethylimipramine in rats results in brisk fever, even when given in small doses (Cranston *et al*. 1972). Similarly, monoamine oxidase inhibitors can result in dramatic fever when taken in overdose, or when taken with tricyclics (Simmons *et al*. 1970). Phenoxybenzamine has been suggested for control of fever in cases in which several antidepressants have been taken in overdose, as it also controls the associated hypertension (Simmons *et al*. 1970).

Atropine is another agent that frequently gives rise to fever when taken in overdose: in up to 20 per cent of such cases the patient is febrile (Shader and Greenblatt 1971). This effect is, once more, likely to be partially centrally mediated, although decreased sweating may be an associated factor. The use of dopamine-blocking agents in combination with anticholinergics may also result in hyperpyrexia, even in therapeutic dosage; this has occurred in patients receiving benztropine together with trifluoperazine, haloperidol, or chlorpromazine, and in patients taking benztropine with chlorprothixene and chlorpromazine (Westlake and Rastegar 1973). This interaction can sometimes pose therapeutic problems, as patients with anticholinergic poisoning are often disturbed and hallucinated. Use of neuroleptics to control these symptoms will obviously worsen the situation. Benzodiazepines should probably be used in these circumstances, and fever reduced by skin cooling.

Other agents may also produce fever partly by central effects. For example, pyrexia is not uncommon when prostaglandins are used to induce termination of pregnancy, either by the intra-amniotic or intravenous route (Fraser and Brash 1974), and it is known that intraventricular administration of prostaglandins in experimental animals is pyrogenic (Milton and Wendlandt 1971). Similarly, injection of H_2-blockers into the third ventricle of chickens causes fever, while injection of H_2-agonists produces a temperature fall (Nistico *et al.* 1978). Conceivably, some of the rare cases of fever caused by cimetidine could be due to this mechanism, although this seems doubtful, as this drug does not cross the blood–brain barrier in significant amounts.

Fever as part of hypersensitivity reactions

There is no doubt that fever is a prominent clinical feature of hypersensitivity (allergic) drug reactions. A drug fever, initially low-grade and subsequently increasing, will often start within 7–10 days of drug administration. It will normally persist as long as the drug is given, but will subside rapidly on discontinuation. Rechallenge will result in recurrence of fever within hours.

Fever may often be the first sign of a hypersensitivity reaction: in a study of 68 cases of drug allergy, of which 31 were fatal, fever was an early feature in almost one-third (Cluff and Johnson 1964). Similarly, in a review of 38 patients with phenytoin hypersensitivity, fever was a prominent feature in 14 cases and the only sign of a reaction in one (Haruda 1979). It is impractical to discuss all drugs that may induce a hypersensitivity reaction, but in several instances fever may be the most prominent feature of the event.

Antituberculous drugs

Fever is a common feature of adverse reactions to antituberculous drugs. In a large study of 1744 cases of tuberculosis treated with various combinations of antituberculous drugs, it was found that adverse reactions occurred in 10.3 per cent of those treated with streptomycin, of which 26.8 per cent were associated with fever; in 8.8 per cent of those treated with *p*-aminosalicylic aid (PAS), of which 43.3 per cent were associated with fever; and in 1.3 per cent of those given isoniazid, of which 59 per cent were febrile (Berte *et al.* 1964). Fever also occurs in patients taking rifampicin and, interestingly, is more frequent in those given the drug intermittently

rather than continuously, in keeping with a hypersensitivity reaction (Zierski 1973).

Antibacterials

Febrile reactions to antibiotics do occur, but are the major feature of only a small number of cases, being more common in association with other manifestations of allergy such as rash and abnormal liver function. In a study of 2877 patients admitted to hospital and given antibiotics it was found that overall 5.4 per cent of patients developed an adverse reaction of some kind, but in only 9 individuals was fever the only or the most prominent feature, 3 of whom had received penicillin, 3 cephalothin, and 1 each ampicillin, oxacillin, and tetracycline (Caldwell and Cluff 1974).

Methyldopa

Fever with methyldopa is well described (Furhoff 1978) and seems to occur in up to 3 per cent of those given the drug. It is the most common adverse reaction associated with methyldopa — of 308 reports in the 1960s and 1970s in Sweden, 166 were of febrile reactions. There appears to be a slight preponderance (60 per cent) of women (Furhoff 1978). Many cases are associated with hepatitis and abnormal liver function tests, reflecting the hypersensitivity nature of the reactions (Klein and Kaminsky 1973).

Miscellaneous drugs

Fever during phenytoin treatment is not uncommon and has been mentioned above; it is frequently simply part of a symptom complex that may include rashes, the Stevens–Johnson syndrome, adenopathy, hepatitis, and blood dyscrasia (Haruda 1979; Stanley and Fallon-Pellici 1978).

Procainamide is another drug that can induce fever as a major symptom of an adverse drug reaction (Hey *et al.* 1965). Transient eosinophilia may occur. Febrile responses to procainamide tend to occur within the first 2–18 days of treatment; the response is probably independent of the subsequent risk of developing the lupus syndrome (Hey *et al.* 1965).

By contrast, those who develop an early febrile reaction to hydralazine may well be rather more likely to develop lupus subsequently (Perry 1973).

Of newer drugs, angiotensin-converting-enzyme inhibitors, such as captopril, may cause fever (Hoorntje *et al.* 1979).

In some cases it is probable that febrile reactions associated with drug hypersensitivity may not be due to the drug *per se*, but to contaminants. For example, antibiotics or egg proteins found in some vaccine products may result in hypersensitivity reactions (see above).

Fever in immunosuppressed patients

A detailed description of this problem is beyond the scope of this chapter. Patients, however, who are immunocompromised by treatment, be it as a result of cancer chemotherapy or an idiosyncratic reaction, are clearly at risk of opportunistic infection, often with associated fever. This problem is dealt with elsewhere in this book (Chapter 23).

Fever as a result of patient idiosyncrasy

Glucose 6-phosphate dehydrogenase deficiency

This enzyme deficiency, dealt with in greater detail elsewhere (see Chapters 3 and 22), is an inherited defect of red cell metabolism (Gross *et al.* 1958). When exposed to a variety of drugs such patients may develop a brisk haemolysis (Carson *et al.* 1956), and this reaction, as with most haemolytic reactions, may be accompanied by a febrile illness (Wallerstein and Aggeler 1964).

Malignant hyperthermia

This condition is one of the most dramatic complications of anaesthesia. It was first described by Saidman and Colleagues (1964), and may occur after exposure to a variety of anaesthetic agents, notably halothane and suxamethonium (Noble *et al.* 1973), although it has been reported with nitrous oxide (Ellis *et al.* 1974), cyclopropane (Lips *et al.* 1982), tubocurarine (Britt *et al.* 1974), isoflurane (McGuire and Easy 1990), and even during epidural anaesthesia with lignocaine and bupivacaine (Kilmanek *et al.* 1976). The syndrome comprises a rapid rise in body temperature (of at least 2°C per hour and up to 1°C every 5–10 minutes), accompanied by some or all of the following: rigidity, hyperventilation, cyanosis, acidosis, hyperphosphataemia, and hyperglycaemia. Initial hyperkalaemia and hypercalcaemia may be followed by hypokalaemia and hypocalcaemia. If the patient is not treated, the temperature may rise to over 42–43°C, and the mortality is 60–70 per cent (Britt and Kalow 1968). In juveniles undergoing anaesthesia in Canada, the frequency of the condition has been estimated to be 1 in 15 000 (WHO 1973).

The disease occurs in patients with an underlying, genetically determined, disorder of muscle; in the first family in which this was recognized, the abnormality was clearly inherited as a dominant characteristic. Further examples of the familial occurrence of malignant hyperpyrexia have been described, and in a review of 115 cases (Britt *et al.* 1969), in 43 cases other members of the family had been affected. In the majority of affected families, resting creatine phosphokinase and aldolase levels may be elevated (Isaacs and Barlow 1970), but this is by no means invariable, and a more accurate prediction of risk can be made by testing muscle biopsy specimens *in vitro*, when an increased sensitivity to anaesthetic agents, potassium, and temperature change can be demonstrated (Moulds and Denborough 1974a,b). In some cases, histological abnormalities comprising the presence of cores in 55 per cent of Type I muscle fibres — 'central core disease' — have been noted (Denborough *et al.* 1973). This is intriguing as similar abnormalities have been described in muscle fibres from Landrace pigs, creatures which also show a susceptibility to develop malignant hyperpyrexia.

It is possible that more than one congenital myopathy may be associated with this syndrome. In a study of all known cases in Australia and New Zealand, it was noted that in 50 per cent the dominant inherited form was likely. In three patients, however, the syndrome appeared to have arisen by spontaneous mutation; a few young males appeared to have a syndrome comprising progressive congenital myopathy, short stature, cryptorchidism, pectus carinatum, lumbar lordosis, and thoracic kyphosis; and a few had myotonia congenita (King *et al.* 1972).

Various treatment strategies have been adopted, and supportive measures including artificial ventilation and cooling, treatment of acidosis, and attention to electrolyte balance are crucial. Of pharmacological treatments, procaine (Harrison 1971), procainamide (Noble *et al.* 1973), and dexamethasone (Ellis *et al.* 1974) have all been advocated. The most effective treatment, however, is undoubtedly intravenous dantrolene sodium. Repeated doses of 1 mg per kg are given at 5 to 10-minute intervals until the syndrome is controlled. A total of 2–3 mg per kg is usually sufficient in humans, but in susceptible pigs up to 10 mg per kg has been given (Hall 1980). This drug should always be immediately available during anaesthesia (Hall 1980).

This subject is also discussed in Chapter 18.

Neuroleptic malignant syndrome (NMS)

A syndrome of uncontrolled heat reaction, similar to malignant hyperpyrexia but in general slightly less dramatic, has been reported following the administration of neuroleptic drugs. The clinical picture comprises hyperthermia, muscle rigidity, fluctuating consciousness, and autonomic disturbances, such as tachycardia, labile blood pressure, incontinence, dyspnoea, and sweating.

NMS tends to occur after physical exhaustion or dehydration, or both, and has been described with haloperidol, thiothixene, and piperazine phenothiazines. The likelihood is that it can be precipitated by most neuroleptics. The syndrome may persist for 5–10 days after discontinuing the drug, much longer if depot preparations have been used. Mortality may approach 20 per cent (Caroff 1980). A case in which hypothyroidism was suspected to have predisposed to the syndrome, induced by thioridazine and haloperidol, has been reported (Moore *et al.* 1990).

It may well be that dopamine receptor modulation is an important factor in the pathogenesis of this condition. The author has seen at least two patients with a similar, but milder, clinical picture following abrupt withdrawal of levodopa.

This subject is also discussed in Chapter 18.

Hypothermia

Hypothermia is usually defined by the presence of a deep body temperature, measured by reliable means, of less than 35°C (Keatinge 1987). Approximately 3 per cent of patients admitted to British hospitals in winter have body temperatures below this level. The majority are elderly, and in most cases, the hypothermia is secondary either to disease, such as stroke or pneumonia, or to drugs (Keatinge 1987). Elderly survivors of accidental hypothermia have been shown to have impaired thermoregulatory reflexes (Collins *et al.* 1977), and in these patients, drugs that further impair thermoregulation, level of consciousness, or central thermoregulatory control, may cause hypothermia. Barbiturates, neuroleptics, and alcohol are common culprits (Keatinge 1987; Caird and Scott 1986). The condition may occur even with relatively small doses in susceptible patients — hypothermia has been reported after as little as a single dose of 5 mg nitrazepam, given to a woman in an environmental temperature of 27°C (Impallomeni and Ezzat 1976).

Concurrent disease may also be a precipitating factor; for example, a single dose of chlorpromazine has produced hypothermia in a hypothyroid patient (Mitchell *et al.* 1959), and certainly benzodiazepines and neuroleptics should be avoided in such patients. Bromocriptine has been held responsible for recurrent falls in temperature (to as low as 35.5°C) in a 59-year-old man suffering from Parkinson's disease (Pfeffer 1990). In addition to direct effects on thermoregulation, drugs may produce the condition by inducing illnesses that are themselves associated with hypothermia, and low body temperatures are not infrequent in those with lactic acidosis induced by phenformin, (Assan *et al.* 1975) and have also been reported in drug-induced hypoglycaemia (Carter 1976). Hypothermia is notoriously common in cases of drug overdosage, and patients with barbiturate or alcohol poisoning, especially if found in cold environments, are frequently very cold (Keatinge 1987).

Drugs affecting cutaneous vasoconstriction can also cause a marked fall in core temperature: thus, any drug blocking sympathetic function will prevent vasoconstriction, increase heat loss, and encourage the development of hypothermia. This has been clearly shown in the case of the ganglion-blocker hexamethonium (Hamilton *et al.* 1954), although this is now largely of historical interest. Prazosin, however, is still widely used, and this drug also appears capable of causing hypothermia (de Leeuw and Birkenhäger 1980), although central mechanisms are likely to be involved as well. Falls in body temperature are also well recognized by anaesthetists, and this is likely to be due to impairment of both peripheral and central thermoregulatory reflexes. The problem is likely to occur at the extremes of age, being particularly important in the neonate. In normal adult patients, heat loss is unlikely to be serious if the ambient temperature is kept over 21°C (Carrie and Simpson 1988). The shivering common after halothane anaesthesia does not seem to be universally associated with significant falls in temperature, and may be part of a generalized muscular reaction (Carrie and Simpson 1988).

Finally, hypothermia may follow the intravenous infusion of large quantities of cold blood or other cold infusion fluids. This is a particular problem in babies (Hey *et al.* 1969), but problems may arise in adults (Boyan 1964), and local cooling of the heart, with resultant arrhythmias, may occur. Use of cold peritoneal dialysis fluid may also result in a fall in core temperature.

The treatment of drug-induced hypothermia follows the same lines as accidental hypothermia of any cause: supportive measures are essential, with attention to fluid and electrolyte balance, glucose homoeostasis, together with gradual rewarming (Keatinge 1987).

Classification of reactions

It is not always possible to classify disorders of thermal regulation into Type A or B reactions. Some reactions, however, such as those caused by drugs with pyrogenic activity, are clearly Type A, whereas others are clearly Type B, a result of patient idiosyncrasy, for example, malignant hyperpyrexia of anaesthesia. In many cases multiple mechanisms may well operate.

References

Assan, R., Heulin, C., Girard, J.R., Lemaire, F., and Attazi, J.R. (1975). Phenformin induced lactic acidosis in diabetic patients. *Diabetes* 24, 791.

Atkins, E. and Bodel, P. (1971). Role of leucocytes in fever. In *Pyrogen and fever* (ed. G. Wostenholme and J. Birch). Churchill Livingstone, Edinburgh.

Atkins, E. and Bodel, P. (1979). Clinical fever: its history, manifestations and pathogenesis. *Fed. Proc.* 38, 57,

Berger, S., Ernst, E.C., and Barza, M. (1976). Comparative incidence of phlebitis due to buffered cephalothin, cephopirin and cephamandole. *Antimicrob. Agents Chemother.* 9, 575.

Bernheim, H.A., Block, L.H., and Atkins, E. (1979). Fever: pathogenesis, pathophysiology and purpose. *Ann. Intern. Med.* 91, 261.

Berte, S.J., Dimase, J.D., and Christianson, C.S. (1964). Isoniazid, para-aminosalicylic acid and streptomycin intolerance in 1744 patients. *Annu. Rev. Respir. Dis.* 90, 598.

Bodel, E., Ralph, P., Wenc, K., and Long, J.C. (1980). Endogenous pyrogen production by Hodgkin's disease and human histiocytic lymphoma cell lives in vitro. *J. Clin. Invest.* 65, 514.

Boyan, C.P. (1964). Cold or warmed blood for massive transfusions? *Am. Surg.* 160, 282.

Britt, B.A. and Kalow, W. (1968). Hyperrigidity and hyperthermia associated with anaesthesia. *Ann. N.Y. Acad. Sci.* 151, 947.

Britt, B.A., Locher, W.G., and Kalow, W. (1969). Hereditary aspects of malignant hyperthermia. *Can. Anaesth. Soc. J.* 16, 89.

Britt, B.A., Webb, G.E., and Leduc, C. (1974). Malignant hyperthermia induced by curare. *Can. Anaesth. Soc. J.* 21, 371.

Caird, F.I. and Scott, P.J.W. (1986). *Drug induced diseases in the elderly.* Elsevier, Amsterdam.

Caldwell, J.R. and Cluff, L.E. (1974). Adverse reactions to antimicrobial agents. *JAMA* 230, 77.

Caroff, S.N. (1980). The neuroleptic malignant syndrome. *J. Clin. Psychiatry* 41, 79.

Carrie, L.E.S. and Simpson, P.J. (1988) *Understanding anaesthesia*, p. 257. Heinemann, London.

Carson P.E., Flanagan, C.L., Ickes, C.E., and Alving, A.S. (1956). Enzymatic deficiency in primaquine sensitive erythrocytes. *Science* 124, 484.

Carter, W.P. (1976). Drug induced hypoglycaemia and hypothermia. *J. Maine Med. Assoc.* 67, 272.

Cluff, L.E. and Johnson, J.E. (1964). Drug fever. *Prog. Allergy* 8, 149.

Collins, S.K.J., Dove, C., and Exton-Smith, A.N. (1977). Accidental hypothermia and compromised temperature homoeostasis in the elderly. *Br. Med. J.* i, 353.

Cooper, K.E., Cranston, W.I., and Honour, A.J. (1967). Observations on the site and mode of action of pyrogens in the rabbit brain. *J. Physiol.* (Lond.) 191, 325.

Cranston, W.I. (1979). Central mechanisms of fever. *Fed. Proc.* 38, 49.

Cranston, W.I., Hellon, R.F., Luff, R.H., and Rawlins, M.D. (1972). Hypothalamic endogenous noradrenaline and thermoregulation in the cat and rabbit. *J. Physiol.* (Lond.) 223, 59.

De Leeuw, P.W. and Birkenhäger, W.H. (1980). Hypothermia: A possible side effect of prazosin. *Br. Med. J.* 281, 1187.

Denborough, M.A., Bennett, X., and Anderson, R. McD. (1973). Central core disease and malignant hyperpyrexia. *Br. Med. J.* i, 272.

Dinarello, G.A., Ward, S.B., and Wolff, S.M. (1973). Pyrogenic properties of bleomycin. *Cancer Chemother. Rep.* 57, 393.

Ekert, H., Colebatch, J.H., and Matthews, R.N. (1972). Short courses of cytosine arabinoside and L-asparaginase in children with acute leukemia. *Cancer* 30, 643.

Ellis, F.R., Clarke, I.M.C., Appleyard, T.N., and Dinsdale, R.C.W. (1974). Malignant hyperpyrexia induced by nitrous oxide and treated with dexamethasone. *Br. Med. J.* iv, 270.

Feldberg, W. and Myers, R.D. (1963). A new concept of temperature regulation by amines in the hypothalamus. *Nature* 200, 1325.

Fraser, I.S. and Brash, I.H. (1974). Comparison of extra and intra-amniotic prostaglandins for therapeutic abortion. *Obstet. Gynecol.* 43, 97.

Furhoff, A.K. (1978). Adverse reactions with methyldopa — a decade's reports. *Acta Med. Scand.* 203, 425.

Gelfand, J.A., Elin, R.J., Berry, F.W., and Frank, M.M. (1976). Endotoxaemia associated with the Jarisch–Herxheimer reaction. *N .Engl. J. Med.* 295, 211.

Groel, J.T. (1963). Amphotericin B reactions. *Am. Rev. Respir. Dis.* 88, 565.

Gross, R.T., Hurwitz, R.E., and Marks, P.A. (1958). An hereditary enzymatic defect in erythrocyte metabolism: Glucose 6-phosphate dehydrogenase deficiency. *J. Clin. Invest.* 37, 1137.

Hall, G.M. (1980). Dantrolene and the treatment of malignant hyperthermia. *Br. J. Anaesth.* 52, 847.

Hamilton, M., Henley, K.S., and Morrison, B. (1954). Changes in peripheral circulation and body temperature after hexamethonium bromide. *Clin. Sci.* 13, 251.

Harrison, G.G. (1971). Anaesthetic-induced malignant hyperpyrexia: a suggested method of treatment. *Br. Med. J.* iii, 454.

Haruda, F. (1979). Phenytoin sensitivity: 39 cases. *Neurology* 29, 1480.

Hayward, J.N. and Boshell, B.R. (1957). Paraldehyde intoxication with metabolic acidosis. Report of two cases, experimental data and a critical review of the literature. *Am. J. Med.* 23, 965.

Hellon, R.F. (1975). Monoamines, pyrogens and cations: their action on central control of body temperature. *Pharmacol. Rev.* 26, 289.

Hey, E.B., Makous, N., and van der Veer, J.B. (1965). Fever and chills as a reaction to procainamide hydrochloride therapy. *Arch. Intern. Med.* 116, 544.

Hey, E.N., Kohlinsky, S., and O'Connel, B. (1969). Heat loss from babies during exchange transfusion. *Lancet* i, 335.

Hoorntje, S.J., Weening, J.J., Kallenberg, C.G.M., Prins, E.R., and Donker, A.J.M. (1979). Serum sickness-like syndrome with membranous glomerulopathy in a patient on captopril. *Lancet* ii, 1297.

Impallomeni, M. and Ezzat, R. (1976). Hypothermia associated with nitrazepam administration. *Br. Med. J.* i, 223.

Ipp, M.M., Gold, R., Greenberg, S., Goldbach, M., Kupfert, B.B., Lloyd, D.D., *et al.* (1987). Acetaminophen prophylaxis of adverse reactions following vaccination of infants with diphtheria–pertussis–tetanus toxoid/polio vaccine. *Pediatr. Infect. Dis.* 6, 721.

Isaacs, H. and Barlow, M.B. (1970). Malignant hyperpyrexia during anaesthesia: a possible association with subclinical myopathy. *Br. Med. J.* i, 275.

Jordan, S.C. and Hampson, F. (1960). Amphetamine poisoning associated with hyperpyrexia. *Br. Med. J.* ii, 844.

Judge, D.J. and Dumard, K.W. (1953). Diphenhydramine (Benadryl) and tripelennamine (Pyribenzamine) intoxication in children. *Am. J. Dis. Child.* 85, 545.

Kakkar, V.V., Franc, C., O'Shea, M.J., Flute, P.T., Howe, C.T., and Clarke, M.B. (1969). Treatment of deep venous thrombosis with streptokinase. *Br. J. Surg.* 56, 178.

Keatinge, W.R. (1987). Cold and drowning. In *Oxford textbook of medicine* (ed. D.J. Weatherall, J.G.G. Ledingham, and D.A. Warrell), p. 6.95. Oxford University Press.

Kilmanek, J., Majewski, W., and Walenick, K. (1976). A case of malignant hyperthermia during epidural anaesthesia. *Anaesth. Resusc. Intens. Ther.* 4, 143.

King, J.O., Denborough, M.A., and Zapf, P.W. (1972). Inheritance of malignant hyperpyrexia. *Lancet*, i, 365.

Klein, H.O. and Kaminsky, N. (1973). Methyldopa fever: recurrence of symptoms with resumption of therapy. *N.Y. State J. Med.* 73, 448.

Laburn, H., Mitchell, D., and Rosendorff, C. (1977). Effects of prostaglandin antagonism on sodium arachidonate fever in rabbits. *J. Physiol.* (Lond.) 267, 559.

Lips, F.J., Newland, M., and Dutton, G. (1982). Malignant hyperthermia triggered by cyclopropane during caesarian section. *Anesthesiology* 56, 144.

McGuire, N. and Easy, W.R. (1990). Malignant hyperthermia during isoflurane anaesthesia. *Anaesthesia* 45, 124.

Mikolich, J.R., Paulson, C.W., and Cross, C.J. (1975). Acute anticholinergic syndrome due to jimson seed ingestion. Clinical and laboratory observations in six cases. *Ann. Intern. Med.* 83, 321.

Milton, A.S. and Wendlandt, S. (1971). Effects on body temperature of prostaglandins of the A, E and F series on injection into the third ventricle of anaesthetised cats and rabbits. *J. Physiol.* (Lond.) 218, 325.

Mitchell, J.R.A., Surridge, D.H.C., and Willison, R.G. (1959). Hypothermia after chlorpromazine in myxoedema psychosis. *Br. Med. J.* ii, 932.

Moore, A.P., Macfarlane, I.A., and Blumhardt, L.D. (1990). Neuroleptic malignant syndrome and hypothyroidism. *J. Neurol. Neurosurg. Psychiatry* 53, 517.

Moulds, R.F.W. and Denborough, M.A. (1974a). Biochemical basis of malignany hyperpyrexia. *Br. Med. J.* ii, 241.

Moulds, R.F.W. and Denborough, M.A. (1974b). Identification of susceptibility to malignant hyperpyrexia. *Br. Med. J.* ii, 245.

Nistico, G., Rotiroti, D., De Sarro, A., and Naccari, F. (1978). Mechanism of cimetidine-induced fever. *Lancet* ii, 265.

Noble, J. and Matthew, H. (1969). Acute poisoning by tricyclic antidepressants: clinical features and management of 100 patients. *Clin. Toxicol.* 2, 403.

Noble, W.H., McKee, D., and Gates, B. (1973). Malignant hyperthermia with rigidity successfully treated with procainamide. *Anesthesiology* 39, 450.

Parks, D.L., Perry, H.O., and Muller, S.A. (1971). Cutaneous complications of pentazocine injections. *Arch. Dermatol.* 104, 231.

Perry, H.M. (1973). Late toxicity to hydralazine resembling systemic lupus erythematosus or rheumatoid arthritis. *Am. J. Med.* 54, 58.

Pfeffer, R.F. (1990). Bromocriptine-induced hypothermia. *Neurology* 40, 383.

Rawlins, M.D. and Cranston, W.I. (1972). Clinical studies on the pathogenesis of fever. In *The pharmacology of thermoregulation*, p. 264. Symposium, San Francisco.

Ruutiainen, J., Panelius, M., and Cantell, K. (1983). Toxic effects of interferon administered intrathecally. *Br. Med. J.* 280, 940.

Sako, W. (1945). Immunisation against pertussis with alum precipitated vaccine. *JAMA* 127, 379.

Saidman, L.J., Havard, E.S., and Eger, E.I. (1964). Hyperthermia during anaesthesia. *JAMA* 190, 1029.

Scott, G.M., Secher, D.S., Flowers, D., Bate, J., Cantell, K., and Tyrell, D.A.J. (1981). Toxicity of interferon. *Br. Med. J.* 282, 1345.

Seabury, J.H. (1961). Experience with amphotericin B. *Chemotherapia* 3, 81.

Seabury, J.H. and Dascomb, H.E. (1958). Experience with amphotericin B for the treatment of systemic mycoses. *Arch. Intern. Med.* 102, 960.

Shader, R.I. and Greenblatt, D.J. (1971). Uses and toxicity of belladonna alkaloids and synthetic anticholinergics. *Sem. Psychiatr.* 3, 449.

Simmons, A.V., Carr, D., and Ross, E.J. (1970). Case of self-poisoning with multiple antidepressant drugs. *Lancet* i, 214.

Stanley, J and Fallon-Pellici, V. (1978). Phenytoin hypersensitivity reaction. *Arch. Dermatol.* 114, 1350.

Tynes, B.S., Otz, J.P., Bennett, I.J.E., and Alling, D.W. (1963). Reducing amphotericin B reactions. A double blind study. *Am. Rev. Respir. Dis.* 87, 264.

Uhl, G., Farber, J., Moench, T., Friday, K., and Light, R.T. (1978). Febrile reactions to pneumococcal vaccine. *N. Engl. J. Med.* 299, 1318.

Wallerstein, R.O. and Aggeler, P.M. (1964). Acute hemolytic anaemia. *Am. J. Med.* 37, 92.

Westlake, R.J. and Rastegar, A. (1973). Hyperpyrexia from drug combination. *JAMA* 225, 1250.

WHO (1973). Pharmacogenetics. *WHO Tech. Rep. Ser.* 524.

Zierski, M. (1973). Side effects under intermittent rifampicin: a general review. *Bull. Un. Int. Tuberc.* 48, 119.

29. Drug-induced sexual dysfunction and infertility

L. BEELEY

The adverse effects of drugs on the reproductive system can be divided into those that impair sexual drive and performance, and those that produce infertility.

Drug-induced sexual dysfunction

Introduction — the pharmacology of normal sexual function

Normal male sexual function depends on the interaction of neurogenic, hormonal, and psychological mechanisms.

Erection is produced by increased blood flow into the erectile tissues of the penis, but the pharmacological basis of this vascular change is not established (Krane *et al.* 1989). Stimulation of sacral parasympathetic pathways produces erection and this has been thought to be mediated through cholinergic vasodilator pathways. There is, however, little evidence that acetylcholine is involved; erection is not prevented by atropine and erectile tissue does not seem to be well supplied with cholinergic nerve fibres. Cholinergic nerves may modulate other neurotransmitter systems rather than act directly on smooth muscle (Krane *et al.* 1989). There is extensive adrenergic innervation of the blood vessels supplying erectile tissue and evidence for both erectile and anti-erectile sympathetic pathways (Brindley 1983*a*). The exact mechanisms involved are unclear; erection can be enhanced by β_2-adrenoceptor stimulation, but the anti-erectile pathway appears to be α-adrenergic. Thus, intracavernosal injection of phenoxybenzamine, an α-adrenoceptor antagonist, can produce erection (Brindley 1983*b*). Vasoconstriction produced by sympathetic stimulation of α-adrenoceptors is thought to bring about detumescence. There is also evidence that non-adrenergic, non-cholinergic relaxation of cavernous smooth muscle plays an essential part in erection, and

vasoactive intestinal polypeptide is one neurotransmitter that may be involved (Ottesen *et al.* 1984). Finally, adequate arterial blood flow in the hypogastric and pudendal arteries is a prerequisite for normal erection.

Ejaculation is preceded by emission of seminal fluid into the urethra and closure of the internal sphincter to prevent backflow of semen into the bladder. Both are mediated by the thoracolumbar sympathetic nerves acting on α-adrenoceptors. Ejaculation itself is a reflex contraction of the bulbar muscles mediated by somatic efferents in the pudendal nerves. Prostaglandins are present in large amounts in seminal fluid. They are known to stimulate penile muscle, and it has been suggested that they may be involved in ejaculation (Bygdeman 1981).

Although reflex erection and ejaculation can both occur after spinal transection, the brain plays an important part in normal sexual function, but neither the pathways concerned nor the neurotransmitters involved have been defined (Brindley 1983*a*; Krane *et al.* 1989).

Libido (sexual desire) is influenced by sex hormones, the emotional and physical health of the individual, and external factors such as availability and attractiveness of the sexual partner. Testosterone is necessary for normal sexual arousal and, although reflexly evoked erection can occur without it, testosterone deficiency is associated with impotence. Hyperprolactinaemia produces loss of libido and impotence when associated with low levels of circulating testosterone (Franks *et al.* 1978). The mechanism for this is not established, but one possibility is that hyperprolactinaemia abolishes the pulsatile release of gonadotrophin-releasing hormone, which reduces luteinizing hormone (LH) release and causes serum testosterone levels to fall (Spark 1983). Normalization of serum testosterone does not always restore potency, and it has been suggested that prolactin may also antagonize the peripheral action of testosterone (Krane *et al.* 1989). Finally, psychological factors have a strong influence on sexual performance.

In women, the neurophysiological mechanisms of sexual function are poorly understood. As in men, activation of the sympathetic system is important and there is evidence that vasoactive intestinal polypeptide may be involved in producing vasodilatation. There is no evidence for involvement of cholinergic innervation (Levin 1980). Dysfunction can be manifest as orgasmic impairment, failure of vaginal lubrication, or vaginismus, or as loss of libido. The role of the sex hormones in female sexual function is also poorly understood (Bancroft 1981). Exogenous androgens are known to enhance sexual responsiveness in women, but the importance of endogenous androgens is disputed. Minimal levels of oestrogen are probably necessary for normal sexual behaviour, but the effect of progesterone is unclear.

Almost all of the published information on drug-induced sexual dysfunction relates to men, and relatively little is known about the effects of drugs on sexual function in women.

Epidemiological aspects

When evaluating reports of adverse effects of drugs on sexual function it is important to be aware of factors that influence studies of these effects: many drugs reputed to affect sexual function are given for disorders that may themselves be associated with impaired sexual function. Thus, sexual problems are frequently attributed to antihypertensive drugs and to drugs used in psychiatry, but even without treatment impotence is more common in hypertensive patients than in a normal control group (Bulpitt *et al.* 1976), and the incidence of sexual dysfunction in untreated psychiatric patients may be as high as 70 per cent, depending on the type of patient studied (Beck 1976; Lief 1977; Beaumont 1978; Nestoros and Lehmann 1979). Also the prevalence of sexual dysfunction in an ill population (Slag *et al.* 1983) is probably higher than the accepted prevalence within the normal population (Kinsey *et al.* 1948). Sexual performance declines with age (Felstein 1980; Bancroft 1982), and both alcohol and smoking may adversely affect it. Many patients are aware that drugs can interfere with their sexual performance and this itself may lead to impotence.

Single case reports are difficult to assess even if a causal relationship seems clear. For example, adequate baseline (pretreatment) information may be lacking and, even if rechallenge with the drug produces recurrence of the sexual problem, this could be due to anticipatory anxiety rather than the pharmacological action of the drug. Controlled studies are therefore necessary to establish a causal relationship, and they are also the only valid way to measure the incidence of sexual adverse effects with particular drugs. As with all epidemiological studies the methods used may influence the results. For example, under-reporting of sexual adverse effects is usual, and a higher incidence will be obtained by using a detailed checklist of specific questions than by asking open-ended questions or relying on spontaneous reporting by the patients. It is important to have appropriate control groups to take account of possible confounding variables. Of these, the disease for which the drug is given, age, smoking, and alcohol intake are probably the most important factors. Very few reported studies have taken either smoking or drinking into consideration.

Finally, interpretation of the literature is not helped by the lack of clear definition by many authors of the terms used. In particular, the term impotence is frequently used to refer to any erectile or ejaculatory problems. This often makes it difficult to be sure exactly what effect the drug is having and to postulate any pharmacological mechanism.

Drugs causing sexual dysfunction

Drug effects on sexual function are generally Type A adverse effects (see Chapter 3): they are predictable or explicable on the basis of the known pharmacology of the drug, and they are dose-related. However, although drugs may predictably interfere primarily with a single component of sexual function the final result may not reflect this. For example, impotence is the most common presenting symptom but it may be the end result of a number of different drug effects — central or peripheral — and the original abnormality may be modified by the effect of secondary anxiety such that a primarily peripheral effect on erection acquires a central component.

Antihypertensive drugs

The prevalence of both impotence and ejaculatory disorders is significantly greater in treated hypertensive patients than in matched controls (Bulpitt and Dollery 1973; Bulpitt *et al.* 1976; Medical Research Council 6Working Party 1981; Hogan *et al.* 1980). In the hypertensive population studied by Bulpitt and others (1976) about 25 per cent of patients reported impotence, as opposed to 17 per cent of untreated hypertensives and 7 per cent of normotensive controls. The prevalence of ejaculatory failure was also about 25 per cent as opposed to 7 per cent in untreated patients and nil in normotensive controls. Hogan and others (1980) reviewed 861 male hypertensive patients and compared them with 177 controls. The prevalence of sexual dysfunction ranged from 9 per cent to 23 per cent depending on the drugs used, compared with 4 per cent in the normotensive controls. Similar figures have been quoted in more recent studies (Bulpitt *et al*. 1989).

Most individual antihypertensive drugs have been reported to cause sexual dysfunction but some are more likely to do so than others.

The adrenergic-neurone blockers bethanidine, debrisoquine, and guanethidine commonly cause both impotence and failure of ejaculation and, in earlier studies done when these drugs were still widely used (Bulpitt and Dollery 1973), the prevalence of sexual dysfunction was higher than with other antihypertensive drugs.

Methyldopa and clonidine are centrally acting α-adrenoceptor agonists that produce their antihypertensive effect by inhibiting sympathetic outflow from the brainstem. Methyldopa has been reported to cause loss of libido, impotence, and ejaculatory failure (Hogan *et al*. 1980; Taylor *et al* 1981; Newman and Salerno 1974; Alexander and Evans 1975). In one study the incidence of sexual dysfunction was 26 per cent (Newman and Salerno 1974) and, in another, 16 out of 30 patients admitted to failure of ejaculation when asked specifically about this (Alexander and Evans 1975). Although reduced sympathetic activity is probably the main cause, the exact mechanisms involved are not clear. Methyldopa can increase serum prolactin concentrations, but hyperprolactinaemia is not always found in patients with methyldopa-induced sexual dysfunction (Taylor *et al*. 1981). The sedative and depressant effects of methyldopa may account for the loss of libido reported. Clonidine has been associated with impotence in some studies (Hogan *et al*. 1980; Onesti *et al*. 1971). As with methyldopa, the mechanism is not clear, but reduced sympathetic activity is the most likely cause. Loss of libido may also occur, from the sedative and depressant effects of this drug.

Impotence is well documented with propranolol (Medical Research Council Working Party 1981; Hogan *et al*. 1980; Burnett and Chahine 1979; Warren and Warren 1977). In a report from the MRC trial of treatment (Medical Research Council Working Party 1981), impotence occurred in 14 per cent of patients after 12 weeks of propranolol therapy, compared with 9 per cent of the control patients; and an incidence of 25 per cent has been reported in patients taking propranolol together with hydralazine and a diuretic (Hogan *et al*. 1980). Reduced penile blood flow has been described in impotent patients taking propranolol and attributed to unopposed α-receptor-mediated vasoconstriction (Forsberg *et al*. 1979). The Committee on Safety of Medicines has had reports of impotence caused by other β-blockers (Griffin 1982), and impotence has been reported in

patients treated with timolol eyedrops (McMahon *et al*. 1979; Fraunfelder and Keyer 1985). Labetalol, which has both α-adrenoceptor and β-adrenoceptor antagonist activity, appears to affect ejaculation rather than erection. In a laboratory study on six volunteers it had no effect on erection but delayed ejaculation in a dose-related manner (Riley *et al*. 1982). It also resulted in a dose-related delay in detumescence, presumably attributable to the α-blocking effect of the drug. Failure of ejaculation has also been reported clinically (Stokes *et al*. 1983). Pure α-adrenoceptor antagonists also seem to produce failure of ejaculation rather than impotence. This is a common adverse effect of phenoxybenzamine (Kedia and Persky 1981), occurring also with indoramin (Pentland *et al*. 1981), but it appears to be uncommon with prazosin (Stessman and Ben-Ishay 1980).

There have been several reports of impotence in patients taking thiazide diuretics (Hogan *et al*. 1980), and the incidence in the MRC trial quoted above (Medical Research Council Working Party 1981) was 16 per cent at 12 weeks. Subsequent studies have suggested, however, that the incidence is much lower than this (Grimm *et al*. 1985; Helgeland *et al*. 1986). The mechanism is unknown. Spironolactone is well known to cause gynaecomastia, and decreased libido and impotence have also been reported (Greenblatt and Koch-Weser 1973; Spark and Melby 1968; Zarren and Black 1975). In one report, 30 per cent of men receiving 400 mg of spironolactone daily developed decreased libido (Spark and Melby 1968), but sexual dysfunction seems to be uncommon in patients on smaller doses. The mechanism is not established. There is no good evidence that spironolactone produces any changes in sex steroid metabolism (Huffman *et al*. 1978), but there is evidence in both animals and man that it acts as an antiandrogen by inhibiting binding of dihydrotestosterone to its receptor (Loriaux *et al*. 1976). Other potassium-sparing diuretics have not been reported to affect sexual function.

In a report from the DHSS Hypertension Care Computing Project (Bulpitt *et al*. 1989) the prevalence of impotence and sexual inactivity was similar with methyldopa, β-blockers, and diuretics, but there was an increased prevalence with hydralazine. There have been few other reports with hydralazine (Ahmad 1980) and sexual dysfunction is not usually an adverse effect of vasodilators. A possible mechanism would be diversion of blood away from the erectile tissues.

Angiotensin-converting-enzyme inhibitors do not appear to produce sexual dysfunction (Croog *et al*. 1986).

Psychotropic drugs

There is little doubt that many psychotropic drugs can

interfere with sexual function. Sexual dysfunction in men is well documented, and recent reports suggest that the sexual response in women can also be affected. Establishing the frequency with which this occurs is made difficult by the fact that sexual problems are common in untreated patients with psychiatric illness. For example, reduced sexual activity has been reported in schizophrenic patients (Nestoros and Lehmann 1979), and loss of libido and impotence are common symptoms of depression (Mitchell and Popkin 1983). Thus, the role of drugs in producing sexual dysfunction in an individual case is often difficult to assess.

Antidepressants

Most of the tricyclic antidepressants have been reported to cause impotence (Mitchell and Popkin 1983; Segraves 1982). This has been attributed to their anticholinergic activity, and in one report it was reversed by bethanecol (Gross 1982). Potentiation of noradrenergic vasoconstriction may, however, be a more important mechanism, and effects on the central nervous system may also be involved. Mazindol, which resembles the tricyclic antidepressants in inhibiting noradrenaline re-uptake into adrenergic neurones but has no anticholinergic activity, has also been reported to cause impotence (McEwen and Meyboom 1983). Interestingly, this too has been reported to be reversed by bethanecol (Yager 1986). The tertiary amines — imipramine, amitriptyline, trimipramine, and clomipramine — are α-adrenoceptor antagonists and can delay or inhibit ejaculation (Mitchell and Popkin 1983; Segraves 1982). The monoamine oxidase inhibitors — phenelzine, tranylcypromine, isocarboxazid — have similar physiological actions to the tricyclic antidepressants, and can also produce both impotence and failure of ejaculation (Segraves 1982). Drugs from both groups of antidepressants have been used successfully to treat premature ejaculation (Mitchell and Popkin 1983).

In women, orgasm is the neuropharmacological equivalent of ejaculation (Shen and Park 1982) and anorgasmia has been reported with amoxapine (a tricyclic antidepressant) (Shen 1982; Gross 1982); with clomipramine (Monteiro *et al.* 1987); and with imipramine (Sovner 1983). In the patient reported by Sovner (1983), substituting desipramine for imipramine restored normal orgasm, which is consistent with the fact that desipramine differs from imipramine in having no α-adrenoceptor antagonist effect. These drugs also differ, however, in that imipramine but not desipramine inhibits neuronal re-uptake of serotonin. That this might be of importance is suggested by reports of reversal of anorgasmia induced by antidepressants with cyproheptadine,

a serotonin antagonist (Riley and Riley 1986*a*). The specific serotonin uptake inhibitor fluoxetine has been associated with several reports of anorgasmia in both men and women, which further supports this suggestion (Lydiard and George 1989; Kline 1989).

There have also been several convincing reports of anorgasmia attributed to monoamine oxidase inhibitors (Barton 1979; Lesko *et al.* 1982; Moss 1983; Pohl 1983) and, at least with phenelzine, this effect seems to be dose-related.

Less is known about the effects of newer antidepressants on sexual function. Some of them lack the peripheral autonomic effects of the tricyclics and monoamine oxidase inhibitors and may therefore be less likely to cause sexual dysfunction. Trazodone has been reported to cause both ejaculatory inhibition (Jones 1984) and anorgasmia (Jani *et al.* 1988), attributed to its α-blocking activity. There have also been several reports of increased libido associated with trazodone (Gartrell 1986; Sullivan 1987).

Antidepressants primarily inhibiting the neuronal uptake of serotonin have been associated with an interesting adverse effect consisting of yawning associated with spontaneous orgasms, with or without clitoral engorgement or ejaculation. This has been reported with clomipramine (McLean *et al.* 1983) and fluoxetine (Modell 1989). It is thought to be a serotonergic effect, and there is evidence in animals that yawning and penile erection are associated (Modell 1989).

Antipsychotic drugs

The phenothiazines (e.g. chlorpromazine, thioridazine) have anticholinergic and α-adrenoceptor antagonist activity. They can cause both impotence and ejaculatory dysfunction (Mitchell and Popkin 1982), and from the limited evidence available the incidence seems to be higher than with antidepressants. Thioridazine is the drug most frequently reported, and this is consistent with the greater peripheral autonomic activity of the piperidine group of phenothiazines. Thus, in one study (Kotin *et al.* 1976), 60 per cent of patients receiving thioridazine reported sexual dysfunction as opposed to 25 per cent of patients taking other antipsychotic drugs. There have been many individual case reports of both impotence and ejaculatory dysfunction in patients taking thioridazine, and isolated reports with chlorpromazine and other antipsychotic drugs, including fluphenazine, trifluoperazine, and chlorprothixene (Mitchell and Popkin 1982). Thioridazine has been used in the treatment of premature ejaculation (Mitchell and Popkin 1982).

Other groups of antipsychotic drugs such as the butyrophenones (e.g. haloperidol) and the diphenylbutylpiperidines (fluspirilene, pimozide) lack the peripheral autonomic effects of the phenothiazines and rarely produce sexual dysfunction. There has, however, been a single well-documented report of impotence apparently produced by treatment with pimozide (Ananth 1982) and impotence has been described in patients on sulpiride (Weizman et al. 1985). All the antipsychotic drugs are dopamine antagonists and many have been shown to produce hyperprolactinaemia (Sacher 1978). Weizman and others (1985) described a group of patients in whom impotence associated with sulpiride was dose-related and correlated with plasma prolactin levels. They cited this as evidence that the hyperprolactinaemia caused the impotence. It may have been, however, that both impotence and hyperprolactinaemia were dose-related. Studies of hypothalamic–pituitary–gonadal function in schizophrenic patients on long-term treatment with phenothiazine have given conflicting results, but there is some evidence that basal testosterone levels and LH secretion may be reduced (Beumont et al. 1974; Apter et al. 1983; Weizman et al. 1985), possibly secondarily to hyperprolactinaemia. There is, however, no convincing evidence these changes play any part in the sexual dysfunction associated with antipsychotic drugs, and the absence of sexual dysfunction with haloperidol suggests peripheral autonomic effects are more important.

There are few reports of sexual dysfunction in women treated with antipsychotic drugs, but one report describes two women who developed anorgasmia with trifluoperazine and thioridazine respectively (Degan 1982), and another describes a woman with anorgasmia due to thioridazine (Shen and Park 1982). It is not surprising that drugs affecting ejaculation in men can produce anorgasmia in women, and it seems likely that this occurs more commonly than it is reported, possibly because women are less likely than men to complain about sexual dysfunction (Shen and Park 1982).

Lithium does not seem to interfere with sexual function in the majority of patients, but there have been a few reports suggesting that lithium may produce impotence and reduced libido (Blay et al. 1982; Kristensen and Jørgensen 1987).

Sexual dysfunction is rarely reported in patients taking benzodiazepines but is probably not uncommon in long-term users. Diazepam has been shown to inhibit orgasm in female volunteers (Riley and Riley 1986b), and inhibition of orgasm and ejaculation have been reported with alprazolam (Sangal 1985; Munjack and Crocker 1986; Uhde et al. 1988). Loss of libido has been reported with lorazepam (Khandelwal 1988), and benzodiazepine

withdrawal has been associated with increased sexual function (Nutt et al. 1986).

The non-benzodiazepine anxiolytic buspirone has been reported to improve impaired sexual function in anxious patients, an improvement that was not correlated with reduction in anxiety and which was attributed to the central pharmacological effects of buspirone, which antagonizes serotonin and enhances dopaminergic and noradrenergic activity (Othmer and Othmer 1987).

Opiates

Opiate addiction is commonly associated with decreased libido and impotence, but sexual activity returns during periods of abstinence (Mendelson and Mello 1982).

Opiates suppress pituitary LH secretion and produce a fall in serum testosterone levels. The precise mechanism for this effect is unknown, but they appear to inhibit the production of gonadotrophin-releasing hormone in the hypothalamus. They also produce hyperprolactinaemia, but the importance of this effect in relation to sexual dysfunction is unclear. Hormone levels return to normal during periods of abstinence.

Cimetidine

Cimetidine has antiandrogen activity. This has been convincingly demonstrated in animals (Winters et al. 1979), but whether it is clinically important in the therapeutic doses usual in man is unclear. Gynaecomastia (Delle Fave et al. 1977; Spence and Celestin 1979; McCarthy 1978) and impotence (Wolfe 1979; Peden et al. 1982; Niv 1986) have been reported occasionally, and a small increase in serum testosterone levels has been reported in some (Peden and Wormsley 1982; van Thiel et al. 1979; Carlson et al. 1981) but not all (Stubbs et al. 1983) studies of endocrine function in patients taking cimetidine. In one study of 22 patients treated with large doses of cimetidine for gastric hypersecretory states (Jensen et al 1983), gynaecomastia occurred in 11 and impotence in 9 patients receiving a mean dose of 5.3 g daily. These effects disappeared when cimetidine was stopped or when the dose was reduced. It seems likely therefore that sexual dysfunction with cimetidine is dose-related, occurring rarely with the doses used for peptic ulcer but more commonly with the large doses required for hypersecretory states. Both gynaecomastia and impotence are attributed to the antiandrogen effect of cimetidine and not to its antihistamine-H_2 properties. Thus, ranitidine does not have these adverse effects (Wang et al. 1983), and patients with cimetidine-induced gynaecomastia and impotence recover when given ranit-idine instead (Peden and Wormsley 1982; Jensen *et al.* 1983).

Anticonvulsants

Reduced sexual activity and impotence have been re-ported in several studies of male epileptics treated with various anticonvulsant regimens (Christiansen *et al.* 1975; Toone *et al.* 1983). This is probably due to changes in sex hormone levels produced by enzyme induction. Free testosterone levels fall and sex-hormone-binding globulin is increased (Toone *et al.* 1983; MacPhee *et al.* 1988). Reduced sexual activity appears to be related to the fall in free testosterone (Christiansen *et al.* 1975; Toone *et al.* 1983). Valproate, which is not an enzyme-inducer, does not affect sex hormone levels or interfere with sexual function (MacPhee *et al.* 1988).

Sex hormones

Loss of libido and impotence occur predictably in men treated with oestrogens. Cyproterone acetate can pro-duce impotence in addition to the reduction in sexual arousal for which it is used, but potency can usually be retained if large doses are avoided.

Analogues of luteinizing-hormone-releasing hormone (LH/FSH-RH), currently being tried in the treatment of prostatic carcinoma, produce impotence by reducing LH and consequently testosterone secretion (*The Lancet* 1983).

A high incidence of impotence has been reported in men treated with high doses of hydroxyprogesterone caproate for benign prostatic hyperplasia (Meiraz *et al.* 1977).

Sexual problems are commonly reported by women taking oral contraceptives. They have been attributed to the progestogen component, but a negative effect of progestogens on sexual function has not been estab-lished, and there are often psychological or other expla-nations for sexual problems in women taking the pill.

Ketoconazole

Ketoconazole inhibits gonadal and adrenal synthesis of androgens and reduces plasma testosterone levels (Allen *et al.* 1983; Pont *et al.* 1982; Schurmeyer and Nieschlag 1982). The clinical importance of this is not yet clear, but gynaecomastia, loss of libido, and impotence have been reported occasionally in men treated with ketoconazole (Schurmeyer and Nieschlag 1982).

Alcohol

The acute effects of alcohol on male sexual performance are well known: erection is impaired with no loss of sexual desire. There are also long-term negative effects on both male and female sexual function (Mandell and Miller 1983). In men, chronic alcoholism is associated with features of hypogonadism (Morgan 1982). Serum testosterone is reduced and there may be loss of libido as well as impotence. The exact mechanism is unknown, but diminished sexual function occurs independently of the presence of alcoholic liver disease. Alcohol has a direct inhibitory effect on testicular steroidogenesis (Anderson and Willis 1981), but effects on the hypo-thalamus, on peripheral testosterone metabolism, and on sex-steroid-binding globulin have also been de-scribed. A neuropathic component to the impotence has been suggested and might be one reason for persistent impotence even after prolonged abstinence.

Other drugs

Impotence has been reported with disopyramide (McHaffie *et al.* 1977; Papadopoulos 1980) and has been attributed to its anticholinergic properties. There is, however, no evidence that impotence is a problem with other anticholinergic drugs. It has been reported with two other antiarrhythmic drugs, verapamil (King *et al.* 1983; Fogelman 1988) and flecainide (Meinertz *et al.* 1984).

There has been a report of impotence with indo-methacin (Miller *et al.* 1989) and of failure of ejaculation with naproxen (Wei and Hood 1980). Impotence in patients receiving non-steroidal anti-inflammatory drugs has been reported to the Committee on Safety of Medi-cines (personal communication) (Table 29.1) but a causal relationship cannot be assumed in such reports. Intracavernous injection of prostaglandin E_1 has been shown to induce penile erection (Schramek and Wald-hauser 1989) and, as mentioned above, it has been suggested that prostaglandins may be involved in ejaculation.

Bromocriptine has been reported to cause impotence in men with Parkinson's disease (Cleeves and Findlay 1987). Both erectile dysfunction and loss of libido associ-ated with menstrual disturbances have been reported with etretinate (Halkier-Sørensen 1987). Impotence and decreased libido have been reported with metoclo-pramide and attributed to the associated hyperprolac-tinaemia (Berlin 1986). Many other drugs have been reported to cause sexual dysfunction but usually in single case reports, and the evidence for a causal relationship is poor. Impotence, with or without decreased libido, has been reported with sulphasalazine (Ireland and Jewell 1989), methotrexate (Blackburn and Alarcon 1989), baclofen, clofibrate, fenfluramine, carbonic anhydrase

TABLE 29.1

TABLE 29.1

Reports to the Committee on Safety of Medicines of sexual dysfunction associated with anti-inflammatory analgesics (1990)

	Impotence	Loss of libido
Azapropazone	3	
Diclofenac	9	2
Diflunisal	1	
Fenbufen	5	4
Flurbiprofen	3	
Ibuprofen	7	4
Indomethacin	6	4
Ketoprofen	2	2
Mefenamic acid	3	
Naproxen	9	2
Phenylbutazone	3	2
Piroxicam	8	4
Sulindac	3	
Tiaprofenic acid	4	1

inhibitors (acetazolamide and dichlorphenamide), and anabolic steroids (*Medical Letter* 1983; Epstein *et al.* 1987).

Sexual dysfunction secondary to testicular damage

Loss of libido and reduced sexual activity are common during treatment in patients with testicular damage due to cancer chemotherapy (Chapman *et al.* 1981; Whitehead *et al.* 1982) (see below). These patients frequently have elevated serum LH concentrations but few have a low testosterone, and sexual dysfunction is not closely correlated with testosterone concentrations. Once treatment has finished, sexual function usually returns to normal and impotence is rare.

Priapism

Drugs probably cause priapism by preventing detumescence. This has been ascribed to α-adrenoceptor antagonist activity, which prevents constriction of the blood vessels supplying erectile tissue. Intracavernosal phenoxybenzamine induces erections in normal men and these are reversed by the α-adrenoceptor antagonist metaraminol (Banos *et al.* 1989). Other neuropharmacological mechanisms, however, may also play a part, and anticholinergic drugs can reverse priapism induced by phenothiazines (Banos *et al.* 1989).

There have been many reports of priapism with phenothiazines (Banos *et al.* 1989), trazodone (Banos *et al.* 1989; Warner *et al.* 1987) and prazosin (Banos *et al.* 1989), and isolated reports with labetalol (Law *et al.* 1980), phenelzine (Yeragani and Gershon 1987), guan-

ethidine and hydralazine (Bhalla *et al.* 1979), nifedipine (Rayner *et al.* 1988), and anticoagulants (Banos *et al.* 1989).

Drugs affecting fertility

Drugs can produce infertility either by a direct effect on the gonads or indirectly by inhibiting pituitary secretion of gonadotrophins.

Drugs directly affecting the gonads

This subject has been reviewed by Gradishar and Schilsky (1988).

Cytotoxic drugs

Many of the drugs used in cancer chemotherapy are toxic to the gonads and can cause infertility. The effects on endocrine function differ in men and women; and the results of toxicity in children may depend on the state of pubertal development at the time of treatment. These three groups will therefore be considered separately.

Adult men

Cytotoxic drugs predominantly affect the germinal epithelium, producing oligospermia or azoöspermia with secondary elevation of plasma FSH levels. Leydig cell function is relatively less affected. Although testosterone levels are usually normal, elevated LH levels are, however, sometimes found, indicating compensated Leydig cell damage (Schilsky *et al.* 1980).

There is increasing evidence that the alkylating agents and procarbazine are more toxic to the testis than other cytotoxic drugs. Both cyclophosphamide and chlorambucil can produce azoöspermia when used as single agents (Schilsky *et al.* 1980; Fairley *et al.* 1972; Buchanan *et al.* 1975; Callis *et al.* 1980). The extent of gonadal damage and the likelihood of recovery depend on the dose and duration of treatment. Irreversible azoöspermia has been reported with both drugs, but recovery can occur even a year or more after treatment has been stopped; and severe damage can be avoided altogether by using small doses.

The combination chemotherapy regimens used to treat Hodgkin's disease produce complete azoöspermia in all patients during treatment (Chapman *et al.* 1981; Whitehead *et al.* 1982), usually after only one or two cycles. Azoöspermia persists in over 80 per cent of patients, but recovery of spermatogenesis has been described and is more likely to occur in patients who are under 30 when treated (Waxman 1983). The two regimens that have been most extensively studied are mustine, procarbazine, and prednisone with either vinblastine or vincristine (MVPP and MOPP). Mustine and procarbazine are thought to be the drugs mainly responsible for infertility, but vincristine and vinblastine may have a potentiating effect (Chapman *et al.* 1981). The combination of cyclophosphamide, vincristine, procarbazine, and prednisone (COPP) is even more toxic than MOPP (Kreuser *et al.* 1987), but the combination of adriamycin, bleomycin, vinblastine, and dacarbazine (ABVD) is less toxic (Kreuser *et al.* 1987).

Regimens that do not contain an alkylating agent are less toxic. In a study of eight men in remission of acute leukaemia 8 months to 8 years after completing treatment (Waxman *et al.* 1983), the four treated for acute myeloid leukaemia with adriamycin, cytarabine, and thioguanine had normal sperm counts. Three, however, of the four treated for acute lymphatic leukaemia with vincristine, adriamycin, and colaspase followed by maintenance therapy with cyclophosphamide, methotrexate, and mercaptopurine had azoöspermia. This was thought to be due to the cyclophosphamide. Return of fertility has also been described after chemotherapy with vinblastine, bleomycin, and cisplatin for disseminated teratoma (Rubery 1983) and after procarbazine, vinblastine, and bleomycin (PVB) treatment of testicular cancer (Kreuser *et al.* 1986).

Methotrexate is less toxic than the alkylating agents, and although prolonged administration of high doses in the treatment of osteosarcoma has produced severe oligospermia during therapy, recovery occurred eventually in all patients (Shamberger *et al.* 1981). The small doses used to treat psoriasis have little or no effect on spermatogenesis in most studies (El-Beheiry *et al.* 1979; Grunnet *et al.* 1977), though reversible oligospermia has been reported (Sussman and Leonard 1980).

Adult women

In women, cytotoxic drugs that affect the ovary produce loss of primordial follicles with failure of both ovulation and endocrine function. Plasma levels of oestradiol and progesterone are low and LH and FSH levels are elevated. There is oligomenorrhoea or amenorrhoea with loss of libido and menopausal symptoms (Shalet 1980).

As in men, the alkylating agents are the most toxic, and ovarian failure has been described after single-agent therapy with cyclophosphamide, chlorambucil, or busulphan (Shalet 1980); after treatment of breast cancer with regimens containing either cyclophosphamide or melphalan (Fisher *et al.* 1979; Koyama *et al.* 1977); and after MVPP combination chemotherapy for Hodgkin's disease (Chapman *et al.* 1979; King *et al.* 1985). The degree of ovarian damage depends not only on the type of drug used and the dose but also on the age of the woman at the time of treatment (Chapman 1982; Fisher

et al. 1979; Koyama *et al.* 1977; Chapman *et al.* 1979), presumably related to the fact that oöcyte numbers decrease with age. Furthermore, ovarian damage appears to be progressive even after treatment has finished (Chapman *et al.* 1979). Thus, pregnancy can occur despite ovarian damage (Chapman 1982) that subsequently progresses to ovarian failure.

Not all cytotoxic drug regimens adversely affect ovarian function. Chemotherapy for chorioncarcinoma, in particular, appears to be compatible with subsequent fertility. In one survey (Rustin *et al.* 1984), 187 women out of 217 who wished to conceive had at least one live birth after completing treatment. All the women had received methotrexate and 37 with a live birth had also received cyclophosphamide. Women who received three or more drugs were, however, less likely to have a live birth, and the highest failure rate occurred with regimens containing actinomycin D or vincristine. In a recent study of 227 women under 35 who had been given adjuvant chemotherapy with doxorubicin, fluorouracil, and cyclophosphamide for breast cancer, there were 35 pregnancies after completion of chemotherapy (Sutton *et al.* 1990).

Children

Early studies suggested that the prepubertal testis was relatively resistant to damage by cytotoxic drugs, but this is probably not true (Shalet 1980). Lendon and others (1978) studied testicular biopsies from 44 boys treated prepubertally with combination chemotherapy for acute lymphatic leukaemia and found a mean reduction of 50 per cent in the tubular fertility index. Cyclophosphamide and cytosine arabinoside produced the most severe damage, but there was evidence that the tubular fertility index improved with increasing time after cessation of therapy. Other studies of postpubertal boys who had received cyclophosphamide or chlorambucil before puberty have also shown a marked reduction in sperm count and increased FSH levels (Shalet 1980). The damage is, however, dose-related and the doses of cyclophosphamide currently used to treat the nephrotic syndrome in childhood appear to have only minor effects on spermatogenesis, insufficient to produce infertility (Trompeter *et al.* 1981).

During puberty the testis may be more susceptible to damage, and combination chemotherapy with MOPP for Hodgkin's disease has been reported to produce both germinal aplasia and Leydig cell failure (Schilsky *et al.* 1980). Regimens that do not contain an alkylating agent are less toxic (Roeser *et al.* 1978); for example, treatment with prednisone, vincristine, methotrexate, and mercaptopurine for acute lymphatic leukaemia in pre-pubertal and pubescent boys does not appear to affect testicular function (Blatt *et al.* 1981). A study of testicular function in 30 adolescent or adult males who had undergone polychemotherapy before or during puberty showed azoöspermia or severe genital cell dysfunction in 20. The alkylating agents, especially MOPP and cyclophosphamide, were the most toxic. Dactinomycin, vincristine, and vinblastine did not appear to have a toxic effect on spermatogenesis (Aubier *et al.* 1987).

The ovaries of prepubertal girls are relatively resistant to cytotoxic drugs, probably because follicular activity is low before puberty. There is good evidence, however, that cytotoxic drugs can produce gonadal damage if enough drug is given. The degree of damage is very variable and the factors that determine susceptibility are not well defined. Normal menstrual function and fertility have been described in women who had received cyclophosphamide for glomerulonephritis in childhood but so also has ovarian damage (da Cunha *et al.* 1979). In one study of children treated for leukaemia (Siris *et al.* 1976), 28 out of 35 girls had normal pubertal development and only three of the others had signs of primary ovarian failure. The main drugs used were methotrexate, vincristine, mercaptopurine, and prednisone, but one of the three patients with ovarian failure had received busulphan. In two other studies of prepubertal girls with acute lymphatic leukaemia (Shalet 1980), combination chemotherapy produced ovarian failure in 3 out of 12 girls; all 3 had received cyclophosphamide. Primary ovarian failure has been reported in three adolescent girls after high-dose melphalan treatment of solid tumours (Kellie and Kingston 1987). An autopsy study (Himelstein-Braw *et al.* 1978) of the ovaries of 31 leukaemic girls showed inhibition of follicle development in most of them. All had been treated with combination chemotherapy regimens which included cyclophosphamide in some but not all patients. The degree of damage was related to duration of treatment. Long-term effects of ovarian damage in childhood are unknown. Impaired follicular development may be reversible, but premature menopause is a possible sequel.

Sulphasalazine

Oligospermia and infertility appear to be quite common in men on long-term treatment with sulphasalazine for inflammatory bowel disease (Birnie *et al.* 1981). These effects are reversible within 2 months of stopping of treatment and reappear rapidly when it is reintroduced.

Semen analysis shows a decrease in sperm density, poor motility, and abnormal sperm morphology with an increased number of large-headed sperm (Toovey *et al.* 1981; Hudson *et al.* 1982). The mechanism by which sulphasalazine produces these effects is unknown.

Sperm motility is reduced during the first 2 months of treatment, which suggests a direct toxic effect on mature spermatozoa (O'Morain *et al.* 1982). Sperm morphology is not, however, significantly impaired until the patients have been taking the drug for more than 2 months, suggesting toxicity at an earlier stage of spermatogenesis (Hudson *et al.* 1982). After withdrawal of treatment, fertility is restored before sperm morphology returns to normal. It has therefore been suggested that the mechanism for infertility may not be the same as that responsible for the abnormal morphology (Hudson *et al.* 1982).

Sulphasalazine is metabolized within the bowel to sulphapyridine and 5-aminosalicylic acid (mesalazine). Only sulphapyridine is absorbed to any great extent and this appears to be the most likely cause of infertility. Thus, in male rats sulphapyridine has the same effect on fertility as sulphasalazine, whereas mesalazine has no effect (O'Morain *et al.* 1982). Also, return of fertility has been reported in patients whose treatment was changed from sulphasalazine to mesalazine (Cann and Holdsworth 1984; Riley *et al.* 1987). As other sulphonamides do not affect fertility in rats and are not known to cause infertility in man, the pyridine component of sulphapyridine is the most likely toxic agent. The increased number of large-headed sperm suggests an interference with DNA synthesis during spermatogenesis and could be due to the antifolate effect of sulphasalazine (Hudson *et al.* 1982).

Antimicrobials

Scattered reports suggest that some antimicrobial agents may interfere with spermatogenesis. Two reports have described a transitory depression of sperm count in men treated with nitrofurantoin (Yunda and Kushniruk 1974). A decreased sperm count was reported in 14 out of 40 men treated with co-trimoxazole (Murdia *et al.* 1978), but this report was subsequently criticized (Guillebaude 1978), and there is no other evidence that either sulphonamides or trimethoprim affect human spermatogenesis. Dapsone has also been reported to cause infertility with recovery after the drug was stopped (Grieve 1979). Niridazole, an antibilharzial remedy, inhibits spermatogenesis in animals. In a study of 20 men with bilharzia, it produced oligospermia with histological evidence of spermatocyte arrest and focal germinal hypoplasia. Recovery had occurred 3 months after the end of treatment (El-Beheiry *et al.* 1982).

Anticonvulsants

Abnormalities of sperm morphology and motility, and

reduced fertility occurred more frequently than expected in one study of epileptic patients taking anticonvulsants (Christiansen *et al.* 1975). Others have not found any significant differences between epileptics and controls (Cohn *et al.* 1982), and the clinical importance of this is unknown.

Drugs inhibiting pituitary secretion of gonadotrophins

Steroid hormones

High doses of testosterone and other androgens produce oligospermia by inhibiting gonadotrophin secretion, mainly that of LH. Oestrogens and some progestogens (19-nortestosterone derivatives) have a similar effect (Neumann *et al.* 1976). A combination of medroxy-progesterone acetate and testosterone enanthate has been shown to produce reversible infertility associated with suppression of sperm function in addition to oligo-spermia or azoöspermia (Wu and Aitken 1989). Schurmeyer and others (1984) described reversible azoösper-mia after treatment with the anabolic steroid nandrolone phenylpropionate in doses only a little higher than those used clinically, and lower than those sometimes used by athletes.

Cyproterone acetate produces a dose-dependent inhibition of spermatogenesis that is due in part to its intratesticular antiandrogen effect and in part to inhibition of pituitary gonadotrophin secretion (Fredricsson and Carlstrom 1981). Infertility is usual with therapeutic doses, but the changes are reversible in the majority of patients, usually within about 5 months, though sometimes longer.

In women, oral contraceptives suppress ovulation by inhibiting gonadotrophin release. Anovulatory cycles may persist for some months after discontinuing the pill, due to delayed recovery of hypothalamic responsiveness (de Lange and Doorenbos 1975). The incidence of post-pill amenorrhoea has been estimated to be about 2 per cent and the duration varies from 2 months to over a year. Women who previously had irregular periods may be at greater risk (de Lange and Doorenbos 1975) but it also occurs in women with previously regular cycles.

Miscellaneous drugs

Diethylstilboestrol

The association of exposure *in utero* to diethylstilboes-trol (DES) and the subsequent development of clear-cell carcinoma of the vagina was first described in 1971. More recently it has become apparent that the spectrum of abnormalities produced by DES is much wider. Many structural abnormalities of the genital tract have been described in both males and females, and there have been reports of diminished reproductive performance (Stillman 1982). This can often be explained by the anatomical abnormalities, but semen analysis has shown reduced sperm counts and low fertility scores in men who were exposed to DES. Actual data on the fertility rates of such men have not been published but the evidence available suggests a relationship between exposure to DES *in utero* and male infertility (Stillman 1982; Stenchever *et al.* 1981).

Alcohol

Oligospermia has been reported in chronic alcoholics, but the incidence, the amount of alcohol required, the mechanism, and the degree to which recovery can occur with abstinence have not been defined (Anderson and Willis 1981; Morgan 1982).

Cannabis

Several studies have reported acute effects of cannabis smoking on spermatogenesis but the importance of this in chronic users of the drug is unknown (Abel 1981).

Smoking

An increased proportion of abnormal sperm has been observed in the semen of smokers attending an infertility clinic (Evans *et al.* 1981). The importance of this finding is unknown, and it was not confirmed by a subsequent report (Rodriguez-Rigau *et al.* 1982).

Drugs affecting sperm motility

Many drugs have been found to inhibit sperm motility *in vitro* (Hong and Turner 1982). They include chlorpromazine (Hong *et al.* 1982); imipramine and other tricyclic antidepressants (Levin *et al.* 1981); lignocaine; tetrahydrocannabinol (a constituent of cannabis); and some β-adrenoceptor antagonists (Hong *et al.* 1982). This effect has been attributed to the membrane-stabilizing properties of these drugs. The concentrations required are far greater than those likely to be achieved during therapeutic use (Hong *et al.* 1982; Mahajan *et al.* 1984), but a preliminary report suggested that propranolol may be an effective vaginal contraceptive (Zipper *et al.* 1983). Lithium has been shown to inhibit sperm motility *in vitro* in concentrations comparable with those achieved in semen after oral administration (Raoof *et al.* 1989).

References

Abel, E.L. (1981). Marihuana and sex: a critical survey. *Drug Alcohol Depend.* 8, 1.

Ahmad, S. (1980). Hydralazine and male impotence. *Chest* 78, 358.

Alexander, W.D. and Evans, J.I. (1975). Side effects of methyldopa. *Br. Med. J.* 2, 501.

Allen, J.M., Kerle, D.J., Ware, H., Doble, A., Williams, G., and Bloom, S.R. (1983). Combined treatment with ketoconazole and luteinising hormone releasing hormone analogue; a novel approach to resistant progressive prostatic cancer. *Br. Med. J.* 287, 1766.

Ananth, J. (1982). Impotence due to pimozide. *Am. J. Psychiatry* 139, 1374.

Anderson, R.A. and Willis, B.R. (1981). Alcohol and male fertility. *Br. J. Alcohol Alcoholism* 16, 179.

Apter, A., Dickermann, Z., Gonen, N., Ass, S., Prager-Lewin, R., Kaufman, H., *et al.* (1983). Effect of chlorpromazine on hypothalamic–pituitary–gonadal function in 10 adolescent schizophrenic boys. *Am. J. Psychiatry* 140, 1588.

Aubier, F., Flamant, F., Brauner, R., Caillaud, J.M., Caussain, J.M. and Lemerle, J. (1987). Male gonadal function after chemotherapy for solid tumours in childhood. *J. Clin. Oncol.* 7, 403.

Bancroft, J. (1981). Hormones and human sexual behaviour. *Br. Med. Bull.* 37, 153.

Bancroft, J. (1982). Erectile impotence — psyche or soma? *Int. J. Androl.* 5, 353.

Banos, J.E., Bosch, F. and Farre, M. (1989). Drug-induced priapism. *Med. Toxicol.* 4, 46.

Barton, J.L. (1979). Orgasmic inhibition by phenelzine. *Am. J. Psychiatry* 136, 1616.

Beaumont, G. (1978). Sexual side-effects of psychotropic drugs. *Br. J. Clin. Pract.* Symposium Suppl. 4, 45.

Beck, A.T. (1976). *Depression: clinical, experimental and therapeutic aspects.* Harper and Row, New York.

Berlin, R.G. (1986). Metoclopramide-induced reversible impotence. *West J. Med.* 144, 359.

Beumont, P.J.V., Corker, C.S., Friesen, H.G., Kolakowska, T., Mandelbrote, B.M., Marshall, J., *et al.* (1974). The effects of phenothiazines on endocrine function. *Br. J. Psychiatry* 124, 420.

Bhalla, A.K., Hoffbrand, B.I., Phatak, P.S., and Reuben, S. (1979). Prazosin and priapism. *Br. Med. J.* 2, 115.

Birnie, G.G., McLeod, T.I.F., and Watkinson, G. (1981). Incidence of sulphasalazine-induced male infertility. *Gut* 22, 425.

Blackburn, W.D. and Alarcon, G.S. (1989). Impotence in three rheumatoid arthritis patients treated with methotrexate. *Arthritis Rheum.* 32, 1341.

Blatt, J., Poplack, D.G., and Sherins, R.J. (1981). Testicular function in boys after chemotherapy for acute lymphoblastic leukaemia. *N. Engl. J. Med.* 304, 1121.

Blay, S.L., Ferraz M.P.T., and Calil, H.M. (1982). Lithium-induced male sexual impairment: two case reports. *J. Clin. Psychiatry* 43, 497.

Brindley, G.S. (1983a). Physiology of erection and management of paraplegic infertility. In *Male infertility.* (ed. T.B. Hargreave), p. 261. Springer-Verlag.

Brindley, G.S. (1983b). Cavernosal alpha-blockade: a new technique for investigating and treating erectile impotence. *Br. J. Psychiatr.* 143, 332.

Buchanan, J.D., Fairley, K.F., and Barrie, J.U. (1975). Return of spermatogenesis after stopping cyclophosphamide therapy. *Lancet* ii, 156.

Bulpitt, C.J. and Dollery, C.T. (1973). Side effects of hypotensive agents evaluated by a self-administered questionnaire. *Br. Med. J.* 3, 485.

Bulpitt, C.J., Dollery, C.T., and Carne, S. (1976). Change in symptoms of hypertensive patients after referral to hospital clinic. *Br. Heart J.* 38, 121.

Bulpitt, C.J., Beevers, G., Butler, A., Coles, E.C., Hunt, D., Munro-Faure, A.D. *et al.* (1989). The effects of antihypertensive drugs on sexual function in men and women: a report from the DHSS Hypertension Care Computing Project. *J. Hum. Hypertension* 3, 53.

Burnett, W.C. and Chahine, R.A. (1979). Sexual dysfunction as a complication of propranolol therapy in men. *Cardiovasc. Med.* 5, 811.

Bygdeman, M. (1981). Effects of prostaglandins on the genital tract. *Acta Vet. Scand.* Suppl. 77, 47.

Callis, L., Nieto, J., Vila, A., and Rende, J. (1980). Chlorambucil treatment in minimal lesion nephrotic syndrome: a reappraisal of its gonadal toxicity. *J. Pediatr.* 97, 653.

Cann, P.A. and Holdsworth, C.D. (1984). Reversal of male infertility on changing treatment from sulphasalazine to 5-aminosalicylic acid. *Lancet* ii, 1119.

Carlson, H.E., Ippoliti, A.F., and Svederloff, R.S. (1981). Endocrine effects on acute and chronic cimetidine administration. *Dig. Dis. Sci.* 26, 428.

Chapman, R.M. (1982). Effect of cytotoxic therapy on sexuality and gonadal function. *Sem. Oncol.* 9, 84.

Chapman, R.M., Sutcliffe, S.B., and Malpas, J.S. (1979). Cytotoxic-induced ovarian failure in women with Hodgkin's disease. *JAMA* 242, 1877.

Chapman, R.M., Sutcliffe, S.B., and Malpas, J.S. (1981). Male gonadal dysfunction in Hodgkin's disease. *JAMA* 245, 1323.

Christiansen, P., Deigaard, J., and Lund, M. (1975). Potens, fertilitet og konshormonudskillelse hos yngre mandlige epilepsilidende. *Ugeskr. Laeger* 137, 2402.

Cleeves, L. and Findley, L.J. (1987). Bromocriptine-induced impotence in Parkinson's disease. *Br. Med. J.* 295, 367.

Cohn, D.F., Homonna, Z., and Paz, G.F. (1982). The effect of anticonvulsant drugs on the development of male rats and their fertility. *J. Neurol. Neurosurg. Psychiatry* 45, 844.

Croog, S.H., Levine, S., Testa, M.A., Brown, B., Bulpitt, C.J., Jenkins, D., *et al.* (1986). The effects of antihypertensive therapy on the quality of life. *N. Engl. J. Med.* 314, 1657.

da Cunha, M.F., Meistrich, M.L., Reid, H.L., and Powell, M.L. (1979). Effect of chemotherapy on human sperm production. *Proc. Am. Assoc. Cancer Res. Am. Soc. Clin. Oncol.* Abstract No. 403.

Degan, K. (1982). Sexual dysfunction in women using major tranquillisers. *Psychosomatics* 23, 959.

de Lange, W.E. and Doorenbos, H. (1975). Sex hormones, anabolic agents and related drugs. In *Meyler's side effects of drugs*. Vol. 8. (ed. M.N.G. Dukes), p. 862. Excerpta Medica, Amsterdam.

Delle Fave, G.F., Tamburrano, G., de Magistris, L., Natoli, C., Santoro, M.L., Carratu, R., *et al.* (1977). Gynaecomastia with cimetidine. *Lancet* 1, 1319.

El-Beheiry, A., El-Mansy, E., and Salama, N. (1979). Methotrexate and fertility in men. *Arch. Androl.* 3, 177.

El-Beheiry, A.H., Kamel, M.N., and Gad, A. (1982). Niridazole and fertility in bilharzial men. *Arch. Androl.* 8, 297.

Epstein, R.J., Allen, E.C. and Lunde, M.W. (1987). Organic impotence associated with carbonic anhydrase inhibitor therapy for glaucoma. *Ann. Ophthalmol.* 19, 48.

Evans, H.J., Fletcher, J., Torrance, M., and Hargreave, T.B. (1981). Sperm abnormalities and cigarette smoking. *Lancet* 1, 627.

Fairley, K.F., Barrie, J.U., and Johnson, W. (1972). Sterility and testicular atrophy related to cyclophosphamide therapy. *Lancet i*, 568.

Felstein, I. (1980). Sexual function in the elderly. *Clin. Obstet. Gynecol.* 7, 401.

Fisher, B., Sherman, B.M., Rockette, H., Redmond, C., Margolese, R., and Fisher, E.R. (1979). L-phenylalanine mustard in the management of premenopausal patients with primary breast cancer. *Cancer* 44, 847.

Fogelman, J. (1988). Verapamil caused depression, confusion and impotence. *Am. J. Psychiatry* 145, 380.

Forsberg, L., Gustavii, B., Hojerback, T., and Olsson, A.M. (1979). Impotence, smoking and β-blocking drugs. *Fertil. Steril.* 31, 589.

Franks, S., Jacobs, H.S., Martin, N., and Nabarro, J.D.N. (1978). Hyperprolactinaemia and impotence. *Clin. Endocrinol.* 8, 277.

Fraunfelder, F.T. and Keyer, S.M. (1985). Sexual dysfunction secondary to topical ophthalmic timolol. *JAMA* 253, 3092.

Fredricsson, B. and Carlstrom, K. (1981). Effects of low doses of cyproterone acetate on sperm morphology and some other parameters of reproduction in normal men. *Andrologia* 13, 369.

Gartrell, N. (1986). Increased libido in women receiving trazodone. *Am. J. Psychiatry* 143, 781.

Gradishar, W. and Schilsky, R. (1988). Effects of cancer treatment on the reproductive system. *CRC Rev. Oncol. Hematol.* 8, 153.

Greenblatt, D.J. and Koch-Weser, J. (1973). Gynaecomastia and impotence. Complications of spironolactone therapy. *JAMA* 223,82.

Grieve, J. (1979). Male infertility due to sulphasalazine. *Lancet* ii, 464.

Griffin, J.P. (1982). Drug-induced sexual dysfunction. In *Iatrogenic diseases* (2nd edn, update 2) (ed. P.F. D'Arcy and J.P. Griffin). p. 193. Oxford University Press.

Grimm, R.H., Cohen, J.D. and McFate Smith, W. (1985). Hypertension management in the Multiple Risk Factor Intervention Trial (MRFIT). *Arch. Intern. Med.* 145, 1191.

Gross, M.D. (1982). Reversal by bethanecol of sexual dysfunction caused by anticholinergic antidepressants. *Am. J. Psychiatry* 139, 1393.

Grunnet, E., Nyfors, A., and Hansen, K.B. (1977). Studies of human semen in topical corticosteroid-treated and methotrexate-treated psoriatics. *Dermatologica* 154, 78.

Guillebaude, J. (1978). Sulpha–trimethoprim combinations and male infertility. *Lancet* ii, 523.

Halkier-Sørensen, L. (1987). Menstrual changes in a patient treated with etretinate. *Lancet* ii, 636.

Helgeland, A., Strommen, R., Hagelund, C.H., *et al.* (1986). Enalapril, atenolol and hydrochlorothiazide in mild to moderate hypertension. *Lancet*. i, 872.

Himelstein-Braw, R., Peters, H., and Faber, M. (1978). Morphological study of the ovaries of leukaemic children. *Br. J. Cancer* 38, 82.

Hogan, M.J., Wallin, J.D., and Baer, R.M. (1980). Antihypertensive therapy and male sexual dysfunction. *Psychosomatics* 21, 234.

Hong, C.Y. and Turner, P. (1982). Drugs and sperm. *Br. Med. J.* 284, 1194.

Hong, C.Y., Chaput de Saintonge, D.M., and Turner, P. (1982). Effects of chlorpromazine and other drugs acting on the central nervous system on sperm motility. *Eur. J. Clin. Pharmacol.* 22, 413.

Hudson, E., Dore, C., Sowter, C., Toovey, S., and Levi A.J. (1982). Sperm size in patients with inflammatory bowel disease on sulphasalazine therapy. *Fertil. Steril.* 38, 77.

Huffman, D.H., Kampmann, J.P., Hignite, C.E., and Azarnoff, D.L., (1978). Gynaecomastia induced in normal males by spironolactone. *Clin. Pharmacol. Ther.* 24, 465.

Ireland, A. and Jewell, D.P. (1989). Sulfasalazine-induced impotence: a beneficial resolution with olsalazine. *J. Clin. Gastroenterol.* 11, 711.

Jani, N.N., Wise, T,N., Kass, E. and Sessler, A. (1988). Trazodone and anorgasmia. *Am. J. Psychiatry* 145, 896.

Jensen, R.T., Collen, M.J., Pandol, S.J., Allende, H.D., Raufman, J-P., Bissonnette, B.M., *et al.* (1983). Cimetidine-induced impotence and breast changes in patients with gastric hypersecretory states. *N. Engl. J. Med.* 308, 883.

Jones, S.D. (1984). Ejaculatory inhibition with trazodone. *J. Clin. Psychopharmacol.* 4, 279.

Kedia, K.R. and Persky, L. (1981). Effect of phenoxybenzamine on sexual function in man. *Urology* 18, 620.

Kellie, S.J. and Kingston, J.E. (1987). Ovarian failure after high-dose melphalan in adolescents. *Lancet* i, 1425.

Khandelwal, S.K. (1988). Complete loss of libido with short-term use of lorazepam. *Am. J. Psychiatry* 145, 1313.

King, D.J., Ratcliffe, M.A. and Dawson, A.A (1985). Fertility in young women and men after treatment for lymphoma. *J. Clin. Pathol.* 38,1247.

King, B.D., Pitchon, R., Stern, E.H., Schweitzer, P., Schneider, R.R., and Weiner, I. (1983). Impotence during therapy with verapamil. *Arch. Intern. Med.* 143, 1248.

Kinsey, A., Pomeroy, W., and Martin, C. (1948). *Sexual behaviour in the human male*, p. 236. W.B. Saunders, Philadelphia.

Kline, M.D. (1989). Fluoxetine and anorgasmia. *Am. J. Psychiatry* 146, 804.

Kotin, J., Wilbert, D.E., Verburg, D., and Soldinger, S.M. (1976). Thioridazine and sexual dysfunction. *Am. J. Psychiatry* 133, 82.

Koyama, H., Wada, T., Nishizawa, Y., Iwanaga, T., Aoki, Y., Tarasawa, T., et al. (1977). Cyclophosphamide-induced ovarian failure and its therapeutic significance in patients with breast cancer. Cancer 39, 1403.

Krane, R.J., Goldstein, I. and de Tejada, I.S. (1989). Impotence. N. Engl. J. Med. 321, 1648.

Kreuser, E.D., Harsch, W. and Hetzel, W.D. (1986). Chronic gonadal toxicity in patients with testicular cancer after chemotherapy. Europ. J. Cancer Clin. Oncol. 22, 289.

Kreuser, E.D., Xiros, N. and Hetzel, W.D. (1987). Reproductive and endocrine gonadal capacity in patients treated with COPP chemotherapy for Hodgkin's disease. J. Cancer Res. Clin. Oncol. 113, 260.

Kristensen, E. and Jørgensen, P. (1987). Sexual function in lithium-treated manic depressive patients. Pharmacopsychiatry 20, 165.

Lancet. (1983). New treatment for prostatic cancer. Lancet ii, 438.

Law, M.R., Copland, R.F.P., Armistead, J.G., and Gabriel, R. (1980). Labetalol and priapism. Br. Med. J. 1, 115.

Lendon, M., Hann, I.M., Palmer, M.K., Shalet, S.M., and Morris Jones, P.H. (1978). Testicular histology after combination chemotherapy in childhood for acute lymphoblastic leukaemia. Lancet ii, 439.

Lesko, L.M., Stotland, N.L., and Sergraves, R.T. (1982). Three cases of female anorgasmia associated with MAOIs. Am. J. Psychiatry 139, 1353.

Levin, R.J. (1980). The physiology of sexual function in women. Clin. Obstet. Gynecol. 7, 213.

Levin, R.M., Amsterdam, J.D., Winokur, A., and Wein, A.J. (1981). Effects of psychotropic drugs on human sperm motility. Fertil. Steril. 36, 503.

Lief, H.I. (1977). Sexual survey No. 5: current thinking on sex and depression. Med. Asp. Hum. Sex. 11, 22.

Loriaux, D.L., Menard, R., Taylor, A., Pita, J.C., and Santen, R. (1976). Spironolactone and endocrine dysfunction. Ann. Intern. Med. 85, 630.

Lydiard, R.B. and George, M.S. (1989). Fluoxetine-related anorgasmy. South. Med. J. 82, 933.

McCarthy, D.M. (1978). Report on the United States experience with cimetidine in Zollinger–Ellison syndrome and other hypersecretory states. Gastroenterology 74, 453.

McEwen, J. and Meyboom, R.H.B. (1983). Testicular pain caused by mazindol. Br. Med. J. 287, 1763.

McHaffie, D.J., Guz, A., and Johnston, A. (1977). Impotence in a patient on disopyramide. Lancet i, 859.

McLean, J.D., Forsythe, R.G. and Kapkin, L.A. (1983). Unusual side effects of clomipramine associated with yawning. Can. J. Psychiatry 28, 569.

McMahon, C.D., Shaffer, R.N., Hoskins, H.B., and Hetherington, J. (1979). Adverse effects experienced by patients taking timolol. Am. J. Ophthalmol. 88, 736.

MacPhee, G.J.A., Larkin, J.G., Butler, E., Beastall, G.H., and Brodie, M.J. (1988). Circulating hormones and pituitary responsiveness in young epileptic men receiving long-term antiepileptic medication. Epilepsia 29, 468.

Mahajan, P., Grech, E.D., Ridgway, E.J., Turner, P., and Pearson, R.M. (1984). Propranolol concentrations in the blood, seminal plasma and saliva in man. Br. J. Clin. Pharmacol. 17, 186P.

Mandell, W. and Miller, C.M. (1983). Male sexual dysfunction as related to alcohol consumption. Alcoholism: Clinical and Experimental Research 7, 65.

The Medical Letter. (1983). Drugs that cause sexual dysfunction. Medical Letter 25, 73.

Medical Research Council Working Party (1981). Adverse reactions to bendrofluazide and propranolol for the treatment of mild hypertension. Lancet ii, 539.

Meinertz, T., Zehender, M.K., Geibel, A., Treese, N., Hofmann, T., Kaspar, W., et al. (1984). Longterm antiarrhythmic therapy with flecainide. Am. J. Cardiol. 54, 91.

Meiraz, D., Margolin, Y., Lev-Ran, A., and Lazebnik, J. (1977). Treatment of benign prostatic hyperplasia with hydroxyprogesterone caproate. Urology 14, 144.

Mendelson, J.H. and Mello, N.K. (1982). Hormones and psychosexual development in young men following chronic heroin use. Neurobehav. Toxicol. Teratol. 4, 441.

Miller, L.G., Rogers, J.C., and Swee, D.E. (1989). Indomethacin-associated sexual dysfunction. J. Fam. Pract. 29, 210.

Mitchell, J.E. and Popkin, M.K. (1982). Antipsychotic drug therapy and sexual dysfunction in men. Am. J. Psychiatry 139, 633.

Mitchell, J.E. and Popkin, M.K. (1983). Antidepressant drug therapy and sexual dysfunction in men: a review. J. Clin. Psychopharmacol. 3, 76.

Modell, J.G. (1989). Repeated observations of yawning, clitoral enlargement, and orgasm associated with fluoxetine administration. J. Clin. Psychopharmacol. 9, 63.

Monteiro, W.D., Noshirvani, H.F., Marks, I.M., and Lelliott, P.T. (1987). Anorgasmia from clomipramine in obsessive–compulsive disorder. Br. J. Psychiatry 151, 107.

Morgan, M.Y. (1982). Sex and alcohol. Br. Med. Bull. 38, 43.

Moss, H.B. (1983). More cases of anorgasmia after MAOI treatment. Am. J. Psychiatry 140, 266.

Munjack, D.J. and Crocker, B. (1986). Alprazolam-induced ejaculatory inhibition. J. Clin. Psychopharmacol. 6, 57.

Murdia, A., Mathur, V., Kothari, L.K., and Singh, K.P. (1978). Sulpha–trimethoprim combinations and male infertility. Lancet ii, 375.

Nestoros, J.N. and Lehmann, H.E. (1979). Neuroleptics and male sexual dysfunction. Int. Drug Ther. Newsletter 14, 21.

Neuman, F., Diallo, F.A., Hasan, S.H., Sechenck, B., and Traore, I. (1976). The influence of pharmaceutical compounds on male fertility. Andrologia 8, 203.

Newman, R.J. and Salerno, H.R. (1974). Sexual dysfunction due to methyldopa. Br. Med. J. 4, 106.

Niv, Y. (1986). Male sexual dysfunction due to cimetidine. Irish Med. J. 72, 252.

Nutt, D., Hackman, A. and Hawton, K. (1986). Increased sexual function in benzodiazepine withdrawal. Lancet ii, 1101.

O'Morain, C.A., Smethurst, P., Hudson, E., and Levi, A.J. (1982). Further studies on sulphasalazine-induced male infertility. Gastroenterology 82, 1140.

Onesti, G., Bock, K.D., Heimsoth, V., Kim, K.E., and Merguet, P. (1971). Clonidine: a new antihypertensive agent. Am. J. Cardiol. 28, 74.

Othmer, E. and Othmer, S.C. (1987). Effect of buspirone on sexual dysfunction in patients with generalised anxiety disorder. *J. Clin. Psychiatry* 48, 201.

Ottesen, B., Wagner, G., Virag, R., and Fahrenkrug, J. (1984). Penile erection: possible role for vasoactive intestinal polypeptide as a neurotransmitter. *Br. Med. J.* 288, 9.

Papadopoulos, C. (1980). Cardiovascular drugs and sexuality. *Arch. Intern. Med.* 140, 1341.

Peden, N.R., Boyd, E.J.S., Browning, M.C.K., Saunders, J.H., and Wormsley, K.G. (1982). Effects of two histamine H$_2$-receptor blocking drugs on basal levels of gonadotrophins, prolactin, testosterone and oestradiol-17β during treatment of duodenal ulcer in male patients. *Acta Endocrinol.* 96, 564.

Peden, N.R. and Wormsley, K.G. (1982). Effect of cimetidine on gonadal function. *Br. J. Clin. Pharmacol.* 14, 565.

Pentland, B., Anderson, D.A., and Critchley, J.A.J.H. (1981). Failure of ejaculation with indoramin. *Br. Med. J.* 284, 1433.

Pohl, R. (1983). Anorgasmia caused by MAOIs. *Am. J. Psychiatry* 140, 510.

Pont, A., Williams, P.L., Loose, D.S., Feldman, D., Reitz, R.E., Bochra, C., and Stevens, D.A. (1982). Ketoconazole blocks adrenal steroid synthesis. *Ann. Intern. Med.* 97, 370.

Raoof, N.T., Pearson, R.M. and Turner, P. (1989). Lithium inhibits sperm motility in vitro. *Br. J. Clin. Pharmacol.* 28, 715.

Rayner, H.C., May, S. and Walls, J. (1988). Penile erection due to nifedipine. *Br. Med. J.* 296, 137.

Riley, A.J. and Riley, E.J. (1986a). The effect of single dose diazepam on female sexual response induced by masturbation. *Sex. Marital Ther.* 1, 49.

Riley, A.J. and Riley, E.J. (1986b). Cyproheptadine and antidepressant-induced anorgasmia. *Br. J. Psychiatry* 148, 217.

Riley, A.J., Riley, E.J., and Davies, H.J. (1982). A method for monitoring drug effects on male sexual response: the effect of single dose labetalol. *Br. J. Clin. Pharmacol.* 14, 695.

Riley, S.A., Lecarpentier, J., Mani, T., Goodman, M.T., Mandal, B.K., and Turnberk, L.A. (1987). Sulphasalazine induced seminal abnormalities in ulcerative colitis: results of mesalazine substitution. *Gut* 38, 1008.

Rodriguez-Rigau, L.J., Smith, K.D., and Steinberger, E. (1982). Cigarette smoking and semen quality. *Fertil. Steril.* 38,115.

Roeser, H.D., Stocks, A.E., and Smith, A.J. (1978). Testicular damage due to cytotoxic drugs and recovery after cessation of therapy. *Aust. N.Z. J. Med.* 8, 250.

Rose, D.P. and Davies, T.E. (1977). Ovarian function in patients receiving adjuvant chemotherapy for breast cancer. *Lancet* i, 1174.

Rubery, E.D. (1983). Return of fertility after curative chemotherapy for disseminated teratoma of testis. *Lancet* i, 186.

Rustin, G.J.S., Booth, M., Dent, J., Salt, S., Rustin, F., and Bagshawe, K.D. (1984). Pregnancy after cytotoxic chemotherapy for gestational trophoblastic tumours. *Br. Med. J.* 288, 103.

Sacher, E.J. (1978). Neuroendocrine responses to psychotropic drugs. In *Psychoparmacology: a generation of progress.* (eds. M.A. Lipton, A. DiMascio, and K.F. Killam), p. 499. Raven Press, New York.

Sangal, R. (1985). Inhibited female orgasm as a side effect of alprazolam. *Am. J. Psychiatry* 142, 1223.

Schilsky, R.L., Lewis, B.J., Sherins, R.J., and Young R.C. (1980). Gonadal dysfunction in patients receiving chemotherapy for cancer. *Ann. Intern. Med.* 93, 109.

Schramek, P. and Waldhauser, M. (1989). Dose-dependent effect and side effect of prostaglandin E$_1$ in erectile dysfunction. *Br. J. Clin. Pharmacol.* 28, 567.

Schurmeyer, T. and Nieschiag, E. (1982). Ketoconazole-induced drop in serum and saliva testosterone. *Lancet* ii, 1098.

Schurmeyer, T., Knuth, U.A., Belkein, L., and Nieschlag, E. (1984). Reversible azoöspermia induced by the anabolic steroid 19-nortestosterone. *Lancet* i, 417.

Segraves, R.T. (1982). Male sexual dysfunction and psychoactive drug use. *Postgrad. Med.* 71, 227.

Shalet, S.M. (1980). Effects of cancer chemotherapy on gonadal function of patients. *Cancer Treat. Rev.* 7, 141.

Shamberger, R.C., Rosenberg, S.A., Scipp, C.A., and Sherins, R.J. (1981). Effects of high-dose methotrexate and vincristine on ovarian and testicular function in patients undergoing postoperative adjuvant treatment of osteosarcoma. *Cancer Treat. Rep.* 65, 739.

Shen, W.W. (1982). Female orgasmic inhibition by amoxapine. *Am. J. Psychiatry* 139, 1220.

Shen, W.W. and Park, S. (1982). Thioridazine-induced inhibition of female orgasm. *Psychiat. J. Univ. Ottawa* 7, 249.

Siris, E.S., Leventhal, B.G., and Vaitukaitis, J.L. (1976). Effects of childhood leukaemia and chemotherapy on puberty and reproductive function in girls. *N. Engl. J. Med.* 294, 1143.

Slag, M.F., Morley, J.E., Elson, M.K., Trence, D.L., Nelson, C.J., Nelson, A.E., et al. (1983). Impotence in medical clinic outpatients. *JAMA* 249, 1736.

Sovner, R. (1983). Anorgasmia associated with imipramine but not desipramine: case report. *J. Clin. Psychiatry* 44, 345.

Spark, R.F. (1983). Neuroendocrinology and impotence. *Ann. Intern. Med.* 98, 103.

Spark, R.F., and Melby, J.C. (1968). Aldosteronism in hypertension. The spironolactone response test. *Ann. Intern. Med.* 69, 685.

Spence, R.W. and Celestin, L.R. (1979). Gynaecomastia associated with cimetidine. *Gut* 20, 154.

Stenchever, M.A., Williamson, R.A., Leonard, J., Karp, L.E., Ley, B., Shy, K., et al. (1981). Possible relationship between in utero diethylstilboestrol exposure and male fertility. *Am. J. Obstet. Gynecol.* 140, 186.

Stessman, J. and Ben-Ishay, D. (1980). Chlorthalidone-induced impotence. *Br. Med. J.* 281, 714.

Stillman, R.J. (1982). In utero exposure to diethylstilboestrol: adverse effects on the reproductive tract and reproductive performance in male and female offspring. *Am. J. Obstet. Gynecol.* 142, 905.

Stokes, G.S., Mennie, B.A., Gellatly, R., and Hill, A. (1983). On the combination of α- and β-adrenoceptor blockade in hypertension. *Clin. Pharmacol. Ther.* 34, 576.

Stubbs, W.A., Delitala, G., Besser, G.M., Edwards, C.R., Labrooy, S., Taylor, R., *et al.* (1983). The endocrine and metabolic effects of cimetidine. *Clin. Endocrinol.* 18, 167.

Sullivan, G. (1987). Increased libido with trazodone. *Am. J. Psychiatry* 144, 967.

Sussman, A. and Leonard, J.M. (1980). Psoriasis, methotrexate and oligospermia. *Arch. Dermatol.* 116, 215.

Sutton, R., Buzadar, A.U. and Hortobagyr, G.N. (1990). Pregnancy and offspring after adjuvant chemotherapy in breast cancer patients. *Cancer* 65, 847.

Taylor, R.G., Crisp, A.J., Hoffbrand, B.I., Maguire, A., and Jacobs, H.S. (1981). Plasma sex hormone concentrations in men with hypertension treated with methyldopa and/or propranolol. *Postgrad. Med. J.* 57, 425.

Toone, B.K., Wheeler, M., Nanjee, M., Fenwick, P., and Grant, R. (1983). Sex hormones, sexual activity and plasma anticonvulsant levels in male epileptics. *J. Neurol. Neurosurg. Psychiatry* 46, 824.

Toovey, S., Hudson, E., Hendry, W.F., and Levi, A.T. (1981). Sulphasalazine and male infertility: reversibility and a possible mechanism. *Gut* 22, 445.

Trompeter, R.S., Evans, P.R., and Barratt, T.M. (1981). Gonadal function in boys with steroid-responsive nephrotic syndrome treated with cyclophosphamide for short periods. *Lancet* i, 1177.

Uhde, T.W., Tancer, M.E., and Shea, C.A. (1988). Sexual dysfunction related to alprazolam treatment of social phobia. *Am. J. Psychiatry* 145, 531.

van Thiel, D.H., Gavaler, J.S., Smith, W.I., and Paul, G. (1979). Hypothalamic–pituitary–gonadal dysfunction in men using cimetidine. *N. Engl. J. Med.* 300, 1012.

Wang, C., Wong, K.L., Lam, K.C., and Lai, C.L. (1983). Ranitidine does not affect gonadal function in man. *Br. J. Clin. Pharmacol.* 16, 430.

Warner, M.D., Peabody, C.A., Whiteford, H.A., and Hollister, L.E. (1987). Trazodone and priapism. *J. Clin. Psychiatry* 48, 244.

Warren, S.C. and Warren, S.G. (1977). Propranolol and sexual impotence. *Ann. Intern. Med.* 86, 112.

Waxman, J. (1983). Chemotherapy and the adult gonad: a review. *J. R. Soc. Med.* 76, 144.

Waxman, J., Terry, Y., Rees, L.H., and Lister, T.A. (1983). Gonadal function in men treated for acute leukaemia. *Br. Med. J.* 287, 1093.

Wei, J. and Hood, J.C. (1980). Naproxen and ejaculatory dysfunction. *Ann. Intern. Med.* 93, 933.

Weizman, A., Maoz, B., Treves, I., Asher, I., and Ben-David, M. (1985). Sulpiride-induced hyperprolactinaemia and impotence in male psychiatric out-patients. *Prog. Neuropsychopharmacol. Biol. Psychiatry* 9, 193.

Whitehead, E., Shalet, S.M., Morris Jones, P.H., Beardwell, C.G., and Deakin, D.P. (1982). Gonadal function after combination chemotherapy for Hodgkin's disease in childhood. *Arch. Dis. Child.* 47, 287.

Winters, S.J., Banks, J.L., and Loriaux, D.L. (1979). Cimetidine is an antiandrogen in the rat. *Gastroenterology* 76, 504.

Wolfe, M.M. (1979). Impotence on cimetidine treatment. *N. Engl. J. Med.* 300, 94.

Wu, F.C.W. and Aitken, R.J. (1989). Suppression of sperm function by depot medroxyprogesterone acetate and testosterone enanthate in steroid male contraception. *Fertil. Steril.* 51, 691.

Yager, J. (1986). Bethanecol chloride can reverse erectile and ejaculatory dysfunction induced by tricyclic antidepressants and mazindol: a case report. *J. Clin. Psychiatry* 47, 210.

Yeragani, V.K. and Gershon, S. (1987). Priapism related to phenelzine therapy. *N. Engl. J. Med.* 317, 117.

Yunda, I.F. and Kushniruk, Y.I. (1974). Effect of nitrofurantoin preparations on spermatogenesis. *Bull. Exp. Biol. Med.* 77, 534.

Zarren, H.S. and Black, P. McL. (1975). Unilateral gynaecomastia and impotence during low dose spironolactone administration in men. *Milit. Med.* 140, 417.

Zipper, J., Wheeler, R.G., Potts, D.M., and Rivera, M. (1983). Propranolol as a novel, effective spermicide: preliminary findings. *Br. Med. J.* 287, 1245.

30. Drug interactions of clinical importance

M. L'E. ORME

Introduction

Information about drugs continues to increase exponentially. Not only do we have many new drugs coming on the market about which expectations as regards safety and efficacy are rising, so that more information is required before they can be marketed, but we also have much more information about the older drugs, as a result of research by interested academics. This increase in information about drugs applies just as much to drug interactions as it does to other areas of pharmacology. Thus the number of reported drug interactions is rising continually and it becomes increasingly difficult to keep abreast of developments in the subject, and to sort out the clinically irrelevant interactions from those that are clinically important.

There is little doubt that the potential for drug interaction is continually present. In most developed countries there are two to three thousand single chemical entities available for prescription and in many cases these are deliberately marketed in combination, so that the number of marketed products (including the combination products) may be in excess of ten thousand. Many of these combination products make little therapeutic sense (e.g. the combination of phenobarbitone and β-adrenoceptor stimulants in asthma therapies) and there is a welcome trend in many countries towards critical review of the need for these products. In addition to prescription-only medicines (POM), there is a wide range of drugs available 'over the counter'. These may be thought of by the patient not as drugs but as tonics, and the prescribing physician may be unaware that the patient is taking these medicaments.

Prevalence of drug interactions

The potential for drug interactions is thus very considerable and there is little doubt that very many patients take several drugs concurrently, so that it is perhaps surprising that adverse drug interactions are not more common. Early studies showed that patients who are admitted to hospital are on average taking 4 or 5 drugs at the same time and one in five patients receives 10 or more during a hospital stay (Crooks and Moir 1974). One patient described by Prescott was given 41 drugs during a single admission (Prescott 1973); another, in the USA, received more than 50 in a 24-hour period (Koch-Weser 1973). The Boston Collaborative Drug Surveillance program studied about 10 000 patients exposed to nearly 84 000 drugs (BCDSP 1972). Out of 3600 adverse drug reactions reported, only 234 (6.5 per cent) were attributable to drug interactions. The overall incidence of adverse drug interactions is hard to estimate, but it is suggested that they are responsible for between 6 and 30 per cent of all adverse drug reactions (BCDSP 1972). In a study of patients on medical wards, 22 per cent of adverse reactions to drugs were due to drug interactions (Borda et al. 1968). In a nursing home population, Blaschke and colleagues (1981) found that 19 per cent of patients were receiving drugs known to interact, while in an outpatient population the figure was 23 per cent (Stanaszek and Franklin 1978). Not all potential drug interactions, however, will necessarily occur in practice. In a study of 64 patients taking debrisoquine, guanethidine, or bethanidine, one-third were taking additional drugs that would have been expected to cause an adverse interaction (Starr and Petrie 1972), yet only three probable interactions were identified. In general practice in Victoria, Australia, Paulet and colleagues (1982) looked at 428 prescriptions and identified 2400 drug combinations. Only 37 possible interactions were detected, none of which was finally thought to be of clinical significance. Thus it would appear that drug interactions tend to be overemphasized.

There is little doubt that the elderly are at particular risk of adverse drug interactions, and the risk also increases as the number of drugs given concurrently rises

(Smith *et al.* 1966; Law and Chalmers 1976; D'Arcy 1982). Other groups of patients at particular risk of adverse drug interactions include patients in intensive care and patients undergoing complicated surgical procedures (Zarowitz *et al.* 1985; May *et al.* 1987; Beers *et al.* 1990).

Clinical importance of drug interactions

The overemphasis on drug interactions has led to the publication in many textbooks of clinical pharmacology and pharmacy of long lists of drug interactions. Why should this be?

1. Many drug interactions are first described in animal studies, often when doses of the drugs used have been much greater than those used clinically. The disposition of many drugs differs in man and animals, and thus drug interactions observed in an animal *in vivo* study may not be encountered in man. Sometimes the opposite is true: rifampicin, a well-known inducer of liver microsomal enzymes in man, is not an inducer in many animal species, notably the rat and rabbit, which are often used in screening studies (Heubel and Netter 1979).

2. Drug interactions are often described initially in *in vitro* studies, either in an isolated tissue or in a test tube. Protein-binding interactions that occur *in vitro* rarely occur in clinical practice (MacKichan 1989). Indeed, it is quite hard to find a clinically relevant drug interaction solely due to displacement from protein binding (as opposed to displacement *plus* inhibition of metabolism). Particular examples are drug interactions involving non-steroidal anti-inflammatory drugs (NSAID), many of which were thought to be due to protein-binding displacement. It has taken a lot of effort and experimental time to show that NSAID do not, in general, cause significant protein-binding displacement in man and that interactions between NSAID and, say, warfarin are unusual (see later) (Orme 1986).

3. Some drug interactions are described initially after a single case report in man. This is becoming less common now that journal editors are becoming increasingly resistant to publishing reports of single clinical cases. Nevertheless, there is a real dilemma here. Following an initial case report of a positive harmful interaction in one patient, two or three studies involving perhaps 20 or 30 individuals may show no evidence of an interaction and there you may think the matter would end. The initial (incorrect) report will continue, however, to be quoted in the literature from time to time, and it is often difficult to get a negative study published. Of course, the positive initial report may be fully confirmed in the later studies,

but the real difficulty arises when subsequent reports show an interaction in 1 out of 10 (or 20) subjects studied: while statistical analysis may well show no evidence of a true interaction, for the one patient affected it may be important. In order to establish the true frequency of the interaction it might be necessary to study a large number of subjects — perhaps several hundred — and this would clearly not be possible. This is a real problem in, for example, the oral contraceptive field, and the debate over interactions with broad-spectrum antibiotics (Back and Orme 1990) (see later).

Definition of 'drug interaction'

In the literature there is considerable confusion over what is or is not a drug interaction. Usually, concern over drug interactions only arises when an adverse event is caused. We should not, however, forget that some drug interactions are beneficial for the patient; and, indeed, two drugs may be deliberately given together for their combined effects (e.g. sulphamethoxazole and trimethoprim; probenecid and penicillin). Even though this aspect of drug interactions is not of prime concern for this book, we shall look at it briefly later in this chapter.

Some drug interactions are reported in the literature when only an additive effect is noted. Thus, the combination of phenobarbitone and alcohol will lead to more sedation than either drug alone; glucocorticoids will compound the hypokalaemia caused by thiazide diuretics. These are not, to my mind, drug interactions but merely the expected results of two drugs having additive effects on a pharmacological endpoint. A true drug interaction is one where the pharmacological outcome is not just a direct result of their two individual effects. Thus synergism may occur where the combined effect of two drugs is considerably greater than the sum of their individual effects. Alternatively, antagonism may result when one drug largely prevents the effect of another. Again, in this latter case I am excluding from discussion all expected antagonistic effects at receptors. Thus it is obvious that a β-receptor antagonist such as propranolol will largely prevent the stimulant effect of a β-agonist such as isoprenaline on β-receptors. This type of 'interaction' will not be discussed further.

Mechanisms of drug interactions

It has become conventional to discuss drug interactions according to the mechanisms involved. These are usually divided into two types; first, pharmacokinetic interactions, in which one drug affects the absorption, distribution, metabolism, or excretion of another; secondly pharmacodynamic interactions in which one drug interferes with the mechanism of action of another drug or affects physiological control processes. Table 30.1 lists the common mechanisms involved. This approach to drug interactions is useful, since if you can understand the mechanism behind any particular interaction you can use this knowledge to predict likely interactions with new drugs. Thus an enzyme-inducing agent, such as rifampicin or phenobarbitone, is likely to induce the metabolism of many drugs that are oxidized or conjugated in the liver and thus diminish their therapeutic effect.

It is worth looking here at each of the mechanisms in turn before looking at some of the drug groups for which drug interactions seem to be especially relevant.

TABLE 30.1
Mechanisms of drug interaction

1. Outside the patient (e.g. in infusion bottle or syringe)
2. In the gastrointestinal tract
3. During distribution of a drug to its site of action
   (e.g. protein-binding displacement)
4. During metabolism of a drug (enzyme inhibition or
   induction)
5. During excretion from the body
6. At the receptor — pharmacodynamic interactions

Pharmacokinetic interactions

Interactions outside the body

It is often forgotten in the hurly-burly of clinical work that drugs may interact before they are even administered to the patient, and this may involve either oral or parenteral routes of drug administration. For a drug given by mouth, much time will have been spent during its development to ensure that no chemical or physical reaction takes place between the constituents of the preparation intended for oral use. Any oral drug formulation may contain up to 25 ingredients which, in addition to the drug itself, may contain binders, fillers (e.g. lactose), colouring and tasting substances, and several other excipients. The pharmaceutical chemists developing the drug will have spent much time ensuring that none of these substances interact with the drug itself, and the stability and purity of the formulation will have been checked over prolonged periods of time and under various adverse storage conditions (e.g. low or high temperature, high humidity).

It is with parenteral mixtures that the clinician has to be particularly careful, and guidance will usually be given by the pharmacists. Additions of one drug to another in an intravenous infusion or syringe should always be avoided if possible. This subject has been reviewed elsewhere (Smith 1984) and pharmacists use as their main source of reference a large 750-page textbook devoted entirely to this subject (Trissel 1988). Problems arise particularly with heparin, penicillin, hydrocortisone, and theophylline when other drugs are added in the infusion bottle.

The following drugs are physically incompatible with heparin: amikacin, amiodarone, diazepam, droperidol, erythromycin, gentamicin, kanamycin, morphine, pentazocine, pethidine, polymyxin, and promethazine; and if one of these is added to a heparin infusion a precipitate forms within 5–10 minutes.

Aminophylline is incompatible in solution with chlorpromazine, and other phenothiazines such as promazine and prochlorperazine; dobutamine; pentazocine; pethidine; and some tetracycline salts. As stated earlier, good clinical practice dictates that no more than one drug should be placed in an infusion bottle or syringe. If it is vital to give two drugs by intravenous injection simultaneously, further advice should be sought. It may be appropriate, if venous access is difficult, to give one drug by injection into the side arm of a running infusion containing the second drug.

Drug interactions during absorption

Many of such interactions have been studied and, as mentioned earlier, not all of them are relevant. Some that have employed a static *in vitro* system have shown what appear to be significant interactions, while others involving an *in vivo* system have shown only minor changes. This subject has been reviewed by Welling (1984) and by Gugler and Allgayer (1990).

It is always going to be difficult to assess the clinical significance of this type of interaction, because of the contrast between kinetic and dynamic effects. Thus it may be relatively easy to show, for example, that an aluminium hydroxide antacid reduces the bioavailability of ketoprofen from 78.3 per cent to 60.9 per cent (Ismail *et al.* 1987) when studied in healthy volunteers. To show the clinical significance of this in patients, however, is likely to be much more difficult. A statistically significant reduction in the bioavailability of warfarin caused by cholestyramine (Robinson *et al.* 1971) is likely to be much more significant clinically than an apparently greater reduction in the bioavailability of penicillin when given with neomycin (Cheng and White 1962); warfarin clearly has a low therapeutic index while penicillin has the opposite property.

TABLE 30.2
*Clinically significant drug interactions occurring
during drug absorption*

1. *Via gastrointestinal motility changes*
   (a) Metoclopramide — enhanced speed of absorption of
       ethanol
       lithium
       paracetamol
   (b) Phenobarbitone-induced reduction of
       griseofulvin levels
2. *Via effects in the lumen of the gut*
   (a) Antacids — reduced absorption of:
       captopril
       ciprofloxacin
       tetracyclines
   (b) Cholestyramine — reduced absorption of
       sulphamethoxazole
       thyroxine
       warfarin
   (c) Tetracycline — reduced absorption of
       iron salts (both drugs show poor absorption)
   (d) Charcoal — reduced absorption of
       carbamazepine
       phenobarbitone
3. *Via damage to gastrointestinal mucosa*
   Cytotoxic drug-induced reduced absorption of
   phenytoin
   verapamil

Drugs may interact during absorption by a variety of mechanisms.

Effect on gastrointestinal motility

Drugs are mainly absorbed from the upper small intestine, where the surface area greatly exceeds that in the stomach. Thus a drug that delays gastric emptying might be expected to delay the absorption of other drugs (Nimmo 1976). In practice, the amount of drug absorbed is not really affected by changes in the gastric emptying rate, although the rate of absorption is affected. Thus metoclopramide, by increasing the rate of gastric emptying, increases the rate of absorption of paracetamol (Nimmo *et al.* 1973) as well as of other drugs such as levodopa and lithium (see Welling 1984). The interaction between metoclopramide and paracetamol is used therapeutically in patients with migraine to speed the onset of the analgesic action of paracetamol. Conversely, propantheline slows the rate of absorption of paracetamol (Nimmo *et al.* 1973) (but not the quantity of drug absorbed); this type of interaction is unlikely, however, to be significant clinically. The reduction in the absorption of griseofulvin induced by phenobarbitone may be therapeutically important and is probably due to an effect on gut motility (Busfield *et al.* 1963).

Luminal effects

Drug absorption interactions may also occur through an effect in the lumen of the gut when one drug may bind by chemical or physical means to another drug. Table 30.2 lists those drugs for which such interactions are thought to be of clinical relevance.

Antacids There is a large literature on drug interactions with antacids, and the subject has been extensively reviewed (Hurwitz 1977; Gugler and Allgayer 1990). The main groups of drugs for which such interactions have been described include antibiotics, β-adrenoceptor blocking drugs, captopril, digoxin, H_2-antagonists, iron salts, NSAID, and theophylline. The literature is confusing, for many of these drugs and most of their interactions are not clinically relevant in most patients. Thus the absorption of diflunisal appears to be reduced by aluminium hydroxide but enhanced by magnesium hydroxide (Verbeeck *et al.* 1979; Tobert *et al.* 1981). Undoubtedly, the interaction between tetracyclines and antacids is significant, since tetracycline forms insoluble chelates with divalent and trivalent ions (Neuvonen 1976), and the absorption of tetracyclines is markedly reduced by aluminium-containing and magnesium-containing antacids. The absorption of the quinolone antibiotics, such as ciprofloxacin and ofloxacin, is also markedly reduced by antacids containing aluminium and magnesium (Höffken *et al.* 1985; Lode 1988), and by ferrous salts given concurrently (Polk *et al.* 1989). The absorption of captopril was significantly reduced by an aluminium–magnesium antacid given concurrently (reduction of the area under the plasma concentration versus time curve [AUC] by 42 per cent), and this resulted in a significantly reduced effect on systolic blood pressure (Mäntylä *et al.* 1984). It is likely that other antacid interactions are only rarely of clinical significance.

Anion-exchange resins — cholestyramine This agent is an anion exchange resin that binds cholesterol and bile acids in the gut and prevents their reabsorption. In addition to binding bile acids, it also binds other antacid drugs that may be administered at the same time. This resin has been shown to reduce the absorption of warfarin (Robinson *et al.* 1971), thyroxine (Northcutt *et al.* 1969), and antibacterials such as sulphamethoxazole (Parsons and Paddock 1975). Other anion-exchange resins, such as colestipol, may also impair drug absorption (Kauffman and Azarnoff 1973), but the problem seems less than with cholestyramine. The solution to this problem is, however, relatively simple. A 2-hour gap should be left between the taking of cholestyramine and the ingestion of other drugs, preferably giving the other drug first. Then an interaction is unlikely to be seen (Welling 1984).

Tetracycline and charcoal   It has already been pointed out that antacids prevent the absorption of tetracycline (Neuvonen 1976). Tetracycline, however, may chelate other ions — in particular iron salts, with the end result of poor absorption of the iron (Neuvonen 1976). This is in fact a double interaction, since both tetracycline and the iron will be poorly absorbed. Again, the interaction can be prevented by giving the iron either 3 hours before or 2 hours after the tetracycline (Gothioni *et al.* 1972).

Charcoal has been implicated in reducing the absorption of certain drugs. Neuvonen and colleagues (1980) showed that this substance could reduce the absorption of phenobarbitone, phenylbutazone, and carbamazepine by up to 95 per cent; charcoal in sufficient quantity to have this effect is rarely given clinically but it could be used to prevent absorption in cases of overdose, were the diagnosis made soon enough.

Damage to gastrointestinal tract

The absorption of some drugs may be reduced due to damage of the small intestine, and this is most likely to be seen with cytotoxic therapy. The absorption of phenytoin (Fincham and Schottelius 1979) and verapamil (Kuhlmann 1985) has been shown to be reduced by 20–35 per cent in patients taking cytotoxic drugs, such as methotrexate, carmustine, and vinblastine, for the treatment of malignant disease. The reduced absorption was accompanied by evidence of loss of therapeutic effect. It is likely that this is an under-reported aspect of drug interaction.

Other mechanisms of drug interaction during the absorption process have been reported, mainly involving alteration of bowel flora, and thus interfering with the deconjugation of drugs and the enterohepatic circulation. This will be discussed at more length during consideration of drugs interacting with oral contraceptive steroids.

Drug interaction during distribution of drugs

Once a drug is absorbed into the body it is then distributed to its site of action, and during this process it may interact with another drug. In practice, the main source of these interactions is displacement from protein-binding sites. While basic drugs are largely bound to acid α_1-glycoprotein in plasma, acidic drugs are bound to albumin. We now recognize that there are several distinct sites to which drugs are bound on the albumin molecule (e.g. warfarin site, diazepam site). If other drugs that bind to the same site are taken, then competition for the binding site occurs and the first drug may be

displaced to circulate free (or unbound) in the plasma. This interaction is readily demonstrated *in vitro* for many drugs, and since the unbound drug is that part which produces the pharmacological effect, it is perhaps natural to assume that enhanced pharmacological effects will occur. The protein-binding displacement interactions have, however, come under closer and closer scrutiny over the last 10–15 years (Sellers 1979; McElnay and D'Arcy 1983), with the conclusion that most are of doubtful clinical importance. Nevertheless, many text books still perpetuate the largely mythical view that protein-binding interactions are of considerable clinical significance. The main reason for this is, I believe, historical. Phenylbutazone was recognized to potentiate the anticoagulant effect of warfarin as long ago as 1959 (Nordoy 1959). Further clinical reports confirmed this within a few years and Solomon and his colleagues (1968) showed that, *in vitro*, phenylbutazone displaced warfarin from protein binding. It was perhaps natural to link the two as cause and effect, and since many other NSAID also displaced warfarin from protein-binding sites on albumin it was assumed that any NSAID would enhance the anticoagulant effect of warfarin. It has

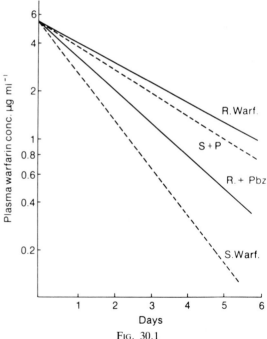

Fig. 30.1

Plasma warfarin concentration decay over a 6-day period after the oral administration of R warfarin and S warfarin to human volunteers before (R. Warf./S. Warf.) and after phenylbutazone (R.+Pbz/S+P) 100 mg thrice daily for 10 days.

Reproduced by kind permission of the authors and of the editor of the *Journal of Clinical Investigation* (1974) 53, 1607.

TABLE 30.3
Non-steroidal anti-inflammatory drugs that interact
with anticoagulants

NSAID	Anticoagulant
Aspirin (high-dose)	Warfarin
Azapropazone	Warfarin
Oxyphenbutazone	Warfarin
Phenylbutazone	Warfarin
	Phenprocoumon
Piroxicam	Acenocoumarin

taken many years to show the true mechanism of this interaction and that most NSAID do not interact adversely with anticoagulants such as warfarin. The interaction between phenylbutazone and warfarin is due to a stereoselective inhibition of the metabolism of warfarin (Sellers 1984). Warfarin as currently marketed consists of a racemic mixture of two enantiomers, R warfarin and S warfarin, S warfarin being five times as potent an anticoagulant as R warfarin. Phenylbutazone inhibits the metabolism of S warfarin and induces that of R warfarin, as shown in Figure 30.1. Thus as far as the kinetics of racemic warfarin are concerned there is no overall change with phenylbutazone but a greater proportion of warfarin in plasma is now the more potent S-warfarin form (Lewis *et al.* 1974; O'Reilly *et al.* 1980). It is now clear that other NSAID do not have this inhibitory effect on warfarin metabolism and therefore that drugs like indomethacin (Vessell *et al.* 1975), naproxen (Jain *et al.* 1979) and diclofenac (Krzywanek and Breddin 1977) do not interact adversely with oral anticoagulants. Care is still needed when NSAID are given to patients on warfarin, because of the increased likelihood of gastrointestinal bleeding. Table 30.3 lists those

NSAIDs that do interact with oral anticoagulants. In each case the mechanism is primarily inhibition of drug metabolism, although displacement from protein binding does play a role.

Current evidence suggests that, for most drugs, if a displacement interaction occurs, then the free concentration of the displaced drug will rise temporarily, but metabolism and distribution will return the free concentration to its previous level and the time this takes will be primarily dependent on the half-life of the displaced drug (MacKichan 1989). The biological significance of the temporary rise in free concentration is not clear but is unlikely to be very much on its own. The total concentration (i.e. free plus bound) of the displaced drug in plasma will fall and this may be of significance if that concentration is being measured for the purpose of therapeutic drug monitoring. Current evidence therefore suggests that for drugs whose metabolism is not inhibited, protein-binding displacement interactions are of *no* clinical significance (MacKichan 1989). If the metabolism of the displaced drug is inhibited at the same time (restrictive clearance), however, then an interaction will be seen. Table 30.4 lists those protein-binding displacement interactions that are thought to be clinically significant because of the combined effect of displacement from protein binding and inhibition of metabolism, leading therefore to sustained higher concentrations of free (unbound) drug.

Drug interactions occurring during metabolism

Many of the clinically relevant drug interactions occur because of alterations in the rate of metabolism of the drug concerned. Most drugs now used in clinical practice

TABLE 30.4
Clinically significant drug interactions involving displacement from protein binding
and decreased free drug clearance

Displaced drug	Interacting drug	Effect	Reference
Carbamazepine	Valproate	Increase in free concentration of carbamazepine Increased toxicity	MacPhee *et al.* 1988
Methotrexate	Salicylate Probenecid	Increase in free methotrexate concentration with increased toxicity	Evans and Christensen 1985
Phenytoin	Valproate	Increased concentration of free phenytoin plus phenytoin toxicity	Rodin *et al.* 1981
Tolbutamide	Sulphaphenazole	Increase in free concentration Increased hypoglycaemia	Christensen *et al.* 1963
Valproate	Salicylate	Increase in free concentration of valproate ?toxicity	Orr *et al.* 1982
Warfarin	Phenylbutazone	see text	Lewis *et al.* 1974 O'Reilly *et al.* 1980

TABLE 30.5
Drugs known to cause enzyme induction in man and to cause significant drug interactions

Barbiturates
Carbamazepine
Dichloralphenazone
Ethanol (chronic use)
Griseofulvin
Phenytoin
Primidone
Rifampicin

TABLE 30.6
Drugs known to be inhibitors of drug metabolism in man and to cause significant drug interactions

Amiodarone
Azapropazone
Cimetidine
Ciprofloxacin
Diltiazem
Disulfiram
Erythromycin
Ethanol (acute)
Isoniazid
Ketoconazole
Oxyphenbutazone
Phenylbutazone
Primaquine
Sulphinpyrazone
Sulphonamides
Valproate
Verapamil

are lipid-soluble and cannot be eliminated as such because they will be reabsorbed across the renal tubule. Metabolic processes convert the lipid-soluble drug to more water-soluble products that can be excreted in the urine or bile. There are two main types of drug metabolic process: phase I reactions involving oxidation, hydrolysis, or reduction; and phase II reactions, which are synthetic reactions involving conjugation of the drug (or its phase 1 product) with, for example, glucuronic acid, sulphate, or glycine. Products of phase II reactions are nearly always pharmacologically inactive, but phase I products are often active either therapeutically or toxicologically (Garattini 1985). The rate of drug metabolism varies widely betweenindividuals but is primarily genetically determined in any one individual. There are many factors that can affect the rate (or route) of drug metabolism (see Chapter 3), but one of the most important is the concomitant administration of other drugs.

The rate of drug metabolism may be increased by the process of enzyme induction, in which the enzyme inducer increases the velocity of the drug metabolic reac-

tion (V_{max}). There is a long list of enzyme inducers that have been detected in animal studies but relatively few are known to be inducers in man. Table 30.5 lists those inducers known to cause problems in man.

The rate of drug metabolism may be reduced by drugs that usually compete for the enzyme site although, rarely, the inhibiting drug may bind to the enzyme site and either inactivate or destroy it. Table 30.6 lists those drugs that are known to inhibit drug metabolism in man and to cause significant interactions. This area has been reviewed extensively elsewhere (Park and Breckenridge 1981).

The field of drug metabolism has advanced considerably in the last few years. The main enzyme responsible for drug oxidation processes is cytochrome P-450. It is now clear that this enzyme consists of many different isoenzymes (Boobis and Davies 1984; Brosen 1990). It is estimated that there may be as many as 200 different P-450 genes in man. The terminology of these different P-450 isozymes is confusing but has recently been revised (Nebert *et al.* 1989). The recommended terminology consists of a roman numeral, then a letter, followed by an arabic numeral. Thus the gene responsible for debrisoquine/sparteine oxidation is designated P-450 II D6. The importance of these isozymes of P-450 for drug interactions is that both enzyme inducers and enzyme inhibitors are likely to be selective in the range of isozymes they affect. This will be the focus of much work in the coming decade. Thus, quinidine, which is a potent inhibitor of P-450 II D6 in human liver studies, has little effect on other P-450 isozymes (Inaba *et al.* 1985). Similarly, primaquine is a potent inhibitor of antipyrine metabolism in man (Back *et al.* 1984a) but has no effect on the metabolism of ethinyloestradiol in spite of a dose size difference approaching 10 000-fold (Back *et al.* 1984b). It is likely that ethinyloestradiol and antipyrine are metabolised by different P-450 isozymes and that primaquine has differential effects on these (Brosen 1990).

Enzyme induction

Some compounds known to be enzyme inducers (e.g. glutethimide and sulphinpyrazone) have been omitted from Table 30.5 because the effect is of little or no clinical importance. Cigarette smoke is also an enzyme inducer but for the purposes of this review it is not considered as a drug. Since the process of enzyme induction requires new protein synthesis, the maximum effect is not seen for 2–3 weeks after starting an enzyme-inducing agent and, similarly, the effect may take some weeks to wear off when the inducing drug is stopped. Rifampicin is unusual in this regard in having a more rapid onset and offset (Park and Breckenridge 1981).

Thus patients taking rifampicin for 2 days for the treatment of nasal carriage of meningococci will experience enzyme induction and interference with other drug therapy (e.g. oral contraceptive steroids — see later). Enzyme induction usually results in the reduction of the pharmacological effect of the induced drug but where the metabolites are active the reverse may occur.

Oral anticoagulants

Oral anticoagulants such as warfarin have their hypoprothrombinaemic effect reduced by enzyme-inducing agents such as carbamazepine, barbiturates, and rifampicin. These interactions have been known for some years and several reviews have been written (Koch-Weser and Sellers 1971; Macleod and Sellers 1976; Serlin and Breckenridge 1983). There should be little need in clinical practice to give an enzyme-inducing agent to patients on warfarin, since benzodiazepines used as sedatives and hypnotics do not cause enzyme induction. Nevertheless, an occasional patient will need, say, both warfarin and carbamazepine and then particular care with anticoagulant control will be needed.

Corticosteroids

Enzyme-inducing agents enhance the metabolic clearance of corticosteroids, such as hydrocortisone (Werk *et al.* 1964), prednisolone (Petereit and Meikle 1977), and dexamethasone (Haque *et al.* 1972). Thus enzyme-inducing agents given to a steroid-dependent asthmatic may induce respiratory problems (Brooks *et al.* 1972); and, similarly, patients with rheumatoid arthritis taking

steroids may be made worse by enzyme-inducing drugs (Brooks *et al.* 1976). Patients with Addison's disease may need increased dosage of corticosteroids to prevent relapse (Edwards *et al.* 1974).

Thus, clinicians need to be aware that if enzyme-inducing agents are given to patients taking corticosteroids a dose increment will be needed, with a subsequent dose reduction when the agent is stopped. When such agents are given to patients taking corticosteroids they may lead to deterioration in renal allograft function, or failure of patients with the nephrotic syndrome to improve (see McInnes and Brodie 1988).

Oral contraceptive steroids

Combined oral contraceptive preparations and progestogen-only preparations lose their contraceptive effect when taken together with an enzyme-inducing agent (Back and Orme 1990). This aspect of drug interaction will be covered separately later on in this chapter.

Cyclosporin

Cyclosporin undergoes extensive metabolism in man and both organ toxicity and immunosuppressive activity appear to be related to cyclosporin concentrations in blood (Canafax and Ascher 1983). Enzyme-inducing agents, such as phenytoin, lower cyclosporin concentrations in blood (see Figure 30.2). This is thought to be due to enzyme induction by phenytoin. Although this interpretation has been questioned by Rowland and Gupta (1987), who feel that the interaction is due to reduced absorption of cyclosporin, there are additional

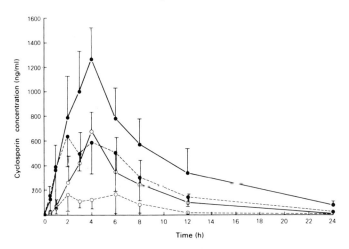

Fig. 30.2

Cyclosporin concentrations measured by high-pressure liquid chromatography before (——) and after (–––) administration of phenytoin (300–400 mg daily) to six volunteers taking cyclosporin. Concentrations are shown both in whole blood (○) and in serum (●).

(Reproduced by kind permission of the authors and of the editor of the *British Journal of Clinical Pharmacology* (1984) 18, 887.)

data (Nation *et al.* 1990) to support the original interpretation of Freeman and his colleagues (1984).

Quinidine

Long-term treatment with enzyme-inducing agents, such as phenytoin or barbiturates, enhances the metabolic clearance of quinidine. Increased dosage of quinidine has been shown to be necessary, and toxicity has been reported when the enzyme-inducing agent was stopped (Chapron *et al.* 1979).

Theophylline

Theophylline is a drug with a low therapeutic index, elimination of which depends largely on metabolism. This being so, it is not surprising to find that drug interactions with theophylline are clinically very important, and the subject has been reviewed extensively (Jonkman and Upton 1984). The elimination of theophylline is markedly enhanced by phenytoin (Marquis *et al.* 1982) and phenobarbitone (Landay *et al.* 1978) such that dosage increments of 30–40 per cent are required to keep the theophylline plasma concentration in the therapeutic range. Rifampicin also increases theophylline metabolic clearance and lowers the plasma concentrations (Hauser *et al.* 1983). It should not be forgotten that tobacco smoking, owing to the hydrocarbons in the smoke, induces drug metabolism, particularly that of theophylline, and the inducing effect may persist for 2–3 months after cessation of smoking (Hunt *et al.* 1976).

Enzyme inhibition

Enzyme inhibition is potentially more important in terms of drug interactions than enzyme induction. The speed of onset is usually more rapid, being determined largely by the half-life of the inhibited drug. Thus for drugs with a short half-life, the effect may be seen within 24 hours of the administration of the inhibiting agent. Table 30.6 lists those drugs that have been shown to be inhibitors of drug metabolism in man and to be responsible for clinically significant drug interactions.

Target areas

Oral anticoagulants The metabolism of warfarin is, as we have seen, inhibited by phenylbutazone, with potentially disastrous effects on anticoagulant control (Lewis *et al.* 1974). A number of other drugs, such as allopurinol, dextropropoxyphene, disulfiram, metronidazole, and sulphonamides, have been reported to inhibit the metabolism of warfarin (McInnes and Brodie 1988). These interactions are only rarely of clinical significance. Cimetidine has been shown to inhibit the

metabolism of warfarin (Serlin *et al.* 1979; O'Reilly 1984) with enhanced anticoagulant effects. In clinical practice cimetidine and warfarin are unlikely to be given together, but where there is a need for a patient to continue warfarin treatment and also to receive an H_2-antagonist then ranitidine is to be preferred, since it does not inhibit warfarin metabolism (Serlin *et al.* 1981; O'Reilly 1984).

Cyclosporin The metabolism of cyclosporin has been shown to be inhibited by ketoconazole, erythromycin, and diltiazem (Ferguson *et al.* 1982; Ptachcinski *et al.* 1985; McInnes and Brodie 1988) and cyclosporin toxicity may then result. No interaction is seen, however, between ciprofloxacin and cyclosporin (Kruger *et al.* 1990).

Theophylline Inhibition of theophylline metabolism is likely to lead to severe adverse effects, particularly cardiac arrhythmias, since the drug is often used to optimum effect by maintaining therapeutic blood levels. A number of drugs have been reported to inhibit theophylline metabolism (Jonkman and Upton 1984), including allopurinol, antibiotics such as ciprofloxacin and troleandomycin, and β-blockers such as propranolol. The two most important drugs in this respect, however, are cimetidine and erythromycin. Cimetidine is a well-known inhibitor of cytochrome P-450 and has been shown to inhibit the metabolism of theophylline producing a 30–50 per cent reduction in its clearance (Jackson *et al.* 1981; Breen *et al.* 1982; Jonkman and Upton 1984). There is little doubt that this is a potentially fatal interaction, since cimetidine may often be given to patients taking theophylline because of the gastric upset the latter tends to cause. Although ranitidine is less likely to cause inhibition of theophylline metabolism, it is not entirely free from blame in this regard (Kirch *et al.* 1984).

Erythromycin is another drug likely to be given concurrently with theophylline that has been shown to inhibit its metabolism. Not all studies have shown this convincingly, and it appears that erythromycin needs to be given for several days before the effect is seen (Jonkman and Upton 1984). In general, the clearance of theophylline is reduced by between 10 and 25 per cent by treatment with erythromycin for 5–7 days, and care will be needed to reduce the dose of theophylline accordingly (Branigan *et al.* 1981; May *et al.* 1982).

Ciprofloxacin is an antibiotic now known to raise concentrations of theophylline, almost certainly by inhibiting its metabolism (Maesen *et al.* 1984).

Phenytoin The pharmacokinetics of phenytoin are such that the drug is sensitive to inhibition of its metabolism by other drugs. Its metabolism is saturable and this effect is noted with concentrations above 10–15 mg per litre (Kutt 1971). The metabolism of phenytoin has been shown to be inhibited by a number of drugs including allopurinol, amiodarone, azapropazone, chloramphenicol, cimetidine, isoniazid, metronidazole, omeprazole, sulphonamides, and valproate (Rodin *et al.* 1981; Nation *et al.* 1990). No particular drug is especially prone to do this, and care should always be taken when prescribing an additional drug to a patient already receiving phenytoin.

Carbamazepine The metabolism of carbamazepine is inhibited by valproate (MacPhee *et al.* 1988) and significant interactions have been reported with chloramphenicol, cimetidine, erythromycin, isoniazid, propoxyphene, and sulphonamides (Vasko 1990). Many of these are now mainly of historical interest, because some of these drugs (e.g. chloramphenicol and sulphonamides) are now used much less frequently than hitherto, but occasional problems are encountered. Recently MacPhee and co-workers showed that verapamil and diltiazem inhibited the metabolism of carbamazepine with an increase of 50 per cent in the concentration of carbamazepine and neurotoxic sequelae. An alternative calcium antagonist, nifedipine, had no such effect (Brodie and MacPhee 1986; MacPhee *et al.* 1986).

Sulphonylureas These interactions, too, are mainly of historical interest, for the reasons given above, since the metabolism of tolbutamide and chlorpropamide has been shown to be inhibited by drugs such as chloramphenicol, dicoumarol, phenylbutazone, and sulphonamides. Although significantly increased hypoglycaemia occurred in some studies, there are few recent reports in this field (McInnes and Brodie 1988).

Inhibiting drugs

Amiodarone This agent is responsible for a number of interactions with digoxin, other antiarrhythmic drugs, and calcium-channel blocking drugs, as well as phenytoin (Lesko 1989). The mechanism is not always inhibition of metabolism (e.g. with digoxin renal clearance may be impaired). Warfarin metabolism, however, is inhibited by amiodarone (Watt *et al.* 1985) and this inhibition affects both R and S warfarin (O'Reilly *et al.* 1987). Amiodarone also inhibits the metabolism of phenytoin and probably also that of quinidine and flecainide.

Cimetidine It has already been shown that cimetidine is an inhibitor of hepatic microsomal drug oxidation and that it achieves this effect by binding to cytochrome P-450. In addition to inhibiting the metabolism of warfarin (Serlin *et al.* 1979), theophylline (Jackson *et al.* 1981), phenytoin (Nation *et al.* 1990), and carbamazepine (Vasko 1990), cimetidine has been shown to inhibit the metabolism of such drugs as chlormethiazole,

diazepam, labetalol, and propranolol (Gerber *et al.* 1985). In the case of these last four drugs it is unlikely that significant clinical problems will be caused. Ranitidine is, in general, viewed as having no effect on drug metabolism, but there are some reported examples of its causing enzyme inhibition involving, notably, fentanyl, metoprolol, and nifedipine, but the clinical significance of these is unclear (Kirch *et al.* 1984).

Ethanol Although chronic ethanol consumption may cause enzyme induction, acute alcohol ingestion has been shown to inhibit drug metabolism. In particular, clearance by conjugation to the glucuronide is particularly affected by alcohol (Lane *et al.* 1985). But normally ethanol levels need to be fairly high, and many studies in which blood ethanol levels have been maintained at 800–1500 mg per litre have shown inhibition of the metabolism of such drugs as diazepam, chlordiazepoxide, and lorazepam (Sellers *et al.* 1980). In general, it is unlikely that any effects will be seen with social drinking, but elimination of drugs following an overdose is likely to be slower if alcohol has also been consumed to excess. Interestingly, excess alcohol protects against liver damage in patients taking an overdose of paracetamol since the oxidation pathway which produces the toxic metabolite is inhibited (Banda and Quart 1982). Of course, chronic alcohol ingestion will make paracetamol hepatotoxicity worse by enzyme induction.

Allopurinol Allopurinol is recognized as a weak inhibitor of drug oxidation in man (Vessell *et al.* 1970). Its clinical relevance in this regard, however, is very minor. There is no effect on theophylline metabolism (Jonkman and Upton 1984) and there is little evidence of any interaction between allopurinol and phenytoin (Nation *et al.* 1990). Allopurinol is important, however, by virtue of its inhibition of xanthine oxidase. Certain cytotoxic drugs such as azathioprine, or its metabolite 6-mercaptopurine, are partly metabolised by xanthine oxidase, and if this enzyme is inhibited by allopurinol the clinical effects of the cytotoxic drugs will be enhanced with haemolysis or bone marrow suppression (Bacon *et al.* 1981). In such patients the dose of azathioprine must be reduced by 75 per cent when allopurinol therapy is started.

Sulphinpyrazone Sulphinpyrazone is an unusual drug since it can induce the metabolism of some drugs (e.g. theophylline) while inhibiting the metabolism of others (e.g. warfarin and tolbutamide). In clinical practice it is only the enzyme inhibition that is of any importance and even here clinical problems are rare, since the drugs are unlikely to be given together. Nevertheless, the combination of sulphinpyrazone and warfarin is not recommended (Miners *et al.* 1982).

Drug interactions during excretion

We have already noted that most drugs are lipid-soluble and hence need metabolising to make them soluble enough in water to be excreted. As a result, not many drugs are sufficiently water-soluble to be excreted unchanged. Interactions during excretion are described for digoxin, lithium, and methotrexate, and these are described elsewhere in this chapter. The effect of diuretics and NSAID leads to a rise in lithium concentration, and methotrexate clearance is reduced by NSAID. The renal tubular system is able both actively to secrete and passively to reabsorb a number of drugs. There are separate active transport systems for acidic and basic drugs in the proximal tubule, and competition for the active transport systems can be expected to occur between drugs secreted by the acidic system and those secreted by the basic system. Table 30.7 lists the drugs secreted by these systems, but the best known interactions are the beneficial interactions between probenecid and penicillin (Kampann *et al*. 1972), and probenecid and indomethacin (Baber *et al*. 1978).

TABLE 30.7
Acidic and basic drugs actively transported into the renal tubular lumen

Acidic	Basic
Acyclovir	Amiloride
Bumetanide	Cimetidine
Cephalosporins	Ethambutol
Frusemide	Procainamide
Indomethacin	Ranitidine
Penicillins	
Phenobarbitone	
Probenecid	
Salicylates	
Sulphonamides	
Thiazide diuretics	

Pharmacodynamic interactions

Pharmacodynamic interactions are less readily classified than those due to changes in pharmacokinetics. In some cases the interaction is due to effects at the receptor but in other cases the interaction is due to an effect on biochemical or physiological mechanisms. As mentioned earlier, interactions that are due to the additive effects of two drugs will not be discussed here.

Interactions at adrenergic nerve endings

Adrenergic-neurone blocking drugs like guanethidine, bethanidine, and debrisoquine lower blood pressure by being pumped into the adrenergic nerve endings by the uptake 1 mechanism and so concentrated there. Tricyclic antidepressant drugs prevent the antihypertensive effects of these drugs by blocking the uptake 1 mechanism (Leishman *et al*. 1963; Skinner *et al*. 1969). This type of interaction is, however, of lesser clinical relevance today, because adrenergic-neurone blocking drugs are rarely now used to treat hypertension.

Interactions with monoamine oxidase inhibitors are still of relevance and we shall examine these later in the chapter.

Direct receptor effects

Clearly agonists at a particular receptor (e.g. a β-adrenoceptor) will interact with antagonists at that receptor but this is entirely expected and requires no further discussion. Spironolactone prevents the healing effects of carbenoxolone on gastric ulcer; and, in turn, carbenoxolone competitively antagonizes the renal effects of spironolactone — both effects probably occurring through an action at the aldosterone receptor (Doll *et al*. 1968).

The hypoprothrombinaemic effects of warfarin are potentiated by clofibrate, quinidine, and dextrothyroxine; and in each case it is proposed that the mechanism is an increased affinity of warfarin for the receptor site (Solomon and Schrogie 1967; Starr and Petrie 1972).

Indirect receptor effects

A number of pharmacodynamic interactions are considered separately, later in the chapter. These include interactions involving monoamine oxidase inhibitors, between NSAID and diuretics, and between NSAID and antihypertensive drugs.

β-Adrenoceptor antagonists and hypoglycaemic agents

In patients treated with insulin or oral hypoglycaemic agents the use of β-adrenoceptor antagonists can produce hypoglycaemia (Reveno and Rosenbaum 1968). In addition, the recognition of hypoglycaemia by a patient may be impaired by β-blockers because of the lack of the usual warning symptoms. Propranolol reduces glycogen breakdown and delays the rise in blood glucose after hypoglycaemia (Davidson *et al*. 1976), while cardioselective drugs such as atenolol have no such effects (Davidson *et al*. 1976). In patients taking propranolol the hypoglycaemic reaction is accompanied by bradycardia rather than the usual tachycardia. In those taking selective β-blockers, such as metoprolol, the heart rate rises and there is little change in blood pressure (Davidson *et al*. 1976). Patients taking insulin or oral hypoglycaemic drugs are thus best advised to take a selective, rather than a non-selective β- blocker, if a drug of this kind is indicated.

β-Adrenoceptor antagonists and other cardioactive drugs

The combination of β-blockers and verapamil has been recognized for some years as deleterious (Krikler and Spurell 1974). Not only is there a combination of the negative inotropic effects of both drugs, resulting in heart failure, but hypotension, atrioventricular block, and asystole have been noted. Other antiarrhythmic agents given concurrently with β-blockers can also produce adverse effects — notably heart failure and hypotension — and examples include nifedipine (Robson and Vishwanath 1982), tocainide (Ibram 1980), disopyramide (Gelipter and Hazell 1980), and lignocaine (Graham et al. 1981).

Spironolactone and potassium chloride

The combination of spironolactone, with its potassium-retaining effect, and potassium chloride is to be avoided, since it has led to hyperkalaemic paralysis and death (McInnes and Ramsay 1987). Indeed, no potassium-retaining diuretic (including triamterene and amiloride) should be given with potassium chloride. In a study by the Boston Collaborative Drug Surveillance Program, hyperkalaemia attributable to spironolactone was found in 5.7 per cent of medical patients not receiving potassium salts. In patients with renal failure also taking potassium salts, that figure rose to 42 per cent (Greenblatt and Koch-Weser 1973). The combination of potassium with potassium-sparing diuretics should always be avoided. Angiotensin-converting-enzyme inhibitors such as captopril also cause a rise in the serum potassium, and problems have arisen when spironolactone was given to patients taking such a preparation (Heel et al. 1980).

Drug interactions with specific drug groups

Drug interactions with oral contraceptive steroids

Oral contraceptive steroids (OCS) are used by some 2 million women in the United Kingdom and by perhaps 60 million women worldwide. Since there has been a trend to lower the dose of steroids in the preparations over the last 10–15 years drug interactions have assumed a greater importance than previously.

Effect of contraceptive steroids on other drugs

OCS do have effects on the metabolism of other drugs, but in general these changes are of minor importance.

The metabolic disposition of some benzodiazepines is affected by OCS, and for those drugs that are metabolised by oxidation OCS inhibit the drug metabolism. Thus, the clearance of diazepam was reduced by 40 per cent when OCS were given (Abernethy et al. 1982). For drugs metabolised by conjugation (e.g. temazepam), the clearance is enhanced by about 50 per cent (Stoehr et al. 1984). Similarly, the clearance of caffeine, metoprolol, prednisolone, and theophylline is reduced in users of OCS, but the changes are relatively small compared with the interindividual variations that are seen in drug metabolism (Back and Orme 1990). Oral contraceptives are reported to enhance the effect of antidepressants and of warfarin, but these changes are not of clinical significance (Breckenridge et al. 1979).

One interesting interaction concerns cyclosporin and ethinyloestradiol, both of which are now known to be metabolised primarily by the same cytochrome P-450 isozyme (P-450 III A4) (Brosen 1990). In a woman treated with cyclosporin, the plasma concentrations rose when the oral contraceptive was started, and this may have been because of competitive inhibition at the P-450 III A4 isozyme (Deray et al. 1987). This interaction may assume greater importance in the future.

Effect of other drugs on oral contraceptive steroids

Antituberculous drugs

Reimers and Jezek described contraceptive failure in 1971 in women taking antituberculous drugs with their OCS. It was quickly realized that the enzyme-inducing agent rifampicin was responsible, and a number of other reports have appeared since then (Orme et al. 1983). Studies showed that rifampicin induced the metabolism both of ethinyloestradiol (Back et al. 1980a) and of the progestogens (Back et al. 1979). From a scientific viewpoint this is interesting because rifampicin induces a cytochrome P-450 isozyme in the liver that is known to be involved in the metabolism of ethinyloestradiol (Guengerich 1988). From a clinical point of view, the degree of induction by rifampicin (up to fourfold or fivefold), the interindividual variation in induction, and the short courses of rifampicin that are usually given, together mean that women taking rifampicin should not rely on OCS for their contraception. This also applies, as mentioned earlier, even to women taking rifampicin only for 2 days to kill nasal meningococci. They should use alternative contraceptive precautions for one month after the course of rifampicin is finished.

Anticonvulsants

A wide variety of anticonvulsants have been reported to cause contraceptive failure when given to women taking

TABLE 30.8
Anticonvulsants and antibiotics involved in alleged interactions in cases of contraceptive failure in women taking oral contraceptive steroids

Anticonvulsants	No. of reports
Carbamazepine	6
Ethosuximide	4
Phenobarbitone	20
Phenytoin	25
Primidone	7
Valproate	1
Antibiotics	
Cephalosporins	2
Co-trimoxazole	5
Erythromycin	2
Metronidazole	3
Penicillins	32
Tetracyclines	12
Trimethoprim	2
Others	5

The data come from reports to the Committee on Safety of Medicines in the United Kingdom received between 1968 and 1984 (see Back *et al.* 1988).

OCS (Coulam and Annegers 1979; Orme *et al.* 1983). Table 30.8 lists those anticonvulsants that have been implicated in reports to the Committee on Safety of Medicines (CSM) in the United Kingdom between 1968 and 1984 (Back *et al.* 1988). Kinetic data are relatively sparse in this field, but phenobarbitone has been shown to cause a fall in the blood level of ethinyloestradiol, presumably by enzyme induction (Back *et al.* 1980*b*). The interaction between ethinyloestradiol and pheno-

barbitone is shown in Figure 30.3. Similarly, carbamazepine and phenytoin have been shown to reduce the plasma concentration of both ethinyloestradiol and progestogens in women taking single doses of OCS (Crawford *et al.* 1990). The degree of change seen in these studies is quite sufficient to cause contraceptive failure, but it is now possible to achieve contraceptive control by using a higher dose OCS preparation. I start with a 50 μg ethinyloestradiol preparation, and if breakthrough bleeding occurs into the second cycle of use the dose can be increased to 80 μg (or if necessary to 100 μg) ethinyloestradiol. Breakthrough bleeding is a reasonable clinical sign of relative oestrogen deficiency. Even though more steroid metabolites will be produced, there is no evidence that these have any pharmacological activity. Alternatively, a standard dose of OCS can be used if sodium valproate is used as the anticonvulsant, since this does not interact with OCS (Crawford *et al.* 1986).

Antibiotics

Broad-spectrum antibiotics have been implicated in causing contraceptive failure in women taking OCS. There are a number of individual case reports in the literature, involving tetracycline, ampicillin, and erythromycin (Orme *et al.* 1983), and 63 pregnancies were reported to the CSM between 1968 and 1984 in women taking antibiotics with their OCS preparation (Back *et al.* 1988). The antibiotics implicated are shown in Table 30.8. In a study of pill method failures recorded in reliable pill takers over a 4-year period (1981 to 1985), Sparrow (1987) in New Zealand found that antibiotics were implicated in 23 per cent of the 163 cases noted.

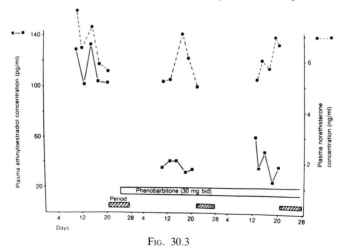

FIG. 30.3
Plasma ethinyloestradiol (■——■) and norethisterone (●---●) concentrations in a patient during a control cycle of oral contraceptive steroid use and during two subsequent cycles of use when the patient was treated with phenobarbitone 30 mg twice daily.
(Reproduced by kind permission of the authors and of the editor of *Contraception* (1980) 22, 495).

Systematic studies with broad-spectrum antibiotics have shown, however, no evidence of any interaction between these antibiotics and OCS. Such antibiotics include ampicillin (Friedman *et al.* 1980; Joshi *et al.* 1980; Back *et al.* 1982), co-trimoxazole (Grimmer *et al.* 1983), and tetracycline and erythromycin (Orme and Back 1986). Indeed, co-trimoxazole significantly increased the blood levels of ethinyloestradiol and made the OCS significantly more effective as judged by a fall in FSH levels, which makes the CSM data in Table 30.8 even harder to understand.

The proposed mechanism involves the enterohepatic circulation of ethinyloestradiol, which is conjugated with sulphate and with glucuronide in the gut wall and liver respectively. These conjugates are excreted in the bile and when they reach the colon they are hydrolysed by gut bacteria (primarily *Clostridia* spp.) to liberate unchanged ethinyloestradiol, which is then reabsorbed into the body. Broad-spectrum antibiotics can be shown to reduce dramatically the ability of faecal microorganisms to hydrolyse ethinyloestradiol (Chapman 1981), and thus ethinyloestradiol conjugates would be expected to be lost in the faeces with a resultant fall in circulating ethinyloestradiol blood levels. It is impossible at the moment to reconcile the two sides of the argument. Most data sheets currently recommend that alternative contraceptive precautions should be taken if a broad-spectrum antibiotics is given to a woman taking OCS. In addition, a number of medicolegal cases involving this interaction have been settled out of court, it being the legal view that, as this is an established interaction, the practitioner is negligent if he or she fails to heed the advice given in data sheets. My own view is that this is a rare interaction but it will be difficult to prove this view conclusively in spite of the weight of scientific data in its favour. The enterohepatic circulation of ethinyloestradiol is probably of very minor importance in most people, as judged from data from women with an ileostomy (Grimmer *et al.* 1986).

Ascorbic acid and paracetamol

Ethinyloestradiol is conjugated with sulphate in the gut wall during absorption and this process accounts for 60 per cent of the first-pass metabolism. Drugs that are given together with ethinyloestradiol and which compete for available sulphate might be expected to result in an increased bioavailability of ethinyloestradiol. This has been shown for ascorbic acid (Back *et al.* 1981) and paracetamol (Rogers *et al.* 1987) with a 50 per cent increase in blood levels of ethinyloestradiol with the former drug. The biological significance of this is not, however, clear and in any case the interaction can be avoided by giving the ascorbic acid or paracetamol 2 hours before (or 2 hours after) the OCS dose.

TABLE 30.9
Clinically important drug interactions with NSAID

Oral anticoagulants (see Table 30.3)
Antihypertensive drugs
Lithium
Loop diuretics
Methotrexate
Phenytoin
Thiazide diuretics
Valproate

Drug interactions with NSAID

Drug interactions with NSAID are becoming increasingly important, particularly as the use of NSAID continues to increase. The clinically relevant interactions with NSAID that have a pharmacokinetic basis, particularly those with anticoagulants, have been covered earlier in the chapter. Many drug interactions have been described with NSAID (see Webster 1985; Orme 1986; Miners 1989; Verbeeck 1990). Many areas of drug interaction such as those with antacids, digoxin, and between NSAID probably have little clinical relevance and the important ones are shown in Table 30.9. One important interaction that involves kinetics is that between NSAID (particularly salicylates) and methotrexate. The renal clearance of methotrexate is reduced by 30–50 per cent if such drugs are given together, and deaths have resulted from this interaction (Singh *et al.* 1986; Thyss *et al.* 1986). If NSAID are given to patients taking methotrexate, the dose of methotrexate should be halved and the patient closely monitored for adverse effects, particularly bone marrow suppression.

Pharmacodynamic interactions with NSAID are increasingly being reported, particularly as far as diuretics and antihypertensive drugs are concerned.

Loop diuretics

The diuretic effect of many drugs is impaired by NSAID. This interaction was first observed between aspirin and spironolactone, but is now chiefly noted with loop diuretics. The reports have primarily involved indomethacin, which has been shown to blunt the diuretic response to frusemide (Patak *et al.* 1975) and to bumetanide (Pedrinelli *et al.* 1980). NSAID are known to cause salt and water retention, but the mechanism is almost certainly more complicated than this. The renal clearance of frusemide is reduced by indomethacin (Smith *et al.*

1979), but it is likely that the mechanism chiefly involves renal prostaglandins. Prostaglandin E_2 is important as a renal vasodilator and becomes particularly relevant in disease states (as opposed to the normal healthy state). Other NSAID such as flurbiprofen (Symmons *et al.* 1983), ibuprofen, and naproxen (Yeung Laiwah and Mactier 1981) inhibit the diuretic effect of frusemide, but sulindac, which spares renal prostaglandins, appears not to do so (Bunning and Barth 1982). It is of interest that the diuretic effect of thiazides is not impaired by indomethacin even though the hypotensive effect is reduced (Favre *et al.* 1983). It is increasingly common to see patients whose heart failure has deteriorated in spite of increased doses of frusemide, and not infrequently the blame lies with the concurrent use of NSAID.

Antihypertensive drugs

Indomethacin was first reported to antagonize the hypotensive effect of β-blockers by Durao and co-workers in 1977. Since then the interaction has been confirmed in controlled studies (Watkins *et al.* 1980; Wing *et al.* 1981). Figure 30.4 shows the effect on blood pressure of giving indomethacin to patients taking bendrofluazide or propranolol (Watkins *et al.* 1980). In addition, indomethacin has been shown to reduce the hypotensive effect of other antihypertensive drugs, such as captopril (Silberbauer *et al.* 1982) as well as other β-blockers, such as oxprenolol (Salvetti *et al.* 1982). There are relatively few data concerning other NSAID, but it does seem to be a class effect rather than restricted to indomethacin, since flurbiprofen has also been shown to inhibit the hypotensive effect of propranolol but not that of atenolol (Webster *et al.* 1983).

Drug interactions with monoamine oxidase inhibitors

Monoamine oxidase inhibitors (MAOI) are effective antidepressant drugs that have had a bad press because of their interaction with food and with other drugs. Nevertheless, some psychiatrists use them regularly and feel that, in the right patient, they are more effective than other antidepressant drugs. MAOI achieve their effect by inhibiting the intraneuronal enzyme monoamine oxidase and, as a result, noradrenaline breakdown in the adrenergic nerve ending is much reduced. This leads to the nerve ending having large stores of noradrenaline ready for release into the synaptic cleft at the behest of either a neuronal discharge or an indirectly acting amine. The action of the directly acting amine noradrenaline is not affected by MAOI, but the hypertensive effects of adrenaline are potentiated by some MAOI (see Chapter 7) to a degree that, while not harmful to healthy patients, may be a hazard to patients with cardiovascular disease. The vasoconstrictor felypressin is not affected by MAOI.

The main indirectly acting amines include amphetamine, tyramine, phenylpropanolamine, and phenylephrine (the last two also have direct effects on α-receptors). Tyramine is normally present in foodstuffs (e.g. cheese, red wine, etc) and is metabolised in the gut wall (as the first-pass effect) to inactive metabolites. The enzyme responsible for this metabolic step, however, is monamine oxidase and in patients taking MAOI such as phenelzine or tranylcypromine the tyramine will be absorbed intact. Amines such as phenylephrine and phenylpropanolamine are present in many cough and cold cures and are readily available over the counter in pharmacies. Thus the ingestion of tyramine (in food)

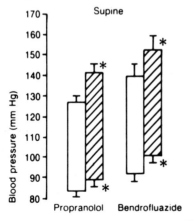
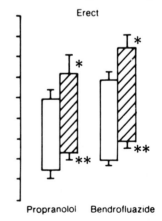

Fig. 30.4

Effect on supine and erect blood pressures of adding either indomethacin (hatched bars) 100 mg daily for 3 weeks, or placebo (open bars) to hypertensive patients receiving treatment with bendrofluazide (n=5) or propranolol (n=8). ★ P<0.05   ★★ P<0.01

Reproduced with permission of the authors and the editor of the *British Medical Journal* (1980) 281, 702).

or phenylpropranolamine leads to a massive release of noradrenaline from adrenergic nerve endings and a syndrome of sympathetic overactivity results with hypertension, headache, excitement, hyperpyrexia, and cardiac arrhythmias (Tollefson 1983). Subarachnoid haemorrhage and death have resulted, and all patients taking MAOI should be instructed explicitly about these problems. Termination of this effect depends upon new enzyme synthesis once the MAOI is stopped, and thus precautions need to continue for 3 weeks after the MAOI is stopped. The problem is encountered with non-selective MAOI. It does not, however, occur with the more selective (Type B) MAOI, such as selegeline when this drug is given in the doses used for Parkinson's disease (5–10 mg daily), though it has been suspected of having caused tyramine-induced hypertension when given in the larger doses (20 mg daily) sometimes given for depression (McGrath et al. 1989).

MAOI also interact with other drugs such as pethidine and tricyclic antidepressants. The danger of this interaction has been underestimated in recent years. It is now clear that, for the antidepressants at least, the drugs that block noradrenaline re-uptake are relatively safe (e.g. imipramine, trimipramine). The danger comes particularly with the use of drugs that selectively block the re-uptake of serotonin, such as clomipramine and fluoxetine (Lader 1990). The combination of MAOI and inhibitors of serotonin re-uptake is potentially lethal. This subject is also discussed in Chapter 7.

Drug interactions between antibiotics

Some of the classical work on drug antagonism was performed with antibiotics. It is now well recognized that it is bad clinical practice to combine a bacteriostatic antibiotic such as tetracycline or chloramphenicol with a bactericidal agent such as penicillin (Lepper and Dowling 1951). The antibiotic effect of gentamicin is reduced by benzylpenicillin and carbenicillin (McLaughlin and Reeves 1971). In contrast, antibiotics may potentiate each other and the most obvious example is the combination of trimethoprim and sulphamethoxazole in co-trimoxazole. The value of the combination in clinical practice in most of the conditions for which it is used is debatable, since most organisms are sensitive to trimethoprim and the addition of the sulphamethoxazole may merely increase the risk of adverse reactions (Lacey et al. 1980). The administration of ethacrynic acid to patients being given low-dose aminoglycoside therapy increases the risk of drug-induced deafness (Mathog and Klein 1969), while loop diuretics such as frusemide increase the risk of nephrotoxicity in patients being given

gentamicin or cephaloridine (Norrby et al. 1976). (See also Chapter 20.)

We have already noted the chelating properties of tetracycline, leading to its poor absorption when given with antacids (Neuvonen 1976); and the poor absorption of both drugs when tetracycline is given to patients taking ferrous salts (Neuvonen 1976). The absorption of ciprofloxacin is much reduced by administration with antacids (Lode 1988) or with ferrous salts (Polk et al. 1989).

Ciprofloxacin is recognized as an enzyme inhibitor (see Drug metabolism section) and it potentiates the effects of theophylline (Maeson et al. 1984), while erythromycin is also known to inhibit the metabolism of theophylline (May et al. 1982). This subject is also discussed in Chapter 23.

Drug interactions with digoxin

Many interactions involving digoxin have been reported (Rodin and Johnson 1988) but most of them are of little clinical significance. By changing electrolyte balance, diuretics can interact adversely with digoxin, although usually the interaction is, mainly, beneficial. Diuretic-induced hypokalaemia increases the risk of digoxin-induced cardiotoxicity (Steiness and Olesen 1976). Thus, patients taking diuretics and digoxin need to have their serum potassium carefully monitored.

The absorption of digoxin is incomplete, and earlier formulations showed marked interindividual variations in absorption. Modern formulations do not have the same problems to any significant degree; thus, many of the drugs that have been believed in the past to have reduced the absorption of digoxin can be regarded as of historical interest only. Cholestyramine and, to a lesser extent, colestipol reduce the absorption of digoxin, but these interactions can be easily avoided by giving the two drugs at least 2 hours apart (Rodin and Johnson 1988). Digoxin was first shown to interact with quinidine in the late 1970s and has been written about extensively since then (Fichtl and Doering 1983). The quinidine-induced rise in plasma digoxin concentrations is usually of the order of twofold to threefold and occurs in 90 per cent of patients (Pedersen et al. 1980). The mechanism is complicated, and quinidine decreases the renal clearance of digoxin (Doering 1979), but it is not clear how much of this effect is due to a change in the renal handling of digoxin and how much to a change in the volume of distribution of digoxin. The interaction is certainly clinically significant and leads to adverse effects (especially cardiotoxicity), and this is more marked in elderly patients (Walker et al. 1983). In many countries (e.g. the

UK), however, quinidine is rarely used as an antiarrhythmic agent and thus the interaction is rarely a problem. Similar interactions have been reported with verapamil (Johnson *et al.* 1987) and amiodarone (Oetgen *et al.* 1984) and both drugs will increase digoxin plasma concentrations by 60–100 per cent. There is no clear evidence that this interaction occurs with other antiarrhythmic or calcium-channel blocking drugs (Rodin and Johnson 1988).

Drug interactions with lithium

There have been several reports of lithium toxicity in patients who were given diuretics as well. Thiazide treatment is associated with a reduction of about 25 per cent in lithium clearance (Petersen *et al.* 1974) and a similar change is seen with loop diuretics (Kerry *et al.* 1980). During long-term diuretic therapy there is increased proximal tubular excretion of sodium and this increases lithium reabsorption. Serum concentrations of lithium will rise by about 30 per cent, leading to toxicity unless a reduction in the dose of lithium is made.

NSAID also interact with lithium and the mechanism is also thought to be due to decreased renal clearance of lithium, with a consequent increase in plasma lithium concentrations. This interaction has been described with several NSAID (Verbeeck 1990), notably indomethacin, ibuprofen (Ragheb *et al.* 1980), and diclofenac (Reimann and Frölich 1980). If patients taking lithium are given NSAID, then the dose of lithium should be decreased by 25 per cent and the plasma concentration of lithium should be checked.

Drug interactions between anticancer drugs

Combination therapy is very common in the field of anticancer drugs and thus interactions are to be expected. This is a specialized field and the reader is referred to a recent review for further information (Balis 1986), and to Chapter 24. We have already noted the problems that may arise when allopurinol is given to patients under treatment with azathioprine or mercaptopurine (Bacon *et al.* 1981), and the reduced renal clearance of methotrexate caused by NSAID (Thyss *et al.* 1986). Both interactions are potentially very serious and have caused major clinical problems in the past.

Beneficial drug interactions

Although the main aim of this book is to deal with adverse drug effects, it should not be forgotten that drugs are often given together for the beneficial effect of the combination. We have come across a number of such examples so far, including probenecid with penicillin or with indomethacin, trimethoprim with co-trimoxazole and, of course, levodopa with carbidopa (a peripheral decarboxylase inhibitor). In the field of hypertension, the combined effect of β-adrenoceptor blocking drugs and diuretics is additive but not synergistic (Freis 1984). Similarly the combined effect of ACE inhibitors, such as captopril, and diuretics is probably synergistic rather than additive (Holland *et al.* 1983). In general, combinations of drugs used for hypertension are additive rather than synergistic (Lam and Shepherd 1990). Other examples of beneficial interactions are shown in Table 30.10.

TABLE 30.10
Examples of beneficial interactions

Salbutamol and theophylline
β-Adrenoceptor antagonists with antianginal and antihypertensive drugs
Levodopa with decarboxylase inhibitor
Levodopa/decarboxylase inhibitor with anticholinergic drug
Sulphonylureas with biguanides
Heparin with aspirin
Opioid analgesics with phenothiazines
Anticoagulants with thrombolytic drugs
Diuretics with potassium sparing diuretics

TABLE 30.11
Drugs at particular risk of interaction

Effect involved	Drugs concerned
Saturable hepatic metabolism	Ethanol Phenytoin Theophylline
Patient dependent on prophylactic effect	Cyclosporin Oral contraceptive steroids
Drug has steep dose–response curve	Chlorpropamide Verapamil
Drug has low therapeutic index	Digoxin Lithium Warfarin
Drug has major toxic effects	Aminoglycosides Cytotoxic drugs Lithium Monoamine oxidase inhibitors

After Brodie and Feely 1988

Conclusions

Drug interactions are an important facet of therapy and, as we have seen, can be beneficial or harmful, leading

TABLE 30.12

*Patients particularly susceptible
to adverse drug reactions*

Elderly patients
Patients taking many drugs
Patients with renal or hepatic disease
Patients with acute illness,
    e.g. anaemia, asthma, heart failure, pneumonia
Patients with unstable disease,
    e.g. cardiac arrhythmias, diabetes mellitus, epilepsy
Patients dependent on long-term drug treatment,
    e.g. Addison's disease, transplant recipients
Patients with more than one prescribing doctor

After Brodie and Feely 1988

either to loss of the therapeutic effect or, particularly, to adverse effects. Some of these effects will be Type A (see Chapter 3) but those that are dangerous are, as we would expect, Type B. Instead of committing numerous lists of drugs to memory, it is possible to instil reason into the subject. First, a knowledge of the mechanism involved allows us to understand the interaction and, one hopes, anticipate similar problems in the future when new but similar drugs appear on the market. Secondly, there are certain areas of drug therapy in which interactions are more likely, either because of the nature of the drugs (e.g. cytotoxic agents) or because the drug has a low therapeutic index. Table 30.11 lists some of the drugs involved here and the reasons for tabulating them. Remembering these drugs will enable us to avoid many of the interactions. Thirdly, certain patients are more susceptible to adverse drug interactions, and the reasons for this are shown in Table 30.12. It is hoped that by remembering these three important points drug interactions will be somewhat less likely to occur in the future.

References

Abernethy, D.R., Greenblatt, D.J., Divoll, M., Arendt, R., Ochs, H.R., Shader, R.I. (1982). impairment of diazepam metabolism by low dose estrogen-containing oral contraceptive steroids. *N. Engl. J. Med.* 306, 791.

Baber, N.S., Halliday, L., Sibeon, R.G., Littler, T., and Orme, M.L'E.. (1978) The interaction between indomethacin and probenecid. A clinical and pharmacokinetic study. *Clin. Pharmacol. Ther.* 24, 298.

Back, D.J. and Orme, M.L'E. (1990). Pharmacokinetic drug interactions with oral contraceptives. *Clin. Pharmacokinet.* 18, 472.

Back, D.J., Breckenridge, A.M., Crawford, F.E., MacIver, M., Orme, M.L'E., Park, B.K., *et al.* (1979). The effect of rifampicin on norethisterone pharmacokinetics. *Eur. J. Clin. Pharmacol.* 15, 193.

Back, D.J., Breckenridge, A.M., Crawford, F.E., Hall, J.M., MacIver, M., Orme, M.L'E., *et al.* (1980a). The effect of rifampicin on the pharmacokinetics of ethinyloestradiol in women. *Contraception* 21, 135.

Back, D.J., Bates, M., Bowden, A., Breckenridge, A.M., Hall, M.J., Jones, H., *et al.* (1980b). The interaction of phenobarbital and other anticonvulsants with oral contraceptive steroid therapy. *Contraception* 22, 495.

Back, D.J., Breckenridge, A.M., MacIver, M., Orme, M.L'E., Purba, H., and Rowe, P.H. (1981). The interaction of ethinyloestradiol with ascorbic acid in man. *Br. Med. J.* 282, 1516.

Back, D.J., Breckenridge, A.M., MacIver, M., Orme, M.L'E., Rowe, P.H., Staiger Ch., *et al.* (1982). The effects of ampicillin on oral contraceptive steroids in women. *Br. J. Clin. Pharmacol.* 14, 43.

Back, D.J., Purba, H.S., Park, B.K., Ward, S.A., and Orme, M.L'E. (1984a). Effect of chloroquine and primaquine on antipyrine metabolism. *Br. J. Clin. Pharmacol.* 16, 497.

Back, D.J., Breckenridge, A.M., Grimmer, S.F.M., Orme, M.L'E., and Purba, H.S. (1984b). Pharmacokinetics of oral contraceptive steroids following the administration of the antimalarial drugs, primaquine and chloroquine. *Contraception* 30, 289.

Back, D.J., Grimmer, S.F.M., Orme, M.L'E., Proudlove, C., Mann, R.D., and Breckenridge, A.M. (1988). Evaluation of Committee on Safety of Medicines Yellow Card reports on oral contraceptive-drug interactions. *Br. J. Clin. Pharmacol.* 25, 527.

Bacon, B.R., Treuhaft, W.H., and Goodman, A.M. (1981). Azathioprine-induced pancytopenia. *Arch. Intern. Med.* 141, 223.

Balis, F.M. (1986). Pharmacokinetic drug interactions of commonly used anticancer drugs. *Clin. Pharmacokinet.* 11, 223.

Banda, P.W. and Quart, B.D. (1982). The effect of mild alcohol consumption on metabolism of acetaminophen in man. *Res. Comm. Chem. Path. Pharmacol.* 38, 57.

BCDSP (Boston Collaborative Drug Surveillance Program) (1972). Adverse drug interactions. *JAMA* 220, 1238.

Beers, M.H., Storrie, M., and Lee, G. (1990). Potential adverse drug interactions in the emergency room. *Ann. Intern. Med.* 112, 61.

Blaschke, T.F., Cohen, S.N., and Tatro, D.S. (1981). Drug-drug interactions and aging. In *Clinical pharmacology in the aged patient* (ed. L.F. Jarvik, D.J. Greenblatt, and D. Harman), p. 11. Raven Press, New York.

Boobis, A.R. and Davies, D.S. (1984). Human cytochromes P-450. *Xenobiotica* 14, 151.

Borda, I.T., Sloane, D., and Jick, H. (1968). Assessment of adverse reactions within a drug surveillance program. *JAMA* 205, 645.

Branigan, T.A., Robbins, R.A., Cady, W.J., Nickols, J.G., and Ueda, C.T. (1981). The effects of erythromycin on the absorption and disposition kinetics of theophylline. *Eur. J. Clin. Pharmacol.* 21, 115.

Breckenridge, A.M., Back, D.J., and Orme, M.L'E. (1979). Interactions between oral contraceptives and other drugs. *Pharmacol. Ther.* 7, 617.

Breen, K.J., Bury, R., Desmond, P.V., Mashford, M.L., Morphett, B., Westwood, B., *et al.* (1982). Effects of cimetidine and ranitidine on hepatic drug metabolism. *Clin. Pharmacol. Ther.* 31, 297.

Brodie, M.J. and Feely, J. (1988). Adverse drug interactions. *Br. Med. J.* 296, 845.

Brodie, M.J. and MacPhee, G.J.A. (1986). Carbamazepine neurotoxicity precipitated by diltiazem. *Br. Med. J.* 292, 1170.

Brooks, P.M., Buchanan, W.W., Grove, M., and Downie, N.W. (1976). Effects of enzyme-induction on metabolism of prednisolone: clinical and laboratory study. *Ann. Rheum. Dis.* 35, 339.

Brooks, S.M., Werk, E.E., Ackerman, S.J., Sullivan, I., and Thrasher, K. (1972). Adverse effects of phenobarbital on corticosteroid metabolism in patients with bronchial asthma. *N. Engl. J. Med.* 286, 1125.

Brosen, K. (1990). Recent developments in hepatic drug oxidation: implications for clinical pharmacokinetics. *Clin. Pharmacokinet.* 18, 220.

Bunning, R.D. and Barth, W.F. (1982). Sulindac — a potentially renal sparing non-steroidal anti-inflammatory drug. *JAMA* 248, 2864.

Busfield, D., Child, K.J., Atkinson, R.M., and Tornich, E.G. (1963). The effect of phenobarbitone on blood levels of griseofulvin in man. *Lancet* ii, 1042.

Canafax, D.M. and Ascher, N.I. (1983). Cyclosporine immunosuppression. *Clin. Pharm.* 2, 515.

Chapman, C.R. (1981). Absorption and metabolism of steroid prodrugs. Unpublished PhD thesis. University of Liverpool.

Chapron, D.J., Numford, D., and Pitogoff, G.I. (1979). Apparent quinidine induced digoxin toxicity after withdrawal of pentobarbital: case of sequential drug interactions. *Arch. Intern. Med.* 139, 363.

Cheng, S.H. and White, A. (1962). Effect of orally administered neomycin on the absorption of penicillin V. *N. Engl. J. Med.* 267, 1296.

Christensen, L.K., Hansen, J.M., and Kristensen, M. (1963). Sulphaphenazole induced hypoglycaemic attacks in tolbutamide treated diabetics. *Lancet* ii, 1298.

Coulam, C.B. and Annegers, J.F. (1979). Do anticonvulsants reduce the efficacy of oral contraceptives. *Epilepsia* 20, 519.

Crawford, P., Chadwick, D., Cleland, J., Tjia, J., Cowie, A., Back, D.J., *et al.* (1986). The lack of effect of sodium valproate on the pharmacokinetics of oral contraceptive steroids. *Contraception* 33, 23.

Crawford, P., Chadwick, D., Martin, C., Tjia, J., Back, D.J., and Orme, M.L'E. (1990). The interaction of phenytoin and carbamazepine with oral contraceptive steroids. *Br. J. Clin. Pharmacol.* 30, 892.

Crooks, J. and Moir, D.C. (1974). The detection of drug interaction in a hospital environment. In *Clinical effects of interaction between drugs* (ed. L.E. Cluff and J.C. Petrie), p. 255. Excerpta Medica, Amsterdam.

D'Arcy P.F. (1982). Drug reactions and interactions in the elderly patient. *Drug Intell. Clin. Pharmacol.* 16, 925.

Davidson, N. McD., Corral, R.J.M., Shaw, T.D.R., and French, C.B. (1976). Observations in man of hypoglycaemia during selective and non-selective beta blockade. *Scott. Med. J.* 22, 69.

Deray, G., Le Hoang, P., Cacoub, P., Assogba, U., Grippon, P., and Baumelou, A. (1987). Oral contraceptive interaction with cyclosporin. *Lancet* ii, 158.

Doering, W. (1979). Quinidine–digoxin interaction: pharmacokinetics, underlying mechanism and clinical implications. *N. Engl. J. Med.* 301, 400.

Doll, R., Langman, M.J.S., and Shawdon, H.H. (1968). Treatment of gastric ulcer with carbenoxolone — antagonistic effect of spironolactone. *Gut* 9, 42.

Durao, V., Prata, M.M., and Goncalves, L.M.P. (1977). Modification of antihypertensive effect of beta-adrenoceptor blocking agents by inhibition of endogenous prostaglandin synthesis. *Lancet* ii, 1005.

Edwards, D.M., Courtenay-Evans, R.J., Galley, J.M., Hunter, J., and Tait, A.D. (1974). Changes in cortisol metabolism following rifampicin therapy. *Lancet* ii, 549.

Evans, W.E. and Christensen, M.L. (1985). Drug interactions with methotrexate. *J. Rheumatol.* 12 (suppl. 12), 15.

Favre, L., Glasson, Ph., Riondel, A., and Valloton, M.B. (1983). Interaction of diuretics and non-steroidal anti-inflammatory drugs in man. *Clin. Sci.* 64, 407.

Ferguson, R.M., Sutherland, D.E.R., Simmons, R.L., and Najarian, J.S. (1982). Ketoconazole, cyclosporin metabolism and renal transplantation. *Lancet* ii, 882.

Fichtl, B. and Doering, W. (1983). The quinidine-digoxin interaction in perspective. *Clin. Pharmacokinet.* 8, 137.

Fincham, R.W. and Schottelius, D.D. (1979). Decreased phenytoin levels in antineoplastic therapy. *Ther. Drug Monit.* 1, 277.

Freeman, D.J., Laupacis, A., Keown, P.A., Stiller, C.R., and Carruthers, S.G. (1984). Evaluation of cyclosporin–phenytoin interaction with observations on cyclosporin metabolites. *Br. J. Clin. Pharmacol.* 18, 887.

Freis, E.D. (1984). Veterans administration cooperative study on nadolol as monotherapy and in combination with a diuretic. *Am. Heart J.* 108, 1087.

Friedman, C.I., Huneke, A.L., Kim, M.H., and Powell, J. (1980). The effect of ampicillin on oral contraceptive effectiveness. *Obstet. Gynecol.* 55, 33.

Garattini, S. (1985). Active drug metabolites. An overview. *Clin. Pharmacokinet.* 10, 216.

Gelipter, D. and Hazell, M. (1980). Interaction between disopyramide and practolol. *Br. Med. J.* 280, 52.

Gerber, M.C., Tejwani, G.A., Gerber, N., and Bianchine, J.R. (1985). Drug interactions with cimetidine: an update. *Pharmacol. Ther.* 27, 353.

Gothioni, G., Neuvonen, P.J., Mattila, M., and Hackman, R. (1972). Iron–tetracycline interaction: effect of time interval between the drugs. *Acta Med. Scand.* 191, 409.

Graham, C.F., Turner, W.N., and Jones, J.K. (1981). Lidocaine–propranolol interactions. *N. Engl. J. Med.* 304, 1301.

Greenblatt, D.J. and Koch-Weser, J. (1973). Adverse reactions to spironolactone: a report from the Boston Collaborative Drug Surveillance Program. *Clin. Pharmacol. Ther.* 14, 136.

Grimmer, M., Allen, W.L., Back, D.J., Breckenridge, A.M., Orme, M.L'E., and Tjia, J. (1983). The effect of co-trimoxazole on oral contraceptive steroids in women. *Contraception* 28, 53.

Grimmer, S.F.M., Back, D.J., Orme, M.L'E., Cowie, A., Gilmore, I., and Tjia, J. (1986). The bioavailability of ethinyloestradiol and levonorgestrel in patients with an ileostomy. *Contraception* 33, 51.

Guengerich, F.R. (1988). Oxidation of 17α ethinyl-estradiol by human liver cytochrome P450. *Molec. Pharmacol.* 33, 500.

Gugler, R. and Allgayer, H. (1990). Effect of antacids on the clinical pharmacokinetics of drugs. An update. *Clin. Pharmacokinet* 18, 210.

Haque, N., Thrasher, K., Werk, E.E., Knowles, M.C., and Sholiton, L.J. (1972). Studies on dexamethasone metabolism in man: Effect of diphenylhydantoin. *J. Clin. Endocrinol. Metab.* 34, 44.

Hauser, A.R., Lee, C., Teague, R.B., and Mullins, C. (1983). The effect of rifampicin on theophylline disposition. *Clin. Pharmacol. Ther.* 33, 254.

Heel, R.C., Brogden, R.N., Speight, T.M., and Avery, G.S. (1980) Captopril — a preliminary review of its pharmacological properties and therapeutic efficacy. *Drugs* 20, 409.

Heubel, F. and Netter, K.F. (1979). Atypical inducing properties of rifampicin. *Biochem. Pharmacol.* 28, 3373.

Höffken, G., Borner, K., Glatzel, P.D., Koeppe, P., and Lode, H. (1985). Reduced enteral absorption of ciprofloxacin in the presence of antacids. *Eur. J. Clin. Microbiol.* 33, 345.

Holland, O.B., von Kuhnert, L., Cambell, W.B., and Anderson, R.J. (1983). Synergistic effect of captopril and hydrochlorothiazide for the treatment of low-renin hypertensive black patients. *Hypertension* 5, 235.

Hunt, S.N., Jusko, W.J., and Yurchak, A.M. (1976). Effect of smoking on theophylline disposition. *Clin. Pharmacol. Ther.* 19, 546.

Hurwitz, A. (1977). Antacid therapy and drug kinetics. *Clin. Pharmacokinet.* 2, 269.

Ibram, H. (1980). Hemodynamic and electrophysiologic interactions between antiarrhythmic drugs and beta blockers with special reference to tocainide. *Am. Heart J.* 100, 1076.

Inaba, T., Jurima, M., Mahon, W.A., and Kalow, W. (1985). *In vitro* studies of two isozymes of human liver cytochrome P-450. Mephenytoin *p*-hydroxylation and sparteine monooxygenase. *Drug Metab. Dispos.* 13, 443.

Ismail, F.A., Khalafallah, N., and Khalil, S.A. (1987). Adsorption of ketoprofen and bumadizone calcium and aluminium containing antacids and its effect on ketoprofen bioavailability in man. *International Journal of Pharmaceutics* 34, 189.

Jackson, J.E., Powell, J.R., Wandell, M., Bentley, J., and Dorr, R. (1981). Cimetidine decreases theophylline clearance. *Am. Rev. Respir. Dis.* 123, 615.

Jain, A., McMahon, F.G., Slattery, J.T., and Levy, G. (1979). Effect of naproxen on steady-state serum concentration and anticoagulant activity of warfarin. *Clin. Pharmacol. Ther.* 25, 61.

Johnson, B.F., Wilson, J., Marwaha, R., Hoch, K., and Johnson, J. (1987). The comparative effects of verapamil and a new dihydropyridine calcium channel blocker on digoxin pharmacokinetics. *Clin. Pharmacol. Ther.* 42, 66.

Jonkman, J.H.G. and Upton, R.A. (1984). Pharmacokinetic drug interactions with theophylline. *Clin. Pharmacokinet.* 9, 309.

Joshi, J.V., Joshi, U.M., Sankhali, G.M., Krishna, U., Mandelkar, A., Chowdhury, V., *et al.* (1980). A study of the interaction of low dose combination oral contraceptive with ampicillin and metronidazole. *Contraception* 22, 643.

Kampmann, J., Hansen, J.M., Siersbaek-Nielsen, K., and Laursen, H. (1972). Effect of some drugs on penicillin half life in blood. *Clin. Pharmacol. Ther.* 13, 516.

Kauffman, R.E. and Azarnoff, D.L. (1973). Effect of colestipol on gastrointestinal absorption of chlorothiazide in man. *Clin. Pharmacol. Ther.* 14, 886.

Kerry, R.J., Ludlow, J.M., and Owen, G. (1980). Diuretics are dangerous with lithium. *Br. Med. J.* 281, 371.

Kirch, W., Hoensch, H., and Janisch, H.D. (1984). Interactions and non-interactions with ranitidine. *Clin. Pharmacokinet.* 9, 493.

Koch-Weser, J. (1973). Drug interactions in cardiovascular therapy. *Am. Heart J.* 90, 93.

Koch-Weser, J. and Sellers, E.M. (1971). Drug interactions with coumarin anticoagulants. *N. Engl. J. Med.* 285, 487 and 547.

Krikler, D.M. and Spurrell, R.A.J. (1974). Verapamil in the treatment of paroxysmal supraventricular tachycardia. *Postgrad. Med. J.* 50, 447.

Kruger, H.V., Schauer, U., Proksh, B., Gobel, M., and Ehninger, G. (1990). Investigation of potential interaction of ciprofloxacin with cyclosporine in bone marrow transplant recipients. *Antimicrob. Agents Chemother.* 34, 1048.

Krzywanek, H.J. and Breddin, K. (1977). Beeinflußt Diclofenac die orale Antikoagulantiensdtherapie und die Plättchenaggregation. *Medizin. Welt.* 28, 1843.

Kuhlmann, J., Woodcock, B., Wilke, J., and Rietbroch, N. (1985). Verapamil plasma concentrations during treatment with cytostatic drugs. *J. Cardiovasc. Pharmacol.* 7, 1003.

Kutt, H. (1971). Biochemical and genetic factors regulating dilantin metabolism in man. *Ann. N.Y. Acad. Sci.* 179, 704.

Lacey, R.W., Lord, V.L., Gunaseberg, H.K.W., Leiberman, P.J., and Luxton, D.E.A. (1980). Comparison of trimethoprim alone and trimethoprim–sulphamethoxazole in the treatment of respiratory and urinary infections with particular reference to the selection of trimethoprim resistance. *Lancet* i, 1270.

Lader, M.H. (1990). Interactions that matter — monoamine oxidase inhibitors. *Prescribers' J.* 30, 48.

Lam, Y.W.F. and Shepherd, A.M.M. (1990). Drug interactions in hypertensive patients. Pharmacokinetic, pharmacodynamic and genetic considerations. *Clin. Pharmacokinet.* 18, 295.

Landay, R.A., Gonzalez, M.A., and Taylor, J.C. (1978). Effect of phenobarbital on theophylline disposition. *J. Allergy Clin. Immunol.* 62, 27.

Lane, E.A., Guthrie, S., and Linnoila, M. (1985). Effects of ethanol on drug and metabolite pharmacokinetics. *Clin. Pharmacokinet.* 10, 228.

Law, R. and Chalmers, C. (1976). Medicines and elderly people. A general practice survey. *Br. Med. J.* i, 565.

Leishman, A.W.D., Matthews, H.L., and Smith, A.J. (1963). Antagonism of guanethidine by imipramine. *Lancet* i, 112.

Lepper, M.M. and Dowling, H.F. (1951). Treatment of pneumococcic meningitis with penicillin compared with penicillin plus aureomycin: studies including observations on an apparent antagonism between penicillins and aureomycin. *Arch. Intern. Med.* 88, 489.

Lesko, L.J. (1989). Pharmacokinetic drug interactions with amiodarone. *Clin. Pharmacokinet.* 17, 130.

Lewis, R.J., Trager, W.F., Chan, K.K., Breckenridge, A., Orme, M.L'E., and Rowland, M., *et al.* (1974). Warfarin. Stereochemical aspects of its metabolism and the interaction with phenylbutazone. *J. Clin. Invest.* 53, 1607.

Lode, H. (1988). Drug interactions with quinolones. *Rev. Infect. Dis.* 10 (suppl. 1), 132.

McElnay, J.C. and D'Arcy, P.F. (1983). Protein binding displacement interactions and their clinical importance. *Drugs* 25, 495.

McGrath, P.J., Stewart, J.W., and Quitkin, F.M. (1989). A possible L-deprenyl-induced hypertension reaction. *J. Psychopharmacol.* 9, 110.

McInnes, G.T. and Brodie, M.J. (1988). Drug interactions that matter. A critical reappraisal. *Drugs* 36, 83.

McInnes, G.T. and Ramsay, L.E. (1987). Pharmacology and clinical use of antimineralocorticoids. In *Pharmacology and clinical uses of inhibitors of hormone secretion and action* (ed. M. Furr and A. Wakeling), p. 233. Baillière, London.

MacKichan, J.J. (1989). Protein binding drug displacement interactions: fact or fiction. *Clin. Pharmacokinet.* 16, 65.

McLaughlin, J.E. and Reeves, D.S. (1971). Clinical and laboratory evidence for inactivation of gentamicin by carbenicillin. *Lancet* i, 261.

Macleod, S.M. and Sellers, E.M. (1976). Pharmacodynamic and pharmacokinetic drug interactions with coumarin anticoagulants. *Drugs* 11, 461.

MacPhee, G.J.A., McInnes, G.T., Thompson, G.G., and Brodie, M.J. (1986). Verapamil potentiates carbamazepine neurotoxicity: a clinically important inhibitory interaction. *Lancet* i, 700.

MacPhee, G.J.A., Mitchell, J.R., Wiseman, L., McLellan, A.R., Park, B.K., McInnes, G.T., *et al.* (1988). Effect of sodium valproate on carbamazepine disposition and psychomotor profile in man. *Br. J. Clin. Pharmacol.* 25, 59.

Maesen, F.P., Teengs, J.P., Baur, C., and Davies, B.T. (1984). Quinolones and raised plasma concentrations of theophylline. *Lancet* ii, 530.

Mäntylä, R., Männistö, P.T., Vuorela, A., Sundberg, S., and Ottoila, P. (1984). Impairment of captopril bioavailability by concomitant food and antacid intake. *Int. J. Clin. Pharmacol. Ther. Toxicol.* 33, 626.

Marquis, J-F., Carruthers, S.G., Spence, J.D., Brownstone, Y.S., and Toogood, J.H. (1982). Phenytoin–theophylline interactions. *N. Engl. J. Med.* 307, 1189.

Mathog, R.H. and Klein, W.J. (1969). Ototoxicity of ethacrynic acid and aminoglycoside antibiotics in uremia. *N. Engl. J. Med.* 280, 1223.

May, D.C., Jarboe, C.H., Ellenburg, D.T., Roe, E.J., and Karibo, J. (1982). The effects of erythromycin on theophyl-

line elimination in normal males. *J. Clin. Pharmacol.* 22, 125.

May, J.R., DiPiro, J.T., and Sisley, J.F. (1987). Drug interactions in surgical patients. *Am. J. Surg.* 153, 327.

Miners, J.O. (1989). Drug interactions involving aspirin (acetylsalicylic acid) and salicylic acid. *Clin. Pharmacokinet.* 17, 327.

Miners, J.O., Foenander, T., Wanwimolruk, S., Gallus, A.S., and Birkett, D.J. (1982). Interaction of sulphinpyrazone with warfarin. *Eur. J. Clin. Pharmacol.* 22, 327.

Nation, R.L., Evans, A.M., and Milne, R.W. (1990). Pharmacokinetic drug interactions with phenytoin. *Clin. Pharmacokinet.* 18, 37, and 131.

Nebert, D.W., Nelson, D.R., Adesnik, M., Coon, M.J., Estabrook, R.W., Gonzalez, F.J., *et al.* (1989). The P-450 superfamily: update on listing of all genes and recommended nomenclature for the chromosomal loci. *DNA* 8, 1.

Neuvonen, P.J. (1976). Interactions with the absorption of tetracyclines. *Drugs* 11, 45.

Neuvonen, P.J. and Elonen, E. (1980). Effect of activated charcoal on absorption and elimination of phenobarbitone, carbamazepine and phenylbutazone in man. *Eur. J. Clin. Pharmacol.* 17, 51.

Nimmo, J., Heading, R.C., Tothill, P., and Prescott, L.F. (1973). Pharmacological evaluation of gastric emptying: Effects of propantheline and metoclopramide on paracetamol absorption. *Br. Med. J.* i, 587.

Nimmo, W.S. (1976). Drugs, disease and gastric emptying. *Clin. Pharmacokinet.* 1, 189.

Nordoy, S. (1959). Combined treatment with phenylbutazone and anticoagulants. *Tidsskr. Nor. Laegeforen.* 79, 143.

Norrby, R., Stenqvist, K., and Elgeford, B. (1976). Interactions between cephaloridine and frusemide in man. *Scand. J. Infect. Dis.* 8, 209.

Northcutt, R.C., Stiel, J.N., Hollifield, J.W., and Stont, E.G. Jr (1969). The influence of cholestyramine on thyroxine absorption. *JAMA* 208, 1857.

Oetgen, W.J., Sobol, S.M., Tri, T.B., Heydorn, W.H., and Rakita, L. (1984). Amiodarone–digoxin interaction. Clinical and experimental observations. *Chest* 86, 75.

O'Reilly, R.A. (1984). Comparative interaction of cimetidine and ranitidine with racemic warfarin in man. *Arch. Intern. Med.* 144, 989.

O'Reilly, R.A., Trager, W.F., Motley, C.H., and Howald, W. (1980). Stereoselective interaction of phenylbutazone with (^{12}C/^{13}C) warfarin pseudoracemates in man. *J. Clin. Invest.* 65, 746.

O'Reilly, R.A., Trager, W.F., Rettie, A.E., and Goulart, D.A. (1987). Interaction of amiodarone with racemic warfarin and its separated enantiomorphs in humans. *Clin. Pharmacol. Ther.* 42, 290.

Orme, M.C.L'E. (1986). Drug interactions. In *Therapeutics in rheumatology* (ed. J.M.H. Moll, H.A. Bird, and A. Rushton), p. 87. Chapman and Hall, London.

Orme, M.L'E. and Back, D.J. (1986). Interactions between oral contraceptive steroids and broad spectrum antibiotics. *Clin. Exp. Dermatol.* 11, 327.

Orme, M.L'E., Back, D.J., and Breckenridge, A.M. (1983). Clinical pharmacokinetics of oral contraceptive steroids. *Clin. Pharmacokinet.* 8, 95.

Orr, J.M., Abbott, F.S., Farrell, K., Ferguson, S., Sheppard, I., and Godolphin, W. (1982). Interaction between valproic acid and aspirin in epileptic children: serum protein binding and metabolic effects. *Clin. Pharmacol. Ther.* 31, 642.

Park, B.K. and Breckenridge, A.M. (1981). Clinical implications of enzyme induction and enzyme inhibition. *Clin. Pharmacokinet.* 6, 1.

Parsons, R.L. and Paddock, G.M. (1975). Absorption of two antibacterial drugs, cephalexin and co-trimoxazole, in malabsorption syndromes. *J. Antimicrob. Chemother.* 1 (suppl.), 59.

Patak, R.V., Mookerjee, B.K., Bentzel, C.J., Hysert, P.E., Babe, M., and Lee, J.B. (1975). Antagonism of the effects of furosemide by indomethacin in normal and hypertensive man. *Prostaglandins* 10, 649.

Paulet, N., Bury, P.C., Needleman, M., and Raymond, K. (1982). Drug interactions. A study and evaluation of their incidence in Victoria. *Med. J. Aust.* i, 80.

Pedersen, K.E., Hastrup, J., and Hvidt, S. (1980). The effect of quinidine on digoxin kinetics in cardiac patients. *Acta Med. Scand.* 207, 291.

Pedrinelli, R., Magagni, A., Arzilli, F., Sassano, P., and Salvetti, A. (1980). Influence of indomethacin on the natriuretic and renin-stimulating effect of bumetanide in essential hypertension. *Clin. Pharmacol. Ther.* 28, 722.

Petereit, L.B. and Meikle, A.W. (1977). Effectiveness of prednisolone during phenytoin therapy. *Clin. Pharmacol. Ther.* 22, 912.

Petersen, V., Hvidt, S., Thomsen, K., and Schon, M. (1974). Effect of prolonged thiazide treatment on renal lithium clearance. *Br. Med. J.* iii, 143.

Polk, R.E., Healy, D.P., Sahai, J., Drwal, L., and Racht, E. (1989). Effect of ferrous sulfate and multivitamins with zinc on absorption of ciprofloxacin in normal volunteers. *Antimicrob. Agents Chemother.* 33, 1841.

Prescott, L.F. (1973). Clinically important drug interactions. *Drugs* 5, 161.

Ptachcinski, R.J., Carpenter, B.J., Burckart, G.J., Venkataramanan, R., and Rosenthal, J.T. (1985). Effect of erythromycin on cyclosporin levels. *N. Engl. J. Med.* 313, 1416.

Ragheb, M., Ban, T.A., Buchanan, D., and Frolich, J.C. (1980). Interaction of indomethacin and ibuprofen with lithium in manic patients under a steady state lithium level. *J. Clin. Psychol.* 41, 397.

Reimann, I.W. and Frölich, J.C. (1980). Effect of diclofenac on lithium kinetics. *Clin. Pharmacol. Ther.* 30, 348.

Reimers, D. and Jezek, A. (1971). Rifampicin und andere Antituberkulostatika bei gleichzeitiger oraler Kontrazeption. *Prax. Klin. Pneumonol.* 25, 255.

Reveno, W.S. and Rosenbaum, H. (1968). Propranolol and hypoglycaemia. *Lancet* i, 920.

Robinson, D.S., Benjamin, D.M., and McCormack, J.J. (1971). Interaction of warfarin and non systemic gastrointestinal drugs. *Clin. Pharmacol. Ther.* 12, 491.

Robson, R.H. and Vishwanath, M.C. (1982). Nifedipine and beta blockade as a cause of heart failure. *Br. Med. J.* 284, 104.

Rodin, E.A., De Sousa, G., Haidukewych, D., Lodhi, R., and Berchou, R.C. (1981). Dissociation between free and bound phenytoin levels in the presence of valproate sodium. *Arch. Neurol.* 38, 240.

Rodin, S.M. and Johnson, B.F. (1988). Pharmacokinetic drug interactions with digoxin. *Clin. Pharmacokinet.* 15, 227.

Rogers, S.M., Back, D.J., Stevenson, P.J., Grimmer, S.F.M., and Orme, M.L'E. (1987). Paracetamol interaction with oral contraceptive steroids: increased plasma concentrations of ethinyloestradiol. *Br. J. Clin. Pharmacol.* 23, 721.

Rowland, M. and Gupta, S.K. (1987). Cyclosporin-phenytoin interaction: re-evaluation using metabolite data. *Br. J. Clin. Pharmacol.* 24, 329.

Salvetti, A., Arzilli, F., Pedrinelli, R., Beggi, P., and Motolese, M. (1982). Interaction between oxprenolol and indomethacin in essential hypertensive patients. *Eur. J. Clin. Pharmacol.* 22, 197.

Sellers, E.M. (1979). Plasma protein displacement interactions are rarely of clinical significance. *Pharmacology* 18, 225.

Sellers, E.M. (1984). Drug displacement interactions: a case study of the phenylbutazone–warfarin interaction. In *Drug protein binding* (ed. M. Reidenberg), p. 257. Praeger Publishers, New York.

Sellers, E.M., Naranjo, C.A., Giles, H.G., Frecker, R.C., and Beeching, M. (1980). Intravenous diazepam and oral ethanol interaction. *Clin. Pharmacol. Ther.* 28, 638.

Serlin, M.J. and Breckenridge, A.M. (1983). Drug interactions with warfarin. *Drugs* 25, 610.

Serlin, M.J., Sibeon, R.G., Mossman, S., Breckenridge, A.M., Williams, J.R.B., Atwood, J.L., et al. (1979). Cimetidine: interaction with oral anticoagulants in man. *Lancet* ii, 317.

Serlin, M.J., Sibeon, R.G., and Breckenridge, A.M. (1981). Lack of effect of ranitidine on warfarin action. *Br. J. Clin. Pharmacol.* 12, 791.

Silberbauer, K., Stanek, B., and Templ, H. (1982). Acute hypotensive effect of captopril in man is modified by prostaglandin synthesis inhibition. *Br. J. Clin. Pharmacol.* 14 (suppl.2), 87S.

Singh, R.R., Malaviya, A.N., Pandey, J.N., Guleria, J.S. (1986). Fatal interaction between methotrexate and naproxen. *Lancet* i, 1390.

Skinner, C., Coull, D.C., and Johnston, A.W. (1969). Antagonism of the hypotensive action of bethanidine and debrisoquine by tricyclic antidepressants. *Lancet* ii, 564.

Smith, D.E., Brater, D.C., Lin, E.T., and Benet, L.Z. (1979). Attenuation of furosemide's diuretic effect by indomethacin: pharmacokinetic evaluation. *J. Pharmacokinet. Biopharmacol.* 7, 265.

Smith, J.W., Seidl, L.G., and Cluff, L.E. (1966). Studies on the epidemiology of adverse drug reactions. V. Clinical factors influencing susceptibility. *Ann. Intern. Med.* 65, 629.

Smith, M. (1984). Drug interactions involving infusion therapy. In *Clinically important adverse drug interactions*, Vol. 2

Nervous system, endocrine system and infusion therapy (ed. J.C. Petrie), p. 329. Elsevier, Amsterdam.

Solomon, H.M. and Schrogie, J.J. (1967). Change in receptor site affinity: a proposed explanation for the potentiating effect of D-thyroxine on the anticoagulant response to warfarin. *Clin. Pharmacol. Ther.* 2, 797.

Solomon, H.M., Schrogie, J.J., and Williams, D. (1968). The displacement of phenylbutazone ^{14}C and warfarin ^{14}C from human albumin by various drugs and fatty acids. *Biochem. Pharmacol.* 17, 143.

Sparrow, M.J. (1987). Pill method failures. *N.Z. Med. J.* 100, 102.

Stanaszek, W.F. and Franklin, C.E. (1978). Survey of potential drug interaction incidence in an outpatient clinic population. *Hosp. Pharm.* 13, 255.

Starr, K.F. and Petrie, J.C. (1972). Drug interactions in patients on long term oral anticoagulant and antihypertensive adrenergic neurone blocking drugs. *Br. Med. J.* iv, 133.

Steiness, E. and Olesen, K.H. (1976). Cardiac arrhythmias induced by hypokalaemia and potassium loss during maintenance digoxin therapy. *Br. Heart J.* 38, 167.

Stoehr, G.P., Kroboth, P.D., Juhl, R.P., Wender, D.B., Phillips, J.P., and Smith, R.B. (1984). Effect of oral contraceptives on triazolam, temazepam, alprazolam and lorazepam kinetics. *Clin. Pharmacol. Ther.* 36, 683.

Symmons, D.P.M., Kendall, M.J., Rees, J.A., and Hind, I.D. (1983). The effect of flurbiprofen on the response to frusemide in healthy volunteers. *Int. J. Clin. Pharmacol. Ther. Toxicol.* 21, 350.

Thyss, A., Milano, G., Kubar, J., Namer, M., and Schneider, M. (1986). Clinical and pharmacokinetic evidence of a lifethreatening interaction between methotrexate and ketoprofen. *Lancet* i, 256.

Tobert, J.A., De Schepper, P., Tjandramaga, T.B., Mullie, A., Buntinx, A.P., Meisinger, M.A.P., *et al.* (1981). Effects of antacids on the bioavailability of diflunisal in the fasting and postprandial states. *Clin. Pharmacol. Ther.* 30, 385.

Tollefson, G.D. (1983). Monoamine oxidase inhibitors: a review. *J. Clin. Psychiatry* 44, 280.

Trissel, L.A. (1988). *Handbook on injectable drugs* (5th edn). American Society of Hospital Pharmacists, Washington.

Vasko, M.R. (1990). Drug interactions. In *Rational therapeutics* (ed. R.L. Williams, D.C. Brater, and J. Mordenti), p. 175. Marcel Dekker, New York.

Verbeeck, R.K. (1990). Pharmacokinetic drug interactions with non steroidal anti-inflammatory drugs. *Clin. Pharmacokinet.* 19, 44.

Verbeeck, R., Tjandramaga, T.B., Mullie, A., Verbesselt, R., and De Schepper, P.J. (1979). Effect of aluminium hydroxide on diflunisal absorption. *Br. J. Clin. Pharmacol.* 7, 519.

Vessell, E.S., Passananti, G.T., and Greene, F.E. (1970). Impairment of drug metabolism in man by allopurinol and nortryptyline. *N. Engl. J. Med.* 283, 1484.

Vessell, E.S., Passananti, G.T., and Johnson, A.O. (1975). Failure of indomethacin and warfarin to interact in normal human volunteers. *J. Clin. Pharmacol.* 15, 486.

Walker, A.M., Cody, R.J., and Greenblatt, D.J. (1983). Drug toxicity in patients receiving digoxin and quinidine. *Am. Heart J.* 105, 1025.

Watkins, J., Abbott, E.C., Hensby, C.N., Webster, J., and Dollery, C.T. (1980). Attenuation of hypotensive effect of propranolol and thiazide diuretics by indomethacin. *Br. Med. J.* 281, 702.

Watt, A.H., Stephens, M.R., Buss, D.C., and Routledge, P.A. (1985). Amiodarone reduces plasma warfarin clearance in man. *Br. J. Clin. Pharmacol.* 20, 707.

Webster, J. (1985). Interactions of NSAIDs with diuretics and beta blockers. Mechanisms and implications. *Drugs* 30, 32.

Webster, J., Hawksworth, G.M., McLean, I., and Petrie, J.C. (1983). Attenuation of the antihypertensive effect of single doses of propranolol and atenolol by flurbiprofen. *Proc. 2nd World Conf. Clin. Pharmacol. Ther.* Abstract No. 2.

Welling, P. (1984). Interactions affecting drug absorption. *Clin. Pharmacokinet.* 9, 404.

Werk, E.E., McGee, J., and Sholiton, L.J. (1964). Effect of diphenylhydantoin on cortisol metabolism in man. *J. Clin. Invest.* 43, 1824.

Wing, L.M.H., Bune, A.J.C., Chalmers, J.P., Graham, J.R., and West, M.J. (1981). The effects of indomethacin in treated hypertensive patients. *Clin. Exp. Pharmacol. Physiol.* 8, 537.

Yeung Laiwah, A.C. and Mactier, R.A. (1981). Antagonistic effect of non-steroidal anti-inflammatory drugs on frusemide induced diuresis in cardiac failure. *Br. Med. J.* 283, 714.

Zarowitz, B., Conway, W., and Popvich, J. (1985). Adverse interactions of drugs in critical care patients. *Henry Ford Hosp. Med. J.* 33, 48.

Index

A

β-Adrenoceptor agonists (*cont.*)
  causing (*cont.*)
    cardiac
      arrhythmias, 110
      ischaemia, 126
    effect on catecholamine tests, 352
    hypoglycaemia, 375
    ketoacidosis, 402
    myalgia, 491
    oedema, pulmonary, 175
α-Adrenoceptor blockers
  causing
    diarrhoea, 236
    hypotension, 158
β-Adrenoceptor blockers
  age effects, 12
  and Peyronie's disease, 501
  causing
    arthralgia, 497
    asthma aggravation, 183
    bladder dysfunction, 557
    bronchospasm, 183
    cardiac
      arrhythmias, 99, 114–15
      depression, 121, 122–3
      ischaemia (withdrawal), 124–5
    cardiomyotoxicity (withdrawal), 118
    diabetic coma, 377–8
    diarrhoea, 236
    effect on
      catecholamine tests, 352
      creatine kinase, 438
      potassium, 410
      thyroid function tests, 149
    fetal/neonatal disorders, 80–1
    gangrene, 521
    hyperglycaemia, 373
    hyperkalaemia, 410
    hyperlipidaemia, 105, 378
    hypertension, 149
    hyperuricaemia, 432
    hypoglycaemia, 374
    hypotension, 158
    lichenoid eruptions, 524
    liver damage, 263
    lupus erythematosus, 502, 504
    myopathy, 554
    neuromuscular blockade, 551, 552
    neuropathy
      orofacial, 220
      peripheral, 546
    ototoxicity, 586
    psoriasiform eruptions, 524
    psychiatric disorders, 602, 603, 604, 622
    Raynaud's phenomenon, 156
    renal damage, 306, 320
    retroperitoneal fibrosis, 318, 500
    seizures, 538
    sexual dysfunction, 775, 782
    skin necrosis, 521
    vasoconstriction, 156
  dangers in phaeochromocytoma, 154
Adriamycin — *see* Doxorubicin
Adverse Drug Reaction Bulletin, 3
Aerosol propellants causing cardiotoxicity, 110
Aerosols,
  causing
    asthma
      aggravation, 182
      deaths, 182–3
    bronchospasm, 182
    epidemic reactions, 182–3

Age
  and
    drug receptors, 30
    renal function, 24
  influence on drug reactions
    β-adrenoceptor blockers, 12
    analgesics, 12
    anticholinergics, 12
    anticoagulants, 12
    antihypertensives, 12
    anti-inflammatories, 11
    antiparkinsonian drugs, 12
    barbiturates, 12
    benzodiazepines, 12
    chloramphenicol, 12
    diazepam, 12
    digoxin, 12
    diuretics, 12
    flurazepam, 12
    heparin, 12
    hypnotics, 12
    metoclopramide, 12
    morphine, 12
    nitrazepam, 12
    novobiocin, 12
    phenothiazines, 12
    phenylbutazone, 12
    propranolol, 12
    streptomycin, 12
    sulphonamides, 12
    tranquillizers, 12
    vitamin K, 12
    warfarin, 12
Agranulocytosis
  drugs causing
    acetazolamide, 647
    allopurinol, 647
    amitriptyline, 647
    amodiaquine, 647
    antibacterials, 647
    anticancer drugs, 647
    anticonvulsants, 647
    antidiabetics, 647
    antihistamines (H₁), 647
    antihistamines (H₂), 647
    antimalarials, 647
    antithyroids, 647
    benzodiazepines, 647
    captopril, 647
    carbamazepine, 647
    carbimazole, 647
    cephalosporins, 647
    chloramphenicol, 647
    chloroquine, 647
    chlorothiazide, 647
    chlorpromazine, 647
    chlorpropamide, 647
    chlorthalidone, 647
    cimetidine, 647
    clindamycin, 647
    co-trimoxazole, 647
    dapsone, 647
    desipramine, 647
    disopyramide, 647
    diuretics, 647
    ethacrynic acid, 647
    Fansidar, 647
    gentamicin, 647
    gold, 647
    H₂-receptor blockers, 647
    hydantoins, 647
    hydralazine, 647

hydrochlorothiazide, 647
imipramine, 647
indomethacin, 647
isoniazid, 647
levamisole, 647
meprobamate, 647
methimazole, 647
methylthiouracil, 647
methyldopa, 647
oxyphenbutazone, 647
paracetamol, 647
pencillamine, 647
penicillins, 647
pentazocine, 647
phenacetin, 647
phenothiazines, 647
phenylbutazone, 647
phenytoin, 647
procainamide, 647
propranolol, 647
propylthiouracil, 647
psychotropics, 647
pyrimethamine, 647
quinidine, 647
quinine, 647
ranitidine, 647
rifampicin, 647
sodium aminosalicylate, 647
streptomycin, 647
sulphadoxine, 647
sulphonamides, 647
sulphonylureas, 647
tetracyclines, 647
thiazides, 647
thiouracils, 647
tocainide, 647
tolbutamide, 647
tricyclics, 647
vancomycin, 647
Akathisia — *see* Dyskinesias
Albumin
  causing emboli, 149
  drugs affecting, 434
Albuterol causing hypomagnesaemia, 424
Alcohol
  causing
    acidosis
      lactic, 378
      metabolic, 400, 401
      respiratory, 399
    anaemia
      megaloblastic, 650
      sideroblastic, 651
    cardiac arrhythmias, 113
    cardiomyotoxicity, 119–20
    chlorpropamide flushing, 36–7
    chromosome damage, 56
    effect on
      acid phosphatase tests, 442
      creatine kinase, 438, 439
      fat metabolism, 390
      folate metabolism, 447
      gastric emptying, 21
      γ-glutamyl transferase, 441
      transferrin, 436
      vitamin A, 448
    enzyme inhibition, 27
    fetal/neonatal disorders, 73–4
    flushing, 36–7, 520
    headache (withdrawal), 539
    hyperlipidaemia, 390

Amiodarone (*cont.*)
  causing (*cont.*)
    pulmonary fibrosis, 191–2
    thrombocytopenia, 648
Amipaque — *see* X-ray contrast media
Amiphenazole causing lichenoid eruptions,
    210, 524
Amitriptyline (*see also* Tricyclic
    antidepressants)
  causing
    agranulocytosis, 647
    cardiac arrhythmias, 105
    colonic perforation, 236
    constipation, 236
    dyskinesias, 540
    effect on
      creatine kinase, 438
      vasopressin, 358
    hyponatraemia, 407
    liver damage, 261
    neuroleptic malignant syndrome, 553
    neuropathy,
      orofacial, 220
      peripheral, 546, 548
    pulmonary oedema, 175
    seizures, 538
    sexual dysfunction, 776
    xerostomia, 216
Ammonium chloride causing acidosis,
    metabolic, 400, 403
Ammonium glycyrrhizinate — *see* Licorice
Amodiaquine
  causing
    agranulocytosis, 647
    anaemia, aplastic, 645
    corneal opacities, 568
    depigmentation of hair, 567
    nail changes, 517
    pigmentation, 210, 519
Amoxapine
  causing
    dyskinesias, 541, 542
    effect on creatine kinase, 438
    hyperglycaemia, 376
    hyperuricaemia, 432
    muscle damage, 318
    myoglobinuria, 318
    pancreatitis, 238
    renal damage, 318
    sexual dysfunction, 776
Amoxycillin
  causing
    erythema multiforme, 522
    erythema, toxic, 522
    hypokalaemia, 414
    liver damage, 267
    pseudomembranous colitis, 668
Amphetamine
  causing
    cardiac
      arrhythmias, 114
      ischaemia, 126–7
    dyskinesias, 542
    effect on
      catecholamine tests, 352
      corticotrophin, 350
      creatine kinase, 438
      thyroid hormone, 346
    fetal/neonatal disorders, 74
    fever, 767
    growth disorders, 499
    headache (withdrawal), 539

hyperthyroidism, 346
muscle damage, 316, 317, 493, 555
mydriasis, 569
myoglobinuria, 318
myopathy, 555
nasal obstruction, 590
neuropathy, peripheral, 546
psychiatric disorders, 603, 605, 606
pulmonary hypertension, 173
renal damage, 313, 318
xerostomia, 216
Amphotericin
  causing
    acidosis, metabolic, 400, 403
    effect on creatine kinase, 438
    fever, 766, 767
    hypokalaemia, 413, 415
    muscle damage, 317, 318
    myoglobinuria, 317
    myopathy, 554
    neuropathy, peripheral, 546, 548
    psychiatric disorders, 605–6
    pulmonary vasculitis, 174
    renal damage, 306, 307, 308
Ampicillin
  and ototoxicity, 582
  causing
    allergy, 693
    chromosome damage, 51
    effect on creatine kinase 438
    erythema multiforme, 207, 522
    fever, 768
    hypokalaemia, 404
    neuromuscular block, 551
    pseudomembranous colitis, 668
    rash in
      glandular fever, 693
      leukaemia, 693
      virus infection, 693
    renal damage, 314, 315
    seizures, 538
    thrombocytopenia, 538
Amsacrine
  causing
    anaemia, aplastic, 645
    Factor X deficiency, 661–2
    infection, 221
Amylase, drugs affecting, 441
Amyl nitrite causing headache, 539
Anabolic steroids
  causing
    dyskinesias, 542
    effect on
      alkaline phosphatase, 440
      amylase, 441
      cholinesterase, 442
      fibrinogen, 437
      γ-glutamyl transferase, 441
      haptoglobin, 436
      prealbumin, 434
      thyroid function tests, 348
      thyroxine-binding globulin, 435
      zinc, 427
    hirsuties, 518
    hoarseness, 595
    liver
      damage, 277, 280, 281
      peliosis, 277
      tumours, 280, 281
    sexual dysfunction, 779
    virilization of larynx, 595

Anaemia, aplastic (pancytopenia)
  drugs causing
    actinomycin, 645
    amidopyrine, 2, 645
    amsacrine, 645
    antibacterials, 645–6
    anticancer drugs, 644–5
    anticonvulsants, 645
    antidepressants, 645
    antidiabetics, 645
    anti-inflammatories, 645
    antimalarials, 645
    antiseptics, 736
    antithyroids, 645, 646
    aspirin, 646
    azathioprine, 645
    BCNU 645
    benoxaprofen, 645, 646
    busulphan, 645
    carbimazole, 645
    carboplatin, 645
    carmustine, 645
    chlorambucil, 645
    chloramphenicol, 11, 36, 645–6
    chlorpromazine, 645
    chlorpropamide, 645
    cisplatin, 645
    co-trimoxazole, 645
    cytarabine, 645
    cytotoxics, 644–5
    doxorubicin, 645
    epirubicin, 645
    etoposide, 645
    fluorouracil, 645
    gold, 645, 646
    hydroxyurea, 645
    indomethacin, 645, 646
    lomustine, 645
    lorazepam, 646
    melphalan, 645
    mepacrine, 645
    mercaptopurine, 645
    methazolamide, 646
    methotrexate, 645
    methylthiouracil, 645
    mitomycin, 645
    mitozantrone, 645
    oxyphenbutazone, 645, 646
    penicillamine, 645, 646
    phenothiazines, 645
    phenylbutazone, 645, 646
    phenytoin, 645
    piroxicam, 645, 646
    plicamycin (mithramycin), 645
    procarbazine, 645
    prothiaden, 645
    propylthiouracil, 645
    psychotropics, 645
    pyrimethamine, 645
    sulindac, 646
    sulphonamides, 645
    sulphonylureas, 645
    thioguanine, 645
    thiotepa, 645
    thiouracils, 645
    trimethoprim, 645
    zidovudine, 646
Anaemia, aplastic (red cell aplasia)
  drugs causing
    azathioprine, 646
    carbamazepine, 646
    chloramphenicol, 646

B

zEthambutol (*cont.*)
  causing (*cont.*)
    hyperuricaemia, 432
    liver damage, 261
    neuropathy
      optic, 545, 570
      peripheral, 546
    taste disorders, 220, 593
Ethamivan causing laryngeal oedema, 595
Ethamsylate causing hypotension, 160
Ethanol — *see* Alcohol
Ethchlorvynol causing porphyria, 429
Ether
  causing
    cardiac depression, 124
    effect on cholinesterase, 442
    malignant hyperthermia, 556
    porphyria, 430
    psychiatric disorders, 609
    seizures, 538
Ethinyloestradiol — *see* Oestrogens
Ethionamide
  causing
    effect on thyroid hormone, 347
    galactorrhoea/gynaecomastia, 355
    hypothyroidism, 347
    liver damage, 251
    salivation, 216
    taste disorders, 220
Ethosuximide
  causing
    chromosome damage, 52
    erythema multiforme, 522
    lupus erythematosus, 502, 523
    psychiatric disorders, 611
Ethotoin causing chromosome damage, 51
Ethylbiscoumacetate
  causing
    effect on vitamin K, 450
    hypouricaemia, 432
Ethylene causing malignant hyperthermia,
  556
Ethylene glycol causing acidosis, metabolic,
  400, 401
Ethylenediamine causing contact dermatitis,
  527
Ethynodiol — *see* Progestogens
Etidronate
  causing
    osteomalacia, 449
    taste disorders, 593
Etofibrate causing hypouricaemia, 432
Etomidate causing adrenal failure, 351
Etoposide
  causing
    anaemia, aplastic, 645
    infections, 221
    liver damage, 269
Etretinate
  causing
    alopecia, 518
    bullous eruptions, 517
    fetal/neonatal disorders, 73
    hyperlipidaemia, 390
    infections, 672
    intracranial hypertension, 540
    liver damage, 273, 278
    photosensitivity, 520
    pseudoporphyria, 520
    psychiatric disorders, 620
'Eve' causing cardiac arrhythmias, 114
Excitement — *see* Behavioural toxicity

Exfoliative dermatitis — *see* Skin eruptions,
  exfoliative
Exophthalmos
  drugs causing
    antithyroids, 567
    lithium, 567
Extrapyramidal disorders — *see* Dyskinesias
Eye
  oedema
    drugs causing
      antithyroids, 567
      corticosteroids, 567
      radioactive-iodine, 567
      vitamin A, 567
  refractive changes
    drugs causing
      acetazolamide, 569
      anticholinergics, 569
      antidiabetics, 569
      antihistamines, 569
      antispasmodics, 569
      insulin, 569
      sulphonamides, 569
      tetracyclines, 569
      thiazides, 569
Eyebrow loss caused by vitamin A, 567
Eyelash depigmentation
  drugs causing
    amodiaquine, 567
    chloroquine, 567
    hydroxychloroquine, 567
Eyelids
  oedema
    drugs causing
      antithyroids, 567
      corticosteroids, 567
      radio-iodine, 567
      vitamin A, 567
  pigmentation
    drugs causing
      chlorpromazine, 567
      phenol, 567
      silver, 567
  retraction
    drugs causing,
      acetylcholine, 567
      choline, 567
      nicotine, 567

F

Factor VIII causing seizures, 539
Factor IX causing thromboembolism, 662
Factor X deficiency caused by amsacrine,
  661–2
Famotidine
  aggravating Sjögren's syndrome, 217
  causing
    salivary gland disorders, 217
    xerostomia, 217
Fanconi syndrome
  drugs causing
    cadmium, 403
    heavy metals, 403
    lead, 403

    mercaptopurine, 402
    mercury, 403
    methyl-3-chrome, 402
    sodium valproate, 403
    solvents, 403
    tetracyclines (degraded), 402, 403
    toluene, 403
    valproate, 403
Fat (*see also* Panniculitis)
  atrophy caused by
    corticosteroids, 500
    insulin, 500
  embolism caused by X-ray contrast media,
    173
  hypertrophy caused by insulin, 500
Fat emulsions
  causing
    effect on bacterial activity, 665
    hypertension, 155
    infections, 665–6
Felodipine
  causing
    effect on plasma protein, 433
    hypercalcaemia, 417
Fenbufen
  causing
    colitis, 235
    effect on aspartate aminotransferase,
      439
    eosinophilia, pulmonary, 185
    pneumonitis, 185
    sexual dysfunction, 779
Fenclofenac
  causing
    effect on
      thyroid function tests, 348–9
      thyroxine-binding globulin, 430
Fenfluramine
  causing
    galactorrhoea/gynaecomastia, 356
    pulmonary hypertension, 173
    psychiatric disorders, 602, 608
    xerostomia, 592
Fenofibrate causing muscle damage, 308
Fenoprofen
  causing
    anaemia, aplastic (red cell aplasia) 646
    renal damage, 320
Fenoterol
  and asthma deaths, 182–3
  causing
    cardiac arrhythmias, 110
    effect on aspartate aminotransferase,
      439
    hypokalaemia, 413
Fentanyl causing respiratory depression, 399
Fertility impairment — *see* Sexual
    dysfunction
Fetal/neonatal disorders
  causing adverse reactions, 37
  drugs studied, suspected, or implicated
    ACE inhibitors, 68, 81, 82
    acetazolamide, 81
    β-adrenoceptor blockers, 80–1
    alcohol, 63, 73–4
    aminopterin, 71
    amiodarone, 82
    amphetamine, 74
    anaesthetics, 66, 76–7
    antacids, 65
    androgens, 72
    anthelmintics, 66

G

H

Intestinal perforation (*cont.*)
  drugs causing (*cont.*)
    potassium, 234
    X-ray contrast media, 752, 753
Intestinal ulceration (*see also* Peptic ulceration)
  drugs causing
    anti-inflammatories, 234
    flucytosine, 234
    gold, 234
    indomethacin, 234
    lithium, 234
    potassium salts, 234
Intracranial hypertension
  drugs causing
    contraceptives, oral, 540
    corticosteroids, 540, 571
    etretinate, 540
    ketamine, 540
    lucoprotein, 540
    minocycline, 571
    nalidixic acid, 540, 571
    nitrofurantoin, 540
    nitrous oxide, 540
    oral contraceptives, 540
    perhexilene, 540
    tetracyclines, 540, 571
    vitamin A, 540, 571
Intralipid — *see* Fat emulsions
Intravenous nutrition
  causing
    effect on
      prealbumin, 434
      retinol-binding protein, 434
    folate deficiency, 447
    infections, 665–6
    vitamin B_1 deficiency, 443
Iocarmate — *see* X-ray contrast media
Iocetamic acid — *see* X-ray contrast media
Iodamide — *see* X-ray contrast media
Iodides
  causing
    allergy, 698, 699, 702, 703
    anaphylaxis, 698
    bullous eruptions,
    effect on
      5-HIAA tests, 359
      thyroid function, 359, 350
      thyroid hormone, 345–7
    erythema multiforme, 207
    erythematous eruptions, 735
    exfoliative dermatitis, 735
    fetal/neonatal disorders, 73, 82
    glottic oedema, 595
    hyperthyroidism, 573
    hypothyroidism, 346
    laryngeal oedema, 595
    pulmonary vasculitis, 173
    purpura, 525, 661
    salivary gland disorders, 217, 594
    salivation, 216
    skin damage, 735
    tissue damage, 734
    vasculitis, pulmonary, 173
Iodipamide — *see* X-ray contrast media
Iodism caused by X-ray contrast media, 748, 754
Iodized oil — *see* X-ray contrast media
Iododerma caused by X-ray contrast media, 748
Iodoform causing stomatitis, 207
Iodoxamate — *see* X-ray contrast media

Ioglycamide — *see* X-ray contrast media
Iohexol — *see* X-ray contrast media
Iopamidol — *see* X-ray contrast media
Iopanoic acid — *see* X-ray contrast media
Iophendylate — *see* X-ray contrast media
Iopromide — *see* X-ray contrast media
Iopydol — *see* X-ray contrast media
Iopydone — *see* X-ray contrast media
Iothalamate — *see* X-ray contrast media
Iotrolan — *see* X-ray contrast media
Iotroxate — *see* X-ray contrast media
Ioversan — *see* X-ray contrast media
Ioxaglate — *see* X-ray contrast media
Iozamic acid — *see* X-ray contrast media
Ipodate — *see* X-ray contrast media
Ipratropium
  causing
    bronchospasm, 180
    viscid sputum, 176
Iproniazid causing liver damage, 262
Iritis and Iris cysts
  drugs causing
    chloroquine, 568
    demecarium, 568
    dyflos, 568
    ecothiopate, 568
Iron
  causing
    effect on zinc, 426
    infections, 666, 668, 669, 672
    intestinal perforation, 234
    nausea and vomiting, 231
    oesophageal ulceration, 595
    pigmentation, 518
    porphyria, 430
Iron–dextran
  causing
    aggravation of rheumatoid arthritis, 498
    infection, 668, 672
Irritability — *see* Behavioural toxicity
Isocarboxazid causing sexual dysfunction, 776
Isoflurane
  causing
    effect on fluoride, 428
    fetal/neonatal disorders, 76
    liver damage, 259
    malignant hyperpyrexia, 556, 769
    psychiatric disorders, 609–10
Isofluophate, effect on cholinesterase, 441
Isoniazid
  and chromosome damage, 53–4
  causing
    acidosis
      metabolic, 400, 401–2
      lactic, 378, 401
    agranulocytosis, 647
    allergy, 701
    anaemia
      aplastic (red cell aplasia), 646
      sideroblastic, 651
    cancer, 681
    effect on
      aspartate aminotransferase tests, 440
      vitamin B_6, 444
    enzyme inhibition, 27
    erythema multiforme, 522
    fetal/neonatal disorders, 67–8
    fever, 768
    flushing, 520
    galactorrhoea/gynaecomastia, 355
    hyperglycaemia, 376
    liver damage, 259–60, 265, 271, 272

lupus erythematosus, 174, 502
neuropathy, peripheral, 28, 546
nicotinic acid deficiency, 443–4
psychiatric disorders, 618–9
purpura, 661
seizures, 538
shoulder–hand syndrome, 498–9
Isopaque — *see* X-ray contrast media
Isoprenaline
  causing
    asthma
      aggravation, 182
      deaths, 182
    cardiac arrhythmias, 110
    cardiomyotoxicity, 118
    effect on
      catecholamine tests, 352
      creatine kinase, 438
      growth hormone, 357
    oral ulceration, 208
    stomatitis, 586
Isosorbide dinitrate
  causing
    halitosis, 221
    psychiatric disorders, 625
Isotretinoin
  causing
    alopecia, 518
    arthralgia/arthritis, 496
    colitis, 235
    conjunctivitis, 568
    corneal opacities, 568
    effect on creatine kinase, 438
    fetal/neonatal disorders, 219, 220, 410, 589
    hyperlipidaemia, 390
    hyperostosis, 496
    infections, 667, 670
    myalgia, 496
    myopathy, 554
    thrombocytopenia, 648

J

Jaundice — *see* Liver damage

K

Kallidinogenase causing hypotension, 215
Kanamycin
  causing
    bronchospasm, 181
    contact dermatitis, 527
    effect on fibrinogen, 437
    fetal/neonatal disorders, 66
    infections, 667
    malabsorption, 235
    neuromuscular block, 541
    ototoxicity, 578, 589
    renal damage, 309

Kathon causing contact dermatitis, 735
Keratitis aggravated by corticosteroids, 568
Kernicterus
  and
    novobiocin, 12
    sulphonamides, 12, 78
    vitamin K, 12
Ketamine
  causing
    hallucinations, 572
    hypertension, 155
    intracranial hypertension, 540
    malignant hyperthermia, 556
    psychiatric disorders, 609
    salivation, 216
    seizures, 538
Ketanserin
  causing
    cardiac arrhythmias, 105, 111–2
    hypertension, 158
Ketoacidosis
  drugs causing
    β-adrenoceptor agonists, 402
    corticosteroids, 402
    pentamidine, 402
    ritodrine, 402
    theophylline, 402
Ketoconazole
  causing
    adrenal failure, 351
    effect on
      acid phosphatase, 442
      thyroid hormone, 347
      sex-hormone-binding globulin, 435
      vitamin D, 359
    enzyme inhibition, 27
    galactorrhoea/gynaecomastria, 353, 354, 355
    hypertension, 150
    hyponatraemia, 417
    hypothyroidism, 347
    liver damage, 263, 268
    sexual dysfunction, 353
Ketoprofen
  causing
    contact dermatitis, 517
    effect on lactic dehydrogenase tests, 439
    renal damage, 320
    sexual dysfunction, 779
Khat causing psychiatric disorders, 607

L

Labetalol
  and Peyronie's disease, 501
  causing
    effect on
      catecholamine tests, 352
      creatine kinase, 438
      phaeochromocytoma, 155
    fetal/neonatal disorders, 81
    headache, 539
    hypertension, 149
    lichenoid eruptions, 524
    liver damage, 263
    lupus erythematosus, 502, 504
    sexual dysfunction, 775, 779

Laboratory tests, drugs causing erroneous
  results, 352, 433, 434, 439, 440, 441,
  442, 743, 751
Labyrinthine disorders — *see* Ototoxicity
Lacrimation, caused by X-ray contrast
  media, 746
Lactic acidosis
  drugs causing
    β-adrenergics, 154
    adrenaline, 378
    alcohol, 378
    biguanides, 378, 400
    catecholamines, 402
    fructose, 378, 401
    glyceryl trinitrate, 401
    isoniazid, 378, 401
    lactulose, 378
    metformin, 378, 400
    nalidixic acid, 378, 402
    nitroprusside, 402
    papaverine, 378, 402
    parenteral nutrition, 401
    phenformin, 378, 400
    polyhydric sugars, 401
    povidone, 402
    prednisolone, 402
    propylene glycol, 401
    ritodrine, 402
    salicylates, 378
    sodium nitroprusside, 378
    sorbitol, 378, 401
    streptozocin, 402
    theophylline, 402
    xylitol, 401
  precipitated by tetracycline, 378
Lactic acid dehydrogenase, drugs affecting,
  439
Lactulose
  causing
    lactic acidosis, 378
    myopathy, 554
Lanolin causing contact dermatitis, 526–7
Laryngeal myopathy caused by inhaled
  steroids, 595
Laryngeal oedema
  caused by
    colaspase, 595
    ethamivan, 595
    iodides, 595
    penicillin, 595
    X-ray contrast media, 595
Laryngospasm
  drugs causing
    antiseptics, 734
    barbiturates, 595
    doxapram, 595
    ethamivan, 595
    thiopentone, 595
    X-ray contrast media, 752
Larynx
  candidiasis (moniliasis) caused by
    corticosteroids, 595
  virilization caused by anabolic steroids, 595
Laxatives — *see* Purgatives
Lead
  causing
    acidosis, metabolic, 400, 403
    anaemia, haemolytic, 650
    effect on
      caeruloplasmin, 436
      plasma proteins, 433
      Fanconi syndrome, 403

growth disorders, 499
    hyperuricaemia, 432
    oral discolouration, 210
    porphyrinuria, 430
  poisoning from
    cosmetics, 427
    herbal remedies, 427
Legionella infections caused by drugs, 669
Lens, contact, stained by rifampicin, 568
Lens opacities — *see* Cataract
Leucopenia — *see* Agranulocytosis
Leukaemia
  ampicillin rashes in, 693
  drugs causing
    anticancer drugs, 684–5
    cytotoxics, 651
    growth hormone, 651
Levamisole
  causing
    agranulocytosis, 647
    arthralgia/arthritis, 498
    thrombocytopenia, 648
  toxicity and HLA status, 11
Levodopa
  causing
    dyskinesias, 219, 540, 544
    effect on
      gastric emptying, 21
      growth hormone, 357
      TRH/TSH, 345
    eye movement disorders, 571
    galactorrhoea/gynaecomastria, 353, 354, 355
    hypertension, 155
    hypokalaemia, 413, 415
    hypotension, 159
    Meige's syndrome, 220
    nausea and vomiting, 231
    neuroleptic malignant syndrome, 543
    psychiatric disorders, 603, 604, 608–9
    respiratory depression, 194
    taste disorders, 220, 593
    xerostomia, 216
Levonorgestrel — *see* Progestogens
LH/FSH/RH analogues causing sexual
  dysfunction, 352, 778
Licorice
  causing
    effect on aldosterone, 352
    hypertension, 150
    hypokalaemia, 35, 413, 414
    myopathy, 554
    paralysis, 35
Lignocaine
  causing
    contact dermatitis, 517
    effect on creatine kinase, 438
    hypotension, 160
    psychiatric disorders, 624
    seizures, 538
    sexual dysfunction, 782
    stomatitis, 206
Limecycline causing oesophageal ulceration,
  594
Lincomycin
  causing
    neuromuscular block, 551, 552
    pseudomembranous colitis, 235, 668
Lipid infusions causing infections,
  665–6, 671
Lipiodol — *see* X-ray contrast media
Lipoproteins, drugs affecting, 387–90

M

Metoprolol
and
   Peyronie's disease, 501
   retroperitoneal fibrosis, 318, 500
   sclerosing peritonitis, 238
causing
   bladder dysfunction, 557
   hyperglycaemia, 374
   liver damage, 263
   psychiatric disorders, 622
Metriphonate, effect on cholinesterase tests, 442
Metrizamide — *see* X-ray contrast media
Metrizoate (iozamic acid) — *see* X-ray
   contrast media
Metronidazole
causing
   effect on aspartate aminotransferase, 440
   eosinophilia, pulmonary, 185
   galactorrhoea/gynaecomastia, 355
   neuropathy, peripheral, 546
   pancreatitis, 237
   pseudomembranous colitis, 668
   renal damage, 313
   taste disorders, 220, 593
Metyrapone
causing
   adrenal failure, 351
   effect on corticotrophin, 350
   hirsuties, 518
   hypotension, 160
Mexiletine
causing
   cardiac arrhythmias, 105
   psychiatric disorders, 122, 624
Mezlocillin causing renal damage, 315
Mianserin
causing
   facial oedema, 222
   liver damage, 262
   thrombocytopenia, 648
Micromelia, drugs causing, thalidomide, 3
Migraine remedies causing peripheral
   vasoconstriction, 156
Milk, cows', causing hypercalcaemia, 416
Milk–alkali syndrome
causing
   hypercalcaemia, 321, 416
   osteosclerosis, 496
   renal calculi, 321
Milrinone causing cardiac arrhythmias, 109
Mineralocorticoids — *see* Corticosteroids
Minocycline
causing
   intracranial hypertension, 540
   ototoxicity, 578, 580
   papilloedema, 571
   pigmentation
      cardiac, 131
      oral, 211
      skin, 518
      teeth, 211
   renal damage, 315
Minoxidil
and lupus erythematosus, 502, 504
causing
   effect on catecholamine tests, 352
   erythema multiforme, 207
   fetal/neonatal disorders, 68
   hirsuties, 518

hypertension (rebound), 149
   thrombocytopenia, 648
Mioprostil causing fetal/neonatal disorders, 71
Miosis caused by morphine, 569
Misonidazole
causing
   neuropathy, peripheral, 548
   ototoxicity, 586
Mistletoe causing liver damage, 282
Mitomycin
causing
   anaemia, aplastic, 645
   chromosome damage, 51
   liver damage, 276
   pneumonitis, 186
   renal damage, 313
   stomatitis, 592
Mitoxantrone
causing
   anaemia, aplastic, 645
   hypomagnesaemia, 425
   infections, 221
Moniliasis — *see* Candidiasis
Monoamine oxidase inhibitors
causing
   bladder dysfunction, 557
   effect on
      adrenal function tests, 351
      catecholamine tests, 352
      5-HIAA tests, 349
      phaeochromocytoma, 154
      prolactin secretion, 356
      vasopressin, 358
   fetal/neonatal disorders, 70
   fever, 767
   galactorrhoea/gynaecomastia, 356
   hyponatraemia, 407
   hypotension, 159
   liver damage, 262
   neuropathy, peripheral, 546
   psychiatric disorders, 615
   sexual dysfunction, 776
Mono-octanoin causing pulmonary oedema, 175–6
Mononucleosis — *see* Infectious
   mononucleosis
MOPP causing sexual dysfunction, 779, 780, 781
Morazone causing nicotinic acid deficiency, 107
Morphine
age effects, 12
causing
   acidosis, respiratory, 399
   effect on
      gastrointestinal motility, 233
      phaeochromocytoma, 154
   fetal/neonatal disorders, 12
   histamine release, 154
   hyperglycaemia, 377
   miosis, 569
   porphyria, 430
   pruritus, 521
   psychiatric disorders, 610
   respiratory depression, 399
   thrombocytopenia, 647
Mouth
allergic reactions, 205–7
hypersensitivity reactions, 205–7
Mouth discolouration — *see* Oral
   discolouration

Mouth ulceration — *see* Oral ulceration
Mouthwashes causing black hairy tongue, 211
MPTP causing dyskinesias, 541
Mucormycosis
drugs causing
   corticosteroids, 671
   desferrioxamine, 671
Muscinol, effect on growth hormone, 357
Muscle damage (fibrosis, necrosis,
   rhabdomyolysis)
drugs causing
   alcohol, 317, 318
   aminocaproic acid, 493
   amoxapine, 318
   amphetamines, 316, 317, 493, 555
   amphotericin, 317, 318
   antibacterials, 493
   barbiturates, 493
   bezafibrate, 317, 318, 492
   carbenoxolone, 317, 318
   chloroquine, 493
   chlorpromazine, 493
   chlorthalidone, 318
   clofibrate, 317, 318
   cocaine, 318, 493
   colchicine, 493
   corticosteroids, 317, 318
   cyclosporin, 493
   cytarabine, 318
   diamorphine, 317
   diphenhydramine, 318, 493
   diuretics, 317, 493
   doxylamine, 318, 493
   emetics, 493
   enflurane, 318
   fenofibrate, 318
   fluoroprednisolone, 317, 318
   gemfibrosil, 317
   haloperidol, 318
   heroin, 317, 318, 493
   lovastatin, 317, 318, 493
   lysergide, 317, 318
   methadone, 493
   methanol, 317, 318
   opiates, 318, 493, 555
   paraphenylenediamine, 555
   pentamidine, 318, 493
   pentazocine, 493
   phenazopyridine, 318
   phencyclidine, 317, 318, 493, 555
   purgatives, 493
   retinoids, 493
   sodium valproate, 318
   streptokinase, 317, 318
   suxamethonium, 318
   terbutaline, 12,14
   theophylline, 318, 493
   toluene, 318
   valproate, 318
   vincristine, 493
Muscle relaxants
causing
   acidosis, respiratory, 399
   malignant hyperthermia, 34–5, 556, 769
   respiratory depression, 399
Muscle spasm, caused by X-ray contrast
   media, 745, 755
Muscle weakness
drugs causing
   anticholinesterases, 573
   pilocarpine, 573

N

Proctitis (*cont.*)
  drugs causing (*cont.*)
    suppositories, 236
    whisky, 236
Procyclidine causing psychiatric disorders, 605
Progestogens
  causing
    carpal tunnel syndrome, 501
    effect on
      albumin, 434
      protein metabolism, 433
      sex-hormone-binding globulin, 435
    fetal/neonatal disorders, 71–2
    hyperglycaemia, 375–6
    liver damage, 270
    masculinization of fetus, 72
    porphyria, 350, 429
    sexual dysfunction, 778
Proguanil
  causing
    anaemia, megaloblastic, 650
    oral ulceration, 209
    stomatitis, 592
Prolactin, drugs affecting secretion — *see* Galactorrhoea/gynaecomastia
Promazine
  causing
    dyskinesias, 540
    liver damage, 266
    seizures, 538
Promethazine
  causing
    fetal/neonatal disorders, 65
    hypertension, 155
    photosensitivity, 520
Propafenone
  and lupus erythematosus, 502, 504
  causing
    cardiac
      arrhythmias, 497
      depression, 122
    hyponatraemia, 407, 409
    taste disorders, 593
Propanidid
  causing
    anaphylaxis, 31
    hypotension, 160
    seizures, 538
Propantheline
  causing
    bladder dysfunction, 557
    effect on gastric emptying, 21
    xerostomia, 216
Propazone causing photosensitivity, 520
Propoxyphene
  causing
    fetal/neonatal disorders, 408–9, 82
    hypoglycaemia, 385
    ototoxicity, 586
Propranolol
  age effects, 12
  and
    Dupuytren's contracture, 501
    lupus erythematosus, 502, 504
    Peyronie's disease, 501
  causing
    asthma aggravation, 183
    bronchospasm, 183
    cardiac ischaemia (withdrawal), 125
    dyskinesias, 541

effect on
  blood lipids, 378
  catecholamine tests, 352
  creatine kinase, 438
  oesophageal motility, 230
  prealbumin, 434
  thyroid-binding globulin, 435
  thyroid function tests, 349
erythema multiforme, 522
fetal/neonatal disorders, 81
headache, 539
hyperglycaemia, 374
hypertension, 149
hyperuricaemia, 432
hypoglycaemia, 373
hypotension, 160
myopathy, 554
neuromuscular block, 552
neuropathy
  orofacial, 220
  peripheral, 546
oesophageal spasm, 230
ototoxicity, 586
psoriasiform eruptions, 524
psychiatric disorders, 622
renal damage, 306
retroperitoneal fibrosis, 318, 500
sexual dysfunction, 775, 782
Propylene glycol
  causing
    acidosis
      lactic, 401
      metabolic, 400, 401
    allergy, 31
    hypersensitivity, 31
    hypotension, 31
    ototoxicity, 582
    renal damage, 311
Propylhexidine causing psychiatric disorders, 607
Propyliodone — *see* X-ray contrast media
Propylthiouracil
  causing
    agranulocytosis, 647
    alopecia, 518
    arthralgia/arthritis, 498
    effect on
      albumin, 434
      amylase, 441
      immunoglobins, 437
      thyroid function tests, 349
      thyroid hormone, 346
    fetal/neonatal disorders, 63
    hypothyroidism, 346
    liver damage, 269, 273
    lupus erythematosus, 502, 504
    neuropathy, peripheral, 546
    ototoxicity, 587
    vasculitis, 519
Prostaglandins
  causing
    bronchospasm, 181
    effect on platelet function, 661
    fetal/neonatal disorders, 71
    fever, 768
    hypotension, 159–60
    psychiatric disorders, 625
Protamine sulphate causing hypotension, 159
Protamine zinc insulin — *see* Insulin
Protein metabolism (*see also* individual plasma proteins), drugs affecting, 433–7
Prothiaden causing anaemia, aplastic, 645

Protozoal infections
  drugs causing
    antilymphocyte globulin, 672
    antilymphoma therapy, 672
    corticosteroids, 671–2
    corticotrophin (ACTH), 672
    desferrioxamine, 672
    docusate calcium, 672
    erythromycin, 672
    immunosuppressants, 672
    iron, 672
    iron–dextran, 672
    methotrexate, 672
    OKT3, 672
    oxytetracycline 672
Pruritus
  drugs causing
    chloroquine, 521
    cocaine, 521
    morphine, 521
    oral contraceptives, 521
    PUVA, 521–2
    X-ray contrast media, 745
Pseudocholinesterase
  abnormalities, 27
  genetic factors, 27
Pseudolupus syndrome due to Venocuran, 504
Pseudomembranous colitis, caused by *Clostridium difficile*, 235, 668
  drugs causing
    amoxycillin, 668
    ampicillin, 668
    antibacterials, 668
    anticancer drugs, 668
    chlorpropamide, 669
    clindamycin, 235, 668
    cytarabine, 668
    lincomycin, 235, 668
    metronidazole, 668
    vancomycin, 668
  treatment with
    metronidazole, 668
    vancomycin, 668
Pseudoporphyria
  caused by
    amiodarone, 430, 517
    anti-inflammatories, 430
    chlorthalidone, 430, 517
    cyclophosphamide, 430
    cyclosporin, 517
    etretinate, 430, 517
    frusemide, 430, 517
    nalidixic acid, 517
    naproxen, 430, 517
    tetracycline, 430, 517
Pseudotumour cerebri — *see* Hypertension, intracranial
Psilocybin causing psychiatric disorders, 616
Psoralens
  causing
    hirsuties, 518
    nail changes, 517
Psoriasiform eruptions — *see* Skin rashes
Psoriasis
  drugs aggravating
    indomethacin, 524
    oxyphenbutazone, 524
    phenylbutazone, 524
Psychiatric reactions, 573, 601–16, 736, 755, 756

S

T

Toxic epidermal necrolysis (Lyell's
    syndrome)
  drugs causing
    allopurinol, 523
    anti-inflammatories, 523
    barbiturates, 523
    captopril, 523
    chloramphenicol, 523
    co-trimoxazole, 523
    dapsone, 523
    gold salts, 523
    hydantoins, 523
    neomycin, 523
    nitrofurantoin, 523
    opium alkaloids, 523
    oxyphenbutazone, 523
    penicillin, 523
    pentamidine, 523
    pentazocine, 523
    phenolphthalein, 523
    phenytoin, 523
    plicamycin (mithramycin), 523
    quinine, 523
    sulphonamides, 523
    tetracyclines, 523
    thiabendazole, 523
Toxic erythema — *see* Erythema
Toxoplasmosis caused by
    immunosuppressants, 672
Trafuril causing contact dermatitis, 528
Tranexamic acid causing
  renal damage, 318
  ureteric clots, 318
Tranquillizers
  age effects, 12
  causing
    galactorrhoea/gynaecomastia, 355
    hyperglycaemia, 376
    hypotension, 159
    hypothermia, 770
    myopathy, 553
    porphyria, 360, 429
    psychiatric disorders, 603
Transferrin, drugs affecting, 436
Tranylcypromine
  causing
    psychiatric disorders, 615
    sexual dysfunction, 776
Traxonax causing hypouricaemia, 432
Trazodone
  causing
    cardiac arrhythmias, 115
    psychiatric disorders, 614–5
    sexual dysfunction, 776, 779
Tremor (*see* Dyskinesias)
Treosulphan causing leukaemia, 685, 686
Triacetyloleandomycin causing liver damage,
  268
Triamcinolone — *see* Corticosteroids
Triamterene
  causing
    anaemia, megaloblastic, 650
    effect on lactic dehydrogenase tests, 439
    hyperkalaemia, 410, 412
    renal
      calculi, 321, 322
      tubular acidosis, 403
Triaziquone causing chromosome damage, 50
Triazolam causing psychiatric disorders, 612
TRH/TSH, drugs affecting 345

Trichlorethylene
  causing
    malignant hyperthermia, 556
    neuropathy, orofacial, 220, 549
    viral infections, 670
Tricyclic antidepressants
  causing
    agranulocytosis, 647
    anaemia, aplastic, 645
    bladder dysfunction, 557
    cardiac arrhythmias, 102, 115
    constipation, 236
    dental caries, 218
    dyskinesias, 219, 540, 541, 542, 552
    effect on
      catecholamine tests, 352
      phaeochromocytoma, 155
      sputum, 176
      vasopressin, 358
    fetal/neonatal disorders, 84
    fever, 767
    folate deficiency, 446
    galactorrhoea/gynaecomastia, 355
    hallucinations, 604
    hyponatraemia, 407
    hypotension, 159
    ileus, 233
    liver damage, 261–2
    neuropathy
      orofacial, 220
      peripheral, 546, 548
    oral ulcers, 666
    parkinsonism, 540
    photosensitivity, 520
    psychiatric disorders, 602, 603, 604
    seizures, 538
    sexual dysfunction, 776, 782
    tremor, 542
    thrombocytopenia, 648
    xerostomia, 216
Tridione — *see* Troxidone
Trifluoperazine
  causing
    dyskinesia, 540, 542
    fever, 767
    galactorrhoea/gynaecomastia, 356
    hyponatraemia, 407, 408
    neuroleptic malignant syndrome, 543
    seizures, 538
    sexual dysfunction, 776
Trifluoperidol causing dyskinesia, 540
Triglycerides, drugs affecting, 387–90
Trihexyphenidyl causing neuromuscular
  block, 551
Tri-iodithyronine, effect on angiotensin-
  converting enzyme, 442
Trimeprazine causing neuroleptic malignant
  syndrome, 543
Trimetaphan, effect on
  phaeochromocytoma, 155
Trimethadione — *see* Troxidone
Trimethoprim (*see also* Co-trimoxazole)
  and chromosome damage, 53
  causing
    acidosis, metabolic, 403
    anaemia, megaloblastic, 650
    erythema multiforme, 522
    fixed drug eruption, 516
    folate deficiency, 445–6
    liver damage, 267
    psychiatric disorders, 618
Trimipramine — *see* Tricyclic antidepressants

Trinitrin — *see* Glyceryl trinitrate
Triorthocresylphosphate causing neuropathy,
  550
Triosil — *see* X-ray contrast media
Triparanol causing myotonia, 556
Tropicamide
  causing
    cerebellar disorders, 573
    confusion, 573
Troxidone
  causing
    fetal/neonatal disorders, 70, 572
    lupus erythematosus, 492
    neuromuscular block, 551
    purpura, 525
Tryptophan, effect on growth hormone, 347
L-Tryptophan
  causing
    eosinophilia–myalgia syndrome, 31–2,
      173, 494–5
    psychiatric disorders, 615
    pulmonary hypertension, 191–2
Tuberculosis, effect of corticosteroids, 669–70
Tubocurarine
  causing
    allergy, 179
    bronchospasm, 179
    effect on
      immunoglobulins, 437
      phaeochromocytoma, 154
    fetal/neonatal disorders, 76
    malignant hyperthermia, 769
Tyramine, effect on phaeochromocytoma, 155

U

Uraemia (*see* Renal damage)
Ureteric obstruction, by
  clots 318, 660
  crystals or calculi, 321–2
  retroperitoneal fibrosis, 318, 500
  retroperitoneal haemorrhage, 318
  ureteric stricture, 326
Uricosurics causing renal calculi, 321
Urinary dysfunction — *see* Bladder
  dysfunction
Urinary incontinence — *see* Bladder
  dysfunction
Urinary obstruction — *see* Bladder
  dysfunction
Urinary retention — *see* Bladder dysfunction
Urinastatin causing hypouricaemia, 432
Urine discolouration caused by X-ray
  contrast media, 754
Urografin — *see* X-ray contrast media
Urokinase causing emboli, 149
Uromine — *see* X-ray contrast media
Urography, adverse effects, 739–49
Urokon — *see* X-ray contrast media
Ursodeoxycholic acid causing liver damage,
  265
Urticaria
  agents causing
    alcohol, 522
    aspirin, 522
    codeine, 522

W

X

Y

Z